Urolithiasis

Jamsheer J. Talati • Hans-Göran Tiselius
David M. Albala • Zhangqun Ye
Editors

Farhat Abbas • M. Hammad Ather
Syed Raziuddin Biyabani • Mahesh Desai
Tyler Luthringer • Amanullah Memon
Kemal Sarica • Ahmed A. Shokeir
Khurram M. Siddiqui
Associate Editors

Urolithiasis

Basic Science and Clinical Practice

Springer

Editors
Jamsheer J. Talati, MBBS, FRCS
Professor Emeritus
Aga Khan University
Department of Surgery
Section of Urology
Karachi, Pakistan

David M. Albala, MD
Associated Medical Professionals
Syracuse
New York, USA

Hans-Göran Tiselius, MD, PhD
Professor Emeritus
Division of Urology
Department of Clinical Science
Intervention and Technology
Karolinska Institutet
Stockholm, Sweden

Zhangqun Ye, MD, PhD
Urology Division
Tongji Hospital
Tongji Medical College, Shanghai, China.
Huazhong University of Science and Technology
Wuhan, Hubei, China

ISBN 978-1-4471-4383-3 ISBN 978-1-4471-4387-1 (eBook)
DOI 10.1007/978-1-4471-4387-1
Springer London Heidelberg New York Dordrecht

Library of Congress Control Number: 2012954241

Printed on acid-free paper

Springer is part of Springer Science+Business Media (www.springer.com)

This book is dedicated to our wives and families to whom we are indebted for their understanding during the preparation of the book…

And to the urological residents, young consultants, faculty, and stone patients of our entire, rapidly evolving world.

Jamsheer Jehangir Talati
Hans-Göran Tiselius
David Mois Albala
Zhangqun Ye

Foreword

The World Health Report of 2010, the biennial flagship publication of the World Health Organization, was devoted to the link between the way health systems are financed and their ability to move closer to the goal of universal coverage [1]. Universal coverage requires all people to have access to quality health services (prevention, promotion, treatment and rehabilitation) when they need them without the risk of incurring severe financial problems linked to paying for care [2, 3]. It is an ambitious goal.

Three inter-related actions to help countries move closer to this goal can be taken in the area of health financing. Countries could raise additional funds for health. They could reduce financial barriers to accessing health services associated with direct out of pocket payments such as user-fees through forms of prepayment with subsequent pooling of resources to spread the financial risks of ill health. They could use the resources they raise as efficiently and equitably as possible. Many countries, rich and poor, have taken steps in one or more of these areas and the World Health Report showed that all countries could take steps to move more rapidly towards the goal of universal coverage.

Clearly the pace at which they can do this varies by country and the resource constraints are particularly severe in low-income countries where the health needs are greatest. Recent work suggests that the low income countries would need immediately an average of US $44 per capita to spend on health, rising to just over $60 in 2015, to have any chance of reaching the health millennium development goals by 2015 [4]. Only $35 is available from domestic and donor funding combined despite a rapid scale up in external assistance for health since the Millennium Declaration was signed in 2000 [5, 6].

These estimates were made based on the costs of ensuring access to a limited range of health services aimed largely at communicable diseases and child and maternal health. Little attention was paid to non-communicable diseases, yet the goal of achieving universal coverage must extend to non-communicable diseases as well. This is increasingly important now that the problems associated with an aging population, the epidemiological transition and chronic diseases are increasing to the extent that the burden of disease associated with them outweighs that of non-communicable diseases even in the low-income countries [7, 8]. The goal of universal coverage must extend to preventing and treating stone disease.

More money for health in poorer countries is critical to achieving this goal, and the gaps between the financial needs and their domestic capacities to raise funds, even with reasonable levels of economic growth, remain large. Although most low-income countries could take steps to increase the availability of their own domestic resources for health, increased external donor support remains critical, something that may be difficult to maintain in the current economic climate of rich countries trying to reduce their budget deficits and their own levels of indebtedness.

More money, however, will not be sufficient by itself. Many countries also need to reduce the financial barriers facing patients when they contemplate seeking and then continuing care it. For example, almost a third of the countries in sub-Saharan Africa raise more than 50 % of their total health resources through direct charges levied on patients at the time they seek care. In India, it is more than 60 % [5]. These direct payments not only ensure that millions of people are not treated, including for stone disease, but they also ensure that millions of those that are treated suffer severe financial problems simply because they became ill and needed to pay for care [9]. Each year, approximately 100 million people are pushed under the poverty line in this way [10].

This can be addressed only by reducing reliance on direct payments levied at the time people obtain care by moving to forms of prepayment and pooling. Various forms of insurance and tax-based funding are the solution and they are being implemented even in lower income countries in the search to reduce the financial barriers to care.

Health financing systems are fundamental to attaining universal coverage, helping to ensure that all people who suffer from stone disease can be identified and treated, and ensuring that appropriate prevention is in place. On the other hand, if there are no health workers with the appropriate training, or no medicines, or no equipment for diagnosis, for example, universal coverage is not possible. That is why this book is so vital. It is about the science of stone disease. It describes the epidemiology, showing how the prevalence, incidence and severity differ substantially across the different parts of the world necessitating different approaches to case finding and treatment.

It describes the causes and natural history of the disease, and then the latest developments in diagnosis, treatment and rehabilitation. As such it is also a practical guide for urologists treating the disease as well as trying to prevent recurrence and limit the impact of illness on the subsequent lives of patients. It helps us to understand what can be done to prevent the disease in the first place.

It also places the science in the context of society and resource constraints. At times it takes the perspective of the health professional, reflecting on how to understand the patient's needs and expectations, and how to practice ethical medicine when the patient or country might not be able to afford the optimal treatment. The clinician's task is to provide exemplary care to as large a population as possible. If the treatment is too expensive, they have to find alternatives. These hard choices can be made only if the urologist is knowledgeable, technically competent, and professional. The book provides a basis for helping clinicians make rational choices in the deployment of technology, including those which are expensive. There are also chapters taking the broader planning or social perspective on how to best finance and manage equipment, including how to reduce costs by sharing equipment.

The information provided in this book will interest researchers seeking to understand disease patterns or the way new technologies relating are developed and disseminated. It will be vital to health professionals seeking to prevent or treat the disease. And it will be important to health planners in their deliberations about how to reduce the burden of stone disease for the resources that are available. All these perspectives are important in their own way, but it is only through the combination of these perspectives that it will be possible to move more rapidly to, and eventually attain, universal coverage everywhere.

Geneva, Switzerland

David B. Evans
Director
Department of Health Systems Financing (HSF)
World Health Organization

Bibliography

1. World Health Organization. WHO|The world health report – health systems financing: the path to universal coverage. 2010. Retrieved from http://www.who.int/whr/2010/en/index.html.
2. World Health Organization. WHA resolution 58.33: sustainable health financing, universal coverage and social health insurance. Fifty-Seventh World Health Assembly. Geneva: World Health Organization; 2005. Retrieved from http://apps.who.int/gb/ebwha/pdf_files/WHA58/WHA58_33-en.pdf.

3. Carrin G, Mathauer I, Evans DB. Universal coverage of health services: tailoring its implementation. Bull World Health Organ. 2008;86(11):857–63.
4. World Health Organization. Constraints to scaling up the health millennium development goals: costing and financial gap analysis. Background document for the taskforce on innovative international financing for health systems, working group 1: constraints to scaling up and costs. 2009. Retrieved from http://www.who.int/choice/publications/d_ScalingUp_MDGs_WHO_finalreport.pdf.
5. World Health Organization. WHO|National Health Accounts. WHO. 2009. Retrieved 1 Nov 2011 from http://www.who.int/nha/en/.
6. Ravishankar N, Gubbins P, Cooley RJ, Leach-Kemon K, Michaud CM, Jamison DT, Murray CJ. Financing of global health: tracking development assistance for health from 1990 to 2007. Lancet. 2009;373:2113–24. doi: 10.1016/S0140-6736(09)60881-3.
7. Boutayeb A, Boutayeb S. The burden of non-communicable diseases in developing countries. Int J Equity Health. 2005;4(1):2.
8. World Health Organization. WHO|The global burden of disease: 2004 update. Geneva: World Health Organization; 2008. Retrieved from http://www.who.int/healthinfo/global_burden_disease/2004_report_update/en/.
9. Wagstaff A. The economic consequences of health shocks: evidence from Vietnam. J Health Econ. 2007;26(1):82–100. doi: 10.1016/j.jhealeco.2006.07.001.
10. Xu K, Evans DB, Carrin G, Aguilar-Rivera AM, Musgrove P, Evans T. Protecting households from catastrophic health spending. Health Affairs. 2007;26(4):972–83. doi: 10.1377/hlthaff.26.4.972.

Preface

Why did four urologists from America, Europe, China, and South Asia get together to edit yet another book on stone disease?

The story winds back to 1997, when one of the current editors, Jamsheer Talati, published jointly, with Roger A. L. Sutton, Farhat Moazzam, and Mushtaq Ahmed, a volume on urolithiasis. This was intended to capture and examine the new developments (of ESWL, laser lithotripsy, minimally invasive operative surgery to name a few) of the preceding two decades, and portray the management of vesical and upper urinary tract calculi. Methodologies were examined for their efficacy and cost effectiveness.

In the foreword to that book, Professor J. E. A. Wickham hoped for a world where technological advancements would be available to all… He wrote:

> Endoscopic stone removal and ESWL have more than justified their place in the surgical armamentarium on the grounds of outstanding efficiency and cost effectiveness as compared with previous methods of open surgery. Such effective new technology, saving as it does much expense, must surely be the way forward for any society, particularly where resources are radically cost contained and difficult to access for the poorer members of the community. Hopefully in the next twenty years economies will have improved so that a full range of interventional therapy for urolithiasis will become available to all populations in all parts of the world.

Fifteen years have passed and that vision has not materialized.

Why?

One would expect that as treatment methods have become "easy" on the patient, and the technology has facilitated the surgeon, our hopes would have been achieved. On the contrary: Urinary stones are still found untreated in all corners of the globe; and the numbers are growing, for various reasons. There is a greater consciousness in the lay public, easier access to services…. But there are also possibly preventable recurrences; and the populations to be served are growing so rapidly. What we see as a result is that though larger segments of population can access sophisticated care, the proportion accessing anything other than open operation in poorer countries yet remains small. Silent stones destroy the kidney. Ignorance of the true prevalence and incidence thwarts planning efforts.

As the disease is seen across the world, we crafted this book with a host of exceptional specialists in each topic, in order to create a consilience of known facts in all fields—epidemiology, basic science, technology, management, prevention, education, ethics, fund raising. The book additionally whispers the need to study geological formations and soils, and to look beyond the urological, deep into society. The book combines all of that with a stimulation of new thinking on the management of this problem, and the need for innovation, stemming from the difficulties of addressing the stone problem effectively in so many parts of the world.

We hope that this book, in addition to assisting urologists in management of stone patients, will stimulate search for answers to critical questions: Are there any simple measures that will eliminate or reduce stone: Will diet and increased water intake vanquish the concreting enemy? What really is the cause of stone? And what is the meaning of the differences in distribution and composition of stones across the world?

To hit hard and eliminate stone disease from all parts of the world is going to be difficult. It will require that the treating physician not only manage the disease effectively but that she or he (i) be cognizant of all the information available and be able to connect all of that in a way that becomes knowledge useful for asking and answering questions on prevention and treatment; and (ii) be creative, and willing to explore the available epidemiological base and the basic science of stone formation to see if there is a new approach to management or a different opportunity for research.

To spread treatment across all parts of the globe, to more than two billion people in India and China alone, is a daunting task. How will we tackle seven billion? But with the entire world looking anew at its financial models of resourcing and spending, it is apt that this book help the readers to try and attempt to find a rational solution for each patient given the resources available; and to find the required resources when they are not easily visible.

How does one teach innovation? And how can one turn a tool into a piece of equipment that can be patented and sold? How does one get expensive equipment when one does not have money? Money is available; there are enough philanthropists to go all around. To engage their attention, trust and confidence have to be built, through exhibition of excellence in management and superlative results. That takes us back to training: It is vital that we train the next generations in concepts and techniques, and then tickle their ability to think through problems. To do so, one needs, once again, information and knowledge.

For governments too it is important that the individual executing stone management be competent and practice accepted, guideline-approved strategies, introduction ever-rising standards that cannot be challenged. Hence the need for consilience and the need to learn from all corners of the world.

What is needed at the end is Equity. This can be achieved through Excellence, Effectiveness, Efficiency, Innovation, Subspecialization, Evidence-based practice, and training that is certified through high-stakes assessment of superlative standards.

Today, the competent lithotomist needs to be more than a cutting edge endoscopist.

Every one—patient, government, administrator, and society—demands competence. Competence is based on professionalism, knowledge and skill. But a physician's responsibility goes beyond that—to see that she or he eliminates the very disease that provides their bread.

Above all therefore it is hoped that this book will stimulate and instigate many urologists to take on the challenge of searching society and their environments for a path leading to the demise of stone disease.

The book attempts to address a major sector of a wide-open plateau of action that the urological trainee and the practicing urologist will need to continue to survey throughout their life. Above all, the book intends to assist the development of a complete Urologist who has many skills in addition to the technical.

Karachi, Pakistan — Jamsheer Talati
Stockholm, Sweden — Hans-Göran Tiselius
Syracuse, NY, USA — David Albala
Wuhan, Hubei, China — Zhangqun Ye

Acknowledgements

The Editors are especially grateful to all contributing authors who have dedicated time and effort despite their busy schedules. For a work of this complexity, the wealth of ideas, guidance, support, critique, and review that we received from our Associate Editors Ahmed Shokeir from Egypt, Kemal Sarica from Turkey, Mahesh Desai from India, Tyler Luthringer from USA, and Farhat Abbas, Hammad Ather, Syed Raziuddin Biyabani, Amanullah Memon, and Khurram Siddiqui, from Pakistan, has been most invaluable.

We are indebted to Ms. Maureen Pierce, whose patience and special expertise as developmental editor provided us continued and intense support in preparation of the manuscript, and in editing, advising, and bringing uniformity to language, text and formats; and to Ms. Diane Lamsback for additional support. The editorial team is also grateful to the larger team from Springer-Verlag—to Nadine Firth and Sarah Cody; to Vinitha Vipin and Stephen Muthu Raj JoeArun; and very specially to Ms. Melissa Morton whose sage advice and suggestions at the very earliest stages of formalization of the ideas for the book gave us courage to build on our earlier thoughts, and helped us develop our Editorial Team.

Our very special thanks are due to the subject expert external reviewers Danette McKinley, John Norcini, Roger A. L. Sutton, Tahira Naru, Zafar Sajjad, Razi Naqvi, and Hussein Sheashaa. Our special thanks also go to James E. Lingeman and Glen Preminger for their support and assistance.

Our thanks are due to the backbone team at the Aga Khan University, where Sean Victor superbly managed the correspondence and the difficult tasks of tracking, computing, correcting, and communicating; Ms. Ashraf Fidai, for the secretarial tasks, Murad Bana for management issues, Aadil Inayat Ali and Aziz Hyder for IT-related and computer support, and Ajmal Rizvi for the graphics and visuals; and to the Aga Khan University (AKU) and Farhat Abbas, Dean AKU, for providing the resources, human capital and time required to make this book possible.

We are grateful to the various publishers who have given permission to use matter published in their journals and books.

Karachi, Pakistan — Jamsheer Jehangir Talati
Stockholm, Sweden — Hans-Göran Tiselius
Syracuse, NY, USA — David Mois Albala
Wuhan, Hubei, China — Zhangqun Ye

Contents

Part I Epidemiology

1 **Epidemiology of Kidney Stones in the European Union** 3
Palle J.S. Osther

2 **Epidemiology of Stone Disease in North America** 13
John D. Denstedt and Andrew Fuller

3 **Epidemiology of Stone Disease in Pakistan** 21
Amanullah Memon, Khursheed Anwar, Nasir Orakzai, M. Hammad Ather, Syed Raziuddin Biyabani, Abdul Razzaq Nasir, Jai Pal Paryani, Farooq Ghani, Khurram Mutahir Siddiqui, Farhat Abbas, Kashif Bangash, Liaqat Ali, Wajahat Aziz, and Jamsheer J. Talati

4 **Epidemiology of Stone Disease in Northern India** 39
Raguram Ganesamoni and Shrawan K. Singh

5 **Epidemiology of Stone Disease in Kerala, South India** 47
Y.M. Fazil Marickar

6 **Epidemiology of Stone Disease in China** 53
Deyi Luo, Hong Li, and Kunjie Wang

7 **Epidemiology of Stone Disease in South America** 61
Fernando Korkes, Nestor Schor, and Ita Pfeferman Heilberg

8 **Epidemiology: South Africa and Sub-Saharan Africa** 67
Allen Rodgers

9 **Epidemiology of Stone Disease in Australia** 73
Ming-Chak Lee and Simon Virgil Bariol

10 **Epidemiology of Stone Disease in Saudi Arabia with an Overview of the Regional Differences** 77
Salah R. El-Faqih

11 **Epidemiology of Stone Disease in Iran** 85
Gholamreza Pourmand and Bita Pourmand

12 **Epidemiology of Stone Disease Over a 40-Year Period in Japan** 89
Yoshihide Ogawa

13 **Epidemiology of Stone Disease in the Russian Federation and Post-Soviet Era** 97
Andrei Novikov, Tair Nazarov, and Vladimir Yu. Startsev

14 **Renal Stone Disease in Different Racial Groups** 107
Jamsheer J. Talati, Naveed Haroon, and Alberto Trinchieri

Part II Etiology

15 **Stone Composition and Morphology: A Window on Etiology** 113
Michel Daudon and Paul Jungers

16 **The Genetics of Kidney Stones** 141
Pietro Manuel Ferraro and Giovanni Gambaro

17 **Familial Clustering of Stone Disease**.................................. 151
Jamsheer Jehangir Talati, Naveed Haroon, and Alberto Trinchieri

18 **Uric Acid Nephrolithiasis: Basic and Clinical Aspects** 155
Khashayar Sakhaee

19 **Oxalate and Urolithiasis**... 165
Ben H. Chew, Dirk Lange, and Roger A.L. Sutton

20 **Anti-inflammatory Proteins in Kidney Stone Matrix** 177
Anwar Ali Siddiqui and Shamim Mushtaq

21 **Physiology of Renal Handling of Citrate** 183
Samra Bashir, Naveed Ahmed Khan, and Anwarul-Hassan Gilani

22 **Urinary Citrate and Stone Disease** 187
Charles Y.C. Pak

23 **Renal Tubular Acidosis and Stone Formation**.......................... 195
Somnuek Domrongkitchaiporn and Wasana Stitchantrakul

24 **Nephrolithiasis and Its Interrelationship with Vitamin D, Parathyroid Hormone, and Calcium**.................................. 199
Aysha Habib Khan

25 **Current Understanding of the Role of Randall's Plaque** 209
Jessica A. Mandeville, Ehud Gnessin, and James E. Lingeman

26 **Melamine-Associated Urinary Stone**.................................. 219
Yao Liang Deng and Cheng Yang Li

27 **Trace Elements in Urolithiasis**... 227
Albrecht Hesse and Roswitha Siener

28 **Infection Stones**... 231
Janet Colli and Raju Thomas

29 **Epidemiological and Etiological Considerations** 237
Hans-Göran Tiselius

Part III Diagnosis

30 **Diagnosis of Urinary Tract Stones: An Overview** 243
Ahmed S. El-Hefnawy and Ahmed A. Shokeir

31 **Diagnosis and Differential Diagnosis of Urinary Tract Stone Disease in Emergency Settings**.. 251
Luo Yang, Hong Li, and Kunjie Wang

32 **The Utilization of Ultrasound in the Diagnosis of Urolithiasis**............. 255
James H. Masterson, Alyson Brinker, Nathan Hawkes, Lee D. Hall, Danielle A. Taysom, Brian K. Auge, and James O. L'Esperance

33 **The Role of Radiological Imaging** 265
Zafar Sajjad

34 **Radiation Exposure in Uroradiology** 271
Maseeh uz Zaman

35 **The Use of Low-Dose CT Scanning** 277
Sean A. Pierre

36 **The Physics of Ultrasound and X-Rays: A Primer for Urologists** 283
K. Razi Naqvi

Part IV Technology and Innovation

37 **The Stone Surgeon/Lithotomists' Armamentarium: Today and Tomorrow** 293
Carl Sarkissian and Manoj Monga

38 **Physics and Technique of Shock Wave Lithotripsy (SWL)** 301
Othmar J. Wess

39 **Laser Lithotripsy Physics** 313
Joel M.H. Teichman, Jinze Qiu, Wook Kang, Kin Foong Chan, and Thomas E. Milner

40 **Bioeffects of Shock Wave Lithotripsy** 327
Ehud Gnessin and James E. Lingeman

41 **History and Development of the Ureteroscope: What Does the Future Hold?** 333
Demetrius H. Bagley and Kelly A. Healy

42 **The Operating Room Technicians' and Nurses' Roles in Urologic Surgery** 343
Mohammad Iqbal and Khurram Mutahir Siddiqui

43 **Innovation in Stone Disease** 347
Brian H. Eisner and Stephen P. Dretler

Part V Management Strategies

44 **The Management of a Patient with an Acute Stone Problem** 353
Ahmed S. El-Hefnawy, Ahmed Abed, and Ahmed A. Shokeir

45 **Open Surgery: Current Status and Techniques** 363
Nagaraja P. Rao

46 **Shock Wave Lithotripsy: Present Indications and Future Prospects** 375
Michael E. Lipkin and Glenn M. Preminger

47 **What You Should Know About Extracorporeal Shock Wave Lithotripsy and How You Can Improve Your Performance** 383
Christian G. Chaussy and Hans-Göran Tiselius

48 **Examples of Clinical Problems that Might Be Encountered in Patients Treated with Extracorporeal Shock Wave Lithotripsy** 395
Hans-Göran Tiselius and Christian G. Chaussy

49 **SWL of Renal and Ureteral Stones: The Chinese Experience** 401
Xizhao Sun, Xiaoming Cong, and Luming Shen

50 **Retrograde Intrarenal Surgery (RIRS)** ... 411
Andreas J. Gross and Christopher Netsch

51 **Percutaneous Nephrolithotomy (PCNL)** ... 417
Mahesh R. Desai and Arvind P. Ganpule

52 **Tubeless Percutaneous Nephrolithotomy** ... 427
Chong H. Choe, James O. L'Esperance, Suzanne R. Gudeman, and Brian K. Auge

53 **Minimally Invasive Percutaneous Nephrolithotomy: The Chinese Approach** ... 433
Guohua Zeng, Wen Zhong, and Zhaohui He

54 **Percutaneous Nephrostomy, Antegrade Stent Placement, and Radiological Control of Post-PCNL Bleeding** ... 439
Tanveer ul Haq and Basit Salam

55 **Management Strategies for Staghorn Stones** ... 445
Markus Margreiter and Michael Marberger

56 **Ureteral Stone Management: An Overview** ... 455
Sutchin R. Patel and Stephen Y. Nakada

57 **Ureteroscopy for Ureteric Stones** ... 463
Gerhard J. Fuchs and Steven G. Koopman

58 **Tricks for Successful Ureteroscopy** ... 473
Zhong Wu and Chen-Chen Feng

59 **Lasers in Stone Disease** ... 481
Anne Sophie Knipper and Andreas J. Gross

60 **Ureteric Stents: Their Use and Abuse** ... 487
Stuart J. Graham and Simon Choong

61 **Ureteric Stenting: Tips and Tricks** ... 503
Syed Muhammad Nazim, Ali Akbar Zehri, and Khurram Mutahir Siddiqui

62 **Transperitoneal Laparoscopic and Retroperitoneoscopic Stone Treatment** ... 509
Marcel Hruza and Jens J. Rassweiler

63 **Role of Robotic-Assisted Surgery in the Management of Urolithiasis** ... 515
Tyler Luthringer, Khurram Mutahir Siddiqui, and David Mois Albala

64 **Management of Urinary Bladder Calculi** ... 519
Jai Pal Paryani and Syed Raziuddin Biyabani

65 **Current Status of Medical Expulsion Therapy for Urinary Calculi** ... 527
Zhangqun Ye and Huan Yang

66 **Dissolution of Stones by Oral and Irrigative Therapy** ... 533
Ruslan Korets, Joseph A. Graversen, and Mantu Gupta

67 **Traditional Chinese Medicine for Treatment of Urinary Stones** ... 539
Xiao He

68 **Patient Safety and the Importance of Informed Consent** ... 543
Robyna Irshad Khan

69 **Anesthesia and Pain Relief for Procedures Performed to Manage Urolithiasis** ... 547
Gauhar Afshan and Aliya Ahmed

Part VI Management of Stones Under Special Circumstances

70 **Shock Wave Lithotripsy, Endourological Intervention, and Hemostatic Defects** ... 557
Bushra Moiz and Syed Raziuddin Biyabani

71 **Cardiac Rhythm Management Devices** ... 563
Azam Shafquat

72 **Stone Disease in Pregnancy** ... 567
Ahmed Mohamed Elshal and Ahmed A. Shokeir

73 **Minimally Invasive Treatment of Calculi in Renal Anomalies** ... 575
Ahmed R. El-Nahas and Ahmed A. Shokeir

74 **Kidney Stones and Chronic Kidney Disease** ... 587
Absar Ali, Quratulain Khan, and Tazeen H. Jafar

75 **Calculus Renal Failure in Pakistan** ... 595
Saiyid Jaffar Ali Naqvi

76 **Urolithiasis in Renal Transplant Donors and Recipients** ... 601
Ahmed M. Harraz and Ahmed A. Shokeir

77 **Primary Hyperoxaluria: The Role and Timing of Liver and Kidney Transplantation** ... 611
Harshal Rajekar and Shrawan K. Singh

Part VII Pediatric Urolithiasis

78 **Metabolic Stone Disease in Children** ... 621
Kemal Sarica

79 **Pediatric Urinary Stone Disease in China** ... 631
Gang Wang

80 **Patient Evaluation and Comparison of Stone-Removing Strategies in Pediatric Patients with Urinary Tract Stones** ... 639
Temuçin Şenkul

81 **Pediatric Vesicle Stone** ... 647
M.S. Ansari, Jatinder Kumar, and Priyadarshi Ranjan

82 **Shock Wave Lithotripsy for Renal Stone in Children** ... 655
M. Hammad Ather

83 **Endourological Approaches to Renal and Ureteric Calculi in Children** ... 659
Zafar Zaidi and Zaheer Alam

Part VIII Prevention of Recurrence

84 **Biochemical Risk Evaluation in Patients with Urolithiasis** ... 671
Hans-Göran Tiselius

85 **Application of Physical Methods to Kidney Stones and Randall's Plaque Characterization** ... 683
Michel Daudon and Dominique Bazin

86 **General and Specific Dietary Advice for the Prevention of Stone Recurrence** ... 709
William G. Robertson

87 **Overview of Stone Prevention Strategies in China** ... 721
Zhiqiang Chen

88 **Management of Hypercalciuria and Oxalates in the Prevention of Stone Recurrence** ... 727
John R. Asplin

89 **Citrate Therapy for Calcium and Uric Acid Stones** ... 735
Ephrem O. Olweny and Margaret S. Pearle

90 **The Importance of Water and Other Fluids in the Prevention of Stone Recurrence** ... 745
Tiziana Meschi, Antonio Nouvenne, and Loris Borghi

91 **Orthophosphates** ... 751
Renata Caudarella

92 **Management of Cystinuria** ... 757
Jan Peter Jessen and Thomas Knoll

93 **The Detection and Management of Primary Hyperparathyroidism in Patients with Urolithiasis** ... 767
Mumtaz Jamshed Khan, Syed Raziuddin Biyabani, Nuzhat Faruqui, and Jamsheer Jehangir Talati

94 **Normocalcemic Hyperparathyroidism: An Illustrative Case Scenario** ... 785
Johar Raza, Jamsheer J. Talati, and Nasir Ud Din Yashkun

95 **How to Perform a Successful Exploration of the Neck for Primary Hyperparathyroidism** ... 791
William R. Lynn and John A. Lynn

Part IX Education, Training, Assessment, and Development

96 **Professional Development and Competence of Physicians** ... 803
Camer W. Vellani

97 **Assessment in Postgraduate Training** ... 807
Zareen Zaidi and John Norcini

98 **Assessment of Competence** ... 819
Edward Matsumoto and Jen Hoogenes

99 **Modern Concepts on Cognito-Psychomotor Skill Development** ... 827
Rebecca L. Tregunna, Matthew F. Bultitude, and Muhammad Shamim Khan

100 **Integration of Competences** ... 837
Munir Ahmed

101 **Education and Training of an Academic Urologic Surgeon** ... 841
Farhat Abbas and Michael Coburn

102 **Advanced Training of a Practicing Urologist in Stone Disease Management** 855
Tamer El-Husseiny and Noor N.P. Buchholz

103 **Across Semantic Turfs: The Need for Broader Education** 863
Syed Nomanul Haq

104 **Stimulating Research and Innovation in Residents** 869
Scott Leslie and Mihir Desai

Part X Equitable Management of Stone Disease

105 **Bringing Sophisticated High-Technology Surgical Care to the Rural Masses: What Is India Doing?** 875
Tehemton E. Udwadia

106 **Bringing Highly Technological Urolithiasis Care to a Billion People: What Is China Doing?** 881
Guo-Min Wang and Jian-Ming Guo

107 **Lithotripter Sharing** 885
André van der Merwe, Nicole Ebinger Mundorff, and Rian Nieuwoudt

108 **Choosing and Purchasing Expensive Medical Equipment: A Hospital Perspective** 891
Nadeem Kamal Mustafa Khan and Farhan Bhayani

109 **Comparative Costs of Various Treatment Strategies and Preventive Measures** 897
Roswitha Siener and Albrecht Hesse

110 **Financial Options for Purchase, Lease, and Hire of Lithotripters** 903
Faridun K. Dadachanji

111 **The Engagement of Philanthropy** 907
Shamsh Kassim-Lakha

112 **The Impact on Health Care of the Recent Global Epidemiological Trends in Urolithiasis** 915
Alberto Trinchieri

113 **Societal Changes and the Etiology of Stone Disease** 921
Dorit E. Zilberman, Tyler Luthringer, Daniel Young, and David M. Albala

Part XI Case Scenarios

114 **Case Scenarios and Interesting Images in Urolithiasis** 931
M. Hammad Ather, Zafar Sajjad, Basit Salam, and M. Nasir Sulaiman

Epilogue 959

Index 961

Contributors

Farhat Abbas, M.B.B.S., FCPS, FRCS, FRCSEd, FEBU, FACS Department of Surgery, Medical College, Aga Khan University, Karachi, Sindh, Pakistan

Ahmed Abed, M.D., M.S. Department of Urology, Urology and Nephrology Center, Mansoura University, Mansoura, Egypt

Gauhar Afshan, FCPS (Pakistan) Department of Anaesthesia, Aga Khan University, Karachi, Sindh, Pakistan

Aliya Ahmed, FFARCS (Ireland) Department of Anaesthesia, Aga Khan University, Karachi, Sindh, Pakistan

Munir Ahmed, M.Sc. (Med Ed. Cardiff), MAcaMed, FRCS, FRCS (Urol) Department of Urology, Kings College of Medicine, University of London, Bromley, Kent, UK

Zaheer Alam, M.B.B.S., MCPS, FCPS Urology Department of Urology, The Indus Hospital, Karachi, Pakistan

David Mois Albala, M.D. Division of Urology, Associated Medical Professionals, Syracuse, NY, USA

Absar Ali, M.D., FACP Department of Medicine, Aga Khan University, Karachi, Sindh, Pakistan

Liaqat Ali, M.B.B.S., FCPS (Urology) Department of Urology, Institute of Kidney Diseases, Peshawar, Khyber PukhtoonKhaw, Pakistan

M.S. Ansari, M.S., MNAMS, MCh, Diplomat National Board Department of Urology and Renal Transplantation, Sanjay Gandhi Postgraduate Institute of Medical Sciences, Lucknow, Uttar Pradesh, India

Khursheed Anwar, M.B.B.S., FRCS, Dip (Urol) Department of Urology, PAEC General Hospital, Islamabad, Pakistan

John R. Asplin, M.D., FASN Department of Medicine, University of Chicago, Litholink Corporation, Chicago, IL, USA

M. Hammad Ather, M.B.B.S., FCPS (Urol), FEBU Department of Surgery, Division of Urology, Aga Khan University, Karachi, Sindh, Pakistan

Brian K. Auge, M.D. Mountain States Urology, St. Luke's Health System, Boise, ID, USA

Wajahat Aziz, M.B.B.S. Department of Urology, Aga Khan University, Karachi, Pakistan

Demetrius H. Bagley, M.D., FACS Department of Urology, Jefferson Medical College, Thomas Jefferson University, Philadelphia, PA, USA

Kashif Bangash, M.B.B.S., FCPS (I) Department of Urology, PAEC General Hospital, Islamabad, Pakistan

Simon Virgil Bariol, M.B.B.S., B.Sc., (Med) FRACS Department of Urology, Westmead Hospital, Westmead, NSW, Australia

Samra Bashir, Ph.D. Department of Biological and Biomedical Sciences, Aga Khan University, Karachi, Sindh, Pakistan

Dominique C. Bazin, Ph.D. Laboratoire de Physique des Solides UMR 8502, Université Paris Sud, Orsay Cedex, France

Farhan Bhayani, B.E. (Mech), MBA, CPM Division of Materials Management, Aga Khan University, Karachi, Sindh, Pakistan

Syed Raziuddin Biyabani, M.B.B.S., FCPS (Urol), FEBU Section of Urology, Department of Surgery, The Aga Khan University, Karachi, Sindh, Pakistan

Loris Borghi, M.D. Department of Clinical and Experimental Medicine, University of Parma, Parma, Italy

Alyson Brinker, B.S. Department of Internal Medicine, Uniformed Services University of the Health Sciences, Bethesda, MD, USA

Noor N.P. Buchholz, M.B.B.S. (D), M.D. (CH), FSSU (CH), FKNMG (NL) Department of Endourology and Stone services, Barts and The London School of Medicine and Dentistry, Barts and the London NHS Trust, West Smithfield, London, UK

Matthew F. Bultitude, M.B.B.S., MRCS, M.Sc., FRCS (Urol) Department of Urology, Guy's and St. Thomas' NHS Foundation Trust, London, UK

Renata Caudarella, M.D. Department of Mineral Metabolism, Fondazione Ettore Sansavini per la Ricerca Scientifica (Health Science Foundation) ONLUS, Lugo, Ravenna, Italy

Kin Foong Chan, Ph.D. VP Engineering, Dermira Inc, Redwood City, CA, USA

Christian G. Chaussy, M.D. Department of Urology, Caritas Medical Center St. Josef, University of Regensburg, Regensburg, Oberpfalz, Germany

Zhiqiang Chen, M.D., Ph.D. Department of Urology, Tongji Hospital, Huazhong University of Science and Technology, Wuhan, Hubei, People's Republic of China

Ben H. Chew, M.D., M.Sc., FRCSC Department of Urology, University of British Columbia, Vancouver, BC, Canada

Chong H. Choe, M.D. Department of Urology, Naval Medical Center, San Diego, CA, USA

Simon Choong, M.B.B.S. (Lon), FRCS (Eng), FRCSEd, MS, FRCS (Urol) The Stone Unit, University College London Hospital, London, UK

Michael Coburn, M.D., FACS Scott Department of Urology, Ben Taub General Hospital, Baylor College of Medicine, Houston, TX, USA

Janet L. Colli, M.D. Department of Urology, Tulane University, New Orleans, LA, USA

Xiaoming Cong, Ph.D. Department of Urology, Nanjing Drum Tower Hospital, The Affiliated Nanjing Drum Tower Hospital of Nanjing University Medical School, Nanjing, Jiangsu, China

Faridun K. Dadachanji, B.A., Economics Advisory Services, Advanced Equities, First Allied Security, San Diego, CA, USA

Michel Daudon, Ph.D. Service des Explorations Fonctionnelles, Tenon Hospital, APHP, Paris, France

Yao Liang Deng, M.D., Ph.D. Department of Urology, The First Affiliated Hospital of Guangxi Medical University, Nanning, Guangxi, China

John D. Denstedt, M.D., FRCSC, FACS Department of Surgery, The University of Western Ontario, London, ON, Canada

Mahesh R. Desai, M.S., FRCS Department of Urology, Muljibhai Patel Urological Hospital, Nadiad, Gujarat, India

Mihir Desai, M.D. Robotic Urological Surgery, USC Institute of Urology, Keck School of Medicine, University of Southern California, Los Angeles, CA, USA

Somnuek Domrongkitchaiporn, M.D. Department of Medicine, Ramathibodi Hospital, Bangkok, Thailand

Stephen P. Dretler, M.D., Department of Urology, Massachusetts General Hospital, Harvard Medical School, Boston, MA, USA

Nicole Ebinger Mundorff, M.D. Department of Urology, University Hospital Basel, Basel, Switzerland

Ahmed M. Elshal, M.Sc., FEBU Department of Urology, Mansoura Urology and Nephrology Center, Mansoura University, Mansoura, Egypt

Brian H. Eisner, M.D. Department of Urology, Massachusetts General Hospital, Harvard Medical School, Boston, MA, USA

Salah R. El-Faqih, MBChB, FRCS (Glasgow), FRCS (England) Department of Surgery (Urology), College of Medicine, King Saud University, Riyadh, Kingdom of Saudi Arabia

Ahmed S. El-Hefnawy, M.D. Department of Urology, Urology and Nephrology Center, Mansoura University, Mansoura, Egypt

Tamer El-Husseiny, MBBCh (Hons), M.Sc. (Urol), MRCS (Ed.) Department of Urology, Queen Elizabeth Hospital Birmingham, University Hospitals Birmingham NHS Foundation Trust, Birmingham, UK

Ahmed R. El-Nahas, M.D. Department of Urology, Urology and Nephrology Center, Mansoura University, Mansoura, Egypt

Ahmed Mohamed Elshal, M.Sc., FEBU Department of Urology, Mansoura Urology and Nephrology Center, Mansoura University, Mansoura, Egypt

David B. Evans, Ph.D. Department of Health Systems Financing (HSF), World Health Organization, Geneva, Switzerland

Nuzhat Faruqui, M.B.B.S., FRCS (Urology), FEBU Section of Urology, Department of Surgery, The Aga Khan University, Karachi, Sindh, Pakistan

Chen-Chen Feng, M.D. Department of Urology, Huashan Hospital, Fudan University, People's Republic of China

Pietro Manuel Ferraro, M.D. Division of Nephrology and Dialysis, Renal Program, Department of Internal Medicine and Medical Specialties, Columbus-Gemelli University Hospital, Rome, Italy

Gerhard J. Fuchs, M.D., FACS Department of Surgery, Minimally Invasive Urology Institute, Cedars-Sinai Medical Center, Los Angeles, CA, USA

Andrew Fuller, M.B.B.S., FRACS Division of Urology, The University of Western Ontario, London, ON, Canada

Giovanni Gambaro, Ph.D. Division of Nephrology and Dialysis, School of Medicine, Columbus-Gemelli University Hospital, Catholic University, Rome, Italy

Raguram Ganesamoni, M.S., MRCS, MCh (Urology) Department of Urology, Postgraduate Institute of Medical Education and Research, Chandigarh, Chandigarh, India

Arvind P. Ganpule, M.S., DNB, MNAMS Department of Urology, Muljibhai Patel Urological Hospital, Nadiad, Gujarat, India

Farooq Ghani, M.D., Ph.D. (Path) USA Department of Pathology, Aga Khan University, Karachi, Pakistan

Anwarul-Hassan Gilani, Ph.D. Department of Biological and Biomedical Sciences, The Aga Khan University Medical College, Karachi, Sindh, Pakistan

Ehud Gnessin, M.D. Department of Urology, Indiana University Health, Indianapolis, IN, USA

Stuart J. Graham, B.Sc., M.B.B.S., FRCSEd, FRCS (Urol) Department of Urology, Whipps Cross Hospital, Barts Health NHS Trust, Leytonstone, London, UK

Joseph A. Graversen, M.D. Department of Urology, Columbia University College of Physicians and Surgeons, New York Presbyterian Hospital Kidney Stone Center, NY, USA

Andreas J. Gross, M.D. Department of Urology, Asklepios Hospital Barmbek, Hamburg, Germany

Suzanne R. Gudeman, M.D. Department of Urology, Naval Medical Center, San Diego, CA, USA

Jian-Ming Guo, M.D., Ph.D. Department of Urology, Zhongshan Hospital, Fudan University, Shanghai, China

Mantu Gupta, M.D. Director of Endourology, Columbia University and NYPH Kidney Stone Center, New York, NY, USA

New York Presbyterian Hospital Kidney Stone Center, New York, NY, USA

Lee D. Hall, M.D. Department of Radiology, Naval Medical Center, San Diego, CA, USA

Syed Nomanul Haq, Ph.D. Social Sciences and Humanities, Lahore University of Management Sciences (LUMS), Lahore, Pakistan

Tanveer ul Haq, M.B.B.S., FCPS, FRCR Department of Radiology, Aga Khan University Hospital, Karachi, Sindh, Pakistan

Naveed Haroon, M.B.B.S. Department of Urology, Aga Khan University, Karachi, Sindh, Pakistan

Ahmed M. Harraz M.D., M.S., MRCS Department of Urology and Nephrology Center, Mansoura University, Mansoura, Egypt

Nathan Hawkes, M.D. Department of Radiology, Naval Medical Center, San Diego, CA, USA

Xiao He, MB Department of Urology, Peking Union Medical College Hospital, Beijing, China

Zhaohui He, M.D. Department of Urology, Minimally Invasive Surgery Center, Guangdong Key Laboratory of Urology, The First Affiliated Hospital of Guangzhou Medical College, Guangzhou, Guangdong, China

Kelly A. Healy, M.D. Department of Urology, Jefferson Medical College, Thomas Jefferson University, Philadelphia, PA, USA

Ita Pfeferman Heilberg, M.D., Ph.D. Nephrology Division, Federal University of São Paulo, São Paulo, Brazil

Albrecht Hesse, Ph.D. Urinary Stone Analysis Centre Bonn, Bonn, Germany

Jen Hoogenes, M.S., Ph.D.(c) Department of Clinical Epidemiology and Biostatistics and Department of Surgery, St. Joseph's Healthcare Hamilton, McMaster University, Hamilton, ON, Canada

Marcel Hruza, M.D. Department of Urology, SLK-Kliniken GmbH, Heilbronn, Germany

Mohammad Iqbal Department of Nursing, Aga Khan University, Karachi, Pakistan

Tazeen H. Jafar, M.D., MPH Department of Medicine, Aga Khan University, Karachi, Sindh, Pakistan

Jan Peter Jessen, M.D. Department of Urology, Sindelfingen-Boeblingen Medical Center, Sindelfingen, Baden-Wuerternberg, Germany

Paul Jungers, M.D. Department of Nephrology, Necker-Enfants Malades Hospital, APHP, Paris, France

Wook Kang American Medical Systems, Minnetonka, MN, USA

Shamsh Kassim-Lakha, MBA Founding President, Aga Khan University and Chairman, Board of Directors of Pakistan Centre for Philanthropy, Islamabad, Pakistan

Aga Khan University, Karachi, Sindh, Pakistan

Aysha Habib Khan, M.B.B.S., FCPS (chemical pathology) Department of Pathology and Microbiology and Medicine, Aga Khan University, Karachi, Sindh, Pakistan

Muhammad Shamim Khan, M.B.B.S., MCPS, FRCS (Urol), FEBU Department of Urology, Guy's and St. Thomas' NHS Foundation Trust, London, UK

Mumtaz Jamshed Khan, M.D., FACS Department of Otolaryngology, Head and Neck Institute, Cleveland Clinic Foundation, Cleveland, OH, USA

Nadeem Kamal Mustafa Khan, B.A., B.Sc. (Econ), FCA Regional CEO, Health Services, Asia, The Aga Khan University Hospital, Karachi, Sindh, Pakistan

Naveed Ahmed Khan, Ph.D. Department of Biological and Biomedical Sciences, Aga Khan University, Karachi, Sindh, Pakistan

Robyna Irshad Khan, FCPS (anaesthesiology), M.B.B.S., MHSc (bioethics) Department of Anesthesia and Intensive Care, Aga Khan University, Karachi, Sindh, Pakistan

Quratulain Khan, M.B.B.S. Department of Medicine, Aga Khan University, Karachi, Sindh, Pakistan

Anne Sophie Knipper, M.D. Department of Urology, Asklepios Hospital Barmbek, Hamburg, Germany

Thomas Knoll, M.D., Ph.D., M.Sc. Department of Urology, Sindelfingen-Boeblingen Medical Center, Sindelfingen, Baden-Wuertternberg, Germany

Steven G. Koopman, M.D. Department of Surgery, Minimally Invasive Urology Program, Cedars-Sinai Medical Center, Los Angeles, CA, USA

Ruslan Korets, M.D. Department of Urology, Columbia University College of Physicians and Surgeons, New York Presbyterian Hospital Kidney Stone Center, NY, USA

Fernando Korkes Division of Urology, ABC Medical School, São Paulo, Brazil

Division of Nephrology, Federal University of São Paulo, São Paulo, Brazil

Jatinder Kumar, M.S. Department of Urology and Renal Transplantation, Sanjay Gandhi Postgraduate Institute of Medical Sciences, Lucknow, Uttar Pradesh, India

Dirk Lange, B.Sc. (Hon), Ph.D. Department of Urologic Sciences, Jack Bell Research Centre, The Stone Centre at Vancouver General Hospital, University of British Columbia, Vancouver, BC, Canada

Ming-Chak Lee, M.B.B.S. Department of Urology, Westmead Hospital, Westmead, NSW, Australia

Scott Leslie, M.D. Robotic Urological Surgery, USC Institute of Urology, Keck School of Medicine, University of Southern California, Los Angeles, CA, USA

James O. L'Esperance, M.D. Department of Urology, Naval Medical Center, San Diego, CA, USA

Cheng Yang Li, M.D., Ph.D. Department of Urology, The First Affiliated Hospital of Guangxi Medical University, Nanning, Guangxi, China

Hammersmith and Ealing Hospitals, London, UK

Hong Li, M.D. Department of Urology, West China Hospital of Sichuan University, Chengdu, Sichuan, China

James E. Lingeman, M.D. Department of Urology, Indiana University Health, Indianapolis, IN, USA

Michael E. Lipkin, M.D. Division of Urology, Department of Surgery, Duke University Medical Center, Durham, NC, USA

Deyi Luo, M.D. Department of Urology, West China Hospital, Sichuan University, Chengdu, Sichuan Province, China

Tyler Luthringer, B.A. Division of Urology, Associated Medical Professionals, Syracuse, NY, USA

John A. Lynn, M.S., FRCS Department of General Surgery, Barnet and Chase Farm Hospital NHS Trust, Bupa Cromwell Hospital, London, UK

Department of Endocrinology, Hammersmith and Ealing Hospitals, London, UK

William R. Lynn, M.B.B.S., B.Sc. (Hons), MRCS Department of General Surgery, Barnet and Chase Farm Hospital NHS Trust, London, UK

Jessica A. Mandeville, M.D. Department of Urology, Indiana University Health, Indianapolis, IN, USA

Amanullah Memon, M.B.B.S., FRCS (Ed) Department of Surgery, Aga Khan University, Karachi, Sindh, Pakistan

Y.M. Fazil Marickar, M.S., MAMS, Ph.D. (Urology), FAMS, FIMSA, DAS, FEMSI Department of Surgery, Azeezia Medical College, Kollam, Kerala, India

Thomas E. Milner, Ph.D. Department of Biomedical Engineering, The University of Texas at Austin, Austin, TX, USA

Michael Marberger, M.D., FRCS (ed) Department of Urology, Medical University of Vienna, Vienna, Austria

Markus Margreiter, M.D., FEBU Department of Urology, Medical University Vienna, Vienna, Austria

James H. Masterson, M.D. Department of Urology, Naval Medical Center, San Diego, CA, USA

Edward Matsumoto, M.D., MEd, FRCSC Division of Urology, St. Joseph's Healthcare, McMaster University, Hamilton, ON, Canada

Tiziana Meschi, M.D. Department of Clinical Sciences, University of Parma, Parma, Italy

Bushra Moiz, M.B.B.S., MCPS (Path), FCPS (Haem) Section of Hematology, Department of Pathology and Microbiology, The Aga Khan University, Karachi, Sindh, Pakistan

Manoj Monga, M.D. Department of Urology, Steven Streem Center for Endourology and Stone Disease, The Cleveland Clinic, Cleveland, OH, USA

Shamim Mushtaq, Ph.D. Department of Biochemistry, National Center for Proteomics, University of Karachi, Karachi, Sindh, Pakistan

Stephen Y. Nakada, M.D. Department of Urology, University of Wisconsin School of Medicine and Public Health, Madison, WI, USA

K. Razi Naqvi, Ph.D. Department of Physics, Norwegian University of Science and Technology (NTNU), Trondheim, Norway

Saiyid Jaffar Ali Naqvi, F.R.C.P. Department of Nephrology, The Kidney Foundation, National Institute of Kidney and Urological Diseases (NIKUD), University of Karachi, Karachi, Pakistan

Abdul Razzaq Nasir, M.B.B.S., FCPS Department of Urology, Bolan Medical College Ouetta, Ouetta, Pakistan

Tair Nazarov, M.D. Department of Urology, Northwestern State Medical University, St. Petersburg, Russian Federation

Syed Muhammad Nazim, M.B.B.S., MCPS, MRCS (Glasgow), FCPS (Urology) Department of Surgery, The Aga Khan University and Hospital Karachi, Karachi, Sindh, Pakistan

Christopher Netsch, M.D. Department of Urology, Asklepios Hospital Barmbek, Hamburg, Germany

Rian Nieuwoudt, Pr.Eng, M.Eng, B.Eng (Stell) Managing Director at Spectra-Medic, AHG Group of Companies, Western Cape, South Africa

John Norcini, Ph.D. Foundation for Advancement of International Medical Education and Research (FAIMER), Philadelphia, PA, USA

Antonio Nouvenne, M.D., Ph.D. Department of Clinical Sciences, University of Parma, Parma, Italy

Andrei Novikov, M.D. Department of Urology, Northwestern State Medical University, St. Petersburg, Russian Federation

Yoshihide Ogawa, M.D., Ph.D. Department of Urology, Tokyo-West Tokushukai Hospital, Akishima City, Tokyo, Japan

Ephrem O. Olweny, M.D. Department of Urology, University of Texas Southwestern Medical Center, Dallas, TX, USA

Nasir Orakzai, M.B.B.S., FRCS Department of Urology, Institute of Kidney Diseases, Peshawar, Khyber PukhtoonKhaw, Pakistan

Palle J.S. Osther, M.D., Ph.D. EAU Section of Urolithiasis (EULIS), Urological Research Center, Fredericia, Denmark

Department of Urology, Fredericia Hospital, Part of Hospital Littlebelt, Institute of Regional Health Services Research, University of Southern Denmark, Fredericia, Denmark

Charles Y.C. Pak, M.D. Internal Medicine, Center for Mineral Metabolism and Clinical Research, University of Texas Southwestern Medical Center at Dallas, Dallas, TX, USA

Jai Pal Paryani, M.B.B.S., FCPS, FEBU Department of Urology, Liaquat University of Medical and Health Sciences, Jamshoro, Sindh, Pakistan

Sutchin R. Patel, M.D. Department of Urology, University of Wisconsin School of Medicine and Public Health, Madison, WI, USA

Margaret S. Pearle, M.D., Ph.D. Department of Urology, University of Texas Southwestern Medical Center, Dallas, TX, USA

Sean A. Pierre, M.D., FRCS (C) Urology Department of Urology, Queen's University, Kingston, ON, Canada

Department of Surgery, Queensway Carleton Hospital, Nepean, ON, Canada

Bita Pourmand, M.D. Department of Urology, Research Development Center, Sina University Hospital, Tehran University of Medical Sciences, Tehran, Iran

Gholamreza Pourmand, M.D. Department of Urology, Research Development Center, Sina University Hospital, Tehran University of Medical Sciences, Tehran, Iran

Glenn M. Preminger, M.D. Department of Urolgical Surgery, Duke University Medical Center, Durham, NC, USA

Duke Comprehensive Kidney Stone Center, Durham, NC, USA

Jinze Qiu, M.A. Department of Biomedical Engineering, The University of Texas at Austin, Austin, TX, USA

Harshal Rajekar, M.S., MRCS, DNB Department of General Surgery, Post Graduate Institute of Medical Education & Research, Chandigarh, Chandigarh, India

Priyadarshi Ranjan, M.S., MCh Department of Urology and Renal Transplantation, Sanjay Gandhi Postgraduate Institute of Medical Sciences, Lucknow, Uttar Pradesh, India

Nagaraja P. Rao, M.B.B.S., ChM, FRCS Ed Formerly Director of Total Stone Management Centre, University Hospital of South Manchester, Manchester, UK

NTR University of Health Sciences, Vijayawada, Andhra Pradesh, India

Pegeia, Paphos, Cyprus

Jens J. Rassweiler, M.D. Department of Urology, SLK Kliniken Heilbronn, University of Heidelberg, Heilbronn, Germany

Johar Raza, M.B.B.S., FCPS (Urol) Section of Urology, Aga Khan University, Karachi, Sindh, Pakistan

William G. Robertson, Ph.D., D.Sc. The Physiology Department, Centre for Nephrology, Royal Free and University College Medical School, London, UK

Allen Rodgers, M.Sc., Ph.D. Department of Chemistry, University of Cape Town, Cape Town, South Africa

Zafar Sajjad, M.B.B.S., MRCP (UK), FRCR Department of Radiology, Aga Khan University, Karachi, Sindh, Pakistan

Khashayar Sakhaee, M.D. Department of Internal Medicine, UT Southwestern Medical Center, Dallas, TX, USA

Basit Salam, M.B.B.S., FCPS Department of Radiology, Aga Khan University Hospital, Karachi, Sindh, Pakistan

Kemal Sarica, M.D., Ph.D. Department of Urology, Yeditepe University, Medical School, Kozyatagi, Istanbul, Turkey

Carl Sarkissian, B.S. Eng Department of Urology, The Cleveland Clinic, Cleveland, OH, USA

Nestor Schor Nephrology Division, Federal University of São Paulo, São Paulo, Brazil

Temuçin Şenkul, M.D. Department of Urology, GATA Haydarpasa Training Hospital Üsküdar, Istanbul, Turkey

Azam Shafquat, M.B.B.S., FHRS Department of Cardiology, King Faisal Specialist Hospital and Research Center, Riyadh, Saudi Arabia

Luming Shen, Ph.D. Department of Urology, Nanjing Drum Tower Hospital, The Affiliated Nanjing Drum Tower Hospital of Nanjing University Medical School, Nanjing, Jiangsu, China

Ahmed A. Shokeir, M.D., Ph.D., FEBU Department of Urology, Urology and Nephrology Center, Mansoura University, Mansoura, Egypt

Anwar Ali Siddiqui, Ph.D. Department of Biological and Biomedical Sciences, Medical College, Aga Khan University, Karachi, Pakistan

Khurram Mutahir Siddiqui, FCPS, FRCS (UK), FEBU Department of Nursing, Section of Urology, The Aga Khan University, Karachi, Pakistan

Roswitha Siener, Ph.D. Department of Urology, University Stone Centre, University of Bonn, Bonn, Germany

Shrawan K. Singh, MS, MCh (Urology) Department of Urology, Postgraduate Institute of Medical Education and Research, Chandigarh, Chandigarh, India

Vladimir Yu. Startsev, M.D. Department of Urology, State Pediatric Medical Academy St. Petersburg, St. Petersburg, Russia

Wasana Stitchantrakul Department of Medicine, Research Center, Ramathibodi Hospital, Mahidol University, Bangkok, Thailand

M. Nasir Sulaiman, M.B.B.S., FRCS, FRCS (Urol) Section of Urology, Department of Surgery, Aga Khan University Hospital, Karachi, Pakistan

Xizhao Sun, M.D. Department of Urology, Nanjing Drum Tower Hospital, The Affiliated Nanjing Drum Tower Hospital of Nanjing University Medical School, Nanjing, Jiangsu, China

Roger A.L. Sutton, DM, FRCP, FRCPC Department of Urological Sciences and Medicine, University of British Columbia, Vancouver, BC, Canada

Jamsheer Jehangir Talati, M.B.B.S., FRCS Section of Urology, Department of Surgery, The Aga Khan University, Karachi, Sindh, Pakistan

Danielle A. Taysom, M.D. Department of Radiology, Naval Medical Center, San Diego, CA, USA

Joel M.H. Teichman, M.D. Department of Urologic Sciences, University of British Columbia, Vancouver, BC, Canada

Raju Thomas, M.D., FACS, MHA Department of Urology, Tulane University, Health Sciences Center, New Orleans, LA, USA

Hans-Göran Tiselius, M.D., Ph.D. Division of Urology, Department of Clinical Science, Intervention and Technology, Karolinska Institutet, Stockholm, Sweden

Rebecca L. Tregunna, M.B.B.S., B.Sc. (Hons.) Department of Urology, Guy's and St. Thomas' NHS Foundation Trust, London, UK

Alberto Trinchieri, M.D., FEBU Department of Urology, A. Manzoni Hospital, Lecco, Italy

Tehemton E. Udwadia, M.S., FCPS, FRCS (Eng), FRCS (Edin), FAMS, FACS (Hon), FICS (Hon), FARSI (Hon) Department of Surgery, Grant Medical College & J.J. Hospital, Mumbai, Maharashtra, India

Department of M.A.S., P.D. Hinduja National Hospital, Mumbai, Maharashtra, India

Parsee General Hospital, Breach Candy Hospital, Mumbai, Maharashtra, India

André van der Merwe, MB Ch B, MRCS (Eng), MRCS (Ed) MMed (Urology), UCT, FC (Urol)SA Department of Urology, Faculty of Health Sciences, University of Stellenbosch and Tygerberg Hospital, Tygerberg, Cape Town, South Africa

Camer W. Vellani, MD (Wales), FRCP (London) Department of Medicine, Aga Khan University, Karachi, Sindh, Pakistan

Gang Wang, M.D., Ph.D. Department of Urology, Peking University First Hospital, Institute of Urology, Peking University, Xicheng District, Beijing, China

Guo-Min Wang Department of Urology, Zhongshan Hospital, Fudan University, Shanghai, China

Kunjie Wang, M.D., Ph.D. Department of Urology, West China Hospital, Sichuan University, Chengdu, Sichuan, China

Othmar J. Wess, Ph.D. Storz Medical AG, Taegerwilen, Thurgau, Switzerland

Zhong Wu, M.D., Ph.D. Department of Urology, Huashan Hospital, Fudan University, Shanghai, People's Republic of China

Huan Yang, M.D., Ph.D. Division of Urology, Tongji Hospital, Tongji Medical College, Huazhong University of Science and Technology, Wuhan, China

Luo Yang, M.D. Department of Urology, West China Hospital of Sichuan University, Chengdu, Sichuan, China

Nasir Ud Din Yashkun, M.B.B.S., FCPS (Histopathology) Department of Pathology, Aga Khan University, Karachi, Sindh, Pakistan

Zhangqun Ye, M.D., Ph.D. Division of Urology, Tongji Hospital, Tongji Medical College, Huazhong University of Science and Technology, Wuhan, China

Daniel Young, M.D. Division of Urology, Duke University Medical Center, Durham, NC, USA

Zafar Zaidi, M.B.B.S., FRCS, FEBU Department of Urology, The Indus Hospital, Karachi, Pakistan

Zareen Zaidi, M.B.B.S., M.D. Foundation for Advancement of International Medical Education and Research (FAIMER), Philadelphia, PA, USA

Maseeh uz Zaman, M.B.B.S., M.S., FCPS, FEBNM, DCBNC, FASNC Department of Radiology, The Aga Khan University Hospital, Karachi, Sindh, Pakistan

Ali Akbar Zehri, M.B.B.S., FCPS (Urology) Section of Urology, Aga Khan Hospital, Dar Es Salaam, Tanzania

Guohua Zeng, M.D., Ph.D. Department of Urology, Minimally Invasive Surgery Center, Guangdong Key Laboratory of Urology, The First Affiliated Hospital of Guangzhou Medical College, Guangzhou, Guangdong, China

Wen Zhong, Ph.D. Department of Urology, Minimally Invasive Surgery Center, Guangdong Key Laboratory of Urology, The First Affiliated Hospital of Guangzhou Medical College, Guangzhou, Guangdong, China

Dorit E. Zilberman M.D. Department of Urology, Chaim Sheba Medical Center, Tel-Hashomaer, Ramat Gan, Israel

Abbreviations

μCT	Micro computed tomography
25(OH)D	Prohormone 25-hydroxyvitamin D
7DHC	7 dehydrocholesterol
ABEUR	Advisory Board of European Urolithiasis Research
ABMS	American Board of Medical Specialties
ABS	American Board of Surgery
ABU	American Board of Urology
ACCP	Amorphous carbonated calcium phosphate
ACE inhibitor	Angiotensin-converting-enzyme inhibitor
ACGME	Accreditation Council for Graduate Medical Education
ACS	American College of Surgery
ADHH	Autosomal dominant hypocalcemia with hypercalciuria
ADHR	Autosomal dominant hypophosphatemic rickets
ADPKD	Autosomal dominant polycystic kidney disease
AGT	Alanine glyoxylate aminotransferase
AHA	Acetohydroxamic acid
AHU	Ammonium acid urate
AIHW	Australian Institute of Health and Welfare
AKU	Aga Khan University
ALARA	As low as reasonably achievable
APDS	Association of Program Directors in Surgery
APTT	Activated partial thromboplastin time
ARB	Angiotensin receptor blocker
ARF	Acute renal failure
ARSI	Association of Rural Surgeons of India
ASI	Association of Surgeons of India
ATP	Adenosine triphosphate
AU	Attenuation units
AUA	American Urological Association
AUA ISE	American Urology Association In-Service Examination
BAUS	British Association of Urological Surgeons
BMD	Bone mineral density
BMI	Body mass index
BNE	Bilateral neck exploration
BPH	Benign prostatic hyperplasia
CanMEDS	Canadian Medical Education Directives for Specialists

CaOx	Calcium oxalate
CaP	Calcium phosphate
CAPD	Continuous ambulatory peritoneal dialysis
CaSR	Calcium sensitive receptor
CASR	Calcium-sensing receptor
CbD	Case-based discussion
CCD	Charge coupled device
CCST	Certificate of completion of specialty training
CEC	Clinical encounter card
CHCPE	Centre for Health Care Policy and Evaluation
CIRF	Clinically insignificant residual fragments
CKD	Chronic kidney disease
CLDN16	Claudin-16
CLL	Cystolitholapaxy
CMS	Centers for Medicare and Medicaid Services
COD	Calcium oxalate dehydrate
COM	Calcium oxalate monohydrate
COT	CaOx trihydrate
CPPS	Chronic pelvic pain syndrome
CPSP	College of Physicians and Surgeons of Pakistan
CRM	Crisis Resource Management
CROES	Clinical Research Office of the Endourological Society
CRT	Cardiac resynchronization therapy
CT	Computed tomography
CTAL	Cortical thick ascending limb
CUA	Chinese Urological Association
DBP	Vitamin D binding protein
DCT	Distal convoluted tubules
DDAVP	De-amino D arginine Vasopressin
DOPS	Direct Observation of Procedural Skills
dRTA	Distal renal tubular acidosis
DSCR	Debt to service coverage ratio
DTPA	Diethylenetriamine pentaacetic acid
DUS	Doppler ultrasonography
EAU	European Association of Urology
ECD	Extracellular domain
ECF	Extracellular fluid
ECG	Electrocardiogram
ECRI	Emergency Care Research Institute
EDS	X-ray energy dispersive spectrometry
EDTA	Ethylenediaminetetraacetic acid
EHL	Electrohydraulic lithotriptor
EMI	Electromagnetic interference
EPAs	Entrustable Professional Activities
ESRD	End-stage renal disease
ESSQ	Endoscopic Surgical Skill Qualification

ESWL	Extracorporeal shockwave lithotripsy
EWTD	European Working Time Directive
FFP	Fresh frozen plasma
FGF23	Fibroblast growth factor 23
FHH	Familial hypocalciuric hypercalcemia
FHHNC	Familial hypomagnesemia with hypercalciuria and nephrocalcinosis
FLS	Fundamentals of Laparoscopy Program
FREDDY laser	Frequency-doubled double pulse ND:YAG laser
FTIR	Fourier transform infrared spectroscopy
FTIRM	FTIR microspectroscopy
F-URS	Flexible uretero-renoscopy
GDNF	Glial-cell-derived neurotrophic factor
GFR	Glomerular filtration rate
GHS rat	Genetic hypercalciuric stone-forming rat
GOALS	Global Operative Assessment of Laparoscopic Skills
GR	Glyoxylate reductase
HAT	Heterodimeric amino acid transporters
HCT	Helical CT
HCUP	Healthcare Cost and Utilization Project
HHRH	Hereditary hypophosphatemic rickets with hypercalciuria
Ho:YAG	Holmium:yttrium-aluminum-garnet
HOX	Hyperoxaluria
HPCS	Healthcare Product Comparison System
HPFS	Health Professional Follow-up Study
HPR	Hydroxypyruvate reductase
IAEA	International Atomic Energy Agency
IAGES	Indian Association of Gastrointestinal Endoscopic Surgery
ICD	Internal cardiac defibrillators
ICRP	International Commission on Radiological Protection
ICSF	Idiopathic calcium oxalate stone formers
IFHH	Idiopathic familial hypocalciuric hypercalcemia
IGNOU	Indira Gandhi National Outreach University
IMCD	Innermedullary collecting ducts
INR	International normalized ratio
IPTH	Intact PTH molecule
IR	Infrared
ITP	Immune-mediated thrombocytopenia
IVP	Intravenous pyelography
IVU	Intravenous urography
JESS	Joint Expert Speciation System
KUB	Kidneys, ureters, and bladder
LED	Light emitting diode
LIBOR	London Interbank Offered Rate
LKT	Liver-kidney transplantation
LMWH	Low molecular weight heparin

LNS	Lesch-Nyhan syndrome
LNT	Linear no-threshold
MAC	Monitored anesthesia care
MAS	Minimal access surgery
MAUS	Melamine-associated urinary stones
MCCQE	Medical Council of Canada Qualifying Examination
MCUG	Micturating cystourethrogram
MET	Medical expulsive therapy
mini PCL	Minimally invasive percutaneous nephrolithotripsy
mini perc	Mini percutaneous nephrolithotomy
Mini-CEX	Mini-Clinical Evaluation Exercise
mini-PAT	Mini-Peer Assessment Tool
MISTELS	McGill Inanimate System for Training and Evaluation of Laparoscopic Skills
MRI	Magnetic resonance imaging
MRU	Magnetic resonance urography
MS	Metabolic syndrome
MSF	Multi-source feedback
MSK	Medullary sponge kidney
mSv	MilliSievert
NAE	Net acid excretion
NAMS	National Hospital Ambulatory Medical Care Survey
NANC	Non-adrenergic non-cholinergic
NASPE/BPEG	North American Society of Pacing and Electrophysiology/British Pacing and Electrophysiology Group
NCCT	Noncontrast computed tomography
NCPHPT	Normocalcemic primary hyperparathyroidism
NGO	Nongovernmental organization
NHANES	National Health and Nutrition Examination Survey
NHANES	National Health and Nutrition Examination Survey
NHS	Nurses' Health Study
NIS	Nationwide Inpatient Samples
NOTSS	Nonoperative technical skills for surgeons
NRPB	National Radiological Protection Board
NSAID	Nonsteroidal anti-inflammatory drug
OAT1	Organic anion transporter 000
OCP	Octacalcium phosphate pentahydrate
OSATS	Objective Structured Assessment of Technical Skills
OSCE	Objective Structured Clinical Examination
PCA	Patient controlled analgesia
PCLN1	Paracellin-1
PCNL	Percutaneous nephrolithotomy
PDE	Phosphodiesterase
PDI	Percussion, inversion therapy and diuresis
PGME	Postgraduate medical education
PH	Primary hyperoxaluria

PH1	Primary hyperoxaluria type I
PH2	Primary hyperoxaluria type II
PHEX	X-linked phosphate-regulating endopeptidase
PHO	Primary hyperoxaluria
PHPT	Primary hyperparathyroidism
PIXE	Proton-induced X-ray emission
PKC	Protein kinase C
PLC	Phospholipase C
PND	Powder neutron diffraction
PNL	Percutaneous nephrolithotripsy
PPi	Inorganic pyrophosphate
PTFE	Polytetrafluoroethylene
PTH	Parathyroid hormone
PUJO	Pelvi-ureteric junction obstruction
PWA	Patients' Welfare Association
QUEST	Queen's Urology Examination Skills Training
RALP	Robotic-assisted laparoscopic pyeloplasty
RBF	Renal blood flow
RC	Renal colic
RCPSC	Royal College of Physicians and Surgeons in Canada
RCT	Randomized controlled trial
RFP	Request for proposal
RIRS	Retrograde intra-renal surgery
RRC	Residency Review Committee
RTA	Renal tubular acidosis
RXR	Retinoid X receptor
RYGB	Roux-en-Y gastric bypass
SAI	Stone age index
SEM	Scanning electron microscopy
SF	Stone formers
SIUT	Sindh Institute of Urology and Transplantation
SPECT	Single photon emission computer tomography
SWL	Shockwave lithotripsy
T2DM	Type 2 diabetes mellitus
TA	Titratable acid
TCO	Total cost of ownership
TDT	Transmission disequilibrium test
THI	Tissue harmonic imaging
THP	Tamm-Horsfall protein
TLC	Thin layer chromatography
TLD	Thermoluminescent dosimeter
TUL	Transurethral ureterolithotripsy
TURP	Transurethral resection of the prostate
UA	Uric acid
UEMS	European Union of Medical Specialists
UFH	Unfractionated heparin

UPJ	Ureteropelvic junction
UPTF1	Urinary prothrombin fragment 1
URS	Ureteroscopy
US	Ultrasonography
USMLE	United States Medical Licensing Examination
UTI	Urinary tract infection
UVB	Ultraviolet B
VCUG	Voiding cystourethrogram
VDR	Vitamin D receptor
VDRE	Vitamin D response elements
VUR	Vesicoureteral reflux
WHO	World Health Organization
XAS	X-ray absorption spectroscopy
XRD	X-ray diffraction
XRF	X-ray fluorescence
ZDF	Zucher diabetic fatty rats
AAMC	Association of American Medical Colleges

Part I

Epidemiology

Epidemiology of Kidney Stones in the European Union

1

Palle J.S. Osther

Abstract

In Europe, prevalence and incidence of urolithiasis have increased markedly during the last decades. There seems to be an age and gender relation of both stone formation and stone composition. Calcium oxalate (CaOx) stones are the most common stone species throughout Europe. With regard to the crystalline forms of CaOx, there seems to be clear age differences, with calcium oxalate dihydrate (COD) occurring significantly more often in young adults compared to calcium oxalate monohydrate (COM), which increases continuously in frequency above the age of 40 years. Infection stones are on retreat in Europe, although there are regional differences, which might reflect differences in health care systems. Uric acid (UA) stone disease is on the rise in parallel with the rising incidence of metabolic syndrome. In general, recurrence rates are still high, and there is a need for more effective preventive measures. New pathophysiological evidence of calcium nephrolithiasis being a micro-environmental disease initiated by interstitial apatite crystal formation (Randall's plaque) may lead to better prevention.

Shockwave lithotripsy (SWL) is the most commonly used method for stone elimination in Europe, although endoscopic procedures due to technological developments are increasingly being used and in some centers, even dominate the treatment scenario. There is still a need for randomized controlled trials both with regard to stone eliminating procedures and preventive measures.

Keywords

Incidence • Urinary stones • Oxalates • Urates • Prevalence • Geographical variation • Stone composition • Urine composition • Staghorn stones • Calcium oxalate stones • Calcium phosphate stones • Infection stones • Uric acid stones • Cystine stones • Practice patterns • Pediatric stones • Age-related stone formation • Recurrence • Stone site

Introduction

It is a general view that kidney stone disease varies in frequency and stone type between different climates and racial groups. Understanding the epidemiology of stone disease is important to determine the significance of the disease at a community level, the associations and risk factors for individuals, and the likelihood of stone recurrence [1]. This section attempts to describe the epidemiology of kidney stone disease within the European Union (EU) including stone compositions, age and gender relationships, risk factors,

P.J.S. Osther, M.D., Ph.D.
EAU Section of Urolithiasis (EULIS),
Urological Research Center, Fredericia, Denmark

Department of Urology,
Fredericia Hospital, Part of Hospital Littlebelt,
Institute of Regional Health Services Research,
University of Southern Denmark, DK-7000 Fredericia, Denmark
e-mail: pjo@urc.nu

J.J. Talati et al. (eds.), *Urolithiasis*,
DOI 10.1007/978-1-4471-4387-1_1, © Springer-Verlag London 2012

and trends in treatment. Because upper urinary tract stone disease is a complex disease, an understanding of the epidemiology, particularly the interactions among different factors, may help lead to approaches that reduce the risk of stone formation [2].

At the beginning of year 2011, the EU with its 27 member states was inhabited by approximately 490 million people [3]. With an overall kidney stone prevalence of 5–10 %, this means that in year 2011 about 25–49 million Europeans suffered from painful kidney stones. Thus, kidney stone disease has a significant impact on the European quality of life and socioeconomics.

Valid contemporary epidemiological data on kidney stone disease is far from available from all EU states. Where specific data is available from specific countries, it will be noted.

Prevalence, Incidence, and Age and Gender Differences

Data from European population-based studies clearly have documented that both prevalence and incidence of upper urinary tract stone disease have increased significantly in the last decades.

Prevalence

In Spain, the annual prevalence increased from 4.16 % (4.5 % in males and 3.8 % in females) in year 1986 [4] to 5.06 % in year 2007 [5]. In Italy, the overall annual prevalence of upper urinary tract stone disease was 4.9 % in females and 6.8 % in males in 1986, increasing to 5.8 and 10.1 % in females and males, respectively, in 1998 [6]. In Germany, the overall prevalence rose from 4 to 4.7 % from 1979 to 2001 (Table 1.1) [7–9].

Incidence

In year 2000, the incidence of urolithiasis in Germany was found to be 1.47 % compared to 0.54 % in 1979 [7, 8]. Significant increases in incidence, although less dramatic, have been noted in Spain and Italy (see Table 1.1) [4–6]. Differences between countries in stone prevalence and incidence may reflect differences in detection rate (clinical-diagnostic procedures), differences in nutritional and environmental factors, as well as differences in approaches to metaphylaxis. Also, regional variations within the same country and between countries may reflect differences in standards of medical care as reflected in a study of a very large series of urinary stone analyses from Germany [10, 11].

Table 1.1 Prevalence and incidence of urolithiasis in two recent European series [5, 7]

	Germany 2000 (%)	Spain 2007 (%)
Prevalence	4.7	5.06
Females	4.0	NA
Males	5.5	NA
Incidence	1.47	0.73
Females	0.63	NA
Males	0.84	NA

Age and Gender

Although rare metabolic conditions causing kidney stone formation are more prevalent in children, it was evident from the aforementioned large German series that children and adolescents have the lowest incidence of stone formation for all compositions [11]. Special issues with regard to kidney stones in children will not be dealt with in this chapter (please refer to Part VII in this book).

Data from both France and Germany show a clear age and gender relation of stone formation [11, 12]. In a French study from 2004, the highest number of calculi was reported in the age groups 40–49 in males compared with 30–39 in females [12]. The overall male/female (M/F) ratio was 2.28. The M/F ratio was highest in young children, whereas it was lowest in teenagers and young adults, as well as in very old subjects [12]. A M/F ratio ≥2 was consistently observed in the age groups between 30 and 79 years, with a maximum occurrence in the 50- to 59-year age group [12]. Data from a 2001 epidemiological survey based on telephone interviews in Germany revealed a prevalence of urolithiasis in individuals above 50 years of age of 9.7 % in males and 5.9 % in females, which corresponds well with the Italian data previously mentioned [6]. This study, which represents the most clear-cut European epidemiological study on incidence and prevalence in recent times, showed a marked increase in stone prevalence in both females and males at the age of 25 and onwards, and particularly in the case of males, this trend was continuous [6]. It was also found that by comparing age distributions of stone patients between years 1979 and 2001 the increase in prevalence and incidence mentioned previously was primarily attributable to the stone occurrence in higher age groups (>50) [6]. On the other hand, it was also found that increasing numbers of younger women are now suffering from urinary stones [6]. The exact reason for this observation is still unclear, but it may be related to diet/metabolic syndrome and/or infections with associated antibiotic treatment related to an earlier sexual debut. In another German study based on analyses of more than 200,000 urinary calculi, it was found that stone formation in females had a peak from ages 60 to 69 years, whereas males showed a stone formation plateau at ages 30–69 years [11]. These figures are slightly different from the French data, which may be due to differences in the distributions of stone compositions between the two countries.

Stone Composition

Distribution of stone compositions in two large contemporary European series is presented in Table 1.2. In both series, there seems to be an age and gender relationship between stone formation and the predominant chemical stone composition [11, 12].

Table 1.2 Distribution of stone compositions in two large contemporary European series

	Germany [11]	France [12]
CaOx (COM/COD)	78 % (NA)	65.2 % (66/34)
CaP	NA	12.7 %
Brushite	1.5 %	1.1 %
Uric acid	11 %	6.9 %
Struvite	6 %[a]	2.2 %
Cystine	0.6 %	1.3 %

CaOx predominantly calcium oxalate, *CaP* predominantly calcium phosphate
[a]Infection stones as a whole

Gender

In the French study of close to 30,000 urinary calculi, it was found that calcium oxalate (CaOx) was by far the most predominant stone component in both genders (64 % in males and 55 % in females) [12]. The CaOx monohydrate form (COM) was significantly more prevalent in males than in females, and COM was 1.9 times more abundant than CaOx dihydrate (COD) in males and 2.8 times more in females [12]. Similar observations have been obtained from Spanish and Italian series [13, 14]. In the large French series, calcium phosphate (CaP) as carbonate apatite was the third most common crystalline species after COM and COD, and CaP was twice as common in females as in males [12]. These data were confirmed in the largest series of stone analyses published to date (Germany) in which calcium-containing calculi were predominant in both genders (84 % in males and 81 % in females) [11]. In this study, incidence of stone composition and age and gender distributions from 1977 to 2006 was evaluated. During this period, the proportion of calcium-containing calculi to the total number of calculi increased from 82 to 86 % in males and from 79 to 84 % in females, and correspondingly, M/F ratio with regard to calcium-containing calculi changed from 1.86/1 in 1977 to 2.7/1 in 2006 [11]. In this large series, there was a tendency toward an increasing frequency of CaP relative to CaOx, and, interestingly, the incidence of brushite increased continuously through the 30 year observation period [11]. The exact reason for this development is not known, but the fact that brushite stones are increasing in frequency represents a clinical challenge, since brushite stones are very hard and effective metaphylaxis is at present not available.

Uric acid (UA) has consistently been shown to be the fourth most common stone component in European series (see Table 1.2) [6, 7, 10–13]. In all series, UA has been found to be more prevalent in males than in females with an M/F ratio approaching 4:1 [11]. In Italian and French series, an increase in UA stone incidence through the last decades has been observed and attributed to the parallel increase in numbers of individuals with metabolic syndrome [6, 12].

The frequency of cystine stones seems to have been fairly constant through the years. In the French series, cystine calculi represented 0–9.6 % of all kidney stones analyzed, depending on age and sex of patients. Peak incidence was observed in the second decade of life in both genders [12]. In the large German series, cystine calculi were noted in 0.4 % of males and 0.7 % of females [11], which correspond well with the Spanish series [5], whereas cystine stones seem to be slightly more prevalent in Denmark and Italy, where cystine was the stone constituent found in 0.9 and 1.9 % of all stones, respectively [6, 15].

The occurrence of stones attributable to infection (magnesium ammonium phosphate [struvite], calcium carbonate apatite, ammonium urate) seems to have decreased through the latest decades, although there may be regional differences within Europe. Infection stones seem to be relatively rare in males and relatively common in females. Both of these trends were evident from the recent German study in which incidence of infection-associated calculi decreased from 4.9 to 3.3 % in males and from 13.5 to 9.2 % in females during the period from 1977 to 2006 [11]. In Spain, the overall proportion of struvite stones to the total number of stones lately has been reported to 3.7 %, an occurrence that corresponds well with the German findings [5, 11].

Age

Data of recent European series clearly show that age has a major influence on stone composition despite the differences according to gender described previously [5, 6, 11, 12]. Among the crystalline forms of CaOx, it was found that COD as a main stone component was five times more prevalent in young adults of both genders compared with that in older age groups, indicating that hypercalciuria is an important etiological factor in young stone-forming patients [12, 16, 17]. In the French series, the contribution of COD as the main component of stones declined by 5 and 3 % in males and females, respectively, every decade from 20 to 80 years [12]. Overall, COD was more common in female patients than in males in the first two decades of life; hereafter the occurrence of COD decreased to below 5 % in females aged >90 years [12]. The proportion of COM as a main component seems to reach a peak in patients with an age between 40 and 70 years, which may be indicative of hyperoxaluria as a main pathogenetic factor in that age group [12, 17].

In males younger than 10 years of age, CaPs have been shown to constitute up to 40 % of cases, hereafter declining to less than 10 % [12]. CaP stones in females—mainly carbonate apatite—were shown to be predominant (31.5 %) in the 20- to 29-year age group, declining to a stable level of 18 % in the age group above 50 years [12]. In the large German series, calcium-containing stones became more common at ages 20 to 29 years, with a peak incidence in females from ages 60 to 69 years and in males from 30 to 69 years [11]. Overall, a tendency was noted that calcium-containing stones became increasingly more common in the middle-age group (40–49 years) during the study period from 1977 to 2006, clearly emphasizing the role of lifestyle changes.

Incidence of UA stone disease seems to rise continuously with age from less than 2 % under the age of 30 to approximately 25 and 40 % above 80 years of age in females and males, respectively [11, 12].

Infection-related calculi appear to be more frequent at the extremes of life [12]. In the large German series, infection calculi were relatively common in young children (<9 years) with a higher rate in boys [11]. Infection stones were most frequent in elderly patients (above 60 years) in both genders; however, as mentioned previously, the overall rate of infection stones in Germany as whole ages decreased significantly in all ages from year 1977 to 2000, which may be attributed to better health care [11].

Regional Variations

The pattern of stone disease within the European Union seems to be rather uniform from country to country. Some heterogeneity has, however, been noted in recent publications. In Italian and French series, an increase in UA stone incidence through the last decades has been observed, which has been attributed to the parallel increase in numbers of individuals with metabolic syndrome [6, 12]. Surprisingly, such an increase was not noted in the large German series [11], which may be due to the fact that the data of this series was based on stone analyses of calculi sampled after spontaneous passage and surgical intervention, thus potentially missing data from stones that were treated by chemolysis [11]. UA stones were, however, more prevalent in the southern region of Germany, which is in accordance with a higher consumption of animal protein in this area compared to other parts of Germany [11]. Since a high consumption of animal protein coincides with a high frequency of metabolic syndrome [18], the European epidemiological data seem to support the metabolic syndrome as a cause of UA nephrolithiasis, probably through a defective ammoniagenesis (insulin resistance) resulting in reduced levels of urine pH [19].

Although infection stones are seen less and less in Europe as a whole, the recent German series revealed distinct differences between the eastern and western parts of Germany [11]. Infection-associated stones were found to be markedly and significantly more common in the area that was formerly the socialist German Democratic Republic (DDR) [11]. The exact reason of this finding is not known. The authors of the chapter speculate that the higher incidence of infection stones in this region may be due to patients coming from other parts of Eastern Europe with lower standards of medical care [11], highlighting that differences in medical care may influence kidney stone epidemiology.

Stone Recurrence

In the German telephone-interview-based study, it was found that approximately 60 % of the stone formers had experienced only one stone episode, 18 % two, 10 % three, and 2 % four episodes [7]. The remaining 10 % had experienced five or more stone episodes. This is in accordance with a Danish series, in which 60 % of the stone population was recorded as first time and 40 % as recurrent stone formers [15]. These figures do not represent exact recurrence rates but rather prevalence of additional stone episodes after the primary event. In a Swedish series, 92 patients with their first stone in 1977 were evaluated 10 years later [20]. Recurrent stone formation during the observation period was observed in 26 % of the patients, with no difference between men and women. This recorded recurrence rate was considerably lower than that reported in a German study on risk factors for recurrence in 134 recurrent stone formers in which 43 % experienced a relapse during a follow-up period of 2 years [21]. The striking difference between these two studies is a reflection of the difference between the study populations. In the Swedish study, the disease course of first-time stone formers and in the German study, the course of recurrent stone formers were evaluated, clearly highlighting the influence of specific risk factors in the epidemiological perspective.

Risk Factors

Our understanding of risk factors for stone formation has increased substantially through the last decades. From an etiological point of view, urolithiasis may be divided in conditions with a definitive metabolic, infection, and anatomical/functional cause of stone formation (MIAF-urolithiasis)

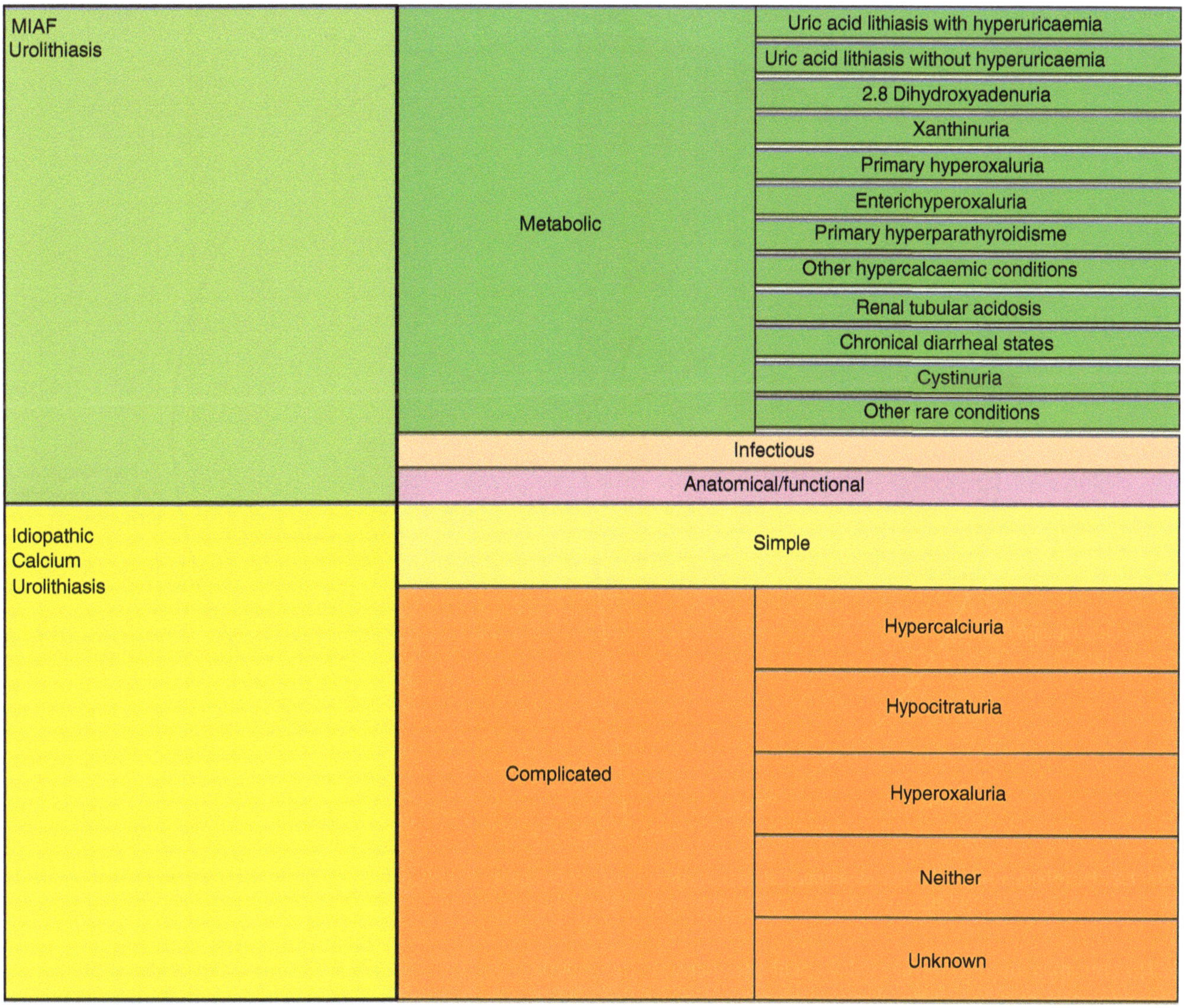

Fig. 1.1 Classification of upper urinary tract stone disease. *MIAF* conditions with overt metabolic, infectious, or anatomical/functional causes of stone formation. MIAF constitutes approximately 15 % of the total stone population [22]

and idiopathic calcium nephrolithiasis, in which specific urinary risk factors for formation of calcium-containing stones may be present [22]. Figure 1.1 presents a classification system based on these two subgroups in which all types of stone diseases may be grouped [22].

MIAF-Urolithiasis

The prevalence of each of the MIAF conditions in a nationwide Danish survey is presented in Fig. 1.2, and the prevalence of metabolic causes is further indicated in Fig. 1.3 [15]. This distribution is in approximate accordance with other published European series [23]. Epidemiological aspects of specific diseases promoting kidney stone formation with special relevance for the European region will be discussed below.

While stone-promoting systemic disease conditions such as primary hyperparathyroidism, renal tubular acidosis, cystinuria, and primary hyperoxaluria type 1 seem to have remained on a stable level in Europe through many years [6, 23, 24], UA stone disease seems to be on a rise in parallel with a rise in incidence of metabolic syndrome [12]. A link between an increased body mass index (BMI) and stone disease has long been recognized [2]. The mechanism of the increased stone risk was not clear, however, until the features of the renal manifestations of insulin resistance were described, thereby connecting UA nephrolithiasis to the metabolic syndrome [25].

In a screening program of close to 40,000 newborns using thin layer chromatography (TLC) in the Spanish Valencian Community, the incidence of subjects at risk of forming cystine stones was found to be 1:1,887 [26], which is considerably higher than the traditional reported incidence of 1:7,000

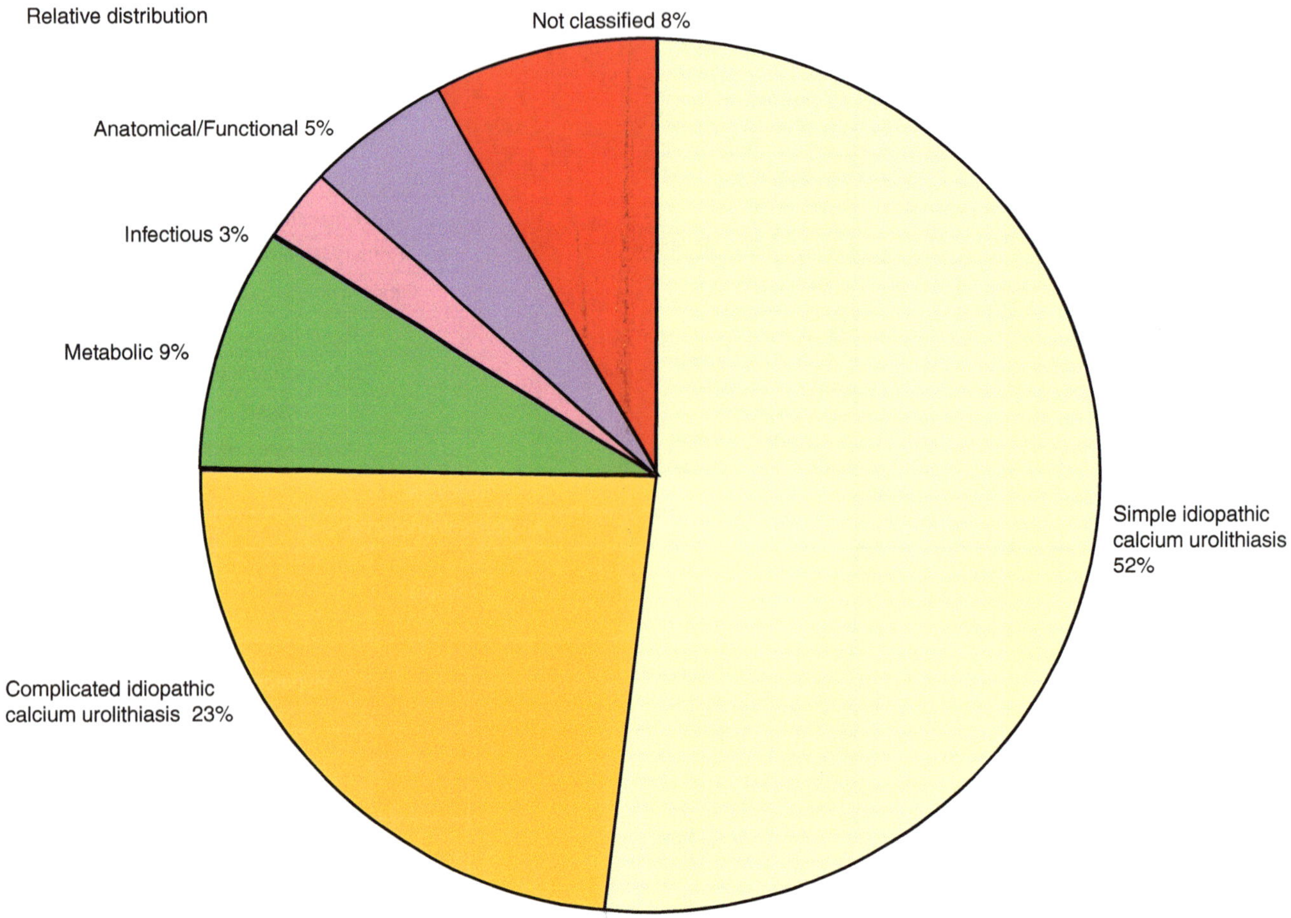

Fig. 1.2 Distribution of MIAF and idiopathic calcium nephrolithiasis in Denmark 2002 (Courtesy of Dr. K. Andreassen, Dr. P. Rosenkilde, Dr. J. Aabech, Dr. A.L. Poulsen and Prof. P.J.S. Osther) (Dansten study) [15]

[27]. This may be due to methodological problems of the screening test or more likely, due to a heterogeneity of the manifestations of the disease and a considerable variation between different populations, the latter of which is poorly documented. Cystinuria is an inherited disorder characterized by abnormal urinary excretion of dibasic amino acids: cystine, ornithine, lysine, and arginine. Mutations in two genes, *SLC3A1* and *SLC7A9*, have been identified. In a comprehensive investigation of the German Study Group for Pediatric Nephrology, an ethnic influence on the distribution of mutations was confirmed by detecting distinct different major mutations between the southern-eastern and western parts of Europe [27]. Whether the different mutation patterns (genotype) result in different clinical expressions of the disease (phenotype) is not known.

Medullary sponge kidney (MSK) is a benign congenital disorder characterized by dilatation of collecting tubules in one or more renal papillae, affecting one or both kidneys [28]. The prevalence of MSK in patients with and without nephrolithiasis was estimated in a Swiss study, in which it was found that the prevalence of MSK in renal stone formers was 8.5 %, which was considerably higher than that in the control population (1.5 %) [29]. The cause of stone formation in MSK may in part be due to urine stasis in the dilated tubules (anatomical or infection factors) and in part functional, since metabolic disorders such as incomplete renal tubular acidosis resulting in hypercalciuria and hypocitraturia have been found in up to 60 % of these cases [30].

In the Danish series (see Fig. 1.2), anatomical/functional causes were found in 5 % of stone formers. Functional refers to the fact that in case of anatomical abnormalities, such as MSK and ureteropelvic junction obstruction, metabolic risk factors such as hypercalciuria and hypocitraturia are often present and contributing to stone formation.

Infection calculi are for sure on retreat in Europe although regional differences as mentioned previously have been documented [11]. In general, infection stones are relatively rare in Europe with a prevalence of around 4 % in males and 10 % in females [11, 12, 31]. The decreasing numbers of staghorn calculi in Europe underlines this observation since urinary tract infections are the most common cause of such calculi [11].

There are no valid European data on the contribution of pharmacological-induced stone formation.

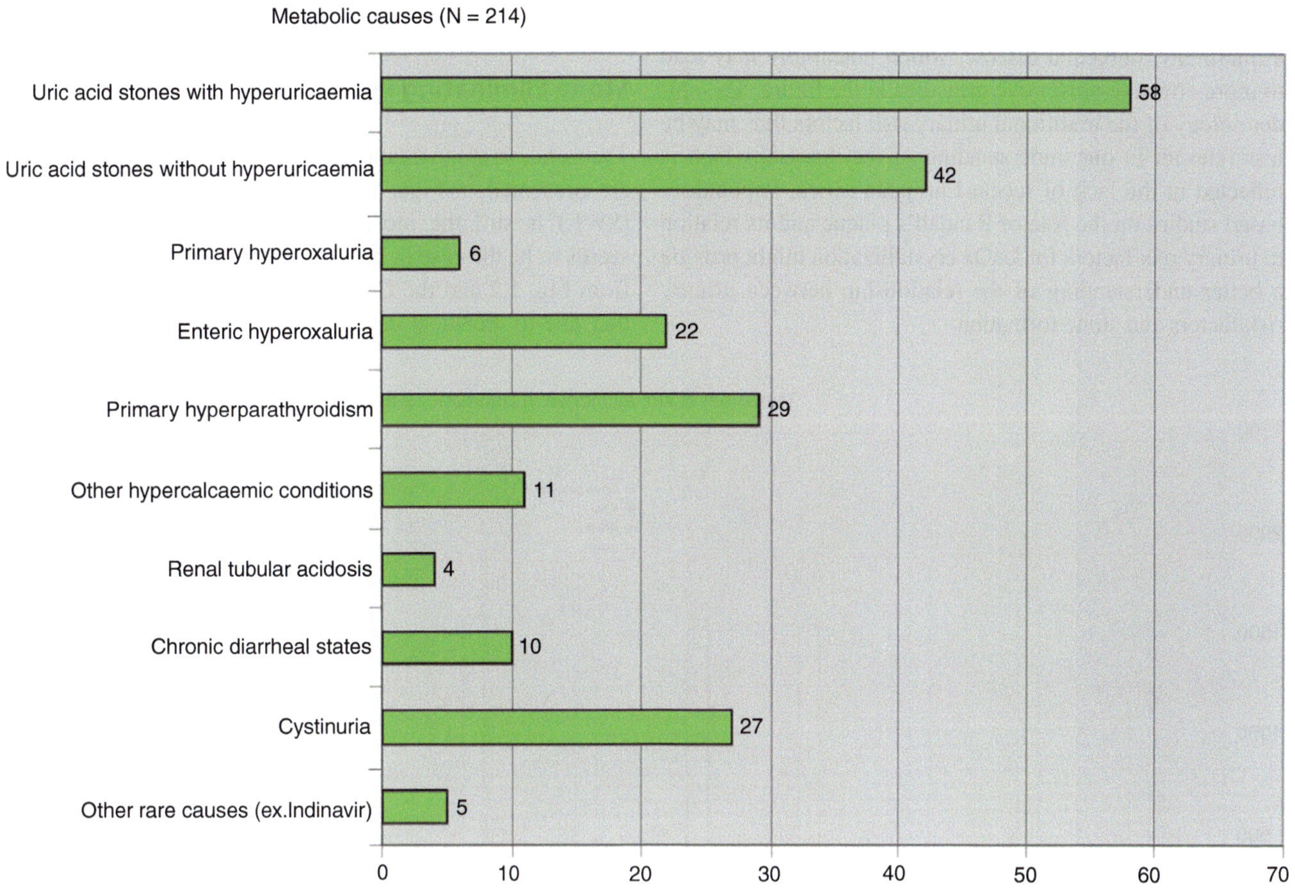

Fig. 1.3 Number of patients with metabolic causes (N=214) in Denmark 2002 (Courtesy of Dr. K. Andreassen, Dr. P. Rosenkilde, Dr. J. Aabech, Dr. A.L. Poulsen and Prof. P.J.S. Osther) (Danstenstudy) [15]

Idiopathic Calcium Nephrolithiasis

The term idiopathic refers to the fact that these patients do not have a specific underlying disease as cause of the stone formation. Specific urinary risk factors have, however, been identified. Alterations of these risk factors jointly result in alterations in ion-activity products of different calcium salts in the urine, thereby altering the risk of crystallization and hence stone formation. As mentioned previously, CaOx stones are by far the most common kidney stone species in Europe. CaOx stones present in forms in which COD or COM are predominant. The French series mentioned previously pointed toward hypercalciuria as the main risk factor in COD and hyperoxaluria in COM stone disease, respectively [12]. In a Spanish series comparing etiological factors of COM and COD urolithiasis, hypercalciuria was clearly associated with COD (71.6 %) compared to COM (34.6 %), whereas hyperoxaluria was found approximately as often in COD (15.7 %) as in COM (11.8 %) stones [13]. In the same series, low urine pH was found more often in COM (39.9 %) than in COD (26.5 %) stones, suggesting that the combination of hyperoxaluria and low urine pH might predispose to COM stone formation. Overall, hypercalciuria, hyperoxaluria, and hypocitraturia seem to be the most prominent individual urinary risk factors for calcium nephrolithiasis in Europe. Data from two recent series are presented in Table 1.3. Recent evidence suggests idiopathic calcium stone formation to be a very complex process that cannot exclusively be explained by increased ion-activity products of potential lithogenic substances in the urine [10]. Both interstitial apatite crystallization and vascular phenomena have been suggested to be involved in the formation of Randall's plaques, which subsequently leads to CaOx stone formation if the right conditions are present in the calyceal urine (i.e., hyperoxaluria) [32–34]. This new insight into the pathophysiology has led to our

Table 1.3 Predominant urinary risk factors for formation of calcium-containing calculi in two recent European series

	Italy [31]	Spain [13]
Hypercalciuria	33.4 %	34.6 % (COM)
		71.6 % (COD)
Hyperoxaluria	22.8 %	11.8 % (COM)
		15.7 % (COD)
Hypocitraturia	26.8 %	13.7 % (COM)
		19.6 % (COD)

understanding of idiopathic calcium nephrolithiasis more as a micro-environmental disease, which potentially may lead to more effective preventive measures in the future. The epidemiology of the traditional urinary risk factors thus may be less relevant in our understanding of the disease, which is reflected in the lack of recent European series. Population-based studies on the role of Randall's plaque and its relation to urinary risk factors for CaOx crystallization might provide a better understanding of the relationship between urinary risk factors and stone formation.

Trends in Kidney Stone Treatment

Stone Eliminating Procedures

The trends in stone treatment in Denmark from 1996 to 2006 are presented in Figs. 1.4 and 1.5. Shockwave lithotripsy (SWL) is still the most prevalent procedure, which also seems to be the case in Italy and Spain (Table 1.4). It is clear from Fig. 1.2 and the German series in Table 1.4, however, that due to technical developments, endoscopic procedures

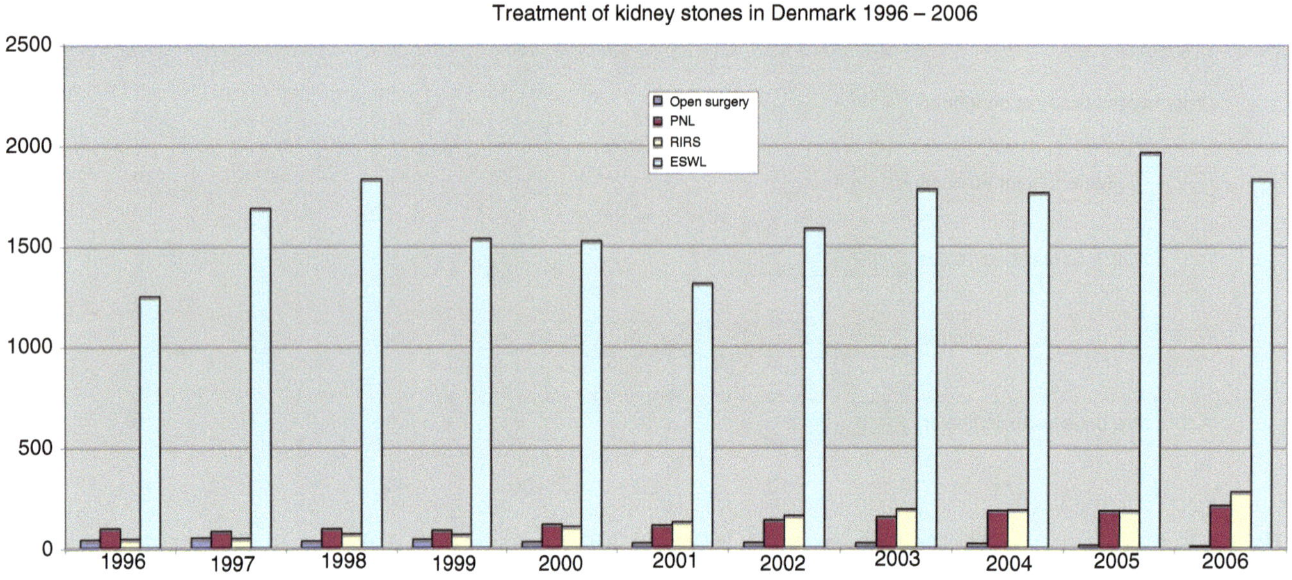

Fig. 1.4 Stone eliminating procedures in Denmark from 1996 to 2006. Danish population is approximately 5.4 million (Courtesy of Dr. Kim Andreassen) (*Source*: Danish National Board of Health)

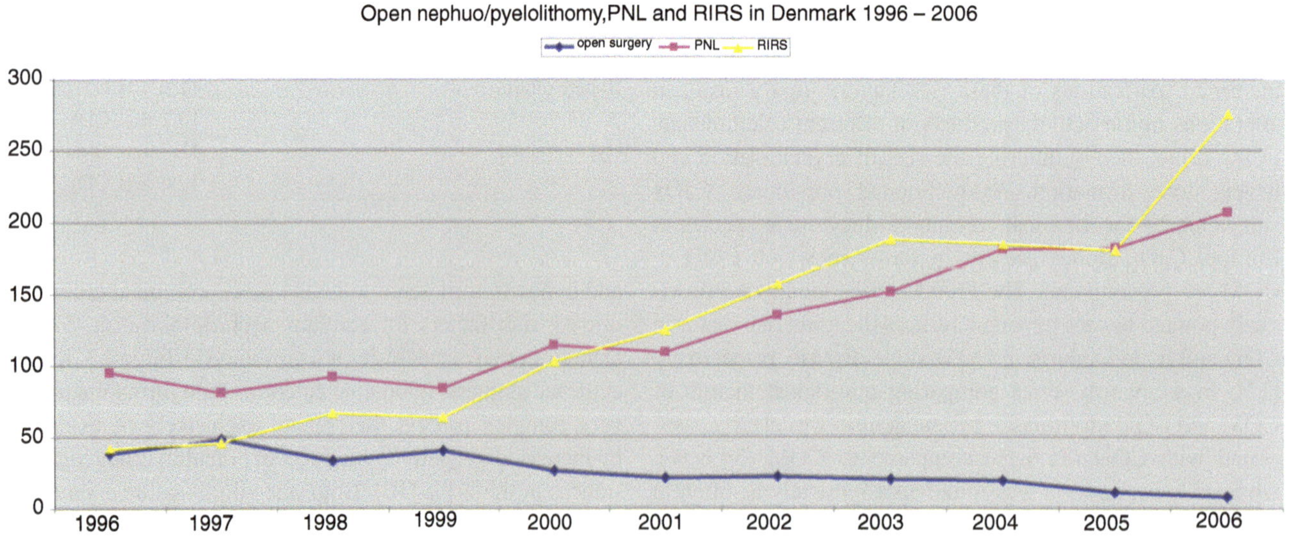

Fig. 1.5 Development of endoscopic and open stone removal procedures in Denmark from 1996 to 2006. *PNL* percutaneous nephrolithotomy, *RIRS* retrograde intrarenal stone surgery. Danish population is approximately 5.4 million (Courtesy of Dr. Kim Andreassen) (*Source*: Danish National Board of Health)

Table 1.4 Distribution of procedures for active stone removal

	Open surgery (%)	PNL (%)	URS (%)	RIRS (%)	SWL (%)
Italy [35]	3	3	14	NA	80
Spain (Alicante)[a]	1	9	29	2	59
Germany (Sindelfingen)[b]	0	14	40	38	8

[a]2011 data from Hospital del Vinalopó, Elche, Alicante, Spain (Courtesy Dr. Juan Galán)
[b]2011 data from Sindelfingen-Boeblingen Medical Center, University of Tübingen, Tübingen, Germany (Courtesy of Prof. Thomas Knoll)

for stone removal are on the rise. Open surgery seems to be limited to very few cases, the majority of which are nephrectomies in cases with non-functioning kidneys. As was the case with the rise in SWL treatments in the 1980s and 1990s, the recent rise in endoscopic stone treatments is basically technology driven rather than evidence based. Also, it cannot be excluded that reimbursement policies affect the treatment scenario in different countries. Well-designed randomized controlled trials comparing different stone eliminating procedures are still a lacking article.

Prevention

Efforts to prevent stone formation in idiopathic calcium nephrolithiasis have so far been insufficient [23]. The reasons for this may be that most preventive measures until now have been based on risk factors identified from whole urine studies. Despite the fact that most stones pass spontaneously or can be removed with non- or slightly invasive methods, the increasing incidence of the disease as well as the increasing recurrence rates, which may be due to the fact that many patients are left with residual stone fragments, calls for serious attention to measures for prevention [7, 23]. From an epidemiological point of view, it is of interest that recent European series have unveiled that selective medical and dietary intervention effectively may reduce the stone-forming potential in recurrent calcium oxalate stone formers [21, 36]. A low-fluid intake and an increased intake of protein and alcohol were identified as the most important dietary risk factors and increased urinary excretion of oxalate as the major urinary risk factor for relapse.

There are no valid European data on the contribution of urinary tract anomalies and pharmacological-induced stone formation.

Conclusion

In Europe, prevalence and incidence of urolithiasis have increased markedly during the last decades. There seems to be an age and gender relation of both stone formation and stone composition. Calcium oxalate stones are the most common stone species throughout Europe. With regard to the crystalline forms of CaOx, there seems to be clear age differences, with COD occurring significantly more often in young adults compared to COM, which increases continuously in frequency above the age of 40 years. Infection stones are on retreat in Europe, although there are regional differences, which might reflect differences in health care systems. UA stone disease is on the rise in parallel with the rising incidence of metabolic syndrome. In general, recurrence rates are still high, and there is a need for more effective preventive measures. New pathophysiological evidence of calcium nephrolithiasis being a micro-environmental disease initiated by interstitial apatite crystal formation (Randall's plaque) may lead to better prevention.

Shockwave lithotripsy is the most commonly used method for stone elimination in Europe, although endoscopic procedures due to technological developments are increasingly being used and in some centers even dominate the treatment scenario. There is still a need for randomized controlled trials both with regard to stone eliminating procedures and preventive measures.

References

1. Hughes P. Kidney stones epidemiology. Nephrology. 2007;12:26–30.
2. Curhan GC. Epidemiology of stone disease. Urol Clin North Am. 2007;34:287–93.
3. European Commission Eurostat Yearbook 2011. http://epp.eurostat.ec.europa.eu/portal/page/portal/eurostat/home/. Accessed on Dec 7, 2012.
4. Rousad A, Pedrajas A. Estudiio epidemiolócico de la urolithiasis en Espana. Asociación Espanola de Urología. Grupo de Urolithiasis; 1986.
5. Sánchez-Martin FM, Millán Rodríguez F, Esquena Fernández S, Segarra Tomás J, Rousaud Barón F, Martínez-Rodríguez F, et al. Incidencia y prevalencia de la urolithiasis en Espana: revision de los datos originales disponibles hasta la actualidad. Actas Urol Esp. 2007;31:511–20.
6. Trinchieri A, Coppi F, Montanari E, Del Nero A, Zanetti G, Pisani E. Increase in the prevalence of symptomatic upper urinary tract stones during the last ten years. Eur Urol. 2000;37:23–5.
7. Hesse A, Brändle E, Wilbert D, Köhrmann K-U, Alken P. Study on the prevalence and incidence of Urolithiasis in Germany comparing the years 1979 vs. 2000. Eur Urol. 2003;44:709–13.

8. Vahlensieck EW, Bach D, Hesse A. Incidence, prevalence and mortality of urolithiasis in the German Federal Republic. Urol Res. 1982;10:161–4.
9. Hesse A, Siener R. Current aspects of epidemiology and nutrition in urinary stones. World J Urol. 1997;15:165–71.
10. Knoll T. Epidemiology, pathogenesis and pathophysiology of urolithiasis. Eur Urol Suppl. 2010;9:802–6.
11. Knoll T, Schubert AB, Fahlenkamp DF, Leusmann DB, Wendt-Nordahl G, Schubert G. Urolithiasis through the ages: data on more than 200,000 urinary stone analysis. J Urol. 2011;185:1304–11.
12. Daudon M, Doré J-C, Jubgers P, Lacour B. Changes in stone composition according to age and gender of patients: a multivariate epidemiological approach. Urol Res. 2004;32:241–7.
13. Galán JA, Conte A, Llobera A, Costa-Bauzá A, Grases F. A comparative study between etiological factors of calcium oxalate monohydrate and calcium oxalate dihydrate urolithiasis. Urol Int. 1996;56:79–85.
14. Trinchieri A, Castelnuovo C, Lizzano R, Zanetti G. Calcium stone disease: a multiform reality. Urol Res. 2005;33:194–8.
15. Andreassen K, Poulsen AL, Olsen PR, Aabeck J, Osther PJ. Classification of urolithiasis in Denmark: A national survey. European Urology Meeting 2007;2(1):126.
16. Maurice-Estepa L, Levillian P, Lacour B, Daudon M. Crystalline phase differentiation in urinary calcium phosphate and magnesium phosphate calculi. Scand J Urol Nephrol. 1999;33:299–302.
17. Daudon M, Labrunie M, Hennequin C, Lacour B, Jungers P. Relative influence of calcium and oxalate urine concentration on the risk of calcium oxalate crystallization. In: Jungers P, Daudon M, editors. Renal stone disease. Crystallization process, pathophysiology, metabolic disorders and prevention. Paris: Elsevier; 1997. p. 72.
18. Azadbakht L, Ezmaillzadeh A. Red meat intake is associated with metabolic syndrome and the plasma C-reactive protein concentration in women. J Nutr. 2009;139:335–9.
19. Traxer O, Lechevallier E, Saussine C, Daudon M, Haymann JP. Metabolic syndrome and urolithiasis. A new concept for the urologist. Prog Urol. 2008;18:828–31.
20. Ahlstrand C, Tiselius HG. Recurrences during a 10-year follow-up after the first renal stone episode. Urol Res. 1990;18:397–9.
21. Siener R, Glatz S, Nicolay C, Hesse A. Prospective study on the efficacy of a selective treatment and risk factors for relapse in recurrent calcium oxalate stone patients. Eur Urol. 2003;44:467–74.
22. Osther PJ, Grenabo L, Haraldsson G, Holmberg G, Lindell O, Mogensen P, et al. Metabolic evaluation and medical management of upper urinary tract stone disease. Guidelines from the Scandinavian Cooperative Group for Urinary Stones. Scand J Urol Nephrol. 1999;33:372–81.
23. Tiselius H-G. Epidemiology and medical management of stone disease. BJU Int. 2003;91:758–67.
24. Trinchieri A, Dormia G, Montanari Z, Zanetti G. Cystinuria: definition, epidemiology and clinical aspects. Arch Ital Urol Androl. 2004;76(3):129–34.
25. Abate N, Chandalia M, Cabo-Chan Jr AV, Moe OW, Sakhaee K. The metabolic syndrome and uric acid nephrolithiasis: novel features of renal manifestation of insulin resistance. Kidney Int. 2004; 65:386–92.
26. Cabello-Tomás ML, Garcia-Gómez AM, Guillén-Domiguez ML. Pilot screening programme for cystinuria in the Valencian Community. Eur J Epidemiol. 1999;15:681–4.
27. Schmidt C, Vester U, Hesse A, Lahme S, Lang F, Zerres K, Eggermann T, and Members of the Arbeitsgemeinschaft Pädiatrische Nephrologie. The population-specific distribution and frequencies of genomic variants in the SLC3A1 and SLC7A9 genes and their application in molecular genetic testing of cystinuria. Urol Res. 2004;32:75–8.
28. Gambaro G, Feltrin GP, Lupo A, Bonfante L, D'Angelo A, Antonello A. Medullary sponge kidney (Lenarduzzi-Cacchi-Ricci disease): a Padua Medical School discovery in the 1930s. Kidney Int. 2006;69:663–70.
29. Laube M, Hess B, Terrier F, Vock P, Jaeger P. Prevalence of medullary sponge kidney in patients with and without nephrolithiasis. Praxis. 1995;84:1224–30.
30. Osther PJ, Bollerslev J, Hansen AB, Engel K, Kildeberg P. Pathophysiology of incomplete renal tubular acidosis in recurrent renal stone formers: evidence of disturbed calcium, bone and citrate metabolism. Urol Res. 1993;2:169–73.
31. Trinchieri A, Rovera F, Nespoli R. Clinical observations on 2086 patients with upper urinary tract stones. Arch Ital Urol Androl. 1996;68:251–8.
32. Evan AP, Lingeman JE, Coe FL, Worcester EM. Randall's plaque of patients with nephrolithiasis begins in basement membranes of thin loops of Henle. J Clin Invest. 2003;111:607–16.
33. Stoller ML, Meng MV, Abrahams HM, Kane JP. The primary stone event: a new hypothesis involving a vascular etiology. J Urol. 2004; 171:1920–4.
34. Tiselius HG. A hypothesis of calcium stone formation: an interpretation of stone research during the past decades. Urol Res. 2011; 39:231–43. Epub 2011 Jan 19.
35. D'Armiento M, Autorino R, De Sio M. PCNL in Italy. Arch Ital Urol Androl. 2010;82:26–9.
36. Siener R, Schade N, Nicolay C, von Unruh GE, Hesse A. The efficacy of dietary intervention on urinary risk factors for stone formation in recurrent calcium oxalate stone patients. J Urol. 2005; 173:1601–5.

2 Epidemiology of Stone Disease in North America

John D. Denstedt and Andrew Fuller

Abstract

Despite recent advances in the surgical techniques and equipment available for the management of urinary lithiasis, the prevalence of this condition continues to increase in the North American population. Associated costs are estimated to exceed 5.3 billion US dollars each year.

Epidemiological studies have implicated a range of contributory dietary, medical, environmental, and genetic factors in the pathophysiology of this disease. Many of these factors are consistent internationally. Despite this, the North American population, with its associated racial, environmental, and socioeconomic diversity, provides unique epidemiological insights. This chapter provides an overview of the risk factors for stone disease as well as incidence and prevalence patterns in a North American context using contemporary data.

Keywords

Incidence • Urinary stones • Oxalates • Urates • Prevalence • Geographical variation • Stone composition • Urine composition • Staghorn stones • Calcium oxalate stones • Calcium phosphate stones • Infection stones • Uric acid stones • Cystine stones • Practice patterns • Pediatric stones • Age-related stone formation • Recurrence • Stone site

Introduction

Despite recent advances in the surgical techniques and equipment available for the management of urinary lithiasis, the prevalence of this condition continues to increase in the North American population. Associated costs are estimated to exceed 5.3 billion US dollars each year [1].

Epidemiological studies have implicated a range of contributory dietary, medical, environmental, and genetic factors in the pathophysiology of this disease. Many of these factors are consistent internationally. Despite this, the North American population, with its associated racial, environmental, and socioeconomic diversity, provides unique epidemiological insights. This chapter provides an overview of the risk factors for stone disease as well as incidence and prevalence patterns in a North American context using contemporary data.

Incidence

Information with regard to incident stone events affecting the North American population in the second half of the twentieth century may be extrapolated from a large population-based study conducted in Rochester, Minnesota [2]. Despite contradictory results in studies from other developed Western nations [3] suggesting a recent increased incidence of urinary lithiasis, these large studies show that the incidence of stone disease has plateaued in North America since the early 1970s.

J.D. Denstedt, M.D., FRCSC, FACS (✉)
Department of Surgery, The University of Western Ontario,
268 Grosvenor Street, London, ON N6A 4V2, Canada
e-mail: john.denstedt@sjhc.london.on.ca

A. Fuller, M.B.B.S., FRACS
Division of Urology, The University of Western Ontario,
London, ON, Canada
e-mail: afuller@sturology.com.au

J.J. Talati et al. (eds.), *Urolithiasis*,
DOI 10.1007/978-1-4471-4387-1_2, © Springer-Verlag London 2012

Table 2.1 Incident symptomatic stone rates in Rochester, MN, USA, by decade

	Women		Men		Total	
Year	Rate (±s.e.)[a]	Cases	Rate (±s.e.)[a]	Cases	Rate (±s.e.)[b]	Cases
1970	43.2 (±14.0)	10	155.1 (±28.5)	31	98.7 (±15.7)	41
1980	53.6 (±13.8)	16	183.7 (±29.3)	42	116.5 (±15.8)	58
1990	92.4 (±16.3)	34	144.0 (±22.3)	44	117.1 (±13.6)	78
2000	68.4 (±12.3)	31	105.0 (±16.8)	40	85.1 (±10.2)	71
Total	*65.8 (±7.0)*	*91*	*140.6 (±11/4)*	*157*	*101.8 (±6.6)*	*248*

Adapted from [2]
[a]Annual age-adjusted rate of new-onset stone disease per 100,000 population
[b]Annual age- and gender-adjusted rate of new-onset stone disease per 100,000 population
Age and gender adjustments based upon US Census 2000 data

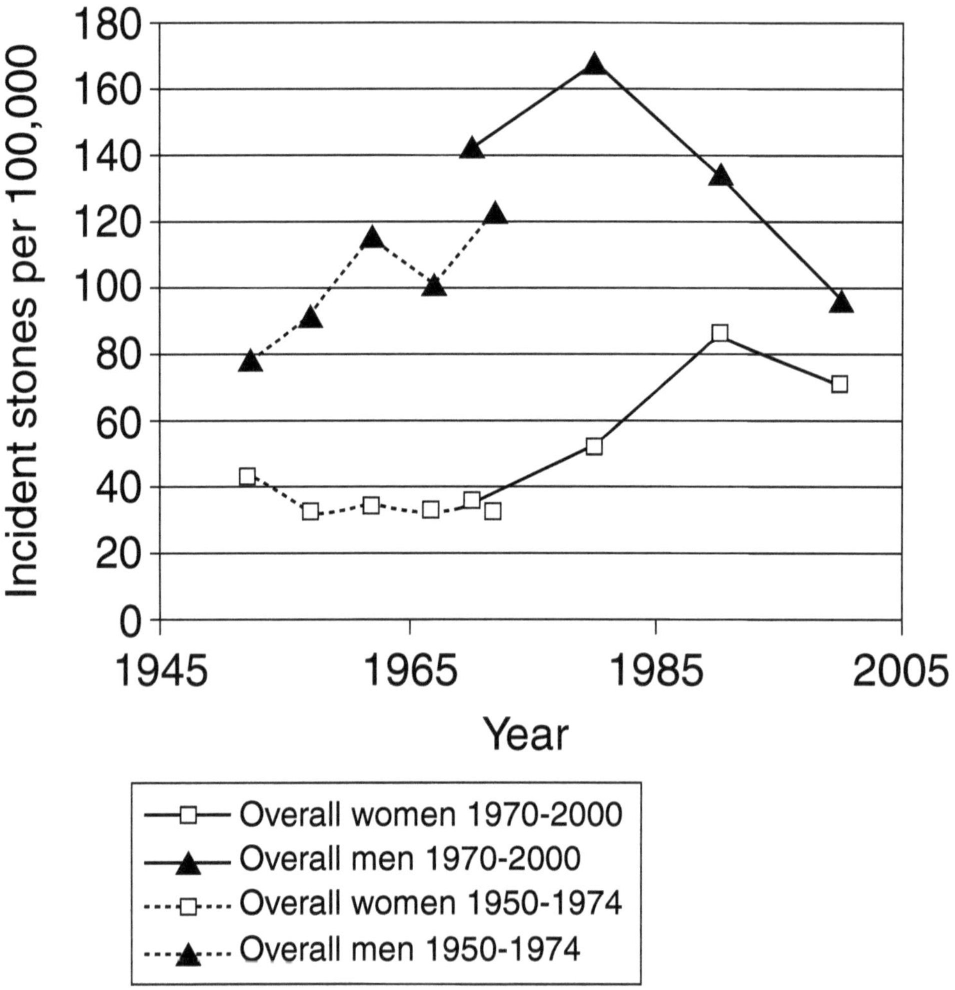

Fig. 2.1 Incident symptomatic stone rates 1950–2000. *Solid lines* depict data from the current Rochester, MN, study (1970–2000). For comparison, the *dotted lines* indicate data from the previous Rochester, MN, USA, study by Johnson et al. (1950–1974) [5]. To facilitate comparison between the two studies, as in the earlier report, all rates are age adjusted to the 1960 US white population (Adapted with permission from Macmillan Publishers Ltd: Kidney International. Lieske et al. [2])

Although stone disease appears to have declined among males since 1970 (Table 2.1), the overall incidence of stone disease has remained stable. This is explained by an increased incidence in females of all ages (Fig. 2.1). The male-to-female ratio reflects this, having declined from 3.1:1 in 1970 to 1.3:1 in 2000 [2]. Peak incidence in females has been shown to occur at a younger age of 20–29 years, compared with 60–69 years for males (see Table 2.1 and Fig. 2.1)

Prevalence

The lifetime risk of stone disease for individuals residing in the USA has been estimated to be 10–15 % and is influenced by racial and environmental factors as well as gender [4, 5]. The United States National Health and Nutrition Examination Survey (NHANES) examined the prevalence of stone disease in a total of 31,479 individuals over two time periods between 1976–1980 and 1988–1994. By incorporating data

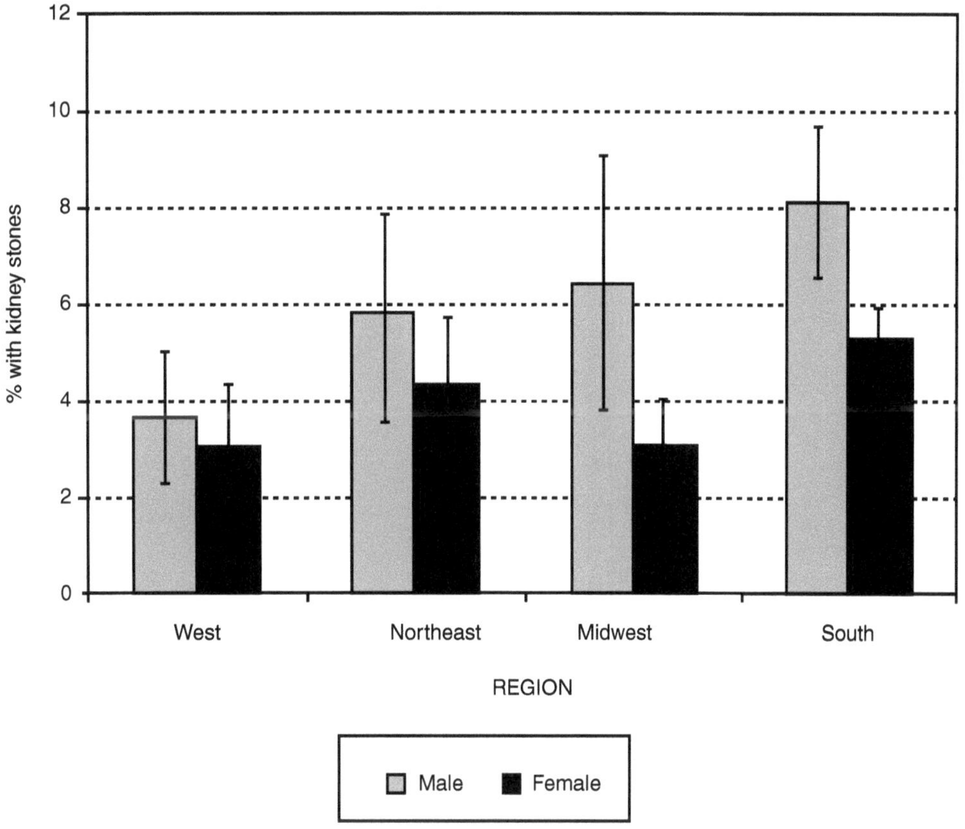

Fig. 2.2 Age-adjusted prevalence of kidney stones in the 1988–1994 United States adult population by gender within regions (Adapted with permission from Stamatelou et al. [6])

from a large community-based survey, the study provides representative information with regard to temporal trends in the prevalence of stone disease. In comparing the two study periods, the prevalence in the United States was noted to have increased from 3.8 to 5.7 % [6]. Such results should be interpreted with a degree of caution, given the emergence of improved technologies for detection and treatment of stone disease between the two periods.

Differences in prevalence according to geographical location have been linked to dehydration and an associated increase in the concentration of lithogenic substances in the urine resulting from warmer climates [7]. Accordingly, the highest rates of stone disease are seen in the Southeastern United States, [8, 9] with the lowest rates in the West and Midwest (Fig. 2.2).

A higher prevalence of stone disease in males is consistent across all age ranges, with a gradual increase in prevalence with age for both male and female patients (see Table 2.2). With regard to ethnicity, African Americans display less than half the prevalence of stone disease when compared with Caucasians [8, 10].

Practice Patterns/Methods of Treatment

The proportion of health care expenditure allocated to the management of urolithiasis continues to increase in North America. In 2000, direct treatment costs were estimated to exceed 2.1 billion dollars [11]. This reflects both an increase in the prevalence of the condition and the emergence of novel minimally invasive treatment options.

Practice patterns within the United States have been captured by several databases, including HCUP (Healthcare Cost and Utilization Project), CMS (Centers for Medicare & Medicaid Services), CHCPE (Centre for Health Care Policy and Evaluation), and NAMS (National Hospital Ambulatory Medical Care Survey).

A total of 617,647 individuals presented to an emergency room with a listed primary diagnosis of urolithiasis in 2000 [11]. This amounts to an estimated rate of 226 cases per 100,000 individuals. The increased availability and acceptance of minimally invasive techniques such as shock wave lithotripsy (SWL) and ureteroscopy led to an increase in ambulatory surgery between 1994 and 1998, with rates of 123/100,000 and 199/100,000, respectively. Accordingly, the mean length of hospital stay decreased for upper tract stones from 2.6 to 2.3 days during the same time period [11].

A reduction in open surgical procedures corresponded with a 60 % increase in ureteroscopic procedures for the period between 1992 and 2000. The rates of percutaneous nephrolithotomy (PCNL) (3–6 %) and SWL (49–54 %) remained essentially unchanged [12]. Although more recent data are lacking, it is likely that the proportion of cases performed ureteroscopically has continued to increase with the

Table 2.2 Percent prevalence and adjusted odds ratio of kidney stone disease history in relation to region of residence, age, race/ethnicity, and use of diuretics among adults 20–74 years of age in 1988–1994 United States population

	Female				Male			
Independent variable	Number	% with stones	Odds ratio[a]	95 % CI	Number	% with stones	Odds ratio[a]	95 % CI
Geographic region								
Northeast	1,066	4.4	0.77	0.5–1.2	840	6.7	0.81	0.5–1.4
South	3,207	5.2	1.0		2,906	7.5	1.0	
Midwest	1,431	3.3	0.57	0.4–0.8	1,226	6.3	0.72	0.4–1.2
West	1,827	3.3	0.57	0.4–0.9	1,658	4.0	0.50	0.3–0.8
Age (years)								
20–39	3,624	2.5	1.0		3,011	2.5	1.0	
40–59	2,294	5.3	1.80	1.2–2.7	2,008	9.5	3.99	2.8–5.7
60–74	1,616	6.0	2.26	1.4–3.6	1,611	11.7	5.08	3.5–7.5
Race/ethnicity								
Caucasian (non-Hispanic)	2,796	4.6	1.0		2,420	7.4	1.0	
African American (non-Hispanic)	2,312	1.7	0.35	0.2–0.5	1,900	1.8	0.24	0.2–0.3
Mexican American	2,094	2.4	0.64	0.5–0.9	2,055	3.0	0.62	0.5–0.9
Diuretic use								
Yes	659	7.6	1.5	1.0–2.5	379	15.6	1.7	1.0–3.2
No	6,878	3.9	1.0		6,248	5.9	1.0	

Adapted from [6]

[a]The odds ratios were estimated using a logistic regression model that included age group, race/ethnicity, geographic region of residence, and use of diuretics as independent variables

advent and dissemination of improved optical systems and ancillary devices.

Stone Composition

Evidence from studies in industrialized countries suggests a significant change in the chemical composition of renal stones during the second half of the twentieth century [13–15]. Calcium oxalate (monohydrate and dihydrate) now accounts for more than 60 % of all stones. This is likely a reflection of alterations in diet, in particular an increase in consumption of foods high in sodium and animal protein. Although many of the larger studies have been conducted in Europe, the results are likely to be representative in a North American context.

Table 2.3 summarizes the distribution of the most frequently encountered stones. While female patients are more likely to form phosphate stones, calcium oxalate stones are more common in male patients [16, 17].

Table 2.3 Distribution of stone types in a North American population

Stone composition	Percentage
Calcium oxalate (monohydrate and dihydrate)	55–61 %
Calcium phosphate	12–13 %
Uric acid	8–14 %
Struvite (magnesium ammonium phosphate)	2–6 %
Cystine	1–6 %

Adapted from [19]

Urinary Parameters

Twenty-four-hour urine analysis remains an important part of the evaluation of the recurrent stone former. Low urine volume (defined as less than 2 L/day) has been implicated in the formation of both calcium- and non-calcium-containing stones, and the inverse relationship between stone formation and urine volume has been proven in observational studies [18]. Up to 92 % of patients with uric acid stones demonstrate low urine output [19]. Although not traditionally recommended, the consumption of caffeinated beverages (tea/coffee) and alcohol (wine/beer) has been shown in observational studies to reduce the subsequent risk of stone formation [20, 21].

Up to 40 % of patients with calcium stone disease have associated hypercalciuria [22]. Hypercalciuria may also be seen in association with uric acid and struvite stones, with rates of 23 and 50 %, respectively [19]. Hyperoxaluria (>45 mg/day; 0.5 mmol/day) is more commonly seen in male calcium stone formers and may affect up to 40 % of such patients. In the North American population, hypocitraturia (<320 mg/day; 1.67 mmol/day) is seen in 5–11 % of patients and in association with all stone types [18, 19].

Predisposing Factors

Medical

Results from the NHANES demonstrated an 80 % increase in the rate of extreme obesity in the USA between 1994 and 2000 [23]. This trend has continued through the first part of the twenty-first century. In addition to increasing the difficulty and complications associated with the treatment of existing stones, comorbid health conditions such as diabetes mellitus, hypertension, and metabolic syndrome have been implicated in the increased prevalence of stones in the North American population [24–27].

Obesity has been shown to negatively impact on urinary parameters, with an increase in the excretion of lithogenic substances, including calcium, oxalate, sodium, and uric acid [28, 29]. The magnitude of this effect is more marked in females, which may account for a recent increased incidence of stone disease in this cohort of patients.

The formation of uric acid stones is commonly seen in those with obesity [30]. Insulin resistance may interfere with renal ammonium production and decrease urine pH [31]. In addition, a diet high in animal protein and purines is often seen in association with obesity and contributes to increased urinary acidity.

A range of other medical conditions, such as gout, inflammatory bowel disease, hyperparathyroidism, and renal tubular acidosis, have a well-established role in the formation of renal stones.

Surgical

In association with the increase in morbid obesity in North America and a frequent failure of individuals to lose weight with lifestyle interventions alone, there was a fivefold increase in the rate of bariatric surgery between 1998 and 2002 [32]. Although weight loss confers significant cardiovascular benefit and reduces the likelihood of metabolic syndrome, modern bariatric surgery has been linked to high rates of hyperoxaluria [33–35]. This has been found to be associated with a significant increase in the formation of calcium oxalate calculi within 5 years of surgery [36]. The mechanism for this remains elusive; however, it is likely to result from a combination of malabsorption and alterations in gut flora.

Genetic

While a clear genetic basis exists for cysteine urolithiasis, the genetic contribution to more common forms of stone disease remains less well defined.

A positive family history confers a 2.5 times increased risk of urolithiasis [37]. The relative contribution of environmental factors such as diet and climate in such families as compared with genetic influence alone requires further investigation.

Dietary/Environmental

As evidenced by the geographic variation in the prevalence of urolithiasis in North America, [8, 9] rates of stone disease are higher in hot, dry climates due to associated dehydration and low urine volumes.

Between the time periods 1976–1980 and 1988–1994, the mean annual temperature (MAT) increased by 0.5 ° C in the United States. The prevalence of stone disease increased during the same time period. The effect of climate change on rates of urolithiasis remains to be precisely defined. Using climate change modeling data, which suggests that mean annual temperatures (MAT) will continue to rise in much of the United States, [38] a 7–10 % increase in the prevalence in stone disease is predicted by 2050 [39]. Figures 2.3 and 2.4 demonstrate predicted changes in the geographical distribution of stone disease, with an expansion of the "stone belt" from the Southeast to the Midwest of the United States.

Several dietary constituents have been implicated in the formation of stones. These are particularly relevant in a North American context, where the diet is generally high in both sodium and animal protein. Animal proteins have been shown to reduce urinary citrate excretion and increase calcium excretion [40]. Likewise, dietary sodium has been shown to induce hypercalciuria [41].

Consumption of high-sugar carbonated beverages has been implicated in the rapid increase in rates of metabolic syndrome, obesity, diabetes, and cardiovascular disease seen within North America. Of all food types, soda is currently the greatest contributor to caloric intake in the United States [42]. Given the overwhelming evidence that obesity predisposes to urolithiasis, it is likely that soda indirectly contributes to stone disease. In addition, such beverages may contribute directly via the metabolism of fructose (the main sweetener used in soda), which increases serum uric acid [43].

The use of vitamin supplements has increased markedly over recent years in Western countries [44–46]. It has been estimated that approximately 40 % of Canadian adults regularly take supplements [47]. A proportion of these preparations contain high doses of vitamin C (ascorbic acid). Due to the metabolism of vitamin C to oxalate, supplementation in excess of the recommended daily intake (90 mg) has been associated with increased oxalate excretion [48] and a 40 % increase in stone formation [24]. In light of these results, patients with a history of calcium oxalate

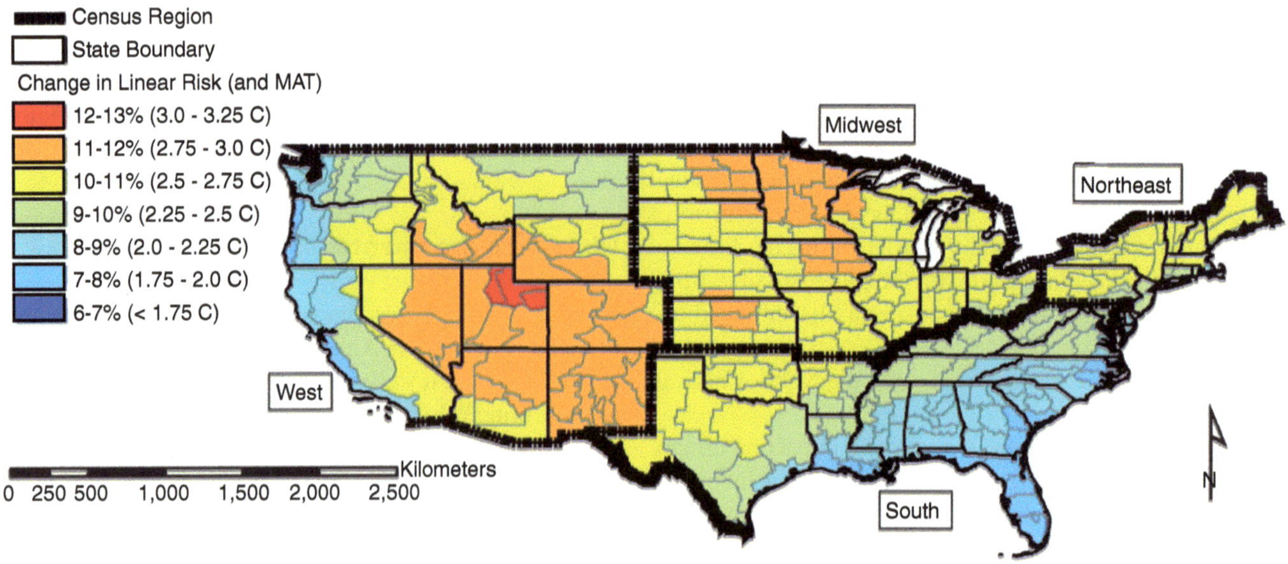

Fig. 2.3 Predicted warming and linear model nephrolithiasis risk change by 2050 for the USA. Strongest warming is in the midcontinent and upper Midwest. *Heavy lines* show the four US census regions, and *light gray lines* show National Oceanic and Atmospheric Administration (NOAA) climate divisions (Adapted with permission from Brikowski et al. [39]. Copyright 2008, National Academy of Sciences, U.S.A.)

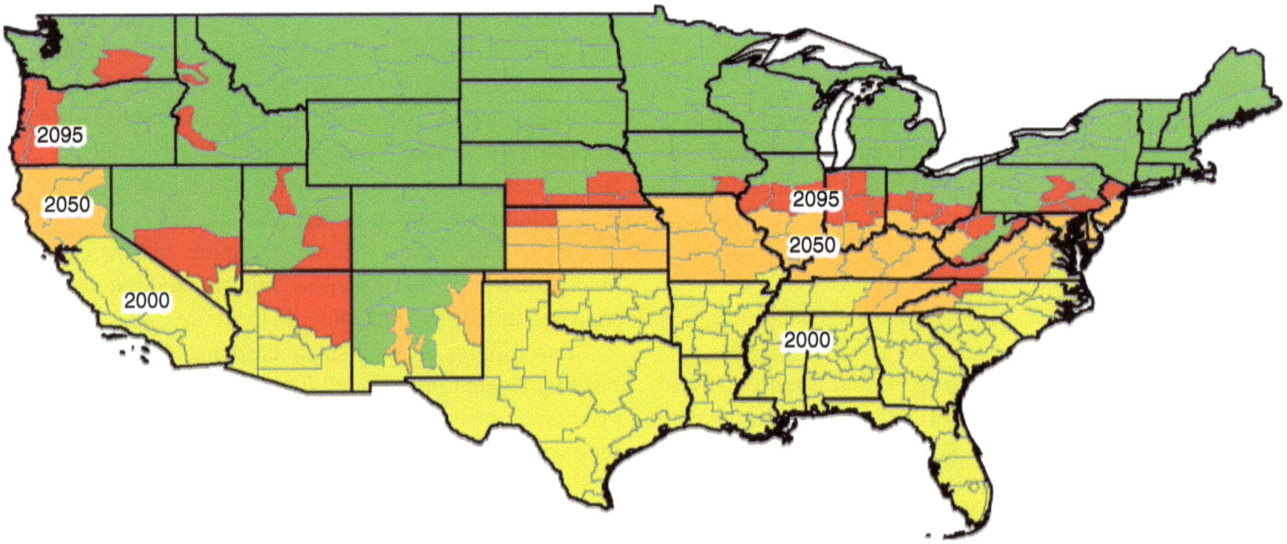

Fig. 2.4 Predicted growth in high-risk stone area (stone belt; risk ratio ≥1.2) vs. time, for 2000 (*yellow*), 2050 (*orange*), and 2095 (*red*), linear model. At 2000, 41 % of the population is within a high-risk zone, 56 % at 2050, and 70 % at 2095, based on year 2000 population distribution (Adapted with permission from Brikowski et al. [39]. Copyright 2008, National Academy of Sciences, U.S.A.)

stone disease should be advised to avoid supplements containing vitamin C.

The importance of adequate dietary calcium in the prevention of osteoporosis for postmenopausal women is well established. In the knowledge that up to 80 % of stones in North America are calcium-containing, the contribution of dietary and supplemental calcium to stone formation has been thoroughly investigated [51]. Contrary to initial beliefs, several studies have convincingly demonstrated an inverse relationship between dietary calcium and risk of stone formation [24, 49, 50]. In light of these results, there appears to be no role for calcium restriction in the context of urolithiasis.

Conclusion

Although the incidence appears to have stabilized in North America over the past three decades, urolithiasis remains a significant health issue, with associated high costs and morbidity. Epidemiological studies have identified new challenges specific to the North American population, particularly in relation to an association between obesity and stone disease.

References

1. Saigal CS, Joyce G, Timilsina AR. Direct and indirect costs of nephrolithiasis in an employed population: opportunity for disease management? Kidney Int. 2005;68:1808–14.
2. Lieske JC, de la Pena Vega LS, Slezak JM, et al. Renal stone epidemiology in Rochester, Minnesota: an update. Kidney Int. 2006; 69(4):760–4.
3. Hesse A, Brandle E, Wilbert D, et al. Study on the prevalence and incidence of urolithiasis in Germany comparing the years 1979 vs. 2000. Eur Urol. 2003;44:709–13.
4. Johnson CM, Wilson DM, O'Fallon WM, et al. Renal stone epidemiology: a 25-year study in Rochester, Minnesota. Kidney Int. 1979;16:624–31.
5. Sierakowski R, Finlayson B, Landes RR, et al. The frequency of urolithiasis in hospital discharge diagnoses in the united states. Invest Urol. 1978;15:438–41.
6. Stamatelou KK, Francis ME, Jones C, et al. Time trends in reported prevalence of kidney stones in the United States: 1976–1994. Kidney Int. 2003;63:1817–23.
7. Pak CY. Etiology and treatment of urolithiasis. Am J Kidney Dis. 1991;18:624–37.
8. Soucie JM, Thun MJ, Coates RJ, et al. Demographic and geographic variability of kidney stones in the United States. Kidney Int. 1994;46:893–9.
9. Curhan GC, Rimm EB, Willett WC, et al. Regional variation in nephrolithiasis incidence and prevalence among United States men. J Urol. 1994;151:838–41.
10. Sarmina I, Spirnak JP. Urinary lithiasis in the black population: an epidemiological study and review of the literature. J Urol. 1987;138:14–7.
11. Pearle MS, Calhoun EA, Curhan GC, et al. Urologic diseases in America project: urolithiasis. J Urol. 2005;173:848–57.
12. Kerbl K, Rehman J, Landman J, et al. Current management of urolithiasis; progress or regress? J Endourol. 2002;16:281–8.
13. Leusmann DB, Blaschke R, Schmandt W. Results of 5035 stone analysis: a contribution to epidemiology of stone disease. Scand J Urol Nephrol. 1990;24:205–10.
14. Daudon M, Donsimoni R, Hennequin C, et al. Sex- and age-related composition of 10617 calculi analyzed by infrared spectroscopy. Urol Res. 1995;23:319–26.
15. Asper R. Epidemiology and socioeconomic aspects of urolithiasis. Urol Res. 1984;12:1–5.
16. Gault MH, Chafe L. Relationship of frequency, age and sex, stone weight and composition in 15,624 stones: comparison of results for 1980 to 1983 and 1995 to 1998. J Urol. 2000;164:302–7.
17. Robertson WG, Peacock M, Heyburn PJ. Clinical and metabolic aspects of urinary stone disease in Leeds. Scand J Urol Nephrol Suppl. 1980;53(suppl):199–206.
18. Curhan GC, Willett WC, Speizer FE, et al. Twenty-four-hour urine chemistries and the risk of kidney stones among women and men. Kidney Int. 2001;59:2290–8.
19. Kourambas J, Aslan P, Teh CL, et al. Role of stone analysis in metabolic evaluation and medical treatment of nephrolithiasis. J Endourol. 2001;15:181–6.
20. Curhan GC, Willett WC, Spiezer FE, et al. Beverage use and risk for kidney stones in women. Ann Intern Med. 1998;128:534–40.
21. Curhan GC, Willett WC, Rimm EB, et al. Prospective study of beverage use and the risk of kidney stones. Am J Epidemiol. 1996;143:240–7.
22. Curhan GC. Epidemiology of stone disease. Urol Clin North Am. 2007;34:287–93.
23. Flegal KM, Carroll MD, Ogden CL, et al. Prevalence and trends in obesity among US adults, 1999–2000. JAMA. 2002;288:1723–7.
24. Taylor EN, Stampfer MJ, Curhan GC. Dietary factors and the risk of incident kidney stones in men: new insights after 14 years of follow-up. J Am Soc Nephrol. 2004;15:3225–32.
25. Taylor EN, Stampfer MJ, Curhan GC. Diabetes mellitus and the risk of nephrolithiasis. Kidney Int. 2005;68:1230–5.
26. Taylor EN, Stampfer MJ, Curhan GC. Obesity, weight gain, and the risk of kidney stones. JAMA. 2005;293:455–62.
27. Cappuccino FP, Strazzullo P, Mancini M. Kidney stones and hypertension: population based study of an independent clinical association. BMJ. 1990;12:1234–6.
28. Taylor EN, Curhan GC. Body size and 24-hour urine composition. Am J Kidney Dis. 2006;48:905–15.
29. Ekeruo WO, Tan YH, Young MD, et al. Metabolic risk factors and the impact of medical therapy on the management of nephrolithiasis in obese patients. J Urol. 2004;172:159–63.
30. Daudon M, Lacour B, Jungers P. Influence of body size on urinary stone composition in men and women. Urol Res. 2006;34:193–9.
31. Abate N, Chandalia M, Cabo-Chan Jr AV, et al. The metabolic syndrome and uric acid nephrolithiasis: novel features of renal manifestation of insulin resistance. Kidney Int. 2004;65:386–92.
32. Santry HP, Gillen DL, Lauderdale DS. Trends in bariatric surgical procedures. JAMA. 2005;294:1909–17.
33. Nelson WK, Houghton SG, Milliner DS, et al. Enteric hyperoxaluria, nephrolithiasis, and oxalate nephropathy: potentially serious and unappreciated complications of Roux-en-Y gastric bypass. Surg Obes Relat Dis. 2005;1:481–5.
34. Asplin JR, Coe FL. Hyperoxaluria in kidney stone formers treated with modern bariatric surgery. J Urol. 2007;177:565–9.
35. Sinha MK, Collazo-Clavell ML, Rule A, et al. Hyperoxaluric nephrolithiasis as a complication of Roux-en-Y gastric bypass surgery. Kidney Int. 2007;72:100–7.
36. Matlaga BR, Shore AD, Magnuson T, et al. Effect of gastric bypass surgery on kidney stone disease. J Urol. 2009;181:2573–7.
37. Curhan GC, Willett W, Rimm E, et al. Family history and risk of kidney stones. J Am Soc Nephrol. 1997;8:1568–73.
38. IPCC4. Climate change 2007: the physical science basis, summary for policy-makers. Fourth climate assessment report (UN Intergovernmental Panel on Climate Change, Geneva), 2007, p. 1–18.
39. Brikowski TH, Lotan Y, Pearle MS. Climate-related increase in the prevalence of urolithiasis in the United States. Proc Natl Acad Sci USA. 2008;105:9841–6.
40. Breslau N, Brinkley L, Hill K, et al. Relationship of animal protein-rich diet to kidney stone formation and calcium metabolism. J Clin Endocrinol Metab. 1998;66:140–6.
41. Muldowney FP, Freaney R, Moloney MF. Importance of dietary sodium in the hypercalciuria syndrome. Kidney Int. 1982;22: 292–6.
42. Block G. Foods contributing to energy intake in the US: data from NHANES III and NHANES 1999–2000. J Food Compost Anal. 2004;17:439–47.
43. Nakagawa T, Hu H, Zharikov S, et al. A causal role for uric acid in fructose-induced metabolic syndrome. Am J Physiol Renal Physiol. 2006;290:F625–31.
44. Millen AE, Dodd KW, Subar AF. Use of vitamin, mineral, nonvitamin, and nonmineral supplements in the United States: the 1987, 1992, and 2000 National Health Interview Survey results. J Am Diet Assoc. 2004;104:942–50.
45. Ervin RB, Wright JD, Kennedy-Stephenson J. Use of dietary supplements in the United States, 1988–94. Vital Health Stat 11. 1999;244:1–14.
46. Slesinski MJ, Subar AF, Kahle LL. Trends in use of vitamin and mineral supplements in the United States: the 1987 and 1992

National Health Interview Surveys. J Am Diet Assoc. 1995; 95:921–3.
47. Guo X, Willows N, Kuhle S, et al. Use of vitamin and mineral supplements among Canadian adults. Can J Public Health. 2009; 1004:357–60.
48. Traxer O, Huet B, Poindexter J, et al. Effect of ascorbic acid consumption on urinary stone risk factors. J Urol. 2003;170:397–400.
49. Curhan GC, Willett WC, Rimm EB, et al. A prospective study of dietary calcium and other nutrients and the risk of symptomatic kidney stones. N Engl J Med. 1993;328:833–8.
50. Curhan GC, Willett W, Speizer F, et al. Comparison of dietary calcium with supplemental calcium and other nutrients as factors affecting the risk for kidney stones in women. Ann Intern Med. 1997;126:497–504.
51. Curhan GC, Willett W, Knight EL, et al. Dietary factors and the risk of incident kidney stones in younger women (Nurses' Health Study II). Arch Intern Med. 2004;164:885–91.

Epidemiology of Stone Disease in Pakistan

3

Amanullah Memon, Khursheed Anwar, Nasir Orakzai, M. Hammad Ather, Syed Raziuddin Biyabani, Abdul Razzaq Nasir, Jai Pal Paryani, Farooq Ghani, Khurram Mutahir Siddiqui, Farhat Abbas, Kashif Bangash, Liaqat Ali, Wajahat Aziz, and Jamsheer J. Talati

Abstract

Urinary tract stones are a common affliction across river, desert, and mountainous regions of Pakistan. A third of the stones have a single component. The commonest stone is composed of oxalate, with phosphate and uric acid as additional components. Calcium oxalate monohydrate is more abundantly present than the dihydrate. Phosphate stones comprise only about 7 % of all stones, and struvite is uncommon. Populations in the north have a greater proportion of pure and predominantly oxalate stones. Rural areas in the south have phosphate stones. The government of British India documented the frequent occurrence of stone in this region from the nineteenth century. The commonest stone was vesical. Noted stone transitions include (1) the marked increase in the discovery of renal stones, (2) the disappearance (except in pockets) of the idiopathic adult vesical stone, and (3) the decrease in children in the proportions of stones that are vesical. Late presentation for treatment and consequent renal destruction are still frequent.

A. Memon, M.B.B.S., FRCS (Ed) (✉)
F. Abbas, M.B.B.S., FCPS, FRCS, FRCSEd, FEBU, FACS
M.H. Ather, M.B.B.S., FCPS (Urol), FEBU
S.R. Biyabani, M.B.B.S., FCPS (Urol), FEBU
K.M. Siddiqui, FCPS, FRCS (UK) FEBU
J.J. Talati, M.B.B.S., FRCS (Ed)
W. Aziz, M.B.B.S.
Section of Urology, Department of Surgery, The Aga Khan University, Stadium Road, 3500, Karachi, Sindh 74800, Pakistan
e-mail: amanullah.memon@aku.edu; farhat.abbas@aku.edu; hammad.ather@aku.edu; raziuddin.biyabani@aku.edu; khurram.siddiqui@aku.edu; jamsheer.talati@aku.edu; wajahat.aziz@aku.edu

K. Anwar, M.B.B.S., FRCS, Dip (Urol)
K. Bangash, M.B.B.S., FCPS (I)
Department of Urology, PAEC General Hospital, Police Lanes, Islamabad 44000, Pakistan
e-mail: khursheedanwar2003@yahoo.com; khursheed_anwar@hotmail.com; drkashifbangash@hotmail.com

N. Orakzai, M.B.B.S., FRCS
L. Ali, M.B.B.S., FCPS (Urology)
Department of Urology, Institute of Kidney Diseases, Hayatabad Medical Complex, Peshawar, Khyber Pukhtoonkhaw, Pakistan
e-mail: n.orakzai@gmail.com; liaqat_99@yahoo.com

A.R. Nasir, M.B.B.S., FCPS
Department of Urology, Bolan Medical College Ouetta, Barwary Road, Quetta 87300, Pakistan
e-mail: nazzaq.nasir@gmail.com

J.P. Paryani, M.B.B.S., FCPS, FEBU
Department of Urology, Liaquat University of Medical and Health Sciences, Jamshoro, Sindh 75500, Pakistan
e-mail: jpsindh@yahoo.com

F. Ghani, M.D., Ph.D. (Path) USA
Department of Pathology, Aga Khan University, Stadium Road, PO Box 3500, Karachi 74800, Pakistan
e-mail: farooq.ghani@aku.edu

J.J. Talati et al. (eds.), *Urolithiasis*,
DOI 10.1007/978-1-4471-4387-1_3, © Springer-Verlag London 2012

Notable is the lack of metabolic abnormality (except for ubiquitous hypocitraturia) in the majority of tested patients. Low calcium excretion and hypovitaminosis D are common. Diet includes unleavened bread, which has lost some of its phytic acid content during preparation, but nevertheless, like nuts and green legumes, has sufficient phytic acid to bind calcium and prevent absorption. Vitamin A supplementation is reported to be adequate. Dietary transitions have begun to affect the urban population and increase their serum uric acid. Practice patterns veer toward open surgery in those public hospitals that do not obtain adequate funds for costly equipment through philanthropy.

Evidence suggests that the transitions in stone frequency, incidence, and site are at least partly due to increased discovery of renal stone because of the availability of investigative technology consequent to economic advancement.

Keywords
Geographical variation • Stone composition • Urine composition • Calcium oxalate stones • Calcium phosphate stones • Infection stones • Uric acid stones • Cystine stones • Aspects on stone removal • Pediatric stones • Age-related stone formation • Recurrence • Stone site • Transitions

Introduction

Pakistan is one of the world's most arid countries [1] but survives because it is "...built around a river"—the Indus and its tributaries—and various groundwater basins [2]. It is a nation in transition that had moved out from poverty. However, with continuing population growth, ignorance, and floods, large sectors have been swept back into an impoverished state. The geographical terrain, culture, dietary habits, earning capacity, and access to health care are extremely varied. This chapter attempts to capture data from the nineteenth and twenty-first centuries (C), from different provinces and settings (rural versus urban).

Figure 3.1 presents a map of the provinces and major cities of Pakistan. There are five provinces in Pakistan. In the south lies Sindh, mostly irrigated desert. Baluchistan's barren mountains lie to the south and west. Khyber-Pukhtoonkhwa, in the northwest, has a heavier intake of red meat. Punjab, the land of five rivers, has a traditional heavy consumption of *lassi*, a drink composed of milk and curds. Gilgit Baltistan lies in the mountainous north, leading to China. Population densities vary widely—from <10 to 50 persons/sq km in Baluchistan to 200–800/sq km in parts of Punjab [3]. A single city, Karachi, in Sindh, holds 18–20 million people—a tenth of the population of Pakistan. It has the most intense hospital documentation support system in the country.

Mountains make hospitals inaccessible. Stone patients in villages may remain undiagnosed from lack of physicians, ultrasound, or X-ray. Statistics present the visible fragment of the disease burden that reaches hospital. Desert populations have greater poverty, a poor economic outlook, malnutrition, little access to milk and water, and suffer vesical stones. The irrigation system, necessary because of lack of rain, has caused salinization. Temperatures range from 50 °C in Jacobabad in northern Sindh in summer to −50 °C in winter in the north.

The information we include in this chapter has been derived from hospital-based published literature as well as from information obtained in response to a questionnaire sent to authors of this chapter.

The Magnitude of the Problem

Data on incidence as a national statistic are not generally available. Rizvi quotes a prevalence of 16 % [4]. Table 3.1 provides examples of incidence derived by extrapolating operating room statistics to population. The incidence (per 100,000) varies from 0.2 to 9.4 in the north [5, 7], to 10.5 in northern Sindh [5], to 200 in southern Sindh [8], and 11.1 to 28 [5, 9] in Baluchistan. The incidence of vesical stones was 0.2 to 1.2/100,000 in Khyber-Pukhtoonkhwa [5] and 7.6 and 9 in Baluchistan and northern Sindh, respectively [6].

From 1933, stone disease operations were frequent in the region that has become Pakistan, with as many as 438, 156, and 266 operations annually for stone in Punjab, North Sindh, and south Sindh [10]. Earlier still, Punjab government documents show that 554 bladder stones were operated in 6 months in 1863 and 2000 each year from 1890 to 1913 [11]. Joshi [12], comparing his 1942 study to notes from Capt. Roberts (1894, published in the *Indian Medical Gazette*), and McCarrison [10] noted a similar frequency over a 50-year span.

A 100 years later, a 1986–1987 study showed the continued prevalence of stones. Dividing Punjab by a jagged line passed through the towns of Sahiwal, Jhang Sarghoda, and

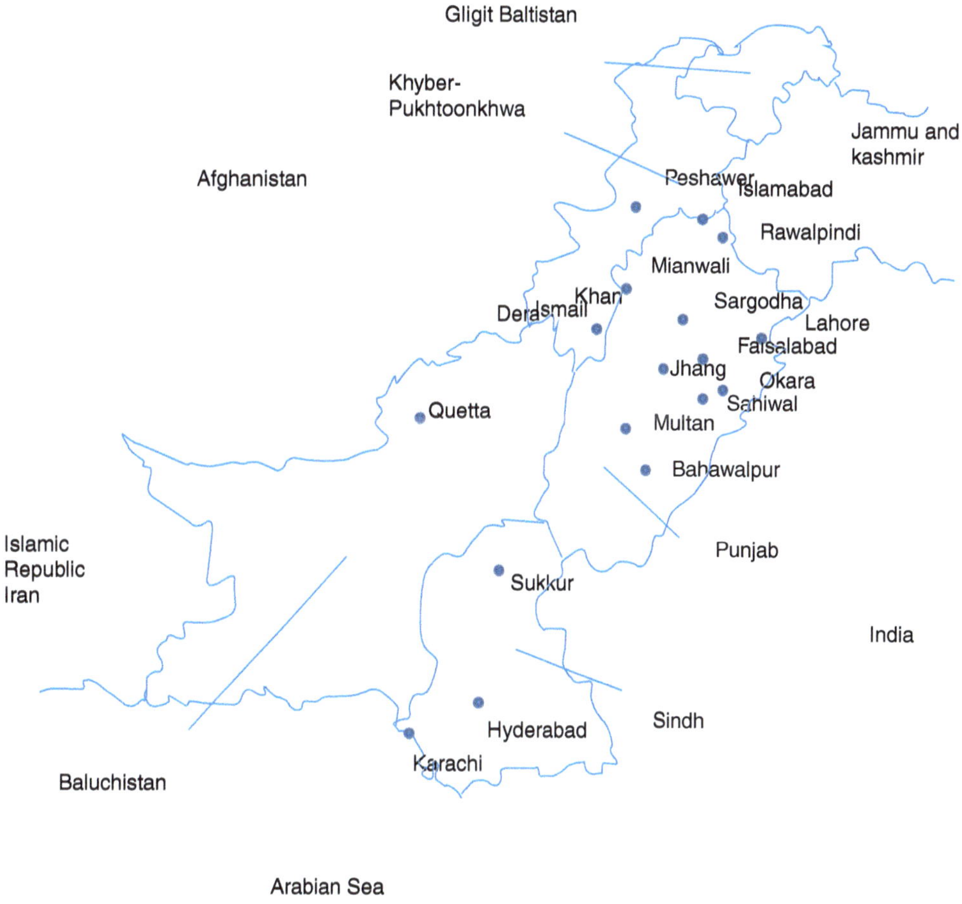

Fig. 3.1 Map of Pakistan, identifying provinces and major cities quoted in the text

Table 3.1 Extrapolating hospital operation room statistics to known population base in the hinterland

Region	Hazara (P-K)	Northern Sindh	Northern Balochistan	Averaged for all three areas
Estimated population of area drained by the institution studied (in millions)	2.855	5.127	3.087	
Vesical stone operations/100,000 population	1.2	9	7.6	6.6
Upper tract stones/colic/100,000	1	1.5	3.5	1.9

Source: Table constructed from information in Ref. [5]

Many in the population in the mountainous area drained by the hospital are unable to reach the hospital for care and hence are not documented in statistics re: incidence. Blanchard calculates an incidence of 7.39/100,000 for the whole country for all stones [6]

Mianwali (see Fig. 3.1), it was noted that 71 % of operations in southwest Punjab were for stone, as compared to 30 % in the northeast Punjab. Vesical stones were four times more common and renal stones twice as common in the southwest as in the northeast Punjab [13]. In 1980–1887, in a hospital in southern Sindh without minimally invasive equipment, 37 % of the urological cases and 11 % of admissions were for stones [14]. In centers of excellence, stone now accounts for 50 % of urological operations.

Pediatric Stone

In the 1990s, 1 in 73 of all hospital admissions and 1 in 24 of pediatric admissions were for urinary stones in a tertiary care hospital in Islamabad [15], distinctly different from the 1 in 1,000 to 1 in 7,600 pediatric admissions in the west in the 1980s [16]. In a primarily ophthalmic care hospital in Taxilla (near Islamabad), cystolithotomies increased sixfold from 1922 to 1990, while the population increased by 3.1 % [17]. In a pediatric urological unit (in 2007), up to 60 % of work is stone-related [18]. In 2010, 35.2 % of stone patients presenting to a public hospital in Baluchistan were <20 years old and 15.4 % <10 years.[1] In Karachi (Sindh), 2.8 % of pediatric stones are seen in ≤1-year-olds, 32.2 % are seen in 1- to 5-year-olds, 39.4 % are seen in 5- to 10-year-olds, and 22.6 % are seen in 10- to 15-year-olds [18].

[1] Personal communication from Dr. Razzaq Nasir, 2011.

Stone Burden and Surgical Workloads

In the 1980s, the overall rate of all surgeries in Pakistan was low, at 124 surgeries/100,000 in the 1980s, which is 1.5–9 % of that in industrialized nations. The burden per surgeon, however, was large, as there are only 0.36 surgeons/100,000 population. This was one-eightieth of the US ratio at that time. As a result, Pakistani surgeons do twice as many operations as those in the United States [6]. Yet, urologist shortages result in a large untreated burden of stone. Each case also has a large stone burden—9.4–16 % are staghorns, and 39.3 % have multiple calculi [19]. A nephrologist is likely to see a stone and obstructive uropathy in 36 % of the patients attending his clinical practice (see also Chap. 75).

Is the Incidence Increasing?

Pakistan's expanding population and health-care systems makes it difficult to determine whether the growing "incidence" of stone is real or an artifact from increased discovery, population growth, and accessibility from improved economics, transport, and roads. Growth rate of the stone burden per hospital is phenomenal. In one public hospital, annual urological operations (50 % of which are for stone) grew from 26,977 to 60,910 and outpatients from 95,740 to 189,660 (2003–2010 period) [20, 21]. In the private sector, clinic visits for urology (of which 50 % of the workload again is for stones) doubled in 12 years (1998–2010) at the Aga Khan University.[2] The workload in these hospitals is because of their excellence and minimally invasive approaches, which attracts patients preferentially.

Clinical Presentation

Stones occur across the life span, becoming rarer after age 60 [22]. From 11 % up to 32 % of stones are seen in children <10 years old [22, 23].

The majority (~65 %) of adult patients present with abdominal pain, 4 26 % with hematuria [22, 24], others with difficult and painful urination, cloudy urine, or (in 5.8 %) with recurrent calculi [24]. Nine percent come after having passed a stone, and 7 % present with urine retention [22].

Urinary Tract Infection (UTI)

From 9.6 to 39 % of stone patients [25] have urinary tract infections (UTI) (see also Chap. 75). In patients who have a UTI, 19 % may have a stone [26].

[2] Statistics from Aga Khan University courtesy of Dr. Raziuddin Biyabani.

Urinary Tract Obstruction

In some regions, as many as 22 % present with severely obstructed urinary tracts, requiring relief before definitive surgery [27], 0.8% [4] to 1.9 % [22] are anuric on presentation, with urology units receiving 10–30 anuric patients a year [28, 29]. One-third of the anuric patients had a solitary kidney, and death was an outcome in 7.5 % [28]. Among those with renal failure and stone, serum creatinine ranged from 3 to 35 mg/dL (265–3,097 μ[mu]mol/L), 33 % were anuric, and 29 % required dialysis. It is remarkable that 72 % of anurics and 49 % of the others with raised serum creatinine improved their creatinine to <2 mg/dL (177 μ[mu] mol/L) at a 2-year follow-up [30].

Silent Stones

Notorious are the silent stones seen in 3–15 % of patients [22, 31, 32]—a rate higher than that in other published studies [33]. In South Asia (India and Pakistan being the most populous countries in this region with approximately 1.38 billion people), 2,619 years of potential life are lost as a result of renal disease. In contrast, the whole world loses 11,415 years [34]. Given the poor access to care, and silent stones, it is not surprising that many still present with pyelonephritis, pyonephrosis, perinephric abscess, xanthogranulomatous pyelonephritis, and anuria.

With improved facilities, late presentations with obstructed renal units and renal failure have been reduced to 1.5 % [25], but from 7.24 to 11.6 % [35, 36] of all chronic renal failure (CRF) in the population is still caused by stone disease.

Presentation in Pediatric Patients

The majority of pediatric patients (51–66 %) present with abdominal pain [32, 37], and 20–33 % have fever [21, 37]. In a public hospital that serves patients in the lower socioeconomic groups, one-third of urine cultures were tested positive, mainly with *Proteus* sp. [32]. On follow-up of infection-free stones, 37.6 % (of 149) developed infection over a period of 3 ± 1.25 years. Fourteen percent of patients with renal failure may have stone(s) in one kidney only; the rest have bilateral disease [18]. When patients have to travel over long distances to reach a hospital, the chances of renal failure increase. At one hospital, two-thirds of the pediatric patients with renal failure had come from distant rural areas—some of them traveling for 20 h at a time [18]. In one unit (SIUT), 8.2 % presented with calculus renal failure, 0.8 % with anuria, and 2.1 % with a unilateral nonfunctioning kidney [25].

Table 3.2 Proportions of stones that are renal ureteric or vesical (from 1998 to 2010)

Year (reference)	Author	City, region	Renal	Ureteric	Vesical	Urethral	UP:LO	Kid: Ure	Free/fee for service
1975 (1971–1975) CHK [98]	Rizvi	Karachi, Sindh	29.5	10.5	56	4	0.66	2.8	Free
1975 SITE female [40]	Yaqin	Karachi, Sindh	73	20	7	0	3.7	3.65	Free
1975 SITE males [40]	Yaqin	Karachi, Sindh	48	23	29	2.5	2.1	2.1	Free
1975 SITE Pediatric [40]	Yaqin	Karachi, Sindh	13	4	76	0.2	3.3	3.25	Free
1983 HFH [17]	Talati	Karachi, Sindh	46.7	23.6	23.6	0	2.33	2	Fee for service
1989 AKU [17]	Talati	Karachi, Sindh	36	43	19.3	1.5	3.76	0.83	Fee for service
1991 AKU [17]	Talati	Karachi, Sindh	51.3	36.8	10.1	1.8	7.4	1.39	Fee for service
1992 AKU [17]	Talati	Karachi, Sindh	62	31	7	0	13.3	2.01	Fee for service
1992 Quetta [9]	Pervez	Quetta, Baluchistan	41	8	51	0	0.96	5.1	Free
1992 Tehsil Hospital Sujjawal [17]	Talati	Sujjawal, Sindh	20.7	2.7	75.1	1.5	0.3	7.67	Free
1996 Mirpurkhas [17]	Talati	Mirpurkhas, Sindh	15.4	10.8	7.3	0.9	0.35	1.43	Free
2003 SIUT Pediatric [42]	Rizvi	Karachi, Sindh	55.2	13.8	31	0	2.23	4	Free
2006 Khyber Teaching Hospital [19]	Ahmed I	Peshawar, Khyber-Pukhtoonkhwa	58.6	24.4	1.7	0	4.88	2.4	Free
2010 Liaquat University of Medical Sciences[a]	Jai Pal	Hyderabad, Sindh			20				Free

[a]Jai Pal, 2011, personal communication

Gender Differences, Stone Site, and Transitions

In general, the gender ratio favors males by 2.1–2.5: 1 [5, 38] but is lower in Khyber-Pukhtoonkhwa at 1.2:1 [19]. Nazir et al. interestingly noted a ratio of 2.8:1 in pediatric patients undergoing extracorporeal shockwave lithotripsy (ESWL) and 3.7:1 for patients undergoing open surgery [39]. In 1933, the gender ratio was documented as 13.2:1. The high male predominance (92.5 %) in those <15 years at that time might have been explained by a dominance of vesical stones. Vesical stones even in 1975 remained predominantly male. In a free hospital for industrial workers' families (viz., Sindh Industrial Trading Estate Hospital Karachi), only 7 % of stones in females were vesical, while 29 % were vesical in males [17]. A review of 2,618 children aged from 3 months to 15 years [18] showed that 64 % were renal stones, 8 % ureteric, and 18 % vesical, whereas the remaining patients had bilateral stones or stones in multiple locations.

Stone Site Transition

Table 3.2 shows the distribution of stones at different times in different units. There are interesting evolutions in the proportions of renal and vesical calculi.

Transitions in Age at Which Vesical Calculi Are Seen

The vesical calculus is usually thought of as a pediatric stone. However, in the 1930s, 7–10 % of all operations in Civil Hospital, a public hospital in Mirpurkhas, Sindh, were mostly for male adults with vesical stones [17]. Adult bladder stones are disappearing selectively from some regions: Since the 1990s, in Mirpurkhas (mid-Sindh), 64 % of bladder stones are now seen in children younger than 10 years [17]. In contrast, in Hyderabad (southern Sindh), even in 2010, 49 % of vesical calculi are in patients >30 years old and 21 % occur in those with an age between 11 and 29 years.[3] Only 30 % of bladder stones were seen in patients younger than 10 years. The adult bladder stone seen in Hyderabad is not the classical obstructed outflow tract stone—only 28 % of stones are associated with benign prostatic hyperplasia (BPH)/stricture. In Baluchistan 1992, the adult pattern persists: 61 % of bladder stones occur in adults (mostly in 20- to 39-year-old patients), while only 3 % are seen in children below the age of 10 [9].

The proportion of upper to lower urinary calculi is distinctively different from that in industrialized countries and appears to be related to earning capacity. In hospitals in Mirpurkhas (mid-Sindh), Sujjawal (southern Sindh), and Taxilla (north Punjab), which are all easily accessible by surrounding rural areas, 1980–1990 saw bladder stones account for 73, 75, and 63.5 % of all operations for stones [17]. In contrast in a free government hospital in an economically advanced, provincial capital (Lahore), in the 1990s, only 15 % of all stone patients had vesical stones [43].

Though the total numbers of vesical stones accessing Aga Khan University (AKU) are small, even at that fee-for-service hospital (in 1997–1999), 74 of 93 patients with vesical stone had no outflow obstruction [44].

In 2010, the burden of vesical stones remained heavy in southern Sindh (in a Hyderabad hospital with excellent

[3]Personal communication from Dr. Jai Pal.

Table 3.3 Proportions of upper to lower urinary tract calculi in the pre- and post-ESWL eras in public and in private hospitals

Private hospitals (HFH and AKU)	Ratio of upper to lower stones		Ratio of renal: ureteric stones		Percentage of stones that are vesical	
	Pre-ESWL Era	Post-ESWL Era	Pre-ESWL era	Post-ESWL era	Pre-ESWL era (%)	Post-ESWL era (%)
HFH 1983	2.33	–	0.85	–	23.6	–
AKU: Pre-ESWL era 1987, Post-ESWL era 1992	3.8	13.3	0.83	2.01	19.3	7.2
	Ratio of upper to: lower stones		Ratio of renal: ureteric		Proportion of stones that are vesical	
Public Hospitals	Pre-ESWL era	Post-ESWL era	Pre-ESWL era	Post-ESWL era	Pre-ESWL era	Post-ESWL era
CHK: Pre-ESWL era 1972–1980	0.95	10.49	10.5	13.1	49 %	7.8 %
SIUT Post-ESWL era 1990–1994						

Data for CHK and SIUT extracted from Tables 3.5 and 3.6 [17]
Legend: *HFH* Holy Family Hospital, *AKU* Aga Khan University, *CHK* Civil Hospital Karachi, *SIUT* Sindh Institute of Urology and Transplantation

rural access) where the renal to vesical stone ratio is 1.5:1, as compared to the 13.3:1 seen at the fee-for-service Aga Khan University, which serves mainly urban populations (Table 3.3).

Factors Affecting the Proportions of Stones that Are Vesical

The changes in proportions of upper to lower calculi might be the result of different socioeconomic conditions, differences in availability of minimally invasive treatment, or other unknown factors.

Stones accounted for 60 % of all operations (1975–1989), at a free hospital serving a larger proportion of the poor and malnourished, but only 23.6 % in a fee-for-service hospital [17] in the same city and at the same time.

The purchase of a lithotripter coincided with a change in proportions of renal calculi to vesical (see Table 3.3). While in 1980s in a free hospital, 60 % of pediatric stones were vesical; by the mid-1990s, only 15 % were such [37].

The apparent transition in stone patterns from purely vesical to renal might also be the result of (1) inability to detect the presence of renal stones in past years; (2) patients' fear of death under anesthetic, which kept them from visiting hospitals; or (3) the lack of sophisticated equipment such as ESWL. Lack of X-ray facilities and ESWL might account for the lower incidence of renal and ureteric calculi that has been reported from 1933 to late in the twentieth century. The child with bladder stone can be identified by a non-medic or the mother—the child is irritable when passing urine and keeps pulling on his penis because of the intense referred pain. The presence of stone can be confirmed by sounding, and the operation done with minimal hospital support sans X-rays or ultrasound.

McCarrison noted a very low incidence of ureteric calculi in the operation statistic. He wrote "Ureteral stone is rare in India" and wisely added, "or it is rarely operated upon." Among the 16,384 calculi removed during the years 1926–1928, there were only 14 ureteral stones. A diagnosis of stone in the ureter was made in other cases, but the patients refused operation [10]. This is probably the reason why the ureteric calculus did not appear as a hospital statistic in the 1930s. Bladder stones can be diagnosed by mothers and laymen because of the characteristic symptoms. The operation is easy and has a low mortality and does not require a sophisticated team.

Practice Patterns

Urologists train and function in widely disparate conditions—with some not having access to equipment for endoscopic or shock wave technology. General surgeons still do urological surgery. The stones are complex and destructive. Patients from out of town require, and demand, definitive single intervention treatment and immediate stone-free status.

The practice patterns (Table 3.4) do not reflect physician choices based on their judgment, knowledge, or technical skill. The inability of the government to buy the highly expensive and costly-to-maintain equipment impedes progress. The practice patterns simply reflect instrument availability, accounting for differences between private hospitals and public hospitals that are not supported by philanthropy (Fig. 3.2).

The proportion of open surgery (Table 3.5) varies from 100 % in a town in the midst of rural Sindh [22] to 19.7 % (1990–2007) in a philanthropy-supported government hospital (SIUT) [25] in Karachi, to <0.3 % in a private sector hospital (Aga Khan University Hospital). In Taxilla, until 1992 [46], all operations except for 3.9 % (which were cystolitholapaxies) were open operations. However, even in those units with ESWL available, ESWL rates varied from 17 to 55 % for treatment of renal stones (see Table 3.5).

The special features of stones in Pakistan are resulting in an open approach for the large stone burden—multiple

Table 3.4 Practice patterns

	ESWL	Open	PCNL	RIRS	URS	ENDO for Ves	Province	Public/private
Ahmed [19]	63.7	96	0	0	0	4	Khyber-Pukhtoonkhwa	Public
Hussain 1990–2009 [25]	55	19.7	6	0	16	4	Karachi Sindh	
Jai Pal[a]	55	27.5	13.7		27	32	Hyderabad Sindh	
Memon 2009 [22]	0	100	0	0	0	0	Nawabshah Sindh	
Orakzai[b]	38.5	31.9	0.3	1.9	13	13	Peshawar Khyber-Pukhtoonkhwa	Both
Razzaq Nasir[c]	17	74.9	0.3	0	5.8	2	Quetta Baluchistan	
Rizvi 2004–2008 [45]	19	30	16		19	16	Karachi Sindh	
Hussain[d] 1990–1995 [25]	68.7	14.4	0		10	6.4		
Hussain[d] 1996–2001 [25]	69.9	11.2	3.6		9.6	2.5		
Hussain[d] 2002–2007 [25]	63.7	16.1	5.1		13	2.3		

Yellow highlight is for pediatric stones only
See Fig. 3.2 for data from Aga Khan University
[a]Jai pal personal communication
[b]Nasir Orakzai personal communication
[c]Razzaq Nasir personal communication
[d]These data demonstrate the trend in use of different modalities of treatment between 1990 and 2007 and are subsets of data from Hussain et al. [25]

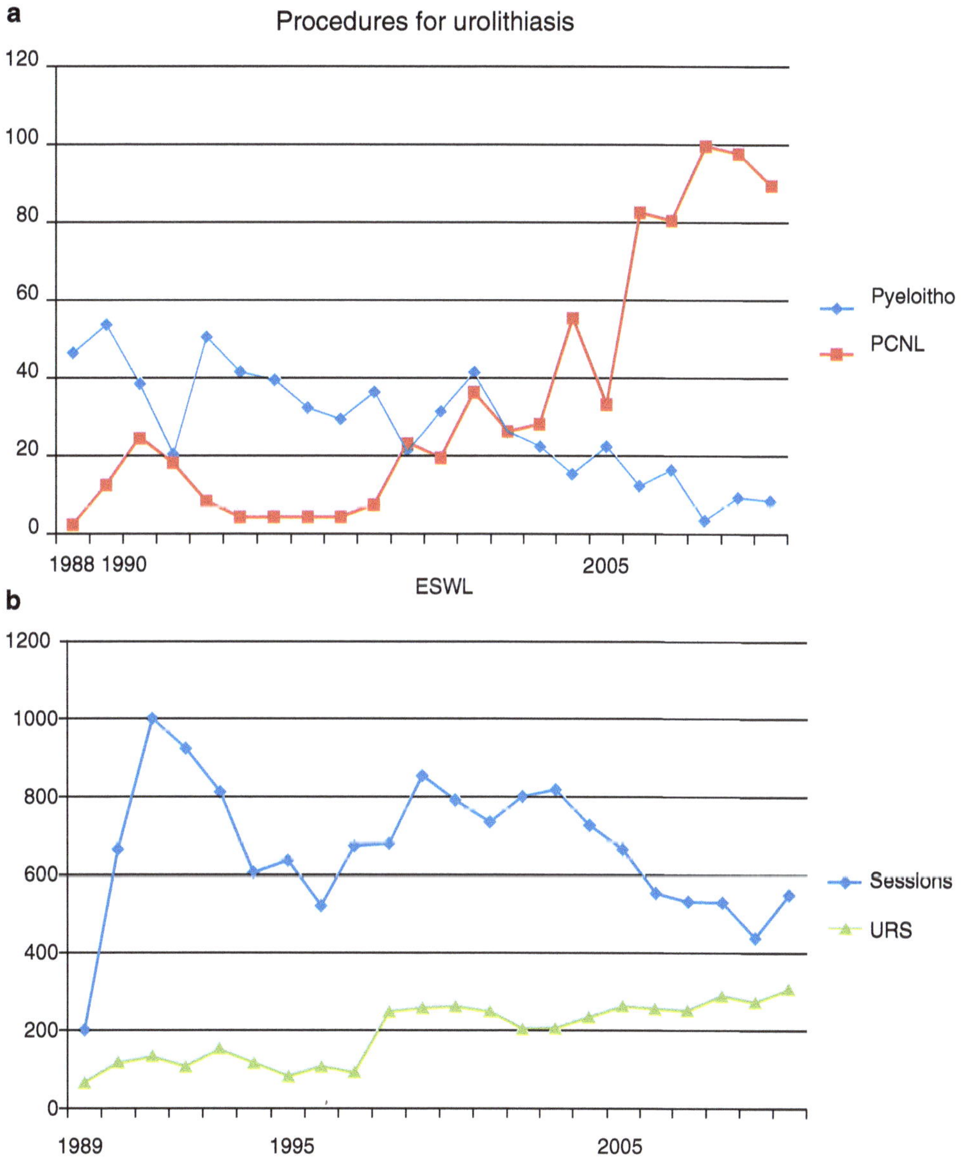

Fig. 3.2 Practice patterns for 1988–2010, Aga Khan University. (**a**) Pyelolithotomies versus PCNL procedures. Note: The scale for (**a**) is in hundreds, (**b**) in tens. (**b**) Number of ESWL sessions compared to ureteroscopy(*URS*)

Table 3.5 Percent composition of stones from different areas

Author and year [reference#]	Geographical location	*N*	Oxalate	P	Uric	Struvite	How many of these are oxalate(O) or urate/uric acid (U)?	UR-P/ UR-P-OX	UR/OX	Cystine
Afzal (53 % pure) 1992 [46]	Taxilla Rawalpindi Islamabad (Khyber-Pukhtoonkhwa)	200	26.5 COM,3 COD	27.5 CaOx-P	13 %	7.5			14.5 % CaOx Uric	0.5
Ahmed I 2006 [19]	(Punjab + Khyber-Pukhtoonkhwa)	852	60	10.5	15	14(triple phos)				0.3
Bukhari thesis 2004 [41]	Quetta (Baluchistan)	80	46 % COM + 19 % COD	11.8 % carbapa-tite + 19 % COD	11.9 % adult 4.1 % Pediatrics 10.7	1.4 M, 7.0 F 3.6 % in adults 5.3 % in peds				
Chand 2009–2010 [23]	Southern Sindh (Sindh)	278	33.1		18.3	7.9	16 % and 22.7 % Mixed	18 + 22.7		
Channa 2005–2006 [47]	Southern Sindh	58	37.9 pure		3.4	10.3	44 OX Ur	44	M:F 2.2:1	
Farooq 1998–2000 [48]	Rahimyar Khan (Punjab)	125	28 % pure	16 % OX + struvite 11.2 % OX + P	6.4 pure				38.4 Mixed ox-urate	
Kanwal [50]	All Pakistan	37[illegible]8	07.6, 35–37 %:inter-mediate	9.40 %	29.9	9.4	S			0.2
Hashmi 1984 [51]	D I Khan (Khyber-Pukhtoonkhwa)	200	60	5, 0x + p = 22	2	9		1		1
Jahangir [49]	Lahore 2003 (Punjab)	60	17							
Tassaduq [52]	Multan (Punjab)	263	22	1.14+ 19	16.7			11	25	
Khalil [53]	Quetta (Baluchistan)	137	25.5	1.4 (13.8 Ca OX + CaP	2.9 (8.7 % ammonium urate)	CaOx + CaP + Mg 1.4			29.1	
Khan JH 2010 [55]	Lahore (Punjab)	50	1600 %	4 ox + P	0 %	12		8	60	(2.1Xanthine)
Newcomb (McCarrison) [10]	Pre-partition India (mainly Punjab + Khyber-Pukhtoonkhwa)	226	5.75	1.32 + 10.17 P-OX	6.63		Urate Oxalate in 34.51 %, Ur OX P 32.74 % P ox in 10.17 %	42	34.5	
Rab 1990 [56]	Khyber-Pukhtoonkhwa	188	58 % Pure	10.4 Caox/p						
Rafique 1992–1999 [57]	Multan (Punjab)	700	26	0.7 (10.4 CaOx + P)	2800 %		CaOX + P + Ur 7.1		21.8 (37 %)	

Author and year [reference#]	Geographical location	*N*	Oxalate	P	Uric	Struvite	How many of these are oxalate(O) or urate/uric acid (U)?	UR-P/ UR-P-OX	UR/OX	Cystine
Rahman [38]	Rawalpindi (Punjab)	428	34 % pure		03 but 37 % contain UA	5	37 % mixed UA containing			0
Rana 1996 [58]		128	52 % pure		27 %					
Rasool M [27] Sial [54]	Dera Ghazi Khan (Punjab)	50	10	0 (20 % CaOx + P)	28 % had >50 % uric acid in the stone	CaOx + CaP + Am = 10 %; No Mg	CaOx + CaP + UR 30		20	
Zafar [59]	Multan (Punjab)	258	33.7	18.9	Am Urate 18.9				22.4	

calculi in 67 %, staghorns in 9–16 % [19], neglected disease, destroyed kidneys, and xanthogranulomatous pyelonephritis. The stated reasons for open surgery in pediatric patients in one series included large stone burden (37 %), anatomical abnormalities (16 %), renal failure (34 %), thin, hydronephrotic cortex (5.8 %), UTI (25 %), failed minimally invasive surgery (18 %), and distance of urological center from residence (23.4 %) [45]. In Pakistan, it is surprising that despite delayed intervention, the nephrectomy rate is low. In Orakzai's[4] series of 999 stone patients, only 1.6 % underwent nephrectomy.

Practice Patterns for Pediatric Patients

In 1994–1995, an era where pediatric ureteroscopes were not available, 36–70 % of pediatric stones, depending on site, were removed by open operation; the rest were treated by ESWL [39, 42]. In 1987–1995, in children, 70 % of renal, 36 % of ureteric, and 68 % of vesical stones were treated by open surgery in the SIUT. ESWL was used for 22 % of renal, 43 % of ureteric and 14 % of vesical stones; percutaneous nephrolithotomy (PCNL) for 7.8 % renal stones, and ureteroscopy (URS) for 18.6 %. Transurethral stone removal was performed in 17.2 % for bladder stones [42]. By 2004–2008, the same unit noted that 70 % were operated through minimally invasive procedures, of which 19 % were by ESWL, 16 % by PCNL, and 18.9 % by URS [45].

Stone Composition

The varying patterns of stone composition from across the country are presented in Table 3.5.

Stones are seldom sent for analysis because of costs, a general lack of conviction of usefulness, difficulty in retrieving fragments, and the few laboratories that offer this service. Most stones are subjected to chemical analysis, while some researchers have used infrared spectroscopy (FTIR) [15, 61–63], thermogravimetric analysis [46] or atomic absorption spectroscopy [64], and laser ablation inductively coupled plasma-mass spectrometry (LA-ICP-MS) [65].

We report separately on upper and lower urinary tract stone composition over the last eight decades because of differences in composition according to site and era.

Single Component Stones

Most stones are complex with at least one predominant component and two other components. One-third (34–36 %) is single component stones [38, 61]. Depending on the region, 16–70 % of stones [10, 46, 58, 61] may be pure single component stones.

Pure, or single component, stones have been variously defined. Some specifically state that this indicates the absence of components other than matrix; others include as pure stones all stone with >59 % of that constituent. The highest percent of single component stones is from the north [10, 51], where 45–70 % percent of stones are pure oxalate. Stones from the north and west show a higher proportion of pure oxalate [46, 51]. Data from the Pakistan Institute of Medical Sciences (PIMS) in the north[5] confirms that *pure* oxalate stones are commoner in the north. In contrast, in southern Sindh (city: Hyderabad), only 37.9 % were pure oxalate [63].

Ureteral calculi (on FTIR) are more often (47 % of the time) single component stones. Renal and vesical stones have a single component in only 22 and 15 %, respectively [61].

The proportion of calcium oxalate monohydrate (COM) to calcium oxalate dihydrate (COD) varies according to region. In the north [46], COM was far more common (26.5 vs. 3 %). In the south [61], COD was present in almost a third as many stones as COM.

Complex Stones

In complex stones, the predominant component in upper urinary tract (UUT) stones is calcium oxalate, most often in combination with phosphate (hydroxyapatite) [61] or uric acid.

The commonest complex stone combinations reported in 1930 by Newcomb [10] are similar to that seen today. However, Newcomb reported fewer (13.7 %) single component stones (6.6 % uric acid, 5.8 % oxalate, and 1.3 % phosphate), but among the mixed stones, urate-oxalate combinations (34.5 %), and urate-oxalate-P (32.7 %) predominated [10]. As of 2010, in PIMS urate-oxalate and phosphate-oxalate stone contribute with 31 and 15 %, respectively.

In UUT stones, Khand found a predominance of COM (present in 75 % of stones) and hydroxyapatite (seen in 51 %) [61]. In LUT stones, ammonium acid urate (AHU) and COM combinations are common, and CaOx-AHU stones were particularly common in children up to 14 years [61].

The difference in the core and shell of stones is shown in Table 3.6.

[4] Personal communication.

[5] Personal communication from Dr. Khursheed Anwar.

Table 3.6 Composition of core and surface of upper and lower urinary tract stone

		Upper urinary tract stone		Lower urinary stone	
		Renal stone		Vesical stone	
Author	Stone component	Core	Surface	Core	Surface
Umar [66]	AHU	64	30	61	37
	CaOX	41	72	35	52
	Uric Acid	3		10	16
	Calcium phosphate apatite	9		7	12
	Struvite	5		6	15
Author	Stone component	Upper urinary tract stone (%)		Lower urinary tract stone (%)	
Khand [61]	COM present in	75		57	
	COD present in	21		17	
	AHU	19		57	
	Hydroxy apatite	50.82		37.25	
	Carbonate apatite	5.74		17.65	
	Uric acid	15		30	
	Single component stone seen in	22 (renal)		47 (ureter)	15

CaOx calcium oxalate, *AHU* ammonium urate, *COM* calcium oxalate monohydrate, *COD* calcium oxalate dihydrate

Phosphate

A significant number of stones have some phosphate (P) mixed with oxalate. At the Aga Khan University Hospital clinical laboratory, stones are received from all over Pakistan. With insights into the analysis of 3,718 stones, Kanwal, Ghani et al. [50] suggested that stones be termed predominantly oxalate (OX) if the OX: P ratio is >10 or predominantly phosphate if the stone contains >50 % of phosphate (an OX/P ratio of <1). In this series, 7.6 % of the stones were predominantly composed of calcium phosphate, 57 % were termed intermediate, and 40 % of male and 29 % of females were classified as predominantly oxalate stone formers. Most series do not use this specific classification. The predominantly phosphate stone is uncommon, but in children, 26 % of the stones are predominantly composed of phosphate versus 6 and 9 % in those 15–39 years and >40 years, respectively. Stones in women have a higher phosphate content and consequently a lower proportion (29 %) of oxalate-dominated stones as compared to male stones (where the predominantly oxalate stone accounts for 40 %) (Table 3.7). Phosphate stones constitute 5 % in Gomal, in district DI Khan in the north (Khyber-Pukhtoonkhwa).

Overall the proportion of phosphate stones has remained unchanged since 1990; when at the AKU urology unit (Karachi, urban, fee-for-service hospital), only 9 % of the stones contained >50 % phosphate [67]. It is likely that the proportion of phosphate stones for Pakistani patients is between 6 and 9 %.

Three exceptions are noted: (1) In hospital accessible by rural population in south Sindh, Khand, noted higher levels of hydroxyapatite in 51 % of UUT and 37 % of LUT stones and carbonate apatite in 6 and 18 % of UUT and LUT stones, respectively [61]. They noted a higher percent of pure phosphate in upper tract calculi in those over 45 years. Similarly, (2) 50 % of 30 bilateral stones in a traditionally agricultural, recently industrialized town, Faisalabad, were phosphate [68]. (3) In PIMS, Khursheed Anwar noted that in complex stones, 23 % had phosphate predominant stones and 26 % had intermediate, oxalate dominant stones (with only 3.5 % having a OX-P ratio of >10).

Table 3.7 The proportions of stones predominantly phosphate or oxalate in an all-Pakistan series of 3,718 stones [50]

	Age groups (years)		
Grouped by	≤15	15–39	≥40
oxalate-to-phosphate ratio	*N* (%)	*N* (%)	*N* (%)
Phosphate(Ox:P ratio <1)	21 (26.6)	46 (9.7)	94 (6.2)
Intermediate (Ox:P ratio 1— <10)	46 (58.2)	252 (53.2)	888 (58.5)
Oxalate (Ox:P ratio >10)	12 (15.2)	176 (37.1)	536 (35.3)

Reproduced by permission of Dr. Farooq Ghani

Struvite

Struvite is detected in 6.4–8.7 % [67, 69] of pediatric stones and in 8–16 % of adult stones [15, 38, 61, 70]. This is in contrast to industrialized countries. Khand noted struvite in 15.6 % of LUT and 2.46 % of UUT stones [61], and Bukhari noted that 23 % of stones in women were struvite. The paucity of struvite in South Asia and the infrequency with which

CaP stones are seen in Asia Minor and Pakistan, than in the Far East (China included) has been noted by Daudon [71].

In summary, as regards phosphate stones, in Pakistan, phosphates other than struvite are seen more commonly in women, in older patients, in bladder stones, and in the patients seeking treatment in hospitals in south of Pakistan, which have direct access for rural patients. Both carbonate and apatite are recorded infrequently.

Uric Acid

From 2 to 38 % [15, 46, 70] of stones are composed of uric acid. The high uric acid stone areas appear to be in:

1. Baluchistan where 27–23 % of women but only 15 % of children and 9.7 % of men had uric acid stones [24]
2. Multan, in Punjab [57, 70], where 28 % of the stones are classified as "pure" uric acid, almost in equal proportion to oxalate stones

Surprisingly, the proportion of uric acid stones is only 2 % in Khyber-Pukhtoonkhwa, a meat-eating province. In contrast, in neighboring Taxilla and Islamabad [46], 16 % of the stones are composed of pure uric acid. This is possibly because of the greater influence of Western lifestyle and diet in Islamabad, the capital of Pakistan.

Most stones have some uric acid within them [72], and while pure uric acid stones in a series might only constitute 3 %, mixed calculi containing uric acid constitute 37 % [38, 56]. On FITR, 15 and 30 % of UUT and LUT stones, respectively, have uric acid [61], and 19 and 57 % of UUT and LUT stones contain ammonium acid urate.

Cystine stones are found in 0.2 % (Kunwal and Ghani) [50] to 0.5 % (Afzal) [46]. *Xanthine* stones are extremely rarely reported except in Khan's series (2.1 %) [15]. Routine screening for cystine is not performed in children or infants, and hence, the real proportion of cystinuria remains unknown.

Because of an extremely complex variety of combinations, Shad [64] attempted to classify stones into 13 distinct combinations. In his series, whitlockite and brushite were also noted among its constituents as were also free amino acids (leucine, isoleucine, tyrosine, glutamic acid, glycine, histidine, threonine, aspartic acid, lysine, alanine, valine, cystine, methionine, phenylalanine, hydroxyproline, arginine, aspartinine, tryptophan).

Trace Elements in Stones

Atomic absorption spectrometric analysis of magnesium and trace elements has shown that the stones contained N, Mg, Ni, Zn, Cu, Fe, Pb, Cr, and Al [73]. Khanum [24] found Ca, Na, Zn, Cu, and Pb in 100 % stones; Mg, Mn, iron, silicone, and titanium in 90 %; Co and Ni in 80 %, and Cr in 74 %. Shad noted that almost all contain Na, K, Mg, Fe, and Zn, but Pb, Ni, Mn, and Cu were not detectable in stones from the Multan area [64]. Chaudhri et al. [65], using laser ablation inductively coupled plasma-mass spectrometry (LA-ICP-MS), demonstrated the interrelationships between spatial distribution of a number of elements—Li, B, Mg, Al, P, Ca, Cr, Mn, Zn, Rb, Sr, Ba, and Pb for different stone types.

Composition of Stones in Pediatric Patients

As in adults, only 36 % of 2,039 stones analyzed from a cohort of 2,618 in a study by Rizvi were single component stones [18, 66]. Khan et al. [15] showed that 50 % of pediatric stones in Rawalpindi/Islamabad were composed of calcium oxalate/phosphate, 26.1 % ammonium urate, 8.7 % of struvite/carbonate apatite, 8.7 % of uric acid, 2.1 % of xanthine, and 4.4 of unidentified components.

Interestingly, ammonium acid urate (AHU) is an important constituent in renal and vesical pediatric stones. On analysis of 2,039 stones, 86.5 % of which were renal, 58 % were found to be composed of AHU, 63 % contained whewellite, 20 % weddellite, 6 % uric acid, 12 % CaP, and 8 % struvite [18]. In this series in renal stones, cystine, xanthine, and protein contributed to 1, 1, and 0.8 %, respectively; two stones each were seen with 2,8 dihydroxyadenine and newberyite and four with whitlockite. On chemical analysis, no difference was found between bladder and kidney stone composition—91 % had Ca, 68.8 % had urate/uric acid, 50 % phosphate, and 43 % oxalate. Iron was found in 40 %, magnesium in 28 %, carbonate in 21 %, sulfate in 10 %, and cystine in 1 %. There were 11 % pure calcium phosphate stones, 9 % pure urate/uric acid stones, 7 % oxalate stones, and 3 % pure carbonate apatite stones.

Metabolic Workup

Analyses of blood and 24-h urinary chemistry are summarized in Table 3.8.

Hypercalcemia is infrequently detected. The majority of serum calcium (S-Ca) levels are generally in the lower range of normal, but Ishaq [78] found that stone formers (SF) had a significantly higher S-Ca (10.6 ± 1.07 mg/dL (2.65 ± 0.27 mmol/L) in SF versus 9.16 ± 0.51 (2.29 ± 0.13 mmol/L) in controls (NSF)—$p = 0.001$). Classical hypercalcemic primary hyperparathyroidism is rare or rarely detected and accounts for only 0.055 % of all operations (67,566) in a tertiary center (AKU) in Karachi [80] and 1.25 % of stone patients [81]. The reason may be that many patients with normocalcemic hyperparathryroidism are being missed, as the screening tool used in Pakistan (with its extant

Table 3.8 Urinary and blood chemistry in stone patients and controls (Mean (SD))

		Serum Ca mmol/L	Serum Urate mmol/24 h	U-ca mmol/24 h	U-urate mmol/24 h	U-Oc mmol/24 h	U-P mmol/24 h
Khand 1994 [74]	Control			3.47 (0.43)		0.26 (0.02)	13.1 (1.67)
	SF			3.47 (0.43)		0.31 (0.03)	27.3 (2.29)
Sutton 1997 [81]	Control			2.75 (1.69)	2.27 (1.20)	0.23 (0.13)	16.8 (8.17)
	SF			4.69 (2.61)	2.72 (1.13)	0.19 (0.10)	22.2 (9.58)
Rizvi 1975 [98]	Control			4.15 (0.66)			
	SF			4.16 (0.66)			
Khanum 1981 [24]	Control	2.48 (0.04)	283 (13)	3.42 (0.18)	1.62	0.44 (0.03)	8.66 (0.52)
	SF	2.481 (0.02)	304 (8) ns	3.77 (0.12)	1.60	0.43 (0.01)	8.75 (0.31)
Khan JA 2003 [76]	Control			5.25 (0.34)		0.40 (0.03)	22.5 (1.97)
	SF			6.65 (0.58)		0.57 (0.05)	16.1 (1.2)
Khan JH 2010 [55]	Control		226 (46)				
	SF		233 (52)				
Ishaq M 2011 [60]	Control		277 (12)		4.98 (0.11)		
	SF		302 (13)		6.05 (5.45)		
Ishaq M 2009 [78]	Control	2.29 (0.13)	226 (46)	1.87 (0.08)			
	SF	2.65 (0.27)	233 (52)	4.18 (0.11)			
Rajput 2007 [84]	Control	2.20 (0.33)	321 (90)	4.48 (2.22)	1.87 (1.03) SD 173.49 mg/24 h		
	SF	2.39 (0.18)	320 (99)	7.19 (4.53)	2.53 (1.08)		

vitamin D deficiency) is a serum calcium measurement. Corrected calcium based on serum albumin has, in our experience, detected an additional 5.8 % hypercalcemic patients, and the difference in reported values of serum calcium and calculated corrected calcium was clinically significant (max difference 2.40 mg/dl, 0.6 mmol/L) [82]. In our experience, in the group of hyper-parathyroid patients operated on, stone disease was present in two-thirds of all patients [80].

Vitamin D deficiency is extant throughout Pakistan. In a small personal series of patients, vitamin D levels measured 17 ± 17 ng/dL. Vitamin A has been measured in one study [24] and was normal 31.13 ± 2.42 in controls and 18.68 ± 1.18 sig $p < 0.01$. In Bahawalpur, hyperuricemia was noted in 15 % of 235 patients [27].

Urinary metabolic workup is done very infrequently. The 24-h urinary analysis detects hyperuricosuria in only 11 %, hypercalciuria in 19 %, and hyperoxaluria in 4 % [81]. *Urinary calcium excretion is low* in the general population and in stone formers. This appears to be an Asian characteristic. Maloney [83] has noted the low urinary calcium levels in Asians living in the United States (mean urinary Ca:146 mg/24 h (3.65 mmol/L)) as compared to US Caucasians (233 mg/24 h (5.83 mmol/L)). Talati, Rizvi, and others have all documented lower urinary calcium levels than in the west (see Table 3.8 blood and urine chemistry). But there are contrary reports:

1. Urinary calcium excretions were found to be higher in SF versus NSF [9, 78], though still <300 mg/day (7.5 mmol/day).
2. In Khyber-Pukhtoonkhwa, Khan noted that the Ca excretion was 266 ± 23.26 mg (6.65 ± 0.58 mmol) in SF versus 210.4 ± 13.76 mg (5.26 ± 0.34 mmol) in controls (NSF), and more importantly, hypercalciuria (>300 mg/24 h (7.5 mmol/24 h)) was present in 76 % of male and 17 % of female stone formers as against only 6 % in controls [76].
3. Shahjehan reported that 31 % were hypercalciuric [72].

Khan et al. noted higher *oxalate* excretions in SF from Khyber-Pukhtoonkhwa (51.26 ± 4.35 mg (0.57 ± 0.05 mmol) versus 35.93 ± 2.54 mg (0.40 + 0.03 mmol)), but the phosphate excretion was lower in stone formers than in controls (500 ± 36.43 (5.23 + 0.38 mmol) versus 696.4 ± 60.97 mg (7.05 ± 0.64 mmol)) [76].

Khan [55] noted no difference in urinary uric acid excretion in a population where 16 % of stones were composed of pure uric and 60 % overall had urates present in 60 % stones. Rajput found hyperuricosuria in 26 % [84], and the mean 24-h urinary excretion of urate was significantly higher (424.31 ± 142.16 mg (2.53 ± 0.85 mmol) versus 314.29 ± 173.49 mg (1.87 ± 1.03 mmol) in controls $p < 0.05$).

Hypocitraturia

Up to 70 % of SF and 72 % of NSF are hypocitraturic (< 320 mg/24 h) [85]. There was no significant difference in urinary citrate excretion between SF and NSF (mean

Table 3.9 Urinary citrate and magnesium excretion

	Khand 1994 [74]		Mithani, Zaidi [79]		Talati [81]	
	Patient		Patient		Patients	
Author, year, ref	Controls		Controls		Controls	
Urinary citrate (mg/24 h)	377±41.3	608.9±54.4	262±197	269±140	325±223	410±43
% hypocitraturic (<320 mg/24h)	76 %		70 %	72 %	55 %	26 %
Urinary Mg	102.6±9.2	95.3±7.3				

262±197 mg/24 h (1.36+1.03 mmol/24 h) versus 269 ± 140 mg/24 h (1.40+0.73 mmol/24 h)) (Table 3.9) [79]. The mean urinary citrate in men 259 mg/24 h (1.35 mmol/24 h) (median value 170 mg, 0.89 mmol) was not significantly lower than in females 265.8 mg/24 h (1.38 mmol/24 h) (median value 255 mg, 1.33. mmol) [79]. Hypocitraturia was present in up to 87 % of the children in whom metabolic studies were done (SIUT) [18]. Khand found that the 24-h urinary citrate was <135 mg (0.70 mmol) in 29 % of SF [74].

In some patients, there appears to be an additional intrinsic defect in the handling of citrate, as 10 % stone formers had low citrate despite an adequate net alkaline absorption (calculated by the method of Oh). Alkali supplementation with citrate increased urinary citrate in 82 % (19/23) of the patients given potassium citrate, while 64 % had improved citrate excretion on administration of sodium bicarbonate. The net alkali absorption increased 94 % in both arms.[6]

Population-Based Study of Urinary Excretion Rates in "Normal" Children

Population-based data on 300 children, aged 4–16 years from Quetta Valley with a body weight of between 11 and 50 kg, showed an average daily urinary volume of 987.5 ± 452.5 mL. Hypercalciuria was noted in 11.5 %; 8.5 % had hyperuricosuria, 2.0 % hyperphosphaturia, 2.5 % hypomagnesuria, 3.5 % hypocitraturia, 6.5 % hypernatriuria, 43.5 % hypokaluria, and 2.1 % hyperoxaluria [86].

Soil, Salinity, Irrigation, and Water

The World Bank draws attention to the salinization resulting from "low rainfall, poor drainage, ancient marine deposits, saline groundwater, and evaporation…(which) combine to create a vast saltsink" [1]. Salinity is increasing and affecting the livelihood of farmers [87].

Joshi has drawn attention to an increase in the number of operations for calculi soon after the building of a dam—the Sukkur Barrage and its related irrigation system in 1933. Sukkur district, which lies above the irrigated area, did not show an increase in stone disease, but in Hyderabad, (in lower Sindh) stone surgery increased from between 492 and 564 operations/year (between 1925 and 1933) to 530 to 709 (1934–1942) after 1933. The increase in numbers of operations was greater than expected from growth of population [12], but it was not sustained. Joshi believed that in arid regions, the percent of MgO is lower (1.27 %) as compared to soil from humid regions (9.29 %). The total soluble matter is 30 %—twice that in humid lands, and calcium oxide is 14 times that in humid land. He also mentions that there is an increase in calcium carbonate in irrigated lands and the calcium magnesium level doubles. Salinity and soil content might possibly have an influence on stone disease.

Socioeconomic, Dietary, and Nutritional Status

Most stone patients are very poor. People with the lowest income have only 22 % share of the total available incomes [88]. Only 44 % have access to sanitation and 65 % to clean water [89].

In 1990, in Abbottabad (Khyber-Pukhtoonkhwa), 88 % of vesical calculi came from rural families, where 68 % earned <US $9/month [75]. In Baluchistan, only 12.5 % of all stone-patient families earned >US $9/month (conversion at 2010 US dollar equivalent), and 22 % earned less than $5.5/month. Seventy percent of stone formers in 1992 in Quetta Baluchistan earned less than PKR 200/month, and not a single stone former or control subject earned >PKR 500/month. In public hospitals in Hyderabad[7] and Karachi (Sindh) of the ~0.7 million stone patients seen in 2009–2010, almost all are poor or would have been unable to access modern technology-based treatment if they had to pay [20].

Poor earnings result in poor health, and 20 % of the population are underweight [90, 91]. In Sindh, 54 % of children are chronically malnourished (as judged by height for age), and 25 % acutely malnourished (weight for height), and 50 % of the 1,878 children surveyed had had diarrhea in the preceding 2 weeks [92]. Of all children, 11.6 % are wasted; 31 % stunted; 41 % underweight, according to the 2001–2002 Government of Pakistan National Nutritional Survey [93]. Not surprisingly, 65 % of 2,618 pediatric

[6] Personal communication from S. Raziuddin Biyabani.

[7] Personal communication, Jai Pal.

patients attending a public sector hospital in Karachi were malnourished and 76 % stunted.

What Do People Eat When They Are So Poor?

For the average Pakistani, 62 % of energy is derived from cereals [94]. In Baluchistan stone formers, their diet was low in protein (74 % of stone formers), Ca (55 %), and fluids (55 %) and high in oxalate (55 %), sodium (39 %), purines (42 %), and refined sugar (41 %) [18]. In pediatric stone patients attending a public hospital in Karachi in 2002, the diet was low in proteins (in 44 %), calcium (in 33 %), and potassium (in 77 %) and high in oxalates in 55 % [69]. The Pakistan Government National Nutrition Survey 2001–2002 reports "an alarming micronutrient deficiency" [93]. However, UNICEF suggests that vitamin A supplementation covered 87 % of the (pediatric) population in 2010.

A diet of unleavened whole wheat bread (which contains phytate, albeit in reduced amounts) is a possible cause of low urinary calcium excretion rates across Pakistan and decreased magnesium absorption. Additionally, milk intake is poor in the mountainous regions of Pakistan—44 to 60 mL/day.

People living in the Thar desert areas of Sindh have periodic bursts of income and achieve a tolerable diet only when they are employed as labor on neighboring area farms. Otherwise, they eat bread made of bajra (pearl millet) and chillies and whey. They cannot afford to drink milk from which the butter and ghee (clarified) butter are made, as they have to sell the ghee to earn a living. The poor near a river cannot eat the fish they catch; it has to be sold to make their living. Poverty, ignorance, and low contraceptive use lead to multiple pregnancies, and the mother's breast does not yield an adequate amount of milk for the *n*th child. The infant who gets little milk grows up deficient in calcium, phosphate, and protein. Vitamin D deficiency is rampant despite the bright sun, raising the question of whether this is caused by ultraviolet (UV) destruction of provitamin D into inert lumisterol [95] or a genetic defect.

Dawson states that calorie intake is improving [75], with an average annual increase of 0.90 % over four decades; a 1 % increase in per capita income increased the daily per capita calorie intake by 0.19 %. Yet food security appeared to be unachievable and remained an "unfulfilled dream" for about 42 million people in 2000/2001 [96].

Current food availability per capita now remains around 2,456 calories/day with 72.5 g protein/day (Pakistant economic report 2009–2010) [97]. The availability of milk, sugar, pulses, and cereals remains similar to 1999 and 2000. Vitamin A and D fortification is mandatory throughout the country but is ignored.

Dawson warned that individuals diversify diets on economic advancement as they substitute more expensive sources of calories for less expensive ones [75]. The part of our population that is becoming increasingly affluent is at risk for rapidly becoming obese as it emerges from a calorie-deficient nutrition. In one study, 18 % of 3,000 Karachi city suburban residents aged 35–70 years developed hyperuricemia [97] in a 5-year follow-up study.

Water intake is low across the country. It is low in relation to the sweating that occurs as farmers work on fields and low in the cities, where there are no public toilets, something that makes shopkeepers and shoppers alike restrict their water intake.

Population growth remains unchecked, and this pushes more people into towns in search of jobs and money. With the urban migration comes a change in diet. In 1951, only 17 % of the population was urban; in the 1990s, 34 % were living in urban areas. In 2010, the megapolis of Karachi contains 26 % of the urban population of Pakistan—10 % of the nation's total population. Overpopulated megacities produce their own marginalized poverty-ridden slums. The lucky citizens get minimum wages compatible with reasonable life, with cash for better diets, carbonated water, and higher protein intake. But there is also a chance for employment and medical insurance by the employer company.

Conclusion

The stones in Pakistan are mostly of calcium oxalate composition and are distributed across the country in irrigated, mountainous, and desert areas. The majority of stones are complex: Calcium phosphate is a minor component in most stones except in the south; pure calcium oxalate stones are more common in the north. Metabolic abnormalities are infrequently looked for and are uncommon when tested for. Pediatric stone disease is still common, as are vesical stones. Transitions in proportions of stones in the bladder, availability and accessibility of medical care, and transitions in diet and economy are being witnessed. Most hospitals still perform a large number of open operations, often by general surgeons, because of manpower and equipment shortages, but the use of URS, PCNL, and ESWL is increasing. Surprisingly, despite neglected stone disease, and significant renal failure as a presentation, the nephrectomy rate is low.

Acknowledgments The authors wish to gratefully acknowledge the assistance of Prof. Shafique ur Rehman and Dr. Noor Ahmed, for provision of data, and Ammara Khan and Mubashir Hussain for researching literature.

References

1. The World Bank. Pakistan's water economy. 2008. http://www.worldbank.org.pk/WBSITE/EXTERNAL/COUNTRIES/SOUTHASIAEXT/PAKISTANEXTN/0,contentMDK:21102841~

pagePK:141137~piPK:141127~theSitePK:293052,00.html. Last accessed 14 Feb 2012.
2. Tamburi AJ. Water management technical report No. 25, a bibliography and literature review of groundwater geology studies in the Indus River Basin. Colorado: Colorado State University, Development PUSoUSAfI. 1973. Report No.: AID/csd-2162 Water Management Research in Arid and Sub-Ilumid Lands of the Less Developed Countries. http://pdf.usaid.gov/pdf_docs/PNAAA335.pdf. Last accessed 9 Apr 2012.
3. Khan FK, editor. Oxford School atlas for Pakistan. 2nd ed. Karachi: Oxford University Press; 2008.
4. Hussain M, Rizvi SA, Askari H, Sultan G, Lal M, Ali B, Naqvi SA. Management of stone disease: 17 years experience of a stone clinic in a developing country. J Pak Med Assoc. 2009;59(12):843–6.
5. Blanchard RJW, Ahmed M. Hospital surgery in rural Pakistan. In: Ahmed M, Blanchard RJW, Elof B, Harrison T, Moazzam F, Suleman S, et al., editors. Surgery for all. Lahore: Ferozsons (Pvt.) Ltd; 1992. p. 49–59.
6. Blanchard RJ, Blanchard ME, Toussignant P, Ahmed M, Smythe CM. The epidemiology and spectrum of surgical care in district hospitals of Pakistan. Am J Public Health. 1987;77(11):1439–45.
7. Rasmussen A, Zaidi AKM. Review of existing data on the mortality and morbidity in Gilgit and Chitral Districts. Publication of a report by Aga Khan University, Karachi; 1988. p. 119.
8. Talati J. Genitourinary surgery in Pakistan. In: Ahmed M, Blanchard RJW, Elof B, Harrison T, Moazzam F, Suleman S, et al., editors. Surgery for All. Lahore: Ferozesons (Pvt.) Ltd; 1992. p. 351–82.
9. Pervez A. Urinary stone survey at Quetta division hospitals with reference to drinking water. Lahore: Punjab University; 1992.
10. McCarrison R. A lecture on the causation of stone in India. Br Med J. 1931;1(3675):1009–15.
11. Khan F. A history of calculous disease of the urinary tract. J Pak Med Assoc. 1973;23:19–24.
12. Joshi LB. Etiology of urinary calculi. Poona: Joshi LB; 1966.
13. Khan FA, Khan JH. Stone survey of the Punjab Hospitals. Pak Postgrad Med J. 1990;1:7–13.
14. Manzar S. Incidence of urolithiasis in Nawabshah, Pakistan. Pak J Surg. 1995;11(2):80–2.
15. Khan MN, Islam S, Afzal S, et al. Urolithiasis in children, a comparison of western and Pakistani data. Pak J Surg. 1991;7:57–60.
16. Walther PC, Lamm D, Kaplan GD. Pediatric urolithiasis, a ten year review. Pediatrics. 1980;65:1068–72.
17. Talati JKF, Drago H, Lall E, Khan MZ, Talati A, Noordzij J. Epidemiology of urolithiasis in Pakistan. In: Talati J, Sutton RAL, Moazam F, Ahmed M, editors. The management of lithiasis: the rational deployment of technology. Dordrecht/London: Kluwer Academics; 1997.
18. Rizvi SAH, Sultan S, Zafar MN, Ahmed B, Faiq SM, Hossain KZ, et al. Evaluation of children with urolithiasis. Indian J Urol. 2007;} 23(4):420–7.
19. Ahmad I, Khattak AH, Jan NA, Durrani SN. Urinary tract calculi: a four years' experience. J Postgrad Med Inst. 2006;20(2):121–5.
20. SIUT. Statistics from the Sindh INstitute of Urology and Transplantation. 2011 [updated 2011; cited]. Available from: http://www.siut.org/services/statistics. Last accessed 9 Apr 2012.
21. Hussain M, Lal M, Ali B, Naqvi SAA, Rizvi SAH. Urolithiasis in sindh: a single centre experience with a review of 10,000 cases. J Nephrol Urol Transplant. 1998;1:10–3.
22. Memon JM, Athar A, Akhund AA. Clinical pattern of urinary stone disease in our setting. Ann King Edward Med Univ. 2009; 15(1):17–20.
23. Chand H, Abbasi KA, Shaikh SA, Paras. Chemical composition of stone in stone passers in Larkana. Pak J Med Health Sci. 2011; 5(2):262–4.
24. Khanum A. A Study on the etiology of urolithiasis. PhD thesis, Karachi University, Karachi, 1981.
25. Hussain M, Rizvi SA, Askari H, Sultan G, Lal M, Ali B, et al. Management of stone disease: 17 years experience of a stone clinic in a developing country. J Pak Med Assoc. 2009;59(12):843–6.
26. Jan H, Akbar I, Kamran H, Khan J. Frequency of renal stone disease in patients with urinary tract infection. J Ayub Med Coll Abbottabad. 2008;20(1):60–2.
27. Rasool M. Urinary stones at Bahawalpur. Prof Med J. 2000;7(4): 529–34.
28. Qayyum A, Anwar MS, Farooq M, Farooq M, Manan A, Khan MS, Shah AA, et al. Calculus related acute renal failure; management strategies. ESCULAPIO – J Serv Inst Med Sci. 2005;1:22–5.
29. Amanullah, Khan G, Lal S, Soomro MI, Jalbani MH. Calculus anuria and its remedy. J Ayub Med Coll. 2010;22(1):112–4.
30. Hussain M, Lal M, Ali B, Ahmed S, Zafar N, Naqvi SA, et al. Management of urinary calculi associated with renal failure. J Pak Med Assoc. 1995;45(8):205–8.
31. Buchholz NP, Abbas F, Afzal M, Khan R, Rizvi I, Talati J. The prevalence of silent kidney stones–an ultrasonographic screening study. J Pak Med Assoc. 2003;53(1):24–5.
32. Rizvi SAH, Naqvi SA, Hussain Z, Shahjehan S. Renal stones in children in Pakistan. Br J Urol Int. 1985;57(6):618–21.
33. Romero V, Akpinar H, Assimos DG. Kidney stones: a global picture of prevalence, incidence, and associated risk factors. Rev Urol. 2010;12(2–3):e86–96.
34. Dirks J, Remuzzi G, Horton S, Schieppati A, Rizvi SAH. Diseases of the kidney and the urinary system. In: Jamison DT, Breman JG, Measham AR, Alleyne G, Claeson M, Evans DB, Jha P, Mills A, Musgrove P, editors. Disease control priorities in developing countries. 2nd edn. Disease control priorities project. Washington D.C.: The International Bank for Reconstruction and Development/The World Bank Group; 2006. p. 695–706.
35. Naqvi SAJ. Nephrology services in Pakistan. Nephrol Dial Transplant. 2000;15(6):769–71.
36. Rizvi SAH, Manzoor K. Causes of chronic renal failure in Pakistan: a single large center experience. Saudi J Kidney Dis Transpl. 2002;} 13(3):376–9.
37. Rizvi SAH, Naqvi SAA, Hussain Z, Hashmi A, Hussain M, Zafar MN, et al. Pediatric urolithiasis: developing nation perspectives. J Urol. 2002;168(4):1522–5.
38. Rahman A, Danish KF, Zafar A, Ahmad A, Chaudhry AR. Chemical composition of non-infected upper urinary tract calculi. Rawal Med J. 2008;33:54–5.
39. Moazam F, Nazir Z, Jafarey AM. Pediatric urolithiasis: to cut or not to cut. J Pediatr Surg. 1994;29(6):761–4.
40. Yaqin H. Urolithiasis in industrial workers. J Pak Med Assoc. 1975;25(10):274–8.
41. Bukhari SI. Mineral composition of renal stones and the effect of citrate on the urinary excretion of Calcium and Oxalate. Thesis, University of Balochistan, Quetta, Balochistan; 2004.
42. Rizvi SAH, Naqvi SA, Hussain Z, Hashmi A, Hussain M, Zafar MN, et al. Management of pediatric urolithiasis in Pakistan: experience with 1,440 children. J Urol. 2003;169(2):634–7.
43. Rashid M, Ahmed W, Gardezi SAR, et al. Composition and epidemiology of urolithiasis. Specialist. 1992;9:219–26.
44. Ather MH, Faruqui N, Abid F, Sulaiman MN. Is there a difference in early perioperative morbidity in transurethral resection of prostate (TURP) versus TURP with cystolitholapaxy and TURP with inguinal herniorrhaphy? Int Urol Nephrol. 2002;33(1):69–72.
45. Rizvi SA, Sultan S, Ijaz H, Mirza ZN, Ahmed B, Saulat S, et al. Open surgical management of pediatric urolithiasis: a developing country perspective. Indian J Urol. 2010;26(4):573–6.
46. Afzal M, Iqbal M, Ahmad H. Thermal analysis of renal stones. J Therm Anal Calorim. 1992;38(7):1671–82.
47. Channa NA, Ghangro AB, Soomro AM, Noorani L. Analysis of kidney stones by FTIR spectroscopy. Journal of LUMHS. 2007;6(2): 66–73.

48. Farooq M, Anwar CHM, Bukhari MA, Hameede A, Mansoor-ul-Haq H. Urinary calculi - biochemical profile of stones removed from urinary tract. Prof Med J. 2007;14(1):6–10.
49. Jahangir M. Correlation of chemical composition of urinary stones. Dissertation (F.C.P.S.), Lahore, 1981, p. 107–16.
50. Kanwal S, Ghani F, Siddiqui I, Habib A. Chemical composition of renal stone and its relationship with age, sex and weight of the renal stone evaluated from 1999 to 2006 at referral laboratory. Karachi: Aga Khan University Faculty Research Assembly. 2007.
51. Hashmi ZA, Bashir G, Nawaz HA. Composition of renal stones: calcium oxalate stones are more common in the North West of Pakistan. J Postgrad Med Inst. 1984;15(2):199–201.
52. Tassaduqe K, Ali M, Salam A, Kanwal L, Afroze N, Masood S, et al. Studies on the chemical composition and presentation of urinary stones in relation to sex and age among human population of Multan, Pakistan. J Med Sci. 1992;3(5):401–10.
53. Khalil NY, Nawaz H, Ahmed S. Urinary calculi: prevalence, types and distribution in urinary tract in Quetta valley and adjacent areas. Professionals. 1998;5(2):197–202.
54. Sial SHJ, Khan ILL, Iqbal S, et al. Chemical analysis of renal calculi from D.G. Khan. Professionals. 1995;2:89–93.
55. Khan JH, Nazir M, Manzoor M, Ahmad Z, Siddiqui I, Mehmood T, et al. Incidence of hyperuricemia in patients of renal calculi and their comparison with chemical analysis of renal stones. Annals of King Edward Medical University. 2010;16(1):27–30.
56. Rab F, Qazi FM, Ahmad R, Zahoorullah, Khan I, Akhtar T. A study of urolithiasis in the North West Frontier Province of Pakistan. J Pak Med Assoc. 1990;40(10):241–3.
57. Rafique M, Bhutta RA, Rauf A, Chaudhry IA. Chemical composition of upper urinary tract calculi in Multan. J Pak Med Assoc. 2000;50(5):145–8.
58. Rana MN, Khan FA. Chemical analysis of 128 stones from the urinary tract. Prog Med. 1976;176(5):45–9.
59. Zafar HM. Prevalence of type of renal stone in Multan Region. J Med Res. 1992;31:13–7.
60. Ishaq M, Laghari MB, Akhund IA, Sabir M. Urinary tract stone disease: serum and urinary calcium in stone formers and non stone formers. Prof Med J. 2011;18(2):243–5.
61. Khand FD, Ansari AF, Khand TU, Memon JM. Analysis of urinary calculi by infrared spectroscopy. J Chem Soc Pak. 1996;18(3):246–9.
62. Zafar MN, Hussain M, Mehdi H, et al. editors. Analysis of urinary calculi by infrared spectroscopy in a Pakistani population (abstract). In: First international symposium of the Institute of Urology and Transplantation, Karachi, 1994.
63. Channa NA, Ghangro A, Soomro AM, Noorani L. Analysis of kidney stones by FTIR spectroscopy. J LUMHS. 2007;6(2):66–73.
64. Shad MA, Ansari TM, Afzal U, Kausar S, Rafique M, Khan MI. Major constituents, free amino acids and metal levels in renal calculi from Multan region. On-line J Biol Sci. 2001;1(11):1063–5.
65. Chaudhri MA, Watling J, Khan FA. Spatial distribution of major and trace elements in bladder and kidney stones. J Radioan Nucl Chem. 2007;271(3):713–20.
66. Umer SA, Sultan S, Zafar MN, Hussain I, Ahmed B, Saulat S, et al. Composition of renal and bladder calculi in pediatric stone formers. J Pediatr Urol. 2009;5(1):S32.
67. Memon A, Talati J. Urolithiasis: composition, symptomology and pathology. In: Talati J, Sutton RAL, Moazam F, Ahmed M, editors. The management of lithiasis: the rational deployment of technology. Dordrecht/London: Kluwer Academics; 1997.
68. Rizvi AM. Bilateral renal stones. Dissertation College of Physicians and Surgeons of Pakistan, Karachi, Pakistan 1987.
69. Rizvi SAH, Naqvi SAA, Hussain Z, Hashmi A, Hussain M, Zafar MN, Sultan S, et al. Pediatric urolithiasis: developing nation perspectives. J Urol. 2002;168(4):1522–5.
70. Zafar MH, Khan MI, Malik NM, et al. Prevalence & type of renal stones in Multan region. Pak J Med Res. 1992;31:13–7.
71. Daudon M, Bounxouei B, Santa Cruz F, da Silva LS, Diouf B, Angwafoo FF, et al. Composition of renal stones currently observed in non-industrialized countries. Prog Urol. 2004;14(6):1151–61.
72. Shahjehan S, Rahman MA. Studies on the etiology of urolithiasis in Karachi. Am J Clin Nutr. 1971;24(1):32–7.
73. Manser WWT, Talati J, Syed AM, Qadeeruddin M, Shireen K, Atomic Absorption Spectrometric analysis if Magnesium and trace elements in urinary tract stones. In: Rao PN, Kavanagh JP, Tiselius HG. Urolithiasis: consensus and controversies. Published by PN Rao and JP Kavanaugh, Lithotriptor unit, South Manchester University Hospitals, Withington Hospital, Manchester M20 8LR, UK, Manchester; 1995.
74. Khand FD, Ansari AF, Khand TU, et al. Is hypocitraturia associated with phosphaturia a potential cause of calcium urolithiasis in first time stone formers? J Pak Med Assoc. 1994;44:179–81.
75. Dawson PJ. Nutrition in Pakistan: estimating the economic demand for calories. Pak J Nutr. 2002;1(1):64–6.
76. Khan JA, Parvaiz S, Shah H. The urinary excretion of calcium, oxalate, inorganic phosphate in normal and renal stone forming patients. Gomal J Med Sci. 2003;1(2):61–3.
77. Rajput AP, Arif A. Impact of drinking water and other causative factors for nephrolithiasis. Pakistan Journal of Medical and Health Sciences. 2007;1(1):37–41.
78. Ishaq M, Laghari MB, Akhund IA, Sabir M. Calcium: serum and urinary, in stone formers and non-stone formers. Prof Med J. 2010;17(4):698–701.
79. Mithani S, Zaidi Z. Comparison of 24 hours urinary citrate levels in urolithiasis patients and healthy controls. J Pak Med Assoc. 2005; 55(9):371–3.
80. Biyabani SR, Talati J. Bone and renal stone disease in patients operated for primary hyperparathyroidism in Pakistan: is the pattern of disease different from the west? J Pak Med Assoc. 1999;49(8): 194–8.
81. Sutton RAL, Talati J, editors. Metabolic and dietary risk factors for urolithiasis. Dordrecht/London: Kluwer Academics; 1997.
82. Talati J, Biyabani SR, Zafar F, Siddiqui J, Zehri A. The significance of correction of serum calcium during evaluation of stone etiology. In: Abstracts of the 2006 annual meeting of the Pakistan Association of Urological Surgeons Peshawar, Peshawar.
83. Maloney ME, Springhart WP, Ekeruo WO, Young MD, Enemchukwu CU, Preminger GM. Ethnic background has minimal impact on the etiology of nephrolithiasis. J Urol. 2005;173(6):2001–4.
84. Rajput AP, Arif A. Impact of drinking water and other causative factors for nephrolithiasis. Pak J Med Health Sci. 2007;1(1): 37–41.
85. Talati J, Siddique AA, Meer O. Urine citrate excretion in stone formers attending a University Hospital in Pakistan. In: 6th European urolithiasis symposium, Stockholm, 1995.
86. Khalil NY, Ahmad S, Khan M, Ali SA, Ali Q, Bukhari SI, et al. Population based data on urinary excretion of various metabolites in children of north western region of Pakistan. J Pak Med Assoc. 1998;48(8):241–2.
87. Tanwir F, Saboor A, Nawaz N. Soil salinity and the livelihood strategies of small farmers: a case study in Faisalabad district, Punjab, Pakistan. Int J Agr Biol. 2003;5(4):440–1.
88. UNICEF. 2010. http://www.unicef.org/infobycountry/pakistan_pakistan_statistics.html. Last accessed 29 Aug 2012.
89. Naqvi NH. Chapter on environment. In: Pakistan economic survey 2009–2010. p. 221–33. www.finance.gov.pk/survey_0910. Last accessed 9 Apr 2012.
90. Khattak MMAK, Khan A, Begum S, Javeria A, Qadir SS. Evaluation of nutritional status of recently hospitalized patients. Pak J Nutr. 2002;1(5):212–6.
91. Shah SM, Selwyn BJ, Luby S, MEchant A, Bano R. Prevalence and correlates of stunting among children in rural Pakistan. Pediatr Int. 2003;45(1):49–53.

92. Ministry of Health, Government of Pakistan. 2003. 2001–2002 national nutrition survey. http://202.83.164.27/wps/portal/Moh/!ut/p/c0/04_SB8K8xLLM9MSSzPy8xBz9CP0os3h_Nx9_SzcPIwP_MAsDA6MQL3NXtxBvIwNzA_2CbEdFAOW90ZM!/?WCM_GLOBAL_CONTEXT=/wps/wcm/connect/MohCL/ministry/home/sahomegeneral/sageneralleft/j_nutrition+program. Accessed 14 Feb 2012.
93. FAO. Nutrition country profile (Pakistan). 2010 [updated 2010; cited]. Available from: http://www.fao.org/ag/agn/nutrition/pak-e.stm. Last accessed 9 Apr 2012.
94. Havinga E, de Kock RJ, Rappoldt MP. The photochemical interconversions of provitamin D, lumisterol, previtamin D and tachysterol. Tetrahedron. 1960;11(4):276–84.
95. Mushtaq K, Gafoor A, Abeduallah. An examination of calorie demand relationship in Pakistan. Pak J Nutr. 2007;6(2):159–62.
96. http://www.economywatch.com/economic-report/pakistan.html. Accessed 14 Feb 2012.
97. Akram M, Asif HM, Usmanghani K, Akhtar N, Jabeen Q, Madni A, et al. Obesity and the risk of hyperuricemia in Gadap Town, Karachi. Afr J Biotechnol. 2011;10(6):996–8.
98. Rizvi SAH. Calculous disease, a survey of 400 patients. J Pak Med Assoc. 1975;25(10):268–74.

Epidemiology of Stone Disease in Northern India

4

Raguram Ganesamoni and Shrawan K. Singh

Abstract

Urinary stone disease is highly prevalent in North India, a part of the stone belt in Asia. Two distinct "stone belts" have been identified in the northwestern region (NW); stone disease is less common in the southern and eastern regions. Calcium oxalate (CaOx) comprises a greater proportion of stones than seen in Western studies. While struvite stones were common in older series from NW, CaOx remains the predominant stone now, even in staghorns. First-degree relatives of stone formers are at higher risk of developing urolithiasis and have significantly higher urinary calcium excretion as compared to the spouses of the stone formers. Urinary tract infection was found to be one of the principal risk factors of urinary stones in North India. Metabolic acidosis is present in up to 45.2 % of stone formers as compared with 10.8 % in non-stone formers. Only dietary calcium correlated significantly with serum and urine calcium in stone formers. Stone patients from North India were shown to have a significantly higher intake of dairy products such as curd and cheese as compared to non-stone cases. Lower concentrations of urinary magnesium, copper, and manganese were noted in stone formers. Zinc excretion was significantly higher in stone formers. A significantly higher urinary urate excretion has been shown among stone formers from Delhi and Rajasthan.

Keywords

Incidence • Urinary stones • Oxalates • Urates • Prevalence • Geographical variation • Stone composition • Urine composition • Staghorn stones • Calcium oxalate stones • Calcium phosphate stones • Infection stones • Uric acid stones • Cystine stones • Practice patterns • Pediatric stones • Age-related stone formation • Recurrence • Stone site

Introduction

Urinary stone disease is highly prevalent in North India, which forms a part of the stone belt in Asia. Although shock-wave lithotripsy and endourological management of stone disease have revolutionized stone management, these modalities have not altered the risk of stone recurrence. The study of distribution and determinants of stone disease can help us in finding new ways of prevention of stone formation and its recurrence. Epidemiological studies including molecular epidemiology help in identification of risk factors for stone disease, which in turn aids in a better understanding of the pathophysiological processes leading to stone formation and how the individual factors interact in the individual stone-forming patient. Since epidemiology of stone disease varies widely in different geographic regions, a careful study of each region is important to guide stone prevention strategies and future research pertinent to the region.

R. Ganesamoni, MS, MRCS, MCh (Urology)
S.K. Singh, MS, MCh (Urology) (✉)
Department of Urology, Postgraduate Institute of Medical Education and Research, Sector 12, Chandigarh, Chandigarh, 160012, India
e-mail: dr_raguramg@yahoo.co.in; shrawanksingh2002@yahoo.com

J.J. Talati et al. (eds.), *Urolithiasis*,
DOI 10.1007/978-1-4471-4387-1_4, © Springer-Verlag London 2012

Incidence and Prevalence

Stone disease has plagued mankind from time immemorial. Sushruta, hailed from Varanasi in North India, the pioneer in stone surgery, described vesicolithotomy about 2,800 years ago [1]. The prevalence of stone disease and the composition of stones vary widely across the world, highlighting the etiological role of different geographic and etiological factors. The overall probability of forming stones differs in various parts of the world and is estimated to 1–5 % in Asia, 5–9 % in Europe, and 13 % in North America [2]. In Asia, a stone-forming belt has been reported to stretch across Sudan, Saudi Arabia, the United Arab Emirates, the Islamic Republic of Iran, Pakistan, India, Myanmar, Thailand, Indonesia, and the Philippines [3]. In India, upper and lower urinary tract stones occur frequently, but the incidence shows wide regional variation [4]. The pattern of occurrence of stone disease in northern India with respect to age and sex is not different from that reported in other regions of the world. Stone disease is more common in males, young adults, and the middle aged. The incidence of endemic bladder calculi was high in children living in rural areas of India until 1980. However, this incidence has decreased in the last few years due to improved socioeconomic status leading to better nutrition and diet. There is a simultaneous increase in upper urinary tract stones [5]. In urban centers, nearly 99 % of stone removal is done endourologically. In rural and semi-urban areas, where still general surgeons treat majority of patients with stone disease, open surgery is still commonly performed.

Geography

The geographic distribution of stone disease tends to roughly follow environmental risk factors; a higher prevalence of stone disease is found in hot, arid, or dry climates such as the mountains, desert, or tropical areas [6]. In India, two distinct "stone belts" have been identified in the northwestern region. One stone belt starts from Amritsar in the North, passes through Delhi and Agra, and ends up in Uttar Pradesh. The other belt starts from Jamnagar in the West Coast and extends inward toward Jabalpur in Central India (Fig. 4.1). Stone disease is less common in the southern and eastern regions of India. Hot climate is considered to be one of the factors for the difference in this distribution [7]. The northwestern parts of India have extremes of temperature (temperature reaches up to 45 ° C or even more during summer), while the southern parts have a relatively uniform warm climate throughout the year. The relative inability of the body to adapt to these changes in weather of different seasons and the lack of drastic changes in fluid intake may play a role in causing the increased incidence of stone disease in northwestern parts of India.

Socioeconomic Status

The incidence of stone disease is more common in lower and middle socioeconomic strata, in particular in those subsisting on a monotonous diet. Endemic bladder stones, which were once common in low socioeconomic groups of eastern Uttar Pradesh and Bihar, probably due to malnutrition and vitamin A deficiency, have become very uncommon now. Low socioeconomic status is associated with lack of health awareness and delay in access to optimal health care. A significant number of patients in North India present with renal insufficiency (15 %) as compared to their counterparts in the West (1.7 %) [8]. Of the 222 million households in India, the absolutely poor households (annual incomes below $1,000) accounted for 15.6 % of them (about 35 million). About 48 % have annual income of more than $2,000. The average family size in India is 4.8 [9]. Though the incidence of stone disease has been found to be higher in lower socioeconomic strata, data regarding average income of stone formers are not available. The burden of healthcare costs frequently pushes people of lower socioeconomic status into further poverty especially if the earning male member of the family is affected.

Site of Occurrence

Similar to Western studies, a reducing trend for bladder calculi has been noted in North India, albeit a little later. The proportion of bladder calculi had significantly decreased from 30.5 % during 1965–1968 to 8.4 % during 1982–1986 [10]. In late 90s also, stones in the bladder have been reported from Satpura belt of Central India and Mumbai in the pediatric age group [11–13] (Fig. 4.2). The consumption of a protein-rich diet has shifted the stone occurrence from the lower to upper urinary tract [6].

Composition

As compared to Western studies where calcium oxalate accounts for 66–72 % of all stones, Indian studies reveal a higher percentage of this stone constituent. Ansari et al. [14] analyzed 1,050 stones (900 renal, 150 ureteric) and found that 977 (93 %) were composed of calcium oxalate, out of which 80 % were calcium oxalate monohydrate and 20 % were calcium oxalate dihydrate. Only a small percentage of the stones contained struvite (1.4 %), apatite (1.8 %), and uric acid (0.95 %). The remaining 2.76 % were mixed stones. A total of 89.9 % of staghorn stones were made of oxalates and only 4.0 % of struvite. This finding is also in contrast to Western studies where staghorn stones more often are composed of struvite. The predominance of

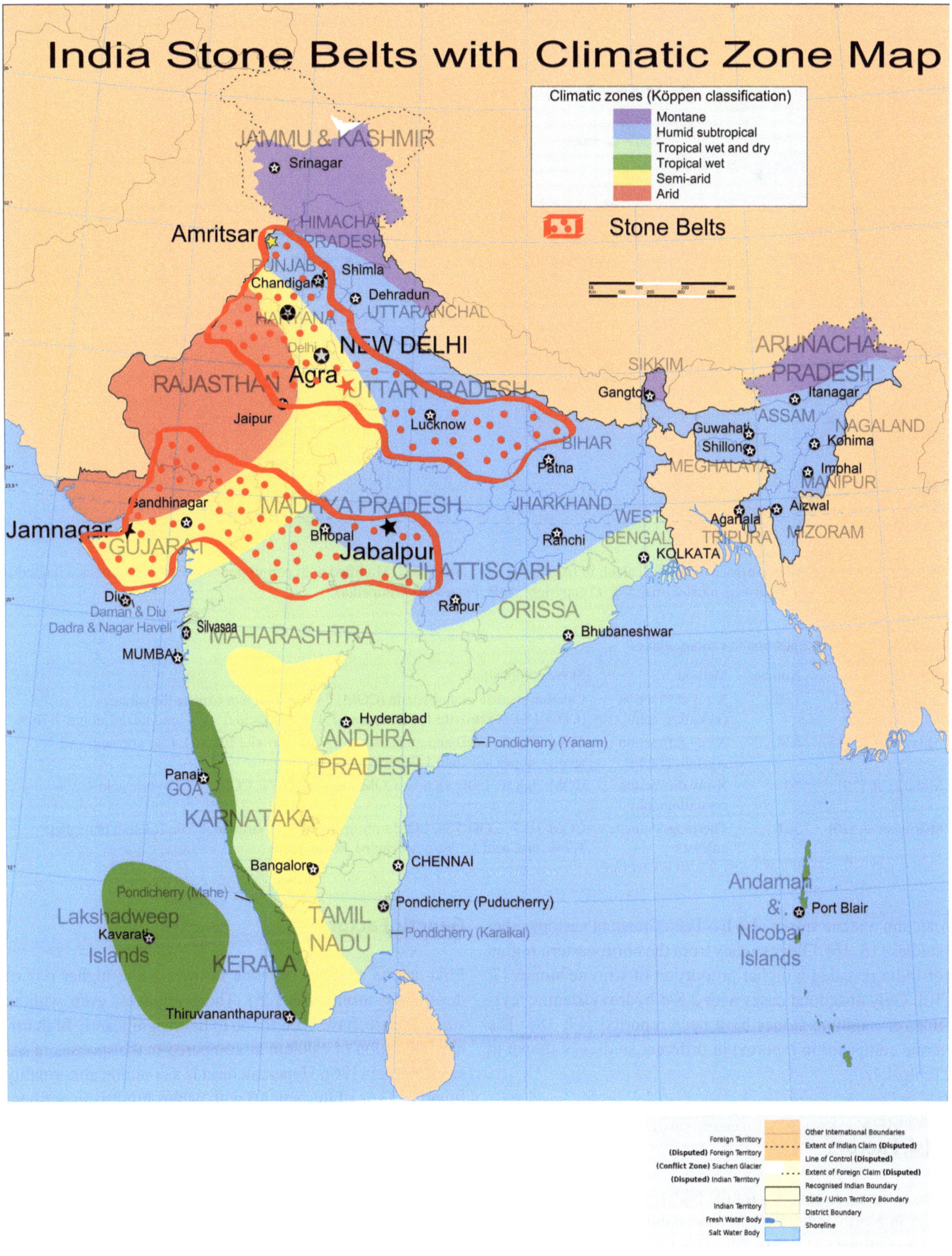

Fig. 4.1 The geographical distribution of the two stone belts in India (Modified with permission from http://commons.wikimedia.org/wiki/File:India_climatic_zone_map_en.svg, © copyright 2007, Saravask)

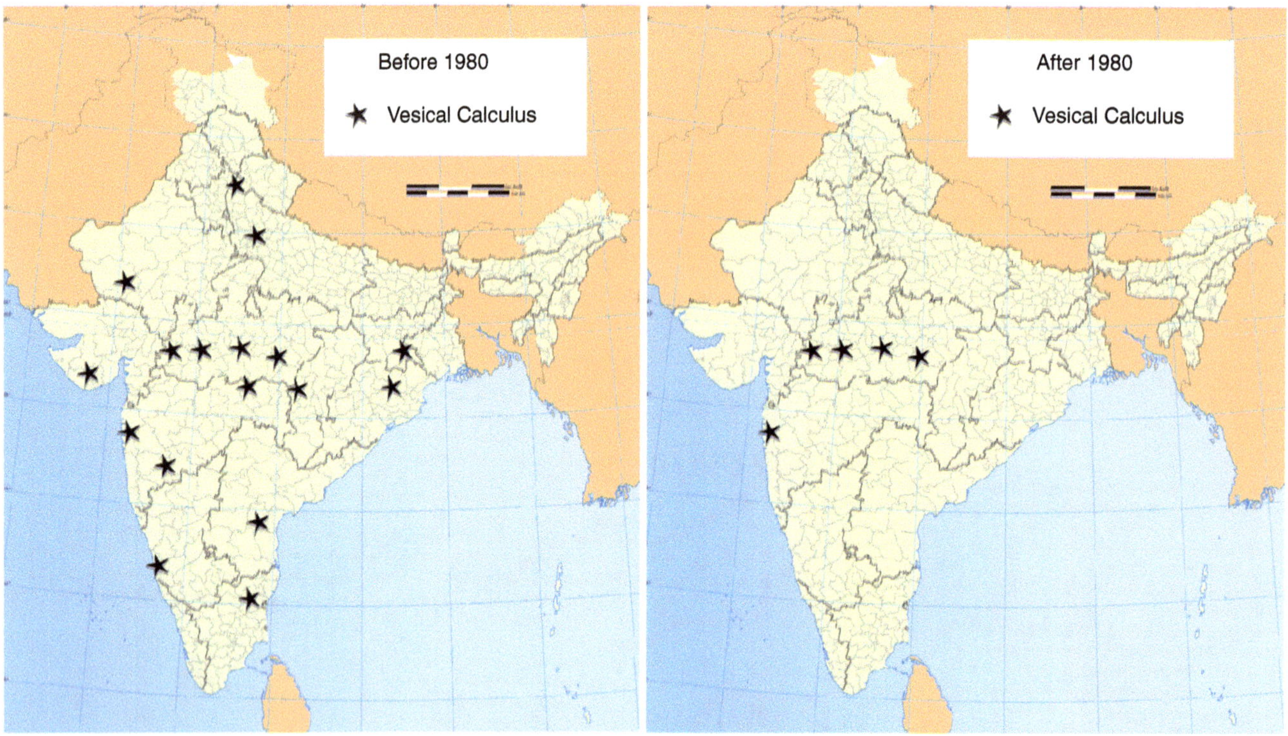

Fig. 4.2 The regions of occurrence of vesical calculi in India before and after 1980 (Modified with permission from http://commons.wikimedia.org/wiki/File:India_Lakshadweep_locator_map.svg. © copyright 2008, PlaneMad/Wikipedia)

Table 4.1 Stone composition in various studies

Author	Number	Method	Stone composition
Ansari et al. [14]	1,050	X-ray diffraction crystallography	Calcium oxalate monohydrate (COM) 74.4 %, calcium oxalate dihydrate (COD)18.6 %, struvite 1.4 %, apatite 1.8 %, uric acid 0.95 %, and mixed stones 2.76 %
Ahlawat et al. [15]	434	X-ray diffraction crystallography	COM 87.3 %, COD and mixed stones 9.7 %, struvite stones 1.4 %, uric acid and apatite stones less than 1 % each
Mittal et al. [19]	80	X-ray diffraction crystallography	COM 70.8 %, COD 18.6 %, COM+uric acid 6 %, COM+COD+uric acid 4.2 %
Sharma et al. [20]	501	Thermogravimetrc analysis	COM 81 %, COD 5 %, COM+phosphate 4.9 %, struvite 2.7 %, calcium phosphate 1.9 %, uric acid 1.2 %, other mixed stones 3.3 %

calcium oxalate stones also has been shown in various other studies [15, 16]. Older studies from the northwestern region of India revealed a higher proportion of struvite stones [7, 10]. Only anecdotal cases with 2,8-dihydroxyadenine, cystine, or xanthine stones have been reported [17, 18]. The stone composition reported in different studies is shown in Table 4.1.

Risk Factors

The various causes cited for the high prevalence of stone disease in North India include food habits, water quality, and the hot climate [11, 21]. The frequency of various urinary risk factors is shown in Table 4.2.

Genetic Factors

First-degree relatives of stone formers are at higher risk of developing urolithiasis [25]. These relatives, even without stone disease, have been found to have significantly high urinary excretion of calcium as compared to the spouses of the stone formers [26]. Hypercalciuria is a common abnormality found in 33 % of the patients with nephrolithiasis in northern India [25]. Intestinal hyper-absorption is predominantly seen in hypercalciuric subjects, and the only hormonal stimulus for the intestinal absorption of calcium is 1, 25 $(OH)_2$ vitamin D_3 and its receptor. The absorption of calcium is associated with vitamin D receptor (VDR) genotype [27]. In a study of VDR genotypes in the North Indian population, it was observed that both normocalciuric nephrolithiasis patients

Table 4.2 Frequency (%) of urinary metabolic abnormality in stone formers from India

	Teotia et al. [22]		Rai et al. [23]	Relan et al. [24]
Urinary risk factors	Male (*n*=5,500)	Female (*n*=3,300)	(*n*=100)	(*n*=150)
Hypercalciuria	26	27	31	38
Hyperoxaluria	29	29	25	–
Hyperuricosuria	18	15	18	15
Hypocitraturia	25	34	–	–
Hypomagnesuria	17	30	–	–
Hyperphosphaturia	30	15	–	–

and hypercalciuric nephrolithiasis patients who had the bb genotype with respect to Bsm I showed higher 24-h urinary calcium excretion than the homozygous BB patients [25].

Systemic Disorders

Diabetes and obesity are known risk factors for urolithiasis. Since the prevalence of these two risk factors is increasing in Indian population [28], urolithiasis may show an upsurge in the future.

Environmental Factors

North India has a hot climate with the Thar Desert located in Rajasthan. A higher incidence of urolithiasis has been demonstrated in tribal people working in a mining environment [29]. One study from the Delhi region of North India could not demonstrate any significant correlation between occupation and stone formation [30]. Lack of access to drinking water or bathroom facilities are real problems in many parts of North India. This may lead to lower fluid intake and a higher risk of stone formation.

Urinary Tract Infection

Urinary tract infection was found to be one of the principal risk factors of urinary stones in North India [7]. The prevalence of positive stone culture has been found to range from 33 to 47 % [30, 31]. Unusual microorganisms like *Ureaplasma urealyticum* have also been isolated from stones [31].

Nanobacteria

Nanobacterium is an extremely small nano-sized microorganism that has been isolated from human renal stones. In a study from Chandigarh, nanobacteria were isolated from 62 % of stones removed by open surgery. These bacteria were shown to be apatite forming. Nanobacteria have been shown to facilitate crystallization and biomineralization, and they thus may play a role in the pathophysiology of renal stone formation [32, 33]. Moynihan's statement that "a gallstone is a tombstone to the memory of the organism within it" probably holds true for renal stone as well [32].

Oxalobacter formigenes

Oxalobacter formigenes is an oxalate-degrading bacterium which has been demonstrated in 65 % of normal individuals and in 30 % of calcium oxalate stone formers from North India [34]. In patients with three or more than three stone episodes, these bacterial colonies were present only in 5.6 % of patients. Oxalate excretion was less in patients colonized with *O. formigenes* as compared to those with no colonization. Hyperoxaluria associated with deficient colonization with *O. formigenes* may be contributing to the risk of urolithiasis in this population.

Metabolic Acidosis

Metabolic acidosis is a risk factor for urolithiasis. It causes calcium mobilization from bone leading to hypercalciuria and decreases urinary excretion of citrate. The incidence of distal renal tubular acidosis defect detected by acid loading test was 22.2 % in a series of recurrent stone formers in North India [35]. The status of metabolic acidosis in idiopathic stone formers has also been studied. Sakthivel et al. found that the prevalence of metabolic acidosis was 45.2 % in stone formers as compared to 10.8 % in non-stone formers [36].

Dietary Factors

Some of the reasons for the high incidence of calcium oxalate stones in northwestern India might be as follows: (1) vegetarian diet (with high oxalate content); (2) high carbohydrate intake (especially rice), which provides an acidic milieu in urine favoring calcium oxalate stone formation; and (3) water quality, its mineral contents, and high fluoride levels [37–39].

In a study from Rajasthan, which has a hot environment, there was no influence of dietary intake of protein, carbohydrate, fat, fiber, calcium, and oxalic acid on urinary excretion of calcium, oxalate, urate, inorganic phosphorus, magnesium, and citrate [40]. But stone formers had higher urinary excretion of oxalate and calcium, lower excretion of citrate, and excreted more saturated urine. A difference in dietary habits does exist between the North and South Indian populations. Tartaric acid content of tamarind, which is used in cooking South Indian dishes such as *sambhar*, might play an inhibitory role against stone formation [41].

Protein

The amount of daily protein intake and the source of protein influence the type and site of stone formed. Endemic bladder calculi are common in regions where dietary protein is derived from plant sources [42]. It has been shown that stone formers from an urban area in India have a significantly higher intake of animal protein curd and cheese in comparison with non-stone-forming subjects [29]. The same study also revealed higher urinary urate excretion in those stone formers.

Calcium

In a study from Delhi, urine calcium correlated significantly to dietary intake of energy, protein, and fats (not carbohydrates) in stone formers only. Only dietary calcium correlated significantly with serum and urine calcium in stone formers. Thus, a dietary contribution of energy, protein, and fat to urinary calcium excretion in stone formers could be possible in this population [43]. Stone patients from North India were shown to have a significantly higher intake of dairy products such as curd and cheese as compared to non-stone cases [29].

Phosphate

In a study from North India, elevated urinary phosphate was shown to be the only factor that was significantly different when stone formers were compared with healthy controls [43]. That the elevated urine phosphate was not significantly correlated with any dietary intake probably indicates that that the metabolism of phosphate rather than its intake plays a role in stone formation [43].

Fluoride

In a study from Rajasthan, a chronic intake of fluoride has been shown to increase the risk of stone formation by a factor of 4.6 [39]. The prevalence of stone disease in endemic area was 750/100,000 as compared to 163/100,000 in non-endemic area for fluorosis. Fluoride is said to be a mild promoter of urinary stone formation by (1) increasing oxalate excretion in urine, by (2) excretion of insoluble calcium fluoride, and by (3) mildly increasing the oxidative burden [39]. The Rajasthani population has been shown to have a high excretion of oxalate, mainly due to defective nutrition [44]. Fluoride may indirectly increase oxaluria by enhancing the absorption of oxalate from the intestine due to low availability of calcium because part of the intestinal calcium is precipitated as calcium fluoride. Since fluoride also possesses the inherent property of being able to bind crystals strongly, which gives more hardness to bone [45], it has been postulated that formation of urinary stones will occur when the aforementioned conditions overwhelm the inhibitory forces present.

Magnesium

In a study from Rajasthan, though magnesium intake was normal in both normal subjects and stone formers, the mean excretion of magnesium was lower than normal in all the groups, suggesting its defective absorption in this population [16]. Lower concentration of urinary magnesium was found in stone formers from Chandigarh, suggesting its inhibitory role in urolithiasis [46].

Trace Elements

Serum levels of zinc, copper, and manganese have been reported to be similar among normal subjects and stone formers. Zinc excretion was significantly higher in stone formers. Copper and manganese excretions in stone formers were significantly lower than in normal subjects [47]. In another study, urinary concentrations of zinc and nickel were found to be significantly lower in stone formers. It suggests that these trace elements might inhibit the crystallization and crystal aggregation [46]. But it is not known whether the urinary excretion of these elements is influenced by dietary intake, environment, or body metabolism.

Drinking Water

In a large survey of 38,805 persons in Rajasthan with analysis of the total hardness of drinking water—Ca, Mg, Na, K, iP, SiO3, SO4, Cl, F, Cu, Zn, and Mn—no association was found between any of these constituents and stone disease [48].

Hyperuricosuria

A significantly higher urinary urate excretion has been shown among stone formers from the Delhi region of North India and Rajasthan [40, 49]. A significantly higher level of serum urate was found in stone patients as compared with non-stone cases, even though the values were within the normal range [49]. Children consuming wheat as a staple diet are at a greater risk of forming a stone because of the increased urine saturation and precipitation of urate [50].

Hypocitraturia

In a study from northwestern India, though urinary citrate excretion was not different between stone formers and normal controls, there was a significant circadian rhythm of urinary citrate excretion in the healthy males. That pattern was absent in stone-forming patients; the acrophase was located near noon in non-stone formers and near midnight in stone formers [13]. In another study of the same population, a significant hypocitraturia was demonstrated [40].

Glycosaminoglycans

Twenty-four hour urinary excretion of glycosaminoglycans (GAGs) was shown to be significantly lower in both male and female stone formers in North India. The 24-h urinary excretion of GAGs was not related to age or sex [51].

Conclusion

Epidemiologic studies of stone disease in North India, though limited in number, does show many important findings that are peculiar to this region. Calcium oxalate, mainly calcium oxalate monohydrate, is the major constituent of stones including staghorn calculi in North India. Fluoride content of water has been shown to be a significant risk factor in endemic regions. The role of nanobacteria and oxalobacter needs to be studied further.

References

1. Das S. Shusruta of India: pioneer in vesicolithotomy. Urology. 1984;23:317–9.
2. Robertson WG. Urinary calculi. In: Nordin BEC, Need AG, Morros HA, editors. Metabolic bone and stone disease. New York. Churchill Livingstone; 1993. p. 249–311.
3. Hussain M, Lal M, Ahmed S, Zafar N, Naqvi SA, Abid-ul-Hassan Rizvi S. Management of urinary calculi associated with renal failure. J Pak Med Assoc. 1995;45:205–8.
4. Colobawalla BN. Incidence of urolithiasis in India. ICMR Tech Rep Ser. 1971;8:42–51.
5. Gupta NP, Kumar A. Endemic bladder stones. In: Rao PN, Preminger GM, Kavanagh JP, editors. Urinary tract stone disease. London: Springer; 2011. p. 239–43. Chapter 20.
6. Abbagani S, Gundimeda SD, Varre S, Ponnala D, Mundluru HP. Kidney stone disease: etiology and evaluation. Int J Appl Pharm Technol. 2010;1:175–82.
7. Pendse AK, Singh PP. The etiology of urolithiasis in Udaipur (western part of India). Urol Res. 1986;14:59–62.
8. Gupta NP, Kochar GS, Wadhwa SN, Singh SM. Management of patients with renal and ureteric calculi presenting with chronic renal insufficiency. Br J Urol. 1985;57:130–2.
9. Data from National Council of Applied Economic Research 2009. www.ncaer.org. Accessed on May 20, 2011.
10. Thind SK, Sidhu H, Nath R, Malakandaiah GC, Vaidyanathan S. Chronological variation in chemical composition of urinary calculi between 1965–68 and 1982–86 in north western India. Trop Geogr Med. 1988;40:338–41.
11. Bakane BC, Nagtilak SB, Patil B. Urolithiasis: a tribal scenario. Indian J Pediatr. 1999;66:863–5.
12. Shah AM, Kalmunkar S, Punekar SV, Billimoria FR, Bapat SD, Deshmukh SS. Spectrum of pediatric urolithiasis in western India. Indian J Pediatr. 1991;58:543–9.
13. Teotia M, Krishna S, Teotia SP. Kidney and vesical stones in children. In: Teotia M, Teotia SP, editors. Nutritional and metabolic bone and stone disease an Asian perspective. New Delhi: CNS Publishers and Distributors; 2008. p. 795–807. Chapter 106.
14. Ansari MS, Gupta NP, Hemal AK, Dogra PN, Seth A, Aron M, et al. Spectrum of stone composition: structural analysis of 1050 upper urinary tract calculi from northern India. Int J Urol. 2005;12:12–6.
15. Ahlawat R, Goel MC, Elhence A. Upper urinary tract stone analysis using X-ray diffraction: results from a tertiary referral centre in northern India. Natl Med J India. 1996;9:10–2.
16. Singh PP, Pendse AK, Rathore V, Dashora PK. Urinary biochemical profile of patients with ureteric calculi in Jodhpur region (north west India). Urol Res. 1988;16:105–10.
17. Sreejith P, Narasimhan KL, Sakhuja V. 2, 8 Dihydroxyadenine urolithiasis: a case report and review of literature. Indian J Nephrol. 2009;19:34–6.
18. Narasimhan KL, Kaur B, Suri D, Mahajan JK. Diagnosis of renal stones with underlying metabolic abnormalities using FTIR spectroscopy. Indian J Pediatr. 2009;76:856.
19. Mittal RD, Kumar R, Mittal B, Prasad R, Bhandari M. Stone composition, metabolic profile and the presence of the gut-inhabiting bacterium *Oxalobacter formigenes* as risk factors for renal stone formation. Med Princ Pract. 2003;12:208–13.
20. Sharma RN, Shah I, Gupta S, Sharma P, Beigh AA. Thermogravimetric analysis of urinary stones. Br J Urol. 1989;64:564–6.
21. Aurora AL, Taneja OP, Gupta DN, Aurora AL, Taneja OP, Gupta DN. Bladder stone disease of childhood. I. An epidemiological study. Acta Paediatr Scand. 1970;59:177–84.
22. Teotia SPS, Teotia M. Environment studies of endemic fluorosis, goiter and stone and their epidemiological interrelationships. Major breakthrough in environmental research and its technical impact on safe drinking water supplies to villages. Technical Project Report. Government of India, Ministry of Environment and Forests; 1990. p. 1–91.
23. Rai RS, Mandal AK, Khullar M, Mehta V, Sharma SK, Singh SK. Hypercalciuria in calcium urolithiasis in northern India: its prevalence, phenotype and mode of inheritance. Bull PGI. 2002;36:102–6.
24. Relan V, Khullar M, Singh SK, Sharmac SK. Urinary risk factors in nephrolithiasis in northern India. Indian J Nephrol. 2004;14:37–40.
25. Relan V, Khullar M, Singh SK, Sharma SK. Association of vitamin d receptor genotypes with calcium excretion in nephrolithiatic subjects in northern India. Urol Res. 2004;32:236–40.
26. Kaul P, Sidhu H, Vaidyanathan S, Thind SK, Nath R. Study of urinary calcium excretion after oral calcium load in stone formers, their spouses and first-degree blood relatives. Urol Int. 1994;52:93–7.
27. Dawson-Hughes B, Harris SS, Finneran S. Calcium absorption on high and low calcium intakes in relation to vitamin D receptor genotype. J Clin Endocrinol Metab. 1995;80:3657.
28. Misra A, Singhal N, Khurana L. Obesity, the metabolic syndrome, and type 2 diabetes in developing countries: role of dietary fats and oils. J Am Coll Nutr. 2010;29(Suppl):289S–301.
29. Barjatiya MK, Singh PP. Zinc and phosphorite mining environment is conducive to urolithiasis. J Renal Sci. 1998;1:10.
30. Baishya RK, Mathew A, Dhawan DR, Desai MR. Renal stone culture: is it relevant? Indian J Pathol Microbiol. 2010;53:901–2.
31. Dewan B, Sharma M, Nayak N, Sharma SK. Upper urinary tract stones & ureaplasma urealyticum. Indian J Med Res. 1997;105:15–21.

32. Khullar M, Sharma SK, Singh SK, Bajwa P, Sheikh FA, Relan V, et al. Morphological and immunological characteristics of nanobacteria from human renal stones of a north Indian population. Urol Res. 2004;32:190–5.
33. Shiekh FA, Khullar M, Singh SK. Lithogenesis: induction of renal calcifications by nanobacteria. Urol Res. 2006;34:53–7.
34. Kumar R, Mukherjee M, Bhandari M, Kumar A, Sidhu H, Mittal RD. Role of *Oxalobacter formigenes* in calcium oxalate stone disease: a study from North India. Eur Urol. 2002;41:318–22.
35. Singh PP, Pendse AK, Ahmed A, Ramavataram DV, Rajpurohit SK. A study of recurrent stone formers with special reference to renal tubular acidosis. Urol Res. 1995;23:201–3.
36. Saktivel MS, Singh SK, Rana SV, Mandal AK. Metabolic role of lactose intolerance in adult patients with renal stone disease in North India. Thesis, Postgraduate Institute of Medical Education and Research, Chandigarh, Dec 2010.
37. Massey LK. Dietary influences on urinary oxalate and risk of kidney stones. Front Biosci. 2003;8:584–94.
38. Masai MH, Ito H, Kotake T. Effect of dietary intake on urinary oxalate excretion in calcium renal stone formers. BJU Int. 1995; 76:692–6.
39. Singh PP, Barjatiya MK, Dhing S, Bhatnagar R, Kothari S, Dhar V. Evidence suggesting that high intake of fluoride provokes nephrolithiasis in tribal populations. Urol Res. 2001;29:238–44.
40. Rajkiran Pendse AK, Ghosh R, Ramavataram DV, Singh PP. Nutrition and urinary calcium stone formation in northwestern India: a case control study. Urol Res. 1996;24:141–7.
41. Singh PP, Hada P, Narula IM, Gupta SK. In vivo effect of tamarind (*Tamarindus indicus* L.) on urolith inhibitory activity in urine. Indian J Exp Biol. 1987;25:863–5.
42. Teotia M, Teotia SP. Endemic vesical stone: nutritional factors. Indian Pediatr. 1987;24:1117–21.
43. Berkemeyer S, Bhargava A, Bhargava U. Urinary phosphorus rather than urinary calcium possibly increases renal stone formation in a sample of Asian Indian, male stone-formers. Br J Nutr. 2007;98: 1224–8.
44. Singh PP, Srivastava DK. Urolithiasis: unbridled furry of oxalate in urinary conduct. Indian J Clin Biochem. 1992;7:75.
45. Burtis CA, Ashwood ER, Teitz NW, editors. Book of clinical chemistry. Philadelphia: Saunders; 1998. p. 1049.
46. Sharma SK, Singh SK, Mandal AK. Study of magnesium and trace elements in renal stones. Br J Urol. 1997;80(suppl):324.
47. Komleh K, Hada P, Pendse AK, Singh PP. Zinc, copper and manganese in serum, urine and stones. Int Urol Nephrol. 1990;22:113–8.
48. Singh PP, Kiran R. Are we overstressing water quality in urinary stone disease? Int Urol Nephrol. 1993;25:29–36.
49. Sinha T, Karan SC, Kotwal A. Increased urinary uric acid excretion: a finding in Indian stone formers. Urol Res. 2010;38:17–20.
50. Wangoo D, Thind SK, Gupta GS, Nath R. Chronobiology of urinary citrate excretion amongst stone-formers and healthy males from north western India. Urol Res. 1991;19:203–6.
51. Sidhu H, Hemal AK, Thind SK, Nath R, Vaidyanathan S. Comparative study of 24-hour urinary excretion of glycosaminoglycans by renal stone formers and healthy adults. Eur Urol. 1989;16:45–7.

Epidemiology of Stone Disease in Kerala, South India

5

Y.M. Fazil Marickar

Abstract

The documented incidence of stone disease in India has been increasing over the years. The stone prevalence rate in Kerala was 2,643 per 100,000 adult inhabitants older than 14 years. The pattern of treatment for stone disease has varied widely over the years. Open surgery was the prime retrieval modality; however, percutaneous nephrolithotomy (PNL) and ureteroscopy (URS) are being increasingly used recently. The majority of stones retrieved were calcium oxalate followed by uric acid. Hyperoxaluria was the most common metabolic abnormality followed by hyperuricemia. Only 0.032 % of patients had specific medical diseases or anatomical defects responsible for stone formation.

Keywords

Urolithiasis • Hyperoxaluria prevalence • Stone retrieval methods • Stone analysis Metabolic abnormalities incidence • Urinary stones • Oxalates • Urates • Prevalence • Geographical variation • Stone composition • Urine composition • Staghorn stones • Calcium oxalate stones • Calcium phosphate stones • Infection stones • Uric acid stones • Cystine stones Practice patterns • Pediatric stones • Age-related stone formation • Recurrence • Stone site

Introduction

There are many problems that complicate the accurate interpretation of epidemiological data regarding urinary stone disease. In a span of 40 years, the epidemiological picture of stone disease has apparently drastically changed [1–7]. In Kerala state, situated at the southern tip of the Indian peninsula (Fig. 5.1), the pattern has changed significantly. The reported incidence of stone disease has increased. This development has been most evident in the pediatric population. The emigration of Keralites to the Gulf countries during these four decades has been accompanied by an associated increase in the number of stone patients [8]. Hospital practice has also seen a change. In the 1970s, there was only one center, the Medical College Hospital at Trivandrum, where there was a urinary stone clinic. In the 1980s, there was a sudden spurt of commissioning of private hospitals across the state. The 1990s saw the emergence of endoscopic procedures and mushrooming of private medical centers all over Kerala with facilities for advanced stone retrieval. Shockwave lithotripsy (SWL), which appeared with a big bang in the state, petered out as a failing procedure due to the high level of residual fragments.

Epidemeology

The population of Kerala on April 14, 2011 was approximately 31,826,053 (extrapolated from a population of 31,948,619 in 2001 and a population of 31,841,374 on February 10, 2010). The prevalence of stone disease (life- time risk) in a population-based study was 26,430 per

Y.M.F. Marickar, MS, MAMS, Ph.D. (Urology), FAMS, FIMSA, DAS, FEMSI
Department of Surgery, Azeezia Medical College, Kollam, Kerala, India
e-mail: fazilmarickar@gmail.com

J.J. Talati et al. (eds.), *Urolithiasis*,
DOI 10.1007/978-1-4471-4387-1_5, © Springer-Verlag London 2012

Fig. 5.1 Map of *Kerala*, India

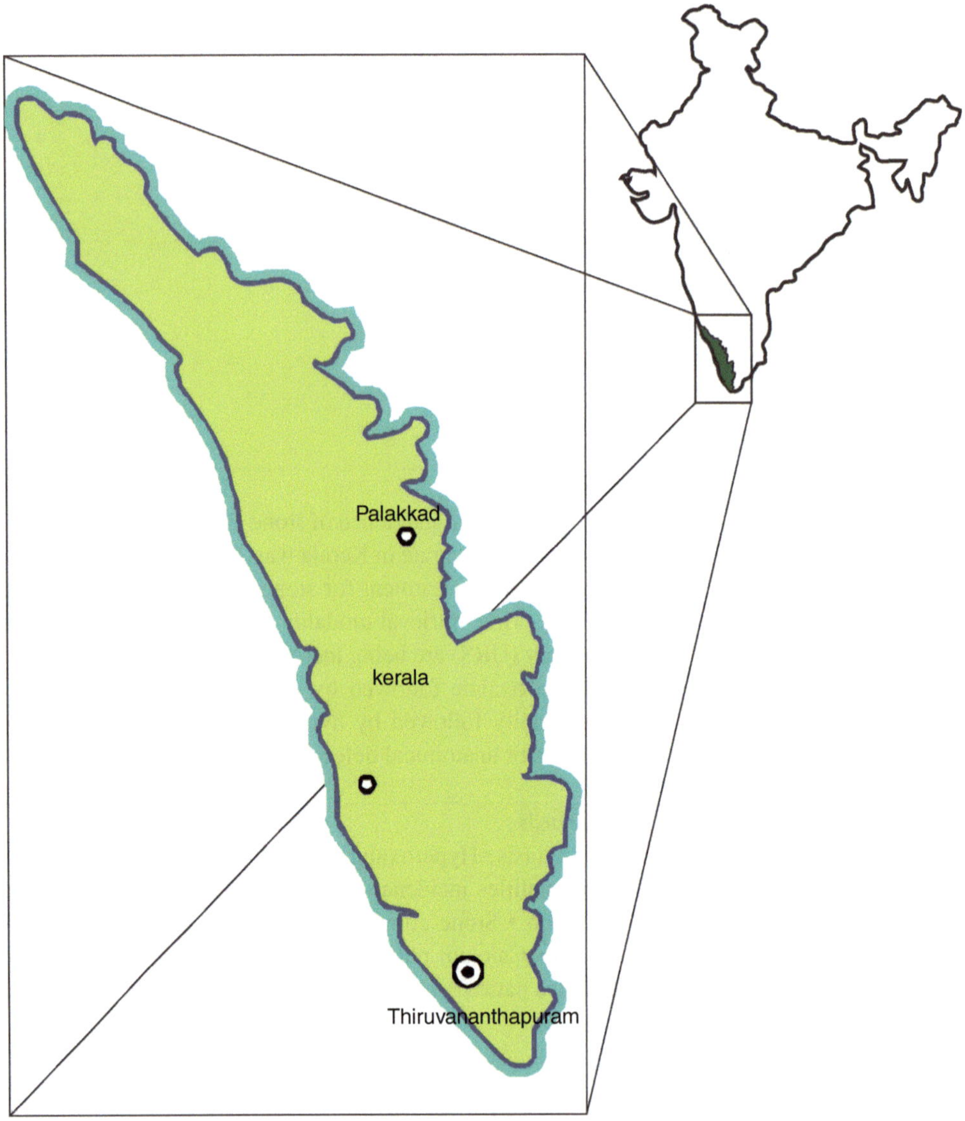

1,000,000 inhabitants above 14 years (32,564 per million males and 15,345 per million females). The incidence of stone disease could be calculated based on the local Medical College Hospital records [9–15]. This incidence ranged from 20.34 per 10,000 hospital admissions in the 1960s to 28.48 per 10,000 hospital admissions in the 2000s. This increase in incidence may not be the whole truth since the advanced equipment available in the corporate hospitals might have attracted many patients because of the available less invasive procedures of SWL and endoscopy. The presentation of patients in the urinary stone clinic conducted by the author (1970–2003 in the Government Medical College and later on in the private sector) would show a general representation of the actual situation because many patients attended the stone clinic even after stone retrieving procedures in other hospitals. The annual number of patients (per million) subjected to active stone removal could be extrapolated from the figures of those attending the stone clinics, to 6,878. The stone retrieval carried out in the stone clinic might have been greater than that in the actual population since there was a pooling of patients also from the surrounding areas. Many patients who had stones removed in other centers came to the stone clinic for metabolic assessment and prophylactic advice.

Stone Retrieval

Approximate distribution (%) of methods for active stone removal for 786 patients undergoing 983 procedures in the last 10 years, as gauged from the author's stone clinic records, is detailed in Table 5.1. This represents surgery performed in multiple centers and is obtained from the records in the stone clinic.

Over the decade 2000–2010, there is a gradual difference in the proportion of patients treated by open surgery

Table 5.1 Procedures for stone removal used on 786 stone patients undergoing 983 procedures

Procedure	Number	Percentage
Open surgery	567	57.7
PNL	178	18.1
URS	184	18.7
RIRS	Nil	0
SWL	54	5.5
Total	*983*	*100*

and less invasive methods because of progressive improvement in availability of instrumentation in both government institutions and private institutions [16]. In a Government Medical College, the open surgical procedures were more common in the earlier part of the decade. The common use of medical expulsion therapy might also reduce the need for ureteroscopy (URS). This is seen in many of the author's patients who pass their ureteric stones following appropriate medical treatment. However, the number of patients reported in the table includes those patients who had URS performed elsewhere and who later were referred to the stone clinic for metabolic assessment and prophylaxis.

Stone Composition

Various methods were utilized for assessing stone composition [17–20]. The information on stone composition presented in Table 5.2 is based on the Fourier transform infrared (FTIR) analysis performed on 700 stone samples.

Metabolic Assessment

One aspect of the study of urinary stones, which has been neglected, is the metabolic assessment. The presence or absence of metabolic investigations has not been directly correlated with the recording of clinical symptoms or radiological growth of stones [21–33]. A total assessment of the patient is necessary for the decision making regarding recurrence prevention. This aspect has remained silent over the years. The advent of citrate therapy in the 1990s produced a spurt in the prescription of different oral citrate preparations. This was done without assessment of urinary citrate levels. Empirical prescriptions led to ineffective prevention of stone formation.

The higher occurrence of stone disease in patients with diabetes mellitus was reported by the author in the 1990s. This fact has been recognized by many other authors later on. The incidence of diabetes in the population of Kerala has been increasing steadily during recent years. This brings to light the fact that lifestyle diseases may play a role in the increasing incidence of stone disease in this part of the world. The risk of lifestyle diseases is reported to be 43 % in Kerala and should be compared with the risk of 14 % in Andhra Pradesh and 25 % in Tamil Nadu, the other South Indian states. Grade I overweight people comprised 15 % of the population in Andhra Pradesh, 18 % in Tamil Nadu, and 22 % in Kerala. The overall prevalence of diabetes in Kerala is about 16.2–50 % higher than in the United States, according to the results of the study published in the *Indian Journal of Medical Research* [34]. It is thus believed that the higher incidence of stone disease in Kerala compared to the neighboring states of South India is linked to the higher socioeconomic status following better educational standards and the influence of Gulf money on the financial and social pattern of living of the Keralites [7].

Table 5.2 Results of Fourier transform infrared (FTIR) analysis of 700 stones calculated from a total of 1,048 different stone constituents

Type of stone	Number	Percentage[a]
Calcium oxalate (COM+COD)	578	55.2
Calcium oxalate+calcium phosphate	104	9.9
Calcium phosphate	34	3.2
Brushite (part of phosphate)	(15)	1.4
Infection stones	12	1.1
MAP+carbonate apatite	Nil	0
Ammonium urate	67	6.4
Uric acid[a]	235	22.4
Cystine	3	0.3
Others	Nil	

[a]Includes 125 pure uric acid stones and 110 mixed with other constituents

Data of metabolic studies carried out in 1,000 patients in the stone clinic during 2007–2010 were compiled to get the figures of urinary metabolic abnormalities; 934 patients had some sort of metabolic abnormality, 97 had a single metabolic abnormality, and 837 had multiple abnormalities. All patients who presented to the stone clinic with proved stone disease (including stones, colic, and crystalluria) were included. The frequency of 24-h urinary and blood metabolic abnormalities encountered in the patients is given in Table 5.3.

Other Causes Contributing to Stone Disease

Various metabolic conditions have been reported to be responsible for stone formation [35–41]. In this chapter, the metabolic conditions thought to have contributed to stone formation in a group of 1,000 patients are detailed below (Table 5.4).

Specific diseases included gout. Anatomical abnormalities included retrocaval ureter, horseshoe kidney, bifid pelvis with narrowing, adult polycystic kidney disease, prostatic enlargement, posterior urethral valve, and malrotated kidneys.

Table 5.3 Metabolic abnormalities in 1,000 patients

Metabolic abnormality	Number	Percentage
Hypercalciuria	113	5.8
Hyperoxaluria	756	39.1
Hypocitraturia	45	2.3
Hyperuricemia	189	9.8
Hypomagnesuria	67	3.5
Low urine pH (less than 5.3)	176	9.1
High urine pH (above 7.0)	32	1.7
Small urine volumes (less than 1,000 mL)	198	10.2
Hyperuricosuria	356	18.4
Total	1,932 abnormalities in 934 patients[a]	

[a]*Note*: 97 had a single metabolic abnormality, whereas 837 had multiple abnormalities

Table 5.4 Other factors that have contributed to stone formation

Sl. No.	Disease	Number	Percentage
1	Specific diseases	27	0.027
2	Pharmacological treatment	Nil	Nil
3	Anatomical abnormalities	5	0.005

Conclusion

The occurrence of stone diseases has been on the rise in Kerala. The high incidence appears to be the ability of Keralites to obtain employment in Gulf countries. Open surgery is being replaced by endoscopic stone retrieval procedures in recent times. The occurrence of metabolic abnormalities related to stone formation is very high in Kerala; the commonest abnormalities are hyperoxaluria and hyperuricosuria.

References

1. Marickar YMF, Joseph D, Abraham PA. Study of urinary stones in Kerala. Indian J Surg. 1976;38:480–4.
2. Marickar YMF, Joseph D, Abraham PA. Study of 192 patients with urinary stones in Kerala. Indian J Surg. 1977;39:144–50.
3. Marickar YMF. Epidemiological aspects of urolithiasis in India. In: Proceedings of the II national conference of the urolithiasis Society of India, Trivandrum, 1983, p. 8–10.
4. Rajendran R, Sachidev K, Thomas J, Marickar YMF. Changing trends in pediatric. Urol Res. 1988;16(3):204.
5. Abraham R, Marickar YMF. Computerised medical record maintenance in urolithiasis. In: Ravikumar R, editor. Proceedings of the 5th Kerala science congress. Trivandrum: SB Press; 1993. p. 259.
6. Jayadevan S, Marickar YMF, Pillai RN. Trend of urolithiasis in Kerala. Inpatient hospital data study. KSJ. 1999;6(1):p25.
7. Marickar YMF, Jayadevan S, Chandran A. Change in demography of stone disease over four decades. In: Gohel MDI, Doris WTAU, editors. Proceedings of the tenth international symposium on urolithiasis. Hong Kong: The Reprographic Unit; 2004. p. 391–3.
8. Roshni SV, Vathsala RK, Moorthy KH, Thomas NE, Aravindakshan C, Marickar YMF. Risk of urolithiasis in gulf returned keralites. In: Ryall RL et al., editors. Urolithiasis II. New York: Plenum Press; 1994. p. 479.
9. Jayadevan S, Marickar YMF, Pillai RN. Statistical survey on urinary stone disease. KSJ. 1998;5(1):31.
10. Jayadevan S, Marickar YMF, Pillai RN. Epidemiological and clinical factors in urolithiasis. KSJ. 1998;5(2):95.
11. Jayadevan S, Marickar YMF, Pillai RN. Incidence and prevalence of urolithiasis. In: Rodgers AL, Hibert BE, Hess B, Khan SR, Preminger GM, editors. Proceedings of the ninth international symposium on urolithiasis, vol. 1, Part 1. University of Cape Town, Cape Town, 2000, p. 392–4.
12. Jayadevan S, Marickar YMF, Pillai RN. Epidemiological and clinical factors in urolithiasis. J Nephrol Urol Transplant. 2001;2(3):90–3.
13. Jacob AT, Marickar YMF. Presentation of urinary stone diseases in Trivandrum. In: Das MR, editor. Proceedings of the fourteenth Kerala science congress. Kerala: St. Joseph Press; 2002. p. 668.
14. Chandran AS, Marickar YMF. Preetha. Hospital incidence and risk factors of urinary stone disease in Kerala – a statistical analysis. In: Valiathan MS, editor. Proceedings of the 15th Kerala science congress. Trivandrum: SB Press; 2003. p. 255–8.
15. Chandran A, Stephen J, Marickar YMF. Epidemiological and clinical factors of urolithiasis in Kerala – a three year study. Urol Res. 2004;33(2):140.
16. Nair N, Varma G, Salim A, Marickar YMF. Retrieval methods in urinary stone. Urol Res. 2008;36(3–4):189.
17. Das P, Marickar YMF. A study of mineral composition of urinary calculi by X-ray diffraction method. Indian J Med Res. 1975;63: 83–92.
18. Sindhu RS, Sapna GI, Marickar YMF. Stone analysis in the out Patient clinic. In: Iyengar PK, editor. Proceedings of the ninth Kerala science congress. Trivandrum: SB Press; 1977. p. 359–61.
19. Marickar YMF, Stephen J, Varma L. Fourier Transform Infrared Analysis (FTIR) vs. Optical microscopy in urinary stone analysis. In: Gohel MDI, Doris WTAU, editors. Proceedings of the tenth international symposium urolithiasis. Hong Kong: The Reprographic Unit; 2004. p. 39–40.
20. Marickar YMF. Does stone composition vary with demographic variables? Urol Res. 2004;33(2):138.
21. Bibilash BS, Vijay A, Marickr YMF. Are urinary stone analysis and metabolic status correlatable. In: Yesodharan EP, editor. Proceeding of the 20th Kerala science congress. Publisher KSCSTE, Thiruvanathapuram, 2008, p. 623–4.
22. Bibilash D, Vijay A, Marickar YMF. Stone composition and metabolic status. Urol Res. 2008;36(3–4):208.
23. Marickar YMF, Salim A, Nair N, Varma G. Investigations for recognizing urinary stone diseases. Urol Res. 2008;36(3–4):185.
24. Marickar YMF, Hyacinth P, Rajamohanan K, Moorthy KH. Citric acid levels in urinary stone patients. In: Proceedings of the II national conference of the urolithiasis society of India, Trivandrum, 1983, p. 102.
25. Hyacinth P, Rajamohanan K, Moorthy KH, Marickar YMF. A study of urolithiasis from 200 patients and 125 urinary stones from Trivandrum area. Arogya. 1984;10:113–7.
26. Marickar YMF, Sachidev K, Rajamohan K, Paul H, Abraham PA. Urine and blood biochemistry – stone patients vs controls in India. Abstracts of the 6th international symposium on urolithiasis and related clinical research, Vancouver, Canada July 24–28. Urol Res. 1988;16(3):180.
27. Thomas NE, Moorthy KH, Roshni SV, Sylaja N, Aravindakshan C, Marickar YMF. Uric acid metabolism in calcium oxalate stone disease. In: Ryall RL et al., editors. Urolithiasis II. New York: Plenum Press; 1994. p. 83.
28. Sindhu S, Vathsala RK, George A, Sachidev K, Marickar YMF. Do stone formers lack inhibitors in urine? Urol Res. 1988;16(3):233.
29. Marickar YMF, Sachidev K, Rajamohanan K, Paul H, Abraham PA. Urine and blood biochemistry - in stone patients and normal

subjects in India. In: Walker VR, Sutton RAL, Cameron EC, Pak CYC, Robertson WG, editors. Urolithiasis. New York: Plenum Press; 1989. p. 721–2.
30. Thomas NE, Moorthy KH, Roshni SV, Sindhu S, Vathsala RK, Sylaja N, et al. Metabolic profile of urinary stone patients in Kerala. In: Proceedings of the VI national conference of the urolithiasis Society of India, Trivandrum 1983.
31. Roshni SV, Moorthy KH, Thomas NE, Sindhu S, Vathsala RK, Sylaja N, et al. Metabolic changes in gulf returned patients. In: Proceedings of the VI national conference of the urolithiasis Society of India, Trivandrum 1983.
32. Abraham A, Ilango S, Sindhu RS, Marickar YMF. Which biochemical parameter is important in which type of stone? In: Das MR, editor. Proceedings of the twelfth Kerala science congress. Thiruvananthapuram: Audio Visual and Reprographic Centre; 1999. p. 327.
33. Marickar YMF, Salim A, Nair N, Varma G. Investigations for recognizing urinary stone diseases. Urol Res. 2009;37(6):349–56.
34. Thankappan KR. Lifestyle diseases the price of Kerala's prosperity. Mail Today, New Delhi, Thursday, February 25, 2010.
35. Rajamohanan K, Hyacinth P, Marickar YMF, Joseph D, Abraham PA. Anatomical anomalies in relation to urinary stone formation. In: Proceedings of the II national conference of the urolithiasis Society of India, Trivandrum, 1983, p. 46–7.
36. Marickar YMF, Moorthy KH, Roshni SV, Thomas NE, Sindhu S, Vathsala RK, et al. Diabetes mellitus - a predisposer to urinary stone disease. In: Proceedings of the VI national conference of the urolithiasis Society of India, Meerut, 1991.
37. Vathsala RK, Moorthy KH, Dhanalekshmy TG, Roshni SV, Aravindakshan C, Marickar YMF. Urolithiasis in diabetes mellitus. In: Ryall RL et al., editors. Urolithiasis II. New York: Plenum Press; 1994. p. 411.
38. Marickar YMF, Thomas NE, Roshni SV, Moorthy KH, Aravindakshan C. Renal tubular acidosis in urinary stone disease. In: Ryall RL et al., editors. Urolithiasis II. New York: Plenum Press; 1994. p. 93.
39. Marickar YMF, Stephen J. Genetic predisposition in urolithiasis. In: Gohel MDI, Doris WTAU, editors. Proceedings of the tenth international symposium on urolithiasis. Hong Kong: The Reprographic Unit; 2004. p. 407–8.
40. Marickar YMF. Cystinuria – the Kerala experience. Urol Res. 2008;36(3–4):219.
41. Marickar YMF. Calcium oxalate stone and gout. Urol Res. 2009;37(6):345–7.

Epidemiology of Stone Disease in China

6

Deyi Luo, Hong Li, and Kunjie Wang

Abstract

Urolithiasis, one of the most common diseases in the genitourinary system, was described as a terrible affliction 7,000 years ago. As modernization and Westernization progress in China, the site, age, gender, geographical, and occupational features of stone formation are gradually changing. In recent years, the overall incidence and prevalence of urinary tract stones in China have increased year by year, with a concomitant sharp reduction in patients with lower urinary tract stones and an increase in patients with upper urinary tract calculi. The prevalence of urinary tract stones is between 1 and 5 %, and the annual new incidence rate is between 1.5 and 2.0/100,000. Clear regional differences are noted in the distribution of urolithiasis in China. The peak onset age lies between 21 and 50, with 67.7–89.6 % patients in that age group. The male-to-female ratio lies between 1:3 and 4:1 in China. The morbidity of urolithiasis is different among the 56 nationalities in China. In recent decades, the composition of urinary stones has changed significantly in China.

Keywords

Epidemiology • China • Urolithiasis • Melamine • Incidence • Urinary stones • Oxalates Urates • Prevalence • Geographical variation • Stone composition • Urine composition Staghorn stones • Calcium oxalate stones • Calcium phosphate stones • Infection stones Uric acid stones • Cystine stones • Practice patterns • Pediatric stones • Age-related stone formation • Recurrence • Stone site

Introduction

Urolithiasis, one of the most common diseases in the genitourinary system, was described as a terrible affliction 7,000 years ago, but it remains a major problem in modern medical science. A gradual increase has been witnessed in the incidence and morbidity of stone disease, to which young people who have their first episodes in their 20s and 30s contribute with a high proportion. Additionally, the site of stone formation has migrated from the lower to the upper urinary tract. A wide spectrum of risk factors—including age, gender, geography, genetics, dietary habits, occupation, and medication—have been recognized, making the pathogenesis of this disease complicated. Therefore, the importance of epidemiological studies of urolithiasis can never be underestimated. Our chapter is focused on the epidemiological characteristics of urolithiasis in China.

Distribution of Urolithiasis in China

Geographical Distribution

There are marked regional differences in the distribution of urolithiasis in China [1]. In general, the incidence of urinary calculi in the South is higher than in the North. From as far back as the 1970s, the statistics regarding the incidence of

D. Luo, M.D. • H. Li, M.D. • K. Wang, M.D., Ph.D. (✉)
Department of Urology, West China Hospital, Sichuan University,
37# Guoxuexiang Street, Chengdu, Sichuan Province 610041, China
e-mail: wangkunjie@gmail.com

J.J. Talati et al. (eds.), *Urolithiasis*,
DOI 10.1007/978-1-4471-4387-1_6, © Springer-Verlag London 2012

urinary calculi showed that the distribution of patients with urinary stones is extremely inhomogeneous in China. Information from large-scale epidemiological data on stone disease is generally lacking. Most of the data on incidence rate is extrapolated from either cross-sectional surveys or from the rate of admissions to area hospitals.

An idea of the incidence can be gauged from the proportion of inpatients with urolithiasis compared to all admissions in urology during the same period. Generally, urolithiasis cases account for less than 14 % North of the Yellow River and about 22–45 % south of the Yangtze River (Fig. 6.1). Heilong Jiang (Fig. 6.2) has the lowest proportion of admissions for urolithiasis, with 2.5 %, while Guizhou has the highest, with 59 %. For the southern provinces—including Jiangxi, Guizhou, Guangxi, Guangdong, Hainan—the incidence of stones is very high [1–7]. In the northern provinces—including Heilong Jiang, Inner Mongolia, Shanxi, Ningxia, Gansu, Qinghai—the incidence of urinary calculi is very low. In 13 provinces of the North, the proportion of patients with urolithiasis (in terms of urological inpatients) during the same period of time was less than 15 %. In eight of these provinces, the incidence was less than 11 %. In 16 provinces of the South, the proportion of patients with urolithiasis was higher than 11 %, especially in six provinces where it was more than 30 %. The incidence of urinary calculi in plain areas is 22.7/100,000.

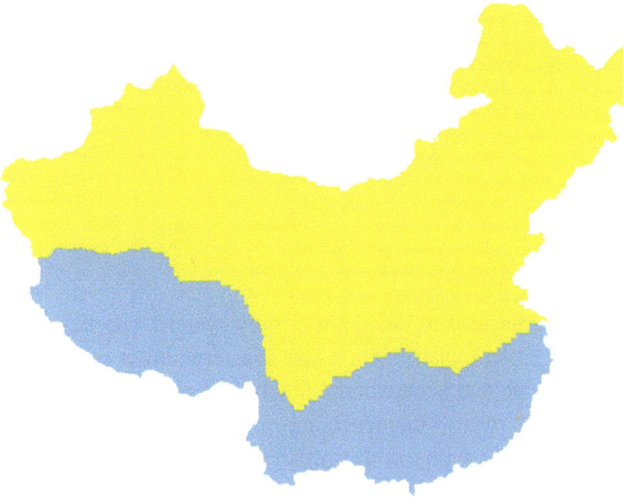

Fig. 6.1 North and south divisions created by the Yangtze river in China

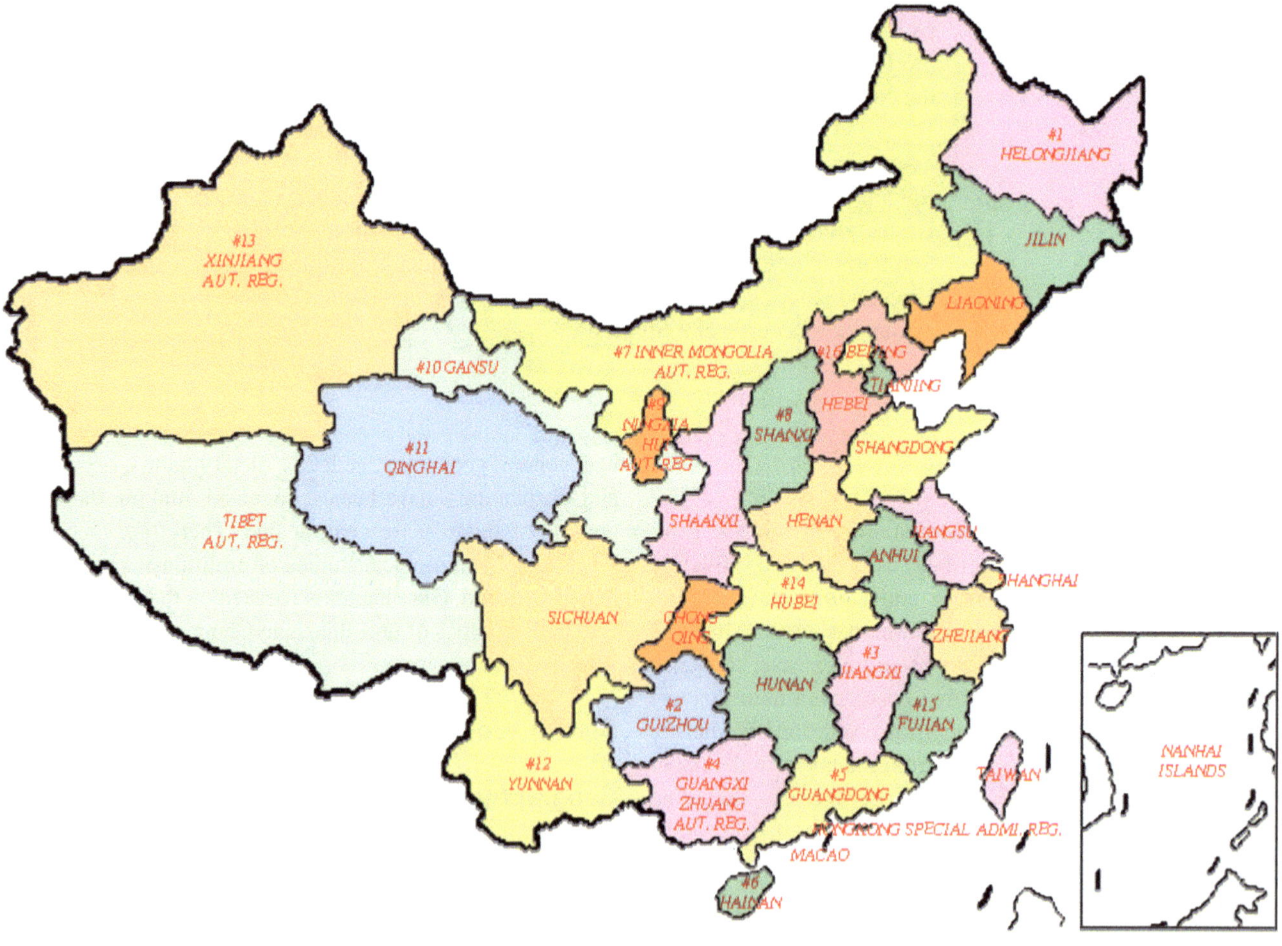

Fig. 6.2 Map of China

The frequency of distribution of urinary stone cases is extremely unbalanced even in high incidence areas. As in Guizhou province, the high incidence areas are mainly distributed in the West to the southeast, while the northeast and southwest have relatively low incidences.

The significant differences in the incidence of urinary calculi between South and North have raised questions as to whether climate conditions and diet play a role for the higher incidence in the South. It is reasonable to hypothesize that the geographical location in the tropical and subtropical regions subjects individuals to climatic conditions of drought. High temperature causes excessive evaporation of water and highly concentrated urine. The increased supersaturation levels of stone salts promote precipitation of crystals and stone formation. In addition, the many hours of sunshine in tropical areas promote synthesis of vitamin D in the body, with an increased urinary excretion of calcium, which is one of the factors that promote stone formation, though the role of vitamin D is far from clear. Additionally, the incidence of urinary calculi also varies seasonally with more patients presenting in the high temperature season.

Age Distribution

The peak onset age of urolithiasis in Chinese patients ranged between 21 and 50, in which group 67.7–89.6 % of all cases were observed [8–14]. According to statistical analysis, Li et al. [9] suggested that the onset of urolithiasis was most common in patients with an age between 31 and 46 years; the 21–30 and 46–50 age groups were in second place, contributing to 22.7–22.5 %, respectively. These three age groups made up 72.8 % of all stone patients. In terms of age distribution for the onset of stone disease, male patients had a single peak between 30 and 50 years, whereas female patients showed a Petronas distribution with peaks at 25–40 and 50–65 years. The prevalence of urolithiasis rises with increasing age, and the disease is most common in the age range of 41–50 years. Of all patients with urolithiasis, 69.9 % were between 31 and 60 years old. That was the peak age for humans suffering from urolithiasis. It may be related to energy consumption, in vivo environment, sex hormones, rapid metabolism, sweating, insufficient drinking, and other factors. Moreover, urolithiasis patients with ages between 50 and 70 years and between 20 and 30 were few, and those younger than 20 and older than 70 were rare. In recent decades, the age distribution of urolithiasis patients has changed significantly as a result of socioeconomic changes (Fig. 6.3a, b). The most important changes were that the prevalence rate of urolithiasis in middle-age persons gradually increased, while the rate in children decreased [15, 16]. In the 1950s, the prevalence of bladder stones in China was 43.8 % and related to malnutrition. By 1976, bladder stones in children were rarely seen in most provinces; the proportion was reduced to 13.2 % of all urinary calculi [1]. As the incidence of urinary stones is affected by diet and drinking habits, childhood exposure to food contaminated with lithogenic substances may result in stone formation. Pediatric stone incidence thus increased during the melamine contaminations of dairy and infant formulas, as well as other food products, in 2008 (see Chap. 26).

Gender Distribution

It is reported that men with urolithiasis are more common than women, with a ratio of 1.3 to 4:1 in China [2–17]. This may be caused by their different diet—men drink alcohol, strong tea, and eat more protein than women do. Also the anatomical differences of the lower urinary tract between genders may be one of the reasons. The incidence rate of idiopathic urolithiasis in men is about one to four times higher than that in women. The lower prevalence in women may be related to a higher urine citrate excretion in women, stimulated by estrogen [18]. Upper urinary tract calculi seem to be a little more common in men than in women. But, lower urinary tract stones are significantly more common in men than in women [9, 10, 13, 15]. Recently, the differences in stone disease between genders have gradually decreased. The prevalence ratio of urolithiasis between men and women in the Guizhou province was 4.6:1 in1977 and 2.8:1 in 1992 [16]. In Rongshui county of Guangxi province [19], the ratio was 7.87:1 in 1977, but decreased to 2.72:1 in 1986. A similar situation is reported in the Dongguan in Guangdong province and Gansu province. The incidence rate for urolithiasis in female patients shows a gradually upward trend [11, 15, 20].

Occupational Distribution

The development of stone disease differs between people with different occupations and social ranks. It is reported that the incidence rate of urolithiasis in farmers, fishermen, service personnel, organizers, and retired persons is relatively high with an average rate of 1.61 %. The incidence rate of urolithiasis in students and technical personnel is relatively low—the average rate is 0.99 %. These differences are, however, not statistically significant [6]. Besides, the morbidity of urolithiasis in people with some special vocations such as for traffic officers, soldiers, surgeons, pilots, and lead-exposed workers is obviously higher than that in a control group [21–23]. In a study by Atan, it was found that the stone disease incidence rate of workers exposed to high temperatures is nine times higher than that in workers exposed to normal temperatures; the metabolic consequences were a low citrate excretion in the urine and small urine volumes. Jiang Lan [24] reported that the incidence rate of urolithiasis

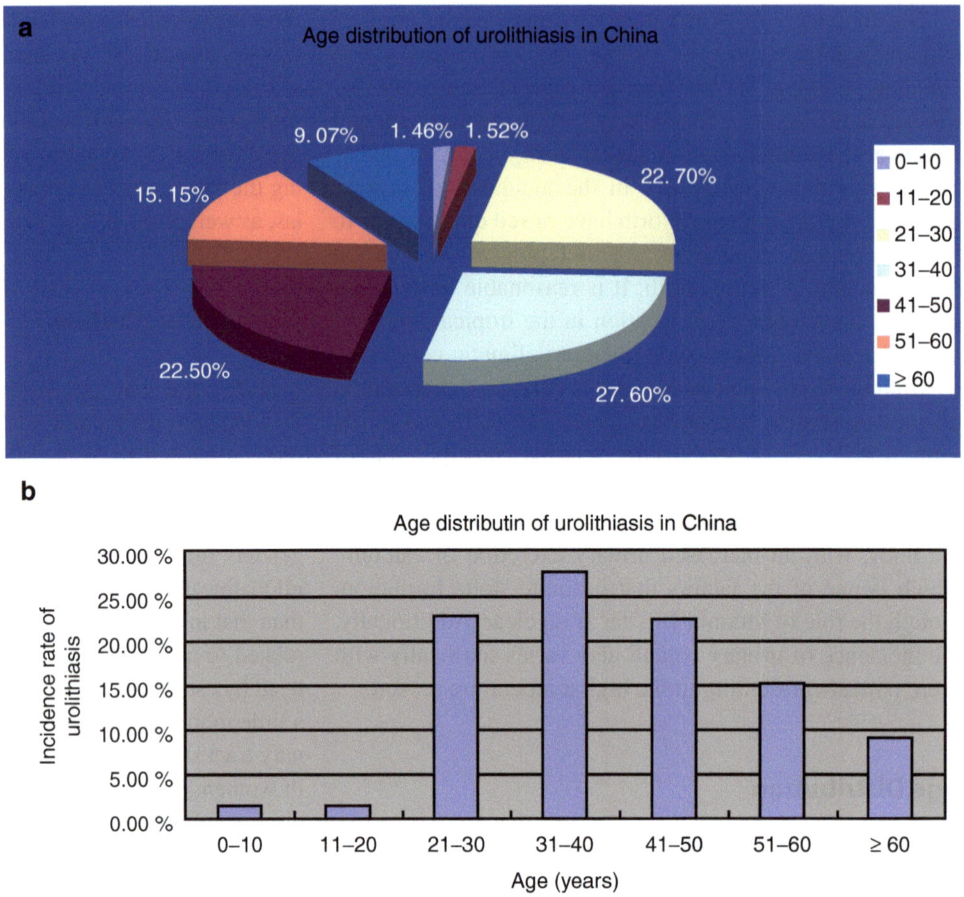

Fig. 6.3 Age distribution of urolithiasis in China by (**a**) pie chart and (**b**) bar chart

in workers exposed to overheating was 13.3 %. However, in the control study group of the support staff for these occupations, the morbidity was only 4.68 %. Furthermore, the longer the exposure to overheating, the higher was the morbidity [25]. The urolithiasis morbidity in cement production workers was 7.11 %, with 7.4 % in males and 6.35 % in females, but in the officers the figure was only 3.91 % [26]. The relationship between the morbidity of the renal calculus and the education levels is negative. Multivariate analysis has shown that the risk of the renal calculus formation increases with age, male gender, and low education level. The investigation in the area of Dongguan, Guangdong province, showed that the morbidity of urolithiasis of intellectual workers is gradually increasing [27]. But it has been reported that the relationship between the morbidity of urolithiasis and the education level is negative [28].

Stone Disease in the Various Nationalities in China

The morbidity of urolithiasis varies considerably among the 56 different nationalities in China [29]. It is reported that the incidence of urolithiasis in the Han nationality is very high: 57.10/100,000. The other rates are: the Miao nationality, 46.50/100,000; the Zhuang nationality, 41.80/100,000; Tong nationality, 40.80/100,000; Yao nationality, 6.80/100,000 in the Rong county [19], Guangxi Zhuang Autonomous Region. The morbidity of urolithiasis of the Yi nationality is the highest, while the Miao nationality is the lowest in Mengzi county Yunnan province [30]. A survey including Han, Tujia, and Miao nationalities showed that the rates were 10.3, 22.5, and 23.1 %, respectively [4]. A study including 2,227 cases of urolithiasis showed 2,167 Uighur patients (97.31 %) and 60 Han patients (2.69 %) in Xinjiang Autonomous Region [31], in conformity with the fact that 95 % are Uighur and 3 % Han. It is supposed that it may be related to the different eating and lifestyle habits, diet structure, and inheritance. At present, the proportionate contribution of genetics and environment to stone formation in these different nationalities yet requires investigation.

Incidence Rate of Urolithiasis

Large-scale epidemiological studies have not been carried out so far. The incidence of urolithiasis was first reported in a census of 12,203 people in Dongguan in Guangdong

Table 6.1 Prevalence of stone disease in different studies

Reference number	15	29	32	33	28	4
Province	Guangdong		Across China	Guizhou		Hubei
City	Dongguan	Shenzhen		Congjiang	Shenzhen	Enshi
Population surveyed	12,203	7,399 >15	188,697	16,424	7,399	799
Prevalence/100	1.16	4.8 6.12M; 4.07 F	0.12%	1.45	4.87	20
Ultrasound used	Yes	Yes	Yes	Yes	Yes	Yes
Year	2008	2004	1982	1989	1999	2008
Reference number	20	20	20	19	19	
Province	Guangdong	Guangdong	Guangdong	Guangxi Zhuang autonomous region	Guangxi Zhuang autonomous region	
City	Dongguan	Dongguan	Dongguan	Rongshui	Rongshui	
Population surveyed	1,565	899	1,776	396	982	
Prevalence/100						
Ultrasound used	Yes	Yes	Yes	Yes	Yes	
Year	1983	1984	1985	1977	1986	
Incidence per 100,000	1.01	1.23	1.4	0.201	0.653	

province; the prevalence was 1.16 % [15]. Xue Si-hu et al. [29] found that the prevalence of kidney stones was 4.87 %, 6.12 % for males and 4.07 % for females. They used ultrasound on a stratified random sample of 7,399 people over the age of 15 in Shenzhen in Guangdong province. Although the survey data lacks information for people under the age of 15, this study provides a more complete and accurate prevalence statistic of urinary stones in China. A study of 188,697 people in North, northeast, northwest, South Central, southwest, and East China detected a prevalence of 0.12 % [32]. In 1989, a survey of 16,424 people of Congjiang county in Guizhou province showed a prevalence of 1.45 % [33]. In 1999, 7,399 people were surveyed in Shenzhen, and 360 cases of patients with renal stones were found; the prevalence was 4.87 % [28]. In 2008, a sample survey of 799 people in Enshi in Hubei province found that the prevalence was 20 % [4]. In recent years, the overall incidence of urinary tract stones and prevalence has increased year by year. In Dongguan, Guangdong province, the urolithiasis new incidence rate of 101/10 million in 1983, and 123/10 million in 1984, rose to 140/10 million in 1985 [20]. In the Rongshui county of Guangxi Zhuang Autonomous Region, the new urolithiasis incidence of 20.2/10 million in 1977 increased to 65.3/10 million in 1986 [19]. Thus, the average of the population prevalence of urinary tract stones was between 1 and 5 %; the annual new incidence rate was 150 to 200/10 million.

In recent years, there has been a sharp reduction in patients with lower urinary tract stones, but a significant increase in patients with upper urinary tract calculi. Upper urinary tract stones occur mainly in the economically developed regions, and lower urinary tract stones mainly in rural areas and other economically backward regions. Recent figures show that about 95 % of the stones are now in the upper urinary tract; lower urinary tract stones comprise about 5 %. Multiple renal or ureteral stones were found on the right side in most cases, simultaneously or successively in more than two organs of the body accounting for 18.2 % of urinary calculi, of which up to 7.5 % had bilateral kidney stones, followed by single kidney and ureteral stones (4.8 %), bilateral ureteral calculi (2.3 %), kidneys, and ureteral stones (1.0 %), unilateral renal and bladder stones (0.5 %), ureter and bladder stones (0.3 %), bladder and urinary tract stones (0.3 %), bilateral renal bladder stones (0.2 %), and kidney and urinary tract stones (0.1 %) [34, 35]. Table 6.1 shows the prevalence of stone disease in different studies.

Chemical Constituents of Calculi

Urinary calculi consist of crystal material and matrix. In most stones, the crystal material comprises oxalate, phosphate, uric acid/urate, and in some rare cases, cystine. The matrix mainly originates from urinary mucoprotein and urine glycosaminoglycans. In recent decades, the composition of urinary stones has changed significantly in China, and the current state of distribution of stones is shown in Fig. 6.4. In Guangzhou, an analysis of 178 cases of urinary calculi shows that between 1870 and 1919, the uric acid/urate stones accounted for 78 % of all stones. From 1960 to 1976, however, calcium oxalate and calcium phosphate accounted for 80 % [21]. It was reported that in Fujian province, Beijing, Guangzhou, and Guizhou province urinary calculi mainly consisted of calcium oxalate and mixed calcium oxalate and calcium phosphate [12, 36–38]. Stones formed in the Dongguan county of Guangdong province, between 1975 and 1978, mainly contained uric acid and mixed urate. A few were composed of magnesium ammonium phosphate. However, in 1984, the main composition of urinary stones was calcium oxalate and mixtures of calcium oxalate and calcium phosphate 1984 [15, 20]. The analysis of 2,129

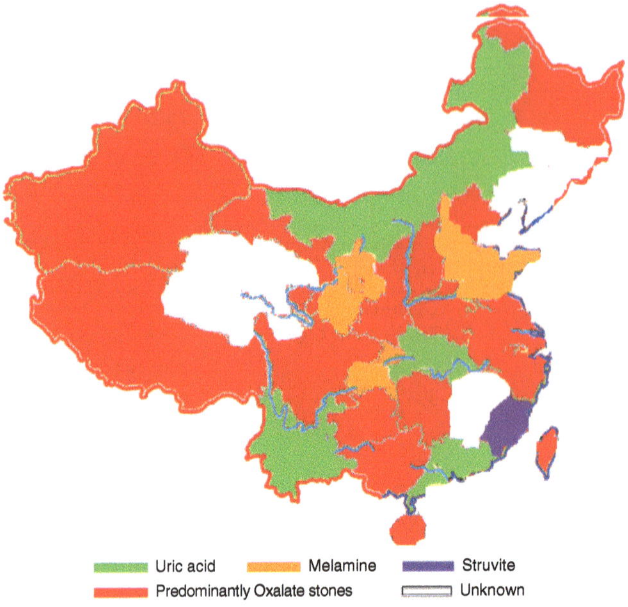

Fig. 6.4 Types of stones in different territories of China

urinary calculi in Nanchang in 2008 and 480 stones in 2010 in south Xinjiang showed that the main component of urinary stones was calcium oxalate [2, 39]. Statistics showed that the composition of upper urinary tract stones commonly was mixtures of calcium oxalate and calcium phosphate, but pure calcium oxalate stones dominated. On the other hand, lower urinary tract stones mainly consisted of calcium oxalate and the calcium phosphate-based mixtures. These results were in accordance with domestic and foreign reports [2, 5, 9, 40]. In addition, the content of ammonium in lower urinary tract stones was higher than that in upper urinary tract stones formed in patients from the Guizhou province and the Guangxi Zhuang Autonomous Region [38, 41]. The idiopathic urinary calculi that had no obvious metabolic explanation contained calcium salts, especially calcium oxalate. Stones accompanying urinary tract infection are mainly composed of magnesium ammonium phosphate. There are also reports that in some areas of China, primary lower urinary tract stones are mainly composed of cystine and the carbonate apatite and are more common in infant malnutrition and urinary tract infection, respectively [42].

Conclusion

In summary, urolithiasis is a commonly encountered disease in the urinary system. Its high recurrence rate can be very disturbing. As the modernization and Westernization progress in China, the site, age, gender, geographical, and occupational features of stone formation are gradually changing. The recent increase of the global incidence may be partially due to the early diagnosis of asymptomatic stones, by means of widespread imaging methods such as ultrasound. Unfortunately, we are still lacking a complete and thorough epidemiological study about urinary stones in China. Further studies in this field are of critical importance for better identification of the risk factors and better prevention of recurrence.

References

1. Wu J, Gu F, Sun C. Urolithiasis. Zhonghua Mi Niao Wai Ke Za Zhi. 1980;1:123.
2. Chen Z, Ji S, Zhu G, et al. Analysis of chemical composition of urinary stones and evaluation of metabolic disturbance in 480 Uighur patients in south Xinjiang. Xian Dai Yu Fang Za Zhi. 2010;20(3):571–9.
3. Zhou Y, Wei L, Liu G, et al. The epidemiology of urinary tract stones in county of Fengcheng from 1989 to 2000. Zhongguo Shi Jian Yi Xue. 2008;3(33):59–60.
4. Liu T, Mou J, Tan S. Study on etiology of the epidemiology of urolithiasis in Enshi region of Hubei province. Shi Jian Yu Fang Yi Xue. 2008;15(3):630–2.
5. Huang T, Long Z, Wu S, et al. Analysis of 3257 urolithiasis inpatients in shunde district. Yi Xue Xin Xi. 2010;4:775–6.
6. Lei J, Chen Z, Cao J, et al. Analysis of risk factor of urinary stone in the residents of Yinchuan county. Zhongguo Gong Gong Wei Sheng Za Zhi. 2008;24(12):1518–9.
7. Fu X, Xi H, Qi J. Analysis of the epidemic features of urolithiasis in Yongzhou county. Zhongguo Gong Gong Wei Sheng Za Zhi. 2006;22(5):586.
8. Zhou J, Li Y, Wang P, et al. Urolithiasis of inpatients in Guizhou province. Zhonghua Wai Ke Za Zhi. 1983;21:761–3.
9. Li Z, Zhang Q, Miu Y, et al. Analysis of 3779 urolithiasis patients. Zhonghua Wai Ke Za Zhi. 1986;24:536–7.
10. Mo S, Ge P, Ye C, et al. The report of 3, 764 urolithiasis patients in Guilin district. Zhonghua Wai Ke Za Zhi. 1985;6:45–8.
11. He J, Liu G. Survey of urolithiasis inpatients in Gansu province. Lin Chuang Mi Niao Wai Ke Za Zhi. 1987;2:51–3.
12. Wei W, Chen S, Liu X, et al. Survey of urolithiasis in Fujian province. Fujian Yi Yao Za Zhi. 1987;9:36–46.
13. Sun W, Ding Z, Zhang J, et al. The age distribution curve and clinical significance of urolithiasis patients in Guangxi region. Zhonghua Mi Niao Wai Ke Za Zhi. 2001;22:100–2.
14. He G, Lin J. Analysis of 1063 urolithiasis cases in Foshan area. Shi Yong Yi Xue Za Zhi. 1996;12:802–3.
15. Mo L. The change of urolithiasis in 25 years in Dongguan area. Zhonghua Wai Ke Za Zhi. 1980;18:333.
16. Shi J, Sun B. Retrospectively analysis of in 15 years in Guizhou province. Zhonghua Mi Niao Wai Ke Za Zhi. 1995;16:599–600.
17. Huang C, Liu J, He Y. Survey and analysis of 6827 urolithiasis in Nanhai western oil companies worker. Zhonghua Mi Niao Wai Ke Za Zhi. 2000;21:623.
18. Blacklock NJ. Urolithiasis: epidemiology. In: Chrisholm GD, editor. Scientific foundations of urology. 3rd ed. Oxford: Heinemann Media Books; 1990. p. 170–5.
19. Yin C. The investigation report of new urolithiasis cases every year nearly 10 years in Rongshui county of Guangxi province. Zhonghua Mi Niao Wai Ke Za Zhi. 1989;10:375–6.
20. Mo L, Deng J, Mu G, et al. The investigation report of new urolithiasis cases by every year in Dongguang county. Zhonghua Mi Niao Wai Ke Za Zhi. 1987;8:177–9.
21. Gu F. Geographical environment and urolithiasis. Zhonghua Wai Ke Za Zhi. 1978;6:323–6.
22. Yu Z, Ren J, Zhang G, et al. Dietary composition and kidney stones. Zhonghua Mi Niao Wai Ke Za Zhi. 1987;8:6–11.

23. Wu Z, Li X, Long X, et al. The investigation for effects of the lead for the incidence of urolithiasis. Dang Dai Yi Shi Za Zhi. 1998;3: 38–9.
24. Jiang L, Zhong X. The investigation for the prevalence of kidney stones in high-temperature operator. Zhongguo Zhi Ye Yi Xue. 2003;30(2):61–2.
25. Li Z, Chen Y. The investigation for the prevalence of kidney stones in cement production workers. Zhi Ye Yu Jiang Kang. 2004;20(12): 141–2.
26. Zeng C. The investigation for the prevalence of urinary stone in welding operator. Shi Yong Yu Fang Yi Xue. 2005;12(4):901.
27. Atan L, Andreoni C, Ortiz V, et al. High kidney stone risk in men working in steel industry at hot temperatures. Urology. 2005;65(5):858–61.
28. Xu S, Cheng J, Zhou H, et al. An epidemiological study of renal calculus in Shenzhen region. Zhonghua Mi Niao Wai Ke Za Zhi. 1999;20:655–7.
29. Liu Y, Wu X. The epidemiological study of urinary stone in China. Zhongguo She Qu Yi Shi. 2005;7(9):4–5.
30. Cao N, Sun L, Tao Z, et al. The study on diet composition for upper urinary tract stone formation I: epidemiological investigation of urolithiasis in Mengzi county. Yun Nan Yi Yao. 1989;80:125–9.
31. Gu C, Xu Z. 2,227 Cases of urinary tract stones at Kashi prefecture-level hospitals in XinJiang. Zhonghua Mi Niao Wai Ke Za Zhi. 1990;11:25.
32. National Survey Consortium urinary system diseases. The investigation report of 18 million people in the incidence of urinary system diseases. Zhonghua Yi Xue Za Zhi. 1982;62:577–80.
33. Sun B, Shi J, Dong H, et al. Epidemiological investigation of urolithiasis in Congjiang county in Guizhou. Guizhou Yi Yao. 1989;13: 231–2.
34. Liu Z, Zhu H, LI Y. Clinical analysis of 214 cases urinary stone disease in Qingyang region. Lanzhou Yi Xue Yuan Xue Bao. 1989;15(4):222–4.
35. Yu H. The relationship between urinary calculi and sleep position. Shaanxi Xin Yi Xue. 1980;9(9):61.
36. Urological Research lab at the First Affiliated Hospital of Beijing Medical University. 1151 Cases of urinary stone composition analysis (196221977). Yi Xue Zi Liao Xuan Bian. 1978;1: 181–2.
37. Zhan H, Mei H, Wang X, et al. Analysis of chemical composition of 4714 cases urinary stones. Zhonghua Shi Yan Wai Ke Za Zhi. 1995;12:316–7.
38. Zhang Y, Cui Z. Analysis of crystal components of 314 cases urinary stones in Guizhou. GuizhouYi Yao. 1982;1:13–5.
39. Li K, Min Y, Du J, et al. 2129 Cases of qualitative analysis of urinary stone composition. Experimental Lab Med. 2008;26(4):450.
40. Ochmanski W, Kmiecik J, Sulowicz W. Analysis of chemical composition of urinary stones. Int Urol Nephro1. 1999;31:743–50.
41. Li S, Wang Z, Bai X. Analysis of chemical composition of 220 cases urinary stones. Guanxi Yi Xue Yuan Xue Bao. 1991;8: 337–40.
42. Ou A, Dai WL, et al. Urinary stone composition analysis and clinical significance (with 401 cases reported). Hua Xi Yi Xue. 2000;15:70–1.

Epidemiology of Stone Disease in South America

7

Fernando Korkes, Nestor Schor, and Ita Pfeferman Heilberg

Abstract

The authors provide an overview of the underlying causes of urolithiasis, rates of metabolic disturbances, stone and demographic characteristics, geographic and seasonal variations, dietary patterns, types of treatment, and approximate costs of stone disease in South America, based on the available data from Brazil and other countries. They conclude that metabolic abnormalities can be found in up to 98 % of stone formers, hypercalciuria, hypocitraturia, and hyperuricosuria being the most common ones. The number of hospital admissions due to urinary stone disease was higher during the summer and in areas of hot and dry weather. Most of the calculi were composed of calcium oxalate. At present, open surgical procedures were substituted for endoscopic and percutaneous procedures, and there is a trend for a continuous increase in the use of flexible devices. The cost of stone disease care is still estimated to be high, but the continuous increase in the access to medical assistance by the population will help to reduce its socioeconomic impact.

Keywords

Epidemiology • Brazil • Urinary calculi • South America • Hypercalciuria • Hypocitraturia Urinary tract stones • Incidence • Urinary stones • Oxalates • Urates • Prevalence • Geographical variation • Stone composition • Urine composition • Staghorn stones • Calcium oxalate stones • Calcium phosphate stones • Infection stones • Uric acid stones • Cystine stones Practice patterns • Pediatric stones • Age-related stone formation • Recurrence • Stone site

Introduction

Epidemiologic data about kidney stone disease in South America are limited, and there is no population-based information on the incidence or prevalence of urolithiasis.

F. Korkes
Division of Urology, ABC Medical School,
São Paulo, Brazil

Nephrology Division, Federal University of São Paulo,
Rua Botucatu, 740, São Paulo 04023-900, Brazil
e-mail: fkorkes@terra.com.br

N. Schor • I.P. Heilberg, M.D., Ph.D. (✉)
Nephrology Division, Federal University of São Paulo,
Rua Botucatu, 740, São Paulo 04023-900, Brazil
e-mail: nestor@nefro.epm.br; ipheilberg@nefro.epm.br

In such a large population as South America (estimated at more than 371,000,000) with distinctive dietary habits and weather conditions and different population characteristics, distinct patterns of urinary stone occurrence are expected to occur. This chapter mainly focuses on the situation in Brazil due to better access to information by the authors. According to the Brazilian Public Health System Database [1], there have been 69,039 hospital admissions directly associated with urinary stone disease during the year of 2010. Urinary stone disease was solely responsible for 0.59 % of all hospital admissions during 2008 in the Brazilian public hospitals [1]. These numbers are impressive, especially if one considers that the majority of treatments for urinary stone disease are performed as outpatient modalities.

J.J. Talati et al. (eds.), *Urolithiasis*,
DOI 10.1007/978-1-4471-4387-1_7, © Springer-Verlag London 2012

Underlying Causes and Metabolic Abnormalities

The most common metabolic disturbances among stone formers are hypercalciuria, hypocitraturia, hyperuricosuria, and hyperoxaluria [2–4]. As the largest South American continent country and the world's fifth largest country, Brazil certainly encompasses significant regional variations due to different local dietary habits and ethnicity from each state. Dietary records obtained from 322 stone-forming (SF) patients from three Brazilian states—Alagoas and Bahia (both in the northeast) and São Paulo (southeast)—revealed a higher consumption of high biological value protein (especially animal protein) and lipid intake by the latter, probably as a result of different dietary habits and/or better socioeconomic status [5, 6]. Additionally, salt intake has also been reported to be higher in another series of SF patients in São Paulo [7]. In a study in the central west region of Brazil, where the average daily temperature is very high and low humidity occurs all year long, a high protein intake (bovine meat) has also been observed [8]. In this area, Almeida and Schor [5] found metabolic disturbances in 98 % of 120 stone-forming patients, with hyperuricosuria being the most frequent one (76 %), followed by hypocitraturia in 43 %, reduced urinary volume in 49 %, idiopathic hypercalciuria and mild hyperoxaluria in 14 %, renal tubular acidosis in 3 %, and cystinuria in 2 %. In another study in a smaller town (Botucatu) in the state of São Paulo [9], 95.5 % of metabolic disturbances were observed among 182 SF patients [6]. The most common disturbances included hypercalciuria (74 %), hypocitraturia (37.3 %), hyperoxaluria (24.1 %), hypomagnesiuria (21 %), hyperuricosuria (20.2 %), hyperparathyroidism (2.4 %), and renal tubular acidosis (0.6 %). The incidence of cystinuria was low in most of the reports [6–8]. Among 648 patients evaluated in Ribeirão Prêto, another city also in the state of São Paulo, hypercalciuria had been detected in 54 % of SF patients, hyperoxaluria in 55 %, and hyperuricosuria in 11 % [9]. In the largest national multicenter study ever conducted in Brazil, 1,320 SF patients were evaluated for metabolic abnormalities [10], revealing that in the southern region of the country, hypercalciuria and hypocitraturia were the most frequent disturbances, observed in 40–60 % and 45–70 % of the patients, respectively. In the northeast, hypercalciuria was also common (22–45 %), but hypocitraturia was less frequent and hyperuricosuria was more common (40–70 %) [10].

In Argentina, among 2,612 SF patients, hypercalciuria had been detected in 58.1 %, hyperuricosuria in 23.9 %, hypocitraturia in 22.7 %, and hypomagnesiuria in 15.9 % [11]. In a series of 212 SF patients evaluated in Uruguay, hypercalciuria has been detected in 36.7 % and hyperuricosuria in 30.7 % [12]. Finally, a large study conducted in Venezuela involving 2,700 SF patients has shown metabolic abnormalities in 87.8 % of patients [13], with hypercalciuria as the most common one (47.2 %), followed by hyperuricosuria in 18.8 % and hypocitraturia in 14.2 %.

Stone Characteristics and Composition

From 648 patients evaluated at the outpatient stone clinic in Ribeirão Prêto, Brazil [9], urinary stones were mostly located in the kidney (74.5 %), followed by the ureter in 23.4 % of cases, and very few in the bladder (2.2 %). Of those patients diagnosed with urinary stone disease, about 25.8 % had been asymptomatic at the time of diagnosis, 32.5 % had one or two episodes of renal colic, and 10.8 % had three or more episodes [9]. In another outpatient stone clinic, staghorn calculi represented 5.8 % of a sample of 630 SF patients of whom 95.6 % were women [14].

In a recent study about stone composition in 325 patients from the northeastern region of Brazil, Da Silva et al. found that 34.7 % were pure stones, of which 59.3 % were composed of calcium oxalate, 23.7 % of uric acid, and 1.8 % of cystine. Struvite represented 7.9 % of the mixed stones [15]. These findings are similar to a worldwide report by Pak et al. [3]. In Argentina, Negri et al. [16] studied 30 patients with pure uric acid stones and concluded that either overweight or obesity and older age were associated with low urine pH in such patients. Impairment in urate excretion associated with increased serum urate had also been found.

Demographic Characteristics

In the series of 799 stone formers evaluated by Negri et al. [19] in Argentina, men predominated over women (57.8 % vs. 42.2 %), similar to what has been reported elsewhere [17]. Among all hospital admissions for urinary stone disease in Brazil in 2010, available information from Public Health Database [1] has shown a similar distribution among the male and female genders (49.9 % vs. 50.1 %). This rate seems not to have changed since 1998. With respect to outpatient evaluations, Vanucchi et al. [9] also did not observe any gender preponderance.

As for age, 62.2 % of public hospital admissions/year in Brazil occurred in patients aged between 20 and 49 years in 2010 [1]. A mean age of 36.9 at the time of the first symptoms of urinary stone disease has been reported for outpatients [9].

According to ethnicity, 63.2 % of patients admitted to public hospitals in Brazil due to urinary stone disease were white, 35.8 % were African descendants, 0.7 % were Asiatic, and 0.2 % were Indians [1]. Considering that whites represent 49.7 % of the Brazilian population whereas 49.5 % are African descendants [18], such findings suggest that, as observed in other countries [17], white subjects tend to have a higher prevalence of urinary stone disease than African descendants, with Asiatics and Indians falling somewhere in between [17].

Geographic Variations

Common climatic characteristics in several areas of South America, such as hot and dry weather, are well-known predisposing factors of urinary stone disease [19]. In such context, genetic factors play an adjunctive role, but may be less important than in other regions of the planet. Nevertheless, 44 % of patients reported family history of stone disease in Ribeirão Prêto, São Paulo [9].

Similar to what has been shown in the United States [20], urinary stone prevalence and metabolic disturbances vary within different regions of Brazil [10] due to distinct dietary habits, weather conditions, and occupations. In fact, the number of hospital admissions due to urinary stone disease in Brazil in 2010 is proportionally higher in the northern regions of the country (Table 7.1, Fig. 7.1) due to the hotter climate in these regions [10].

Table 7.1 Representative distribution of the Brazilian population different regions (% of total population) and hospital admission due to urinary stone disease in 2010 [1, 18]

	Hospital admissions due to urinary stone disease [1]		Brazilian population [18]	
	n	%	Millions	%
North	3,707	5.37	15.80	8.28
Northeast	13,590	19.68	53.07	27.82
Central west	8,655	12.54	14.26	7.48
Southeast	31,266	45.29	80.30	42.10
South	11,821	17.21	27.30	14.31
Total	*69,039*	*100*	*190.73*	*100*

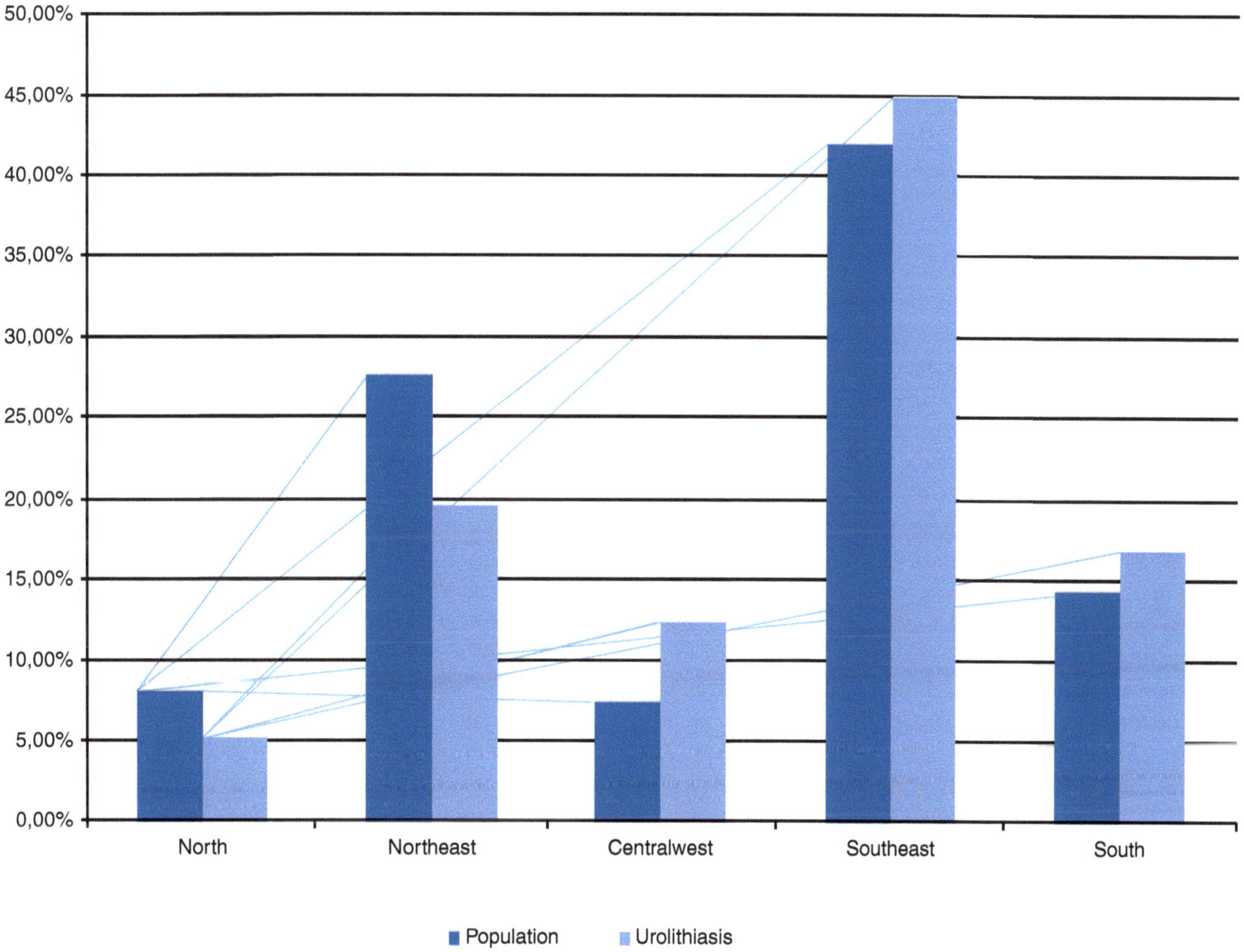

Fig. 7.1 Representative distribution of Brazilian population according to regions (% of total population) and hospital admission due to urinary stone disease in 2010 (% of total admissions) [1, 18]

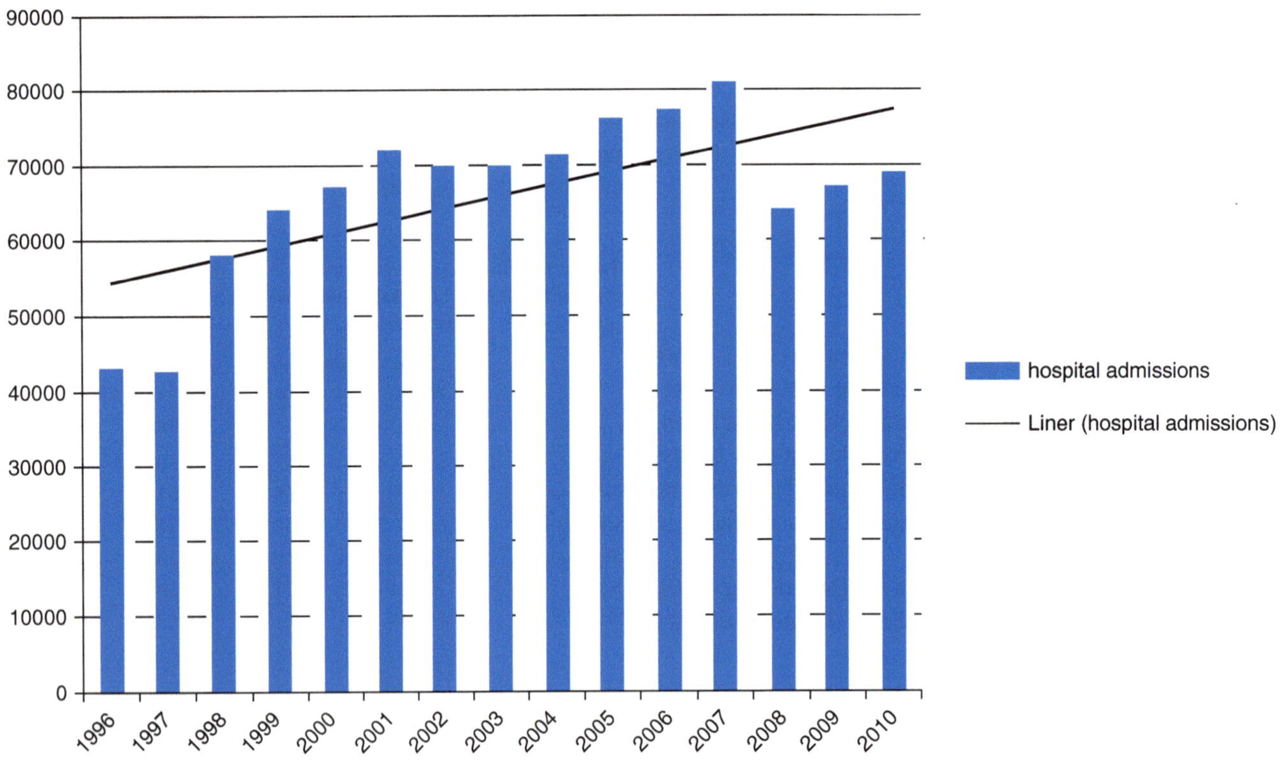

Fig. 7.2 Distribution of hospital admissions due to urinary stone disease from 1996 to 2010 [1]

Seasonal Variation

Hospital admissions due to urinary stone disease, as aforementioned, vary according to the weather conditions [10], explaining at least in part the geographic variation disclosed all over the country. In Brazil, there are two distinctive periods of the year according to the average temperature. Indeed, hospital admissions for urinary stone disease were 10 % higher during the hot compared to the colder months [1]. When data from 1996 to 2010 were compared, hospital admissions due to urinary stone disease increased in more than 60 % during that period (43,176–69,309, Fig. 7.2). These findings differ from those observed in other countries. Mandel et al. have reported a constant hospital discharge rate for urinary stone disease during the last decades in the US veterans' population [21]. Pearle et al. have noticed that rates of inpatient hospitalizations for a diagnosis of urolithiasis decreased by 15 % between 1994 and 2000 [22]. The epidemiological changes in Brazil may be ascribed to several factors such as continuous increase in the size of population, better data reporting, better access to public medical assistance, or increase in the incidence of urinary stone disease as reported by other investigators in other parts of the world [17].

Treatment

Follow-up is definitely a major problem when treating patients with urinary stone disease, with respect to either treatment of preexisting calculi or prevention. In the series of Ribeirão Prêto, São Paulo [13], only 45 % of the patients completed the laboratorial exams as requested. After 3 years, only 20 % of patients were still adhering to treatment [9]. Among the 648 patients, extracorporeal shock wave lithotripsy (SWL) was required in 20 % of the cases, of whom 21 % required two sessions, 29.4 % three, and 10.7 % four or more sessions. In 6.7 % of the patients, an intervention had to be undertaken [9]. In one center for stone treatment in São Bernardo do Campo, a district in São Paulo, the number and modalities of treatment [23] have been in accordance with the ones previously reported by Pak et al. in a worldwide multicenter study [3]. SWL was the most common procedure for stone removal, used in 74.7 % of cases. Ureteroscopy was required in 16.1 % and percutaneous stone removal in 7.7 %, and, when surgery was required, the laparoscopic route was the most commonly applied method, in 1.5 % of these patients [23]. There is a trend for an increasing use of flexible devices, in cases that were previously treated by SWL or percutaneous surgery.

However, as a developing country, Brazilian access to medical assistance is not universal yet, rendering some peculiarities more prone to occur. In a series of 37 staghorn calculi treated in the town of Botucatu in São Paulo, Amaro et al. [14] have reported 27 % of nephrectomies, while the remaining patients underwent percutaneous stone removal [14]. Additionally, when evaluating the ureteroscopic surgery performed in Brazil, a high incidence of large and impacted ureteral stones can still be observed [24, 25], which may end up in kidney losses and higher complication rates. Hopefully, with the recent increased access to medical assistance in the population, these problems are continuously being reduced at present.

Costs

Urolithiasis has a significant economic impact because of its high prevalence and recurrence rates. Additionally, its incidence peaks during the working ages. In 2010 in Brazil, public hospital admissions due to urolithiasis were responsible for 236,402 days lost at work, and the mean length of hospital stay was around 3.4 days. Considering that this information represents only the treatment on an inpatient basis, one can estimate that the real number is even higher. Inpatient admissions for urolithiasis were associated with 201 deaths in the public health system in 2010, with a mortality rate of approximately 0.29 %. In the same year, according to the public health database, US $17.5 million has been spent on hospital admissions due to urolithiasis, with a mean cost per patient of US $253.54. Although numbers associated with outpatient treatment and emergency care are not available in this country, if one considers the same proportion of cases as treated in the USA [26], it could be estimated that the Brazilian Public Health System spends more than US $37 million/year on the treatment of urinary stones (US $17.5 million for inpatient care, US $10.9 million for outpatient care, and US $8.8 million fort emergency care). If we extrapolate from these numbers, we could estimate yearly expenses of at least US $80 million for the treatment of urinary stone disease in Brazil. This represents 0.03 % of the national annual costs for health care.

In a referral center for stone treatment in Ribeirão Prêto, São Paulo, a city with about 500,000 inhabitants, there were 2,648 consultations per year. In the same period of time, there were 333 hospital admissions directly related to urinary stone disease, leading to 3.37 % of the total cost for hospital admissions in the public health system in that specific region [9].

If days lost at work are considered as well, these costs are higher. These numbers demonstrate that urinary stone disease represent a significant amount of total health care costs. Therefore, it should not only be considered as a disease, but as an important public health issue. Strategies to prevent urinary stone disease and its complications should be undertaken to reduce these costs.

Conclusion

Based on available data from Brazil and other South American countries, we conclude that metabolic abnormalities can be found in up to 98 % of stone formers, hypercalciuria, hypocitraturia, and hyperuricosuria being the most common ones. Hospital admissions are higher during the summer and in areas of hot weather. The number of endoscopic and percutaneous procedures is continuously increasing, but the cost of stone disease for the Public Health System is still estimated to be high in South American countries.

References

1. DATASUS. Department of Informatics of SUS. Brasília: Health Ministery; 2011 [cited 2011 03/12/2011]. Available from: http://www2.datasus.gov.br/DATASUS/index.php. Accessed on March 12, 2011
2. Heilberg IP. Update on dietary recommendations and medical treatment of renal stone disease. Nephrol Dial Transplant. 2000; 15(1):117–23.
3. Pak CY, Resnick MI, Preminger GM. Ethnic and geographic diversity of stone disease. Urology. 1997;50(4):504–7.
4. Heilberg IP, Schor N. Renal stone disease: causes, evaluation and medical treatment. Arq Bras Endocrinol Metabol. 2006;50(4):823–31.
5. Almeida WS, Schor N. Epidemiological and metabolic evaluation in renal stone patients living in a specific region of Brazil. Int Braz J Urol. 2001;27(5):432–9.
6. Amaro CR, Goldberg J, Amaro JL, Padovani CR. Metabolic assessment in patients with urinary lithiasis. Int Braz J Urol. 2005; 31(1):29–33.
7. Giugliani R, Ferrari I. Metabolic factors in urolithiasis: a study in Brazil. J Urol. 1980;124(4):503–7.
8. Giugliani R, Ferrari I, Greene LJ. Frequency of cystinuria among stone-forming patients in region of Brazil. Urology. 1986;27(1):38–40.
9. Vannucchi MTI, Geleilete TJM, Bessa EL. Urolithiasisin public health services – aprevention protocol for outpatients. J Bras Nefrol. 2003;25(4):165–71.
10. Heilberg IP, Teixeira SH, Novoa CG, Barros E, Ferreira Filho SR, Melo MEA, et al. The Brazilian multicentric study of nephrolithiasis (MULTILIT). In: Pak CYC, Resnick MI, Preminger GM, editors. Urolithiasis 1996 – proceedings of the 8th international symposium on urolithiasis. Dallas: Millet the Printer; 1996. p. 498–9.
11. del Valle E, Spivacow R, Zanchetta JR. Metabolic changes in 2612 patients with nephrolithiasis. Medicina (B Aires). 1999;59(5 Pt 1): 417–22.
12. Ventura J, Fernandez J, Gauronas W, Szpinak B, Olaizola I, Zampedri L, et al. Uruguai. In: Schor N, Heilberg IP, editors. Calculose renal – fisiopatologia, diagnóstico e tratamento. São Paulo: Sarvier Ltda; 1995. p. 350–3.
13. Weisinger JR, Bellorin-Font E, Sylvia V, Hum-Pierres J, Paz-Martinez V. An ambulatory metabolic study of calcium urolithiasis

in Venezuela. In: Schuville PO, editor. Urolithiasis and related clinical research. New York: Plenum Press; 1985. p. 275–8.
14. Amaro CR, Goldberg J, Agostinho AD, Damasio P, Kawano PR, Fugita OE, et al. Metabolic investigation of patients with staghorn calculus: is it necessary? Int Braz J Urol. 2009;35(6):658–61. discussion 62–3.
15. da Silva SF, Silva SL, Daher EF, Silva Junior GB, Mota RM, da Silva CA B. Determination of urinary stone composition based on stone morphology: a prospective study of 325 consecutive patients in an emerging country. Clin Chem Lab Med. 2009;47(5):561–4.
16. Negri AL, Spivacow FR, Del Valle EE, Forrester M, Rosende G, Pinduli I. Role of overweight and obesity on the urinary excretion of promoters and inhibitors of stone formation in stone formers. Urol Res. 2008;36(6):303–7.
17. Curhan GC. Epidemiology of stone disease. Urol Clin North Am. 2007;34(3):287–93.
18. Instituto Brasileiro de Geografia e Estatística (IBGE). Ministério do Planejamento, Orçamento e Gestão – Governo Federal do Brasil; 2010. Available from: http://www1.ibge.gov.br/home/.Accessed on Feb. 28, 2011
19. Fakheri RJ, Goldfarb DS. Ambient temperature as a contributor to kidney stone formation: implications of global warming. Kidney Int. 2011;79(11):1178–85.
20. Soucie JM, Coates RJ, McClellan W, Austin H, Thun M. Relation between geographic variability in kidney stones prevalence and risk factors for stones. Am J Epidemiol. 1996;143(5):487–95.
21. Mandel NS, Mandel GS. Urinary tract stone disease in the united states veteran population. I. Geographical frequency of occurrence. J Urol. 1989;142(6):1513–5.
22. Pearle MS, Calhoun EA, Curhan GC. Urologic diseases in America project: urolithiasis. J Urol. 2005;173(3):848–57.
23. Lucio II JS, Korkes F, Lopes-Neto AC, Silva EG, Mattos MHE, Pompeo ACL. Steinstrasse predictive factors and outcomes after extracorporeal shockwave lithotripsy. Int Braz J Urol. 2011;37(4):477–82.
24. Korkes F, Lopes-Neto AC, Mattos MH, Pompeo AC, Wroclawski ER. Patient position and semi-rigid ureteroscopy outcomes. Int Braz J Urol. 2009;35(5):542–7. discussion 8–50.
25. Brito AH, Mitre AI, Srougi M. Ureteroscopic pneumatic lithotripsy of impacted ureteral calculi. Int Braz J Urol. 2006;32(3):295–9.
26. Lotan Y. Economics and cost of care of stone disease. Adv Chronic Kidney Dis. 2009;16(1):5–10.

Epidemiology: South Africa and Sub-Saharan Africa

8

Allen Rodgers

Abstract

Epidemiological data on urolithiasis in sub-Saharan Africa are scarce because research resources throughout most of the continent are poor. South Africa is an exception in this regard. Stone disease has been reported in several countries. Epidemiological factors in these regions are not unusual. However, in a few countries the disease is extremely rare. The absence of stones can be attributed to epidemiological factors in all regions except South Africa, where stone rarity arises because of racial differences between the white and black population groups. Routine urinary biochemical risk factors cannot account for this phenomenon. However, the protective capacity of urinary proteins may play a role in this regard.

Keywords

Incidence • Urinary stones • Oxalates • Urates • Prevalence • Geographical variation • Stone composition • Urine composition • Staghorn stones • Calcium oxalate stones • Calcium phosphate stones • Infection stones • Uric acid stones • Cystine stones • Practice patterns • Pediatric stones • Age-related stone formation • Recurrence • Stone site

Introduction

The scarcity of epidemiological data on urolithiasis in Africa has been previously described and has been attributed to a general lack of resources and facilities for conducting research surveys [1]. Literature searches yield very little information. However, scrutiny of the few articles that have been published suggests that the nature of the disease can be broadly placed into three main categories: endemic pediatric bladder stones, upper urinary tract calcium oxalate (CaOx) stones, and stone absence or rarity. The distribution of these categories is summarized in the color-coded map shown in Fig. 8.1. (Although Algeria and Egypt are not "sub-Saharan" countries, they are presented on the map for the interest of readers.) It is immediately apparent that in South Africa the seemingly contradictory categories of stone occurrence and stone rarity both occur. Unlike Nigeria and Southern Sudan where stone rarity has been attributed to epidemiological factors (low calcium in drinking water, low consumption of dairy products, and labor-intensive lifestyle on the one hand, and low climatic temperatures, high relative humidity, low urinary calcium, and high urinary volume on the other), in South Africa it is attributed to race. Research resources and facilities in South Africa are of a high standard. As such, reliable data are available on the epidemiology of the disease in this country (see Fig. 8.1).

In 1961 Wise and Kark reported a remarkable statistic concerning the number of cases of urinary calculi occurring in King Edward VIII Hospital, Durban, South Africa, during the period 1951–1959 [2]. They found that 483,450 black patients had been admitted for a variety of disorders but that only seven (0.0014 %) were admitted for urolithiasis. This finding supported an earlier report by Vermooten who had found only 4 cases in 91,000 admissions [3]. Although there has not been any similar study since then on stone incidence

A. Rodgers M.Sc., Ph.D.
Department of Chemistry, University of Cape Town,
Private Bag, Rondebosch 7701, Cape Town, South Africa
e-mail: allen.rodgers@uct.ac.za

J.J. Talati et al. (eds.), *Urolithiasis*,
DOI 10.1007/978-1-4471-4387-1_8,

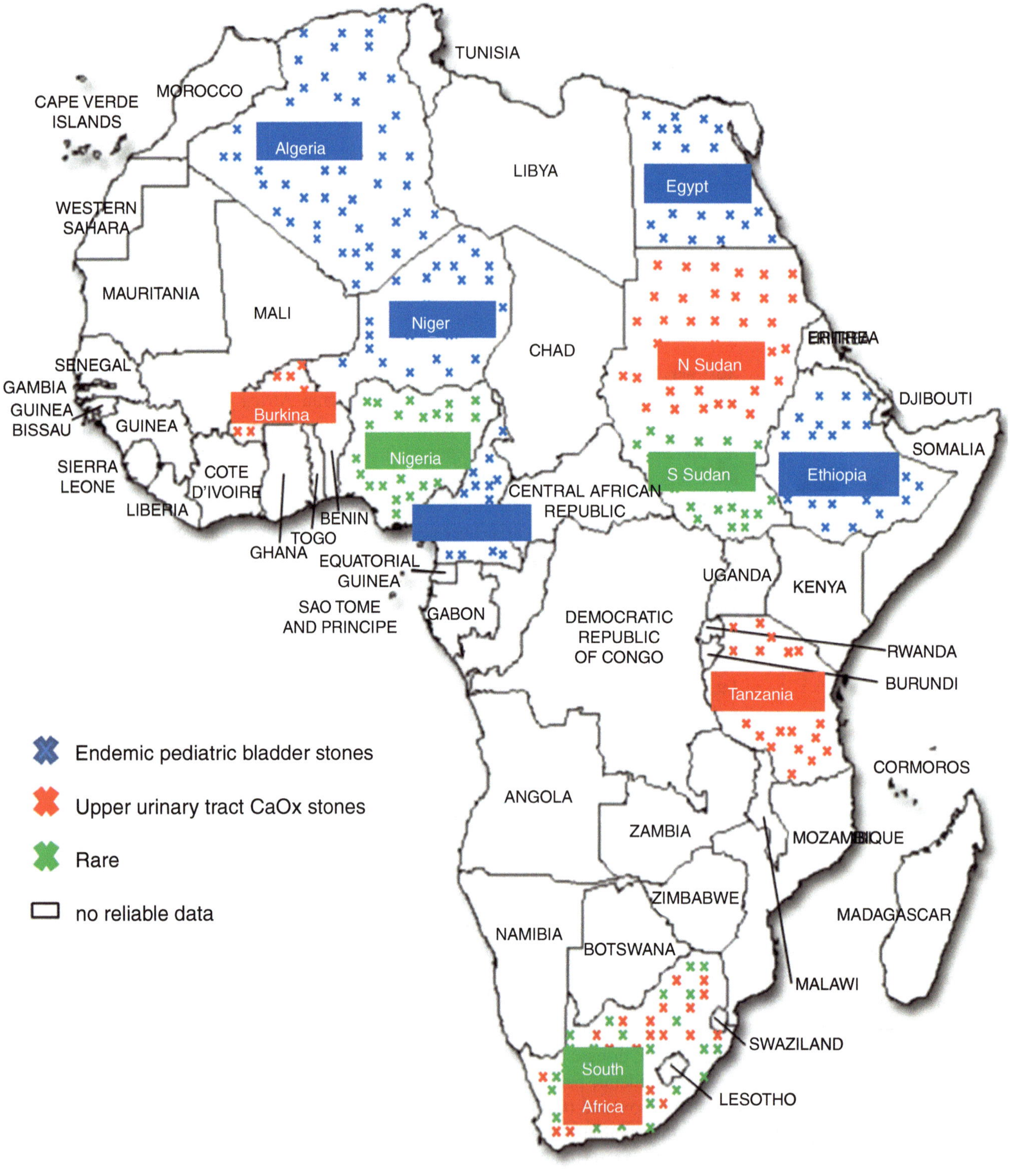

Fig. 8.1 Distribution of urinary stone disease in Africa

per se in the black population, the rarity of the disease in this population group is widely accepted today.

The existence of two population groups—one of which is stone prone while the other is relatively stone free—has presented a unique opportunity for South African researchers to investigate this phenomenon with a view to understanding lithogenic and anti-lithogenic risk factors in urolithiasis.

Interestingly, there is evidence of another race group in South Africa showing an opposite stone trait to that of the black group. In the Department of Urology at the Nelson

Table 8.1 Summary of percentage compositional analysis in South African stone collections

Authors	Gray et al. (1982) [5]	Beukes et al. (1987) [6]	Sutor (1972) [7]	Kerr et al. (1993) [8]	Rodgers (2011) [present study]
Location	Durban	Bloemfontein	Cape Town	Durban	Cape Town
Number of stones	300	1,002	49	5,065	3,737
CaOx	74.4	65.2	43.0	70.8	60.8
CaP	4.3	10.1	4.0	5.8	4.6
Urate/uric acid	18.3	16.0	4.0	9.9	11.5
CYS	1.3	0.7	2.0	0.2	0.8
STR	4.0	6.1	0.0	2.2	9.2

Mandela School of Medicine in Durban, 227 patients with a confirmed diagnosis of renal stone disease were admitted for treatment in 1997 [4]. Of these, 156 (70 %) were Indians, suggesting an unusually high incidence of this disease in this population group

This chapter aims to consolidate the various studies that have been conducted on urolithiasis in South Africa and to present new unpublished data in the hope that a coherent and meaningful overview may be obtained.

Stone Analysis

Several major stone collections have been analyzed [5–8]. A summary of the results of these studies is given in Table 8.1. For the purposes of simplifying the data, stone compositions have been consolidated into five main groups: calcium oxalate (CaOx), calcium phosphate (CaP), urate/uric acid, cystine (CYS), and struvite (STR). Mixtures involving two or more of these components have not been included in the table. Remarkably, one of the studies managed to accumulate 108 stones from black patients, albeit that it was over a period of 15 years and 23 of them were composed of struvite, indicating urinary infection as their cause [6]. The composition of these stones was not significantly different to that of the white group. The table also includes unpublished data from the present author's own laboratory.

Comparison of the results of these studies is somewhat difficult and probably futile, since the categorization of stone types varies from one study to another. It is not obvious how any one type has been defined, nor is it apparent how mixed compositions have been dealt with. A further difficulty is that the stones have been collected from different regions, each of which may have its own peculiar demographic characteristics. Thus, rigorous comparison of the studies is not feasible. However, some generalizations may be permitted. CaOx stones appear to be less common in the Cape Town area than in the other two centers, while the opposite is true for STR stones. The occurrence of CaP is high in the Bloemfontein study, while urate is high in the latter study as well as in the early Durban study. There are no other features regarding interregional comparisons. On a time scale, there is a suggestion that the occurrence of pure CaOx and pure urate stones may be decreasing. Perhaps these components are appearing more frequently in stones of mixed composition.

Urine Analysis

Studies on the pathogenesis of urolithiasis involve urine analysis as one of the first steps in the work-up of patients. In the case of stone rarity in South Africa's black population, comparison of the urinary biochemical risk factors for stone formation has been an obvious starting point. Surprisingly, there have been only two studies that have compared urine composition in healthy white and healthy black subjects. One was published in 1967 [9], while the other has not yet been published and involves data from the present author's own laboratory.

The usefulness of the early study [9] for assessing the relative risk of stone formation is severely limited by virtue of the absence of urinary oxalate values. Besides the crucial importance of this variable as an independent risk factor, its absence prevents the calculation of the relative supersaturation of CaOx, which is widely regarded as a powerful composite risk indicator. Nevertheless, other interesting features are apparent in the study: urinary calcium, citrate, and pH are all significantly lower in the black group (2.03 ± 1.4 mmol/24 h vs. 3.45 ± 1.85 mmol/24 h; 1.87 ± 1.24 mmol/24 h vs. 2.74 ± 1.10 mmol/24 h; and 6.0 ± 0.57 vs. 6.2 ± 0.49, respectively). While the lower urinary calcium in black subjects is consistent with the lower stone incidence in this group relative to the white group, the lower urinary citrate and pH are counterintuitive, as both of these are indicative of a relatively *higher* risk of CaOx stone formation in the former group. Moreover, although the urinary calcium is significantly lower in the black group, it nevertheless lies within the normal range for healthy males [10] Thus, while it might account (to some extent) for a *lower* stone incidence in this group compared to whites, it does not account for its near absence from the group in general.

Values for the aforementioned three variables as well as those for oxalate and the relative supersaturation of CaOx, determined in the present author's own laboratory, are given in Table 8.2. While urinary calcium is significantly lower in

Table 8.2 Urinary risk factors in healthy black and white males: present study

	Healthy black males (HBM)	Healthy white males (HWM)	*p* values
	n=264	*n*=413	HBM versus HWM
Ca (mmol/24 h)	2.58 (±0.090)	3.36 (±0.100)	<0.001
Ox (mmol/24 h)	0.28 (±0.008)	0.24 (±0.006)	<0.001
Cit (mmol/24 h)	2.60 (±0.078)	2.62 (±0.061)	ns
pH	6.19 (±0.028)	6.25 (±0.021)	ns
RS CaOx	3.76 (±0.204)	3.83 (±0.168)	ns

black subjects (in agreement with the findings of Modlin [9]), there were no statistically significant differences in urinary citrate and pH. However, surprisingly and counter intuitively, urinary oxalate was found to be significantly *higher* in black subjects. Furthermore, notwithstanding this higher oxalate excretion in blacks, the relative supersaturation of CaOx in this group showed no difference to that in the white group.

These results demonstrate that the traditional urinary risk factors for urinary CaOx stone formation cannot account for the rarity of this disease in black South Africans.

Other studies have compared urine compositions in healthy black volunteers with those in black and white stone formers [11] and between Asian and white stone formers [4]. In the former study, demographic, serum, urinary, and dietary risk factors were measured in healthy black volunteers (BN) and in white and black stone formers (WSF and BSF, respectively). Remarkably, the researchers were able to recruit 22 black stone formers in this study over a period of 10 years. They found that urinary calcium in black stone formers was significantly higher than in BN and significantly lower than in WSF. Besides serum calcitriol being higher in BSF compared to WSF, no other risk factors were found to be different. Thus, the authors were not able to hypothesize about protective factors in the urine of black individuals.

In the latter of the two aforementioned studies [4], the authors investigated metabolic risk factors in 82 white and 58 Indian stone-forming patients (Ind). The only differences that they identified were a significantly higher incidence of complete renal tubular acidosis type 1 and a lower urine output in Ind. The authors suggest that these two factors may explain the higher prevalence of urinary stone disease in this group.

While the results of these two studies [4, 11] are interesting, they do not provide any insights concerning the mystery surrounding the rarity of stones in the black group.

Since traditional urinary biochemical risk factors have not been able to account for this phenomenon, the possible role of urinary proteins has been investigated in this context. Evidence in support of this notion has been identified. Crystal matrix extract, rich in urinary prothrombin fragment 1 (UPTF1) and derived from the urines of both groups, was tested for their inhibitory activity toward CaOx nucleation in synthetic urine [12]. The extract from the urine of black subjects was found to be superior in this regard. In a follow-up study, the inhibitory capacity of pure UPTF1 from each group was tested in the ultrafiltered urine from which it was derived. A synergistic relationship was observed, with the optimum activity being that produced by the protein-urine combination in black subjects [13]. In another study, urinary albumin derived from black subjects was shown to be a more powerful inhibitor of CaOx crystallization than that obtained from the urine of white subjects [14]. These studies suggest that the inhibitory capacity of urinary proteins may be a key factor in explaining the racial difference in stone incidence in South Africa's black and white population groups.

Conclusion

The profile of urinary stone disease in South Africa continues to offer unique opportunities for gaining insights into the pathogenesis and management of this disease. Research on the question of the black population's apparent natural protection toward this disease has shown that achieving these insights is not easy. Despite this, efforts must continue. A population group in which stone disease is extremely rare cannot be ignored as it may yet reveal meaningful answers to the questions about this disease in general.

References

1. Rodgers A. The riddle of kidney stone disease: lessons from Africa. Urol Res. 2006;34:92–5.
2. Wise RO, Kark AE. Urinary calculi and serum calcium levels in Africans and Indians. S Afr Med J. 1961;35:47–50.
3. Vermooten V. The occurrence of renal calculi and their possible relation to diet. JAMA. 1937;109:857–9.
4. Abdel Goad EH, Bereczky ZB. Metabolic risk factors in patients with renal stones in KwaZulu Natal: an inter-racial study (Asians and Whites). BJU Int. 2004;93:120–3.
5. Gray D, Laing M, Nel F, Naude JH. Composition of urinary calculi collected in the Durban area. S Afr Med J. 1982;61:121–5.
6. Beukes GJ, De Bruyn H, Vermaak WJH. Effect of epidemiological factors on the composition and racial distribution of renal calculi. Br J Urol. 1987;60:1–5.
7. Sutor DJ. Composition of urinary calculi by X-ray diffraction. Collected data from various localities. Parts XII-XIV. Northern Ireland, South Africa and Kuwait. Br J Urol. 1972;44:287–91.

8. Kerr A, Laing M, Nel F. Fifteen years and 5000 X-ray patterns later: renal stone analysis at the University of Natal, Durban. S Afr J Sci. 1993;89:528–30.
9. Modlin M. The aetiology of renal stone: a new concept arising from studies on a stone-free population. Ann R Coll Surg Engl. 1967; 40:155–78.
10. Hesse A, Classen A, Knoll M, Timmerman F, Vahlensieck W. Dependence of urine composition on the age and sex of healthy subjects. Clin Chim Acta. 1986;160:79–86.
11. Whalley NA, Martins MC, Van Dyk RC, Meyers AM. Lithogenic risk factors in normal black volunteers, and black and white recurrent stone formers. BJU Int. 1999;84:243–8.
12. Durrbaum D, Rodgers A, Sturrock E. A study of crystal matrix extract and urinary prothrombin fragment 1 from a stone-prone and stone-free population. Urol Res. 2001;29:83–8.
13. Webber D, Rodgers A, Sturrock E. Synergism between urinary prothrombin fragment 1 and urine: a comparison of inhibitory activities in stone-prone and stone-free population groups. Clin Chem Lab Med. 2002;40:930–6.
14. Rodgers A, Mensah P, Schwager S, Sturrock E. Inhibition of calcium oxalate crystallization by commercial human serum albumin and human urinary albumin isolated from two different race groups: evidence for possible molecular differences. Urol Res. 2006; 34:373–80.

Epidemiology of Stone Disease in Australia

9

Ming-Chak Lee and Simon Virgil Bariol

Abstract

Despite the significant morbidity and considerable financial burden associated with stone disease, there is a surprising lack of published epidemiological data on renal stone disease in Australia. This is unfortunate, given our country's unique racial diversity, geography, climate, and diet. Collating data from government hospital admissions in 2006–2007 showed an estimated annual incidence of upper urinary tract calculi of 131 cases/100,000, and this rate has remained steady over the past decade. This contrasts the upward trend in the number of stone procedures performed over the same period and the increasing use of endoscopic interventions compared with other stone treatment techniques.

Keywords

Urinary tract stone • Aborigines • Epidemiology • Oxalate • Hypercalciuria • Incidence Urinary stones • Oxalates • Urates • Prevalence • Geographical variation • Stone composition • Urine composition • Staghorn stones • Calcium oxalate stones • Calcium phosphate stones • Infection stones • Uric acid stones • Cystine stones • Practice patterns • Pediatric stones • Age-related stone formation • Recurrence • Stone site

Introduction

Renal colic is a common presentation to hospital emergency departments worldwide. Studies from the United States have shown an annual incidence of stone disease between 70 and 120 cases/100,000 at a financial cost in excess of US $2 billion in 2000 [1]. The lifetime risk of kidney stones is 12 % in men and 6 % in women with a higher prevalence in Saudi Arabia and lower rates in Asian and European countries [2, 3].

Despite the significant morbidity and the considerable financial cost associated with this condition, there is surprisingly little published epidemiological data on stone disease in Australia. This is particularly unfortunate since data from other developed nations may not necessarily be applicable to Australia, given the country's unique racial diversity, geography, climate, and diet. Local epidemiological data, therefore, is vital to public health planning and, in particular, service provision and resource allocation. The importance of comprehensive and up-to-date local epidemiological data was highlighted in a recent paper by McNeill et al. [4]. The study found an unacceptable disparity in waiting times for stone treatment between private and public patients, which was instrumental in convincing the New South Wales health department to fund more laser units in public hospitals [4].

In 2007, Australia had an estimated population of 21.2 million people [5]. Data collected from the Australian Institute of Health and Welfare (AIHW) on public and private hospital admissions during 2006–2007 showed an annual incidence of upper urinary tract calculi of 131 cases/100,000 [6]. This rate has essentially remained static over the past decade (Fig. 9.1).

The lifetime risk of stone disease in Australia is presently unknown due to the lack of comprehensive data collection. Also, while there are some statistics on treatment rates for stone disease in Australia, the use of multistep interventions

M.-C. Lee, M.B.B.S.
S.V. Bariol, M.B.B.S., B.Sc., (Med) FRACS (✉)
Department of Urology, Westmead Hospital,
Cnr Hawkesbury and Darcy Road, Westmead, NSW 2145, Australia
e-mail: ming_chak@hotmail.com; bariols@bigpond.net.au

J.J. Talati et al. (eds.), *Urolithiasis*,
DOI 10.1007/978-1-4471-4387-1_9, © Springer-Verlag London 2012

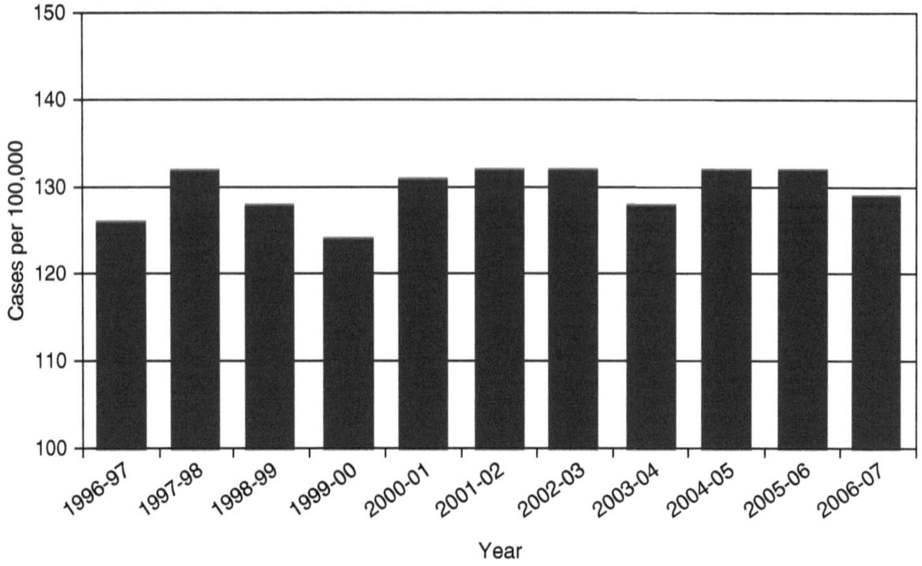

Fig. 9.1 Incidence of upper urinary tract stones in Australia from 1996 to 2007

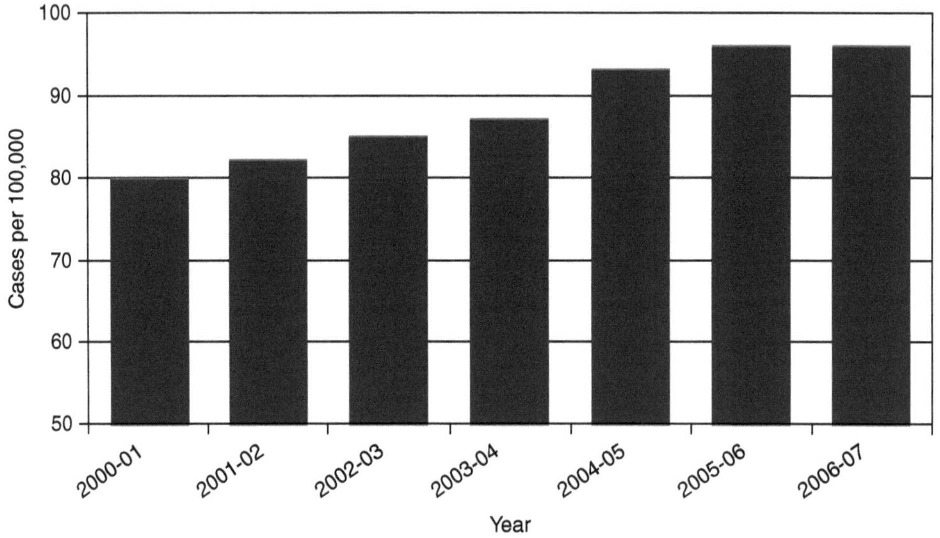

Fig. 9.2 Rate of intervention for upper urinary tract stones in Australia from 2000 to 2007

and combination therapy has made it difficult to determine the percentage of patients subjected to active stone management. In addition, complex and disparate coding practices between health services make it almost impossible to retrieve and analyze public hospital data accurately. Nonetheless, collating Medicare Australia data for non-public hospital procedures claimable by registered providers and Australian Institute of Health and Welfare (AIHW) figures for urological interventions in public hospitals has shown a combined annual stone treatment rate of 96 cases/100,000 in 2006–2007 [7, 8]. This rate of active management has increased significantly in the past decade (Fig. 9.2). Given the relatively stable incidence of symptomatic stone disease, the rising treatment rates are likely to be at least in part the result of an increasingly complex therapeutic pathway for patients presenting with stone disease.

The preferred option for active stone removal has also undergone a dramatic shift in the past decade. The percentage of endoscopic interventions performed in Australia has increased substantially from 66 % in 2000 to 75 % in 2007, which has been at the expense of all other stone management therapies (Fig. 9.3) [7, 8].

Regarding treatment numbers however, shock wave lithotripsy has remained steady while the number of percutaneous, open, and laparoscopic uretero- and nephrolithotomy procedures has decreased [9]. Even after taking into account Australia's population growth, there has been a considerable increase in the annual number of stone removal interventions performed, with endoscopic procedures contributing substantially to this trend (Fig. 9.4). Further study, however, is required to determine whether this is caused by an increasing incidence of stone disease

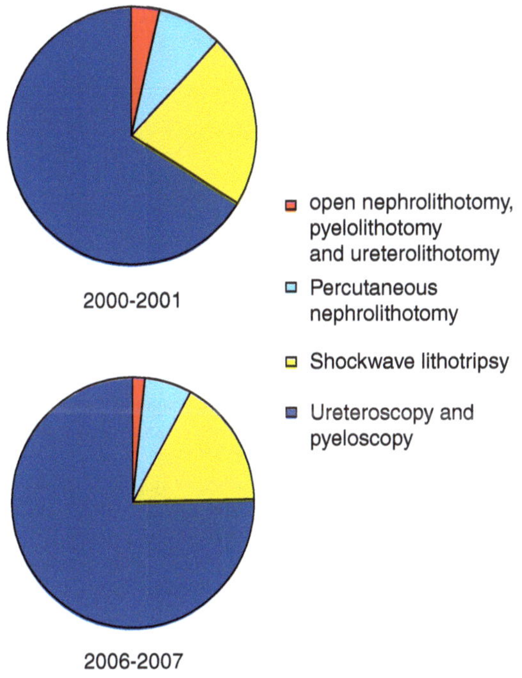

Fig. 9.3 Proportional comparison of active stone treatment modalities between 2000–2001 and 2006–2007

or higher retreatment rates with the advent of less invasive therapies.

Unfortunately data concerning metabolic investigations in Australian stone formers is far less contemporary. Lavan et al. reported the results of stone analysis and thorough metabolic assessments in 619 consecutive patients attending a tertiary stone clinic in Sydney more than 30 years ago [10]. Abnormalities in calcium metabolism were identified in 197 patients (32 %) including hypercalciuria in 178 patients (29 %) and hypercalcemia in 24 patients (4 %) of which 19 had histologically demonstrated primary hyperparathyroidism. In addition, cystinuria was detected in 4 patients (<1 %), and medullary sponge kidney was diagnosed in 16 patients (3 %). The study was performed in the early 1970s when compound or phenacetin-containing analgesics were still widely used in Australia. Interestingly, of the 53 patients who had nephrocalcinosis, 15 had a history of heavy analgesic use. Regarding chemical composition, mixed calcium oxalate and phosphate stones were the most common, and calcium was present in all but 14 of the 255 stones analyzed [10].

Baker et al. reviewed the incidences of various stone types analyzed in South Australia between 1977 and 1991 [11]. They reported calcium oxalate (with or without phosphate) in 68 %, uric acid in 17 %, infection stones (magnesium ammonium phosphate) in 12 %, and pure calcium phosphate in 3 %. The study also noted a significant increase in the incidence of uric acid stones in the summer and autumn months, while infection stones occurred less frequently in spring and summer. No seasonal variation was detected in the incidence of calcium oxalate stones [11].

A discussion of stone disease epidemiology in Australia would be incomplete without consideration of our indigenous

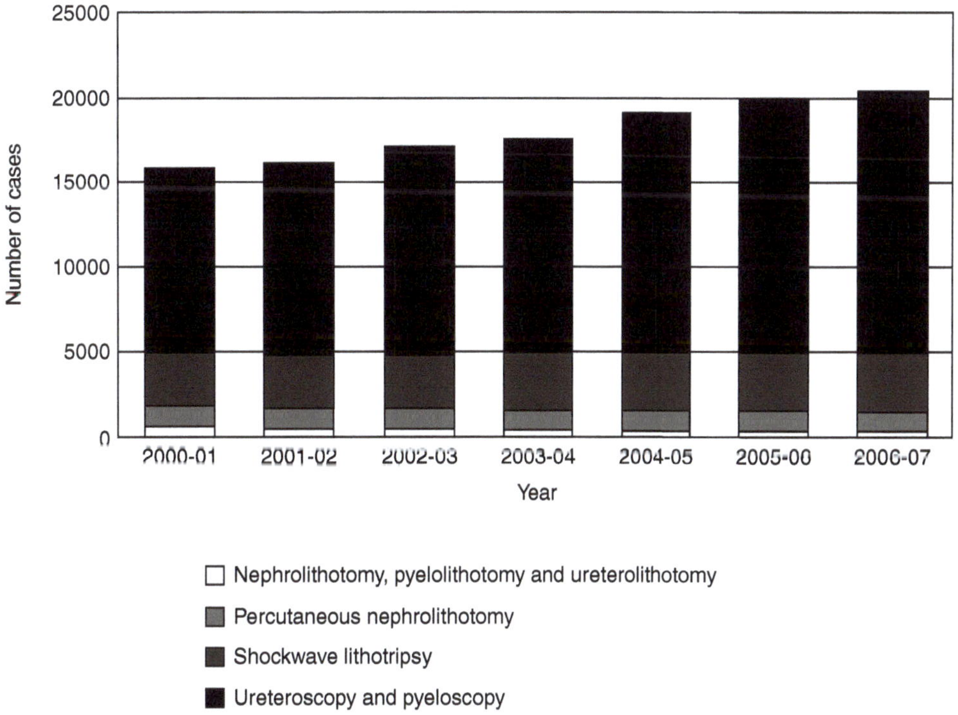

Fig. 9.4 Comparison of treatment modalities for upper urinary tract stones in Australia from 2000 to 2007

population and in particular Aboriginal children. In the central Australian town of Alice Springs with a large Aboriginal population, a study by Farago examined the incidence of kidney stones in 774 patients referred for urinary tract investigation between January 1982 and December 1985 [12]. The study showed that stone disease was surprisingly uncommon in Aboriginal adults, but more frequent in non-Aboriginal adults and Aboriginal children. Of the patients referred for imaging, 14 % of non-Aboriginal adults had urinary stones, compared with only 8 % of Aboriginal adults. In addition, while no non-Aboriginal children had urolithiasis, 7 % of the Aboriginal children had stones, including 12 children less than 3 years of age. The findings were curious in that the high incidence of stone disease in non-Aboriginal adults was thought to be due to the arid conditions experienced in Alice Springs, yet despite the lower water intake and higher exposure to those same climatic influences, the incidence in Aboriginal adults was lower. It was suggested that the Aboriginal population may have some endogenous protection against stone formation, which makes the higher incidence in Aboriginal children and infants particularly alarming. The calculi were predominantly uric acid in composition, but occurred in the upper urinary tract unlike bladder stones seen in children from developing countries [13]. As this is confined to Aboriginal children in desert areas of Central Australia and the hot tropical north, environmental factors appear to be an important factor in stone formation. However, dietary factors including carbohydrate intolerance causing chronic metabolic acidosis have also been postulated [14].

Conclusion

In summary, although widespread population-based studies are currently lacking, the incidence of stone disease in Australia would appear similar to other Western countries and has been stable over the past decade. The management of stone disease has evolved with a higher proportion of less invasive procedures, but possibly at the expense of an increasing number of urological procedures being performed annually.

References

1. Pearle MS, Calhoun EA, Curhan GC. Urologic diseases in America project: urolithiasis. J Urol. 2005;173:848–57.
2. Brener ZZ, Winchester JF, Salman H, Bergman M. Nephrolithiasis: evaluation and management. South Med J. 2011;104(2):133–9.
3. Curhan GC. Epidemiology of stone disease. Urol Clin North Am. 2007;34:287–93.
4. McNeill F, McNeill J, Brooks AJ. Management of kidney stone disease in New South Wales: an observational study. Med J Aust. 2008;189:596–7.
5. Australia Bureau of Statistics. Australian historical population statistics. Data cube: excel spreadsheet cat. No. 3105.0.65.001, last viewed 4 Apr 2011. 2008. http://www.abs.gov.au/AUSSTATS/abs@.nsf/DetailsPage/3105.0.65.0012008?OpenDocument.
6. Australian Institute of Health and Welfare. Australian hospital statistics 1996–2007. Canberra: AIHW; 2010. Data cube, last viewed 4 Apr 2011, http://www.aihw.gov.au/principal-diagnosis-data-cubes/
7. Australian Institute of Health and Welfare. Australian hospital statistics 2000–2007. Canberra: AIHW; 2010. Data cube, last viewed 4 Apr 2011, http://www.aihw.gov.au/procedures-data-cubes/
8. Medicare Australia. Medicare item reports. Canberra, last viewed 4 Apr. 2011. https://www.medicareaustralia.gov.au/statistics/mbs_item.shtml.
9. Lee MC, Bariol SV. Changes in stone management in Australia. BJU Int. 2011;52:29–33.
10. Lavan JN, Neale FC, Posen S. Urinary calculi. Clinical, biochemical and radiological studies in 619 patients. Med J Aust. 1971;2:1049–61.
11. Baker PW, Coyle P, Bais R, Rofe AM. Influence of season, age and sex on renal stone formation in South Australia. Med J Aust. 1993;159:390–2.
12. Farago C. Urolithiasis in the Aboriginal and non-Aboriginal children and adults of central Australia. Australas Radiol. 1987;21:300–3.
13. Carson PJ, Brewster DR. Unique pattern of urinary tract calculi in Australian Aboriginal children. J Paediatr Child Health. 2003;39:325–8.
14. Baldwin DN, Spencer JL, Jeffries-Stokes CA. Carbohydrate intolerance and kidney stones in children in the Goldfields. J Paediatr Child Health. 2003;39:381–5.

Epidemiology of Stone Disease in Saudi Arabia with an Overview of the Regional Differences

10

Salah R. El-Faqih

Abstract

In Saudi Arabia, urolithiasis is an upper urinary tract disease with predominance of calcium oxalate and uric acid/urate stones. The environmental temperature is high and water intake inadequate. Stone patients have low urinary volume, pH, and calcium, but high oxalate and urate excretion. Endemic bladder stones have disappeared. Lifetime risk of a stone episode is 50 times higher than in the West. Stones are predominantly calcium oxalate (82 %) all urate/uric acid (11.5 %). Phosphate stones are only found in 5.8 %. Diet is rich in purine and oxalate; hyperoxaluria, hypocalciuria, and hypouricosuria are common.

While diabetes is seen in 25–30 % of the population, the linkage with stone disease has not been examined. In Iraq, bladder stones are seen in 15 %. In Jordan, 17.7 % are calcium phosphate. In Iran and Turkey, patients have a strong family history of stones. In Iran the gender ratio is low (1.15:1 as compared to 4:1). A metabolic cause is found in 75 % of pediatric patients.

Keywords

Incidence • Urinary stones • Oxalates • Urates • Prevalence • Geographical variation • Stone composition • Urine composition • Staghorn stones • Calcium oxalate stones • Calcium phosphate stones • Infection stones • Uric acid stones • Cystine stones • Practice patterns Pediatric stones • Age-related stone formation • Recurrence • Stone site

Introduction

The prevalence of urolithiasis is widely variable in different parts of the world, and big differences in urinary stone disease pattern have been reported from different geographical areas [1]. In the Kingdom of Saudi Arabia, the treatment of urinary tract stones remains to form a major part of the urological surgery practice, and they do constitute a major health problem. The pattern of urinary tract stone disease has undergone a continuous change over the years with a higher prevalence of upper urinary tract stones in adults and less lower tract stones in children. The endemic bladder stones have almost disappeared in many regions of the world; and in Saudi Arabia they are extremely rare nowadays [2]. The changing socioeconomic conditions are believed to have contributed to the change in the incidence as well as in the composition of urinary stones [3]. The lithogenic factors that lead to the stone formation and the change in stone disease pattern seem to be multifactorial, where lifestyle and dietary factors play an important role [4, 5].

S.R. El-Faqih, MBChB, FRCS (Glasgow), FRCS (England)
Department of Surgery (Urology), College of Medicine,
King Saud University, P.O. Box 7805, Riyadh, 11472,
Kingdom of Saudi Arabia
e-mail: srelfaqih@hotmail.com

J.J. Talati et al. (eds.), *Urolithiasis*,
DOI 10.1007/978-1-4471-4387-1_10,

Prevalence

In Saudi Arabia, it has been estimated that the expected lifetime risk of a stone episode is at least 50 % higher than in the West, and by the age of 60–70 years, 20 % of men have experienced at least one stone episode in their lives [2, 6]. Data from the Gulf states, including Saudi Arabia, indicate that the problem is essentially an upper tract disease affecting adults—where it may reach an epidemic scale—rather than a lower urinary tract endemic stone disease [2]. The male-to-female ratio is approximately 4:1, and the stones are mainly composed of calcium oxalate and/or uric acid. In fact, the high age-specific expectancy of stone formation in Saudi males has been shown to extend over the entire age range, including children, and idiopathic calcium stone formation in Saudi children is twice as common as in children in the West, with a high proportion of uric acid and urate stones and less struvite stones [7]. These differences may be attributed to dietary habits and lifestyle factors.

Stone Composition

Knowledge of the stone composition may be of great importance as it may help to delineate the possible underlying lithogenic factors and accordingly help in advising the stone formers about preventive measures. In the Saudi Arabian adult population, upper urinary tract stones predominate; the majority of these stones (81.5 %) are composed of calcium oxalate, with uric acid and urate on second place (11.5 %). It is striking that calcium phosphate stones constitute only 5.8 % with less than half of them (2.3 %) being struvite stones. This stone composition is different from what is seen in the West, particularly regarding the low incidence of infection stones [8].

Urine Composition

Metabolic studies in Saudi Arabia have shown striking differences among both stone formers and normal subjects as compared with the West [2]. In the Saudi population studied, there was a lower urinary volume, lower pH, and lower calcium and citrate, while on the other hand, the excretion of oxalate and urate was high (Table 10.1). So the urine in Saudi subjects, in other words, is supersaturated with calcium oxalate and uric acid but has a lower level of calcium. These urinary findings correlate very well with the pattern of stone composition in this country [2].

Table 10.1 Comparison of 24-h urine biochemistry in normal and stone-forming men in the United Kingdom (UK) and Saudi Arabia (KSA)

	UK		KSA	
	Normal	S-F[a]	Normal	S-F
Urine volume (L)	1.6	1.76	1.25	1.56
Urine pH	6.04	6.00	5.82	5.68
Calcium (mmol)	6.0	8.8	3.2	4.6
Oxalate (mmol)	0.33	0.43	0.53	0.69
Uric acid (mmol)	2.9	3.3	4.7	4.8
Citrate (mmol)	3.3	3.1	1.0	–

Adapted from Robertson et al. [2]
[a]*S-F* stone-formers

Diet and Urine Composition

The differences in urine composition could be a reflection of the differences in the dietary habits that influence the excretion of stone-forming substances in urine [3]. Studies on Saudi subjects, stone formers and non-stone formers, have shown that the Saudi diet includes larger quantities of purine and oxalate-rich food stuffs and less calcium than in the West (Table 10.2), that is why hypercalciuria is an uncommon finding in Saudi stone formers [9].

Hyperoxaluria, in fact, is likely to be more important than hypercalciuria regarding the risk of stone formation in Saudi stone formers [9, 10]. Hyperuricosuria, on the other hand, has been reported even in Saudi non-stone-forming subjects in whom the mean 24-h urinary urate content is higher than what is reported in the West [11]. The high urinary oxalate/calcium ratio and high acid load when combined with the reported low urinary volume make the circumstances ripe for calcium oxalate and uric acid stone formation, and this explains their high prevalence. This urine composition may influence the medical treatment of recurrent stones formers. Calcium citrate has been suggested as a treatment of recurrent idiopathic stone formers; it will not cause hypercalciuria because of the already existing low levels of urinary calcium, while in the meantime citrate will have the added benefit of alkalizing the urine, which will reduce the risk of calcium oxalate and the risk of uric acid stone formation [8].

Drinking Water

The relation between the type of drinking water and stone formation has been extensively investigated in the literature. Studies in Saudi Arabia did not show any evidence to relate

Table 10.2 Daily dietary intakes in male calcium stone-formers from the United Kingdom (UK), the United States (USA), and Saudi Arabia (KSA)

	UK	USA	KSA
Animal protein (g)	61	85	87
Calcium (mmol)	24.5	25.0	13.0
Oxalate (mmol)	1.4	2.4	3.8
Purine (mg)	190	257	268
Oxalate/calcium ratio	0.06	0.10	0.29

Adapted from Robertson et al. [2]

stone formation to drinking of hard, tap, or underground water. On the contrary, drinking of soft water alone was associated with a high prevalence of urolithiasis [11].

Climate Conditions and Fluid Intake

In Saudi Arabia the hot weather prevails in most parts of the country and extends over many months of the year. The sweating, dehydration, and documented low urinary volume may contribute significantly to urine supersaturation and stone formation and are regarded as a strong risk factor [2]. Many studies have supported this, not only in native patients, but also in expatriates who spend some time in the region. The association between renal colic episodes and the exposure to dry, hot conditions has been well documented in the region [12–14]. In fact, renal colic was very common in American troops operating in Iraq with documented stone passage in 28 % of that group of patients [15]. The stone development can occur rapidly, with some appearing 90 days after deployment in hot and dry climate [16]; hence, the universal advice to our stone formers is to increase their fluid intake and increase their urine volume to at least 2 L/day.

Diabetes and Obesity

The relationship between renal stones and diabetes mellitus is well-known. Urine from diabetic stone formers has been shown to contain more oxalate and to have lower pH levels than nondiabetic stone formers [17]. The prevalence of diabetes in the adult Saudi population is among the highest in the world and has been estimated to range between 25 and 30 % of population [18], and obesity is running at an epidemic rate with a prevalence of 35 % of the population [19]. Although dietary habits of idiopathic stone formers have been thoroughly investigated in Saudi Arabia, neither has the relation between diabetes and obesity and stone formation been addressed, nor has the role of daily intake of fat been studied.

Urolithiasis in the Region

There are worldwide regional differences in the prevalence of urinary stone disease. These regional variations affect the frequency of developing a stone as well as the composition of the stone. Even in the same country, urinary stone disease may differ from one area to another due to differences in lithogenic factors [20–22].

In Iraq, studies have shown geographical differences between various provinces with a male-to-female ratio ranging from 2:1 to 4:1 [22] with a predominance of calcium oxalate and uric acid stones. There is a predominance of upper urinary tract stones, but the incidence of bladder stones is still relatively high at 15 %, and infection stones are still common in females [22, 23].

In Kuwait, the majority of urinary tract stones is in the upper tract with an average annual incidence of 23.9 in a population of 100,000. The stones are predominantly calcium oxalate (72 %), but uric acid and urate stones account for 15 %. The urine composition is similar to what has been reported in Saudi Arabia with high urinary oxalate and urate [24].

In the United Arab Emirates, the studies show results almost identical to the pattern seen in stone-forming patients in Saudi Arabia [3, 25].

In Jordan, in a study of 486 stone formers, it was found that upper urinary tract stones predominate with a male-to-female ratio of 3:1. Calcium oxalate stones were most common (64.8 %), followed by calcium phosphate (17.7 %), and uric acid (13 %)—a spectrum of stones different from what is seen in Saudi Arabia [26].

In Iran, the data are variable, and this may reflect cultural, lifestyle, and dietary differences in various regions of Iran, and the prevalence is variable with an overall annual pooled incidence rate of 136/100,000 inhabitants [27]. A study from Kerman showed a prevalence of 1.9 %, and the authors attributed this to the geographical location of the Kerman province [28]. This study also showed a very strong family history among stone formers. It is also of interest to note that the male-to-female ratio was as low as 1.15:1 [29].

In Turkey, the annual incidence was reported to be 1.7 % and the male-to-female ratio 1:1, with a strong family history, and the urinary stone disease showed a trend toward a geographical distribution within the country [30]. The prevalence is lower in Black Sea and Central Anatolia and Eastern Anatolia Regions than in Aegean and Southeastern Anatolia regions. The reason for this is not clear, but the population movement toward the western part of the country over the past years may have contributed to this regional distribution [30]. The stones predominantly were composed of calcium oxalate (57 %) and uric acid (8 %), and upper urinary tract stones dominanated [31].

In Algeria, although upper tract stones predominate (77 %), bladder stones are still relatively common. It is interesting to notice that although the pattern of stone disease is changing toward what is seen in the industrial countries with the majority of stones being composed of calcium oxalate, urinary tract infection remains a significant cause of stone formation where struvite stones constitute nearly 29 % of all renal stones. Uric acid stones were found in 8.8 % of the cases in a series of 1,354 stones studied [32].

Childhood Urolithiasis in Saudi Arabia

Despite the high incidence of urinary stone disease in Saudi Arabia, childhood urolithiasis remains an uncommon problem. Nevertheless, in a country where 40 % of the population belongs to the pediatric age group, it remains an important clinical problem that deserves attention for prevention as well as treatment. This is particularly important as an identifiable cause may be found in about 75 % of children with urinary tract stones [33]. Pediatric patients tend to form stones in a recurrent pattern with high recurrence rates, an important point to consider in investigation and treatment of stone-forming children [34].

Data from different parts of the world and in our region has shown a shift in the pattern as well as in the etiology of pediatric urolithiasis [35]. In Saudi Arabia it has been estimated that urolithiasis in children constitutes less than 1 % of all stones and is predominantly of upper urinary tract type. The endemic bladder stones have almost totally disappeared [7, 35, 36]. The mean age at diagnosis is 12 years, and the male-to-female ratio is 2:1. The incidence of urinary tract infection is variable in different studies but has been demonstrated in 10–17 % of the patients [7, 36]. *Escherichia coli* was the commonest pathogen isolated, which is in contrast to many reports of the association between *Proteus* infection and stone formation. *Proteus* strains were not isolated in the population studied in Saudi Arabia [7, 36].

In a study of 85 stone-forming children, 60 % had formed idiopathic stones. It is worth mentioning that nearly 12 % of those children had hypercalciuria in contrast to the adult population of stone formers from the same region in whom the incidence of hypercalciuria was much lower (4.6 %) [7]. Metabolic causes were implicated in 10 % of the patients, mainly in the form of cystinuria and primary hyperoxaluria [7]. Analysis of stone composition showed less struvite, but a predominance of calcium oxalate (35 %) and an interestingly high incidence of uric acid stones of 30 %, a figure that is much higher than the 1.3–7.6 % reported in the Western countries. There were no definite metabolic abnormalities detected in this group of uric acid stone-forming children [7]. Nevertheless, it is very important to emphasize the need for metabolic screening of all stone-forming children because a urinary tract infection, which is very common in these children, can mask underlying metabolic causes, which are now very common and may be the most common cause [37].

The idiopathic (endemic) bladder stones have almost totally disappeared and are considered to be extremely rare, and most of the bladder stones seen were secondary to a definite underlying cause [7, 36].

Childhood Urolithiasis in the Region

In Kuwait, similar figures were reported with a predominance of calcium oxalate stones as well as a high proportion of uric acid stones. Metabolic causes are implicated as the main lithogenic factors, while diet and environmental factors are believed to play a trivial role [38].

In Jordan, childhood urolithiasis constitutes 1.85 % of all stones with the average age of occurrence at 14 years and with a male-to-female ratio in this age group at 2:1. 1.2 % of the stones were composed of cystine [26].

In Iraq, although data on stone composition in children are scarce, studies have shown an early age of occurrence, with the majority of cases diagnosed below the age of 5. There was a high male-to-female ratio of 2.8:1 with a strong family history of stone formation. Metabolic disorders were demonstrated in 52 % of the children, while urinary tract infection was implicated in 25.5 % of patients. Although the majority of stones were found in the upper urinary tract, endemic bladder stones were found in 11 % of the stone-forming children, a proportion which is much higher than in Saudi Arabia [39, 40].

In Iran, it is mainly an upper tract disease with a mean age of occurrence at 3.3 years and a strong family history. The reported incidence of bladder stones was low (3.3 %), and metabolic risk factors were common [41, 42].

In Yemen, although there are very few studies, it is interesting to note the high incidence of uric acid or urate component in as many as 75 % of the childhood stones—this may be related to dietary causes [43].

It is interesting to note that studies from North African countries (Egypt [44], Sudan [45], Tunisia [46], Algeria [47], and Morocco [48]) have shown similar profiles of childhood urolithiasis with predominantly upper urinary tract stones. Calcium oxalate was the major constituent together with the uric acid and urate, but the incidence of struvite stones and endemic bladder stones is still significantly higher than that seen in Saudi Arabia. Metabolic causes ranged from 6 to 20 %, as a reflection of cultural, lifestyle, and dietary habits.

In Turkey, it is mainly an upper tract disease with a male-to-female ratio of 2.3:1. Metabolic abnormalities accounted for 33 % of the stones, and there was a 26 % incidence of infection stones [49].

With the advances in imaging techniques, it is now possible to detect urinary stones in children without exposure to radiation. Ultrasound has been proven to be efficient and very sensitive in childhood urinary stone detection [50]. The convenience and high sensitivity of ultrasound make it readily available and are of great help in early detection of childhood urolithiasis in the absence of specific symptoms of stone disease in this age group [7, 36]. Furthermore early recognition and subsequent treatment of metabolic abnormalities will reduce interventions and will minimize the damage inflected on stone-bearing kidneys in children [51].

Urinary Stone Management in Saudi Arabia

In spite of the extensive metabolic research on stone formation, we are not closer to understanding why stones form or how we successfully can prevent their recurrence after removal. Accordingly stone removal, which can now be done with minimal invasiveness, remains the mainstay of management of patients with urinary tract stones.

The simultaneous introduction of extracorporeal shockwave lithotripsy (SWL) [52], percutaneous nephrolithotripsy (PCNL) [53], and transurethral ureterorenoscopy (URS) [54] in the early 1980s has nearly eliminated the need of open surgery for stones at all locations in the urinary tract in adults and children alike. With the ready availability of these treatment modalities, clinicians have become less critical in terms of indications for intervention.

In Saudi Arabia, urology departments were at the forefront, and institutions have acquired these new technologies and adopted the new treatment modalities early on in their course of development. Scientific papers from various Saudi urological institutions have been published from 1980s, and many institutions have integrated stone management centers, and some run endourology and SWL postgraduate fellowship programs, based on the vast experience of stone management in the country [55, 56].

For simple renal stones of less than 2 cm in diameter, SWL monotherapy, in our experience, as well as that of others, proved to be very successful with more rapid stone clearance for renal pelvic stones than for calyceal stones [55, 57]. The modifications of lithotriptors made the treatment very convenient, and the modification of shockwave delivery improved the results [58]. The introduction of internal ureteral stenting has further expanded the indications of SWL for renal stones, and it is now possible to treat larger stones with SWL in the presence of an internal stent, but stents are not without morbidity. Studies from the author's institution have shown that the morbidity of internal stents in association with SWL treatment is time related; it increases after 6 weeks of indwelling time [59].

In the author's experience, PCNL monotherapy is the best option for complicated renal stones with the highest stone free rate, while shockwave monotherapy proved to be significantly less successful and requires multiple sessions with a high rate of residual fragments [56]. In fact the combination of SWL and PCNL (sandwich) therapy coupled sometimes with internal ureteral stents has further increased the success rate and reduced the intervention morbidities and the need for multiple punctures [56]. The ready availability and adaptation of those modalities have nearly eliminated the need for open renal stone surgery in Saudi Arabia.

The success of SWL in the kidney has expanded its use to the upper ureter and then to the whole ureter. The studies from Saudi Arabia have shown very good results of SWL monotherapy for stones in the whole ureter [60]. The introduction and evolution of URS with intracorporeal lithotriptors and laser have proved to be successful for removal of ureteric stones with very high stone-free rates [61], but obviously it is an invasive technique and not without morbidity, which sometimes can be serious [62]. On the other hand, the very high success rate, coupled with the low morbidity of URS, in management of lower ureteric stones has led us to start a debate already in 1987 on what is the best treatment for distal ureteric stones—SWL or URS [63]. Until now, this debate has not been properly settled. For large bladder stones we have advocated the use of SWL prior to endoscopic evacuation. This will reduce the operating time and reduce the transurethral endoscopic manipulations [64].

In children, pediatric urologists in Saudi Arabia have adopted the aforementioned noninvasive modalities of SWL and various endourologic techniques with excellent results, and with the introduction of miniature endourologic equipments, open surgery even for the hardest of stones is an extreme rarity [65, 66].

Economics and Impact on Healthcare Systems

Urinary stone disease is a common urological problem, and it can affect people of all ages, children, adolescents, young adults, and the elderly, and it is an important healthcare problem in its effects as well as its treatment [67]. The advances in noninvasive treatment of urinary tract stones over the past 30 years have shifted the emphasis away from the thorough metabolic investigations. Although the noninvasive modalities of SWL and endourologic techniques are very efficient in removing the stones, they offer nothing to prevent the stone formation at a time when we know that it is a recurring disease. Accordingly, comprehensive metabolic workup for idiopathic stone formers is required so that the treatment and prevention go hand-in-hand as complimentary measures [68]. Such an approach may help to minimize the risk of stone formation as a cause of chronic kidney disease and reduce the cost and burden on the healthcare system.

Conclusion

In Saudi Arabia, urolithiasis is an upper urinary tract disease with predominance of calcium oxalate and uric acid/urate stones and with less struvite stones even in children. The findings in urine comprise a low volume, low pH, and low calcium, but high oxalate and high urate excretion. Dietary, climate, and lifestyle factors may have contributed to these abnormalities.

In spite of the fact that stones can now be efficiently removed without open surgery in almost all patients, adults and children alike, it is very important to emphasize the need of thorough metabolic studies for idiopathic stone formers in general and for children in particular.

References

1. Trinchieri A. Epidemiology and socioeconomic aspects of urolithiasis. Arch Ital Urol Androl. 1996;68:203–49.
2. Robertson WG, Walker VR, Hughes H, Husain I, El-Faqih SR. Renal stone disease in the middle east. In: Hatano M, editor. Nephrology, vol. 1. Tokyo: Springer; 1991. p. 815–22.
3. Hussain I, Badsha SA, Al Ali IH, Walton M, Saheb A, Jafree S. A survey of urinary stone disease in Abu Dhabi. Emir Med J. 1979;1: 17–33.
4. Robertson WG. Renal stones in the tropics. Semin Nephrol. 2003;23(1):77–87.
5. Robertson WG. Renal stones: an update with particular reference to their cause and treatment in the Arabian Peninsula. K KAU Med Sci. 1995;4:3–15.
6. Robertson WG, Hughes H. Epidemiology of urinary stone disease in Saudi Arabia. In: Ryall R, Bais R, Marshall VR, Rofe AM, Smith LH, Walker VR, editors. Urolithiasis 2. New York/London: Plenum Press; 1994. p. 453–5.
7. Al-Rasheed SA, El-Faqih SR, Husain I, Abdurrahman M, Al-Mugeirin MM. The aetiology and clinical pattern of childhood urolithiasis in Saudi Arabia. Int Urol Nephrol. 1995;27(4):349–55.
8. Husain I, El-Faqih SR. Renal stone in the tropics: epidemiology, pathogenesis and current choices in non-surgical treatment. Asian J Surg. 1995;18(1):12–9.
9. Robertson WG, Nisa M, Husain I, et al. The importance of diet in the etiology of primary calcium an uric acid stone formation – the Arabian experience. In: Walker VR, Sutton RAL, Cameron ECB, Pak CYC, Robertson WG, editors. Urolithiasis. New York: Plenum Press; 1989. p. 725–39.
10. Robertson WG, Qunibi W, Husain I, et al. The calculation of stone risk in the urine of middle-eastern men and western expatriates living in Saudi Arabia. In: Walker VR, Sutton RAL, Cameron ECB, Pak CYC, Robertson WG, editors. Urolithiasis. New York: Plenum Press; 1989. p. 669–71.
11. Abdel-Halim RE, Baglaf AO, Sibaei Al, Merzibani M, Hadrami MS, Noorwali A, et al. Urolithiasis in the Western Region of Saudi Arabia: a clinical, biochemical and epidemiological study. Riyadh: King Abdul Aziz City for Science and Technology; 1996. p. 74–278.
12. Khan AS, Rai ME, Gandapur G, Pervaiz A, Shah AH, Hussain AA, Siddiq M. Epidemiological risk factors and composition of urinary stones in Riyadh Saudi Arabia. J Ayub Med Coll Abbottabad. 2004;16(3):56–8.
13. Nouri-Majalan N, Baghianimoghadam B, Amiri N, Moghaddasi-Moosavi S. Metabolic abnormalities in patients with recurrent stone formation in a hot territory. Bratisl Lek Listy. 2010;111(2):79–82.
14. Boscolo-Berto R. Seasonal variations of renal colics and urolithiasis: is this the time for a shared benchmark to study the phenomenon? Urol Res. 2010;38(6):523–4.
15. Pugliese JM, Baker KC. Epidemiology of nephrolithiasis in personnel returning from operation freedom. Urology. 2009;74(1):56–60.
16. Evans K, Costabile RA. Time to development of symptomatic urinary calculi in a high environment. J Urol. 2005;173:858–61.
17. Eisner BH, Porten SP, Bechis SK, Stoller ML. Diabetic kidney stone formers excrete more oxalate and have longer urine pH than nondiabetic stone formers. J Urol. 2010;183(6):2244–8.
18. Alqurasgi KA, Aljabri KS, Bokhari SA. Prevalence of diabetes mellitus in a Saudi community. Ann Saudi Med. 2011;31(1):19–23.
19. Al-Nozha MM, Al-Mazrou YY, Al-Maatouq MA, Arafah MR, Khalil MZ, Khan NB, et al. Obesity in Saudi Arabia. Saudi Med J. 2005;26(5):824–9.
20. Knoll T. Epidemiology, pathogenesis, and pathophysiology of urolithiasis. Eur Urol Suppl. 2010;9:802–6.
21. Abdel-Halim RE. Urolithiasis in adults: clinical and biochemical aspects. Saudi Med J. 2005;26(5):705–13.
22. Afaj AH, Sultan MA. Mineralogical composition of the urinary stones from different provinces in Iraq. ScientificWorldJournal. 2005;21(5):24–38.
23. Qaader DS, Yousif SY, Mahdi LK. Prevalence and etiology of urinary stones in hospitalized patients in Baghdad. East Mediterr Health J. 2006;12(6):853–61.
24. El-Reshaid K, Mughal H, Kappor M. Epidemiological profile, mineral metabolic pattern and crystal crystallography of urolithiasis in Kuwait. Eur J Epidemiol. 1997;13(2):229–34.
25. Nasir SJ. The mineralogy and chemistry of urinary stones from the United Arab Emirates. Qatar Univ Sci J. 1999;18:189–202.
26. Alsheyab F, Hani IB, Mosameh Y. Chemical composition of urinary calculi in North Jordan. J Biol Sci. 2007;7(7):1290–2.
27. Basiri A, Shakhssalim N, Khoshdel AR, Naghavi M. Regional and seasonal variation in the incidence of urolithiasis in Iran: a place for obsession in case finding and statistical approach. Urol Res. 2009; 37(4):197–204.
28. Ketabchi AA, Aziziolahi GA. Prevalence of symptomatic urinary calculi in Kerman, Iran. Urol J. 2008;5(3):156–60.
29. Safarinejad MR. Adult urolithiasis in a population-based study in Iran: prevalence, incidence and associated risk factors. Urol Res. 2007;35:73–82.
30. Muslumanoglu AY, Binbay M, Yuruk E, Akman T, Tepeler A, Esen T, et al. Updated epidemiologic study of urolithiasis in Turkey. I: changing characteristics of urolithiasis. Urol Res. 2011;39:309–14.
31. Yapanoglu T, Demirel A, Adanur S, Yuksel H, Polat O. X-ray diffraction analysis of urinary tract stones. Turk J Med Sci. 2010;40(3):415–20.
32. Djelloul Z, Djelloul A, Bedjaoui A, Kaid-Omar Z, Attar A, Daudon M, Addou A. Urinary stones in Western Algeria: study of the composition of 1,354 urinary stones in relation to their anatomical site and the age and gender of the patients. Prog Urol. 2006;16(3): 328–35.
33. Milliner DS, Murphy ME. Urolithiasis in paediatric patients. Mayo Clin Proc. 1993;68(3):241–8.
34. Noe HN. Hypercalciuria and pediatric stone recurrences with and without structural abnormalities. J Urol. 2000;164(3 Pt 2):1094–6.
35. El-Faqih SR, Husain I, et al. Renal stone in the middle east: epidemiology and pathogenesis. In: Talati J, editor. The management of lithiasis: the rational deployment of technology. Dordrecht/Boston/ London: Kluwer Academic Publishers; 1997. p. 41.
36. Al-Rasheed S, Al Jurayyan AM, Al Nasser MN, Al Mugeiren MM, Al-Salloum AA, Petterson BA. Nephrolithiasis in children and adolescents in the South Western region in Saudi Arabia. Saudi J Kidney Dis Transpl. 1995;6(4):396–9.
37. Coward RJM, Peters CJ, Duffy PG, Corry D, Kellet MJ, Choong S, et al. Epidemiology of paediatric renal stone disease in the UK. Arch Dis Child. 2003;88:962–5.
38. Al-Eisa AA, Al-Hunayyan A, Gupta R. Pediatric urolithiasis in Kuwait. Int Urol Nephrol. 2002;33(1):3–6.
39. Ali SH, Rifat UN. Etiological and clinical patterns of childhood urolithiasis in Iraq. Pediatr Nephrol. 2005;20(10):1453–7.

40. Aboud MJ, Kadhim MM. Review for urolithiasis in patients attending the paediatric surgery unit at Al-Qadisiya Governorate, Iraq. N Iraqi J Med. 2010;6(3):17–23.
41. Mortazavi F, Mahbubi L. Clinical features and risk factors of pediatric urolithiasis. Iran J Ped. 2007;17(2):129–33.
42. Sepahi MA, Heidari A, Shajari A. Clinical manifestation and etiology of renal stones in children less than 14 years age. Saudi J Kidney Dis Transplant. 2010;21(1):181–4.
43. Holman E, Khan AM, Flasko T, Toth C, Salah MA. Endoscopic management of pediatric urolithiasis in a developing country. Urology. 2004;63:159–62.
44. Aggour A, Ziada AM, Abdelhamid AZ, Abdelrahman S, Morsi A. Metabolic stone composition in Egyptian children. J Pediatr Urol. 2009;5(2):132–5.
45. Elfadil GA, Ibrahim ME, Ahmed SAM. Metabolic constituents of urinary stone composition in Sudanese children. Egypt Acad J Biol Sci. 2010;2(2):21–5.
46. Alaya A, Nouri A, Najjar MF. Urolithiasis in Tunisian children: a study of 100 cases. Saudi J Kidney Dis Transplant. 2009;20(6):1096–100.
47. Harrache D, Mesri A, Addou A, Semmoud A, Lacour B, Daudon M. Urolithiasis in children in West Algeria. Ann Urol (Paris). 1997;31(2):84–8.
48. Qussama A, Kzaiber F, Mernari B, Semmoud A, Daudon M. Analysis of calculi by infrared spectroscopy in children from the Moroccan mid-Atlas region. Ann Urol (Paris). 2000;34(6):384–90.
49. Bak M, Ural R, Agin H, Serdaroglu E, Calkavur S. The metabolic etiology of urolithiasis in Turkish children. Int Urol Nephrol. 2009;41(3):453–60.
50. Al Rasheed SA, Al Mugeiren MM, Al-Faqih SR, Hussein I, Muzrakchi A. Ultrasound detection rate of children urilithiasis. Ann Trop Paediatr. 1992;12(3):317–20.
51. Gurgoze MK, Sari MY. Results of medical treatment and metabolic risk factors in children with urolithiasis. Pediatr Nephrol. 2011; 26:933–7.
52. Chaussy C, Schmiedt E, Jocham D, Brendel W, Forssmann B, Walther V. First clinical experience with extracorporeally induced destruction of kidney stones by shock waves. J Urol. 1982;127:417–20.
53. Alken P, Hutschenreiter G, Gunther R, Marberger M. Percutaneous stone manipulation. J Urol. 1981;125:463–6.
54. Perez-Castro Ellendt E, Martinez-Pineiro JA. Ureteral and renal endoscopy. A new approach. Eur Urol. 1982;8:117–20.
55. Husain I, El-Faqih SR, Ekman P, Seraj P. Extracorporeal lithotripsy in the management of renal stone. Emir Med J. 1986;4:108–15.
56. El-Faqih SR. Non-surgical management of complicated renal stone. Emir Med J. 1988;6:7–10.
57. Talic RF, El-Faqih SR. Extracorporeal shock wave lithotripsy for lower pole nephrolithiasis: efficacy and variable that influence treatment outcome. Urology. 1998;51(4):544–7.
58. Madbouly K, El-Tiraifi AM, Seida M, El-Faqih SR, Atassi R, Talic RF. Slow versus fast shock wave lithotripsy rate for urolithiasis: a prospective randomized study. J Urol. 2005;173(1):127–30.
59. El-Faqih SR, Shamsuddin AB, Chakrabarti A, Atassi R, Kardar AH, Osman MK, et al. Polyurethane internal ureteral stents in treatment of stone patients: morbidity related to indwelling times. J Urol. 1991;146:1487–91.
60. Farsi HM, Mosli HA, Alzemaity M, Behnesy AA, Ibrahim MA. In situ extracorporeal shock wave lithotripsy (SWL) for the management primary ureteric calculi in children. J Pediatr Surg. 1994;29(10):1315–6.
61. Tayib A. Low power laser in the management of ureteral stones. Saudi Med J. 2010;31(3):289–92.
62. Ekman P, Husain I, Sharma ND, El-Faqih SR. Transurethral ureteroscopy. Safety guide wire as an aid to a more aggressive approach. Br J Urol. 1987;60:23–7.
63. El-Faqih SR, Husain I, Ekman PE, Sharman ND, Chakrabarty A, Talic R. Primary choice of intervention for distal ureteric stone: ureteroscopy or SWL ? Br J Urol. 1988;62:13–8.
64. Husain I, El-Faqih SR, Shamsuddin AB, Atassi R. Primary extracorporeal shock wave lithotripsy in management of large bladder calculi. J Endourol. 1994;8:183–6.
65. Farsi HM, Mosli HA, Alzimaity M, Bahnassay AA, Ibrahim MA. In situ extracorporeal shock wave lithotripsy for primary ureteric calculi. Urology. 1994;43(6):776–81.
66. Callaway TW, Lingardh G, Basata S, Sylven M. Percutaneous nephrolithotomy in children. J Urol. 1992;148(3 Pt 2):1067–8.
67. Trinchieri A. Epidemiological trends in urolithiasis: impact on our healthcare system. Urol Res. 2006;34:151–6.
68. Robertson WG. Is prevention of stone recurrence financially worthwhile? Urol Res. 2006;34:157–61.

11 Epidemiology of Stone Disease in Iran

Gholamreza Pourmand and Bita Pourmand

Abstract

Iran is a country of great variation in geography and climate. The urolithiasis prevalence rate is 5.7 %, and the incidence is 145/100,000. The gender ratio (M:F) is 1.15–1.38:1. Stone recurrence occurs in 36 %. The most common coexisting diseases are hypertension (15.8 %) and diabetes (11.4 %). Stone disease is more common in the uneducated; 13.6 % are obese and 37.1 % overweight. The commonest stone components are whewellite (81.5 %), apatite (69 %), weddellite (40.7 %), and ammonium acid urate (24.4 %). In one study, infection stone comprised 6.5 % of all stones.

Keywords

Incidence • Urinary stones • Oxalates • Urates • Prevalence • Geographical variation • Stone composition • Urine composition • Staghorn stones • Calcium oxalate stones • Calcium Phosphate stones • Infection stones • Uric acid stones • Cystine stones • Practice patterns Pediatric stones • Age-related stone formation • Recurrence • Stone site

Introduction

Kidney stones (or renal calculi from Latin *ren*, *renes*, "kidney" and *calculi*, "pebbles") form in the kidneys from dissolved urinary minerals. Renal stones have been found in Egyptian mummies [1], and their history dates back to 4,800 years. Many historical and distinguished persons like Napoleon, Muzaffar al-Din Shah, and Roger Moore (to name a few) have suffered from this disease throughout human history.

The urolithiasis prevalence rate has been variably reported to be in the range of 3.5–18.5 % [2]. The most common stone constituents are calcium, oxalate, protein, carbohydrate, and phosphate (Fig. 11.1). The following influencing factors can play a role in kidney stone formation: environment, diet, gender (men outnumber women by ratios roughly between 1.5 and 2.1 or more), geography, fluid intake, climate and season (within most countries, warmer climates are associated with more stones), occupation (stones have been repeatedly associated with "hot" or outdoor occupations such as lifeguards), culture (intra-family marriages, religious customs, and traditional rituals), and associated diseases (obesity, diabetes, hypertension, gout, possible role of *Oxalobacter formigenes* or nanobacteria).

Among the most widely accepted risk factors of urolithiasis—including age, race and ethnicity, education, body mass index (BMI), hypertension, medication, mean annual temperature, annual sunlight level, and ultraviolet radiation—a few have been studied in Iran.

Geographical Specifications of Iran

Iran is an Asian country located in the Middle East with the total area of 1,648,195 km^2 and a population of 72 million. The Caucasus Mountains are located in the north of the country and the Persian Gulf as well as tropical regions in

G. Pourmand, M.D. (✉) • B. Pourmand, M.D.
Department of Urology, Research Development Center, Sina University Hospital, Tehran University of Medical Sciences, Imam Khomeini Street, Hassan Abad Sq., Tehran, Iran
e-mail: gh_pourmand@yahoo.com; bita_pourmand@yahoo.com

J.J. Talati et al. (eds.), *Urolithiasis*,
DOI 10.1007/978-1-4471-4387-1_11, © Springer-Verlag London 2012

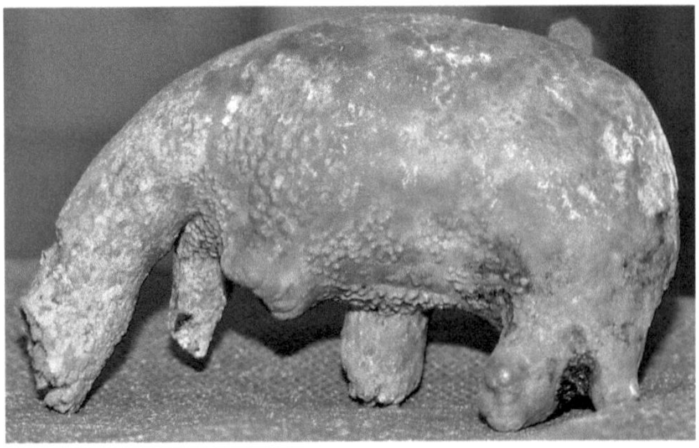

Fig. 11.1 Example of a large Iranian kidney stone

the southern part. Therefore, this vast country has a very wide range of climatic conditions from freezing mountainous areas to hot deserts; there is a great difference between temperature and humidity in various parts of Iran. Consequently, two of the widespread influencing factors of urolithiasis, namely, climate and geographical location, are present in this region. It can be presumed that there is a remarkable potential for residents of Iran to form kidney stones.

Temperature differences reach 19 °C (in September) or 26.3 °C (in February) and humidity differences may be as great as 98 %.

Urolithiasis in Iranian Clinical Research

The first study was conducted on 8,413 persons randomly selected from 30 provinces of Iran [3]. The prevalence of urinary stones was 5.7 % (436 patients). In the two age groups 15–29 and 60–69 years, the prevalence was 0.9 and 8.2 %, respectively. The male-to-female ratio was 1.15:1. The annual incidence of urolithiasis was 145.1/100,000 in 2005 (the population under study is 8,413 persons). The majority of patients (56 %) experienced their first stone episode. Stone recurrences were observed in 36 % of patients in the 30- to 39-years age group. The average cumulative recurrence rates after 1, 5, and 10 years were 16, 32, and 53 %, respectively.

Iran is a multiethnic country with Arab, Fars, Kurdish, Turkish, etc., ethnicities; however, ethnicity did not have a significant effect on the prevalence.

The regional distribution was more prevalently found in south central (Kerman and Hormozgan provinces) and southwest (Fars, Boushehr, Khoozestan, Ilam, and Chaharmahal-va-Bakhtiari provinces) of the country. The mentioned provinces are among the ones receiving a great deal of sunlight. As expected, sunlight was a factor of prevalence increment. Increased production of 25-hydroxycholecalciferol in the skin, after conversion to 1.25-dihydroxy-vitamin D, increases the intestinal absorption of calcium.

Overweight, defined as a BMI above 25, was considered a risk factor for forming kidney stones by 72 % of male and 61 % of female cases of the study.

Obesity, use of diuretics, hypertension, unemployment, tea, cola, meat, positive family history of urinary stones, and higher temperature are positively associated with urolithiasis, while consumption of coffee, dairy products, and cereals as well as the educational level had a negative association. Fish, vegetable, and fruit consumption did not show any specific impact.

The annual incidence of stone formation in industrialized regions is generally considered to be 150–200 cases/100,000 [4]. The prevalence of urolithiasis in Iran (5.7 %) does not match the prevalence rates of the neighboring countries but almost equals the rates of Western Europe. Some of the countries with similar rates are Japan (7 %) [5], USA (8 %) [6], Germany (4.7 %) [5], and Korea (3.5 %) [7].

The second study, a nationwide multicenter epidemiologic study, was carried out on 12 ecologic zones across Iran during four seasons from September 2006 to August 2007 [8]. From among the 117,956 referrals to the radiologic centers, 6,089 image-proven cases were picked.

Factors investigated in this study were age, gender, race, geographic location, education, body mass index, and hypertension. First presentation, old symptomatic, old asymptomatic, and incidentally detected cases were 39.5, 36.2, 11.5, and 7.3, respectively.

The male-to-female ratio was 1.38:1 with the mean age of 41.5 ± 16.3 years and the peak incidence range of 55–65 years.

The diagnosis was primarily based on KUB (kidneys, ureters, and bladder) X-ray examinations (28.1 %), ultrasonography (85.3 %), and intravenous pyelography (IVP, 18.6 %). It was discovered that the most common coexisting diseases were hypertension (15.8 %) and diabetes (11.4 %). The number of uneducated cases outweighed the educated (24.5 %). Moreover, most cases were current smokers (20 %).

BMI was not a significant factor as only 13.6 % of the patients were obese; 37.1 and 49.3 % were overweight and normal/underweight, respectively. The incidence rate was 407/100,000, and the disease was more likely to present in the autumn.

It could be concluded that the prevalence of the disease was 5.7 % with an incidence of 1,360/one million. It was also found that west-central and southwest were the geographically stone-predominant regions of the country.

Joint Research Between Tehran University and Autonoma University, Spain

The mineral composition of 103 stones from Iran was determined by polarization microscopy and infrared spectroscopy, and the most common components were whewellite (81.5 %), apatite (69 %), weddellite (40.7 %), and ammonium acid urate (24.4 %). Ectopic ossification was found in 2.9 % of the stone nuclei.

Twenty-five patients were from children, who had formed both ammonium acid urate and calcium oxalate stones. This suggests that a high proportion of the Iranian children with urolithiasis have nutritional disorders [9].

Tehran University and University of Bonn, Germany (2004)

In this study, 241 patients comprising 145 males with the mean age of 40.4 years and 96 females with a mean age of 42.5 years were studied. The mean calculus weight and number were 4.28 g and 4.33, respectively [10].

There were 34 (14.1 %) pure calculi comprising carbonate apatite (2), weddellite (6), brushite (1), ammonium monohydrate (2), uric acid (19), struvite (1), and cystine (3). In 207 (85.6 %) patients, the stones had a mixed composition.

Joint Research with Microbiology Department of Public Health School of TUMS

The prevalence of infected stones in the urinary tract was studied in 168 patients including 116 males and 52 females with the mean age of 37 years. Seven cases with positive urine cultures had infected stones (6.4 %), 6 cases with non-infected stones grew organisms (3.8 %), and infected stones comprised 6.5 % of all stones [11].

Proteus mirabilis and *Pseudomonas aeruginosa* were the most commonly encountered bacteria (18 %). Urease-positive bacteria were observed in 54 % of the infected stones and 6 % of noninfected stones. Urine and stone samples explained that only 14.5 % had the same type of bacteria.

In 2006, urinary proteins were evaluated in a case-controlled study conducted in 100 calcium stone formers. The mean age of patients with at least two episodes of calcium stone formation was 38.6±10.3 years. The control group included 100 healthy individuals with a mean age of 33.8±9.7 years. There was a significant positive correlation between urinary citrate and promoters of stone formation, including urinary calcium, oxalate, and urate in the control group. The Tamm-Horsfall protein level in urine of stone formers was not quantitatively different from that of healthy individuals, but the level increased in association with bacteriuria. Albumin and transferrin might play a presumptive role in stone formation [12].

Conclusion

In order to make comprehensive plans for reducing the prevalence of stone formation, each country needs to determine the factors affecting stone formation. Iran has various climatic conditions and lifestyles; also, temperature and humidity are subject to great differences in various regions. Since 30 years, multidimensional studies have been conducted on epidemiologic aspects and chemical analysis as well as on the relationship between stones and associated diseases, age, weight, sex, etc. The prevalence of the disease is currently estimated to be 5.7 % and its male-to-female ratio shows a slight increase.

Like other parts of the world, calcium oxalate is the most common stone and most others are mixed ones. In one study, infection stones comprised 6.5 % of all stones. The most prevalent microorganisms in infection stone diseases are *Proteus mirabilis* and *Pseudomonas aeruginosa*. In tropical regions, it is probable that exposure to more sunlight, influences stone formation. Tamm-Horsfall protein excretion was increased in patients whose stones were accompanied by bacteriuria.

Based on the study of inhibitors and promoters of urinary stones as well as epidemiologic factors, countries would be able to prepare protocols for preventing stone formation.

References

1. Cotte M, Walter P, Tsoucaris G, Dumas P. Studying skin of an Egyptian mummy by infrared microscopy. Vib Spectrosc. 2005;38(1–2):159–67.
2. Hesse A, Siener R. Current aspects of epidemiology and nutrition in urinary stone disease. World J Urol. 1997;15(3):165–71.
3. Muslumanoglu AY, Binbay M, Yuruk E, Akman T, Tepeler A, Esen T, et al. Updated epidemiologic study of urolithiasis in Turkey. I: changing characteristics of urolithiasis. Urol Res. 2011;39(4):309–14.
4. Rodgers A, Hibbert B, Hess B, Khan S, Preminger G. Urolithiasis 2000. In: Proceedings of the ninth international symposium on urolithiasis. University of Capetown, South Africa, 2000, p. 667.
5. Iguchi M, Umekawa T, Katoh Y, Kohri K, Kurita T. Prevalence of urolithiasis in Kaizuka City, Japan – an epidemiologic study of urinary stones. Int J Urol. 1996;3(3):175–9.
6. Curhan G, Rimm E, Willett W, Stampfer M. Regional variation in nephrolithiasis incidence and prevalence among United States men. J Urol. 1994;151(4):838–41.
7. Kim H, Jo MK, Kwak C, et al. Prevalence and epidemiologic characteristics of urolithiasis in Seoul, Korea. Urology. 2002;59(4):517–21.
8. Ziaee SAM, Basiri A, Nadjafi-Semnani M, Zand S, Iranpour A. Extracorporeal shock wave lithotripsy and transureteral lithotripsy in the treatment of impacted lower ureteral calculi. Urol J. 2009;3(2):75.
9. Cifuentes JM, Pourmand G. Mineral composition of 103 stones from Iran. Br J Urol. 1983;55(5):465–8.
10. Pourmand G, Alidaee MR, Rasuli S, Maleki A, Mehrsai A. Do cigarette smokers with erectile dysfunction benefit from stopping? A prospective study. BJU Int. 2004;94(9):1310–3.
11. Pourmand M, Saeedi K, Pourmand G, Ghaemi E. The prevalence of infected stones in the urinary tract and their relationship to urease positive bacteria. J Nephrol Urol Transplant. 2000;1(1):5–8.
12. Pourmand G, Nasseh H, Sarrafnejad A, et al. Comparison of urinary proteins in calcium stone formers and healthy individuals: a case-control study. Urol Int. 2006;76(2):163–8.

Epidemiology of Stone Disease Over a 40-Year Period in Japan

12

Yoshihide Ogawa

Abstract

Calcium-containing stones are the most common form of nephrolithiasis and account for about 80% of all renal stones. This condition most often occurs in the fifth to sixth decades of life and is more common in men than women (M:F ratio, 2.25:2.62). A hospital-based survey performed in Japan over a 40-year period (1965–2005) showed an increase in the annual incidence of urolithiasis (from 437 to 1,340/million) and its lifetime prevalence (from 4.0 to 10.8%). Shockwave lithotripsy is the mainstay for treatment of stones in the upper urinary tract (90.9%), followed by transurethral ureterolithotripsy, percutaneous nephrolithotomy, and open surgery.

Reviewing the 40-year period, accumulated evidence suggests the importance of lifestyle modification by correcting a Westernized diet, insufficient fluid intake, and poor physical activity for prevention of urolithiasis.

Keywords

Incidence • Urinary stones • Oxalates • Urates • Prevalence • Geographical variation • Stone composition • Urine composition • Staghorn stones • Calcium oxalate stones • Calcium phosphate stones • Infection stones • Uric acid stones • Cystine stones • Practice patterns • Pediatric stones • Age-related stone formation • Recurrence • Stone site

Introduction

Kidney stones arise from the growth of crystals into stones via a process that requires local tissue damage associated with inflammation and/or mechanical stress, the presence of macromolecules in the urine to promote formation of crystal aggregates and adhesion to epithelial cells, and supersaturation of the urine with certain salts (which varies with a circadian rhythm). Urolithiasis tends to recur, but its recurrence can be prevented by altering these factors. However, the only current well-established conservative management of calcium oxalate stones is reduction of urinary supersaturation by correcting both hyperoxaluria and hypercalciuria and by increasing the urinary levels of citrate and magnesium. The extent of saturation may also be influenced by the urine volume, so dietary habits, daily activities, and environmental factors all exert an important effect on urinary saturation. It takes several years for an aggregate of crystals to grow large enough to cause symptoms. Calculi will not grow in undersaturated urine, but most people usually excrete urine that is supersaturated, so there is positive "energy" for precipitation of crystals and for the subsequent growth of crystal aggregates into stones. This "energy" is higher in the early morning and after dehydration.

Stones usually form in one of the kidneys, so stasis of urine and anatomical variations may also play an important role. Physical exercise and early mobilization after bed rest along with a moderate diet and a high fluid intake may be essential for prevention of recurrent urolithiasis.

Y. Ogawa, M.D., Ph.D.
Department of Urology, Tokyo-West Tokushukai Hospital,
3-1-1 Matsubara-cho, Akishima City, Tokyo 196-0003, Japan
e-mail: yoshihide.ogawa@tokushukai.jp

J.J. Talati et al. (eds.), *Urolithiasis*,
DOI 10.1007/978-1-4471-4387-1_12, © Springer-Verlag London 2012

Table 12.1 The annual incidence and lifelong prevalence of stone disease in Japan between 1965 and 2005[a]

	1965	1975	1985	1995	2005
Population in Japan	99.2	111.9	121.0	125.6	127.8
M/F (× million)	48.7/50.5	55.1/56.8	59.5/61.6	61.6/64.0	62.3/65.4
Annual incidence	437	534	657	809	1340
M/F (per million)	638/243	757/317	916/408	1175/461	1920/793
M:F ratio	2.62	2.39	2.25	2.55	2.42
Elderly ratio M:F	9.0/10.4%	10.5/13.0%	12.6/16.9%	18.1/22.9%	25.3/30.4%
(60 years and older)	9.7%	11.8%	14.8%	20.5%	27.9%
Life-time prevalence (M/F %)	4.7/2.1%	5.7/2.7%	7.1/3.6%	9.4/4.1%	15.1/6.8%
Estimated total no. of stone pt. M/F	53,502/20,420	54,751/22,909	79,962/35,538	106,094/41,606	119,149/52,106
Annual incidence of lower UT stones M/F (per million)	47	42	42	59	91
	85/11	73/13	73/12	98/22	141/44

[a]The elderly population (60 years or older) has been increasing during this period

Incidence and Prevalence of Urolithiasis

Japanese people are relatively homogenous from an ethnical point of view and have lived in a similar fashion for a long period. Vesical calculus was common before World War II, but there has been an upsurge in the incidence of upper urinary tract stones since 1935 [1]. A gradual diet-dependent stone wave (Steinwelle) was noted around that time, but dramatic Westernization of Japanese lifestyle occurred rapidly after World War II. The current national health insurance system was introduced in 1961. Calcium-containing stones in the upper urinary tract have increased in incidence since the war along with dietary and environmental changes. Advances in treatment and imaging techniques may also have contributed to a progressive increase in detection and hence the incidence and prevalence of urolithiasis. These trends will therefore probably persist in the near future.

The annual incidence of upper urinary tract stones has increased steadily in Japan from an estimated 437/million (638 in men and 243 in women) in 1965 to 1,340/million (1,920 in men and 793 in women) in 2005 [2]. The annual incidence of upper urinary tract stones has increased 2.3- to 5.4-fold in men and 2.0- to 17.4-fold in women of all age groups except for those under 30 years old. The incidence among men peaks in the fifth and sixth decades of life, while that among women peaked during the third decade in 1965, but after that during the sixth decade. The lifetime prevalence has increased from 4.7% for men and 2.1% for women in 1965 to 15.1% for men and 6.8% for women in 2005, with urolithiasis being more common in men than women during the period (M:F ratio, 2.25:2.62) [2–6] (Table 12.1).

The annual incidence of lower urinary tract stones has increased from 47/million (85 for men and 11 for women) in 1965 to 91/million (141 and 44, respectively) in 2005. The incidence peaks during the ninth decade of life or older [7]. The incidence of lower urinary tract stones is higher in the elderly population, unlike the incidence of upper urinary tract stones, suggesting that its increase is associated with the aging of the Japanese population. The percentage of elderly persons (60 years old) in the total Japanese population has increased from 9.7% in 1965 to 27.9% in 2005.

Stone Removal (SWL, TUL, AND PNL)

The introduction of shock wave lithotripsy (SWL) in Japan markedly altered interventional management of stone disease, and thereafter the benefits of SWL have been recognized throughout this country. Innovative procedures, including percutaneous nephrolithotomy (PNL) and transurethral ureterolithotripsy (TUL), were introduced in the early 1980s, and open lithotomy decreased markedly after that time. These advances in endourology and SWL revolutionized the treatment of urolithiasis, with SWL rapidly taking over from PNL, TUL, and open stone removal (Table 12.2). The total number of patients with upper urinary tract stones (both initial and recurrent episodes) was estimated to be 73,922 in 1965 and 171,255 in 2005 [1, 2, 6]. The total number of patients treated by SWL was estimated to be 43,982 in 1990; 57,787 in 1995; and 62,113 in 2005 [2, 6]. The first extracorporeal shock wave lithotripter in Japan was installed in 1984, and the cost of SWL therapy has been covered by national health insurance since 1988. The number of lithotripters in Japan has shown an explosive increase from 13 in 1986 to 258 in 1990, 528 in 1995, 912 in 2008, and 944 in 2011 [6, 8]. A decrease in the number of patients treated/institution (from 171 in 1990 to 109 in 1995) and the slow recent increase of lithotripters (from 912 in 2008 to 944 in 2011) may indicate that the number of lithotripters has reached saturation [6].

Clinical experience over a 20-year period has proven the safety, reliability, and reproducibility of SWL. More than 90% of patients who need active treatment are eligible

Table 12.2 Treatment of upper urinary tract stones in Japan from 1965 to 2005[a]

	1965–1980	1985	1990	1995	2005
Pt. no. reported	32,779	44,038	59,600	82,022	96,477
Estimated total no.	73,922	77,660	115,500	147,700	171,255
Active treatment	22.4%	23.6%	42.5%	42.9%	39.9%
Expectant treatment	77.6%	76.4%	57.5%	57.1%	60.1%
Lithotripter (year)	0	13 (1986)	258	528	912 (2008)
SWL with/without PNL/TUL (%)	0	18.9%	89.6%	91.2%	90.9%
Estimated pt. no.		1,765	43,982	57,787	62,113
PNL and/or TUL (%)	0	28.0%	7.5%	7.2%	8.3%
Estimated pt. no		2,619	3,682	4,562	5,671
Open surgery	100%	53.1%	2.9%	1.6%	0.8%
Estimated pt. no.	16,672	4,960	1,424	1,014	547

[a]Advances in endourology and SWL have revolutionized the treatment of urolithiasis, with SWL rapidly overtaking PNL, TUL, and open procedures for stone removal. The number of lithotripters has increased rapidly in Japan, and SWL is the mainstay of treatment for stone disease

Table 12.3 Composition of upper urinary tract calculi in Japan from 1965 to 2005[a]

Composition (M/F%)	1965	1975	1985	1995	2005
Ca containing	83.7/71.3	83.7/71.3	84.5/75.0	86.1/82.5	92.1/90.3
CaOx	35.1/17.9	35.1/17.9	37.9/23.4	47.4/31.7	74.9/63.1
CaP	4.2/9.1	4.2/9.1	2.9/7.7	1.5/5.4	6.5/12.8
CaOx + CaP	44.4/44.3	44.4/44.3	43.7/43.9	37.2/45.4	10.7/14.4
Infection stone	7.5/23.3	7.5/23.3	5.2/18.3	2.7/10.5	1.4/5.1
Urate	4.6/1.4	4.6/1.4	5.7/1.4	5.6/2.7	5.5/2.2
Cystine	1.6/1.1	1.6/1.1	1.0/1.1	1.4/1.9	0.7/1.6
Others	2.6/2.9	2.6/2.9	3.6/4.2	4.2/2.4	0.3/0.7

[a]The percentage of calcium-containing stones and uric acid or urate stones has increased gradually, while infection stones have decreased

Table 12.4 Composition of lower urinary tract calculi in Japan from 1965 to 2005[a]

Composition (M/F%)	1965	1975	1985	1995	2005
Calcium containing	50.7/42.7	50.7/42.7	55.0/41.7	58.8/42.9	70.6/41.5
Infection stone	26.2/39.8	26.2/39.8	20.4/44.8	14.2/54.3	13.7/53.3
Uric acid/urate	11.3/2.1	11.3/2.1	13.9/2.9	20.0/0.0	15.4/4.4
Cystine	1.4/1.7	1.4/1.7	0.7/0.7	0.7/0.0	0.3/0.7
Others	10.4/13.7	10.4/13.7	10.0/9.9	6.2/2.8	0.0/0.0

Calcium-containing stones and uric acid or urate stones have increased gradually, while infection stones have decreased

for SWL and, when combined with endourological procedures, more than 95% of patients were able to benefit from this method in 2005 and thus avoided open surgery. Some urologists have become more aware of the limitations and morbidity of SWL (hypertension, renal damage, and diabetes over the long term), and there has been a trend for decreased use of SWL while TUL procedures have increased. The mean annual numbers of patients undergoing SWL, TUL, and PNL during the period from 2007 to 2009 were estimated to 96,967 (85.4%), 14,691 (12.9%), and 1,875 (1.7%), respectively, according to the Japanese Urological Association (JUA) questionnaire survey in teaching hospitals [9]. From a survey conducted by the Japanese Society of Endourology and SWL [8], the number of patients receiving SWL, TUL, and PNL in 2009 was estimated to 105,567 (78.7%), 26,392 (19.7%), and 2,103 (1.6%), respectively.

Stone Composition

Data from a total of 88,975 stones were accumulated from surveys between 1965 and 2005, and analysis showed that 82.7% (M/F 85.2/76.1%) were composed of calcium oxalate and/or calcium phosphate, 7.8% (M/F 4.0/17.6%) of struvite with or without carbonate apatite, 4.4% (M/F 5.5/1.5%) of uric acid or urate, and 1.1% (M/F 1.1/1.2) of cystine (Tables 12.3 and 12.4) [2]. The incidence of stones containing calcium has increased by 8.4% in men and 19.0% in women over that period, while the incidence of infection stones has decreased by 6.1% in men and 18.2% in women. The incidence of uric acid/urate stones is higher in men and that of infection stones is higher in women [2].

Regarding calcium-containing stones, analysis of a small series of 1,816 stones showed that pure stones comprised

58.4% of the total, with calcium oxalate stones accounting for 40–21% monohydrate (whewellite), 6.6% dihydrate (weddellite), and 12.4% combined monohydrate and dihydrate—and calcium phosphate stones accounting for 5.1%. The other 41.6% of the stones consisted of calcium oxalate mixed with other components. Thus, calcium oxalate stones, predominantly in the form of whewellite, showed a high prevalence among pure calculi, while the predominant combinations among mixed calculi were weddellite+calcium phosphate (53%) or weddellite/whewellite+calcium phosphate (47%) and whewellite+uric acid/urate (72%) or weddellite/whewellite+uric acid/urate (28%) [10].

Regarding uric acid/urate stones, a series of 69,949 stones included 3,625 uric acid stones (5.2%), 53 ammonium acid urate stones (0.08%), and 36 sodium urate stones (0.05%) [11].

Infection stones are usually formed of struvite and carbonate apatite, which were reported to account for 174 out of 2,724 stones (6.4%), but their ratio and frequency were not reported precisely [12]. Magnesium ammonium phosphate-containing stones accounted for approximately 20% of all stones before 1960 [13]. Analysis of 735 patients with stone disease revealed recurrence in 38.6% of patients with magnesium ammonium phosphate calculi and 38.9% with mixed magnesium ammonium phosphate-calcium oxalate calculi [14].

Composition of lower urinary tract calculi in Japan between 1965 and 2005 showed that calcium-containing stones and uric acid or urate stones among men had increased gradually, while infection stones had decreased. Calcium-containing stones in the lower urinary tract had remained constant, while uric acid/urate and infection stones showed a relatively slight increase among women (see Table 12.4) [7].

Geographical Variation of Calculi

In Japan, there was a "kidney stone belt" located in the Kinki (Kyoto and Osaka), Shikoku, and Hokkaido districts in 1985, with stones being less common in eastern Tohoku, northern Kanto, and Kyushu districts (Fig. 12.1) [5]. Calcium stones were more prevalent, and infection stones were less frequent

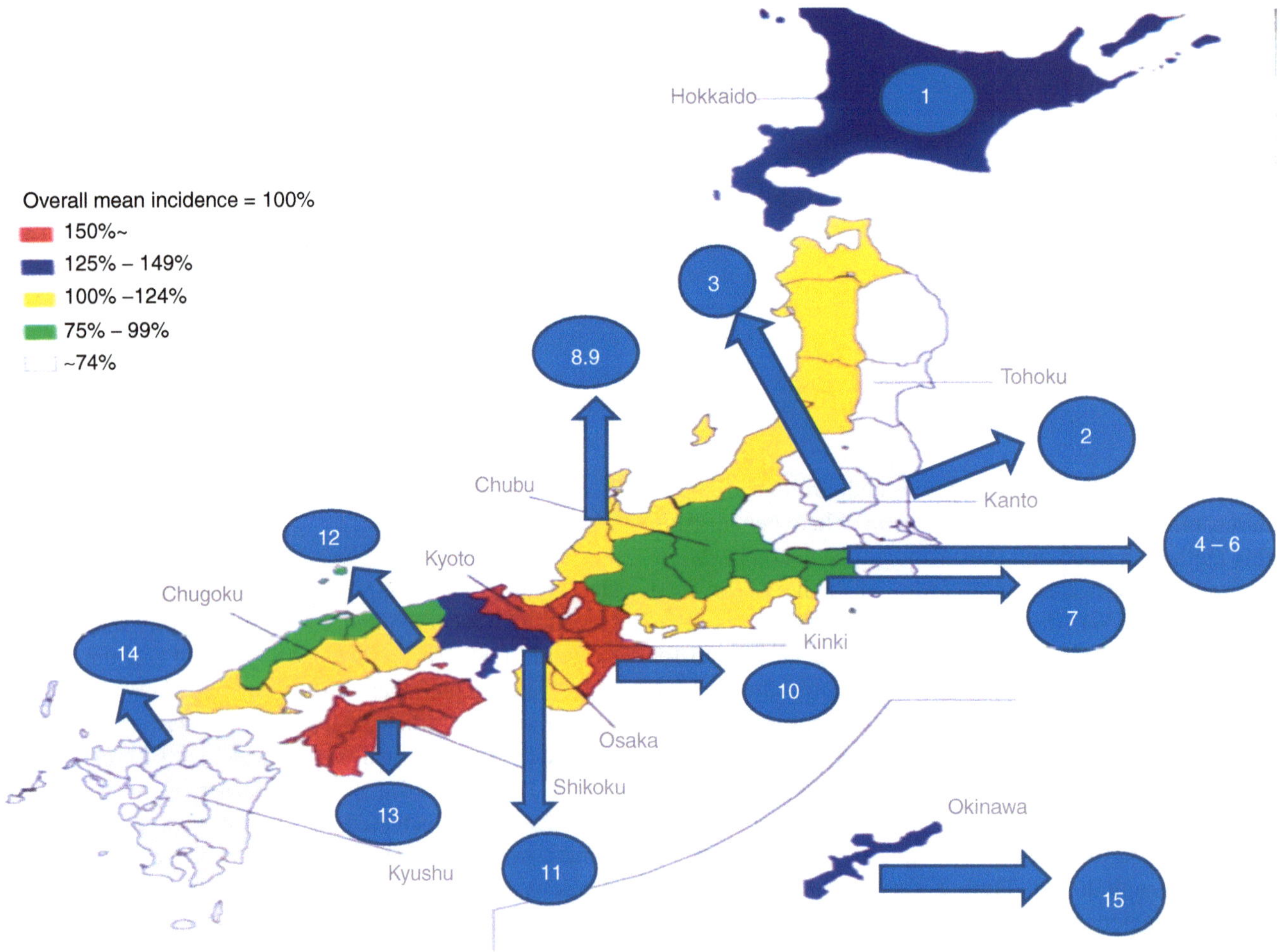

Fig. 12.1 Geographical distribution of the annual incidence of urolithiasis in Japan. The incidence is higher in the Kinki, Shikoku, and southern Chubu and Chugoku districts, while it is lower in eastern Kanto and Tohoku. This pattern has not changed during the last 20 years

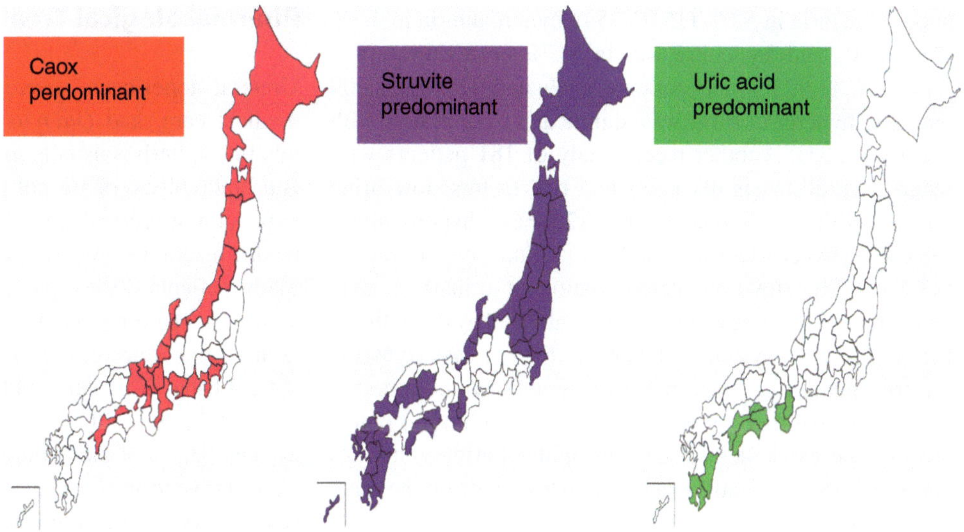

Fig. 12.2 Geographical distribution of stone composition in Japan. Calcium stones are more prevalent (percentage of calcium stones >79%) in urban areas (Tokyo and Osaka area) than in rural districts, while infection stones show the reverse distribution (percentage of struvite stones >10%). Uric acid stones were more prevalent (percentage of uric acid stones >7%) in southern Kyushu, Shikoku, and the southern Kinki district

Table 12.5 Stone composition at different places: reported stone composition from representative areas in Japan[a]

	CaOx (%)	CaOx + CaP (%)	CaP (%)	Struvite (%)	UA/Urate	Cystine (%)	Reference
1 M/F	43.8/33.3	40.6/50.0	0/7.0	1.6/2.4	7.8/4.8		Okuyama et al. [15]
2	34.8	39.6	13.7	3.4	6.0	1.7	Yazaki et al. [16]
3 M/F	19.9/8.4	66.6/56.9	0.4/2.0	8.4/29.0	3.6/2.7	0.8/1.0	Takasaki [13]
4	36.3	38.9	11.6	6.6	4.8	1.8	Matsushita et al. [17]
5	27.4	43.5	6.9	14.1	5.2	2.0	
6	39.8	43.1	9.6	1.6	2.9	0.6	Ishihara [18]
7 M/F	34.0/12.6	52.1/51.6	0.2/1.3	8.1/30.2	3.6/0	1.1/2.5	Odajima [19]
8	23.1	60.4	4.3	3.1	8.5	0.3	Yamaguchi [20]
9	32.3	36.7	1.0	22.1	6.0	1.6	Ikeda [21]
10	43.0	38.7	2.6	3.6	9.1	1.6	Kawamura et al. [23]
11	24.7	54.6	6.2	6.4	6.1	1.1	Koide [24]
12	28.2	46.9	9.7	6.9	5.3		Ueda [25]
13	19.6	47.4		13.4	15.4		Fujita [26]
14	23.2	52.5	0.2	14.6	5.2	1.3	Ikeda [27]
15	40.0	35.4	5.1	3.7	15.8	0	Hossain et al. [10]

[a]The data show variations in relation to time and institutional characteristics

in urban areas (Tokyo and Osaka) than in rural districts. In 1985, uric acid stones were more prevalent in southern Kyushu, Shikoku, and the southern Kinki district (Fig. 12.2) [5]. There have been many reports on the composition of calculi from various local areas at different times, as shown in Fig. 12.1 and Table 12.5 [10, 13, 15–27]. The reported findings vary with time and are not compatible with the nationwide results [29–32].

Etiological Factors

The causes of urolithiasis were investigated from 4 studies in a total of 67,972 stone patients [4, 5, 12, 17]. In 80% of patients, stones were either "idiopathic" or the cause was not evaluated. Excluding such cases, the most frequent etiological factors among the other 13,527 patients (20%) were metabolic and endocrine disorders in 6,555 (48.5%), followed by urinary stasis in 4,394 (32.5%), urinary tract infection in 2,996 (22.1%), immobilization in 979 (7.2%), and drugs in 217 (1.6%). Metabolic and endocrine disorders included hypercalciuria (21.4%), hyperparathyroidism (5.0%), hypercalcemia (0.4%), hypophosphatemia (6.9%), hypomagnesiuria (2.0%), gout or hyperuricemia (42.7%), hyperuricosuria (10.8%), hyperoxaluria (2.7%), hypocitraturia (0.5%), cystinuria (5.2%), and renal tubular acidosis (1.3%) [4, 5, 12, 17]. Assessment of 531 cases of hypercalciuria showed that it was subdivided into idiopathic (22.2%), absorptive (46.3%), renal leak (27.5%), and hypophosphatemic (4.0%) [5].

However, these data are relatively old and measurement of citrate and oxalate was not common at that time. The nationwide survey on urolithiasis in 2005 showed that hypercalcemia was seen in 2.0% (155/7,750 patients), hyperuricemia was in 13.5% (1067/7,905), hypercalciuria in 6.7% (181/2,695), hyperuricosuria in 5.6% (154/2,754), hyperoxaluria in 4.3% (73/1,693), and hypocitraturia in 8.2% (138/1,681) in a series of 11,923 stone patients evaluated [2]. In 1,709 patients, hyperuricosuria was significantly correlated with obesity [2, 31]. Another recent study of 181 patients with recurrent urolithiasis disclosed five risk factors: low urine output (43.6%), hypercalciuria (20.4%), hyperoxaluria (58.6%), hyperuricosuria (31.5%), and hypocitraturia (33.7%) [33]. However, determination of urinary oxalate and citrate is not done routinely or reimbursed by the national health insurance system in Japan, so it is not easy to assess the true pattern of these risk factors nationwide. Another problem is that there is no international definition or cutoff level for these risk factors, so the meaning of urinary findings varies between institutions and is hard to discuss on the same standard level.

Although based on a small series of studies (222 spot urine and 188 24-h urine samples), the following points are worth noting. Hypercalciuria and hyperoxaluria have a major influence on urinary calcium oxalate saturation, and are fairly common (30 and 40%) in critically supersaturated urine, less common (22.4 and 8.6%) in metastably supersaturated urine, and not detected in undersaturated urine. In contrast, hypocitraturia and hypomagnesiuria are often associated with undersaturation and are more common (63.8–80%) at any level of saturation. It is hard to predict the level of calcium-oxalate saturation by using single urine variables and no other urine variable than urinary saturation gives an appropriate indication of the risk of stone formation. Therefore, the saturation level of either early morning urine or a 24-h urine specimen appears to be the best predictor of stone risk [34–37].

Urinary pH is another important lithogenic factor and is closely associated with the crystallization of some special types of stones (uric acid and cystine stones). When urine is acidic (low pH), salting out of these substances occurs and crystals form. The consumption of meat is often associated with a decrease of urinary pH. Mean pH of 24-h urine decreased over a 20-year period (1985–2005) from 6.0 to 5.5 in women and from 5.8 to 5.4 in men according to a longitudinal study of 225,826 individuals (168,042 men and 57,784 women) [38]. This trend was associated with an increased occurrence of the metabolic syndrome in the Japanese population (M/F 25.3/10.6% in 2008). The obesity rate (BMI >25) was 24.8% in 1995 and 31.7% in 2009 among Japanese men aged 20–60 years, while it was 26.0% in 1995 and 21.8% in 2009 among women, suggesting that obesity is still increasing among men but is decreasing gradually among women.

Long-term use of some drugs in 81 patients, such as acetazolamide (59.3%), steroids (28.4%), phenindione (1.2%), vitamin D (2.5%), and PAS-Ca (1.2%), is associated with stone formation [4, 12].

Pharmacological Treatment

Ureteral stones cause severe pain that forces patients to seek medical care, and *Quercus salicina* extract (urocalun 1–2 tab. tid) or herb is usually given to promote stone expulsion. But alpha-blockers are not generally prescribed to promote expulsion of ureteral stones because they are not covered by health insurance. As soon as their pain subsides, however, many patients do not pay attention to the management of stones or make regular visits to the stone clinic. Recurrent stone-formers are usually followed up regularly on an outpatient basis. The nationwide survey on urolithiasis in 2005 showed that more than 10,000 stone patients were followed up, and 63.1% of them underwent mainly dietary education. Stone prevention is considered strongly in patients who have risk factors for increased stone activity, including stone formation before age 30 years, family history of stones, multiple stones at presentation, some special stones (uric acid and cystine), and residual stones after surgical treatment. In reality, medical treatment, including thiazide diuretics (used for 0.4% of patients), allopurinol (3.6%), citrate salts (5.7%), and magnesium salts (0.2%), is still not effectively utilized [30, 31]. Potassium sodium hydrogen citrate (uralyt-U 1 tab or 1 g tid or qid) has been commercially available since 1988 in Japan and annual consumption of uralyt-U was 50% in 1990, 65% in 1995, 65% in 2000, and 85% in 2005 in comparison with that in 2010 (195 million tablets and 46.5 t granules = approximately $40 million/year). Urocalun (*Quercus salicina* extract) has been commercially available since 1969 in Japan, and annual consumption of urocalun was 42% in 1975, 109% in 1985, 99% in 1995, 102% in 2005 in costwise comparison with that in 2010 ($ 8 million); approximately 50 million tablets were prescribed in 1995 and 2000, and 63 million tablets in 2010, showing a mild fluctuation in a period from 1985 to 2010.

Anatomical Abnormalities

Abnormalities of the urinary tract have been reported to cause urolithiasis in 4.6–6.6% of cases by causing pooling or stasis of urine [5, 12]. Such abnormalities may be congenital or acquired [39]. Anatomical abnormalities of urinary tract that can increase the risk of stone formation include horseshoe kidney, obstruction of the ureteropelvic junction (UPJ), dilatation of the collecting system, and calyceal diverticulum. Sponge kidney disease (tubular ectasia) has been reported in 2.0% of men and 2.5% of women with urolithiasis, duplication of the pelvis and ureter in 1.5 and 2.7%, ureteral stricture in 2.1 and 2.5%, and lower urinary tract obstruction in 2.5 and 0.2%, in men and women, respectively [17]. In stone forming patients, the prevalence of sponge kidney disease was reported to be 1/5,000–20,000, while that of calyceal diverticulum was 1/300, horseshoe kidney 1/600–1/1,800, stricture of the ureterovesical junction 1/308 and vesicoureteral reflux 1/500 1/1,000. UPJ strictures were very common (1/100–1/200) [40].

Conclusion

Both historical and current epidemiological data provide a variety of pathophysiological information about urolithiasis. Dietary and environmental changes have been remarkable and have led to an increasing incidence of stone disease over a 40-year period in Japan. Despite ethnic homogeneity, there are some regional differences in the incidence of urolithiasis and stone composition. The available evidence with regard to the importance of changing dietary habits for the prevention of kidney stones emphasizes the need of further steps back to the traditional Japanese diet. Faced with an increased occurrence of the metabolic syndrome due to the current unbalanced diet, we also must reevaluate the classical preventive measures for urolithiasis such as alkaline magnesium salts and pyridoxine (potential association with oxalate metabolism and citrate excretion) [41]. Dietary advice and increased fluid intake are cheap and simple interventions for this preventable renal condition.

References

1. Inada T, Miyazaki S, Omori T, Nihira H, Hino T. Statistical study on urolithiasis in Japan. Urol Int. 1958;7(1–3):150–65.
2. Yasui T, Iguchi M, Suzuki S, Kohri K. Prevalence and epidemiological characteristics of urolithiasis in Japan: national trends between 1965 and 2005. Urology. 2008;71(2):209–13.
3. Inada T. Study of urinary calculi. Nippon Hinyokika Gakkai Zasshi. 1966;57(9):917–29.
4. Yoshida O. Epidemiology of urolithiasis in Japan. Nippon Hinyokika Gakkai Zasshi. 1979;70:975–83.
5. Yoshida O, Okada Y. Epidemiology of urolithiasis in Japan: a chronological and geographical study. Urol Int. 1990;45(2):104–11.
6. Yoshida O, Terai A, Ohkawa T, Okada Y. National trend of the incidence of urolithiasis in Japan from 1965 to 1995. Kidney Int. 1999;56(5):1899–904.
7. Yasui T, Iguchi M, Suzuki S, Okada A, Itoh Y, Tozawa K, et al. Prevalence and epidemiologic characteristics of lower urinary tract stones in Japan. Urology. 2008;72(5):1001–5. Epub 2008 Sep 25.
8. Arakawa T. Present status and perspectives of treatment for urolithiasis in Japan. Jpn J Endourol SWL. 2009;22:142–7.
9. JUA education committee. Questionnaire study of teaching hospitals: teaching workshop 2010. Jpn J Urol. 2010;101(Suppl):S15–7.
10. Hossain RZ, Ogawa Y, Hokama S, Morozumi M, Hatano T. Urolithiasis in Okinawa, Japan: a relatively high prevalence of uric acid stones. Int J Urol. 2003;10(8):411–5.
11. Okada Y. Epidemiological studies on rare urinary calculi in Japan. Hinyokika Geka. 1990;3(8):939–44.
12. Koide T. Urolithiasis. Nippon Rinsho. 1993;51(Suppl):450–6. Review.
13. Takasaki E. Chronological variation in the chemical composition of upper urinary tract calculi. J Urol. 1986;136(1):5–9.
14. Takasaki E. An observation on the composition and recurrence of urinary calculi. Urol Int. 1975;30(3):228–36.
15. Okuyama M, Nishihara M, Kunieda M, Fujii H, Kato Y, Yamaguchi S, et al. Epidemiological characteristics of urolithiasis in Okhotsk coast area in Hokkaido. Hinyokika Kiyo. 2004;50(9):599–603.
16. Yazaki T, Umeyama T, Kikuchi K, Shimazui T, Uchida K, Iizumi T, Takeshima H, Nemoto S, Ishikawa S, Ishikawa H, et al. Study of urinary tract stone – correlation of urinary tract stones analyzed at Tsukuba University with clinical manifestations. Nippon Jinzo Gakkai Shi. 1985;27(1):103–11.
17. Matsushita K, Ishikawa H, Sasaki M, Shinoda M, Nagakura K, Koyama Y, et al. Clinical observation of urinary calculi at the Department of Urology, Keio University. Nihon Hinyokika Gakkai Zasshi. 1982;73(8):1005–10.
18. Takayasu H, Ogawa A, Ueno A, Miyashita A, Kawamura T, Higashihara E, et al. Statistical analysis of urolithiasis. Nippon Hinyokika Gakkai Zasshi. 1978;69(4):436–42.
19. Ishihara Y, Tanifuji T, Higaki Y, Yoshida H, Imamura K. The clinical study of 794 patients with an upper urinary tract stone analyzed by infrared spectroscopy. Hinyokika Kiyo. 1987;33(3):344–52.
20. Odajima K, Mashimo S, Omata T, Arakawa T, Seiichi K, Yoshizawa K, et al. Statistical analysis of urolithiasis. Hinyokika Kiyo. 1987;33(3):353–6.
21. Yamaguchi K, Ohkawa M, Orito M, Fuse H, Nakashima T, Tokunaga S, et al. A clinical survey of urinary calculi in terms of stone compositions. Nippon Jinzo Gakkai Shi. 1988;30(4):375–83.
22. Ikeda R, Suzuki K, Tanaka T, Taniguchi T, Shiraiwa K, Ben A, et al. Statistical analysis on 1,500 urinary calculi by using microcomputer. Hinyokika Kiyo. 1984;30(2):183–9.
23. Kawamura J, Yamasaki Y, Tochigi H, Tajima K, Yanagawa M, Hori N, et al. Epidemiologic study on urolithiasis in Mie prefecture. 1. Present status in 1985. Hinyokika Kiyo. 1986;32(9):1225–30.
24. Kawamura J, Yanagawa M, Tochigi H, Komeda Y, Okabe S, Kinoshita N, et al. Epidemiologic study on urolithiasis in Mie prefecture. 2. Present status in 1988. Hinyokika Kiyo. 1991;37(3):235–42.
25. Koide T, Oka T, Takaha M, Sonoda T. Urinary tract stone disease in modern Japan. Stone incidence, composition and possible causes in Osaka district. Eur Urol. 1986;12(6):403–7.
26. Ueda H. Epidemiological and clinical studies of urolithiasis in Okayama. Nishi Nippon Hinyoukika. 1986;48:107–15.
27. Fujita T, Watanabe H, Ike N, Kondou K. Epidemiological studies on upper urinary tract urolithiasis in Kochi. Jin To Touseki. 1987;(Suppl):355–360.
28. Ikeda M, Ohmori A, Sakamoto K. Upper urinary tract calculi: twenty years' experience in the urology department of Fukuoka University Hospital. Nishi Nippon Hinyoukika. 1994;56:998–1001.
29. Yoshida O, Nonomura M. Epidemiology of urolithiasis. Jin To Touseki. 1987;(Suppl):21–25.
30. Okada Y, Yoshida O. Epidemiology of urolithiasis. In: Ohkawa T, editor. MOOK urology: No. 8 Urolithiasis. Tokyo: Kanehara Shuppan; 1994. p. 47–56.
31. Iguchi M. Epidemiology. In: Ogawa Y, editor. Nephrolithiasis and urolithiasis. Tokyo: Igakushoin; 2007. p. 23–9.
32. Iguchi M. Epidemiology of urolithiasis. In: Kohri K, editor. All about urolithiasis. Tokyo: Igakushoin; 2008. p. 8–11.
33. Yoshimura K, Koide T. Urolithiasis. Nippon Rinsho. 2002;60 Suppl 1:553–9.
34. Yagisawa T, Hayashi T, Yoshida A, Kobayashi C, Okuda H, Ishikawa N, et al. Comparison of metabolic risk factors in patients with recurrent urolithiasis stratified according to age and gender. Eur Urol. 2000;38(3):297–301.
35. Ogawa Y, Yonou H, Hokama S, Oda M, Morozumi M, Sugaya K. Urinary saturation and risk factors for calcium oxalate stone disease based on spot and 24-hour urine specimens. Front Biosci. 2003;1(8):a167–76.

36. Ogawa Y, Hatano T. Risk factors in urinary calcium oxalate stone formation and their relation to urinary calcium oxalate supersaturation. Int J Urol. 1996;3(5):356–60.
37. Ogawa Y. Impact of sodium-potassium citrate on the diurnal variations in urinary calcium oxalate and calcium phosphate saturation levels in normal individuals. Br J Urol. 1994;73(2):136–41.
38. Ogawa Y. Circadian rhythms of urinary saturation levels of calcium oxalate and calcium phosphate in normal male individuals. Hinyokika Kiyo. 1993;39(9):785–9.
39. Tsuji H. Urinary pH and metabolic syndrome. Ningen Dock. 2007;22(3):55–60.
40. Ogawa Y, Hatano T. Genetic aspects of urolithiasis. Mol Urol. 1997;1:65–83.
41. Okada Y, Yoshida O. Anomalies of the upper urinary tract. Nippon Rinsho. 1993;51:457–67.
42. Ogawa Y, Hossain RZ. Vitamin B6 deficiency. In: Kohri K, editor. All about urolithiasis. Tokyo: Igakushoin; 2008. p. 178–9.

Epidemiology of Stone Disease in the Russian Federation and Post-Soviet Era

13

Andrei Novikov, Tair Nazarov, and Vladimir Yu. Startsev

Abstract

The incidence of urolithiasis is very high in all countries of the post-Soviet area. Nowadays stone formation is also highly endemic in areas of the Central Asian republics. The main reasons for stone formation on Russia territory are urodynamic disorders and urinary tract infection, pyelonephritis, and metabolic pathologies. We have noted an improvement of diagnosis and treatment of urolithiasis due to successful scientific and technological development. Due to the results of our evaluation, a special epidemiological program based on the problems of urolithiasis will be developed in Russia in the near future. Our common aim is to join more effective treatment of patients with different forms of kidney stones and prevention of this difficult disease.

Keywords

Urolithiasis • Urinary stones • Russian Federation • Oxalates • Urates annual incidence • Prevalence • Geographical variation • Stone composition • Urine composition • Calcium oxalate stones • Calcium phosphate stones • Infection stones • Uric acid stones • Cystine stones • Practice patterns • Pediatric stones • Age-related stone formation • Recurrence • Stone site

Introduction

The absolute count of officially registered patients with genitourinary system diseases in Russia increased from 12,397,693 to 15,257,971 between 2002 and 2007. The number of registered cases per 100,000 population also increased from 8,675.6 to 10,728 during the same period.

A. Novikov, M.D. (✉) • T. Nazarov, M.D.
Department of Urology,
Northwestern State Medical University,
41, Kirochnaya Str., St. Petersburg 191015, Russia
e-mail: novikov_urol@mail.ru; tair-nazarov@yandex.ru,
tair-nazarov@mail.ru

V.Yu. Startsev, M.D.
Department of Urology,
State Pediatric Medical Academy St. Petersburg,
2, Lytovskaya Str., St. Petersburg 194100, Russia
e-mail: vlad_startsev@mail.ru

The absolute count of registered cases of urolithiasis in the Russian Federation increased from 629,453 in 2002 to 663,374 in 2004. It declined slightly to 656,911 in 2005, but in 2006 increased again to 687,457 cases. In 2007 and 2008, there was a further increased incidence to 691,620 and 704,373, respectively. The number of registered cases in a population of 100,000 rose from 440.5 in 2002 to 463.7 in 2004. In 2005, it declined slightly to 462.7, but again rose to 481.6 in 2006. In 2007 and 2008, the incidence was further increased to 599.3 and 609.3, respectively (Figs. 13.1, 13.2, 13.3, and 13.4).

The maximum frequency index of urolithiasis (for a population of 100,000) was documented in 2002–2008 in the Far Eastern Federal District. The index increased over the period from 529.9 to 714.7. The lowest frequency index (360.6) was recorded 2002 in the Ural Federal District. Low indices were also recorded in the Southern Federal District in 2003, 2004, 2005, 2006, 2007, and 2008 (370.9, 385.5, 386.4, 378.2, 492.94, and 510.3, respectively).

J.J. Talati et al. (eds.), *Urolithiasis*,
DOI 10.1007/978-1-4471-4387-1_13, © Springer-Verlag London 2012

Fig. 13.1 Prevalence of urolithiasis in Russia population in 2002–2008 (in abs.)

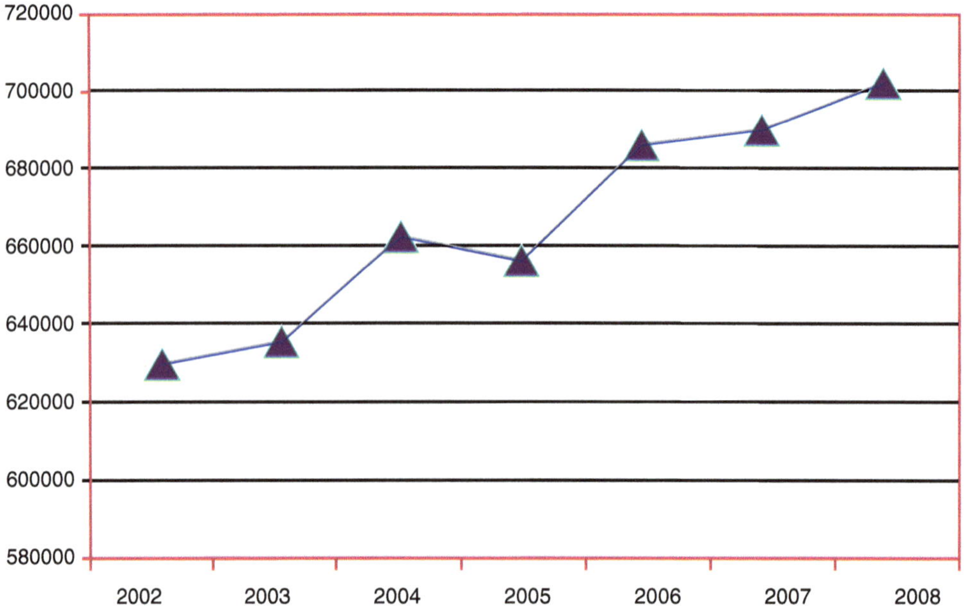

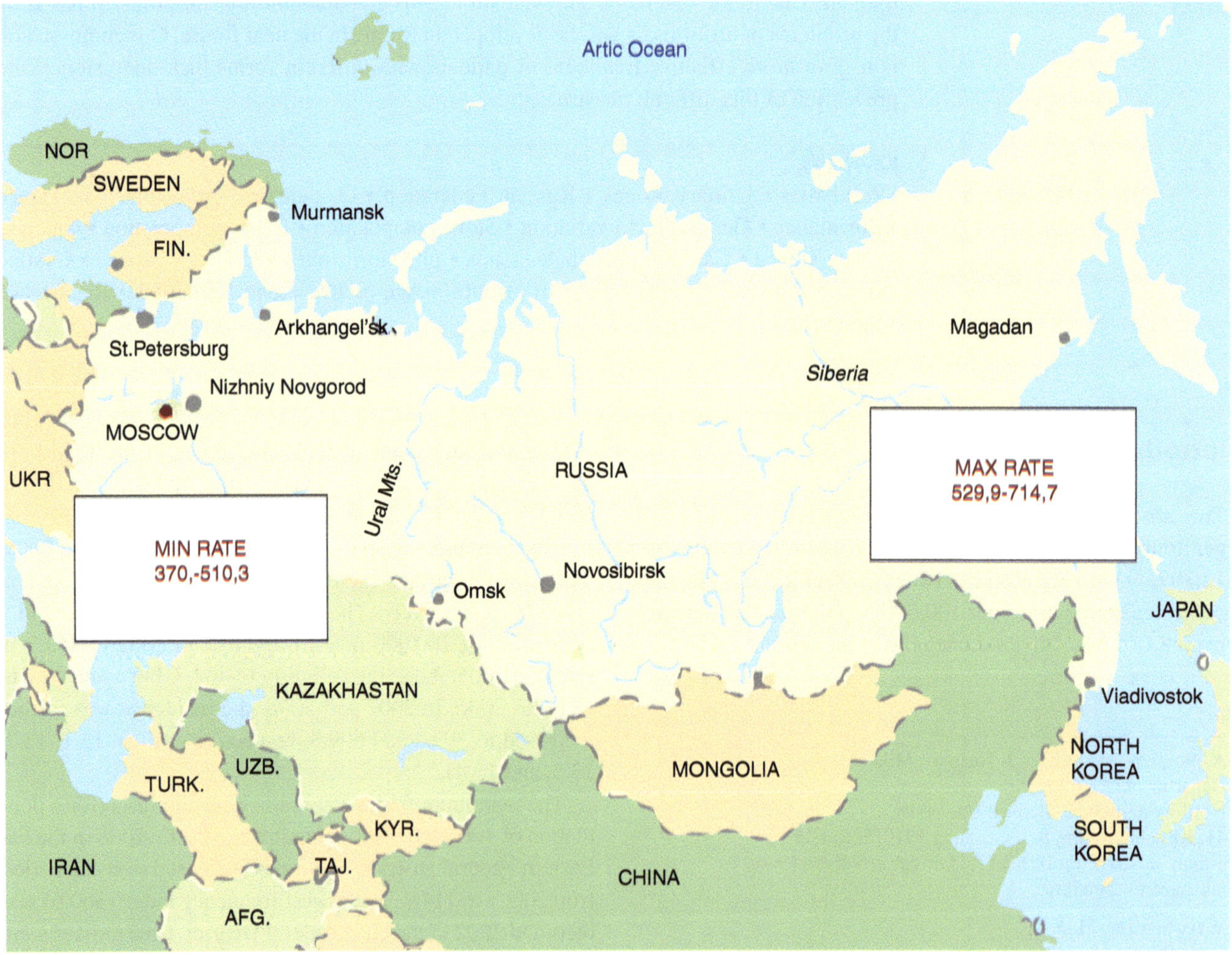

Fig. 13.2 Official statistics about the incidence of urolithiasis on Russia territory in 2002–2008 (per 100,000 people)

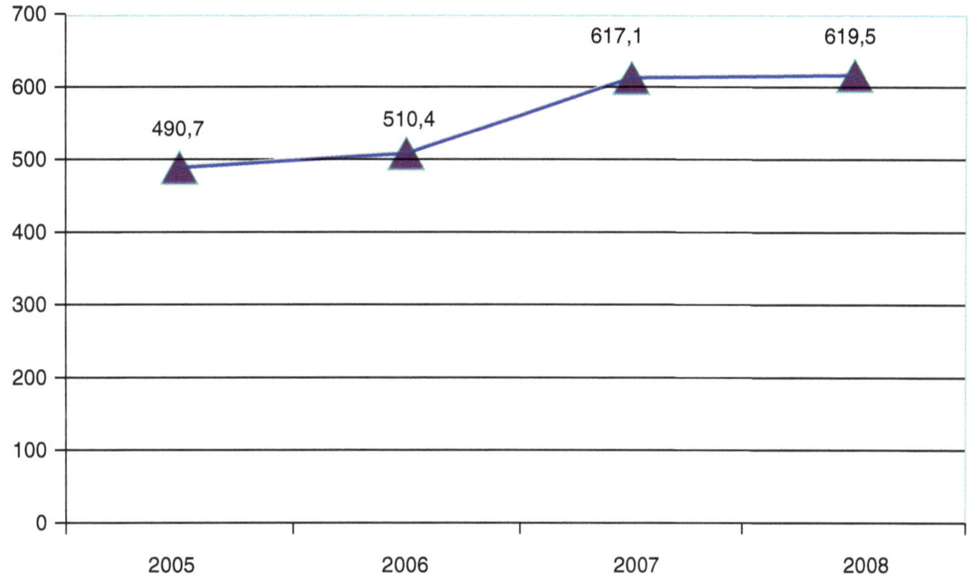

Fig. 13.3 Prevalence of urolithiasis in northwest region of Russia in 2005–2008 (per 100,000 people)

In region-wise analysis, the maximum frequency index of urolithiasis (per 100,000) was recorded in 2002 and 2008 in Altai Krai 1014.1 and 1483.4, respectively. In 2003, 2004, and 2005, the maximum index was observed in the Magadan region with values 1142.2, 1216.2, 1081.3, 1147.7, and 972.7, respectively. Minimum indices of 176.5 and 172.2 were registered in 2002 and 2005 in the Evenk Autonomous Okrug, in 2003 in Karachay-Cherkessia (150.6), in 2004 in the Republic of Kalmykia (180.3), in 2006 in the Agin-Buryat Autonomous Okrug (191.3), and in 2007 and 2008 in the Jewish Autonomous Oblast (237.6 and 252.7, respectively). All those data in comparison with the incidence of the prostate diseases are shown in Table 13.1.

Prevalence and Characteristics of the Mineral Composition of Urinary Stones in St. Petersburg: A 7-Year Retrospective Analysis

In accordance with review of the international scientific literature, the incidence of urolithiasis varies greatly in different countries, with averages of 1–5 % in Asia, 5–9 % in Europe, 13 % in North America, and 20 % in Saudi Arabia [1, 2]. Epidemiological studies in 10 countries show a certain similarity of the geographical distribution of urolithiasis, in terms of the chemical composition of stones [3–5]. However, the chemical composition of bladder stones has its own peculiarities in every country. Moreover, it is known that the clinical and metabolic characteristics of urolithiasis can fluctuate significantly by lapse of time in any particular region [6, 7].

These differences are considered to depend on environmental factors, national dietary habits, and socioeconomic conditions [8, 9]. The goal of the research was to explore specific characteristics of urolithiasis and prevalence of its metabolic types, based on the results from a 7-year retrospective analysis of the mineral compounds of ureteral calculi obtained from patients in St. Petersburg (Fig. 13.5).

Data and Methods

The data for study were provided by the results of a 7-year retrospective analysis of 750 cases of stones removed surgically or fragmented by contact and extracorporeal lithotripsy or just spontaneously passed in urolithiasis patients residing in St. Petersburg. To determine the mineral composition of urinary calculi, X-ray diffraction phase analysis (XRD) and infrared spectroscopy (IR spectroscopy) were used as the most informative methods of examination. The crystal-chemical structure of the stones was defined by XRD (diffractometer "DRON-3"). IR spectroscopic analysis (spectrometer "Specord-75 IR") made it possible to detect and to identify organic and inorganic substances without crystal structure.

Results

Among all the studied crystallites, some types occurred more frequently: botryoidal, spheroidal, and ellipsoidal. Some crystallites had dendritic irregular shape; few of them had cloddy shape with outgrowths or uneven surface. The kidney stones were likely to have intricate shapes. Stones found in the kidney had a dendritic morphology with a main stone body and many outgrowths. Urinary stones can be different in color with variations from brown to white, due to their composition. The examined stones had a size range between 7 and 5 cm, and each weighed less than 30 g. It was

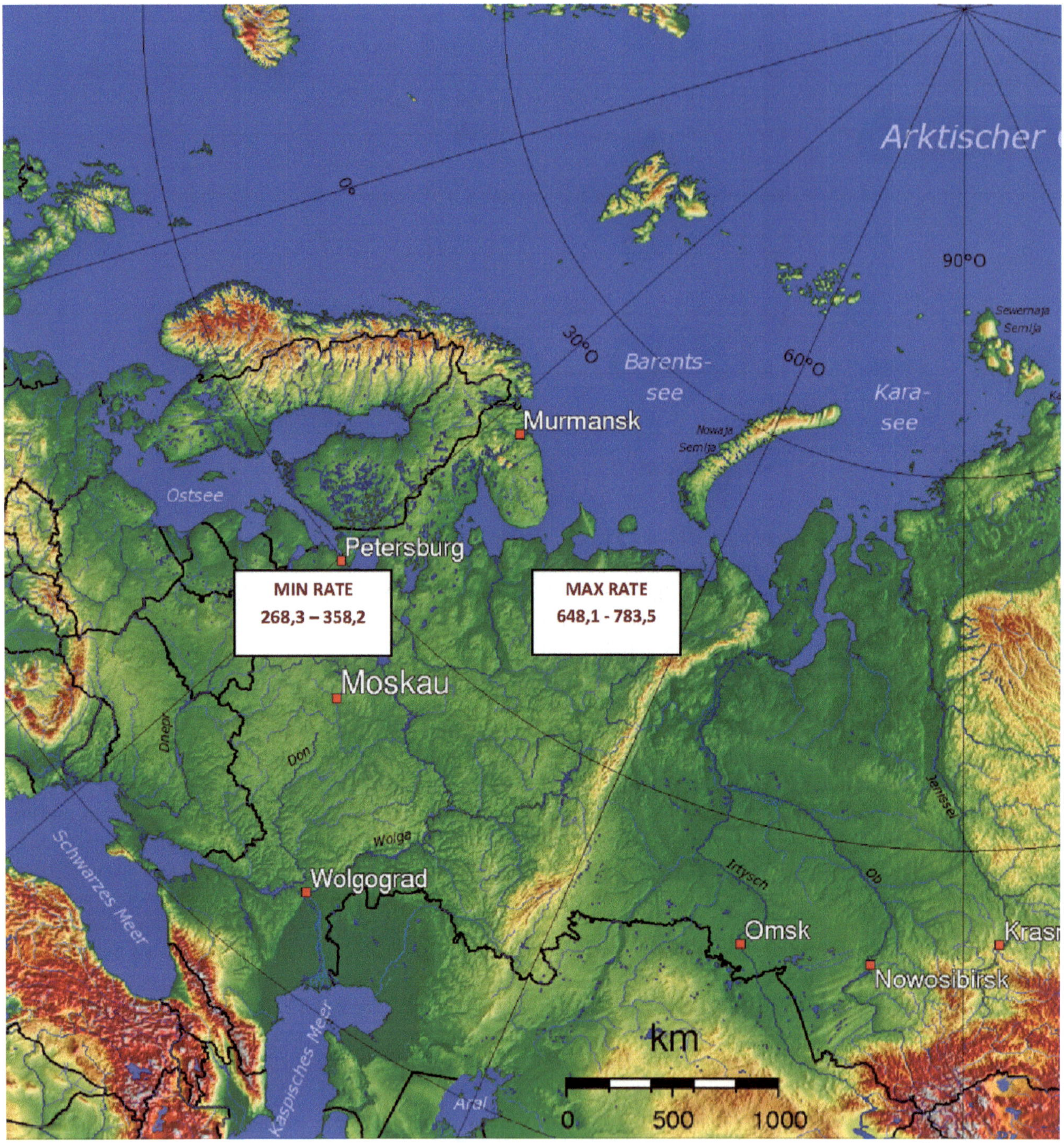

Fig. 13.4 Official statistics about the incidence of urolithiasis in the northwest region of Russia (per 100,000 people). *Minimum rate*: 268.3–358.2. *Maximum rate*: 648.1–783.5 (Modified with permission from http://upload.wikimedia.org/wikipedia/commons/3/3d/Russland_topo.png)

noticed that large stones formed in men twice as often as in women. Four types of stones were identified according to the mineral composition: oxalate stones, phosphate stones, uric acid/urate stones, and cystine stones. The stones of mixed composition were subsumed to the particular group based on their prevailing components. Oxalate stones occurred in 66 % of the cases, phosphate stones in 20.8 %, uric acid/urate stones in 10.5 %, and cystine stones in 2.7 % (Table 13.2). The sex distribution of the patients is shown in Fig. 13.6.

Monomineral stones were found in 278 patients (37.1 %) and compound stones in 472 patients (62.9 %) (Fig. 13.7).

Oxalate stones occurred more frequently in men (35.9 %) than in women (30 %) and phosphate stones more often in women (12.4 % vs. 8.5 %). Uric acid/urate and cystine stones were found in men 2.2 and 2.9 times more often than in women. Among all the collected calculi, 20 mineral compounds were encountered most frequently: calcium oxalates (whewellite, weddellite), calcium phosphates (apatite, struvite), and urates (uric acid). In some rare cases, brushite, cystine, and xanthine

Table 13.1 The incidence expressed in total numbers and frequency index of urolithiasis in the federal subjects of Russian Federation

Officially registered patients (adults)				
	Urolithiasis			
	Absolute count per 100 000 population			
	2007	2008	2007	2008
Federal subjects of the Russian Federation	691,620	704,373	599.3	609.3
Central Federal District	192,060	193,563	615.6	619.9
Belgorod Oblast	6,733	6,446	539.4	514.1
Bryansk Oblast	7,846	7,784	732.1	726.8
Vladimir Oblast	6,234	6,771	515.6	560.7
Voronezh Oblast	11,045	11,464	578.6	600.8
Ivanovo Oblast	4,801	4,972	530.5	550.3
Kaluga Oblast	5,121	5,424	612.5	648.3
Kostroma Oblast	2,621	2,736	456.1	476.7
Kursk Oblast	5,239	5,456	545.4	568.6
Lipetsk Oblast	5,006	5,074	517.9	524.9
Moscow Oblast	25,055	26,268	448.5	468.4
Oryol Oblast	5,563	5,280	817.6	776.2
Ryazan Oblast	6,951	7,460	711.7	764.6
Smolensk Oblast	5,914	5,658	718.4	689.1
Tambov Oblast	5,584	5,923	606.2	644.3
Tver Oblast	4,966	5,240	432.8	457.5
Tula Oblast	8,148	8,053	614.2	608.6
Yaroslavl Oblast	9,797	9,261	890.8	842.0
Moscow	65,436	64,293	730.8	716.5
Northwestern Federal District	69,346	69,657	617.1	619.5
Republic of Karelia	3,792	3,853	671.6	681.4
Komi Republic	6,161	6,113	796.7	791.0
Arkhangelsk Oblast	6,242	5,769	606.1	560.4
Nenets Autonomous Okrug	350	417	1125.1	1335.0
Vologda Oblast	4,163	4,361	418.3	438.0
Kaliningrad Oblast	3,403	3,398	440.9	439.3
Leningrad Oblast	4,615	4,936	335.5	358.2
Murmansk Oblast	4,928	5,056	707.4	726.1
Novgorod Oblast	4,994	4,570	923.6	846.6
Pskov Oblast	2,674	2,680	454.1	456.5
Saint Petersburg	28,374	28,921	727.3[a]	740.4
North Caucasian Federal District				
Southern Federal District	87,810	91,290	492.9	510.3
Republic of Adygea	1,648	1,735	467.1	490.7
Republic of Dagestan	8,896	9,762	480.4	521.1
Republic of Ingushetia	3,091	3,612	957.4	1101.0
Kabardino-Balkar Republic	2,857	2,390	418.8	348.7
Republic of Kalmykia	903	848	420.6	394.5
Karachay-Cherkess Republic	866	860	263.5	261.3
Republic of North Ossetia-Alania	2,513	2,395	459.0	435.9
Chechen Republic	3,044	3,241	406.3	426.7
Krasnodar Krai	18,431	19,328	444.6	464.3
Stavropol Krai	9,896	9,697	454.9	444.3
Astrakhan Oblast	5,282	5,880	668.9	740.2
Volgograd Oblast	13,129	12,712	613.0	593.5
Rostov Oblast	17,254	18,830	491.0	536.0

Officially registered patients (adults)				
Federal subjects	Urolithiasis			
	Absolute count per 100 000 population			
	2007	2008	2007	2008
Volga Federal District	144,455	147,898	588.5	601.7
Republic of Bashkortostan	21,028	22,116	659.5	691.0
Mari El Republic	2,296	2,352	405.6	415.1
Republic of Mordovia	4,843	4,992	695.8	717.7
Republic of Tatarstan	18,777	17,905	623.0	591.5
Udmurt Republic	5,269	6,045	431.4	494.4
Chuvash Republic	5,565	5,271	541.1	511.3
Perm Krai	14,551	13,775	667.1	631.4
Kirov Oblast	4,556	4,898	389.8	419.8
Nizhny Novgorod Oblast	13,156	13,802	469.8	493.4
Orenburg Oblast	12,667	12,345	748.9	728.8
Penza Oblast	5,902	5,763	510.5	498.5
Samara Oblast	18,421	20,957	703.2	799.0
Saratov Oblast	10,600	10,428	497.6	489.3
Ulyanovsk Oblast	6,824	7,249	629.4	668.3
Urals Federal District	51,133	53,499	519.7	542.3
Kurgan Oblast	2,284	2,599	293.5	334.6
Sverdlovsk Oblast	15,617	15,684	434.0	435.3
Tyumen Oblast	20,422	20,838	781.3	791.6
Khanty-Mansi Autonomous Okrug	5,992	6,327	520.2	544.4
Yamalo-Nenets Autonomous Okrug	4,206	4,106	1032.1	1000.0
Chelyabinsk Oblast	12,810	14,378	449.7	504.0
Siberian Federal District	103,839	104,429	66:5.5	668.2
Altai Republic	761	804	506.9	532.2
Buryat Republic	2,785	3,095	381.3	422.4
Tuva Republic	685	615	330.9	295.2
Republic of Khakassia	3,962	4,263	934.7	1002.5
Altai Krai	29,874	30,360	1458.7	1483.4
Zabaykalsky Krai	3,679	3,826	431.8	448.4
Krasnoyarsk Krai	13,765	14,169	595.6	611.5
Irkutsk Oblast	12,065	11,910	615.0	606.0
Kemerovo Oblast	13,892	13,247	608.2	579.2
Novosibirsk Oblast	10,607	10,792	490.6	498.5
Omsk Oblast	7,874	7,452	482.6	456.4
Tomsk Oblast	3,890	3,896	462.2	461.5
Far Eastern Federal District	36,369	36,949	704.2	714.7
Sakha Republic	3,407	3,630	492.6	522.5
Kamchatka Krai	1,534	1,685	549.4	603.1
Primorsky Krai	12,139	11,919	745.0	731.4
Khabarovsk Krai	7,204	7,682	631.9	672.4
Amur Oblast	7,044	7,211	1023.6	1048.0
Magadan Oblast	1,538	1,296	1147.7	972.7
Sakhalin Oblast	2,821	2,834	673.4	676.5
Jewish Autonomous Oblast	346	369	237.6 ~	252.7
Chukotka Autonomous Okrug	336	323	891.5	857.1

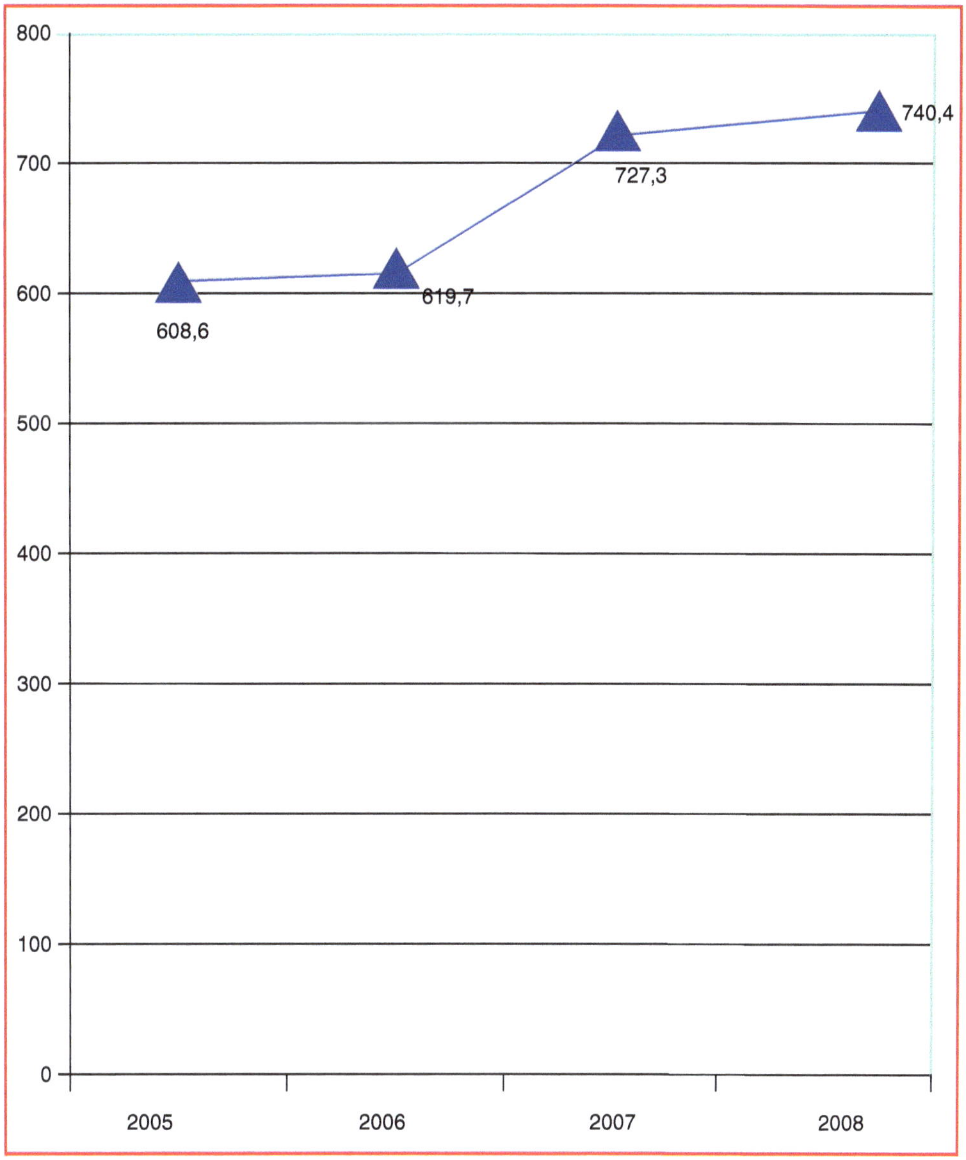

Fig. 13.5 Dynamics of the prevalence of urolithiasis in St. Petersburg in 2005–2008 (per 100,000 people)

were detected. The analyses showed that for calcium oxalate, whewellite was present much more frequently (38.7 %) than weddellite (6.8 %) and calculi of uric acid most frequently contained anhydrous uric acid (16.6 %).

Thus, both the incidence of urolithiasis and its transformations, observed in St. Petersburg in recent years, are similar to the situation in other countries. The obtained data can provide a background for further epidemiological studies. In addition, these results show that data from international epidemiological studies can be used to develop measures to prevent the spread of urolithiasis. This information can also be used to evaluate efficacy of therapeutic and preventive measures aimed at reducing the incidence of urolithiasis. The data presented indicate the need to carry out on urban, regional, and federal levels a special epidemiological program for effective treatment and prevention of urolithiasis.

Table 13.2 Recorded mineral composition of urinary calculi in inhabitants of St. Petersburg ($n=750$)

	Breakdown of patients with urolithiasis	
Type of mineral	Absolute number	%
Oxalates	495	66.0
Phosphates	156	20.8
Uric acid/urate	79	10.5
Cystine	20	2,7
Total	750	100

Epidemiology of Urolithiasis in the Countries of the Former Soviet Union (Post-Soviet Area)

Urolithiasis is one of the most common urological diseases—more than 2–3 % of the working age population has

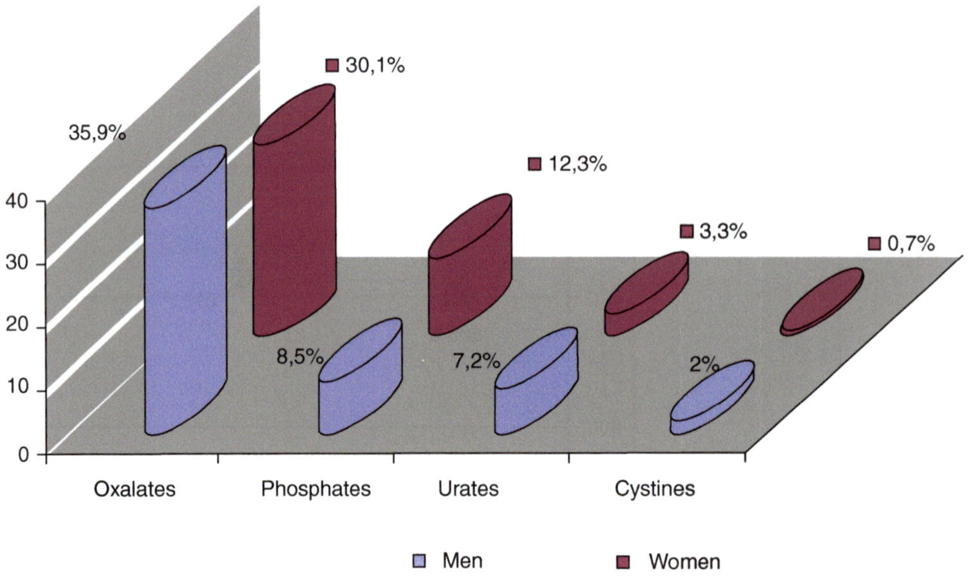

Fig. 13.6 Sex distribution of the patients with urinary stones

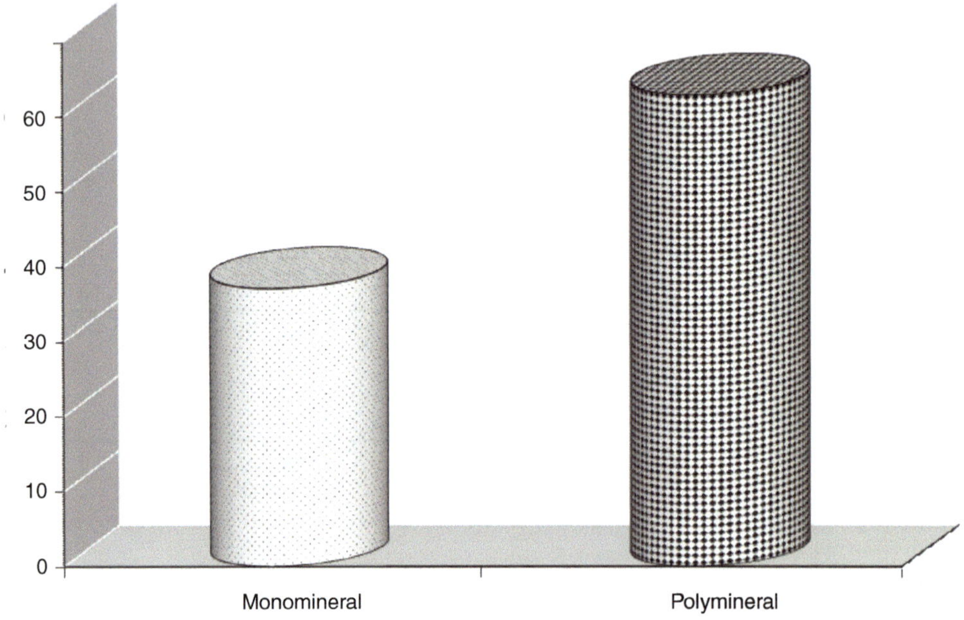

Fig. 13.7 Chemical composition of urinary stones in patients from St. Petersburg

urolithiasis. Of all patients in urological hospitals, 30–40 % have urolithiasis [6, 10].

From the work published by Mirkasimova, Grebenshchikova, and others, it was suggested to assign high priority to epidemiology in the USSR [11]. In the 1980s, the annual incidence rate in a population of 100,000 was 17 in Moscow Oblast, 53 in Ukraine, 48 in Kyrgyzstan, 24 in Turkmenistan, 30 in Uzbekistan, and 35 in the South Caucasus republics. It is worth noting that in the Central Asian republics nonresidents have urolithiasis much more frequently (81.3 %) than aboriginal inhabitants (18.7 %) [12].

In 2006, the Ukraine had the highest incidence of urolithiasis, with 658 cases in a population of 10,000 [13]. In the Republic of Belarus, there were 103 patients with urolithiasis per 10,000 in 2004 [14], while Tajikistan had 256 patients per 10,000 in 2005 [15]. All authors proclaim a progressive increase in the incidence of urolithiasis during recent years. This phenomenon is associated with improved diagnosis of urolithiasis with advent of diagnostic sonography.

The incidence of urolithiasis is largely dependent on climatic factors [16]. Urolithiasis remains endemic in the regions with hot and dry climate. This is the reason why the Central Asian republics and the South Caucasus republics have a particularly high incidence of urolithiasis. Causes for kidney stone formation in arid zones are increased endogenous production of vitamin D in consequence of prolonged high insulation and dehydration with increasing urate concentration [17]. International spread of urolithiasis can also be determined by other external causative factors. Researchers Arshba and Izashvili found that there were 11.6 patients with urolithiasis per 10,000 inhabitants in eastern Georgia and 6.6 patients in western Georgia. Tsintsadze assumed that this fact was explained by unequal concentration of molybdenum in green edible plants used for food. Pogosyan considered the hyperlithogenesis to be a consequence of silicon shortage—silicon, which exhibits characteristics of protective colloids, can keep crystalloids in fluid condition (crystalloid solution) [11].

Nowadays, available literature on composition of urinary stones is provided only by the Belarusian and Ukrainian authors. Thus, Pasechnikov [13] reports that oxalate and uric acid/urate stones are most common in the Ukraine, and approximately 85 % of urinary calculi contain calcium oxalate. The most common types of urinary stones in the Republic of Belarus [14] are oxalate stones (one-third of all stones), uric acid/urate stones (30 %), and phosphate stones (27 %).

According to Voshchula [14], 34 % of the patients with urolithiasis in the Republic of Belarus were females, and 66 % were males. The increased number of female patients with urolithiasis (female urolithiasis proliferation) in recent years was associated with local causal factors such as urodynamic disorders, urinary tract infection, and pyelonephritis. The predominance of male patients is frequently explained by metabolic disorders. Another reason why men have more urinary stones than women is benign prostatic hyperplasia, which can be a pathogenetic factor of urinary stone formation. A so-called sex ratio (the quotient between men and women with urolithiasis) that is greater than unity was recorded by other authors [6].

In addition to the data from Ukrainian authors [18], the relapse rate of stone formation during the first 3 years reached 53 %. As many as 90–95 % of the relapses occurred within the first year. Long-term observation revealed that the recurrence rate might be as high as 77 %. Recurrence preventive treatment to correct metabolic disorders in patients with urolithiasis may reduce the relapse rate by 15 % within a 10-year observation period [14]. Long-term follow-up care is necessary for patients with urolithiasis to avoid various complications [19]. In 35.4 % of the patients, various types of complications occurred in combinations. One of the most common complications was calculus pyelonephritis, which accounted for approximately 88.9 % of all complications.

Conclusion

Urolithiasis is an important and urgent medical problem in all countries of the former Soviet Union. Recently, kidney stones in Russia and in the countries of the former Soviet Union have had a strong tendency to increase. Changes in the morbidity of urolithiasis in all countries of the former Soviet Union are largely the same. The areas of Central Asian republics are well known to have a high endemic rate of stone formation. Men are more prone to forming stones than are women. The main reasons for stone formation in the territory of the Russian Federation are: urodynamic disorders, urinary infection, pyelonephritis, and various metabolic pathologies. Despite the large number of recurrent kidney stones, we observe improvements in the diagnosis and treatment of urolithiasis due to the successful scientific and technologic development.

In the near future, a special epidemiological program based on the problems of urolithiasis will be developed in Russia and all countries of the former Soviet Union to join more effective treatment and prevention of this disease.

References

1. Pak CY, Resnick MI, Preminger GM. Ethnic and geographic diversity of stone disease. Urology. 1997;50(4):504–7.
2. Ramello A, Vitale C, Marangella M. Epidemiology of nephrolithiasis. J Nephrol. 2000;13(3):45–50.
3. Arias Fúnez F, et al. Epidemiology of urinary lithiasis in our unit. Clinical course in time and predictive factors. Arch Esp Urol. 2000;53(4):343–7.
4. Tiselius HG. Epidemiology and medical management of stone disease. BJU Int. 2000;91:758–67.
5. Nazarov T. Features of current urolitiasis of men. In: The 6th world congress on che aging male, Tampa, 14–24 Feb 2008, p. 17.
6. Nazarov T. Physical and chemical and biochemical parameters of urine in pathogenesis urolithiasis. In: 12th European symposium on urolithiasis. Final program and book of abstracts, Lisbon, 4–7 July 2007, p. 27.
7. Nazarov T, et al. Diagnostic value of physical and biochemical parametres of urine in metophylaxis Urolithiasis. In: 13th European symposium on urolithiasis. Final program and book of abstracts, Genuia, 15–17 Oct. 2009, p. 83.
8. Bartoletti RCT, Mondaini N, et al. Epidemiology and risk factors in urolithiasis. Urol Int. 2007;79(1):3–7.
9. Yasui T, et al. Prevalence and epidemiologic characteristics of lower urinary tract stones in japan. Urology. 2008;72(5):1001–5.
10. Dzeranov NK, Lopatkin NA. Clinical guidelines. In: Urolithiasis. Moscow: "Overley"; 2007. p. 296
11. Tiktinsky OL, Alexandrov VP. Urolithiasis. "Piter": AVP; 2000. p. 346.
12. Tinaliev MT. Epidemiology of urolithiasis in kyrgyzstan. Urol Nefrol (Mosk). 1983;3:26–31.
13. Pasechnikov SP. Modern aspects of citrate therapy in urolithiasis. Ukrainian scientific magazine "Health of man" Kiev, 2007. p. 109–13.
14. Voshchula VI. Urolithiasis: etiotropic and pathogenetic treatment and prophylactic. Minsk: VEVER; 2006. p. 268.
15. Kadirov ZA, et al. Abilities of modern methods of laboratory analyses in estimation of degree of severity and incidence of urolithiasis in Tajikistan. Clinical laboratory diagnostic; 2008. p. 17–21.
16. Polienko AK, Sevost'ianova OA, Moiseev VA. Epidemiology of urolithiasis. Urology. 2005;5:68–71.
17. Kolpakov IS. Urolithiasis. Moscow: "Medicine"; 2006. p. 222.
18. Dzyurak VS. Urolithiasis: pathogenesis, diagnostic, treatment. Magazine of the physician; 1998. p. 2–4.
19. Nazarov T, et al. Retrospective analysis of diagnostic and treatment in urgent condition of patients with urolithiasis. Medical magazine of Nizhny Novgorod. 2006. p. 112–6.

Renal Stone Disease in Different Racial Groups

14

Jamsheer J. Talati, Naveed Haroon, and Alberto Trinchieri

Abstract

A study of racial differences in stone type and metabolic abnormalities over time suggests a convergence to a common pattern across the world. This conclusion is supported by studies of individuals of different races who cross over into another geographical and cultural milieu. Nevertheless, gender differences do exist, and some distinctive geographical differences in idiopathic stone patterns remain. The relative influence of genetic and environmental factors in the genesis of stone remains unknown, but appears to favor the hypothesis that the apparent racial differences arise from environmental and dietary influences.

Keywords

Racial differences • Gender differences • African • Metabolic abnormalities • Urolithiasis • Stone composition

Introduction

A review of the literature suggests a number of racial differences in stone composition and metabolic disorders. This chapter attempts to examine that evidence. What emerges is that most of the stated differences in the spatial distribution of stone disease may well be due to environmental factors such as geographical terrain, climate, and diet. This chapter explores the evidence for this but does not address the transitions in incidence of vesical stones or the genetic abnormalities that determine stone formation—topics that are dealt with elsewhere in this book (see Chaps. 3 and 16).

J.J. Talati, M.B.B.S., FRCS (✉) N. Haroon, M.B.B.S.
Section of Urology, Department of Surgery,
Aga Khan University, Stadium Road,
Karachi, Sindh 74800, Pakistan
e-mail: jamsheer.talati@aku.edu; naveed.haroon@aku.edu

A. Trinchieri, M.D., FEBU
Department of Urology, A. Manzoni Hospital,
Via Dell'Eremo 9/11, Lecco 23900, Italy
e-mail: a.trinchieri@ospedale.lecco.it

Accumulating evidence leads us to believe that dietary and environmental factors may be more important than ethnicity in the etiology of calculi. As example, Maloney et al. [1] found only minor differences in stone composition, or proportions of patients with metabolic disorders in different racial groups, within a country.

Earlier, racial predisposition for nephrolithiasis had been claimed by comparing prevalence and incidence data in populations resident in their countries of origin. The drawback of so doing is that the differences might have been influenced by climate and terrain. For example, the high (20 %) lifetime prevalence in Saudi Arabia (see Chap. 10) could well be caused by higher environmental temperatures and poor water intake.

Other studies have collected data from different races within the same country. Such data are more useful because these findings are less biased by interfering factors such as lifestyle and climate. In such data also, there is the possibility that the frequency of stones (in such multiracial communities) may simply be reflecting the population demography or socioeconomic differences of racial groups. As example, in Hussain et al.'s studies in Malaysia, most of the urinary tract stones were observed in the Malays as compared to the Chinese people, whereas in a neighboring country, Singapore,

J.J. Talati et al. (eds.), *Urolithiasis*,
DOI 10.1007/978-1-4471-4387-1_14, © Springer-Verlag London 2012

most of the stone formers are Chinese [2]. As Hussain's study shows, it is the frequency of the distributions of ethnic groups in the total population of Malaysia and Singapore that is reflected in the relative contribution of ethnic groups to the stone-forming populations in the two regions.

A cautious interpretation of data is required, especially as frequency of stones ascertained from hospital-based data (in a multiracial community) could also reflect different degrees of access to medical care. This is a particularly important confounder, as illustrated in the example that follows, when attempting to find out if truly the black races are less prone to urolithiasis.

Differences Between Black and Caucasian Populations

A significant body of information seems to show racial difference in stone-forming propensity between blacks and Caucasians. Most of the published data compare black and white populations within either the USA or within South Africa.

The earliest reports on racial differences were from Africa. Vermooten [3] found only two urolithiasis patients in a million admissions in South Africa, as compared to one urolithiasis white South African patient per 460 admissions. In the 1970s, Esho [4] reported on the low frequency of stones in Nigeria—45 stone patients among 636,735 patients seen in the clinics of Lagos University Teaching Hospital. Additionally, there were only 2 stones in 5,022 autopsies, thus reducing the risk that calculations from clinical cases were missing out on the silent stones. Mbonu reported that stone frequency remained low (13/100,000) [5] even in the 1980s, with most of the stones being associated with infection and obstruction.

The rarity of finding a stone patient in hospital [3] could have been partly accounted for by poor access to care. However, a lower incidence of stone continues to be reported in sub-Saharan Africa in 1984, where Mbuno et al. [5] saw only 81 cases of urolithiasis in 5 years.

Differences Between Blacks and Caucasians in the USA

In the USA, some initial investigations described a higher incidence of nephrolithiasis in whites than in blacks [6, 7], although other studies demonstrated no differences between the two races [8, 9]. Until the end of the last century, blacks were hospitalized for nephrolithiasis less frequently than whites, and nephrolithiasis accounted for the hospitalization of 0.45–0.89 % in whites and 0.14–0.23 % in blacks [10]. However, it should be considered that the black population, for socioeconomic reasons, could prefer home remedies rather than the more expensive hospital services. In the US black population, the male/female ratio was lower or even inverse of that in the white population. The most common type of calculi was infection stones, which accounted for 45 % of the total and were particularly frequent in females (49 %). Calcium stones were proportionally less commonly represented in blacks (32 %) than in whites, while uric stones (20 %) were relatively more common; the occurrence of cystine stones (1 %) was comparable with that observed in the white population [10]. Taylor noted that on average, black women excreted 65 mg (1.6 mmol) less urinary calcium/day and 4 mg (0.04 mmol) more oxalate than Caucasians [11].

More recently, an increase in the incidence of stone disease in the black populations has been observed [12] in conjunction with the increased amount of food consumed and the associated low intake of vegetables. Both factors might aggravate the risk of stone formation [13].

Differences Between Blacks and Caucasians in South Africa

Data from South Africa (SA) shows a great difference in renal stone incidence between blacks and whites [5]. This difference between prevalence rates in black and Caucasian populations in SA can be explained by the more marked socioeconomic differences between the two races in SA compared with the USA, the different dietary intakes, and the relative infrequency with which the black population (being less well-off) ask for medical advice.

However, while black subjects from peri-urban settlements do report energy intakes below the recommended dietary allowance [14, 15], recent data [16] show that a shift in dietary intake toward the Western diet is occurring among urban blacks. In the urban population, no relevant difference of dietary patterns was demonstrable between black and white healthy subjects other than a higher percentage of energy obtained from carbohydrates for black subjects [17]. There are areas of continuing poorer nutrition in the black population [14], but a recent population-based survey confirmed that urbanization of Africans influences the nutrition and health transition in SA, involving a risk of subsequent emergence of diseases previously uncommon among blacks [16, 18].

Differences in Metabolic Abnormalities and Stone Types

As stated, Maloney et al. [1] concluded that ethnicity does not influence stone formation. He based this conclusion on the fact that all racial groups demonstrated a similarity in the incidence of underlying metabolic abnormalities, suggesting that dietary and environmental factors may be more important than ethnicity in the etiology of stone disease. In particular, hypocitraturia, hyperuricosuria, hyperoxaluria, gouty diathesis, and high sulfate levels were equally represented among all ethnic groups.

- Taylor, however, did note that on average, black women excreted 65 mg (1.6 mmol) less urinary calcium ($p<0.001$) and 4 mg (0.04 mmol) more oxalate [11].
- Similarly, there is a difference in calcium excretion in Pakistanis as compared to US citizens. Hypercalciuria is infrequent, and urinary calcium as well as citrate is lower in stone patients and controls in Pakistan (Chap. 3) as compared to the USA. This may simply reflect lower vitamin D levels and the use of phytate-rich foods in Pakistan and the liberal consumption of milk and milk products in the USA.

The following are some other specific examples of greater differences in metabolic abnormalities:

- Japan has an unusually high rate of primary hyperparathyroidism (PHPT) for an industrialized country—10 % (see Chap. 12)—which contrasts with the lower rate of detection in Pakistan, where the lower incidence might be explained by the masking of hypercalcemia because of vitamin D deficiency.
- Eisner et al. observed that Asian-Pacific Islander stone formers excreted greater amounts of urate and less citrate than white patients [21] .
- Landau observed that the incidence of uric acid stones in Israel is greater in Bedouin than in Jewish children (1.02 vs. 0.13 cases/1,000 inhabitants), which they linked with the higher urate excretion (mean urate excretion index 0.8 ± 0.39 (0.048 ± 0.023 mmol/L) vs. 0.55 ± 0.26 mg/dL (0.033 ± 0.015 mmol/L) glomerular filtration rate (GFR), respectively) [22].
- In northeast Thailand, periodic paralysis and a familial form of distal RTA are well known. Incomplete distal RTA is seen in about 8 % of the patients. However, recent evidence suggests that many of the cases are sporadic [23, 24].
- Aboriginal people of Canada were found to have a prevalence rate approximately one-third of that seen in the non-aboriginal (nonnative) population—with 0.858 renal stone episodes in a population of 1,000 nonnative persons compared with 0.222 in aboriginal people [25].

Differences in Stone Composition

There are many examples of racial differences in stone composition. There is lack of clarity whether these findings are time trends or true racial/genetic differences. For example:

- Purine stones are four times more frequent in Tahitian men than in North African men [26].
- Stones in Australian Aborigines [27] are usually composed of uric acid/urate, usually occur in the upper urinary tract, and develop at an early age. They are not associated with anatomic anomalies or abnormal urate production/metabolism. Carson [27] notes that this pattern of urolithiasis is distinctive and different from the global pattern of endemic bladder stones in young children in developing countries and predominantly calcium stones in the upper tracts of older children and adults in affluent industrialized countries. These observations raise the possibility that the stones are genetically determined.
- Cystine stones account for 1.3 % of adult stones in China [28]—a similar rate to elsewhere in the world (0.5–2 %). However, the pediatric cystine stone incidence is 12.5 % (see Chap. 79), higher than in the rest of the world, raising issues of different rates of maturation of enzymes responsible for resolution of cystinuria.
- The frequency of calcium phosphate stones is particularly low in boys in developing countries (8.3 vs. 45.1 % in France, $p<0.0001$) [26].
- Struvite stones are uncommon in Pakistan (Chap. 3), Saudi Arabia [26], and in India where 90 % of staghorn stones are composed of calcium oxalate and only 1.4 % contain struvite [29].
- In Japan, struvite accounts for 32 % of staghorn stones (an additional 22 % containing phosphate) [30]. In the Tajima area, in the northern part of Hyogo Prefecture, from 1991 to 1993, struvite accounted for only 4.5% with 90 % composed of calcium oxalate and calcium phosphate [31].

Differences in Gender Distribution: Are They Indicative of Genetic Factors?

Sex ratios until recently always have favored males. Men are known to be more commonly afflicted in the white and Asian populations where they comprise 62 and 64 % of the stone-forming populations, respectively. In Hispanics [32] and blacks, a reversed gender distribution was noted with women accounting for 68 and 60 % of the stone formers, respectively. In the black population, the male to female (M:F) ratio was lower or even inverse than in the white population. In Nigeria today, the M:F ratio is 5:1 [5].

Conclusion

Much of the difference in prevalence of idiopathic nephrolithiasis in different racial groups seems to be related to demographics and socioeconomic conditions of the various populations. The effects of race are confounded by differences in diet. Mobility of citizens throws one racial group into the eating patterns of a completely different nature and leads to a homogenization of the results of 24-h urinary metabolic workup.

It will most likely emerge that renal stone patients from different racial groups demonstrate marginal differences in underlying metabolic abnormalities and stone types—a situation that reflects differences in their dietary pattern. Further investigation might reveal that the underlying genetic and environmental processes leading to stone formation are the same right across the world.

References

1. Maloney ME, Springhart WP, Ekeruo WO, Young MD, Enemchukwu CU, Preminger GM. Ethnic background has minimal impact on the etiology of nephrolithiasis. J Urol. 2005;173:2001–4.
2. Talati J. Familial clustering and sex incidence of urolithiasis. In: Talati J et al., editors. The management of lithiasis. Dordrecht: Kluwer Academic Publishers; 1997. p. 69–75.
3. Vermooten V. The occurrence of renal calculi and their possible relation to diet: as illustrated in the south African negro. JAMA. 1937;109(11):857–9.
4. Esho JO. Experience with urinary calculus disease in Nigerians as seen at the Lagos University Teaching Hospital. Niger Med J. 1976; 6(1):18–22.
5. Mbonu O, Attah C, Ikeakor I. Urolithiasis in an African population. Int Urol Nephrol. 1984;16(4):291–6.
6. Quinland WS. Urinary lithiasis: review of thirty-three cases in Negroes. J Urol. 1945;53:791–804.
7. Pierce LW, Bloom B. Observations in urolithiasis among American troops in a desert area. J Urol. 1945;54:466–70.
8. Dodson AI, Clark JR. Incidence of urinary calculi in American negroes. JAMA. 1946;37:1063–6.
9. Mason JC, Miles BJ, Belville WD. Urolithiasis and race: another viewpoint. J Urol. 1985;134:501.
10. Sarmina I, Spirnak JP, Resnick MI. Urinary lithiasis in the black population: an epidemiological study and review of the literature. J Urol. 1987;138:14–7.
11. Taylor EN, Curhan GC. Differences in 24-hour urine composition between black and white women. J Am Soc Nephrol. 2007;18:654–9.
12. Stamatelou KK, Francis ME, Jones CA, Nyberg LM, Curhan GC. Time trends in reported prevalence of kidney stones in the United States: 1976–1994. Kidney Int. 2003;63:1817–23.
13. Kant AK, Graubard BI, Kumanyika SK. Trends in black-white differentials in dietary intakes of U.S. adults, 1971–2002. Am J Prev Med. 2007;32:354–5.
14. Modlin M, Davies PJ, Crawford D. Dietary structure and urinary composition in a stone-free population. In: Smith LH, Robertson WG, Finlayson B, editors. Urolithiasis: clinical and basic research. New York: Plenum Press; 1981. p. 337.
15. Rodgers A, Allie-Hamdulay S, Pinnock D, Baretta G, Trinchieri A. Risk factors for renal calcium stone formation in South African and European young adults. Arch Ital Urol Androl. 2009;81:171–4.
16. Charlton KE, Bourne LT, Steyn K, Laubscher JA. Poor nutritional status in older black South Africans. Asia Pac J Clin Nutr. 2001;10:31–8.
17. MacKeown JM, Pedro TM, Norris SA. Energy, macro- and micronutrient intake among a true longitudinal group of south African adolescents at two interceptions (2000 and 2003): the Birth-to-Twenty (Bt20) study. Public Health Nutr. 2007;10:635–43.
18. Bourne LT, Lambert EV, Steyn K. Where does the black population of South Africa stand on the nutrition transition? Public Health Nutr. 2002;5:157–62.
19. Tibazarwa K, Ntyintyane L, Sliwa K, Gerntholtz T, Carrington M, Wilkinson D, et al. A time bomb of cardiovascular risk factors in South Africa: results from the heart of Soweto study "heart awareness days." Int J Cardiol. 2009;132:233–9.
20. Kruger HS, Venter CS, Vorster HH, THUSA Study. Physical inactivity as a risk factor for cardiovascular disease in communities undergoing rural to urban transition: the THUSA study. Cardiovasc J S Afr. 2003;14:16–23.
21. Eisner BH, Porten SP, Bechis SK, Stoller ML. The role of race in determining 24-hour urine composition in white and Asian/Pacific Islander stone formers. J Urol. 2010;183(4):1407–11.
22. Landau P, Tovbin D, Shalev H. Pediatric urolithiasis in southern Israel: the role of uricosuria. Pediatr Nephrol. 2000;14:1105–10.
23. Stitchantrakul W, Kochakarn W, Ruangraksa C, Domrongkitchaiporn S. Urinary risk factors for recurrent calcium stone formation in Thai stone formers. J Med Assoc Thai. 2007;90:688–98.
24. Phakdeekitcharoen B, Ruangraksa C, Radinahamed P. Hypokalaemia and paralysis in the Thai population. Nephrol Dial Transplant. 2004;19:2013–8.
25. Pylypchuk G, Unger D, Wiser L, O'Reilly K, Weckworth P. Racial influence in renal stone disease: a Saskatchewan story. Can J Urol. 1995;2(3):159–63.
26. Daudon M, Bounxouej B, Santa Cruz F, Leite da Silva S, Diouf B, Angwafoo 3rd FF, et al. Composition of renal stones currently observed in non-industrialized countries. Prog Urol. 2004;14(6):1151–61.
27. Carson PJ, Brewster DR. Unique pattern of urinary tract calculi in Australian Aboriginal children. J Paediatr Child Health. 2003; 39(5):325–8.
28. Jing Z, GuoZeng GW, Ning J, JiaWei Y, Yan G, Fang Y. Analysis of urinary calculi composition by infrared spectroscopy: a prospective study of 625 patients in eastern China. Urol Res. 2007;38(2):111–5. zjurol@yahoo.cn.
29. Ansari MS, Gupta NP, Hemal AK, Dogra PN, Seth A, Aron M, Singh TP, Specturn of stone composition: structural analysis of 1050 upper urinary tract calculi from northern India, Int J Urol 2005;12(1):12–6.
30. Akaqashi K, Tanda H, Kato S, Ohnishi S, Nakajima H, Nanbu A, Nitta T, Koroku M, Sato Y, Hanzawa T, Characteristics of patients with Staghorn Calculi in our experience, Int J Urol 2004;11(5): 276–81.
31. Takahashi T, Yamane A, Okasho K, Yoshikawa T, Sawazaki H, Wataru S, Taki Y, Takeuchi H, Incidence of upper urinary tract stone during 15 years in Tajima Area Japan: a hospital based study, Urol Res. 2009;37(6):305–10.
32. Michaels EK, Nakagawa Y, Miura N, Pursell S, Ito H. Racial variation in gender frequency of calcium urolithiasis. J Urol. 1994;152 (6 Pt 2):2228–31.

Part II

Etiology

Stone Composition and Morphology: A Window on Etiology

15

Michel Daudon and Paul Jungers

Abstract

Physical methods, namely, X-ray diffraction (XRD) and Fourier transform infrared spectroscopy (FTIR) reliably identify specific forms of nephrolithiasis involving a single component such as cystine, 2,8-dihydroxyadenine, xanthine, uric acid, struvite, and drugs as well as common-type stones made of calcium oxalate (CaOx) and/or calcium phosphate. However, for the latter, these methods do not provide etiologic information in clinical practice because a same-stone composition may be the result of very different lithogenic processes. A comprehensive stone analysis method combining morphological examination followed by XRD or FTIR analysis of the core, middle layers, and surface of calculi provides a more complete contribution to etiologic diagnosis than compositional analysis alone. Using this method, stones may be classified into 7 types subdivided in 22 subtypes. Among CaOx stones, type Ic COM calculi are pathognomonic of primary hyperoxaluria. Among calcium phosphate stones, a peculiar morphology of carbapatite stones (type IVa2) is closely associated with distal tubular acidosis, whereas in primary hyperparathyroidism calculi are predominantly made of carbapatite mixed with weddellite or of brushite (type IVd). Ammonium urate calculi of type IIId are found in patients with low phosphate intake and chronic diarrhea due to laxative abuse or in children with endemic urolithiasis. Uric acid calculi are mainly suggestive of low urine pH related to insulin resistance as observed in metabolic syndrome or type 2 diabetes or in case of colon resection. Among common, idiopathic CaOx stones, predominance of whewellite (type I morphology) is mainly associated with high urinary oxalate concentration, whereas predominance of weddellite (type II morphology) is associated with hypercalciuric states. This method is of decisive interest for early diagnosis—and therefore proper treatment—of severe diseases such as primary hyperoxaluria and 2,8-dihydroxyadeninuria.

Keywords

Stone analysis • Crystalline phases • Morphology • Etiology • Infrared spectroscopy • Classification • Tubular acidosis • Primary hyperparathyroidism • Primary hyperoxaluria • Hypercalciuria • Hyperoxaluria • Infection stones

M. Daudon, Ph.D. (✉)
Service des Explorations Fonctionnelles, Tenon Hospital, APHP, 4 Rue de la Chine, Paris 75020, France
e-mail: michel.daudon@tnn.aphp.fr

P. Jungers, M.D.
Department of Nephrology, Necker-Enfants Malades Hospital, APHP, 149 Rue de Sèvres, Paris 75015, France
e-mail: pl.jungers@gmail.com

Introduction

Among physical methods, X-ray diffraction (XRD) and Fourier transform infrared spectroscopy (FTIR) are now universally used for stone analysis. They identify stone constituents and provide semiquantitative evaluation of their respective proportions within a calculus. These physical

J.J. Talati et al. (eds.), *Urolithiasis*,
DOI 10.1007/978-1-4471-4387-1_15, © Springer-Verlag London 2012

methods reliably identify specific forms of nephrolithiasis involving a single component such as cystine, 2,8-dihydroxyadenine, xanthine, uric acid, struvite, or drugs, as well as stones made of calcium oxalate (CaOx) and/or calcium phosphate. They allow assessing the relative proportion of components in mixed stones made of several crystalline phases such as CaOx monohydrate (COM), CaOx dihydrate (COD), carbapatite, or brushite.

However, because XRD or FTIR analysis is often performed on a powdered sample of the whole stone, no indication is given as to the respective location (core or peripheral layers) of the diverse constituents in the case of mixed stones, even if the stone is large enough to allow a separate analysis of its different parts. Additionally, a similar composition, for instance, CaOx as main component, may be the result of diverse lithogenic processes, including diet imbalance, low diuresis, genetic, or acquired diseases. Moreover, the same crystalline phase, for instance, COM as the main component, may correspond to very different etiopathogenic conditions, such as primary hyperoxaluria, enteric hyperoxaluria, or idiopathic CaOx nephrolithiasis [1, 2]. In contrast, COD stones are clearly related to hypercalciuria in a high proportion of cases [1–3]. The corresponding stones exhibit quite a distinct morphology easily identified both in surface and section.

On the other hand, the initial nucleation process may be very different from the biochemical factors responsible for the further stone growth. All these considerations suggest that stone analysis should provide information on chemical composition, identification of crystalline phases, as well as their location within the stone.

Stone Composition

Analytical Aspects

Urinary calculi result from a long-term exposure to supersaturated urine. Because the urine composition is constantly varying according to dietary and drinking habits, the stones may contain several components, some of them being often found in very low proportion. In other cases, the pathological conditions responsible for stone formation may induce urine supersaturation regarding several chemical compounds that may crystallize simultaneously in urine and that will be present together in the stone. Indeed, more than 100 chemical and crystalline forms have been identified in urinary calculi (Table 15.1). Among them, 15 are frequent (more than 1 % of stones), the other ones being considered as rare but often related to specific lithogenic conditions. From an epidemiological point of view, calcium oxalate is now the most common chemical component of urinary stones throughout the world. However, it is associated in a majority of cases to other crystalline phases as minor components that may have a clinical relevance.

Today, chemical methods are yet extensively used for stone analysis. However, chemical methods fail to identify rare purine stones resulting from genetic disorders such as 2,8-dihydroxyadenine [4–6] or drug-induced calculi [7–9]. Moreover, they are unable to provide reliable information on crystalline phases present in calcium stones. Only physical methods are able to identify such a diversity of components [10, 11]. For this purpose, several techniques were proposed in routine practice [12], including X-ray powder diffraction [13–18], infrared spectroscopy [19–25], Raman spectroscopy, [26–30], or thermal analysis [31–34]. Among these techniques, X-ray powder diffraction was the first technique applied to stone analysis [35]. Nevertheless, because of constraints for installing such equipment in a lab and due to some limitations in detecting very minor components and poorly crystallized material, it was progressively superseded by infrared spectroscopic techniques, which are easier to perform. Today, the other techniques are used for stone analysis in a limited number of labs. Infrared spectrometers are set up in numerous countries through the world, and more than 100,000 stones are analyzed each year by that technique. However, only a few books presenting reference spectra are available in the literature [27, 29, 36, 37]. Because of a lack of references, especially for mixtures, the accurate interpretation of infrared spectra may be difficult in a number of cases, leading to inappropriate interpretation of stone composition as observed in quality control surveys recently performed in Western countries [38, 39].

Clinical Aspects

When considering calcium oxalate stones, the expected cause for a 97 % COM stone nucleated on a carbapatite Randall's plaque, which represents only 3 % of the stone mass, is completely different from a 90 % COD stone including 10 % carbapatite randomly distributed. In the first case, the stone growth is the result of mild hyperoxaluria as a consequence of oxalate-rich food consumption and/or low diuresis, the nucleation of the stone being induced by calcium oxalate crystal deposit on a papillary calcification made of carbapatite and possibly related to transient (past) hypercalciuria [40, 41]. In the second case, nucleation and further growth of the stone may be related to persistent hypercalciuria, the origin of which remaining to be determined by appropriate metabolic investigations.

Among calcium stones, carbapatite is the second most common crystalline phase. Because carbapatite is highly dependent on pH, it must be expected that carbapatite-rich stones are developed in poorly acidic and often alkaline urine, which is suggestive for either urinary tract infection (UTI) or metabolic disorders responsible for chronically elevated urine pH, associated, or not, with hypercalciuria [42–44]. Carbapatite is rarely pure in human stones and the other crystalline phases present as minor components may help to orient diagnosis. For example, carbapatite associated with COD is highly suggestive of hypercalciuria and should induce the search for primary hyperparathyroidism [45]. In contrast, carbapatite associated with COM is more often related to medullary sponge kidney and other causes of urine stasis. Carbapatite associated with other calcium phosphates such as amorphous carbonated calcium phosphate (ACCP) and/or whitlockite must orient to a possible chronic urinary tract infection at the origin of the stone [46]. Carbapatite associated with brushite and/or octacalcium phosphate pentahydrate (OCPP) is commonly a marker of hypercalciuria, the presence of OCPP being suggestive of an active and recent lithogenic process [47]. In the case carbapatite is associated with any proportion of struvite, a UTI by urea-splitting bacteria can be asserted [46, 48]. At last, using infrared spectroscopy as a routine method for stone analysis, it is possible to determine the carbonation rate of carbapatite, which may be relevant to orient toward an infection stone in the absence of struvite in the stone [49].

In the case of purine stones, pure uric acid is suggestive of low urine pH related to metabolic syndrome and obesity [50], type 2 diabetes [51–54], or hydroelectrolytic diarrhea.

Table 15.1 Components identified in urinary calculi

Mineral components	Organic components	Drugs
Calcium phosphates	***Calcium oxalates***	***Inhibitors of proteases***
Hydroxyapatite (calcium hydroxyphosphate)	Whewellite (calcium oxalate monohydrate)[a]	Indinavir monohydrate
		Atazanavir
Carbapatites (carbonated calcium hydroxyphosphates)[a]	Weddellite (calcium oxalate dihydrate)[a]	Nelfinavir
Octacalcium phosphate	Caoxite (calcium oxalate trihydrate)	Amprenavir
Pentahydrate[a]	***Other oxalate salts***	***Antinucleosidic drugs***
Amorphous carbonated calcium	Humboldtine (Iron (II) oxalate dihydrate)	Efavirenz
Phosphates[a]	***Calcium citrate***	***Quinolones***
Brushite (dicalcium phosphate dihydrate)[a]	Tricalcium dicitrate	Oxolinic acid
Whitlockite (calcium magnesium phosphate hydrate)[a]	Tetrahydrate[a]	Flumequine
Magnesium phosphates	***Purines***	Ciprofloxacin (magnesium salt)
Bobierrite (trimagnesium phosphate octahydrate)	Anhydrous uric acid[a]	Norfloxacin (magnesium salt)
Trimagnesium phosphate pentahydrate	Uric acid monohydrate	***Aminopenicillins***
Newberyite (dimagnesium phosphate trihydrate)	Uric acid dihydrate[a]	Amoxicillin trihydrate
Magnesium ammonium phosphates	Amorphous uric acid	Ampicillin trihydrate
Struvite (magnesium ammonium phosphate hexahydrate)[a]	Ammonium hydrogen urate[a]	***Cephalosporins***
Dittmarite (magnesium ammonium phosphate monohydrate)	Sodium hydrogen urate monohydrate[a]	Ceftriaxone (calcium salt)
Hannayite (Magnesium ammonium hydrogenophosphate octahydrate)		***Sulfamides***
Zinc phosphate	Calcium hydrogen urate hexahydrate	*N*-acetylsulfamethoxazole chlorhydrate
Hopeite (zinc phosphate tetrahydrate)	Magnesium hydrogen urate hexahydrate	Sulfadiazine
Calcium carbonates	Potassium hydrogen urate	*N*-acetylsulfadiazine
Calcite (anhydrous calcium carbonate)	Sodium potassium urate	*N*-acetylsulfaguanidine
Aragonite (anhydrous calcium carbonate)	Dipotassium urate	*N,N*-diacetylsulfaguanidine
Vaterite (anhydrous calcium carbonate)	Disodium urate	*N*-acetylsulfaperine
Hydroxycalcite (calcium carbonate monohydrate)	Xanthine	*N*-acetylsulfapyridine
Calcium sulfate	Hypoxanthine	*N*-acetylsulfisoxazole
Gypsum (calcium sulfate dihydrate)	Hydroxy-8-adenine	***Allopurinol***
Silicium-containing minerals	Dihydroxy-2,8-adenine	Oxypurinol
Amorphous silica (opaline silica)	Methyl-1-uric acid	***Amino-4-quinoleines***

(continued)

Table 15.1 (continued)

Mineral components	Organic components	Drugs
Cristobalite (silicon dioxide)	***Pyrimidines***	Glafenic acid
	Potassium orotate	Hydroxy-2 glafenic acid
	Amino acids	Hydroxy-4 glafenic acid
	Cystine[a]	Antrafenic acid
	Tyrosine	Floctafenic acid
	Leucine	***Pteridines***
	Proteins	Triamterene
	Albumin[a]	4¢-hydroxytriamterene
	Uropontin[a]	4¢-hydroxytriamterene sulfate
	Bikunin	***Guaifenesin***
	Nephrocalcin	Calcium beta-(2-methoxyphenoxy) lactate
	Retinol-binding protein	***Others***
	Beta-2-microglobulin	Nitrofurantoin
	Alpha-1-microglobulin	Aciclovir
	Glycosaminoglycans	Ephedrine
	Hyaluronic acid	Norephedrine
	Heparan sulfate[a]	Pseudoephedrine
	Chondroitin sulfate	Hydroxyphenazopyridine sulfate
	Lipids	***Drugs and exogenous organic compounds***
	Cholesterol	Silicon (stents)
	Tripalmitin	Polyester (ligature)
	Tristearin	Polyethylene (ligature)
	Triolein	Polyglactic acid (ligature)
	Calcium palmitate	Polyamides (ligatures)
	Calcium stearate	Polyurethanes (stents)
	Cholesteryl palmitate	
	Cholesteryl stearate	
	Fatty acids	
	Miscellaneous	
	Homogentisic acid	

[a]Components commonly found in more than 1 % of urinary tract stones

In contrast, ammonium hydrogen urate is highly suggestive of hyperuricosuria with high ammonium excretion or local production (due to urinary tract infection by urea-splitting bacteria), and urine pH is normal to high [55, 56]. If urine pH is normal, the main cause of ammonium hydrogen urate is commonly chronic diarrhea, either as a consequence of laxative abuse [57–59] or in the context of low protein and dairy product consumption associated with cereal-rich food, the latter profile corresponding to the so-called endemic urolithiasis [55, 60, 61]. In the case urine pH is high (above 7), urinary tract infection by urease-producing bacteria should be looked for.

Epidemiological Considerations

Stone disease was reported as constantly increasing during the past 30 years in most industrialized countries where successive epidemiological surveys have been performed [62–65]. Urolithiasis affects between 5 and 12 % of the general population and two times more often males than females. Of note, a trend to a decrease of the male-to-female ratio has been recently reported in the United States [66, 67] and Japan [68].

Regarding the stone composition, the data reported in the literature are commonly based on the main component identified in each calculus. Such an approach is relevant at the population level because it reflects the main risk factors of stone formation for that population. However, it may hide specific conditions of stone formation revealed by crystalline phases present in minor proportions in the stones [69]. So, the results of stone analysis should provide a wide spectrum of information for a good assessment of epidemiological data and risk factors involved in stone formation, including:

- The frequency of the main components
- The occurrence of all identified components

Table 15.2 Distribution of stone composition (expressed as main components) observed in Europe and United States

Authors	Herring [15]	Brien et al. [70]	Daudon et al. [71]
Year	1962	1982	1995
Country	United States	Germany	France
No. of calculi	10,000	10,000	10,438
Stone composition (%)			
Calcium oxalates	73.1	71.8	66.0
Calcium oxalate monohydrate	31.7	57.4	42.8
Calcium oxalate dihydrate	41.4	14.4	23.2
Calcium phosphates	8.3	8.8	16.6
Struvite	9.2	5.3	2.8
Ammonium hydrogen urate	<0.1	0.3	0.6
Uric acid	7.2	11.4	10.1
Cystine	0.9	0.3	1.2
Other	1.2	2.1	2.7

- The composition of nucleus
- The main associations found in the stones

Such a panel of data should allow a more accurate knowledge of urolithiasis in a given country and a better comparison between published series.

Epidemiological Data in Adult Patients

In industrialized countries, it was extensively reported that calcium oxalate stones were the most common among urinary calculi, accounting for more than 70 % of all stones in large series published from the beginning of the 1960s [14, 15, 64, 70]. Indeed, significant differences in the distribution of stone components (especially between crystalline phases) have been observed from country to country due to different risk factors in the studied populations (Table 15.2) [15, 70, 71].

However, in most countries throughout the world, calcium oxalate was found as the main component of a majority of urinary calculi [72–77].

Influence of Gender

Several endogenous and exogenous factors may influence significantly the stone composition. For example, calcium phosphate is more frequent in female patients while calcium oxalate and uric acid are usually more frequent in males. In our experience, based on the analysis of more than 31,000 urinary calculi analyzed from the beginning of the twenty-first century, calcium oxalate was found as main component in 74.9 % of stones in men and 57.9 % in women, COD representing 22.9 % of stones in men and 13.4 % in women (Table 15.3). In contrast, calcium phosphate stones were found almost three times more often in female than in male stone formers (27.1 vs. 9.7 %, $p<0.00001$) with a still higher difference between genders for carbapatite (24.1 % in females and only 7 % in males). Struvite stones appeared as a very small group in both genders (2.4 % in females, 1 % in males). If we consider that struvite is a specific marker for UTI by urease-producing bacteria, its identification in a stone is very important from a medical point of view. Indeed, when considered the percentage of stones containing any proportion of struvite, infection-related stones clearly appeared 3.5–5 times more frequent (12 % in females, 3.6 % in males). Regarding uric acid stones, they represented 11.2 % of all stones in men and 7 % in women. Cystine stones were found in 1.2 % of cases in men and 2.1 % in women. Lastly, ammonium hydrogen urate was scarcely observed as a main component of calculi in France as well as in other industrialized countries (0.2 % in our experience without any significant difference between genders) [16, 78–80], while it was reported more frequently in other countries [72, 76, 81, 82].

Considering now the occurrence of stone components, data summarized in Table 15.4 clearly provide evidence that most stones contain at least two components and that some of them may be as frequent as calcium oxalate but are commonly found in minor proportion. This is the case of calcium phosphate, especially carbapatite, which is often neglected in the statistical data of large series of stones and which is actually found in 79.3 % of the stones in France while its frequency as a main component is only 12.3 % (see Table 15.3). That point is very important for identifying the cause of stone formation or the epidemiological changes in stone composition within a group of stone formers. In fact, a high proportion of urinary stones are initiated by a chemical phase that is not present during the further growth of the stone. The initial phase, despite its very small proportion within the stone, is clinically relevant because it is the marker of the metabolic or environmental conditions involved in stone nucleation. In the absence of such a nucleator, the stone could be not formed. As a consequence, the selective analysis of the stone nucleus is an important step in the identification of the lithogenetic process in a patient. In our experience, carbapatite was found at the origin of the stone in a high proportion of cases, namely, 46 % (52 % in men and 43 % in women). However, the carbapatite content of the stones was less than 5 % in 50 % of cases.

Table 15.3 Frequency (%) of the main components identified in stones from French adult patients ($N=31{,}430$, period 2001–2010)

	Males		Females		Total	
Main component	Number	%	Number	%	Number	%
Calcium oxalates	16,413	74.9	5,687	57.9	22,100	69.7
Calcium oxalate monohydrate	*11,392*	*52.0*	*4,370*	*44.5*	*15,762*	*49.7*
Calcium oxalate dihydrate	*5,021*	*22.9*	*1,317*	*13.4*	*6,338*	*20.0*
Calcium phosphates	2,129	9.7	2,659	27.1	4,788	15.1
Carbapatite	*1,532*	*7.0*	*2,363*	*24.1*	*3,895*	*12.3*
Brushite	*515*	*2.35*	*182*	*1.85*	*697*	2.2
OCP	*42*	*0.2*	*34*	*0.35*	*76*	*0.2*
ACCP	*17*	*0.1*	*44*	*0.45*	*61*	*0.2*
Whitlockite	*23*	*0.1*	*36*	*0.4*	*59*	*0.2*
Struvite	228	1.05	238	2.4	469	1.5
Presence of struvite	*795*	*3.6*	*1,174*	*12.0*	*1,969*	*6.2*
Uric acids	2,464	11.2	692	7.05	3,156	9.9
Uric acid anhydrous	*2,066*	*9.4*	*604*	*6.15*	*2,670*	*8.4*
Uric acid dihydrate	*398*	*1.8*	*88*	*0.9*	*486*	*1.5*
Ammonium urate	39	0.2	33	0.3	72	0.2
Cystine	254	1.2	206	2.1	460	1.45
Proteins	227	1.0	144	1.5	371	1.2
Drugs	45	0.2	23	0.2	68	0.2
Miscellaneous	107	0.5	100	1.0	207	0.65

Table 15.4 Occurrence (%) of stone components observed in France according to the gender of adult patients

	Males	Females
Calcium oxalate	93.0	87.8
Whewellite (COM)	90.2	84.8
Weddellite(COD)	58.8	54.4
Carbapatite (CA)	77.8	82.7
Brushite	3.9	3.6
Octacalcium phosphate, $5H_2O$	2.3	3.9
Whitlockite	3.0	6.3
ACCP	7.4	18.8
Struvite	3.5	11.9
Uric acids	14.4	9.6
Ammonium hydrogen urate	2.6	5.4
Sodium hydrogen urate, $1H_2O$	1.2	0.5
Sodium potassium urate	<0.1	<0.1
Dipotassium urate	<0.1	0.1
Cystine	1.2	2.0
Opal	0.1	<0.1

Influence of Age

Stone composition varies with age, as a consequence of changes in lithogenic risk factors in children and in adult patients as well. As underlined by Robertson [83], changes in stone composition may be observed in both genders during the lifetime. For example, in adults, uric acid stones are infrequent in young European stone formers and become the prevalent category in oldest patients [84] in relation to the increase of body mass index and of the type 2 diabetes occurrence [50, 53]. In contrast, among calcium oxalate stones, weddellite is more common in young than in old patients [84, 85].

Differences Between Countries

Although calcium oxalate appears as the main component in a majority of stones for most countries, some differences are observed according to the studied population group. Some examples can be described for illustrating that point (Tables 15.5 and 15.6). As shown in the tables, calcium oxalate stones were especially frequent in Asia Minor and less frequent in Polynesia. Among crystalline phases, the occurrence of COD stones was high in South America and low in sub-Saharan Africa. Ammonium urate was more frequent in the core of stones from Southeast Asia by comparison with other geographic areas. Uric acid was especially frequent in stones from male patients living in Polynesia, while the occurrence of carbapatite was high in female patients in the same region. MAP stones were more frequent in male and female stone formers who lived in sub-Saharan Africa by comparison to other parts of the world. Such variations in stone composition reflect different stone risk factors in the studied populations.

Epidemiological Data in Pediatric Stone Formers

One of the main differences between industrialized and developing countries is the proportion of pediatric stones,

Table 15.5 Occurrence (%) of main components in urinary calculi from male patients in developing countries grouped according to the geographic area [86]

Geographic area		CaOx	COM	COD	CaP	MAP	Purines	UA	AmUr	Cys	Others
Asia Minor	Global	**84.6**	**63.5**	21.1	**1.0**	**1.0**	11.5	9.6	1.9	0	2.9
	Core	**68.9**	**58.6**	10.3	**14.9**	**1.2**	12.7	9.2	3.5	0	2.3
Southeast Asia	Global	71.9	58.4	13.5	**9.0**	3.4	11.3	7.9	**3.4**	0	4.4
	Core	51.2	42.9	8.3	16.7	**1.2**	19.0	7.1	**11.9**	0	11.9
South America	Global	71.7	38.4	**33.3**	2.6	5.1	18.0	15.4	2.6	0	2.6
	Core	52.8	**22.2**	**30.6**	19.4	2.8	16.7	13.9	2.8	0	8.3
North Africa	Global	71.3	55.5	15.8	8.6	6.4	**8.6**	8.6	0	0.8	4.3
	Core	42.7	35.8	**6.9**	**35.9**	6.1	**7.7**	**6.9**	**0.8**	0.8	6.8
Sub-Saharan Africa	Global	67.2	59.0	**8.2**	3.3	**16.4**	9.9	**6.6**	3.3	0	3.3
	Core	58.9	51.8	7.1	17.9	**8.9**	10.7	7.1	3.6	0	3.6
Polynesia	Global	**50.6**	**29.9**	20.7	6.9	4.6	**35.7**	**34.5**	1.2	0	2.3
	Core	**39.7**	27.7	12.0	20.5	2.4	**33.7**	**27.7**	6.0	0	3.7

Stones were from the following countries: Asia Minor (Turkey, Pakistan), Southeast Asia (China, Laos, Vietnam), South America (Brazil, Paraguay), North Africa (Algeria, Morocco, Tunisia), Black Africa (Cameroon, Mali, Senegal), and Polynesia (Tahiti)
Abbreviations: *CaOx* calcium oxalates, *COM* calcium oxalate monohydrate, *COD* calcium oxalate dihydrate, *CaP* calcium phosphates, *MAP* struvite, *UA* uric acids, *AmUr* ammonium hydrogen urate, *Cys* cystine

Table 15.6 Occurrence of main components in urinary calculi from female patients in developing countries grouped according to the geographic area [86]

Geographic area		CaOx	COM	COD	CaP	MAP	Purines	UA	AmUr	Cys	Others
Asia Minor	Global	**81.1**	**81.1**	**0**	13.5	2.7	**0**	**0**	**0**	0	2.7
	Core	**48.3**	**48.3**	**0**	41.4	**0**	6.9	6.9	**0**	0	3.4
Southeast Asia	Global	68.7	59.3	9.4	25.0	6.3	**0**	**0**	**0**	0	0
	Core	44.4	44.4	0	37.0	3.7	**3.7**	**0**	3.7	0	11.2
South America	Global	58.6	41.2	**17.4**	28.3	8.7	2.2	2.2	**0**	2.2	0
	Core	36.8	26.3	**10.5**	44.8	7.9	5.3	0	5.3	2.6	2.6
North Africa	Global	64.6	58.3	6.3	14.6	**2.1**	8.4	6.3	2.1	0	10.4
	Core	40.0	37.5	2.5	45.0	2.5	13.4	6.7	6.7	0	6.7
Sub-Saharan Africa	Global	34.3	34.3	**0**	**8.6**	**31.4**	**11.4**	5.7	**5.7**	0	8.6
	Core	34.6	34.6	**0**	**19.2**	**30.8**	**19.3**	3.9	**15.4**	0	3.9
Polynesia	Global	**25.3**	**16.0**	9.3	**58.7**	4.0	9.3	**9.3**	0	0	2.7
	Core	**20.0**	**18.5**	1.5	**55.4**	10.8	12.3	**9.2**	3.1	0	1.5

Stones were from the following countries: Asia Minor (Turkey, Pakistan), Southeast Asia (China, Laos, Vietnam), South America (Brazil, Paraguay), North Africa (Algeria, Morocco, Tunisia), Black Africa (Cameroon, Mali, Senegal), and Polynesia (Tahiti)
Abbreviations: *CaOx* calcium oxalates, *COM* calcium oxalate monohydrate, *COD* calcium oxalate dihydrate, *CaP* calcium phosphates, *MAP* struvite, *UA* uric acids, *AmUr* ammonium hydrogen urate, *Cys* cystine

which is very low in the former and often very high in the latter. Another significant difference is the composition of stones in children. Among 1,621 stones from French children aged between 2 months and 17 years old, we found that 38.5 % were predominantly made of calcium oxalate, while 43.4 % were calcium phosphate. Among the latter, 15.5 % contained any proportion of struvite (Table 15.7). Thus, in our experience, when considering stones mainly composed of struvite (7.6 %) and those predominantly composed of calcium oxalate or calcium phosphate or ammonium urate but also containing any minor proportion of struvite, we found that at least 26.2 % of all pediatric stones were related to UTI by urea-splitting microorganisms.

In our experience, purine stones were rather infrequent in French children. They included ammonium hydrogen urate (found as the main component of 3.4 % of calculi), uric acid (2.0 %), dihydroxyadenine (0.3 %), and xanthine (0.1 %).

Cystine was the main component of 4.1 % of stones, while drugs including silica and antiseptics were found in 0.6 % of cases.

Of interest, a significant difference was found between boys and girls concerning the distribution of the main components (see Table 15.7). For example, calcium oxalate counted for 32.3 % of stones in boys and 50.1 % in girls. In contrast with the data from adult patients, calcium phosphate stones were more frequent in boys (49.4 %) than in girls (31.3 %), and struvite was present as a main component in 8.1 % of stones in male and 6.6 % in female patients. Accordingly, struvite was identified in any proportion more frequently in boys (30.1 %) than in girls (18.2 %).

Table 15.7 Frequency of main components found in urinary calculi from French children stone formers ($N=1,621$)

	Boys		Girls		Total	
Main component	Number	%	Number	%	Number	%
Calcium oxalates	351	32.3	273	50.1	624	38.5
Calcium oxalate monohydrate	*178*	*16.4*	*127*	*23.8*	*305*	*18.8*
Calcium oxalate dihydrate	*173*	*15.9*	*146*	*27.3*	*319*	*19.7*
Calcium phosphates	537	49.4	167	31.3	704	43.4
Carbapatite	*451*	*41.5*	*128*	*24.0*	*579*	*35.7*
Brushite	*31*	*2.8*	*18*	*3.4*	*49*	*3.0*
OCPP	*14*	*1.3*	*7*	*1.3*	*21*	*1.3*
ACCP	*27*	*2.5*	*10*	*1.9*	*37*	*2.3*
Whitlockite	*14*	*1.3*	*4*	*0.7*	*18*	*1.1*
Struvite	88	8.1	35	6.6	123	7.6
Presence of struvite	*328*	*30.1*	*97*	*18.2*	*425*	*26.2*
Purines	71	6.6	23	4.3	94	5.8
Uric acids	*25*	*2.3*	*8*	*1.5*	*33*	*2.0*
Ammonium urate	*41*	*3.8*	*14*	*2.6*	*55*	*3.4*
Dihydroxyadenine	*4*	*0.4*	*1*	*0.2*	*5*	*0.3*
Xanthine	*1*	*0.1*	*0*	*0*	*1*	*<0.1*
Cystine	32	2.9	34	6.4	66	4.1
Drugs	8	0.7	2	0.4	10	0.6

In developing countries, only few data based on sufficiently large series of stones analyzed by physical methods are available. During the past century, it was commonly reported that stone disease mainly affected children and, among them, preferentially boys with a sex ratio M/F often >10 and that stone composition was predominantly uric acid and/or ammonium hydrogen urate and phosphates, while calcium oxalate was poorly represented [87]. In parallel, the location of the stones was the lower urinary tract in a large majority of cases [88, 89]. At the end of the twentieth century, significant changes were observed in the stone profile of these countries [86, 87]. An increase of calcium oxalate content in the stones was observed and also a change in stone location from the bladder to the kidney. The ratio between children and adult stone formers progressively decreased, and in parallel, the male-to-female sex ratio varied in the same way. In Table 15.8 are summarized data from several countries regarding stone composition in children. The data provide evidence that calcium oxalate is actually the most frequent component. However, some differences still exist according to the series as concern the frequency of ammonium urate. That compound was found as the main crystalline phase of pediatric stones in 5 % of cases in Armenia and in more than 25 % of cases in Turkey. On the other hand, a significant proportion of calcium oxalate stones have been initiated by an ammonium urate nucleus. In our experience [86], ammonium urate was found at the beginning of the stone in about 40 % of pediatric stones collected in various developing countries, while carbapatite was found as the core of calculi in 43 % of stones formed in French children.

Influence of Age

As in adults, the patient's age may influence the composition of stones, as a result of changes in the risk factors involved in stone formation. For example, in infants born and living in industrialized countries, calcium phosphate is the main component of most stones as a result of urinary tract infection, while in children aged more than 5 years old, calcium oxalate becomes the prevalent form of stones. Uric acid and/or ammonium hydrogen urate are more frequent in young children than in older ones, in part as a result of tubular immaturity in infants, which may induce high levels of uricosuria and purine crystallization.

In developing countries, urinary calculi developed in infant and young children often are initiated by ammonium hydrogen urate as a result of multiple factors: diarrhea episodes and/or urinary tract infection, cereal-rich regimen, and low phosphate intake [60, 90, 93]. *Biological consequences of these conditions are a low diuresis and a high urine concentration of both uric acid and ammonium ions while urinary sodium and potassium content is decreased (digestive losses), thus favoring ammonium urate supersaturation and crystallization.*

Today, in an increasing proportion of cases, ammonium urate is surrounded by layers of calcium oxalate as a consequence of chronic low diuresis and oxalate-rich vegetables

Table 15.8 Stone composition reported in pediatric population from developing countries

Authors	Sarkissian et al. [90]	Rizvi et al. [89]		Marrakchi et al. [91]	Meiouet and El Kabbaj [92]
Year	2001	2003		2008	2010
Country	Armenia	Pakistan		Tunisia	Morocco
Stone localization	UUT+LUT	UUT	LUT	UUT+LUT	UUT+LUT
No. of calculi	198	527	245	187	222
Stone composition (%)					
Calcium oxalate	62	47.5	45	61.5	51.8
Calcium oxalate monohydrate	–	45	39	49.2	43.2
Calcium oxalate dihydrate	–	2.6	6	12.3	8.6
Calcium phosphate	7	15.1	10	18.8	9.5
Ammonium hydrogen urate	5	26.7	28	6.4	15.3
Uric acid	7	4.7	8	5.9	2.2
Struvite	17	5.5	8	7.0	14.9
Cystine	2	0.2	0	5.3	4.0
Others	–	–	–	2.1	2.3

consumption. Thus, in some countries, the occurrence of ammonium hydrogen urate as main component is low [90] by comparison to other countries [93–96]. In children aged more than 5 years, calcium oxalate is the commonest form of urinary calculi in both genders.

Of note, urinary calculi resulting from an inherited disorder and made of calcium oxalate, cystine, or dihydroxyadenine are commonly discovered in children aged more than 5 years.

Proposed Methodology for a Comprehensive Stone Analysis

A comprehensive stone analysis must be able to provide information for identifying the cause of the stone disease. To achieve this goal, several kinds of information should be collected from the analysis:

- Nature and proportion of crystalline phases
- Distribution of the crystalline phases within the stone
- Composition of the stone nucleus or stone core when available
- Identification of specific lithogenic process such as stone formation from a Randall's plaque, crystalline conversion, and dodecahedral crystals of weddellite
- Morphological data suggestive of specific lithogenic conditions or pathologies at the origin of the stone

As shown in Fig. 15.1a–h, the same crystalline phase appears under a diversity of morphological features that are often related to very different etiological conditions. Therefore, we advocate a comprehensive stone analysis method combining morphological examination followed by XRD or FTIR analysis of the core, middle layers, and surface of the stone. That morpho-constitutional analysis of stones provides a more reliable contribution to etiologic diagnosis of stone disease than compositional analysis alone.

Thus, the stone analysis should include two steps:

1. The first step, based on an optical examination through a moderately growing stereomicroscope, is to collect data on stone morphology. In most cases, that first examination is especially useful to identify stone nucleus and the different stages of the further stone growth. During the optical examination of the stones, the samples judged relevant for the comprehensive analysis may be chosen for further identification of their accurate composition based on the use of other physical methods. That first step is also of a valuable help in the case only chemical methods are available for identifying stone components because morphological examination allows identifying most of the common crystalline species found in the stones.
2. The second step is the use of a physical method (infrared spectroscopy or X-ray diffraction) capable of providing more reliable information on the stone composition, relevant from a clinical point of view, and sensitive enough to analyze separately small parts such as the core, the inner layers, and the periphery of the stone. In routine practice, Fourier transform infrared spectroscopy based on signal transmission is the most appropriate method because it offers the opportunity to analyze very small samples (less than 100 μmug if required) and to provide an accurate spectrum of all mineral or organic components, whatever their crystalline state.

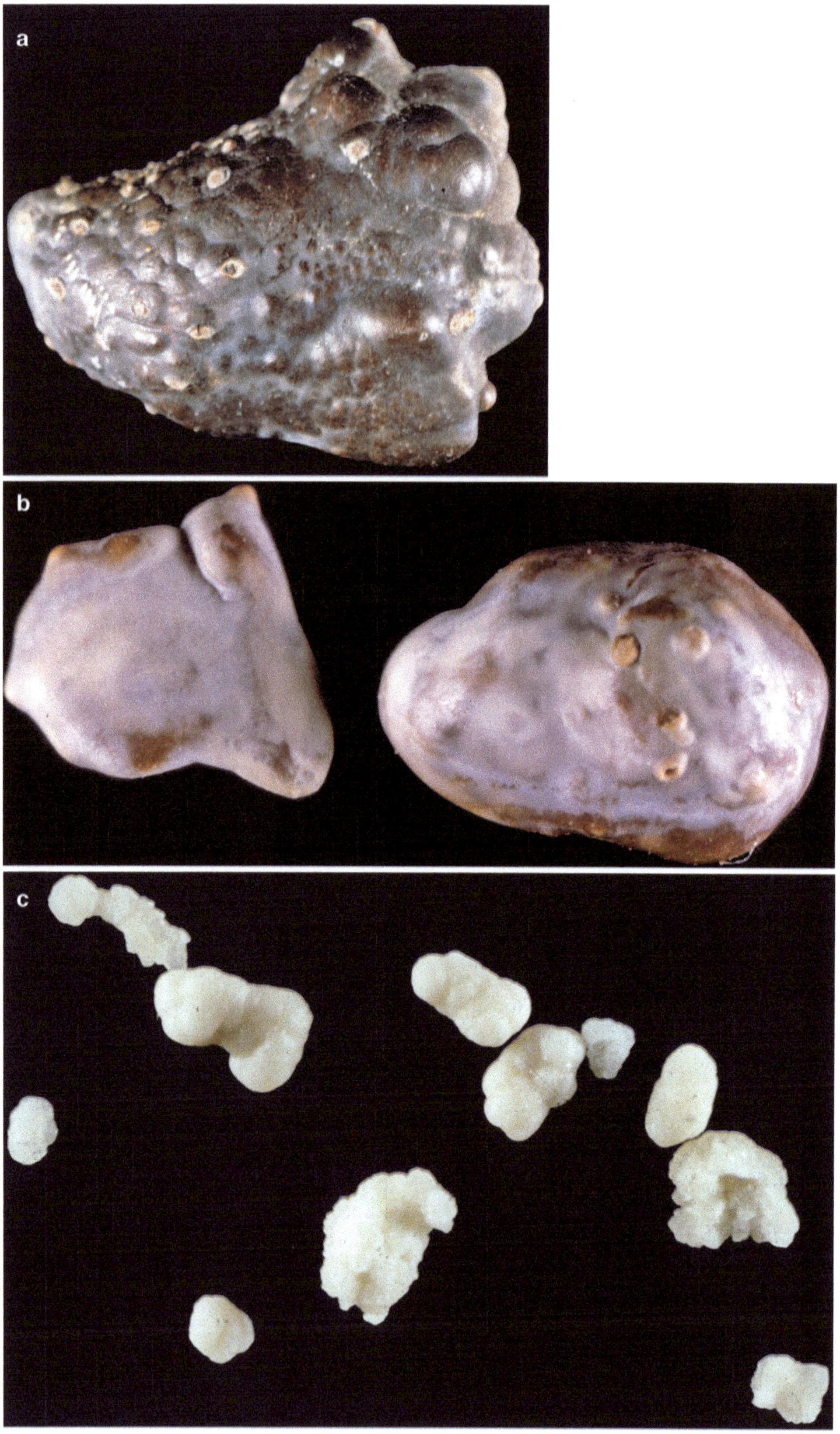
a
b
c

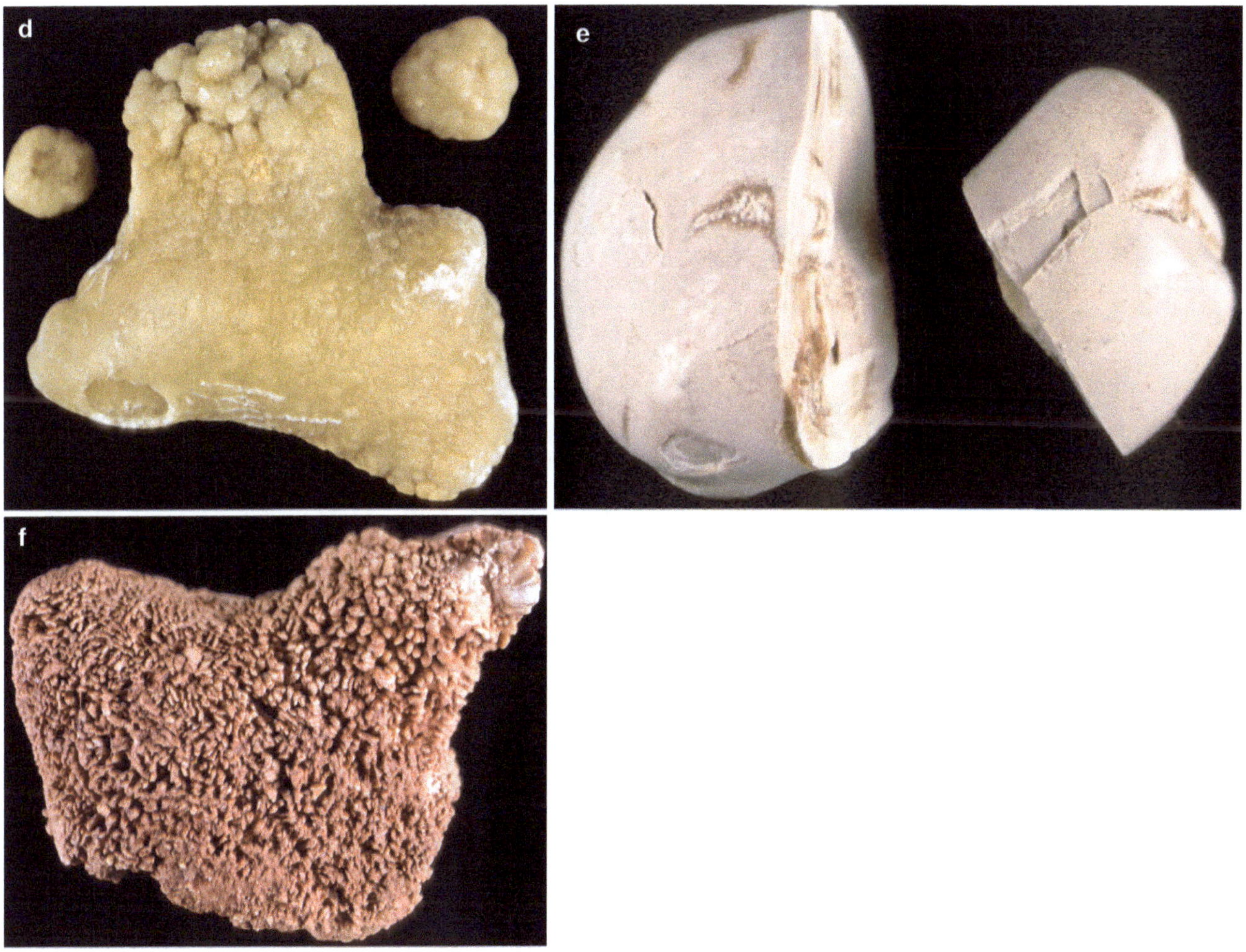

Fig. 15.1 (continued)

Fig. 15.1 Different subtypes of calculi made of pure or nearly pure whewellite illustrating the clinical interest of stone morphology examination to orient diagnosis. (**a**) Common whewellite stone with a *dark-brown* surface (subtype Ia). Such calculi essentially result from intermittent mild hyperoxaluria induced by oxalate-rich food consumption or as a consequence of low diuresis (high urine oxalate concentration). The *dark color* may be considered a sign of a "quiescent" stone. (**b**) Whewellite stone with a *dark-brown* surface (subtype Ia) extensively coated by a very recent layer of small whewellite crystals as a result of a recent peak of oxalate concentration in urine. Such aspect may be considered as a marker of an "active" stone. (**c**) Whewellite stones (subtype Ic) spontaneously passed in a young child aged 3 years. Note the white color which is a marker of a very active lithogenic process as a result of a heavy hyperoxaluria as observed in the case of primary hyperoxaluria type 1. (**d**) Whewellite stones (subtype Ic) as pieces of a staghorn nephrolithiasis in a child aged 7 years presenting with primary hyperoxaluria. The light color of the stone and the budding aspect are highly suggestive of that inherited disease. (**e**) Whewellite stone fragments presenting a light smooth surface as a consequence of continuous rubbing of the stone against other calculi confined in the same anatomical site due to an anomaly of the urinary tract such as a caliceal diverticulum or a pelvis junction syndrome. Such morphology corresponds to the subtype Id of the stone classification. (**f**) Whewellite stone with an uncommon morphology resulting from a crystalline conversion of caoxite (the initial phase) to whewellite. Such calculi are very rare. They have been observed in patients suffering heavy hyperoxaluria from genetic or iatrogenic origin associated with an abnormal stabilization of caoxite in urine as a consequence of an altered urine inhibition. Most cases of such whewellite stones were described in patients suffering cardiovascular diseases and long-term treated with the association of two drugs: piridoxilate and pentaerythritol tetranitrate. (**g**) Whewellite stones (subtype Ie) with a heterogeneous surface as a result of various hyperoxaluric states in a patient suffering from Crohn's disease with subsequent extended ileal resection, steatorrhea, and high oxalate absorption by the colon mucosa. (**h**) Example of a whewellite stone (subtype Ia) developed from a Randall's plaque. Such calculi are the result of secondary nucleation of calcium oxalate from a papillary calcium phosphate deposit. Typically, such calculi have a locally depressed surface, which corresponds to the papillary print and containing a whitish small deposit (*arrow*), commonly made of carbapatite (Randall's plaque), initially formed within the interstitium of the deep medullar part of the kidney and growing up to the papillary epithelium. Carbapatite Randall's plaque could be the consequence of transient hypercalciuric states, while subtype Ia whewellite developed from the plaque is highly suggestive for a secondary lithogenic process related to a mild hyperoxaluria

Fig. 15.1 (continued)

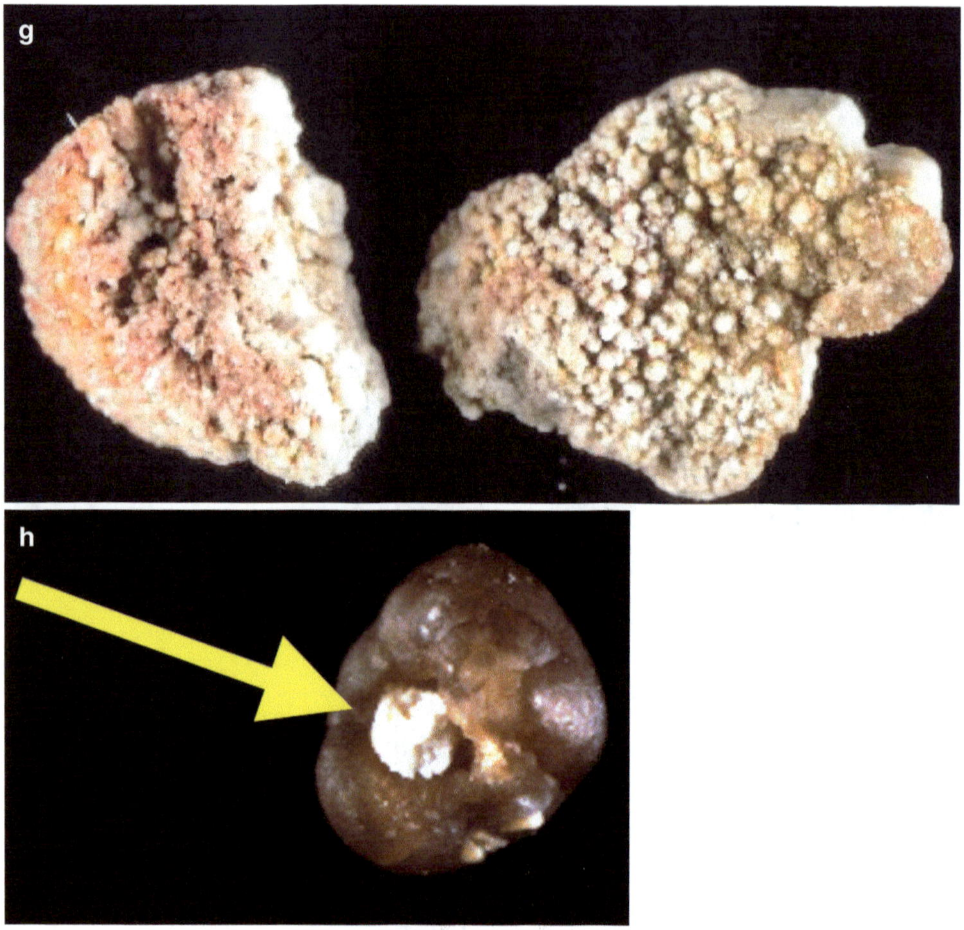

Morpho-Constitutional Classification of Stones

Morpho-Constitutional Stone Analysis Method

The method adopted for morpho-constitutional analysis was reported in detail elsewhere [2]. In short, it consists of examining by means of a stereomicroscope (magnification ×10 to ×40) the morphology of stone surface and section, with special attention paid to identify the nucleus (or core) and the inner organization of the stone. The main points to be recorded are size and form of the stone, color and aspect (smooth, rough, budding, etc.) of its surface, presence of an umbilication, structure of the section (well organized with concentric layers and/or radiating organization, or loose and poorly organized), aspect, and location of the nucleus. Thereafter, each part of the calculus (nucleus, midsection, and surface) is processed for analysis by FTIR, and the global proportion of components is determined on a powdered sample of the whole stone.

In stones of specific composition such as cystine, 2,8-dihydroxyadenine, xanthine, struvite, or drug-containing calculi [9], morphologic examination is of limited interest if physical methods such as FTIR or X-ray diffraction are used for identifying stone composition. In contrast, in the case of stones analyzed by chemical methods, morphological examination is of crucial importance to suspect a specific uncommon composition, especially with respect to components that cannot be reliably identified by usual chemical reactions. As often reported in the literature, 2,8-dihydroxyadenine [5, 6] is commonly mistaken with uric acid by chemical methods. However, stone morphology is very different (see Fig. 15.16) and may immediately orient toward this specific type of stone [4].

Morphological Classification of Stones

Because a same chemical component, such as CaOx, calcium phosphate, or uric acid, presents under several different forms, distinct morphological aspects may be individualized, which reflects different etiopathogenic conditions.

By morphological examination, urinary calculi may be classified into 7 main types and 22 subtypes, as summarized in Figs. 15.2, 15.3, 15.4, 15.5, 15.6, and 15.7 with photographs illustrating the corresponding morphology of both surface and section of the stones. Briefly, type I was assigned to whewellite and type II to weddellite stones. All trioxypurines (uric acids and urates) were grouped together in the type III and all calcium and magnesium phosphates were

Subtype	Main crystalline phase	Main morphological characteristics	Surface	Section
Ia (n = 8151) (18.0%)	Whewellite	Mamillary surface. Section made of concentric layers with radiating organization. Color: brown. Frequent umbilication and Randall's plaque indicative of papillary origin	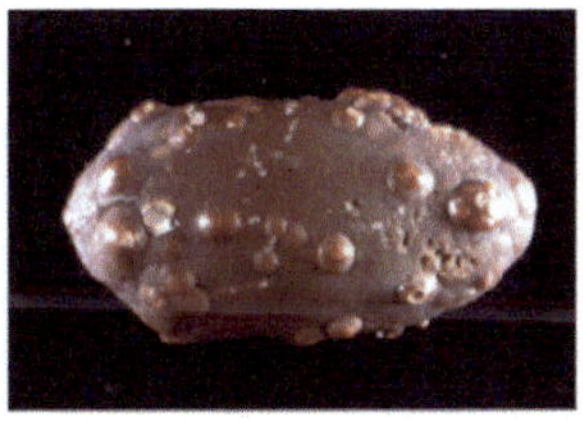	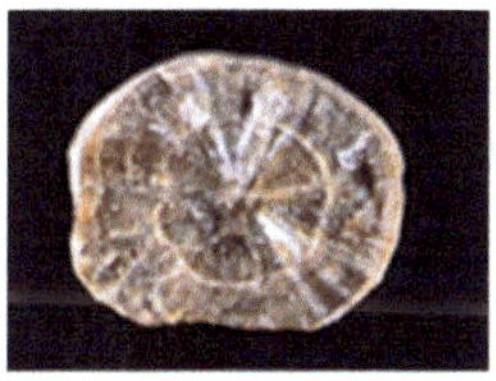
Ib (n = 458) (1.0%)	Whewellite	Mamillary and rough surface. No umbilication. Unorganized section. Color: brown to dark brown	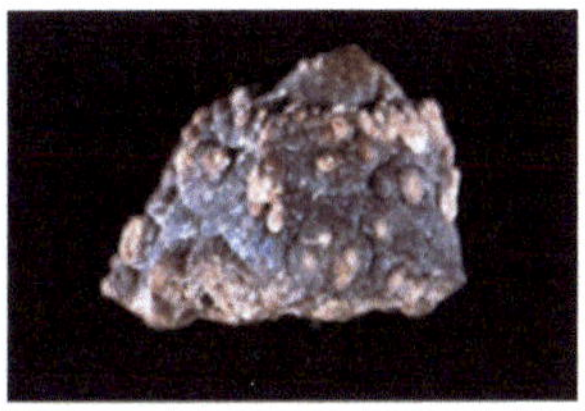	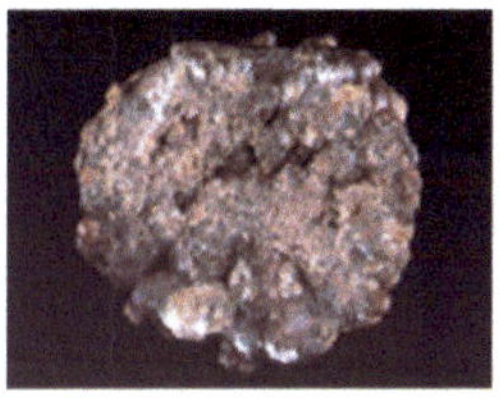
Ic (n = 88) (0.2%)	Whewellite	Budding surface. Finely granular and poorly organized section. Light color, cream to pale yellow-brown	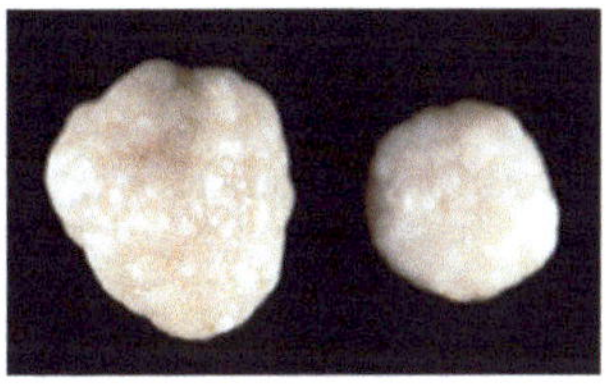	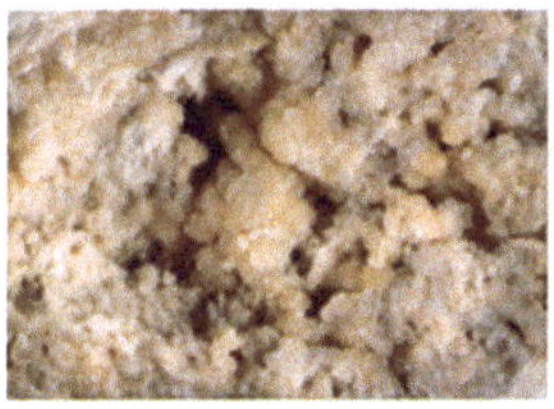
Id (n = 379) (0.8%)	Whewellite	Smooth surface. Compact section made of thin concentric layers. Color: beige or pale brown	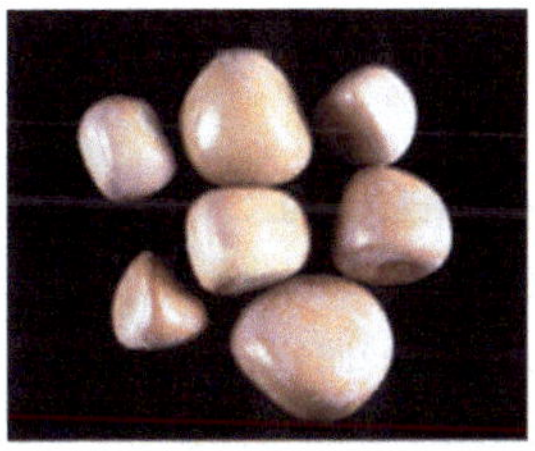	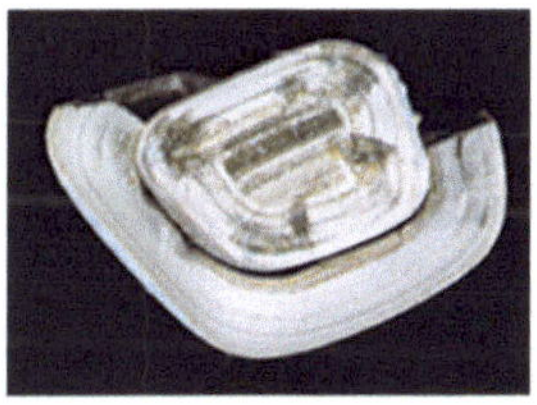
Ie (n = 170) (0.4%)	Whewellite	Locally budding, mamillary or rough surface. Section: locally unorganized or radiating structure. Color: pale yellow-brown to brown	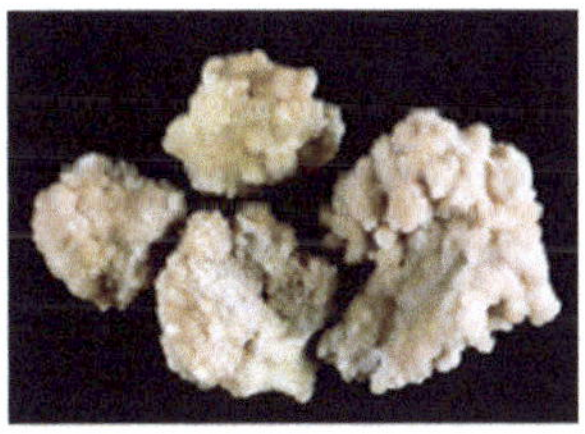	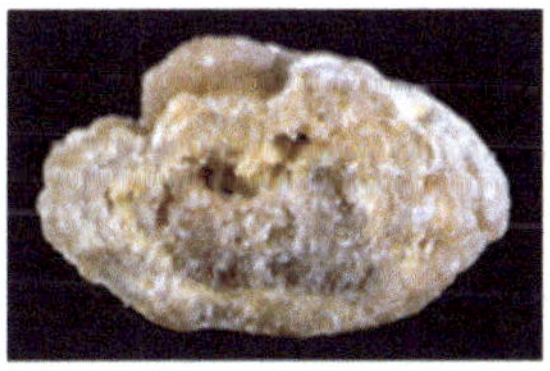

Fig. 15.2 Type I stones, composed of calcium oxalate monohydrate (*COM*) or whewellite

Subtype	Main crystalline phase	Main morphological characteristics	Surface	Section
IIa (n = 2807) (6.2%)	Weddellite	Spiculated surface showing aggregated bipyramidal crystals with sharp angles and edges. Section showing loose radial crystallization. Color: pale yellow-brown	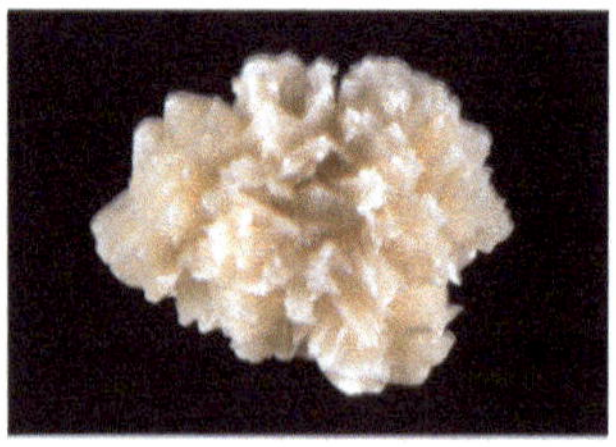	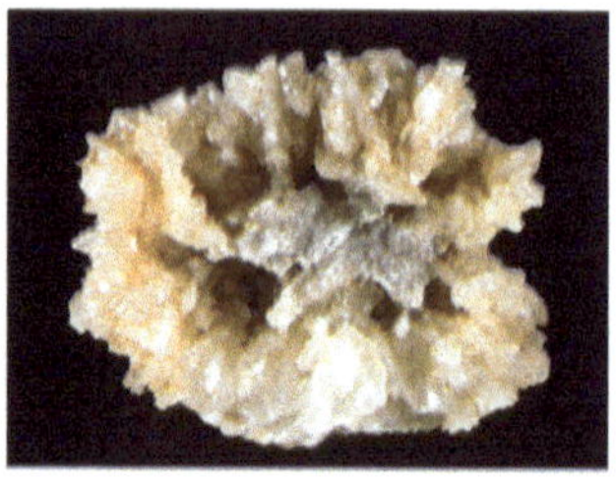
IIb (n =1220) (2.7%)	Weddellite	Spiculated surface showing aggregated bipyramidal crystals with blunt angles and ridges. Section showing compact unorganized crystallization. Color: pale yellow-brown	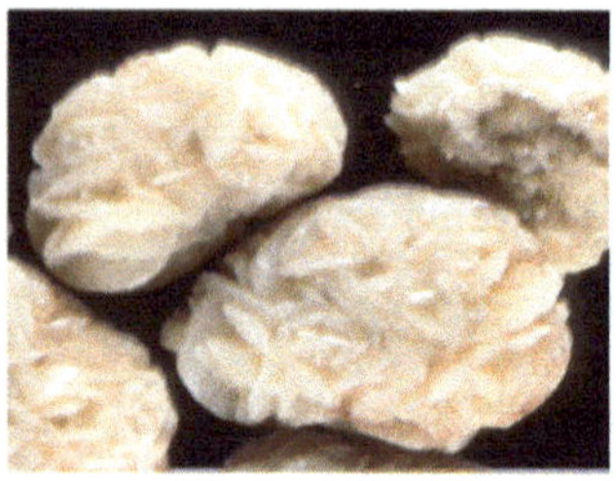	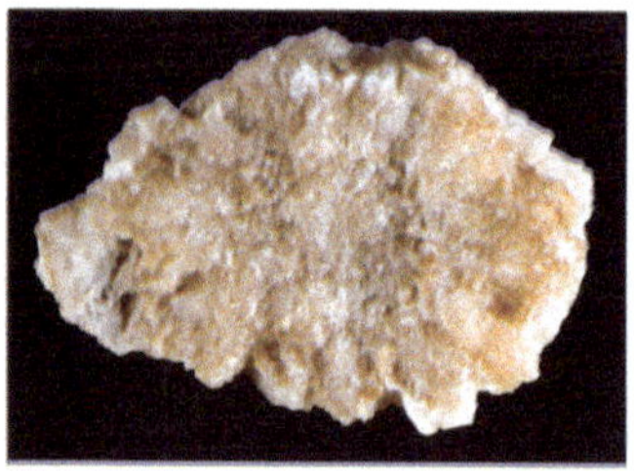
IIc (n = 28) (0.06%)	Weddellite	Rough surface. Section: unorganized core with diffuse concentric structure in periphery. Color: gray-beige to dark yellow-brown	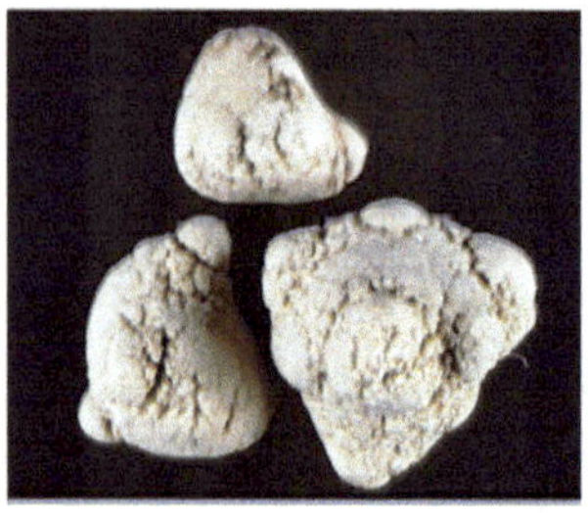	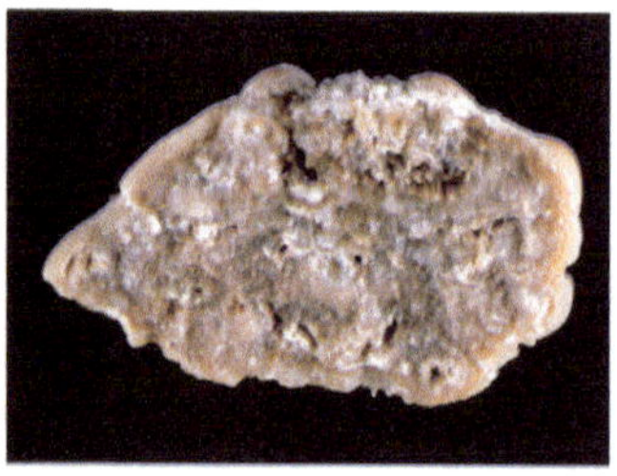

Fig. 15.3 Type II stones, mainly composed of calcium oxalate dihydrate (*COD*) or weddellite

Subtype	Main crystalline phase	Main morphological characteristics	Surface	Section
IIIa (n = 711) (1.6%)	Uric acid anhydrous	Homogeneous smooth surface. Section: concentric structure with radiating organization. Color: typically orange	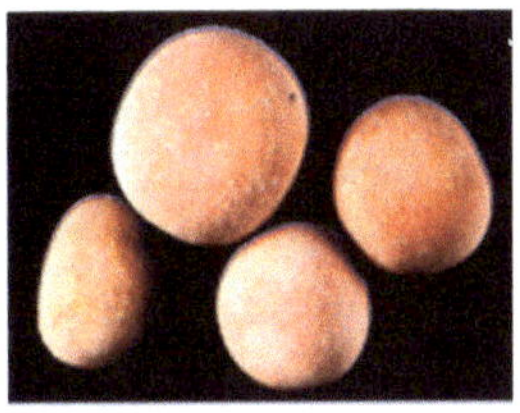	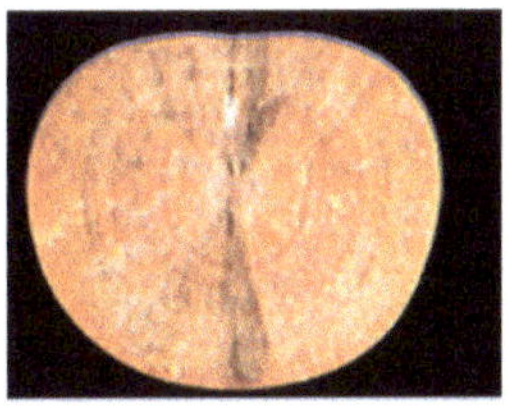
IIIb (n = 2506) (5.5%)	Uric acide dihydrate (± uric acid anhydrous	Embossed, rough and porous surface. Heterogeneous color from beige to brown–orange. Poorly organized section with frequent porous areas. Color: orange	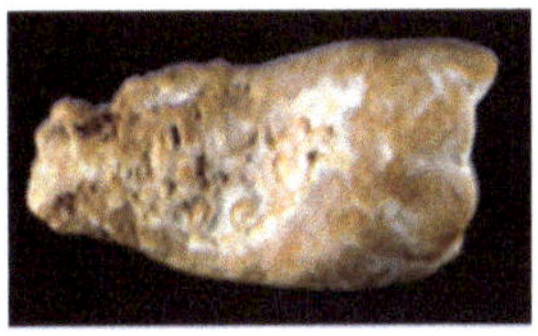	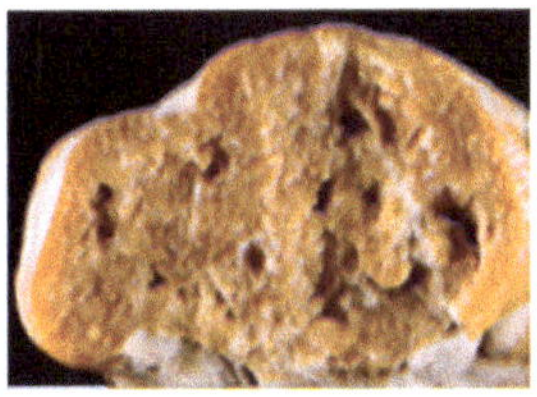
IIIc (n = 146) (0.3%)	Urate salts, including ammonium hydrogen urate	Homogeneous rough and locally porous surface. Beige to grayish. Unorganized porous section. Color: whitish to grayish	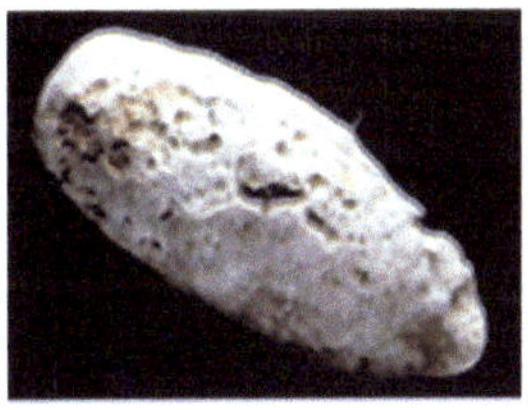	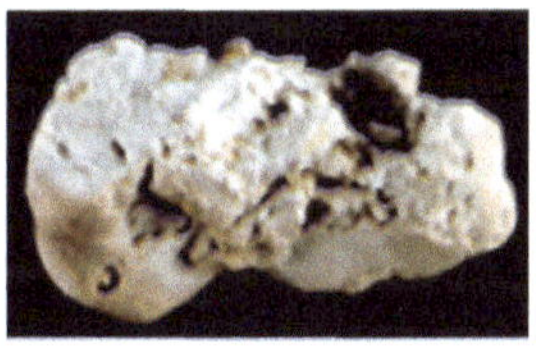
IIId (n = 33) (0.07%)	Ammonium hydrogen urate	Heterogeneous embossed, rough and porous surface. Color: grayish to brown. Section made of altornated layers, thick and brownish or thin and grayish, locally porous	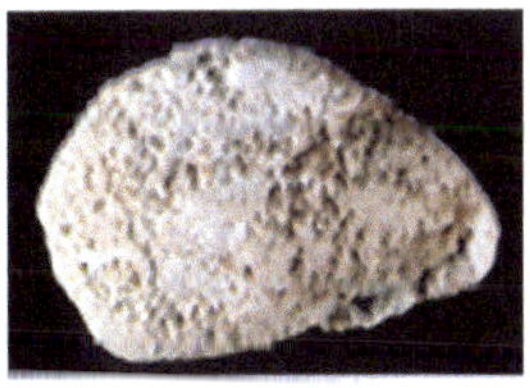	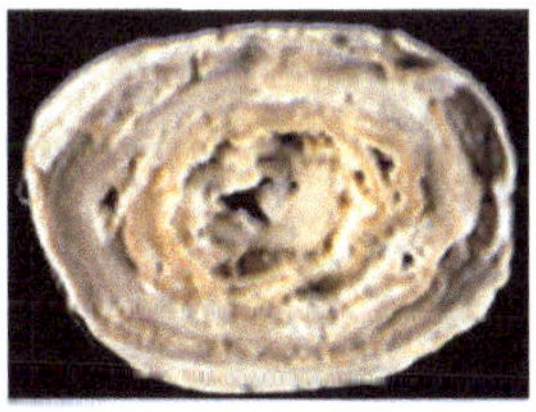

Fig. 15.4 Type III stones, mainly composed of uric acids or urate salts

Subtype	Main crystalline phase	Main morphological characteristics	Surface	Section
IVa1 (1179) (2.6%)	Carbapatite	Rough homogenous surface. Section: poorly organized, or diffuse concentric layers. Color: whitish to beige	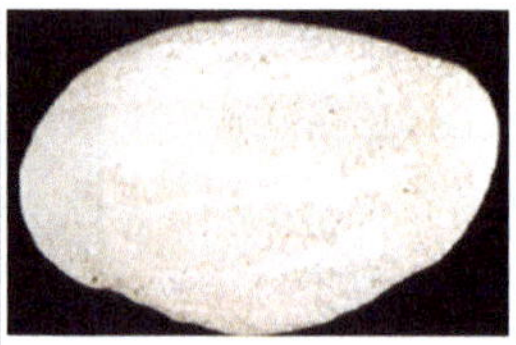	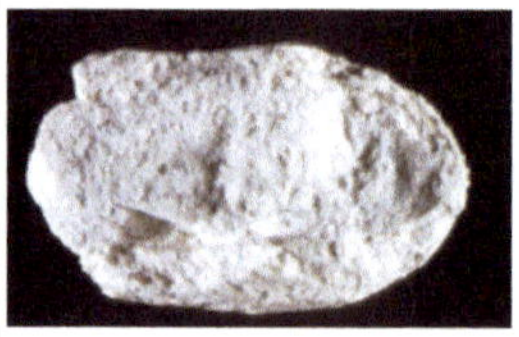
IVa2 (n = 249) (0.55%)	Carbapatite	Embossed and varnished surface with small cracks. Glazed appearance. Section made of alternated layers, thick brown-yellow and thin beige. Often, multiple nuclei.	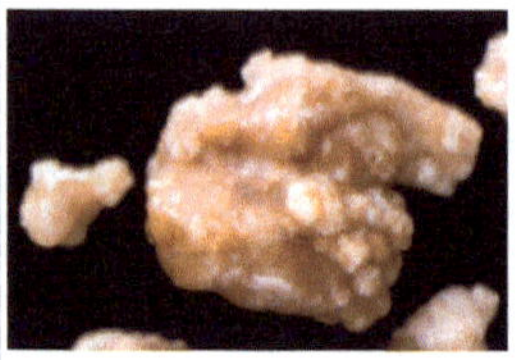	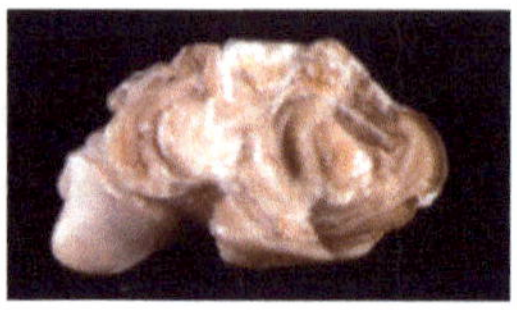
IVb (n=1669) (3.7%)	Carbapatite + struvite	Heterogeneous, both embossed and rough surface. Heterogeneous color, cream to dark brown. Section made of irregularly alternating thick, whitish, and thin, brown-yellow layers.	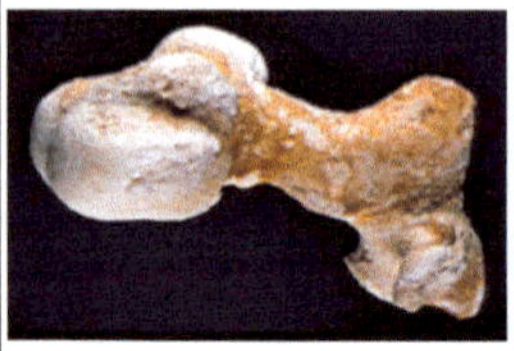	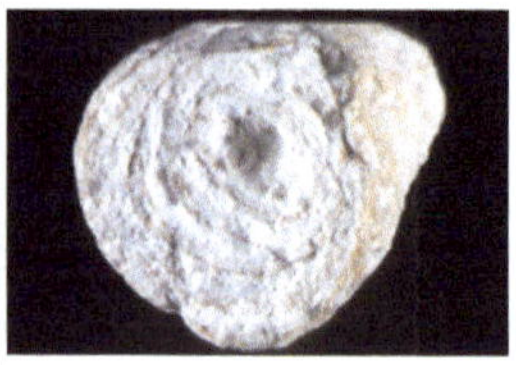
IVc (n = 528) (1.2%)	Struvite	Homogenous surface made of amalgamate crystals with blunt angles and edges. Section: crude radial crystallization. Color: whitish.	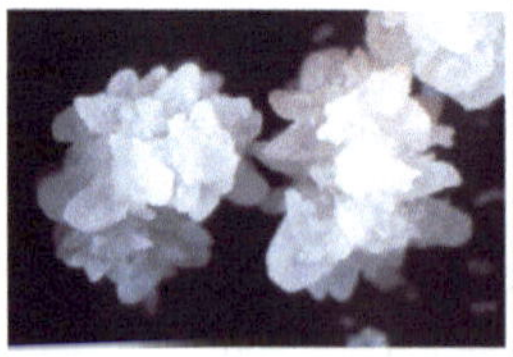	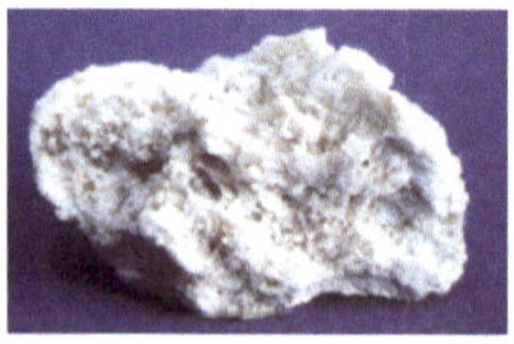
IVd (n = 610) (1.4%)	Brushite	Finely rough or dappled surface. Section made of concentric layers with radial crystallization. Color: whitish to beige.	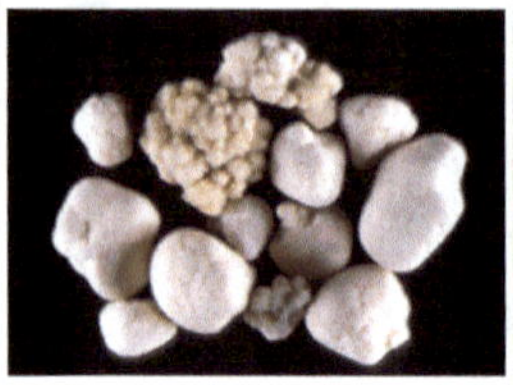	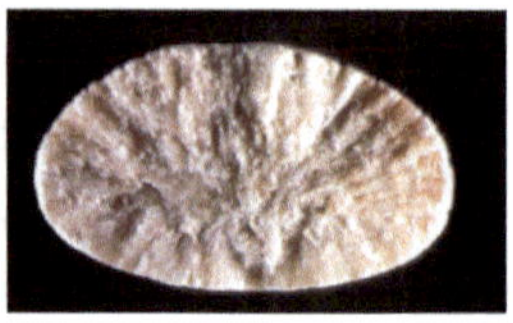

Fig. 15.5 Type IV stones, mainly composed of calcium and/or magnesium phosphates

Subtype	Main crystalline phase	Main morphological characteristics	Surface	Section
Va (n = 527) (1.2%)	Cystine	Rough surface. Section: poorly organized, sometimes radiating organization. Color: yellowish	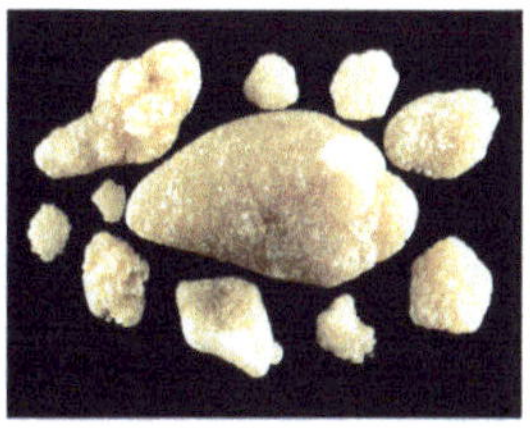	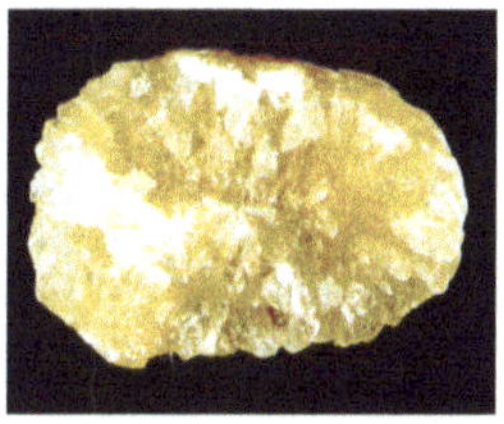
Vb (n = 62) (0.1%)	Cystine	Smooth surface. Section: concentric layers in periphery, unorganized core. Color: cream to yellowish	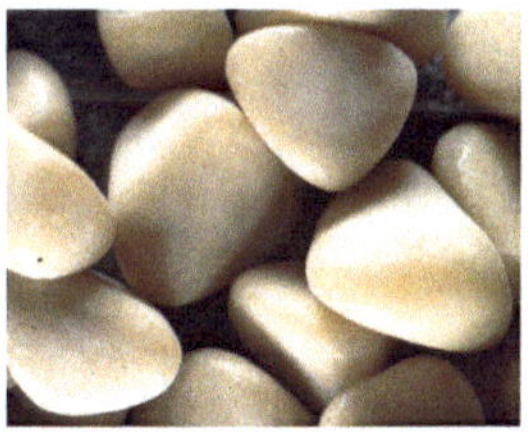	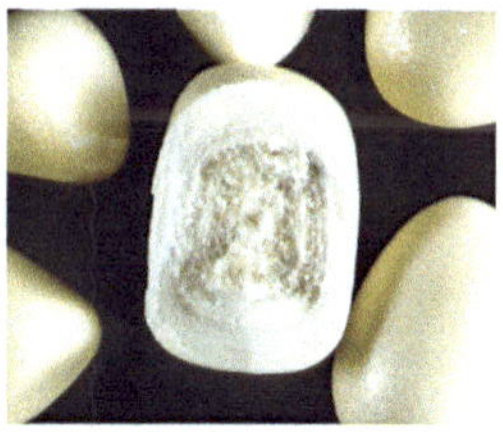

Fig. 15.6 Type V stones, composed of cystine

included in the type IV. Type V was assigned to cystine stones and type VI to protein-rich calculi. Finally, type VII was assigned to all stones containing rare components such as rare purines and drugs. The figures indicate the respective frequency of the various types and subtypes as observed among 45,298 calculi analyzed at our laboratory over the past 20 years. The relative frequency of the various types may be different in other populations.

As shown in Figs. 15.2, 15.3, 15.4, 15.5, 15.6, and 15.7, nearly half of stones (48.5 %) were of homogenous composition, corresponding to a single type of the classification (that means pure stones or stones containing minor components accounting for less than 10 % of the stone mass), whereas the other half (51.5 %) were of mixed structure, as shown in Table 15.9.

Factors Influencing Stone Morphology

The morphology of stones, for a given chemical composition, depends on a number of factors, especially the size and shape of constitutive crystals [97]. As an example, uric acid and struvite, which often present as large crystals and aggregates in urine, lead to rapidly growing and poorly organized stones, whereas COM stones, made of small crystals, exhibit a dense, well-organized structure.

Kinetics of crystal growth significantly influences the stone structure. The well-organized inner structure with concentric layers and radiating crystallization of COM calculi (see Fig. 15.2, subtype Ia) suggests an intermittent stone growth such as observed in idiopathic CaOx stone formers, whereas the heavy, permanent hyperoxaluria as observed in patients with primary hyperoxaluria type 1 results in the formation of pure COM calculi with a poorly organized structure (see Fig. 15.2, subtype Ic).

Surface color of stones also reflects kinetics of lithogenesis or peculiar lithogenic conditions. A dark color of COM stones reflects incorporation of macromolecules and pigments into the stone during a slow lithogenic process. In contrast, thin whitish layer at the surface of a dark-brown whewellite stone (Fig. 15.8a, b) reflects the recent deposition of COM crystals favored by a transient period of high urine oxalate concentration [97]. Confinement within a cavity (such as a diverticulum) or hydronephrosis results in a smooth, plane, and often poorly pigmented surface of stones (see Fig. 15.2, subtype Id), the light color resulting in this case from rubbing of stones against each other.

Relationships Between Stone Composition, Morphology, and Etiology

Calcium Oxalate Stones

CaOx presents in three distinct crystalline forms, namely, CaOx monohydrate (COM) or whewellite, CaOx dihydrate (COD) or weddellite, and CaOx trihydrate (COT) or caoxite, which reflect different lithogenic conditions.

Idiopathic Calcium Oxalate Stones

Common stones made predominantly of COM or COD present with a quite distinct morphology. Common COM stones

Subtype	Main crystalline phase	Main morphological characteristics	Surface and section
VIa (n = 39) (0.1%)	Proteins	Matrix calculi. Homogeneous surface. Unorganizad section. Color: cream to pale brown.	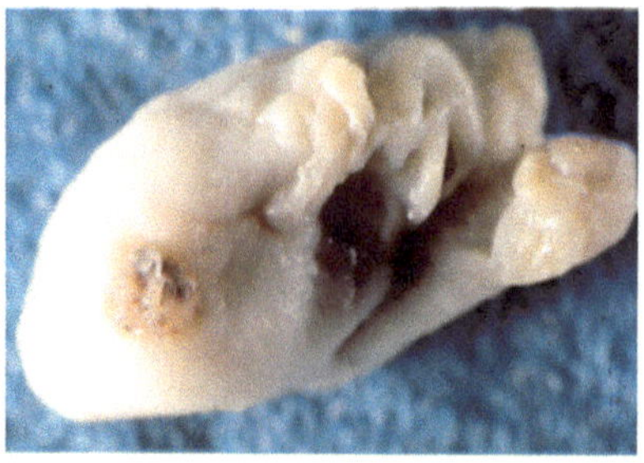
VIb (n = 345) (n = 0.8%)	Proteins and drugs or metabolic compounds	Heterogeneous, irregularly rough surface. Locally scaled. Section: crude and diffuse foliated structure. Color: dark brown to black. Other components often present in these stones may alter the structure and the color.	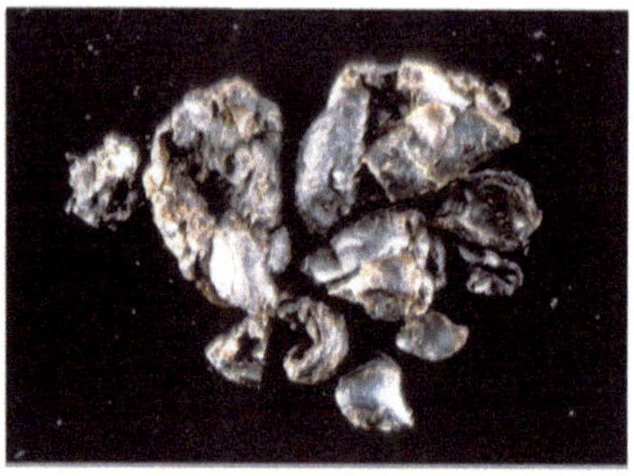
VIc (n = 71) (0.2%)	Proteins and whewellite	Homogeneous, smooth surface with clefts and scales. Color dark brown. Section made of a dark brown protein shield surrounding a loose, unorganized light core containing whewellite crystals mixed with proteins.	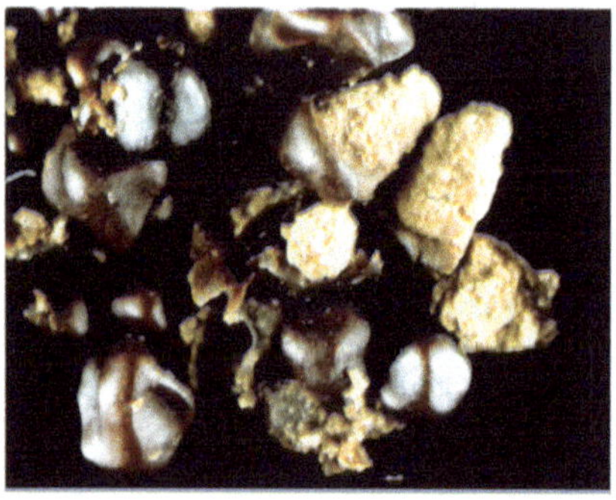

Fig. 15.7 Type VI stones, containing pure or abundant proteins

Table 15.9 Urinary calculi of mixed types

Mixed types	No. of stones (%)
Ia+IIa or Ia+IIb	9,243 (20.4)
IIa+IVa1 or IIb+IVa1	5,417 (12.0)
Complex type I+II+IV	2,701 (6.0)
Ia+IIIb	658 (1.4)
Ia+IVa	534 (1.2)
IIa+IVb	257 (0.6)
Other mixed types	3,171 (7.0)
Total	21,981 (48.5)

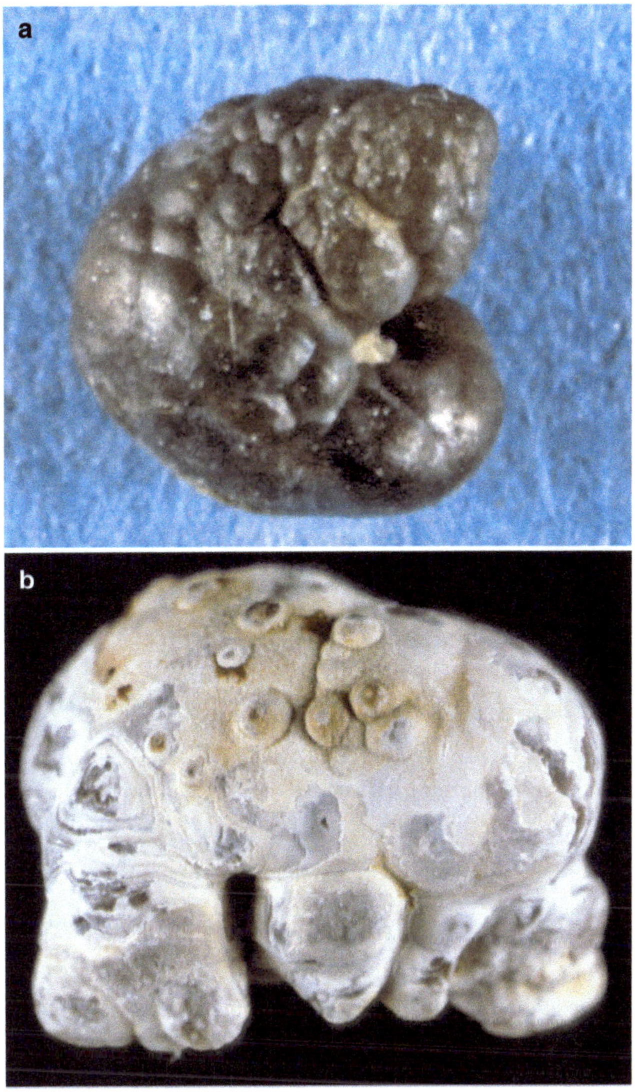

Fig. 15.8 (**a**) *Dark-brown* COM stone as a result of urine pigments progressively deposited at the surface of COM crystals. The *dark color* of COM stones is suggestive of a slow growth. When the surface exhibits a *dark color*, it can be concluded the stone is not metabolically active. (**b**) Whitish to grayish thin layer corresponding to a recent deposit of COM crystals at the surface of a *dark-brown* calculus. Such a finding suggests the stone was in an active phase at the time it was removed or spontaneously passed

exhibit a smooth, wrinkled, or mammillary dark-brown surface (see Fig. 15.2), while COD calculi have a prickly, light yellowish-brown surface (see Fig. 15.3). Within the group of CaOx stones, COD calculi are mostly found in hypercalciuric conditions [85, 97, 98], whereas COM calculi rather result from high urinary oxalate concentration without excessive calcium level [98]. Combination of both hypercalciuria and high oxalate concentration results in the formation of large aggregates and mixed-type (COM and COD) calculi (Fig. 15.9).

Primary Hyperoxaluria and "Type Ic" Calculi

As previously mentioned, calculi from patients with primary hyperoxaluria (PH), which are made of pure COM, exhibit a quite different morphology than that observed for common COM stones, with a pale-yellowish surface and a loose, unorganized section (see Fig. 15.2, subtype Ic). Scanning electron microscopy confirmed the differences in crystalline structure between common-type and PH1 calculi [99]. All 88 stones from patients with PH1 analyzed in our laboratory had this Ic morphologic aspect, which appears to be virtually pathognomonic for the disease. Therefore, this peculiar morphology of pure COM stones should immediately orient to the diagnosis of this severe disease, thus prompting comprehensive laboratory evaluation and early institution of proactive therapeutic strategy.

Enteric Hyperoxaluria

In enteric hyperoxaluria, as observed in ileal resection for Crohn's disease, jejunoileal bypass for obesity, or bariatric surgery, stones exhibit a more heterogeneous structure than in the aforementioned conditions, with alternately poorly organized areas and locally concentric layers with radiating

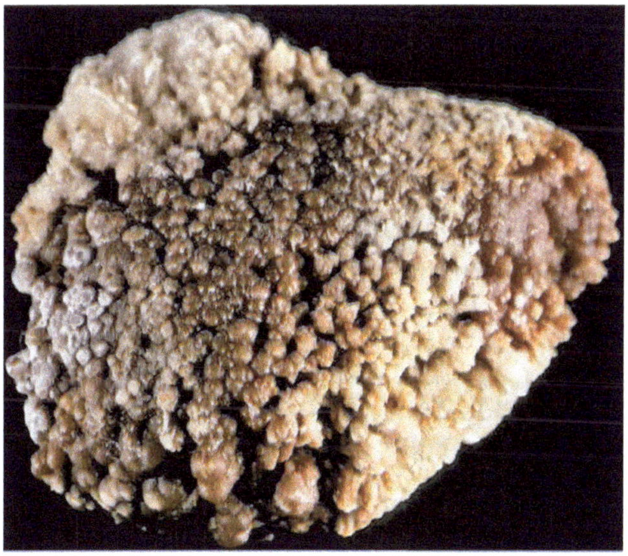

Fig. 15.9 CaOx stone composed of a mixture of COM and COD indicative of both hypercalciuria and hyperoxaluria, commonly of dietary origin

organization (see Fig. 15.2, subtype Ie). The color variations from poorly to well-organized layers also reflect changes in the kinetics of stone growth. However, in a limited number of cases, due to severe and repeated hyperabsorption of oxalate by the colon mucosa, a heavy hyperoxaluria may be observed, which is responsible for massive crystalluria of whewellite leading to the formation of calculi which resemble subtype Ic. Thus, such a morphological type should be always considered as highly suggestive for a severe lithogenic process, which is in addition a frequent cause for kidney failure.

Calcium Oxalate Dihydrate Stones

Hypercalciuria is identified as a major lithogenic factor in COD calculi. In our experience, about 85 % of all stones mainly composed of COD are associated with hypercalciuria. However, some morphological features may orient more specifically toward some urine abnormalities. Commonly, COD presents in stones as octahedral (bipyramidal) crystals. However, in case they appear as dodecahedral crystals (Fig. 15.10), they are especially indicative for a heavy hypercalciuria, urine calcium concentration being often found higher than 10 mmol/L.

In other cases, COD may present as large octahedral crystals, the size of which being higher than 2.5 mm (Fig. 15.11). In such cases, hypercalciuria is often associated with other biochemical disorders such as hyperoxaluria and hypocitraturia.

Finally, calcium oxalate stones composed by a mixture of COM and COD, which is a common finding, are suggestive of intermittent urine abnormalities from a dietary origin such as hypercalciuric and/or hyperoxaluric states related to:

- Low diuresis due to low water intake or high water losses (hot climates, intestinal losses, etc.)
- High consumption of salt or animal proteins that are known to induce hypercalciuria in genetically predisposed patients
- Oxalate-rich vegetable intake

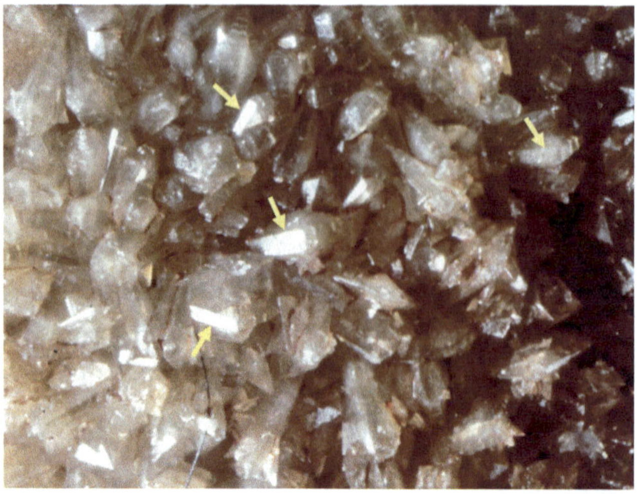

Fig. 15.10 Detail of the surface of a type IIa stone made of COD. Note the presence of dodecahedral crystals of COD (*arrows*), which are currently a marker of heavy hypercalciuria responsible for stone formation

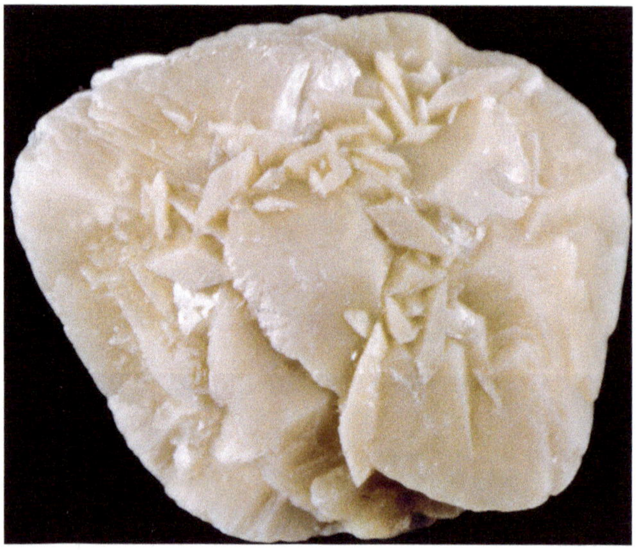

Fig. 15.11 Type IIb stone mainly composed of COD as very large crystals suggesting that hyperoxaluria, in addition to hypercalciuria, is involved in the stone formation

Umbilicated Calculi and Randall's Plaque

As first described by Alexander Randall in 1936 [100, 101], CaOx stones developed on papillary calcium deposits exhibit a characteristic morphology with a visible concave dip ("umbilication") containing a small calcium phosphate deposit at their surface (Fig. 15.12), a material similar to that present in the Randall's plaque [102]. Therefore, calculi exhibiting an umbilication, the footprint of a papilla, are likely to have been formed at the tip of a papilla on a Randall's plaque as also reported 20 years ago by Cifuentes-Delatte et al. [103, 104] and more recently by our group [22, 105].

Detailed morphologic examination of umbilicated stones identifies two different types of material deposited in the umbilication. In typical CaOx calculi detached from a Randall's plaque, the deposit visible in the umbilication is made of carbapatite with COM being the mineral layer apposed closest to the plaque, embedded in proteins [106]. In our experience, nearly half of CaOx umbilicated calculi developed on a Randall's plaque are made of pure COM, whereas the other half are made of mixed COM and COD, with COM consistently being the first layer at the contact of carbapatite (Fig. 15.13) [107].

In a minority of cases, the morphology and composition of the material found in the umbilication is different, including other calcium phosphates such as amorphous carbonated calcium phosphate (ACCP), whitlockite or brushite, or purines, mainly sodium hydrogen urate (Fig. 15.14) and more rarely uric acid, thus indicating a different metabolic origin of the stone [22, 107]. In such cases, a typical Randall's

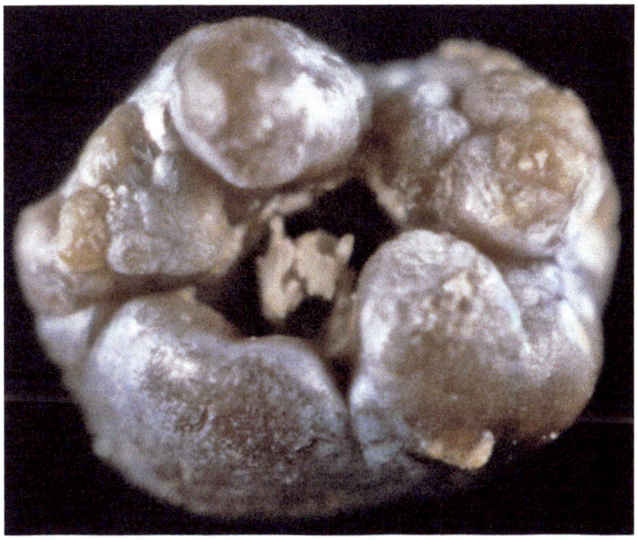

Fig. 15.12 Typical umbilicated COM stone with "Randall's plaque" composed of carbapatite within the cavity

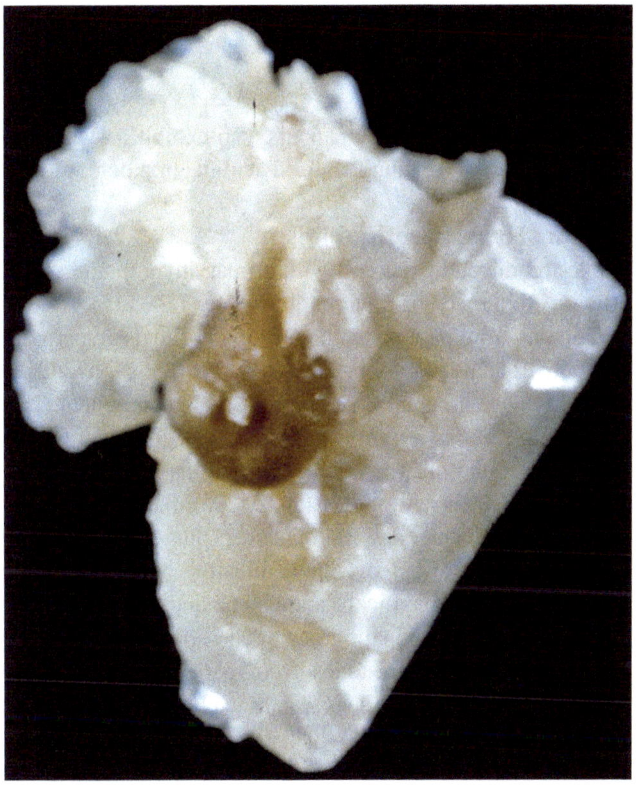

Fig. 15.13 Example of COD calculus developed from a Randall's plaque. Note the first layers around the plaque are made of *dark brown* COM, even when the stone is mainly composed of COD resulting from hypercalciuria

plaque may be present, but it seems not to be necessary for inducing stone formation at the surface of a renal papilla.

In our series, the proportion of umbilicated stones was especially high among COM stones (39.6 %), while it was only 8.6 % among COD calculi ($p<0.0001$). Table 15.10 summarizes the proportions of umbilicated stones found among spontaneously passed calculi of various compositions. About 60 % of all spontaneously passed COM stones exhibited an umbilication and a Randall's plaque, the corresponding proportion being only 16 % for COD calculi. Interestingly, 6 % of uric acid and 2.5 % of calcium phosphate stones that were spontaneously passed exhibited an umbilicated structure with a Randall's plaque as the nidus of the stone. For comparison, the occurrence of Randall's plaque identified from stone analysis was about 12.5 % in Spain [104] and in Balearic Islands [108]. Of note, several reports based on ureteroscopic examination of the renal papillae of stone formers underlined the high occurrence of Randall's plaques in the kidneys, varying from 57 % in France [69] to 75–80 % in the United States [109].

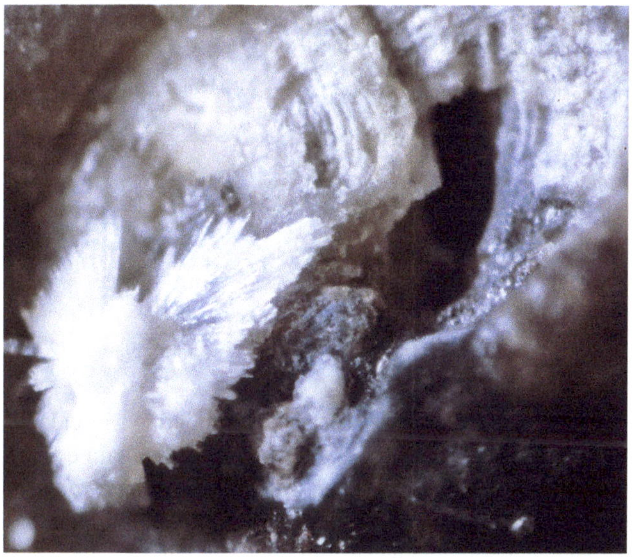

Fig. 15.14 Another example of umbilicated stone initiated on the papilla from an aggregate of needle-shaped crystals composed of sodium hydrogen urate monohydrate. Sodium hydrogen urate crystals are mixed with carbapatite, which suggests a Randall's plaque has probably initiated the stone process

Hypercalciuria was reported as a possible factor for Randall's plaque formation [40, 41]. When the papillary deposit is composed of sodium urate needles, other etiological factors must be sought such as high sodium and urate excretion, which are often found. However, as seen in Fig. 15.14, sodium urate may be admixed with carbapatite in the plaque, thus suggesting a multifactorial etiology of the stone.

Calcium Phosphate Stones

Stones predominantly made of calcium phosphate are a very heterogeneous group. Phosphate stones have diverse crystalline composition and morphology, which reflect distinct etiopathogenic conditions.

Table 15.10 Frequency of umbilication and Randall's plaque among spontaneously passed calculi collected between 1997 and 2007

Main stone component	Number of stones	Umbilication	
		Number	%
COM	7,323	4,482	61.2
COD	2,823	468	16.6
Uric acid	1,432	96	6.7
Carbapatite	1,262	29	2.3
Brushite	162	4	2.5
Cystine	156	1	0.6
Overall	13,158	5,080	38.6

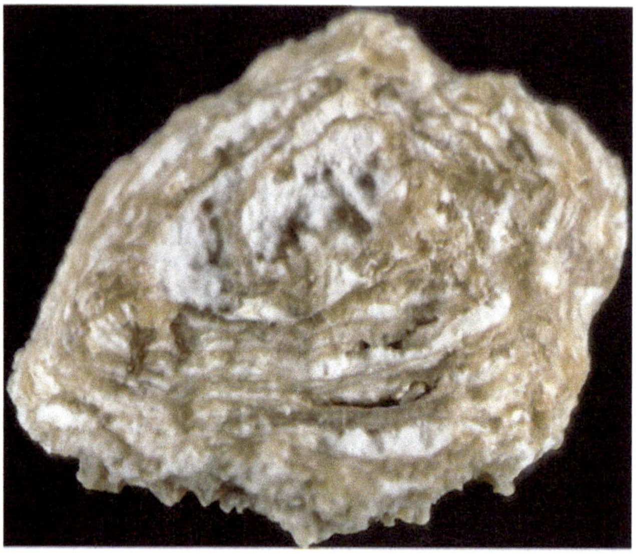

Fig. 15.15 Example of a typical stone section of a stone formed in patients suffering primary hyperparathyroidism. The stone is made of a mixture of weddellite and carbapatite. Its morphology is IIa+IVa1. About 50 % of stones developed in primary hyperparathyroidism exhibit such morphology

The commonest crystalline phases identified in calcium phosphate stones are carbapatite (often as the main component), amorphous carbonated calcium phosphate, octacalcium phosphate pentahydrate, and brushite. Whitlockite, a mixed calcium and magnesium phosphate, is less frequently encountered. Of note, brushite presents as large, aggregated rod-shaped crystals giving a peculiar morphology to calculi (see Fig. 15.5, subtype IVd), whereas all other phases of calcium phosphates are composed of tiny particles made of nanocrystals less than 15 nm in size [107].

Common Calcium Phosphate Stones

More frequent in female than in male adult patients [84, 110], common calcium phosphate stones exhibit a homogeneous whitish and rough surface made of very small crystals of carbapatite. The section is often poorly organized, exhibiting only loose concentric layers, the color of which resembles that of the surface (see Fig. 15.5, subtype IVa1). Although mainly composed of carbapatite, these stones often contain several other crystalline phases of calcium phosphate, the identification of which is of interest for stone etiology. Of note, calcium phosphate is often admixed with CaOx, either COM or COD or both as in medullary sponge kidney [98].

Distal Renal Tubular Acidosis (dRTA)

Patients with dRTA were known to form calculi mainly composed of carbapatite [44, 111], and a recent study has shown apatite plugging of Bellini's ducts in five patients with dRTA [112]. Morphologic examination of phosphatic stones made of carbapatite revealed a peculiar morphology (type IVa2) in patients with congenital or acquired distal tubular acidosis [22]. These calculi are characterized by a light yellow-brown, glazed surface with an aspect of cracks and an inner structure made of irregular whitish and yellow-brown concentric layers (see Fig. 15.5, subtype IVa2). In our experience, 51 (89.5 %) of 57 patients with a Sjögren syndrome and nephrolithiasis had stones exhibiting this IVa2 morphology [97], a finding in agreement with observation by other authors of a close association between Sjögren syndrome, distal tubular acidosis, and carbapatite stones [113]. Of note, we observed that some stones produced by MSK patients also exhibit a IVa2 morphology, thus suggesting localized acidification defects.

Primary Hyperparathyroidism

Stones produced by patients with primary hyperparathyroidism are often made of calcium phosphate [114, 115]. Among 267 stones from patients with confirmed primary hyperparathyroidism analyzed at our laboratory [45], 36 % had COD and 32 % had carbapatite as the single main component. This composition is in keeping with the recent findings of Evan et al. who found in five patients with primary hyperparathyroidism and recurrent phosphate stone formation both typical Randall's plaques and Bellini's ducts plugged with apatite covered with CaOx [116]. Of note, in only 5 out of 267 stones (1.9 %), we found a typical Randall's plaque at the surface of the stone. A low carbonation rate of carbapatite (8 % in average) was recorded in stones from patients with primary hyperparathyroidism. Other crystalline phases were found as main component of stones, namely, COM (in 16 %) and brushite (in 14 %). Stones mainly composed of COM always exhibit a heterogeneous morphology. In contrast, primary hyperparathyroidism is very infrequent in case of stones with type I morphology (0.02 %). In half of our 267 cases, stone morphology was a mixture of types II (COD) and IVa1 (carbapatite) (Fig. 15.15). Worthy of note, 14 % of our patients with primary hyperparathyroidism had stones mainly composed of brushite, an infrequent form of calcium phosphate stones (see Fig. 15.5, subtype IVd), and reciprocally 11 % of patients with brushite stones were diagnosed with primary hyperparathyroidism.

Carbonation Rate

Carbapatite is a carbonate-containing calcium phosphate. The carbonate content results from the substitution of several sites in the crystal lattice of apatite by carbonate ions, which may replace either phosphate ions (sites A) or hydroxyl ions (site B). Moreover, the peripheral hydrated layer of apatite crystals may also contain a variable proportion of carbonate ions. As a consequence, all biological apatites are carbonate apatite or carbapatite. The carbonation rate of carbapatite may be assessed by measuring the ratio of the peaks corresponding to asymmetric stretching bands of carbonate ion at 1,420 cm^{-1} and of phosphate ion at 1,035 cm^{-1}. In our experience, the carbonation rate of carbapatite was usually less than 10 % in carbapatite stones of metabolic origin, whereas most carbapatite stones resulting from urinary tract infection (UTI) by urea-splitting microorganisms had a carbonation rate of 15–33 % [46]. Thus, a high carbonation rate of carbapatite is suggestive of a past or present participation of UTI in the lithogenic process [49].

Purine Stones

Two different types of surface and inner structure may be observed in uric acid stones and in ammonium urate stones.

Uric Acid Stones

Common uric acid stones exhibit a smooth or slightly rough, orange surface and are mainly composed of uric acid anhydrous. The inner structure reveals concentric layers with a radiating organization of the crystals (see Fig. 15.4, subtype IIIa). Such stones are often found in the bladder of elderly men with prostate hypertrophy.

The morphology of uric acid kidney stones formed by patients with the metabolic syndrome or diabetes type 2 is different. The surface is heterogeneous, simultaneously rough and embossed, and locally porous; the color ranges from beige to red orange. The inner structure is unorganized and porous, with sometimes poorly organized layers in the periphery (see Fig. 15.4, subtype IIIb). This type of stone usually contains high proportions of uric acid dihydrate.

Ammonium Urate

The commonest form observed in Western countries corresponds to calculi with a homogenous rough surface with local porous areas. The color is usually grayish, sometimes pale yellow. The inner structure is commonly loose, unorganized, and locally porous, the color being the same as in the surface. Such type of ammonium urate (see Fig. 15.4, subtype IIIc) is found mainly in two pathological conditions: local production of ammonium ions from urea in patients with UTI by urea-splitting bacteria or increased urine pH by therapeutic alkalinization aimed at dissolving radiolucent stones presumably made of uric acid.

A distinct morphology of ammonium urate stone (see Fig. 15.4, subtype IIId) is observed in cases of base loss due to chronic diarrhea in anorectic patients with laxative abuse and low phosphate intake, resulting in compensatory increase in urinary ammonia excretion [57, 59]. Stones observed in this condition are of very dark color with purplish shades.

A similar mechanism is operating in children (mainly boys) with endemic bladder urolithiasis in developing countries. Stones exhibit a very heterogeneous surface with rough, embossed, and porous areas, beige to brownish in color. The inner structure is grossly concentric, made of alternate thick and thin layers, the former being compact and brownish, whereas the latter are loose and locally porous, beige in color.

Correlations Between Stone Morphology and Etiopathogenic Factors

Morphological typing helps to orient etiological diagnosis because of the strong relationships found between stone structure and composition and etiopathogenic factors involved in the lithogenetic process. These correlations are based on clinical and laboratory data recorded in parallel with stone analysis [2, 46, 97, 98].

Etiopathogenic Orientations Given by Morphologic Classification of Stones

Table 15.11 summarizes the main diagnostic orientations provided by the morphologic typing of stones. Several types are especially useful from a clinical point of view because they are highly suggestive of severe diseases and they help for a rapid detection of such pathological conditions. For example, among calcium stones, subtype Ic stones must prompt to look for heavy hyperoxaluria and especially primary hyperoxaluria type 1. Mixed subtypes Ia + IIa or Ia + IIb are commonly related to moderate hyperoxaluria and hypercalciuria, the cause of which being essentially of dietary origin. Among calcium phosphates, subtype IVa2 stones are especially related to distal tubular acidosis or medullary sponge kidney. Among purine calculi, ammonium urate stones exhibiting a IIId morphology result in most cases from digestive problems, while IIIc stones mainly result from hyperuricosuria associated with UTI by urease-splitting bacteria. Stone morphology can help for detecting unusual composition. For example, in case of routine stone analysis by chemical methods in routine practice, an initial examination of stone morphology may help to detect unusual composition (drugs, rare purine stones, etc.). Figure 15.16a–c illustrate that point, showing that dihydroxyadenine (a compound of genetic origin not identified by chemical methods

Table 15.11 Main correlations between morphological stone types and etiopathogenic factors

Type	Main component	Common etiological factor	Subtype	Specific etiology
I	Whewellite	Hyperoxaluria	Ia	Randall's plaque, low diuresis, excessive urine oxalate concentration
				Medullary sponge kidney (MSK)
			Ib	Moderate hyperoxaluria, stasis, crystalline conversion from COD to COM
			Ic	Primary hyperoxaluria type I
			Id	Anatomic anomaly, obstruction with multiple stones
			Ie	Enteric hyperoxaluria
II	Weddellite	Hypercalciuria	IIa	Idiopathic hypercalciuria (IH)
			IIb	IH + moderate hyperoxaluria
			IIc	Hypercalciuria + anatomic anomaly + multiple stones and obstruction
III	Uric acid	Low urine pH and/or hyperuricosuria	IIIa	Stasis, bladder stone in patients presenting with benign prostate hypertrophy
			IIIb	Low renal ammoniagenesis, metabolic syndrome, type 2 diabetes
	Urates	Hyperuricosuria + normal or alkaline pH	IIIc	Alkaline therapy, urinary tract infection by urea-splitting microorganisms
	Ammonium urate		IIId	Chronic diarrheas, loss of electrolytes, low phosphorus intake, laxative abuse
IV	Carbapatite	Permanent high urine pH (>6.2)	IVa1	UTI (ACCP, WK or MAP in the stone), IH
				Incomplete distal tubular acidosis (DTA)
		Tubular acidification defect	IVa2	Severe DTA (inherited or acquired, Sjögren syndrome), MSK
	Carbapatite	UTI	IVb	UTI (ACCP, WK or MAP in the stone)
				Incomplete DTA, long-term treatment with carbonic anhydrase inhibitors
				Primary hyperparathyroidism
	Struvite	UTI by urea-splitting microorganisms	IVc	UTI by urea-splitting microorganisms
	Brushite	Hypercalciuria	IVd	IH, primary hyperparathyroidism, incomplete DTA, low citrate excretion, past history of infectious chronic pyelonephritis
V	Cystine	High urine cystine excretion	Va	Inherited cystinuria
			Vb	Inherited cystinuria + insufficient alkaline diuresis + default of dietary advices
VI	Proteins	UTI	VIa	Infectious chronic pyelonephritis
			VIb	Infectious chronic pyelonephritis by urea-splitting microorganisms, some drug-containing nephrolithiasis (triamterene, quinolones, etc.), proteinuria, etc.
		Kidney failure	VIc	Chronic hemodialysis + calcium and vitamin D supplementation + moderate hyperoxaluria
VII	Drugs	Drug-containing stones		Long-term treatment by the drug

ACCP amorphous carbonated calcium phosphate, *COM* calcium oxalate monohydrate, *COD* calcium oxalate dihydrate, *WK* whitlockite, *MAP* magnesium ammonium phosphate hexahydrate (struvite), *DTA* distal tubular acidosis, *UTI* urinary tract infection

that mistake it for uric acid) does not have the same morphological characteristics as uric acid and could be suspected by a simple stereomicroscopic examination.

Quantitative Associations Between Etiology and Morpho-Constitutional Analysis of Urinary Stones

Table 15.12 summarizes the quantitative relationships found between some morphological types of stones, irrespective to their crystalline composition, and specific etiopathogenic conditions. Thus, strong correlations between hypercalciuria and type II stones were observed. In case of primary hyperparathyroidism, stones with a mixed type II + IVa1 or with a IVd subtype counted for 72.7 % of cases.

In patients suffering enteric hyperoxaluria, subtype Ie stones were present in 82.5 % of cases, whereas calcium oxalate stones had a type Ia morphology in 88 % of patients presenting with dietary hyperoxaluria.

Sjögren syndrome and inherited distal tubular acidosis are known to induce CaP stones. However, such a composition is not typical for these pathological conditions. In contrast, CaP

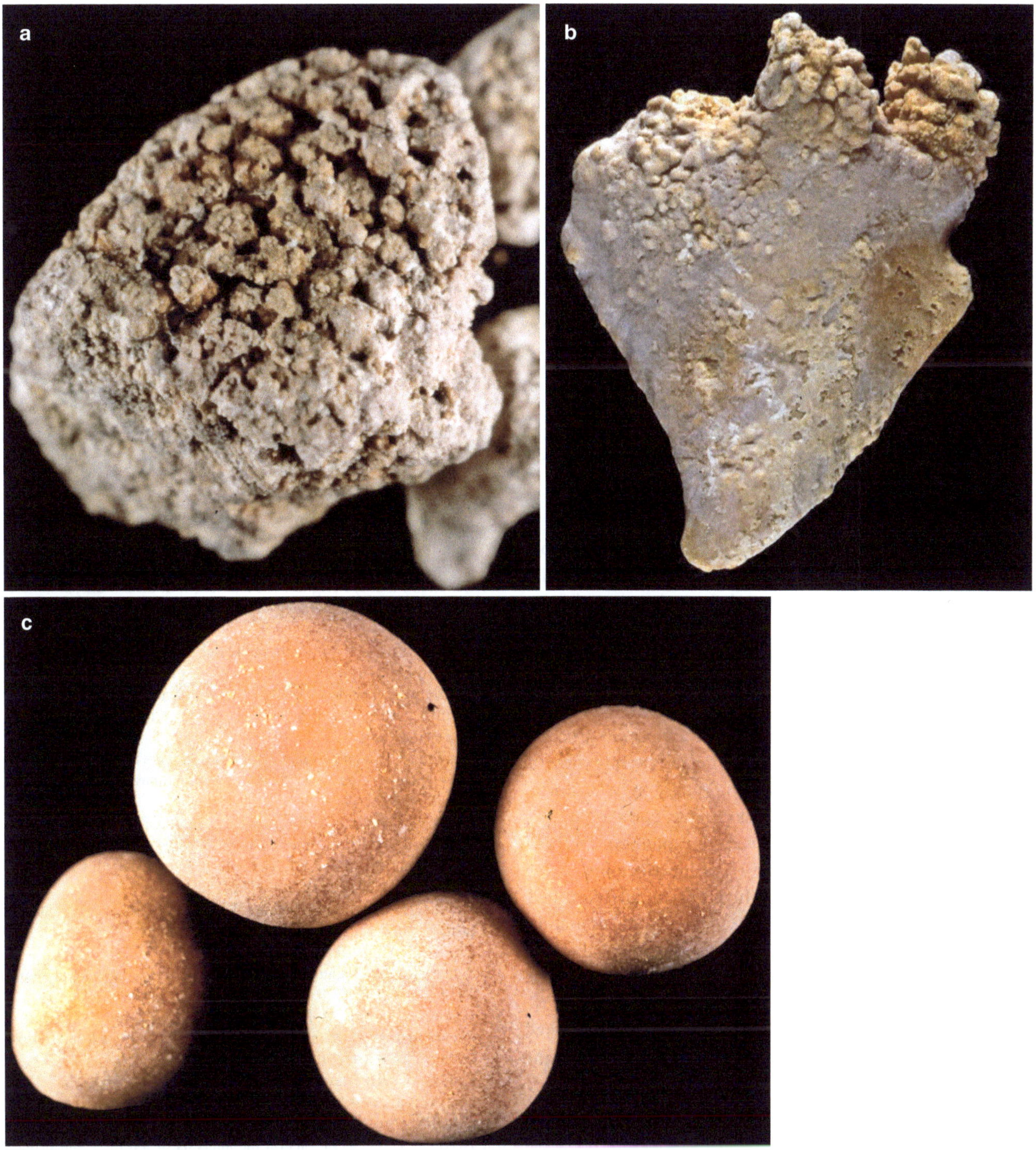

Fig. 15.16 (**a**) 2,8-dihydroxyadenine stone, a specific marker of adenine phosphoribosyltransferase deficiency. (**b**) Pyelic stone made of uric acid presenting a type IIIb morphology. (**c**) Multiple uric acid stones with a type IIIa morphology removed from the bladder. The morphological characteristics and the color are very different for these three types of stones

stones exhibiting a subtype IVa2 morphology were observed in more than 89 % of cases among 84 patients suffering either Sjögren syndrome or genetic distal tubular acidosis.

Among patients suffering type 2 diabetes, females are especially at risk to develop uric acid stones exhibiting a subtype IIIb (37 % vs. 13 % in the absence of diabetes, $p<0.00001$). Finally, in patients who had chronic diarrhea and ammonium urate stones in the urinary tract, we found that stone morphology exhibited a subtype IIId in more than 91 % of cases.

Table 15.12 Relationships between stone morphology and etiopathogenic conditions

Pathogenic conditions	No. of cases	Stone morphology	Frequency (%)
Idiopathic hypercalciuria	850	Type IIa	83.2
		Mixed type IIa+Ia	10.8
Primary hyperparathyroidism	267	Mixed type IIa/b+IVa1	58.3
		Type IVd	14.4
		Type IVa1	12.4
		Type IIa	11.7
Idiopathic hyperoxaluria	342	Type Ia	88.1
Primary hyperoxaluria type 1	88	Type Ic	100
Enteric hyperoxaluria	63	Type Ie	82.5
Sjögren syndrome	57	Type IVa2	89.5
Inherited distal tubular acidosis	27	Type IVa2	89.2
Type 2 diabetes in stone formers			
Male patients	669	Type IIIb	30.9[a]
Female patients	193	Type IIIb	37.0[a]
Diarrhea and low phosphate intake	46	Type IIId	91.3

[a]Type IIIb stones were found in 23.7 % of male stone formers and in only 13 % of female stone formers without diabetes matched for age

Conclusion

Routine morpho-constitutional analysis of stones by morphologic examination combined with FTIR or X-ray diffraction considerably improves information gained from stone analysis to identify the cause of stone disease. Indeed, stones with the same chemical composition exhibit distinct morphological characteristics according to their cause, which determines the degree of metabolic abnormalities and the kinetics of the lithogenic process. The most striking example is the unique morphology of stones produced by patients with primary hyperoxaluria, which is pathognomonic for this etiology and should contribute to early diagnosis and management of this rare, but very severe disease. Selective FTIR identification of the composition of core (or umbilication), middle part, and surface of every stone allows to identify the initiating lithogenic process (in the nucleus or in the Randall's plaque) and the factors which subsequently contributed to stone growth. In conclusion, the proposed morpho-constitutional method of urinary stone analysis, which moreover is rapid and cheap, provides clinically relevant orientations for targeted etiologic evaluation.

References

1. Daudon M, Réveillaud RJ. Whewellite and weddellite: toward different etiopathogenesis. Interest of the morphological typing of the stones. Nephrologie. 1984;5:195–201 (in French).
2. Daudon M, Bader CA, Jungers P. Urinary calculi: review of classification methods and correlations with etiology. Scanning Microsc. 1993;7:1081–106.
3. Asplin JR, Lingeman J, Kahnoski R, Mardis H, Parks JH, Coe FL. Metabolic urinary correlates of calcium oxalate dihydrate in renal stones. J Urol. 1998;159:664–8.
4. Bouzidi H, Lacour B, Daudon M. 2,8-dihydroxyadenine nephrolithiasis: from diagnosis to therapy. Ann Biol Clin (Paris). 2007;65:585–92.
5. Ceballos-Picot I, Perignon JL, Hamet M, et al. 2,8-dihydroxyadenine urolithiasis, an underdiagnosed disease. Lancet. 1992;339:1050–1.
6. Simmonds HA. 2,8-dihydroxyadenine lithiasis. Clin Chim Acta. 1986;160:103–8.
7. Couzigou C, Daudon M, Meynard JL, et al. Urolithiasis in HIV-positive patients treated with atazanavir. Clin Infect Dis. 2007;45:e105–8.
8. Daudon M, Estépa L, Viard JP, Joly D, Jungers P. Urinary stones in HIV-1-positive patients treated with indinavir. Lancet. 1997;349:1294–5.
9. Daudon M, Jungers P. Drug-induced renal calculi: epidemiology, prevention and management. Drugs. 2004;64:245–75.
10. Daudon M, Réveillaud RJ. Methods of urinary calculus analysis: a critical review. Adv Nephrol. 1986;15:219–44.
11. Hesse A, Kruse R, Geilenkeuser WJ, Schmidt M. Quality control in urinary stone analysis: results of 44 ring trials (1980–2001). Clin Chem Lab Med. 2005;43:298–303.
12. Schneider HJ. Technik der Harnsteinanalyse. Leipzig: Thieme; 1974.
13. Bastian PJ, Lorken M, Euler H, Lummen G, Bastian HP. Results of the evaluation of 85,337 urinary stone analyses. Aktuelle Urol. 2008;39:298–304.
14. Leusmann DB, Blaschke R, Schmandt W. Results of 5035 stone analysis: a contribution to epidemiology stone disease. Scand J Urol Nephrol. 1990;24:205–10.
15. Herring LC. Observations on the analysis of ten thousand urinary calculi. J Urol. 1962;88:545–56.
16. Mandel N, Mandel I, Fryjoff K, Rejniak T, Mandel G. Conversion of calcium oxalate to calcium phosphate with recurrent stone episodes. J Urol. 2003;169:2026–9.
17. Otnes B, Montgomery O. Method and reliability of crystallographic stone analysis. Invest Urol. 1980;17:85–92.
18. Prien EL, Frondel C. Studies in urolithiasis. I. The composition of urinary calculi. J Urol. 1947;57:949–91.
19. Beischer D. Analysis of renal calculi by infrared spectroscopy. J Urol. 1955;73:653–9.
20. Berthelot M, Cornu G, Daudon M, Helbert M, Laurence C. Computer-aided infrared analysis of urinary calculi. Clin Chem. 1987;33:2070–3.

21. Daudon M, Protat MF, Réveillaud RJ. Analysis of calculi by infrared spectroscopy. Advantages and limits of the method. Ann Biol Clin. 1978;36:475–89 (in French).
22. Estepa L, Daudon M. Contribution of Fourier transform infrared spectroscopy to the identification of urinary stones and kidney crystal deposits. Biospectroscopy. 1997;3:347–69.
23. Maurice-Estepa L, Levillain P, Lacour B, Daudon M. Infrared analysis of urinary stones: a trial of automated identification. Clin Chem Lab Med. 1999;37:1043–52.
24. Tsay YC. Application of infrared spectroscopy to urinary calculi. J Urol. 1961;86:838–54.
25. Volmer M, Wolthers BG, Metting HJ, de Haan TH, Coenegracht PM, van der Slik W. Artificial neural network predictions of urinary calculus compositions analyzed with infrared spectroscopy. Clin Chem. 1994;40:1692–7.
26. Daudon M, Protat MF, Réveillaud RJ, Jaeschke-Boyer H. Infrared spectrometry and Raman microprobe in the analysis of urinary calculi. Kidney Int. 1983;23:842–50.
27. Hidalgo A, Santos M, Carmina P, Garcia-Ramos JV, Bellanato J, Cifuentes Delatte L. Analisis de calculos urinarios por espectroscopia infraroja y Raman. Madrid: Instituto de Optica (Daza de Valdes) C.S.I.C; 1983.
28. Hong TD, Phat D, Plaza P, Daudon M, Dao NQ. Identification of urinary calculi by Raman laser fiber optics spectroscopy. Clin Chem. 1992;38:292–8.
29. Nguyen Quy D, Daudon M. Infrared and Raman spectra of calculi. Paris: Elsevier; 1997.
30. Sudlow K, Woolf A. Identification of renal calculi by their Raman spectra. Clin Chim Acta. 1991;203:387–93.
31. Kaloustian J, El-Moselhy TF, Portugal H. Determination of calcium oxalate (mono- and dihydrate) in mixtures with magnesium ammonium phosphate or uric acid: the use of simultaneous thermal analysis in urinary calculi. Clin Chim Acta. 2003;334:117–29.
32. Rose GA, Woodfine C. The thermogravimetric analysis of renal stones (in clinical practice). Br J Urol. 1976;48:403–12.
33. Sharma RN, Shah I, Gupta S, Sharma P, Beigh AA. Thermogravimetric analysis of urinary stones. Br J Urol. 1989;64:564–6.
34. Tozuka K, Konjiki T, Sudo T. Study of passed stones by means of X-rays, infrared and thermal analyses. J Urol. 1983;130:1119–22.
35. Saupe E. Rontgendiagramme von menschlichen Korkengeweben und Konkrementen. Fortsch Geb Rontgenst. 1931;44:204–11.
36. Hesse A, Sanders G. Atlas f infrared spectra for the analysis of urinary concrements. Stuttgart: Georg Thieme; 1988.
37. Oliver LK, Sweet RV. A system of interpretation of infrared spectra of calculi for routine use in the clinical laboratory. Clin Chim Acta. 1976;72:17–32.
38. Krambeck AE, Lingeman JE, McAteer JA, Williams Jr JC. Analysis of mixed stones is prone to error: a study with US laboratories using micro CT for verification of sample content. Urol Res. 2010;38:469–75.
39. Siener R, Buchholz N, Daudon M, et al. Quality assessment of urinary stone analysis: results of a multicenter study of laboratories in Europe. Eur Urol Suppl. 2011;10:463 (A).
40. Evan AP, Lingeman JE, Coe FL, et al. Randall's plaque of patients with nephrolithiasis begins in basement membranes of thin loops of Henle. J Clin Invest. 2003;111:607–16.
41. Kuo RL, Lingeman JE, Evan AP, et al. Urine calcium and volume predict coverage of renal papilla by Randall's plaque. Kidney Int. 2003;64:2150–4.
42. Daudon M, Bouzidi H, Bazin D. Composition and morphology of phosphate stones and their relation with etiology. Urol Res. 2010;38:459–67.
43. Gault MH, Parfrey PS, Robertson WG. Idiopathic calcium phosphate nephrolithiasis. Nephron. 1988;48:265–73.
44. Gault MH, Chafe LL, Morgan JM, et al. Comparison of patients with idiopathic calcium phosphate and CaOx stones. Medicine (Baltimore). 1991;70:345–59.
45. Bouzidi H, de Brauwere D, Daudon M. Does urinary stone composition and morphology help for prediction of primary hyperparathyroidism? Nephrol Dial Transplant. 2011;26:565–72.
46. Maurice-Estepa L, Levillain P, Lacour B, et al. Crystalline phase differentiation in urinary calcium phosphate and magnesium phosphate calculi. Scand J Urol Nephrol. 1999;33:299–305.
47. Méria P, Hadjadj H, Jungers P, Daudon M, and Members of the Urolithiasis Committee of the French Urological Association. Stone formation and pregnancy: pathophysiological insights gained from morphoconstitutional stone analysis. J Urol. 2010;183:1412–6.
48. Griffith DP, Osborne CA. Infection (urease) stones. Miner Electrolyte Metab. 1987;13:278–85.
49. Carpentier X, Daudon M, Traxer O, Jungers P, Mazouyes A, Matzen G, Véron E, Bazin D. Relationships between the carbonation rate of carbapatite, morphological characteristics of calcium phosphate stones and etiology. Urology. 2009;73:968–75.
50. Daudon M, Lacour B, Jungers P. Influence of body size on urinary stone composition in men and women. Urol Res. 2006;34:193–9.
51. Daudon M, Jungers P. Mellitus diabetes and calculi. Feuillets de Biologie. 2001;42:37–9 (in French).
52. Daudon M, Lacour B, Jungers P. High prevalence of uric acid calculi in diabetic stone formers. Nephrol Dial Transplant. 2005;20:468–9.
53. Daudon M, Traxer O, Conort P, Lacour B, Jungers P. Type 2 diabetes increases the risk for uric acid stones. J Am Soc Nephrol. 2006;17:2026–33.
54. Pak CY, Sakhaee K, Moe O, et al. Biochemical profile of stone-forming patients with diabetes mellitus. Urology. 2003;61:523–7.
55. Klohn M, Bolle JF, Reverdin NP, Susini A, Baud CA, Graber P. Ammonium urate urinary stones. Urol Res. 1986;14:315–8.
56. Miano R, Germani S, Vespasiani G. Stones and urinary tract infections. Urol Int. 2007;79 Suppl 1:32–6.
57. Dick WH, Lingeman JE, Preminger GM, Smith LH, Wilson DM, Shirrell WL. Laxative abuse as a cause for ammonium urate renal calculi. J Urol. 1990;143:244–7.
58. Hara N, Koike H. A case of ammonium urate urinary stone. Hinyokika Kiyo. 2004;50:351–3 (in Japanese).
59. Kato Y, Hou K, Saga Y, Yamaguchi S, Yachiku S, Kawakami N. Ammonium acid urate stone due to laxative abuse: a case report. Hinyokika Kiyo. 2004;50:799–803 (in Japanese).
60. Kamoun A, Daudon M, Abdelmoula J, et al. Urolithiasis in Tunisian children: a study of 120 cases based on stone composition. Pediatr Nephrol. 1999;13:920–5.
61. Thambi Dorai CR, Dewan PA, Boucaut HA, Ehrlich J. Urolithiasis in Australian aboriginal children. Aust N Z J Surg. 1994;64:99–101.
62. Hesse A, Brandle E, Wilbert D, Kohrmann KU, Alken P. Study on the prevalence and incidence of urolithiasis in Germany comparing the years 1979 vs. 2000. Eur Urol. 2003;44:709–13.
63. Stamatelou KK, Francis ME, Jones CA, Nyberg LM, Curhan GC. Time trends in reported prevalence of kidney stones in the United States: 1976–1994. Kidney Int. 2003;63:1817–23.
64. Yoshida O, Okada Y. Epidemiology of urolithiasis in Japan: a chronological and geographical study. Urol Int. 1990;45:104–11.
65. Trinchieri A. Epidemiological trends in urolithiasis: impact on our health care systems. Urol Res. 2006;34:151–6.
66. Lieske JC, Pena de la Vega LS, Slezak JM, et al. Renal stone epidemiology in Rochester, Minnesota: an update. Kidney Int. 2006;69:760–4.
67. Scales Jr CD, Curtis LH, Norris RD, et al. Changing gender prevalence of stone disease. J Urol. 2007;177:979–82.
68. Yoshida O, Terai A, Ohkawa T, Okada Y. National trend of the incidence of urolithiasis in Japan from 1965 to 1995. Kidney Int. 1999;56:1899–904.
69. Daudon M, Traxer O, Williams JC, Bazin DC. Randall's plaques. In: Rao PN, Preminger GM, Kavanagh JP, editors. Urinary tract stone disease. London: Springer; 2011. p. 103–12.
70. Brien G, Schubert G, Bick C. 10000 analysis of urinary calculi using X-ray diffraction and polarizing microscopy. Eur Urol. 1982;8:251–6.

71. Daudon M, Donsimoni R, Hennequin C, Fellahi S, Le Moël G, Paris M, Troupel S, Lacour B. Sex- and age-related composition of 10,617 calculi analyzed by infrared spectroscopy. Urol Res. 1995; 23:319–26.
72. Balla AA, Salah AM, Khattab AH, et al. Mineral composition of renal stones from the Sudan. Urol Int. 1998;61:154–6.
73. Chou YH, Li CC, Wu WJ, et al. Urinary stone analysis of 1,000 patients in southern Taiwan. Kaohsiung J Med Sci. 2007;23:63–6.
74. Daudon M, Traxer O, Lechevallier E, Saussine C. Epidemiology of urolithiasis. Prog Urol. 2008;18:802–14 (in French).
75. Jing Z, GuoZeng W, Ning J, JiaWei Y, Yan G, Fang Y. Analysis of urinary calculi composition by infrared spectroscopy: a prospective study of 625 patients in eastern China. Urol Res. 2010;38:111–5.
76. Prasongwatana W, Bovornpadungkitti S, Chotikawanich E, Pachitrat K, Suwanatrai S, Sriboonlue P. Chemical components of urinary stones according to age and sex of adult patients. J Med Assoc Thai. 2008;91:1589–94.
77. Tanthanuch M, Apiwatgaroon A, Pripatnanont C. Urinary tract calculi in southern Thailand. J Med Assoc Thai. 2005;88:80–5.
78. Kuruma H, Arakawa T, Kubo S, et al. Ammonium acid urate urolithiasis in Japan. Int J Urol. 2006;13:498–501.
79. Schneider HJ, Berg C. Epidemiologische aussagen zum harnsteinleiden auf der grundlage von 100,000 harnsteinanalysen. Unter besonderer berücksichtigung der rezidive. Fortschr Urol Nephrol. 1981;17:33–9.
80. Suzuki K, Yamashita Y, Matuzaki J. Clinical assessment of ammonium acid urate urinary calculi. Hinyokika Kiyo. 2010;56:5–9 (in Japan).
81. Kheradpir MH, Armbruster T. Childhood urolithiasis in Iran :a comparative study on the calculi composition of 121 cases. Z Kinderchir. 1985;40:163–9.
82. Pandeya A, Prajapati R, Panta P, Regmi A. Assessment of kidney stone and prevalence of its chemical composition. Nepal Med Coll J. 2010;12:190–2.
83. Robertson WG, Peacock M, Heyburn PJ. Clinical and metabolic aspects of urinary stone disease in Leeds. Scand J Urol Nephrol Suppl. 1980;53:199–206.
84. Daudon M, Doré JC, Jungers P, Lacour B. Changes in stone composition according to age and gender of patients: a multivariate epidemiological approach. Urol Res. 2004;23:241–7.
85. Trinchieri A, Castelnuovo C, Lizzano R, Zanetti G. Calcium stone disease: a multiform reality. Urol Res. 2005;33:194–8.
86. Daudon M, Bounxouei B, Santa Cruz F, et al. Composition of renal stones currently observed in non-industrialized countries. Prog Urol. 2004;14:1151–61 (in French).
87. Asper R. Epidemiology and socioeconomic aspects of urolithiasis. Urol Res. 1984;12:1–5.
88. Johnson O. Vesical calculus in Ethiopian children. Ethiop Med J. 1995;33:31–5.
89. Rizvi SA, Naqvi SA, Hussain Z, et al. Management of pediatric urolithiasis in Pakistan: experience with 1,440 children. J Urol. 2003;169:634–7.
90. Sarkissian A, Babloyan A, Arikyants N, Hesse A, Blau N, Leumann E. Pediatric urolithiasis in Armenia: a study of 198 patients observed from 1991 to 1999. Pediatr Nephrol. 2001;16:728–32.
91. Marrakchi O, Belhaj R, Bahlous A, et al. La lithiase urinaire chez l'enfant Tunisien. Etude à propos de 187 cas. Prog Urol. 2008;18: 1056–61.
92. Meiouet F, El Kabbaj S. Composition of urinary calculi in Moroccan children and interest of morpho-constitutional analysis in the etiology of pediatric urolithiasis. In: Pediatric nephrology symposium. Marrakech, 25–27 Nov 2010.
93. Alaya A, Nouri A, Najjar MF. Prevalence and composition of urolithiasis in a Tunisian pediatric population. Prog Urol. 2009;19: 395–400.
94. Angwafo III FF, Daudon M, Wonkam A, Kuwong PM, Kropp KA. Pediatric urolithiasis in sub-Saharan Africa: a comparative study in two regions of Cameroon. Eur Urol. 2000;37:106–11.
95. Oussama A, Kzaiber F, Mernari B, Semmoud A, Daudon M. Analysis of calculi by infrared spectroscopy in children from the Moroccan mid-atlas region. Ann Urol (Paris). 2000;34:384–90 (in French).
96. Rizvi SAH, Naqvi SAA, Hashmi ZHA, et al. Pediatric urolithiasis: developing nation perspectives. J Urol. 2002;168:1522–5.
97. Daudon M, Jungers P, Bazin D. Stone morphology: implication for pathogenesis. In: Evan AP, Lingeman JE, McAteer JA and Williams JC Jr, editors. Renal stone disease 2, American Institute of Physics conference proceedings. Melville; 2008, 1049, p. 199–215.
98. Daudon M, Jungers P. Clinical value of crystalluria and quantitative morphoconstitutional analysis of urinary calculi. Nephron Physiol. 2004;98:31–6.
99. Daudon M, Jungers P, Bazin D. Peculiar morphology of stones in primary hyperoxaluria. N Engl J Med. 2008;359:100–2.
100. Randall A. An hypothesis for the origin of renal calculus. N Engl J Med. 1936;214:234–7.
101. Randall A. The origin and growth of renal calculi. Ann Surg. 1937;105:1009–27.
102. Matlaga BR, Williams Jr JC, Kim SC, et al. Endoscopic evidence of calculus attachment to Randall's plaque. J Urol. 2006;175:1720–4.
103. Cifuentes Delatte L, Minon-Cifuentes JL, Medina JA. Papillary stones: calcified renal tubules in Randall's plaques. J Urol. 1985; 133:490–4.
104. Cifuentes Delatte L, Minon-Cifuentes J, Medina JA. New studies on papillary calculi. J Urol. 1987;137:1024–9.
105. Daudon M. Epidemiology of nephrolithiasis in France. Ann Urol. 2005;39:209–31 (in French).
106. Evan AP, Coe FL, Lingeman JE, et al. Mechanism of formation of human CaOx renal stones on Randall's plaque. Anat Rec (Hoboken). 2007;290:1315–23.
107. Daudon M, Traxer O, Jungers P, et al. Stone morphology suggestive of Randall's plaque. In: Evan AP, Lingeman JE, Williams JC Jr, editors. Renal stone disease, American Institute of Physics conference proceedings. Melville; 2007, 900, p. 26–34.
108. Grases F, Costa-Bauza A, Ramis M, Montesinos V, Conte A. Simple classification of renal calculi closely related to their micromorphology and etiology. Clin Chim Acta. 2002;322:29–36.
109. Matlaga BR, Coe FL, Evan AP, Lingeman JE. The role of Randall's plaques in the pathogenesis of calcium stones. J Urol. 2007; 177:31–8.
110. Gault MH, Chafe L. Relationship of frequency, age, sex, stone weight and composition in 15,624 stones: comparison of results for 1980 to 1983 and 1995 to 1998. J Urol. 2000;164:302–7.
111. Konnak JW, Kogan BA, Lau K. Renal calculi associated with incomplete distal renal tubular acidosis. J Urol. 1982;128:900–2.
112. Evan AP, Lingeman J, Coe F, et al. Renal histopathology of stone-forming patients with distal renal tubular acidosis. Kidney Int. 2007;71:795–801.
113. Eriksson P, Denneberg T, Tiselius HG. Risk factors of calcium stone formation in patients with primary Sjogren's syndrome. Urol Res. 1996;24:39–43.
114. Pak CY, Poindexter JR, Adams-Huet B, et al. Predictive value of kidney stone composition in the detection of metabolic abnormalities. Am J Med. 2003;115:26–32.
115. Parks JH, Coe FL, Evan AP, Worcester EM. Clinical and laboratory characteristics of calcium stone-formers with and without primary hyperparathyroidism. BJU Int. 2009;103:670–8.
116. Evan AE, Lingeman JE, Coe FL, et al. Histopathology and surgical anatomy of patients with primary hyperparathyroidism and calcium phosphate stones. Kidney Int. 2008;74:223–9.

The Genetics of Kidney Stones

16

Pietro Manuel Ferraro and Giovanni Gambaro

Abstract

Nephrolithiasis is a common condition. The most common types of kidney stones contain calcium (most often calcium oxalate or calcium phosphate), representing 90 % of all stones.

The etiology of calcium nephrolithiasis is multifactorial, involving nutritional, environmental, and genetic determinants. Genetics play a role in defining the metabolic "milieu" from which kidney stones may form. Monogenic stone-forming conditions are rare but very interesting as "models" to highlight the genetic component of idiopathic nephrolithiasis. Among the others, a tendency to form stones may derive from anomalies of the calcium-sensing receptor, adenylyl cyclase, vitamin D receptor, claudin, chloride channels, phosphatidylinositol 4,5-bisphosphate 5-phosphatase, sodium/phosphate transporter, carriers involved in the pathogenesis of distal renal tubular acidosis, genes involved in renal morphogenesis, and medullary sponge kidney.

Keywords

Genetics • Hypercalciuria • Kidney stones • Mendelian inheritance • Vitamin D • Renal tubular acidosis • Medullary sponge kidney • Calcium-sensing receptor • Cystinuria • Hyperuricosuria • Primary hyperoxaluria

Introduction

Nephrolithiasis is a common condition whose incidence is rising in Westernized countries. The prevalence of kidney stones in American adults increased from 3.8 % in the years 1976–1980 to 5.2 % in the years 1988–1994 [1]. The most common types of kidney stone contain calcium (most often calcium oxalate or calcium phosphate), representing 90 % of all stones, while the rest are composed of uric acid (7 %), cystine (1 %), and other constituents.

The etiology of this disorder is multifactorial, involving a complex interaction of nutritional, environmental, and genetic determinants. The nutritional factors include dietary intake of calcium, salt, animal proteins, fructose, and other nutrients and hydration, while exposure to sun, drugs, and other medical conditions (such as obesity, hypertension, diabetes mellitus, cystic fibrosis, or gout) also play a role in stone formation. These conditions may interact with metabolic abnormalities such as hypercalciuria, hyperphosphaturia, hyperoxaluria, hyperuricosuria, cystinuria, or a urine acidification defect and thus lead to kidney stone formation. A role of genetics in creating this metabolic "milieu" can be hypothesized too. Monogenic stone-forming conditions are rare but have nonetheless proved invaluable for identifying

P.M. Ferraro, M.D. (✉)
Division of Nephrology and Dialysis, Renal Program, Department of Internal Medicine and Medical Specialties, Columbus-Gemelli University Hospital, Via G. Moscati 31, Rome 00168, Italy
e-mail: manuel.ferraro@hotmail.com

G. Gambaro, Ph.D.
Division of Nephrology and Dialysis, School of Medicine, Columbus-Gemelli University Hospital, Catholic University, Rome, Italy
e-mail: giovanni.gambaro@rm.unicatt.it

J.J. Talati et al. (eds.), *Urolithiasis*,
DOI 10.1007/978-1-4471-4387-1_16, © Springer-Verlag London 2012

candidate genes that might explain the genetic component of the much more frequent "idiopathic" or multifactorial nephrolithiasis.

There is plenty of evidence to support the role of genetics in kidney stone disease. Individuals who form stones have a higher prevalence of relatives with nephrolithiasis than those who do not [2], although family history alone is not enough to distinguish between inherited and environmental factors. That a genetic component exists has been unquestionably demonstrated by studies on twins, which have confirmed that a predisposition to kidney stones is inheritable—as emerges from an analysis of the Vietnam Era Twin (VET) Registry, showing that the rate of kidney stones in monozygotic twins was higher (32 %) than in dizygotic twins (17 %) [3].

Hypercalciuric Nephrolithiasis

The most common metabolic abnormality found in stone formers is hypercalciuria, defined as a urinary calcium excretion in excess of 0.1 mmol/kg/24 h, or 300 mg (7.5 mmol) per 24 h in males and 250 mg (6.25 mmol) per 24 h in females. About 40 % of calcium stone formers are hypercalciuric, and vice versa, individuals with hypercalciuria have a higher prevalence of kidney stones than normocalciuric subjects [4]. The cutoff used to define hypercalciuria as a risk factor for stones is debatable, however, and criticized because urinary calcium excretion is a quantitative trait that follows a Gaussian distribution: while some people labeled as hypercalciuric never develop stones, not all stone formers are hypercalciuric. It is now commonly accepted that urinary calcium excretion is at least partly under genetic control. While some authors have considered idiopathic hypercalciuria as a monogenic condition with a Mendelian autosomal dominant inheritance, analyses on the proportion of hypercalciuric first-degree relatives of probands in different unrelated families, which is in the range of 10–40 % [5–7], support the hypothesis of a polygenic mode of transmission and an interaction with environmental factors. This is further supported by statistical modeling on 221 French-Canadian families selected because they had at least two members with calcium nephrolithiasis. The best fit for the inheritance of hypercalciuria was shown by a mixed codominant/polygenic model, which gave a heritability score of 58 % with a polygenic component of 11 % [8]. This estimated percentage variance of urinary calcium excretion, justified by the influence of multiple genes, is consistent with two other studies that reported a heritability of calcium excretion of 47 % [9] and 52 % [10], respectively.

Hypercalciuria is classically divided into three categories: *absorptive hypercalciuria*, in which the intestine would absorb an abnormal amount of calcium, giving rise to a tendency for high calcium levels and consequently to secondary hypercalciuria; *resorptive hypercalciuria*, due to the loss of calcium from the bony skeleton leading to hypercalciuria; and *renal leak hypercalciuria*, caused by a tubular defect with an impaired calcium reabsorption from the ultrafiltrate and hypercalciuria regardless of calcium ingestion, serum levels, and body stores. Several observations have actually led to the conviction that hypercalciuria is a single, common disorder [11–13], namely, the coexistence of different categories of hypercalciuria in some families [5, 6], the possibility of a change of category some years after the first diagnosis [14], and the different phenotypes induced on administering 1,25-dihydroxy-vitamin D, depending on dietary calcium intake [13].

The candidate genes that may contribute to hypercalciuria and calcium nephrolithiasis have been suggested by the known genetic abnormalities found in the rare monogenic Mendelian conditions whose phenotype includes calcium nephrolithiasis.

Calcium-Sensing Receptor

The CaSR gene, located on chromosome 3q21.1, encodes a 1078 amino acid protein, a plasma membrane G-protein-coupled receptor expressed mainly in the parathyroid gland, specific segments of the renal tubule, bone, intestine, and C-cells in the thyroid gland. The CaSR acts as a sensor of extracellular calcium levels. In the parathyroid gland, its activation stimulates the secretion of parathyroid hormone, which in turn takes effect on the tubule by stimulating phosphaturia, stimulating the conversion of 25-hydroxy-vitamin D to 1,25-dihydroxy-vitamin D and promoting calcium reabsorption in the distal convoluted tubule. In conditions characterized by a loss of CaSR function, the set point for PTH secretion is higher and the individuals affected consequently fail to show a hypercalciuric response to hypercalcemia, leading to a picture of familial hypocalciuric hypercalcemia (FHH). Conversely, gain-of-function CaSR mutations or polymorphisms result in autosomal dominant hypocalcemia with hypercalciuria (ADHH) and kidney stones. Females homozygous for the CaSR-activating polymorphism R990G have shown a significantly higher urinary calcium excretion than heterozygous women or women homozygous for the 990R allele [14]. The ADHH phenotype is characterized by asymptomatic hypercalcemia (though some patients may have carpopedal spasms and seizures), hyperphosphatemia, and hypomagnesemia. This picture differs from hypoparathyroidism and pseudohypoparathyroidism in that patients with ADHH have low-normal PTH levels. More than 40 CaSR gene mutations have been associated with ADHH [15]. Another phenotype of the CaSR-activating mutation is Bartter's syndrome type V. In this autosomal dominant condition, the findings common in

ADHH (hypercalciuric nephrolithiasis) are associated with the typical salt-wasting picture secondary to ROMK channel inhibition, presumably caused by CASR activation in the basolateral membrane of the thick ascending limb [16].

Even loss of function mutations of the CASR gene might cause hypercalciuria, based on evidence that CaSR activation in the collecting duct leads to a reduction of the water permeability of this segment of the nephron induced by the antidiuretic hormone, with a consequent urine dilution that minimizes the risk of stone formation [17]. A reduced action of the CaSR in this pathway may cause urine supersaturation and nephrolithiasis. The whole CaSR gene was recently mapped in a cohort of 463 calcium stone formers and 213 healthy controls: two variant alleles (rs7652589 and rs1501899) were found significantly more frequently in the normocitraturic stone formers than in the controls. A correlation also emerged between the CATTCA haplotype and the stone-forming condition: this haplotype includes the 5'UTR region and the two promoters of the CaSR gene, and homozygotes and heterozygotes for the CATTCA haplotype were significantly more associated with normocitraturic kidney stones (with odds ratios of 3.8 and 1.7, respectively, by comparison with individuals not carrying the CATTCA haplotype) [18].

Soluble Adenylyl Cyclase

Linkage studies performed on three families with apparently autosomal dominant idiopathic hypercalciuria showed a significant LOD score for a locus on chromosome 1q23.3-q24, encoding SAC, which is a protein acting as a divalent cation and bicarbonate sensor [19]. SAC exists in both cytosolic and membrane-bound forms, and its activity promotes the generation of cyclic adenosine monophosphate (cAMP). The mechanisms by which mutations in the structure and function of this protein induce renal stones have yet to be elucidated.

Vitamin D Receptor (VDR)

The involvement of vitamin D in the pathogenesis of calcium stones is suggested by a number of observations, such as the usually increased intestinal calcium absorption in subjects with nephrolithiasis. A study has also shown that circulating lymphocytes from patients with hypercalciuria have a higher VDR expression [20]. Scott et al. investigated the linkage of the VDR locus to idiopathic calcium stone formation in a cohort of 47 French-Canadian families [21], finding an association between nephrolithiasis and polymorphic loci in chromosome 12q12-q14, the region containing the VDR gene. Sequencing of the VDR gene revealed no mutations, however, but only conservative substitutions. The authors concluded that a gene in the candidate locus other than VDR might be associated with hypercalciuria. It is noteworthy that the 12q12-q14 locus contains the 1,α-hydroxylase gene, whose product protein is implicated in vitamin D production, but a study conducted on 36 families with probands suffering from hypercalciuric stone disease failed to identify any association between the 1,α-hydroxylase gene and nephrolithiasis [22].

Claudin

Individuals with an autosomal recessive form of familial hypomagnesemia with hypercalciuria and nephrocalcinosis (FHHNC) show mutations in a gene on chromosome 3q27 encoding claudin-16 (CLDN16), which is also called paracellin-1 (PCLN1). This protein of 305 amino acids is expressed at tight junctions of the thick ascending limb of Henle and has a central role in paracellular calcium and magnesium reabsorption.

A particular form of FHHNC, characterized by severe ocular involvement, has been found in one Swiss and eight Spanish/Hispanic families: although these patients showed no mutations in the CLDN16 gene, they had mutations on chromosome 1p34.2 instead, which is a region encoding claudin-19, a tight junction protein expressed in the kidney and eye [23].

Chloride Channel 5

Dent disease is an X-linked recessive disorder characterized by low-molecular-weight proteinuria, hypercalciuria, nephrocalcinosis, nephrolithiasis, and renal failure [24]. It is caused by mutations on the gene encoding the chloride/proton antiporter CLCN5, located on chromosome Xp11.22. CLCN5 is mainly expressed in the proximal tubule, the thick ascending limb of Henle, and the intercalated cells of the collecting duct. CLCN5 mutations lead to impaired chloride transport and acidification of the endosomal lumen and ultimately to abnormal solute reabsorption by the renal tubule.

Other conditions characterized by CLCN5 mutations include X-linked recessive nephrolithiasis and X-linked recessive hypophosphatemic rickets. These conditions can all be termed as "X linked hypercalciuric nephrolithiasis" or "Dent disease complex."

Finally, one Turkish patient with a CLCN5 gene mutation has reportedly shown a picture of Bartter-like syndrome with hypokalemia, metabolic alkalosis and secondary hyperreninemic hyperaldosteronism with a normal blood pressure, associated with hypercalciuria, nephrocalcinosis, and renal stones; this phenotype has been labeled "Bartter's syndrome type VI" [25].

Phosphatidylinositol 4,5-Bisphosphate 5-Phosphatase

This enzyme, encoded by the OCRL1 gene on chromosome Xq25, controls the phosphatidylinositol signaling pathway by hydrolyzing the 5-phosphate of a series of second messengers, e.g., inositol 1,4,5-trisphosphate, inositol 1,3,4,5-tetrakisphosphate, phosphatidylinositol 4,5-bisphosphate, and phosphatidylinositol 3,4,5-trisphosphate. OCRL1 occurs in lysosomes and endosomes in renal proximal tubular cells: in the presence of OCRL1 gene mutations, inositol polyphosphates (and phosphatidylinositol 4,5-bisphosphate in particular) accumulate in the renal proximal tubular cells, disrupting lysosomal and endosomal functions. The clinical picture of such an X-linked recessive disorder, named Lowe's oculocerebrorenal syndrome, is characterized by a proximal tubular loss of bicarbonate, phosphate, and amino acids; hypercalciuria; renal stones; and rickets. Renal dysfunction develops in the first years of life. Extrarenal manifestations include mental retardation, muscle hypotonia, and cataracts.

In 2005, 13 cases were described with a Dent disease phenotype (low-molecular-weight proteinuria, hypercalciuria, and nephrocalcinosis or nephrolithiasis, or hematuria, or hypophosphatemia, or renal insufficiency). None of these subjects had CLCN5 gene mutations, while five had an inactivating mutation of the OCRL1 gene; unlike patients with Lowe syndrome, they had no ocular abnormalities or metabolic acidosis; three patients were mentally retarded. The syndrome has been defined as Dent disease type 2 [26].

Sodium/Phosphate Transporter

Renal stone formation occurs in subjects with impairment of phosphate transporters. The loss of phosphate stimulates the synthesis of calcitriol, which in turn causes hyperabsorption of phosphate and calcium from the intestine, sustaining elevated levels of urinary calcium and phosphate excretion [27]. Mutations in NPT2a, a gene on chromosome 5q35 encoding a sodium/phosphate cotransporter expressed on the renal proximal tubular brush border, have been described in patients with hypophosphatemia, reduced tubular phosphate reabsorption, and kidney stones or bone demineralization [28].

Patients with autosomal recessive hereditary hypophosphatemic rickets with hypercalciuria (HHRH) carry homozygous or compound heterozygous mutations of the NPT2c gene on chromosome 9q34, which encodes a similar sodium/phosphate transporter.

It is worth noting that both NPT2a and NPT2c appear to be regulated by the X-linked phosphate-regulating endopeptidase homolog (PHEX) and the fibroblast growth factor 23 (FGF23); mutations of the former have been shown to cause a form of X-linked hypophosphatemia [29], while mutations of the latter occur in autosomal dominant hypophosphatemic rickets (ADHR) [30].

Serine/Threonine Kinase

A distinct family of serine/threonine kinases characterized by the absence of a lysine residue in the kinase domain (with no lysine [K] kinases, WNK) has been described. Mutations in WNK1 and WNK4 genes are linked to pseudohypoaldosteronism type II (Gordon's syndrome) with hyperkalemia, metabolic acidosis, normal glomerular filtration rate, and low renin levels. Subjects carrying a particular mutation of WNK4 (Q565E) have an abnormally high urinary calcium excretion, while those with WNK1 mutations have urinary calcium excretion levels comparable with controls [31, 32]. WNK4 is a multifunctional protein that regulates renal ion transport; in particular, it regulates the activity of the thiazide-sensitive Na^+-Cl^- cotransporter (NCC), the ROMK channel, and the osmolarity-sensitive Ca^{2+}-permeable channels TRPV4 and TRPV5 (transient receptor potential cation channel subfamily V members 4 and 5), and it also modulates paracellular Cl^- permeability. The hypercalciuric effects of the Q565E WNK4 mutation may be explained by the enhanced NCC-mediated Na^+ transport or by direct effects on the TRPV carriers [33].

Locus on 9q33.2-q34.2

In 2005, a Spanish kindred with an apparently autosomal dominant form of hypercalciuric nephrolithiasis underwent a genome-wide study that revealed mutations on chromosome 9q33.2-q34.2 [34]. This region contains approximately 170 genes, and the gene responsible for the syndrome has yet to be identified.

Genes Causing Distal Renal Tubular Acidosis

This condition is characterized by a derangement in the acid–base balance that is physiologically assured by bicarbonate reabsorption and acid excretion in the tubule. In primary distal renal tubular acidosis (dRTA), the kidney is unable to restore the acid–base homeostasis after an acid load because of an impaired bicarbonate reabsorption or hydrogen ion secretion in the distal nephron. This often leads to hypercalciuria, along with nephrocalcinosis, nephrolithiasis, and hyperchloremic metabolic acidosis. It is most likely secondary to the bone buffering of acids, which increases calcium mobilization from bone [35].

Both autosomal dominant and recessive types of inheritance have been described for this condition. A form of autosomal dominant dRTA has been observed in subjects with gene SLC4A1 mutations on chromosome 17q21-q22, encoding the erythrocyte anion exchanger AE1, which acts on the erythrocyte membranes as an exchanger of chloride and bicarbonate. AE1 is also expressed in the intercalated cells of the collecting ducts: subjects with inactivating AE1 mutations have a typical picture of dRTA with hypercalciuria and kidney stones [36]. AE1 mutations are also associated with an autosomal recessive form of dRTA with hemolytic anemia or ovalocytosis [37, 38].

A form of autosomal recessive dRTA is seen in subjects with progressive sensorineural deafness [39], who have mutations of the ATP6B1 gene on chromosome 2cen-q13, encoding the B subunit of the apical proton pump (H^+-ATPase) that mediates acid secretion in the collecting duct. The protein is also expressed in the cochlea and endolymphatic sac, a region that requires active hydrogen secretion to maintain the right endolymph pH.

Another form of autosomal recessive dRTA with normal hearing can be caused by mutations of the ATP6N1B gene on chromosome 7q33-q34, encoding a kidney-specific accessory subunit expressed in the distal nephron [40].

Medullary Sponge Kidney: The Case for Genes of Renal Morphogenesis

Medullary sponge kidney (MSK) is a condition characterized by cystic anomalies in the precalyceal ducts and defects in urinary acidification and concentration [41]. MSK patients have been reported to often develop nephrolithiasis [42]. This condition has been described in subjects with developmental disorders such as Beckwith-Wiedemann syndrome (whose hallmark features are exomphalos, macroglossia, and gigantism) and congenital hemihypertrophy. Although MSK is thought to be a sporadic condition, there is evidence to suggest that genetic inheritance may have a role and cases of apparently autosomal dominant transmission have been reported [43]. The issue was investigated systematically in a large cohort of MSK patients by Fabris et al. [44], who clearly demonstrated that over 50 % of MSK cases are indeed familial and the evidence supports a Mendelian, autosomal dominant inheritance. A mutation analysis recently performed on 55 patients with MSK found a heterozygosity for two novel variants of the glial-cell-derived neurotrophic factor (GDNF), c.-45G>C and c.-27+18G>A, in eight patients. Five of these eight cases were found to be familial, and the allele variants co-segregated with the disease in a dominant pattern of inheritance. A further case-controlled analysis confirmed these alleles as being significantly associated with MSK [45]. Together with its receptor, the rearranged during transfection (RET) gene, GDNF plays a pivotal part in renal morphogenesis, enabling the proper differentiation and signaling of the "ureteric bud/metanephric blastema" interface. The link between GDNF-dependent abnormal renal morphogenesis and nephrolithiasis/nephrocalcinosis in MSK is not known. One hypothesis is that an abnormal nephrogenesis would cause the mistargeting of a number of epithelial carriers. This could explain why so many different tubular handlings are abnormal in MSK. Patients carrying the GDNF variants certainly reveal a more severe distal tubular acidification derangement [45].

Hyperoxaluria

Since the majority of kidney stones consist of calcium oxalate, the metabolism of oxalate plays a major part in the pathogenesis of nephrolithiasis as well as in calcium metabolism. As concerns the latter, conditions characterized by an enhanced urinary oxalate excretion stem from various factors, such as dietary intake, intestinal absorption, intestinal microbiota, endogenous metabolism, and tubular handling. The importance of genetics in hyperoxaluric conditions is well known.

Primary hyperoxaluria type I (PH1) is an autosomal recessive condition characterized by an abnormally high urinary oxalate excretion (>1.0 mmol/1.73 m^2/24 h) and calcium oxalate stones, caused by mutations of the AGXT gene on chromosome 2q36-q37, which encodes alanine-glyoxylate aminotransferase, a liver-specific enzyme, low levels of which give rise to glyoxylate accumulation and conversion to oxalate, which is then excreted by the kidneys in abnormally large quantities [46].

Primary hyperoxaluria type II (PH2) is caused by mutations in the GRHPR gene on chromosome 9cen, encoding the glyoxylate reductase/hydroxypyruvate reductase gene [47]. As in the case of PH1, impairment in the glyoxylate metabolic pathway may lead to the accumulation of this substance, its conversion into oxalate and hyperoxaluria.

Another "non-PH1/PH2" form of primary hyperoxaluria has been described that involves no AGXT or GRHPR mutations. One of the candidate genes for this condition is SLC26A6, a gene on chromosome 3p21.3 encoding a chloride-oxalate exchanger expressed in the gut and renal tubules. The involvement of this gene in human hyperoxaluria derives from a model of *Slc26a6 (−/−)* mice, in which hyperoxaluria and nephrolithiasis secondary to net intestinal hyperabsorption of oxalate have been described, though a similar condition has not been described in humans as yet [48].

Cystinuria

This autosomal recessive condition can be caused by a defect of a cystine/amino acid transporter, comprising a first heavy subunit (rBAT) and a second light subunit (bo, +AT) associated with the first to form the active transporter [49]. Mutations may occur in the SLC3A1 gene on chromosome 2p16.3, encoding the heavy subunit of the carrier, or in the SLC7A9 gene on chromosome 19q13.1, encoding the light subunit [50]. Around 25 % of patients with cystinuria have no SLC3A1 or SLC7A9 mutations, however, suggesting a role for other as yet unknown genes.

Hyperuricosuria

Uric acid stones are a relatively common cause of nephrolithiasis, but again (as in calcium nephrolithiasis), the inherited Mendelian forms are quite rare. Monogenic conditions leading to hyperuricemia and hyperuricosuria include Lesch-Nyhan syndrome (LNS), featuring mental retardation with self-destructive biting, cerebral palsy, choreoathetosis, and uric acid stones. This condition is caused by a defect in the HPRT gene on chromosome Xq26-q27.2, encoding hypoxanthine-guanine phosphoribosyltransferase. While a complete loss of function of this enzyme leads to a clinical picture of LNS, a partial deficiency has been described in subjects with Kelley-Seegmiller syndrome, which is characterized by renal stones and uric acid nephropathy, without the neurological signs of LNS.

URAT1 gene mutations on chromosome 11q13, encoding a urate-anion exchanger expressed mainly in the proximal tubular epithelium, have been reported in patients with hypouricemia and nephrolithiasis, reflecting an impaired tubular urate reabsorption [51].

In 2001, a genome-wide study performed on a small population of individuals with a seemingly autosomal dominant inheritance of uric acid stones showed that two chromosomal regions (10q21-q22 and 20q13.1-13.3) were significantly associated with stone formation [52].

Genes Responsible for Other Conditions

Citrate is a natural inhibitor of urinary stones, and states in which urinary citrate is reduced are a risk factor for nephrolithiasis. Conditions causing chronic acidosis lead to a compensatory increase in tubular citrate absorption; for instance, distal renal tubular acidosis may coincide with both hypercalciuria and hypocitraturia. The main citrate transporter in the kidney is a sodium-dependent carrier encoded by the SLC13A5 gene on chromosome 17p13-p12. No mutations of this gene have been described in subjects with kidney stones to date.

Inorganic pyrophosphate (PPi) is a potent calcification inhibitor. The expression of the PPi carrier ANKH has been demonstrated in human renal collecting ducts [53], but there is no evidence that mutations or polymorphisms at this site are associated with nephrolithiasis.

Tamm-Horsfall protein (THP), or uromodulin, is the most abundant protein in urine. It is synthesized in the thick ascending limb of Henle's loop. Patients with mutations of the UMOD gene on chromosome 16p12.3 have a complex picture of hyperuricemia and gout, or medullary cystic kidney disease, but no renal stones. On the other hand, patients with nephrolithiasis excrete higher than normal amounts of an abnormally sialylated THP [54]. These findings suggest a role for the genes regulating THP maturation in nephrolithiasis.

Interaction Between Genes and Environment in Nephrolithiasis

An interaction between a "polygenic" predisposition (due to mutations or functional variants in several genes regulating calcium homeostasis) and environmental factors is thought to be essential for the onset of a hypercalciuric trait and idiopathic calcium oxalate stone formation [55]. This view is supported by evidence that nephrolithiasis occurs more frequently in subjects with a family history of stones: a familial aggregation for stones has been reported, ranging from 16 to 50 % [56, 57]. Familial clustering may also be explained by nongenetic factors, such as dietary habits, an impression supported by the fact that changes in eating habits may change both the incidence and the chemical composition of stones [58]. Most studies nonetheless support the conviction that a genetic predisposition has a fundamental role in stone formation. A study by Bianchi et al. showed that calcium excretion correlated between parents and progeny and between siblings, but not between spouses (who presumably share the same dietary habits) [59]; the authors concluded that half the variance in urinary calcium excretion is attributable to additive genetic factors, a finding confirmed by several others [8–10].

Although the issue has not been investigated, we speculate that the common form of uric acid nephrolithiasis might also be driven by a combination of environmental and genetic factors.

Figure 16.1 summarizes the interactions between genes and the environment in nephrolithiasis.

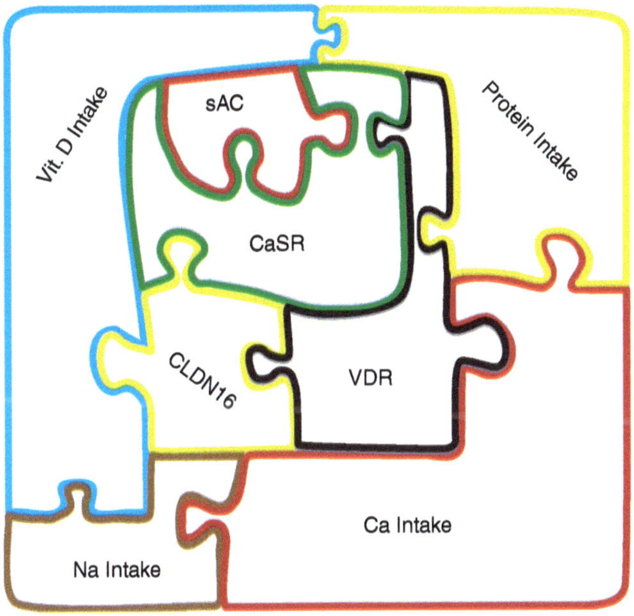

Fig. 16.1 Schematic representation of the main characteristics of hypercalciuric nephrolithiasis. Idiopathic hypercalciuria is a polygenic disorder (represented by the various genes forming the inner part of the puzzle and possibly by many others, both known and still unknown), in which the contribution of each gene may vary, but their global contribution to the pathogenesis of the disease is approximately 50 %, according to a number of studies—the other 50 % being determined by environmental (mainly nutritional) factors

From Monogenic Disorders to Idiopathic Nephrolithiasis

Mutations of the majority of the previously mentioned genes responsible for monogenic disorders involving nephrolithiasis have been sought in patients with common nephrolithiasis, but the hypothesis that mutations or allele variants of candidate genes might give rise to a greater susceptibility to stone formation in these individuals has rarely been confirmed. An extensive review of the published evidence of the role of candidate genes in idiopathic hypercalciuria is available [24].

As a side note, studying the genetics of idiopathic nephrolithiasis comes up against several methodological difficulties. The classical approaches used to identify diseases causing loci in Mendelian diseases (i.e., linkage analysis and positional cloning) are useless when applied to such a complex disease with a seemingly polygenic pattern of inheritance as idiopathic nephrolithiasis, because they rely on the relative contribution to the disease of a susceptibility gene. Researchers have resorted to case–control association studies, in which the frequency of a selected allele variant is compared in affected and unaffected individuals. A weakness of this kind of study lies in the need for an a priori hypothesis that is clearly limited, in the case of idiopathic nephrolithiasis, by our incomplete understanding of its pathogenesis. Findings from case–control studies are also often not confirmed by meta-analyses [60]. There is little justification for seeking just one or a few single nucleotide polymorphisms (SNPs) in a given gene by means of association studies in a disease as complex as idiopathic nephrolithiasis, whereas haplotype studies may be more likely to produce more robust results with this experimental design.

Different family-based strategies have been developed to reduce the inconsistencies and biases raised by population stratification in case–control association studies. One of the strongest designs is the transmission disequilibrium test (TDT), which investigates the probands and their parents (i.e., the disequilibrium in allele transmission from parents to probands). The source of controls is thus represented by the parents, and the effects of the environment are reduced because eating habits are often similar in the same family. Another family-based study uses the sib-pair design, the purpose of which is to determine whether siblings tend to express the same disease phenotype when they share the same inherited allele; this type of study avoids the difficulties often encountered in obtaining information from parents.

Conclusion

The main features of genetic forms of nephrolithiasis are presented in this chapter. This may serve as a basis to understand the genetic component of idiopathic nephrolithiasis as well as its multifactorial pathogenesis.

References

1. Stamatelou KK, Francis ME, Jones CA, et al. Time trends in reported prevalence of kidney stones in the united states: 1976-1994. Kidney Int. 2003;63:1817–23.
2. Curhan GC, Willett WC, Rimm EB, et al. Family history and risk of kidney stones. J Am Soc Nephrol. 1997;8:1568–73.
3. Goldfarb DS, Fischer ME, Keich Y, et al. A twin study of genetic and dietary influences on nephrolithiasis: a report from the Vietnam Era Twin (VET) registry. Kidney Int. 2005;67:1053–61.
4. Lerolle N, Lantz B, Paillard F, et al. Risk factors for nephrolithiasis in patients with familial idiopathic hypercalciuria. Am J Med. 2002;113:99–103.
5. Nicolaidou P, Themeli S, Karpathios T, et al. Family pattern of idiopathic hypercalciuria and its subtypes. J Urol. 1996;155:1042–4.
6. Harangi F, Méhes K. Family investigations in idiopathic hypercalciuria. Eur J Pediatr. 1993;152:64–8.
7. Lerolle N, Coulet F, Lantz B, Paillard F, Houillier P, Soubrier F, Gattegno B, Jeunemaître X, Ronco P, Rondeau E. No evidence for point mutations of the calcium-sensing receptor in familial idiopathic hypercalciuria. Nephrol Dial Transplant. 2001;16:2317–22.
8. Loredo-Osti JC, Roslin NM, Tessier J, et al. Segregation of urine calcium excretion in families ascertained for nephrolithiasis: evidence for a major gene. Kidney Int. 2005;68:966–71.

9. Falchetti A, Vezzoli G, Gambaro G. Genetics of primary hypercalciuria. Clin Cases Miner Bone Metab. 2004;1:27–33.
10. Hunter D, De Lange M, Snieder H, et al. Genetic contribution to bone metabolism, calcium excretion, and vitamin D and parathyroid hormone regulation. J Bone Miner Res. 2001;16:371–8.
11. Vezzoli G, Soldati L, Gambaro G. Hypercalciuria revisited: one or many conditions? Pediatr Nephrol. 2008;23:503–6.
12. Aladjem M, Barr J, Lahat E, et al. Renal and absorptive hypercalciuria: a metabolic disturbance with varying and interchanging modes of expression. Pediatrics. 1996;97:216–9.
13. Maierhofer WJ, Lemann Jr J, Gray RW, et al. Dietary calcium and serum 1,25-(OH)2-vitamin D concentrations as determinants of calcium balance in healthy men. Kidney Int. 1984;26:752–9.
14. Vezzoli G, Terranegra A, Arcidiacono T, et al. R990G polymorphism of calcium-sensing receptor does produce a gain-of-function and predispose to primary hypercalciuria. Kidney Int. 2007;71: 1155–62.
15. Hendy GN, D'Souza-Li L, Yang B, et al. Mutations of the calcium-sensing receptor (CASR) in familial hypocalciuric hypercalcemia, neonatal severe hyperparathyroidism, and autosomal dominant hypocalcemia. Hum Mutat. 2000;16:281–96.
16. Vargas-Poussou R, Huang C, Hulin P, et al. Functional characterization of a calcium-sensing receptor mutation in severe autosomal dominant hypocalcemia with a Bartter-like syndrome. J Am Soc Nephrol. 2002;13:2259–66.
17. Sands JM, Naruse M, Baum M, et al. Apical extracellular calcium/polyvalent cation-sensing receptor regulates vasopressin-elicited water permeability in rat kidney inner medullary collecting duct. J Clin Invest. 1997;99:1399–405.
18. Vezzoli G, Terranegra A, Arcidiacono T, et al. Calcium kidney stones are associated with a haplotype of the calcium-sensing receptor gene regulatory region. Nephrol Dial Transplant. 2010;25: 2245–52.
19. Reed BY, Heller HJ, Gitomer WL, et al. Mapping a gene defect in absorptive hypercalciuria to chromosome 1q23.3-q24. J Clin Endocrinol Metab. 1999;84:3907–13.
20. Zerwekh JE, Yu XP, Breslau NA, et al. Vitamin D receptor quantitation in human blood mononuclear cells in health and disease. Mol Cell Endocrinol. 1993;96:1–6.
21. Scott P, Ouimet D, Valiquette L, et al. Suggestive evidence for a susceptibility gene near the vitamin D receptor locus in idiopathic calcium stone formation. J Am Soc Nephrol. 1999;10:1007–13.
22. Scott P, Ouimet D, Proulx Y, et al. The 1 alpha-hydroxylase locus is not linked to calcium stone formation or calciuric phenotypes in French-Canadian families. J Am Soc Nephrol. 1998;9:425–32.
23. Konrad M, Schaller A, Seelow D, et al. Mutations in the tight-junction gene claudin 19 (CLDN19) are associated with renal magnesium wasting, renal failure, and severe ocular involvement. Am J Hum Genet. 2006;79:949–57.
24. Gambaro G, Vezzoli G, Casari G, et al. Genetics of hypercalciuria and calcium nephrolithiasis: from the rare monogenic to the common polygenic forms. Am J Kidney Dis. 2004;44:963–86.
25. Besbas N, Ozaltin F, Jeck N, et al. CLCN5 mutation (R347X) associated with hypokalaemic metabolic alkalosis in a Turkish child: an unusual presentation of Dent's disease. Nephrol Dial Transplant. 2005;20:1476–9.
26. Hoopes Jr RR, Shrimpton AE, Knohl SJ, et al. Dent disease with mutations in OCRL1. Am J Hum Genet. 2005;76:260–7.
27. Priè D, Friedlander G. Genetic disorders of renal phosphate transport. N Engl J Med. 2010;362:2399–409.
28. Prié D, Huart V, Bakouh N, et al. Nephrolithiasis and osteoporosis associated with hypophosphatemia caused by mutations in the type 2a sodium-phosphate cotransporter. N Engl J Med. 2002;347:983–91.
29. Sabbagh Y, Jones AO, Tenenhouse HS. PHEXdb, a locus-specific database for mutations causing X-linked hypophosphatemia. Hum Mutat. 2000;16:1–6.
30. Econs MJ, McEnery PT. Autosomal dominant hypophosphatemic rickets/osteomalacia: clinical characterization of a novel renal phosphate-wasting disorder. J Clin Endocrinol Metab. 1997;82: 674–81.
31. Mayan H, Munter G, Shaharabany M, et al. Hypercalciuria in familial hyperkalemia and hypertension accompanies hyperkalemia and precedes hypertension: description of a large family with the Q565E WNK4 mutation. J Clin Endocrinol Metab. 2004;89: 4025–30.
32. Achard JM, Warnock DG, Disse-Nicodème S, et al. Familial hyperkalemic hypertension: phenotypic analysis in a large family with the WNK1 deletion mutation. Am J Med. 2003;114:495–8.
33. Jiang Y, Ferguson WB, Peng JB. WNK4 enhances TRPV5-mediated calcium transport: potential role in hypercalciuria of familial hyperkalemic hypertension caused by gene mutation of WNK4. Am J Physiol Renal Physiol. 2007;292:F545–54.
34. Wolf MT, Zalewski I, Martin FC, et al. Mapping a new suggestive gene locus for autosomal dominant nephrolithiasis to chromosome 9q33.2-q34.2 by total genome search for linkage. Nephrol Dial Transplant. 2005;20:909–14.
35. Fabris A, Bernich P, Abaterusso C, et al. Bone disease in medullary sponge kidney and effect of potassium citrate treatment. Clin J Am Soc Nephrol. 2009;4:1974–9.
36. Bruce LJ, Cope DL, Jones GK, et al. Familial distal renal tubular acidosis is associated with mutations in the red cell anion exchanger (Band 3, AE1) gene. J Clin Invest. 1997;100:1693–707.
37. Wrong O, Bruce LJ, Unwin RJ, et al. Band 3 mutations, distal renal tubular acidosis, and southeast Asian ovalocytosis. Kidney Int. 2002;62:10–9.
38. Tanphaichitr VS, Sumboonnanonda A, Ideguchi H, et al. Novel AE1 mutations in recessive distal renal tubular acidosis. Loss-of-function is rescued by glycophorin a. J Clin Invest. 1998;102:2173–9.
39. Karet FE, Finberg KE, Nelson RD, et al. Mutations in the gene encoding B1 subunit of H^+-ATPase cause renal tubular acidosis with sensorineural deafness. Nat Genet. 1999;21:84–90.
40. Smith AN, Skaug J, Choate KA, et al. Mutations in ATP6N1B, encoding a new kidney vacuolar proton pump 116-kD subunit, cause recessive distal renal tubular acidosis with preserved hearing. Nat Genet. 2000;26:71–5.
41. Gambaro G, Feltrin GP, Lupo A, et al. Medullary sponge kidney (Lenarduzzi-Cacchi-Ricci disease): a Padua Medical School discovery in the 1930s. Kidney Int. 2006;69:663–70.
42. Cameron S. Medullary sponge kidney. In: Davison AM, Cameron JS, Grunfeld J-P, Ponticelli C, Ritz E, Winearls CG, van Ypersele C, editors. Oxford textbook of clinical nephrology. 3rd ed. Oxford: Oxford University Press; 2004. p. 2495–501.
43. Kuiper JJ. Medullary sponge kidney in three generations. N Y State J Med. 1971;71:2665–9.
44. Fabris A, Lupo A, Ferraro PM, et al. The medullary sponge kidney is frequently an inherited disorder: a systematic analysis of a large cohort. In: XLVII ERA-EDTA congress, Munich, 25–28 June 2010.
45. Torregrossa R, Anglani F, Fabris A, et al. Identification of GDNF gene sequence variations in patients with medullary sponge kidney disease. Clin J Am Soc Nephrol. 2010;5(7):1205–10.
46. Cochat P, Deloraine A, Rotily M, et al. Epidemiology of primary hyperoxaluria type 1. Nephrol Dial Transplant. 1995;10 Suppl 8:3–7.
47. Williams HE, Smith Jr LH. Hyperoxaluria in L-glyceric aciduria: possible pathogenic mechanism. Science. 1971;171:390–1.
48. Monico CG, Weinstein A, Jiang Z, et al. Phenotypic and functional analysis of human SLC26A6 variants in patients with familial hyperoxaluria and calcium oxalate nephrolithiasis. Am J Kidney Dis. 2008;52:1096–103.
49. Dello Strologo L, Pras E, Pontesilli C, et al. Comparison between SLC3A1 and SLC7A9 cystinuria patients and carriers: a need for a new classification. J Am Soc Nephrol. 2002;13:2547–53.

50. Botzenhart E, Vester U, Schmidt C, et al. Cystinuria in children: distribution and frequencies of mutations in the SLC3A1 and SLC7A9 genes. Kidney Int. 2002;62:1136–42.
51. Tanaka M, Itoh K, Matsushita K, et al. Two male siblings with hereditary renal hypouricemia and exercise-induced ARF. Am J Kidney Dis. 2003;42:1287–92.
52. Ombra MN, Forabosco P, Casula S, et al. Identification of a new candidate locus for uric acid nephrolithiasis. Am J Hum Genet. 2001;68:1119–29.
53. Carr G, Sayer JA, Simmons NL. Expression and localisation of the pyrophosphate transporter, ANK, in murine kidney cells. Cell Physiol Biochem. 2007;20:507–16.
54. Jaggi M, Nakagawa Y, Zipperle L, et al. Tamm-Horsfall protein in recurrent calcium kidney stone formers with positive family history: abnormalities in urinary excretion, molecular structure and function. Urol Res. 2007;35:55–62.
55. Srivastava T, Schwaderer A. Diagnosis and management of hypercalciuria in children. Curr Opin Pediatr. 2009;21:214–9.
56. Resnick M, Pridgen DB, Goodman HO. Genetic predisposition to formation of calcium oxalate renal calculi. J Am Soc Nephrol. 1997;278:1313–8.
57. Gambaro G, Marchini F, Piccoli A, et al. The abnormal red-cell oxalate transport is a risk factor for idiopathic calcium nephrolithiasis: a prospective study. J Am Soc Nephrol. 1996;7:608–12.
58. Trinchieri A. Epidemiology of urolithiasis. Arch Ital Urol Androl. 1996;68:203–49.
59. Bianchi G, Vezzoli G, Cusi D, et al. Abnormal red-cell calcium pump in patients with idiopathic hypercalciuria. N Engl J Med. 1988;319:897–901.
60. Ioannidis JP, Ntzani EE, Trikalinos TA, et al. Replication validity of genetic association studies. Nat Genet. 2001;29:306–9.

Familial Clustering of Stone Disease

17

Jamsheer Jehangir Talati, Naveed Haroon, and Alberto Trinchieri

Abstract

Across the world, from 15 to 68 % of patients with stone may have a family history of stone in their first-degree relatives. A family history is associated with an earlier onset of disease and a greater chance of recurrence. The lifetime risk (to age 75) for a brother of the propositi is ~50 %. The reason for a high frequency of stone in the immediate family might be consanguinity, dietary, or environmental. If genetic factors are present, the inheritance appears polygenetic rather than monogenetic.

Keywords

Family history • Urinary tract stone • Monogenetic inheritance • Polygenetic inheritance • Environmental • Lifetime risk

Introduction

A high incidence of renal stones has been frequently reported among family members of patients with nephrolithiasis. Trinchieri et al. [1] reported a 25 % rate of positive family history in patients forming calcium stones and a 43 % in patients forming uric acid/urate stones. Resnick [2] drew attention to specific findings that there was a more frequent association of family history with calcium oxalate stones than with calcium phosphate stones. In 1960, McGeown et al. [3] compared patients hospitalized for calcium stone disease with a control group of patients hospitalized for other pathologies, showing that family history for renal stones was more frequently positive among stone patients than among the controls that were grouped by sex and age.

Subsequent studies confirmed the finding of a more frequent positive family history in renal stone formers. Churchill [4] observed a more frequent positive family history among renal stone formers (39 %) than among controls (20 %), although the difference was only significant for female patients and controls. Trinchieri [5] observed a higher incidence of nephrolithiasis among relatives in the first degree of urolithiasis patients (37.4 %) than among controls (12.8 %) and confirmed that the tendency to positive family history was greater among female patients (45 %) than among males (31 %).

In another survey, Ljunghall [6], reviewing 380 recurrent patients in a stone clinic, reported that 55.4 % (64.7 % females and 51 % males) had a history of stone in the family. Among the ordinary stone patients, 18 % of the fathers and 8 % of the mothers also had formed renal stones. The corresponding figures for female stone patients with renal tubular defects were 40 and 33 %, respectively.

After the first observations from Europe and North America, an increased risk of stone formation in presence of

J.J. Talati, M.B.B.S., FRCS (✉) N. Haroon, M.B.B.S.
Section of Urology, Department of Surgery, Aga Khan University, 3500, Stadium Road, Karachi, Sindh 74800, Pakistan
e-mail: jamsheer.talati@aku.edu; naveed.haroon@aku.edu

A. Trinchieri M.D., FEBU
Department of Urology, A. Manzoni Hospital, Via Dell'Eremo 9/11, Lecco 23900, Italy
e-mail: a.trinchieri@ospedale.lecco.it

J.J. Talati et al. (eds.), *Urolithiasis*,
DOI 10.1007/978-1-4471-4387-1_17, © Springer-Verlag London 2012

a family history of renal stones was confirmed by several studies from other countries in the world [7–12]. Hussain et al. in a study on Malaysian renal stone patients, quoted in Talati et al. [8] in Kelantan province, demonstrated that 33 % of renal stone formers had a first-degree relative with stone. The influence of family history on kidney stone formation was described as even greater (up to 50 %) in some pediatric stone populations [10, 11]. In a study conducted in Pakistan, 52 % of stone patients and 18 % of controls had at least one other first-degree relative with a history of stone disease [8].

Apart from speculating about the effect of genetic and environmental influences in stone disease, there are also clinical reasons why we should enquire into the familial incidence of stone in all patients who seek our advice, especially in stone belt countries. The presence of a positive family history for renal stones (in patients presenting with other diseases) increases the risk of stone formation in male relatives of the proband, who may never have experienced a previous stone incident, and the association between family history and the risk of stone formation is stronger in men aged<60 years [13]. Curran's study revealed a 2.57 increased relative risk for stone if a family member had presented a stone. A patient in a stone-producing family is likely to get stone disease at a younger age [12], and Resnick [2] calculated that for a male living to 75 years, the lifetime risk for brothers of the propositi (the proband) approached 50 %, indicating the need for prophylactic interventions in family members. Additionally, with a family history of stone, one is more likely to form stones under extreme conditions (such as fighting a desert war) [14].

The frequency of stones in the first-degree relatives of propositi is listed in Table 17.1, and the percent of parents and siblings of propositi affected by stone are mentioned in Table 17.2.

For the patient presenting with one or several stones, it is useful to know if there is a family history, because not only will he or she likely be younger but will also suffer risk of more frequent recurrences [12]. Ljunghall [6] suggested that the greater the number of recurrences, the more likely was the possibility that a relative also formed stones. Fortunately, the risk of single or multiple stone recurrences was independent of whether propositi had recurrent stones or multiple stones [2]. Badr [18] (from studies of in a population from Iran) also concluded that there was no relation between the number and size of the calculi and the family history.

When Coe screened 73 relatives of patients with hypercalciuria, 36 % of them had hypercalciuria. Stones formed in 43 % of the 44 first-degree relatives [22].

For all of these reasons, it is worth exploring how frequently stone disease is detected in family members of stone patients and also worth the effort to try to unravel whether the cause is genetic or environmental. Residents should record the pedigree of families as part of their intelligent initial history and physical.

Table 17.1 Reported frequency of first-degree relatives of stone patients affected by stone disease

Country	Year	Author	% of propositi SF having a relative with a history of stone (versus controls)
Argentina	2008	Spivacow [10]	32.9
Czech	1987	Kruzek [15]	23.6 (7.8)
England	1983	Robertson [16]	14.8 (9.1)
India	2009	Marickar [17]	16.2
Iran	2007	Badr [18]	28.6
Iran	2008	Ketabchi [9]	14.9 (6.5)
Italy	1987	Trinchieri [1]	37 % [45 % of females and 31 % males]
Kuwait	1997	El-Reshaid [19]	53
Malaysia	1997	Hussain [8]	33
New Zealand	2009	Davidson [7]	20
Pakistan	1997	Talati [8]	52 (18)
Sweden	1985	Ljunghall [6]	55 % [64 % females and 51 % males]
Thailand	2009	Sritippayawan [20]	21.1
Turkey	2010	Koyuncu [12]	27.4
Turkey	2010	Ertan [21]	68.2 % [27 % of stone patients from consanguineous marriages]

Methodologies Employed in Various Studies

The studies we reviewed use different approaches to obtain data. Most are based on questionnaires given to patients with stone disease. Some questionnaires were administered to patients in special stone clinics (which tend to attract the recurrent stone former as was the case in Ljunghall's stone

Table 17.2 Percent of parents and siblings of propositi and controls affected by stone disease

	Resnick		Talati		Ljunghall	Marickar	McGeown
	Propositi	Control	Propositi	Control	Propositi	Propositi	Propositi
Fathers	15.1	4.1	14	05	7.5 % of parents	18 %	31
Mothers	11.3	4.0	09	01		8	05.6
Brothers	20.5	7.0	16	03	4.5 % of siblings	08 %	47.8
Sisters	8.2	4.1	07	03			0.7

clinic study [6]). Some studies have analyzed population data obtained for other reasons. For example, in another investigation, Ljunghall [23] reviewed 2,500 middle-aged men in a general survey, noting differences in family history. Curhan [13] reviewed a database of 37,999 male participants in a health professional follow-up study.

Most questionnaire-based studies rely on recall. The accuracy of the results depends on awareness of stone disease in other relatives. There is a risk to underestimate the incidence of stones in the family because stone patients may be ignorant of his relatives who have a stone. Furthermore, some of them may be harboring silent stones. In fact, the incidence of silent stones is around 3–15 % in Pakistan (see chapter 3). A more accurate picture would emerge if all family members had an ultrasound examination carried out. However, as stones occur over such a wide age range, even such studies can fail to give information about previous neglected stone episodes.

All of this points to the likelihood that the reported frequency of stone in family members is an underestimate.

Is Familial Clustering Due to Genetic or Dietary Factors?

While studies clearly demonstrate a role for family history as a risk factor for idiopathic calcium stone disease, a definitive conclusion cannot be reached on whether the mechanism of familial clustering is attributable to genetic or environmental factors.

In fact, it can be argued that the relatives of stone patients (not spouses) not only share some of the genetic pattern but (and this would now be true for the spouse as well) are also exposed to the same environmental, dietary, and climatic factors.

To assess the effect of this potential problem, some studies have assessed the incidence of lithiasis also in acquired relatives (wives and husbands) who, at least for a certain period of time, share the same environmental conditions but have a different genetic pattern.

McGeown [3] demonstrated that spouses of stone formers are not affected by the disease more than controls, but spouses of patients with positive family history are more frequently affected by the disease (8.8 %) than spouses of patients with negative family history (3.3 %).

According to Resnick et al. [2], the incidence of stones was significantly greater among the male relatives (fathers and brothers) of renal stone patients than among their spouses, while there was a similar but not statistically significant trend among female relatives. Trinchieri et al. [5] also confirmed that family history for stones was more frequent in stone patients than among their wives and husbands (38.9 % versus 18.4 %).

Furthermore, the increased risk of stone formation in subjects with positive family history of stone disease appeared to be independent of their dietary intake of calcium [13].

Biyabani et al. demonstrated that, surprisingly, urinary citrate:urinary creatinine ratios showed a greater variation between siblings (667.4 + 200) than between propositi and unrelated individuals (13.2 + 180) [24].

A prevalent role of genetic factors should involve an enhancement of the tendency to family clustering of stone disease in populations with high incidence of marriages between blood relatives.

In Andalusia, Torres [25] studied a gypsy population with a high incidence of marriages between blood relatives (26.9 %) compared with the remaining population (4.1 %). In the gypsy population, the incidence of stone disease was lower than in the non-gypsies (1.14 % versus 4.34 %), but in gypsies with lithiasis, family history for stones was more frequent (26.9 %) than in the remaining Andalusian population (4.1 %). On the contrary, in Pakistan, where consanguineous marriages are quoted as up to 60 % of all marriages, consanguineous marriage between parents of renal stone formers was observed in only 16 % [8]. This may be because the hospital care (a fee-for-service hospital) was accessed by a greater proportion of literate and upwardly mobile populations, with a lower incidence of inbreeding. Despite this, the frequency of positive family history in that cohort was 52 %.

Monogenetic or Polygenic Inheritance

The way in which the genetic predisposition for idiopathic calcium nephrolithiasis is transmitted has been the subject of a number of hypotheses. Resnick et al. [2] considered both monogenic and polygenic mechanisms, but on the basis of classical concepts of genetics, they excluded monogenic mechanisms, dominant, recessive, autosomal, or X-related.

In contrast, the hypothesis of polygenic transmission appears more plausible. Such a hypothesis requires that the frequency of the disease is the same in the two sexes. Hence, the greater incidence in males must be explained in some way; perhaps there is a higher onset "threshold" for females. The greater prevalence of the disease among patients' female relatives further supports the polygenic hypothesis, because the onset of the disease in the gender less frequently affected (female) requires a more marked genetic alteration, so the genetic risk among relatives must be higher.

It must be noted here that the risk in male relatives appears to be higher in Pakistani populations: 6 % of patients have a brother affected by stone disease, while only 2.6 % have a similarly affected sister. Interestingly, even in this population of all the possible sisters or brothers, 1.6 % or 1.4 %, respectively, are afflicted by stone. Four percent of patients had a paternal uncle and 4 % a maternal uncle affected, but only

0.83 % had a maternal aunt and none had a paternal aunt affected. When all families where a father and son were affected were considered collectively, 36 % of all the sons in that cohort were affected by stone disease. Similarly in families where a father and daughter were affected, 26 % of all daughters were affected. Badr [18] (in a population from Iran) found that 71 % of the affected family members were siblings.

Goodman et al. [26] developed a statistical model hypothesizing that the presence of 3 loci correlated with the polygenetic mechanism of hereditary predisposition with two codominant alleles for each of them.

The identification of these genetically determined metabolic alterations has yet to be made.

Potential hereditary defects could act through increased excretion of lithogenic solutes (calcium, oxalate) or a lack of crystallization inhibitors or an excess of crystallization promoters.

Conclusion

As familial clustering is seen across the world and the risk for stone formation in relatives of stone formers is higher, family history should be recorded in each patient. Whether the relatives of propositi should be screened, and if so how often, remains an unanswered question. The relative contribution of polygenetic and environmental influences also remains unresolved for most of the "idiopathic stone" formers.

References

1. Trinchieri A, Mandressi A, Luongo P, Mazza L, Zaatar C, Pisani E. Recurrence and family history of renal stone disease. Contrib Nephrol. 1987;58:30–3.
2. Resnick M, Pridgen DB, Goodman HO. Genetic predisposition to formation of calcium oxalate renal calculi. N Eng J Med. 1968;278(24):1313–8.
3. McGeown MG. Heredity in renal stone disease. Clin Sci. 1960;19:465–71.
4. Churchill DN, Maloney CM, Bear J, Bryant DG, Fodor G, Gault MH. Urolithiasis–a study of drinking water hardness and genetic factors* 1. J Chronic Dis. 1980;33(11–12):727–31.
5. Trinchieri A, Mandressi A, Luongo P, Coppi F, Pisani E. Familial aggregation of renal calcium stone disease. J Urol. 1988;139(3):478.
6. Ljunghall S, Danielson BG, Fellström B, Holmgren K, Johansson G. Family history of renal stones in recurrent stone patients. Br J Urol. 1985;57(4):370–4.
7. Davidson PJ, Sheerin IG, Frampton C. Renal stone disease in Christchurch, New Zealand. Part 1: presentation and epidemiology. N Z Med J. 2009;122(number 1297):49–56.
8. Talati J. Familial clustering and sex incidence of urolithiasis. Dev Nephrol. 1997;38:69–78.
9. Ketabchi AA, Aziziolahi GA. Prevalence of symptomatic urinary calculi in Kerman, Iran. Urol J. 2008;5(3):156–60.
10. Spivacow FR, Negri AL, del Valle EE, Calviño I, Fradinger E, Zanchetta JR. Metabolic risk factors in children with kidney stone disease. Pediatr Nephrol. 2008;23(7):1129–33.
11. Alpay H, Ozen A, Gokce I, Biyikli N. Clinical and metabolic features of urolithiasis and microlithiasis in children. Pediatr Nephrol. 2009;24(11):2203–9.
12. Koyuncu HH, Yencilek F, Eryildirim B, Sarica K. Family history in stone disease: how important is it for the onset of the disease and the incidence of recurrence? Urol Res. 2010;38(2):105–9.
13. Curhan GC, Willett WC, Rimm EB, Stampfer MJ. Family history and risk of kidney stones. J Am Soc Nephrol. 1997;8(10):1568.
14. Pugliese JM, Baker KC. Epidemiology of nephrolithiasis in personnel returning from operation Iraqi freedom. Urology. 2009; 74(1):56–60.
15. Kruzek VVM. Familial incidence of urolithiasis in Czechoslovakia, abstracts of 13th urolithiasis symposium. Urol Res. 1987;15:115.
16. Robertson WG, Peacock M, Baker M, et al. Epidemiological studies on urinary stone disease in Leeds. In: Rayall RL, Brockis JG, Marshall VR, et al., editors. Urinary stone disease. Edinburgh: Churchill–Livingstone; 1984. p. 8–9.
17. Fazil Marickar YM, Salim A, Vijay A. Pattern of family history in stone patients. Urol Res. 2009;37(6):331–5.
18. Ahmadi Asr Badr Y, Hazhir S, Hasanzadeh K. Family history and age at the onset of upper urinary tract calculi. Urol J. 2009; 4(3):142–6.
19. El-Reshaid K, Mughal H, Kapoor M. Epidemiological profile, mineral metabolic pattern and crystallographic analysis of urolithiasis in Kuwait. Eur J Epidemiol. 1997;13(2):229–34.
20. Sritippayawan S, Borvornpadungkitti S, Paemanee A, Predanon C, Susaengrat W, Chuawattana D, et al. Evidence suggesting a genetic contribution to kidney stone in northeastern Thai population. Urol Res. 2009;37(3):141–6.
21. Ertan P, Tekin G, OÖger N, Alkan S, Horasan GD. Metabolic and demographic characteristics of children with urolithiasis in western Turkey. Urol Res. 2011;39(2):105–10.
22. Coe FL, Parks JH, Moore ES. Familial idiopathic hypercalciuria. N Eng J Med. 1979;300(7):337–40.
23. Ljunghall S. Family history of renal stones in a population study of stone formers and healthy subjects. Br J Urol. 1979;51(4):249–52.
24. Biyabani R, Talati J, Mithani S. Comparative study of urinary citrate excretion in siblings and unrelated individuals in the general population, 25th SIU world congress Singapore book of abstracts; 2000. p. 283.
25. Torres RC, Fernández ME, Zuluaga GA, Gálvez AL, Del Rio SS. An epidemiological study of renal lithiasis in gypsies and others in Spain. J Urol. 1984;131(5):853.
26. Goodman HO, Brommage R, Assimos DG, Holmes RP. Genes in idiopathic calcium oxalate stone disease. World J Urol. 1997; 15(3):186–94.

Uric Acid Nephrolithiasis: Basic and Clinical Aspects

18

Khashayar Sakhaee

Abstract

Of the kidney-stone-forming population, 8–10 % are comprised of uric acid nephrolithiasis. The major pathophysiologic mechanism for uric acid stone formation is unduly acidic urine. At a urinary pH below 5.0, the concentration of sparingly soluble uric acid increases and promotes uric acid precipitation. Unduly acidic urine is likely due to decreased ammonium excretion and/or increased endogenous acid production. The underlying mechanism of these abnormalities has been linked to the metabolic syndrome but may also be associated with renal fat accumulation in the kidney (lipotoxicity). Although low urinary pH is necessary, it alone may not be sufficient to cause uric acid crystallization. Therefore, it is plausible that the lack of an *inhibitor* or the presence of a *promoter* of stone formation may play a role in uric acid nephrolithiasis.

Keywords

Nephrolithiasis • Uric acid • Metabolic syndrome • Urine pH

Introduction

Uric acid (UA) nephrolithiasis comprises 8–10 % of all kidney stones [1, 2]. The principal identifiable pathogenetic abnormality is unduly acidic urine, which titrates urate to highly insoluble UA [3, 4]. However, it has recently been shown that the prevalence of UA stones is significantly higher in certain subsets of stone formers such as those with type 2 diabetes mellitus (T2DM) and/or obesity [5–9]. More specifically, unduly low urine pH, the major abnormality responsible for UA stone formation, has been directly related to a number of features of the metabolic syndrome (MS) [10]. Given that obesity is becoming a worldwide pandemic [11], UA nephrolithiasis has emerged as a primary heath concern.

K. Sakhaee, M.D.
Department of Internal Medicine, Charles and Jane Pak Center for Mineral Metabolism and Clinical Research,
UT Southwestern Medical Center,
5323 Harry Hines Blvd., Dallas, TX 75390-8885, USA
e-mail: khashayar.sakhaee@utsouthwestern.edu

Epidemiology of Uric Acid Nephrolithiasis and Its Link to the Metabolic Syndrome

Although UA stone prevalence varies among different regions of the world, its distribution is highest in the Middle East and in certain European countries [12, 13]. The incidence of UA stone disease is also high in Pakistan (28 %), Israel (22 %), Japan (16 %), and immigrant Chinese decedents in San Francisco, California (15 %) [14–17]. Additionally, the prevalence of UA nephrolithiasis and gout among the Southeast Asian Hmong immigrant population in the United States is significant [18, 19]. In northeastern Thailand, a geographical region adjacent to the Hmong homeland of Laos but with an ethnically distinct population, approximately 20 % of kidney stones are UA in nature [20]. Consanguinity, specific dietary habits and the adoption of Western behavior may be responsible for the high incidence of UA stone disease in the Hmong population. However, such a relationship has not been fully explored. Indeed, a high prevalence of obesity and hypertension (phenotypes associated with UA nephrolithiasis in Western

J.J. Talati et al. (eds.), *Urolithiasis*,
DOI 10.1007/978-1-4471-4387-1_18, © Springer-Verlag London 2012

society) [7–10, 21–25] are present in this population, specifically among the Hmong youth born in the United States [26, 27].

Physicochemical Properties of Uric Acid

Urinary UA solubility is limited to 96 mg/L. Since UA excretion in humans generally exceeds 600 mg/day, this poses a great risk for UA precipitation [4]. Given that UA is a weak acid (pK_a of 5.35 at 37 °C), urinary pH plays an important determinant role in UA solubility [28]. Unduly acidic urine (urinary pH$\leq$5.5) leads to the precipitation of sparingly soluble UA, increasing the predisposition for UA nephrolithiasis [29]. In addition, UA crystals may indirectly increase the propensity for mixed UA and calcium oxalate stone formation due to heterogeneous nucleation and epitaxial crystal growth processes (Fig. 18.1) [30–32]. Moreover, UA solubility in the urinary milieu is influenced by electrolyte composition and the fact that solubility of monopotassium urate is several folds higher than monosodium urate [32, 33]. The latter physicochemical property has a principal role in the treatment of UA stone formers due to the superiority of potassium alkali treatment to sodium alkali treatment [34].

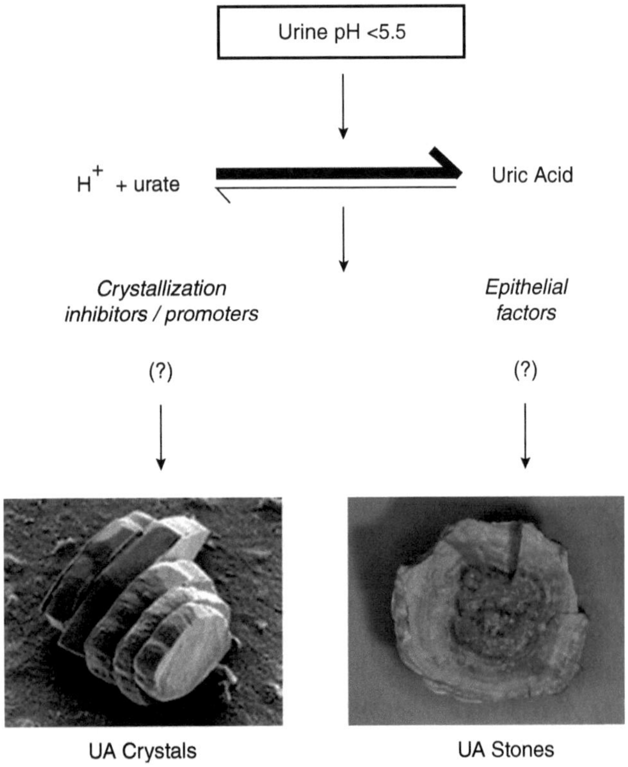

Fig. 18.1 Physicochemical scheme of uric acid stone formation

Although unduly acidic urine is the most important physicochemical factor in UA stone formation, normal urine is often metastably supersaturated with respect to UA. This suggests the presence of urinary inhibitors of UA crystallization. Furthermore, it has previously been shown that unduly acidic urine, an invariant feature in subjects with UA nephrolithiasis, is also present in a subset of patients with T2DM without kidney stones [25]. This heterogeneity indicates that aciduria alone may be necessary but is not sufficient to cause UA nephrolithiasis. Therefore, it is plausible that the lack of an *inhibitor* or the presence of a *promoter* may, in part, account for the difference in propensity for stone formation. Besides pH-dependent solubility, existing literature is scarce on factors that might be involved in UA stone formation. In vitro experiments have identified macromolecules that inhibit adhesion of UA crystals to renal epithelial cells, indirectly supporting the inhibitory role of these compounds against UA precipitation [35].

Uric Acid Homeostasis

UA is the end product of purine metabolism in higher mammals. In this species, serum UA concentrations and urinary UA excretions are high due to the absence of the hepatic enzyme uricase, which converts UA to a more soluble compound, allantoin [36]. Three main mechanisms that may influence UA production include de novo synthesis, dietary purine intake, and tissue catabolism. In de novo synthesis, inosinic acid is produced by the incorporation of ribose and phosphate into the backbone of glycine. Inosinic acid gives rise to UA. Dietary purine leads to UA production by providing ribonucleic acid and purine bases such as adenine and guanine [37]. De novo synthesis and tissue catabolism are responsible for 50 % of the daily urate load, with the remainder coming from dietary sources [37]. In addition, 25 % of synthesized UA is excreted through the intestinal tract by intestinal uricolysis and the remaining 75 % by the kidney [38].

Renal Uric Acid Handling

Approximately 5 % of circulating urate is bound to plasma protein. Therefore, urate is freely filtered in the renal glomerulus, and urate excretion approximates 5–10 % of the filtered load in humans [39]. A three-compartmental model of urate handling has been proposed to include filtration, reabsorption, and secretion [40]. A fourth component, postsecretory reabsorption, has been suggested; however, its role is not fully accepted [41]. Most complexities in the understanding of renal UA handling originate from the heterogeneous nature in different species and the bidirectional transport mechanisms across the renal tubular cell [36]. Basic studies in various species have primarily measured net UA transport yet lack distinction between reabsorption and secretion [42, 43]. Despite previous limitations, recent advances have been made in the identification of major proteins involved in renal UA transport.

Urate-anion exchanger, URAT1, is an apical membrane electroneutral urate-anion exchanger protein responsible for urate reabsorption [44]. The mutation of this transporter protein has been associated with hypouricemia and hyperuricosuria in human subjects [44]. Urate transporter-channel, UAT, is an electrogenic uniporter, which has been shown to have a role in urate secretion from the cell into the lumen. Due to its wide tissue expression, UAT has been proposed to act in a "housekeeping" function for urate efflux. UAT is expressed in the apical membrane of the renal proximal tubular cell and facilitates urate secretion into the tubular lumen [45, 46]. Organic anion transporter 1 (OAT1) has been localized to basolateral membrane of the proximal convoluted tubule [47, 48]. OAT1 is an electroneutral urate/organic anion exchanger with a wide range of substrate affinities [49]. It has been suggested that this transporter is responsible for peritubular uptake of urate and ultimately its secretion. No genetic mutation has been reported with the lack of expression of this transporter. OAT3 has also been localized to the basolateral membrane of the proximal convoluted tubule as well as other parts of the nephron including the thick ascending limb of Henle, distal tubule, connecting tubule, and collecting duct cells [49]. Although the urate transport function of OAT3 has not been fully elucidated, its localization to the proximal tubular nephron suggests its role in both UA secretion and reabsorption.

Pathophysiology and Etiologic Causes of Uric Acid Nephrolithiasis

Three principal pathophysiologic mechanisms responsible for UA stone formation are low urine volume, hyperuricosuria, and an unduly acidic urinary environment (Fig. 18.2). The etiologic mechanism(s) for UA stone formation are complex and diverse. These may be genetic [23, 50, 51] or acquired [52–54]. However, the MS has emerged as the most prevalent cause of UA stone formation [7–10, 21–25].

Low Urinary Volume

Low urine volume is one of the main contributing factors of UA stone formation since the urinary environment is known to become supersaturated with respect to UA salt. This may occur with chronic diarrhea and/or excessive sweating [52, 53]. Under these conditions low urine volume is associated with excessively acidic urine due to gastrointestinal (GI) alkali loss or abundant acid production [52, 53].

Hyperuricosuria

Both genetic and environmental factors play an important role in the development of hyperuricosuria. In certain circumstances, such as primary gout, both dietary and genetic influences contribute to increased serum UA concentrations and ultimately increased urinary UA excretion. However, these abnormalities may not be detected in all gouty patients [21, 55]. In rare genetic disorders including X-linked hypoxanthine-guanine phosphoribosyl transferase deficiency, X-linked phosphoribosyl pyrophosphate synthetase overactivity, and autosomal recessive glucose-6-phosphatase activity, hyperuricosuria and hyperuricemia are invariant features [51]. Therefore, these genetic abnormalities mostly present during childhood and potentially lead to increased risk of kidney stones, renal failure, and gout. In addition, a specific genetic disorder involving a mutation of URAT1 (encoded by SLC22A12) has been shown to present with hyperuricosuria (typically >900 mg/day), hypouricemia (serum UA concentration of approximately 1 mg/dL), risk of kidney stone formation (in roughly 10 % of affected subjects), and exercise-induced acute renal failure [56, 57]. Acute kidney injury shown by biopsy has been due to acute tubular necrosis without evidence of intratubular UA crystal deposition [58]. The exact mechanism of acute renal injury has not been fully established.

Low Urine Volume	Low Urinary pH	Hyperuricosuria
• Diarrheal State	• Idiopathic Uric Acid Nephrolithiasis	• Congenital Disorders
• Strenuous Physical Exercise	• Primary Gout	• Primary Gout
	• Diarrhea	• Uricosuric Drugs
	• Strenuous Physical Exercise	• Myeloproliferatice Disorder
	• High Animal Protein Intake	• High Animal Protein Intake

Fig. 18.2 Pathogenesis and etiologies of uric acid nephrolithiasis

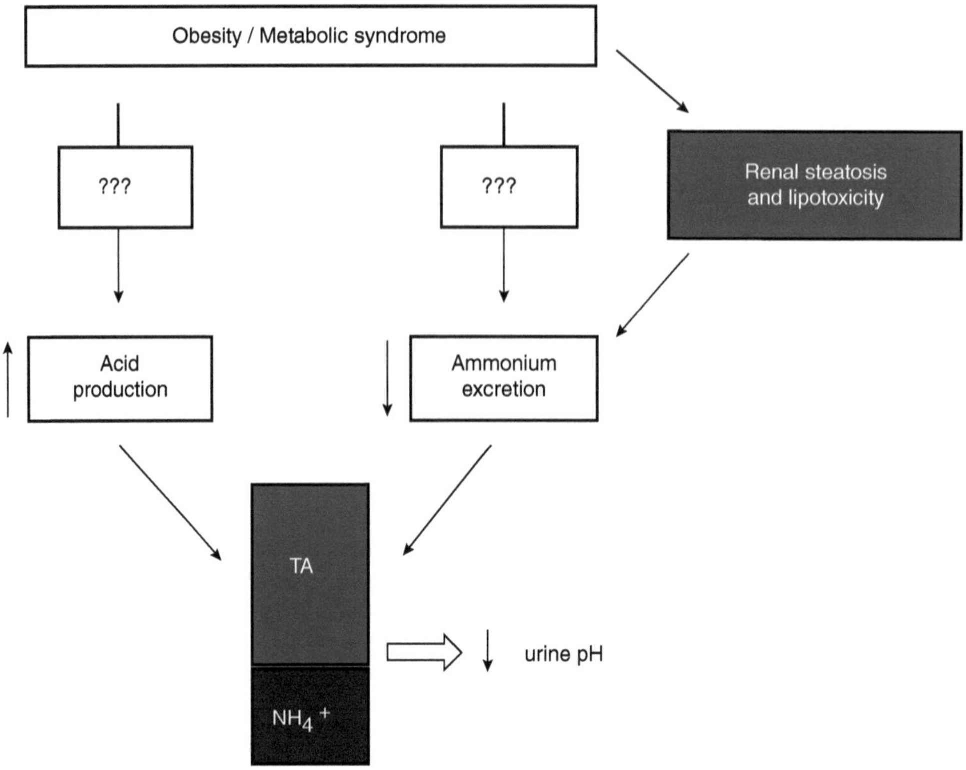

Fig. 18.3 Proposed model for the pathophysiologic mechanism(s) of low urinary pH

However, it has been suggested that the attenuated antioxidant effect of UA to counteract the increased free radicals released with strenuous physical exercise may be responsible [59, 60].

Environmental risk factors may secondarily lead to UA overproduction as well as significant hyperuricosuria. This may occur with overindulgence in purine-rich foods or as a result of increased tissue breakdown seen in malignancies and following chemotherapy. Some drugs such as probenecid, high-dose salicylate, and use of radiocontrast materials may also lead to increased risk of UA stone formation due to significant hyperuricosuria [4].

Acidic Urinary pH

In UA stone formers, the most important and invariant feature is overly acidic urine, which increases the urinary content of undissociated UA and consequently increases the propensity for UA precipitation [21, 61]. It has recently been shown that UA stone formers share similar characteristics with the MS [21, 24]. Cross-sectional studies in normal non-stone-forming subjects and kidney stone formers have shown an inverse relationship between urinary pH, body weight, and increasing features of the MS [10, 23]. Major progress over the past decade has been made in the disclosure of two major etiologic factors that result in low urine pH: (1) Impaired ammonium (NH_4^+) excretion and (2) increased endogenous acid production (Fig. 18.3) [21, 24].

Impaired NH_4^+ Excretion

NH_4^+ is a high-capacity urinary buffer (pK_a of 9.2) that, under normal circumstances, effectively buffers most urinary protons, while the remaining are buffered by titratable acid (TA). In UA nephrolithiasis with defective NH_4^+ excretion, most protons are buffered by TA to maintain an acid–base homeostasis [21, 62]. However, this occurs at the expense of low urine pH, which is conducive for UA precipitation. Defective NH_4^+ excretion has been shown to occur at a steady state while on a fixed metabolic diet. In addition, this defect is further amplified by a single-dose acid load of NH_4^+ chloride [21]. Moreover, it has been shown that defective NH_4^+ excretion is not specific to UA stone formers but may be considered a general feature of the MS and T2DM [10, 23–25].

Cellular Basis of Low Urinary pH: Role of Renal Lipotoxicity

The renal proximal tubule plays a principal role in both synthesis and secretion of NH_4^+ [63, 64]. NH_4^+ produced by the proximal tubule is transported across the luminal membrane of the proximal tubular cell either directly as NH_4^+ or as non-ionic diffusion of NH_3. Sodium-hydrogen exchanger NHE3 is crucial for this transport activity since it functions both as a Na^+/NH_4^+ exchanger and in luminal H^+ secretion required for the trapping of diffused NH_3 in the renal proximal tubular lumen [63–68].

Cellular mechanism(s) linking the MS to the development of UA stones have recently been examined. In obesity, diabe-

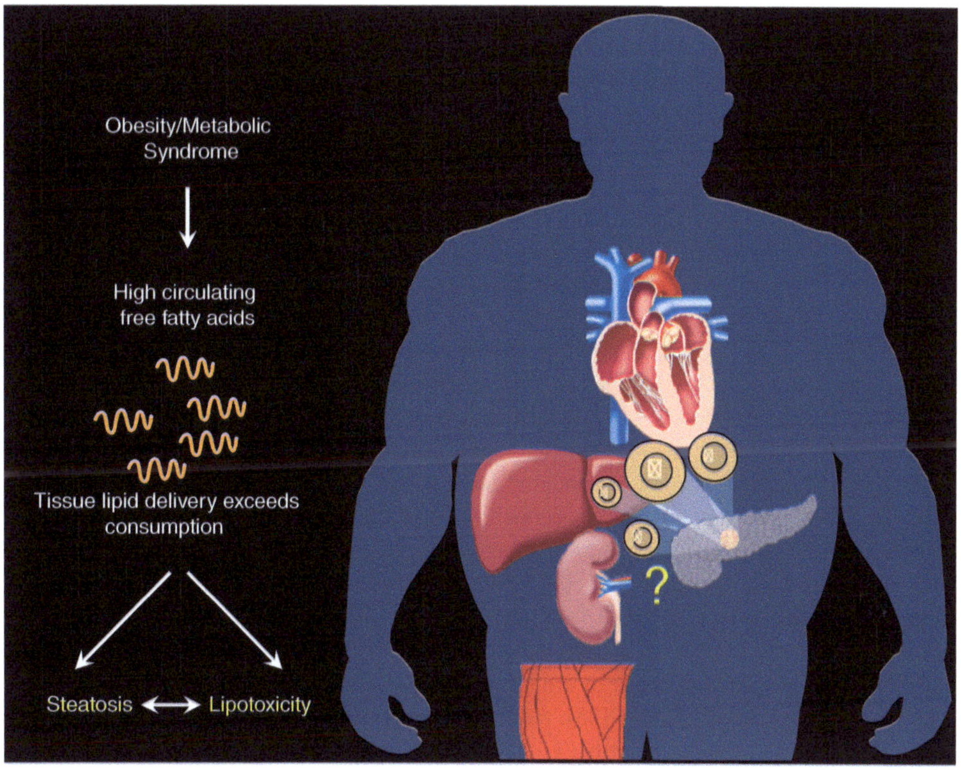

Fig. 18.4 Organ steatosis in obesity and the metabolic syndrome. The "β" symbols in the figure represent pancreatic beta cells

tes, and the MS, there is an imbalance between caloric intake and caloric utilization. This disequilibrium leads to fat accumulation in non-adipocyte tissue [69]. The process of fat redistribution, "lipotoxicity," has been shown to affect cardiac myocytes, pancreatic (beta) β-cells, skeletal muscle cells, and parenchymal liver cells (Fig. 18.4) [69–74]. Triglyceride itself does not exert any cellular damage on the target organs. However, its toxic by-products—including nonesterified fatty acid, fatty acyl-CoA, diacylglycerol, and ceramides—may play a potential role in cellular injury [75, 76]. Proximal tubular cells are particularly susceptible to lipotoxicity due to the increased filter load of free fatty acid [76, 77]. Supporting evidence can be found in recent studies using Zucker diabetic fatty (ZDF) rats, an established animal model of obesity and the MS [78] and cellular models of opossum proximal tubular cell cultures showing the causative role of renal steatosis in the pathogenesis of urinary acidification defects [79]. When compared to lean control rats, ZDF rats showed higher renal triglyceride content, diminished urinary NH_4^+ and pH, as well as lower levels of brush-border membrane NHE3 activity and protein [79]. In addition, the direct effect of fat accumulation was demonstrated in opossum kidney cell lines incubated with a mixture of long-chain fatty acids. This study showed that intracellular lipid accumulation leads to a dose-dependent decrease in expression of NHE3 activity and protein and decrease in NH_4^+ secretion [79]. To further establish the contribution of renal fat accumulation and acidification defects in ZDF rats, treatment with thiazolidinediones was shown to restore urinary profiles to levels comparable to the controls and was accompanied by a reduction in renal triglyceride accumulation [80].

Insulin receptors are detected in various segments of the nephron [81, 82]. In addition, in vitro studies have shown that insulin has stimulatory function on both renal NH_4^+ synthesis [83, 84] and secretion via NHE3 [65]. Since NHE3 plays an important part in the transport or trapping of NH_4^+, insulin resistance may potentially lead to defective renal NH_4^+ excretion. At the present time, abnormalities in insulin signaling pathways have not been studied in this population. However, a causal relationship between peripheral insulin resistance, urinary NH_4^+ excretion, and low urinary pH was demonstrated in a hyperinsulinemic euglycemic clamp study illustrating that urinary NH_4^+ excretion increases in lean normal subjects yet does not change in patients with UA nephrolithiasis [22].

Increased Endogenous Acid Production

Metabolic balance studies have demonstrated increased net acid excretion (NAE) in UA stone formers and in diabetic non-stone formers compared to normal controls [21, 25]. Given that NAE matches net acid production, these studies suggest that net acid production is higher in UA nephrolithia-

Table 18.1 Differential diagnosis of UA stones

Stone type	Biochemical profiles pH	UA	$FE_{uric\ acid}$	Calcium	Serum UA	Response to alkali treatment
UA stones	↓	↔	↓	↔	↑	+
Xanthine stones	↔	↑↔	↔	↔	↓	–
2,8-dihydroxyadenine	↔	↔	↔	↔	↔	–
Mixed UA/CaOx stones	↓↔	↑↔	↓↔	↑↔	↑↔	+
Hyperuricosuric calcium stones	↔	↑	↔	↔	↔	+

↑ increased, ↓ decreased, ↔ normal/no change, + positive response, – negative response

sis and T2DM [21, 25]. To date, no studies have explored the source and nature of these putative acid anions. However, as a footprint measure of possible organic acid overproduction, the aforementioned studies calculated the differences between all measured urinary cations and anions. Yet, the urinary anion gap among these groups did not reach significant [21, 25]. The discrepancy between NAE and urinary anion gap suggests that increased NAE in these patients is potentially due to net GI alkali loss. Although GI alkali absorption was not directly measured, net GI alkali absorption (calculated as the difference in urinary cations–anions) was low in patients with T2DM [25]. Additional metabolic balance studies are needed to further elucidate the potential role of net GI alkali loss in this population.

Diagnosis

General Diagnosis

The first step taken in the diagnosis of UA stones is establishment of stone analysis. If UA stone composition is confirmed, this should be followed by the exclusion of acquired causes of UA nephrolithiasis such as diarrheal state, strenuous physical exercise, high animal protein intake, myeloproliferative disorders, and/or uricosuric medications. Natural history of the illness may also be an indicator of this diagnosis since patients with rare hereditary enzymatic uric acid pathway mutations typically present with significant hyperuricemia (serum UA > 10 mg/d:), hyperuricosuria (urinary UA > 1000 mg/day), aggressive stone formation, renal failure, and mostly childhood presentation [51]. Presentation with hypouricemia, hyperuricosuria, increased risk of kidney stones, and exercise-induced acute renal failure may represent a genetic mutation in the URAT1 transporter [56, 57]. Hyperuricemia and reduced fractional excretion of UA associated with familial juvenile gouty nephropathy, medullary cystic kidney disease type 2, and renal failure represent a mutation in the gene encoding for uromodulin [85].

A thorough metabolic evaluation is needed in all subjects, including full blood chemistries and 24-h urine profiles. Urine biochemical profiles should include total volume, pH measured by electrode, creatinine, sodium, potassium, calcium, magnesium, oxalate, citrate, sulfate, and chloride. This evaluation will account for the contribution of dietary and metabolic aberrations. Urinary sulfate is a surrogate marker of acid ash intake (found in meat and meat products). Such a diet will increase urinary UA and lower urine pH by providing high amounts of purine and acid load. Net GI alkali absorption will determine the contribution of dietary alkali versus acid [25]. Computerized tomography is usually necessary in symptomatic patients with hematuria, pain, and abnormal renal function.

Differential Diagnosis

The most neglected diagnostic step by practicing physicians is the distinction between hyperuricosuric calcium stone formers and UA stone formers [86, 87]. Urinary pH is a distinctive diagnostic test to distinguish between these two disorders, with urinary pH ≤ 5.5 in UA stone formers and ≥ 5.5 in hyperuricosuric calcium stone formers (Table 18.1). Low urine pH may be the only abnormal finding in patients with UA nephrolithiasis [21]. The only radiolucent kidney stones that should be differentiated between UA stones are the rare occurrences of 2,8-dihydroxyadenine and xanthine stones (see Table 18.1) [29, 88]. 2,8-Dihydroxyadenine stones are the result of a genetic abnormality detected in patients with adenine phosphoribosyl transferase deficiency, and xanthine stones may occur with allopurinol treatment and in inherited disorders such as Lesch-Nyhan syndrome or hereditary xanthinuria.

Treatment

Conservative Treatment

Lifestyle modifications play an important role in the management of all kidney stone formers, including patients with UA nephrolithiasis. Attainment of sufficient fluid intake for dilution of the stone-forming constituents has a primary role. It is recommended that the patient drinks 3 L of fluid to maintain

Table 18.2 Comparison of potassium alkali treatment versus sodium alkali treatment in UA nephrolithiasis

	Potassium alkali	Sodium alkali
Urinary pH	↑	↑
Urinary citrate	↑	↑
Urinary calcium	↓	↑ ↔
Inhibitory effect against CaOx	↑↑	↑ ↔
Prevention of UA stones	↑↑	↑↑
Prevention of calcium stones	↑↑	↑

↑ increased, ↑↑ highly significant increase, ↓ decreased, ↔ normal/no change

2 L of urine per day. Additional fluid repletion is necessary for individuals who work in hot atmospheric conditions and those who perform strenuous physical exercise [53]. In some instances, instruction is given to limit meat and meat product intake in order to avoid a purine-rich diet.

Pharmacological Treatment

Low urine pH is the principle and invariable stone risk parameter for the development of UA nephrolithiasis. Treatment with alkali salts has been shown to effectively raise urine pH and ultimately prevent the incidence of stone disease [34, 89, 90]. Although both potassium and sodium alkali treatments have been shown to equally raise urinary pH, potassium alkali treatment is specifically advantageous since potassium alkali reduces urinary calcium excretion, therefore decreasing the risk of calcium oxalate stone formation, which has been shown to occur with sodium alkali treatment in this population [34, 90] (Table 18.2). Sodium alkali may be substituted in individuals with impaired renal function and in those with GI intolerance to potassium salt. The recommended daily dosage of alkali depends upon the size of the patient and dietary intake of acid ash. Typically, practicing physicians monitor treatment by changes in urinary pH. The customary recommended initial dose is 30–60 mEq/day. Urinary pH should be monitored after 6 months of treatment in order to avoid a rise in pH above 6.7, which may increase the risk of calcium phosphate stone formation [91]. In other instances, one may use urinary NH_4^+ as a marker of sufficient alkalinization. In this case, 50 % reduction of urinary NH_4^+ excretion following alkali treatment is suggestive of sufficient neutralization. In rare instances, carbonic anhydrase inhibitor (Diamox®, DuraMed, Cincinnati, OH) can be used to allow for urinary alkalinization. However, this treatment may pose a risk since the development of systemic metabolic acidosis and hypocitraturia, in association with highly alkaline urine, may increase the risk of calcium phosphate stones [92–94].

Allopurinol treatment is commonly prescribed in hyperuricosuric UA nephrolithiasis. This treatment is indicated in female subjects with urinary uric acid >600 mg/day and in male subjects >700–800 mg/day on an ad-lib diet. Allopurinol is also the principal tool in patients with gout, in genetic UA metabolism disorders, and in conditions associated with increased tissue catabolism. The adverse effects of this medication are minimal. However, it should be used with caution in patients with renal impairment [95]. Febuxostat (Uloric®, Takeda, Deerfield, IL) is a newly released purine analog inhibitor of xanthine oxidase with a primary indication in patients with hyperuricemia and gout. However, its effectiveness in lowering urinary UA has not been confirmed in the UA stone-forming population.

Conclusion

With the worldwide epidemic of obesity, it is expected that UA stone prevalence will progressively increase. Previous studies have linked the increase in UA nephrolithiasis with the MS, obesity, and T2DM [5, 7–9]. Major progress has been made in the understanding of the pathophysiological mechanism(s) of UA stone formation. Two distinct defects elucidated by careful metabolic studies include defective urinary NH_4^+ excretion and increased acid production [10, 21–25, 61, 96–98]. Experimental studies using ZDF rats and opossum kidney cell cultures reported that renal steatosis and reduced NHE3 activity are responsible for decreased NH_4^+ secretion [79, 80]. Furthermore, ZDF rat treatment with thiazolidinediones, a therapy that is known to reduce non-adipose tissue steatosis, reduced renal triglyceride accumulation and restored urinary acidification profiles in this animal model [80]. Ongoing double-blind, placebo-control studies are underway to detect whether the use of this agent is associated with the restoration of urinary acidification parameters in patients with UA nephrolithiasis.

Acknowledgements The author would like to acknowledge Hadley Armstrong Palmer for her primary role in the preparation and editorial review of this manuscript.

The author was supported by the National Institutes of Health Grant R01-DK81423.

References

1. Mandel NS, Mandel GS. Urinary tract stone disease in the United States veteran population. II. Geographical analysis of variations in composition. J Urol. 1989;142(6):1516–21.
2. Lieske JC, de la Vega LS, Gettman MT, Slezak JM, Bergstralh EJ, Melton III LJ, et al. Diabetes mellitus and the risk of urinary tract stones: a population-based case–control study. Am J Kidney Dis. 2006;48(6):897–904.

3. Henneman PH, Wallach S, Dempsey EF. The metabolism defect responsible for uric acid stone formation. J Clin Invest. 1962;41:537–42.
4. Asplin JR. Uric acid stones. Semin Nephrol. 1996;16(5):412–24.
5. Pak CY, Sakhaee K, Moe O, Preminger GM, Poindexter JR, Peterson RD, et al. Biochemical profile of stone-forming patients with diabetes mellitus. Urology. 2003;61(3):523–7.
6. Ekeruo WO, Tan YH, Young MD, Dahm P, Maloney ME, Mathias BJ, et al. Metabolic risk factors and the impact of medical therapy on the management of nephrolithiasis in obese patients. J Urol. 2004;172(1):159–63.
7. Daudon M, Lacour B, Jungers P. High prevalence of uric acid calculi in diabetic stone formers. Nephrol Dial Transplant. 2005; 20(2):468–9.
8. Daudon M, Traxer O, Conort P, Lacour B, Jungers P. Type 2 diabetes increases the risk for uric acid stones. J Am Soc Nephrol. 2006; 17(7):2026–33.
9. Daudon M, Lacour B, Jungers P. Influence of body size on urinary stone composition in men and women. Urol Res. 2006;34(3):193–9.
10. Maalouf NM, Cameron MA, Moe OW, Adams-Huet B, Sakhaee K. Low urine pH: a novel feature of the metabolic syndrome. Clin J Am Soc Nephrol. 2007;2(5):883–8.
11. World Health Organization. Global Database on Body Mass Index. 2012. Available from: http://apps.who.int/bmi/index.jsp?introPage=intro_2.html. Last accessed 1 Nov 2012.
12. Atsmon A, DeVries A, Frank M. Uric acid lithiasis. Amsterdam: Elsevier; 1963.
13. Hesse A, Schneider HJ, Berg W, Hienzsch E. Uric acid dihydrate as urinary calculus component. Invest Urol. 1975;12(5):405–9.
14. Rafique M, Bhutta RA, Rauf A, Chaudhry IA. Chemical composition of upper renal tract calculi in Multan. J Pak Med Assoc. 2000;50(5):145–8.
15. Herbstein FH, Kleeberg J, Shalitin Y, Wartski E, Wielinski S. Chemical and x-ray diffraction analysis of urinary stones in Israel. Isr J Med Sci. 1974;10(12):1493–9.
16. Hossain RZ, Ogawa Y, Hokama S, Morozumi M, Hatano T. Urolithiasis in Okinawa, Japan: a relatively high prevalence of uric acid stones. Int J Urol. 2003;10(8):411–5.
17. Fay R. Calculus disease of upper urinary tract in San Francisco Chinese. Urology. 1981;18(2):123–6.
18. Portis AJ, Hermans K, Culhane-Pera KA, Curhan GC. Stone disease in the Hmong of Minnesota: initial description of a high-risk population. J Endourol. 2004;18(9):853–7.
19. Portis AJ, Laliberte M, Tatman P, Moua M, Culhane-Pera K, Maalouf NM, et al. High prevalence of gouty arthritis among the Hmong population in Minnesota. Arthritis Care Res (Hoboken). 2010;62(10):1386–91.
20. Prasongwatana V, Sriboonlue P, Suntarapa S. Urinary stone composition in North-East Thailand. Br J Urol. 1983;55(4):353–5.
21. Sakhaee K, Adams-Huet B, Moe OW, Pak CY. Pathophysiologic basis for normouricosuric uric acid nephrolithiasis. Kidney Int. 2002;62(3):971–9.
22. Abate N, Chandalia M, Cabo-Chan Jr AV, Moe OW, Sakhaee K. The metabolic syndrome and uric acid nephrolithiasis: novel features of renal manifestation of insulin resistance. Kidney Int. 2004;65(2):386–92.
23. Maalouf NM, Sakhaee K, Parks JH, Coe FL, Adams-Huet B, Pak CY. Association of urinary pH with body weight in nephrolithiasis. Kidney Int. 2004;65(4):1422–5.
24. Cameron MA, Maalouf NM, Adams-Huet B, Moe OW, Sakhaee K. Urine composition in type 2 diabetes: predisposition to uric acid nephrolithiasis. J Am Soc Nephrol. 2006;17(5):1422–8.
25. Maalouf NM, Cameron MA, Moe OW, Sakhaee K. Metabolic basis for low urine pH in type 2 diabetes. Clin J Am Soc Nephrol. 2010;5(7):1277–81.
26. Munger RG, Gomez-Marin O, Prineas RJ, Sinaiko AR. Elevated blood pressure among Southeast Asian refugee children in Minnesota. Am J Epidemiol. 1991;133(12):1257–65.
27. Himes JH, Story M, Czaplinski K, Dahlberg-Luby E. Indications of early obesity in low-income Hmong children. Am J Dis Child. 1992;146(1):67–9.
28. Finlayson B, Smith LH. Stability of first dissociable proton of uric acid. J Chem Engl Data. 1974;19:94–7.
29. Riese RJ, Sakhaee K. Uric acid nephrolithiasis: pathogenesis and treatment. J Urol. 1992;148(3):765–71.
30. Coe FL, Kavalach AG. Hypercalciuria and hyperuricosuria in patients with calcium nephrolithiasis. N Engl J Med. 1974;291(25):1344–50.
31. Pak CY, Hayashi Y, Arnold LH. Heterogeneous nucleation with urate, calcium phosphate and calcium oxalate. Proc Soc Exp Biol Med. 1976;153(1):83–7.
32. Pak CY, Waters O, Arnold L, Holt K, Cox C, Barilla D. Mechanism for calcium urolithiasis among patients with hyperuricosuria: supersaturation of urine with respect to monosodium urate. J Clin Invest. 1977;59(3):426–31.
33. Wilcox WR, Khalaf A, Weinberger A, Kippen I, Klinenberg JR. Solubility of uric acid and monosodium urate. Med Biol Eng. 1972;10(4):522–31.
34. Sakhaee K, Nicar M, Hill K, Pak CY. Contrasting effects of potassium citrate and sodium citrate therapies on urinary chemistries and crystallization of stone-forming salts. Kidney Int. 1983;24(3): 348–52.
35. Koka RM, Huang E, Lieske JC. Adhesion of uric acid crystals to the surface of renal epithelial cells. Am J Physiol Renal Physiol. 2000;278(6):F989–98.
36. Rafey MA, Lipkowitz MS, Leal-Pinto E, Abramson RG. Uric acid transport. Curr Opin Nephrol Hypertens. 2003;12(5):511–6.
37. Seegmiller JE, Laster L, Howell RR. Biochemistry of uric acid and its relation to gout. N Engl J Med. 1963;268:712–6, 64–73, 821–7.
38. Roch-Ramel F, Guisan B. Renal transport of urate in humans. News Physiol Sci. 1999;14:80–4.
39. Maesaka JK, Fishbane S. Regulation of renal urate excretion: a critical review. Am J Kidney Dis. 1998;32(6):917–33.
40. Gutman AB, Yu TF. A three-component system for regulation of renal excretion of uric acid in man. Trans Assoc Am Physicians. 1961;74:353–65.
41. Diamond HS, Paolino JS. Evidence for a postsecretory reabsorptive site for uric acid in man. J Clin Invest. 1973;52(6):1491–9.
42. Kramp RA, Lassiter WE, Gottschalk CW. Urate-2-14C transport in the rat nephron. J Clin Invest. 1971;50(1):35–48.
43. Roch-Ramel F, Diezi-Chomety F, De Rougemont D, Tellier M, Widmer J, Peters G. Renal excretion of uric acid in the rat: a micropuncture and microperfusion study. Am J Physiol. 1976; 230(3):768–76.
44. Enomoto A, Kimura H, Chairoungdua A, Shigeta Y, Jutabha P, Cha SH, et al. Molecular identification of a renal urate anion exchanger that regulates blood urate levels. Nature. 2002;417(6887):447–52.
45. Leal-Pinto E, Tao W, Rappaport J, Richardson M, Knorr BA, Abramson RG. Molecular cloning and functional reconstitution of a urate transporter/channel. J Biol Chem. 1997;272(1):617–25.
46. Lipkowitz MS, Leal-Pinto E, Rappoport JZ, Najfeld V, Abramson RG. Functional reconstitution, membrane targeting, genomic structure, and chromosomal localization of a human urate transporter. J Clin Invest. 2001;107(9):1103–15.
47. Tojo A, Sekine T, Nakajima N, Hosoyamada M, Kanai Y, Kimura K, et al. Immunohistochemical localization of multispecific renal organic anion transporter 1 in rat kidney. J Am Soc Nephrol. 1999;10(3):464–71.
48. Kojima R, Sekine T, Kawachi M, Cha SH, Suzuki Y, Endou H. Immunolocalization of multispecific organic anion transporters, OAT1, OAT2, and OAT3, in rat kidney. J Am Soc Nephrol. 2002;13(4):848–57.
49. Sekine T, Cha SH, Endou H. The multispecific organic anion transporter (OAT) family. Pflugers Arch. 2000;440(3):337–50.

50. Mineo I, Kono N, Hara N, Shimizu T, Yamada Y, Kawachi M, et al. Myogenic hyperuricemia. A common pathophysiologic feature of glycogenosis types III, V, and VII. N Engl J Med. 1987; 317(2):75–80.
51. Moe OW, Abate N, Sakhaee K. Pathophysiology of uric acid nephrolithiasis. Endocrinol Metab Clin North Am. 2002;31(4): 895–914.
52. Grossman MS, Nugent FW. Urolithiasis as a complication of chronic diarrheal disease. Am J Dig Dis. 1967;12(5):491–8.
53. Sakhaee K, Nigam S, Snell P, Hsu MC, Pak CY. Assessment of the pathogenetic role of physical exercise in renal stone formation. J Clin Endocrinol Metab. 1987;65(5):974–9.
54. Reddy ST, Wang CY, Sakhaee K, Brinkley L, Pak CY. Effect of low-carbohydrate high-protein diets on acid–base balance, stone-forming propensity, and calcium metabolism. Am J Kidney Dis. 2002;40(2):265–74.
55. Alvarez-Nemegyei J, Medina-Escobedo M, Villanueva-Jorge S, Vazquez-Mellado J. Prevalence and risk factors for urolithiasis in primary gout: is a reappraisal needed? J Rheumatol. 2005;32(11): 2189–91.
56. Tanaka M, Itoh K, Matsushita K, Wakita N, Adachi M, Nonoguchi H, et al. Two male siblings with hereditary renal hypouricemia and exercise-induced ARF. Am J Kidney Dis. 2003;42(6):1287–92.
57. Ichida K, Hosoyamada M, Hisatome I, Enomoto A, Hikita M, Endou H, et al. Clinical and molecular analysis of patients with renal hypouricemia in Japan-influence of URAT1 gene on urinary urate excretion. J Am Soc Nephrol. 2004;15(1):164–73.
58. Ohta T, Sakano T, Igarashi T, Itami N, Ogawa T. Exercise-induced acute renal failure associated with renal hypouricaemia: results of a questionnaire-based survey in Japan. Nephrol Dial Transplant. 2004;19(6):1447–53.
59. Peden DB, Hohman R, Brown ME, Mason RT, Berkebile C, Fales HM, et al. Uric acid is a major antioxidant in human nasal airway secretions. Proc Natl Acad Sci USA. 1990;87(19):7638–42.
60. Vollaard NB, Shearman JP, Cooper CE. Exercise-induced oxidative stress:myths, realities and physiological relevance. Sports Med. 2005;35(12):1045–62.
61. Pak CY, Sakhaee K, Peterson RD, Poindexter JR, Frawley WH. Biochemical profile of idiopathic uric acid nephrolithiasis. Kidney Int. 2001;60(2):757–61.
62. Sakhaee K. Recent advances in the pathophysiology of nephrolithiasis. Kidney Int. 2009;75(6):585–95.
63. Nagami GT. Ammonia production and secretion by the proximal tubule. Am J Kidney Dis. 1989;14(4):258–61.
64. Nagami GT. Renal ammonium production and excretion. In: Seldin DW, Giebisch G, editors. The kidney: physiology and pathophysiology. Philadelphia: Lippincott Williams & Wilkins; 2000. p. 1995–2014.
65. Nagami GT. Luminal secretion of ammonia in the mouse proximal tubule perfused in vitro. J Clin Invest. 1988;81(1):159–64.
66. Bobulescu IA, Di Sole F, Moe OW. Na^+/H^+ exchangers: physiology and link to hypertension and organ ischemia. Curr Opin Nephrol Hypertens. 2005;14(5):485–94.
67. Bobulescu IA, Moe OW. Na^+/H^+ exchangers in renal regulation of acid–base balance. Semin Nephrol. 2006;26(5):334–44.
68. Kinsella JL, Aronson PS. Interaction of NH_{44} and Li^+ with the renal microvillus membrane Na^+–H^+ exchanger. Am J Physiol. 1981;241(5):C220–6.
69. Lee Y, Hirose H, Ohneda M, Johnson JH, McGarry JD, Unger RH. Beta-cell lipotoxicity in the pathogenesis of non-insulin-dependent diabetes mellitus of obese rats: impairment in adipocyte-beta-cell relationships. Proc Natl Acad Sci USA. 1994;91(23):10878–82.
70. Szczepaniak LS, Nurenberg P, Leonard D, Browning JD, Reingold JS, Grundy S, et al. Magnetic resonance spectroscopy to measure hepatic triglyceride content: prevalence of hepatic steatosis in the general population. Am J Physiol Endocrinol Metab. 2005; 288(2):E462–8.
71. Bachmann OP, Dahl DB, Brechtel K, Machann J, Haap M, Maier T, et al. Effects of intravenous and dietary lipid challenge on intramyocellular lipid content and the relation with insulin sensitivity in humans. Diabetes. 2001;50(11):2579–84.
72. McGavock JM, Victor RG, Unger RH, Szczepaniak LS. Adiposity of the heart, revisited. Ann Intern Med. 2006;144(7):517–24.
73. Szczepaniak LS, Dobbins RL, Metzger GJ, Sartoni-D'Ambrosia G, Arbique D, Vongpatanasin W, et al. Myocardial triglycerides and systolic function in humans: in vivo evaluation by localized proton spectroscopy and cardiac imaging. Magn Reson Med. 2003;49(3): 417–23.
74. McGarry JD. Banting lecture 2001: dysregulation of fatty acid metabolism in the etiology of type 2 diabetes. Diabetes. 2002; 51(1):7–18.
75. Unger RH. Lipotoxic diseases. Annu Rev Med. 2002;53:319–36.
76. Weinberg JM. Lipotoxicity. Kidney Int. 2006;70(9):1560–6.
77. Birn H, Christensen EI. Renal albumin absorption in physiology and pathology. Kidney Int. 2006;69(3):440–9.
78. Clark JB, Palmer CJ, Shaw WN. The diabetic Zucker fatty rat. Proc Soc Exp Biol Med. 1983;173(1):68–75.
79. Bobulescu IA, Dubree M, Zhang J, McLeroy P, Moe OW. Effect of renal lipid accumulation on proximal tubule Na^+/H^+ exchange and ammonium secretion. Am J Physiol Renal Physiol. 2008;294(6): F1315–22.
80. Bobulescu IA, Dubree M, Zhang J, McLeroy P, Moe OW. Reduction of renal triglyceride accumulation: effects on proximal tubule Na^+/H^+ exchange and urinary acidification. Am J Physiol Renal Physiol. 2009;297(5):F1419–26.
81. Meezan E, Freychet P. Specific insulin receptors in rat renal glomeruli. Ren Physiol. 1980;3(1–6):72–8.
82. Nakamura R, Emmanouel DS, Katz AI. Insulin binding sites in various segments of the rabbit nephron. J Clin Invest. 1983;72(1): 388–92.
83. Krivosikova Z, Spustova V, Dzurik R. Participation of P-dependent and P-independent glutaminases in rat kidney ammoniagenesis and their modulation by metabolic acidosis, hippurate and insulin. Physiol Res. 1998;47(3):177–83.
84. Chobanian MC, Hammerman MR. Insulin stimulates ammoniagenesis in canine renal proximal tubular segments. Am J Physiol. 1987;253(6 Pt 2):F1171–7.
85. Hart TC, Gorry MC, Hart PS, Woodard AS, Shihabi Z, Sandhu J, et al. Mutations of the UMOD gene are responsible for medullary cystic kidney disease 2 and familial juvenile hyperuricaemic nephropathy. J Med Genet. 2002;39(12):882–92.
86. Sorensen CM, Chandhoke PS. Hyperuricosuric calcium nephrolithiasis. Endocrinol Metab Clin North Am. 2002;31(4):915–25.
87. Pak CY, Poindexter JR, Peterson RD, Koska J, Sakhaee K. Biochemical distinction between hyperuricosuric calcium urolithiasis and gouty diathesis. Urology. 2002;60(5):789–94.
88. Cameron JS, Moro F, Simmonds HA. Gout, uric acid and purine metabolism in paediatric nephrology. Pediatr Nephrol. 1993;7(1):105–18.
89. Freed SZ. The alternating use of an alkalizing salt and acetazolamide in the management of cystine and uric acid stones. J Urol. 1975;113(1):96–9.
90. Pak CY, Sakhaee K, Fuller C. Successful management of uric acid nephrolithiasis with potassium citrate. Kidney Int. 1986;30(3):422–8.
91. Coe FL, Evan A, Worcester E. Kidney stone disease. J Clin Invest. 2005;115(10):2598–608.
92. Gordon EE, Sheps SG. Effect of acetazolamide on citrate excretion and formation of renal calculi. N Engl J Med. 1957;256(26):1215–9.
93. Lamb EJ, Stevens PE, Nashef L. Topiramate increases biochemical risk of nephrolithiasis. Ann Clin Biochem. 2004;41(Pt 2): 166–9.
94. Kuo RL, Moran ME, Kim DH, Abrahams HM, White MD, Lingeman JE. Topiramate-induced nephrolithiasis. J Endourol. 2002;16(4):229–31.

95. Becker MA, Schumacher Jr HR, Wortmann RL, MacDonald PA, Eustace D, Palo WA, et al. Febuxostat compared with allopurinol in patients with hyperuricemia and gout. N Engl J Med. 2005; 353(23):2450–61.
96. Sakhaee K. Uric acid nephrolithiasis: pathogenesis, diagnosis, and treatment. In: Pearle M, Nakada S, editors. Urolithiasis: medical and surgical management. London: Informa Healthcare; 2009. p. 93–104.
97. Sakhaee K. Uric acid metabolism and uric acid stones. In: Rao NP, Preminger GM, Kavanaugh J, editors. Urinary tract stone disease. London: BC Decker Publisher, Springer; 2011.
98. Sakhaee K. Medical management: uric acid and cystine stones. In: Rao NP, Preminger GM, Kavanaugh J, editors. Urinary tract stone disease. London: Publisher, Springer; 2011.

Oxalate and Urolithiasis

19

Ben H. Chew, Dirk Lange, and Roger A. L. Sutton

Abstract

Calcium oxalate is the major component of 70–80 % of renal calculi. Both of these components have both dietary and endogenous sources. Oxalate is found in many plant foods but is particularly rich in certain foods such as spinach, certain nuts, green leafy vegetables, and fruits. Hyperoxaluria occurs in 18 % of kidney stone patients, and treatment has been to reduce intake of oxalate-containing foods or co-ingesting calcium-containing foods or supplements in an attempt to have calcium and oxalate bind together to stay in the gastrointestinal tract. Oxalate absorption occurs all along the intestinal tract and recently shown to be transported from the bloodstream into the lumen of the gastrointestinal tract (i.e., secreted). Small intestine and proximal colon are thought to be the secretory portion, and the distal colon is thought to absorb oxalate into the body. This may prove to be an important mechanism to reduce systemic levels of oxalate in future studies. The intestinal bacterium, *Oxalobacter formigenes*, has been shown to degrade oxalate from dietary foodstuffs and is found less commonly in stone-forming patients. There are any other oxalate-degrading bacteria, but many of these do not rely solely on oxalate as their main food source. There is much room for investigation in this area as only a small amount of the complete intestinal flora can be identified using traditional microbiologic techniques. Probiotic preparations involving many different types of bacteria have met with limited success in clinical trials to reduce hyperoxaluria. There are many subtypes of *O. formigenes* and it is unknown which would be the best to recolonize kidney stone patients. Enteric hyperoxaluria increases the bioavailability of oxalate in patients with extensive small-bowel resection or enteric bypass surgery for obesity. Primary hyperoxaluria is a rare genetic disorder whereby the defective liver enzyme peroxisomal AGT1 results in a failure to convert glyoxylate to glycine or glycolate resulting in an increased conversion to oxalate. Treatment is challenging and typically requires a combined hepatic and renal transplantation.

Keywords

Oxalate • Nephrolithiasis • Calcium • Primary hyperoxaluria • Hypercalciuria • Hyperoxaluria

B.H. Chew, M.D., M.Sc., FRCSC• R. A. L. Sutton, DM, FRCP, FRCPC
Department of Urologic Sciences, University of British Columbia, Vancouver, BC, Canada
e-mail: ben.chew@ubc.ca

D. Lange, B.Sc., (Hon), Ph.D. (✉)
Department of Urologic Sciences, Jack Bell Research Centre, The Stone Centre at Vancouver General Hospital, University of British Columbia,
2660 Oak Street, Vancouver, BC, V6H 3Z6, Canada
e-mail: dirk.lange@stonecentrevgh.ca

Introduction

Calcium oxalate is the major component of 70–80 % of renal calculi. A minority of calcium stones result from specific disease entities, most of which cause an increase in the urinary excretion of calcium or oxalate. For example, about 5 % of renal stones are caused by primary hyperparathyroidism, and a smaller proportion results from severe hyperoxaluria caused by inherited enzyme defects (primary hyperoxaluria)

J.J. Talati et al. (eds.), *Urolithiasis*,
DOI 10.1007/978-1-4471-4387-1_19,

or by major bowel disease or resection (enteric hyperoxaluria). The majority of calcium oxalate stone formers do not have any identifiable underlying disease – that is, idiopathic stones. Oxalate is the anion of the simplest dicarboxylic acid: oxalic acid $(COOH)_2$. The clinical importance of oxalate is the extreme insolubility of its calcium salt, calcium oxalate, in water (0.0071 g/l at 37°) [1]. Hyperoxaluria, found in 18 % of stone patients [2], may be defined as a urinary oxalate excretion that exceeds two standard deviations above the mean for normal subjects (approximately 500 umol or 45 mg/day).

Oxalate in the Diet

Oxalate is present in many foods in various concentrations and when ingested is absorbed into the bloodstream. Oxalate is also a metabolic waste product of a variety of precursors, mainly amino acids and ascorbic acid. The excretion of oxalate is mainly via the urine, but there is also some capacity for excretion into the intestinal lumen. Oxalate is widespread in foods of vegetable origin, including green leaves, fruits, vegetables, and nuts. Not all of the oxalate detected in foods by chemical analysis is bioavailable, or available for absorption from the gut; for example, some may be in the form of calcium oxalate, rather than more soluble salts [3–7]. Data on the oxalate content of foods have been available for many years, but because of problems with analysis, and with the assessment of bioavailability [8–10], older data are often unreliable. Recently, using improved analytical methods, more useful data on dietary sources of oxalate have become available [11–14]. Some examples of foods that have only recently been recognized to contain substantial amounts of oxalate include soy-based foods [15, 16], cranberry juice concentrate [17], and star fruit [18, 19]. Practically, the patient requires a list of foods that are known to contain significant quantities of absorbable oxalate, or have been shown to significantly increase the urinary excretion of oxalate, so that the intake of these foods can be minimized or avoided. Very detailed information on the oxalate content of food can be found on the Web site of the Oxalosis and Hyperoxaluria Foundation.[1]

The average daily oxalate content of a usual Western diet is estimated to be 100–150 mg [5, 13, 20, 21] but may be as high as 1,000 mg in individuals who consume high-oxalate foods [22]. Between 5 and 15 % of the oxalate ingested in food may be absorbed [4–6, 13, 23, 24]; the intestinal absorption of oxalate may be greater in stone formers than in nonstone formers [2, 3, 20, 23–26], but this has not been a consistent finding [6]. Traditionally it was believed that only 15 % of the oxalate excreted in the urine was derived from dietary oxalate, but recent studies have shown that this proportion can be as high as 50 % [2, 3, 20, 25–27]. This has obvious implications in terms of the benefit to be expected from effective dietary oxalate restriction.

The immediate metabolic precursors of oxalate (L-glycerate, hydroxypyruvate, glycolate, or glyoxylate) may also be present in food, but their contribution to the urinary oxalate is unknown [28–31].

Intestinal Handling of Oxalate

Sites and Mechanisms

Oxalate absorption can occur in the stomach [32, 33], the small intestine, and the colon [4]. From a theoretical analysis of the changing pH and calcium concentrations along the gastrointestinal tract, and their predicted effects on oxalate solubility and passive oxalate absorption, Jaeger and Robertson concluded that the stomach may be a major site of oxalate absorption but that net absorption probably also occurs in the small intestine and the colon [34]. The transport of oxalate from the blood to the intestinal lumen, more marked in the small intestine than the colon, was demonstrated in the rat, using ^{14}C labeled oxalate in 1973 [35]. Since 80 % of an intravenous dose of radiolabeled oxalate can be recovered unchanged in the urine in normal humans, the magnitude of the intestinal secretory flux has been assumed to be fairly small [36, 37].

The mechanisms involved in intestinal oxalate transport have recently been reviewed by Hatch and Freel [38, 39]. Oxalate absorption may involve both paracellular and transcellular routes; active transcellular transport in experimental animals can proceed in either absorptive or secretory directions, and there is heterogeneity between intestinal segments. In general, in experimental studies on isolated intestine, small intestine and proximal colon spontaneously secrete oxalate, while the distal colon actively absorbs oxalate [40].

The active transport of oxalate involves anion exchange proteins, including Slc26a6, which is expressed on the apical membrane in renal tubule and intestine and has been shown to mediate chloride-oxalate exchange in the mouse [41]. Of particular interest in relation to hyperoxaluria and renal stones, Slc26a6 null mice, lacking this transporter, have recently been shown to have a defect in the secretory flux of oxalate in the duodenum [42] and distal ileum [43] so that net transport is in the absorptive rather than secretory direction. Plasma and urinary oxalate are increased, and many of these mice have calcium oxalate stones in the bladder as well as some intratubular crystals in the kidney [42]. It is not yet clear whether an impairment of the intestinal secretory flux of oxalate could lead to a significant increase in net oxalate absorption in man. Although the role of successive intestinal segments in oxalate absorption in normal humans is not

[1] www.ohf.org

known with certainty, the peak urinary excretion after an oral oxalate load occurs within about 4 h, suggesting that most absorption occurs in the upper intestine [27, 44–47].

Effect of Dietary Calcium and Calcium Supplements

Many studies have shown that increased calcium ingestion in the diet decreases oxalate absorption [48–54]. This is presumed to result from the precipitation of insoluble calcium oxalate in the gut lumen that is excreted in the stool. Studies using ^{13}C-labeled oxalate [55] have shown that oxalate absorption decreases progressively as dietary calcium is increased from 200 to 1,200 mg/day; further increases in dietary calcium have a smaller effect on oxalate absorption. This interrelationship between calcium intake and oxalate absorption has been offered as an explanation for the rather robust inverse relationship between dietary calcium intake and stone prevalence observed in epidemiological studies [56]. However, the same authors did not find an increased prevalence of hyperoxaluria in patients who formed stones compared with those who did not [57].

The recognition that a low dietary calcium intake can promote calcium oxalate stone formation has led to the abandonment of the traditional advice to restrict calcium intake [56, 58]. Some investigators have even suggested the widespread use of dietary calcium supplements [59]. However, others have cautioned against the use of calcium supplements as preventative treatment for recurrent calcium stones [60]. The timing of administration of calcium supplements (relative to meals) and the choice of calcium salt are probably important: calcium supplements given with meals have the potential to reduce oxalate absorption, whereas calcium given separately from food may increase the urinary calcium excretion without decreasing oxalate [61, 62]. Calcium supplements have been reported to increase stone prevalence in some studies [63] but not in others [56, 64]. Calcium citrate may have advantages over other calcium salts such as calcium carbonate in part because of the associated increase in urine citrate [65]. Calcium carbonate has also been reported to cause some increase in urinary citrate [66].

Pak et al. compared the urine composition in normocalciuric and hypercalciuric stone patients on a normal- and a low (400 mg)-calcium diet together with oxalate restriction. They did not observe an increase in urinary oxalate when the dietary calcium was reduced. They concluded that an increase in urinary oxalate can be prevented by restricting oxalate in the diet and that restriction of dietary calcium and oxalate results in a fall in calcium oxalate saturation in hypercalciuric patients [67]. In the study of stone patients by Borghi and colleagues [58], which compared traditional dietary calcium restriction with a normal calcium intake plus salt and protein restriction, both groups were advised to avoid high-oxalate foods. However, the urinary oxalate excretion was significantly lower in the normal-calcium group than in the calcium-restricted group, and the patients with a normal calcium intake also had a significantly lower frequency of stone recurrence.

In summary, calcium supplements may help to reduce the urinary oxalate excretion and, in some patients, may reduce the risk of recurrence of idiopathic calcium stones, though this is not well supported by clinical trials. Calcium supplements may be particularly beneficial in patients with hyperoxaluria in whom the urinary calcium is not high, particularly if the dietary intake of calcium is below the recommended daily allowance. They should be used with caution in patients known to have intestinal calcium hyperabsorption [65]. Calcium citrate may be the calcium salt of choice. Calcium supplements should be given with meals, and it may be prudent to begin with a low dose such as 100–150 mg calcium. It is possible that liquid calcium preparations or dairy products might be more effective than calcium in solid or pill form, since it would be predicted that a liquid preparation might mix more effectively with food, allowing the calcium to bind oxalate more efficiently. Milk or milk products have been shown to reduce oxalate absorption from tea [68] and from spinach [69].

Both calcium and oxalate concentrations in the urine probably peak after meals, and it may be at these times that calcium oxalate saturation is highest and the risk of stone growth the greatest. It may be more relevant to study the blunting of postprandial oxalate peaks by calcium supplements than to study the averaged effect over 24 h. In that context, a recent study suggests that the postprandial rise in urinary calcium excretion results from a reduction in renal tubular calcium reabsorption rather than an increase in the filtered load [70]. There is an urgent need for prospective studies of the value of calcium supplementation for the prevention of recurrence of idiopathic calcium oxalate stones and for practical guidelines on optimal levels of calcium supplementation.

Bacterial Oxalate Degradation in the Intestine

Bacteria capable of utilizing oxalic acid as a sole source of carbon were first recognized almost a century ago [71]. Many species of oxalate-degrading bacteria have subsequently been identified, particularly in soil but also in feces [1]. Oxalate-degrading organisms were identified in human feces in 1940 [72]. In 1980, Dawson et al. [73] isolated from rumen contents of sheep and cattle a previously unknown anaerobic bacterium with substrate specificity for oxalate, *Oxalobacter formigenes*. This organism rapidly proliferates when dietary oxalate increases and allows livestock to tolerate oxalate levels in their diet that would otherwise be lethal [74]. Other oxalate-degrading bacteria have been identified in human feces, for example, *Enterococcus faecalis* [75]. The evidence from human and animal studies that *Oxalobacter* plays a significant role in the intestinal handling of oxalate has recently been reviewed in detail by Hatch and Freel [40].

Humans lack the enzymes required to degrade oxalate and prevent its systemic absorption in the intestine. To overcome the lack of certain metabolic enzymes, the human intestinal microflora has evolved to contain bacterial species with genomes that encode enzymes that humans do not possess. Hodgkinson presented data showing that less than 50 % of the oxalate in a normal diet of 130 mg/day could be accounted for by absorption or excretion in the feces [1]. The remainder was presumed to be destroyed by bacterial degradation in the colon.

Components of intestinal microflora have the ability to degrade oxalate, including several lactic acid bacterial species [76]. In a study of children suffering from recurrent urolithiasis or nephrocalcinosis, treatment with *Lactobacillus* species led to a reduction in urinary oxalate excretion [77]. Treatment of six adult patients with secondary hyperoxaluria with a lactic acid bacterial mixture consisting of *Lactobacillus acidophilus*, *L. plantarum*, *L. brevis*, *Streptococcus thermophilus*, and *B. infantis* [78] led to a significant reduction in urinary oxalate excretion. More recently, patients suffering from intestinal oxalate hyperabsorption showed a significant reduction in urinary oxalate levels following treatment with a probiotic mixture consisting of *Streptococcus thermophilus*, three strains of *Bifidobacterium* species (*B. breve*, *B. longum*, and *B. infantis*), and four strains of *Lactobacillus* species (*L. acidophilus*, *L. plantarum*, *L. paracasei*, and *L. delbrueckii* subsp. *bulgaricus*) [79]. Patients with the greatest increase in urinary oxalate following an 80-mg oral oxalate challenge showed the most substantial decrease in urinary oxalate after taking the probiotic for 4 weeks. Even after another 4-week washout period, this effect did carry on after another 80-mg oxalate challenge, but not to the same degree as when patients ingested the probiotic daily. Patients who absorbed moderate amounts of oxalate after the oral challenge did not show as large a drop in urinary oxalate in response to the probiotics. Fecal culture for *O. formigenes* revealed that it was present in only 2 of the 11 patients studied at any time during the study; furthermore, these 2 patients did not exhibit any difference in oxalate absorption or excretion compared to the rest of the group. These two patients did not appear to benefit from being colonized with *O. formigenes* with respect to the amount of oxalate they absorbed [79].

Stone-forming patients without hyperoxaluria who were given an oxalate-rich diet and a mixture of *Lactobacillus casei* and *Bifidobacterium breve* showed variable effects on urinary oxalate levels. A reduction in urinary oxalate levels was only observed in 50 % of patients, and the overall mean decrease was not significant [80]. In contrast, patients with mild hyperoxaluria given similar probiotic treatments did not have a reduction in either urinary oxalate excretion or calcium oxalate supersaturation [81]. Similarly, a randomized double-blind, placebo-controlled trial involving the administration of Oxadrop, a mixture of four lactic acid bacterial species, to patients with idiopathic and enteric hyperoxaluria did not show any effect of the probiotic mixture to reduce urinary oxalate levels [82]. The ability of these bacterial species to utilize several compounds including carbohydrates and amino acids as carbon and energy sources may account for their limited contribution to oxalate degradation. Furthermore, these bacteria do not exclusively reside in the large intestine, further lessening their potential impact on hyperoxaluria. This may explain the unresponsiveness of hyperoxaluric patients to probiotic bacteria; supplemental lactic acid bacteria in the gut do not decrease high systemic levels of oxalate.

In contrast, *O. formigenes* is a commensal bacterium of the human large intestine that utilizes oxalate as its only energy source, and colonization with *O. formigenes* has been associated with a reduced risk of recurrent kidney stone formation, as several studies have indicated that the number of patients colonized by *O. formigenes* is lower (26–46 %) compared to non-stone-forming controls (60–77 %) [83, 84]. A correlation has also been reported between reduced *O. formigenes* colonization and hyperoxaluria [84]. Stone formers who lack *O. formigenes* have higher numbers of stone episodes compared to those that are colonized. Antibiotic use appears to be important in the loss of *O. formigenes* colonization; none of the patients who previously received antibiotics were colonized versus 74 % of patients who were not on antibiotics and were colonized. The fact that 73 % of the colonized patients had three or more stone episodes suggests that factors other than *O. formigenes* colonization status contribute importantly to recurrent stone formation. Despite these studies questioning the importance of *O. formigenes* in determining oxalate excretion, the fact that colonized stone formers have been shown to have lower urinary oxalate levels compared to non-colonized patients does suggest that *O. formigenes* may play an important role.

O. formigenes is believed to prevent a rise in oxalate absorption following the consumption of high-oxalate foods by breaking the oxalate down in the intestine, thus preventing its absorption. In addition to promoting oxalate consumption in the gut, *O. formigenes* has recently been shown to increase intestinal oxalate secretion by triggering reverse movement of oxalate from the blood back into the intestine for degradation. Therefore, it may also be a potential treatment for patients with primary hyperoxaluria [85].

The ability of *O. formigenes* to decrease urinary oxalate levels via degradation of dietary oxalate has been shown in rat animal models in which animals were naturally colonized or had *O. formigenes* introduced via daily administration. These studies indicate a possible role for *O. formigenes* in the treatment of enteric hyperoxaluria. In addition to this, recent studies have suggested that the presence of *O. formigenes* stimulates secretion of oxalate from the systemic circulation back into the intestinal lumen for subsequent degradation [43, 86]. Although the exact mechanism for this phenomenon has not been identified, it is hypothesized that the intestinal degradation of oxalate by *O. formigenes* contributes to the maintenance of a transepithelial gradient that favors passive (no energy requirement) paracellular (between cells) movement of oxalate from the blood into the intestinal lumen. The ability of *O. formigenes* to degrade intestinal oxalate and to stimulate secretion of systemic oxalate into the lumen of the gut suggests that recolonization of patients lacking this bacterium and suffering from hyperoxaluria and associated recurrent stone disease may represent a promising treatment.

The use of oral *O. formigenes* to break down simultaneously administered dietary oxalate was studied in four volunteers, who after an overnight fast ingested a high-oxalate meal with or without concomitant ingestion of *O. formigenes*. Urinary oxalate was approximately 40 % lower in the individuals co-ingesting *O. formigenes* [87].

O. formigenes has also shown promise to decrease urinary oxalate and calcium oxalate supersaturation levels following recolonization of patients suffering from hyperoxaluria type 1 [88]. Seven of eleven patients with normal renal function showed decreased urinary oxalate levels following a 4-week treatment with *O. formigenes*. This beneficial effect was, however, only short-lived, as long-term posttreatment follow-up of 1–2 years showed that persistent intestinal colonization is not achieved in most patients. In a single patient, colonization was maintained and resulted in the normalization of urinary oxalate excretion over time [89]. Overall these results indicate that recolonization of individuals lacking *O. formigenes* is a promising treatment option; however, further characterization of the determinants of intestinal colonization is required in order to make it applicable to all patients.

Colonization with *Oxalobacter* is detected by culture and/or DNA analysis of stool samples. Between 60 and 80 % of most healthy populations test positive [90–92]. Most children up to the age of 8 are colonized, but only 75 % of healthy adults are colonized [91]. The administration of antibiotics can eradicate *Oxalobacter* colonization [93, 94].

Enteric Hyperoxaluria

The term enteric hyperoxaluria implies hyperoxaluria secondary to (usually severe) bowel disease: most commonly extensive small-bowel resection for Crohn's disease or small-bowel bypass surgery for obesity [95–97].

Paradoxically, in these disorders, in which most nutrients are malabsorbed, dietary oxalate is hyperabsorbed, and it is believed that the excess urinary oxalate in enteric hyperoxaluria is entirely of dietary origin [96, 98].

The primary hyperoxalurias, together with enteric hyperoxaluria, are responsible for the most severe cases of hyperoxaluria. In any patient with a daily urinary oxalate exceeding 1,000 umol, one of these underlying causes is likely.

Enteric hyperoxaluria was first recognized in the early 1970s [99]. It is recognized that enteric hyperoxaluria can complicate intestinal malabsorption of any cause, provided at least a portion of the colon is intact [100]. Enteric hyperoxaluria does not occur in patients with an ileostomy.

The pathogenesis of enteric hyperoxaluria is believed to involve the binding of calcium in the intestinal lumen to fatty acids, reducing the amount of calcium that is available to complex oxalate. As a result, the bioavailability of oxalate increases. Both fatty acids and malabsorbed bile acids increase permeability of the colon to oxalate and thus absorption [100, 101]. Other stone-inducing risk factors associated with bowel disease include reduced urine volume due to diarrhea and low urine citrate secondary to bicarbonate loss in the stool and metabolic acidosis. Conversely, urinary calcium is often very low due to calcium and vitamin D malabsorption, which would help reduce the risks of stone formation. There has been much debate regarding the importance of urinary oxalate versus calcium in contributing to the risk of calcium oxalate stones [102]. There is also in vitro evidence that the molar ratio of calcium to oxalate may be relevant: ratios approaching unity cause more crystal formation than normal ratios of 5:1 [103].

Enteric hyperoxaluria and aggressive calcium oxalate stone formation are common in the wake of small-bowel bypass surgery for obesity [104]. Stones have been reported in 20–30 % of these patients. Newer bariatric surgical procedures such as Roux-en-Y gastric bypass surgery produce less severe hyperoxaluria and stone disease, but this remains a problem [105]. By contrast, enteric hyperoxaluria does not appear to result from the gastric banding procedure [106].

The medical management of stones associated with enteric hyperoxaluria can be problematic. Theoretically, removal of oxalate from the diet should correct the hyperoxaluria, but in practice only modest reductions in urinary oxalate generally result from the usual advice regarding avoidance of high-oxalate foods. Other measures that have been used include a high fluid intake, reduction in dietary fat intake within the limits of dietary requirements, and cholestyramine (2–4 g with each meal), which binds oxalate and fatty acids and reduces urinary oxalate. Calcium supplements taken with each meal bind oxalate and reduce its absorption. However, urinary calcium may increase modestly, and there are no clear guidelines regarding optimal levels of calcium supplementation. Potassium citrate or sodium bicarbonate may be given to improve the hypocitraturia. No formal clinical trials have been undertaken to validate these forms of treatment for enteric hyperoxaluria.

In extreme cases of enteric hyperoxaluria secondary to small-bowel bypass, if renal impairment develops, accompanied with increasing serum oxalate levels and oxalosis, surgical reversal of the bypass may be necessary to correct oxalate hyperabsorption. These patients are often very resistant to reversal because of the fear of regaining their previous excessive weight.

Hyperoxaluria in the Idiopathic Calcium Oxalate Stone Former

Identification

Hyperoxaluria is usually defined as a 24-h urinary excretion of oxalate greater than 500 umol or 45 mg. Severe hyperoxaluria (greater than 1,000 umol/day) is suggestive of either primary (genetic) or enteric hyperoxaluria. The difficulties associated with the determination of oxalate in urine samples have been reviewed recently [34]. The processing of the samples, especially acidification sufficient to ensure the dissolution of calcium oxalate crystals, is particularly important. Another potential problem leading to underestimation of urinary oxalate in patients with stones in situ could be the depletion of urinary minerals as a result of their accretion into rapidly growing stones [107].

Not only is there substantial day-to-day variation in oxalate excretion in subjects on free diets, but there are also considerable fluctuations in the urinary oxalate concentration during the day, which are not captured by analyzing a 24-h collection. There may be peaks in urinary oxalate concentration, for example, following the ingestion of high-oxalate foods, when renal tubular oxalate secretion may occur [6]. These could be of particular importance in triggering stone growth, and their identification would require the analysis of appropriately timed "spot" urine samples, which is not a routine part of the metabolic investigation of stone patients.

Notwithstanding these reservations surrounding the measurement of the 24-h urine content of oxalate, this remains the standard approach to the identification and monitoring of hyperoxaluria.

There has been a long-standing debate regarding the relative importance of increases in the urinary excretion of oxalate and calcium. Small increases in oxalate excretion may contribute disproportionately to the level of calcium oxalate saturation in the urine and to calcium oxalate crystalluria and stones [50, 108]. Interventions designed to lower urinary oxalate should not be restricted to patients with arbitrarily defined hyperoxaluria. These measures may be appropriate, for example, in patients whose urinary oxalate exceeds the 70th (rather than 95th) percentile (i.e., in excess of 41 mg (910 umol) per day in men or 31 mg (690 umol) per day in women [109]) and perhaps in all calcium oxalate stone formers in whom other approaches have failed to prevent recurrences of stone formation.

Pathogenesis

Increasing fluid intake [110], decreasing urinary calcium [111] and uric acid [112] excretion, and increasing citrate excretion [113] have been shown to reduce stone recurrences in recurrent calcium oxalate stone formers. However, there have been no studies that demonstrate a reduction in stone recurrences from measures designed to reduce urinary oxalate excretion alone, in patients with either a normal or an increased oxalate excretion. The finding of hyperoxaluria in a calcium oxalate stone former should prompt the physician to identify the cause. The possible mechanisms include:

1. Increased dietary content of bioavailable oxalate
2. Enhanced fractional intestinal oxalate absorption, which could result from decreased oxalate binding by calcium in the intestinal lumen, related to a low calcium intake, from an increase in the intestinal absorptive flux of oxalate or a decrease in its intestinal secretory flux (including occult enteric hyperoxaluria)
3. Decreased bacterial oxalate degradation in the intestinal lumen
4. Increased intake of ascorbic acid or increased conversion of ascorbate to oxalate
5. Increased intake, or conversion to oxalate, of other precursors such as protein, glycolate, hydroxyproline, and certain sugars
6. Increased net tubular secretion of oxalate [114]
7. Increased endogenous oxalate production due to genetic enzyme defects from occult PH1, PH2, or PH3

Although "renal hyperoxaluria," secondary to a disorder of renal oxalate handling and analogous to so-called renal hypercalciuria, has occasionally been postulated, the existence of such an entity as a cause of sustained hyperoxaluria is unlikely. If renal oxalate wasting occurred, it would result in a low serum oxalate level, but not sustained hyperoxaluria, unless it coexisted with of one of the aforementioned mechanisms to account for increased oxalate generation or absorption.

Dietary Management

Hyperoxaluria in excess of 45 mg (1,000 umol) per day requires the careful exclusion of enteric hyperoxaluria (due to extensive bowel disease or small-bowel resection or bypass for obesity) and primary hyperoxaluria. Enteric hyperoxaluria usually results from obvious bowel disease or resection or bypass. The exclusion of primary hyperoxaluria will be considered in detail later in this chapter.

In the idiopathic calcium oxalate stone former with less severe hyperoxaluria, it is usual to seek dietary causes first and attempt to correct them. Ascorbic acid supplements should be discontinued. The patient should be advised to take a normal calcium intake of 1,000–1,200 mg/day. The diet history may help to identify a large intake of high-oxalate foods, and the patient should be given advice on the major dietary sources of oxalate and advised to avoid or moderate them. Numerous studies have shown that reduction in dietary oxalate results in a reduction in urinary oxalate excretion, but in practice the effect is often small [26, 81]. If the intake of meat protein is high, advice on restriction to 10 oz or less per day should be provided. Until the role of dietary hydroxyproline as a precursor of urinary oxalate is clarified, it may be prudent to recommend moderation in gelatin intake.

After the patient has followed this diet for at least 2 weeks, the urinary calcium and oxalate should be rechecked. If the oxalate remains high and the urinary calcium excretion is not increased, or if the dietary calcium intake is below the recommended dietary allowance (1,000–1,200 mg/day), consideration may be given to calcium supplementation and/or redistribution of calcium intake to coincide with meals that may contain significant quantities of oxalate.

As discussed previously, this may be achieved by taking a calcium supplement equivalent to 100–150 mg calcium (e.g., 1/3 cup of milk or 1/4 cup of calcium-fortified milk) with main meals. Additional calcium may be given if the total intake is still below 1,000 mg/day or if the urinary oxalate remains high and hypercalciuria does not occur. Calcium citrate may have special advantages as a calcium supplement in calcium oxalate stone formers because of the beneficial effect of the accompanying increase in urinary citrate. Further monitoring of the urinary calcium and oxalate may be required to obtain the optimum balance of dietary oxalate and calcium. As noted previously, there is a need for guidelines regarding optimal levels of calcium supplementation in these patients, as there is a risk that increases in urinary calcium could more than offset any reduction in oxalate. In a patient who develops hypercalciuria, salt intake should be moderated, and if necessary, a low dose of a thiazide diuretic or indapamide may be added to control the hypercalciuria.

Monitoring of the 24-h urinary urea (or sulfate) and sodium will reveal whether the patient is adhering to the recommended meat protein and salt restriction. There has been evidence that supplemental pyridoxine in addition to dietary advice has been able to reduce elevated 24-h urinary oxalate levels to normal levels [115].

Primary Hyperoxaluria (PH)

If the aforementioned dietary approach fails to normalize urinary oxalate excretion, the possibility that the patient has mild PH presenting as apparent idiopathic hyperoxaluria should be considered. A positive family history, as well as an early age of onset of stone disease, may be suggestive. The majority of PH patients present in late childhood/early adolescence, but milder variants occur and may present in later life with hyperoxaluria and/or renal calculi or renal failure [116].

Three types of primary hyperoxaluria (PH) are currently recognized. In type I primary hyperoxaluria (PH1), the defective enzyme is hepatic peroxisomal AGT1, coded by the AGXT gene located on chromosome 2; the hyperoxaluria is usually accompanied by increased urinary glycolate. In the less common type II primary hyperoxaluria (PH2), mitochondrial glyoxylate reductase is defective, due to mutations of the GRHPR gene (located on chromosome 9), and the hyperoxaluria is usually accompanied by increased urinary L-glycerate. Some patients with the primary hyperoxaluria phenotype do not have mutations of either AXGT or GRHPR gene, so it had been assumed for some time that defects in other genes might also cause primary hyperoxaluria [117]. Very recently a new type of PH, PH3, has been described, which results from a defect in the DHDPSL gene found on chromosome 10 [118]. Although this gene's function is not completely known, it is theorized to encode for 4-hydroxy-2-oxoglutarate aldolase involved in the final step of hydroxyproline metabolism, thus resulting in excessive oxalate levels if defective [118].

In PH1 and PH2, failure to convert glyoxylate to glycine or glycolate results in its increased conversion to oxalate and consequent hyperoxaluria [119]. The determination of urinary glycolate and L-glycerate may be helpful in leading to the diagnosis of PH1 and PH2, respectively. However, 25–30 % of patients with PH1 do not have an increase in urinary glycolate [120], and a normal urinary L-glycerate has been reported in PH2 [121]. Studies of the activities of the relevant enzymes in a liver biopsy have been the definitive diagnostic test, but (noninvasive) genetic testing can now identify common mutations that occur in these diseases [117, 122–124]. Milliner presented an evidence-based algorithm for the diagnosis of hyperoxalurias in 2005 [117]. At that time, screening for the three most common mutations of the AGXT gene provided a definitive diagnosis (identifying homozygotes or compound heterozygotes) in 34 % of liver biopsy documented cases of PH1, while screening for the single commonest mutation of the GRHPR gene provided a definitive diagnosis in 25 % of cases of PH2. Research laboratories can sequence the entire genes to identify other mutations, potentially reducing further the need for liver biopsy.

Approximately 25–30 % of PH1 patients show an improvement or even complete normalization of the urinary oxalate excretion when treated with pharmacological doses of pyridoxine (vitamin B6), the cofactor for AGT1 [125], but the dose requirement of pyridoxine is very variable. While doses as low as 25 mg/day have provided some response [126], other patients may require as much as 10 mg/kg/day [125]. Because of these uncertainties, and because certain mutations are associated with pyridoxine responsiveness [122], it is preferable to make a genetic diagnosis before embarking on a therapeutic trial with pyridoxine. Long-term treatment with pyridoxine and neutral orthophosphate has been reported to be effective in preserving renal function in PH1 patients [125]. Treatment with supplemental pyridoxine only provides effective treatment in 25–30 % of PH1 patients [125, 127].

When suspected clinically, primary hyperoxaluria may be confirmed by liver biopsy or, less invasively, by searching for the commoner mutations of the causative genes or even by complete gene sequencing [117, 128–130]. Many mutations of the AGXT gene have been identified, and recently it has been reported that two of these, G170R, the commonest mutation, and F152I, are predictive of responsiveness to pyridoxine [122]. These mutations cause mis-targeting of AGT1 to the mitochondria rather than the peroxisomes [131].

Other mainstays of conservative therapy to reduce the precipitation of calcium oxalate in the kidney and delay end-stage renal disease are to maintain high volumes of fluid intake, urinary alkalinization, and administer pyridoxine to those patients who respond to it [132]. Renal replacement therapy should be started when the glomerular filtration rate (GFR) becomes less than 30 ml/min/1.73 m^2 [133]. Renal replacement therapy should be instituted with transplantation or hemodialysis. Renal transplantation is more effective at reducing systemic oxalate levels; if hemodialysis is required before transplantation, it may be necessary to utilize hemodialysis 5–6 days a week in addition to nightly peritoneal dialysis in order to maintain adequate removal of daily oxalate production [133]. Transplanting the kidney alone results in potential recurrence of disease in patients with PH1. Combining renal and hepatic transplantation provides a lower risk of disease recurrence and should be considered the mainstay in patients with PH1, which provides an 80 % 5-year patient survival rate [134]. In the less severe PH2, the role of liver transplantation is much less clear. The understanding and treatment of PH has improved over the last two decades. Early diagnosis and initiating treatment before renal failure has improved therapy for PH. This has recently been well reviewed by Hoppe et al. [134].

Conclusion

Possible Future Strategies

Improved understanding of the origins of urinary oxalate could lead to novel therapeutic strategies. For example, if hydroxyproline is confirmed to be an important source of glyoxylate and oxalate, it has been suggested that analogues of hydroxyproline might be developed that could block hydroxyproline transport into, or metabolism by, mitochondria [31, 135]. Since 40 % of the urinary oxalate is normally derived from ascorbate, interventions aimed at decreasing the conversion of ascorbic acid to oxalate might be worth exploring. Pyridoxamine has recently been shown to reduce endogenous oxalate levels in rats, perhaps by reacting with intermediates of oxalate biosynthesis such as glycolaldehyde and glyoxylate and decreasing their conversion to oxalate [136–139]. Pyridoxamine is used as a nutritional supplement; further studies are required to determine its usefulness in treating hyperoxaluria.

References

1. Hodgkinson A. Oxalic acid in biology and medicine. London: Academic; 1977.
2. Penniston KL, Nakada SY. Effect of dietary changes on urinary oxalate excretion and calcium oxalate supersaturation in patients with hyperoxaluric stone formation. Urology. 2009;73(3):484–9.
3. Pais Jr VM, Holmes RP, Assimos DG. Effect of dietary control of urinary uric acid excretion in calcium oxalate stone formers and non-stone-forming controls. J Endourol. 2007;21(2):232–5.
4. Knight J, Holmes RP, Assimos DG. Intestinal and renal handling of oxalate loads in normal individuals and stone formers. Urol Res. 2007;35(3):111–7.
5. Holmes RP, Ambrosius WT, Assimos DG. Dietary oxalate loads and renal oxalate handling. J Urol. 2005;174(3):943–7. discussion 7.
6. Holmes RP, Assimos DG. The impact of dietary oxalate on kidney stone formation. Urol Res. 2004;32(5):311–6.
7. Brinkley LJ, Gregory J, Pak CY. A further study of oxalate bioavailability in foods. J Urol. 1990;144(1):94–6.
8. Chai W, Liebman M. Effect of different cooking methods on vegetable oxalate content. J Agric Food Chem. 2005;53(8):3027–30.
9. Chai W, Liebman M, Kynast-Gales S, Massey L. Oxalate absorption and endogenous oxalate synthesis from ascorbate in calcium oxalate stone formers and non-stone formers. Am J Kidney Dis. 2004;44(6):1060–9.
10. Chai W, Liebman M. Assessment of oxalate absorption from almonds and black beans with and without the use of an extrinsic label. J Urol. 2004;172(3):953–7.
11. Massey LK. Food oxalate: factors affecting measurement, biological variation, and bioavailability. J Am Diet Assoc. 2007;107(7):1191–4. quiz 1195–6.
12. Kynast-Gales SA, Massey LK. Food oxalate: an international database. J Am Diet Assoc. 2007;107(7):1099.
13. Holmes RP, Kennedy M. Estimation of the oxalate content of foods and daily oxalate intake. Kidney Int. 2000;57(4):1662–7.
14. Hoenow RH, Hesse A. Comparison of extraction methods for the determination of soluble and total oxalate in foods by HPLC-enzyme-reactor. Food Chem. 2002;78:511–21.
15. Al-Wahsh IA, Horner HT, Palmer RG, Reddy MB, Massey LK. Oxalate and phytate of soy foods. J Agric Food Chem. 2005;53(14):5670–4.
16. Massey LK, Palmer RG, Horner HT. Oxalate content of soybean seeds (*Glycine max*: Leguminosae), soyfoods, and other edible legumes. J Agric Food Chem. 2001;49(9):4262–6.
17. Terris MK, Issa MM, Tacker JR. Dietary supplementation with cranberry concentrate tablets may increase the risk of nephrolithiasis. Urology. 2001;57(1):26–9.

18. Fang HC, Chen CL, Lee PT, et al. The role of oxalate in star fruit neurotoxicity of five-sixths nephrectomized rats. Food Chem Toxicol. 2007;45(9):1764–9.
19. Chen CL, Fang HC, Chou KJ, Wang JS, Chung HM. Acute oxalate nephropathy after ingestion of star fruit. Am J Kidney Dis. 2001; 37(2):418–22.
20. Siener R, Schade N, Nicolay C, von Unruh GE, Hesse A. The efficacy of dietary intervention on urinary risk factors for stone formation in recurrent calcium oxalate stone patients. J Urol. 2005; 173(5):1601–5.
21. Siener R, Ebert D, Nicolay C, Hesse A. Dietary risk factors for hyperoxaluria in calcium oxalate stone formers. Kidney Int. 2003;63(3):1037–43.
22. Zarembski PM, Hodgkinson A. The oxalic acid content of English diets. Br J Nutr. 1962;16:627–34.
23. Hesse A, Schneeberger W, Engfeld S, Von Unruh GE, Sauerbruch T. Intestinal hyperabsorption of oxalate in calcium oxalate stone formers: application of a new test with [13C2]oxalate. J Am Soc Nephrol. 1999;10 Suppl 14:S329–33.
24. Voss S, Hesse A, Zimmermann DJ, Sauerbruch T, von Unruh GE. Intestinal oxalate absorption is higher in idiopathic calcium oxalate stone formers than in healthy controls: measurements with the [(13) C2]oxalate absorption test. J Urol. 2006;175(5):1711–5.
25. Massey LK. Dietary influences on urinary oxalate and risk of kidney stones. Front Biosci. 2003;8:s584–94.
26. Holmes RP, Goodman HO, Assimos DG. Contribution of dietary oxalate to urinary oxalate excretion. Kidney Int. 2001;59(1):270–6.
27. Krishnamurthy MS, Hruska KA, Chandhoke PS. The urinary response to an oral oxalate load in recurrent calcium stone formers. J Urol. 2003;169(6):2030–3.
28. Harris KS, Richardson KE. Glycolate in the diet and its conversion to urinary oxalate in the rat. Invest Urol. 1980;18(2):106–9.
29. Schnedler N, Burckhardt G, Burckhardt BC. Glyoxylate is a substrate of the sulfate-oxalate exchanger, sat-1, and increases its expression in HepG2 cells. J Hepatol. 2011;54(3):513–20.
30. Yu L, Jiang J, Zhang C, et al. Glyoxylate rather than ascorbate is an efficient precursor for oxalate biosynthesis in rice. J Exp Bot. 2010; 61(6):1625–34.
31. Knight J, Jiang J, Assimos DG, Holmes RP. Hydroxyproline ingestion and urinary oxalate and glycolate excretion. Kidney Int. 2006;70(11):1929–34.
32. Cerqueira VD, Riet-Correa G, Barbosa JD, et al. Colic caused by *Panicum maximum* toxicosis in equidae in northern Brazil. J Vet Diagn Invest. 2009;21(6):882–8.
33. Hautmann RE. The stomach: a new and powerful oxalate absorption site in man. J Urol. 1993;149(6):1401–4.
34. Jaeger P, Robertson WG. Role of dietary intake and intestinal absorption of oxalate in calcium stone formation. Nephron Physiol. 2004;98(2):p64–71.
35. Dobson DM, Finlayson B. Oxalate transport from plasma to intestinal lumen in the rat. Surg Forum. 1973;24:540–2.
36. Elder TD, Wyngaarden JB. The biosynthesis and turnover of oxalate in normal and hyperoxaluric subjects. J Clin Invest. 1960;39:1337–44.
37. Hodgkinson A, Wilkinson R. Plasma oxalate concentration and renal excretion of oxalate in man. Clin Sci Mol Med. 1974;46(1):61–73.
38. Hatch M, Freel RW. The roles and mechanisms of intestinal oxalate transport in oxalate homeostasis. Semin Nephrol. 2008;28(2): 143–51.
39. Hatch M, Cornelius J, Allison M, et al. *Oxalobacter* sp. reduces urinary oxalate excretion by promoting enteric oxalate secretion. Kidney Int. 2006;69(4):691–8.
40. Hatch M, Freel RW. Intestinal transport of an obdurate anion: oxalate. Urol Res. 2005;33(1):1–16.
41. Jiang Z, Grichtchenko II, Boron WF, Aronson PS. Specificity of anion exchange mediated by mouse Slc26a6. J Biol Chem. 2002; 277(37):33963–7.
42. Jiang Z, Asplin JR, Evan AP, et al. Calcium oxalate urolithiasis in mice lacking anion transporter Slc26a6. Nat Genet. 2006;38(4):474–8.
43. Freel RW, Hatch M, Green M, Soleimani M. Ileal oxalate absorption and urinary oxalate excretion are enhanced in Slc26a6 null mice. Am J Physiol Gastrointest Liver Physiol. 2006;290(4):G719–28.
44. Barilla DE, Notz C, Kennedy D, Pak CY. Renal oxalate excretion following oral oxalate loads in patients with ileal disease and with renal and absorptive hypercalciurias. Effect of calcium and magnesium. Am J Med. 1978;64(4):579–85.
45. Marangella M, Fruttero B, Bruno M, Linari F. Hyperoxaluria in idiopathic calcium stone disease: further evidence of intestinal hyperabsorption of oxalate. Clin Sci (Lond). 1982;63(4):381–5.
46. Prenen JA, Boer P, Dorhout Mees EJ. Absorption kinetics of oxalate from oxalate-rich food in man. Am J Clin Nutr. 1984;40(5):1007–10.
47. Lindsjo M, Danielson BG, Fellstrom B, Ljunghall S. Intestinal oxalate and calcium absorption in recurrent renal stone formers and healthy subjects. Scand J Urol Nephrol. 1989;23(1):55–9.
48. Zarembski PM, Hodgkinson A. Some factors influencing the urinary excretion of oxalic acid in man. Clin Chim Acta. 1969;25(1):1–10.
49. Marshall RW, Cochran M, Hodgkinson A. Relationships between calcium and oxalic acid intake in the diet and their excretion in the urine of normal and renal-stone-forming subjects. Clin Sci. 1972;43(1):91–9.
50. Robertson WG, Hughes H. Importance of mild hyperoxaluria in the pathogenesis of urolithiasis – new evidence from studies in the Arabian peninsula. Scanning Microsc. 1993;7(1):391–401.
51. Jaeger P, Portmann L, Jacquet AF, Burckhardt P. Influence of the calcium content of the diet on the incidence of mild hyperoxaluria in idiopathic renal stone formers. Am J Nephrol. 1985;5(1):40–4.
52. Massey LK, Sutton RA. Modification of dietary oxalate and calcium reduces urinary oxalate in hyperoxaluric patients with kidney stones. J Am Diet Assoc. 1993;93(11):1305–7.
53. Lemann Jr J, Pleuss JA, Worcester EM, et al. Urinary oxalate excretion increases with body size and decreases with increasing dietary calcium intake among healthy adults. Kidney Int. 1996;49(1):200–8.
54. Hess B, Jost C, Zipperle L, Takkinen R, Jaeger P. High-calcium intake abolishes hyperoxaluria and reduces urinary crystallization during a 20-fold normal oxalate load in humans. Nephrol Dial Transplant. 1998;13(9):2241–7.
55. von Unruh GE, Voss S, Sauerbruch T, Hesse A. Dependence of oxalate absorption on the daily calcium intake. J Am Soc Nephrol. 2004;15(6):1567–73.
56. Curhan GC, Willett WC, Rimm EB, Stampfer MJ. A prospective study of dietary calcium and other nutrients and the risk of symptomatic kidney stones. N Engl J Med. 1993;328(12):833–8.
57. Curhan GC, Willett WC, Speizer FE, Stampfer MJ. Twenty-four-hour urine chemistries and the risk of kidney stones among women and men. Kidney Int. 2001;59(6):2290–8.
58. Borghi L, Schianchi T, Meschi T, et al. Comparison of two diets for the prevention of recurrent stones in idiopathic hypercalciuria. N Engl J Med. 2002;346(2):77–84.
59. Williams CP, Child DF, Hudson PR, et al. Why oral calcium supplements may reduce renal stone disease: report of a clinical pilot study. J Clin Pathol. 2001;54(1):54–62.
60. Heller HJ, Doerner MF, Brinkley LJ, Adams-Huet B, Pak CY. Effect of dietary calcium on stone forming propensity. J Urol. 2003;169(2):470–4.
61. Curhan GC, Willett WC, Speizer FE, Spiegelman D, Stampfer MJ. Comparison of dietary calcium with supplemental calcium and other nutrients as factors affecting the risk for kidney stones in women. Ann Intern Med. 1997;126(7):497–504.
62. Domrongkitchaiporn S, Sopassathit W, Stitchantrakul W, et al. Schedule of taking calcium supplement and the risk of nephrolithiasis. Kidney Int. 2004;65(5):1835–41.
63. Curhan GC. Dietary calcium, dietary protein, and kidney stone formation. Miner Electrolyte Metab. 1997;23(3–6):261–4.

64. Curhan GC, Willett WC, Knight EL, Stampfer MJ. Dietary factors and the risk of incident kidney stones in younger women: Nurses' Health Study II. Arch Intern Med. 2004;164(8):885–91.
65. Sakhaee K, Poindexter JR, Griffith CS, Pak CY. Stone forming risk of calcium citrate supplementation in healthy postmenopausal women. J Urol. 2004;172(3):958–61.
66. StitchantrakulW,SopassathitW,PrapaipanichS,Domrongkitchaiporn S. Effects of calcium supplements on the risk of renal stone formation in a population with low oxalate intake. Southeast Asian J Trop Med Public Health. 2004;35(4):1028–33.
67. Pak CY, Odvina CV, Pearle MS, et al. Effect of dietary modification on urinary stone risk factors. Kidney Int. 2005;68(5):2264–73.
68. Savage GP, Charrier MJ, Vanhanen L. Bioavailability of soluble oxalate from tea and the effect of consuming milk with the tea. Eur J Clin Nutr. 2003;57(3):415–9.
69. Brogren M, Savage GP. Bioavailability of soluble oxalate from spinach eaten with and without milk products. Asia Pac J Clin Nutr. 2003;12(2):219–24.
70. Worcester EM, Gillen DL, Evan AP, et al. Evidence that postprandial reduction of renal calcium reabsorption mediates hypercalciuria of patients with calcium nephrolithiasis. Am J Physiol Renal Physiol. 2007;292(1):F66–75.
71. Bassalik K. Uber die Verarbeitung der Oxelsaure durch Bacillus extorquens n. sp. Jahrbucher Wissenschaftliche Botanik. 1913;53:255.
72. Barber HH, Gallimore EJ. The metabolism of oxalic acid in the animal body. Biochem J. 1940;34(2):144–8.
73. Dawson KA, Allison MJ, Hartman PA. Isolation and some characteristics of anaerobic oxalate-degrading bacteria from the rumen. Appl Environ Microbiol. 1980;40(4):833–9.
74. Allison MJ, Cook HM. Oxalate degradation by microbes of the large bowel of herbivores: the effect of dietary oxalate. Science. 1981;212(4495):675–6.
75. Hokama S, Honma Y, Toma C, Ogawa Y. Oxalate-degrading *Enterococcus faecalis*. Microbiol Immunol. 2000;44(4):235–40.
76. Turroni S, Vitali B, Bendazzoli C, et al. Oxalate consumption by lactobacilli: evaluation of oxalyl-CoA decarboxylase and formyl-CoA transferase activity in *Lactobacillus acidophilus*. J Appl Microbiol. 2007;103(5):1600–9.
77. Rogowska-Kalisz A, Tkaczyk M, Bilinska W, Nowicki M. The results of conservative treatment of oxalate urolithiasis in children. Pol Merkur Lekarski. 2003;15(85):51–4.
78. Campieri C, Campieri M, Bertuzzi V, et al. Reduction of oxaluria after an oral course of lactic acid bacteria at high concentration. Kidney Int. 2001;60(3):1097–105.
79. Okombo J, Liebman M. Probiotic-induced reduction of gastrointestinal oxalate absorption in healthy subjects. Urol Res. 2010;38(3): 169–78.
80. Ferraz RR, Marques NC, Froeder L, et al. Effects of *Lactobacillus casei* and *Bifidobacterium breve* on urinary oxalate excretion in nephrolithiasis patients. Urol Res. 2009;37(2):95–100.
81. Lieske JC, Tremaine WJ, De Simone C, et al. Diet, but not oral probiotics, effectively reduces urinary oxalate excretion and calcium oxalate supersaturation. Kidney Int. 2010;78(11):1178–85.
82. Goldfarb DS, Modersitzki F, Asplin JR. A randomized, controlled trial of lactic acid bacteria for idiopathic hyperoxaluria. Clin J Am Soc Nephrol. 2007;2(4):745–9.
83. Sidhu H, Holmes RP, Allison MJ, Peck AB. Direct quantification of the enteric bacterium *Oxalobacter formigenes* in human fecal samples by quantitative competitive-template PCR. J Clin Microbiol. 1999;37(5):1503–9.
84. Troxel SA, Sidhu H, Kaul P, Low RK. Intestinal *Oxalobacter formigenes* colonization in calcium oxalate stone formers and its relation to urinary oxalate. J Endourol. 2003;17(3):173–6.
85. Balch G, Metcalfe C. Developmental effects in Japanese medaka (*Oryzias latipes*) exposed to nonylphenol ethoxylates and their degradation products. Chemosphere. 2006;62(8):1214–23.
86. Hatch M, Freel RW, Vaziri ND. Regulatory aspects of oxalate secretion in enteric oxalate elimination. J Am Soc Nephrol. 1999;10 Suppl 14:S324–8.
87. Duncan SH, Richardson AJ, Kaul P, et al. *Oxalobacter formigenes* and its potential role in human health. Appl Environ Microbiol. 2002;68(8):3841–7.
88. Hoppe B, Beck B, Gatter N, et al. *Oxalobacter formigenes*: a potential tool for the treatment of primary hyperoxaluria type 1. Kidney Int. 2006;70(7):1305–11.
89. Hoppe B, von Unruh G, Laube N, Hesse A, Sidhu H. Oxalate degrading bacteria: new treatment option for patients with primary and secondary hyperoxaluria? Urol Res. 2005;33(5): 372–5.
90. Goldkind D, Cave DR, Jaffin B, Robinson W, Bliss SM. A new factor in enteric hyperoxaluria. *Oxalobacter formigenes*. Am J Gastroenterol. 1985;80:860.
91. Sidhu H, Enatska L, Ogden S, et al. Evaluating children in the Ukraine for colonization with the intestinal bacterium *Oxalobacter formigenes*, using a polymerase chain reaction-based detection system. Mol Diagn. 1997;2(2):89–97.
92. Han JZ, Zhang X, Li JG, Zhang YS. The relationship of *Oxalobacter formigene*s and calcium oxalate calculi. J Tongji Med Univ. 1995; 15(4):249–52.
93. Sidhu H, Hoppe B, Hesse A, et al. Absence of *Oxalobacter formigenes* in cystic fibrosis patients: a risk factor for hyperoxaluria. Lancet. 1998;352(9133):1026–9.
94. Mittal RD, Kumar R, Bid HK, Mittal B. Effect of antibiotics on *Oxalobacter formigenes* colonization of human gastrointestinal tract. J Endourol. 2005;19(1):102–6.
95. Parks JH, Worcester EM, O'Connor RC, Coe FL. Urine stone risk factors in nephrolithiasis patients with and without bowel disease. Kidney Int. 2003;63(1):255–65.
96. Trinchieri A, Lizzano R, Castelnuovo C, Zanetti G, Pisani E. Urinary patterns of patients with renal stones associated with chronic inflammatory bowel disease. Arch Ital Urol Androl. 2002; 74(2):61–4.
97. Yuan CY, Juang YB, Juan CC, Tseng CH. Hyperoxaluria, nephrolithiasis, nephrocalcinosis and renal failure after massive resection of the small intestine: report of a case. J Formos Med Assoc. 1992; 91(9):917–20.
98. McConnell N, Campbell S, Gillanders I, Rolton H, Danesh B. Risk factors for developing renal stones in inflammatory bowel disease. BJU Int. 2002;89(9):835–41.
99. Smith LH, Fromm H, Hofmann AF. Acquired hyperoxaluria, nephrolithiasis, and intestinal disease. Description of a syndrome. N Engl J Med. 1972;286(26):1371–5.
100. Dobbins JW, Binder HJ. Importance of the colon in enteric hyperoxaluria. N Engl J Med. 1977;296(6):298–301.
101. Kathpalia SC, Favus MJ, Coe FL. Evidence for size and charge permselectivity of rat ascending colon. Effects of ricinoleate and bile salts on oxalic acid and neutral sugar transport. J Clin Invest. 1984;74(3):805–11.
102. Pak CY, Adams-Huet B, Poindexter JR, et al. Rapid communication: relative effect of urinary calcium and oxalate on saturation of calcium oxalate. Kidney Int. 2004;66(5):2032–7.
103. Evan AP, Lingeman JE, Worcester EM, et al. Renal histopathology and crystal deposits in patients with small bowel resection and calcium oxalate stone disease. Kidney Int. 2010;78(3): 310–7.
104. Park AM, Storm DW, Fulmer BR, et al. A prospective study of risk factors for nephrolithiasis after Roux-en-Y gastric bypass surgery. J Urol. 2009;182(5):2334–9.
105. Sinha MK, Collazo-Clavell ML, Rule A, et al. Hyperoxaluric nephrolithiasis is a complication of Roux-en-Y gastric bypass surgery. Kidney Int. 2007;72(1):100–7.

106. Semins MJ, Asplin JR, Steele K, et al. The effect of restrictive bariatric surgery on urinary stone risk factors. Urology. 2010; 76(4):826–9.
107. Laube N, Pullmann M, Hergarten S, Schmidt M, Hesse A. The alteration of urine composition due to stone material present in the urinary tract. Eur Urol. 2003;44(5):595–9.
108. Robertson WG, Peacock M. The cause of idiopathic calcium stone disease: hypercalciuria or hyperoxaluria? Nephron. 1980;26(3): 105–10.
109. Coe FL, Evan A, Worcester E. Kidney stone disease. J Clin Invest. 2005;115(10):2598–608.
110. Borghi L, Meschi T, Amato F, et al. Urinary volume, water and recurrences in idiopathic calcium nephrolithiasis: a 5-year randomized prospective study. J Urol. 1996;155(3):839–43.
111. Ettinger B, Citron JT, Livermore B, Dolman LI. Chlorthalidone reduces calcium oxalate calculous recurrence but magnesium hydroxide does not. J Urol. 1988;139(4):679–84.
112. Ettinger B, Tang A, Citron JT, Livermore B, Williams T. Randomized trial of allopurinol in the prevention of calcium oxalate calculi. N Engl J Med. 1986;315(22):1386–9.
113. Barcelo P, Wuhl O, Servitge E, Rousaud A, Pak CY. Randomized double-blind study of potassium citrate in idiopathic hypocitraturic calcium nephrolithiasis. J Urol. 1993;150(6):1761–4.
114. Bergsland KJ, Zisman AL, Asplin JR, Worcester EM, Coe FL. Evidence for net renal tubule oxalate secretion in patients with calcium kidney stones. Am J Physiol Renal Physiol. 2011;300(2):F311–8.
115. Ortiz-Alvarado O, Miyaoka R, Kriedberg C, et al. Pyridoxine and dietary counseling for the management of idiopathic hyperoxaluria in stone-forming patients. Urology. 2011;77(5):1054–8.
116. Coulter-Mackie MB, White CT, Hurley RM, Chew BH, Lange D. Primary Hyperoxaluria Type 1. In: Pagon RA, Bird TD, Dolan CR, Stephens K, editors. GeneReviews [Internet]. Seattle (WA): University of Washington, Seattle; 1993- 2002 Jun 19 [updated 2009 Aug 11]. PMID: 20301460.
117. Milliner DS. The primary hyperoxalurias: an algorithm for diagnosis. Am J Nephrol. 2005;25(2):154–60.
118. Belostotsky R, Seboun E, Idelson GH, et al. Mutations in DHDPSL are responsible for primary hyperoxaluria type III. Am J Hum Genet. 2010;87(3):392–9.
119. Danpure CJ. Primary hyperoxaluria. In: Sriver CR, Beaudet AL, Sly WS, Valle D, editors. The metabolic and molecular bases of inherited disease. 8th ed. New York: McGraw-Hill, Health Professions Division; 2001.
120. Danpure CJ: Primary Hyperoxaluria. In *The metabolic and molecular bases of inherited disease*. 8th edition. Edited by Scriver CR, Beaudet AL, Sly WS, Valle D. New York: McGraw-Hill; 2001: 3323–3367.
121. Rumsby G, Sharma A, Cregeen DP, Solomon LR. Primary hyperoxaluria type 2 without L-glycericaciduria: is the disease underdiagnosed? Nephrol Dial Transplant. 2001;16(8):1697–9.
122. Monico CG, Olson JB, Milliner DS. Implications of genotype and enzyme phenotype in pyridoxine response of patients with type I primary hyperoxaluria. Am J Nephrol. 2005;25(2):183–8.
123. van Woerden CS, Groothoff JW, Wijburg FA, et al. Clinical implications of mutation analysis in primary hyperoxaluria type 1. Kidney Int. 2004;66(2):746–52.
124. Rumsby G, Williams E, Coulter-Mackie M. Evaluation of mutation screening as a first line test for the diagnosis of the primary hyperoxalurias. Kidney Int. 2004;66(3):959–63.
125. Milliner DS, Eickholt JT, Bergstralh EJ, Wilson DM, Smith LH. Results of long-term treatment with orthophosphate and pyridoxine in patients with primary hyperoxaluria. N Engl J Med. 1994;331(23):1553–8.
126. Yendt ER, Cohanim M. Response to a physiologic dose of pyridoxine in type I primary hyperoxaluria. N Engl J Med. 1985;312(15):953–7.
127. Kopp N, Leumann E. Changing pattern of primary hyperoxaluria in Switzerland. Nephrol Dial Transplant. 1995;10(12):2224–7.
128. Williams EL, Acquaviva C, Amoroso A, et al. Primary hyperoxaluria type 1: update and additional mutation analysis of the AGXT gene. Hum Mutat. 2009;30(6):910–7.
129. Coulter-Mackie MB, Lian Q, Applegarth DA, et al. Mutation-based diagnostic testing for primary hyperoxaluria type 1: survey of results. Clin Biochem. 2008;41(7–8):598–602.
130. Coulter-Mackie MB, Rumsby G. Genetic heterogeneity in primary hyperoxaluria type 1: impact on diagnosis. Mol Genet Metab. 2004;83(1–2):38–46.
131. Purdue PE, Takada Y, Danpure CJ. Identification of mutations associated with peroxisome-to-mitochondrion mistargeting of alanine/glyoxylate aminotransferase in primary hyperoxaluria type 1. J Cell Biol. 1990;111(6 Pt 1):2341–51.
132. Chand AQ, Kaskel FJ. Pediatrics: timely diagnosis of primary hyperoxaluria type 1. Nat Rev Nephrol. 2009;5(12):670–1.
133. Hoppe B, Beck BB, Milliner DS. The primary hyperoxalurias. Kidney Int. 2009;75(12):1264–71.
134. Jamieson NV. A 20-year experience of combined liver/kidney transplantation for primary hyperoxaluria (PH1): the European PH1 transplant registry experience 1984–2004. Am J Nephrol. 2005;25(3):282–9.
135. Knight J, Holmes RP. Mitochondrial hydroxyproline metabolism: implications for primary hyperoxaluria. Am J Nephrol. 2005; 25(2):171–5.
136. Cellini B, Montioli R, Paiardini A, Lorenzetto A, Voltattorni CB. Molecular insight into the synergism between the minor allele of human liver peroxisomal alanine: glyoxylate aminotransferase and the F152I mutation. J Biol Chem. 2009;284(13): 8349–58.
137. Cellini B, Bertoldi M, Montioli R, Paiardini A, Borri Voltattorni C. Human wild-type alanine: glyoxylate aminotransferase and its naturally occurring G82E variant: functional properties and physiological implications. Biochem J. 2007;408(1):39–50.
138. Scheinman JI, Voziyan PA, Belmont JM, et al. Pyridoxamine lowers oxalate excretion and kidney crystals in experimental hyperoxaluria: a potential therapy for primary hyperoxaluria. Urol Res. 2005;33(5):368–71.
139. Chetyrkin SV, Kim D, Belmont JM, et al. Pyridoxamine lowers kidney crystals in experimental hyperoxaluria: a potential therapy for primary hyperoxaluria. Kidney Int. 2005;67(1):53–60.

Anti-inflammatory Proteins in Kidney Stone Matrix

20

Anwar Ali Siddiqui and Shamim Mushtaq

Abstract

Kidney stone disease (nephrolithiasis) is an ancient and globally common health problem. Identification of novel therapeutic molecules for better outcome and successful prevention of the occurrence of stones are crucially essential. The pathogenesis of calcium oxalate stone formation is a multistep process and in core includes nucleation, crystal growth, crystal aggregation, and crystal retention. Promoters of stone formation and inhibitors may exist in the same milieu, trying to win over each other. Proteins have the lion's share in the renal stone genesis and considered to have potential role in nephrolithiasis. Many proteins are known to inhibit stone formation, by adsorbing to the surface of the crystal, thereby inhibiting crystal growth and aggregation. However, the stimuli for these events are not completely known. Recent investigations have identified low molecular weight anti-inflammatory proteins including myeloperoxidase, defensin, and calgranulin. However, the presence of a well-formed stone itself initiates an inflammatory response, leading to release of these proteins and further amplification of stone formation process. This chapter provides a brief overview of anti-inflammatory proteins and their role in nephrolithiasis.

Keywords

Nephrolithiasis • Inflammation • Anti-inflammatory proteins • Myeloperoxidase • Defensin • Calgranulin • MCP-1 • Calcium oxalate • Hyperoxaluria • Crystal aggregation

Introduction

Exploration of the role of anti-inflammatory proteins in urolithiasis is attracting considerable interest. A number of inflammatory and anti-inflammatory proteins have been identified to play a role in the initiation of the process of urolithiasis. The roles of various proteins as inhibitors and promoters have been extensively discussed in a recent publication [1–3]. This chapter focuses on anti-inflammatory proteins and their possible role in the process of lithogenesis.

Kidney Stones' Matrix Constituents

Kidney stones are composed of two phases—crystalline mineral and noncrystalline organic matrix phases—while crystals often are of several different types found in a protein matrix. Different mechanisms for the formation of a range of renal stone types have been proposed [1]. Based on the rate of occurrence, the most prevalent types of crystals, seen in >80 % of stones, are either the monohydrate or dihydrate forms of calcium oxalate (CaOx), seen in varying combinations with other constituents. Uric acid, magnesium, ammonium phosphate (struvite), and cystine stones are less frequent [4–6].

A.A. Siddiqui, Ph.D. (✉)
Department of Biological and Biomedical Sciences, Medical College, Aga Khan University, Stadium Road, Karachi, 74800, Pakistan
e-mail: anwar.siddiqui@aku.edu

S. Mushtaq, Ph.D.
Department of Biochemistry, National Center for Proteomics, University of Karachi, Karachi, Sindh, Pakistan

J.J. Talati et al. (eds.), *Urolithiasis*,
DOI 10.1007/978-1-4471-4387-1_20, © Springer-Verlag London 2012

Organic matrix is a central part of all kidney stones [7], constituting 2–10 % of total dry weight [8–10]. All types of organic biomolecules (proteins, lipids, and carbohydrates) have been identified in the organic matrix of kidney stones; however, protein is the major component within organic matrix, representing about 0.3–8 % of the dry weight of stones [11–13].

A better understanding of the components of stone matrix and their interactions on the molecular level is therefore necessary for gaining an insight into the early stages of the formation of the stone nidus. To date, exact pathogenic mechanisms of kidney stone formation remain poorly understood, though a variety of factors have been identified. These are considered to influence the formation of renal stones and are generally grouped into two categories:

1. Those present in urine that alter the rate of crystal nucleation, agglomeration, and growth—comprising various salts, proteins, glycoproteins, and phospholipids
2. Cellular surface components having inherent properties that promote the adherence and/or uptake of nascent crystals by renal epithelial cells

Kidney stones are a complex and common disorder for which a variety of risk factors has been identified. Several studies have focused on the physical-chemical characteristics of these risk factors to further elucidate the underlying mechanism of the stone genesis.

Kidney stone formation is highly influenced by the physical-chemical processes governing nucleation, crystal growth, and aggregation of soluble salts—mainly calcium oxalate (CaOx). The most intriguing question that remains unanswered is that despite the fact that these processes invariably occur in a large majority of humans, not all of them have the tendency to form stones. Multiple theories have been put forward, and various external factors in diet and the environment have been identified as promoters and inhibitors of stone genesis. However, none so far has been able to gain the status of a solitary proven etiological factor. Nevertheless, it is a widely accepted fact that a combination of various factors in a particular environmental condition contributes to the enhancement of the process of urolithogenesis by initiating the crystallization and aggregation of calcium oxalate crystals. A large number of inhibitors and promoter proteins of crystallization leading to stone genesis have been reported [14]. In vitro experiments suggest that a selective imbalance between inhibitor and promoter concentrations result in increased crystallization of calcium oxalate. This happens more commonly in the susceptible group where it leads to crystallization in the renal tubules and crystal deposition in kidneys.

Identification of molecules that are either inhibitors or promoters from the matrix of kidney stones, as well as the urine of stone formers, could help in designing new approaches in the prevention, treatment, and prophylaxis of stone. Much of the recent research focuses on the role of various nontraditional risk factors, such as oxidative stress, role of proteins, and genetic polymorphism that influence the process of urolithiasis.

Proteins associated with renal stones are often classified in three categories, as those playing a role in causation, as effectors, and as bystanders [15–17].

Anti-inflammatory Proteins and Their Possible Roles in Noninfection Kidney Stones

Crystal deposition is a relatively common occurrence in the kidneys and is often associated with inflammation. In turn, a number of crystals have been shown to invoke an inflammatory response in diverse cell types. Calcium phosphate (CaP) and calcium oxalate (CaOx) are two main noninfectious stone crystal phases that may induce kidney cell damage and inflammation [18–22].

A few reports have substantiated the viewpoint that renal epithelial cell injury or inflammation promotes crystal attachment to epithelial cells [23–25]. This interaction changes the property of affected cells and leads to unmasking of attachment sites beneath or between cells [26]. The main difficulties in explaining the molecular mechanism of the crystal-membrane interaction arise from the complex structure of the cell membrane. It is therefore not surprising that the interaction between renal tubular cell membrane components and calcium oxalate crystals is now thought to be an important phenomenon in the development of kidney stones. The adherence and uptake of crystals appears to be crystal specific, greater for calcium oxalate than for calcium phosphate [27, 28].

In the event of an injury or inflammation, phosphatidylserine being a negatively charged membrane phospholipid would appear to be a preferred binding site [29]. Injury and inflammation cause further enrichment of cell membranes with phosphatidylserine, which in turn increases calcium oxalate crystal binding by renal epithelial cells (Fig. 20.1).

Various reports [30–32] support the notion that in hyperoxaluric cell damage, macrophages migrate toward the site of inflammation, releasing cytokines and some anti-inflammatory proteins—particularly monocyte chemoattractant protein-1 (MCP-1), which is also expressed by renal cells—where they play an active or passive role in stone genesis [33, 34]. Besides other anti-inflammatory proteins, three low molecular weight proteins—namely, myeloperoxidase-A (MPO-A), (alpha)α-defensin, and calgranulin—found in the inner core of CaOx stones have been identified as new components of stones [35].

Myeloperoxidase (MPO)

Myeloperoxidase is a recent addition to this group of stone-related proteins. It is associated with many renal diseases and

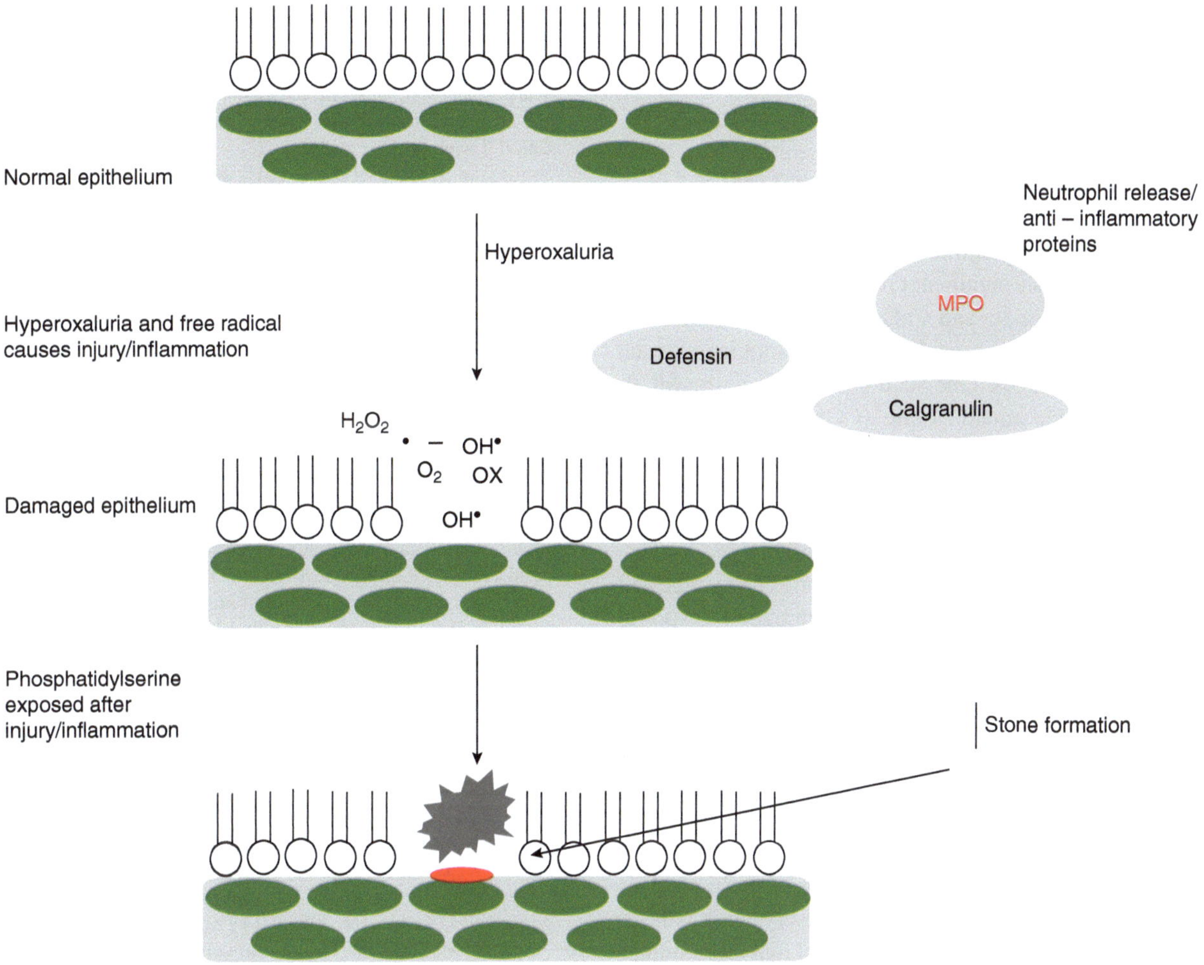

Fig. 20.1 Role of anti-inflammatory proteins. The proposed model depicting hyperoxaluria-/free radicals-induced injury and inflammation leads to release of anti-inflammatory proteins. Calcium oxalate crystals bind to negatively charged phosphatidylserine perhaps alone or in association with cationic anti-inflammatory protein and make a complex, which modulates (positively or negatively) their adhesion to renal cells. *MPO* myeloperoxidase

inflammation. Presence of MPO in CaOx stones could also be a result of CaOx crystal-induced injury or released by the leukocytes in response to the inflammation occurring in renal epithelial cells [35–37]. This initial injury creates a high possibility of interaction between the cationic MPO and the anionic side of the membrane exposed by injury or inflammation. Hyperoxaluria further intensifies the formation of MPO and exacerbates CaOx aggregates at the already exposed epithelial membrane.

Defensin

Defensin is also a cationic and non-glycosylated anti-inflammatory protein [38]. Presence of its fragments in the inner core of CaOx stones [15], particularly in the presence of MPO and persistent hyperoxaluria, suggests that it may also bind to membrane phospholipids, exposed after inflammation, thereby contributing in nucleation of stone genesis with higher affinity for oxalate ions.

Calgranulin (Calprotectin)

Calgranulin is a 28-kDa member of S100 family of small-size calcium-binding acidic proteins, ubiquitously found in various organs. Recently S100 protein has been isolated from human urine [39] and CaOx stones [18]. In vivo, purified urinary calgranulin inhibits both CaOx crystals' growth and aggregation. It has also been identified in the matrix of infection or struvite stones [16]. Its exact role in promotion or inhibition of stone has not been established. Its highly acidic nature enables it to bind cationic molecules, which get integrated into stones, suggesting a linkage with cationic proteins, but its first freight are salts, if such are present in supersaturated urine (e.g., hyperoxaluria).

With the recent advent of more sensitive and powerful techniques, a number of new proteins have been identified that might be involved in initiating the process of urolithiasis by promoting calcium oxalate crystallization and aggregation. Among these are the anti-inflammatory proteins such as myeloperoxidase, defensin, and calgranulin, which are recent additions with a strong potential to act as initiators of urolithiasis.

Monocyte Chemoattractant Protein-1 (MCP-1)

It was hypothesized that inflammation following crystal-induced injury plays a significant role in CaOx stone genesis [40, 41] and that oxalate and CaOx crystals stimulate renal epithelial cells to produce cytokines and chemokines, which attract the macrophages. One such chemokine is the MCP-1. Calcium oxalate monohydrate (COM) crystal induces MCP-1 production in the renal tubules and has been proposed to be important in the progression of hyperoxaluric urolithiasis [42, 43].

In 2008, Michael and his group identified 158 proteins that have a potential role in stone formation. They suggested stone formation induces a cellular inflammatory response and the protein components of this response contribute to the abundant stone matrix proteome [32].

Conclusion

An array of secreted, surface-associated molecules and stone matrix anti-inflammatory proteins have been suggested as promoters of crystal attachment to cells. However, our understanding of the role of these proteins in stone formation and retention of the crystal is still far from complete. One challenge is the fact that most studies on the role of proteins involved in formation of stones are based on experimental findings in hyperoxaluric animals. Under those conditions the tubular urine is often highly supersaturated with calcium oxalate, a situation that seems less likely in humans—whether stone-forming patients or normal subjects. Whether the described proteins have a similar effect on calcium phosphate remains a subject for future research.

References

1. Bushinsky DA. Renal lithiasis. In: Humes HD, editor. Kelly's textbook of internal medicine. 4th ed. New York: Lippincott Williams & Wilkins; 2000. p. 1243–8.
2. Forterre S, Raila J, Kohn B, Brunnberg L, Schweigert FJ. Protein profiling of organic stone matrix and urine from dogs with urolithiasis. J Anim Physiol Anim Nutr (Berl). 2006;90(5–6):192–9.
3. Selvam R, Kalaiselvi P. Oxalate binding proteins in calcium oxalate nephrolithiasis. Urol Res. 2003;31(4):242–56.
4. Pak CYC, Poindexter JR, Adams-Huet B, Pearle MS. Predictive value of kidney stone composition in the detection of metabolic abnormalities. Am J Med. 2003;115:26–32.
5. Bushinsky DA. Calcium nephrolithiasis. In: Favus MJ, editor. Primer on the metabolic bone diseases and disorders of mineral metabolism. 6th ed. Washington, D.C.: American Society of Bone and Mineral Research; 2006. p. 456–60.
6. Brien G, Schubert G, Bick C. 10,000 analyses of urinary calculi using X-ray diffraction and polarizing microscopy. Eur Urol. 1982;8:251–6.
7. Warpehoski MA, Buscemi PJ, Osborn DC, Finlayson B, Goldberg EP. Distribution of organic matrix in calcium oxalate renal calculi. Calcif Tissue Int. 1981;33:211–22.
8. Srinivasan S, Kalaiselvi P, Varalakshmi P. Epitaxial deposition of calcium oxalate on uric acid rich stone matrix is induced by a 29 kDa protein. Clin Chim Acta. 2006;364:267–74.
9. Roberts SD, Resnick MI. Glycosaminoglycans content of stone matrix. J Urol. 1986;135:1078–83.
10. Ibrahim A, Shaker Y, Hawary M, Fayek K, et al. Immunochemical studies of serum, urine, and calculus proteins in urolithiasis. Clin Physiol Biochem. 1985;3:16–22.
11. Boyce WH. Organic matrix of human urinary concretions. Am J Med. 1968;45:673–83.
12. Williams Jr JC, Zarse CA, Jackson ME, Witzmann FA, McAteer JA. Variability of protein content in calcium oxalate monohydrate stones. J Endourol. 2006;20:560–4.
13. Lian JB, Prien Jr EL, Glimcher MJ, Gallop PM. The presence of protein-bound gamma-carboxyglutamic acid in calcium containing renal calculi. J Clin Invest. 1977;59:1151–7.
14. Ryall R. The possible roles of inhibitors, promoters and macromolecules in the formation of calcium kidney stones. In: Rao NKJ, Preminger G, editors. Urinary tract stone disease. London: Springer; 2011. p. 31–60.
15. Atmani F, Glenton PA, Khan SR. Identification of proteins extracted from calcium oxalate and calcium phosphate crystals induced in the urine of healthy and stone forming subjects. Urol Res. 1998; 26(3):201–7.
16. Ryall RL. Macromolecules and urolithiasis: parallels and paradoxes. Nephron Physiol. 2004;98(2):p37–42.
17. Aihara K, Byer KJ, Khan SR. Calcium phosphate-induced renal epithelial injury and stone formation: involvement of reactive oxygen species. Kidney Int. 2003;64(4):1283–91.
18. Asselman M, Verkoelen CF. Crystal-cell interaction in the pathogenesis of kidney stone diseases. Curr Opin Urol. 2002;12(4):271–6.
19. Befus AD, Mowat C, Gilchrist M, Hu J, Solomon S, Bateman A. Neutrophil defensins induce histamine secretion from mast cells: mechanisms of action. J Immunol. 1999;163:947–53.
20. Bennett J, Dretler SP, Selengut J, Orme-Johnson WH. Identification of the calcium-binding protein calgranulin in the matrix of struvite stones. J Endourol. 1994;8(2):95–8.
21. Bigelow MW, Wiessner JH, Kleinman JG, Mandel NS. Calcium oxalate crystal membrane interactions: dependence on membrane lipid composition. J Urol. 1996;155:1094–8.
22. Green ML, Freel RW, Hatch M. Lipid peroxidation is not the underlying cause of renal injury in hyperoxaluric rats. Kidney Int. 2005; 68(6):2629–38.
23. Habibzadegah-Tari P, Byer KG, Khan SR. Oxalate induced expression of monocyte chemoattractant protein-1 (MCP-1) in HK 2 cells involves reactive oxygen species. Urol Res. 2005;33:440–7.
24. Habibzadegah-Tari P, Byer KG, Khan SR. Reactive oxygen species mediated calcium oxalate crystal-induced expression of MCP-1 in HK-2 cells. Urol Res. 2006;34:26–36.
25. Hillegass LM, Griswold DE, Brickson B, Albrightson-Winslow C. Assessment of myeloperoxidase activity in whole rat kidney. J Pharmacol Methods. 1990;24(4):285–95.
26. Iida S, Peck AB, Johnson-Tardieu J, et al. Temporal changes in mRNA expression for bikunin in the kidneys of rats during CaOx nephrolithiasis. J Am Soc Nephrol. 1999;10:986–96.
27. Karlsson KA. Animal glycosphingolipids as membrane attachment sites for bacteria. Annu Rev Biochem. 1989;58:309–50.
28. Khan SR. Crystal-induced inflammation of the kidneys: results from human studies, animal models, and tissue-culture studies. Clin Exp Nephrol. 2004;8(2):75–88.

29. Khan SR. Tubular cell surface events during nephrolithiasis. Curr Opin Urol. 1997;7:240–7.
30. Umekawa T, Chegini N, Khan SR. Oxalate ions and calcium oxalate crystals stimulate MCP-1 expression by renal epithelial cells. Kidney Int. 2002;61:105–12.
31. Umekawa T, Tsuji H, Uemura H, Khan SR. Superoxide from NADPH oxidase as second messenger for the expression of osteopontin and monocyte chemoattractant protein-1 in renal epithelial cells exposed to calcium oxalate crystals. BJU Int. 2009;104(1):115–20.
32. Merchant ML, Cummins TD, Wilkey DW, Salyer SA, Powell DW, Klein JB, Lederer ED. Proteomic analysis of renal calculi indicates an important role for inflammatory processes in calcium stone formation. Am J Physiol Renal Physiol. 2008;295(4):F1254–8.
33. Liang L, Chen J, Vittal R, Selvanayagam ZE, McAteer JA, Deng L, Tischfield J, Chin KV, Sahota A. Expression profiling of crystal-induced injury in human kidney epithelial cells. Nephron Physiol. 2006;103(1):53–62.
34. Lieske JC, Swift H, Martin T, Patterson B, Toback FG. Renal epithelial cells rapidly bind and internalize calcium oxalate monohydrate crystals. Proc Natl Acad Sci USA. 1994;91:6987–91.
35. Mushtaq S, Siddiqui AA, Naqvi ZA, et al. Identification of myeloperoxidase, α-defensin and calgranulin in calcium oxalate renal stones. Clin Chim Acta. 2007;384:41–7.
36. Malle E, Woenckhaus C, Waeg G, Esterbauer H, Gröne EF, Gröne HJ. Immunological evidence for hypochlorite-modified proteins in human kidney. Am J Pathol. 1997;150(2):603–15.
37. Mandel N. Crystal-membrane interaction in kidney stone disease. J Am Soc Nephrol. 1994;5:S37–45.
38. Pillay SN, Asplin JR, Coe FL. Evidence that calgranulin is produced by kidney cells and is an inhibitor of calcium oxalate crystallization. Am J Physiol. 1998;275(2 Pt 2):F255–61.
39. Robertson WG, Peacock M, Nordin BE. Inhibitors of the growth and aggregation of calcium oxalate crystals in vitro. Clin Chim Acta. 1973;43(1):31–7.
40. Sarica K, Yagci F, Bakir K, Erbagci A, Erturhan S, Uçak R. Renal tubular injury induced by hyperoxaluria: evaluation of apoptotic changes. Urol Res. 2001;29(1):34–7.
41. Selvam R. Calcium oxalate stone disease: role of lipid peroxidation and antioxidants. Urol Res. 2002;30:35–47.
42. Sheng X, Jung T, Wesson JA, Ward MD. Adhesion at calcium oxalate crystal surfaces and the effect of urinary constituents. Proc Natl Acad Sci USA. 2005;102(2):267–72.
43. Umekawa T, Chegini N, Khan SR. Increased expression of monocyte chemoattractant protein-1 (MCP-1) by renal epithelial cells in culture on exposure to calcium oxalate, phosphate and uric acid crystals. Nephrol Dial Transplant. 2003;18:664–9.

Physiology of Renal Handling of Citrate

21

Samra Bashir, Naveed Ahmed Khan, and Anwarul-Hassan Gilani

Abstract

Citrate is a weak organic acid, which is formed endogenously in the Krebs cycle or may be ingested with diet. Dietary citrate gets absorbed almost completely from the intestine and is rapidly metabolized in the liver and kidneys; therefore, Krebs cycle is the primary source of plasma and urinary citrate under normal conditions. As physiological pH is far above the pK_a value of citrate, most of it exists in plasma as citrate^{3-}, which filters freely from glomeruli. Urinary excretion of citrate is predominantly determined by the rate of proximal tubule reabsorption, which takes place in a pH- and Na^+-dependent manner through luminal membrane Na^+-dicarboxylate cotransporter. Citrate reabsorbed from luminal fluid as well as taken from peritubules is metabolized inside proximal tubular cells. Acid-base balance, urinary divalent cations, potassium depletion, starvation, chronic diarrhea, and malabsorption are important modulators of citrate excretion.

Keywords

Citrate • Renal handling • Tubular reabsorption • Na^+-dependent dicarboxylate transporter Krebs cycle • Hypocitraturia • Renal tubular acidosis

Introduction

Urinary citrate plays an important role in preventing the formation of kidney stones and inhibits nephrolithiasis by forming soluble complexes with calcium and by inhibiting crystal nucleation, growth, and agglomeration [1]. Low urinary citrate is a well-accepted risk factor for calcium nephrolithiasis. The incidence of hypocitraturia among calcium stone formers from various studies ranges from 20 to 60 %. Increased urinary citrate excretion in hypocitraturic calcium stone formers by means of alkaline therapy has been recommended to decrease the risk for recurrent calcium stone formation [2].

Citrate Metabolism

Approximately 4 g of dietary citric acid is consumed by an adult per day, which is nearly completely absorbed from the intestine both in normal individuals and in patients with idiopathic hypocitraturia [3]. Biochemically intracellular citrate is a central component of the tricarboxylic acid cycle (Krebs cycle) in which adenosine triphosphate (ATP) is produced from glucose and other metabolic fuels [1]. Dietary citrate is rapidly utilized predominately in the liver and kidneys. Therefore, plasma citrate levels (approximately 0.1 mM) appear relatively independent of diet, and plasma citrate is derived primarily from endogenous production [4]. However, an oral citrate load does increase plasma citrate [3].

Citrate is the most abundant organic anion found in urine. Normal urinary excretion of citrate is at least 200 mg

S. Bashir, Ph.D. (✉) • N.A. Khan, Ph.D.
Department of Biological and Biomedical Sciences,
Aga Khan University,
Stadium Road, Karachi, Sindh, 74800, Pakistan
e-mail: samra.bashir@aku.edu; naveedahmed.khan@aku.edu

A.-H.Gilani, Ph.D.
Department of Biological and Biomedical Sciences,
The Aga Khan University Medical College,
Karachi, Sindh, 74800, Pakistan
e-mail: anwar.gilani@aku.edu

J.J. Talati et al. (eds.), *Urolithiasis*,
DOI 10.1007/978-1-4471-4387-1_21,

or 1 mmol (192 mg) per day but averages more than 500 mg/day in most individuals [1]. Due to rapid metabolism, ingested citrate cannot cause a direct increase in urine citrate. But if plasma citrate can increase, as stated previously, this would increase filtered load. Citrate, however, serves as a source of dietary alkali as it is metabolized into bicarbonate, which increases serum, and particularly urine pH and thus urine citrate content by decreasing proximal tubular reabsorption [1, 5]. Usually oral citrate, 60 mEq (20 mmol) per day (range 30–110 mEq; 10–37 mmol), normalizes urinary citrate excretion in patients with hypocitraturia [3].

Renal Filtration and Reabsorption of Citrate

Citric acid is a tricarboxylic acid with pKa values of 2.9, 4.3, and 5.6; therefore, in plasma and, to a lesser extent, in urine, it exists predominately as citrate^{3-} [4]. In this form, it circulates in plasma unbound to protein and filters freely from glomerulus [3]. In humans, 65–90 % of the filtered citrate is reabsorbed mainly through proximal convoluted tubules and to a lesser extent through proximal straight tubules. As significant tubular secretion of citrate has not been demonstrated, citrate excreted in urine represents 10–35 % of the filtered load left after tubular reabsorption [4], as shown in Fig. 21.1. Citrate reabsorbed from the lumen of the renal tubules represents a major fraction of the citrate consumed in renal oxidative metabolism, with peritubular uptake of citrate accounting for the remainder (up to 30–40 %) [6, 7]. Tubular uptake of citrate is an active process as it maintains citrate concentration in proximal tubular cells 3–4 times higher than in plasma [8].

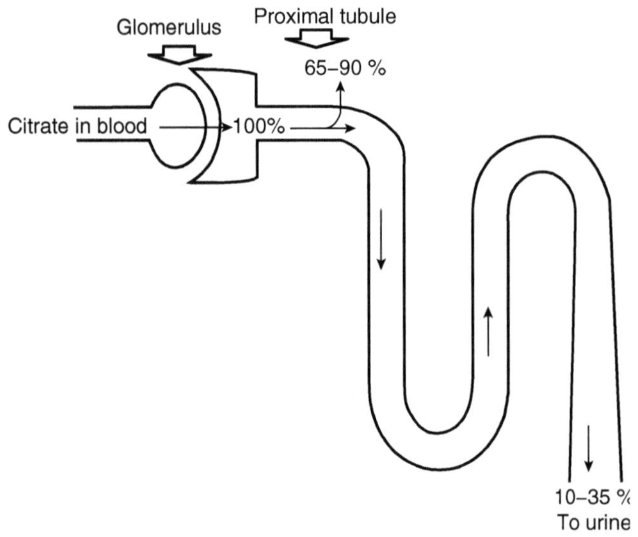

Fig. 21.1 Hypothetical diagram of citrate handling by renal tubule

Tubular Transport of Citrate

Experiments using brush border and basolateral membrane vesicles have revealed the mechanisms involved in tubular transport of citrate (Fig. 21.2). Tubular reabsorption of citrate involves an apical Na^+-dependent dicarboxylate cotransporter (NaDC-1), which predominantly transports the dicarboxylate form of citrate and several other Krebs cycle intermediates [9]. The transport is an electrogenic process coupling $3Na^+$ with each divalent anion. The predominant transportation of divalent form underlies the pH-dependence of this mechanism as relative proportion of citrate^{2-}, normally constituting 10 % of the free plasma citrate, varies under the physiological range of pH [4]. Transportation of interstitial fluid citrate across the basolateral membrane is not well studied in human proximal tubular cells. It has been suggested that it probably involves a tricarboxylate transporter that, similar to the apical transporter, transports citrate^{3-} in a Na^+-dependent manner. Transportation is, however, electroneutral as $3Na^+$ are transported with a trivalent anion and pH independent [10].

Renal Metabolism of Citrate

Citrate that is reabsorbed from the lumen or taken up through the basolateral membrane undergoes metabolism in proximal tubular cells [1], as shown in Fig. 21.2. Most of the citrate enters the mitochondria and is utilized by incorporating into Krebs cycle through mitochondrial aconitase, which catalyzes the first step leading to the oxidation of citrate with liberation of CO_2 and H_2O, providing approximately 10 % of renal oxidative metabolism [11]. Some of the citrate is acted upon by cytosolic adenosine triphosphate citrate lyase, which catalyzes the conversion of citrate and CoA into oxaloacetate and acetyl-CoA. Acetyl-CoA produced through this process is used in the synthesis of fatty acids and cholesterol [12].

Regulators of Citrate Excretion

Because the filtered load of citrate remains relatively constant, proximal tubular citrate reabsorption predominately regulates urinary citrate excretion [13]. Acid-base homeostasis is the most important physiological determinant of tubular reabsorption and thus urinary citrate excretion. Net gastrointestinal alkali absorption and titratable acid in urine have been identified as independent factors determining urinary citrate levels [2]. Following an acid load, both the transport and metabolic processes are upregulated leading to hypocitraturia; in contrast, an alkali load increases citrate excretion, by regulating only the metabolic process [13]. Since citrate is predominately transported as citrate^{2-}, a

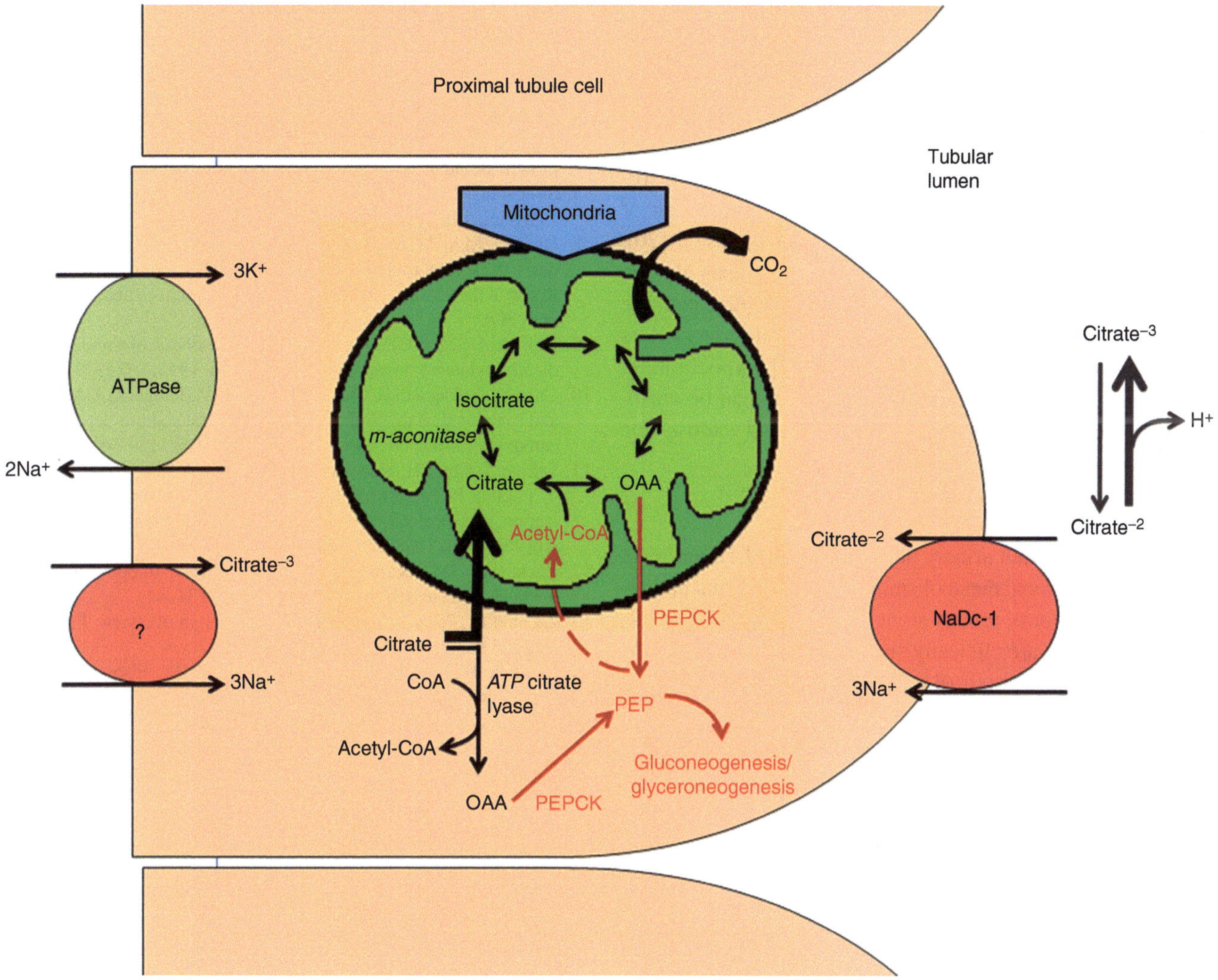

Fig. 21.2 Illustration of the mechanism of tubular transport across apical and basolateral membranes of proximal tubular cells and renal metabolism of citrate. *NaDC-1* sodium-dependent dicarboxylate transporter 1, *CoA* coenzyme A, *m-aconitase* mitochondrial aconitase, *OAA* oxaloacetate, *PEP* phosphoenolpyruvate, *PEPCK* phosphoenolpyruvate carboxykinase

lower pH that increases citrate^{2-} concentration will increase citrate reabsorption, for example, citrate^{2-} concentration rises about threefold as luminal pH falls from 7.4 to 6.9 [1]. Metabolic acidosis causes an increase in the activities of cytoplasmic enzyme ATP citrate lyase and mitochondrial aconitase [14, 15]. Both of these pathways converge on phosphoenolpyruvate carboxykinase (PEPCK), whose activity is also increased in metabolic acidosis [6]. PEPCK promotes these pathways by preventing accumulation of oxaloacetate, an anionic intermediate of the Krebs cycle and the product of citrate lyase-mediated reaction. PEPCK generates PEP from oxaloacetate to be subsequently used in gluconeogenesis and glyceroneogenesis or to reenter the Krebs cycle as acetyl-CoA, as shown in Fig. 21.2 [16]. The abovementioned metabolic changes result in increased renal cell citrate oxidation, decreased intracellular citrate concentration, and increased citrate reabsorption [1]. The opposite sequence of events occurs with alkali feeding. Metabolic acidosis also increases NaDC-1activity and thus citrate transportation across apical membrane [6].

Renal tubular acidosis, particularly distal renal tubular acidosis, has been recognized for decades as a cause of recurring calcium stones. Hypocitraturia has been recognized as a sole cause of calcium stones in some patients with renal tubular acidosis. Low urinary citrate also occurs with other causes of chronic acidosis or chronic acid loads. Diet high in animal protein is prone to cause stones due to low urinary pH and citrate content. Carbonic anhydrase inhibitors including acetazolamide and topiramate can lower urinary citrate via their acid-base effect and increase risk of stone formation [1, 17].

Chronic potassium depletion, low urinary calcium and magnesium, chronic diarrhea, malabsorption, low intestinal alkaline absorption, and low urine volume are additional causes of hypocitraturia [2, 18]. Potassium depletion increases activity of luminal membrane NaDC-1 transporter, decreases intracellular pH, and increases H^+ secretion into tubular lumen causing hypocitraturia [2, 19]. Divalent cations (e.g., Ca^{++} and Mg^{++}) cause increased citrate excretion possibly due to formation of complexes with citrate, although involvement of some additional mechanisms has also been suggested [20]. Starvation reduces urine citrate excretion perhaps due to increased citrate transport consistent with an adaptive increase in the number of the luminal membrane citrate transporters and systemic acidosis during starvation [12, 19]. Hypocitraturia related to chronic diarrhea and malabsorption can be attributed to potassium and magnesium depletion and acidosis due to bicarbonate loss in stool [3, 12].

Conclusion

Citrate is the main urinary organic anion and a significant substrate for renal metabolism. Being an important endogenous inhibitor of urinary stone formation, changes in citrate excretion are clinically significant. Citrate is actively reabsorbed into proximal renal tubule through a Na^+- and pH-dependent transporter. Changes in acid-base homeostasis and other clinical derangements affecting citrate transport into renal tubule and renal metabolism lead to changes in urinary citrate content.

References

1. Hamm LL, Hering-Smith KS. Pathophysiology of hypocitraturic nephrolithiasis. Endocrinol Metab Clin North Am. 2002;31:885–93.
2. Domrongkitchaiporn S, Stitchantrakul W, Kochakarn W. Causes of hypocitraturia in recurrent calcium stone formers: focusing on urinary potassium excretion. Am J Kidney Dis. 2006;48:546–54.
3. Goldberg H, Grass L, Vogl R, Rapoport A, Oreopoulos DG. Urine citrate and renal stone disease. CMAJ. 1989;141:217–21.
4. Hamm LL. Renal handling of citrate. Kidney Int. 1990;30:728–35.
5. Pak CYC, Skurla C, Brinkley L, Sakhaee K. Augmentation of renal citrate excretion by oral potassium citrate administration: time course, dose frequency schedule, and dose response relationship. J Clin Pharmacol. 1984;24:19–26.
6. Aruga S, Wehrli S, Kaissling B, Moe OW, Preisig PA, Pajor AM, et al. Chronic metabolic acidosis increases NaDC-1 mRNA and protein abundance in rat kidney. Kidney Int. 2000;58:206–15.
7. Simpson DP. Citrate excretion: a window of renal metabolism. Am J Physiol. 1983;244:F223–34.
8. Hediger MA, Mount DB, Rolfs A, Romero MF. The molecular basis of solute transport. In: Brenner BM, editor. Brenner and Rector's the kidney, vol. I. 7th ed. Philadelphia: Saunders; 2004. p. 261–308.
9. Pajor AM. Sequence and functional characteristic of a renal sodium/dicarboxylate co transporter. J Biol Chem. 1995;270:5779–85.
10. Chen X, Tsukaguchi H, Chen XZ, Berger UV, Hediger MA. Molecular and functional analysis of SDCT2, a novel rat sodium-dependent tricarboxylate transporter. J Clin Invest. 1999;103:1159–68.
11. Sekine T, Cha SH, Hosoyamada M, Kanai Y, Watanabe N, Furuta Y, Fukuda K, Igarashi T, Endou H. Cloning, functional characterization, and localization of a rat renal Na^+-dicarboxylate transporter. Am J Physiol. 1998;275:F298–305.
12. Zuckerman JM, Assimos DG. Hypocitraturia: pathophysiology and medical management. Rev Urol. 2009;11:134–44.
13. Zacchia M, Preisig P. Low urinary citrate: an overview. J Nephrol. 2010;23 suppl 16:S49–56.
14. Melnick JZ, Preisig PA, Moe OW, Srere PA, Elshourbagy NA, Alpern RJ. Renal cortical mitochondrial aconitase is regulated in hypo- and hypercitraturia. Kidney Int. 1996;54:160–5.
15. Melnick JZ, Srere PA, Elshourbagy NA, Moe OW, Preisig PA, Alpern RJ. Adenosine triphosphate citrate lyase mediates hypocitraturia in rats. J Clin Invest. 1997;101:170–7.
16. Yang J, Kalhan SC, Hanson RW. What is the metabolic role of phosphoenolpyruvate carboxykinase? J Biol Chem. 2009;284:27025–9.
17. Mirza N, Marson AG, Pirmohamed M. Effect of topiramate on acid–base balance: extent, mechanism and effects. Br J Clin Pharmacol. 2009;68:655–61.
18. Unwin RJ, Capasso G, Shirley DG. An overview of divalent cation and citrate handling by the kidney. Nephron Physiol. 2004;98:15–20.
19. Pajor AM, Sun N. Characteristics of the rabbit renal Na^+-dicarboxylate co-transporter using antifusion protein antibodies. Am J Physiol. 1996;271:C1808–16.
20. Hering-Smith KS, Gambala CT, Hamm LL, Gilani AH. Citrate and succinate transport proximal tubule cells. Am J Physiol Renal Physiol. 2000;278:F492–8.

Urinary Citrate and Stone Disease

22

Charles Y.C. Pak

Abstract

Citrate plays an important role in calcium oxalate stone formation. Hypocitraturia has now been found in topiramate therapy, bariatric surgery, and high-protein low-carbohydrate diet. Citrate indirectly reduces urinary saturation of stone-forming calcium salts by complexing calcium and reducing ionized calcium fraction in urine; its direct effect on nucleation, crystal growth, and agglomeration is minor or uncertain. Hypocitraturia can be readily corrected by potassium citrate treatment. This treatment also increases urinary pH.

The physicochemical effects of increased urinary citrate and pH from potassium citrate treatment when critically examined by estimating urinary saturation of brushite and calcium oxalate reveal that potassium citrate treatment does not increase urinary saturation of brushite and more dramatically decreases the saturation of calcium oxalate.

Keywords

Urinary citrate • Potassium citrate • Brushite • Calcium oxalate • Topiramate • Atkins diet Bariatric surgery • Physicochemical action of citrate

Introduction

Citrate plays an important role in formation of calcium-containing kidney stones in three ways. First, hypocitraturia is commonly encountered among patients with stones due to a variety of metabolic and dietary disturbances. Second, citrate ion is an inhibitor of crystallization of stone-forming salts—calcium oxalate and calcium phosphate. Third, preponderant evidence has accumulated showing that correction of hypocitraturia by potassium citrate produces physicochemical and clinical improvement.

This topic has been thoroughly covered in prior reviews. This chapter will focus on new findings reported during the past decade with respect to the aforementioned areas of citrate research.

C.Y.C. Pak, M.D.
Center for Mineral Metabolism and Clinical Research, University of Texas Southwestern Medical Center at Dallas, 5323 Harry Hines Blvd., Dallas, TX 75390-8571, USA
e-mail: charles.pak@utsouthwestern.edu

Causes of Hypocitraturia

Hypocitraturia is due to a variety of metabolic and dietary-environmental disturbances (Table 22.1). Metabolic disturbances include distal renal tubular acidosis [1], acquired metabolic acidosis from topiramate [2], hypokalemia from potassium-losing diuretic therapy (resulting in reduced intracellular pH), and excessive intestinal alkali loss in chronic diarrheal conditions. Dietary-environmental factors include strenuous physical exercise (resulting in lactic acidosis) [3],

Table 22.1 Causes of hypocitraturia

Metabolic causes
Distal renal tubular acidosis
Acquired metabolic acidosis from topiramate therapy
Hypokalemia from diuretic therapy
Roux-en-Y gastric bypass surgery
Dietary-environmental causes
Strenuous physical exercise
Excessive sodium intake
Atkins high meat-low carbohydrate diet

J.J. Talati et al. (eds.), *Urolithiasis*,
DOI 10.1007/978-1-4471-4387-1_22, © Springer-Verlag London 2012

salt abuse (leading to bicarbonaturia) [4], and exaggerated intake of sulfur-containing animal proteins (conferring acid load) [5]. The common denominator is intracellular acidosis in the renal proximal tubular cells [6], which impairs citrate lyase and aconitase and activates citrate cotransporter. The recently described causes of hypocitraturia topiramate therapy, gastric bypass surgery for morbid obesity, and high-animal protein low-carbohydrate diet are further elaborated below.

Topiramate Therapy

Topiramate is a neuromodulatory agent widely used for prevention of seizures and migraine. By inhibiting renal carbonic anhydrase, it has the capacity to produce metabolic acidosis. Thus, it has been shown to produce hypocitraturia, high urinary pH, and modest hypercalciuria [7]. Short-term trials have not shown increased incidence of kidney stones. However, a higher incidence of stones is likely with chronic use. A preliminary study revealed a prevalence of 10.7 % during long-term use [2].

Bariatric Surgery for Morbid Obesity

It is well known that intestinal bypass surgery and inflammatory disease of the small bowel could produce renal stones by causing hypocitraturia (from intestinal alkali loss and ensuing metabolic acidosis) and hyperoxaluria (from fat malabsorption). The Roux-en-Y gastric bypass (RYGB) surgery has now become widely popular for the control of morbid obesity, since it is less invasive and is attendant with fewer complications than intestinal bypass surgery. Although no overt metabolic acidosis ensues after RYGB surgery, moderate-severe hypocitraturia and hyperoxaluria have been reported [2, 8, 9]. A recent study reported a twofold increase in stone incidence [10].

Despite hypocitraturia and hyperoxaluria, urinary calcium is also reduced in patients with RYGB surgery, probably owing to impaired intestinal calcium absorption [11, 12]. Thus, urinary saturation of calcium oxalate has been shown to be only modestly increased [13].

Supplementation with calcium and vitamin D is now commonplace after RYGB surgery to overcome parathyroid stimulation and bone loss from impaired calcium absorption [14]. A potential concern of this supplementation is increased urinary calcium, which could provoke stone formation.

High-Animal Protein Low-Carbohydrate Diet (Atkins Diet)

Atkins diet rich in animal proteins and low in carbohydrate is commonly used for weight reduction. The physiological and physicochemical effect of this diet was investigated under a constant metabolic diet in ten obese subjects [15].

During the first 2 weeks of induction diet, a considerable acid load was delivered, indicated by increased net acid excretion and reduced urinary citrate (Fig. 22.1). Commensurate with these changes, urinary calcium rose and pH decreased. The reduced pH opposed the hypocitraturic and hypercalciuric effects. Thus, the urinary saturation of calcium oxalate, recalculated as supersaturation index (SI) by using the JESS computer program [16], increased only modestly. Other effects probably contribute to the stone-provoking action of high-animal protein diet, such as the urate induction of calcium oxalate crystallization [17].

Physicochemical Action of Citrate

Citrate ion is an important "inhibitor" of the crystallization of stone-forming salts: calcium oxalate and calcium phosphate. Most of the inhibitor activity is derived indirectly from formation of citrate complexes of calcium, which reduces the ionized calcium concentration and hence the saturation of calcium salts. Citrate ion might also have a direct inhibitory action, independent of its reduction of calcium oxalate saturation.

Citrate Complexation of Calcium

Total citrate is a sum of ionized fractions (H_2Cit^-, $HCit^{2-}$, and Cit^{3-}) and non-ionized fraction (Cit). The ionized forms of citrate react with calcium ion (Ca^{2+}) to form soluble calcium-citrate complexes: $CaH_2Cit^+ + CaHCit + CaCit^-$. There might be other calcium-citrate complexes, such as calcium phosphocitrate.

Total calcium is also a sum of ionized and non-ionized fractions; the latter include calcium-citrate complexes. Thus, the amount of Ca^{2+} is reduced in the presence of citrate. The process by which increased urinary citrate reduces urinary saturation of calcium oxalate is described as follows.

Urinary saturation of calcium oxalate is defined by activity product (alpha) αCa^{2+} (alpha) αOx^{2-}, where α (alpha) is ionic activity and Ca^{2+} and Ox^{2-} are calcium and oxalate ions. α(alpha) is equal to the activity coefficient, γ (gamma), times the concentration of ionized calcium [Ca^{2+}] or oxalate [Ox^{2-}]. γ (gamma) is a complex inverse function of ionic strength.

Thus, urinary saturation of calcium oxalate or activity product is given by

$$\alpha Ca^{2+} \cdot \alpha Ox^{2} = \gamma\left[Ca^{2+}\right] \cdot \gamma\left[Ox^{2-}\right].$$

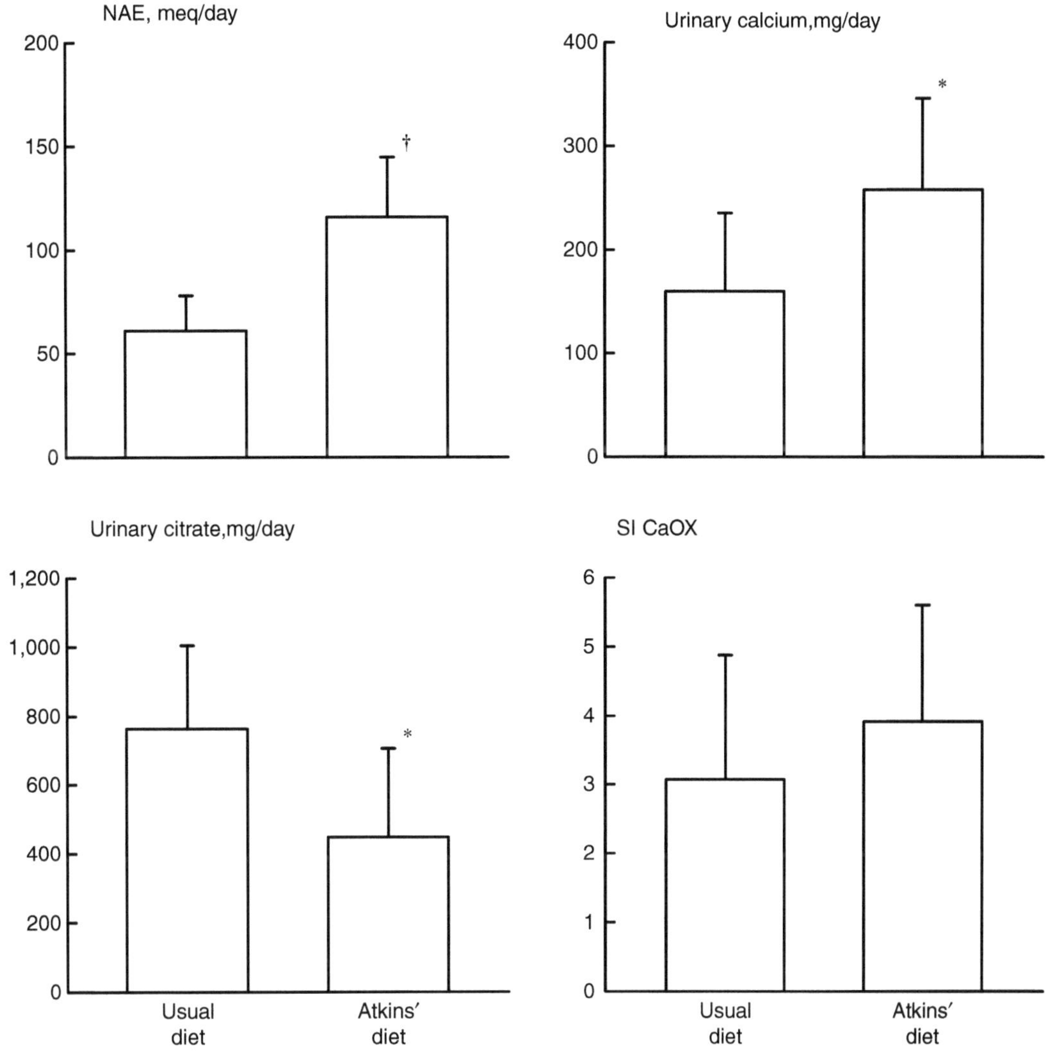

Fig. 22.1 Effect of high-protein low-carbohydrate diet (Atkins diet) on urinary net acid excretion, calcium, citrate, and supersaturation index. *NAE* net acid excretion. *SI* supersaturation index, a measure of urinary saturation calculated by JESS program. *Vertical bars* indicate mean + SD. * $p < 0.05$ and † $p < 0.001$ from the usual diet

In the presence of citrate, [Ca^{2+}] is reduced by formation of soluble complexes with citrate. Urinary saturation or activity product, expressed as (alpha) αCa^{2+} · (alpha) α Ox^2, is therefore reduced by citrate (Fig. 22.2).

By the same process, increased urinary citrate reduces urinary saturation of brushite ($CaHPO_4 \cdot 2H_2O$), a precursor phase of hydroxyapatite (see Fig. 22.2). However, a rise in urinary citrate is often associated with increased urinary pH, which might override the effect of the former (to be described).

Effect of Citrate on Crystal Growth and Crystal Agglomeration

Earlier studies indicated that citrate is a potent inhibitor of crystal growth of calcium phosphate. A recent study [18] revealed that this action of citrate is modest and that most of its inhibition of crystal growth probably ensues from its reduction in urinary saturation of calcium phosphate resulting from complexation of calcium. Earlier, citrate was shown to inhibit spontaneous nucleation of calcium oxalate [19]. Most of this action was ascribed to citrate complexation of calcium. Overall, citrate's inhibition of crystal growth and spontaneous nucleation is probably largely due to the reduction in saturation of calcium salts by formation of calcium-citrate complexes.

Using a method based on kinetic criteria rather than visual detection, Kok et al. [20] reported that calcium oxalate agglomeration was inhibited by citrate. We recently confirmed this finding [21]. The mechanism by which citrate inhibits agglomeration of calcium oxalate crystals has not been clarified.

In summary, citrate inhibits crystallization of calcium salts mostly by lowering their saturation rather than by a direct action. Conversely, urinary environment deficient in citrate is conducive to the crystallization of stone-forming calcium salts.

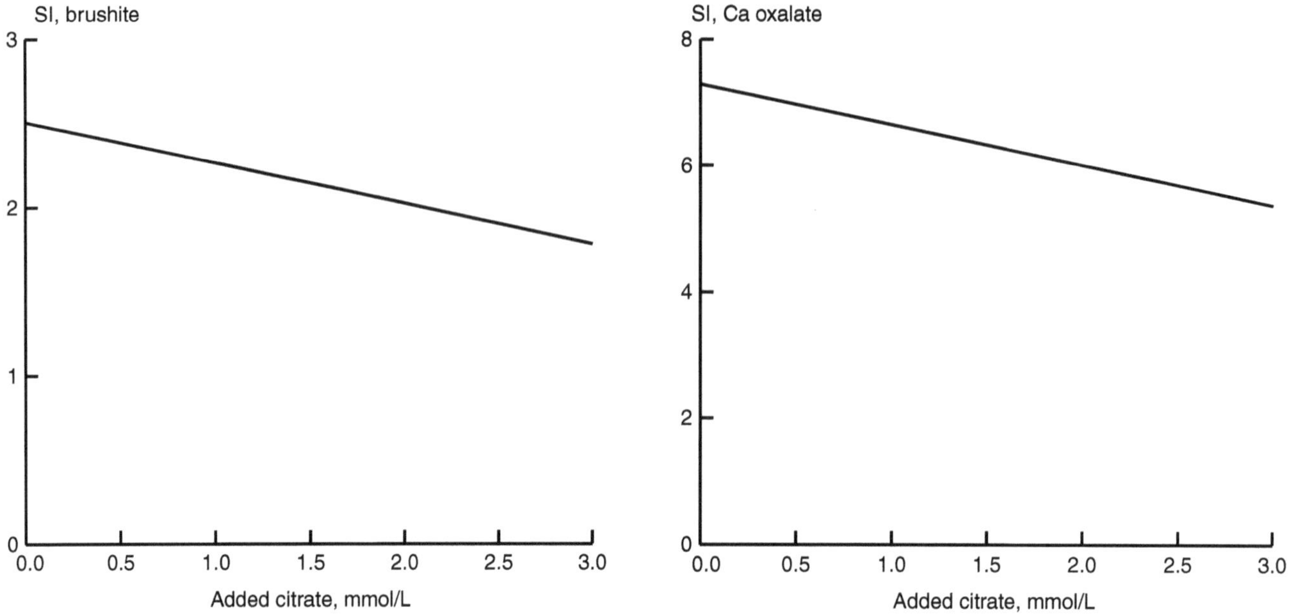

Fig. 22.2 Effect of increasing urinary citrate on urinary saturation of calcium oxalate and brushite. Citrate was added in varying amounts to achieve a wide range of urinary citrate, while other components were kept the same. SI of brushite and calcium oxalate were then computed

Action of Potassium Citrate

Potassium citrate is well known to correct hypocitraturia and is widely used in the management of calcium oxalate nephrolithiasis [22, 23]. The mode of action of potassium alkali has been extensively reported previously and will only be briefly described. Instead, the discussion will focus on newer findings.

Physiological Action of Potassium Citrate

By providing an alkali load, potassium citrate increases urinary citrate and pH by its renal action. Potassium bicarbonate shares the above physiological action of potassium citrate, but is not available commercially. Unlike sodium citrate or bicarbonate, potassium citrate or bicarbonate reduces urinary calcium excretion [24, 25]; this effect is modest and transient. The physicochemical action of potassium citrate is not only due to increased urinary citrate but also to increased urinary pH.

Physicochemical Action of Potassium Citrate

The relative effect of citrate and pH on urinary saturation of brushite and calcium oxalate depends on the exact software program used for the computation of activity products. Several computer programs have been introduced to compute soluble complexes, pH-dependent dissociations and ionic strength, permitting calculation of activity product of brushite and calcium oxalate in urine. They differ from each other, with respect to the exact complexes implicated and the values for formation constants assigned to the complexes. Two computer programs are currently in use.

Equil2 Program

Relative saturation (RSR) by Equil2 program [26] is the most popular and widely adopted among computer programs. RSR represents the ratio of activity product computed in urine and the thermodynamic solubility product (activity product in synthetic solutions at steady state), where activity products are computed by using the Equil2 program.

JESS Program

In 2006, SI or supersaturation index by JESS program [16] was introduced. It takes into consideration additional complexes—mainly calcium phosphocitrate and calcium dihydrogen phosphate dimer. SI is displayed as the ratio of activity product in urine divided by thermodynamic solubility product, both calculated by the JESS program.

Comparison of Equil2 Versus JESS Program

Recently, SI and RSR of brushite and calcium oxalate computed from same urine samples were carefully compared with the activity product ratio (APR), a semiempirical method based on actual growth or dissolution of synthetic solid phase in urine [27, 28]. SI corresponded closely with APR for both brushite and calcium oxalate (Fig. 22.3). However, RSR overestimated APR by nearly twofold. Thus,

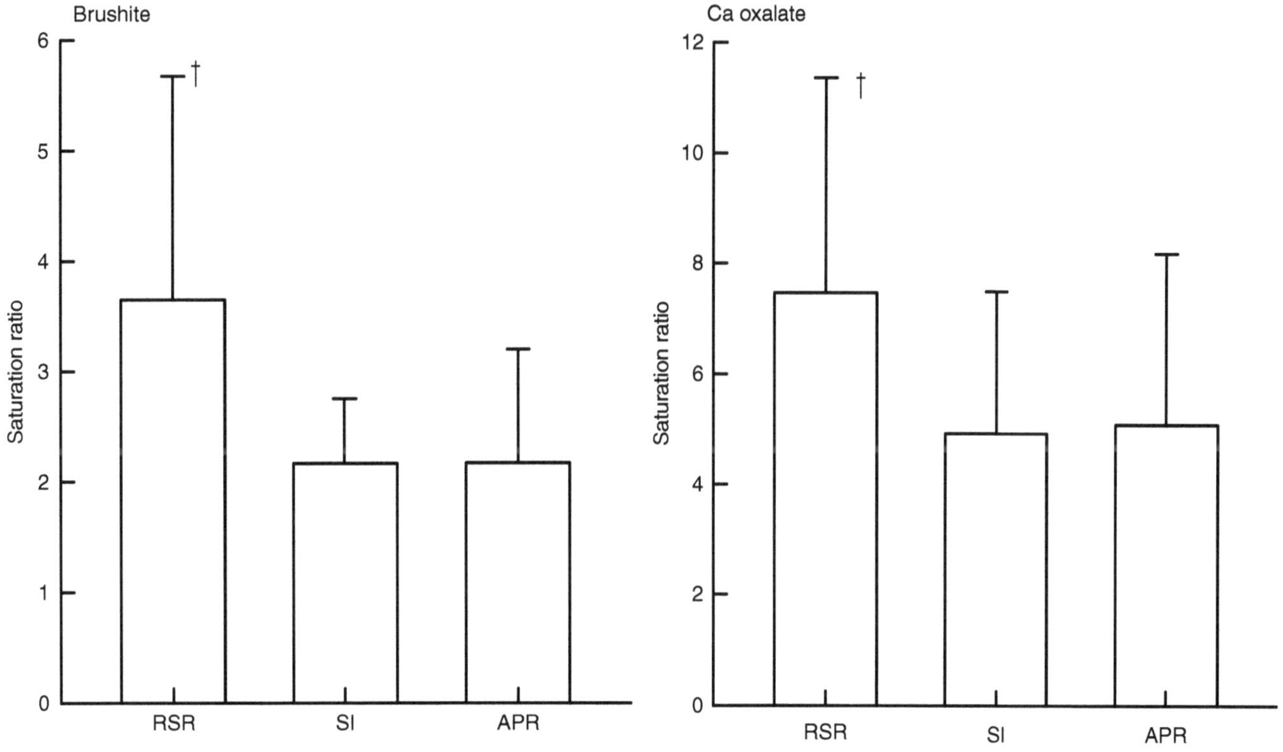

Fig. 22.3 Comparison of RSR and SI of brushite and calcium oxalate versus APR. In same urine samples, RSR and SI of brushite and calcium oxalate were computed by Equil2 and JESS programs, and APR was experimentally obtained from the growth or dissolution of synthetic brushite and calcium oxalate added to whole urine. *Vertical bars* indicate mean + SD. † = $p < 0.001$ from APR

by accommodating additional complexes of calcium (such as calcium phosphocitrate and calcium dihydrogen phosphate dimer), SI accurately estimated urinary saturation of stone-forming calcium salts. Conversely, RSR overestimated urinary saturation of calcium salts, by failing to consider such complexes.

Varying Effects of pH on SI and RSR of Calcium Oxalate

The physicochemical effect of citrate ion was described earlier (see Fig. 22.2). The increased urinary citrate from potassium citrate alone reduces saturation of calcium salts by complexing calcium and thereby lowering ionized calcium concentration. However, potassium citrate also increases urinary pH; this action often overrides that of the increased citrate excretion.

The formation of additional calcium complexes mentioned previously (by JESS but not by Equil2) becomes more prominent at higher pH. In 24-h urine samples collected from 12 subjects, urinary pH alone was varied over a wide range, while other components were kept the same; SI and RSR were then computed (data from Pak et al. [18]).

The dependence of urinary RSR of brushite (calculated by Equil2) on urinary pH is shown in Fig. 22.4 (left, dashed line). Brushite saturation increased dramatically as pH was raised. A rise in pH enhances the dissociation of phosphate, increasing ionized phosphate fractions. At the same time, it decreases the ionized calcium fraction from the formation of soluble complexes of calcium. When Equil2 program was used, the reduction in ionized calcium was modest, since this program did not accommodate additional complexes. Thus, the effect of increased phosphate dissociation predominated.

In contrast, the rise in SI brushite was modest with increasing pH (solid line, left Fig. 22.4). By using the JESS program, the reduction in ionized calcium fraction was more prominent owing to accommodation of additional complexes, attenuating the effect of dissociation of phosphate.

The dependence of urinary RSR of calcium oxalate on urinary pH is displayed in Fig. 22.4 (left, dashed line). RSR of calcium oxalate decreased only slightly with a rise in pH. In the usual pH range of urine, oxalate is nearly fully dissociated. By the Equil2 program, the decline in ionized calcium fraction is modest, balancing the effect of oxalate dissociation. However, SI declined dramatically with increasing pH (solid line), reflective of a sharp decline in ionized calcium fraction from accommodation of additional calcium complexes by the JESS program.

Thus, by accommodating additional pH-dependent complexes of calcium, SI probably more accurately reveals the effect of increased pH. A rise in urinary pH produces only a modest rise in urinary saturation of brushite and substantially reduces urinary saturation of calcium oxalate.

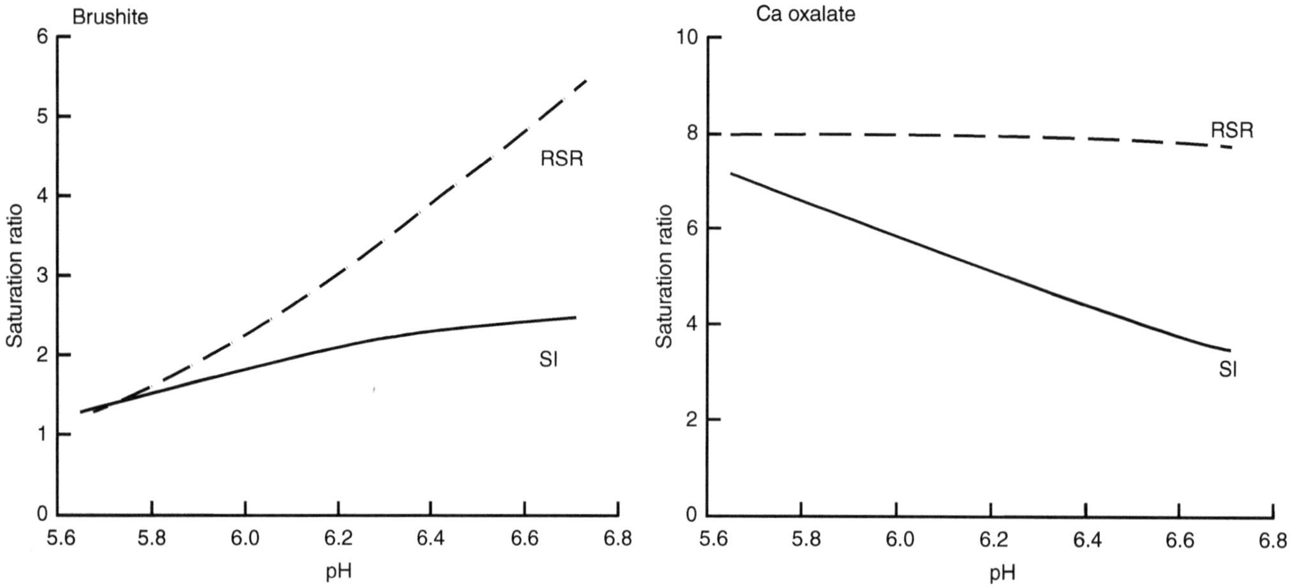

Fig. 22.4 Effect of change in urinary pH on RSR and SI of brushite and calcium oxalate. Urinary pH was adjusted over a wide range while other components were kept the same

Effect of Potassium Citrate Treatment on Urinary RSR and SI of Brushite and Calcium Oxalate

The in vivo effect of potassium citrate therapy will now be considered. As noted before, potassium citrate treatment increases urinary citrate as well as pH.

Based largely on results with RSR, there has been a concern that this treatment could cause or aggravate calcium phosphate stone formation by overly increasing urinary saturation of brushite. This concern was reinforced by the finding of increasing calcium phosphate fraction on stone analysis [29].

To provide clarification, RSR and SI of brushite and calcium oxalate were retrieved or calculated from five long-term trials in idiopathic calcium oxalate nephrolithiasis with potassium citrate [30–34] and one trial with an analogous potassium alkali, potassium-magnesium citrate [35]. Figure 22.5 (top) displays changes in RSR of brushite and calcium oxalate before and after treatment with potassium alkali. RSR brushite increased steeply following potassium citrate treatment in five of six trials (top left), due to predominance of dissociation of phosphate (from increased pH) over calcium complexation (from increased citrate and pH). Conversely, RSR calcium oxalate declined modestly in all six trials during treatment (top left), owing to complexation of calcium (from increased citrate and pH).

Compared to RSR, SI brushite increased only modestly, with a slight rise in four and a decline in two trials, during potassium citrate treatment (bottom left, Fig. 22.5). Moreover, SI calcium oxalate declined in all six trials, more so than RSR (bottom right). As previously enumerated, this difference between the effects of RSR and SI was probably due to the failure of the former method to accommodate additional pH-dependent complexes of calcium.

The findings with SI are probably more valid, since SI yields a more accurate measure of urinary saturation of brushite and calcium oxalate than RSR (see Fig. 22.3). Thus, the fact that potassium citrate does not increase urinary saturation of calcium phosphate by using the SI method allays concern over potential complication of calcium phosphate stones during this treatment. Moreover, a more marked reduction in urinary saturation of calcium oxalate by SI indicates that this treatment might be more effective against calcium oxalate stone formation than previously believed.

Conclusion

Citrate plays an important role in calcium oxalate stone formation. Hypocitraturia has now been found in topiramate therapy, bariatric surgery, and high-protein low-carbohydrate diet. Citrate indirectly reduces urinary saturation of stone-forming calcium salts by complexing calcium and reducing ionized calcium fraction in urine; its direct effect on nucleation, crystal growth, and agglomeration is minor or uncertain. Hypocitraturia can be readily corrected by potassium citrate treatment. This treatment also increases urinary pH.

The physicochemical effects of increased urinary citrate and pH from potassium citrate treatment were critically examined by estimating urinary saturation of brushite and calcium oxalate with the traditional Equil2 program and the recently introduced JESS program. Compared to results derived with the Equil2 program, the JESS program revealed that potassium citrate treatment

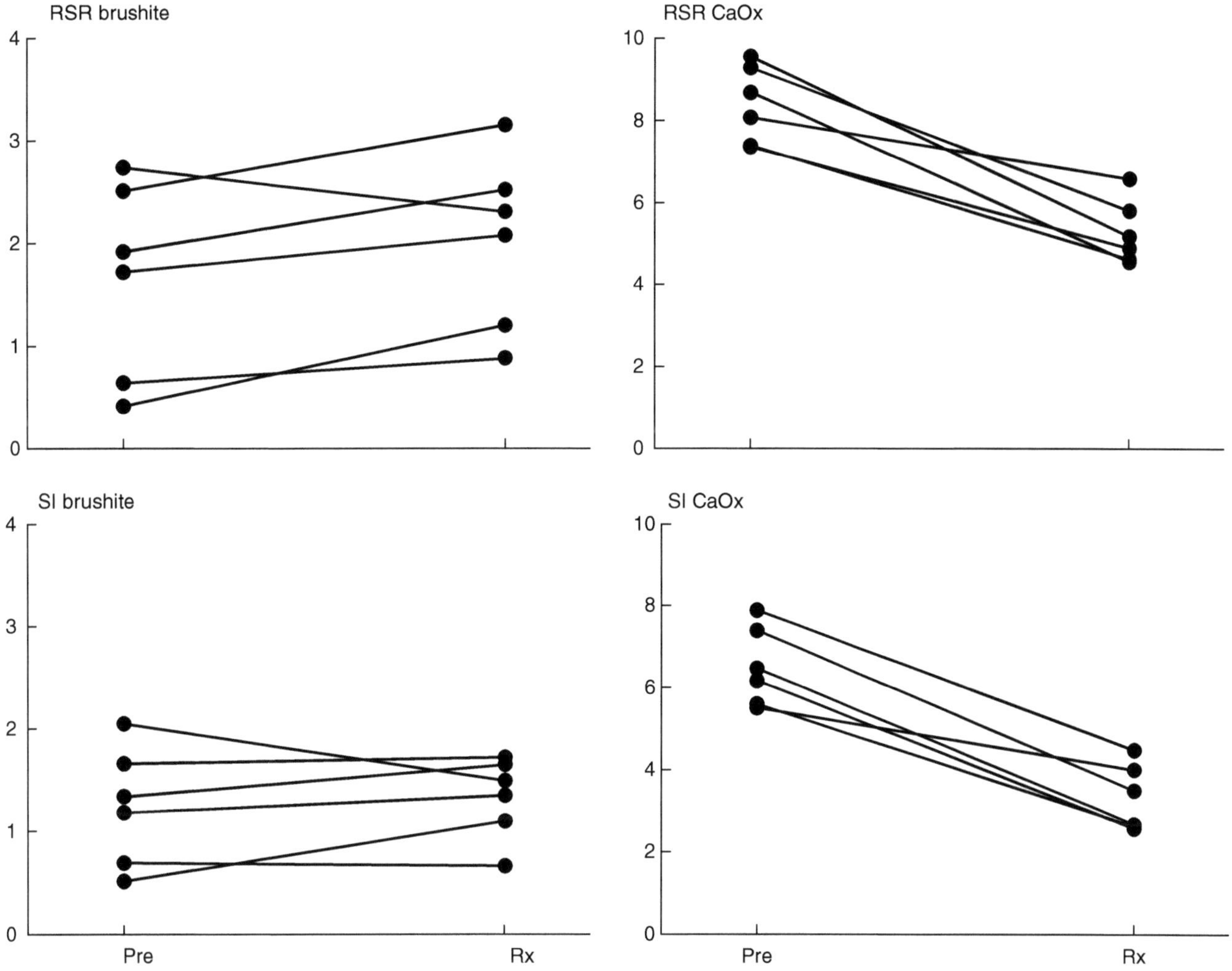

Fig. 22.5 Effect of long-term potassium citrate treatment on RSR and SI of brushite and calcium oxalate. Each *line* represents a separate trial. *Pre* pretreatment, *Rx* potassium citrate treatment

does not increase urinary saturation of brushite and more dramatically decreases the saturation of calcium oxalate.

The JESS program more accurately estimates urinary saturation of calcium salts by accommodating additional pH-dependent complexes of calcium. Thus, potassium citrate probably does not increase the risk for calcium phosphate crystallization, and it is probably more effective in reducing the risk for calcium oxalate crystallization than previously thought.

References

1. Preminger GM, Sakhaee K, Skurla C, Pak CYC. Prevention of recurrent calcium stone formation with potassium citrate therapy in patients with distal renal tubular acidosis. J Urol. 1985;134:20–3.
2. Maalouf NM, Langston JP, Van Ness PC, Moe OW, Sakhaee K. Nephrolithiasis in topiramate users. Urol Res. 2011;39(4):303–7.
3. Sakhaee K, Nigam S, Snell P, Hsu MC, Pak CYC. Assessment of the pathogenetic role of physical exercise in renal stone formation. J Clin Endocrinol Metab. 1987;65:974–9.
4. Sakhaee K, Harvey JA, Padalino PK, Whitson P, Pak CYC. Potential role of salt abuse on the risk for kidney stone formation. J Urol. 1991;150:310–2.
5. Coe FL, Moran E, Kavalich AG. The contribution of dietary purine over-consumption to hyperuricosuria in calcium oxalate stone formers. J Chronic Dis. 1976;29:793–800.
6. Moe OW, Preisig PA. Dual role of calcium in mammalian urine. Curr Opin Nephrol Hypertens. 2005;15:419–24.
7. Welch BJ, Graybeal D, Moe OW, Maalouf NM, Sakhaee K. Biochemical and stone-risk profiles with topiramate treatment. Am J Kidney Dis. 2006;48:555–63.
8. Asplin JR, Coe FL. Hyperoxaluria in kidney stone formers treated with modern bariatric surgery. J Urol. 2007;177:565–9.
9. Park AM, Storm DW, Fulmer BR, et al. A prospective study of risk factors for nephrolithiasis after Roux-en-Y gastric bypass surgery. J Urol. 2009;182:2334–9.
10. Matlaga BR, Shore AD, Magnuson T, et al. Effect of gastric bypass surgery on kidney stone disease. J Urol. 2009;181:2573–7.
11. Riedt CS, Brolin RE, Sherrell RM, Field MP, Shapses SA. True fractional calcium absorption is decreased after Roux-en-Y bypass surgery. Obesity. 2006;14:1940–8.
12. Tondapu P, Provost B, Adams-Huet B, et al. Comparison of the absorption of calcium carbonate and calcium citrate after Roux-en-Y gastric bypass. Obes Surg. 2009;19:1256–61.

13. Maalouf NM, Tondapu P, Guth ES, Livingston EH, Sakhaee K. Hypocitraturia and hyperoxaluria after Roux-en-Y gastric bypass surgery. J Urol. 2010;183:1026–30.
14. Bruno C, Fulford AD, Potts JR, et al. Serum markers of bone turnover are increased at six and 18 months after Roux-en-Y bariatric surgery: correlation with the reduction in leptin. J Clin Endocrinol Metab. 2010;95:159–66.
15. Reddy ST, Wang CY, Sakhaee K, Pak CYC. Effect of low-carbohydrate, high-protein diets on acid–base balance, stone-forming propensity, and calcium metabolism. Am J Kidney Dis. 2002;40:265–74.
16. Rodgers A, Allie-Harmdulay S, Jackson G. Therapeutic action of citrate in urolithiasis explained by chemical speciation: increase in pH is the determinant factor. Nephrol Dial Transplant. 2006;21:361–9.
17. Grover PK, Ryall RI, Marshall VR. Dissolved urate promotes calcium oxalate crystallization; epitaxy is not the cause. Clin Sci. 1993;85:303–7.
18. Pak CYC, Rodgers K, Poindexter JR, Sakhaee K. New methods for assessing crystal growth and saturation of brushite in whole urine: effect of pH, calcium, and citrate. J Urol. 2008;180:1532–7.
19. Nicar MJ, Hill K, Pak CYC. Inhibition by citrate of spontaneous precipitation of calcium oxalate in vitro. J Bone Miner Res. 1987;2:215–20.
20. Kok DJ, Papapoulos SE, Bijvoet OLM. Excessive crystal agglomeration with low citrate excretion in recurrent stone-formers. Lancet. 1986;1:1056–8.
21. Sakhaee K, Griffith C, Pak CY. Biochemical control of bone loss and stone-forming propensity by potassium-calcium citrate after bariatric surgery. Surg Obes Relat Dis. 2011;8(1):67–72.
22. Pak CYC, Fuller CJ, Sakhaee K, Preminger GM, Britton F. Long-term treatment of calcium nephrolithiasis with potassium citrate. J Urol. 1985;134:11–9.
23. Barcelo P, Wuhl O, Servitge E, Rousaud A, Pak CY. Randomized double-blind study of potassium citrate in idiopathic hypocitraturic calcium nephrolithiasis. J Urol. 1993;150:1761–4.
24. Sakhaee K, Nicar MJ, Hill K, Pak CYC. Contrasting effects of potassium citrate and sodium citrate therapies on urinary chemistries and crystallization of stone-forming salts. Kidney Int. 1983;24:348–52.
25. Lemann Jr J. Relationship between urinary calcium and net acid excretion as determined by dietary protein and potassium: a review. Nephron. 1999;81(Supp 1):18–25.
26. Werness PG, Brown CM, Smith LH, Finlayson B. Equil2: a basic computer program for the calculation of urinary saturation. J Urol. 1985;134:1242–4.
27. Pak CYC, Moe OW, Maalouf N, et al. Comparison of semi-empirical with computer-derived methods for estimating urinary saturation of brushite. J Urol. 2009;181:1423–8.
28. Pak CYC, Maalouf NM, Rodgers K, Poindexter JR. Comparison of semi-empirical with computer-derived methods for estimating urinary saturation of calcium oxalate. J Urol. 2009;182:2951–6.
29. Parks JH, Worcester EM, Coe FL, Evan AP, Lingeman JE. Clinical implications of abundant calcium phosphate in routinely analyzed kidney stones. Kidney Int. 2004;66:777–85.
30. Pak CYC, Fuller CJ. Idiopathic hypocitraturic calcium oxalate nephrolithiasis successfully treated with potassium citrate. Ann Intern Med. 1986;104:33–7.
31. Pak CYC, Peterson R. Successful treatment of hyperuricosuric calcium oxalate nephrolithiasis with potassium citrate. Arch Intern Med. 1986;146:863–8.
32. Pak CY, Heller HJ, Pearle MS, et al. Prevention of stone formation and bone loss by combined dietary and pharmacological intervention. J Urol. 2003;169:465–9.
33. Pak CYC, Sakhaee K, Fuller CJ. Successful management of uric acid nephrolithiasis with potassium citrate. Kidney Int. 1986;30:422–8.
34. Pak CY. Citrate and renal calculi. Miner Electrolyte Metab. 1987;13:257–66.
35. Ettinger B, Pak CY, Citron JT, et al. Potassium-magnesium citrate is an effective prophylaxis against calcium oxalate nephrolithiasis. J Urol. 1997;158:2069–73.

23 Renal Tubular Acidosis and Stone Formation

Somnuek Domrongkitchaiporn
and Wasana Stitchantrakul

Abstract

Distal renal tubular acidosis (RTA) syndrome is a condition caused by the acidification defect in collection tubule. The syndrome is characterized by a persistent hyperchloremic, normal plasma anion gap and metabolic acidosis in patients with relatively normal glomerular filtration rate (GFR). Hypokalemia is also common. Most patients are associated with recurrent calcium oxalate or calcium phosphate stone formation and nephrocalcinosis. Metabolic bone disease and growth retardation are common complications. Occasionally, patients may present with hypokalemic paralysis. The treatment aims to provide adequate alkaline therapy to neutralize the daily acid production. All the associated complications should be prevented. Monitoring of urinary parameters such as calcium-to-creatinine or citrate-to-creatinine ratio is essential to ensure appropriate dosage of alkaline therapy.

Keywords

Renal tubular acidosis • Renal stone • Alkaline therapy • Periodic paralysis • Citrate Osteopenia • Osteomalacia

Introduction

Renal tubular acidosis (RTA) syndromes are characterized by a persistent hyperchloremic normal plasma anion gap and metabolic acidosis in patients with relatively normal glomerular filtration rate (GFR). The RTA syndromes have been classified into three main categories: proximal RTA or type 2, hyperkalemic RTA or type 4, and distal RTA or type 1 [1]. Proximal RTA is caused by a defect of HCO_3^- reabsorption in the proximal tubule and is characterized by a decreased renal HCO_3^- threshold and HCO_3^- leakage in the urine. In hyperkalemic RTA, or type 4, metabolic acidosis is caused by impaired ammonia genesis and lower rate of NH_4^+ excretion. However, the ability to acidify urine is still intact. The hallmark of distal RTA is a defect of the collecting duct to acidify the urine appropriately during acidosis. The defect in acidification results in impaired NH_4^+ and titratable acid excretion and consequently, a positive acid balance in the body. High urine pH and hypokalemia are typically present in addition to a normal gap metabolic acidosis. The chronic positive acid balance causes calcium, magnesium, and phosphate wasting. Recent evidence also suggests that downregulation of calcium and magnesium transport proteins in the kidney contributes to calcium and magnesium wasting [2]. Renal production of citrate is also decreased in response to acidosis, resulting in hypocitraturia. The alterations in urine constituents are favorable to recurrent renal stone formation and nephrocalcinosis [3]. By contrast, both proximal RTA and hyperkalemic RTA are rarely associated with recurrent renal stone formation. Therefore, this chapter will be limited only to the pathophysiology and treatment of distal RTA.

S. Domrongkitchaiporn, M.D. (✉)
Department of Medicine, Ramathibodi Hospital,
Rama 6, Bangkok, 10400, Thailand
e-mail: rasdr@mahidol.ac.th

W. Stitchantrakul
Department of Medicine, Research Center,
Ramathibodi Hospital, Mahidol University,
Bangkok, Thailand

J.J. Talati et al. (eds.), *Urolithiasis*,
DOI 10.1007/978-1-4471-4387-1_23, © Springer-Verlag London 2012

Pathogenesis

The pathogenesis of classic distal RTA could result from (1) defective apical H^+ATPase, or H^+K^+-ATPase; (2) defective basolateral HCO_3^-/Cl^- exchanger; (3) H^+ leak pathway; and (4) defective intracellular carbonic anhydrase. The defects can be acquired or inherited and either autosomal dominant or recessive. The autosomal dominant form is associated with mutation in AE1 gene, which encodes basolateral HCO_3^-/Cl^- exchanger in the collecting duct [4]. Two different recessive mutations in the gene encoding B1-subunit of H^+-ATPase have been described. One defect is associated with sensorineural deafness and the other has normal hearing [4]. The inherited forms usually present early in childhood. In addition, an unusually high incidence of distal RTA has been reported in northeastern Thailand [5]. A defect in AE1 gene encoding HCO_3^-/Cl^- exchanger in association with ovalocytosis has been reported in some families with autosomal recessive transmission [6]. However, the molecular defect in the majority of cases in Thailand is still uncertain.

Clinical Manifestation

Most RTA patients present with recurrent renal stone formation. The stone-forming activity tends to be more severe and has an earlier age of onset compared to those among other stone formers. A high frequency of calcium phosphate stone has been reported from stone analysis [7]. However, calcium oxalate stone is still the most common stone type found in distal RTA patients. Bilateral nephrocalcinosis is a common associated finding detected on plain X-ray of the kidneys or on ultrasonogram. Unlike idiopathic calcium stone formers, a large proportion of patients with complete distal RTA have nephrocalcinosis, often very extensive, as well as stones.

Typically, serum electrolytes show hypokalemic, normal gap acidosis. A finding of serum bicarbonate less than 10 mEq/L is not uncommon. The urine pH is inappropriately high. Urinary citrate is markedly decreased compared to those with other causes of hypocitraturia [8]. The majority of patients have the normal serum creatinine level. However, distal RTA children with long-standing disease may develop chronic kidney disease later in life [9].

Patients with severe disease may present with proximal muscle weakness and nonspecific musculoskeletal pain. The musculoskeletal complications result mainly from a long-standing hypokalemia and respond rapidly to potassium repletion. Although it is uncommon, distal RTA patients, both adults and children, may present with acute periodic paralysis [10]. Respiratory failure has also been reported [11]. Most patients had recognized proximal muscle weakness in both lower extremities and myalgia for some time before an attack. The development of flaccid paralysis tends to progress over a few days. The paralysis reverses only after potassium repletion. The presentation is sometimes very similar to that of idiopathic hypokalemic periodic paralysis, which is also common in the northeast of Thailand. Most patients with idiopathic hypokalemic paralysis are male, whereas the majority of distal RTA patients with acute paralysis are female. The finding of normal gap acidosis in patients with acute flaccid paralysis should suggest a physician look for distal RTA as the underlying cause. Most adult RTA patients also have low bone mineral density due to suppressed bone formation and increased bone resorption. A histomorphometric study of iliac crest bone biopsy from distal RTA patients demonstrated a histologic feature more compatible with adynamic bone disease than osteomalacia. Only mild elevation in osteoid thickness was found [12]. Children with RTA also suffer from failure to thrive and have a short stature due to chronic acidosis [13].

Among patients with the partial defects in tubular acidification, or incomplete RTA, blood pH is within the normal range, and serum electrolytes are normal. However, in the face of acute acid load, the patients fail to excrete the acid efficiently, and consequently the urine pH is inappropriately high or greater than 5.5. Most incomplete RTA patients also suffer from recurrent renal stone formations and osteopenia [14, 15]. In a community-based survey in a province in the northeast of Thailand, incomplete RTA was found in 6.4 % of the population [16]. A high incidence of incomplete RTA had also been reported among patients referred for evaluation of osteopenia [17]. This subgroup of patients may develop severe osteopenia without history of stone formation or the presence of nephrocalcinosis. Therefore, renal tubular acidification function test should be considered as a part of the investigation to determine underlying causes of recurrent renal stone formation and osteoporosis.

Diagnosis

Distal RTA is characterized by the inability to lower urinary pH maximally (<5.5) under the stimulus of systemic acidosis. The impaired secretion of NH_4^+ is secondary to this defect. In general, HCO_3^- reabsorption is still intact. Distal RTA should be suspected in patients with a hyperchloremic, normal gap, metabolic acidosis without an evidence of gastrointestinal HCO_3^- losses, taking acetazolamide or topiramide, or ingesting exogenous acid. Urine pH in combination with the urinary excretion of NH_4^+ should be evaluated to assess the distal tubular acidification function [18]. Although urinary ammonium excretion can be measured directly in most laboratories, an estimation of ammonium excretion derived from concentration of electrolytes in the urine, $Na^+ + K^+ - Cl^-$, is more practical [19]. The urine anion gap becomes progressively more negative as NH_4^+ excretion increases. A positive urine anion gap in the face of systemic acidosis is suggestive of inappropriate excretion of ammonium salt, indicating the renal tubular acidification defect. The next step is to determine the ability of the kidney to acidify the urine. The failure to lower urine pH below 5.5 during spontaneous systemic acidosis (blood pH < 7.35), or after an ammonium chloride (NH_4Cl) load, establishes the diagnosis of distal RTA. In isolated distal RTA, fractional excretion of bicarbonate at normal plasma HCO_3^- concentration should not exceed 5 % of the filtered load. A greater fractional excretion of bicarbonate indicates an additional defect in proximal tubule, impaired HCO_3^- reabsorption. More details of diagnostic tests to confirm the diagnosis and to distinguish distal RTA from other forms of RTA are available elsewhere [1].

Incomplete RTA should be suspected in patients with recurrent calcium stone formation, especially calcium phosphate stone, and persistent high urine pH (>6). The diagnosis of incomplete RTA requires NH_4^+ loading test, as the patients do not develop acidosis spontaneously. Ammonium chloride, 0.1 mg/kg, is given orally to induce metabolic acidosis, and monitoring of urine pH should be done for at least 6 h. If the patient fails to lower urine pH to less than 5.5 while the blood pH is lower than 7.35, the diagnosis of incomplete RTA can be made. The ammonium chloride test is unpleasant for the patient. An alternative, more palatable furosemide test has been described [1]. After infusion of 1 mg/kg body weight of furosemide, a normal subject should be able to acidify urine (pH < 5.5) within 2–3 h. A failure to acidify urine suggests distal renal tubular acidosis. However, the failure to acidify urine after furosemide administration does not always indicate irreversible renal tubular defect. The elevated urine pH may result from low sodium excretion without renal acidification defect. It should also be noted that a high urine pH may result from urinary tract infection with urea-splitting organisms.

Treatment

The aims of treatment are not only to correct the biochemical abnormalities but to fundamentally prevent all complications of long-standing systemic acidosis, including recurrent renal stone formation, nephrocalcinosis, osteopenia, growth retardation, and chronic kidney disease. After systemic acidosis is corrected, serum bicarbonate rises to normal level, urine citrate increases, and urine calcium and phosphate fall. Alkaline therapy also reduces urinary potassium excretion. Therefore, hypokalemia is corrected spontaneously without the need of the potassium supplements in most patients with mild to moderate potassium depletion. In case of severe depletion, alkaline therapy should be given in the form of potassium salt (e.g., potassium bicarbonate or potassium citrate). However, a rapid elevation of blood pH with alkaline therapy may precipitate hypokalemia. Thus, in extreme circumstance, when patients present with severe hypokalemia and flaccid paralysis or respiratory depression, intravenous potassium supplement may be necessary and should be administered prior to alkaline therapy. Sodium bicarbonate can exacerbate hypokalemia and be potentially life threatening in acute situations if given alone. In general, therefore, potassium alkali is preferred, though cost can be an issue.

Monitoring of urinary constituents after the initiation of alkaline therapy is necessary for all RTA patients. Solely raising serum bicarbonate to a normal level may not be adequate. Many patients who have achieved normal serum bicarbonate level are still hypocitraturic and hypercalciuric. The dosage of an alkaline supplement should be adjusted until urinary citrate-to-creatinine or calcium-to-creatinine ratio returns to normal. The monitoring of both parameters is valuable to ensure adequate alkaline therapy in this group of patients [20].

An unavoidable side effect of alkaline supplementation is the elevation of urinary pH, and a worsening of calcium phosphate supersaturation. Patients on alkaline therapy, therefore, should be monitored to ensure a reduction in the risk of calcium phosphate stone formation. In adult patients with distal RTA, 1–3 mEq/kg/day of an alkaline supplement should be adequate to neutralize the production of metabolic acid [21]. In growing children, a higher amount of alkaline, 2–5 mEq/kg/day, may be required to completely correct most of the urinary abnormalities [20]. In young infants, as much as 5–8 mEq/kg/day of alkaline may be needed [22]. All forms of alkaline therapy are equally effective in terms of the correction of metabolic acidosis. However, potassium salts are preferred to sodium salts. In addition to potassium repletion, potassium salts can avoid the calciuric effect of sodium [23].

Among patients with incomplete RTA, alkaline therapy also corrects hypercalciuria and hypocitraturia, reduces the risk of renal stone formation, and increases bone mineral density. Lesser amounts of alkaline are required compared to classic distal RTA patients. Monitoring of the urinary citrate-to-creatinine or calcium-to-creatinine ratio is recommended to ensure optimal treatment in this group of patients in whom overt acidosis is not present in a routine serum electrolyte determination [20].

The severity of acidosis depends on the ability of renal excretion of acid and also the rate of endogenous acid production. Accordingly, an increased dietary intake of fruits and vegetables should be advised to be another source of an alkaline supplement to the body. Dietary modification is particularly helpful in patients with incomplete form as most of them have low-grade metabolic acidosis. Lifelong medications can be avoided if all the abnormal urine constituents can be successfully corrected by the modification of diet alone.

Conclusion

Correction of systemic acidosis with alkaline therapy will not only lower the frequency of stone formation but also correct osteopenia and abnormal bone histology. A controlled study has demonstrated a dramatic improvement in bone mineral density and bone histologic findings in RTA patients 1 year after continuous potassium citrate supplementation [24]. Growth rate also markedly increased in those children with RTA, who were treated before puberty [20]. Long-term alkaline therapy may also prevent further deposition of calcium in renal parenchymal tissue and renal injury. However, significant reduction of nephrocalcinosis has never been reported. Long-term treatment with sodium thiosulfate has also failed to reverse nephrocalcinosis [25].

Unfortunately, in children with hereditary transmitted forms, the associated hearing loss does not respond to alkaline therapy. Distal RTA is a permanent disease. Alkaline therapy does not restore the tubular function. Therefore, lifelong treatment should be maintained. However, the prognosis is excellent if the treatment has begun early in life or in the early stage of disease and appropriate amounts of alkaline supplements are prescribed. Patient education must be an essential part of the treatment to provide understanding of the disease and to ensure lifelong compliance.

References

1. Soriano JR. Renal tubular acidosis: the clinical entity. J Am Soc Nephrol. 2002;13:2160–70.
2. Nijenhuis T, Renkema K, Hoenderop J, Bindels R. Acid-base status determines the renal expression of Ca^{2+} and Mg^{2+} transport proteins. J Am Soc Nephrol. 2006;17:617–26.
3. Batlle DC, Sehy JT, Roseman MK, Arruda JA, Kurtzman NA. Clinical and pathophysiological spectrum of acquired distal renal tubular acidosis. Kidney Int. 1981;20:389–96.
4. Karet F. Inherited distal renal tubular acidosis. J Am Soc Nephrol. 2002;13:2178–84.
5. Nilwarangkur S, Nimmannit S, Chaovakul V, Susaengrat W, Ong-aj-Yooth S, Vasuvattakul S, et al. Endemic primary distal renal tubular acidosis in Thailand. Q J Med. 1990;74:289–301.
6. Vasuvattakul S, Yenchitsomanus PT, Vachuanichsanong P, Thuwajit P, Kaitwatcharachai C, Laosombat V, et al. Autosomal recessive distal renal tubular acidosis associated with Southeast Asian ovalocytosis. Kidney Int. 1999;56:1674–82.
7. Backman U, Danielson BG, Johansson G, Ljunghall S, Wikström B. Incidence and clinical importance of renal tubular defects in recurrent renal stone formers. Nephron. 1980;25:96–101.
8. Nilwarangkur S, Malasit P, Nimmannit S, Susaengrat W, Ong-Aj-Yooth S, Vasuvattakul S, et al. Urinary constituents in an endemic area of stones and renal tubular acidosis in northeastern Thailand. Southeast Asian J Trop Med Public Health. 1990;21:437–41.
9. Caldas A, Broyewr M, Dechaux M, Kleinknecht C. Primary distal tubular acidosis in childhood: clinical study and long-term follow-up of 28 patients. J Pediatr. 1992;121:233–41.
10. Bresolin NL, Grillo E, Fernandes VR, Carvalho FL, Goes JE, da Silva RJ. A case report and review of hypokalemic paralysis secondary to renal tubular acidosis. Pediatr Nephrol. 2005;20:818–20.
11. Kalita J, Nair PP, Kumar G, Misra UK. Renal tubular acidosis presenting as respiratory paralysis: report of a case and review of literature. Neurol India. 2010;58:106–8.
12. Domrongkitchaiporn S, Pongsakul C, Sirikulchayanonta V, Stitchantrakul W, Ongphiphadhanakul B, Radinahamed P, et al. Metabolic bone disease in distal renal tubular acidosis. Kidney Int. 2000;59:1086–93.
13. Chang CY, Lin CY. Failure to thrive in children with primary distal type renal tubular acidosis. Acta Paediatr Taiwan. 2002;43:334–9.
14. Osther PJ, Bollerslev J, Hansen AB, Engel K, Kildeberg P. Pathophysiology of incomplete renal tubular acidosis in recurrent renal stone formers: evidence of disturbed calcium, bone and citrate metabolism. Urol Res. 1993;21:169–73.
15. Preminger GM, Sakhaee K, Skurla C, Pak CYC. Prevention of recurrent calcium stone formation with potassium citrate therapy in patients with distal renal tubular acidosis. J Urol. 1985;134:20–3.
16. Pongchaiyakul C, Domrongkitchaiporn S, Stitchantrakul W, Chailurkit L, Rajatanavin R. Incomplete renal tubular acidosis and bone mineral density: a population survey in an area of endemic renal tubular acidosis. Nephrol Dial Transplant. 2004;19:3029–33.
17. Weger M, Deutschmann H, Weger W, Kotanko P, Skrabal F. Incomplete renal tubular acidosis in 'primary' osteoporosis. Osteoporos Int. 1999;10:325–9.
18. Wrong O. Distal renal tubular acidosis: the value of urinary pH, PCO_2 and NH_4^+ measurements. Pediatr Nephrol. 1991;5:249–55.
19. Batlle DC, Hizon M, Cohen E, Gutterman C, Grupta R. The use of the urinary anion gap in the diagnosis of hyperchloremic metabolic acidosis. N Engl J Med. 1988;318:594–9.
20. Domrongkitchaiporn S, Khositseth S, Stitchantrakul W, Tapaneya-olarn W, Radinahamed P. Dosage of potassium citrate in the correction of urinary abnormalities in pediatric distal renal tubular acidosis patients. Am J Kidney Dis. 2002;39:383–91.
21. DuBose TD, McDonald GA. In: DuBose TD, Hamm LL, editors. Acid-base and electrolyte disorders: a companion to Brenner and Rector's the kidney. Philadelphia: WB Saunders; 2002. p. 189–206.
22. RodríguezSoriano J, Vallo A, Castillo G, Oliveros R. Natural history of primary distal renal tubular acidosis treated since infancy. J Pediatr. 1982;101:669–76.
23. Lemann Jr J, Gray RW, Pleuss JA. Potassium bicarbonate, but not sodium bicarbonate, reduces urinary calcium excretion and improves calcium balance in healthy men. Kidney Int. 1989;35:688–95.
24. Domrongkitchaiporn S, Pongskul C, Sirikulchayanonta V, Stitchantrakul W, Leeprasert V, Ongphiphadhanakul B, et al. Bone histology and bone mineral density after correction of acidosis in distal renal tubular acidosis. Kidney Int. 2002;62:2160–6.
25. Agroyannis BJ, Koutsikos DK, Tzanatos HA, Konstadinidou IK. Sodium thiosulphate in the treatment of renal tubular acidosis I with nephrocalcinosis. Scand J Urol Nephrol. 1994;28:107–8.

Nephrolithiasis and Its Interrelationship with Vitamin D, Parathyroid Hormone, and Calcium

24

Aysha Habib Khan

Abstract

Calcium is a major component of 85 % of renal stones. The incidence of renal stone diseases is increasing, possibly consequent to the widespread use of calcium supplementation. A genetic contribution with defects in the regulation of renal calcium excretion has been suggested as a cause of renal stone disease. The parathyroid hormone (PTH) and vitamin D axis plays a key role in the calcium and phosphate homeostasis. The parathyroid gland responds with rapid changes of PTH in response to fluctuations in the extracellular calcium concentration, thereby regulating minute-to-minute normalization of serum ionized calcium, through stimulation of renal tubular calcium reabsorption and bone resorption. On a more chronic basis, PTH also stimulates the conversion of 25-hydroxyvitamin D to 1,25-dihydroxyvitamin D (calcitriol) in the proximal renal tubular cells, thereby stimulating intestinal calcium absorption. Hypersecretion of parathyroid hormone results in hypercalcemia thus predisposing the individual to development of nephrolithiasis.

Vitamin D is recognized as an important hormone in health and disease. There has been an increasing appreciation of the complexity and importance of its regulation, functions, and supplementation. The use of calcium and vitamin D supplementation, though safe, has been shown to be associated with an increase in the incidence of renal lithiasis.

Abnormalities related to vitamin D deficiency and parathyroid hormone disorders in the general population are reported globally with an increased incidence of cardiovascular disease, diabetes, metabolic syndrome, and cancer rates, which is linked to protracted exposure to abnormal internal milieu such as occurs with vitamin D deficiency. This chapter reviews the recent advances and interrelationship in the understanding of calcium, vitamin D, and PTH axis as they affect the process of stone formation in the kidney in health and diseases.

Keywords

Renal stone • Calcium • Vitamin D • Parathyroid hormone (PTH)

Introduction

Renal stone disease affects 5 % of adults and the incidence seems to be increasing over the last decades [1]. In the United States, the lifetime prevalence of kidney stones in adult women increased to 37 % between 1996–1980 and 1988–1994 [2]. This increase corresponds to the widespread use of calcium supplementation in the treatment of osteoporosis [3, 4].

A.H. Khan, MBBS, FCPS (chemical pathology)
Department of Pathology and Microbiology and Medicine,
Aga Khan University, Stadium Road,
Karachi, Sindh, 74800, Pakistan
e-mail: aysha.habib@aku.edu

J.J. Talati et al. (eds.), *Urolithiasis*,
DOI 10.1007/978-1-4471-4387-1_24, © Springer-Verlag London 2012

A kidney stone can only form in urine that is supersaturated with respect to the specific components of the stone. The underlying metabolic abnormalities include hypercalciuria, hyperphosphaturia, hyperoxaluria, hypocitraturia, hyperuricosuria, cystinuria, a low urinary volume, and a defect of urinary acidification. High concentrations increase free ion activities, while the presence of inhibitors of crystallization decreases ionization.

Calcium (Ca) is a major component of 85 % of renal stones, largely as either calcium oxalate or phosphate. A genetic contribution and defects in the regulation of renal calcium excretion have been suggested as causes of renal stone disease. Hypercalciuric nephrolithiasis may occur as a monogenic disorder or as a polygenic trait. Studies of monogenic forms of hypercalciuric nephrolithiasis (e.g., Bartter syndrome, Dent's disease, autosomal dominant hypophosphatemia, hereditary hypophosphatemic rickets with hypercalciuria, and familial hypomagnesaemia with hypercalciuria) have provided insights into the renal tubular pathways that regulate calcium reabsorption and predispose to kidney stones [5–7].

The parathyroid hormone (PTH) and vitamin D (25-(OH) D) axis plays a key role in calcium and phosphate homeostasis. The parathyroid gland responds with rapid changes of PTH in response to fluctuations in the extracellular calcium concentration, thereby providing minute-to-minute regulation of serum ionized calcium through stimulation of renal tubular calcium reabsorption and bone resorption. On a more chronic basis, PTH also stimulates the conversion of 25-(OH) D to calcitriol (1,25-$(OH)_2$D) in proximal renal tubular cells, thereby stimulating intestinal calcium absorption [8, 9].

Over the last decade, research has given insight into many new areas of vitamin D action [10–20]. Vitamin D is now recognized as an important hormone in health and disease; there has been an increasing appreciation of the complexity and importance of its regulation. Recently, newer strategies and recommendations have been put forward for dietary and supplementary intake of vitamin D and calcium in the light of the existing pandemic of vitamin D deficiency and concern for treatment of osteoporosis [21, 22]. Calcium and vitamin D supplementation, though safe, has been accompanied by an increase in the incidence of renal lithiasis [4]. In addition, hypersecretion of parathyroid hormone results in hypercalcemia, thus predisposing the individual to the development of nephrolithiasis [23].

Basic animal and clinical data have shown important and complex roles of vitamin D and PTH in maintaining a variety of essential regulatory functions in health. Abnormalities of these in the general population are reported globally, including that of vitamin D deficiency and secondary hyperparathyroidism. The general population has also been shown to have an increased incidence of cardiovascular disease, diabetes, metabolic syndrome, and cancer rates, which is linked to protracted exposure to abnormal internal milieu such as occurs with vitamin D deficiency. It is beyond the scope of this chapter to give a comprehensive review of the biology of both hormones. This chapter reviews the recent advances and interrelationship in the understanding of calcium, vitamin D, and PTH axis as they affect the process of stone formation in the kidney in health and diseases.

Vitamin D: Production, Metabolism, Transport, and Mechanism of Action

Production of Vitamin D

Vitamin D (calciferol) exists in two forms in nature: vitamin D_3 (cholecalciferol) and vitamin D_2 (ergocalciferol) in animal sources and plant sources, respectively. The main food sources of vitamin D are fatty fish, cod-liver oil, and to a lesser extent eggs. However, natural sources are generally unable to provide the recommended intake of vitamin, and food sources are variably fortified with vitamin D_3 or D_2 to fulfill body requirements [9].

The main source of vitamin D is provided by synthesis in skin, when exposed to ultraviolet B (UVB) rays in sunlight. UVB irradiation of 7-dehydrocholesterol (7DHC) within wavelengths of 290–310 nm produces previtamin D, which undergoes a thermally induced isomerization to vitamin D_3, lumisterol, and tachysterol. Vitamin D_3 so produced in the skin is stored in the plasma membrane of basal epidermal keratinocytes. Prolonged exposure to UVB does not produce toxic amounts of D_3, as previtamin D_3 is photolabile and easily isomerized to functionally inert lumisterol and tachysterol. In sunny countries, therefore, no more than 10–20 % of the initial previtamin D_3 concentrations may ultimately end up as vitamin D_3 [9, 24, 25].

Metabolism of Vitamin D

Vitamin D is biologically inert and is carried in blood, bound to vitamin D-binding protein (DBP). The first hydroxylation by cytochrome P450 enzymes takes place in the liver, giving rise to prohormone 25-hydroxyvitamin D (25-(OH)D). The 25-hydroxylation is not tightly regulated; the principal determinant of its rate is the circulating level of vitamin D. These enzymes have high capacity for substrate [26]. 25-(OH)D is then released into circulation to be carried to the proximal tubular epithelial cells of the kidney [9, 24, 25].

In the kidney, megalin-bound DBP carrying 25-(OH)D is taken by endocytic internalization into the proximal tubular epithelial cells from the tubular lumen [27, 28]. There it undergoes 1α(alpha)-hydroxylation to produce 1,25-$(OH)_2$D, which is the naturally occurring ligand for the vitamin D receptor

(VDR). The kidney is the richest source of 1α-hydroxylase enzyme (CYP27B1). The regulation of CYP27B1 in the proximal renal tubular cells is controlled by parathyroid hormone (PTH) and fibroblast growth factor 23 (FGF-23) [29, 30]. This enzyme is also found in a number of extrarenal sites including parathyroid cells, immune cells, and a variety of normal and malignant epithelia where it provides $1,25\text{-(OH)}_2D$ for intracrine or paracrine access to VDR in these cells. The activity of extrarenal CYP27B1 is governed by the availability of extracellular substrate 25-(OH)D to the enzyme and is immune to control by either PTH or FGF-23 [31, 32].

In the kidney, another enzyme 24-hydroxylase (CYP24) converts $1,25\text{-(OH)}_2D$ to $1,24,25\text{-(OH)}_3D$ and $24,25\text{-(OH)}_2D$. The 24-hydroxylated products are biologically inert and under feedback control of $1,25\text{-(OH)}_2D$ itself, thus providing negative feedback control of the amount of $1,25\text{-(OH)}_2D$ made in and released from the kidney [26].

Transport of Vitamin D

Vitamin D must be transported from its site of production in the skin and absorption from gut to the liver for 25-hydroxylation and then from liver to sites where 1α-hydroxylation by CYP27B1 can take place. Further for the genomic actions, $1,25\text{-(OH)}_2D$ is transported to tissues containing cells expressing VDR.

DBP is the specific chaperon for transport of vitamin D and its metabolites in serum. The serum DBP is a member of the albumin family of proteins, having high capacity and high affinity for 25-hydroxylated metabolites. It is synthesized in the liver and is freely filterable into the urine. It has a serum half-life of 2.5–3.0 days and is largely reclaimed from the urine after filtration. Reclamation is achieved by DBP being bound to megalin and cubulin, which are embedded in the plasma membrane of the proximal renal tubular epithelial cells, with eventual transcellular transport and return to the circulation through intracellular DBP chaperons [33].

Vitamin D_3 is rapidly deposited in adipose tissue where it becomes a long-term store, which is difficult to dislodge. Hence, one has to be cautious about giving patients large amounts of vitamin D, especially by intramuscular injections.

The main circulating form of vitamin D is 25-(OH)D. It is the best measure of vitamin D status. It has a long half-life (3 weeks). On the contrary, $1,25\text{-(OH)}_2D$ is present in small quantities and has a shorter half-life (4–6 h), but has 1,000 times greater affinity for VDR as compared to 25(OH)D [9].

Mechanism of Action

It is suggested that there exists a plasma membrane-anchored receptor for DBP. This receptor is endocytically internalized with intracellular chaperons moving $1,25\text{-(OH)}_2D$ to VDR. VDR functions as a heterodimer with the retinoid X receptor (RXR) for activation of vitamin D target genes. Once formed, the complex interacts with specific DNA sequences—the vitamin D response elements (VDRE)—within the promoter of target genes, resulting in either activation or suppression of transcription [34–37].

In the body, VDR is widespread, but the classic actions of $1,25\text{-(OH)}_2D$ involving regulation of calcium and phosphate occurs through VDR present in bone, gut, and kidney. In these actions, $1,25\text{-(OH)}_2D$ acts in concert with PTH and FGF-23, controlling regulation of CYP27B1 gene expression in proximal tubular cells at the level of transcription, with PTH as the major stimulator and FGF-23 as inhibitor of CYP27B1 gene, respectively. $1,25\text{-(OH)}_2D$ in turn suppresses PTH production directly by a transcriptional mechanism and indirectly by increasing serum calcium levels [38–41]. $1,25\text{-(OH)}_2D$ also increases the level of calcium-sensing receptor (CaSR) in the parathyroid gland further enhancing negative influence of calcium and $1,25\text{-(OH)}_2D$ on PTH secretion [42–44].

FGF-23, on the other hand, inhibits production of $1,25\text{-(OH)}_2D$ by the kidney while increasing the expression of CYP24, whereas $1,25\text{-(OH)}_2D$ stimulates FGF-23 production, which then downregulates CYP27B1 expression, thus completing the feedback loop. FGF-23 levels are also regulated through diet, with dietary Pi supplementation increasing and restriction suppressing FGF-23 levels [29, 30, 45, 46].

Calcium, Vitamin D, and Parathyroid Hormone: Physiological Aspects

Calcium Homeostasis: Role of Calcium-Sensing Receptor (CaSR)

Calcium concentration is maintained within narrow limits (1.1–1.3 mM) through an intricate homeostatic system made up of parathyroid glands, calcitonin-secreting C cells (of the thyroid gland), kidney, bone, and intestine. The key components of this system are the Ca-sensitive cells that work through the calcium-sensitive receptor (CaSR) to sense small perturbations in calcium concentration from normal and return calcium to its normal levels [47–49].

The principal structural domains in the CaSR protein include an amino acid extracellular domain (ECD), a seven membrane-spanning motif, and a carboxy-terminal(C-) tail. Within its intracellular loops and C-tail, the human CaSR harbors five predicted protein kinase C (PKC) sites. Activation of PKC diminishes CaSR-mediated stimulation of phospholipase C (PLC), conferring negative feedback regulation of CaSR-mediated stimulation of PLC [47, 50].

Parathyroid gland expresses the highest levels of CaSR mRNA and protein. Low calcium concentration stimulates PTH secretion, gene expression, and cellular proliferation. The increased PTH level enhances bone resorption liberating calcium and phosphate from the bone, enhances renal calcium reabsorption, and inhibits phosphate reabsorption. It also enhances activity of 1-alpha-hydroxylase to increase conversion of 25-(OH)D to 1,25-$(OH)_2D$, which then promotes intestinal calcium and phosphate reabsorption and increased reabsorption of filtered calcium along the nephron to restore ECF calcium to normal and to inhibit further production of PTH and 1,25-$(OH)_2D$ [47, 50, 51].

The opposite sequence of events occurs when extracellular fluid (ECF) calcium is raised. There is stimulation of renal CaSR, which suppresses the release of PTH and 1,25-$(OH)_2D$ thus decreasing skeletal calcium release and intestinal calcium reabsorption, thereby restoring the elevated ECF calcium to normal.

Physiology of Calcium Absorption and Transport in the Renal Tubule

The kidney plays a key role in calcium homeostasis, and PTH has a major role in fine adjustment of this important renal function.

Only free calcium and the calcium in complex with anions are filtered through the glomerulus. Proximal tubules reabsorb 60–70 % of the filtered calcium primarily through the paracellular pathway, which is governed by various physical forces affecting passive cation transport. A small fraction undergoes active absorption across the cells [52–54].

In medullary and cortical thick ascending limbs (TAL), approximately 20 % of calcium is absorbed through a cellular and paracellular route. Basal calcium absorption proceeds through the paracellular pathway, where its rate of movement is determined by prevailing electrochemical driving forces, which in turn are established by the extent of sodium absorption. The cellular component of calcium absorption in the thick limbs is regulated by PTH in the cortical TAL and by calcitonin in the medullary TAL [55, 56].

The distal convoluted tubules (DCT) and collecting tubules (CT) reabsorb 8–10 % of the filtered load. This absorption is active being stimulated by PTH and follows a transcellular route [55, 56].

Role of Parathyroid Hormone in Renal Calcium Absorption and Transport

Calcium reabsorption is actively regulated in the distal nephron according to the needs in the cortical TAL, DCT, and connecting segment under the influence of PTH. An increase in ionized calcium decreases PTH secretion, which in turn decreases tubular calcium reabsorption and increases calcium excretion thus restoring normocalcemia. The high serum calcium also contributes to calciuresis via CaSR [56].

In addition to its effect on calcium reabsorption, PTH inhibits mainly proximal tubular but also distal tubular reabsorption of phosphorus by inhibiting sodium-phosphate cotransporters in the luminal membrane of the proximal tubule.

PTH stimulates the synthesis of 1-alpha-hydroxylase in the proximal tubules and thus increases the conversion to 1,25-$(OH)_2D$. It also decreases the activity of 24-hydroxylase enzyme that inactivates 1,25-$(OH)_2D$. This is a particularly important action of PTH in maintaining calcium homeostasis in states of vitamin D deficiency [57, 58].

At both sites, PTH binds to the PTH receptor (PTHR) and enhances Ca reabsorption. In CTAL, this occurs by increasing the activity of Na/K/2Cl cotransporter that drives NaCl reabsorption and stimulates paracellular calcium and magnesium reabsorption. The CaSR is also present in the CTAL where increased ECF calcium activates phospholipase A2, reducing the activity of Na/K/2Cl cotransporter and that of an apical K channel thus decreasing paracellular calcium reabsorption. Raised ECF calcium antagonizes the effect of PTH in this nephron segment, and ECF calcium can in fact participate in this way in the regulation of its own homeostasis. Inhibition of NaCl reabsorption and loss of NaCl in the urine may contribute to the volume depletion seen in severe hypercalcemia [59–64].

In the DCT, CaSR modulates PTH-enhanced calcium reabsorption in response to extracellular calcium by modulating expression of key vitamin D inducible genes involved in transcellular transport in this segment of the nephron, like transient receptor potential channel (TRPV5); calbindin D_{28K} and the basolateral calcium pump; PMCA1b and sodium-calcium exchanger, NCX1. PTH markedly stimulates calcium reabsorption in the DCT primarily by augmenting NCX1 activity through a cyclic AMP-mediated mechanism [65, 66].

Role of Vitamin D in Renal Calcium Absorption and Transport

The active form of vitamin D, 1,25-$(OH)_2D$, enhances the actions of PTH on calcium transport in distal tubule cells by increasing PTH receptor mRNA and binding activity in distal tubule cells, by inducing the synthesis of calbindins and TRPV5 in the distal tubules.

It has been suggested that calbindin-D_{28k} stimulates the high-affinity system in the distal luminal membrane, and calbindin-D_{9k} enhances the ATP-dependent calcium transport of the basolateral membrane. An apical calcium channel,

TRPV5, which is co-localized with the calbindins and induced by 1,25-$(OH)_2D$, has been identified in the DCT and CT. Calbindin-D_{28k} is directly associated with TRPV5 and controls TRPV5-mediated calcium influx [27, 65, 67].

Vitamin D has been reported to increase or decrease renal phosphate reabsorption depending on the parathyroid status.

In calcium homeostasis, a major indirect function of 1,25-$(OH)_2D$ is to enhance mobilization of calcium stores when dietary calcium is sufficient to maintain a normal ECF calcium. As with PTH, 1,25-$(OH)_2D$ enhances osteoclastic bone resorption by binding to receptors in the preosteoblastic stromal cell and stimulating the RANK/RANKL system to enhance the proliferation, differentiation, and activation of the osteoclastic system from its monocytic precursors. Endogenous and exogenous 1,25-$(OH)_2D$ have also been reported to have an anabolic role in vivo [68].

Calcium, Vitamin D, and Parathyroid Hormone: Role in Lithogenesis

Calcium is a major component of 85 % of kidney stones, largely as either calcium oxalate or calcium phosphate. Risk factors leading to calcium nephrolithiasis include low urinary volume, hypercalciuria, hyperoxaluria, hypocitraturia, and hyperuricosuria. High urinary calcium concentrations, which may be due to increased calcium excretion, low urinary volume, or both, produce supersaturation of urine with calcium salts in the DT and urine, leading to crystal formation. Dietary calcium has a protective role on stone formation by increasing the calcium oxalate binding in the gut thus decreasing absorption of oxalate.

Vitamin D Replacement Therapy and Stone

Associative studies have described various disease states with deficiency of vitamin D and improved patient outcomes with the use of vitamin D therapies. Calcium along with vitamin D has been recognized as a necessary supplement for the prevention of osteoporotic fracture in postmenopausal women. However, calcium and vitamin D supplementation is not always benign, and a 17 % increase in the formation of new stones has been reported in the Women's Health Initiative CaD supplementation trial, suggesting a possible causative role for CaD supplementation use [4]. There are limited randomized, controlled trials as to the best practice in the timing, dosage, and follow-up of administration of vitamin D and its implication in the production of nephrolithiasis. Nonetheless, it is expected that improved understanding will come through applying recent development of both basic science and translational work evolving in the field. New insights on the role of vitamin D-PTH axis are being identified in the pathophysiology of the diseases associated with nephrolithiasis.

Idiopathic Hypercalciuria

In industrialized nations with a heavy intake of calcium, the single most common cause of calcium oxalate stones is hypercalciuria, seen in one third of the patients [2]. Hypercalciuria is an accepted cause of stones in industrialized countries with calcium-rich diets fortified with vitamin D [4]. Idiopathic hypercalciuria (IH) is the commonest metabolic abnormality in patients with renal calcium stones, characterized by excess calcium excretion above 250 mg/day (6.25 mmol) in women and 300 mg/day (7.5 mmol) in men with no identifiable metabolic cause and normal calcium levels [5, 69]. IH can be found in up to 40 % of stone formers, but has an incidence of <10 % in the overall population. Patients with hypercalciuria have a family history of nephrolithiasis in 69 % suggesting a genetic basis of the disease. But IH has a complex polygenic trait. Ninety percent of IH patients never form a kidney stone, but in these patients, a further increase in urine calcium oxalate supersaturation from calcium supplements would enhance the risk of stone formation [7, 70, 71].

In IH, a generalized increase in calcium turnover is seen caused by dysregulation of calcium transport in intestine, kidney, and bone, giving rise to major subtypes of IH: absorptive, renal leak, and resorptive hypercalciuria, respectively [72, 73]. Radiolabeled calcium studies have demonstrated an excessive absorption of calcium by the intestine in almost all patients with IH. While studies assessing the net calcium absorption using controlled diets demonstrate that urine calcium is higher than net absorption, suggesting that some of the urine calcium is being derived from bone, leading to abnormal bone mineral wasting in IH [74].

The pathogenic mechanism is linked to high 1,25-$(OH)_2D$ levels seen in IH patients as compared to controls. 1,25-$(OH)_2D$ is believed to upregulate expression of calcium transport proteins in the intestine including the apical calcium channel, TRPV6. In addition, an altered tissue vitamin D response has been reported by several studies [75, 76]. Studies on VDR levels have also suggested an increased number of VDR in patients with IH. Genetic hypercalciuric stone-forming (GHS) rats, like humans with IH, have a systemic abnormality in calcium homeostasis. Though 1,25-$(OH)_2D$ levels are normal in GHS rats, significantly high levels of VDR are found in bone, kidney, and intestine compared to normal rats, explaining the increased sensitivity to 1,25-$(OH)_2D$ in tissues of GHS rats [74, 77, 78]. In the gut, vitamin D-responsive genes are expressed at increased levels in response to small doses of 1,25-$(OH)_2D$ with consequent increased expression of protein related to calcium homeostasis such as TRPV6 in the gut, calbindins, and CaSR [79, 80].

In genetic hypercalciuric stone-forming (GHS) rats, an increased number of vitamin D receptors may be the underlying mechanism. Studies have reported an increased number of VDR in monocytes of humans with IH.

Primary Hyperparathyroidism

Primary hyperparathyroidism is reported as the most common cause of hypercalcemia in many surveys. Together with malignancy it accounts for 90 % of hypercalcemic patients. It is a relatively common endocrine disorder, with an incidence as high as 1 in 500 to 1 in 1,000 [81–84].

Primary hyperparathyroidism (PHPT) is caused by parathyroid adenoma in 80 % of the cases. Less commonly, it is caused by hyperplasia of all four parathyroid glands [85]. The pathophysiology of primary hyperparathyroidism relates to the loss of normal feedback control of PTH by extracellular calcium and a reduced sensitivity to extracellular calcium [86, 87]. The clonal origin of most parathyroid adenomas suggests a defect at the level of gene controlling growth of the parathyroid cell or the expression of PTH. Patients with primary hyperparathyroidism have been discovered in whom the PTH gene is rearranged to a site adjacent to the cell cycle regulator, cyclin D1 gene, leading to over expression. Other genes that are under study for a possible role in the development of primary hyperparathyroidism are the CaSR gene, VDR gene, and RET [88, 89].

Introduction of multichannel analyzers in the 1970s by which serum calcium and phosphorus levels were routinely measured resulted in the detection of many asymptomatic hyperparathyroid patients with mild hypercalcemia. This method identified several asymptomatic hypercalcemic individuals with primary hyperparathyroidism and a four- to fivefold increase in incidence. Nowadays, lack of overt elevation of calcium has been shown in many patients with primary hyperparathyroidism, and this phenomenon is well known in literature as normocalcemic primary hyperparathyroidism (NCPHPT) based on normal serum total calcium levels [90, 91].

In early 1970s, a more rapid growth of adenomas was linked to deficiency of vitamin D. PHPT patients with bone disease had a greater degree of vitamin D deficiency and threefold greater PTH values than PHPT patients with stone disease. An inverse correlation between 25-(OH)D and PTH in healthy as well as patient populations is widely recognized nowadays [92]. An inverse correlation between 25-(OH)D and parathyroid gland weight has been reported by Rao et al., while the correlation between 1,25-$(OH)_2$D and PTH was not significant [93]. These results suggest stimulation of parathyroid adenoma growth by suboptimal vitamin D status. Presence of 1-alpha-hydroxylase has been demonstrated in parathyroid cells suggesting a direct effect of 25-(OH)D on PTH secretion and parathyroid gland growth. Decreased 25-(OH)D levels in primary hyperparathyroidism are also linked to increased conversion to 1,25-$(OH)_2$D [93].

Vitamin D deficiency/insufficiency is nowadays regarded as pandemic. Studies from China and India reported an association of large parathyroid adenomas with vitamin D deficiency and insufficiency. Silverberg reported improvement in osteitis fibrosa, decrease in levels of PTH, and reduction in parathyroid adenoma weights after improving the vitamin D status. The bone disease was more severe in those with concomitant vitamin D deficiency regardless of the clinical severity of primary hyperparathyroidism [94]. Second, vitamin D deficiency and insufficiency seem to be more prevalent in patients with primary hyperparathyroidism than in geographically matched populations. Coexisting vitamin D deficiency may cause the serum calcium level to fall into the normal range, which can lead to diagnostic uncertainty. In such patients, it is particularly important to rule out vitamin D insufficiency, which can lower serum calcium levels into the normal range. Reevaluation of these individuals after optimization of 25-(OH)D levels, and/or after correction of other secondary causes of hyperparathyroidism, is necessary to secure the diagnosis [95–97].

Tertiary Hyperparathyroidism

Hypercalcemic hyperparathyroidism due to autonomous function of parathyroid tissue is usually the outcome of long-standing secondary hyperparathyroidism and is characterized by a lack of suppression of PTH by calcium or vitamin D analogues. CaSR underexpression results in an increase in parathyroid hormone secretory set point and a depletion of VDR [98, 99]. The most common cause of tertiary hyperparathyroidism is long-standing chronic kidney disease. It can also occur in patients with X-linked hypophosphatemic rickets and adult-onset (autosomal) dominant hypophosphatemic rickets/osteomalacia in which long-term treatment with phosphate and vitamin D stimulates parathyroid secretion producing hypercalcemic hyperparathyroidism. High-dose oral phosphate increases plasma phosphate, causing a transient decrease in ionized calcium and a decrease in 1,25-$(OH)_2$D levels [100, 101]. A similar picture is observed in oncogenic osteomalacia treated with phosphate and vitamin D. FGF-23 also plays a role by suppressing 1,25-$(OH)_2$D production [30, 102].

1,25-$(OH)_2$D-Induced Hypercalcemia

Vitamin D intoxication is caused by increased ingestion of one of its metabolites, or as a result of inappropriate overproduction of 1,25-$(OH)_2$D by lymphoproliferative and granulomatous disorders like sarcoidosis and tuberculosis, or by overexpression of the enzyme 1-alpha-hydroxylase. This results in intestinal hyperabsorption of calcium, hypercalciuria, and finally hypercalcemia.

In case of intoxication by regular vitamin D, the pathogenesis is not completely clear. Despite marked increases in concentration of 25-(OH)D, serum levels of active vitamin D are normal. The postulated mechanism includes competition by high serum 25-(OH)D for binding sites on VDR or DBP. In addition, extrarenal activation of 25-(OH)D by local 1-alpha-hydroxylase in bone and intestine can give rise to hypercalcemia [103].

In granulomatous disorder, the overproduction is not under feedback control. The production of active vitamin D depends on availability of substrate. A positive correlation is seen in these conditions between 25-(OH)D and 1,25-$(OH)_2$D [103–105].

Conclusion

The bulk of the epidemiologic evidence underscores the importance of vitamin D and PTH in the development of nephrocalcinosis and renal stones. In addition, studies to determine the impact of fixed dosage regimens of vitamin D, versus targeting values, in large populations would be beneficial in the face of the emerging newer role of vitamin D-PTH axis.

References

1. Serio A, Fraioli A. Epidemiology of nephrolithiasis. Nephron. 1999;81 Suppl 1:26–30.
2. Stamatelou KK, Francis ME, Jones CA, Nyberg LM, Curhan GC. Time trends in reported prevalence of kidney stones in the United States: 1976–1994. Kidney Int. 2003;63(5):1817–23.
3. Jackson RD, LaCroix AZ, Gass M, Wallace RB, Robbins J, Lewis CE, et al. Calcium plus vitamin D supplementation and the risk of fractures. N Engl J Med. 2006;354(7):669–83.
4. Wallace RB, Wactawski-Wende J, O'Sullivan MJ, Larson JC, Cochrane B, Gass M, et al. Urinary tract stone occurrence in the Women's Health Initiative (WHI) randomized clinical trial of calcium and vitamin D supplements. Am J Clin Nutr. 2011;94(1):270–7.
5. Frick KK, Bushinsky DA. Molecular mechanisms of primary hypercalciuria. J Am Soc Nephrol. 2003,14(4):1082–95.
6. Cameron MA, Sakhaee K, Moe OW. Nephrolithiasis in children. Pediatr Nephrol. 2005;20(11):1587–92.
7. Moe OW, Bonny O. Genetic hypercalciuria. J Am Soc Nephrol. 2005;16(3):729–45.
8. Potts JT. Parathyroid hormone: past and present. J Endocrinol. 2005;187(3):311–25.
9. Holick MF. Vitamin D deficiency. N Engl J Med. 2007;357(3): 266–81.
10. Liu PT, Stenger S, Li H, Wenzel L, Tan BH, Krutzik SR, et al. Toll-like receptor triggering of a vitamin D-mediated human antimicrobial response. Science. 2006;311(5768):1770–3.
11. Gombart AF, Borregaard N, Koeffler HP. Human cathelicidin antimicrobial peptide (CAMP) gene is a direct target of the vitamin D receptor and is strongly up-regulated in myeloid cells by 1,25-dihydroxyvitamin D_3. FASEB J. 2005;19(9):1067–77.
12. Provvedini DM, Tsoukas CD, Deftos LJ, Manolagas SC. 1,25-dihydroxyvitamin D_3 receptors in human leukocytes. Science. 1983;221(4616):1181–3.
13. Clark SA, Stumpf WE, Sar M, DeLuca HF, Tanaka Y. Target cells for 1,25 dihydroxyvitamin D_3 in the pancreas. Cell Tissue Res. 1980;209(3):515–20.
14. Rook GA, Steele J, Fraher L, Barker S, Karmali R, O'Riordan J, et al. Vitamin D_3, gamma interferon, and control of proliferation of Mycobacterium tuberculosis by human monocytes. Immunology. 1986;57(1):159–63.
15. Wang TT, Nestel FP, Bourdeau V, Nagai Y, Wang Q, Liao J, et al. Cutting edge: 1,25-dihydroxyvitamin D_3 is a direct inducer of antimicrobial peptide gene expression. J Immunol. 2004;173(5):2909–12.
16. Weber G, Heilborn JD, Chamorro Jimenez CI, Hammarsjo A, Torma H, Stahle M. Vitamin D induces the antimicrobial protein hCAP18 in human skin. J Invest Dermatol. 2005;124(5):1080–2.
17. Medzhitov R. Recognition of microorganisms and activation of the immune response. Nature. 2007;449(7164):819–26.
18. Kreutz M, Andreesen R, Krause SW, Szabo A, Ritz E, Reichel H. 1,25-dihydroxyvitamin D_3 production and vitamin D_3 receptor expression are developmentally regulated during differentiation of human monocytes into macrophages. Blood. 1993;82(4):1300–7.
19. Penna G, Adorini L. 1 Alpha,25-dihydroxyvitamin D_3 inhibits differentiation, maturation, activation, and survival of dendritic cells leading to impaired alloreactive T cell activation. J Immunol. 2000;164(5):2405–11.
20. Penna G, Amuchastegui S, Giarratana N, Daniel KC, Vulcano M, Sozzani S, et al. 1,25-Dihydroxyvitamin D_3 selectively modulates tolerogenic properties in myeloid but not plasmacytoid dendritic cells. J Immunol. 2007;178(1):145–53.
21. Boonen S, Lips P, Bouillon R, Bischoff-Ferrari HA, Vanderschueren D, Haentjens P. Need for additional calcium to reduce the risk of hip fracture with vitamin d supplementation: evidence from a comparative metaanalysis of randomized controlled trials. J Clin Endocrinol Metab. 2007;92(4):1415–23.
22. Tang BM, Eslick GD, Nowson C, Smith C, Bensoussan A. Use of calcium or calcium in combination with vitamin D supplementation to prevent fractures and bone loss in people aged 50 years and older: a meta-analysis. Lancet. 2007;370(9588):657–66.
23. Fraser WD. Hyperparathyroidism. Lancet. 2009;374(9684):145–58.
24. Holick MF, MacLaughlin JA, Clark MB, Holick SA, Potts Jr JT, Anderson RR, et al. Photosynthesis of previtamin D_3 in human skin and the physiologic consequences. Science. 1980;210(4466):203–5.
25. Holick MF, Uskokovic M, Henley JW, MacLaughlin J, Holick SA, Potts Jr JT. The photoproduction of 1 alpha,25-dihydroxyvitamin D_3 in skin: an approach to the therapy of vitamin-D-resistant syndromes. N Engl J Med. 1980;303(7):349–54.
26. Omdahl JL, Bobrovnikova EA, Choe S, Dwivedi PP, May BK. Overview of regulatory cytochrome P450 enzymes of the vitamin D pathway. Steroids. 2001;66(3–5):381–9.
27. Hoenderop JG, Nilius B, Bindels RJ. Epithelial calcium channels: from identification to function and regulation. Pflugers Arch. 2003;446(3):304–8.
28. Hoenderop JG, van Leeuwen JP, van der Eerden BC, Kersten FF, van der Kemp AW, Merillat AM, et al. Renal Ca^{2+} wasting, hyperabsorption, and reduced bone thickness in mice lacking TRPV5. J Clin Invest. 2003;112(12):1906–14.
29. Perwad F, Azam N, Zhang MY, Yamashita T, Tenenhouse HS, Portale AA. Dietary and serum phosphorus regulate fibroblast growth factor 23 expression and 1,25-dihydroxyvitamin D metabolism in mice. Endocrinology. 2005;146(12):5358–64.
30. Shimada T, Hasegawa H, Yamazaki Y, Muto T, Hino R, Takeuchi Y, et al. FGF-23 is a potent regulator of vitamin D metabolism and phosphate homeostasis. J Bone Miner Res. 2004;19(3):429–35.

31. Hewison M, Burke F, Evans KN, Lammas DA, Sansom DM, Liu P, et al. Extra-renal 25-hydroxyvitamin D_3-1alpha-hydroxylase in human health and disease. J Steroid Biochem Mol Biol. 2007; 103(3–5):316–21.
32. Zierold C, Darwish HM, DeLuca HF. Two vitamin D response elements function in the rat 1,25-dihydroxyvitamin D 24-hydroxylase promoter. J Biol Chem. 1995;270(4):1675–8.
33. Cooke NE, Haddad JG. Vitamin D binding protein (Gc-globulin). Endocr Rev. 1989;10(3):294–307.
34. Christakos S, Dhawan P, Liu Y, Peng X, Porta A. New insights into the mechanisms of vitamin D action. J Cell Biochem. 2003; 88(4):695–705.
35. DeLuca HF. Overview of general physiologic features and functions of vitamin D. Am J Clin Nutr. 2004;80(6 Suppl):1689S–96.
36. Rachez C, Freedman LP. Mechanisms of gene regulation by vitamin D(3) receptor: a network of coactivator interactions. Gene. 2000;246(1–2):9–21.
37. Sutton AL, MacDonald PN. Vitamin D: more than a "bone-a-fide" hormone. Mol Endocrinol. 2003;17(5):777–91.
38. Li YC, Pirro AE, Amling M, Delling G, Baron R, Bronson R, et al. Targeted ablation of the vitamin D receptor: an animal model of vitamin D-dependent rickets type II with alopecia. Proc Natl Acad Sci USA. 1997;94(18):9831–5.
39. Sneddon WB, Barry EL, Coutermarsh BA, Gesek FA, Liu F, Friedman PA. Regulation of renal parathyroid hormone receptor expression by 1, 25-dihydroxyvitamin D_3 and retinoic acid. Cell Physiol Biochem. 1998;8(5):261–77.
40. Lambers TT, Weidema AF, Nilius B, Hoenderop JG, Bindels RJ. Regulation of the mouse epithelial Ca2(+) channel TRPV6 by the Ca(2+)-sensor calmodulin. J Biol Chem. 2004;279(28):28855–61.
41. Demay MB, Kiernan MS, DeLuca HF, Kronenberg HM. Sequences in the human parathyroid hormone gene that bind the 1,25-dihydroxyvitamin D_3 receptor and mediate transcriptional repression in response to 1,25-dihydroxyvitamin D_3. Proc Natl Acad Sci USA. 1992;89(17):8097–101.
42. Brown AJ, Zhong M, Ritter C, Brown EM, Slatopolsky E. Loss of calcium responsiveness in cultured bovine parathyroid cells is associated with decreased calcium receptor expression. Biochem Biophys Res Commun. 1995;212(3):861–7.
43. Brown AJ, Zhong M, Finch J, Ritter C, Slatopolsky E. The roles of calcium and 1,25-dihydroxyvitamin D_3 in the regulation of vitamin D receptor expression by rat parathyroid glands. Endocrinology. 1995;136(4):1419–25.
44. Hauache OM. Extracellular calcium-sensing receptor: structural and functional features and association with diseases. Braz J Med Biol Res. 2001;34(5):577–84.
45. Larsson T, Marsell R, Schipani E, Ohlsson C, Ljunggren O, Tenenhouse HS, et al. Transgenic mice expressing fibroblast growth factor 23 under the control of the alpha1(I) collagen promoter exhibit growth retardation, osteomalacia, and disturbed phosphate homeostasis. Endocrinology. 2004;145(7):3087–94.
46. Burnett SM, Gunawardene SC, Bringhurst FR, Juppner H, Lee H, Finkelstein JS. Regulation of C-terminal and intact FGF-23 by dietary phosphate in men and women. J Bone Miner Res. 2006; 21(8):1187–96.
47. Brown EM, MacLeod RJ. Extracellular calcium sensing and extracellular calcium signaling. Physiol Rev. 2001;81(1):239–97.
48. Brown EM. Mechanisms underlying the regulation of parathyroid hormone secretion in vivo and in vitro. Curr Opin Nephrol Hypertens. 1993;2(4):541–51.
49. Brown EM, Gamba G, Riccardi D, Lombardi M, Butters R, Kifor O, et al. Cloning and characterization of an extracellular Ca(2+)-sensing receptor from bovine parathyroid. Nature. 1993;366(6455):575–80.
50. Berridge MJ, Bootman MD, Roderick HL. Calcium signalling: dynamics, homeostasis and remodelling. Nat Rev Mol Cell Biol. 2003;4(7):517–29.
51. Brown EM. Extracellular Ca^{2+} sensing, regulation of parathyroid cell function, and role of Ca^{2+} and other ions as extracellular (first) messengers. Physiol Rev. 1991;71(2):371–411.
52. Ng RC, Rouse D, Suki WN. Calcium transport in the rabbit superficial proximal convoluted tubule. J Clin Invest. 1984; 74(3):834–42.
53. Bomsztyk K, George JP, Wright FS. Effects of luminal fluid anions on calcium transport by proximal tubule. Am J Physiol. 1984;246(5 Pt 2):F600–8.
54. Ullrich KJ, Rumrich G, Kloss S. Active Ca^{2+} reabsorption in the proximal tubule of the rat kidney. Dependence on sodium- and buffer transport. Pflugers Arch. 1976;364(3):223–8.
55. Bourdeau JE, Burg MB. Effect of PTH on calcium transport across the cortical thick ascending limb of Henle's loop. Am J Physiol. 1980;239(2):F121–6.
56. Suki WN, Rouse D. Hormonal regulation of calcium transport in thick ascending limb renal tubules. Am J Physiol. 1981;241(2):F171–4.
57. Silver J, Elstein D. Regulation of 25-OH-D3 1 alpha-hydroxylase and 24-hydroxylase activities along the rat nephron and in isolated kidney cells. Miner Electrolyte Metab. 1985;11(3):173–7.
58. Okazaki T, Igarashi T, Kronenberg HM. 5'-flanking region of the parathyroid hormone gene mediates negative regulation by 1,25-(OH)2 vitamin D_3. J Biol Chem. 1988;263(5):2203–8.
59. Ba J, Friedman PA. Calcium-sensing receptor regulation of renal mineral ion transport. Cell Calcium. 2004;35(3):229–37.
60. Maiti A, Beckman MJ. Extracellular calcium is a direct effecter of VDR levels in proximal tubule epithelial cells that counter-balances effects of PTH on renal Vitamin D metabolism. J Steroid Biochem Mol Biol. 2007;103(3–5):504–8.
61. Hebert SC, Brown EM, Harris HW. Role of the Ca(2+)-sensing receptor in divalent mineral ion homeostasis. J Exp Biol. 1997; 200(Pt 2):295–302.
62. Thebault S, Hoenderop JG, Bindels RJ. Epithelial Ca^{2+} and Mg^{2+} channels in kidney disease. Adv Chronic Kidney Dis. 2006; 13(2):110–7.
63. Hoenderop JG, van der Kemp AW, Hartog A, van Os CH, Willems PH, Bindels RJ. The epithelial calcium channel, ECaC, is activated by hyperpolarization and regulated by cytosolic calcium. Biochem Biophys Res Commun. 1999;261(2):488–92.
64. Hoenderop JG, De Pont JJ, Bindels RJ, Willems PH. Hormone-stimulated Ca^{2+} reabsorption in rabbit kidney cortical collecting system is cAMP-independent and involves a phorbol ester-insensitive PKC isotype. Kidney Int. 1999;55(1):225–33.
65. Wasserman RH, Fullmer CS. Vitamin D and intestinal calcium transport: facts, speculations and hypotheses. J Nutr. 1995;125(7 Suppl):1971S–9.
66. Pannabecker TL, Chandler JS, Wasserman RH. Vitamin-D-dependent transcriptional regulation of the intestinal plasma membrane calcium pump. Biochem Biophys Res Commun. 1995;213(2): 499–505.
67. Peng JB, Chen XZ, Berger UV, Vassilev PM, Tsukaguchi H, Brown EM, et al. Molecular cloning and characterization of a channel-like transporter mediating intestinal calcium absorption. J Biol Chem. 1999;274(32):22739–46.
68. Raisz LG, Trummel CL, Holick MF, DeLuca HF. 1,25-dihydroxycholecalciferol: a potent stimulator of bone resorption in tissue culture. Science. 1972;175(23):768–9.
69. Scheinman SJ. Nephrolithiasis. Semin Nephrol. 1999;19(4): 381–8.
70. Schwarz RD, Dwyer NT. Pediatric kidney stones: long-term outcomes. Urology. 2006;67(4):812–6.
71. Resnick M, Pridgen DB, Goodman HO. Genetic predisposition to formation of calcium oxalate renal calculi. N Engl J Med. 1968;278(24):1313–8.
72. Henneman PH, Benedict PH, Forbes AP, Dudley HR. Idiopathic hypercaicuria. N Engl J Med. 1958;259(17):802–7.

73. Coe FL, Parks JH, Moore ES. Familial idiopathic hypercalciuria. N Engl J Med. 1979;300(7):337–40.
74. Bushinsky DA. Recurrent hypercalciuric nephrolithiasis – does diet help? N Engl J Med. 2002;346(2):124–5.
75. Maierhofer WJ, Gray RW, Cheung HS, Lemann Jr J. Bone resorption stimulated by elevated serum 1,25-(OH)2-vitamin D concentrations in healthy men. Kidney Int. 1983;24(4):555–60.
76. Adams ND, Gray RW, Lemann Jr J, Cheung HS. Effects of calcitriol administration on calcium metabolism healthy men. Kidney Int. 1982;21(1):90–7.
77. Bushinsky DA, Frick KK, Nehrke K. Genetic hypercalciuric stone-forming rats. Curr Opin Nephrol Hypertens. 2006;15(4):403–18.
78. Bushinsky DA, Asplin JR, Grynpas MD, Evan AP, Parker WR, Alexander KM, et al. Calcium oxalate stone formation in genetic hypercalciuric stone-forming rats. Kidney Int. 2002;61(3):975–87.
79. Li XQ, Tembe V, Horwitz GM, Bushinsky DA, Favus MJ. Increased intestinal vitamin D receptor in genetic hypercalciuric rats. A cause of intestinal calcium hyperabsorption. J Clin Invest. 1993;91(2):661–7.
80. Yao J, Kathpalia P, Bushinsky DA, Favus MJ. Hyperresponsiveness of vitamin D receptor gene expression to 1,25-dihydroxyvitamin D_3. A new characteristic of genetic hypercalciuric stone-forming rats. J Clin Invest. 1998;101(10):2223–32.
81. Melton 3rd LJ. The epidemiology of primary hyperparathyroidism in North America. J Bone Miner Res. 2002;17 Suppl 2:N12–7.
82. Phitayakorn R, McHenry CR. Incidence and location of ectopic abnormal parathyroid glands. Am J Surg. 2006;191(3):418–23.
83. Wermers RA, Khosla S, Atkinson EJ, Hodgson SF, O'Fallon WM, Melton 3rd LJ. The rise and fall of primary hyperparathyroidism: a population-based study in Rochester, Minnesota, 1965–1992. Ann Intern Med. 1997;126(6):433–40.
84. Adami S, Marcocci C, Gatti D. Epidemiology of primary hyperparathyroidism in Europe. J Bone Miner Res. 2002;17 Suppl 2:N18–23.
85. Mundy GR, Cove DH, Fisken R. Primary hyperparathyroidism: changes in the pattern of clinical presentation. Lancet. 1980; 1(8182):1317–20.
86. Thakker RV. Diseases associated with the extracellular calcium-sensing receptor. Cell Calcium. 2004;35(3):275–82.
87. Khosla S, Ebeling PR, Firek AF, Burritt MM, Kao PC, Heath 3rd H. Calcium infusion suggests a "set-point" abnormality of parathyroid gland function in familial benign hypercalcemia and more complex disturbances in primary hyperparathyroidism. J Clin Endocrinol Metab. 1993;76(3):715–20.
88. Farnebo F, Enberg U, Grimelius L, Backdahl M, Schalling M, Larsson C, et al. Tumor-specific decreased expression of calcium sensing receptor messenger ribonucleic acid in sporadic primary hyperparathyroidism. J Clin Endocrinol Metab. 1997;82(10):3481–6.
89. Garner SC, Hinson TK, McCarty KS, Leight M, Leight Jr GS, Quarles LD. Quantitative analysis of the calcium-sensing receptor messenger RNA in parathyroid adenomas. Surgery. 1997;122(6):1166–75.
90. Silverberg SJ, Shane E, Jacobs TP, Siris E, Bilezikian JP. A 10-year prospective study of primary hyperparathyroidism with or without parathyroid surgery. N Engl J Med. 1999;341(17):1249–55.
91. Mazzaglia PJ, Berber E, Kovach A, Milas M, Esselstyn C, Siperstein AE. The changing presentation of hyperparathyroidism over 3 decades. Arch Surg. 2008;143(3):260–6.
92. Mansoor S, Habib A, Ghani F, Fatmi Z, Badruddin S, Siddiqui I, et al. Prevalence and significance of vitamin D deficiency and insufficiency among apparently healthy adults. Clin Biochem. 2010;43(18):1431–5.
93. Rao DS, Agarwal G, Talpos GB, Phillips ER, Bandeira F, Mishra SK, et al. Role of vitamin D and calcium nutrition in disease expression and parathyroid tumor growth in primary hyperparathyroidism: a global perspective. J Bone Miner Res. 2002;17 Suppl 2:N75–80.
94. Silverberg SJ, Shane E, Dempster DW, Bilezikian JP. The effects of vitamin D insufficiency in patients with primary hyperparathyroidism. Am J Med. 1999;107(6):561–7.
95. Jesudason D, Need AG, Horowitz M, O'Loughlin PD, Morris HA, Nordin BE. Relationship between serum 25-hydroxyvitamin D and bone resorption markers in vitamin D insufficiency. Bone. 2002;31(5):626–30.
96. Vieth R, Ladak Y, Walfish PG. Age-related changes in the 25-hydroxyvitamin D versus parathyroid hormone relationship suggest a different reason why older adults require more vitamin D. J Clin Endocrinol Metab. 2003;88(1):185–91.
97. Malabanan A, Veronikis IE, Holick MF. Redefining vitamin D insufficiency. Lancet. 1998;351(9105):805–6.
98. Grzela T, Chudzinski W, Lasiecka Z, Niderla J, Wilczynski G, Gornicka B, et al. The calcium-sensing receptor and vitamin D receptor expression in tertiary hyperparathyroidism. Int J Mol Med. 2006;17(5):779–83.
99. Kebebew E, Duh QY, Clark OH. Tertiary hyperparathyroidism: histologic patterns of disease and results of parathyroidectomy. Arch Surg. 2004;139(9):974–7.
100. Knudtzon J, Halse J, Monn E, Nesland A, Nordal KP, Paus P, et al. Autonomous hyperparathyroidism in X-linked hypophosphataemia. Clin Endocrinol (Oxf). 1995;42(2):199–203.
101. Rivkees SA, El-Hajj-Fuleihan G, Brown EM, Crawford JD. Tertiary hyperparathyroidism during high phosphate therapy of familial hypophosphatemic rickets. J Clin Endocrinol Metab. 1992;75(6):1514–8.
102. Huang QL, Feig DS, Blackstein ME. Development of tertiary hyperparathyroidism after phosphate supplementation in oncogenic osteomalacia. J Endocrinol Invest. 2000;23(4):263–7.
103. Lips P. Relative value of 25(OH)D and 1,25(OH)2D measurements. J Bone Miner Res. 2007;22(11):1668–71.
104. Barbour GL, Coburn JW, Slatopolsky E, Norman AW, Horst RL. Hypercalcemia in an anephric patient with sarcoidosis: evidence for extrarenal generation of 1,25-dihydroxyvitamin D. N Engl J Med. 1981;305(8):440–3.
105. Davies M, Mawer EB, Hayes ME, Lumb GA. Abnormal vitamin D metabolism in Hodgkin's lymphoma. Lancet. 1985;1(8439): 1186–8.

Current Understanding of the Role of Randall's Plaque

25

Jessica A. Mandeville, Ehud Gnessin, and James E. Lingeman

Abstract

The mechanisms by which urinary calculi develop in humans are not entirely understood. In the 1930s, Randall described white plaques on the papillae of cadaveric kidneys from patients with calculi and postulated that this was the site of stone formation in all stone formers. His theory was not well received and for many years was abandoned. It is now known that in certain subsets of stone formers (idiopathic calcium oxalate stone formers), stone formation does occur by overgrowth on Randall's plaque. However, many other types of stone formers do not demonstrate evidence of classic Randall's plaque and must therefore possess a different mechanism for stone formation. Careful endoscopic assessment and renal tissue biopsies from unique stone-forming patients (i.e., those with cystinuria, primary hyperparathyroidism, renal tubular acidosis, and primary hyperoxaluria) has revealed evidence of crystalline plugging within dilated ducts of Bellini with associated inflammation and cell injury. These findings are not identified in idiopathic calcium oxalate stone formers and lead one to believe that alternate pathways to the development of nephrolithiasis must be at play. In this chapter we review the composition and anatomic location of Randall's plaque as well as describe the stone-plaque interface and mechanism of stone overgrowth. Additionally, we review the specific endoscopic and histologic abnormalities in stone-forming patients with cystinuria, brushite stone disease, gastric bypass, ileostomy, primary hyperparathyroidism, renal tubular acidosis, and primary hyperoxaluria and propose potential mechanisms for stone formation.

Keywords

Randall's plaque • Nephrolithiasis • Calcium oxalate • Cystinuria • Brushite • Primary hyperparathyroidism • Renal tubular acidosis • Primary hyperoxaluria • Ducts of Bellini

Introduction

Original Description of Randall's Plaque

In the late 1930s, Alexander Randall proposed that kidney stones grew on the renal papilla attached to underlying deposits or "plaques." Randall examined more than 1,100 cadaveric kidneys, by opening the renal pelvis and carefully examining each papilla with a lens. During these evaluations, he observed white-colored areas on the papillary tips in approximately 20.5 % of the renal units. These white plaques appeared to lie underneath the surface of the urothelium, and

J.A. Mandeville, M.D. • E. Gnessin, M.D. • J.E. Lingeman, M.D. (✉)
Department of Urology, Indiana University Health,
1801 North Senate Boulevard, Suite 220,
Indianapolis, IN 46202, USA
e-mail: jmandevi@iuhealth.org; egnessin@iupui.edu;
jlingeman@iuhealth.org

J.J. Talati et al. (eds.), *Urolithiasis*,
DOI 10.1007/978-1-4471-4387-1_25,

further evaluation of these papillary lesions with light microscopy suggested that they were located within the interstitium of the kidney. Chemical analysis of the plaques revealed the presence of calcium, nitrogen, carbon dioxide, and phosphorous [1, 2].

In addition to the presence of the calcium-containing plaques, Randall also noted that in some of the renal units, small stones were firmly attached to the areas of plaque. After further evaluating the attached stones, he observed that these calculi appeared to be growing from the interstitial calcium plaque. Additionally, some areas of plaque were noted to have no overlying urothelium and were therefore exposed to urine within the calyx. Finally, he identified some detached stones that had phosphate-containing areas on their surface, which could have potentially represented prior sites of attachment to calcium plaques [1, 2].

Despite the importance of these findings, Randall's theory that stones formed attached to papillary plaques was not widely accepted for several reasons. First, he did not have the necessary technology to determine the exact mineral composition of the papillary plaques nor the composition of mineral at the plaque-stone interface. Second, he proposed that *all* types of kidney stones formed by overgrowth on plaques. His theory was widely disregarded, and it was not until recently that his ideas were reevaluated with regard to the formation of kidney stones. It is now quite clear that Randall's plaque plays an important part in calculus formation in a certain subset of stone formers, namely, idiopathic calcium oxalate stone formers (i.e., calcium oxalate stone formers without evidence of systemic, stone-forming diseases such as primary hyperparathyroidism, distal renal tubular acidosis, sarcoidosis, bowel disease/resection/bypass, or medullary sponge kidney) [1, 2].

Current Understanding of Randall's Plaque

Plaque Location

Evan et al. have extensively studied Randall's plaque in a wide variety of stone formers using a papillary mapping and biopsy protocol [3]. Their initial studies of idiopathic calcium oxalate stone formers (ICSF) revealed that lesions consistent with Randall's plaque were identified at the time of endoscopy in 100 % of these patients. In contrast, in a group of non-stone-forming patients undergoing renal surgery for other indications (i.e., renal neoplasm), no visible Randall plaques were identified. The plaques of the ICSF patients were irregular in appearance and located on the papillary tips, near the openings of ducts of Bellini (Fig. 25.1a). Most plaques appeared to be sub-urothelial; however, occasional plaques seemed to lack urothelial layers. Initial evaluation of the biopsy specimens with light microscopy revealed that the plaques were always in the interstitium of the kidney and followed the thin loops of Henle up the inner medulla. Further evaluation with electron microscopy demonstrated deposits ranging in size from 50 nm to deposits that formed dense bands, which completely surrounded loops of Henle (Fig. 25.1b). Interestingly, the great majority of tubular cells associated with surrounding plaque deposits showed no evidence of cellular damage or injury. Occasionally, in tubules completely encased by dense crystalline deposits, some cells appeared to be damaged, as evidenced by detachment from the basement membrane and cytoplasmic vacuolization [3]. If the non-stone-forming patients in whom no Randall plaques were visualized, either extremely few or no Yasue-positive deposits were identified.

To further characterize the initial site of crystal deposition in the formation of plaques, biopsy specimens of tissue immediately adjacent to regions of Randall's plaque were evaluated in order to identify the most minimal sites of crystal deposition. Light microscopy revealed very small Yasue-positive (calcium substitution staining) deposits primarily surrounding the thin loops of Henle. Further evaluation with transmission electron microscopy demonstrated that the deposits were located within the basement membrane of the thin loops of Henle and vasa recta, and, regardless of deposit size, the basement membranes of the thin loops of Henle were always involved. Again, no obvious deleterious changes within the cells of the loops of Henle were identified [3].

Plaque Composition

To precisely identify the crystalline composition of the plaque deposits, Evan et al. performed infrared and X-ray diffraction analyses. In all instances, infrared analysis of the Yasue-positive deposits revealed the presence of calcium phosphate in the form of hydroxyapatite. This finding was subsequently confirmed by X-ray diffraction analysis in all cases [3].

Calcium Oxalate Stone Growth on Plaques in ICSF Patients

In 2006, Matlaga and associates reported on the endoscopic findings of stone attachment to Randall's plaque in ICSF patients. In their series of 24 kidneys from 23 ICSF patients, they identified Randall's plaque in 100 % of renal units and found stones attached to areas of underlying plaque in 48 % (Fig. 25.2a, b) [4]. Additionally, Williams and colleagues have used microcomputed tomography (μ[mu]CT)—a technique that distinguishes mineral composition based on differences in X-ray attenuation—to evaluate stones from ICSF patients confirmed as being attached to plaque at the time of surgical intervention. In their initial study of μ(mu)

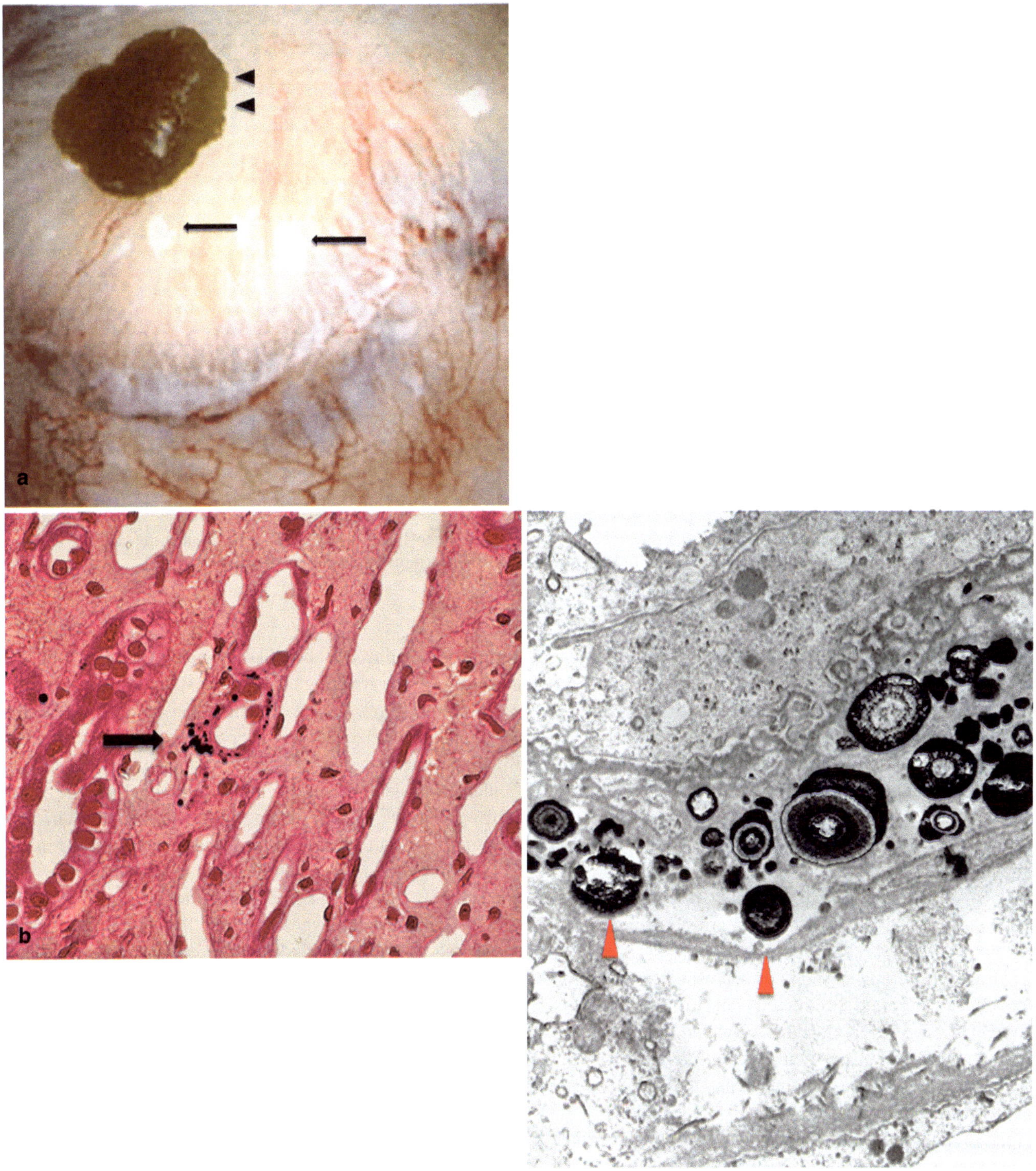

Fig. 25.1 (**a**) Endoscopic view of an ICSF patient. Multiple Randall's plaques are identified (*single arrows*). Additionally, an attached stone is present (*double arrowheads*). (**b**) Light microscopic view (*single black arrow*) and transmission electron microscopic view (*red arrowheads*) of Yasue-positive deposits with the basement membranes of thin loops of Henle

CT evaluation of a small series of attached stones, apatite deposits were identified in all of the predominantly calcium oxalate stones studied and in some instances were identified within concave, stone-surface patches, which could have represented the site of plaque attachment [5]. Because the stone orientation in relation to papillary plaque was not known at the time of μ(mu)CT analysis, this study could not confirm that these stones grew attached to plaque, but it was important in further driving efforts to confirm the accuracy of Randall's theory in ICSF patients.

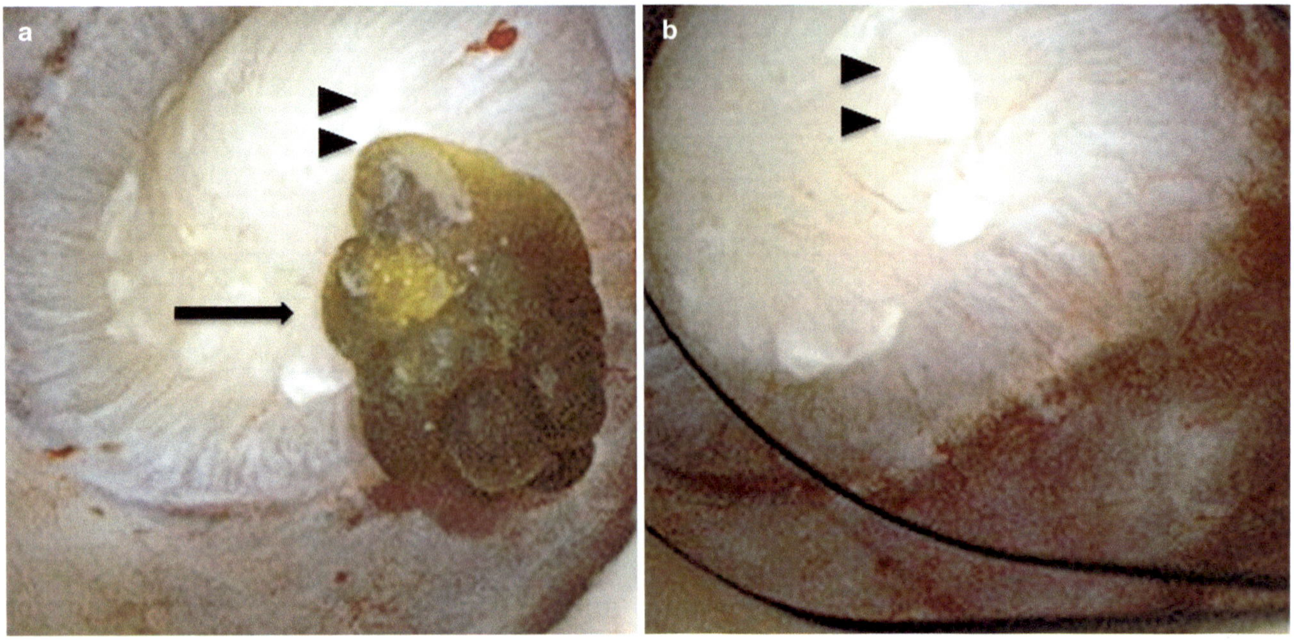

Fig. 25.2 (**a**) Typical attached stone in an ICSF patient (*single arrow*). Randall's plaque is noted on the papilla around the stone (*double arrowheads*). (**b**) Same papilla as in (**a**), after the stone has been manipulated with a Nitinol basket. The area of plaque to which the stone was attached is easily identified (*double arrowheads*)

While the endoscopic observation of stone attachment to Randall's plaque in ICSF stone patients has lent some proof to Randall's original theory of stone growth, it does not provide any understanding of how the process might occur—i.e., the mechanism by which a calcium oxalate stone actually forms on a plaque. It has previously been proposed that elevated urine calcium and reduced urine volume lead to the formation of Randall's plaques in human renal papillae [6]. To date, the process by which these plaques grow toward the surface of the papilla and eventually become exposed to urine via loss of urothelial integrity remains largely unknown.

However, through a series of sophisticated immunohistochemical, infrared spectrometry and μ(mu)CT analyses, Evan et al. have begun to shed new light on the processes that may be occurring at the stone-plaque interface [7]. At the time of exposure to intraluminal urine, the plaque becomes exposed to a number of urinary proteins, including Tamm-Horsfall protein (THP) and osteopontin. These proteins, which are both prevalent in human urine, have an affinity for apatite crystals and appear to form a layer (possibly with other, as yet undetermined proteins) that covers the surface of the exposed plaque. Subsequently, amorphous apatite crystals form within this new protein-matrix layer, a process that appears to be driven by urinary supersaturation of calcium phosphate. Additional urinary proteins are then able to attach to the apatite crystals, forming yet another protein-matrix layer. This again allows for another burst of calcium phosphate crystallization. This process appears to repeat itself, generating a ribbon-like morphology of protein and apatite crystals covering the area of exposed plaque [7].

At some point, apatite crystallization appears to overtake the inhibitory effects of urinary proteins and apatite crystals begin to extend into the collecting system lumen. Eventually, calcium oxalate with or without additional apatite overgrowth begins, again driven by urinary supersaturation. While it has not been precisely determined why the initial crystal type to attach to the exposed plaque is apatite, it is most likely due to the fact that the protein-matrix layer initially formed on the exposed plaque has an affinity for calcium phosphate crystals [7]. The findings of Evan and colleagues, along with the previous work of Kuo, outlining the relationship between elevated urinary calcium and papillary plaque coverage, are important in the urologists' understanding of the appropriate therapies for managing ICSF patients with hypercalciuria [6, 7]. These findings certainly strengthen the argument for urinary calcium reduction with agents such as thiazide diuretics in these patients, as this may reduce plaque abundance and will decrease the urinary supersaturation of calcium oxalate, which eventually drives stone formation.

Unattached Stones in ICSF Patients

In 2009, Miller and colleagues evaluated stones that appeared to be unattached from the renal papilla at the time of percutaneous or ureteroscopic interventions in ICSF patients [8].

In their analysis, 21 stones that were found free within the collecting system were compared to an additional 90 stones that were identified as being attached to renal papillae. Micro-CT technology was used to characterize the composition and ultrastructure of the attached and unattached stones. Of the 21 unattached stones analyzed, 12 showed clear evidence of prior attachment to renal papillae, with each containing a mucus-covered, concave region on only one surface, which by μ(mu)CT analysis contained apatite. The remaining nine unattached stones did not contain mucus-covered, concave, apatite-containing regions on a surface and instead had uniform, dark-brown surfaces. Analysis with μ(mu)CT revealed uniform surfaces with X-ray attenuation values consistent with calcium oxalate monohydrate. However, all nine stones demonstrated subsurface regions that contained apatite. This study provided further evidence to support the fact that most, if not all, stones form attached to papillary plaques in ICSF patients. While it could not be proven from this study, it is certainly possible that the unattached stones without surface apatite had previously grown attached to papillae and at some point became detached [8].

Prior to the study by Miller and colleagues, earlier work by Cifuentes et al. focusing on spontaneously passed stones revealed the presence of surface plaque in 72.4 % of the stones analyzed. Additionally, 13 of the stones with surface plaques contained calcified renal tubules, suggesting that the origin was from a papillary tip [9]. While there are still some aspects of stone formation on Randall's plaques that remain a mystery, the combined results of all of the aforementioned studies provide strong evidence that this is indeed the mechanism by which stone formation occurs in ICSF patients.

Stone Formation in Non-ICSF Patients

While there is strong evidence to support Randall's theory of calcium oxalate stone growth on interstitial plaques in ICSF patients, far less is known about the mechanisms of calculus formation in other stone-forming disease states. Patients with conditions such as cystinuria, brushite stone disease, gastric bypass for obesity, ileostomy for bowel disease, primary hyperparathyroidism (HPT), distal renal tubular acidosis (RTA), and primary hyperoxaluria (HOX) may display evidence of papillary interstitial plaques but additionally have other more dominant and unique papillary features, which suggest that alternate pathways to stone formation are at play.

Tubular Deposits/Ductal Plugging

Coe and colleagues have extensively studied the papillary features of seven additional distinct groups of stone formers (including cystinuria, brushite, gastric bypass, ileostomy, HPT, RTA, and HOX) as well as those of non-stone formers [10]. While some of these stone-forming phenotypes demonstrate endoscopic and histopathologic evidence of papillary interstitial plaques, they all additionally demonstrate tubular deposits of varying crystalline composition—a finding that is uniformly absent in ICSF patients. An additional unique finding that is distinct from ICSF patients is the fact that stone formers with tubular deposits demonstrate evidence of inflammatory response with destruction of epithelial cells and interstitial fibrosis [10].

Differentiating Tubular Deposits from Randall's Plaque

Endoscopically, tubular deposits appear quite different than classic Randall's plaques. Tubular deposits are yellow-colored, suburothelial lesions that often protrude out of the openings of largely dilated ducts of Bellini. Histologically, tubular deposits are located within innermedullary collecting ducts (IMCD) and ducts of Bellini as opposed to the interstitial location of Randall's plaque. Again, tubular deposits appear to be destructive in nature as there is evidence of inflammation and tubular cell injury and death. To date, it has not yet been proven that tubular deposits serve as anchors for stone growth; however, it seems clear that processes different from that of stone overgrowth on plaque are at play in the aforementioned stone-forming disease states, and this is an aspect of the pathology of nephrolithiasis that is actively being researched [10].

Stone-Forming Phenotypes

The papillary and histologic findings of seven distinct stone-forming phenotypes are described as follows (See Table 25.1 for a summary of the endoscopic and histopathological findings identified in the carious stone formers.).

Cystinuria

Endoscopic evaluation of the papillae of cystine stone formers reveals many dilated ducts of Bellini with plugs composed of cystine crystals, which on some occasions project into the collecting system. Randall's plaque may be identified in amounts equivalent to those found in non-stone formers (Fig. 25.3) [10, 11]. Analysis of papillary biopsies demonstrates dilation of IMCDs along with epithelial cell injury within the loops of Henle and IMCDs. Apatite crystals are identified within the loops of Henle and IMCDs, while the large plugs identified within the dilated ducts of Bellini are always composed of cystine. Evan and colleagues have proposed a hypothesis to account for these findings and suggest

Table 25.1 Relative amount of plaque coverage, papillary damage, and stone growth on plaque identified in the various stone phenotypes

Stone disease	Plaque presence	Papillary damage[a]	Stones on plaque
Idiopathic calcium oxalate stone former	++	–	++
Cystinuria	–	+	–
Brushite	++	+++	–
Gastric bypass	–	+	–
Ileostomy	+	+	–
Primary hyperparathyroidism	Variable	++	+/–
Renal tubular acidosis	–	+++	–
Primary hyperoxaluria	–	++	–

[a]Papillary damage is determined based on degree of pitting, papillary retraction, duct of Bellini dilation and deposits within ducts of Bellini noted during endoscopy and papillary mapping

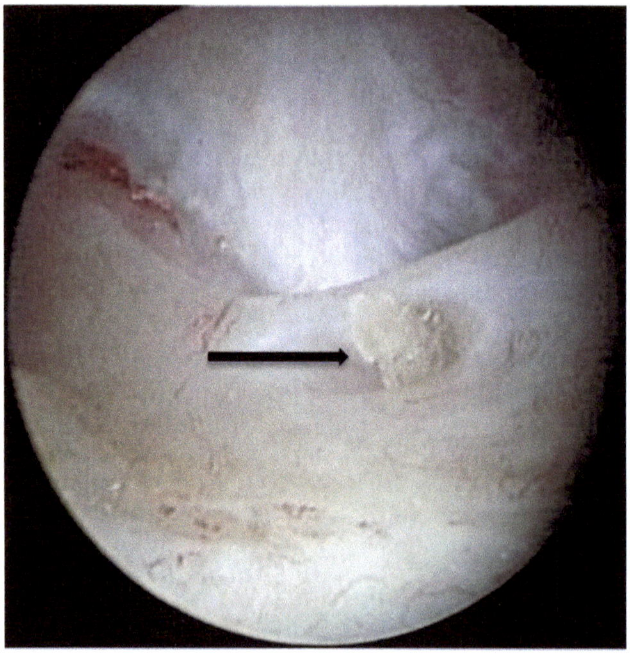

Fig. 25.3 Endoscopic view of a papilla in a patient with cystinuria. There is minimal identifiable Randall's plaque. There is a large cystine plug within a dilated duct of Bellini (*single arrow*)

that cystine crystallizes within the ducts of Bellini, resulting in cell injury and obstruction of individual nephrons. These changes could then potentially lead to loss of fluid pH regulation in IMCDs and subsequently allow for apatite crystallization [10–12].

Brushite Stone Formers

Brushite stone formers typically have a significant degree of hypercalciuria and alkaline urine and tend to have aggressive stone disease [13]. Evan and colleagues have endoscopically and histologically studied a cohort of brushite stone formers [14]. Endoscopically, these patients have unique-appearing papillae in which three different types of deposits are

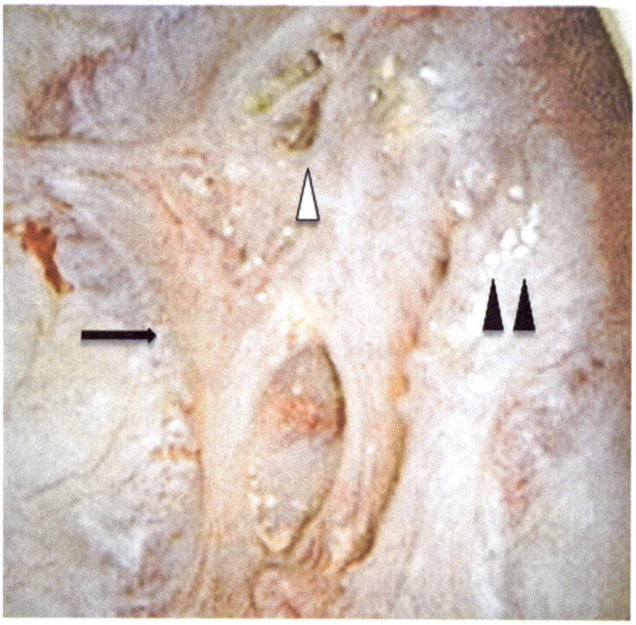

Fig. 25.4 Endoscopic view of a papilla in a brushite stone former. The papilla is quite abnormal, with areas of retraction and pitting (*single black arrow*). Areas of Randall's plaque are present (*double black arrowheads*). Dilated ducts of Bellini with plugs are also identified (*single white arrowhead*)

identified. Typical-appearing Randall's plaque is noted in this cohort of patients, yet stone overgrowth on these plaques is not observed. Also, yellow deposits arising from dilated ducts of Bellini (which project into the lumen of the collecting system) and suburothelial deposits (typically along the sides of the papillae) within the lumens of IMCDs are present. An additional abnormal endoscopic finding in brushite stone formers includes retraction of papillae and papillary pitting, which is typically associated with dilated ducts of Bellini. The prevalence of plugging and papillary changes is variable among this group of stone formers, but it is often severe (Fig. 25.4).

Histologically, there is evidence of extensive cell injury and interstitial fibrosis around the crystal-filled collecting ducts. Similar signs of interstitial fibrosis, tubular atrophy, and glomerulosclerosis are noted within cortical tissue samples as well. Mineral analysis of the tubular deposits in brushite patients reveals mostly apatite, although calcium oxalate may be found in small amounts on some occasions [10, 11, 14].

Gastric Bypass

Patients who undergo jejunoileal bypass for the management of obesity are at risk for forming calcium oxalate stones due to the metabolic abnormalities induced by the procedure. These patients develop fat malabsorption, intestinal saponification of calcium and magnesium, decreased binding of calcium and oxalate in the gut, and subsequent hyperoxaluria. Additionally,

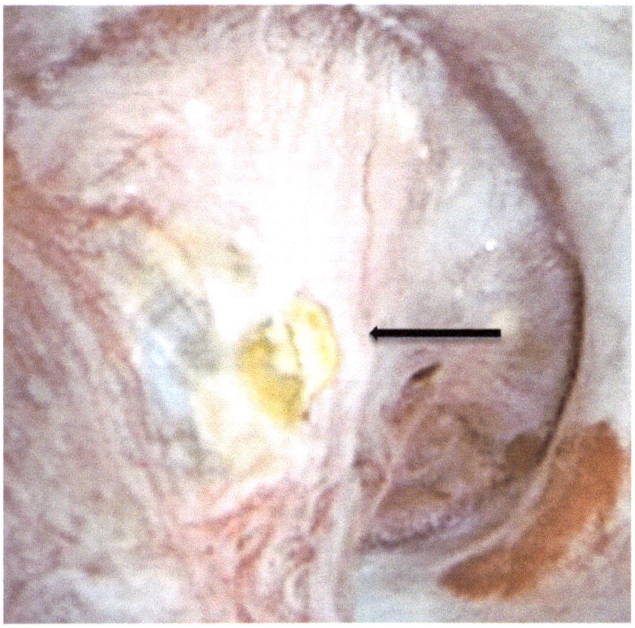

Fig. 25.5 Endoscopic view of a papilla in a patient who has undergone bariatric surgery. No Randall's plaques are identified. Note the nodular plug emanating from a largely dilated duct of Bellini (*single arrow*)

they are prone to low-volume, acidic urine, again due to malabsorption.

Evan and associates have studied patients who have undergone intestinal bypass and subsequently developed calcium oxalate stones as a unique cohort [3]. Interestingly, when evaluated endoscopically, these patients do not demonstrate evidence of typical Randall's plaque. Instead, nodular yellow deposits project off of the papillary urothelium in close proximity to the openings of ducts of Bellini (Fig. 25.5). Histologically, no interstitial apatite deposits are present. Crystals appear to be attached to the apical surfaces of collecting duct cells or fill the ducts completely, and there is associated cell injury and death. Analysis of the crystals within the IMCDs and ducts of Bellini reveals the majority to be apatite. This is a rather puzzling finding due to the fact that these patients generally have acidic urine with high calcium oxalate content, which does not promote supersaturation of apatite, a mineral that typically forms in an alkaline environment (see later discussion on mechanisms for tubular plaque formation) [3, 10, 11].

Ileostomy Patients

Ileostomy patients are prone to significant GI losses, low urine volume, and highly acidic urine. These patients lack a colon and therefore do not readily absorb oxalate. Therefore, the stone type to which they are most prone is uric acid. Endoscopically, these patients are also noted to harbor Randall's plaque and tubular deposits. They generally do not demonstrate evidence of stone overgrowth on plaque, although this may be seen on occasion. Microscopically, the tubular deposits are identified within the thin limbs of the loops of Henle and within the collecting ducts. Again, there is associated cellular injury and fibrosis. This cohort of patients represents another paradox, in that their tubular deposits are composed of apatite and/or ammonium acid urate, both minerals that form in an alkaline environment [10, 15].

Primary Hyperparathyroidism

Patients with HPT are prone to forming both calcium oxalate and calcium phosphate (hydroxyapatite and brushite) stones and represent a unique cohort of stone formers. These patients have also been extensively studied by Evan and colleagues [16]. The renal papillae in these patients demonstrate a significant amount of variability with regard to plaque coverage. In some patients, Randall's plaque is found in amounts similar to that of non-stone formers, while in others, large quantities of Randall's plaque with attached stones are identified. In all patients with HPT, at least some of the papillae demonstrate evidence of tubular deposits and ductal plugging, but again, the degree to which this occurs is variable. Additionally, papillary changes including pitting and retraction are noted in varying degrees (Fig. 25.6) [16].

Histopathology reveals plugging of ducts of Bellini and IMCDs with crystals as well as associated cell injury/death and interstitial fibrosis. In some instances, the ductal plugging extends to the outer medullary collecting ducts (OMCDs) and cortical collecting ducts. In all patients studied by Evan and colleagues, the crystalline composition of the plugged ducts was uniformly apatite. The constellation of endoscopic and histopathologic findings in HPT patients is quite similar to those seen in brushite stone formers. However, to date, HPT patients are the only stone formers that have been noted to have both tubular deposits and stone overgrowth on Randall's plaque. The finding of abundant Randall's plaque in patients with HPT could in part be due to the associated induced hypercalciuria, a urinary parameter associated with plaque abundance. Unfortunately, to date, the papillary studies of HPT patients have been performed on those who have already undergone curative treatment for their hyperparathyroidism. Therefore, marked hypercalciuria and elevated urinary pH (parameters that are prominent in brushite and RTA patients) had not been documented prior to endoscopic surgery in this cohort and therefore cannot be presumed to be the cause for ductal plugging with apatite [16].

Renal Tubular Acidosis

Patients with distal RTA possess a defect in hydrogen ion secretion in the distal nephron, which results in metabolic acidosis, hypocitraturia, and persistently alkaline urine. Due to the alkaline nature of their urine, they are prone to developing calcium phosphate stones (apatite), although some patients may form stones that contain varying amounts of

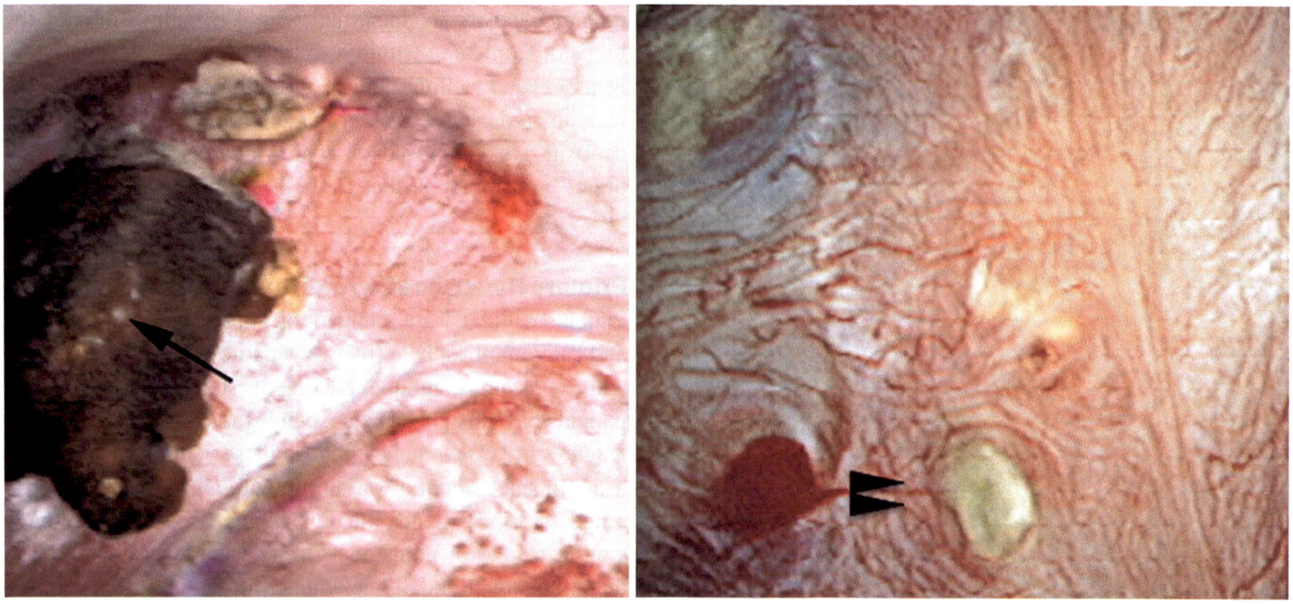

Fig. 25.6 Endoscopic view of a papilla in a patient with HPT. On *the left*, an attached calcium oxalate stone is present (*single arrow*). On *the right*, a plugged duct of Bellini is identified (*double arrowheads*)

calcium oxalate. Patients with this condition frequently have aggressive stone disease and demonstrate radiographic evidence of nephrocalcinosis.

Evan and colleagues have also studied the surgical pathology and histopathology in this unique cohort of stone formers [17]. Endoscopically, a broad spectrum of abnormalities are noted, with some patients demonstrating minimally abnormal papillae and others demonstrating severe pitting of the papillae and numerous dilated ducts of Bellini with protruding mineral plugs. Additionally, suburothelial densities are often encountered (Fig. 25.7). When the urothelium overlying these densities is unroofed, small stones within cavities are identified. These stones are actually isolated within the parenchyma. At the time of endoscopic intervention in these patients, the great majority of stones identified on radiographic films are identified within the collecting system and are amenable to surgical removal [17].

Analysis of papillary biopsies from these patients reveals apatite deposition (combined with trace amounts of calcium oxalate in rare instances) within IMCDs and ducts of Bellini with associated interstitial fibrosis and epithelial cell loss. In these patients the degree of fibrosis is extensive and is often found surrounding tubules that do not contain mineral deposits. Cortical biopsies reveal a range of glomerular diseases, but changes of interstitial fibrosis are generally mild [17].

Primary Hyperoxaluria

Patients with HOX have disorders of glyoxalate metabolism that are inherited in an autosomal recessive fashion. These abnormalities result in excessive oxalate production and urinary excretion, which in turn leads to calcium oxalate nephrolithiasis. These patients can potentially go on to develop end-stage renal disease (ESRD) and numerous other complications associated with dystrophic calcification of calcium oxalate.

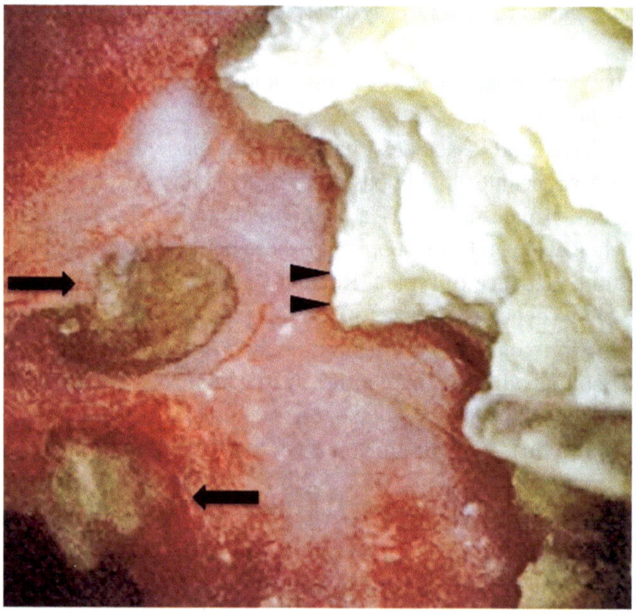

Fig. 25.7 Endoscopic view of a patient with RTA undergoing PNL. Note the large crystalline plugs within dilated ducts of Bellini (*single arrows*). No significant Randall's plaque coverage is identified. A large calyceal stone that has been partially treated is seen on the right (*double arrowheads*)

This cohort of patients has been less well studied due to the rarity of the disease. However, endoscopic and pathologic evaluations of kidneys in HOX patients with ESRD have been performed [10]. Endoscopically, HOX patients have minimal Randall's plaque in amounts similar to that seen in non-stone-forming patients. However, these patients do demonstrate papillary tubular deposits within ducts of Bellini and IMCDs. Analysis of tubular deposits reveals abundant calcium oxalate, a unique finding when compared to other stone-forming phenotypes in which ductal deposits are identified. In patients with HOX and ESRD, deposits can be identified in all segments of the nephron. As in other stone formers with ductal plugging, interstitial fibrosis and cell death is observed [10]. Table 25.1 summarizes the degree of plaque coverage, papillary damage, and stone growth on plaque in all of the aforementioned stone phenotypes.

Mechanisms of Ductal Deposit and Stone Formation

The process by which patients with prominent tubular deposits and ductal plugging form stones is not yet well understood and is currently the subject of active and elegant research. It is clear, however, that the pathway to stone formation must be different than that which occurs in ICSF, as patients with the aforementioned phenotypes (with the exception of some patients with HPT) do not demonstrate evidence of stone overgrowth on Randall's plaque. It is quite likely that different processes are occurring within the tubular deposit phenotypes [10].

If one reviews Finlayson's hypothesis that calcium oxalate is formed too slowly and in too small an amount to plug a renal tubule without an anchoring site, it would seem to hold true (with the exception of HOX patients who have exceedingly high oxalate excretion) based on the findings in the previously described stone formers [18]. Given the fact that tubular deposits are found in ducts of Bellini and IMCDs, one would expect that this is related to the urinary supersaturation of various crystals (i.e., calcium phosphate or calcium oxalate). This would explain why patients who do not form stones and have low supersaturations of calcium oxalate and calcium phosphate demonstrate no evidence of deposits. Calcium phosphate supersaturation in patients with cystinuria (likely as a result of alkaline therapy), brushite stone disease, RTA, and HPT are quite high, and it is possible that this results in deposits secondary to free solution nucleation. This free solution theory of ductal plugging also seems appropriate in HOX patients in whom the urinary supersaturation of calcium oxalate is exceedingly high when compared to all other stone formers [10].

However, how can one explain the finding of apatite and/or ammonium acid urate plugging in patients with ileostomy, when these patients have extremely low urinary pH and low calcium phosphate supersaturation? How can gastric bypass patients, who have high calcium oxalate supersaturation and low calcium phosphate supersaturation, develop apatite plugs within their ducts? Somehow, it must be the case that tubule fluid pH is higher than that of the bulk urine, at least in some ducts of Bellini and IMCDs. How and why these localized defects in tubular urine acidification arise is not well understood and studies assessing the pH of bulk urine, normal ducts, and abnormal (plugged) ducts in ileostomy patients are currently underway [10].

Conclusion

One final and important distinguishing feature between the stone phenotypes in which tubular deposits are prominent and ICSF patients is the fact that patients with tubular deposits demonstrate evidence of interstitial fibrosis, cellular injury, and death, while ICSF patients do not demonstrate any evidence of tissue damage. The postulated mechanisms by which tissue damage occurs in the various types of stone formers are diverse. What is important is that these stone formers must be considered as being at risk for developing renal dysfunction at some point in their lifetime. Therefore, it is important that these patients are monitored closely and any metabolic abnormalities that they harbor must be managed aggressively. Additionally, the fact that these patients have cellular injury associated with tubular deposits makes one consider the possibility that aggressive stone removal, including removal of tubular plugs, may lead to a reduction in renal tissue damage in the future.

References

1. Evan AP. Physiopathology and etiology of stone formation in the kidney and urinary tract. Pediatr Nephrol. 2010;25:831–41.
2. Randall A. The etiology of primary renal calculus. Int Abstr Surg. 1940;71:209–40.
3. Evan AP, Lingeman JE, Coe FL, et al. Randall's plaque of patients with nephrolithiasis begins in basement membranes of thin loops of Henle. J Clin Invest. 2003;111:607–16.
4. Matlaga BR, Williams JC, Kim SC, et al. Endoscopic evidence of calculus attachment to Randall's plaque. J Urol. 2006;175:1720–4.
5. Williams JC, Matlaga BR, Kim SC, et al. Calcium oxalate calculi found attached to the renal papilla: preliminary evidence for early mechanisms in stone formation. J Endourol. 2006;20:885–90.
6. Kuo RL, Lingeman JE, Evan AP, et al. Urine calcium and volume predict coverage of renal papilla by Randall's plaque. Kidney Int. 2003;64:2150–4.
7. Evan AP, Coe FL, Lingeman JE, et al. Mechanism of formation of human calcium oxalate renal stones on Randall's plaque. Anat Rec. 2007;290:1315–25.
8. Miller NL, Williams JC, Evan AP, et al. In idiopathic calcium oxalate stone formers, unattached stones show evidence of having originated as attached stones on Randall's plaque. BJU Int. 2009;105:242–5.
9. Cifuentes Delatte L, Minon-Cifuentes JL, Medina JA. Papillary stones: calcified renal tubules in Randall's plaques. J Urol. 1985;133:490–4.

10. Coe FL, Evan AP, Lingeman JE, et al. Plaque and deposits in 9 human stone diseases. Urol Res. 2010;38:239–47.
11. Miller NL, Evan AP, Lingeman JE. Pathogenesis of renal calculi. Urol Clin North Am. 2007;34:295–313.
12. Evan AP, Coe FL, Lingeman JE, et al. Renal crystal deposits and histopathology in patients with cystine stones. Kidney Int. 2006; 69:2227–35.
13. Krambeck AE, Handa SE, Evan AP, et al. Profile of the brushite stone former. J Urol. 2010;184:1367–71.
14. Evan AP, Lingeman JE, Coe FL, et al. Crystal-associated nephropathy in patients with brushite nephrolithiasis. Kidney Int. 2005;67:576–91.
15. Evan AP, Lingeman JE, Coe FL, et al. Intra-tubular deposits, urine and stone composition are divergent in patients with ileostomy. Kidney Int. 2009;76:1081–8.
16. Evan A, Lingeman JE, Coe FL, et al. Histopathology and surgical anatomy of patients with primary hyperparathyroidism and calcium phosphate stones. Kidney Int. 2008;74:223–9.
17. Evan AP, Lingeman J, Coe F, et al. Renal histopathology of stone forming patients with distal renal tubular acidosis. Kidney Int. 2007;71:795–801.
18. Finlayson B, Reid F. The expectation of free and fixed particles in urinary stone disease. Invest Urol. 1978;15:442.

Melamine-Associated Urinary Stone

26

Yao Liang Deng and Cheng Yang Li

Abstract

Melamine-associated urinary stones (MAUS) have emerged as a new urologic disease. This chapter reviews the renal toxicity of melamine in animals and human beings, especially regarding urinary stone formation and its clinical features and management.

Keywords

Melamine • Urinary stone • Human being • Treatment

Introduction

Melamine is a chemical used primarily for the production of melamine resins typically by reaction with formaldehyde [1,2]. Food or milk contaminated with melamine could cause biotic toxicity, and the most common toxicity is renal toxicity, including urinary stone formation, renal tubular necrosis, and acute renal failure (ARF). The melamine-associated urinary stone (MAUS) has emerged as a new urologic disease, about which, until now, there is still a very limited clinical and experimental experience.

What Is Melamine?

Melamine is one of three triazines, which are nitrogen-containing organic heterocyclic compounds. Its molecular formula is $C_3N_6H_6$ or $C_3N_3(NH_2)_3$, and its molecular weight is 126.12. In industrial use, it is combined with formaldehyde to produce melamine resin, a very durable thermosetting plastic, and melamine foam, a polymeric cleanser. Other commercial products containing melamine include countertops, dry erase boards, fabrics, glues, housewares, and flame retardants.

Beginning in 1958, melamine has been used in fertilizers and is occasionally offered as a nonprotein nitrogenous source for feeding cattle. But it was shown to be an ineffective nonprotein nitrogen source for animals because of its slow hydrolysis in ruminants. This chemical should never have been added into any kind of foods or drinks. Melamine caught the public attention for the epidemic of "pet food-induced nephrotoxicity in North America" in 2007 [1, 2]. In March 2007, numerous cases of acute renal failure in dogs and cats were associated with the ingestion of a variety of dog and cat pet foods. One of the main contaminants was melamine, which was added to the food to give falsely high protein content.

Metabolism of Melamine in Animals and Its Toxicity

Data from animal studies showed that melamine is not metabolized by animals and is rapidly eliminated in the urine. More than 90 % of ingested melamine is excreted within 24 h. The half-life of melamine excretion in animal studies ranged from 2.7 to 4.0 h [3, 4]. The levels of melamine in blood, liver, or plasma are similar [3]. The volume of distribution of melamine in pigs is 0.61 ± 0.04 L/kg, and it is not extensively distributed to most organ tissues [4].

A variety of toxic effects from melamine have been studied in animals. The most common toxicity is renal toxicity, which is also the area of most concern to nephrologists.

Y.L. Deng, M.D., Ph.D. (✉) • C.Y. Li, M.D., Ph.D.
Department of Urology, The First Affiliated
Hospital of Guangxi Medical University,
Shuang Yong Road, No. 6, Nanning, Guangxi 530021, China
e-mail: dylkf317@163.com

J.J. Talati et al. (eds.), *Urolithiasis*,
DOI 10.1007/978-1-4471-4387-1_26, © Springer-Verlag London 2012

Toxicity can be classified as acute or chronic. Acute toxicity leads to renal failure and death. The lethal dose of melamine that would result in death in 50 % of the tested animals (LD50) in rats is 3.161 g/kg body wt [5] and in rabbits is >1 g/kg body wt [6]. The chronic renal toxicity includes urinary stone formation and chronic kidney damage. The carcinogenicity of melamine in animals was also determined. Occurrence of urinary bladder tumors in male rats correlates well with stone formation and exposure to high dosages [5].

In the "pet food-induced nephrotoxicity" event, not only was melamine present but also another toxic compound—cyanuric acid—which gave rise to a very high mortality in these animals. Cyanuric acid (s-triazine-2,4,6-triol) is structurally related to melamine. Melamine combined with cyanuric acid results in acute renal failure in cats within 48 h after ingestion. In combination, the toxic dosage in their diet is as low as 0.2 % melamine and 0.2 % cyanuric acid; whereas, in contrast, no evidence of renal failure can be detected in groups taking up to 1 % of either melamine or cyanuric acid alone in their diet for 10 days [7]. The toxicity is size dependent, with cats affected more than dogs and small dogs affected more than large ones [1, 8]. The mortality of combined melamine and cyanuric acid is as high as 74 % in dogs and 61 % in cats [2].

Urinary Stone Formation in Animals

The most commonly reported chronic renal toxicity of melamine is stone formation. Incidence ranges from 5 to 100 % depending on the dosage of melamine, gender, and amount of water intake [5, 9]. The incidence of stone formation increases with daily exposure to melamine. The lowest possible daily dosage of melamine that results in bladder stone formation is as low as 750 ppm for 13 weeks [5].

The dose-response curve for the induction of urolithiasis in weanling rats is extremely steep. This suggests formation of stone occurs in supersaturated urine, but not in urine that is under saturated [10].

A study performed on mice with exposure to 13 weeks of melamine showed that male mice are much more affected than females, despite similar body weights. Relative risk of stone formation in males is twice as great as in females [5].

A study of exposure to melamine for 36 weeks in rats demonstrated the incidence of stone formation was reduced by increasing the amount of fluid intake [9].

In our study [11], rats received melamine in the diet for 12 weeks followed by a 4-week period without chemicals. Results confirmed that a 3.0 % (w/w) dose level of melamine in the diet induced urinary stone formation and kidney lesion (Figs. 26.1 and 26.2a–d). Withdrawal of melamine resulted in reduction in size of urinary stones and improvement of kidney lesions.

Analysis of the stones' composition demonstrated either a combination of melamine and uric acid or melamine in a matrix of protein, uric acid, and phosphate [12].

Outbreak of Urinary Stones in Children Consuming Melamine-Tainted Milk

Urinary stones are relatively uncommon in children, and the incidence accounts for 2.0–2.7 % of all urinary stones in human beings. The most common factor that induces childhood urinary stone is metabolic abnormalities [13, 14], and the next common factors are urinary tract infection and urinary system deformities. Melamine is a newly identified cause of urinary stones. Infants and young children in some areas of China developed urinary stones after being fed with milk powder that was tainted with melamine in 2008. An estimated 300,000 children have been affected. Of the children, 99.2 % were younger than 3 years, although more children who were older than 3 years were reported afterward. The highest content of melamine in the milk powder products for infants and young children is 2,563 mg/kg milk powder. The number of patients with MAUS accounts for about 1.39 % of the total number of children who have a history of consuming the melamine-tainted milk powder products [15].

Clinical Features and Diagnosis

Many infants and young children with MAUS without obstruction are virtually asymptomatic and only picked up after ultrasound of the kidneys. A small proportion of patients may have symptoms or signs like crying, vomiting, and hematuria. Careful parents may find turbid urine or even fine sand gravel-like stones in the patients' urine. There was a very small proportion (2.5 %) of the individuals who developed ARF caused by urinary tract stone obstruction [16]. The overt manifestations of obstructive renal failure are oliguria or anuria; severe patients may have convulsions, edema, or hypertension. Mortality was recorded in four cases.

Urinalysis of exposed children revealed microscopic hematuria with or without proteinuria. Melamine can be detected in the urine of the affected children by biochemical test or the presence of fan-shaped crystals.

MAUS in humans are characteristic. Analysis of stone composition mainly demonstrated melamine and uric acid (Fig. 26.3). These stones basically do not contain calcium. They are soft in nature and can be broken up easily (Fig. 26.4). They usually occur bilaterally, and multiple stones are often present [17]. Most of the stones are usually <1 cm in diameter.

Imaging examinations for MAUS have certain characteristics. MAUS were generally radiolucent, and plain X-ray films (kidneys, ureters, and bladder [KUB]) failed to show

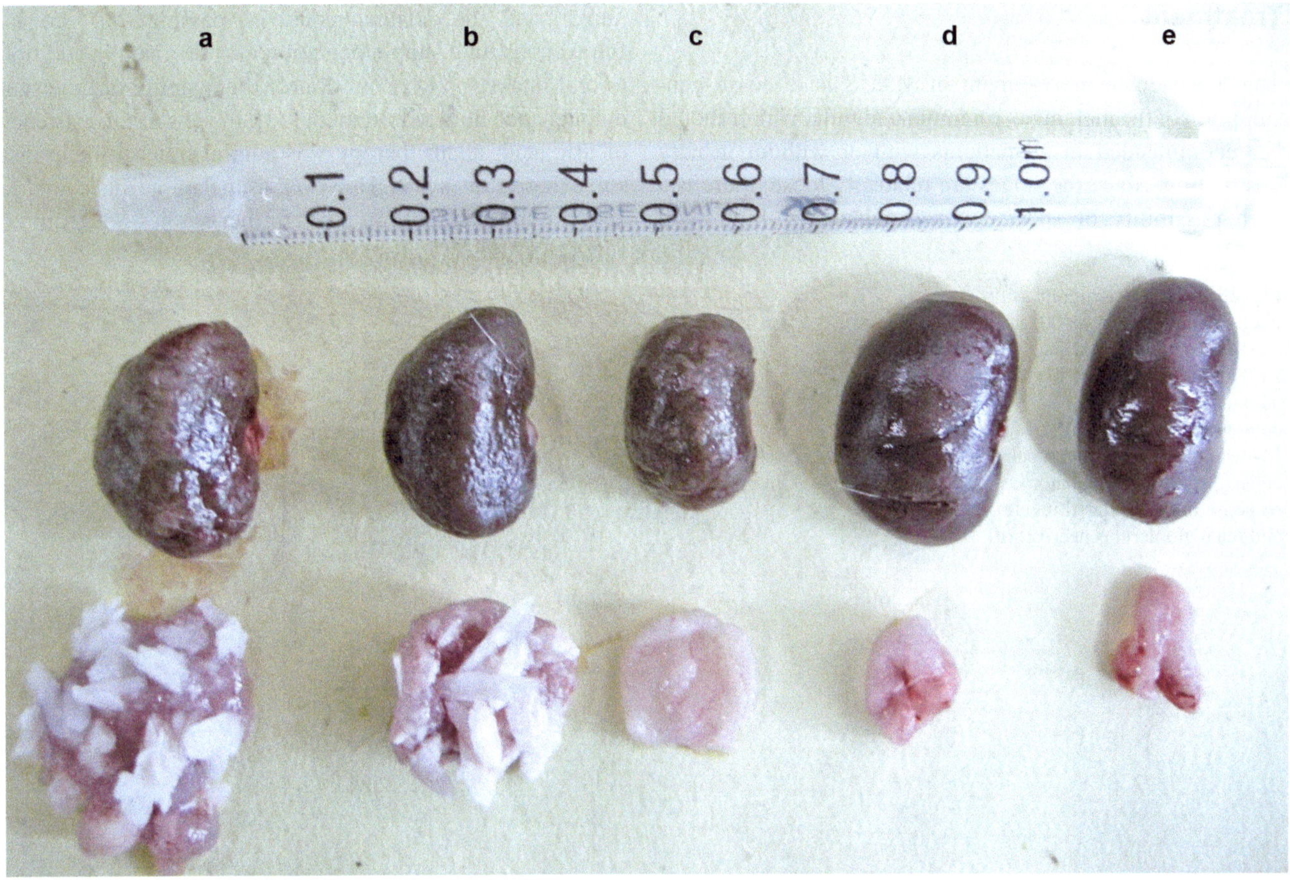

Fig. 26.1 Kidneys and bladders of rats administered melamine (3 % W/W in the diet for 1 month) (**a–c**) and control rats fed a normal diet (**d, e**), showing the formation of bladder stones (**a, b**) and kidney damage (**a–c**)

their presence. However, some of the patients showed low-density images of the lump-like stones in KUB, which may be due to increased resolution of the digitalized photographs and relatively shorter anteroposterior diameter of the abdomen of infants and young children [15]. At the same time, it is also possible that larger stones might also contain a certain amount of calcium at the edges as suggested by the stronger echogenicity around the stones.

Ultrasound screening is a simple and easy measure to detect the urinary stones and urinary obstruction (Fig. 26.5). The echo intensity properties of the stones are similar to those of uric acid stones. The lump-like stones had weaker echogenicity than calcium-containing stone. Most of the larger MAUS are oval in shape, and the whole echogenicity of the stones can be shown (i.e., the central part of the stone and its posterior edge). Weak or no echo image is shown behind the image of the stones. Some of the stones show strong shell-like echogenicity for the edges, and the central parts are hypoechoic. Up to 40 % of MAUS are gravel-like and could be shown more clearly under high-frequency transducer. The echogenicity for gravel-like stones have an appearance of aggregated fine gravel without particular shape, and there are no or weak shadows posterior to the stone echogenicity. Stones of single granules were shown as strong point-like echogenicity 0.1–0.3 cm in diameter; there were no acoustic shadows, but there was a sign of comet tail.

Intravenous urography (IVU) remains the modality of choice for the visualization of the entire urinary tract and especially the urothelium covering the pyelocalyceal systems, ureters, and bladder. The examination provides both anatomic and renal physiologic/functional information. MAUS appears as filling defects; hydronephrosis and hydroureter were shown above the obstructive sites in IVU. Plain computed tomography (CT) scan is able to identify structures in more detail and can pick up smaller stones of density different from the surrounding tissues (Fig. 26.6). But in view of the large radiation dose of X-ray for children (noncontrast CT scan is estimated to entail 200 times the radiation dose of a plain chest X-ray, depending on the machine and patient's size), ultrasound is the preferred first-line examination.

The diagnosis of MAUS is not difficult in most of the cases. Highlights for diagnosis of MAUS are as follows:

- History of consuming melamine-contaminated milk powder
- Clinical manifestations of obstructive renal failure in infants and young children
- Features of the imaging examinations
- Analysis of the composition of the expelled urinary stones demonstrated melamine

Treatment

The first step in management of MAUS is to cease consumption of the melamine-contaminated milk, which should be recommended in all patients with or without urinary obstruction. Since the stones are relatively loose, there is a high possibility of spontaneous expulsion. A high fluid intake will be advantageous in passing out stones. Intravenous fluid supplementation may be given in addition to oral intake, up to about double the quantity of the usual maintenance fluid requirement [18]. In view of the existence of uric acid, alkali therapy was administrated to help dissolve these stones [19]. However, as melamine and cyanuric acid are more soluble in acid, further studies are required

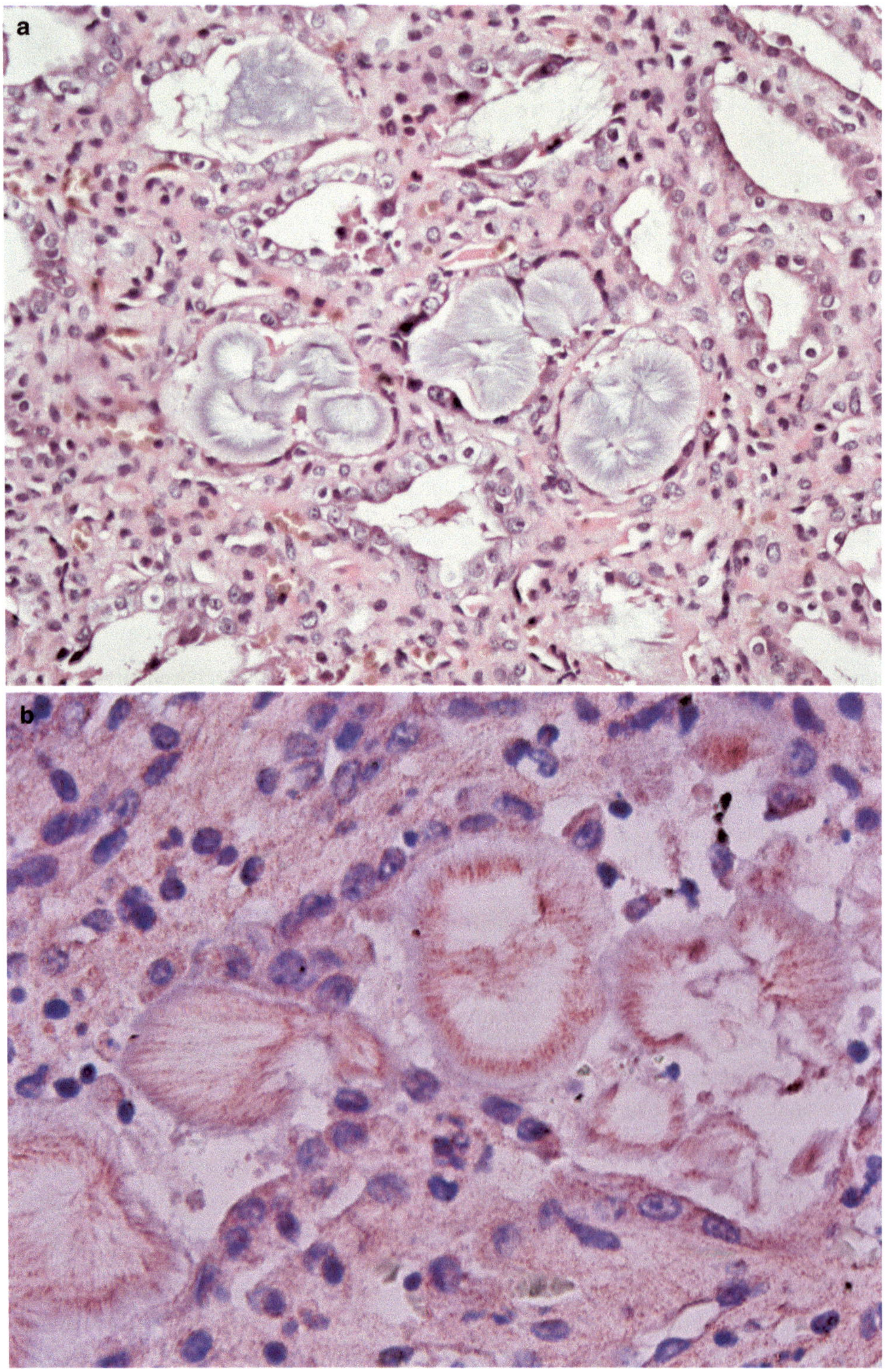

Fig. 26.2 Photomicrographs of H&E-stained (**a**, **c**, **d**, ×400) and 72 h Oil Red O–stained (**b**, ×1,000) kidney sections of rats administrated melamine, demonstrating crystals deposit (**a**, **b**), distended tubules and tubular cells injury (**b**), inflammatory response in renal interstitium (**c**), and renal glomerulus necrosis (**d**)

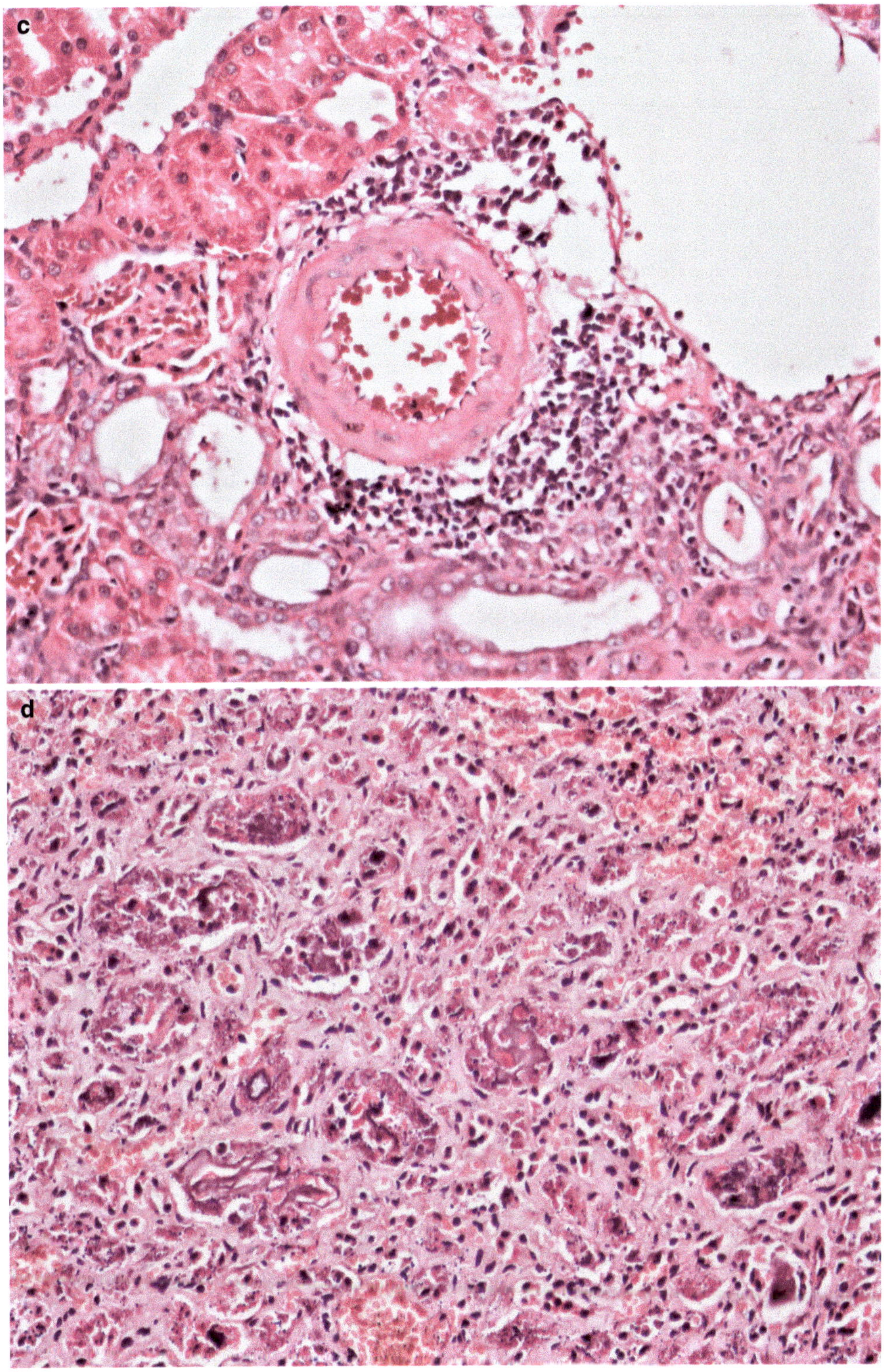

Fig. 26.2 (continued)

before making a recommendation and that may well depend on the actual composition of the stones.

If conservative medical therapy fails or the patient advances to an ARF due to obstruction, interventional approaches will become essential. Experiences from Chinese clinics suggest that cystoscopy or ureteroscopy for retrograde ureteral catheterization or renal puncture for nephrostomy should be chosen first. Those approaches need special facilities and equipments and generally provide reliable results. Secondly, to remove the stones, extracorporeal shock wave

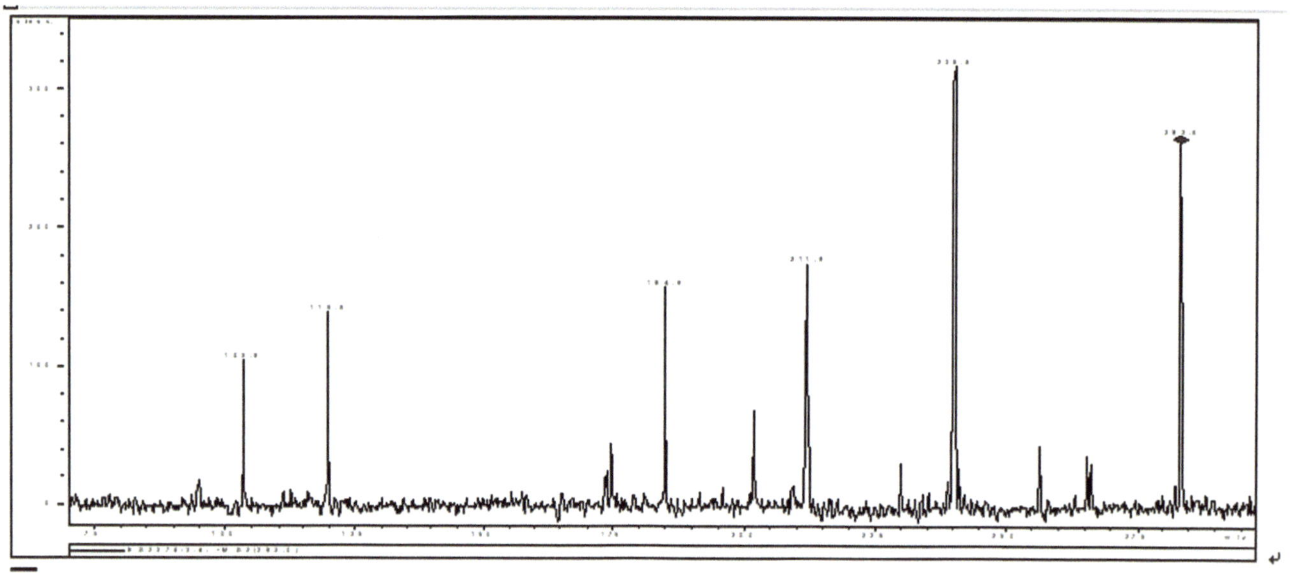

Fig. 26.3 ESI-MS^2 for the composition of urinary stones from infants being fed with milk powder tainted with melamine, demonstrated melamine and uric acid

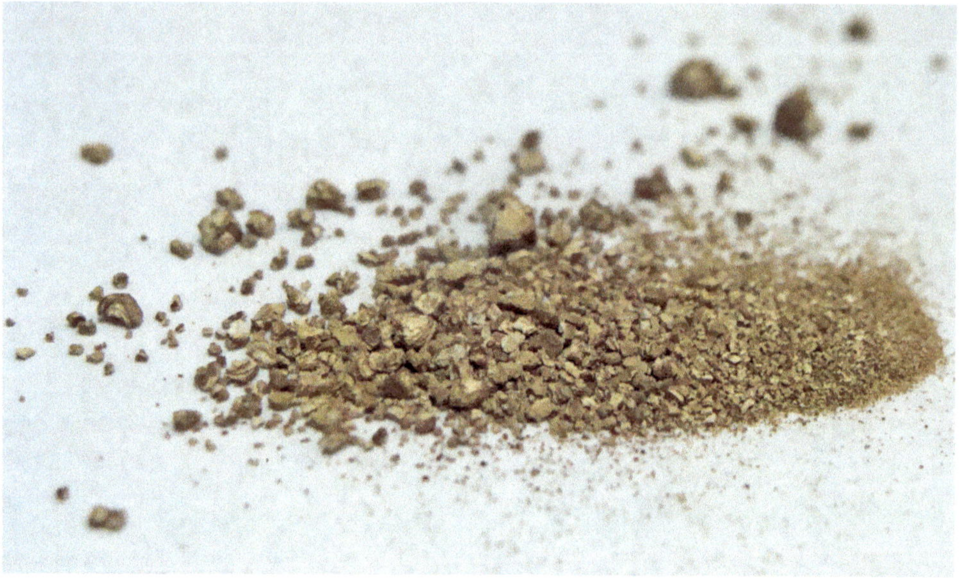

Fig. 26.4 The expelled melamine-associated urinary stone from infant being fed with milk powder tainted with melamine. The surface of the stone is *brown* and the inner part is *white*

lithotripsy (ESWL), minimally invasive percutaneous nephrolithotripsy (mini-PCNL), or even open lithectomy can be considered as the second-line treatment [18]. Data showed that there was no significant difference in the efficacy of different therapeutic approaches for relieving renal failure [20]. It was suggested that the primary principle for selecting different interventional approaches to relieve the obstruction is safety and efficacy and the next one should consider about minimal injury to the infants and children. Selection of the approaches should be based on comprehensive consideration of the disease status, technical skills of the physicians or surgeons, and the medical facilities and equipments [20].

Outcome

After passage or removal of the stones, renal function recovered even in those with renal failure, and the urinary obstructions did not proceed. In the 1-year-long follow-up in our study, we found that children who suffered from MAUS

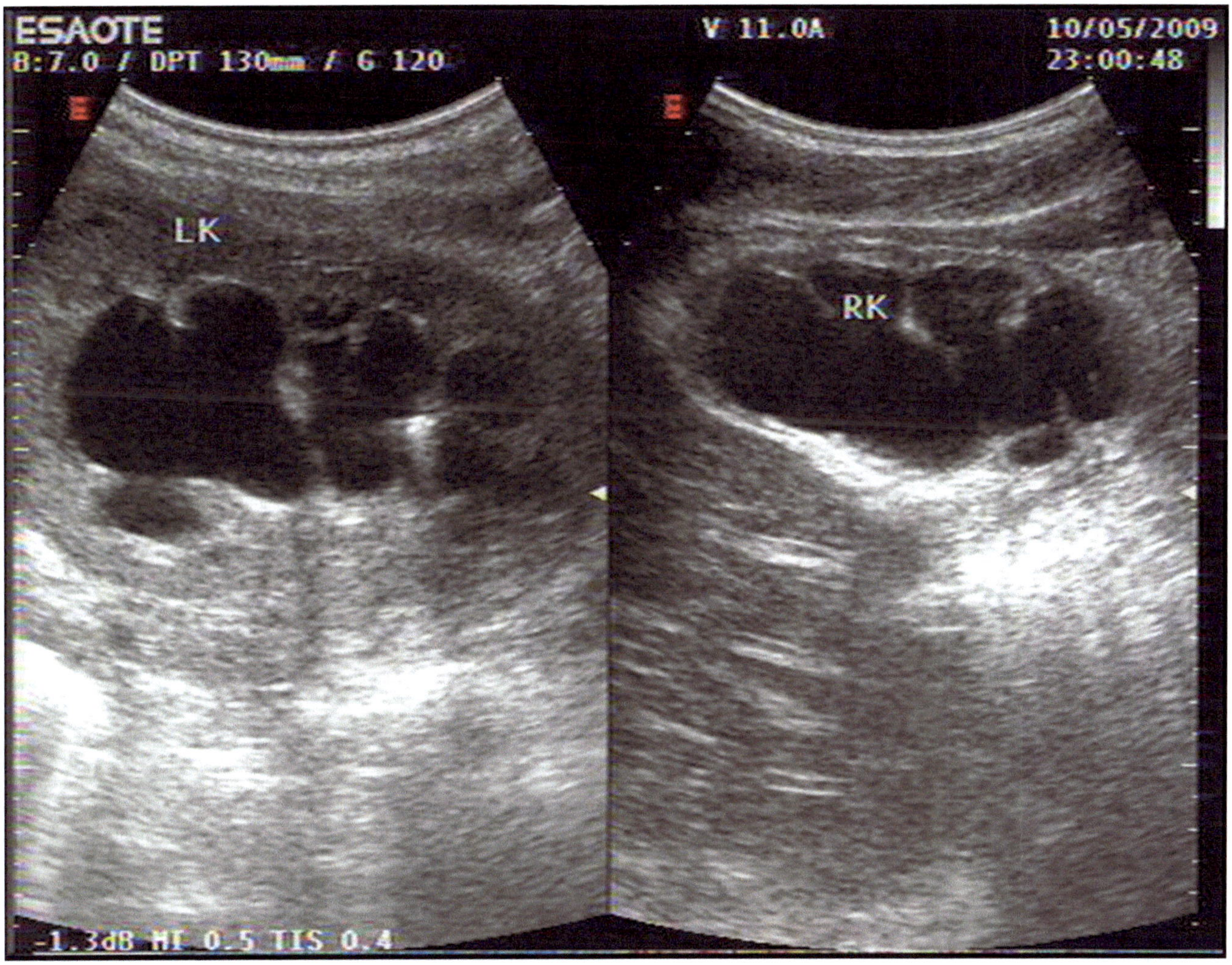

Fig. 26.5 Urinary system ultrasonogram of a 5-year-old boy being fed with milk powder tainted with melamine. Hydronephrosis was detected in both kidneys. There is a 0.8- × 0.6-cm stone in the right side of pyelocalyceal system. The patient was diagnosed with bilateral ureteric and renal stones

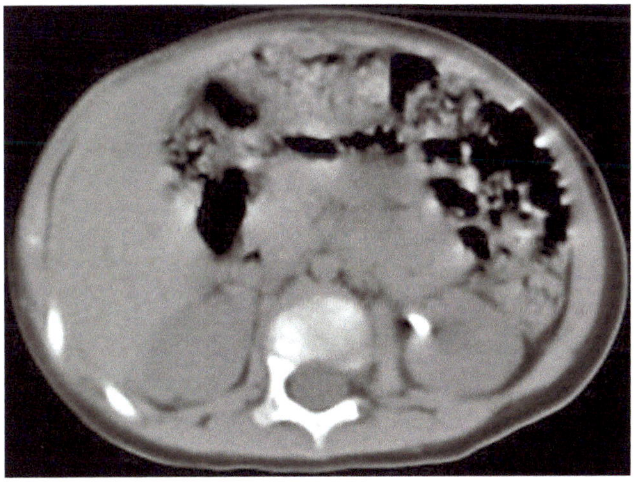

Fig. 26.6 CT scan of a patient with a melamine stone

recovered well; there was no evidence of long-term renal damage, and no recurrence of urinary stones was found. Three children failed to expel the stones by conservative medical therapy; the stones remained in situ, but the sizes decreased. No urothelial tumor was found. Long-term follow-up studies of these children are warranted to assess more comprehensively the public health impact of consuming milk products contaminated with melamine.

Conclusion

Melamine stones are a new entity caused by addition of the toxic product to milk.

The formation of melamine-associated urinary stones in humans is somewhat different from the crystallization in renal tubules that occurs in animals. It is postulated that the crystals so formed serve as nidus for deposition of other chemicals like uric acid and in the process give rise to stone formation. The missing link is the role of cyanuric acid or other analogues, which may explain the pathogenesis. Such analogues actually inhibit hepatic uric acid oxidase, an effect that increases circulating uric acid levels [1] that may explain the composition of stones containing uric acid. Much work still needs to be carried out on this condition.

References

1. Dobson RL, Motlagh S, Quijano M, Cambron RT, Baker TR, Pullen AM, et al. Identification and characterization of toxicity of contaminants in pet food leading to an outbreak of renal toxicity in cats and dogs. Toxicol Sci. 2008;106:251–62.
2. Burns K. Researchers examine contaminants in food, deaths of pets: survey, case definition, studies implicate combination of melamine and cyanuric acid. J Am Vet Med Assoc. 2007;231:1632–44.
3. Mast RW, Jeffcoat AR, Sadler BM, Kraska RC, Friedman MA. Metabolism, disposition and excretion of [14C]melamine in male Fischer 344 rats. Food Chem Toxicol. 1983;21:807–10.
4. Baynes RE, Smith G, Mason SE, Barrett E, Barlow BM, Riviere JE. Pharmacokinetics of melamine in pigs following intravenous administration. Food Chem Toxicol. 2008;46:1196–200.
5. Melnick RL, Boorman GA, Haseman JK, Montali RJ, Huff J. Urolithiasis and bladder carcinogenicity of melamine in rodents. Toxicol Appl Pharmacol. 1984;72:292–303.
6. Screening information data set (SIDS) for high production volume chemicals, Organisation for Economics Cooperation and Development, United Nations Environment Programme (UNEP) Publications. Nairobi; 2002. Available at: http://www.inchem.org/documents/sids/sids/108781.pdf. Accessed 18 Dec 2008.
7. Puschner B, Poppenga RH, Lowenstine LJ, Filigenzi MS. Assessment of melamine and cyanuric acid toxicity in cats. J Vet Diagn Invest. 2007;19:616–24.
8. Reimschuessel R, Gieseker CM, Miller RA, Ward J, Boehmer J, Rummel N, et al. Evaluation of the renal effects of experimental feeding of melamine and cyanuric acid to fish and pigs. Am J Vet Res. 2008;69:1217–28.
9. Ogasawara H, Imaida K, Ishiwata H. Urinary bladder carcinogenesis induced by melamine in F344 male rats: correlation between carcinogenicity and urolith formation. Carcinogenesis. 1995;16:2773–7.
10. Heck HD, Tyl RW. The induction of bladder stones by terephthalic acid, dimethyl terephthalate, and melamine (2,4,6-triamino-s-triazine) and its relevance to risk assessment. Regul Toxicol Pharmacol. 1985;5:294–313.
11. Li CY, Deng YL, Chen L, Long FZ, Tao ZW, Meng DD, et al. Development of urinary calculus formation and renal injury in rats administered melamine. Chin J Pathophysiol. 2010;26:2217–21.
12. World Health Organization. Melamine and cyanuric acid: toxicity, preliminary risk assessment and guidance on levels in food. World Health Organization; 2008. Available at: http://www.who.int/foodsafety/fs_management/Melamine.pdf. Accessed 18 Dec 2008.
13. Spivacow FR, Negri AL, del Valle EE, Calvino L, Fradinger E, Zanchetta JR. Metabolic risk factors in children with kidney stone disease. Pediatr Nephrol. 2008;23:1129–33.
14. Cameron MA, Sakhaee K, Moe OW. Nephrolithiasis in children. Pediatr Nephrol. 2005;20:1587–92.
15. Jia LQ, Shen Y, Wang XM, He LJ, Xin Y, Hu YX. Ultrasonographic diagnosis of urinary calculus caused by melamine in children. Chin Med J. 2009;122:252–6.
16. Preliminary fact sheet concerning urinary stone relating to Melamine-tainted milk formula in children. The Ministry of Health of the People's Republic of China; 2008. Available at: http://www.moh.ov.cn/publicfiles/business/htmlfiles/mohbgt/s3582/200809/37783.htm. Accessed 18 Dec 2008.
17. Recommendation on diagnosis and treatment of children consuming melamine tainted product. The Ministry of Health of the People's Republic of China; 2008. Available at: http://www.moh.gov.cn/publicfiles///business/cmsresources/mohyzs/cmsrsdocument/doc2317.doc. Accessed 18 Dec 2008.
18. Hospital Authority Expert Group on MTMP related disorders. Updated guidelines for assessment and treatment of melamine tainted milk product related disorders (version 3). Hospital Authority website: http://ha.home/qns/mtmp/man.htm. Accessed 12 Nov 2008.
19. Sanlu infant milk formula incident public consultation guidelines. Chinese Center for Disease Control and Prevention website: http://www.chinacdc.net.cn/n272442/n272530/n3226631/index.html. Accessed 11 Nov 2008.
20. Sun N, Shen Y, Sun Q, Li XR, Jia LQ, Zhang GJ, et al. Diagnosis and treatment of melamine-associated urinary calculus complicated with acute renal failure in infants and young children. Chin Med J. 2009;122:245–51.

Trace Elements in Urolithiasis

27

Albrecht Hesse and Roswitha Siener

Abstract

Trace elements are essential substances, whose content in the human tissue is less than 50 ppm (50 mg/kg). These elements, such as zinc, copper, nickel, iron, and strontium, are able to form poorly soluble salts with oxalate and phosphate ions. No pure urinary stones consisting of these compounds are known so far. However, the incorporation of zinc phosphate (hopeite) in layers in a struvite stone has been described. Organic stones, such as uric acid, contain only small amounts of trace elements. Compared to calcium oxalates, the concentration of zinc and other trace elements is higher in calcium phosphate stones. Trace elements can contribute to the stabilization of calcium oxalate dihydrate (weddellite), an unstable compound. The disintegration of calcium oxalate monohydrate (whewellite) by shock wave lithotripsy (SWL) is supposed to be improved by the incorporation of trace elements. An incorporation of trace element compounds in layers or also the replacement of calcium in the crystal lattice of whewellite can be responsible for this effect. In conclusion, depending on the stone type and according to their occurrence in urine, trace elements are incorporated into a urinary stone and can affect its properties.

Keywords

Trace elements • Urinary calculi • Whewellite • Weddellite • Carbonate apatite • Crystal structure • Zinc • Iron • Strontium • Fluorine

Introduction

Trace elements are inorganic nutritional components whose essentiality in humans has been experimentally proven in amounts of less than 50 mg/day, whose content in the tissue is less than 50 ppm ($<50\times10^{-6}$ g/g wet weight) and whose function is biochemically ensured [1]. Essential trace elements in humans are chromium (Cr), cobalt (Co), copper (Cu), fluorine (F), iron (Fe), iodine (I), manganese (Mn), molybdenum (Mo), nickel (Ni), selenium (Se), and zinc (Zn) [1].

All other elements, whose essentiality has been proven by semisynthetic rations in animal studies over several generations and for which deficiency symptoms were found under these extreme conditions, without knowing their special functions, are called ultra trace elements [1]. Aluminum (Al), antimony (Sb), arsenic (As), barium (Ba), bismuth (Bi), boron (B), bromine (Br), cadmium (Cd), caesium (Cs), germanium (Ge), lead (Pb), lithium (Li), mercury (Hg), rubidium (Rb), samarium (Sm), silicon (Si), strontium (Sr), thallium (Tl), titanium (Ti), and tungsten (W) are counted among ultra trace elements [1]. All inorganic bodily components can induce intoxications, if ingested in large amounts, by inhibition of the effect of essential substances, by interactions with other elements, or by redistribution of essential substances in the body, which can cause diseases [1].

A. Hesse, Ph.D. (✉)
Urinary Stone Analysis Centre Bonn,
Theaterplatz 14, D-53177 Bonn, Germany
e-mail: beratung@harnsteinanalysezentrum-bonn.de,
albrecht-hesse@web.de

R. Siener, Ph.D.
Department of Urology, University Stone Centre, University of Bonn,
Sigmund-Freud-Strasse 25, D-53105 Bonn, Germany
e-mail: roswitha.siener@ukb.uni-bonn.de

J.J. Talati et al. (eds.), *Urolithiasis*,
DOI 10.1007/978-1-4471-4387-1_27, © Springer-Verlag London 2012

Stone Types with Trace Elements

Trace elements such as Zn, Cu, Ni, Al, Sr, Cd, and Pb are able to form poorly soluble salts with phosphate and oxalate ions. Due to the low concentrations of these elements in urine, these substances usually do not form stones. However, it is conceivable that these phosphates and oxalates are incorporated into the corresponding urinary stones. Using standard methods for urinary stone analysis—infrared spectroscopy (IR) and X-ray diffraction (XRD)—compounds of phosphates and oxalates, respectively, with trace elements are mostly not detected as urinary stone type [2, 3]. Proportions of less than 1 % in a urinary stone are usually not detectable by these methods. Pure urinary stones consisting of trace element compounds have not yet been described. However, trace elements can be found in different concentrations in all types of urinary stones.

Importance of Individual Trace Elements for Urolithiasis

Due to the poor solubility of compounds of some trace elements with phosphate and oxalate, respectively, the formation of urinary stones is conceivable, but in view of the low concentrations in urine, practically not relevant. The occurrence of trace elements in the urinary stone types repeatedly gave rise to investigations on the importance of these elements in urinary stone pathogenesis [4–6]. Generally, it has become apparent that the content of trace elements in kidney stones is minimal, compared to the amounts that are consumed daily and excreted in urine.

Zinc

Zn has an important function in body growth (DNA and RNA polymerase) and in the function of cell membranes and erythrocytes. Zinc phosphate—$Zn_3(PO_4)_2 \cdot 4H_2O$; hopeite—was described as embedded substance in a struvite/carbonate apatite urinary stone [7]. Zinc in elemental form was found in higher concentrations in calcium-containing but also in organic urinary stones compared to other trace elements [8–14]. Calcium phosphate calculi contained more Zn than calcium oxalates [10, 14]. By contrast, brushite stones contain significantly less Zn than carbonate apatite calculi [14]. These findings suggest that Zn can form a salt with phosphate but that the formation conditions (i.e. acidic pH range) for brushite whose structure differs from that of carbonate apatite are less suitable.

Weddellite calculi contain more Zn than whewellite stones [9–11, 14–16]. It has been experimentally determined that Zn and other elements are jointly responsible for the stabilization of weddellite [10, 17]. The separate analysis of core and shell of urinary stones revealed higher concentrations of Zn in the core of mixed calcium oxalate/apatite stones than in pure calcium oxalate or struvite stones, respectively [18, 19]. It was concluded from the higher Zn content of the stone core that Zn and other trace elements (Cu, Sr) could play a role in the formation of the nucleus. Bazin et al. could not confirm the higher Zn concentration of the core versus outer layers of the stone [14].

Zn concentrations were found to be higher in urinary stones collected from smokers than in stones from nonsmokers. However, urinary Zn concentration did not differ between both groups [20]. No association could be established between smoking, trace elements, and urinary stone formation. Determination of Zn in the urine of stone patients compared to healthy subjects revealed both, increased 24 h urinary Zn excretion on the one hand [8, 21–24] but also significantly decreased Zn excretions on the other hand [13, 25]. Other authors did not find significant differences in Zn excretion between healthy subjects and stone formers [11, 16]. An increased Zn excretion is probably not causally related to the genesis of urinary stones, but rather the result of an increased epithelialization for which Zn is required. Crystallization experiments showed a change in calcium oxalate crystal structures in the presence of Zn [25]. The crystal growth rate did not change in other experiments [26]. However, Zn was found to inhibit the crystal growth of calcium oxalate [27] and calcium phosphate when present at physiologic concentrations [26].

Some elements appear to interfere with whewellite stone fragility [28]. Whewellite stones with higher Zn content (Fe and Mn also play a role) fragmented more easily by SWL [29]. Thus a reduction of trace elements (Zn) concentrations of a renal stone might make the stone harder to fragment. The incorporation of the trace elements into the crystal lattice and also the incorporation of compounds of trace elements in layers into the stone probably facilitate the fragmentation of urinary stones.

Iron

Fe is a frequent trace element with a variety of functions in the human body. All studies found a much lower content of Fe in non-calcium than in calcium-containing stones [10, 11, 14, 15]. The higher Fe content could result from the inhibitory properties of Fe^{3+} on calcium oxalate crystallization [30, 31]. The presence of Fe in calcium oxalate stones may result from trapping of Fe ions at the crystal surface or in the crystal lattice [14, 32]. An increased 24 h urinary Fe excretion was found in calcium oxalate stone patients compared with healthy subjects [13, 21].

Strontium

Sr forms poorly soluble complexes with phosphate and oxalate that can be incorporated into the urinary stone. Moreover, Sr can replace Ca in the crystal lattice. Especially high concentrations of Sr were recorded in calcium phosphate stones [11, 14, 15].

Other Trace Elements

The cited authors determined quantitatively a large number of trace elements in urinary stones, urine, and also in serum. However, an association with stone formation can be established only in a few cases. The occurrence of some of the trace elements is increased in calcium-containing stones, and only a few of them accumulate in organic stones, especially uric acid stones (As, Sb) [11]. Long-term Cd exposure leads to renal damage and a higher incidence of calcium stones [33, 34].

In an area with drinking water fluoridation for caries prophylaxis in Germany, significantly increased fluorine concentrations were determined in whewellite and weddellite calculi compared to stones of an area without drinking water fluoridation. The F content was higher in weddellite than in whewellite stones. Moreover, the F content was increased in carbonate apatite, struvite, and uric acid stones in the fluoridated area. The F content resulted in an increased degree of crystallization and hence in an increased strength of carbonate apatite [9, 35].

For the stabilization of the individual urinary stone phases, such as weddellite [14, 17] and uric acid dihydrate [36], specific urinary components are responsible. As pure chemical compounds, these urinary stone substances are very unstable and transform into the stable crystal phases whewellite or uric acid, respectively, with elimination of water. Trace elements, major elements such as magnesium, and also high molecular substances contribute to the stabilization of weddellite and uric acid dihydrate.

Conclusion

Trace elements are ingested with food. Environmental influences and workplace exposures can increase the intake of specific trace elements. A large number of trace elements are essential for specific metabolic processes, temporarily stored and excreted via the kidneys. This can result in the accidental incorporation of trace elements into urinary stones but also affect crystal formation or change the properties of urinary stones. As stated by Grases and colleagues, "When considering all different aspects discussed, it is evident that the importance of trace elements in urolithogenesis is not a mineralogical or crystallographic problem, so their role must be of another kind" [25].

References

1. Deutsche Gesellschaft für Ernährung, Österreichische Gesellschaft für Ernährung, Schweizerische Gesellschaft für Ernährungsforschung, Schweizerische Vereinigung für Ernährung (German, Austrian and Swiss Societies of Nutrition). Referenzwerte für die Nährstoffzufuhr (Reference values for nutrient intake). Frankfurt: Umschau Braus; 2000.
2. Hesse A, Sanders G. Atlas of infrared spectra for the analysis of urinary concrements. Stuttgart/New York: Thieme; 1988.
3. Hesse A, Kruse R, Geilenkeuser WJ, Schmidt M. Quality control in urinary stone analysis: results of 44 ring trials (1980–2001). Clin Chem Lab Med. 2005;43:298–303.
4. Eusebio E, Elliott JS. Effect of trace metals on the crystallization of calcium oxalate. Invest Urol. 1967;4:431–5.
5. Sutor DJ. Growth studies of calcium oxalate in the presence of various ions and compounds. Br J Urol. 1969;41:171–8.
6. Scott R, East BW, Janczyszyn J, Boddy K, Yates AJ. Concentration and distribution of some minor and trace elements in urinary tract stones: a preliminary study. Urol Res. 1980;8:167–9.
7. Parsons J. Zinc phosphate identified as a constituent of urinary calculi. Science. 1953;118:217–8.
8. Schneider HJ, Straube G, Anke M. Zinc in urinary calculi (German). Z Urol Nephrol. 1970;63:895–900.
9. Hesse A, Dietze HJ, Berg W, Hienzsch E. Mass spectrometric trace element analysis of calcium oxalate uroliths. Eur Urol. 1977;3:359–61.
10. Levinson AA, Nosal M, Davidman M, Prien EL, Prien EL, Stevenson RG. Trace elements in kidney stones from three areas in the United States. Invest Urol. 1978;15:270–4.
11. Joost J, Tessadri R. Trace element investigations in kidney stone patients. Eur Urol. 1987;13:264–70.
12. Durak I, Yasar A, Yurtarslani Z, Akpoyraz M, Tasman S. Analysis of magnesium and trace elements in urinary calculi by atomic absorption spectrophotometry. Br J Urol. 1988;62:203–5.
13. Atakan IH, Kaplan M, Seren G, Aktoz T, Gül H, Inci O. Serum, urinary and stone zinc, iron, magnesium and copper levels in idiopathic calcium oxalate stone patients. Int Urol Nephrol. 2007;39:351–6.
14. Bazin D, Chevallier P, Matzen G, Jungers P, Daudon M. Heavy elements in urinary stones. Urol Res. 2007;35:179–84.
15. Wandt MAE, Underhill G. Covariance biplot analysis of trace element concentrations in urinary stones. Br J Urol. 1988;61:474–81.
16. Hofbauer J, Steffan I, Höbarth K, Vujicic G, Schwetz H, Reich G, Zechner O. Trace elements and urinary stone formation: new aspects of the pathological mechanism of urinary stone formation. J Urol. 1991;145:93–6.
17. Hesse A, Berg W, Schneider HJ, Hienzsch E. A contribution to the formation mechanism of calcium oxalate urinary calculi. II. In vitro experiments concerning the theory of the formation of whewellite and weddellite urinary calculi. Urol Res. 1976;4:157–60.
18. Lin SM, Tseng CL, Yang MH. Determination of major, minor and trace elements in urinary stones by neutron activation analysis. Int J Rad Appl Instrum A. 1987;38:635–9.
19. Singh VK, Rai AK, Rai PK, Jindal PK. Cross-sectional study of kidney stones by laser-induced breakdown spectroscopy. Lasers Med Sci. 2009;24:749–59.
20. Slojewski M, Czerny B, Safranow K, Drozdzik M, Pawlik A, Jakubowska K, Olszewska M, Golab A, Byra E, Chlubek D, Sikorski A. Does smoking have any effect in urinary stone composition and the distribution of trace elements in urine and stones? Urol Res. 2009;37:317–22.
21. Elliot JS, Ribeiro ME. The urinary excretion of trace metals in patients with calcium oxalate urinary stone. Invest Urol. 1973;10:253–5.
22. Hesse A, Schneider HJ, Berg W. Die Bedeutung von Spurenelementen in der Harnsteingenese. Zbl Pharm. 1978;117:753–6.

23. Trinchieri A, Mandressi A, Luongo P, Longo G, Pisani E. The influence of diet on urinary risk factors for stones in healthy subjects and idiopathic renal calcium stone formers. Br J Urol. 1991;67:230–6.
24. Rangnekar GV, Gaur MS. Serum and urinary zinc levels in urolithiasis. Br J Urol. 1993;71:527–9.
25. Grases F, Ruiz J, Costa-Bauza A, Coll R, Conte A. Zinc, copper and oxalocalcic urolithiasis. Urol Int. 1993;50:205–8.
26. Meyer JL, Angino EE. The role of trace metals in calcium urolithiasis. Invest Urol. 1977;14:347–50.
27. Grases F, Genestar C, Millan A. The influence of some metallic ions and their complexes on the kinetics of crystal growth of calcium oxalate. J Crystal Growth. 1989;94:507–12.
28. Küpeli S, Arikan N, Durak I, Sarica K, Akpoyraz M, Karalezli G. Efficiency of extracorporeal shockwave lithotripsy on calcium-oxalate stones: role of copper, iron, magnesium and zinc concentrations on disintegration of the stones. Eur Urol. 1993;23:409–12.
29. Turgut M, Unal I, Berber A, Demir TA, Mutlu F, Aydar Y. The concentration of Zn, Mg and Mn in calcium oxalate monohydrate stones appears to interfere with their fragility in ESWL therapy. Urol Res. 2008;36:31–8.
30. Meyer JL, Thomas WC. Trace metal-citric acid complexes as inhibitors of calcification and crystal growth. II. Effects of Fe(III), Cr(III) and Al(III) complexes on calcium oxalate crystal growth. J Urol. 1982;128:1376–8.
31. Munoz JA, Valiente M. Effects of trace metals on the inhibition of calcium oxalate crystallization. Urol Res. 2005;33:267–72.
32. Loutfi A, van Reen R, Hamid GA. Studies on bladder stone disease in Egyptian children. V. Composition of bladder stones. J Egypt Med Assoc. 1974;57:124–36.
33. Friberg L. Health hazards in the manufacture of alkaline accumulators with special reference to chronic cadmium poisoning: a clinical and experimental study. Acta Med Scand. 1950;138 Suppl 240: 1–124.
34. Scott R, Patterson PJ, Burns R, Ottoway JM, Hussain FER, Fell GS, Dumbuya S, Iqbal M. Hypercalciuria related to cadmium exposure. Urology. 1978;11:462–5.
35. Hesse A, Müller R, Schneider HJ, Taubert F. Analytic experiments on the significance of the fluorine content of urinary calculi (German). Urologe A. 1978;17:207–10.
36. Hesse A, Schneider HJ, Berg W, Hienzsch E. Uric acid dihydrate as urinary calculus component. Invest Urol. 1975;12:405–9.

Infection Stones

28

Janet Colli and Raju Thomas

Abstract

Infection stones composed of struvite result from urinary infection by urease-splitting organisms. These produce ammonia and alkalinize the urine. Infection and stone growth cannot be eliminated without the meticulous clearance of all stone fragments. Acetohydroxamic acid is effective in limiting urease production by bacteria and eliminating infection in these patients, but such therapy can cause serious side effects.

Keywords

Infection stones • Struvite • pH • Urease-producing bacteria • Urinary ammonium levels Urinary infection • PCNL/PNL • SWL • Open surgery

Introduction

Staghorn calculi are usually defined as large calculi that occupy the renal pelvis and at least two of the calyceal system within a kidney. Staghorn calculi can be relatively simple or complex, based on configuration of the renal calyces and status of infundibuli (Fig. 28.1a–c).

Infection stones are also known as struvite stones and are composed of magnesium, ammonium, and phosphate, mixed in with carbonate. These struvite stones form only in the presence of bacteria that produce urease. The common urease-producing bacteria that can populate the urinary tract are *Proteus*, *Klebsiella*, *Pseudomonas*, and *Enterococci*. The theory behind stone formation is that splitting of urea by the aforementioned bacteria results in alkaline urine and thus stone formation. Another suggested theory is that such bacterial infection may induce formation of these stones by increasing adherence of crystals. There is said to be an association between nonurease bacteria and struvite stones because of the production of urinary matrix substances that increase crystal adherence to the renal epithelium.

In patients who are prone to such stones, the urine ammonia levels are above 30 mM/24 h and urine pH above 7.0. However, some infection stones begin as calcium oxalate stones that become infected with a urease-producing bacterium.

It is now widely accepted that prompt intervention in management of staghorn calculi is critical. Published reports by Blandy and Singh, 1976, show that urosepsis and renal insufficiency follow when the stones are managed conservatively and nephrectomy and dialysis ensued in about 50 % of patients with a high mortality rate of 25 % [1].

Signs and Symptoms

Struvite calculi account for most of the staghorn calculi. They can grow relatively quickly and fill the pelvis and extend into the renal collecting system. These stones are easily diagnosed on radiological findings, and most of these are radiopaque unless the composition of matrix is proportionately higher. Because women are susceptible to urinary tract infections, struvite infection and staghorn calculi are more common in women. The other etiological factors are presence of a foreign body within the renal collecting systems as

J. Colli, M.D. (✉)
Department of Urology, Tulane University,
1430 Tulane Avenue, SL-42, New Orleans, LA, 70112-2699, USA
e-mail: jcolli1@tulane.edu

R. Thomas, M.D., FACS, MHA
Department of Urology, Tulane University, Health Sciences Center,
1430 Tulane Avenue, SL-42, New Orleans, LA, 70112-2699, USA
e-mail: rthomas@tulane.edu

J.J. Talati et al. (eds.), *Urolithiasis*,
DOI 10.1007/978-1-4471-4387-1_28, © Springer-Verlag London 2012

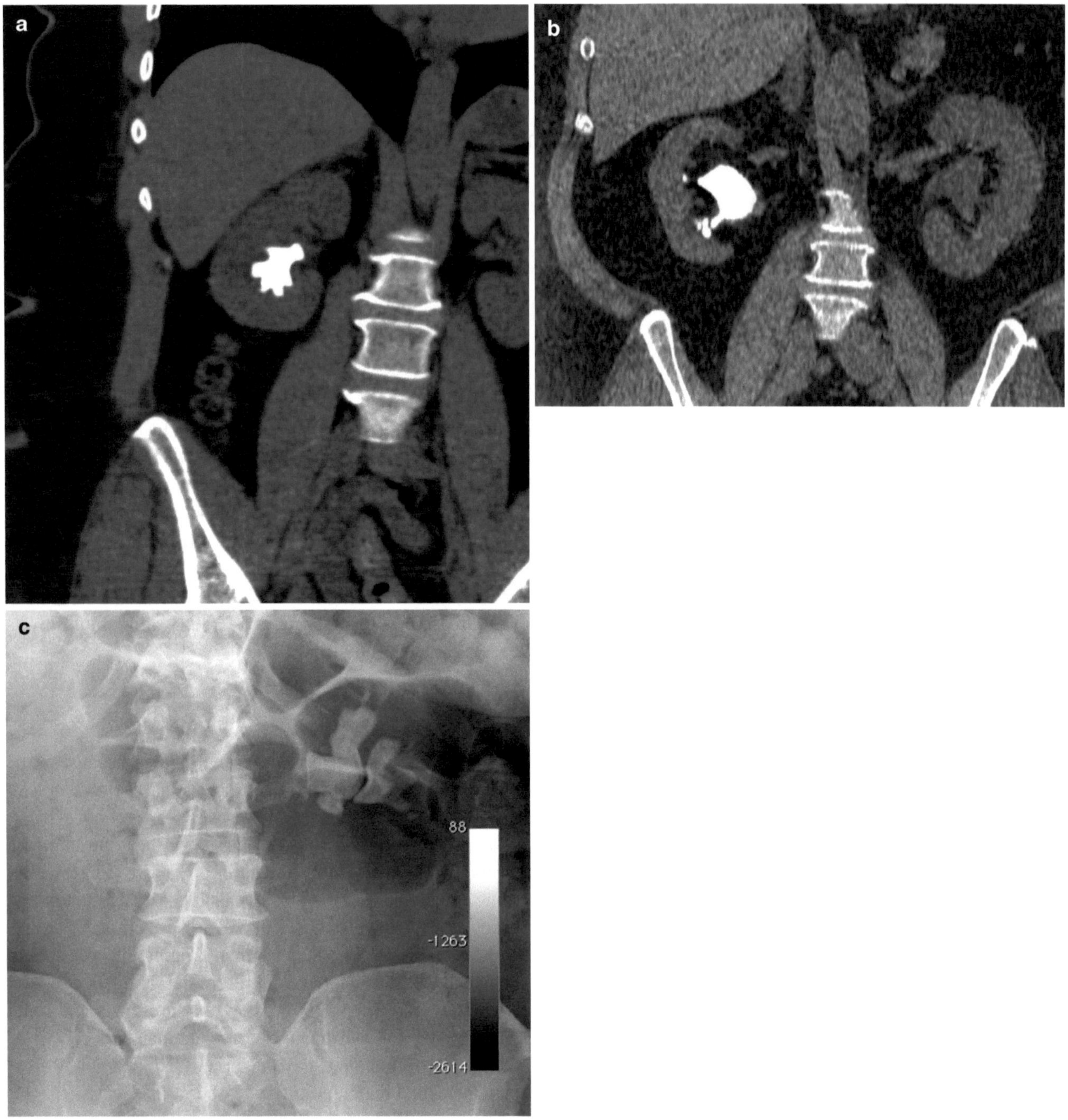

Fig. 28.1 (**a**, **b**) Relatively simple staghorn calculi. (**c**) Complex staghorn calculus

well as a diagnosis of neurogenic bladder. Comarr reported that 8 % of patients with spinal cord injury developed infection stones [2]. Another group susceptible to infection stones are those who have indwelling urinary catheters and those undergoing urinary diversion.

Clinical Presentation

Patients with struvite infection stones present with flank pain, fever, dysuria, and frequency of urination; and if the patient has an active urinary tract infection, the patient can present with fever and mimic an acute abdomen. Associated symptoms include weakness and loss of appetite. The question of whether metabolic abnormalities are present in these patients has been debated. Resnick reported that a significant proportion of patients with infections stones do have metabolic disorders. While Lingeman and colleagues have concluded, upon reviewing the literature, that metabolic abnormalities are present in patients with struvite and calcium oxalate stones but not in patients with pure infection struvite stones.

Rarely, patients progress from the struvite stones to a condition known as xanthogranulomatous pyelonephritis, which can destroy the renal parenchymal and can even mimic certain renal tumors, on radiographic imaging.

Diagnostic Work-Up

Today, the diagnostic work-up of choice would be a computed tomography (CT) scan without and with intravenous contrasts if the serum creatinine level permits contrast use [3]. This work-up will give an anatomic view of both kidneys and also if there is a parenchymal involvement with any XGP process. Also any abscess location within the kidney can be identified.

A clean catch of midstream urine for analysis and culture in men and a catheterized analysis in women is recommended so as to obtain a correct understanding of the antibiotics to which the bacteria is susceptible.

Prior to any definitive treatment, appropriate antibiotic therapy is recommended so as to prevent any risk of urosepsis. The other routine work-up recommendations are a complete blood count, a metabolic panel, etc. These may be part of routine pre-anesthesia clearance work-up. A nuclear medicine MAG-3 renal scan can evaluate the functional status of the involved kidney.

Treatment

The technological advances over the past 20 years or so have truly revolutionized the management of staghorn calculi.

The goal of treatment for management and removal of the staghorn calculi is to render the kidney as stone-free as possible. Any residual fragments will act as a nidus, and it is not surprising to find recurrences of the stones, unless the kidney is made stone-free. Nevertheless, open surgery is still considered a viable approach to manage complex staghorn calculi. Though the procedure of anatrophic nephrolithotomy has been overshadowed by the percutaneous lithotripsy procedures, and often a combination of SWL (extracorporeal shock wave lithotripsy) is utilized to render the patient stone-free, the open surgical approach with the idea to split open the kidney and remove the stone in its entirety is still a procedure to be considered when truly indicated, especially in the complex renal staghorn calculi.

However, today one would consider percutaneous nephrostolithotripsy (PCNL) as the procedure of choice for the stones, and often multiple percutaneous tracts are needed to render the patient stone-free (Fig. 28.2). In complex staghorn calculi, with multiple calyceal involvement, not only are multiple percutaneous tracts needed, but often multiple treatment sessions are required (Fig. 28.3a–c) [4–6].

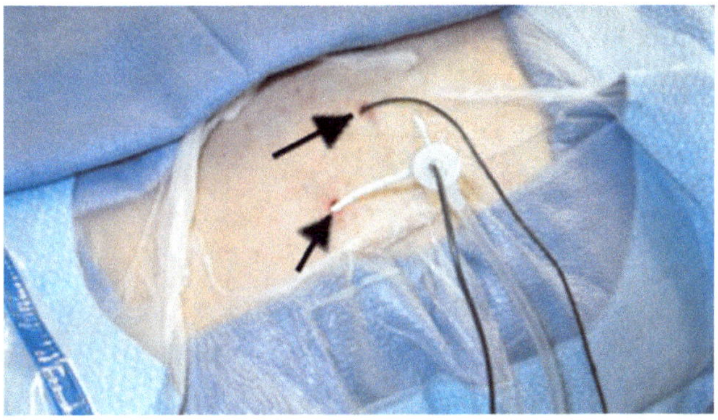

Fig. 28.2 Two percutaneous tracts in place prior to dilatation for PCNL. Nephrostomy tracts (*arrows*)

Often, especially after the introduction of flexible nephroscopy and ureteroscopy equipment, these can also be used as an adjuvant treatment and holmium laser can be used to fragment these stones.

Often, based on the complexity of the occupation of the calyceal systems, all three technological procedures, namely, percutaneous lithotripsy, in combination with ureteroscopic retrograde holmium laser lithotripsy, or in combination with ESWL, may be required for optimizing treatment. Lingeman has reported remarkable success with PCNL: 92 % of kidneys with partial staghorn calculi and up to 91 % with complete staghorn calculi were rendered stone-free with a combination of PCNL and SWL [7, 8].

The nephrolithotripsy procedure, followed by rigorous lavage with Renacidin™ of the renal pelvis to remove all fragments of the infectious stones, has reduced recurrence rates from 40 to 2 % during a 7-year follow-up [9]. Such adjuvant treatments are used infrequently today.

Results

A multivariate analysis shows that the PCNL has the highest rate of stone-free status, but use of other technologies such as SWL and ureteroscopy in conjunction with SWL may be most conducive to stone-free status.

If an infection stone has been identified, then we will classify treatment options as:

1. ESWL for small calculi
2. Large stone in the renal pelvis: PCNL +/– ESWL
3. Incomplete staghorn could be PCNL and ESWL (stone burden mainly in renal pelvis, see Fig. 28.1a)
4. Complete staghorn with favorable anatomy: Multiple tract PCNL +/– ESWL (Fig. 28.1b)
5. Giant complicated staghorn: open surgical anatrophic nephrolithotomy
6. XGP with poorly, functioning kidney therapy would be nephrectomy

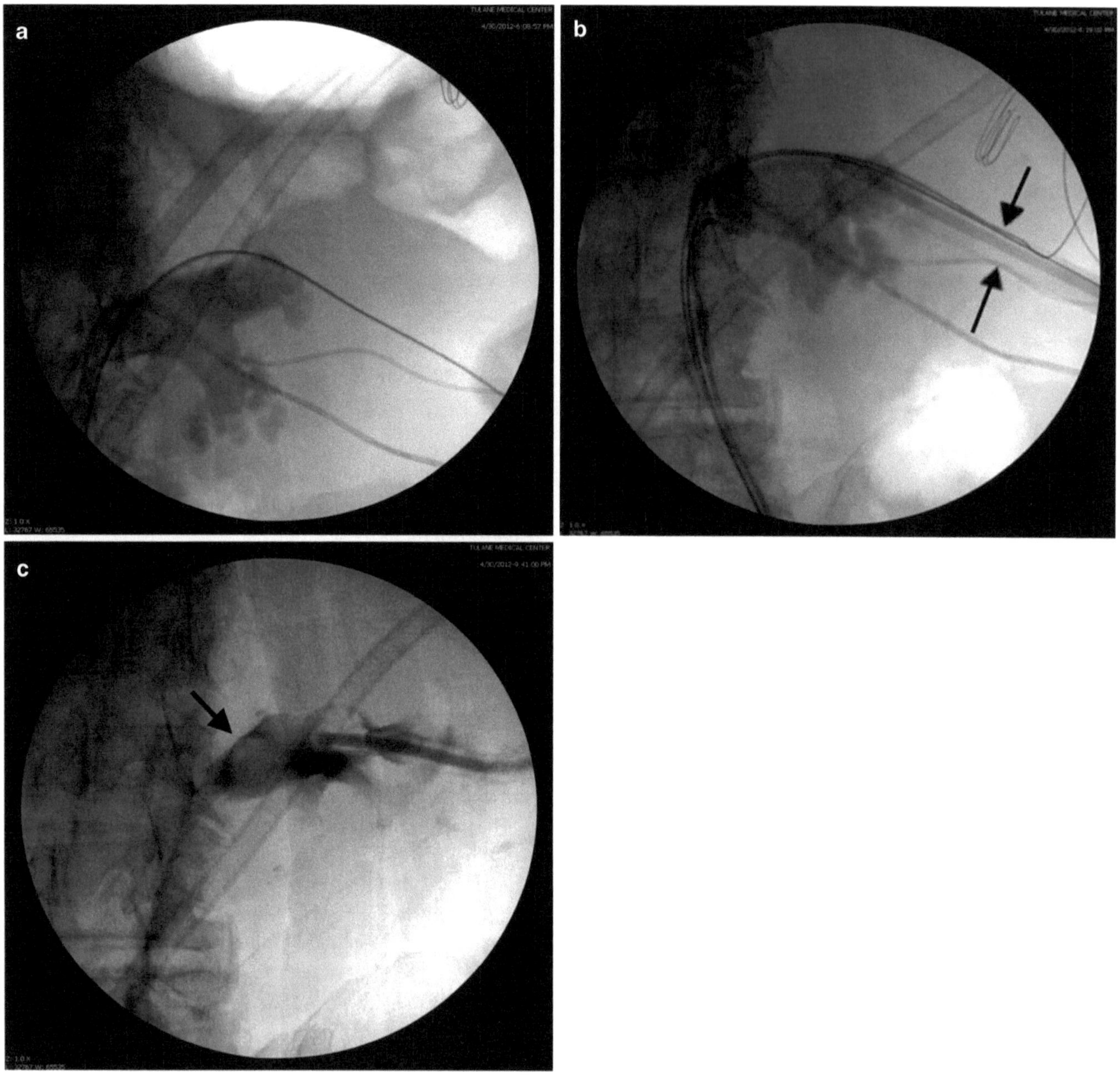

Fig. 28.3 (**a**) Multiple percutaneous tracts in place, prior to dilatation of any tract. (**b**) Access sheet in place in upper pole calyx (see *arrows*). (**c**) Nephrostogram showing nephrostomy tube in place after PCNL. Balloon in renal pelvis (see *arrow*)

Long-term antibiotic therapy has proven to be ineffective in eradicating infection and does not substitute for complete removal of even the smallest particulate of the stone.

Follow-Up Management

Postsurgical follow-up includes evaluation of the renal function as well as periodic check of the urine to make sure there is no recurrence of urea-splitting bacterial infection.

Conclusion

Prompt diagnosis of patients with urinary tract infection and staghorn calculi is most critical. Adequate work-up to diagnose and stage the staghorn calculi is important. Using modern technology and a combination of PCNL +/− URS +/− SWL and +/− open surgical intervention can render the patient stone-free. However, periodic evaluation of the kidney and appropriate imaging study will be able to give us more information about the status of the involved renal unit. Moreover, diagnosing and preventing recurrent urinary tract infection is important.

References

1. Blandy JP, Singh M. The case for a more aggressive approach to staghorn stones. J Urol. 1976;115:505.
2. Comarr AE, Kawaicki GR, Bors E. Renal calculosis in patients with traumatic cord lesions. J Urol. 1962;85:647–56.
3. Miller OF, Rineer SK, Reichard SR, et al. Prospective comparison of unenhanced spiral computed tomography and intravenous urogram in the evaluation of acute flank pain. Urology. 1998;52:982–7.
4. Munver R, Delvecchio FC, Newman GE, Preminger GM. Critical analysis of supracostal access for percutaneous renal surgery. J Urol. 2001;166(4):1242–6.
5. Gupta R, Kumar A, Kapoor R, et al. Prospective evaluation of safety and efficacy of the supracostal approach for percutaneous nephrolithotomy. BJU Int. 2002;90(9):809–13.
6. Segura JW, Patterson DE, LeRoy AJ, et al. Percutaneous removal of kidney stones: review of 1,000 cases. J Urol. 1985;134(6):1077–81.
7. Lingeman JE. Results of 313 staghorn treatments. In: Presented at 4th symposium on SWL: state of the art, Indianapolis, 1988.
8. Chaussy C, Brendel W, Schmiedt E. Extracorporeally induced destruction of kidney stones by shock waves. Lancet. 1980;2(8207):1265–8.
9. Mulvaney WP. The clinical use of renacidin in urinary calcifications. J Urol. 1960;84:206–12.

Epidemiological and Etiological Considerations

29

Hans-Göran Tiselius

Abstract

This chapter summarizes and discusses some aspects of stone disease from an epidemiological and etiological point of view. The discussion is based on selected data that have been given in the various preceding chapters. In view of what we know so far and regarding recent findings in calcium stone formation, attempts are made to predict in which direction stone research best should move. Improved methods to identify risk factors of stone formation might thus give us a basis for more efficient prevention tools for patients with recurrent stone formation.

Keywords

Epidemiology • Etiology • Stone composition • Risk factors • Future research

Introduction

It is evident from the various epidemiology chapters in this volume that stone disease is a worldwide health problem that causes a great burden to the health care system in terms of management as well as cost. There are, accordingly, few geographical areas and populations in which formation of urinary stones and its clinical consequences is not an important part of the daily urological practice. Previous reports have shown that absence of stone disease is encountered among Eskimos [1], coast inhabitants of Japan [2], and black people in South Africa [3]. In all other populations, there is a considerable annual incidence and prevalence. Such data are, however, very difficult to obtain and accordingly great variations for instance in terms of incidence, are obvious from the numbers presented from various regions. There are several factors that influence this statistical information. Important factors are how the health care is organized and how the stone problems are recorded and collected for the whole population or for a representative subgroup of stone-forming patients. Moreover, different authors might have used different definitions of both annual incidence and prevalence. Nevertheless, the data found above comprise an approximate although useful guide to the dimension of the problem.

But it stands to reason that all this information accordingly has to be interpreted with caution. For details regarding the incidence rates, the reader should refer to the individual chapters. The rounded-off numbers of lifetime risk as well as prevalence reported from different parts of the world are summarized in Table 29.1. This information is of relevance not only for health economists but the data also provide valuable clues to underlying etiologic factors. It is of interest to note that in many regions there seems to be a reduction of the male dominance in the stone-forming populations.

In the industrialized part of the world, bladder stones have been a rarity since a long time, whereas this condition obviously still exists in some regions. But also, in populations with a well-recognized high frequency of bladder stones has a remarkable decrease been noted. With increased affluence, stone disease has moved upwards from the bladder to the upper urinary tract, and today almost all stones are encountered in the kidneys or ureters.

Although calcium oxalate stones undoubtedly constitute the major problem (Table 29.2), unfortunately for that type of

H.-G. Tiselius, M.D., Ph.D.
Division of Urology, Department of Clinical Science, Intervention and Technology, Karolinska Institutet, Stockholm SE-141 86, Sweden
e-mail: hans-goran.tiselius@telia.com, hans-goran.tiselius@ki.se

J.J. Talati et al. (eds.), *Urolithiasis*,
DOI 10.1007/978-1-4471-4387-1_29, © Springer-Verlag London 2012

stone, it has been most difficult to get a satisfactory and complete explanation. The general conclusion is, however, that calcium oxalate stones are the result of a concert action of several important factors. It is highly interesting that pure calcium phosphate stones only are seen in a relatively small number of patients, despite the common presence of calcium phosphate salts in urine, commonly recorded hypercalciuria (Table 29.3), and periods during the day with a high pH. It is probable that a substantial number of stones classified as calcium oxalate stones also have a small content of calcium phosphate but that information is usually absent from most reports of stone composition (see Table 29.2). It is probably the accuracy of the analytical methods that are important in this regard.

Table 29.1 An overview of prevalence and male/female quotients in different geographical regions

Geographical regions	Prevalence (%)	Quotient men/women
Europe	5–10	2.7–4.1
North America	10–15[a] 6 (3–8)	1.3
Pakistan	~12	1.2–2.5
Southern India (Kerala)	3	
China		1.3–4.0
Brazil		1.00
Argentina		1.37
KSA	20[a]	4.0
Iran	6	1.15
Japan	15[a] 7	2.42
Russia	0.5–1.5	
Turkey		1.0

[a]Lifetime risk
The numbers extracted from the various chapters have been rounded off

Whereas calcium oxalate stone disease apparently is increasing, there is a clear trend that the frequency of infection stones is decreasing [4]. This is probably the result of appropriate early recognition and treatment of urinary tract infections. Cystine stones, on the other hand, have remained rather constant with a low frequency and small geographical variations. These stones are usually encountered in not more than maximally 2–3 % of all stone formers.

Uric acid (and most of these stones are composed of uric acid and should not be termed urate stones [5]) is a stone constituent that discloses the greatest geographical variation. The occurrence of uric acid stones is more common in regions with a warm climate. But uric acid stones also show an increased frequency in other parts of the world as a consequence of the wide-spread metabolic syndrome [6–8]. Ammonium urate stones occur and are also reported in several series of stone analyses. Such stones form as a consequence of high concentrations of urinary urate and a simultaneous urinary tract infection with urease-producing microorganisms [9].

Detailed information on urine composition is not available from all geographical areas, most certainly because the collection and analysis of representative and reliable urine samples is a both difficult and expensive procedure. When such information is available, analysis almost always has been carried out in selected groups of stone-forming patients. Standardized laboratory methods are necessary and so is the appropriate handling of the urine. Despite these obstacles, there is a lot of information on frequencies of hypercalciuria, hyperoxaluria, hypocitraturia, hypomagnesuria, hyperuricosuria, and small urine volumes (see Table 29.3). Also in this regard can we see a pronounced variation, but there is a com-

Table 29.2 An overview of stone composition (%) in different geographical regions

Geographical region	CaOx	CaOx+CaP	CaP	Infection stone	Uric acid	AmUr	Cystine
Europe	65–78		13	4–10	7–11	–	0.6–1.3
North America	55–61		12–13	2–6	8–14	–	1–6
Pakistan	38–70		–	6–16	2–38	–	0.2
Northern India	93	2.8 (?)	1.8	1.4	0.95	–	–
Southern India (Kerala)	56	10	3.3	1.2	23	6.5	0.3
China	80			–	–	–	–
Brazil	59	~7 (?)	–	8	24	–	1.8
Africa (south)	43–74		4.0–10.1	0–9.2	4–18	–	0.2–2.0
Australia	68		3	12	17	–	–
KSA	82		–	3.5	2.3	12	–
Kuwait	72		–	–	15		–
Iran	65		–	1	8	24	1.4
Jordan	65		18		13	–	–
Algeria	62 (?)			29	9	–	–
Japan	63–75	11–14	6.5–13	1.4–5.1	2.2–5.5		0.7–1.6
Russia	66		21		11		2.7
South Africa	43–74		4–10	4–9	4–18	–	0.2–1.3
Turkey	57		–	–	8	–	–

The question marks (?) indicate that the given number is an approximate conclusion of presented data and thus has to be interpreted with care

Table 29.3 An overview of urine abnormalities (%) in different geographical regions

Geographical region	U-Ca high	U-Ox high	U-Cit low	U-Mg low	U-Vol small	U-Ur high	U-pH low
Europe	33–72	23	27				
North America	40	40	5–11		92[a]		
Pakistan	19–76	~4[b]	55–76			11–26	
Brazil	14–74	14–70	37–43	21	49	20–76	
Argentina	58		23	16		24	
Uruguay	37					31	
Venezuela	47		14			19	
Australia	29						
N. India							
S. India	7.2	48.0	2.9	4.3	12.6	12.0	11.2
South Africa							

[a]Less than 2,000 mL/24 h
[b]From Karachi only

mon general pattern showing that a high urinary calcium, low urinary citrate, high urinary oxalate, and small urine volumes are important risk factors. It is of note, however, that urinary calcium generally seems to be low in Asian populations. The regionally very common occurrence of hyperuricosuria, commonly associated with small urine volumes, is probably very well reflecting the high frequency of uric acid stone formation.

With this background and with recent progress in the understanding of calcium oxalate stone pathology [10–12], it is relevant to ask the question: In which direction should calcium stone research move? There is probably no easy and straightforward answer to that question, but we definitely need a better understanding and identification of the crucial factor or factors that initiate stone formation. That kind of information is necessary for development of successful and tolerated/accepted methods for recurrence prevention. The therapeutic tools should be designed so that patient compliance is better than that we see today [9]. There are a number of aspects that might be rewarding in this regard.

Analysis of urine for estimating the supersaturation with CaOx is fundamental. For detection of specific individual risk periods during the day, urine should probably be collected and analyzed in a different way than in the 24 h or other long-term urine samples that so far have been our routine [13, 14]. We also need some simple and cheap methods for measuring the level of calcium oxalate supersaturation in urine [15].

Measurements of urine pH in fresh (or reasonably fresh) urine are most certainly highly important [11, 16]. In view of the considerable diurnal variation, this variable has seldom been measured in an appropriate way. It would indeed be desirable to have a device for accurate pH-measurements in minute urine volumes (for instance directly in the urine stream) in a way similar to what was provided with the Urimho device [17] used many years ago for conductivity measurements in urine. With the advanced technology that we have today, development of such a device should not be too complicated.

Efforts to pharmacologically influence the initial step in stone formation should be carefully investigated and evaluated. Treatment directed toward elimination of peaks of risk periods should be dictated by findings in the diurnal risk pattern.

If a suitable pharmacological approach eventually will show the need of several agents, it seems desirable to have them all combined in one pill. All other solutions are likely to seriously decrease patient compliance.

These were some personal aspects based on findings in the literature and my own experience. Other approaches might be even more rewarding, but we need to realize that stone initiation and stone development is not a continuous process. Therefore, dynamic thinking and a dynamic treatment approach are necessary components of rational recurrence prevention. Whichever way we go, our efforts should result in a treatment that efficiently can counteract calcium oxalate stone formation. It is also of utmost importance that such treatment programs are well tolerated by the patients and free of side effects in order to allow for a good compliance. Moreover, all such treatment efforts should be cost-effective.

Primary prevention, prophylactic treatment in its proper sense was reasonably discussed [18], and I agree with the authors that such an approach is not possible or necessary in most areas, but it might be a solution for some geographical areas and populations in which there is an extremely high incidence and prevalence of stone formation.

Conclusion

For the future, it is essential to take additional steps in an optimal recording of patient data—in a structured and standardized way—so that reliable epidemiological and etiological information can be obtained. Hopefully, it thereby will become possible to decide on the recurrence preventive effect in large patient populations treated in different ways.

References

1. Sinclair HM. The relative importance of essential fatty acids of the linoleic and linolenic families: studies with an Eskimo diet. Prog Lipid Res. 1982;20:897–9.
2. Okagawa Y. Epidemiology of stones in Japan. Jap J Urol. 1979; 70:975–83.
3. Rodgers A. The riddle of kidney stone disease: lessons from Africa. Urol Res. 2006;34:92–5.
4. Knoll T, Schubert AB, Fahlenkamp D, Leusmann DB, Wendt-Nordahl G, Schubert G. Urolithiasis through the ages: data on more than 200,000 urinary stone analyses. J Urol. 2011;185:1304–11.
5. Tiselius HG. Solution chemistry of supersaturation. In: Coe FL, Favus MJ, Pak CYC, Parks JH, Preminger GM, editors. Kidney stones: medical and surgical management. Philadelphia: Lippincott-Raven Publishers; 1996. p. 33–64.
6. Hara S, Tsuji H, Ohmoto Y, Amakawa K, Hsieh SD, Arase Y, et al. High serum uric acid level and low urine pH as predictors of metabolic syndrome: a retrospective cohort study in a Japanese urban population. Metabolism. 2012;61:281–8.
7. Asplin JR. Obesity and urolithiasis. Adv Chronic Kidney Dis. 2009; 16:11–20.
8. Strohmaier WL, Wrobel BM, Schubert G. Overweight, insulin resistance and blood pressure (parameters of the metabolic syndrome) in uric acid urolithiasis. Urol Res. 2012;40:171–5.
9. Tiselius H-G, Alken P, Buck C, Gallucci M, Knoll T, Sarica K, et al. Guidelines on urolithiasis. European Association of urology guidelines. 2009 ed. Arnhem: European Association of Urology; 2009.
10. Evan AP, Lingeman JE, Worcester EM. Role of interstitial apatite plaque in the pathogenesis of common calcium oxalate stone. Semin Nephrol. 2008;28:111–9.
11. Tiselius HG. A hypothesis of calcium stone formation: an interpretation of stone research during the past decades. Urol Res. 2011; 39:231–43.
12. Coe FL, Evan AP, Worcester EM, Lingeman JE. Three pathways for human kidney stone formation. Urol Res. 2010;38:147–60.
13. Robert M, Roux JO, Bourelly F, Boularan AM, Guiter J, Monnier L. Circadian variations in the risk of urinary calcium oxalate stone formation. Br J Urol. 1994;74:294–7.
14. Ahlstrand C, Larsson L, Tiselius H-G. Variations in urine composition during the day in patients with calcium oxalate stone disease. J Urol. 1984;131:77–81.
15. Grases F, Costa-Bauzá A, Prieto R, Arrabal M, De Haro T, Lancina J, et al. Urinary lithogenesis risk tests: comparison of a commercial kit and a laboratory prototype test. Scand J Urol Nephrol. 2011; 45:312–8.
16. Tiselius HG, Lindbäck B, Fornander AM, Nilsson MA. Studies on the role of calcium phosphate in the process of calcium oxalate crystal formation. Urol Res. 2009;37:181–92.
17. Tiselius HG. Calcium oxalate crystallization properties in urine with different specific electrical conductivities. J Urol. 1992;148:990–4.
18. Lotan Y, Pearle MS. Cost-effectiveness of primary prevention strategies for nephrolithiasis. J Urol. 2011;186:550–5.

Part III

Diagnosis

Diagnosis of Urinary Tract Stones: An Overview

30

Ahmed S. El-Hefnawy and Ahmed A. Shokeir

Abstract

Diagnosis of urinary tract stones starts with careful history taking. In case of presence of recurrent attacks of renal colic and stone disease, the recommended diagnostic approach is to start with plain radiography and ultrasonography. Non-contrast computed tomography is currently the diagnostic image modality of choice and has replaced intravenous pyelography especially in case of atypical presentation or when history of stone disease is absent. Contrast-enhanced computed tomography or intravenous pyelography should be done if further intervention is planned. T2-weighted magnetic resonance imaging (MRI) is useful particularly in pregnant women. Each patient with urolithiasis (no difference between high- or low-risk groups) should undergo basic biochemical workup.

Keywords

Renal colic • Stone • Urolithiasis • Diagnosis • Management • Metabolic workup

Introduction

The diagnosis of urolithiasis has undergone considerable evolution in recent years. This chapter addresses the various clinical, laboratory, and radiological tests that are necessary for diagnosis of urolithiasis. In addition, it highlights indications and basic metabolic workup that should be done in patients with urolithiasis.

Clinical Presentation

The main presentation of patients with urolithiasis is renal colic, which results from obstruction of the urinary tract due to stone impaction either at the calyceal neck or at more distal sites of constriction (pelviureteral junction, crossing of the ureter over the iliac vessels, and ureterovesical junction) [1].

A.S. El-Hefnawy, M.D. • A.A. Shokeir, M.D., Ph.D., FEBU (✉)
Department of Urology, Urology and Nephrology Center, Mansoura University, Mansoura, Egypt
e-mail: a_s_elhefnawy@yahoo.com; ahmed.shokeir@hotmail.com

Renal colic is typically characterized by abrupt onset of episode that occurs during the night or early morning hours. The localization of pain begins in the area of the flank, courses laterally around the abdomen, and generally radiates to the area of the groin and testicle in the male or to the labia majora in the female [2]. Renal colic may be associated with gastrointestinal symptoms because of the proximity of adjacent organs and due to reflex stimulation of celiac ganglion.

Position of ureteric stone could be judged by the site of referred pain. If the stone is lodged in the upper ureter, the pain radiates to the testis since the nerve supply of this organ is similar to that of the kidney and upper ureter (T11–12). When stone obstructs the mid-ureter, pain on the right side is referred to the right lower quadrant of the abdomen (resembles appendicitis), on the left side over the lower left quadrant (resembles diverticulitis). Stones of the lower pelvic ureter are frequently presented with irritative lower urinary tract symptoms including urgency, frequency, and suprapubic discomfort. Migration of the stone down to the intramural part of the ureter gives pain that may radiate to the tip of the penis in the male [3]. Renal colic should be differentiated from other non-calculous conditions with similar presentation. In females, gynecological processes that need to be

J.J. Talati et al. (eds.), *Urolithiasis*,
DOI 10.1007/978-1-4471-4387-1_30, © Springer-Verlag London 2012

considered include ovarian torsion, ovarian cyst, and ectopic pregnancy. In men, symptoms of pathology arising in the scrotum such as tumor, epididymitis, or prostatitis may mimic the symptoms of distal ureteral stones [4]. Renal pain may be confused with pain resulting from irritation of the costal nerves, most commonly T10–12. Such pain has a similar distribution from the costovertebral angle across the flank toward umbilicus. Unlike renal pain, the intensity of radicular pain may be altered by changing position. Furthermore, such pain is not colicky in nature [3].

Renal colic is almost always felt on the same side of stone. Clark and Norman have described a phenomenon —"mirror pain"—in which the pain is felt on the contralateral side of stone [5]. Atypical presentation of renal colic may also occur in patients with horseshoe kidneys or renal ectopia. Sometimes non-obstructing stones may be asymptomatic and are found incidentally on image studies or during the evaluation of micro-hematuria. Stone migration along the course of the ureter is sometimes associated with attacks of hematuria. In some instances, gross hematuria may be the only presenting complaint. In staghorn stones, urinary tract infections could be the warning sign. In case of bilateral silent stones, renal insufficiency could be the first presentation.

To sum up the contribution of the most significant clinical diagnostic factors, a clinical diagnostic score showed that acute abdominal pain of short duration (≤12 h), loin or renal tenderness, and hematuria (erythrocytes ≤ 10) are the most significant predictors of acute renal colic [6, 7].

Physical Examination

There is no pathognomic sign of urolithiasis. Patients with renal pain are usually moving around, holding their flanks. Severe renal colic may be associated with tachycardia and elevated blood pressure. Concomitant urinary tract infection can lead to fever. Abdominal examination may reveal moderate, deep flank tenderness on palpation [8]. Digital rectal examination may locate impacted stone in posterior urethra.

Urine Analysis

Pyuria is a common finding in urolithiasis either in presence or absence of infection. Gross or microscopic hematuria is another common finding and occurs in approximately 90 % of patients; however, the absence of hematuria does not exclude the presence of stones [9]. An acidic urine pH promotes uric acid or cystine stones, whereas an alkaline pH favors the crystallization of calcium- and phosphate-containing stones [10]. Identification of urine crystals may reflect an active phase of urinary lithiasis and indicates the type of existing calculus. Tetrahedral "envelopes" are seen in calcium oxalate dihydrate stones; hourglass crystals may be seen in calcium oxalate monohydrate stones, while hexagonal crystals confirm cystinuria. Uric acid crystals may be amorphous or seen as irregular plates. Microscopic appearance of rectangular "coffin-lid" crystals may indicate presence of struvite calculi [11].

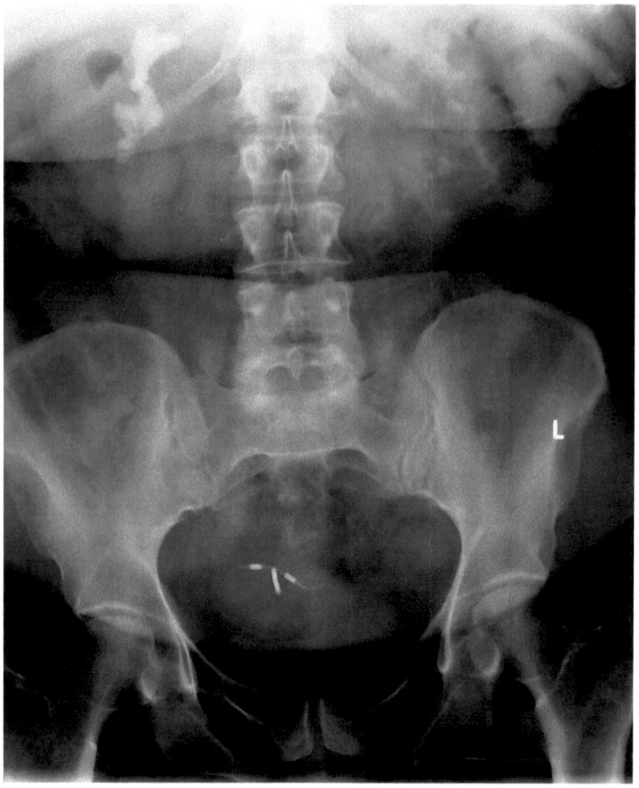

Fig. 30.1 Plain abdominal radiograph demonstrating radio-opaque staghorn stone of right kidney

Imaging Studies

Plain Kidneys-Ureters-Bladder Radiographs (KUB)

For a long time, plain X-ray KUB (kidneys-ureters-bladder) has been traditionally considered as the ideal radiological method and first choice in case of suspected urolithiasis. X-ray KUB has the ability to detect most urinary stones (75–90 % are radio-opaque) [2] and, in addition, gives an idea of its composition, through an assessment of the degree of radio-opacity (Fig. 30.1). Calculi that contain calcium are radiodense [12]. Calcium phosphate (apatite) stones are the most radio-opaque and have a density similar to that of bone [13]. However, the sensitivity and specificity of X-ray KUB range from 44 to 77 % and from 80 to 87 %, respectively [14].

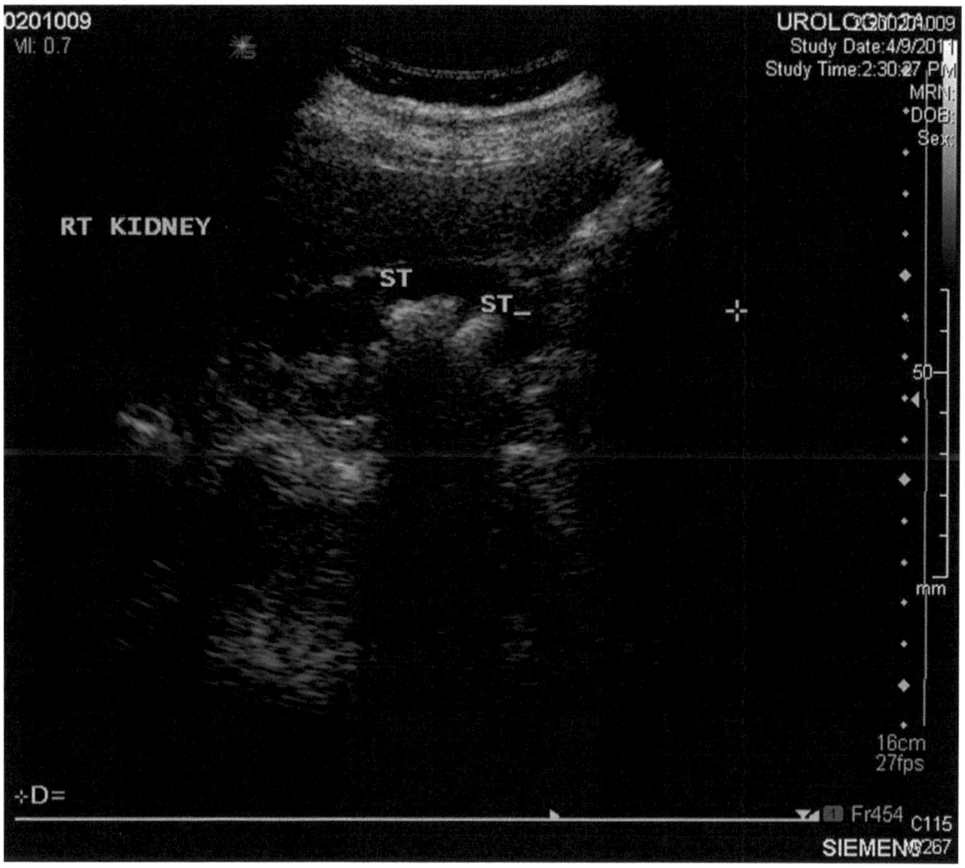

Fig. 30.2 Renal US demonstrates multiple echogenic foci with acoustical shadowing in middle and lower calyx of right kidney

There are many limitations that lessen the usefulness of X-ray KUB. Calculi of pure uric acid, xanthine, dihydroxyadenine, indinavir, triamterene, or matrix can be considered truly radiolucent and cannot be detected by X-ray KUB. Even radio-opaque calculi are frequently obscured by stone or bowel gas, and ureteral stones overlying the bony pelvis or transverse processes of vertebrae are occasionally difficult to identify. Common abdominal calcifications can mimic the appearance of urolithiasis. Therefore, X ray KUB should not be performed if a non-contrast-enhanced computed tomography (NCCT) is being considered [15]. It is recommended to use X-ray KUB for following the course of patients with known radio-opaque stones [16].

Ultrasonography (US)

Ultrasonography (US) has many advantages that make it ideal as a method of initial evaluation and for further follow-up of patients with renal stones. It is noninvasive; the equipment is portable and is relatively inexpensive [17]. An additional advantage is that it does not require either radiographic contrast media or ionizing radiation, making it an attractive screening modality in pregnancy and renal impairment [3, 18].

Grayscale US can identify stones located in the calyces, pelvis, pelvi-ureteric junction, and ureterovesical junction, as well as dilatation of the upper urinary tract. Renal calculi are markedly echogenic and produce acoustic shadowing (Fig. 30.2). Pyelocaliectasis is considered to be an indirect sign of renal obstruction. Nevertheless, dilatation of the collecting system depends on the size and location of the stone, and the duration and the degree of obstruction. It takes many hours for frank pyelocaliectasis to develop after sudden, even complete, obstruction [7]. For renal stones >5 mm, ultrasound has a sensitivity of 96 % and a specificity of nearly 100 % [19]. For all stone locations, the sensitivity and specificity of ultrasound reduce to 78 and 31 %, respectively [19, 20]. Mos and colleagues reported 73 % sensitivity for detection of ureteral calculi. Transrectal US may aid in the identification of distal ureteric stones [21]. Serafini and coworkers reported accurate assessment of a variety of distal ureteral pathologies including distal calculi by placement of high-frequency, high-resolution probes within the vagina [22]. A recent report demonstrated that 80 % of stones located in the distal 4 cm of distal ureteral length could be detected using 6–10 MHz transrectal/transvaginal end-fire probe [23].

However, the operator-dependent nature of US, poor accuracy when measuring the size of the stone, and inability to locate ureteral stones are limiting factors. Also, a

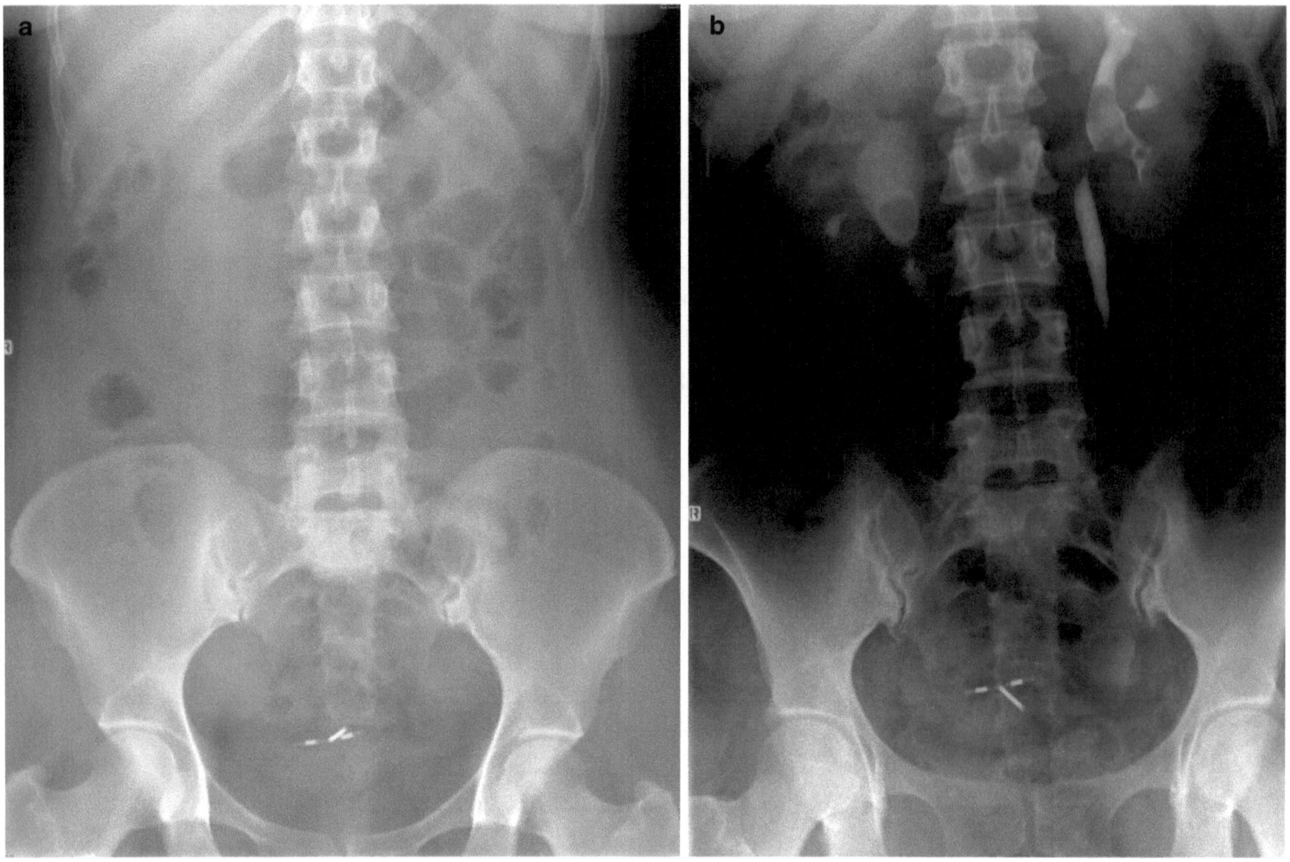

Fig. 30.3 (**a**) KUB demonstrates presence of intrauterine contraceptive device and no evidence of calcular shadows. (**b**) IVU demonstrating filling defects from radiolucent stones in both renal pelvis

false-positive diagnosis of obstruction could occur in patients with pyelonephritis and vesicoureteric reflux, and obstruction could be reported because of residual dilatation after relief of obstruction or dilatation because of over distension of the bladder. The combination of abdominal radiography and grayscale US through demonstration of calculi or pyelocaliectasis is very useful [24]. Using this combination of modalities could detect up to 79 % of ureteric calculi [25].

Doppler ultrasonography (DUS) is used in the diagnosis of obstructive uropathy through measurement of the renal resistive index. Several studies have used the difference between the resistive index of obstructed and non-obstructed kidneys, and satisfactory results have been obtained [26–28]. We have shown that a resistive index difference of at least 0.04 gives a sensitivity of 90 % and a specificity of 100 % in the diagnosis of renal colic [28]. Nevertheless, in patients with solitary kidneys or those with bilateral renal obstruction, albeit clinically uncommon, a change in resistive index is of no value. The diagnostic accuracy of this index may be decreased if the patients are given nonsteroidal anti-inflammatory drugs (NSAIDs) [29]. Therefore, it is recommended to do DUS before giving NSAIDs and during the attack of pain.

Intravenous Urogram (IVU)

Intravenous urogram (IVU) has been proposed in the past as the "gold standard" for detection of urinary obstruction as it provides both anatomical and functional data that are considered necessary before decision of management plan. Radiolucent stones are detected as filling defects within collecting systems once the urinary tract fills with contrast (Fig. 30.3a, b). However, accuracy of IVU (as an emergency measure) was not found to be superior to KUB in case of acute flank pain due to a "shutting down" effect [30]. Other limitations include inability to obtain proper bowel preparation to aid in imaging because of the acute nature of the study, the need to assess renal function before contrast injection, inability to visualize some stones (e.g., uric acid), and the time-consuming nature of the study.

The contrast media used in IVU have potential adverse effects, notably allergic reactions and nephrotoxicity. For patients with reported allergic reactions or who may be at risk, some precautions should be followed: (1) low-molecular nonionic contrast medium should be used; (2) a corticosteroid (e.g., prednisolone 30 mg) administered between 12 and 2 h before the contrast medium is injected; and (3) the corticosteroid could be combined with an intramuscular injection

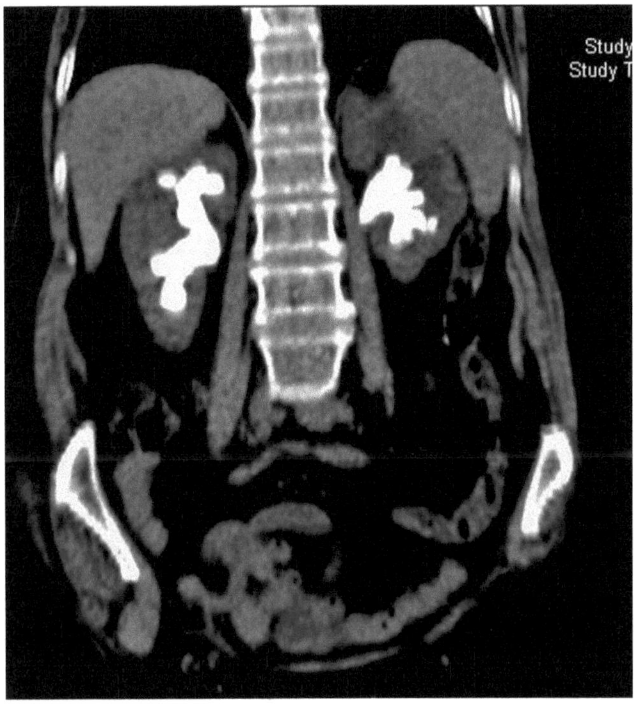

Fig. 30.4 NCCT reformatted image demonstrates bilateral renal staghorn stones

of an antihistamine agent (e.g., clemastine 2 mg), given 1 h before administration of contrast medium [31, 32].

Intravenous administration of contrast medium may result in a reduced renal perfusion and toxic effect on tubular cells. The vasoconstriction of glomerular afferent arterioles causes a reduced glomerular filtration rate (GFR) and increased renal vascular resistance. Nephrotoxicity caused by contrast medium is diagnosed by the demonstration of an increase of 25 % or at least a 44 μmol/L rise in the level of serum creatinine during the 3 days that follow intravascular administration of the agent when there is no alternative explanation [33]. Risk factors to develop contrast nephropathy include increased serum creatinine, diabetes, age over 70 years, dehydration, congestive heart failure, and concurrent treatment with nephrotoxic drugs. These risks may be minimized by adequately hydrating the patient, minimizing the amount of contrast material that is infused, and increasing the time interval between consecutive contrast studies. It is better to avoid the use of contrast media when an alternative imaging modality can provide equivalent information.

Computed Tomography (CT)

With the introduction of spiral CT, non-contrast CT studies (NCCT) are rapidly becoming the standard means of evaluating patients presenting to emergency departments with acute flank pain (Fig. 30.4). This method carries many advantages including rapid performance and the fact that there is no need to inject contrast. In addition, CT can detect non-urological abnormalities, such as acute appendicitis or ovarian cyst, which could present with acute colic-mimicking pain of ureteral stone. Uric acid and xanthine stones are radiolucent on plain films but can be detected by NCCT. However, indinavir stones cannot be detected on NCCT [34].

It has been reported that unilateral ureteral dilation in association with perinephric stranding of fat was the most accurate predictor of ureteral stone with positive and negative predictive values of 99 and 95 %, respectively [35]. In a prospective study that included 109 patients who presented with acute flank pain, CT showed a sensitivity of 96 %, a specificity of 96 %, and an overall accuracy of 96 % [28]. In a more recent study, sensitivity of NCCT was 100 % for detection of stone location in patients with compromised renal function [25].

Several reports have evaluated NCCT in predicting stone composition. Nakada and colleagues have found significant difference between the Hounsfield measurement of uric acid calculi (mean 344 ± 152 HU) and the Hounsfield measurement of calcium oxalate (mean 652 ± 490 HU) [36]. Micro-CT has been shown to identify the mineral composition of urinary stones [37]. Micro-CT X-ray attenuation values were measured for mineral that was positively identified by infrared microspectroscopy (FT-IR). Micro-CT X-ray attenuation units (AU) were collected for six minerals that could be found in regions that appeared to be pure, including uric acid (3,515–4,995 AU), struvite (7,242–7,969 AU), cystine (8,619–9,921 AU), calcium oxalate dihydrate (1,3815–1,5797 AU), calcium oxalate monohydrate (1,6297–18,449 AU), and hydroxyapatite (21,144–23,121 AU). These AU values did not overlap. Recently, simultaneous dual-energy (DE) multidetector CT was introduced to improve stone composition [38, 39]. Reported results are promising; however, it is still based on in vitro models.

There are a number of potential pitfalls in the interpretation of CT. Phleboliths in the pelvis can often be seen along the normal anatomical course of the ureter and can mimic ureteral stones. The ring sign is helpful for distinguishing stones from phleboliths. A gonadal vein can sometimes be confused with a dilated ureter and can be distinguished by following the superior course of the structure in question. The main disadvantage of NCCT compared to IVP is its inability to evaluate renal function. Recent studies have shown that contrast-enhanced spiral CT has a high accuracy when calculating selective renal function, an advantage additional to the delineation of accurate anatomical details in patients with chronic obstructive uropathy [40]. However, the radiation exposure from CT is generally high [41–43], which contraindicates its use during pregnancy (Table 30.1).

To minimize risk of radiation exposure, low-dose CT (see Chap. 35) has been recently used [44]. Poletti showed that in

Table 30.1 Dose of radiation per image modality

Image modality	Dose of radiation (mSv)
KUB	0.5–1
IVU	1.3–3.5
Regular-dose NCCT	4.5–5
Low-dose NCCT	0.97–1.7
Enhanced CT	25–35

CT computed tomography, *IVU* intravenous urography, *KUB* kidneys-ureters-bladder radiograph, *NCCT* non-contrast-enhanced computed tomography

patients with a body mass index (BMI) < 30, low-dose CT had a sensitivity of 86 % for detecting ureteric stones <3 mm and 100 % for detecting calculi >3 mm [45]. In a meta-analysis of prospective studies by Niemann, low-dose CT diagnosed urolithiasis with a pooled sensitivity of 0.966 (95 % CI: 0.950–0.978) and specificity of 0.949 (95 % CI: 0.920–0.97) [46].

Magnetic Resonance Urography (MRU)

In some clinical conditions, such as pregnancy, patients that have undergone multiple prior CT exams and, in patients with vague clinical presentation, an imaging alternative to CT should be employed [47]. In addition, MR nephrouretero-gram has the ability to provide quantitative analysis of renal function that has the potential to direct clinical management in the setting of obstructing calculi.

Although MRI is relatively insensitive for the direct detection of urinary calculi, using rapid, single-shot T2-weighted sequences with and without fat saturation provides an abdominopelvic MRI that can detect the sequelae of clinically active stone disease in addition to alternate inflammatory conditions that may mimic the symptoms of renal colic. In a prospective study comparing NCCT, MRU, and combined US and KUB for diagnosis of ureteral obstruction, Shokeir and colleagues have reported that the sensitivity of MRU for detecting urinary stones was 69.2 % [25]. When combined with KUB and US, the sensitivity of MRI in detecting stones was 90 % [48]. Detecting urinary stones by MRU depends on secondary signs because stones are not represented directly, as on a plain X-ray or CT. Hence, it is impossible to detect parenchymal stones by MRU, but pelvic or ureteral stones can be visualized because they are surrounded by fluid and produce a filling defect within the high signal intensity of the urine. These filling defects may be mimicked by physiological peristalsis of the ureter [25].

Guidelines for Diagnosis

Patients with history of previous attacks of renal colic and stone disease should initially be evaluated by abdominal radiography; NCCT is reserved for undiagnosed problems.

Table 30.2 Basic urine and blood analysis for metabolic workup in emergency stone patient

Urine
Urinary sediment/dipstick test out of spot urine sample
Red cells
White cells
Nitrite
Urine pH level by approximation
Urine culture or microscopy
Blood
Serum blood sample
Creatinine
Uric acid
Ionized calcium
Sodium
Potassium
Blood cell count
CRP
If intervention is likely or planned: coagulation test (PTT and INR)

CRP C-reactive protein, *INR* international normalized ratio, *PTT* partial thromboplastin time

Patients with no history of stone disease or with atypical clinical presentation should be initially evaluated by NCCT. IVP or enhanced CT is carried out after NCCT in undiagnosed cases or when endoscopic or open intervention is decided upon. If NCCT is not available, evaluation should include abdominal radiography and ultrasonography followed, if necessary, by IVP. Abdominal radiography and ultrasonography are suitable methods for follow-up of the patients. In pregnant women, ultrasonography with Doppler assistance is of particular importance, and MRU could add great help.

Metabolic-Related Diagnostic Methods

Besides image studies, each patient with urolithiasis (no difference between high- and low-risk groups) should undergo biochemical workup.

The last European panel consensus (Vienna, 2011) [49] has recommended basic analysis for every emergency stone patient (Table 30.2).

Only high-risk stone formers are obliged to undergo a specific metabolic evaluation. High-risk groups include recurrent stone formers, strong family history of stones, intestinal disease (particularly chronic diarrhea), pathological skeletal fractures, osteoporosis, history of urinary tract infection with calculi, personal history of gout, renal insufficiency, stone composed of (cystine, uric acid, or struvite) solitary kidney, and in case of anatomic abnormalities [11]. For the initial specific metabolic workup, the patient should be stone-free. A minimum of 20 days is recommended between stone expulsion or removal and 24-h urine collection [50].

Specific metabolic evaluation generally requires the collection of two consecutive 24-h urine samples [51]. The collecting bottles should be either prepared with 5 % thymol in isopropanol (10 mL for a 2-L bottle) or stored at a cool temperature (<8 °C or less) during the collection period [50].

Alternatively, spot urine samples can be used, particularly when it may be difficult to carry out 24-h collections; e.g., in younger children [52]. Spot urine studies normally index the excretion rates to creatinine [52, 53]. However, results based on spot urine may vary with collection time and the patient's gender, body weight, and age.

There are several risk indices to detect the crystallization risk for calcium oxalate or calcium phosphate in the urine; e.g., APCaOxindex [54, 55] and EQUIL [56]. Joint Expert Speciation System (JESS) is another approach that is based on an extensive database of physiochemical constants [57]. However, the clinical validation of these risk indices in terms of recurrence prediction or therapy improvement is still ongoing, and the benefit remains controversial [49].

Conclusion

Standard evaluation of patients with urolithiasis includes thorough history taking and adequate physical examination and supported by appropriate imaging procedure. Ultrasonography is the primary screening modality. NCCT has become the standard for diagnosis of acute flank pain and has higher sensitivity than IVU. Contrast-enhanced CT or IVU should be done if further intervention is planned. Basic metabolic workup should be done regardless of the degree of risk after the first presentation with stone disease. However, there are different views on this, and the reader is referred to Part VIII of this book, which explores strategies on prevention of recurrence.

References

1. Travaglini F, Bartoletti R, Gacci M, Rizzo M. Pathophysiology of reno-ureteral colic. Urol Int. 2004;72(1):20–3.
2. Teichman JM. Clinical practice. Acute renal colic from ureteral calculus. N Engl J Med. 2004;350(7):684–93.
3. Shokeir AA. Renal colic: pathophysiology, diagnosis and treatment. Eur Urol. 2001;39(3):241–9.
4. Rucker CM, Menias CO, Bhalla S. Mimics of renal colic: alternative diagnoses at unenhanced helical CT. Radiographics. 2004;24 Suppl 1:S11–28.
5. Clark AJ, Norman RW. "Mirror pain" as an unusual presentation of renal colic. Urology. 1998;51(1):116–8.
6. Eskelinen M, Ikonen J, Lipponen P. Usefulness of history-taking, physical examination and diagnostic scoring in acute renal colic. Eur Urol. 1998;34(6):467–73.
7. Shokeir AA. Renal colic: new concepts related to pathophysiology, diagnosis and treatment. Curr Opin Urol. 2002;12(4):263–9.
8. Serinken M, Karcioglu O, Turkcuer I, Ozkan HI, Keysan MK, Bukiran A. Analysis of clinical and demographic characteristics of patients presenting with renal colic in the emergency department. BMC Res Notes. 2008;1:79.
9. Bove P, Kaplan D, Dalrymple N, Rosenfield AT, Verga M, Anderson K, et al. Reexamining the value of hematuria testing in patients with acute flank pain. J Urol. 1999;162(3 Pt 1):685–7.
10. Wagner CA, Mohebbi N. Urinary pH and stone formation. J Nephrol. 2010;23 Suppl 16:S165–9.
11. Pietrow PK, Preminger GM. Evaluation and management of urinary lithiasis. In: Wein AJ, Kavoussi LR, Novick AC, Partin AW, Peters CA, editors. Campbell–Walsh urology, vol. II. 9th ed. Philadelphia: Saunders Elsevier; 2007. p. 1393–431. Chap 43.
12. Lalli AF. Symposium on renal lithiasis. Roentgen aspects of renal calculous disease. Urol Clin North Am. 1974;1:213–27.
13. Roth R, Finlayson B. Observations on the radiopacity of stone substances with special reference to cystine. Invest Urol. 1973;11: 186–9.
14. Heidenreich A, Desgrandschamps F, Terrier F. Modern approach of diagnosis and management of acute flank pain: review of all imaging modalities. Eur Urol. 2002;41(4):351–62.
15. Kennish SJ, Bhatnagar P, Wah TM, Bush S, Irving HC. Is the KUB radiograph redundant for investigating acute ureteric colic in the non-contrast enhanced computed tomography era? Clin Radiol. 2008;63(10):1131–5.
16. Portis AJ, Sundaram CP. Diagnosis and initial management of kidney stones. Am Fam Physician. 2001;63(7):1329–38.
17. Moş C, Holt G, Iuhasz S, Moş D, Teodor I, Hălbac M. The sensitivity of transabdominal ultrasound in the diagnosis of ureterolithiasis. Med Ultrason. 2010;12(3):188–97.
18. Patlas M, Farkas A, Fisher D, Zaghal I, Hadas-Halpern I. Ultrasound vs CT for the detection of ureteric stones in patients with renal colic. Br J Radiol. 2001;74(886):901–4.
19. Varma G, Nair N, Salim A, Marickar YM. Investigations for recognizing urinary stone. Urol Res. 2009;37(6):349–52.
20. Middleton WD, Dodds WJ, Lawson TL, Foley WD. Renal calculi: sensitivity for detection with US. Radiology. 1988;167(1):239–44.
21. Holmes 3rd DR, Robb R. Trans-urethral ultrasound (TUUS) imaging for visualization and analysis of the prostate and associated tissues. Stud Health Technol Inform. 2000;70:126–32.
22. Serafini G, Gandolfo N, Gandolfo N, Gazzo P, Martinoli C, Derchi LE. Transvaginal ultrasonography of nongynecologic pelvic lesions. Abdom Imaging. 2001;26(5):540–9.
23. Cantoro D, Galosi AB, Conti A, Muzzonigro G. Distal ureter studied with endocavitary end-fire probe: application in adult urology ultrasonographic clinic. Arch Ital Urol Androl. 2010;82(4):211–4.
24. Dalla Palma L, Pozzi Mucelli R, Stacul F. Present-day imaging of patients with renal colic. Eur Radiol. 2001;11(1):4–17.
25. Shokeir AA, El-Diasty T, Eassa W, Mosbah A, El-Ghar MA, Mansour O, Dawaba M, El-Kappany H. Diagnosis of ureteral obstruction in patients with compromised renal function: the role of noninvasive imaging modalities. J Urol. 2004;171(6 Pt 1): 2303–6.
26. Shokeir AA, Abdulmaaboud M. Resistive index in renal colic: a prospective study. BJU Int. 1999;83(4):378–82.
27. Shokeir AA, Mahran MR, Abdulmaaboud M. Renal colic in pregnant women: role of renal resistive index. Urology. 2000;55(3): 344–7.
28. Shokeir AA, Abdulmaaboud M. Prospective comparison of nonenhanced helical computerized tomography and Doppler ultrasonography for the diagnosis of renalcolic. J Urol. 2001;165(4):1082–4.
29. Shokeir AA, Abdulmaaboud M, Farage Y, Mutabagani H. Resistive index in renal colic: the effect of nonsteroidal anti-inflammatory drugs. BJU Int. 1999;84(3):249–51.
30. Elton TJ, Roth CS, Berquist TH, Silverstein MD. A clinical prediction rule for the diagnosis of ureteral calculi in emergency departments. J Gen Intern Med. 1993;8:57–62.
31. Morcos SK, Thomsen HS, Webb JA, Contrast Media Safety Committee of the European Society of Urogenital Radiolology.

Prevention of generalized reactions to contrast media: a consensus report and guidelines. Eur Radiol. 2001;11(9):1720–8.
32. Thomsen HS, Morcos SK. Contrast media and the kidney: European Society of Urogenital Radiology (ESUR) guidelines. Br J Radiol. 2003;76(908):513–8.
33. Tiselius HG, Alken P, Buk C, Gallucci M, Knoll T, Sarica K, et al. EAU guidelines on urolithiasis. Diagnostic procedures. The edition presented at EAU annual congress. Guidelines Office, Arnhem, The Netherlands. 2008. p. 9–19.
34. Wu DS, Stoller ML. Indinavir urolithiasis. Curr Opin Urol. 2000;10(6):557–61.
35. Smith RC, Rosenfield AT, Choe KA, Essenmacher KR, Verga M, Glickman MG, Lange RC. Acute flank pain: comparison of non-contrast-enhanced CT and intravenous urography. Radiology. 1995;194(3):789–94.
36. Nakada SY, Hoff DG, Attai S, Heisey D, Blankenbaker D, Pozniak M. Determination of stone composition by noncontrast spiral computed tomography in the clinical setting. Urology. 2000;55(6): 816–9.
37. Zarse CA, McAteer JA, Sommer AJ, Kim SC, Hatt EK, Lingeman JE, et al. Nondestructive analysis of urinary calculi using micro computed tomography. BMC Urol. 2004;4(1):15.
38. Boll DT, Patil NA, Paulson EK, Merkle EM, Simmons WN, Pierre SA, et al. Renal stone assessment with dual-energy multidetector CT and advanced postprocessing techniques: improved characterization of renal stone composition – pilot study. Radiology. 2009;250(3):813–20.
39. Ferrandino MN, Pierre SA, Simmons WN, Paulson EK, Albala DM, Preminger GM. Dual-energy computed tomography with advanced postimage acquisition data processing: improved determination of urinary stone composition. J Endourol. 2010;24(3): 347–54.
40. El-Ghar ME, Shokeir AA, El-Diasty TA, Refaie HF, Gad HM, El-Dein AB. Contrast enhanced spiral computerized tomography in patients with chronic obstructive uropathy and normal serum creatinine: a single session for anatomical and functional assessment. J Urol. 2004;172(3):985–8.
41. Thomson JM, Glocer J, Abbott C, Maling TM, Mark S. Computed tomography versus intravenous urography in diagnosis of acute flank pain from urolithiasis: a randomized study comparing imaging costs and radiation dose. Australas Radiol. 2001;45(3):291–7.
42. Kluner C, Hein PA, Gralla O, Hein E, Hamm B, Romano V, et al. Does ultra-low-dose CT with a radiation dose equivalent to that of KUB suffice to detect renal and ureteral calculi? J Comput Assist Tomogr. 2006;30(1):44–50.
43. Van Der Molen AJ, Cowan NC, Mueller-Lisse UG, Nolte-Ernsting CC, Takahashi S, Cohan RH, CT Urography Working Group of the European Society of Urogenital Radiology (ESUR). CT urography: definition, indications and techniques. A guideline for clinical practice. Eur Radiol. 2008;18(1):4–17.
44. Jellison FC, Smith JC, Heldt JP, Spengler NM, Nicolay LI, Ruckle HC, et al. Effect of low dose radiation computerized tomography protocols on distal ureteral calculus detection. J Urol. 2009; 182(6):2762–7.
45. Poletti PA, Platon A, Rutschmann OT, Schmidlin FR, Iselin CE, Becker CD. Low-dose versus standard-dose CT protocol in patients with clinically suspected renal colic. AJR Am J Roentgenol. 2007;188(4):927–33.
46. Niemann T, Kollmann T, Bongartz G. Diagnostic performance of low-dose CT for the detection of urolithiasis: a meta-analysis. AJR Am J Roentgenol. 2008;191(2):396–401.
47. Kalb B, Sharma P, Salman K, Ogan K, Pattaras JG, Martin DR. Acute abdominal pain: is there a potential role for MRI in the setting of the emergency department in a patient with renal calculi? J Magn Reson Imaging. 2010;32(5):1012–23.
48. Abou El-Ghar ME, Shokeir AA, Refaie HF, El-Diasty TA. MRI in patients with chronic obstructive uropathy and compromised renal function: a sole method for morphological and functional assessment. Br J Radiol. 2008;81(968):624–9.
49. Türk C, Knoll T, Petrik A, Sarica K, Straub M, Seitz C. Guidelines on urolithiasis. Arnhem: European Association of Urology; 2011. Chapter 11, Section 1.
50. Shekarriz B, Stoller ML. Uric acid nephrolithiasis: current concepts and controversies. J Urol. 2002;168(4 Pt 1):1307–14.
51. Tiselius HG. Aetiological factors in stone formation. In: Davison AM, Cameron JS, Grunfeld J-P, Kerr DN, Ritz E, Winearls CG, editors. Oxford textbook of clinical nephrology. 3rd ed. Oxford: Oxford University Press; 2005. p. 1201–23.
52. Coe FL, Evan A, Worcester E. Kidney stone disease. J Clin Invest. 2005;115(10):2598–608.
53. Welch BJ, Graybeal D, Moe OW, Maalouf NM, Sakhaee K. Biochemical and stone-risk profiles with topiramate treatment. Am J Kidney Dis. 2006;48(4):555–63.
54. Wilcox WR, Khalaf A, Weinberger A, Kippen I, Klinenberg JR. Solubility of uric acid and monosodium urate. Med Biol Eng. 1972;10(4):522–31.
55. Pak CY, Waters O, Arnold L, Holt K, Cox C, Barilla D. Mechanism for calcium urolithiasis among patients with hyperuricosuria: supersaturation of urine with respect to monosodium urate. J Clin Invest. 1977;59(3):426–31.
56. Mattle D, Hess B. Preventive treatment of nephrolithiasis with alkali citrate – a critical review. Urol Res. 2005;33(2):73–9.
57. Rodgers AL, Allie-Hamdulay S, Jackson GE. JESS: what can it teach us? In: Evan AP, Lingeman JE, Williams Jr JC, editors. Proceedings of renal stone disease 1st annual international urolithiasis research symposium, 203 November 2006, Indianapolis, Indiana. Melville/New York: American Institute of Physics; 2007. p. 183–91. ISBN 878-0-7354-0406-9.

Diagnosis and Differential Diagnosis of Urinary Tract Stone Disease in Emergency Settings

31

Luo Yang, Hong Li, and Kunjie Wang

Abstract

Renal or ureteric pain is usually so characteristic that diagnosis is often instantaneous. However, it is always prudent to differentiate it from other more serious causes of abdominal pain, herpes, pain from intercostal nerve irritation, and musculoskeletal pain.

Keywords

Renal pain • Ureteric colic • Abdominal muscle guarding • Pancreatitis • Cholecystitis Appendicitis • Ovarian cyst torsion • Ectopic pregnancy • *Herpes zoster* • Emergency room

Introduction

Flank pain suggestive of renoureteral colic is a common presentation in the emergency room. Flank pain has many causes and is not always due to ureteral obstruction, and there are many different contexts in which a stone patient will visit the emergency room (ER). The patient may attend an ER because of flank pain, fever, dysuria, retention, anuria, sepsis, pyonephrosis, pyelonephritis, or recurrent urinary tract infection (UTI). At times when adequate physician care is not available, a patient with anuria may present to ER with pulmonary edema because of inappropriate and overzealous intravenous fluid administration by their family physician. In this chapter, we describe the diagnosis and differential diagnosis of renal colic—the main presenting feature in the majority of renal stone patients attending ER.

Clinical Presentation and Diagnosis

Typical renal colic is a colicky pain felt in the flank, which radiates often to the ipsilateral lower abdomen, groin, inside of the thigh, testes, and glands in males or labium in females. It is often assoteciad with tenderness in the flank and costovertebral angle [1–3]. Upper ureteral obstruction often results in pain radiating to the external genitalia, whereas if the obstruction is in the middle ureter, it may radiate to the lower abdomen; however, lower ureteral obstruction results in trigonal irritation and suprapubic discomfort [1–8] and lower urinary tract symptoms.

Hematuria is commonly associated with acute ureteral obstruction due to stones. However, the degree of hematuria does not correlate with degree of obstruction. Absence of microscopic hematuria does not rule out presence of urolithiasis.

Nausea and vomiting are the result of a significant autonomic response to the ureteral colic. Associated infection may manifest as cold sweat, fever, weak pulse, and hypotension [1–3].

History and Physical Examination

Careful inquiry into the nature of the pain, its location, radiation, aggravating cause, and past history of stone or family history of stone assist in making the diagnosis. Additionally, the significance of physical examination cannot be overstated. Presence of costovertebral angle tenderness is typically seen with ureteral and renal stones. The main purpose of examination is to exclude other disease leading to abdominal and lumbar back pain [1–7]. A menstrual history and vaginal examination can be most useful.

L. Yang, M.D. • H. Li, M.D. • K. Wang, M.D., Ph.D. (✉)
Department of Urology, West China Hospital of Sichuan University, 37# Guoxuexiang Street, Chengdu, Sichuan Province 610041, China
e-mail: wangkunjie@gmail.com

J.J. Talati et al. (eds.), *Urolithiasis*,
DOI 10.1007/978-1-4471-4387-1_31, © Springer-Verlag London 2012

At times, there is difficulty in differentiating pain arising in the lumbar musculoskeletal complex from renal colic. The latter seldom radiates to the thigh, though on occasions it may radiate to the medial thigh. Pain associated with herniation of lumbosacral disc emfremium pain radiates down the back of the leg and is aggravated by movement. Straight leg raising might be limited, and movement in bed causes pain.

The preceding chapter has described the investigatory procedures that help diagnose the cause of the pain. We would like to draw attention to the following points:

1. While hematuria and leukocyturia are often present, their absence does not exclude urolithiasis, as the incidence of hematuria in renal colic is about 8 % [9, 10], and the sensitivity and specificity of diagnosis of renal colic by urinalysis are 69 and 27 %, respectively [11].
2. While ultrasound is a low-cost and quick imaging method, it cannot detect stones in the ureter with ease; although hydronephrosis may suggest ureteral stone. Its advantage is that radiolucent stones can be detected and that it is a first choice for the pregnant woman in ER and for those with renal failure. However, the diagnostic rate of ultrasound is only 50 % [9, 12, 13]. The ultrasound can pick up tumors [14]—in some cases rare tumors [15]—which might have bled and resulted in clot colic.
3. The sensitivity and specificity of an X-ray KUB in the diagnosis of urolithiasis are 69 and 82 % [16]. KUB X-rays miss radiolucent and small stones, especially when the abdomen is ill prepared, as it is in situations where the patient attends an ER.
4. The intravenous urogram is of limited value today, though it can identify filling defects signifying stones or necrosed papillae and other reasons for urinary obstruction such as ureteropelvic obstruction or ureteric stricture [11].
5. Today, non-contrast computed tomography (NCCT) is the first choice, with a sensitivity and specificity of 90 % [7, 10, 13, 16–19] far beyond that of ultrasound and KUB.

Differential Diagnosis

Ureteric colic can often mimic pain due to other intra-abdominal pathologies. Table 31.1 lists the common conditions with which renal colic might be confused and their distinctive features.

Emergency Diagnosis in Primary Care Settings

On a home visit, a carefully taken history and physical examination of a patient with a sudden lumbar pain and tenderness in the costospinal (costovertebral) angle could support a diagnosis of renal colic. If there is a high probability that the pain is from renal colic, the physician can start the appropriate medication at the patient's home. If an accurate diagnosis cannot be reached, the patient should be referred to an emergency room at a hospital.

In the physician's clinic, it might be possible to do some laboratory examinations, such as urine analysis, to determine whether there is hematuria. If possible, an ultrasonograph should be done, as it may show a stone in the urinary tract or hydronephrosis or loss of one of the ureteric jets in case of unilateral obstruction of the ureter.

If a patient is seen in a village setting, with limited availability of medical equipment, the main complaint of the patient and the physical examination are the mainstays on which a diagnosis is made, and the treatment planned is

Table 31.1 The differential diagnosis of renal/ureteric colic

Abdominal causes			
S. no.	Pathology	Silent features on history and examination	Investigations
1.	Cholelithiasis/ biliary colic	Severe, sharp colicky pain localized to right upper quadrant and epigastric region of abdomen +ve Murphy's sign Absence of urinary symptoms	U/S abdomen: presence of gall stones, thickened gall bladder wall with peri-cholecystic fluid Normal urinalysis and KUB
2.	Acute pancreatitis	Steady, gnawing pain localized to epigastrium and right upper quadrant, radiates directly to back with associated nausea and vomiting Absence of urinary symptoms	Raised serum amylase and lipase Normal urinalysis CT scan abdomen and pelvis with pancreatic protocol shows swollen and inflamed pancreas with peri-pancreatic fluid
3.	Splenic abscess and infarct	Severe left upper quadrant pain Usually occurs in patients with atrial fibrillation or other conditions of peripheral embolism and hypercoagulable states, e.g., sickle-cell disease, polycythemia vera Absence of urinary symptoms	CT scan abdomen with CT angio Normal urinalysis

Abdominal causes			
S. no.	Pathology	Silent features on history and examination	Investigations
4.	Acute appendicitis	Initial central (periumbilical) pain that shifts to the right iliac fossa in the region of McBurney's point	Normal urinalysis (in case of pelvic appendicitis, microscopic hematuria can occur)
		Rebound tenderness and Rovsing's and psoas signs	A focused abdominal CT scan shows inflamed appendix with absence of ureteric stone
		Mimics right-sided colic due to mid-ureteric stone	Ultrasound is useful in diagnosing appendicitis [1, 2, 20]
5.	Diverticular disease	Left lower quadrant pain, dull or colicky in nature with no radiation to the genitalia	CT scan abdomen and pelvis shows presence of diverticulae with thickened bowel wall
		No urinary S/S if uncomplicated	Barium enema + colonoscopy (contraindicated in acute inflammation)
		Mimics left-sided colic due to mid-ureteric stone	Normal urinalysis
6.	Adnexal pathologies (cysts/neoplasm of ovary)	Chronic deep-seated pelvic pain with:	
	Salpingo-oophoritis	Dysmenorrhea	Tumor markers
	Endometriosis	Dyspareunia	U/S pelvis
	Pelvic inflammatory disease	Infertility	Urinalysis
	Ectopic pregnancy	History of TB or chronic GU infection	B-HCG
		Abdominal pain (initially R or L lower quadrant), diffuse if ruptured with generalized peritoneal signs	
		Menstrual cycle abnormalities (missed or late periods)	
		Vaginal bleeding	
		Shock if ruptured	
7.	Mesenteric lymphadenitis	Young children with fever, and abdominal pain aggravates with movements and accompanied by GI upsets	Normal urinalysis
		Absence of urinary S/S	CT abdomen and pelvis shows mesenteric lymphadenopathy >5 mm
8.	Mesenteric ischemia	Elderly patients with known cardiovascular comorbidities and atherosclerotic disease Symptoms of diffuse abdominal pain, toxic look with minimal abdominal signs	CT scan abdomen angiography
9.	Renal tuberculosis and renal tumors	When bleeding occurs, these patients usually present with a distending type of pain Obstruction with blood clots can mimic renal colic	The ultrasound and plain abdominal film or NCCT can assist in diagnosis
Extra-abdominal causes			
10.	Basal (lobar) pneumonia/pleurisy	High-grade fever with lower chest/upper abdominal pain (mimics pyelonephritis)	CXR (patch of consolidation)
		Associated with cough, SOB, pleuritic pain aggravated with deep breathing	Blood and sputum for C/S
		Lack of urinary symptoms	
		Abnormal chest auscultation	
11.	*Herpes zoster* (lower thoracic/upper lumbar sensory nerve root)	Sharp excruciating neuralgic pain radiates along the distribution of nerve anteriorly	
		Eruption of a patch of vesicles (shingles) 4–6 days after pain	
		Absence of urinary S/S	
12.	Musculoskeletal pain (painful rib syndrome, radicular pain, etc.)	Pain radiates anteriorly and goes to legs	Normal urinalysis and CT KUB/ultrasound
		Aggravates with changing position	MRI shows compression of nerve root
		No urinary symptoms	
		Absence of GI symptoms	

Source: Table prepared by Dr. Syed Muhammad Nazim

according to the doctor's experience, which often helps in making an accurate diagnosis.

Who Should Diagnose and Treat Renal Colic?

In the typical case, a family doctor can make the diagnosis of renal colic, as can also the physicians in the ER, on the basis of symptoms and the examinations, assisted at times with a NCCT. A urologic nurse who has rich experience in stone disease emergency work can also make the right diagnosis. If the primary physician cannot make a reasonably certain diagnosis, he/she must ask for a urologist's immediate help.

Conclusion

In most cases, the diagnosis of ureteric colic and renal pain is instantaneous and certain, especially in patients with a past history of stone disease. However, a careful physician will make sure that he/she does not miss any of the other differential diagnoses (see Table 31.1). In patients with a known history of colic, the NCCT has the best sensitivity and assists the physician in confirming the diagnosis, but the acute nature of pain and its intensity requires a clinical diagnosis and immediate pain relief.

References

1. Gerber GS, Brendler CB. Evaluation of the urologic patient: history, physical examination, and urinalysis. In: Campbell's urology. 8th ed. Philadelphia: W.B. Saunders; 2002. p. 133.
2. Guo Z, Na Y. The main symptoms of urinary system. In: Na Y, Guo Z, eds. Pract Urol. 1st ed. Beijing: The People's Medical Publishing House; 2009. p. 3.
3. McAninch JW. Symptoms of disorders of the genitourinary tract. In: Tanagho EA, McAninch JW, editors. Smith's urology. 17th ed. New York: Lange Medical Books/McGraw-Hill; 2008. p. 30–8.
4. Boost KA, Zwissler B. Emergency checklist: renal colic. MMW Fortschr Med. 2009;151(45):39.
5. Lazio MP, Costello HH, Courtney DM. A comparison of analgesic management for emergency department patients with sickle cell disease and renal colic. Clin J Pain. 2010;26(3):199–205.
6. Walther S, Hilburger M, Bader MJ, Stief CG, Strittmatter F. Urolithiasis. MMW Fortschr Med. 2010;152(16):42–5, quiz 46.
7. Alshamakhi AK, Barclay LC, Halkett G, et al. CT evaluation of flank pain and suspected urolithiasis. Radiol Technol. 2009;81(2): 122–31.
8. Tuma J. CME ultrasound diagnosis 31. Renal colic: and the anamnesis? Praxis. 2009;98(22):1261, quiz 1262.
9. Haroun AA, Hadidy AM, Mithqal AM, Mahafza WS, Al-Riyalat NT, Sheikh-Ali RF. The role of B-mode ultrasonography in the detection of urolithiasis in patients with acute renal colic. Saudi J Kidney Dis Transpl. 2010;21(3):488–93.
10. Prunel P, Verhoest G, Boudry G, Rohou T, Bouget J, Patard JJ, et al. Impact of low-dose CT in the diagnosis and treatment of renal colic in emergency department. Prog Urol. 2010;20(9):633–7.
11. Hazhir S, Badr YA, Darabi JN. Comparison of intranasal desmopressin and intramuscular tramadol versus pethidine in patients with renal colic. Urol J. 2010;7(3):148–51.
12. Elgamasy A, Elsherif A. Use of Doppler ultrasonography and rigid ureteroscopy for managing symptomatic ureteric stones during pregnancy. BJU Int. 2010;106(2):262–6.
13. Gedvilas D, Argatu D, Lukosevicius S, Basevicius A. Aorto-caval fistula clinically presenting as left renal colic. Findings of multislice computed tomography. Medicina (Kaunas). 2008;44(8):619–22.
14. Song J. The diagnosis and differential diagnosis of renal colic. Chin Pract Med. 2010;31:60–1.
15. Bauer RM, Siegert S, Nordhaus C, Staehler M. Epidermoid cyst of the kidney: a rare cause of recurrent renal colic. Urologe A. 2010;49(4):540–2.
16. Rish KA. Diagnostic value of combine with abdominal ultrasound in diagnosis of in Jordan. Mary Slessor J Med. 2005;5(1):57–60.
17. Eray O, Cubuk MS, Oktay C, Yilmaz S, Cete Y, Ersoy FF. The efficacy of urinalysis, plain films, and spiral CT in ED patients with suspected renal colic. Am J Emerg Med. 2003;21(2):152–4.
18. Khalid NS. The value of combined urinalysis and abdominal ultrasound in diagnosing renal colic in aqaba region. JRMS. 2003; 10(2):41–3.
19. Katz DS, Scheer M, Lumerman JH, Mellinger BC, Stillman CA, Lane MJ. Alternative or additional diagnoses on unenhanced helical computed tomography for suspected renal colic: experience with 1000 consecutive examinations. Urology. 2000;56(1):53–7.
20. An R. The diagnosis and treatment of renal colic. J Clin Doct. 2008;5:14–6.

The Utilization of Ultrasound in the Diagnosis of Urolithiasis

32

James H. Masterson, Alyson Brinker, Nathan Hawkes, Lee D. Hall, Danielle A. Taysom, Brian K. Auge, and James O. L'Esperance

Abstract

Ultrasound uses high-frequency sound waves to image internal structures. Ultrasound probes generally range from 2 to 20 MHz, with higher frequencies allowing greater resolution and lower frequencies allowing greater tissue penetration. As an imaging modality for urolithiasis, ultrasound is sensitive (81–96 %) and specific (100 %) for detection of renal stones and holds the additional benefit of not exposing the patient to radiation. To obtain the best diagnostic accuracy, patients should be rolled as necessary to improve viewing of the kidneys. A transvaginal exam may be performed to locate a distal ureteral stone. On ultrasound, renal calculi are visualized as curvilinear, echogenic foci with posterior acoustic shadowing. The use of tissue harmonics can help enhance shadowing of small stones. Renal ultrasound remains an effective means for detecting renal stones. Although computed tomography (CT) is more sensitive and readily available, ultrasound should be considered in evaluating renal colic in pregnant women, children, and patients in which a nonradiation technique is preferred.

Ultrasound is also used for percutaneous access for nephrolithotripsy or antegrade ureteroscopy and should be performed by radiologists or surgeons well versed in the procedure. A small amount of contrast diluted 50:50 is then injected through the needle to opacify the collecting system under fluoroscopy. Ideally, only echogenic-tipped needles should be used for puncture. If unavailable, roughening the needle with a scalpel will greatly improve visualization of the needle on the ultrasound image.

Keywords

Ultrasound • Percutaneous access • Urolithiasis • Echogenic needle tips • Antegrade ureteroscopy • Percutaneous nephrolithotomy (PCNL)

J.H. Masterson, M.D. (✉) • J.O. L'Esperance, M.D.
Department of Urology, Naval Medical Center, San Diego, 34800 Bob Wilson Drive, San Diego 92134, CA, USA
e-mail: james.masterson@med.navy.mil; james.lesperance@med.navy.mil

A. Brinker, B.S.
Department of Internal Medicine, Naval Medical Center, 620 John Paul Jones Circle, Portsmouth, VA 23708, USA

N. Hawkes, M.D. • L.D. Hall, M.D. • D.A. Taysom, M.D.
Department of Radiology, Naval Medical Center, San Diego, 34800 Bob Wilson Drive, San Diego, CA 92134, USA
e-mail: nathan.hawkes@med.navy.mil; lee.hall2@med.navy.mil; danielle.taysom@med.navy.mil

B.K. Auge, M.D.
Mountain States Urology, St. Luke's Health System, 510 N 2nd Street, Boise, ID 83702, USA
e-mail: brianauge@me.com

J.J. Talati et al. (eds.), *Urolithiasis*,
DOI 10.1007/978-1-4471-4387-1_32, © Springer-Verlag London 2012

Introduction

Ultrasound uses high-frequency sound waves to image internal structures. Piezoelectric crystals are used to create sound waves when charged with an electric voltage. The same crystals then convert reflected sound waves into an electric signal. This electric signal is then converted into an image. Ultrasound probes generally range from 2 to 20 MHz, with higher frequencies allowing greater resolution and lower frequencies allowing greater tissue penetration. With a frequency range of 2–20 MHz, the resolution ranges from 1 to 0.1 mm [1].

Sound waves reflect more easily at air-tissue and bone-tissue interfaces. This loss of sound wave propagation causes difficulties in viewing structures deep to bowel, lung, and bone.

Imaging Modalities for Urolithiasis

Urolithiasis can be evaluated by multiple imaging modalities including computed tomography (CT), plain radiography of kidneys, ureters, and bladder (KUB), intravenous pyelography (IVP), and ultrasound [2, 3]. CT has the highest sensitivity and specificity for urolithiasis (97 and 100 %) but exposes the patient to radiation [4]. In children, the estimated increased risk is 1:500 for a fatal cancer due to the CT radiation [5]. A KUB detects 60–70 % of stones but also exposes the patient to radiation. An IVP detects 70–90 % of stones and requires radiation, intravenous contrast administration, and optimized technique to maximize evaluation. The combination of plain radiography and IVP has 98 % sensitivity [6]. Ultrasound is sensitive (81–96 %) and specific (100 %) for detection of renal stones while also having the benefit of not exposing the patient to radiation [6–8]. The ability to detect a stone is related to size but not related to stone location or size of the patient [6]. Recent evidence suggests that ultrasound may overestimate the size of stones by 1.9 mm [9]. This may become significant in choosing a treatment. Generally, stones larger than 1 cm are not suspected to spontaneously pass, whereas stones less than 1 cm may be treated with medical expulsive therapy [10].

Ultrasound is the modality of choice when imaging a pregnant woman or child with a suspected urolith to obviate the risk of radiation [8, 11–13]. Because ultrasound requires a high degree of technical proficiency, it can be more time intensive. In a busy emergency room (ER), a CT scanner is much more expeditious and should generally be used as a first-line approach for suspected urolithiasis [11, 14].

Diagnosis of Urolithiasis by Ultrasound

Diagnosis of urolithiasis can be done with transabdominal and transvaginal sonographic imaging (Fig. 32.1a–c) [15]. Curvilinear ultrasound probes are generally used for transabdominal viewing [16]. The curved array allows for a wider viewing angle to facilitate viewing between the bony rib cage. This is at the cost of lateral resolution especially in viewing deeper tissue. A linear probe would give better resolution but may be difficult to manipulate through the "windows" of the rib cage [1]. Cavitary probes are used for transvaginal viewing. These are traditionally used to view the uterus and ovaries; however, they also serve to effectively view the distal ureters as they course behind and into the bladder. An oscillating probe sweeps each sector independently. This allows for a more compact probe than the curvilinear probe and gives as wide a viewing window [17].

Performing the Exam

Patients suspected of urolithiasis may undergo an ultrasound exam of both kidneys and bladder. This allows for comparison of the left and right kidneys as well as evaluation for ureteral jets at the bladder. The patient should hydrate before the exam with either IV fluid or 400 mL of water by mouth. This will optimize sensitivity for detecting hydronephrosis and ureterectasis [15]. The optimal viewing of the kidneys is with the patient in the supine position. During the exam, the patient should be rolled as necessary to improve viewing of the kidneys [15] (Figs. 32.2 and 32.3). A transvaginal exam may be performed to locate a distal ureteral stone. This is best performed with a visible bladder, which is a different technique than routine pelvic ultrasound done with an empty bladder. This technique may be ideal in a gravid patient with a distended abdomen and contraindication for a CT scan (Fig. 32.4) due to the pregnancy. This technique can be difficult to interpret due to bowel gas shadowing and pelvic fat obscuring the stone.

Ultrasound Features of Renal Calculi

On ultrasound, renal calculi are visualized as curvilinear, echogenic foci with posterior acoustic shadowing (Table 32.1). Stones may have a similar echogenicity to renal sinus fat and may be obscured but can usually be detected by posterior acoustic shadowing. The use of tissue harmonics can help enhance shadowing of small stones. Hydronephrosis is easily detected by ultrasound and suggests obstructive renal calculi

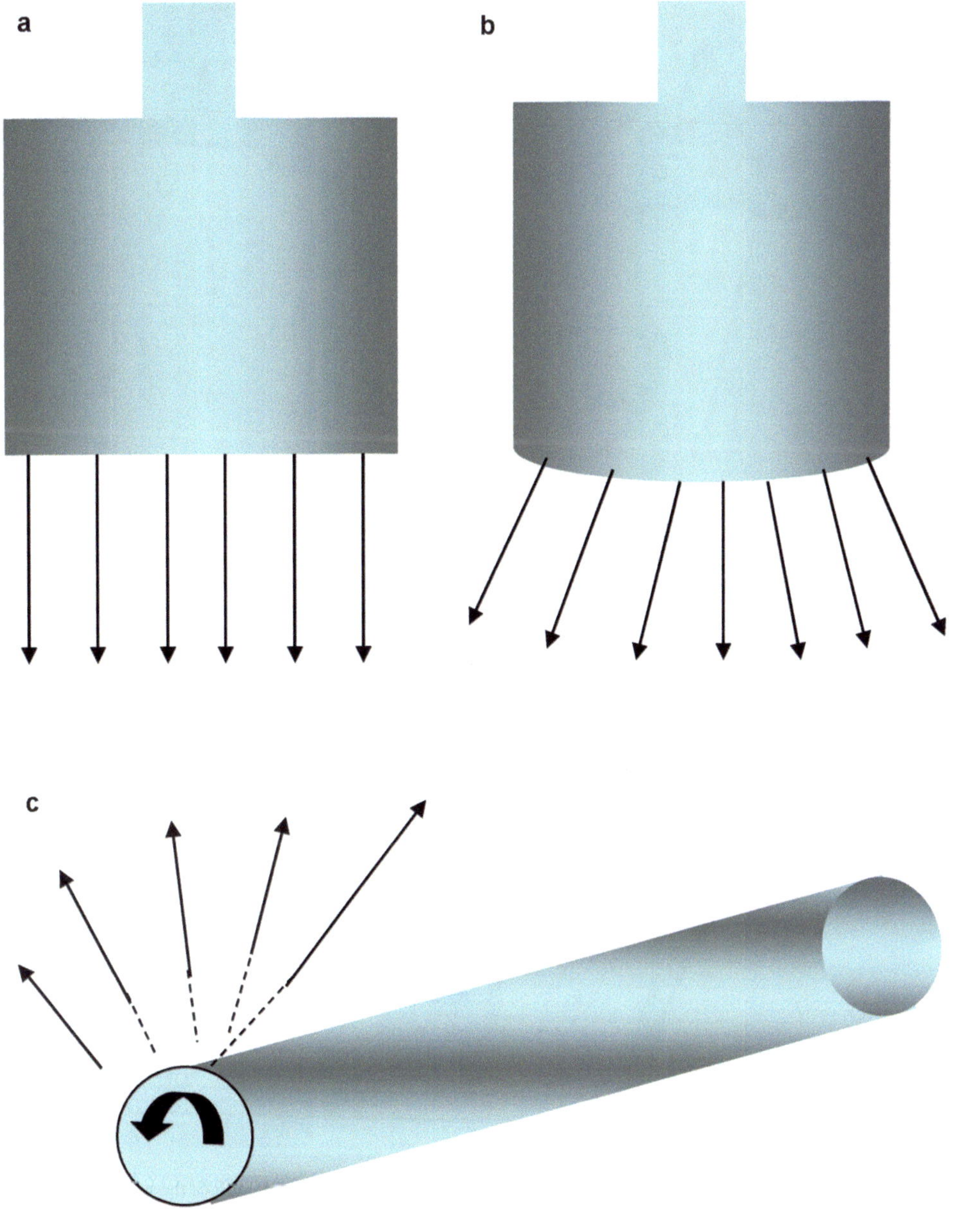

Fig. 32.1 (**a**) A linear probe provides a square viewing window. (**b**) A curvilinear probe allows for viewing between bony ribs and wider viewing angle at the loss of lateral resolution. (**c**) An oscillating probe is similar to a curvilinear probe but allows for a more compact probe head, at a slight loss of real-time viewing

[18]. The use of color Doppler can produce a twinkling artifact—a series of alternating colors behind a stone [19]. Also, applying color Doppler at the bladder can reveal ureteral jets indicating at least partial patency of the ureter [20–22]. Our institution's protocol requires monitoring the bladder for at least 5–10 min before determining absence of ureteral jets. The absence of ureteral jets does not specifically indicate the system is obstructed [22]. Technical factors related to Doppler use, decreased urine production, and decreased ureteral motility are all possible causes for an absent ureteral jet [22]. Pulse wave Doppler can be used to determine the resistive index (RI) with a high-resistive index indicating a high resistance to blood flow (Figs. 32.5, 32.6, and 32.7). This may assist in identifying obstruction in the setting of a non-dilated collecting system. RI is calculated as (peak systolic velocity-end diastolic velocity)/peak systolic velocity. A value greater than 0.7 is considered abnormal. This has a sensitivity of 45 % and a specificity of 91 %. A difference greater than 0.04 between the left and right kidneys is 95 % sensitive and 100 % specific for obstruction [23].

A transvaginal ultrasound can be used to more closely examine the distal ureters [24]. However, bowel gas, unfamiliarity with the procedure, and an empty bladder can confound interpretation of images.

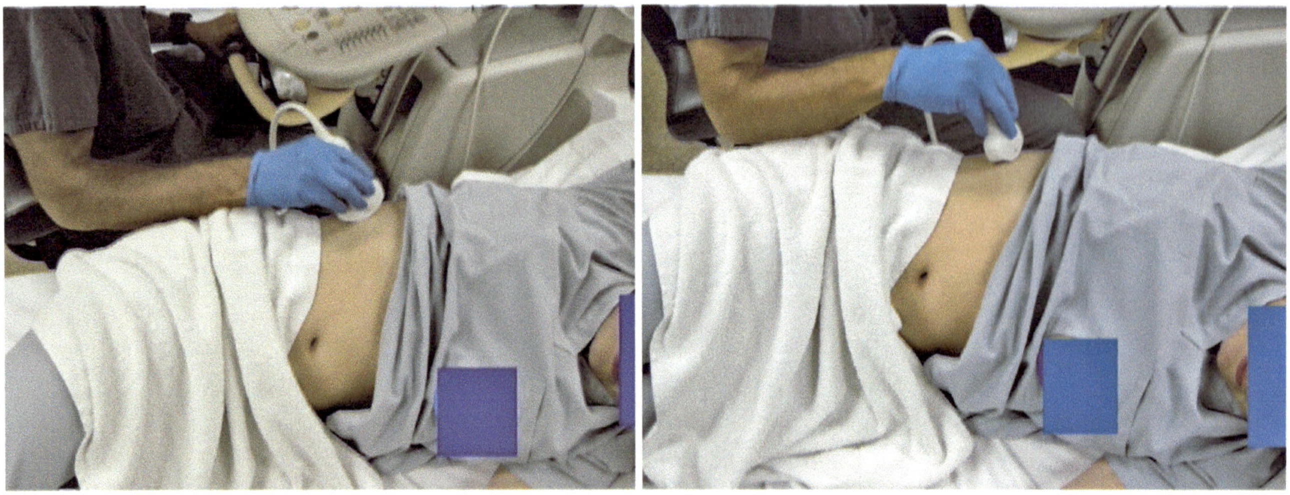

Fig. 32.2 Examining the kidneys. The optimal viewing window is determined by individual anatomic location of the kidneys and body habitus. The picture on the *left* demonstrates sagittal imaging. Note that proper anatomic position is displayed by placing the probe notch cephalad during sagittal imaging and to the *left* during transverse imaging (*right*)

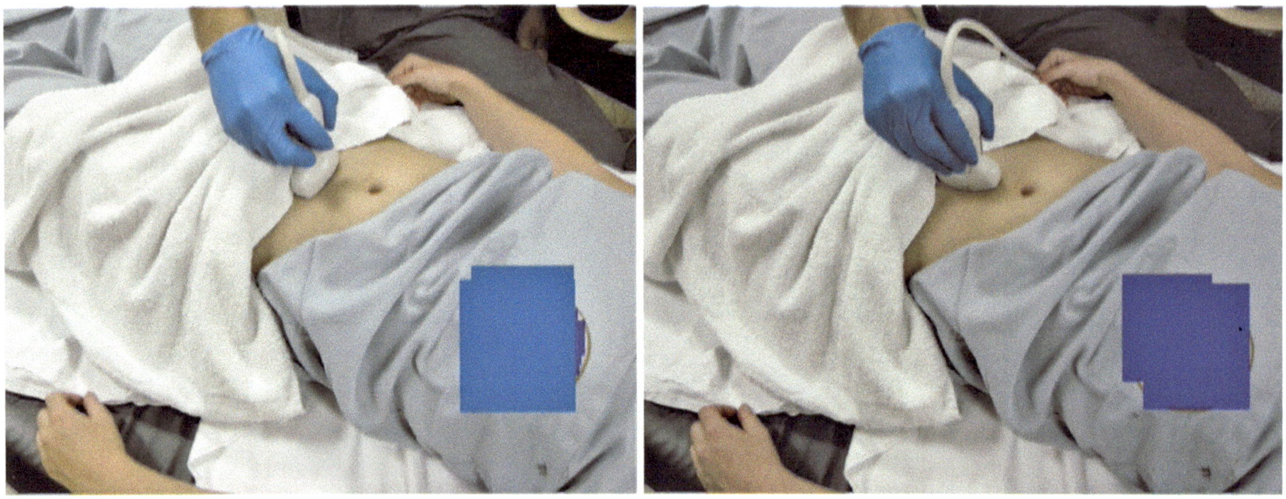

Fig. 32.3 Examining the bladder. Note *the image on the left* shows transverse imaging with the curvilinear probe positioned at the bladder base superior to the pubic symphysis and angled caudally. The notch is on the left of the probe. This projects proper anatomic orientation on the monitor. *The image to the right* demonstrates longitudinal imaging of the bladder. The probe notch is maintained at cephalad

Percutaneous Access for Nephrolithotripsy or Antegrade Ureteroscopy

Per the American Urological Association (AUA) guidelines, the indications to perform a percutaneous nephrolithotomy (PCNL) or antegrade ureteroscopy are listed as follows [10, 25, 26]:

- Staghorn renal stones or stone greater than 2 cm
- Proximal ureteral stone greater than 15 mm

In patients with kidneys that have an abnormal lie, rotation, or form, complete "on table" clearance with PCNL should be considered because kidney drainage is likely impaired. Due to the distorted anatomy, ultrasound-guided percutaneous access should be performed by surgeons well versed in the procedure [27].

Urologists may request interventional radiology to obtain percutaneous access of the collecting system or perform the access themselves. Access can be gained with three different methods. The first is a blind stick into the kidney, opacification of the collecting system with contrast, and then using fluoroscopy, obtain a better access point. The second is to place a ureteral open-ended stent, opacify the collecting system, through the stent, and then gain access under fluoroscopic control [28]. The third method is through an ultrasound-guided needle placement into the collecting system (Fig. 32.8a, b) [28]. This

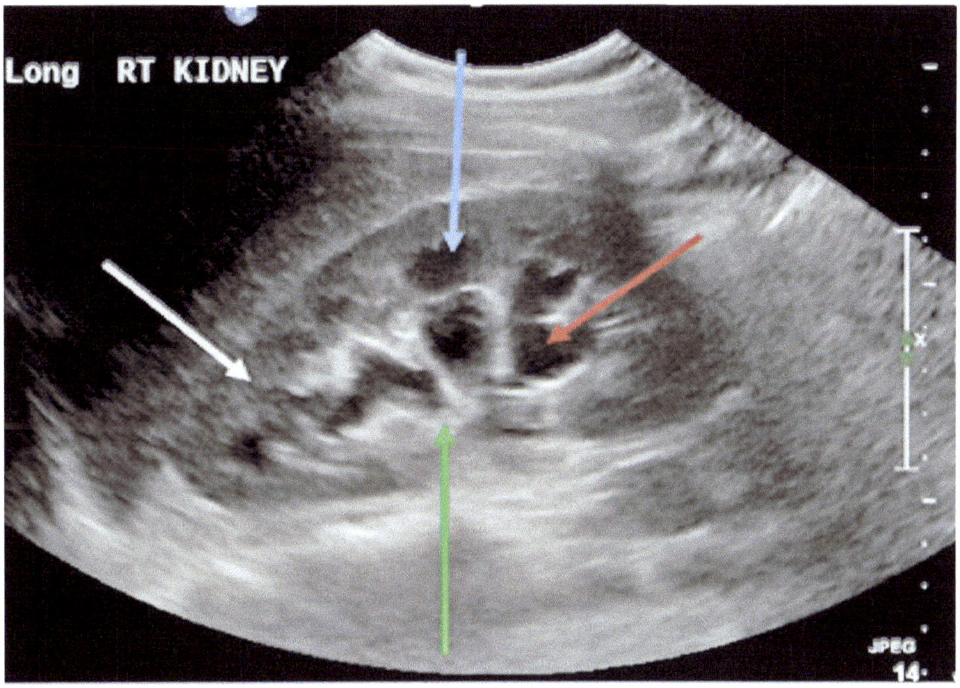

Fig. 32.4 This is a longitudinal view of the kidney. Cephalad—*left of the screen*; caudal—*right of the screen*; superficial—*top of the screen*; deep—*bottom of the screen*. Note the kidney with a moderate degree of hydronephrosis: *red arrow*—dilated renal pelvis; *green arrow*—sinus fat—hyperechoic region surrounding the renal pelvis; *blue arrow*—medullary pyramid; *white arrow*—renal cortex

Table 32.1 Ultrasound indicators of a urinary stone

Curvilinear echogenic focus with shadowing [2, 16]
Pelviectasis or hydronephrosis [18, 30–31]
Absence of ureteral jet(s) [15, 24]
Twinkling artifact posterior to stone when using color Doppler [15, 19]
Resistive index greater than 0.7 [15, 23]
Difference in resistive index >0.04 between the right and left kidneys [23]

chapter will deal solely with the ultrasound portion of the procedure.

The patient is prepped and draped in the prone position over a fluoroscopic table. If the stone is visible on fluoroscopy, the C-arm is iso-centered in both lateral and AP views. The initial landmarks are at the intersection of four fingerbreadths lateral to the spine and immediately inferior to the rib cage. Obviously, depending on renal anatomy and desired calyx, this may be adjusted.

The stone and kidney are viewed either longitudinally or horizontally. The optimal position for transducer placement depends on the stone location, body habitus, and operator preference. The skin and tissue along the projected path is then infiltrated with a local anesthetic. A small nick with an 11-blade is made in the skin at the inferior edge of the probe. The needle is then advanced under fluoroscopic guidance through a renal calyx into the collecting system [29]. Color Doppler may be used to avoid renal vasculature [26]. A small amount of urine is extracted and sent for culture. A small amount of contrast diluted 50:50 is then injected through the needle to opacify the collecting system under fluoroscopy. A small amount of air could also be injected to provide differentiation between the posterior (clear on fluoro) and anterior (opacified) calyces. At this point, the procedure is best continued under fluoroscopy.

Using a curvilinear probe, advancement of the needle will appear distorted given the sector view the probe provides. Also, even if using an echogenic tip, the needle tip will become attenuated as it proceeds deeper through tissue. There are several techniques to overcome these challenges.

Ideally, only echogenic-tipped needles should be used. If the needle does not have the roughened appearance of an echogenic tip, spending a few minutes roughening the needle with a scalpel will greatly assist the procedure by improving visualization of the needle on the ultrasound image (Fig. 32.9).

Also, at our institution, care is taken when infiltrating local anesthesia. This should be done under ultrasound with multiple angles and passes of a long 25-gauge needle. A pass should be made into the kidney as well. This allows visualizing the ideal path for the larger prepackaged 21-gauge needle.

Always remember to only move the needle or the probe at a time. Do not move both simultaneously. If searching for the needle with the probe, move the probe to the suspected area and then pause. During that pause, wiggle the needle. This will make it more visible on ultrasound.

When the cortex of the kidney is encountered, the patient is asked to hold their breath. This allows the kidney to stop moving due to respirations. A quick jab will then seat the

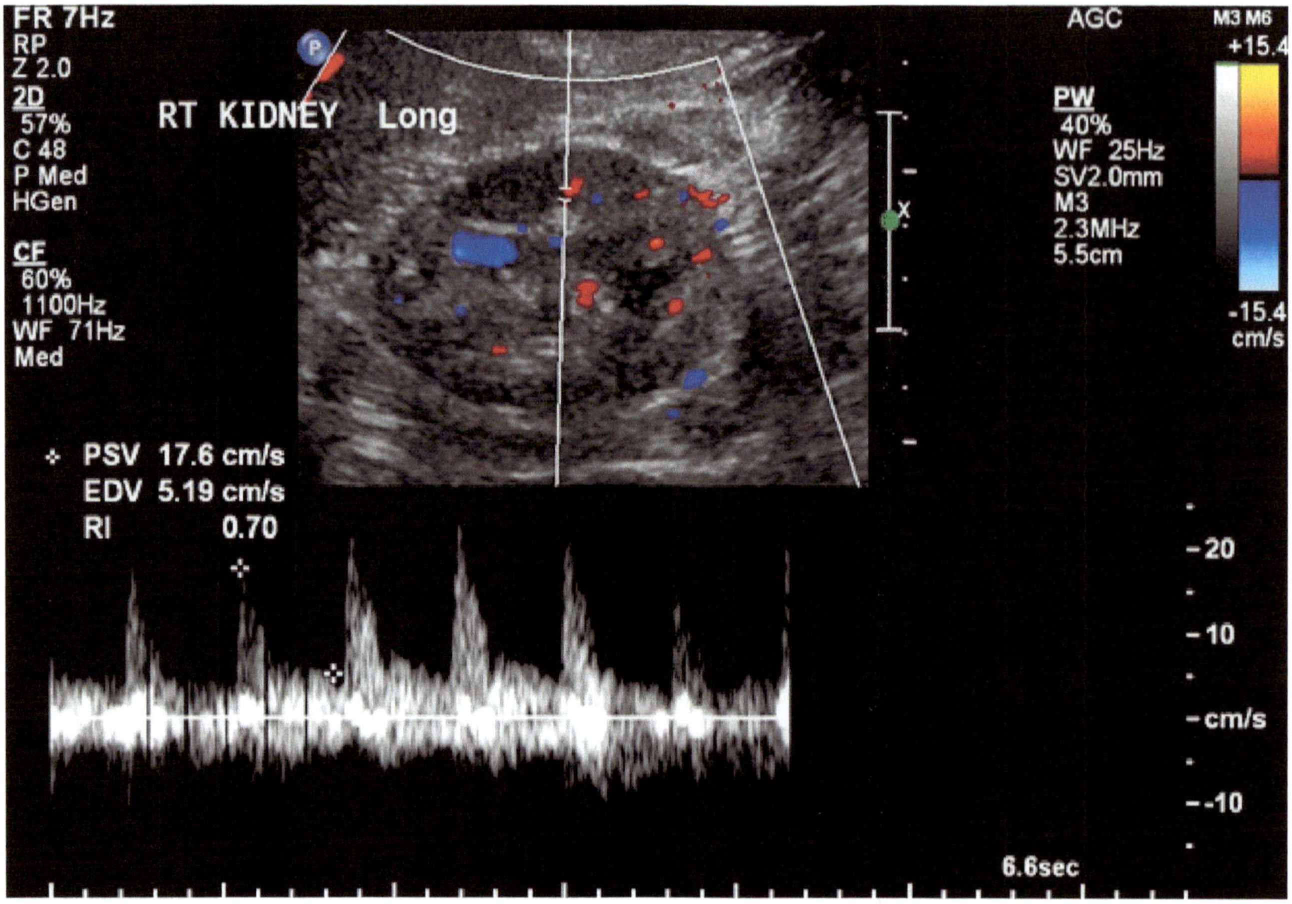

Fig. 32.5 View of the right kidney using pulse wave Doppler. Note the waveform with peak systolic velocity (*PSV*) and end diastolic velocity (*EDV*) indicated. The resistive index (*RI*) is calculated as (PSV – EDV)/PSV = (17.6 – 5.19)/17.6, with the result 0.70 in this example. This indicates upper limits of normal resistance

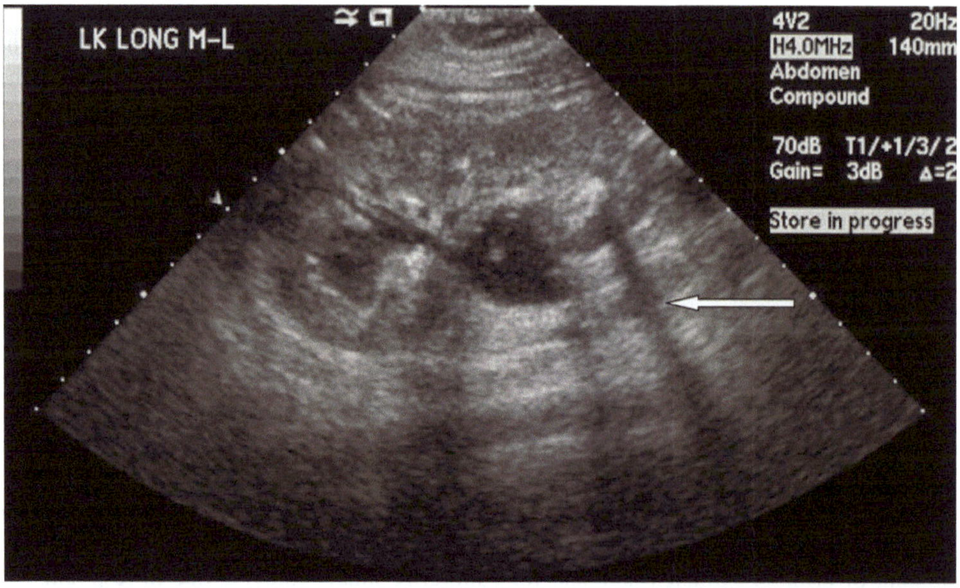

Fig. 32.6 Longitudinal view of a kidney with multiple calcifications. Note the extensive shadowing deep to the calcifications. The *white arrow* indicates shadowing behind an inferior pole calcification

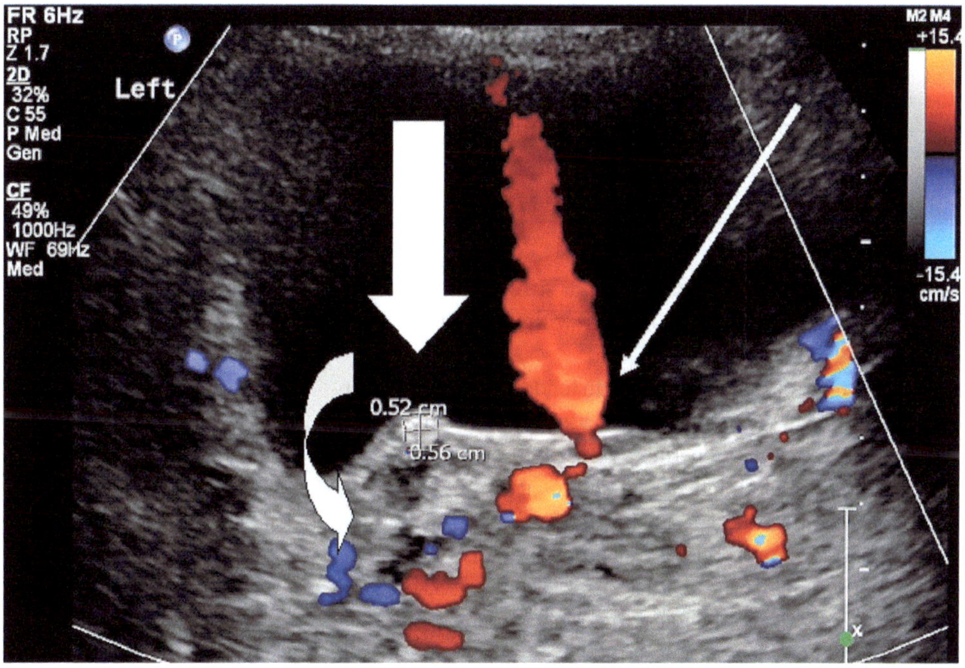

Fig. 32.7 Transverse view of a full bladder in a patient with right flank pain. Note the following signs: left ureteral jet (*thin arrow*), right ureteral orifice calcification (*thick arrow*), posterior shadowing (*curved arrow*)

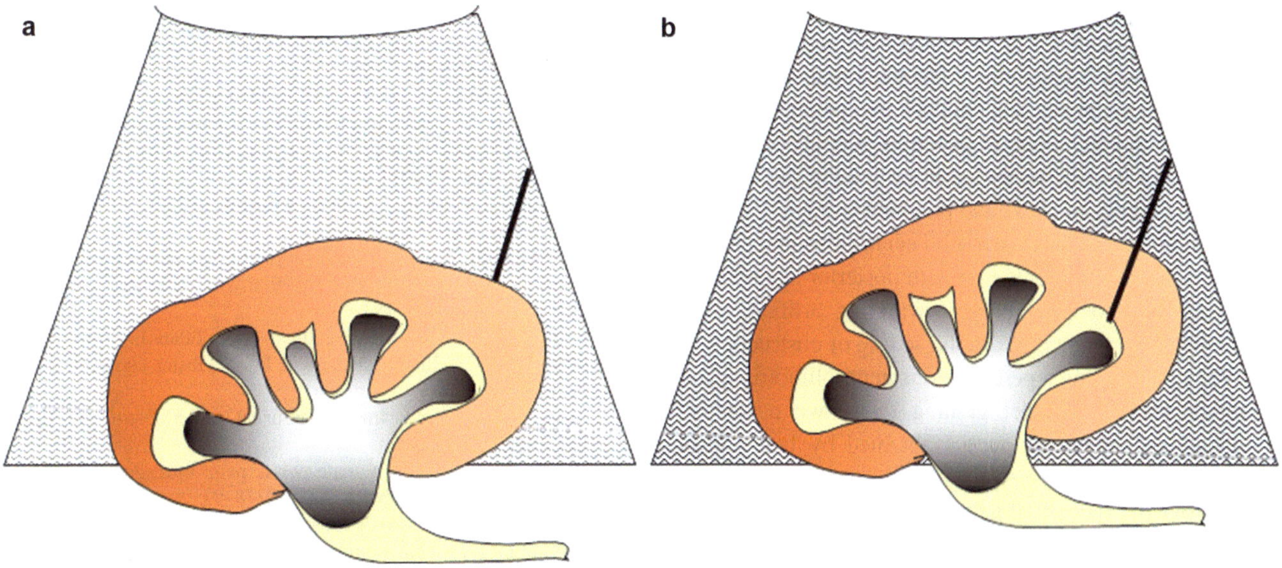

Fig. 32.8 Diagram of percutaneous access. (**a**) As the needle becomes visible, advance to the cortical margin superior to a pyramid. (**b**) Have the patient hold his breath and enter the parenchyma with a quick jab

needle in the kidney. The patient may again breathe, and the needle should freely move superiorly and inferiorly with respirations. The needle is then advanced into the collecting system. You may ask the patient to momentarily hold their breath as needed. Keep in mind that the needle may not be visible, especially in more obese patients.

The mandril or stylet is removed, and the needle is slowly drawn back while simultaneously withdrawing through a syringe. Once urine is aspirated, inject a small amount of contrast under fluoroscopy.

Another method to avoid difficulty in locating the needle under ultrasound as it is advancing is to use an attachable needle guide. This fits onto the transponder and allows for more controlled needle advancement.

Use caution when injecting a dilute mixture of contrast. If the renal pelvis has not been penetrated, the contrast will obscure the fluoroscopy images. For this reason, we initially use a 50:50 mixture to improve washout if the contrast is not injected into the collecting system. If it is injected in the collecting system, this will also ensure that the stone is not

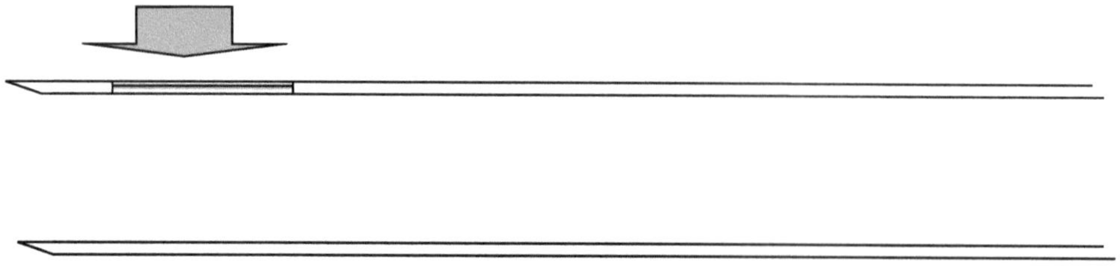

Fig. 32.9 If the needle does not have an echogenic tip (*arrow in top image*), a scalpel can be used to roughen the distal tip of a non-echogenic needle tip (*bottom image*)

masked. By not masking the stone, a second puncture may be performed under fluoroscopy with the stone easily visible.

If the renal pelvis is severely distended, a more concentrated contrast, 80:20, can be used. This will ensure opacification of the collecting system without injecting too much fluid into an already distended renal pelvis.

Using the ultrasound probe during access attempts reduces the likelihood of perforating the colon, liver, or spleen. If the physician is not overly distracted by Doppler US, consider using it to identify and avoid large renal vessels while placing the initial needle.

Conclusion

Renal ultrasound is an effective means for detecting renal stones. Although CT is more sensitive and readily available, ultrasound should be considered in evaluating renal colic in pregnant women, children, and patients in which a nonradiation technique is preferred. A transvaginal ultrasound is a helpful technique in evaluating the distal ureters, especially in obese and pregnant women. Ultrasound findings that are consistent with nephroliths or uroliths are a curvilinear echogenic foci with posterior acoustic shadowing, dilated renal pelvis, twinkling artifact, and an increased resistive index in the setting of obstruction. When performing a percutaneous nephrolithotripsy, urologists should consider gaining their own access with ultrasound or having access obtained by interventional radiology. There are several subtle techniques that can improve the success of gaining access safely.

Acknowledgements The views expressed in this article are those of the authors and do not reflect the official policy or position of the US Department of the Navy, US Department of Defense, or the United States Government.

We appreciate the valuable assistance HM2 Todd Brook and HM1 Rashard Scott provided in obtaining photographs.

References

1. Adam A, Dixon AK. Chapter 1 "Ultrasound and General Principles". In: Adam A (editor). Grainger & Allison's diagnostic radiology. 5th ed. Philadelphia: Churchill Livingstone/Elsevier; 2008.
2. Diament MJ, Malakzadeh M. Ultrasound and the diagnosis of renal and ureteral calculi. J Pediatr. 1986;109:980–3.
3. Richmond J. Radiological diagnosis of kidney stones. Nephrology. 2007;12:S34–6.
4. Westphalen AC, Hsia RY, Maselli JH, Wang R, Gonzales R. Radiological imaging of patients with suspected urinary tract stones: national trends, diagnoses, and predictors. Acad Emerg Med. 2011;18:S31.
5. Kokorowski PJ, Hubert K, Nelson CP. Evaluation of pediatric nephrolithiasis. Indian J Urol. 2010;26:531–5.
6. Middleton WD, Dodds WJ, Lawson TL, Foley WD. Renal calculi: sensitivity for detection with US. Radiology. 1988;167(1):239–44.
7. Ather MH, Jafri AH, Sulaiman MN. Diagnostic accuracy of ultrasonography compared to unenhanced CT for stone and obstruction in patients with renal failure. BMC Med Imaging. 2004;4:2.
8. Hwang K, Mason MD, Peters CA. Clinical practice: surgical approaches to urolithiasis in children. Eur J Pediatr. 2011; 170:681–8.
9. Ray AA, Ghiculete D, Pace KT, Honey RJD. Limitations to ultrasound in the detection and measurement of urinary tract calculi. Urology. 2010;76:295–300.
10. Preminger Gea. AUA/EAU 2007 guideline for the management of ureteral calculi. Available at: http://www.auanet.org/content/guidelines-and-quality-care/clinical-guidelines.cfm?sub=uc2011. Accessed Aug 20, 2011.
11. Caterson RJ, Pokorny CS. Investigating the patient with renal colic. Med Today. 2001;2:52–5.
12. Chadwick DJ, Kasthuri RS. Plain radiograph and renal tract ultrasound in the management of children with renal tract calculi [1]. Clin Radiol. 2001;56:783.
13. Buchholz N, Biyabani R, Sulaiman MN, Talati J. Urolithiasis in pregnancy – a clinical challenge. Eur J Obstet Gynecol Reprod Biol. 1998;80:25–9.
14. Ames CD, Older RA. Imaging in urinary tract obstruction. Braz J Urol. 2001;27:316–25.
15. Bau A, Atri M. Acute female pelvic pain: ultrasound evaluation. Semin Ultrasound CT MRI. 2000;21:78–93.
16. Smith RJ, Horrow MM. Ultrasonographic evaluation of acute urinary tract and male genitourinary pathology. Ultrasound Clin. 2011;6:195–213.
17. Stoylen A. Basic ultrasound, echocardiography and Doppler for clinicians. Available at: http://folk.ntnu.no/stoylen/strainrate/ultrasound/. Accessed Nov 2010.
18. Goertz JK, Lotterman S. Can the degree of hydronephrosis on ultrasound predict kidney stone size? Am J Emerg Med. 2010;28: 813–6.
19. Davran R. The usefulness of color Doppler twinkling artifact in the diagnosis of urinary calculi. Eur J Radiol. 2009;71:378.
20. Delair SM, Kurzrock EA. Clinical utility of ureteral jets: disparate opinions. J Endourol. 2006;20:111–4.
21. Pepe P, Motta L, Pennisi M, Aragona F. Functional evaluation of the urinary tract by color-Doppler ultrasonography (CDU) in 100 patients with renal colic. Eur J Radiol. 2005;53:131–5.
22. Burke BJ, Washowich TL. Ureteral jets in normal second- and third-trimester pregnancy. J Clin Ultrasound. 1998;26:423–6.

23. Shokeir AA, Mahran MR, Abdulmaaboud M. Renal colic in pregnant women: role of renal resistive index. Urology. 2000;55:344–7.
24. McAleer SJ, Loughlin KR. Nephrolithiasis and pregnancy. Curr Opin Urol. 2004;14:123–7.
25. Preminger Gea. AUA 2005 guideline for the management of staghorn calculi (validated in 2009). Available at: http://www.auanet.org/content/guidelines-and-quality-care/clinical-guidelines.cfm?sub=sc2011. Accessed Aug 20, 2011.
26. Lu M, Pu X, Gao X, Zhou X, Qiu J, Si-Tu J. A comparative study of clinical value of single B-mode ultrasound guidance and B-mode combined with color Doppler ultrasound guidance in mini-invasive percutaneous nephrolithotomy to decrease hemorrhagic complications. Urology. 2010;76:815–20.
27. Ganpule AP, Desai MR. Urolithiasis in kidneys with abnormal lie, rotation or form. Curr Opin Urol. 2011;21:145–53.
28. Osman M, Wendt-Nordahl G, Heger K, Michel MS, Alken P, Knoll T. Percutaneous nephrolithotomy with ultrasonography-guided renal access: experience from over 300 cases. BJU Int. 2005;96:875–8.
29. Haussegger K, Portugaller H. Percutaneous nephrostomy and antegrade ureteral stenting: technique-indications-complications. Eur J Radiol. 2006;16:2016–30.
30. Herbst M, Rosenberg G, Bomann S, Moore C. Accuracy of point-of-care ultrasound for hydronephrosis in patients with suspected renal colic. Acad Emerg Med. 2011;18:S173.
31. de Souza LRMF, Goldman SM, Faintuch S, et al. Comparison between ultrasound and noncontrast helical computed tomography for identification of acute ureterolithiasis in a teaching hospital setting. Sao Paulo Med J. 2007;125:102–7.

The Role of Radiological Imaging

33

Zafar Sajjad

Abstract

X-ray-based imaging modalities of plain films and computerized tomography (CT) are the common modalities used to detect urinary tract calculi. Plain films on their own have a low sensitivity and specificity for the detection of renal stones. Intravenous urograms (IVUs), which are obtained by intravenously injecting iodine-containing organic compounds prior to taking X-ray images, were the mainstay of radiological detection. Several problems were associated with the use of these iodinated compounds. The advent of helical CT has obviated their need in the majority of patients. CT scanning detects renal calculi with a high degree of accuracy. Exposure to ionizing radiation is a concern that needs to be addressed and dose-reduction measures should be employed whenever feasible.

Keywords

X-rays • Computerized tomography (CT) • Non-contrast computed tomography (NCCT) Renal calculi • Diagnosis

Introduction

Imaging plays an integral part in the diagnosis and management of urinary tract calculi. This chapter will attempt to introduce the role of imaging using X-ray-based modalities.

Imaging Modalities for Renal Tract Stones

Plain Abdominal Films

Plain films are a good and low-cost way to image renal tract stones. This is because a large percentage of renal tract stones contain calcium and are therefore visible on plain films. Historically up to 90 % of the urinary stones are considered radio-opaque [1]. The actual detection rates, however, vary greatly. The sensitivity of plain films for the detection of urinary stones ranges between 45 and 59 %, with specificity ranging between 71 and 77 % [1–4]. This low sensitivity is attributed to obscuration of the areas of interest by overlying bowel shadows and bony structures such as transverse processes of lumbar vertebrae. The low specificity, on the other hand, is attributed to non-urological opacities such as calcified gall stones, fecaliths, phleboliths, and calcified lymph nodes [1]. Surprisingly, there is little evidence that preparing the bowel prior to plain film adds significantly to the detection rates; therefore, bowel preparation is not recommended as a routine prerequisite for plain abdominal films (Fig. 33.1) [5].

Plain films, commonly labeled kidneys-ureters-bladder (KUB) X-rays, play a central role in the management of known radio-opaque stones. It is widely used for treatment planning and follow-up. The radio-opacity of a stone cannot always be ascertained from the scout film on non-contrast computed tomography (NCCT). While the Hounsfield units will give an indication as to whether the stone will be visible during percutaneous nephrolithotomy or ureteroscopy on the

Z. Sajjad, M.B.B.S., MRCP(UK), FRCR
Department of Radiology, Aga Khan University,
Stadium Road, Karachi, Sindh 74800, Pakistan
e-mail: zafar.sajjad@aku.edu

J.J. Talati et al. (eds.), *Urolithiasis*,
DOI 10.1007/978-1-4471-4387-1_33, © Springer-Verlag London 2012

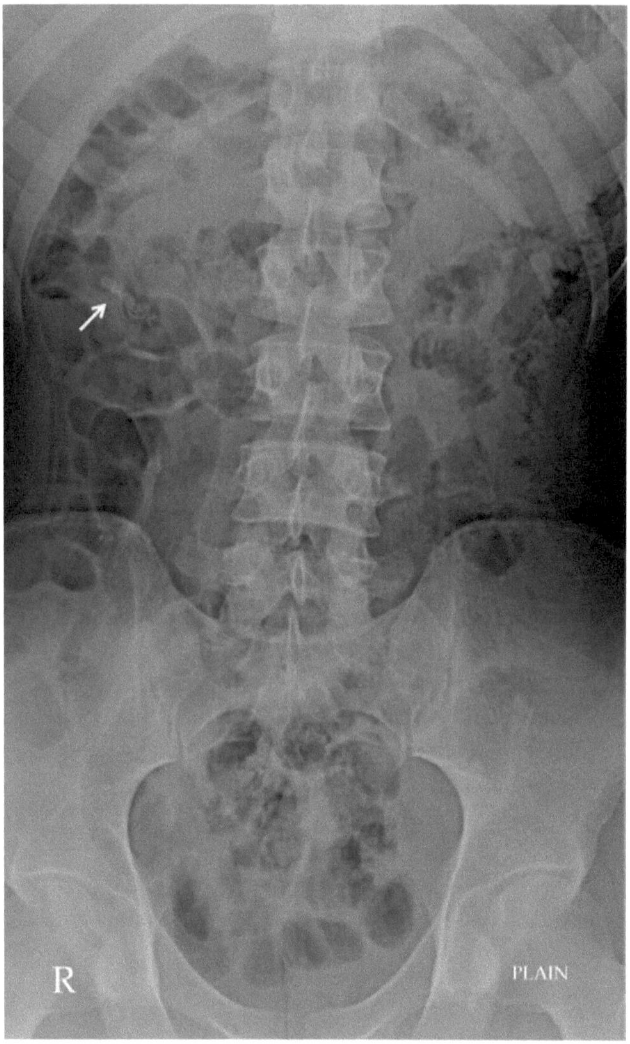

Fig. 33.1 Plain supine abdominal film in a patient with renal colic. The multiple stones in the right renal area (*white arrow*) are difficult to visualize owing to significant amount of overlying bowel gas. Neither renal outline could be seen. Situations such as this are common and difficult to overcome. Additional imaging (usually with CT) is required to confirm the presence of stones

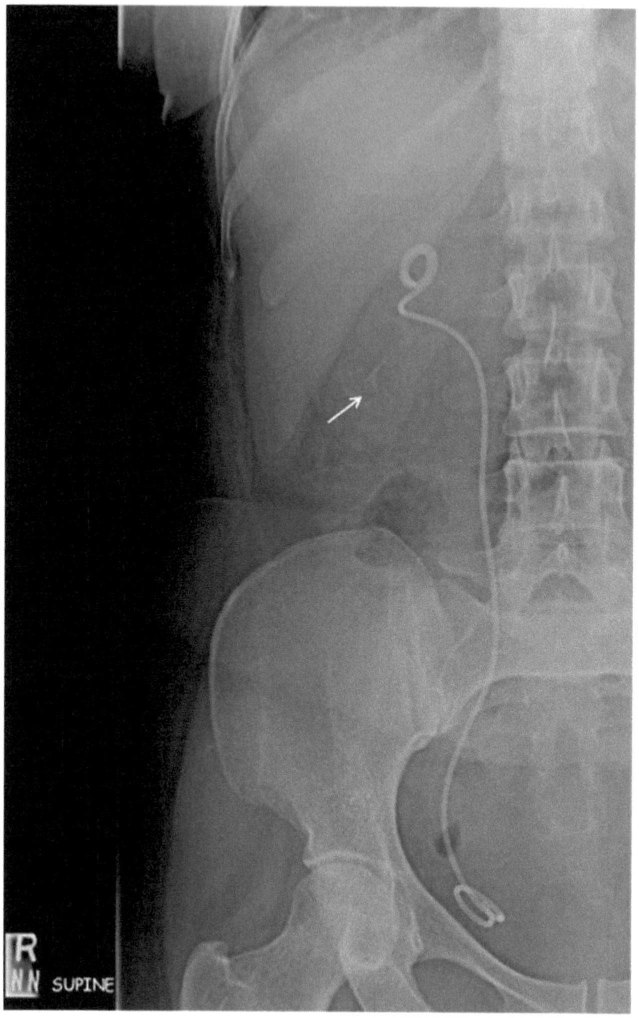

Fig. 33.2 Hemi-KUB. Post-lithotripsy follow-up. A right-sided double J stent is in place. Tiny residual calculi at the right lower pole (*arrow*). The required information regarding the position of the stent and the residual stone burden is obtained at a significant reduction in radiation dose

image intensifier, the surgeon is likely to ask for a KUB film for this assessment. The KUB X-ray is also used to assess the status of patients managed conservatively [6].

Reducing Radiation Exposure When Multiple Follow-Up X-Rays Are Required Following SWL of Renal Stones

Patients usually require several X-ray examinations as part of their treatment, say with shockwave lithotripsy (SWL) or medical expulsion therapy. As the diagnosis has been established by earlier X-rays, and the stone burden already known, there is a rationale for carrying out a more focused study in an attempt to minimize radiation exposures. The most commonly applied strategy is the use of the so-called hemi-KUB. In this procedure, only one side of the abdomen is imaged. The coverage needs to extend across the midline a little over to the other side as the vesicoureteric junction is very close to the midline (the trigone being only 1.5″ × 1.5″ × 1.5″ in a distended bladder and 1″ × 1″ × 1″ otherwise). The reduction in radiation is less than 50 %, because of other considerations, but certainly the patient receives a reduced dose (Fig. 33.2) [7].

Intravenous Urogram (IVU)

An intravenous urogram (IVU) is a series of X-ray images obtained after an intravenous injection of a water-soluble contrast agent that is preferentially excreted via the kidneys.

Table 33.1 Risk factors for the development of contrast-mediated nephropathy (CMN)[a]

Prior renal impairment	Raised serum creatinine especially due to diabetic nephropathy
Dehydration	Especially in children and the elderly
Congestive cardiac failure	
Age	>70 years
Concurrent administration of nephron-toxic drugs	NSAIDs, etc.
Diabetes mellitus	Especially if taking biguanides (Metformin)

[a]Modified from European Society of Urogenital Radiology guidelines for avoiding CMN

The contrast agents most commonly used are organic iodides such as diatrizoate. These agents are broadly divided into high-osmolar agents with typical osmolality more than 1.5 osm/kg (e.g., diatrizoate), low-osmolar agents with typical osmolality of around 0.67 osm/kg (e.g., iohexol), and iso-osmolar agents with osmolality of 0.36 osm/kg (e.g., iotrolan). The cost and safety profile are inversely related, with the high-osmolar agents being the cheapest and the iso-osmolar agents being the safest. The general global trend has been to move toward the low- and iso-osmolar agents [8].

All of the aforementioned agents contain iodine in variable amounts. All agents are nephrotoxic to variable degrees, and all agents are associated with allergic reactions. The incidence of both nephrotoxicity and allergic reactions is highest with high-osmolar agents and lowest with iso-osmolar agents. The iso-osmolar agents are, however, very viscous and need special handling with contrast warmers, etc. to allow manageable injection profiles.

Nephrotoxicity of these agents is a major consideration, especially in patients whose renal function may be impaired by the underlying stone disease. Measures to reduce the risk of nephrotoxicity include identification of the patients at risk (Table 33.1), avoiding the use of high-osmolar agents, using the lowest dose (which would give the desired result) and adequate hydration prior to the administration of the contrast agent. The risk of renal damage is increased in those with pre-existing renal failure and those using nephrotoxic drugs concurrently. The use of so-called renal protective agents such as *N*-acetylcysteine is not established [9]. When a rise in serum creatinine occurs, it is transient and nephrotoxicity seldom results in end-stage renal failure in patients who had a previously normal serum creatinine.

A serum creatinine is not considered mandatory before an intravenous pyelography (IVP), though most often the urologist would have had this investigation done. It is therefore worthwhile looking at available serum creatinine reports and modifying protocol accordingly.

Patients with known atopy or reactive airways disease are at an increased risk of allergic reactions and may require pretreatment with steroids. The risk of a fatal anaphylactoid reaction after the injection of a standard dose of low-osmolar contrast agent is estimated at 0.9/100,000 contrast administrations [10]. While iso-osmolar contrast solutions (often termed nonionic contrast) have a lower risk of mild to moderate reactions, the risk of fatal reactions is the same for both ionic and nonionic contrast [11]. The reaction may be immediate or delayed, sometimes after the patient has reached home.

The contrast agent starts to be excreted by the kidney immediately after intravenous injection. Usually a standard dose of 50 ml of a low-osmolar contrast agent with an iodine content of 300–370 mg/ml is used in adults. In patients with normal renal function and no obstruction, the peak opacification of the upper tracts is obtained between 7 and 12 min after injection. The standard IVU series comprises of a control film, a cross kidney film immediately after the injection of the contrast agent (nephrographic phase), followed by cross kidney films at 5 and 10 min (pyelographic phase). A full-length film is taken when the ureters are being opacified, usually between 10 and 15 min. Further films and views may be needed as required to sort out particular questions in individual patients. The additional views include, but are not limited to, prone images, oblique images, and delayed films if one or both kidneys demonstrate delayed contrast excretion. The information derived from the IVP will be dependent on the availability of a radiologist to review each film as it is developed.

Ureteric stones are particularly well demonstrated on IVU examinations. These are shown as asymmetric or delayed excretion of contrast or filling defects. Occasionally, a continuous column of contrast within the ureters (which when unobstructed show peristalsis and are therefore never visible in their entirety) draws attention to the obstruction by a ureteric stone. When the direct visualization and the secondary signs are combined, the sensitivity of the IVU is reported to be 90 % (Fig. 33.3) [12].

Until fairly recently, the IVU was the mainstay for the assessment of urinary calculi, especially those lying in the ureter. The development of non-contrast CT pyelography has dethroned IVU, which is now seldom used in this context. Significant drawbacks in the routine application of the IVU include the contrast-related issues and the relatively long examination times, particularly in the presence of renal tract obstruction when delayed films may be required for several hours [13]. The IVU is a radiologist-intensive investigation.

Computed Tomography

In computed tomography (CT), a mechanical gantry containing an X-ray tube and a bank of detectors rotates around the patient. Data are collected as the gantry rotates. Using mathematical calculations and computer modeling, the data is

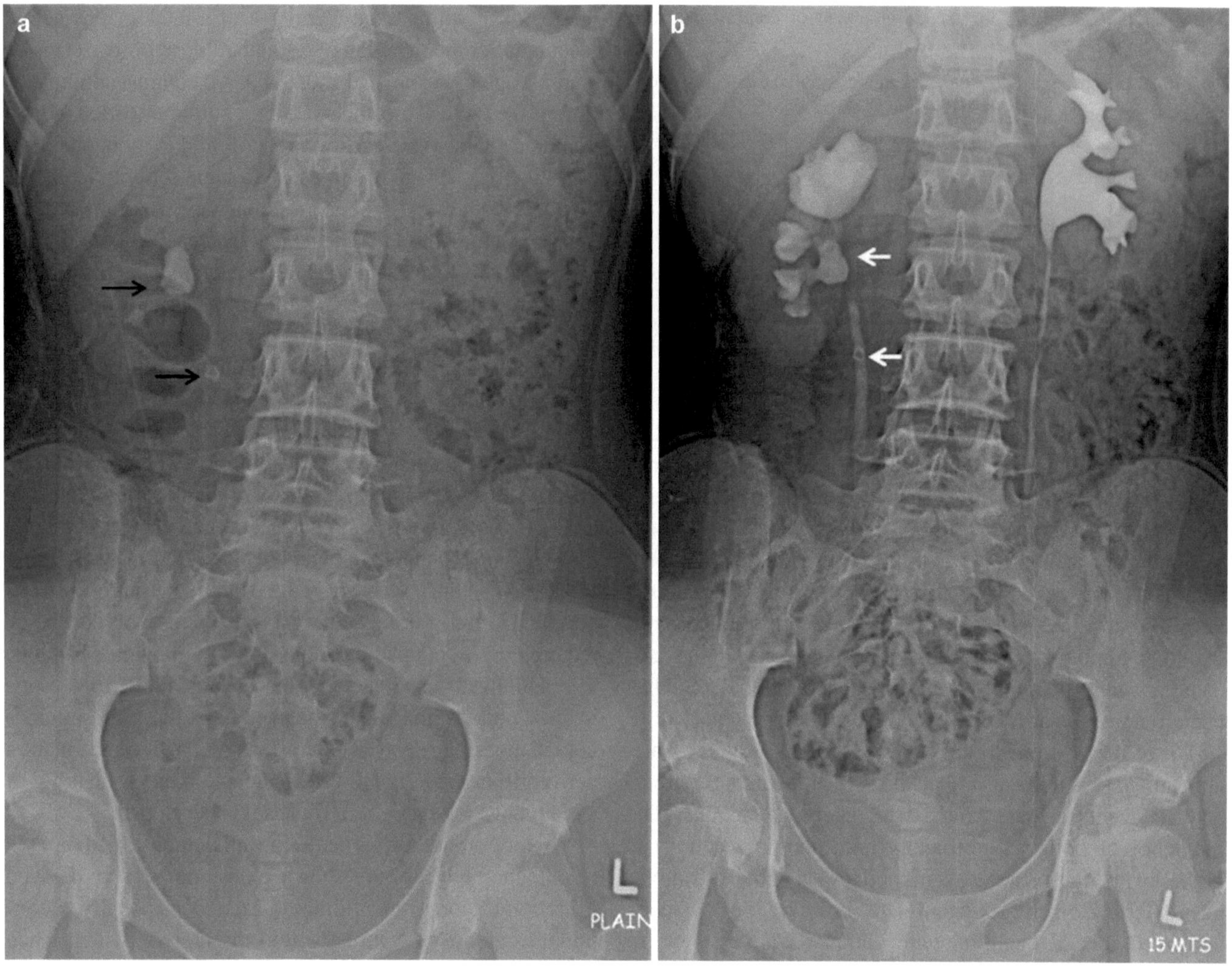

Fig. 33.3 Two films from an IVU series. (**a**) Control film obtained prior to the injection of contrast. This demonstrates two calcified opacities. The large opacity lies over the right renal area (*upper black arrow*). The smaller opacity (*lower black arrow*) lies in line of the right ureter. The left renal area is overlapped by bowel gas shadows. (**b**) Film taken 15 min after intravenous injection of an iodinated contrast medium. The large opacity simulates contrast in the pelvis and without the presence of the control film may be misinterpreted (*upper white arrow*). The right ureteric calculus is clearly seen (*lower white arrow*). The left-sided collecting system is normal. The case highlights some of the shortcomings of the IVU. Renal pelvic and calyceal calculi may be completely undetectable on post-contrast images

reconstructed to give an image. The CT scan is exquisitely sensitive to changes in density in the body. The stones that are lucent on plain films are clearly visualized on CT scans. In the early models of the scanners, the gantry rotated while the patient remained stationary. Only one axial image could be obtained at a time. After each acquisition, the patient was moved to the next image position, and the processes were repeated. This method of obtaining the CT is called incremental CT. As the images are acquired in suspended respiration to eliminate movement artifact, this meant that to cover the entire urinary tract it took many images, and therefore, many separate breath holds. This led to two artifacts: slice misregistration and partial volume averaging. Both led to small stones being missed. The early CT scanners were therefore not suitable for stone detection [14].

The introduction of the helical CT into clinical practice in 1989 revolutionized CT scanning. During a helical scan, continuous image acquisition takes place as the patient is moved through the scanner. This allows a large area to be covered in a short time. As it was now possible to acquire volume data from the diaphragm to the pelvis in a single breath hold, both slice misregistration and partial volume effects were eliminated.

Smith et al. [15] published their paper comparing unenhanced CT with IVU in the context of acute flank pain in 1995. This has set the tone for the imaging of renal tract

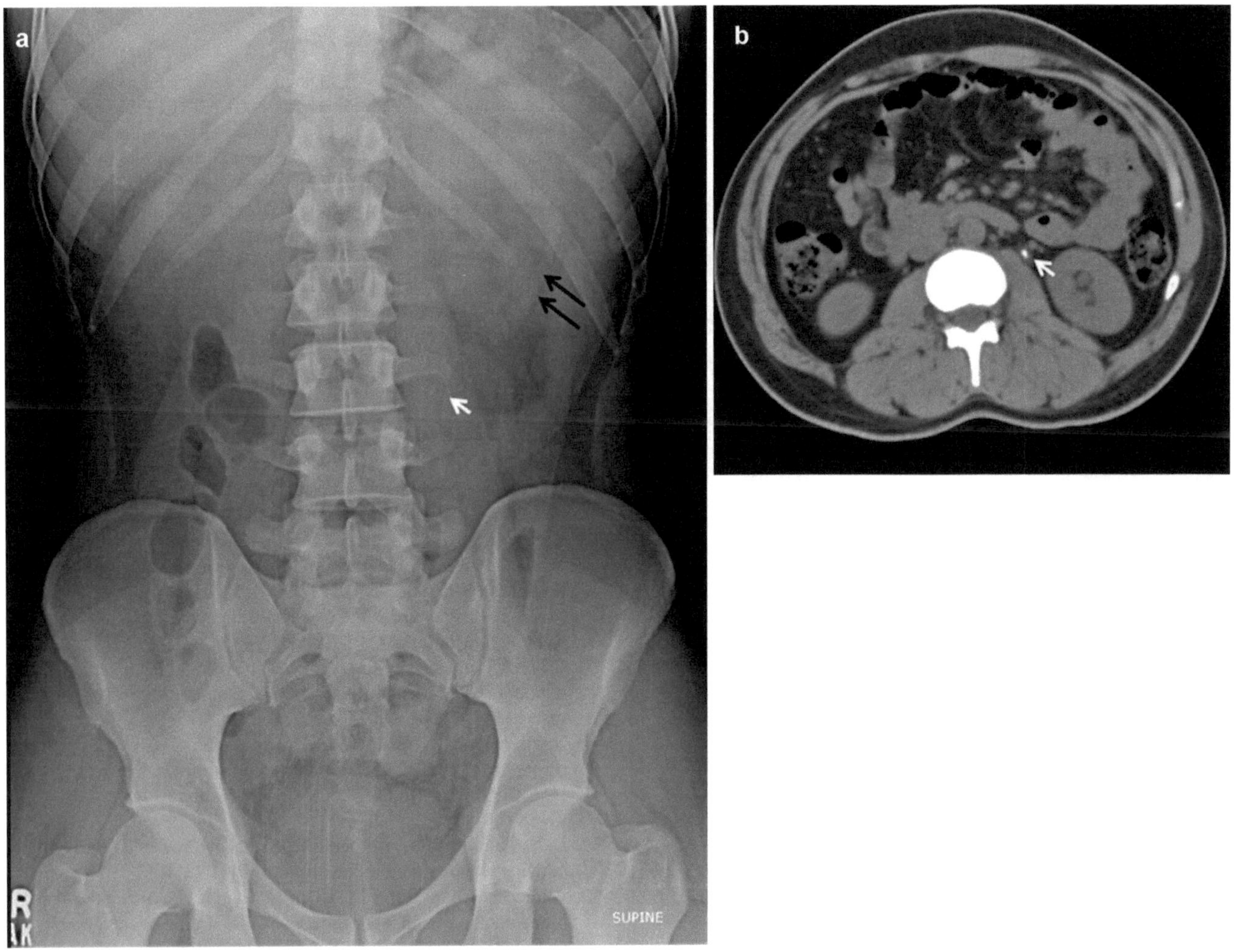

Fig. 33.4 (**a**) Plain abdominal film. Despite the absence of the overlying bowel the small left ureteric calculus (*white arrow*) is difficult to see. Had it overlapped the transverse process of a lumbar vertebra it would have been virtually invisible. The renal outlines (*black arrows*) are clearly defined. (**b**) On the accompanying axial CT scan image, carried out 45 min after the plain film, the ureteric calculus (*white arrow*) is clearly identified. Note the absence of any secondary signs around the kidney

stones. With a sensitivity of 95–100 % and specificity of 94–96 %, this has become a vital part of stone imaging [1]. In addition to the high sensitivity and specificity, there are several practical advantages to using unenhanced CT. The need for contrast and its associated problems is eliminated, the scan time is short, there is no need for delayed imaging; and CT demonstrates lesions other than renal tract stones that may be the cause of the symptoms and radiolucent stones. Although not widely applied in clinical settings, CT has the ability to distinguish between the different types of stones based on their density, internal structure, and energy absorption [6, 14].

The procedure is simple. No preparation is required. A full bladder is helpful but not mandatory. Images are acquired in a single breath hold from the top of the diaphragm to the lower margin of the ischial tuberosity. Images are reviewed ideally on an electronic terminal where the display densities can be manipulated. Both direct visualization of stones and indirect signs of ureteral obstruction are sought (Figs. 33.4 and 33.5).

The radiation received during a CT can be reduced by various means, including the low-dose CT, a topic that is discussed in some detail by Pierre in Chap. 35.

Conclusion

CT KUB has revolutionized the imaging of renal stones. Modern CT scanners offer a high degree of sensitivity and specificity with an excellent safety profile. As the patients with renal stones require repeated studies, cumulative radiation burden should be kept in mind when deciding upon the appropriate imaging method.

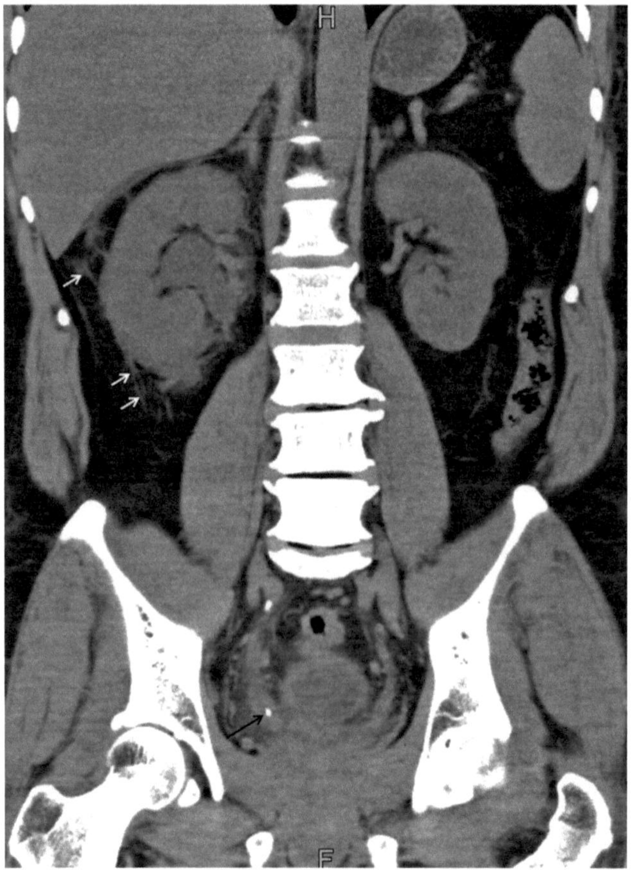

Fig. 33.5 Coronal CT image from a patient with right-sided renal colic. Not only is the calculus in the right distal ureter clearly visualized (*black arrow*), the secondary signs of perinephric fat stranding (*white arrows*) are also present. In the absence of direct visualization of the calculus (the calculus either having been passed or too small to resolve), these secondary sign are extremely useful and may be used to confirm the diagnosis of renal colic as the cause of a patient's symptoms

References

1. Portis AJ, Sunddaram CP. Diagnosis and initial management of kidney stones. Am Fam Physician. 2001;63(7):1329–38.
2. Levine JA, Neitch J, Verga M, Darymple N, Smith RC. Ureteral calculi in patients with flank pain: correlation of plain radiography with unenhanced helical CT. Radiology. 1997;204:27–31.
3. Mutgi A, Williams JW, Nettle M. Renal colic: utility of the plain abdominal roentgenogram. Arch Intern Med. 1991;151:1589–92.
4. Haddad MC, Sharif HS, Shahed MS, et al. Renal colic: diagnosis and outcome. Radiology. 1992;184:83–8.
5. Bailey SR, Tyrrell PNM, Hale M. A trial to assess the effectiveness of bowel preparation prior to intravenous urography. Clin Radiol. 1991;44(5):335–7.
6. Sandhu C, Anson KM, Patel U. Urinary tract stones – part I: role of radiological imaging in diagnosis and treatment planning. Clin Radiol. 2003;58:415–21.
7. Talati J, Khan S, Biyaban R, Khan RA, Naz I, Abbas F, et al. Reduction of radiation exposure to patients in the follow-up of shockwave lithotripsy. BJU Int. 2000;85:404–7.
8. Katzberg RW. Urography into the 21st century: New contrast media, renal handling imaging characteristics and nephotoxicity. Radiology. 1997;204:297–312.
9. Morcos SK. Prevention of contrast media nephrotoxicity – the story so far. Clin Radiol. 2004;59(5):381–9.
10. Caro JJ, Trindade E, McGregor M. The risks of death and of severe nonfatal reactions with high- vs low-osmolality contrast media: a metaanalysis. AJR Am J Roentgenol. 1991;156:825–32.
11. Namasivayam S, Kalra MK, Torres WE, Small WC. Adverse reactions to intravenous iodinated contrast media: a primer for radiologists. Emerg Radiol. 2006;12:210–5. doi:10.1007/s10140-006-0488-6.
12. Dalla Palma L, Pozzi-Mucelli R, Stacul F. Present day imaging of patients with renal colic. Eur Radiol. 2001;11:4–17.
13. Ahmed F, Abdul Zafar M, Khan N, Haider Z, Ather MH. A paradigm shift in imaging for renal colic – is it time to say good bye to an old trusted friend? Int J Surg. 2010;8(3):252–6.
14. Heidenreich A, Desgrandschamps F, Terrier F. Modern approach of diagnosis and management of acute flank pain: review of all imaging modalities. Eur Urol. 2002;41(4):351–62.
15. Smith R, Rosenfield AT, Choe KA, Essenmacher KR, Verga M, Glickman MG, et al. Acute flank pain: comparison of non-contrast-enhanced CT and intravenous urography. Radiology. 1995;194:789–94.

Radiation Exposure in Uroradiology

34

Maseeh uz Zaman

Abstract

Over the last two decades, there has been an increase in the use of radiation-based imaging during investigation and management of urolithiasis. This raises concerns regarding radiation exposure to patients, technologists, and physicians. The effective dose received by the individual determines the risk of stochastic effects of ionizing radiations. Dose-dependent or deterministic effects are fairly uncommon in medical imaging. The International Atomic Energy Agency (IAEA) has recommended that clinicians justify and optimize radiation-based procedures to minimize the radiation exposures. Various practical steps along with modification in imaging protocols have been advised in this regard. Radiation exposure to the conceptus (the embryo or fetus and all the tissues that surround it during pregnancy) in a pregnant or possibly pregnant female is a matter of great concern due to rare but possible detrimental effects. Risk for these detrimental effects of radiation upon conceptus and fetus can be calculated by a medical physicist based upon the age of conceptus at the time of said examination and a reasoned estimate of absorbed dose.

Keywords

Kidneys-ureters-bladder (KUB) • Computed tomography (CT) • CT KUB • Fluoroscopy Stochastic effect • Effective dose • Pregnancy • Preventive measures

Introduction

It has been more than a century since X-rays were used to detect renal stones. X-ray-based imaging modalities like conventional X-rays used for the kidneys-ureters-bladder (KUB) film and the intravenous urogram, computerized tomography (CT), and fluoroscopy are now an integral part of the management of various urological diseases, including urolithiasis. Today, the multislice CT is the most sensitive and specific imaging test for urolithiasis and is increasingly being used for the detection and follow-up of calculi. In addition, fluoroscopy is being increasingly used for various procedures like nephrostomy, insertion of stents, and stone removal. Because of the frequent use of radiological procedures, there has been a growing concern about the radiation exposure to patients (especially those in the pediatric age group), technologists, radiologists, and urologists [1].

The biological effects of ionizing radiations, like X-rays, may be deterministic or stochastic. Deterministic effects are dose-dependent, and after a threshold, the severity of effects (e.g., erythema and skin ulceration) increases with the amount of dose delivered. Stochastic effects are those that occur both as a result of predictable estimates as well as by chance or random occurrences. Stochastic effects of irradiation are not dose-dependent, but the probability of adverse effects (e.g., cancer and genetic effects) increases with the magnitude of the dose. For example, in diagnostic radiology, it is the stochastic effect that is considered when designing radiation protection measures, because the radiation dose in most fluoroscopy and diagnostic procedures is

M. uz Zaman, M.B.B.S., M.S., FCPS, FEBNM, DCBNC, FASNC
Nuclear Medicine Section, Department of Radiology,
The Aga Khan University Hospital,
Stadium Road, Karachi, Sindh 74800, Pakistan
e-mail: maseeh.uzzaman@aku.edu

J.J. Talati et al. (eds.), *Urolithiasis*,
DOI 10.1007/978-1-4471-4387-1_34, © Springer-Verlag London 2012

quite low. However, few reports of erythema and ulceration (deterministic effects) following fluoroscopy procedures have been published [2, 3].

Presently, there has been a steady rise in the number of diagnostic and interventional urological procedures (primarily CT and fluoroscopy) resulting in higher radiation doses to patients and staff over time. Therefore, there is a greater need for educating and training medical staff, students, and other health-care professionals in the principles of radiation protection. Recent guidelines of the International Commission on Radiological Protection (ICRP) recommend reduction of exposure risk by proper application of the fundamental principles of justification, optimization of protection, and conformation to recommended dose limits [4].

The Concept of Effective Dose

The effective dose (ED) is a measure of the delivered radiation dose that is related to the probability of stochastic effects from exposure to low doses of ionizing radiation [5]. The measurement of exposure, calculation of the dose of radiation absorbed by tissue exposed to indirect and direct ionizing radiation, and the effect of that exposure become necessary as we continue to increase our use of radiological investigations in urolithiasis management. For biological tissues, doses are reported in sieverts (in the SI system), 1 Sv (100 rem in the old system) being equivalent to 1 J/kg. In some countries, the radiation badges still measure dose in rem.

The ICRP recommends not to exceed an effective dose of 20 mSv/year on average over a defined period of 5 years, as the dose limit for radiation workers [6]. Similarly, the annual limit for equivalent dose to different organs is specified—for the lens of the eye it is 150 millisievert (mSv), to the skin it is 500 mSv, and for the extremities it is 500 mSv for the staff [6]. For patients undergoing radiation-based investigation or therapy, there is no recommended dose limit, but urologists and radiologists need to ascertain if the procedure is justifiable on the basis of medical benefits outweighing the radiation risk. Nevertheless, for both patients and staff, the radiation dose should be as low as reasonably achievable (ALARA) [7]. Fortunately, most medical staff are exposed to much less than this level of radiation exposure. Table 34.1 shows mean radiation dose (in millisievert) received by patients in different urological procedures.

Table 34.1 Typical radiation doses to patients in urological procedures [8]

Procedure	Mean effective dose (mSv) values
Abdominal radiography (AP)	0.7
Intravenous urogram (6 films)	2.5
Micturating cystourethrogram (MCUG)	1.2
Cystography	1.8
Lithotripsy	1.3
Nephrostomy	3.4
Percutaneous nephrolithotomy (PCNL)	4.5
Ureteric stenting	4.7
CT abdomen	10[a]
Renal angiogram	2–30

[a]The table mentions the mean effective dose, but the range for a noncontrast CT might more accurately be stated to range up to 20.1–66.3 mSv. The number of phases, anatomic coverage/phase, and scanning parameters all contributed to this variation in dose [9]

Risk of Radiation Effects

The prediction and calculation of future radiation-induced biological damage is difficult and controversial. If one uses the linear no-threshold model (LNT), one accepts the assumption that the risk is directly proportional to the dose at all dose levels and presumes that the summation of small exposures will have the same effect as one large exposure equivalent to the total of the smaller doses of irradiation received over time. The LNT therefore predicts higher exposure risk. Calculated alternatively, using the threshold model, one presumes that the effects of small doses are negligible. Other models predict an even lower risk by presuming that very small doses might be beneficial. There is continuing debate as to which is the correct model to use. Additionally, the risk of radiation effects at low dose is itself still debatable, as the majority of these estimates have been derived from the risks at high doses (calculated from the effects in the atom bomb survivors in Japan) by extrapolating that risk, linearly, to lower doses. This too might lead to an overestimation of the radiation risk.

Compounding the issue is the fact that the risk of late manifestations of stochastic radiation effects is greater in children than in adults due to their longer lifespan. In pediatric uroradiology, patient size is an important factor as radiation dose absorbed increases exponentially with the thickness of the body part being imaged. Thus, an obese child would absorb a higher dose than a thin child. In the year 2000, the National Radiological Protection Board (NRPB) of the United Kingdom (UK) published reference doses for pediatric patients of different body mass indices to make the calculation of radiation dose more accurate [10]. According to Almen and Mattson, a dose of 2.2 mSv during a micturating cystourethrogram (MCUG) procedure in a child would lead to a greater risk of cancer: 1 in 3,200 over a patient's lifetime [11]. However, the dose incurred in MCUG is extremely unlikely to give deterministic effects.

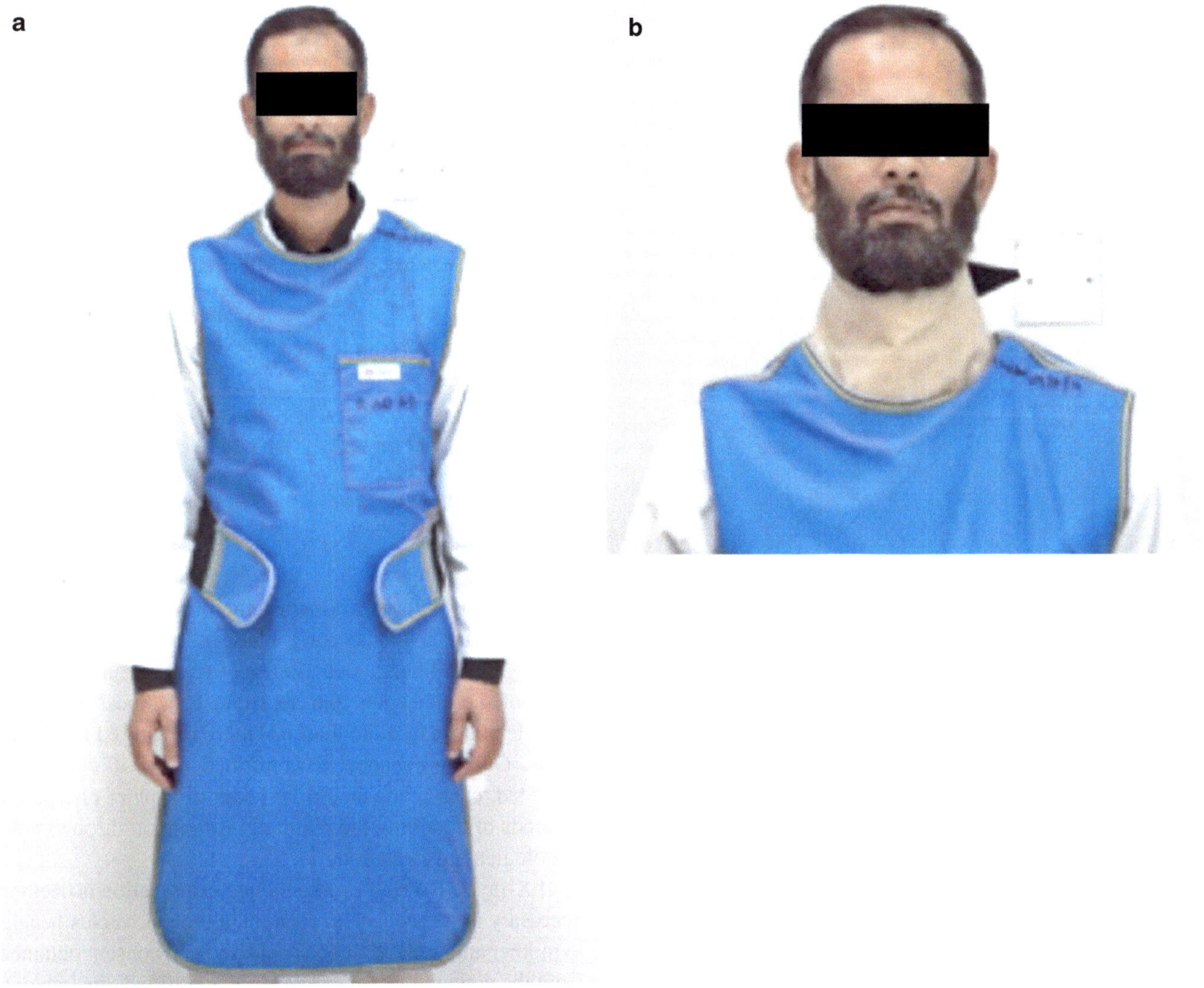

Fig. 34.1 Lead shielding (**a**) apron and (**b**) thyroid shield worn to minimize radiation exposure to operator

Risks from Fluoroscopy

Fluoroscopy is commonly used during urological interventions. It is imperative that urologists, interventional radiologists, urology residents, anesthesiologists, and operating room staff should be aware of the radiation doses they might receive. The practice of carrying personal dosimeters, such as thermoluminescent dosimeters (TLD), for dose measurement also reminds them of the importance of protection from unnecessary radiation and also dispels unfounded fears. Although collimation of the X-ray beam prevents direct radiation exposure to the urologist and assisting personnel, it is not often remembered that the patient, while absorbing radiation during the procedure, becomes a secondary source of exposure through radiation scatter [12]. The extremities and head of the operators receive higher doses, whereas the trunk, which is shielded by a lead apron (Figs. 34.1a, b and 34.2), receives much lower radiation doses [13]. As expected, the length of fluoroscopy exposure influences the effective dose received. With a mean fluoroscopic screening time of 2–6 min, the radiation dose to the fingers is significantly low (0.14–0.28 mSv) [14–16]. However, significantly high radiation dose to fingers occurs with a mean fluoroscopy time of 22 min [17].

Radionuclide Imaging Procedures

Nuclear medicine procedures are sensitive functional imaging tools that use administration of tracer quantity of technetium-99m labeled DTPA, MAG-3, and DMSA (diethylene triamine pentaacetic acid, mercapto acetyl triglycine, dimercapto succinic acid, respectively). These procedures provide reliable information about the perfusion, cortical

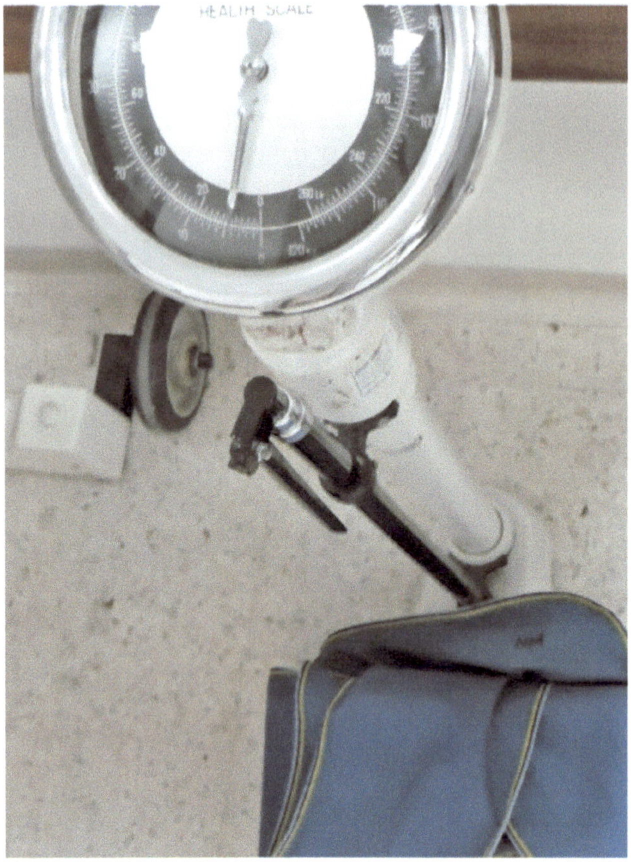

Fig. 34.2 The lead apron is heavy and can weigh as much as 4.5 kg

uptake, clearance, cortical scarring, and also differential renal function. The effective doses from a Tc-99m DTPA, Tc-99m MAG-3, and Tc-99m DMSA studies are 3.1 mSv [18], 5.6 mSv [19], and 1 mSv [20]. Parathyroid imaging with Tc-99m MIBI (methoxy isobutyl isonitrile) is a sensitive tool to localize a functioning parathyroid adenoma in native or ectopic site. An effective dose received by a patient from one examination is 0.33 mSv/mCi (1.8–6.7 mSv) [19]. Frequent voiding in 4–6 h after the procedure significantly reduces the effective dose, primarily by minimizing the dose to urinary bladder [21].

Pregnancy and Radiation Exposure in Uroradiology

Radiation exposure to a pregnant or potentially pregnant patient from medical imaging procedure is a matter of great concern due to possible detrimental effects of ionizing radiation to a developing embryo and fetus. Every woman in her reproductive age should be screened for the possibility of pregnancy, so as to minimize the number of unexpected exposures to pregnant patients. As per recommendation of the ICRP, radiation-based examination of the lower abdomen and pelvis in women of reproductive age should be confined to the 10-day interval following the onset of menstruation ("10-day rule"). In the early phase of pregnancy (before organogenesis starts), radiation may result in undetectable death of the conceptus and abortion. It has been observed that a fetal dose of more than 100 mGy is required for this to occur. Once pregnancy is confirmed or if it cannot be excluded, every care should be taken to explore alternative methods of obtaining the required information through non-radiological investigations.

If X-ray, CT scan, or radionuclide examination is deemed necessary in a pregnant women, then the risk versus benefit to mother and fetus must be considered and consent obtained from the patient. Once the procedure is justified, the imaging physician and technologist should follow the protocol to optimize the study and minimize radiation. The American College of Radiology has published detailed guidelines in this regard, which is beyond the scope of this chapter [22].

In spite of detailed screening for pregnancy in women in reproductive age, there is always a possibility that a patient may come to know that she is pregnant days or weeks after a radiation-based procedure has been conducted upon her. In the vast majority of cases, potential risks are very low and risk assessment can be calculated by a medical physicist based upon the age of conceptus at the time of the examination and a reasonable estimate of absorbed dose to the conceptus [22].

Table 34.2 Measures to reduce radiation dose to patients, operator, and staff [8]

Measures to reduce patient's dose	Measures to reduce operator's and staff dose
1. Control fluoroscopy time and use last-image-hold to review findings	1. 0° or 30° angulations (toward operator) of primary beam
2. Use proper collimation and reduce field size and field overlap	2. Keep hands out of beam
3. Use pulsed fluoroscopy and low frame rate	3. Protective well-fitted lead apron (0.35 mm lead aprons and thyroid shields for the operating surgeon/radiologist and 0.25 mm lead aprons for other operating room staff [23] (Fig. 34.1)
4. Maximize distance between X-ray tube and patient	4. Leaded glasses
5. Minimize distance between patient and image receptor	5. Use movable shields

Measures to Attain as Low as Reasonably Achievable Dose

All staff within the operating field should work together to achieve as low as reasonably achievable (ALARA) dose by adhering to good practices. Table 34.2 outlines the measures to ensure lower radiation exposure to patients, operator, and staff.

Conclusion

Radiation-based imaging modalities have been playing a pivotal role in the diagnosis and treatment of various urological diseases. However, over the last few years, concerns have been raised over the issues of radiation exposures especially in the pediatric population. A policy of justification and optimization for use of these radiation-based procedures could reduce the unjustified exposure to staff, physicians, and patients substantially.

References

1. King S, Pitcher EM, Smail MA. Optimizing medical radiation exposures for uroradiological procedures, with special emphasis on paediatric imaging. BJU Int. 2002;89:510–6.
2. US Food and Drug Administration. Avoidance of serious X-ray induced skin injuries to patients during fluoroscopically guided procedures. Med Bull. 1994;24:7–17.
3. Vano E, Arranz L, Sastre JM, Moro C, Ledo A, Garate MT, et al. Dosimetric and radiation protection considerations based on some cases of patient skin injuries in interventional cardiology. Br J Radiol. 1998;71(845):510–6.
4. International Commission on Radiological Protection. Recommendations of the International Commission on Radiological Protection: ICRP publication 105. Ann ICRP. 2007;37:6.
5. Martin CJ. Effective dose: how should it be applied to medical exposures? Br J Radiol. 2007;80:639–47.
6. International Commission on Radiological Protection [homepage on the Internet]. Summary recommendation [cited 2008 Feb 1]. http://www.icrp.org/docs/Summary_B-scan_ICRP_60_Ann_ICRP_1990_Recs.pdf. Accessed 8 Feb 2012.
7. Kumar P. Radiation safety issues in fluoroscopy during percutaneous nephrolithotomy. Urol J. 2008;5:15–23.
8. http://rpop.iaea.org/RPOP/RPoP/Content/InformationFor/HealthProfessionals/6_OtherClinicalSpecialities/Urology/index.htm#URFAQ08. Accessed 9 May 2011.
9. Vrtiska TJ, Hartman RP, Kofler JM, Bruesewitz MR, King BF, McCollough CH. Spatial resolution and radiation dose of a 64-MDCT scanner compared with published CT urography protocols. Am J Roentgenol. 2009;192(4):941–8. http://www.ajronline.org/content/192/4/941.full.
10. Hart D, Wall BF, Shrimpton PC, Bungay DR, Dance DR. Reference doses and patient size in pediatric radiology. NRPB report 318. National Radiological Protection Board; 2000.
11. Almen A, Mattson S. The radiation dose to children from X-ray examinations of the pelvis and the urinary tract. Br J Radiol. 1995;68:604–13.
12. Giblin JG, Rubenstein J, Taylor A, Pahira J. Radiation risk to urologist during endourologic and a new shield that reduces exposure. Urology. 1996;48(4):624–7.
13. Niklason LT, Marx VM, Chan H. Interventional radiologist: occupational radiation doses and risk. Radiology. 1993;187:729–33.
14. Bowsher WJ, Blott P, Whitfield HN. Radiation protection in percutaneous nephrolithotomy. Br J Urol. 1992;69:231–3.
15. Law J, Inglis JA, Tolley DA. Radiation dose to urological surgeons during X-ray fluoroscopy for percutaneous stone extraction. Br J Radiol. 1989;62:185–7.
16. Kumari G, Kumar P, Wadhwa P, Aron M, Gupta NP, Dogra PN. Radiation exposure to the patient and operating room personnel during percutaneous nephrolithotomy. Int Urol Nephrol. 2006;38:207–10.
17. Rao PN, Faulkner K, Sweeney JK, Asbury DL, Sambrook P, Blacklock NJ. Radiation dose to patient and staff during percutaneous nephrolithotomy. Br J Urol. 1987;59:508–12.
18. National Council on Radiation Protection and Measurements. Exposure of the US population from diagnostic medical radiation. NCRP Report 100. National Council on Radiation Protection and Measurements, Bethesda; 1989.
19. International Commission on Radiation Protection. Radiation dose to patients from radiopharmaceuticals: Addendum to ICRP 53. ICRP Publication 80. New York: Pergamon Press; 1999.
20. Vestergren E, Jacobsson L, Lind A. Administered activity of Tc-99m DMSA for kidney scintigraphy in children. Nucl Med Commun. 1998;19:695–701.
21. Stabin M, Taylor Jr A, Eshima D, Wooter W. Radiation dosimetry for technetium-99m-MAG3, technetium-99m-DTPA, and iodine-131-OIH based on human biodistribution studies. J Nucl Med. 1992;33:33–40.
22. http://www.acr.org/SecondaryMainMenuCategories/quality_safety/guideline/dx/pregnancy.aspx. Accessed 8 Feb 2012.
23. Links A. Medical and dental guidance notes. A good practice guide on all aspects of ionizing radiation protection in the clinical environment. J Radiol Prot. 2002;22:334.

The Use of Low-Dose CT Scanning

35

Sean A. Pierre

Abstract
Imaging modalities such as ultrasound do not have the sensitivity and specificity of computed tomography (CT) scan in the accurate assessment of urolithiasis. However, concerns regarding the exposure of patients to multiple investigatory CT scans, given the radiation exposure associated with such examinations, have led to definition of protocols that reduce radiation exposure while achieving similar diagnostic efficiency as standard CT scanning. With improved CT protocols using the information obtained during a CT scan, less radiation is required to provide adequate information on urinary stone disease.

Keywords
Calculi • Low-dose computed tomography (CT) • Ionizing radiation • Radiation exposure X-ray • Tissue • Urinary • Beam collimation width • Post-data acquisition protocols

Introduction

Given that there is a definite association between ionizing radiation and the incidence of various forms of cancer, the use of ionizing radiation-based testing in medical imaging in tests such as computed tomography (CT) has become a contentious issue. Non-contrast helical CT is currently the gold standard for the diagnosis and assessment of urolithiasis, and the use of this modality has significantly increased over the past 20 years [1]. Concerns have been raised regarding the exposure to the ionizing radiation associated with this test, especially because of the often chronic/recurrent nature of urolithiasis, and the need for repeat imaging. A study looking at radiation exposure over the course of an acute urinary calculus episode and for 1 year after the episode showed that 20 % of patients received more than the recommended yearly limit for radiation exposure during their management [2].

S.A. Pierre, M.D., FRCS (C) Urology
Department of Urology, Queen's University, Kingston, ON, Canada

Department of Surgery, Queensway Carleton Hospital, 3045 Baseline Road, Nepean, ON K2H 8P4, Canada
e-mail: spierre@hotmail.com

J.J. Talati et al. (eds.), *Urolithiasis*,
DOI 10.1007/978-1-4471-4387-1_35, © Springer-Verlag London 2012

Various strategies have been implemented to try to reduce the dose of ionizing radiation patients are exposed to during the evaluation, treatment, and follow-up of urolithiasis. Low-dose CT scanning represents one of these approaches.

Background

Radiation exposure is generally quantified using the standard international (SI) unit of gray (Gy), where 1 Gy is equal to 1 J of radiation absorbed per kilogram of tissue. Prior to this, the typical unit for radiation exposure was the rad (*r*adiation *a*bsorbed *d*ose); 1 Gy is equivalent to 100 rads. However, neither of these units takes into account the fact that different tissues have different responses to radiation, usually related to the type of radiation being administered (and, to a lesser extent, specific tissue characteristics). The unit used to better reflect the proportional estimate of tissue damage (often referred to as "biological harm"), essentially the "effective dose" or "dose equivalent," is the sievert (Sv). The conversion from gray to sievert involves multiplication of the former by a "weighting factor," which takes into account different tissue characteristics. Most radiation exposures involved in the medical field are in the range of millisieverts (mSv).

Radiation exposure is an accepted risk factor for the development of malignancy [3–8]. It has been challenging to correlate the amount of radiation exposure to the likelihood of developing a malignancy due to the lack of human-based data. The majority of the data used to determine this risk has been extrapolated from the outcomes of the survivors of the atomic bombings at Hiroshima and Nagasaki [9–13] and on studies of workers in the nuclear industry [14–18]. The general applicability of these data has been brought into question in more recent times, given that the populations examined were certainly exposed to much higher radiation doses over a longer period of time than most patients undergoing radiologic testing involving ionizing radiation. The International Commission on Radiation Protection currently recommends that radiation exposure not exceed 20 mSv/year over a 5-year period or 50 mSv in any single year [19–21].

The average exposure of an individual at sea level from background cosmic radiation is estimated to be 1–3 mSv/year (depending on location on the earth). A single airline flight rarely exceeds 1 mSv [8, 22], even in the presence of solar flares, which can increase radiation exposure.

The factors contributing to the ionizing radiation dose associated with a CT scan include the X-ray energy level (represented by the tube voltage and tube current), the beam collimation width (or "pitch" representing the size of each "slice" on the CT scan), and the volume of tissue being scanned (or "scan length"). These help limit the phenomena that influence the accuracy of CT in accurately assessing the presence and volume of urolithiasis present (volume artifact, beam hardening, motion artifact). Higher radiation doses allow for decreased "noise" in the *data* acquired during the test since they are more likely to penetrate material and be picked up by the detector, rather than be reflected. However, lower-energy photons allow for more discrimination between materials of differing densities (essentially different attenuation) and thus decrease the noise in the *image* acquired.

What Is It and Why Do It?

Given the increased utilization of medical imaging studies using ionizing radiation, multiple strategies have been developed to decrease patient exposure to ionizing radiation. In the management of the patient with urolithiasis, imaging modalities that do not use ionizing radiation (ultrasound, magnetic resonance imaging) simply do not have the sensitivity and specificity of CT, and as such are used mainly as adjuncts to try to minimize radiation exposure after the diagnosis has been definitively made.

Low-dose CT scan represents an attempt to achieve the same diagnostic efficiency as standard CT scanning using a lower dose of ionizing radiation to get the same image data [23]. This is usually done by decreasing the current of the CT scanner from the usual values of 120–160 to 70–120 mA and/or by decreasing the tube voltage from 120–140 to 80–100 kVp.

As previously mentioned, the beam collimation width or pitch can also be changed to decrease radiation exposure. Increasing the beam collimation width by 50 % results in a 33 % decrease in radiation exposure. Unfortunately, this significantly decreases the sensitivity of CT for urinary calculi, especially smaller calculi [24]. Typically, beam collimation widths from 1.5 to 5 mm are used to detect urinary calculi, but with each mm increase in beam collimation width, there is a decrease in the sensitivity and specificity of CT for urinary calculi.

The average radiation exposure of a patient who has had a standard dose CT of the abdomen and pelvis ranges from 10 to 20 mSv. Low-dose CT scan has been able to decrease that exposure to the range of 2.5–5 mSv [2]. This is actually in the range of exposures for a kidneys-ureters-bladder (KUB)/plain film of the abdomen and pelvis (0.1–2 mSv) with much greater accuracy in detection of urolithiasis.

For most stones greater than 3 mm in size, low-dose CT has similar diagnostic efficiency as standard CT [25–28]. In addition, secondary signs of urolithiasis (e.g., hydronephrosis, perinephric stranding) are just as readily detected with low-dose CT parameters as with standard CT parameters, which would help in situations where the calculus itself is not definitively identified (Figs. 35.1 and 35.2).

Disadvantages

Because of the increased noise with the use of low-dose CT scan, there have been concerns with respect to the accuracy of diagnosis of urolithiasis using a low-dose CT scan strategy, primarily because of the increased noise associated with this approach. Most studies suggest that most calculi greater than 3 mm in size will be detected with low-dose CT scan [23]; those that are not, with no evidence of hydronephrosis, are thought to be stones that would pass easily in any case and are less of a significant clinical issue. There has also been evidence to suggest that small ureteral calculi are more likely to be missed on low-dose CT as compared to standard CT (Figs. 35.3, 35.4, 35.5, and 35.6) [23].

Many of the studies done to compare standard-dose CT with low-dose CT have used computer-based models to "add" noise to standard-dose CT scans and then have had the tests read by qualified professionals [25, 29]. This has been accepted as a valid method for comparing the two modalities, although some still believe that the gold standard would be performing the two types of CT scan in the same patient at the same time; this, however, would increase the radiation exposure of the patient. Alternatively, cadaver studies have been done using both standard- and low-dose CT protocols on the same cadaver; these studies have also been used to support the validity of computer-based models to accurately compare standard CT to low-dose CT [30].

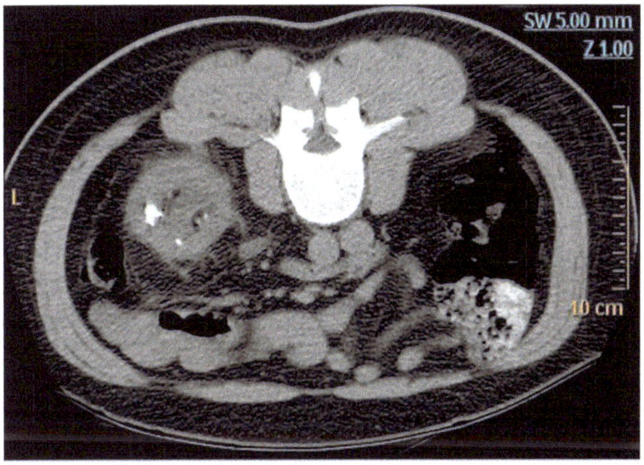

Fig. 35.1 Renal calculus, larger than 3 mm, standard radiation dose (Ferrandino M. et al., Duke University, Durham, North Carolina)

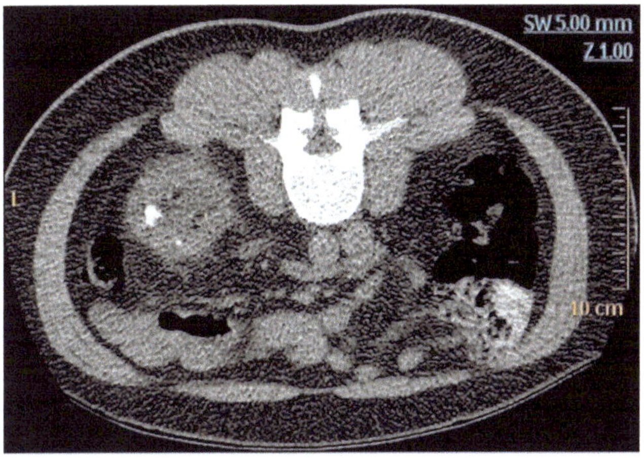

Fig. 35.2 Renal calculus, larger than 3 mm, 56 % radiation dose reduction (Ferrandino M. et al., Duke University, Durham, North Carolina)

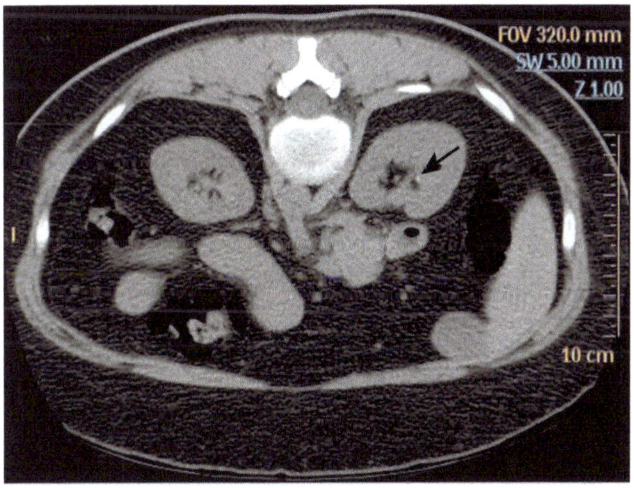

Fig. 35.3 Renal calculus, less than 3 mm, standard radiation dose (Ferrandino M. et al., Duke University, Durham, North Carolina)

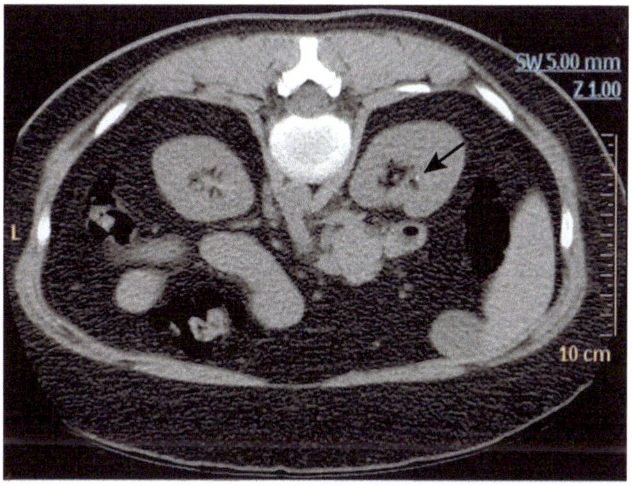

Fig. 35.4 Renal calculus, less than 3 mm, 19 % radiation dose reduction (Ferrandino M. et al., Duke University, Durham, North Carolina)

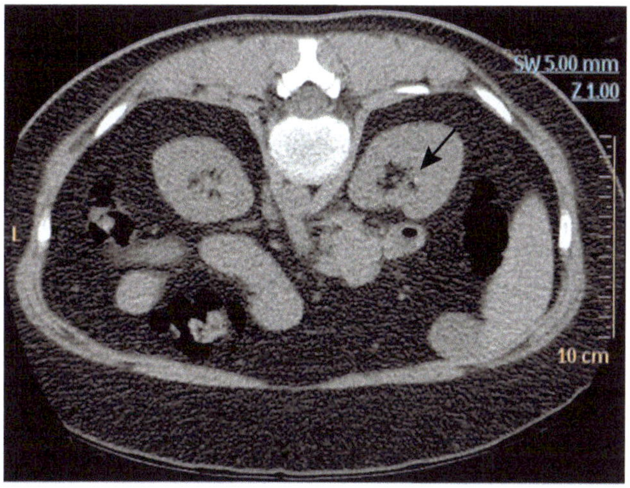

Fig. 35.5 Renal calculus, less than 3 mm, 38 % radiation dose reduction (Ferrandino M. et al., Duke University, Durham, North Carolina)

In morbidly obese patients, the fat attenuation of the X-ray radiation usually makes for images with a significant amount of "noise" artifact; indeed, the effect is much like that of a low-dose CT scan itself. Low-dose CT is therefore expected to have an even lower sensitivity for small urinary tract stones in the morbidly obese patient population [31, 32]. Optimizing the CT parameters to try to achieve reasonable quality images with as low radiation exposure as possible would help address this issue.

The decrease in image quality seen with the presence of metal in the abdomen and pelvis (e.g., hip replacements, lumbar vertebral rods) is exacerbated with low-dose CT, as the effect of the "noise" generated by the scattering of the X-ray radiation by the metal is much more difficult to correct for with low-dose CT.

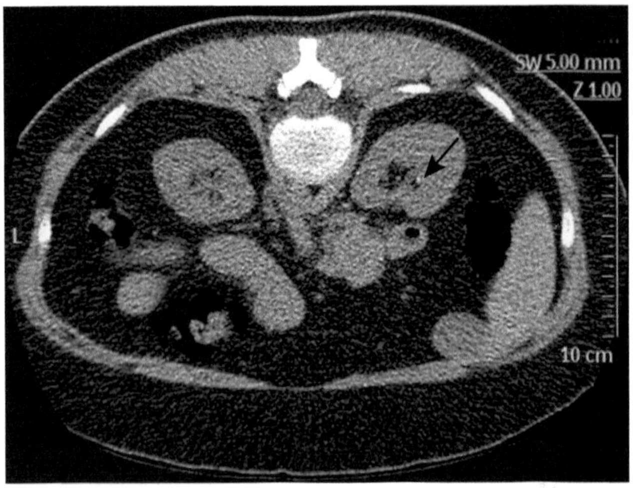

Fig. 35.6 Renal calculus, less than 3 mm, 56 % radiation dose reduction (Ferrandino M. et al., Duke University, Durham, North Carolina)

Conclusion

ALARA (as low as reasonably achievable) and Image Gently approaches to medical imaging represent the overall philosophy of the radiation community to try to decrease patient radiation exposure while not compromising patient management.

A number of different strategies are incorporated into this philosophy. Improved post-data acquisition protocols represent improvements in the computer interpretation of the information garnered during a CT scan so that less radiation is required to give similar quality images. Modifications to the imaging strategy itself, such as better demarcation of the regions of interest (decreased scan length), along with timing of scans to decrease the number of passes (the so-called "double-pump" strategy for multiphasic CT abdomen and pelvis for gross hematuria evaluation), can also decrease the radiation exposure associated with each CT scan. Nonionizing radiation alternatives (e.g., MR urography) are also being investigated for their ability to give information comparable to the CT-based alternatives.

The renewed respect for the amount of radiation patients are exposed to has driven a renewed focus on the use of CT-based technologies in patient care so as to ensure continued effectiveness of diagnosis and follow-up, without significantly increasing the risk of potential secondary malignancy.

References

1. Brenner DJ, Hall EJ. Computed tomography – an increasing source of radiation exposure. N Engl J Med. 2007;357(22):2277–84.
2. Ferrandino MN, Bagrodia A, Pierre SA, Scales Jr CD, Rampersaud E, Pearle MS, et al. Radiation exposure in the acute and short-term management of urolithiasis at 2 academic centers. J Urol. 2009; 181(2):668–72, discussion 73.
3. Brenner D, Elliston C, Hall E, Berdon W. Estimated risks of radiation-induced fatal cancer from pediatric CT. AJR Am J Roentgenol. 2001;176(2):289–96.
4. Brenner DJ, Doll R, Goodhead DT, Hall EJ, Land CE, Little JB, et al. Cancer risks attributable to low doses of ionizing radiation: assessing what we really know. Proc Natl Acad Sci USA. 2003; 100(24):13761–6.
5. Brenner DJ, Sachs RK. Estimating radiation-induced cancer risks at very low doses: rationale for using a linear no-threshold approach. Radiat Environ Biophys. 2006;44(4):253–6.
6. Eisenberg MJ, Afilalo J, Lawler PR, Abrahamowicz M, Richard H, Pilote L. Cancer risk related to low-dose ionizing radiation from cardiac imaging in patients after acute myocardial infarction. CMAJ. 2011;183(4):430–6.
7. Griffey RT, Sodickson A. Cumulative radiation exposure and cancer risk estimates in emergency department patients undergoing repeat or multiple CT. AJR Am J Roentgenol. 2009;192(4):887–92.
8. Morgan WF, Schwartz JL. Environmental Mutagen Society symposium on 'Risks of low dose, low dose rate exposures of ionizing radiation to humans'. Int J Radiat Biol. 2007;83(7):491–9.
9. Shimizu Y, Kato H, Schull WJ, Preston DL, Fujita S, Pierce DA. Studies of the mortality of A-bomb survivors. 9. Mortality, 1950–1985: part 1. Comparison of risk coefficients for site-specific cancer mortality based on the DS86 and T65DR shielded kerma and organ doses. Radiat Res. 1989;118(3):502–24.
10. Preston DL, Shimizu Y, Pierce DA, Suyama A, Mabuchi K. Studies of mortality of atomic bomb survivors. Report 13: solid cancer and noncancer disease mortality: 1950–1997. Radiat Res. 2003; 160(4):381–407.
11. Preston DL, Pierce DA, Shimizu Y, Cullings HM, Fujita S, Funamoto S, et al. Effect of recent changes in atomic bomb survivor dosimetry on cancer mortality risk estimates. Radiat Res. 2004; 162(4):377–89.
12. Shimizu Y, Pierce DA, Preston DL, Mabuchi K. Studies of the mortality of atomic bomb survivors. Report 12, part II. Noncancer mortality: 1950–1990. Radiat Res. 1999;152(4):374–89.
13. Pierce DA, Preston DL. Radiation-related cancer risks at low doses among atomic bomb survivors. Radiat Res. 2000;154(2):178–86.
14. Zablotska LB, Ashmore JP, Howe GR. Analysis of mortality among Canadian nuclear power industry workers after chronic low-dose exposure to ionizing radiation. Radiat Res. 2004;161(6): 633–41.
15. Colgan PA, Currivan L, Fenton D. An assessment of annual whole-body occupational radiation exposure in Ireland (1996–2005). Radiat Prot Dosimetry. 2008;128(1):12–20.
16. Howe GR, Zablotska LB, Fix JJ, Egel J, Buchanan J. Analysis of the mortality experience amongst U.S. nuclear power industry workers after chronic low-dose exposure to ionizing radiation. Radiat Res. 2004;162(5):517–26.
17. Wing S, Richardson DB. Age at exposure to ionising radiation and cancer mortality among Hanford workers: follow up through 1994. Occup Environ Med. 2005;62(7):465–72.
18. Cardis E, Vrijheid M, Blettner M, Gilbert E, Hakama M, Hill C, et al. The 15-country collaborative study of cancer risk among radiation workers in the nuclear industry: estimates of radiation-related cancer risks. Radiat Res. 2007;167(4):396–416.
19. Wrixon AD. New ICRP recommendations. J Radiol Prot. 2008; 28(2):161–8.
20. Wrixon AD. New recommendations from the International Commission on Radiological Protection – a review. Phys Med Biol. 2008;53(8):R41–60.
21. Wallo A, Domotor S, Vazquez G. U.S. Department of energy policies, directives, and guidance for radiological control and release of property. Health Phys. 2006;91(5):526–8.

22. Kojo K, Helminen M, Leuthold G, Aspholm R, Auvinen A. Estimating the cosmic radiation dose for a cabin crew with flight timetables. J Occup Environ Med. 2007;49(5):540–5.
23. Zilberman DE, Tsivian M, Lipkin ME, Ferrandino MN, Frush DP, Paulson EK, et al. Low dose computerized tomography for detection of urolithiasis – its effectiveness in the setting of the urology clinic. J Urol. 2011;185(3):910–4.
24. McCollough CH, Primak AN, Braun N, Kofler J, Yu L, Christner J. Strategies for reducing radiation dose in CT. Radiol Clin North Am. 2009;47(1):27–40.
25. Paulson EK, Weaver C, Ho LM, Martin L, Li J, Darsie J, et al. Conventional and reduced radiation dose of 16-MDCT for detection of nephrolithiasis and ureterolithiasis. AJR Am J Roentgenol. 2008;190(1):151–7.
26. Heneghan JP, McGuire KA, Leder RA, DeLong DM, Yoshizumi T, Nelson RC. Helical CT for nephrolithiasis and ureterolithiasis: comparison of conventional and reduced radiation-dose techniques. Radiology. 2003;229(2):575–80.
27. Poletti PA, Platon A, Rutschmann OT, Schmidlin FR, Iselin CE, Becker CD. Low-dose versus standard-dose CT protocol in patients with clinically suspected renal colic. AJR Am J Roentgenol. 2007;188(4):927–33.
28. Kim BS, Hwang IK, Choi YW, Namkung S, Kim HC, Hwang WC, et al. Low-dose and standard-dose unenhanced helical computed tomography for the assessment of acute renal colic: prospective comparative study. Acta Radiol. 2005;46(7):756–63.
29. Frush DP, Slack CC, Hollingsworth CL, Bisset GS, Donnelly LF, Hsieh J, et al. Computer-simulated radiation dose reduction for abdominal multidetector CT of pediatric patients. AJR Am J Roentgenol. 2002;179(5):1107–13.
30. Jellison FC, Smith JC, Heldt JP, Spengler NM, Nicolay LI, Ruckle HC, et al. Effect of low dose radiation computerized tomography protocols on distal ureteral calculus detection. J Urol. 2009; 182(6):2762–7.
31. Mulkens TH, Daineffe S, De Wijngaert R, Bellinck P, Leonard A, Smet G, et al. Urinary stone disease: comparison of standard-dose and low-dose with 4D MDCT tube current modulation. AJR Am J Roentgenol. 2007;188(2):553–62.
32. Tartari S, Rizzati R, Righi R, Deledda A, Terrani S, Benea G. Low-dose unenhanced CT protocols according to individual body size for evaluating suspected renal colic: cumulative radiation exposures. Radiol Med. 2010;115(1):105–14.

The Physics of Ultrasound and X-Rays: A Primer for Urologists

36

K. Razi Naqvi

Abstract
Imaging applications of ultrasound and X-rays and the principles underlying tomography and X-ray crystallography are explained within a common framework, using the vocabulary of waves and rays, without assuming prior knowledge of these concepts on the part of the reader.

Keywords
Radiography • Tomography • Tomosynthesis • Ultrasonography • Contrast enhancement • Tissue harmonic imaging

Introduction

A discussion of sound and light is a natural starting point for describing diagnostic applications of ultrasound and X-rays. The sensation of sound or light is produced when some energy is transported from a source of sound or light to the sensing element (the ear or the eye or some other detector). Both sound and light are transported by means of wave motion. Sound waves can propagate only through oscillations of the particles of a medium. When the medium is a liquid or soft tissue, these oscillations occur along the direction of propagation, and the wave is said to be longitudinal. Light waves are called electromagnetic waves because they consist of oscillations of two fields (electric and magnetic) that are perpendicular (or transverse) to each other and to the direction of propagation.

K.R. Naqvi, Ph.D.
Department of Physics,
Norwegian University of Science and Technology,
Hoegskoleringen 5, Trondheim NO-7491, Norway
e-mail: razi.naqvi@ntnu.no

Terminology

If we consider a bead that is going round a circular wire loop at a constant speed and hold the loop such that our eyes are in the plane of the loop, the bead would appear to move simply back and forth along a straight line with a nonuniform speed. An illustration of this may be found in the four Galilean moons of Jupiter, which are large enough to be seen through an inexpensive telescope. These moons move uniformly around Jupiter in near-circular coplanar orbits, but since we see these orbits edgewise, we get the impression that the moons simply go back and forth across the face of the planet to one end of the apparent route and back behind the planet to the other end of the route. "Back and forth" movement of this type is called *simple harmonic motion*. In other words, simple harmonic motion is uniform circular motion seen edgewise; mathematically, one would describe it as the projection of uniform circular motion on the diameter of the circle. If one could view the Galilean moons along a direction perpendicular to the plane of the orbits, no moon would ever be out of sight, and the orbits would look circular.

J.J. Talati et al. (eds.), *Urolithiasis*,
DOI 10.1007/978-1-4471-4387-1_36, © Springer-Verlag London 2012

The time taken by the bead to describe one rotation is also the *period* of the simple harmonic motion. If we denote this time by P and its reciprocal by ν, the angular velocity comes out to be

$$\omega = 2\pi/P = 2\pi\nu.$$

Simple harmonic oscillation leads to the concept of sinusoidal waves and provides the basic terminology of wave motion. If ξ denotes a physical quantity of interest (e.g., the density of the medium), a sinusoidal wave of amplitude ξ_0 traveling along the positive χ direction can be described by the equation

$$\xi = \xi_0 \sin 2\pi(kx - \omega t + \phi) = \xi_0 \sin\left[2\pi\left(\frac{x}{\lambda} - \frac{t}{P} + \frac{\phi}{2\pi}\right)\right].$$

where λ is the "space period," or the wavelength, and ϕ is the phase. For a single wave, the phase may be chosen arbitrarily, but the phase difference between two waves will remain invariant to this choice. The velocity of propagation υ is related to λ and ν as follows:

$$v = \nu\lambda.$$

Non-sinusoidal waves can be described as superpositions of sinusoidal waves of different frequencies and amplitudes.

Change in Frequency

A change in the frequency of a wave can provide useful information. We will consider two mechanisms for such changes.

A medium is said to interact linearly with an incident sinusoidal wave of frequency ν when the emerging wave is a sinusoid of the same frequency (but not necessarily the same amplitude or phase). When the interaction is nonlinear, the emerging wave is a superposition of sinusoidal waves of the fundamental frequency ν and its higher harmonics (2ν, 3ν,...). The efficiency of generating a wave of frequency $n\nu$ is proportional to the nth power of the intensity of the beam; this means that the third and higher harmonics may be ignored for our applications and that the second harmonic will be narrower than the fundamental since the intensity of the latter is highest in the central portion.

Even if the frequency of the waves emitted by a source is held constant, the frequency measured by a detector will be higher (or lower) if the source is moving toward (or away from) the detector; the phenomenon is known as the Doppler effect, and the change in frequency is called Doppler shift [1].

Rays and Waves: Specular and Diffuse Reflection

It is more convenient, when one is dealing with a beam of light or sound whose wavelength is very much smaller than the dimensions of obstacles in the path of the beam, to describe the laws governing the behavior of waves in terms of rays, using geometrical terminology (geometrical optics/acoustics). Reflection and refraction, which come under this category, take place when a ray encounters an interface (boundary) between two different media; for our purpose, the refractive index of a medium may be taken as its principal propagation property. In speaking of reflection, it is important to distinguish between *specular* reflection from a perfectly smooth surface and *diffuse* reflection from a granular or rough surface. In the former case, all rays of a parallel beam incident on the surface obey the familiar laws of reflection from a surface and therefore reflect as a parallel beam; in the latter case, though the laws of reflection are obeyed locally, the granularity of the surface will send reflected rays in various directions, resulting in a diffuse scattering of the originally parallel rays of light or sound. We will consider diffuse reflection and scattering as the limit of reflection from randomly oriented surface elements [2].

A surface is said to be acoustically/optically plane if the protrusions and depressions that determine its unevenness are much smaller than the wavelength of sound/light. Since the irregularities in a common ground glass plate are larger than the wavelength of light, one normally sees a diffuse reflection. However, at grazing incidence, the effective size of the ridges and valleys becomes smaller than the wavelength of light, and a specular reflection may be seen even from frosted glass [3].

If one is trying to focus energy that is propagated by a wave train, the smallest diameter into which the energy can be concentrated is of the order of a wavelength. If one is using a wave train to delineate an object, the best resolution that can be achieved is of the order of a wavelength.

The normal range of human hearing is between 20 Hz and 20 kHz, and sounds with frequencies above about 20 kHz are called ultrasound. The speed of sound in tissue is similar to that in water, namely, 1.5 km/s, so that at a frequency of 1.5 MHz, which is the order of frequency normally used, the wavelength in tissue is about 1 mm. Ultrasound is generated by converting electrical oscillations into the mechanical vibrations of a piezoelectric crystal, and it is detected by the converse process (the generation of an electrical signal by a piezoelectric material when it is subjected to a pressure fluctuation). Ultrasound is a nonionizing radiation and is considered safe at the low power levels that are used in medical applications.

Electromagnetic waves whose wavelengths lie in the 400–700 nm range are visible to a normal eye. X-rays have wavelengths in the 0.01–10 nm range; those used for diagnostic purposes, with wavelengths in the 0.01–0.1 nm range, are called hard X-rays because of their large penetrating power. X-rays are generated inside an evacuated tube where electrons, emitted by an incandescent cathode, are accelerated toward a metallic anode held at a high potential with respect to the cathode. When the energetic electrons hit the target, X-rays are generated by two different processes, producing discrete lines and a continuum. X-ray lines are produced when the incident electrons ionize one of the two innermost *K*-shell electrons in the atoms of the anode. The vacancy thus created in each *K*-shell is filled by a transition of an electron from a higher shell, accompanied by the release of the energy difference between the two shells in the form of an X-ray line. Hard X-rays, which originate from transitions whose terminal state is the first quantum state, are called the *K*-series, whose lines are designated in decreasing order of their wavelength, as K_α, K_β, and K_γ. When the K_α is emitted, a vacancy is created in the *L*-shell, which in turn is filled by the transition of an electron from the *M*-shell, accompanied by the emission of a soft X-ray line. Continuous X-rays are emitted when the incident electrons are scattered by the strong electric field of the nuclei of the anode atoms.

X-rays are an ionizing form of radiation, and radiologists must take appropriate measures to protect themselves and the patients from unnecessary exposures. The ionizing ability of X-rays is used for their detection. Röntgen was able to detect X-rays because he noticed a glow on a nearby fluorescent screen, and a few days later, he used a photographic film for producing a radiograph of his wife's hand. These methods and their modern digital adaptations are still widely used in radiological examinations [4]; no loss of generality will be incurred by assuming in the following discussion that a photographic film is used as the image forming medium.

Law of Exponential Attenuation

Let a collimated beam of ultrasound or X-rays (of a certain frequency) be incident on a homogeneous slab of thickness *s*, and let I_0 and I denote the intensity of the incident and emergent beams, respectively. The law of attenuation of intensity, which is derivable from purely geometrical considerations, can be expressed as follows:

$$I = I_0 e^{-\mu s} = I_0 e^{-s/l}.$$

where μ (the attenuation coefficient) and $l = 1/\mu$ (the attenuation length) depend on the substance considered and on λ, the incident wavelength. The quantity l is the mean distance a ray will travel before it suffers absorption or scattering; the quantity $A = \mu s$ will be called attenuance. The transmittance $T = I/I_0$ represents the probability that a ray will emerge from the slab along its original path, and $U = 1 - T$ is the probability that a ray will be absorbed or scattered within the slab; if the attenuance A is large compared to unity (as would be the case for the passage of hard X-rays through a kidney stone), T will be close to zero, and if A is small compared to unity, U will be close to A (since $e^X = 1 + X + X^2/2 + \ldots$). If the slab happens to be inhomogeneous, which is true for our problems, the aforementioned considerations will still hold, but μ will now represent an average over the different materials in the path of the beam.

For ultrasound, μ is approximately proportional to ν (*nu*); this is why higher frequencies (shorter wavelengths), which would lead to better spatial resolution, cannot be used for imaging purposes. For X-rays, μ is approximately proportional to $\lambda^3 Z^4$, where Z is the atomic number of the attenuating material; this implies that an organ with a high-Z material will have a large attenuance, but the attenuance of tissue (a low-Z substance) will be small.

Radiography

The standard arrangement for producing a radiograph is depicted in Fig. 36.1. A divergent beam of X-rays emerging from a suitably sized aperture is made to pass through *S*, the specimen to be examined. At first, we will ignore scattering and assume that an X-ray is either absorbed or transmitted along its original path and that *S* contains three bodies, one of which, labeled *a*, is opaque (or a perfect absorber) and the other two, labeled *b* and *c*, are imperfect absorbers. Those areas of the film that receive no X-rays will turn out, after chemical development, to be white, whereas those which do receive some radiation will appear as gray or black depending on the dose delivered to particular regions of the film. The shadow of object *a* will be white, sharp, and of nearly equal size; object *b*, which is partly transmitting and farther away from the film, will cast a gray shadow, with indistinct outlines and larger than actual size. In order to view obstacle *c*, which cannot be detected with this arrangement (because its shadow is blocked by obstacle *a*), the line of sight must be changed. A radiograph is a representation of the mean attenuation offered by all the material through which X-rays have passed; furthermore, it is a projection on a flat surface of everything in every plane between the anode and the film. One view is an isolated observation and prone to misinterpretation.

We must now take account of scattering, which presents an extremely severe problem in radiography. When scattering is present, some X-rays (represented by ray 2 in Fig. 36.1) will be deviated from their original paths and strike the film in regions that would be inaccessible in the absence of scattering. Consequently, the areas that would be darker (lighter) in the absence of scattering will become less dark (and less

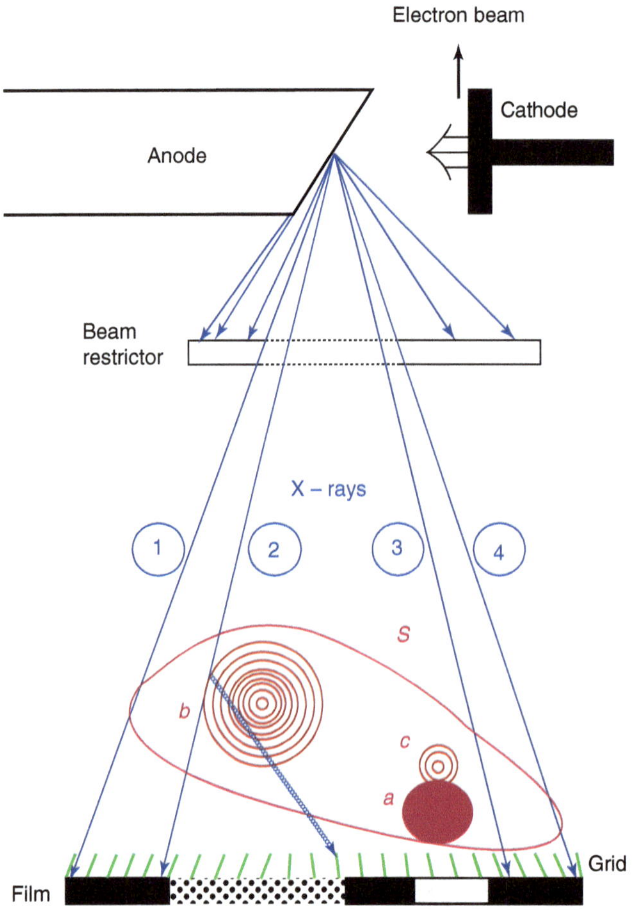

Fig. 36.1 Schematic representation of the arrangement used for producing a radiograph. A divergent beam of X-rays is made to pass through *S* (the specimen under examination), and the transmitted beam is intercepted by an X-ray-sensitive detecting surface (shown here as a photographic film). The purpose of the grid is explained in the text. Of the four rays shown have, only ray 2 suffers some scattering

bright, respectively) on account of scattering. Recording a radiograph in the presence of scattering is analogous to photographing an object that is placed behind a frosted glass wall or in an extremely dense fog. It is possible to mitigate against scattering by using an arrangement that prevents scattered rays from reaching the film. This can be achieved by interposing a grid of judiciously aligned thin strips of lead (or some other strongly absorbing metal), which preferentially absorb the X-rays that are deflected from their original paths. The shadow cast by the grid itself can be eliminated by a rapid movement of the grid during the exposure [5], or by using appropriate software, if one is using digital imaging [6].

Tomography

The prefix *tomo* is derived from the Greek word for slice. The technique of focal plane (or conventional) tomography makes use of the fact that if a radiograph is formed by superposing different views, each of which is taken by moving the X-ray source and the film according to a definite scheme, only a desired layer will be kept in sharp focus, and other layers will be blurred out. The photographic analogue of this strategy is the use of a large aperture for obtaining a narrow depth of field, an arrangement in which the region of interest is kept in sharp focus, whereas other regions are out of focus and fuzzy. The main shortcomings of conventional tomography can be overcome by using digital tomosynthesis, where digital images are superposed and refined through software [7].

In conventional tomography the beam of X-rays passes through a large volume (containing the slice to be examined), and the information from the unwanted region of the irradiated volume can at best be blurred out. It is preferable to use a narrow X-ray beam and view a thin slice at different angles; by restricting the measurements to the paths contained only in the slice of interest, one does not collect information pertaining to other parts of the body. The patient is positioned within a gantry that houses an X-ray source and several detectors, and each measurement gives an average attenuation coefficient for the path traversed by the beam. Several measurements are made after appropriate translations and rotations of the source and detectors. If a sufficient number of views or projections are taken, the distribution of attenuation coefficients within each layer may be determined. The patient is moved and another slice is viewed. The reconstruction of the image of a slice from its projections is, of course, a process of considerable mathematical complexity, now routinely performed by a computer; hence the name computed tomography (CT), but it is worth bearing in mind that the use of a computer is neither necessary (in principle) nor unique to this method. Generally, the slices are either overlapping or contiguous, though some protocols call for gaps between the slices.

In contrast to the sequential data acquisition in conventional CT (CCT), a relatively slow technique, helical CT (HCT) scanners have a gantry that rotates continuously in the same direction. During scanning, data acquisition is combined with continuous movement of the patient through the gantry. The path of the X-rays through the body can be described as a spiral or helix, which accounts for the name of the technique. HCT enables both an improved efficiency of existing CT applications and the development of new applications such as CT angiography and virtual endoscopy. Consequently, HCT is going to replace CCT in all body regions and has become the preferred method for examining urinary organs [8].

The outstanding performance of CT (sequential as well as helical) should not be allowed to obscure the fact that patients examined by this technique are subjected to higher doses of radiation than those used in conventional radiography [9].

Ultrasonography

Ultrasonography relies on sending an intense ultrasonic pulse (hereafter the primary pulse) and detecting the faint echo reflected from the object under investigation; the biosonar of an echolocating bat utilizes the same principle [10], but its performance cannot yet be rivaled by the equipment available to medical workers. A probe held against the skin is used both for transmitting the outgoing pulse and for receiving the reflected pulse.

The primary pulse suffers attenuation as it travels through the body; in addition, it undergoes a partial reflection whenever it encounters an interface, and the reflections give rise to the first and subsequent echoes. Each echo is also attenuated as it makes its way to the transducer, where its strength and the round-trip time (or delay) are recorded. The average speed of sound through tissue is used for converting the delays into distances between the source and the reflecting interfaces (and thereby into depths, or the locations of the interfaces within the body). It has become customary to display each echo (above a certain threshold) as a spot on a linear axis (showing depth), the brightness of the spot being proportional to the intensity of the echo; this mode of display is called B-mode display.

A standard ultrasonic pulse-echo image is produced by sweeping a single transducer (or an array of a few transducers) across the patient's body or by using an annular array of transducers and displaying all the echoes on a screen. The maximum possible scanning speed of acoustic imaging systems is limited by the speed of sound in tissue, the maximum depth of tissues of interest, and the detail required for the image, which determines the number of lines/scan.

Ultrasound images are often acquired between ribs or through layers of surface fat, which produce undesired distortions and echoes. Tissue harmonic imaging (THI), which focuses on detecting echoes of the second harmonic wave, reduces this problem because the second harmonic beam is created not close to the body surface but at a depth of a few centimeters, where the primary beam is more focused [11]. A better spatial resolution is an additional advantage of using a higher frequency for imaging.

The diagnostic potential of ultrasonic scans can be enhanced by combining measurements of Doppler shifts of the echoes, which allows one to monitor, for example, blood flow while one is imaging the vessels through which the blood is flowing [1].

Contrast Enhancing Methods

Two physical characteristics of an image determine its diagnostic value: contrast and definition. In photography, the corresponding terms are "exposure" and "focus." A radiograph records T, the probability that a pencil of rays would leave the body without deviating from its original path, and objects will be visible only if they differ in attenuance from their surroundings. A radiograph can easily distinguish between bone (since calcium is a high-Z element) and soft tissue (which is composed of low-Z elements). The average atomic number of hollow structures can be increased by filling the cavity with a high-Z liquid; this is the physical basis of using iodinated contrast media.

Since the acoustic attenuation coefficient does not depend on tissue density, an ultrasonograph differs from a radiograph or a CT scan. Highly dense tissues, such as bone or kidney stones, readily reflect echoes and, therefore, appear bright white on an ultrasound image, just as in a radiograph; however, since air (such as in the bowel) is also a good reflector, the edge of the bowel appears white on an ultrasound image. A chance discovery in the late 1960s (that air microbubbles enhanced the ultrasound signal) provided the incentive for the development of contrast-enhanced ultrasound imaging [12, 13].

The contrast in a conventional radiograph arises from differences in the value of A in adjoining regions. Since localized areas of disease almost always appear in soft tissues, which have all similar low values of μ, the contrast is poor because the radiographer has to deal with differences in small quantities. This difficulty can be overcome by using a method where differences in the speed of X-rays (or the refractive index of the tissue) create the contrast. When X-rays pass through a weakly attenuating object, the emergent and the incident rays differ not only in amplitude but also in phase. The fact that the difference between the phase shifts introduced by two media is significantly larger than the difference in their values of μ has been used for developing a phase-based alternative to the conventional attenuation-based radiography: The technique is called X-ray phase-contrast imaging or refractive index radiology; the method has been evaluated for the imaging of renal cell carcinoma and prostate cancer [14].

X-Ray Diffraction by Crystals

Scattering of X-rays by a crystalline sample could be represented as a "reflection" by successive planes of atoms in the crystal. Figure 36.2 depicts a set of parallel planes (separated by a distance d) in the crystal structure and a beam of X-rays (of wavelength λ) incident at an angle θ. Some of the rays will be "reflected" from the upper layer of atoms, the angle of reflection being equal to the angle of incidence. Some of the rays will be absorbed; some others will be "reflected" from the second layer and so on with successive layers. All the waves "reflected" by a single crystal plane will be in phase, but those "reflected" from different planes will in

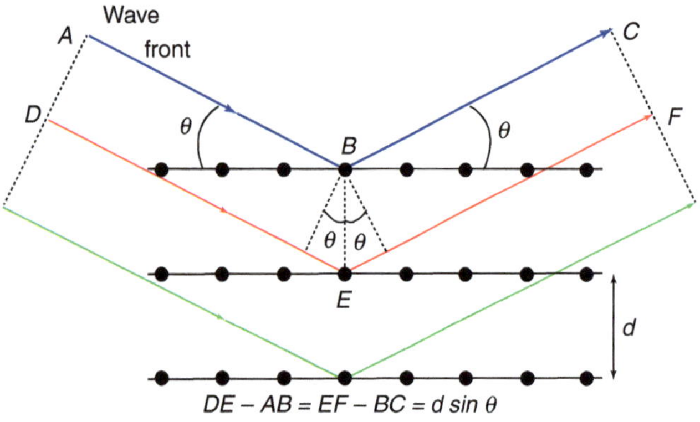

Fig. 36.2 Reflection of X-rays from atomic planes in a crystal

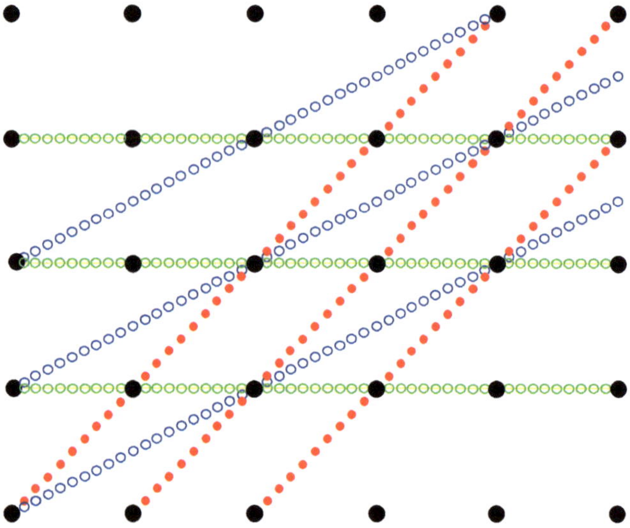

Fig. 36.3 Three possible families of atomic planes in a crystal

general have different phases. Only under certain strict conditions will all the "reflected" waves be in phase and will therefore reinforce one another, leading to sharp interference maxima. The condition is that the path difference Δ between the waves "reflected" from successive planes must be an integral number of wavelengths, $n\lambda$; it can be easily verified that

$$\Delta = 2d\sin\theta.$$

Given λ and the value of θ for which the relation $2d\sin\theta = n\lambda$

(Bragg condition) is satisfied, one can calculate d. For a particular crystal structure, one can have many families of atomic planes with different values of d (Fig. 36.3). By varying θ and detecting maxima arising from other families, one can derive structural information about the scattering crystal.

The X-ray data for the most common components of human kidney stones are known [15]; the data for the specimen under test are matched against the standard lines, and lines that cannot be matched represent other crystalline components in the sample.

X-ray diffraction analysis uses the known wavelength of the incident X-ray to deduce the value of d for a given value of θ. Conversely, if d and θ are known, the wavelength of the incident X-ray can be determined. By allowing non-monochromatic X-rays to fall on a known crystal, the arrangement shown in Fig. 36.2 can be used for analyzing the spectral distribution of the source and for isolating X-rays of the desired wavelength; some arrangements for phase-contrast X-ray imaging make use of this principle [16].

Conclusion

The technical capabilities of imaging systems based on X-rays and ultrasound have gone through a revolution in the last few decades, but the basic principles that determine the formation of a good image have not changed. The foundations of medical imaging and X-ray crystallography have been reviewed with an eye toward urological applications and without delving into mathematical details. More relevant information may be found in the references, which have been selected primarily for their pedagogical value.

References

1. Boote EJ, Doppler US techniques: concepts of blood flow detection and flow dynamics. RadioGraphics. 2003;23:1315–27.
2. Naqvi KR, Merzlyak MN, Melø TB. Absorption and scattering of light by suspensions of cells and subcellular particles: an analysis in terms of Kramers-Kronig relations. Photochem Photobiol Sci. 2004;3:132–7.
3. Fakhruddin H. Specular reflection from a rough surface. The Physics Teacher. 2003;41:206–7.
4. Tubiana M. From Bertha Roentgen's hand to current medical imaging: one century of radiological progress. Eur Radiol. 1997;7:1507–13.
5. Barnes GT. Contrast and scatter in x-ray imaging. RadioGraphics. 1991;11:307 23.
6. Foos DH, Yorkston J, Wang X. Grid suppression in imaging. US application 20110033101, 2011.
7. Sone S, Kasuga T, Sakai F, Aoki J, Izuno I, Tanizaki Y, et al. Development of a high-resolution digital tomosynthesis system and its clinical application. RadioGraphics. 1991;11:807–22.
8. Schreyer HH, Uggowitzer MM, Ruppert-Kohlmayr A. Helical CT of the urinary organs. Eur Radiol. 2002;12:575–91.
9. Mettler FA, Huda W, Yoshizumi TT, Mahesh M. Effective doses in radiology and diagnostic nuclear medicine: a catalog. Radiology. 2008;248:254–63.
10. Suga N. Biosonar and neural computation in bats. Sci Am. 1990;262(6):34–41.

11. Powers J, Kremkau F. Medical ultrasound systems. Interface Focus. 2011;1:477–89.
12. Goldberg BG, Liu J-B, Forsberg F. Ultrasound contrast agents: a review. Ultrasound Med Biol. 1994;20:319–33.
13. Tang M-X, Mulvana H, Gauthier T, Lim AKP, Cosgrove DO, Eckersley RJ, et al. Quantitative contrast-enhanced ultrasound imaging: a review of sources of variability. Interface Focus. 2011;1: 529–39.
14. Yoon CY, Sung DJ, Lee JH, Kim AR, Oh CW, Je JH, et al. Imaging of renal and prostate carcinoma with refractive index radiology. Int J Urol. 2007;14:96–103.
15. Mandel I, Mandel N. Structure and compositional analysis of kidney stones. In: Stoller ML, Meng MV, editors. Urinary stone disease: a practical guide to medical and surgical management, chap. 5. Totowa, NJ: Humana; 2007. p. 69–81.
16. Zhou S-A, Brahme A. Development of phase-contrast X-ray imaging techniques and potential medical applications. Phys Medica. 2008;24:129–48.

Part IV

Technology and Innovation

The Stone Surgeon/Lithotomists' Armamentarium: Today and Tomorrow

37

Carl Sarkissian and Manoj Monga

Abstract

Advancements over the past three decades in endourological instrumentation have transformed the stone surgeon's armamentarium. This chapter reviews the most significant recent advancements and commonly used tools for conducting ureteroscopy and percutaneous nephrolithotomy. Based on in vitro and clinical studies, we provide a comparative assessment of numerous devices, including properties and critical design characteristics that support improved functionality and outcomes. Additionally, we focus on changing trends and clinical challenges associated with medical devices used for treating stone disease.

Keywords

Operating room organization • Guidewire • Access sheath • Ureteral balloon dilator Ureteral occluding device • Stone retrieval devices/baskets • Flexible ureteroscope • Intracorporeal lithotrite • Endoirrigation systems • Instrumentation

Introduction

The field of endourology is characterized by continuous technological innovation that has revolutionized methods of treatment and diagnosis in numerous medical fields. The trend toward less invasive treatments with the use of semi-rigid and flexible ureteropyeloscopy has dramatically improved patient outcomes and hospitalization costs and constantly challenges endourologists to be familiar with an increasingly large armamentarium for implementing the leading treatment methodologies.

C. Sarkissian, B.S. Eng
Department of Urology, The Cleveland Clinic,
9500 Euclid Avenue, Mailcode Q9-1, Cleveland, OH 44195, USA
e-mail: sarkisc@ccf.org

M. Monga, M.D. (✉)
Department of Urology, Steven Streem Center
for Endourology and Stone Disease, The Cleveland Clinic,
9500 Euclid Avenue, Mailcode Q10-1, Cleveland, OH 44195, USA
e-mail: mongam@ccf.org

Operating Room Setup and Patient Preparation

Strategic design and layout of the operating room is essential for ensuring safe and efficient utilization of equipment. Often mounted on articulating ceiling-supported arms, the light source, lithotrite generator, and video and C-arm monitors are positioned on one side of the patient to simplify viewing for the surgeon and to provide room for movement of the C-arm on the opposite side (Fig. 37.1). C-arm image intensifiers should include software with last image hold memory, image processing, text/graphics, and additional functions to quickly view images on demand [1].

Once anesthetized, the patient is placed in the lithotomy position, with a slight extension of the leg on the intended treatment side for preventing acute compartment syndrome [2]. Typically, we utilize pneumatic compression boots to promote circulation and reduce the risk of deep vein thrombosis [3]. If potential for a percutaneous approach is uncertain, a prone split-leg position may simplify additional necessary procedures.

J.J. Talati et al. (eds.), *Urolithiasis*,
DOI 10.1007/978-1-4471-4387-1_37,

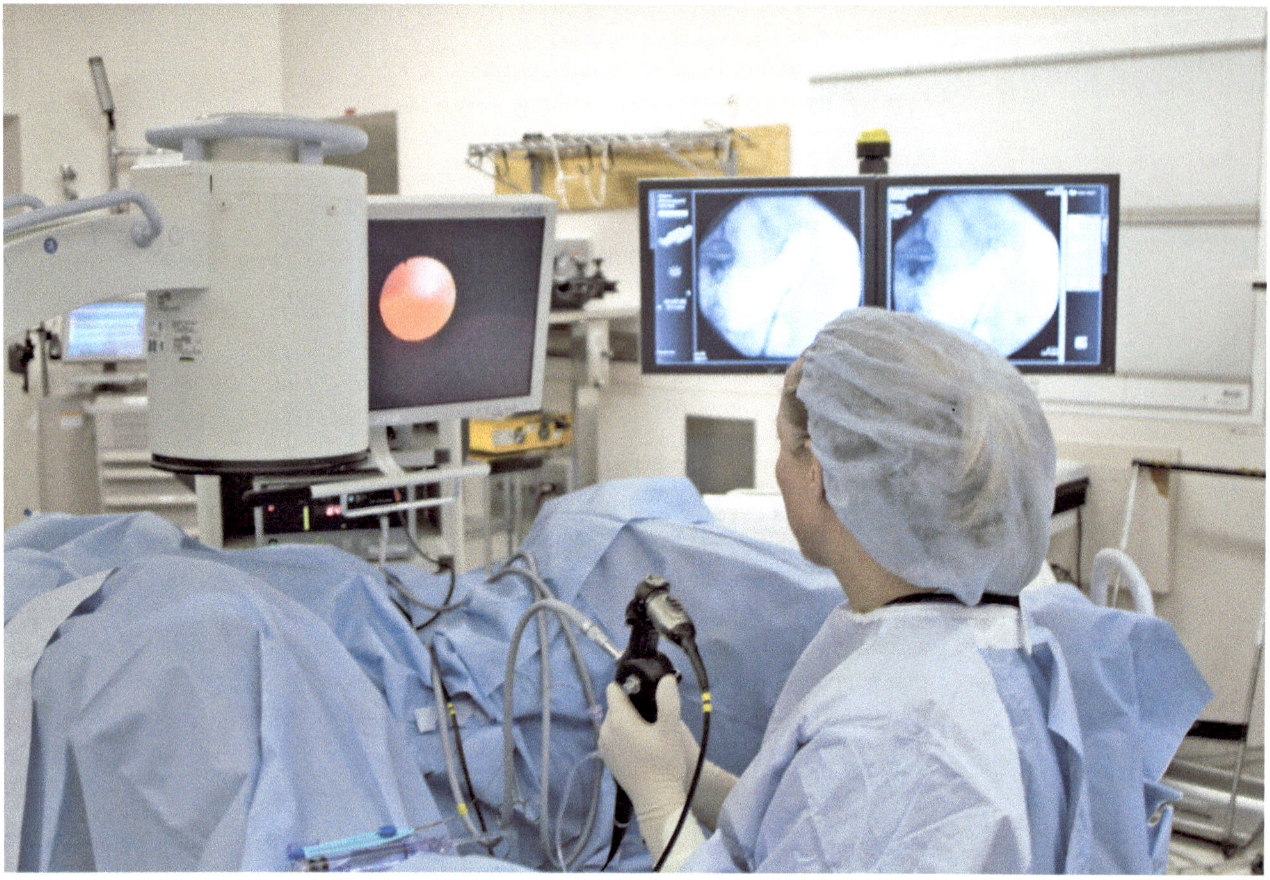

Fig. 37.1 Typical operating room layout. To simplify viewing for the surgeon, the light source, lithotrite generator, and video and C-arm monitors are positioned on one side of the patient. This setup also provides room for movement of the C-arm on the opposite side

Initial Access

Guidewires

Guidewires provide a means of obtaining access through the tortuous paths of the upper urinary tract and are often utilized as a safety instrument alongside the ureteroscope to allow for stent insertion in the event of ureteral perforation or procedural complications. The diameter, commonly 0.035 or 0.038 , was historically the leading factor in guidewire choice; however, the development of superelastic alloys, hydrophilic polymer coatings, and new designs has led to smaller diameter wires of all types [4].

Ideal guidewires are designed with a lubricious tip that easily bends when encountering an obstruction, reducing the likelihood of tissue perforation [5]. Guidewires vary with regard to tip length and configuration (straight, angled, J-shaped) to aide in the passage of impacted ureteral stones and strictures [6]. When significant resistance is encountered, a 5-F open-ended catheter may be used to facilitate a retrograde pyelogram for revealing irregularities of the upper urinary tract anatomy. In such instances, angled-tip guidewires can be used in conjunction with a torque device for guiding the wire through the correct path.

Hydrophilic polytetrafluoroethylene (PTFE)-coated wires reduce the force required for advancement and risk of ureteral trauma; however, an equilibrium of lubricity is necessary to prevent inadvertent loss of access to the upper urinary tract [4, 6]. The core wire portion of a guidewire provides the rigidity necessary to prevent buckling and kinking of the shaft during advancement and manipulation within the urinary tract while supporting stabilization and straightening of the ureter [7, 8]. For coaxial passage of stents, access sheaths, and catheters, the authors often employ rigid wires such as the Amplatz Super Stiff (Boston Scientific, Natick, MA, USA), which has been demonstrated to reduce the risk of buckling when compared to nine other commercially available wires [4]. Recent advancements with superelastic alloys provide the ability to gradually vary rigidity of the core wire from the shaft to the tip, which may improve torquability and pushability characteristics for greater control and safety [7, 9]. Although some authors suggest that the use of a safety wire complicates routine ureteroscopic procedures and induces unnecessary wear on fragile scopes, their use is still advocated for complex cases and when simultaneous basketing is intended [10–12].

Ureteral Access Sheaths

Simplifying repetitive access to the upper urinary tract with access sheaths has been demonstrated to reduce operative time [13], maintain low intrarenal pressure [14], and increase stone-free rates for flexible ureteroscopy [15]. Current access sheaths consist of an outer sheath and inner dilator that may be backloaded over a super-stiff guidewire and advanced up to the ureteral orifice, easing dilation and advancement of the outer sheath into the ureter.

Access sheaths range from 20 to 55 cm in length, with shorter lengths for females and longer lengths for when access up to the proximal ureter and renal pelvis is required [16]. The most common diameter is a 12/14 F; however, depending on the diameter of the ureteroscope and patient anatomy, other sizes may be more appropriate.

Sheath placement is sometimes hindered by buckling or kinking, for which in vitro [17, 18] and randomized clinical studies [19] have suggested the Cook Flexor (Cook Urological, Bloomington, IN, USA) and the Gyrus ACMI Uropass (Gyrus ACMI, Southborough, MA, USA) to be the most resistant when compared to several other commercially available devices. The increased acceptance of access sheath use may be attributed to the development of rigid low-profile sheaths that promote efflux of irrigant fluid around the ureteroscope, maximizing visibility and reducing the risk of ureteral trauma, especially when large calculi require repetitive basketing [16].

Ureteral Balloon Dilators

When encountering a tight ureteral orifice due to ureteral stricture or spasm, the inability to place a ureteral access sheath may advocate ureteral balloon dilatation. Balloon material, configuration, and dimensions contribute to differences within this class of devices, which ideally achieve and maintain maximum expansion despite constrictive forces. An in vitro study evaluating the effect of inflation pressure and compressive forces on expansion revealed 7 of the 14 devices evaluated averaged over 100 % of the expected maximum at burst pressure, with the Cook Ascend AQ (Cook Urological) demonstrating the least variability [20]. Such findings advocate careful use to prevent complications, especially when extensive dilation is used in the lower ureter, which can affect renal function [21]. Postoperative discomfort following ureteral dilation with a balloon dilator has been shown to be significantly more than with an access sheath, further encouraging their use for only the most challenging cases [13].

Intracorporeal Lithotrites

The introduction of lithotrites may be traced back numerous centuries ago; however, their dramatic transformation over recent decades has led to the ability to safely remove large renal calculi in a minimally invasive fashion [22]. Methods of stone comminution have transitioned from mechanical crushing, to electrohydraulic (ELH), pneumatic, pulsed-dye, and ultrasonic lithotrites, to finally, the current gold standard: laser lithotripsy [23].

Pneumatic lithotrites are limited by the surgical method (percutaneous access or semirigid scopes) and increase the risk of retrograde stone migration. However, pneumatic probes provide an economical alternative, and portable CO_2 cartridge powered devices have even been developed for convenience [24].

Ultrasonic/ballistic combinational lithotrites, such as the Swiss Lithoclast (Electro Medical Systems, Dallas, TX, USA), consist of a rigid hollow tube that vibrates at ultrahigh frequencies to induce stone fragmentation. Fragmentation efficiency of these devices is somewhat dependent on stone composition [25]. However, their ability to simultaneously suction out fragments precludes the need for significant stone basketing during percutaneous procedures.

The success and widespread use of holmium:yttrium-aluminum-garnet (Ho:YAG) lasers for lithotripsy may be attributed to the thin and flexible optical fibers optimal for passing through the working channel of flexible ureteroscopes while increasing stone fragmentation ability for all stone types [26]. The precisely focused and directed 2,100-nm light beam results in high optical energy absorption in water that limits energy propagation to a distance of 0.5–1.0 mm, minimizing the risk of ureteral damage [26–28]. Stone ablation with Ho:YAG lasers involves a photothermal process with direct energy absorption by the stone. A vaporization bubble is created that destabilizes and decomposes all stone types [26, 29], attenuating stone retropulsion [30] and producing significantly smaller fragments than ultrasonic, pulsed-dye, or electrohydraulic lithotripsy for easier postoperative stone passage [31]. Furthermore, clinical trials have demonstrated improved stone-free rates for holmium laser lithotripsy when compared to pneumatic [32] and EHL [33] lithotrites.

A downside of laser lithotripsy is the risk of optical fiber fracture that can damage flexible ureteroscopes. Although 365-μm laser fibers have demonstrated greater durability and stone fragmentation efficiency [34], studies indicate 200-μm fibers minimize the reduction in deflection capabilities with flexible ureteroscopes when compared to 365-μm diameter fibers [35, 36].

Ureteral Occluding Devices

Ureteral occlusion devices are most advocated in cases involving a high risk of stone migration, such as considerable hydroureteronephrosis and use of pneumatic lithotripsy, or when access to flexible scopes is limited for upper tract retrieval. Occluding devices are available in a variety of forms, including gel-based and mechanical balloon devices, though mechanical wire-based devices have gained recognition over the past decade. The most successfully reported wire-based devices include the Stone Cone (Boston Scientific, Boston, MA) [37] and NTrap (Cook Urological, Spencer, IN) [38] and most recently the Accordion (Percutaneous Systems, Mountain View, CA) [39].

The 2.8-F Cook NTrap (Cook Urological) utilizes retractable 7-mm-wide net, with 24 interwoven wires that have been demonstrated to prevent the passage of plastic beads larger than 1.5 mm [40]. The Stone Cone (Boston Scientific) consists of concentric stainless steel and nitinol coils coated in PTFE that remain within an outer sheath until being deployed past the stone, expanding to either 7 or 10 mm in diameter. Clinical evaluations of the Stone Cone and NTrap have both demonstrated increased stone-free rates when compared to a control group [38, 41, 42]; however, the in vivo performance of the Accordion has yet to be reported.

Thermosensitive water-soluble polymers, such as the BackStop, have also been safely used for preventing stone migration during laser and pneumatic lithotripsy [43]. Using a 3-F ureteral catheter, the polymer is injected above the stone, where it transitions to a gel phase at body temperature [44]. After sufficient fragmentation, irrigation with cold saline liquefies the polymer, while residual gel dissolves in urine within 2 h [44].

Current ureteral occluding devices require additional procedures prior to lithotripsy, adding to the complexity and upfront costs associated with ureteroscopic stone extraction. The decision to use such tools must take into consideration the additional risk of ureteral perforation associated with deployment.

Stone Retrieval Devices

The evolution of stone retrieval devices has coincided with the increasing relevance of ureteroscopy with stone extraction. The ductility, responsiveness, and kink resistance of nitinol have contributed to the trend toward nitinol-based designs that have demonstrated improved retrieval and release capabilities in vitro [45, 46] as well as an increased range of deflection with flexible scopes [48]. Basket designs include single or paired wires; spherical, helical, and tipless designs; and complex woven wire net configurations [47, 48]. Three- and four-prong graspers, as well as alligator- or rat-tooth forceps, are suggested to provide a safer alternative to more complex basket designs due to the reliable release capabilities when manipulating a stone that is larger than anticipated [49]. However, the large size and weak hold of such devices can also make them problematic.

Basket design dramatically affects the ability to capture, contain, and disengage stones, as well as safety for different situations. Tipless baskets have been demonstrated in vitro to improve retrieval over tipped designs of stones in caliceal and ureteral models and are also suggested to pose less risk of tissue perforation [45, 50]. Helical baskets have been demonstrated to provide significantly greater radial dilation forces that may aid in stone extraction when ureteral stricture or edema complicates stone identification and entrapment [51]. Of 13 baskets tested, the 1.5-F Cook N-Circle was the only to demonstrate linear opening and closing mechanisms that may facilitate stone capture and visualization; however, such small diameter baskets may lack the radial force necessary to expand a narrow lumen [52].

Additional design features include articulating stone baskets, such as the Bard Dimension (Bard Urological, Covington, GA), which incorporates a basket deflecting mechanism intended to ease the capture of hard-to-reach caliceal stones and facilitate reliable stone release. When laser lithotripsy prior to stone acquisition cannot be accomplished, devices such as the 1.9-F Escape (Boston Scientific) or 1.5-F Sacred Heart Halo may be used, as they both allow for the simultaneous passage of a 200-μm laser fiber [53]. Additionally, the 1.5-F Sacred Heart Halo allows for rotation of an engaged stone by the use of a wheel on the handle for enhanced manipulation. When lithotripsy results in small fragments, weaved net configurations, such as that of the Cook N-Compass (Cook Urological), may provide an advantage of capturing multiple fragments 1 mm or less in size.

Flexible Ureteroscopes

Although the first report of an actively deflectable ureteroscope was in 1971 [54], it was not until the 1980s when a working channel and irrigation system were included that these devices became increasingly used for diagnosis and treatment of upper urinary tract diseases as a result of improved visibility, maneuverability, and instrument compatibility [55].

Active deflection over 270° for improving access to lateral and inferior caliceal infundibula [56] may be achieved with a dual-lever mechanism for increasing unidirectional deflection (Dur8-E; Gyrus ACMI, Southborough, MA) or bidirectional deflection (Flexvision U-500; Stryker, San Jose, CA). A unilever system, such as that presented by the Wolf Viper (Richard Wolf Endoscopy, Vernon Hills, IL), also offers 270° of bidirectional deflection, furthering ergonomic design of flexible ureteroscopes [57]. Dual-channel flexible ureteroscopes, such as the Wolf Cobra (Richard Wolf Endoscopy), have demonstrated improved deflection and irrigation while simultaneously providing the ability to stabilize tissue or stones while conducting tissue ablation or lithotripsy with a laser fiber through the secondary channel [58].

Active deflection can be reduced by passage of working channel instruments and laser fibers by as much as 52 % [36], amplifying the loss of deflection due to fatigue of angulation wires contained within the device. Fatigue of deflection mechanisms is commonly noted as the reason for repair, for which current devices may require as often as every 6–15 procedures [59], further adding to the significant financial investment required for these devices [60]. Consequently, semi-disposable flexible ureteroscopes have been developed, such as the PolyScope, which incorporates a disposable 8-F sheath with a 3-F working channel that is advanced over a reusable 10,000-pixel fiber-optic shaft [61]. This design eliminates the need for sterilization between cases and reduces wear and tear within working channels and the subsequent risk of irrigation leakage into fiber-optic bundles and corrodible deflection mechanisms [61].

Miniaturization of flexible ureteroscopes from greater than 9 to 7.4 F has eased ureteral introduction and reduced the need for ureteral dilation [62] and overall postoperative patient morbidity [63]. Downscaling components has also challenged instrument longevity [64], especially fragile optical fibers that affect image resolution, brightness, and contrast [65]. We are currently entering a new era of digital flexible ureteroscopes, which have replaced optical fibers with a charge-coupled device (CCD) chip, increasing deflection capabilities and eliminating drawbacks associated with optical fiber wear [66]. Standard xenon light sources requiring light cables have also been exchanged for cheaper and cooler wireless light-emitting diode (LED) technology, lessening scope weight and improving ergonomics.

A clinical evaluation of the digital DUR-D (Gyrus ACMI) revealed significantly reduced operative time and a similar rate of success when compared to a Karl Storz Flex-X2 fiber-optic ureteroscope [67]. An in vitro assessment of optical characteristics between digital (Olympus URF-V) and fiber-optic (Olympus URF-P3) devices revealed the digital model to have significantly improved resolution and color reproduction, as well as a 5.3 times larger image size [68]. The enhanced visibility of digital ureteroscopes will aid in the diagnosis and treatment of upper urinary tract abnormalities; however, significant time is still required before this technology becomes widely affordable for institutions.

Endoirrigation Systems

Endoirrigation systems are essential for dilating the ureter and upper collecting system to facilitate instrument passage and clear vision throughout endoscopic procedures. The presence and caliber of instruments in the working channel can dramatically affect flow through the scope and sometimes completely impede flow altogether [69]. Passive gravity-based systems rely on hydrostatic pressure to continuously deliver irrigant fluid and are commonly used in conjunction with a tourniquet or pressure-bag compression system to help maintain adequate flow.

Active hand- and foot-pump systems are used for delivering controlled irrigation. The single-action pump (Boston Scientific) is a 10-mL vacuum syringe utilizing a one-way valve that automatically refills the syringe after each pump. The Peditrol (EMS Medical Systems, Stroud, UK) is a foot-pump device with a 3-mL syringe attached to the pedal, which automatically refills from a gravity bag [70]. An in vitro study compared passive gravity systems to active hand- and foot-pump devices with regard to the likelihood of causing stone migration and determined the single-action pump exerted the least force on the stone of the hand-held devices, suggesting a reduced likelihood of causing stone migration [71]. An automated irrigation/suction system (ENDO FMS UROLOGY; Future Medical Systems USA, Glen Burnie, M.D.) has also been developed for controlling pressure and flow rate for which an initial report suggests improved working space and visibility over standard gravity pressure systems [72].

Conclusions and Future Innovations

Development of instrumentation will strive to improve stone-free rates, simplify procedures, and reduce costs and overall patient morbidity. Robotic-assisted ureteroscopy systems have already demonstrated clinical success and provide a clear ergonomic advantage for a surgeon, which serves to decrease the learning curve for a variety of surgical procedures [73]. In addition to increasing the surgeon's range of motion and precision, robotics may improve efficiency of tasks by providing the surgeon quick access to all surgical duties and advanced three-dimensional imaging within a single console while also remaining a safe distance from the radiation field [73]. As the rate of technological innovation continues to increase, surgeons are presented with a perpetually improving means of challenging current treatment methods and revealing the incredible potential for the field of endoscopy.

References

1. Sabnis RB, Mishra S, Sharma R, Desai MR. Preoperative planning and designing of a fluorocompatible endourology operating room. J Endourol. 2009;23(10):1579–85.
2. Meyer RS, White KK, Smith JM, Groppo ER, Mubarak SJ, Hargens AR. Intramuscular and blood pressures in legs positioned in the hemilithotomy position: clarification of risk factors for well-leg acute compartment syndrome. J Bone Joint Surg Am. 2002;84-A:1829–35.
3. Forrest JB, Clemens JQ, Finamore P, Leveillee R, Lippert M, Pisters L, et al. AUA best practice statement for the prevention of deep vein thrombosis in patients undergoing urologic surgery. J Urol. 2009;181(3):1170–7. http://www.auanet.org/content/media/dvt.pdf.
4. Clayman M, Uribe CA, Eichel L, Gordon Z, McDougall EM, Clayman RV. Comparison of guidewires in urology. Which, when, and why. J Urol. 2004;171(6):2146–50.
5. Pedro RN, Hendlin K, Weiland D, Ramani A, Kohler TS, Anderson K, et al. In vitro evaluation of ureteral perforation forces. Urology. 2007;70(3):592–4.
6. Liguori G, Antoniolli F, Trombetta C, Biasotto M, Amodeo A, Pomara G, et al. Comparative experimental evaluation of guidewire use in urology. Urology. 2008;72(2):286–9.
7. Schroder J. The mechanical properties of guidewires. Part 1: stiffness and torsional strength. Cardiovasc Intervent Radiol. 1993;16(1):43–6.
8. Ekman P, Husain I, Sharma ND, Al-Fagih SR. Transurethral ureteroscopy: safety guidewire as an aid to a more aggressive approach. BJU. 1987;60(1):23–7.
9. Sutou Y, Yamacuchi K, Suzuki M, Furakawa A, Omori T, Takagi T, et al. High maneuverability guidewire with functionally graded properties using new superelastic alloys. Minim Invasive Ther Allied Technol. 2006;15(4):204–8.
10. Eandi J, Hu B, Low RK. Evaluation of the impact and need for use of a safety guidewire during ureteroscopy. J Endourol. 2008;22(8):1653–8.
11. Dickstein RJ, Kreshover JE, Babayan RK, Wang DS. Is a safety wire necessary during routine flexible ureteroscopy. J Endourol. 2010;24(10):1589–92.
12. Abrahams HM, Stoller ML. The argument against the routine use of ureteral access sheaths. Urol Clin North Am. 2004;31(1):83–7.
13. Kourambas J, Byrine RR, Preminger GM. Does a ureteral access sheath facilitate ureteroscopy? J Urol. 2001;165(3):789–93.
14. Landman J, Kenkatesh R, Ragab M, Rehman J, Lee DI, Morrissey KG, et al. Comparison of intrarenal pressure and irrigant flow during percutaneous nephroscopy with an indwelling catheter, ureteral occlusion balloon, and ureteral access sheath. Urology. 2002;60(4):584–7.
15. L'esperance JO, Ekeruo WO, Scales C, Marguet CG, Springhart WP, Maloney ME, et al. Effect of ureteral access sheath on stone-free rates in patients undergoing ureteroscopic management of renal caculi. J Urol. 2005;66(2):252–5.
16. Monga M, Bhayani S, Landman J, Conradie M, Sundaram C, Clayman R. Ureteral access for upper urinary tract disease: the access sheath. J Endourol. 2001;15(8):831–4.
17. Monga M, Gawlik A, Durfee W. Systematic evaluation of ureteral access sheaths. J Urol. 2004;63(5):834–6.
18. Pedro RN, Hendlin K, Durfee WK, Monga M. Physical characteristics of next-generation ureteral access sheaths: buckling and kinking. J Urol. 2007;70(3):440–2.
19. Monga M, Best S, Venkatesh R, Ames C, Lieber D, Vanlangendock R, et al. Prospective randomized comparison of 2 ureteral access sheaths during flexible retrograde ureteroscopy. J Urol. 2004;172(2):572–3.
20. Hendlin K, Lund B, Dockendorf K, Ramani A, Monga M. Radial dilation of ureteral balloons: comparative in vitro analysis. J Endourol. 2005;19(5):575–8.
21. Selmy G, Houssouna M, Begin LR, Coolsaet BOL, Elhilali M. Effect of balloon dilation of ureter on upper tract dynamics and ureteral wall morphology. J Endourol. 1993;7(3):211–9.
22. Herr HW. Crushing the stone: a brief history of lithotripsy, the first minimally invasive surgery. BJU Int. 2008;102(4):432–5.
23. Marguet CG, Sung JC, Springhart WP, L'Esperance JO, Zhou S, Zhong P, et al. In vitro comparison of stone retropulsion and fragmentation of the frequency doubled, double pulse ND:YAG laser and the holmium:YAG laser. J Urol. 2005;173(5):1797–800.
24. Nerli RB, Koura AC, Prabha V, Kamat G, Alur SB. Use of LMA Stonebreaker as an intracoporeal lithotrite in the management of ureteral calculi. J Endourol. 2008;22(4):641–3.
25. Krambeck AE, Miller NL, Humpheys MR, Nakada SY, Denstedt JD, Razvi H, et al. Randomized controlled, multicenter clinical trial comparing a dual-probe ultrasonic lithotrite with a single-probe lithotrite for percutaneous nephrolithotomy. BJU Int. 2010;107(5):824–8.
26. Teichman JMH, Vassar GJ, Glickman RD. Holmium:yttrium-aluminum-garnet lithotripsy efficiency varies with stone composition. Urology. 1998;52(3):392–7.
27. Vassar GJ, Teichman JMH, Glickman RD. Holmium:YAG lithotripsy efficiency varies with energy density. J Urol. 1998;160(2):471–6.
28. Nazif OA, Teichman J, Glickman RD, Welch AJ. Review of laser fibers: a practical guide for urologists. J Endourol. 2005;18(9):818–29.
29. Dushinski JW, Lingeman JE. High-speed photographic evaluation of holmium laser. J Endourol. 1998;12(2):177–81.
30. Lee H, Ryan RT, Teichman JMH, Kim J, Choi B, Arakeri NV, et al. Stone retropulsion during holmium:YAG lithotripsy. J Urol. 2003;169(3):881–5.
31. Teichman JMH, Vassar GJ, Bellman GC, Bishoff JT. Holmium:YAG lithotripsy yields smaller fragments than lithoclast, pulsed dye, or electrohydraulic lithotripsy. J Urol. 1998;159(1):17–23.
32. Jeon SS, Hyun JH, Lee KS. A comparison of holmium:YAG laser with Lithoclast lithotripsy in ureteral calculi fragmentation. Int J Urol. 2005;12(6):544–7.
33. Teichman JM, Rao RD, Rogenes VJ, Harris JM. Ureteroscopic management of ureteral calculi: electrohydraulic versus holmium:YAG lithotripsy. J Urol. 1997;158(4):1357–61.
34. Calvano CT, Moran ME, White MD, Borhan-Manesh A, Mehlhaff BA. Experimental utilization of the holmium laser in a model of ureteroscopic lithotripsy: energy analysis. J Endourol. 1999;13(2):113–5.
35. Kuo RL, Aslan P, Zhong P, Preminger GM. Impact of holmium laser settings and fiber diameter on stone fragmentation and endoscope deflection. J Endourol. 1998;12(6):523–7.
36. Poon M, Beaghler M, Baldwin D. Flexible endoscope deflectability: changes using a variety of working instruments and laser fibers. J Endourol. 1997;11(4):247–9.
37. Maislos SD, Volpe M, Albert PS, Raboy A. Efficacy of the stone cone for treatment of proximal ureteral stones. J Endourol. 2004;18(9):862–4.
38. Wang CJ, Huang SW, Chang CH. Randomized trial of NTrap for proximal ureteral stones. J Urol. 2011;77(3):553–7.
39. Vejdani K, Eisner BH, Pengune W, Stoller ML. Effect of laser insult on devices used to prevent stone retropulsion during ureteroscopic lithotripsy. J Endourol. 2009;23(4):705–7.
40. Holley PG, Sharma SK, Perry KT, Turk TM. Assessment of novel ureteral occlusion device and comparison with stone cone in prevention of stone fragment migration during lithotripsy. J Endourol. 2005;19(2):200–3.

41. Eisner BH, Dretler SP. Use of the stone cone for prevention of calculus retropulsion during Holmium:YAG laser lithotripsy: case series and review of the literature. Urol Int. 2009;82(3):356–60.
42. Farahat YA, Elbahnasy AM, Elashry OM. A randomized prospective controlled study for assessment of different ureteral occlusion devices in prevention of stone migration during pneumatic lithotripsy. J Urol. 2011;77(1):30–5.
43. Rane A, Bradoo A, Rao P, Shivde S, Elhilali M, Anidjar M, et al. The use of a novel reverse thermosensitive polymer to prevent ureteral stone retropulsion during intracorporeal lithotripsy: a randomized controlled trial. J Urol. 2010;183(4):1417–21.
44. Sacco D, McDougal WS, Schwarz A. Preventing migration of stones during fragmentation with thermosensitive polymer. J Endourol. 2007;21(5):504–7.
45. Zeltser IS, Bagley DM. Basket design as a factor in retention and release of calculi in vitro. J Endourol. 2007;21(3):337–42.
46. Netsch C, Herrera G, Gross AJ, Bach T. In vitro evaluation of Nitinol stone retrieval baskets for flexible ureteroscopy. J Endourol. 2011;25(7):1217–20.
47. Monga M, Hendlin K, Lee C, Anderson JK. Systematic evaluation of stone basket dimensions. Urology. 2004;63(6):1042–4.
48. Salimi N, Mahajan A, Don J, Schwartz B. A novel stone retrieval basket for more efficient lithotripsy procedures. J Med Eng Technol. 2009;33(2):142–50.
49. Rosette JJ, Skrekas T, Segura JW. Handling and prevention of complications in stone basketing. Eur Urol. 2006;50:991–9.
50. Lukasewycz S, Hoffman N, Botnaru A, Deka PM, Monga M. Comparison of tipless and helical baskets in an in vitro ureteral model. Urology. 2004;64(3):435–8.
51. Hendlin K, Lee C, Anderson K, Monga M. Radial dilation force of tipless and helical stone baskets. J Endourol. 2004;18(10):946–7.
52. Korman E, Hendlin K, Monga M. Small diameter nitinol stone baskets: radial dilation force and dynamics of opening. J Endourol. 2011;25:1537–40. doi:10.1089/end.2010.0585. Epub 2011 Mar 25.
53. Kesler SS, Pierre SA, Brison DI, Preminger GM, Munver R. Use of the Escape nitinol stone retrieval basket facilitates fragmentation and extraction of ureteral and renal calculi: a pilot study. J Endourol. 2008;22(6):1213–7.
54. Takayasu H, Aso Y, Takagi T, Go T. Clinical application of fiber-optic pyeloureteroscope. Urol Int. 1971;26(2):97–104.
55. Multescu R, Geavlete B, Georgescu D, Geavlete P. Conventional fiberoptic flexible ureteroscope versus fourth generation digital flexible ureteroscope: a critical comparison. J Endourol. 2010;24(1):17–21.
56. Bagley DH. Intrarenal access with the flexible ureteropyeloscope: effect of active and passive deflection. J Endourol. 1993;7(3):221–4.
57. Holden T, Pedro R, Hendlin K, Durfee W, Monga M. Evidence-based instrumentation for flexible ureteroscopy: a review. J Endourol. 2008;22(7):1423–6.
58. Ortiz Alvarado O, Haberman K, Chotikawanich E, Monga M. The Cobra dual-channel flexible ureteroscope: novel function, novel applications. J Endourol Part B Videourol. 2010. doi:10.1089/vid.2010.0002.
59. Afane JS, Olweny EO, Bercowsky E, Sundaram CP, Dunn MD, Shalhav AL, et al. Durability of flexible ureteroscopes: a single center evaluation of the durability and function of the new endoscopes smaller than 9F. J Urol. 2000;164(4):1164–8.
60. Carey RI, Gomez CS, Maurici G, Lynne CM, Leveillee RJ, Bird VG. Frequency of ureteroscope damage seen at tertiary care center. J Urol. 2006;176(2):607–10.
61. Bader MJ, Gratzke C, Walther S, Schlenker B, Tilki D, Hocaoglu Y, et al. The PolyScope: a modular design, semidisposable flexible ureterorenoscope system. J Endourol. 2010;24(7):1061–6.
62. Hudsen RG, Conlin M, Bagley D. Ureteric access with flexible ureteroscopes: effect of the size of the ureteroscope. BJU Int. 2005;95(7):1043–4.
63. Grasso M, Bagley D. Small diameter, actively deflectable, flexible ureteropyeloscopy. J Urol. 1998;160(5):1648–53.
64. Monga M, Best S, Venkatesh R, Ames C, Lee C, Kuskowski M, et al. Durability of flexible ureteroscopes: a randomized prospective study. J Urol. 2006;176(1):137–41.
65. Knudsen B, Miyaoka R, Shah K, Holden T, Turk TM, Pedro RN, et al. Durability of the next generation flexible fiberoptic ureteroscopes: a randomized prospective multi-institutional clinical trial. Urology. 2010;75(3):534–8.
66. Multescu R, Geavlete GD, Geavlet P. Convention fiberoptic flexible ureteroscope versus fourth generation digital flexible ureteroscope: a critical comparison. J Endourol. 2010;24(1):17–21.
67. Binbay M, Yuruk E, Akman T, Ozgor F, Seyrek M, Ozkuvanci U, et al. Is there a difference in outcomes between digital and fiberoptic flexible ureterorenoscopy procedures? J Endourol. 2010;24(12):1929–34.
68. Zilberman DE, Lipkin ME, Ferrandino MN, Simmons WN, Mancini JG, Raymundo ME, et al. The digital flexible ureteroscope: in vitro assessment of optical characteristics. J Endourol. 2011;25(3):519–22.
69. Bach T, Geavlete B, Herrmann TR, Gross AJ. Working tools in flexible ureterorenoscopy – influence on flow and deflection: what does matter? J Endourol. 2008;22(8):1639–43.
70. Blew B, Dagnone AJ, Pace KT, Honey RJ. Comparison of peditrol irrigation device and common methods of irrigation. J Endourol. 2005;19(5):562–5.
71. Hendlin K, Weiland D, Monga M. Impact of irrigation systems on stone migration. J Endourol. 2008;22(3):453–8.
72. Lechevallier E, Luciani M, Nahon O, Lay F, Coulange C. Transurethral ureterorenolithotripsy using new automated irrigation/suction system controlling pressure and flow compared with standard irrigation: a randomized pilot study. J Endourol. 2003;17(2):97–101.
73. Desai MM, Grover R, Aron M, Ganpule A, Joshi SS, Desai MR, et al. Robotic flexible ureteroscopy for renal calculi: initial clinical experience. J Urol. 2011;186(2):563–8.

Physics and Technique of Shock Wave Lithotripsy (SWL)

38

Othmar J. Wess

Abstract

Extracorporeal shock wave lithotripsy (SWL) is a gentle and noninvasive treatment procedure suitable for a wide range of kidney and ureteral stones. The technique makes use of extremely short transient (<1 μs) pressure pulses with pressure amplitudes up to 100 MPa (1,000 bars). Brittle stone material breaks into small pieces, whereas biological tissue passes shock waves without significant damage. Different shock wave generation principles (electrohydraulic, piezoelectric and electromagnetic) are presented, and basic shock wave parameters are discussed with regard to stone fragmentation and side effects. Modern lithotripsy devices utilize fluoroscopic and/or echographic imaging methods for stone localization and targeting. As with all sophisticated technologies, SWL requires comprehensive technical and anatomical skills to fully benefit from this exciting treatment method.

Keywords

Shock waves • Extracorporeal lithotripsy • Shock wave lithotripsy (SWL) • Kidney stones • Electrohydraulic • Piezoelectric • Electromagnetic

Introduction

On February 7, 1980, in Munich, Germany, for the first time, kidney stones were successfully fragmented within a patient's body by externally generated shock waves. The mechanical energy of shock waves was transmitted through the intact skin and concentrated on the stone without significant damage of the tissue. The granular fragments were flushed out of the body in natural way, eliminating the need for invasive surgery. This date marks the beginning of a new era characterized by application of acoustic energy for noninvasive stone fragmentation and clearing [1, 2]. The revolutionary finding was that shock waves may pass through living tissue without significant injury or side effects while being simultaneously strong enough to fragmentize hard urinary stones. The key reasons are the following: first, elasticity of living tissue, which may pass high transient pressures up to 100 MPa (1,000 bars) and more; second, the liberation of transient forces predominantly at acoustic interfaces with different acoustic characteristics (acoustic impedance); and third, the possibility to couple acoustic energy with low intensity into the body and concentrate (focus) it on the region of interest, the stone to be fragmented. This option allows the stone to be exposed to sufficient shock wave power for fragmentation while, simultaneously, all other tissue areas, which are passed by the shock waves, are only affected insignificantly.

To date, stones in the entire urinary tract are susceptible to shock wave fragmentation only limited by the occasionally huge amount of fragments to be passed via naturalis through the urinary tract.

O.J. Wess, Ph.D.
Storz Medical AG,
Lohstampfestrasse 8, Product Development, Taegerwilen,
Thurgau 8274, Switzerland
e-mail: wess.othmar@storzmedical.com

Electronic supplementary material The online version of this chapter (doi:10.1007/978-1-4471-4387-1_38) contains supplementary material, which is available to authorized users.

J.J. Talati et al. (eds.), *Urolithiasis*,
DOI 10.1007/978-1-4471-4387-1_38, © Springer-Verlag London 2012

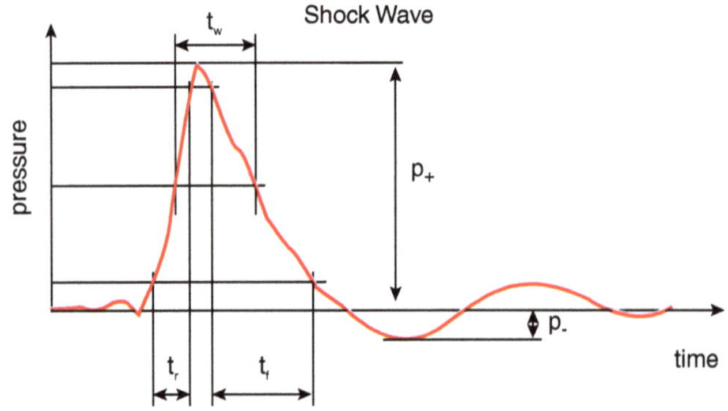

Fig. 38.1 Time profile of a medical shock wave (p_+ peak positive pressure, p_- peak negative pressure, t_r rise time, t_w pulse width, t_f fall time)

Nature of Shock Waves

Medically used shock waves are mechanical waves featuring extremely high-pressure amplitudes in the range of 10–100 MPa (100–1,000 bars). They require an elastic medium such as gas, fluids, or soft tissue for propagation and cannot be transmitted through vacuum. Shock waves appear in nature as explosive noise generated by atmospheric lighting or by detonation of explosive material. A typical pressure–time profile of a shock wave in water is shown in Fig. 38.1. Usually, medical shock waves are generated in water propagating with approximately the speed of sound (1,500 m/s eq. 5,400 km/h). Due to the very high-pressure amplitudes, however, normal linear propagation conditions are exceeded so that the highest pressure components travel slightly faster than lower pressure components resulting in a steepening of the pressure ascend of the wave as shown in Fig. 38.2. Shock waves in gaseous or fluid mediums propagate as longitudinal waves featuring particle movements in direction of propagation and reverse. As acoustic waves in general, shock waves may be reflected, refracted, diffracted, or strayed when passing inhomogeneities with respect to acoustic features (acoustic impedance) of the medium. Shock waves may be focused for energy concentration at specific regions within human bodies in order to expose selected target areas such as tissue under treatment or kidney and ureteral stones.

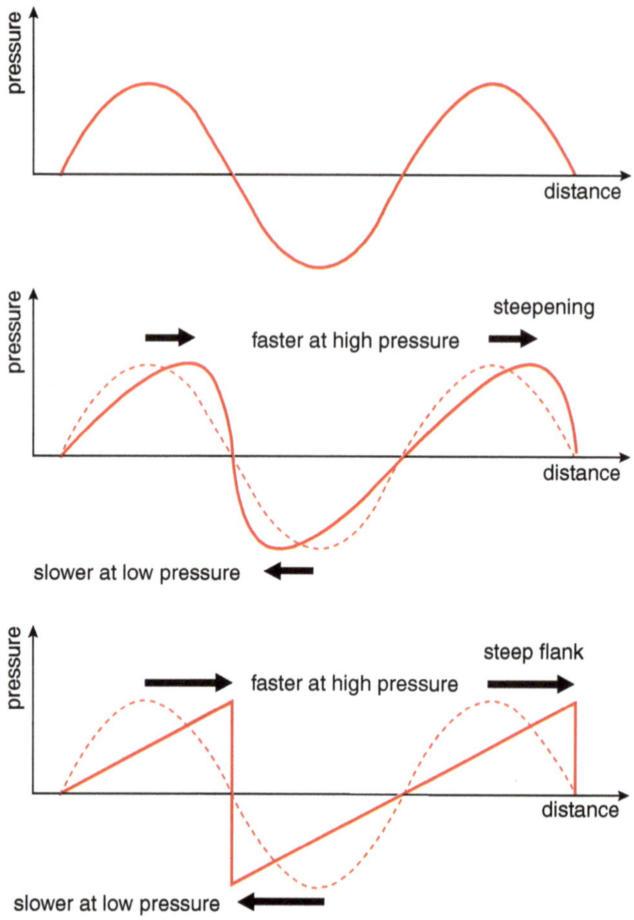

Fig. 38.2 Steepening of pressure rise. The pressure rise is compressed to shorter rise times due to nonlinear propagation (faster with higher pressure, slower with lower pressure). At high-pressure amplitudes, shock fronts with steep rise develop with travel distance

Shock Wave Generation Methods

Electrohydraulic Shock Wave Generation

Shock waves may be generated by explosive processes, primarily, expanding faster than the speed of sound in a particular medium such as water. Instead of explosive material, the first clinically used method was based on a high-energy electrical discharge across a 1-mm spark gap ignited in a water bath. A capacitor bank was charged by approximately 20,000 V (20 kV) and discharged across the electrode generating a rapidly expanding plasma channel (spark). This plasma channel pushed the surrounding water by pressures of more than 100 MPa, which propagated into the medium. Figure 38.3 shows a series of high-speed photographs (frame rate 10^7 frames/s) with a lighting spark between two electrode tips and a spherically expanding shock wave displayed with shadow photographic technique. Electrical discharge generates shock waves in its physical meaning from the origin on since the expanding velocity of the spark channel is slightly higher than speed of sound. After a few millimeters of travel, electrohydraulically generated shock waves are slowed down to normal propagation velocity (approximately 1,500 m/s). They may be reflected by acoustic mirrors and focused onto the target position of the stone.

The primary shock wave generated by this method is a spherically expanding wave, which propagates with the speed of sound into the surrounding medium. The energy is dissipated by expansion and needs to be concentrated on the target stone for fragmentation. Concentration is done by

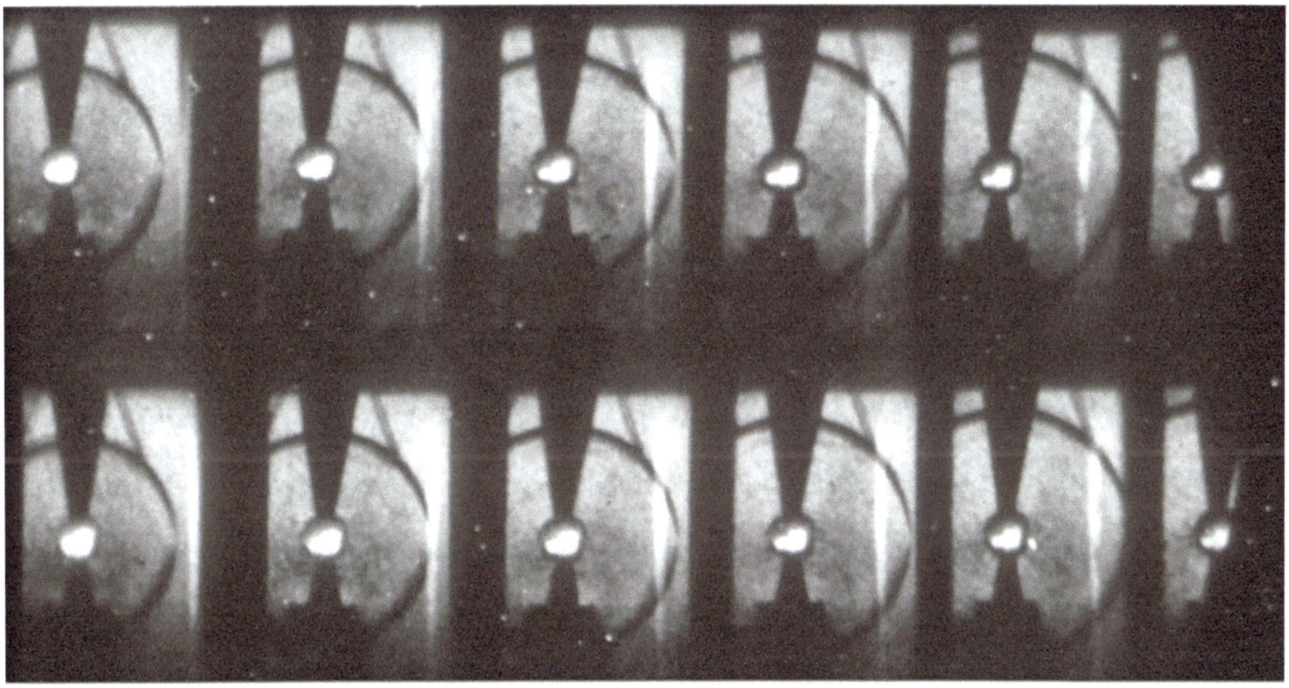

Fig. 38.3 HF photography of spark and shock wave generated in water (10^7 frames/s). A spark is ignited between two electrode tips in a distance of approximately 1 mm. The plasma channel between the tips expands with supersonic velocity and generates a spherical shock wave. The shock wave separates from the plasma channel as soon as the expansion velocity of the spark channel drops below the propagation velocity in water (1,500 m/s)

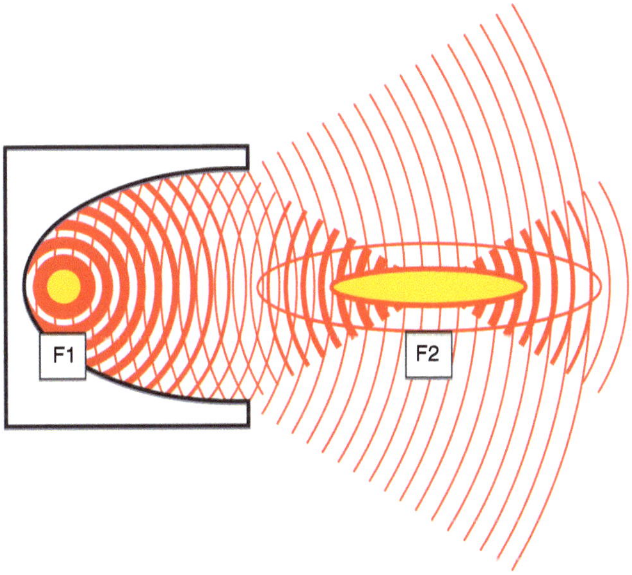

Fig. 38.4 Spherical shock waves generated in the first focal spot *F1* of a semi-ellipsoid arc partly concentrated on an area around *F2*, the second focal spot of the ellipsoidal structure. Part of the primary spherical wave is radiated as dissipating wave without being focused

reflection of the spherical wave at the surface of a hollow ellipsoidal metal reflector (see Fig. 38.4).

The spark gap is placed at the first focal spot of the ellipsoid, and the primarily diverging wave is concentrated at the second focal point in a distance. By cutting the ellipsoidal structure at an intermediate level, this second focal spot can be placed outside the metal structure to be aimed from outside the human body at the target stone within the body.

This pioneering type of shock wave generation and focusing has been very successful and motivated engineers to further develop shock wave techniques to overcome some of the disadvantages of the electrohydraulic principle such as frequent change of worn-out electrodes, fluctuations of energy output, and excessive noise.

A subgroup of electrohydraulic generators, called "electroconductive shock wave generators," makes use of a conductive fluid between the electrode tips in order to reduce energy fluctuations of sequential shocks.

Piezoelectric Shock Wave Generation

A more reproducible method of shock wave generation is based on the piezo effect, which is widely used in ultrasound diagnostic devices. Making use of the piezo effect, a large number of piezo ceramic elements are activated simultaneously by applying an electrical tension of several kilovolts (kV). According to the electrical excitation, the elements expand, and the displacement of the surface generates a pressure wave that propagates into the adjacent medium. Piezoelectric elements can be arranged on the inner surface of a spherical calotte to generate a spherical wave directed to the center of the calotte. A piezoelectric shock wave generator is shown in Fig. 38.5.

Whereas the electrohydraulically generated shock waves originate from a tiny small point-shaped area between the electrode tips with extremely high pressure and high energy density, piezoelectrically generated shock waves are emitted by a relatively large area with low energy density. In order to provide sufficient energy for stone fragmentation within the focal zone, a relatively large area of active piezo ceramic elements (several hundred square centimeters) is required. The acoustic energy is generated as (non-shock wave) pressure pulse and concentrated to a small area at the center of the calotte. It becomes a shock wave by steepening on its travel to the focus as shown in Fig. 38.2.

Piezoelectric shock wave generators avoid the need for frequent and costly change of electrodes as in the electrohydraulic case and last several million shocks. Due to its complexity, an exchange of the total shock wave head is more expensive. Another advantage of piezoelectric generators is the reproducibility of each single shock and the precise control of the shock wave parameters. The fragmentation power of piezo elements is relatively low. It requires quite a large active area to yield sufficient energy for stone fragmentation. There are attempts to make use of a sandwich structure of two active areas: one at the inner surface of the spherical calotte and another at the outer surface. A slight delay of activation between the two active spheres allows for a certain pulse shaping. By this technique, the size of the large calottes may be reduced to more convenient dimensions. Nevertheless, the overall fragmentation power seems to be inferior to other techniques.

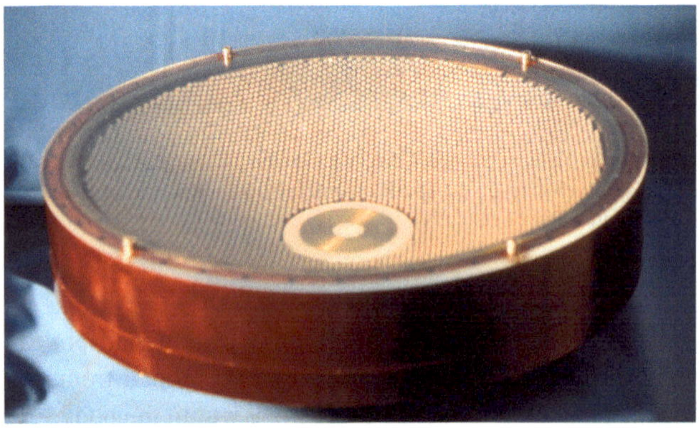

Fig. 38.5 Piezo-calotte. Numerous piezo elements are arranged on a spherical bowel and activated simultaneously to generate a self-focussing spherical pulse wave

Electromagnetic Shock Wave Generation

The method of electromagnetic shock wave generation is based on the physical principle of electromagnetic induction, as used, for example, in loudspeakers. A strong pulse current running through an electrical coil generates repelling forces in a conducting membrane attached to the coil separated only by a thin insulation foil. The conducting membrane is activated by eddy currents and pushed toward the adjacent medium (water). Although the displacement of the membrane measures only a fraction of a millimeter, the surrounding water is compressed, and the according pressure distortion is radiated as pressure wave into the medium (Fig. 38.6a, b).

Two different configurations are used in modern shock wave lithotripsy (SWL) devices. The traditional electromagnetic generator utilizes a flat coil/membrane arrangement

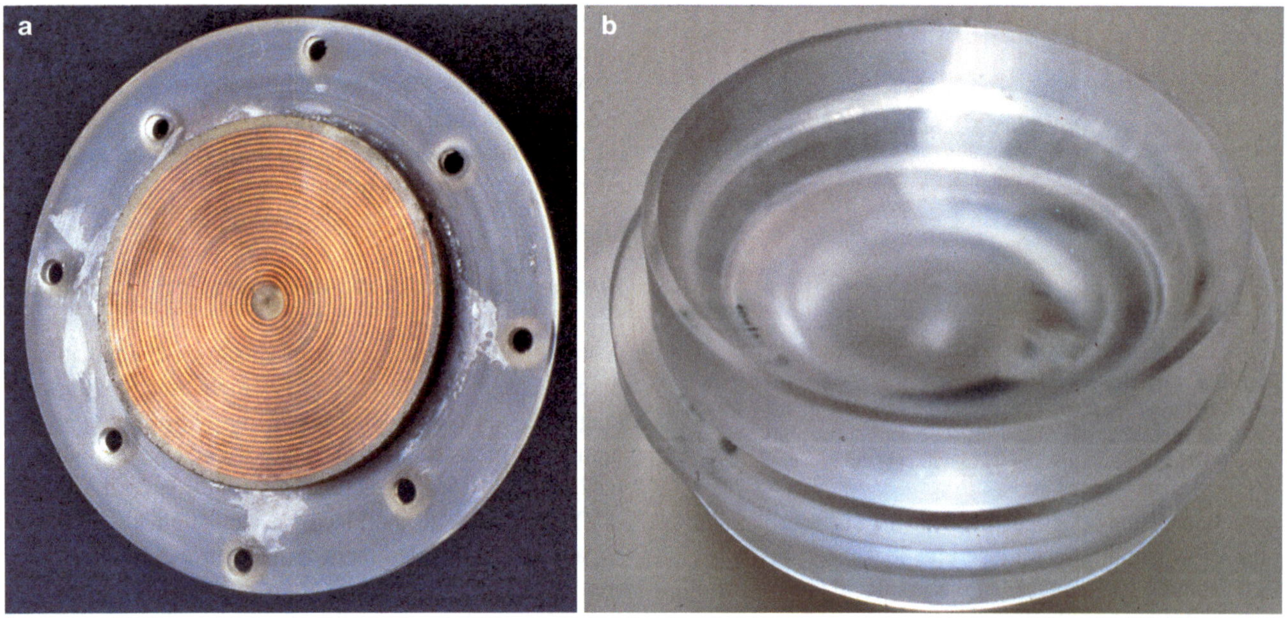

Fig. 38.6 Flat coil/acoustic lens configuration. The electrical flat coil (**a**) is covered by an insulation foil and a conducting membrane. Primary plane acoustic waves are focused with the aid of an acoustic lens (**b**)

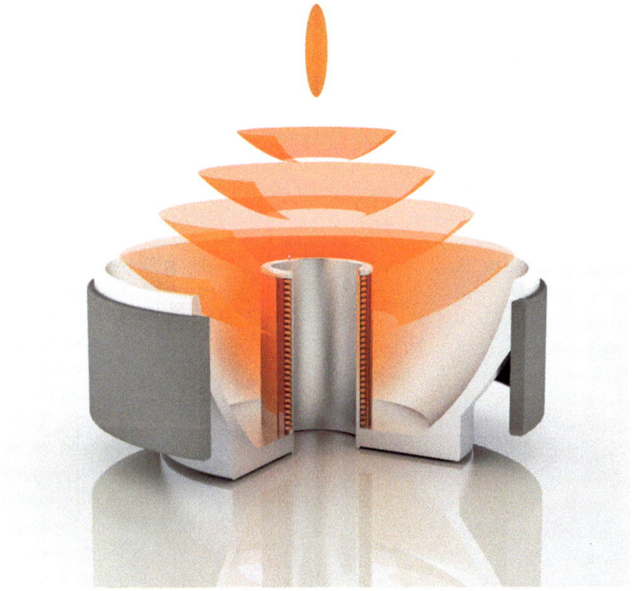

Fig. 38.7 Cylinder source. The electrical cylinder coil is covered by an insulation foil and a conducting membrane. The primary cylindrical wave is reflected and focused by a rotational parabolic reflector. The hollow center may be used for in-line fluoroscopic or ultrasonic stone localization

that focuses a primarily plane pressure wave by aid of an acoustical lens. The most advanced configuration has a cylindrical coil/membrane and a special rotational parabolic reflector for focusing the primarily cylindrical pressure wave to a precise focal spot (Fig. 38.7). As in the case of piezoelectric generators, pressure waves generated by electromagnetic principle turn into shock waves by steepening when concentrated in the focal zone. The coil configuration provides a central opening for high-precision in-line integration of X-ray or ultrasound localization devices.

The cylinder configuration does not require acoustical lenses and offers widest apertures for gentle energy transmission into the body and largest focal depth for treatment of obese patients with extraordinary stone-to-skin distances.

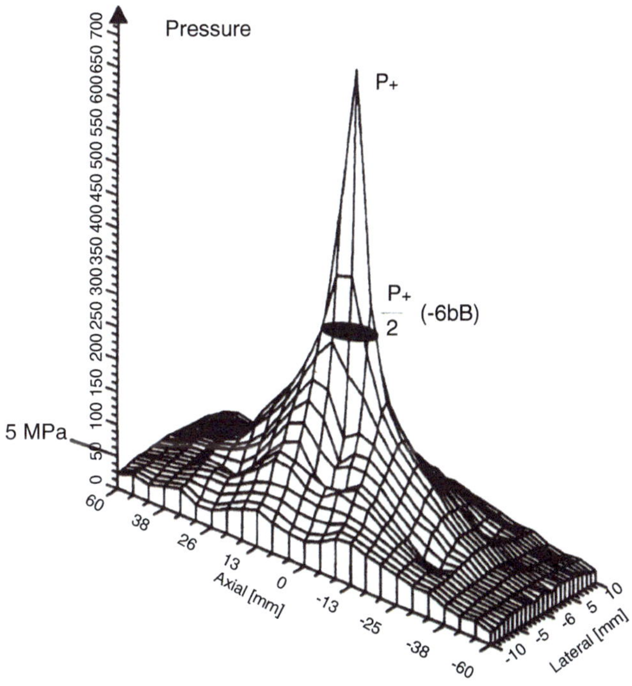

Fig. 38.8 Spatial pressure field. The –6-dB zone is characterized by 50 % of the actual peak pressure p_+. The area exceeding the pressure of 5 MPa may change with energy settings (different peak pressure)

Physical Characteristic of Shock Waves

Medically used shock wave devices may be characterized by the type of shock wave generator and the spatial and temporal parameters of the shock wave field. Aperture diameters, focus distances, lateral and axial focus dimension, peak pressure, and energy flux density are parameters affecting fragmentation power of a shock wave device as well as pain sensation and risk of side effects [3–6].

Pressure

The shock wave field is measured by taking time-pressure records $p(t)$ point by point, scanning a small hydrophone through the three-dimensional shock wave field. For each spatial position, the peak pressure p_+ and the time profile $p(t)$ of the pressure curve are taken, including rise time and time duration of each single pulse as shown in Fig. 38.1. Shock waves in medicine feature typically peak pressures of 10–100 MPa (100–1,000 bars) and sometimes more. Rise times are in the range of <10–100 ns (nanosecond), depending on the type of generation. Time duration of the pressure curve is approximately 0.5 μs (microsecond). Pulse length in water/tissue is <1 mm. Each shock wave pulse is associated with negative (tensile) wave components in the range of 10 % of the peak pressure p_+.

–6 dB Focal Zone and 5 MPa Treatment Zone

Shock waves are coupled over a wide surface area into the body and are concentrated (focused) to a treatment area with intensified energy. The transmission pathway is protected against high acoustic energy reducing side effects while, simultaneously, effective treatment and possible side effects are restricted to the region of interest, the treatment zone. The therapeutic shock wave field thus shows a central peak of highest pressure p_+ and a continuously declining pressure around as shown in Fig. 38.8.

Taking the peak pressure p_+ as reference, a three-dimensional zone may be defined with pressure values being equal or greater than ½ p_+, the so-called –6-dB isobar. This zone is usually taken as focal zone of a lithotripter. Please note that

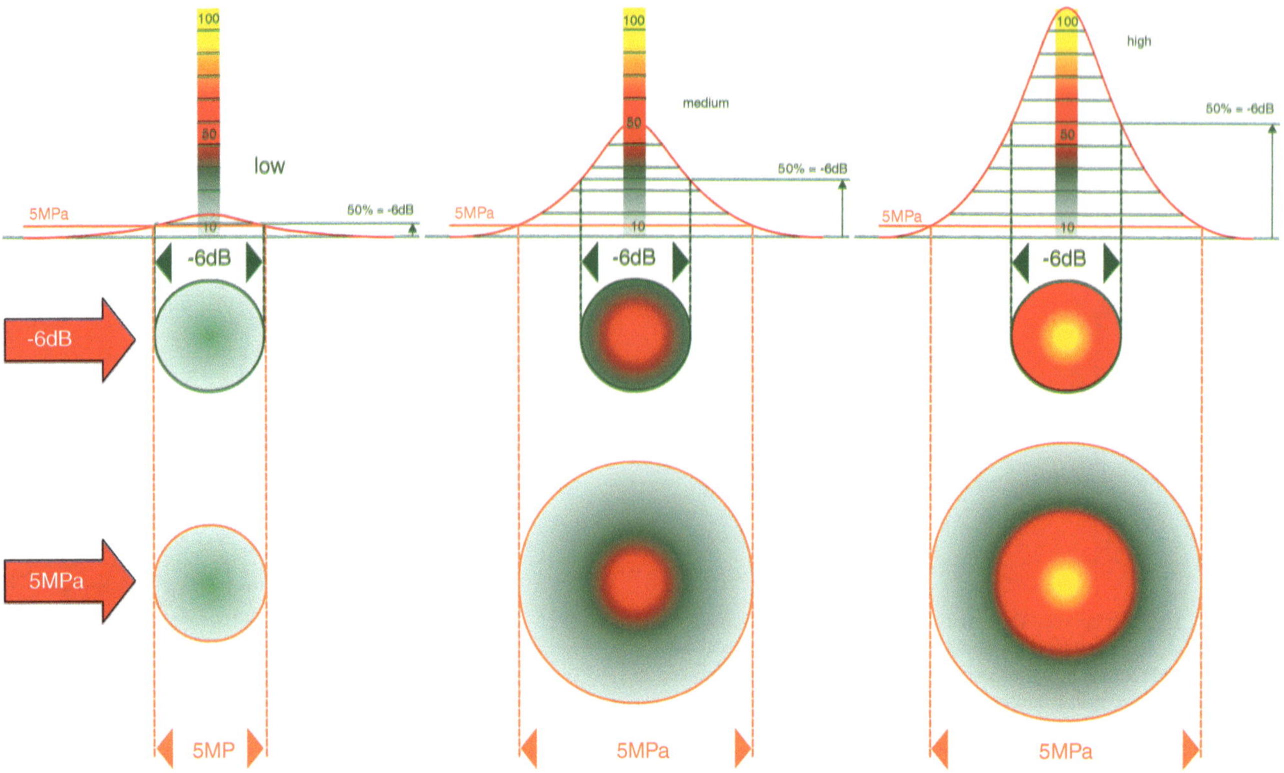

Fig. 38.9 A –6-dB focus zone versus 5-MPa treatment zone at different energy settings. With increasing energy the treatment area, defined by the 5-MPa zone, increases accordingly whereas the dimensions of the physical focus zone (–6 dB) may stay independent in size from the selected energy setting. Nevertheless, the energy content (see text) of the focus zone may vary significantly

this focus definition does not reflect the dimensions of the treatment area itself. It only relates, per physical definition, to the peak pressure. The peak pressure p_+ may vary between different devices and settings significantly without affecting the focal size. Therefore, the –6-dB focal zone simply reflects the degree of energy concentration, but is neither a measure to characterize the power of the shock wave field nor the area within which a shock wave field may break stones.

To enable a comparison between different energy settings and different devices, one may define the zone within a fixed isobar—of, for example, 5 MPa—as an area of therapeutic (fragmentation) efficiency. Even though the definition of 5 MPa seems to be arbitrary, it reflects the influence of the energy setting on the spatial dimensions of the effective zone (Fig. 38.9).

Energy

Although $p(t)$ being the primary parameter of a three-dimensional shock wave field, it does not correlate directly with the fragmentation efficiency, the main goal of a shock wave lithotripter. Shock wave energy (not only pressure) is needed to break stones. The energy may be calculated for a given area A by taking pressure curves $p(t)$ within the area A and acoustical parameters of the propagation medium density (ρ) and sound velocity (c), according to the formula:

$$E = A/\rho c \int p^2(t)\mathrm{d}t\,(\text{energy})$$

The acoustical energy of a shock wave pulse is given in millijoules (mJ). As a rule, several hundreds or thousands of shock wave pulses are emitted per treatment, so that the total emitted energy is yielded by multiplication with the number of pulses.

Only that portion of the shock wave field that hits the stone will contribute to stone fragmentation. For characterization of different lithotripsy devices, a medium-sized stone with a circular cross section with a diameter of 12 mm is taken for reference by convention. The energy within this cross-sectional area A gives a comparable number for the fragmentation power of a lithotripter device.

Published data on the energy content of the –6-dB focal zone are just physical parameters that do not characterize the fragmentation power of a lithotripter (see chapter "-6dB Focal Zone and 5 MPa Treatment Zone").

Energy Flux Density (ED)

As previously mentioned, the therapeutic effect of shock waves depends on how much shock wave energy is deposited on the stone. The part that is missing the stone cannot contribute to fragmentation. Therefore, not only energy values are of interest but also the energy flux density (ED), a measure for the spatial energy concentration (energy E/area A):

$$E/A = 1/\rho c \int p^2(t)\mathrm{d}t = \text{ED (energy flux density)}$$

The energy flux density (ED) is given in millijoules per square millimeter (mJ/mm^2).

The total amount of shock wave energy delivered to the stone may be calculated by integration of the energy flux density over the cross-sectional area of the stone.

The parameters previously described are usually sufficient to characterize a shock wave field for medical applications.

Shock wave devices that work with different generation principles can differ in relation to the listed parameters. The "quality" of the shock waves used in the treatment zone, however, seems to be independent from the generation principle. In other words, the measurement of the above parameters in the treatment zone does not allow any fundamental conclusions to be drawn about the type of generation. Electrohydraulically generated shock waves are not better or worse than piezoelectrically or electromagnetically generated shock waves, although secondary parameters such as accuracy of repetition, dose control, energy range, and operating costs for consumables may differ significantly.

Note that the parameters discussed previously Ohysical Characteristics of Shock Waves are usually measured in water. Due to the inhomogeneities in living tissue, however, deviations from the straight propagation of shock waves occur. With increasing depth in the body, the peak pressure as well as ED values may significantly be reduced by realistic anatomical conditions. Accordingly, focal dimensions (−6-dB focus) may be significantly (up to 10 mm) expanded depending on individual anatomical conditions [7].

Medical Shock Wave Effects

Wanted Effects

Although shock waves feature extremely high pressures for very short time duration, elasticity of living tissue allows for transmission of high-pressure waves usually without significant lesions. Shock wave-specific forces are generated at acoustic interfaces characterized by different acoustic impedances (density $\rho \times$ propagation velocity c). Since water, where shock waves are usually generated, and soft tissue feature similar acoustic impedances, shock wave forces at the water/skin interfaces are small as well as at interfaces between different soft tissues. At the interface between kidney and stone, however, a significant impedance mismatch creates strong forces by incident and reflected waves. Fragmentation forces are generated at front and rear surface of the stone when shock waves are transmitted and reflected (Fig. 38.10a). Erosion and spallation (Hopkinson effect) at rear surface are observed (Fig. 38.10b). There are different additional fragmentation effects discussed such as squeezing, fatigue by development of micro rupture lines, and others including cavitation effects [8–12].

Cavitation is an important mechanism for stone fragmentation. The tensile trail of shock waves tears open small cavitation bubbles (Fig. 38.11). They may collapse by generating a needlelike water jet when close to an acoustic interface such as the stone surface. Those microjets are directed toward the interface and may have the velocity of gun bullets of several hundred m/s. The impact of these high-velocity microjets contributes to erosion and is an important factor of stone fragmentation.

Shock waves were introduced into medicine primarily for noninvasive stone fragmentation. Meanwhile, however, another important shock wave effect was discovered. Shock wave stimulation of soft tissue results in regeneration and improved blood supply and is widely used in a variety of medical indications, mainly for treatment of chronic pain diseases such as chronic pelvic pain syndrome (CPPS), orthopedic pain diseases, and cardiology.

Unwanted Effects

As with any medical method, there are always side effects (Paracelsus 1493–1541). Fortunately, shock waves are associated with predominately beneficial features, but certain unwanted side effects may occur. The stone-breaking power of shock waves may cause tissue lesions mainly by cavitation effects. The mentioned microjets may punch small vessels and cause microbleedings, which may, rarely, result in significant hematomas (Fig. 38.12). Administration of anticoagulation drugs has to be thoroughly controlled.

Since shock waves may affect the nervous system as well as the cardiac excitation system, according effects such as cardiac interference are possible risks. Due to a major mismatch of acoustic impedances of soft tissue and gas-containing organs (lungs, intestine), significant forces may be generated at interfaces to such organs. Therefore, these organs should be kept free from shock wave exposure, at least from the high energetic focal area. Bony structures exposed to shock waves will distort shock wave propagation, avoiding successful stone fragmentation. Last, but not least, shock wave application for stone treatment causes pain. Depending on the shock wave generation methods and treatment strategy, pain killers or even general anesthesia may be appropriate.

How to Apply Shock Waves

As a general rule, the mentioned benefits (stone fragmentation, less invasiveness etc.) have to be balanced against rare,

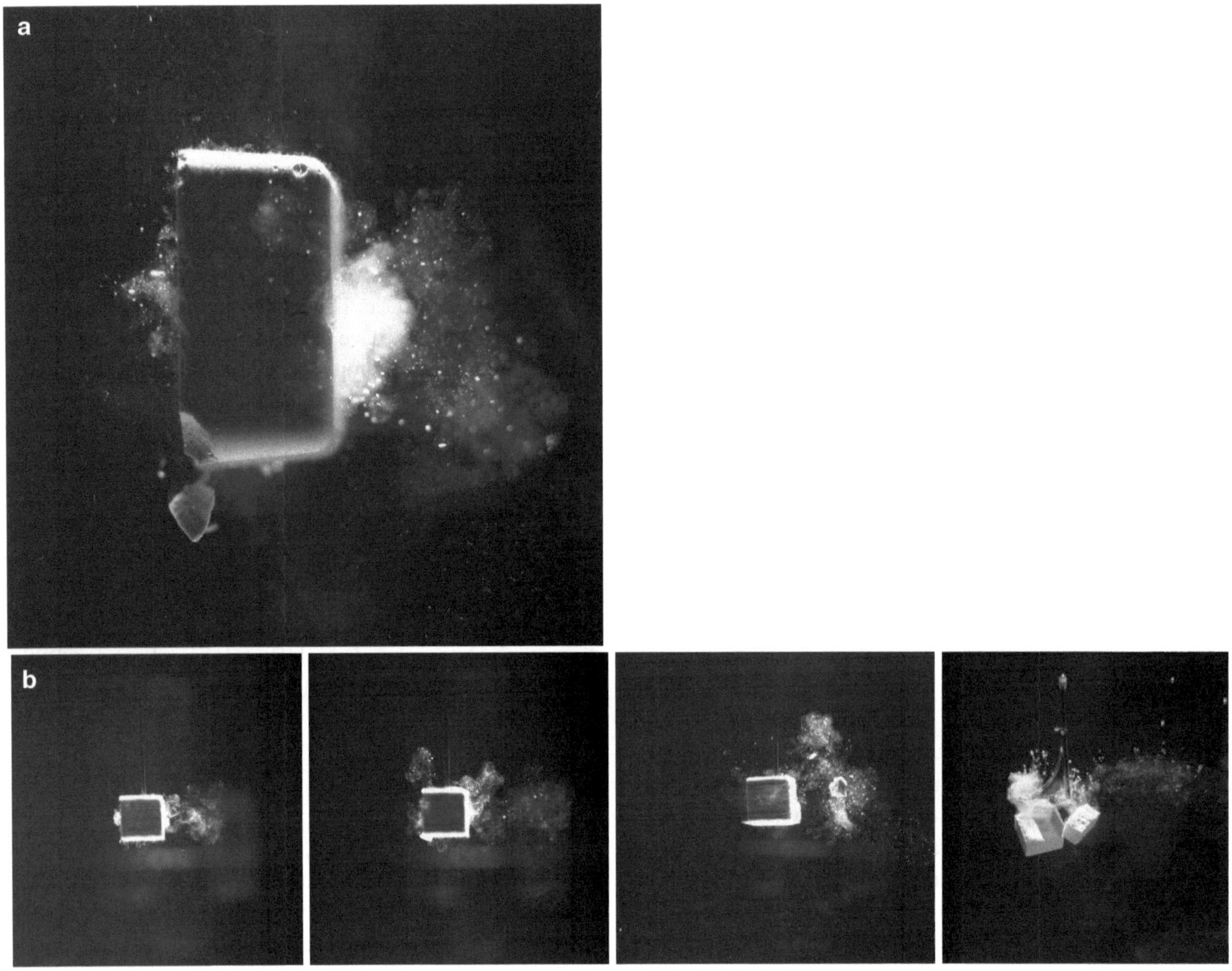

Fig. 38.10 (**a**) An artificial stone of plaster (3 × 3 × 1.5 cm) is hit from the right by a focused shock wave. The front surface (*right*) is eroded and a crater develops. The whole stone is shattered and pieces break off the corner. (**b**) Sequential shock waves (incident from *right*) hit a 1-cm cube of plaster. At the rear surface (*left*), spallation due to the Hopkinson effect is seen, and pieces are expelled from the front surface until the stone breaks completely

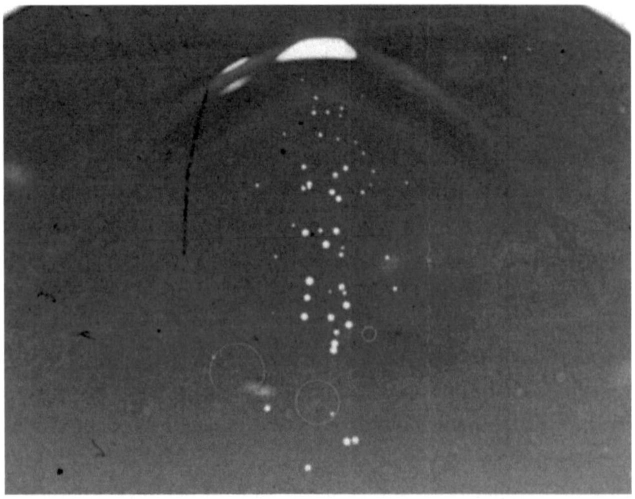

Fig. 38.11 The shock wave at top propagated from the *bottom to top* (approximately 75 mm) within 50 μs and generated a cloud of cavitation bubbles. The time history of bubble expansion and the following collapse can be deduced from their spatial location. Bubbles immediately behind the shock front were just generated and growing. *Bubbles in the middle* have been generated approximately 30 μs before when the shock front passed this area. They reached maximal diameters and start to collapse. At the lower third, they collapsed completely after 40–50 μs and create spherically expanding secondary shock waves (*circles at lower part of the image*)

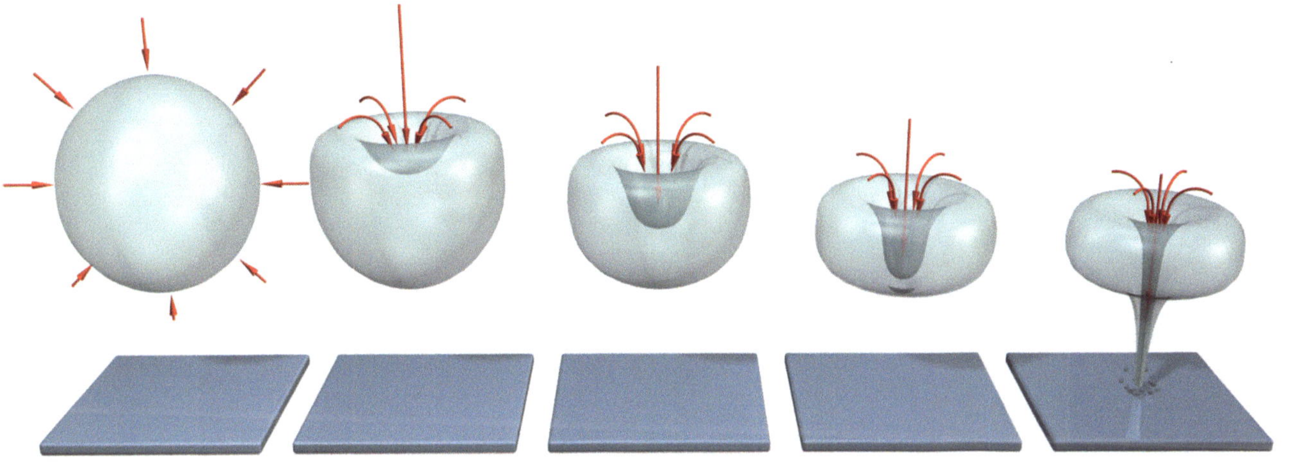

Fig. 38.12 Collapse of a cavitation bubble (schematic) close to an acoustic interface (stone surface). Due to asymmetric streaming conditions at the interface, an asymmetrical collapse occurs and generates a microjet directed toward the interface. Microjets featuring velocities up to several hundred m/s affect the interface and contribute to erosion and stone fragmentation as well as tissue lesions

but possible side effects (tissue lesions, pain, hematoma etc.). Two aspects have to be considered: (1) skills and diligence of the operating personnel and (2) technical concepts and configurations of the shock wave sources.

First: The operator needs medical training for exact diagnosis of stone diseases and in-depth anatomical knowledge to proper selection of the appropriate shock wave passage to the stone and optimal patient positioning. It does not suffice to see the stone at the predetermined position by the localization device if the transmission pathway through the tissue is obstructed by bony or gaseous structures. If necessary, the position of the patient has to be corrected repeatedly. Since with extracorporeal lithotripsy shock wave energy is generated outside the body, it needs to be transmitted to the body without significant losses. The coupling area of a shock wave head at the surface of the patient may include air bubbles that will significantly reduce effective energy coupling even if the bubbles seem to be insignificantly small. Great care is required to perform the coupling process to satisfaction. These skills and sufficient experience of the operator are mandatory. They were not always given in the past and could cause low success rates not to be accused to the device.

Second: From a technical point of view, the configuration of the shock wave field can be optimized to provide sufficient amount of acoustic energy for stone fragmentation preferably only at the location of the stone and to keep the energy exposure low anywhere else. The same rationale holds true also for the area where beneficial (fragmentation) as well as impairing cavitational effects may occur. The technical solution is a shock wave head with a wide aperture for soft and pain-free energy transmission and an appropriately sized treatment zone, not too big to affect tissue excessively around the stone and not too small to make positioning difficult. In spite of the differences between treatment zone and focal zone (see previous), the ability of a device to focus precisely is preferred if stone localization is frequently checked. There is no consensus about the optimal size of the treatment zone. Larger treatment zones may facilitate positioning but lack generous power reserves for excessively hard stones when needed. Additionally, even at lower energy settings, an increased tissue area is exposed to significant shock wave energy far beyond the dimensions of the stone treated. Whenever the power setting of a device is sufficient for stone fragmentation, a certain risk, usually small, to generate tissue lesions cannot be excluded. Single shock wave devices such as the MODULITH® SLX-F2 (STORZ MEDICAL), therefore, offer switchable focus capabilities for an individually matched treatment strategy regarding size and hardness of stones, localization, pain sensation, and other parameters.

Device Concepts

Routine lithotripsy procedures demand for ergonomic device concepts consisting of a shock wave generator, localization modality such as ultrasound and/or X-ray, a patient support, and positioning structure. Ultrasound localization provides real time control of stone location and progress of fragmentation but requires according skills of the operator that are not common in all countries. Fluoroscopic targeting seems to be preferred more widely. Both localization modalities may be applied in-line, out of the center of the shock wave source,

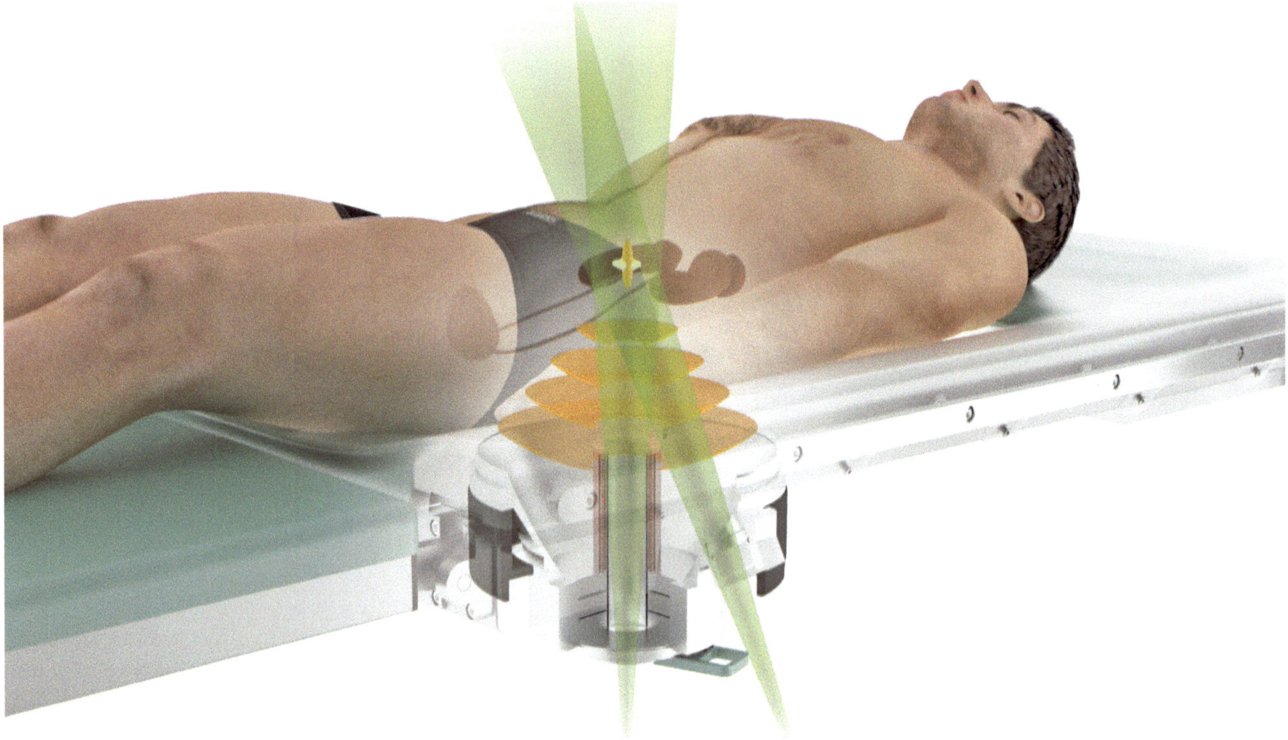

Fig. 38.13 In-line localization. Fluoroscopy or ultrasound localization arranged in-line with shock wave propagation enables precise control of stone position and quality of shock wave passage

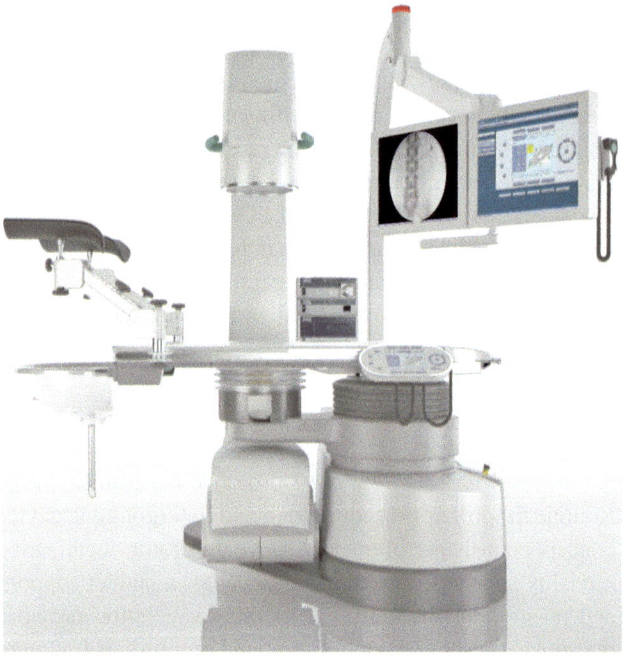

Fig. 38.14 Multifunctional urological workstation for lithotripsy, endourology, and percutaneous nephrolithotomy (*PCNL*)

meaning coaxially with the direction of shock wave propagation, or off-line, meaning outside the therapy head. The in-line configuration enables direct control of the coupling area as well as the transmission area within the body allowing for optimized treatment selection with respect to coupling direction and quality of energy transmission (Fig. 38.13).

For busy stone centers with large numbers of SWL patients, dedicated lithotripsy workstations, just for lithotripsy purposes, may be the best choice. Today's multifunctional workstations include highly flexible patient support and positioning systems as well as high-quality fluoroscopic imaging and localization devices to enable endourologic and percutaneous stone treatment procedures on the same device. A modern multifunctional workstation is shown in Fig. 38.14.

Conclusion

Extracorporeal shock wave lithotripsy is an efficient and gentle stone treatment method less invasive than percutaneous or transureteral procedures. Although SWL techniques seem to feature low risks and simple operation, excellent SWL results require special operational skills as well as technical and anatomical knowledge in order to gain full benefit of modern lithotripsy technology.

Acknowledgement The author worked from 1979 till 1987 in the field of extracorporeal shock wave lithotripsy for Dornier Medizintechnik GmbH, Münich, Germany, and from 1988 till 2009 for STORZ MEDICAL AG, Taegerwilen, Switzerland. Since 2010, he is consultant for STORZ MEDICAL AG.

References

1. Chaussy C, Brendel W, Schmiedt E. Extracorporeally induced destruction of kidney stones by shock waves. Lancet. 1980;2:1265.
2. Chaussy C, Schmiedt E, Jocham D. Extracorporeal shock wave lithotripsy (ESWL) for treatment of urolithiasis. Urology. 1984;23:59–66.
3. Wess O, Ueberle F, Dührßen R-N, Hilcken D, Krauß W, Reuner T, et al. Working group technical developments – consensus report. In: Chaussy C et al., editors. High energy shock waves in medicine. Stuttgart: Thieme Verlag; 1997. p. 63–71.
4. Rubin JI, Arger PH, Pollack HM, Banner MP, Coleman BG, Mintz MC, et al. Kidney changes after extracorporeal shock wave lithotripsy: CT evaluation. Radiology. 1987;162:21.
5. Kaude JV, Williams CM, Millner MR, Scott KN, Finlayson B. Renal morphology and function immediately after extracorporeal shock wave lithotripsy. AJR Am J Roentgenol. 1985;145:305–13.
6. Matlaga B, McAteer J, Connors B, Handa R, Evan A, Williams J, et al. Potential for cavitation-mediated tissue damage in shockwave lithotripsy. J Endourol. 2008;22:121–6.
7. Wess O, Stojan L, Rachel U. Untersuchungen zur Präzision der Ultraschallortung in vivo am Beispiel der extrakorporal induzierten Lithtripsie. 2. Konsensus Workshop der Deutschen Gesellschaft für Stosswellenlithotripsie: Die Stosswelle, Forschung und Technik. Chaussy C, Eisenberger F, Jocham D, Wilbert D, editors. Attempto Verlag Tübingen GmbH ISBN 3-89308-228-X, Medizin und Technik; 1995. p. 37–44.
8. Lokhandwalla M, Sturtevant B. Fracture mechanics model of stone comminution in ESWL and implications for tissue damage. Phys Med Biol. 2000;45:1923–40.
9. Zhong P, Xi XF, Zhu SL, Cocks FH, Preminger GM. Recent developments in SWL physics research. J Endourol. 1999;13:611–7.
10. Crum LA. Cavitation microjets as a contributory mechanism for renal calculi disintegration in ESWL. J Urol. 1988; 140:1587–90.
11. Eisenmenger W. The mechanisms of stone fragmentation in ESWL. Ultrasound Med Biol. 2001;27:683–93.
12. Sapozhnikov OA, Maxwell AD, MacConaghy B, Bailey MR. A mechanistic analysis of stone fracture in lithotripsy. J Acoust Soc Am. 2007;121:1190–202.

Laser Lithotripsy Physics

39

Joel M.H. Teichman, Jinze Qiu, Wook Kang, Kin Foong Chan, and Thomas E. Milner

Abstract

Lasers can be used as intracorporeal lithotriptors for urinary calculi. Laser lithotripsy generally involves one of two mechanisms: photoacoustic or photothermal lithotripsy. Photoacoustic lithotripsy produces large fragments but has difficulty in fragmenting calcium oxalate monohydrate, cystine, and brushite stones. Photothermal lithotripsy produces small fragments and is effective in fragmenting all stone compositions. Photothermal lithotripsy, such was with the holmium:YAG laser, tends to be slow compared to photoacoustic lithotripsy. The physics of photothermal lithotripsy is reviewed with the objective to enhance fragmentation efficiency and minimization of retropulsion.

Keywords

Laser • Lithotripsy • Holmium • Photoacoustic • Photothermal • Urinary calculus • Calcium oxalate monohydrate • Cystine

Introduction

A laser is a relatively pure form of optical energy, i.e., light. The word "laser" is an acronym for Light Amplification by Stimulated Emission of Radiation. A basic laser consists of a gain medium in a resonant optical cavity. The gain medium is an excitable material, gas, solid, or liquid, capable of releasing photons when its electrons are excited, "stimulated," or "pumped" by an external energy source. This external energy source can be electric current, chemical energy, or another light source. Since the gain medium is usually a homogeneous substance, electrons are stimulated to uniform, higher energy orbitals and release photons with identical energy when they return to their more stable, lower energy orbitals. This process results in the emission of light at a single wavelength. Thus, lasers are fundamentally different than ordinary light from a household lightbulb or the sun's rays that emit multiple wavelengths.

Amplification is usually achieved by placing the gain medium in a resonant cavity, the simplest of which is a box with two reflective surfaces on opposite ends. Imagine that the reflective surfaces act as mirrors on opposite sides and that there is no possible escape for the photons. Stimulated

J.M.H. Teichman, M.D. (✉)
Department of Urologic Sciences, University of British Columbia, 1081 Burrard Street, Vancouver, BC V6Z 1Y6, Canada
e-mail: urosec@providencehealth.bc.ca

J. Qiu, M.A. • T. E. Milner, Ph.D.
Department of Biomedical Engineering, The University of Texas at Austin, Austin, TX 78712, USA

W. Kang
American Medical Systems, Minnetonka, MN, USA

K.F. Chan, Ph.D. (✉)
VP Engineering, Dermira Inc, 2055 Woodside Road Ste 270, Redwood City, CA 94061, USA
e-mail: kin@dermira.com, kfchan@alumni.utexas.net

J.J. Talati et al. (eds.), *Urolithiasis*,
DOI 10.1007/978-1-4471-4387-1_39, © Springer-Verlag London 2012

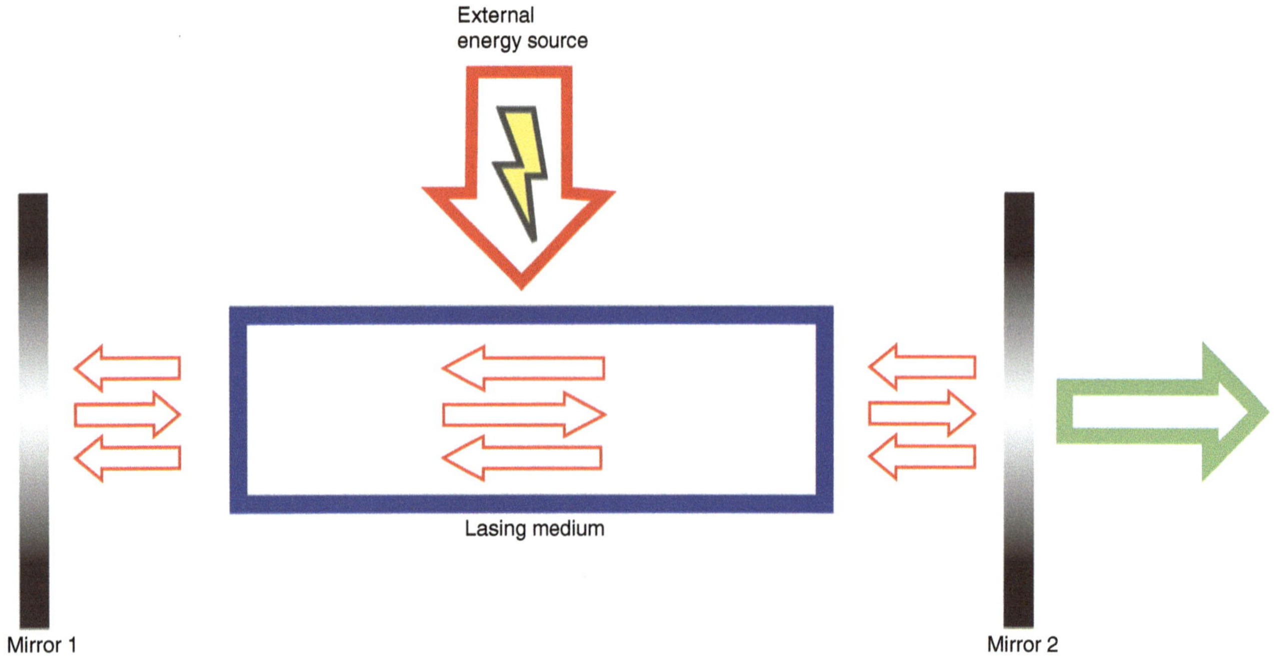

Fig. 39.1 Standard laser consists of a lasing medium, energized by an external energy source such as a flashlamp. Light oscillates between the mirrors, increasing in energy with each passage. Mirror 2 is partly transparent and the laser beam emerges as a high-quality, collimated beam of laser energy (Reprinted with permission from Teichman et al. [1])

light emission is thus reflected back and forth in the resonator through the gain medium providing further excitation and emission, with each stimulated photon having the opportunity to collide into a non-stimulated atom, in a binomial expansion, until it reaches a certain balance and the signal saturates. Furthermore, the opposite position of the mirrors produces radiation that is directional and in phase. The end result is the production of highly uniform, collimated light of a single wavelength of in-phase photons (Fig. 39.1).

In practice, the mirrors on the opposite ends of the gain medium consist of one total reflector and one partial reflector. The total reflector is ideally a 100 % reflective mirror, while the partial reflector allows a portion of the light in the resonator to escape and is the output end of the laser cavity where the laser beam is emitted. This arrangement allows for continuous emission of laser energy and is appropriately referred to as a continuous wave laser. Alternatively, the light can be released in a pulsed fashion by various mechanisms. One example is a Q-switched laser, which uses a Venetian blind or shutter mechanism to intermittently release light. Another example is a mode-locked or phase-locked laser, which takes advantage of constructive and destructive interference in the resonant cavity to produce extremely short laser light pulses. The pulse duration has important implications for the mechanics of lithotripsy. Among pulsed lasers used for lithotripsy either commercially available or available for research applications, pulse durations vary from femtoseconds to microseconds. In general, lasers for kidney stone applications are conveniently categorized on the basis of their pulse durations as ultrashort (less than 500 ns), short (1–10 μs), and long pulse (greater than 250 μs).

The first lithotripsy lasers produced used a synthetic ruby crystal as a gain medium and a flashlamp as an energy "pump"[2]. Subsequently, multiple gain media with different pumping mechanisms have been devised to deliver laser energy of different wavelengths at different energy settings. Lasers used in medical applications differ from industrial lasers in that their construction requires them to be mobile, to be readily serviced, and to withstand the rigors of clinical use.

Gas lasers are among the oldest laser types for medical applications. These lasers use a gas such as carbon dioxide as the gain medium [3]. CO_2 lasers produce laser light with a wavelength of 10,600 nm. They are the highest power continuous wave lasers that are currently available and also quite efficient. CO_2 laser light is highly absorbed by water and thus has a narrow depth of penetration. As a result, CO_2 lasers have been useful in treating penile and vulvar lesions such as superficial squamous cell carcinoma and ablative skin resurfacing but are yet to benefit stone fragmentation because fiber-optic delivery of 10.6-μm wavelengths necessary for intracorporeal lithotripsy either suffers losses in the fiber or limitations of hollow waveguides in an aqueous environment [4–6].

Dye lasers use an organic dye such as coumarin as the gain medium and are usually flashlamp pumped [7]. These lasers are both tunable (meaning the emitted wavelength can be changed) and also produce short pulse durations with resultant high peak pressures. The coumarin dye laser has a

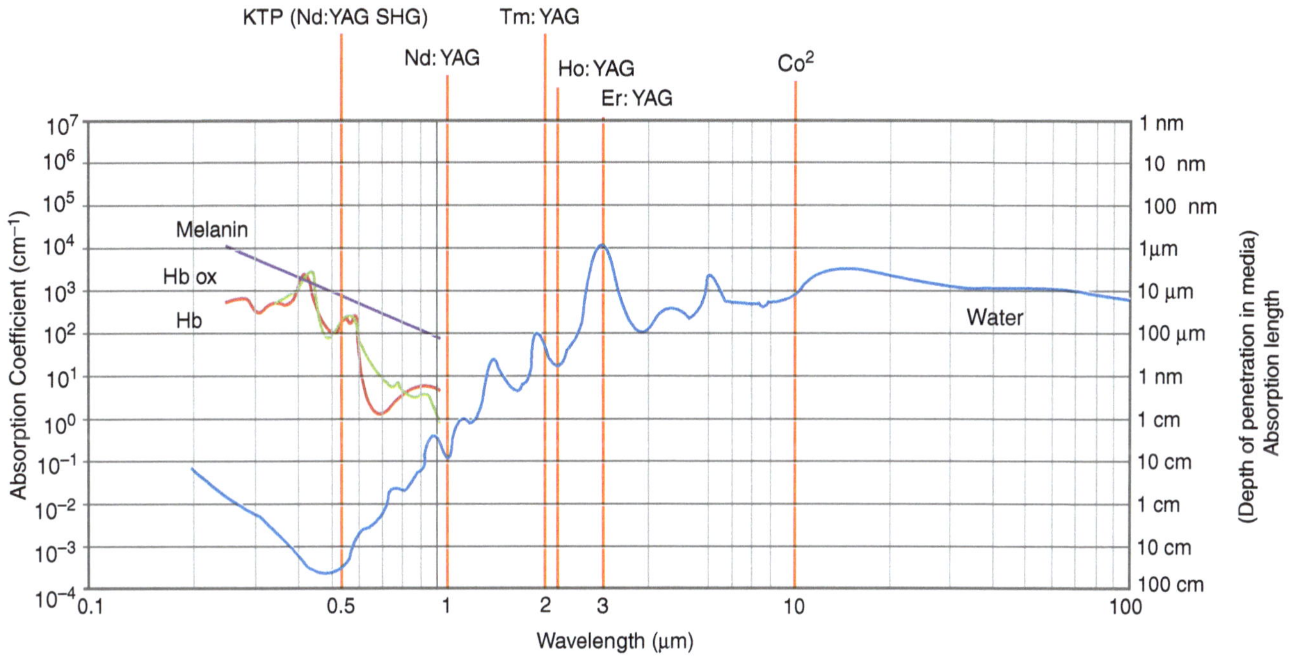

Fig. 39.2 Optical absorption coefficients of different skin components are displayed in the figure from UV to infrared spectrum. A secondary scale is displayed on the right side to show the depth of optical penetration (Adapted with permission from Teichmann et al. [10]. Copyright Springer-Verlag 2007)

wavelength of 504 nm, which is well absorbed by hemoglobin. Any excess or stray energy at 504 nm that "pass points" the stone and strikes the ureter is absorbed by hemoglobin and dissipated through blood flow, acting as an "energy sink," providing a high margin of safety during lithotripsy [8]. While they are safe, efficient lithotriptors, they tend to produce large fragments and are poorly capable of fragmenting hard stones such as cystine, brushite, or calcium oxalate monohydrate stones [8, 9].

Solid-state lasers use a solid gain medium. The solid gain medium is often composed of a crystalline host material doped with ions, which can be excited to the desired energy levels. These lasers commonly produce high output power in the near-infrared spectrum. A common laser crystal is yttrium aluminum garnet (YAG). Lasers using YAG doped with neodymium, holmium, erbium, and thulium have been produced and studied for application in urology. Of these, the long-pulse (pulse duration 250–350 μs) holmium:YAG (Ho:YAG) laser has become the dominant laser currently used for lithotripsy, due to its versatility and safety profile. Another solid-state laser lithotriptor is the FREDDY (frequency-doubled double-pulse Nd:YAG) laser. This laser uses a KTP crystal in the resonator of a Nd:YAG laser to produce and emit laser light at both 1,064 and 532 nm simultaneously.

Diode lasers use a semiconductor. A thin wafer crystal is doped with a thin layer of holes and electrons creating a charge bias across the semiconductor. Typically, the energy source is electrical. Diodes are most commonly used in nonmedical applications such as barcode scanners and CD and DVD players. In medicine, the most common clinical diode lasers operate at 800–980 nm and are used primarily for soft tissue applications. Recent experiments of diode lasers at 1.9 μm show potential application for kidney stones. The relative absorptions of hemoglobin, melanin, and water of radiation from various laser types are shown in Fig. 39.2.

Laser-Tissue Interaction

When laser energy strikes tissue, there are three possible interactions: photochemical, photothermal, and photomechanical interactions [11]. Photochemical interactions occur when laser light facilitates or catalyzes chemical reactions in tissues. This process is usually achieved by administering a photosensitive dye, which accumulates in a desired tissue. This process, known as photodynamic therapy, takes advantage of a particular dye's ability to produce singlet oxygen when stimulated by light of a certain wavelength, which can then rapidly react with any nearby biomolecules. Photosensitizers to stones have rarely been attempted for laser lithotripsy, and success has been limited. Photochemical laser mechanisms are not used for lithotripsy currently.

Photothermal interaction occurs when direct irradiation of tissues or materials by the laser light leads to vaporization and even ablation or fragmentation of tissues. Photothermal lithotripsy can occur either by direct absorption of photons by the stone crystalline structure and disruption of the lattice or by water within the lattice rapidly heating and producing fast vapor flow that in turn disrupts the lattice ("explosive vaporization" as occurs when one microwaves popcorn). Photothermal interaction is the dominant mechanism when long-pulse laser (approximately 2–500 μs/pulse) is applied [12]. For example, the free-running Ho:YAG and erbium:YAG lasers fragment stones by photothermal mechanism. Efficient fragmentation or ablation through photothermal interaction is often associated with thermal confinement, where the laser energy is delivered within a pulse duration, usually <10 ms, shorter than the time it takes for heat to diffuse away from the immediate irradiated zone, causing adequate thermal buildup within the tissue for rapid vaporization [13].

Photomechanical laser ablation occurs when the production of transient stress waves occurs from the deposition of laser energy on a tissue, material, or its surroundings, which then leads to cell death or ablation in tissues and lithotripsy in stones. The pulsed dye and FREDDY lasers are examples of photomechanical lasers [13–15]. During laser lithotripsy using short-pulse lasers (typically less than 10 μs), transient stress waves can be caused by three distinct mechanisms: thermoelastic expansion, recoil due to ejection of ablated material, and by expansion of materials undergoing phase change [12, 13]. Thermoelastic expansion waves are generated when a tissue or material expands due to transient heating by laser energy. This expansion produces a pressure wave, which travels in all directions, but is reflected at the surface of the material producing a negative pressure wave traveling inward from the surface. If the negative pressure wave is strong enough, mechanical disruption may occur—a process known as spallation. Spallation occurs when a material undergoes rapid heating or cooling. This rapid temperature cooling may produce irregular fragmentation. Secondly, when tissue ablation causes material to be ejected, conservation of momentum causes a recoil pressure wave, which may produce stress fracture deep into the actual surface of ablation [16]. Lastly, and most importantly in lithotripsy using short-pulse lasers (<1 μs), laser-induced phase changes produce significant transient pressure waves that can fragment urinary calculi [12]. One example of such a phase change is the production of plasma. Plasma is considered a fourth state of matter. It is produced by the vaporization of ions that exist in a cloud of shared, free electrons. Due to plasma's instability, rapid plasma expansion and contraction produces pressure waves capable of inducing stress fractures in the matrix of a stone. Plasma occurs with extremely short pulse durations, typically <500 ns, such as achieved with Q-switched lasers [12]. Lasers that fragment stone via plasma mechanisms produce extremely high peak pressures at the tip of the optical fiber by virtue of the ultrashort pulse duration. Another example of phase-change-induced pressure waves is the formation of cavitation bubbles, and cavitation occurs typically for lasers with pulse durations between 500 ns and 1 μs (although may continue to occur for pulse durations up to 10 μs). A cavitation bubble is caused by the rapid spherical expansion of laser-induced water vapor at the laser fiber tip [12]. The spherical bubble then rapidly collapses in the noncompressible surrounding water several hundred milliseconds later. When collapse occurs, it releases the energy stored from its generation in an instant, creating very strong pressure waves, which strain the crystal matrix of stones leading to fragmentation [12, 14]. Fragmentation due to plasma formation may produce larger fragments compared to laser-induced cavitation bubbles [12]. An exception to this trend toward larger fragments is the fragmentation of stone material from femtosecond lasers, which are currently only available in research laboratories [17]. Femtosecond ablation of hard material, such as stones, is characterized by tiny fine debris. Cavitation bubbles produce a characteristic pressure transient pattern. An initial pressure transient is caused by cavitation bubble expansion, followed by bubble collapse after the end of the pulse duration. After bubble collapse, there is a higher pressure transient caused by the release of bubble energy, leading to fragmentation. The amplitude (force) of the pressure transient is related to the maximal bubble radius (raised to the power of three) [12]. Thus, photomechanical laser lithotripsy is characterized by initial pressure transient (bubble expansion), termination of the laser pulse, bubble collapse, a second pressure transient, and subsequent lithotripsy [12, 13]. The time course differs from photothermal lithotripsy, so that photomechanical (cavitation-induced) lithotripsy produces an expanding spherical vapor bubble that after collapse produces mechanical energy that transmits to the stone and causes lithotripsy; photothermal lithotripsy produces direct irradiation of the stone and lithotripsy [12, 13]. In general, efficient fragmentation or ablation through photomechanical interaction is often associated with stress confinement, where the laser energy was delivered within a pulse duration, usually <1 μs, shorter than the time it takes for mechanical stress to propagate away from the immediate irradiated zone, causing a rapid buildup of pressure and heat within the tissue and often generating a shock wave that causes physical dissociation of the target tissue or crystalline structure.

The distribution of laser energy in tissues is important in determining the applications of a particular laser. The choice of laser wavelength depends on the optical properties of the target tissue [11]. If the tissue causes a large amount of photon scattering, less radiation is absorbed per unit tissue volume and the optical penetration is diminished. If there is minimal scattering, the only limit to penetration of laser irradiation is laser absorption by the material. If a tissue absorbs a particular wavelength well and has a low scatter, the spatial confinement will be high (high fluence). In other words, the depth of penetration is small. Conversely, a poorly absorbing material with high scatter will lead to a deep depth of penetration or low fluence [11]. The width of the laser beam also affects the confinement of laser energy. A wide beam deposits its energy over a large surface area producing a lower fluence at the same depth within the tissue than that of a narrow laser beam of the same power level [15, 16]. Finally, tissue pigmentation can affect laser distribution in tissues. Pigments preferentially absorb some wavelengths and can confine laser energy to their locations [18] (see Fig. 39.2).

Physics of Laser Lithotripsy

The ideal laser lithotripsy device produces predictable fragmentation of all stone compositions, is simple to operate and efficient, and has a wide safety margin for surrounding tissues, so there is maximal stone fragmentation with minimal collateral damage. As a general rule, photomechanical lasers have high safety margin for lithotripsy with efficient fragmentation (fast fragmentation in a short amount of time); photothermal lasers have an acceptable (but lower) safety margin with less efficient fragmentation (slower fragmentation over a longer period of time) [13]. However, photothermal lasers produce smaller fragments and fragment all stone compositions compared to photomechanical lasers [19].

Pulsed dye lasers were among the first lasers to be used clinically in lithotripsy [8, 9, 12]. Coumarin green pulsed dye lasers operate at 504–540 nm, a wavelength highly absorbed by hemoglobin (see Fig. 39.2). They fragment stones by a photomechanical mechanism [11, 13, 14]. A key component to the effective photomechanical lithotripsy of pulsed dye lasers is the short (<1 μs) pulse duration. Cavitation bubble collapse is important in dye laser lithotripsy. One advantage of this mechanism is that it obviates the need to have the laser in direct contact with the stone, since the laser-induced shock wave from cavitation bubble collapse propagates in all directions from the fiber tip and can thus be placed anywhere close to the stone to cause fragmentation. In fact, placing the fiber directly on the stone limits cavitation bubble expansion, thereby limiting the amplitude of the resultant shock wave and inhibits lithotripsy [14]. Maximal bubble expansion and therefore maximal cavitation and consequent laser-induced shock wave amplitude are achieved with a separation distance of 1 mm between fiber tip and the stone surface. Pressure transients can exceed 300 bars. Another advantage of this system is the inherent safety of these lasers. Dye laser light at 504 nm is well absorbed by hemoglobin, which acts as a laser and heat sink and protects local tissues from thermal injury (see Fig. 39.2). However, these lasers are limited by several factors. They tend to produce large, heterogeneous fragments [17]. Also, fragment ejection and high transient pressure waves can cause significant retropulsion of the stone, making lithotripsy more time-consuming and potentially more difficult [15]. Finally, fragmentation results with hard stones such as brushite, calcium oxalate monohydrate, and cystine are disappointing [20]. A common clinical scenario is to perform retrograde ureteroscopy or ureteronephroscopy for a ureteral or renal stone, respectively, that has failed shock wave lithotripsy. This scenario implies a selection bias toward durile stones (hard stones that tend not to fragment with mechanical energy) such as calcium oxalate monohydrate, brushite, or cystine that comes to endoscopic lithotripsy. It is therefore clinically relevant that the laser lithotripsy device be capable of fragmenting these durile compositions.

With ultrashort laser pulse duration (<500 ns), high peak pressures are produced by the temporal confinement of laser energy. This temporal confinement is especially important in the production of plasma as a lithotripsy mechanism, which requires large amounts of energy [21, 22]. Q-switched alexandrite and Nd:YAG lasers have been attempted for lithotripsy, but a practical limitation is that the high peak power causes fiber tip destruction and shards of optical fiber can be created within the ureter [23, 24]. Femtosecond laser lithotripsy has been described in vitro. These lasers are capable of fragmenting all stone compositions, including durile compositions such as calcium oxalate monohydrate and cystine. However, there is no practical means to deliver femtosecond laser energy through an optical fiber for clinical lithotripsy currently [17, 25, 26].

The FREDDY laser fragments stones by a similar photomechanical mechanism. By incorporating a KTP crystal in the resonator of a Nd:YAG laser, the FREDDY laser produces laser wavelengths of 532 and 1,064 nm, with pulse durations of 0.3–1.5 μs. At these pulse durations, the light at 532-nm wavelength induces plasma formation, which is further enhanced by the light at 1,064 nm, leading to high-energy pressure transients [27–29]. This laser design is cost-effective and has a high safety margin [30, 31]. Although also effective for lithotripsy, the FREDDY laser is less effective in fragmenting hard calculi [32, 33].

The Ho:YAG laser fragments stones using a photothermal mechanism [34]. Most Ho:YAG lasers generate light of a wavelength of 2.12 μm and operate at a pulse duration of 250–350 μs, significantly longer than pulse dye lasers. This long pulse duration precludes any significant stress confinement, so vapor bubble expansion and collapse are irregular in shape (i.e., not spherical), so that bubble collapse occurs at multiple loci at different times with no significant pressure transients created [35]. Time-resolved imaging studies and transient pressure wave studies of Ho:YAG lasers failed to show a significant photomechanical effect [14, 30, 36]. The pressure transients from Ho:YAG are typically between 8 and 20 bars, significantly lower than the pressure transients produced by photomechanical lasers (>300 bars) [12, 14, 30]. Most reports of clinical Ho:YAG lithotripsy employ pulse energies of <1.0 J. In tests of pulse energies at 2.0 J, the pressure transients are still in a modest range of

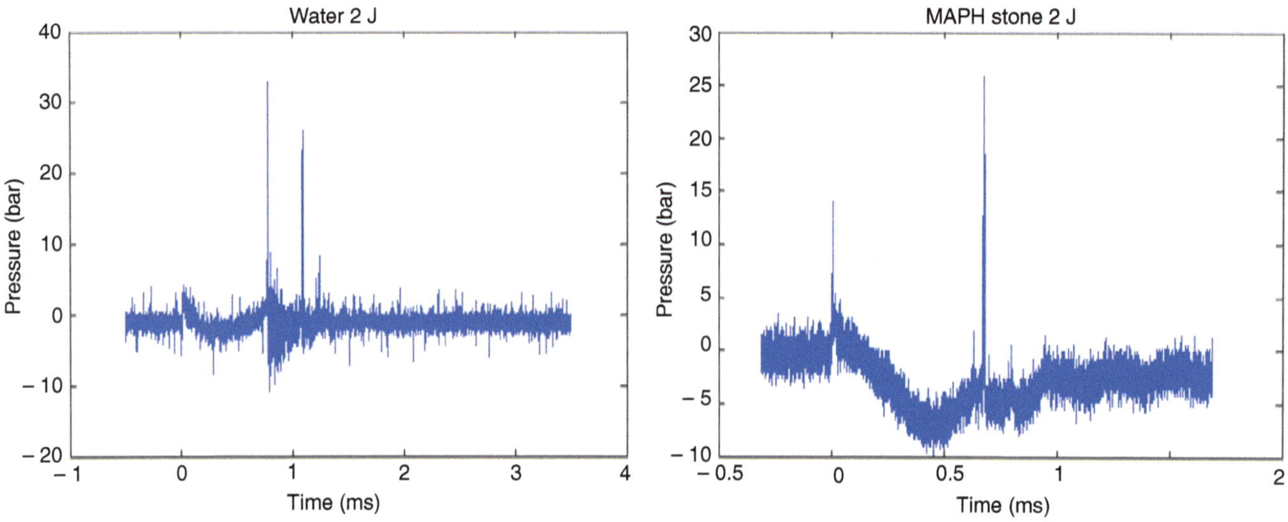

Fig. 39.3 Pressure transients in still water and contact MAPH stone lithotripsy: The optical fiber used has a core diameter of 365 μm

20–40 bars, well below the much higher pressures achieved with photomechanical lasers (Fig. 39.3).

In a series of experiments, Vassar et al. demonstrated the photothermal mechanism of the Ho:YAG laser [30]. Each of the experiments showed evidence either of direct energy absorption by the stone or paucity of pressure transients. When hydrated and dehydrated stones were irradiated in air or water, the dehydrated stones in air showed the more fragmentation. This finding indicates lack of photomechanical effect, due to the lack of aqueous medium for plasma and cavitation bubble-induced pressure transients. It also shows that water literally impedes lithotripsy as it absorbed (and dissipated) energy from direct absorption by the stone. High-speed imaging also shows the dynamics of Ho:YAG laser lithotripsy: An initial period of up to 60 μs is required to vaporize the water between the fiber tip and the stone surface, after which the energy is more efficiently coupled through vapor to the stone—called the "Moses effect" (as if Moses parted the water on flight from Egypt) [13, 14, 30]. Again, this phenomena shows how water absorbs and dissipates long-pulse Ho:YAG energy compared to photomechanical lithotripsy where water is required to produce a cavitation bubble. During Ho:YAG lithotripsy, fragment ejection begins 60-μs into a 250-μs pulse, while the laser continues to emit. This time course whereby lithotripsy occurs during the pulse (rather than after the pulse) is consistent with direct energy absorption as opposed to cavitation bubble collapse dynamics. Another finding is that the Ho:YAG laser produces more lithotripsy when oriented at 90° to the stone surface (normal incidence), indicating that direct irradiation is relevant, and energy density is critical to reach criterion threshold for ablation; when the laser fiber tip is placed in contact with the stone surface but oriented parallel to the stone surface (90-degree laser incidence), a large vapor bubble forms, but no ablation occurs [37]. In contrast to photomechanical lasers, the angle of orientation between the fiber tip and stone makes little difference in fragmentation. Indeed, other studies show that incident angle is correlated to Ho:YAG lithotripsy efficiency [38–40]. Further evidence of photothermal mechanism included the production of thermal breakdown products during lithotripsy with the Ho:YAG laser and enhanced lithotripsy when stones were irradiated at room temperature versus cold [30].

The impact of pulse duration is integral to mechanism. In an important experiment, Jansen et al. fired a holmium:YAG laser through an optical fiber in still water (no stone) varying the pulse duration and used high-speed images to document the vapor bubble dynamics for each pulse duration [35]. At 500-ns pulse duration (using a Q-switch), large spherical cavitation bubbles were created, which collapsed to a single locus, releasing significant ripples (pressure transients) in the water. As the laser pulse duration was expanded, the vapor bubble became less spherical and the collapse events occurred at multiple loci, producing less ripples in water. As the pulse duration was lengthened to 260 μs, the bubble became pear shaped and collapsed asymmetrically with no ripples seen. Thus, the long-pulse Ho:YAG laser used currently does not create any significant photomechanical effect (Fig. 39.4) [15, 37]. There is roughly a linear correlation between the pulse energy applied and the volume of ablation crater created with long-pulse Ho:YAG lithotripsy (Fig. 39.5).

Ho:YAG lasers do exhibit some limitations. The generation of small, powderized fragments means less efficient lithotripsy and longer procedure times [41]. This inefficiency can be overcome by simply increasing the energy or frequency settings, but the higher efficiency comes at the cost of more retropulsion, higher risk of collateral tissue damage, and tip degradation with energy settings >1.0 J [42]. Several

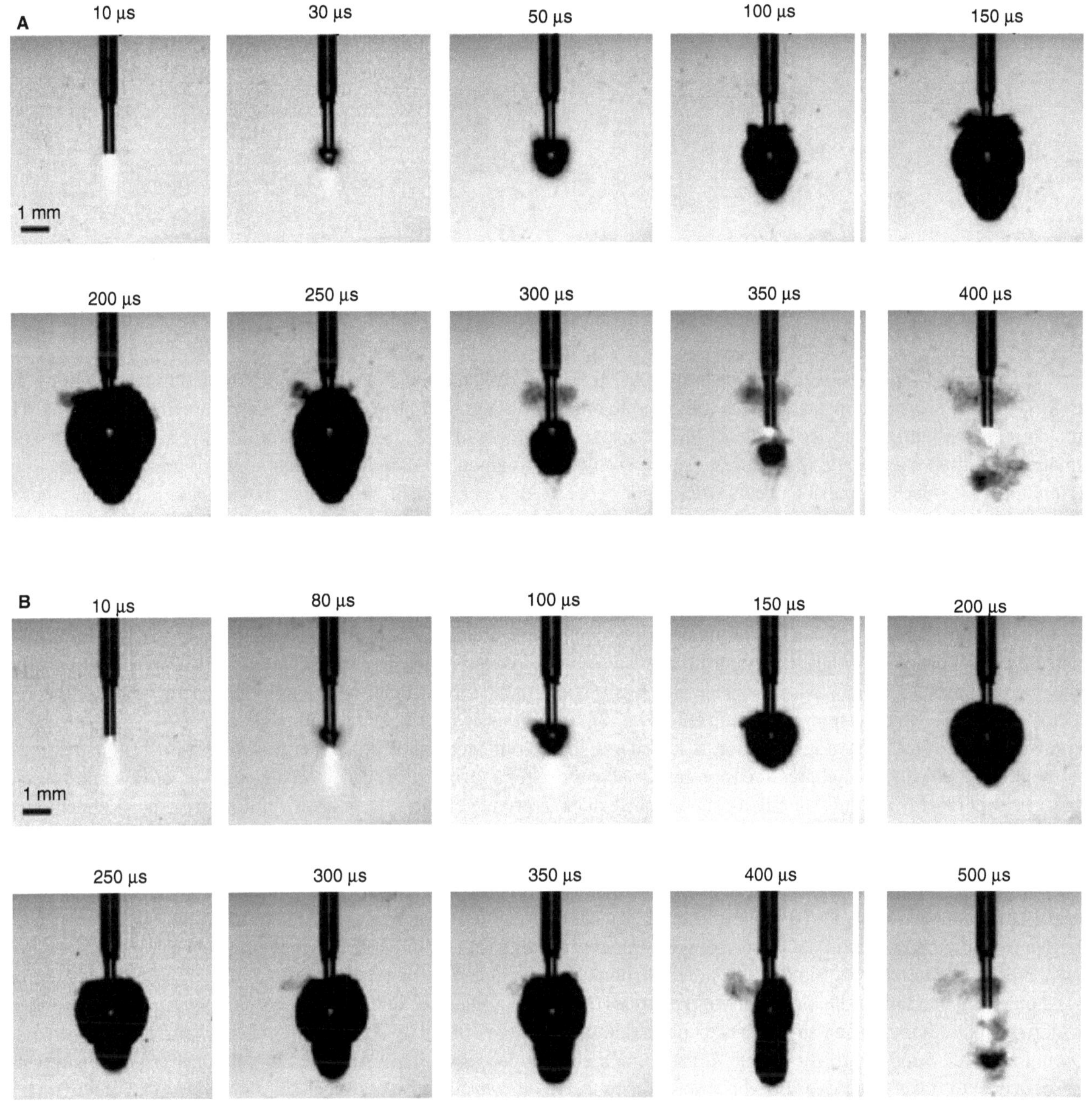

Fig. 39.4 Compilation of bubble expansion and collapse at room temperature for two pulse durations: (**a**) short pulse, (**b**) long pulse. Fiber diameter 365 µ, energy 800 mJ. Elapsed time after initiation of pulse shown above each image (Reprinted with permission from Kang et al. [16]. Copyright 2006 Wiley-Liss, Inc., a subsidiary of John Wiley & Sons, Inc)

experiments have demonstrated that use of higher pulse energies with the Ho:YAG laser produces more lithotripsy for a given dosimetry (i.e., the same total energy). One experiment showed that when stones were stabilized in vitro with forceps, maximal fragmentation was achieved with 2.0-J pulse energy settings compared to lower pulse energy settings despite the same total energy exposure. In another set of in vitro experiments, this same phenomenon was observed: more lithotripsy at 2.0-J pulse energy compared with lower pulse energies. However, at low pulse energies (0.2–0.5 J), lithotripsy produces tiny stone debris (less than 1 mm), whereas at high pulse energies (1–2 J), more "chunks" larger than 1 mm were produced. And when stones were not constrained, higher pulse energy produced more retropulsion and correspondingly decreased fragmentation. Thus, laser lithotripsy efficiency is largely a balance between fragmentation per time, maintaining small dust fragments and reducing retropulsion.

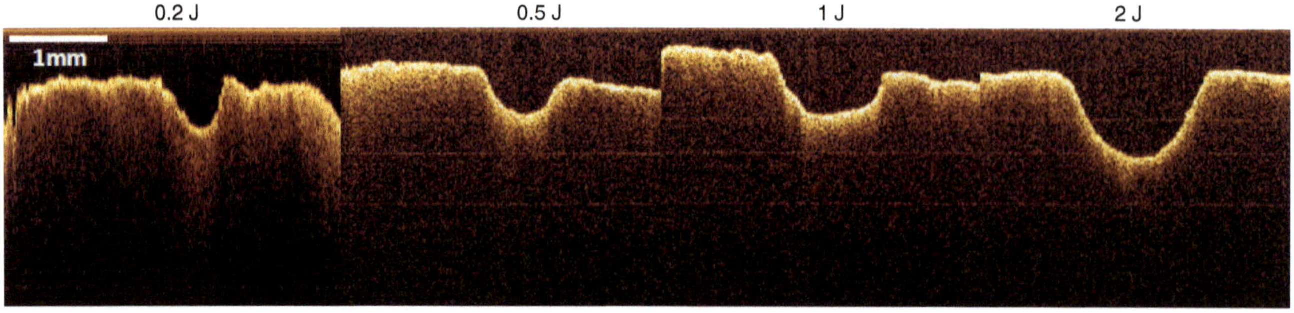

Fig. 39.5 Cross-sectional optical computed tomography images of ablation craters: The demonstrated stone is uric acid

Retropulsion is an occasional issue with Ho:YAG lithotripsy at normal energy settings but is less compared to other intracorporeal lithotripsy devices such as electrohydraulic lithotripsy, pulsed dye lasers, or pneumatic devices. With holmium:YAG, stone retropulsion occurs from vapor bubble expansion and collapse, the momentum imparted by debris ejection [15]. Lee et al. showed that fragments always eject at a right angle from the stone surface, regardless of the incident angle [15]. A large-diameter fiber creates a wide, shallow crater, allowing for greater *x*-axis vectors of plume ejection and increased retropulsion. In contrast, a small fiber creates narrow, deep craters, with more *y*-axis vectors ejecting less *x*-axis vector debris, so retropulsion is minimized (Fig. 39.6). Another strategy to minimize retropulsion is to prolong the pulse duration. Since the recoil pressure is proportional to the radiant power (energy per pulse duration), shorter pulse durations with high energy density produce higher retropulsion. In addition, faster debris ejection along with stronger momentum during shorter pulse durations even augments recoil pressure and retropulsion (Fig. 39.7). Experimentally, extended long pulse duration holmium:YAG lasers achieve less retropulsion/pulse and less retropulsion/unit of stone ablation [15, 44]. Some commercially available holmium:YAG lasers offer a "normal" pulse duration and an "extended" pulse duration. During Ho:YAG laser lithotripsy, bubble formation and collapse frequently take place due to light absorption by surrounding irrigation. Kang et al. demonstrated that short pulse durations yield faster rate of bubble generation in association with higher collapse pressure than long pulse durations (Fig. 39.8) [15]. Stronger pressure transients as well as high-speed liquid jet formation account for more stone retropulsion during short-pulse (350-μs electrical pulse duration, 170-μs FWHM, or optical duration) lithotripsy compared to extended-pulse (700-μs electrical pulse duration, 320-μs FWHM, or optical duration) lithotripsy. Although the exact role of bubble dynamics has not been determined, a fiber tip should always make contact with stone surface to minimize any energy loss by water absorption and its secondary effect of bubble collapse on stone retropulsion. Overall, stone retropulsion during laser lithotripsy can be reduced by increasing the pulse duration and implementing smaller-diameter fibers.

What are the most efficient power settings to employ for Ho:YAG lithotripsy? There are competing objectives. The single most important objective is to achieve as much stone fragmentation with a given amount of power or time. From this perspective, increasing pulse energy (keeping power constant) achieves maximum fragmentation [15, 45, 46]. However, increasing pulse energy produces greater retropulsion and therefore decouples the fiber tip from the stone surface, so increasing energy is absorbed by water (rather than the stone). As a result, increasing pulse energy settings risk reduced lithotripsy efficiency. If stones are prevented from retropulsion, then increasing pulse energy settings increase lithotripsy efficiency, although fragment sizes are larger compared to low pulse energy settings [44, 45]. Interestingly, for a given pulse energy, an increased repetition rate does not produce more retropulsion but does increase fragmentation. Thus, the optimal power setting depends on the outcome desired: Low pulse energy at a fast repetition rate produces fine, powderized fragmentation debris but overall a slower fragmentation rate compared to using high pulse energy settings at risk of larger fragmentation chunks [45].

One way to overcome some of the limitations of current photothermal lithotripsy is to use lasers with wavelengths more efficiently absorbed by renal calculi. Experiments with free-electron lasers showed that lithotripsy is more efficient at wavelengths between 2.9 and 3.1 μm as compared to 2.1 μm (Ho:YAG wavelength) [16]. The erbium:YAG laser has a wavelength of 2.9–2.94 μm, making it a potentially more efficient lithotriptor than the Ho:YAG laser. Similar to the Ho:YAG laser, experiments have shown the Er:YAG laser operates with a paucity of photomechanical effects, has similar vapor bubble characteristics, and ablates multiple stone types with symmetric ablation craters [47, 48]. Er:YAG and Ho:YAG lasers were compared experimentally at similar energy levels. Er:YAG lasers produced more lithotripsy than Ho:YAG lasers but with marginally larger fragments at 50 mJ. However, when Ho:YAG lasers were ramped up to 500 J, the amount of lithotripsy was similar to the Er:YAG laser at 50 J. Although there was some difference at the same energy output, similar amounts of lithotripsy can be achieved by simply increasing the Ho:YAG power and frequency settings. But

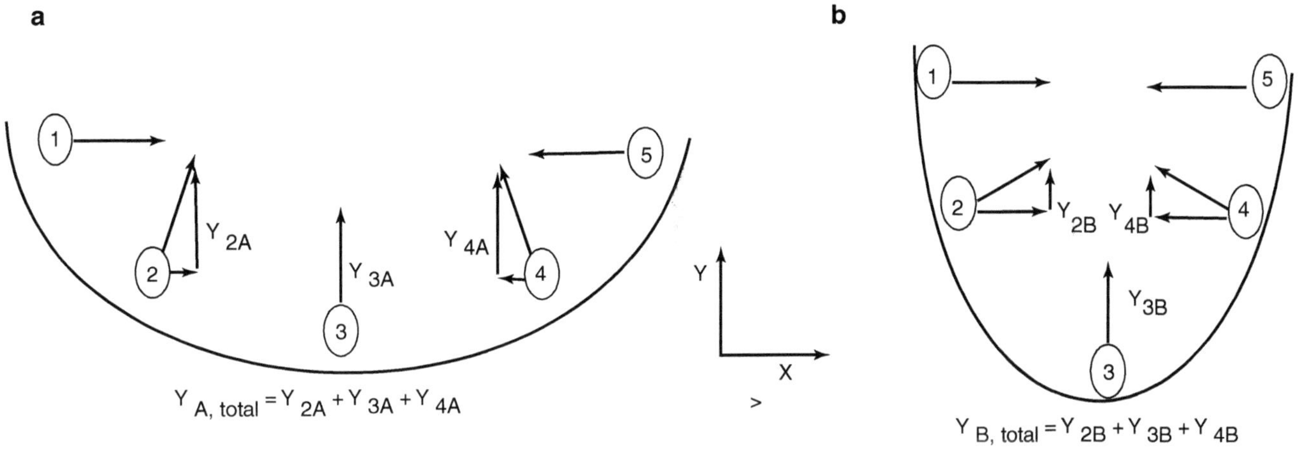

Fig. 39.6 Diagram of ejection of ablated stone particles from a wide versus narrow laser fiber. (**a**) Wide and shallow crater. (**b**) Narrow and deep crater. Note the total vector in the Y direction greater for the wider crater (Reprinted with permission from Lee et al. [43]. Copyright Elsevier 2003)

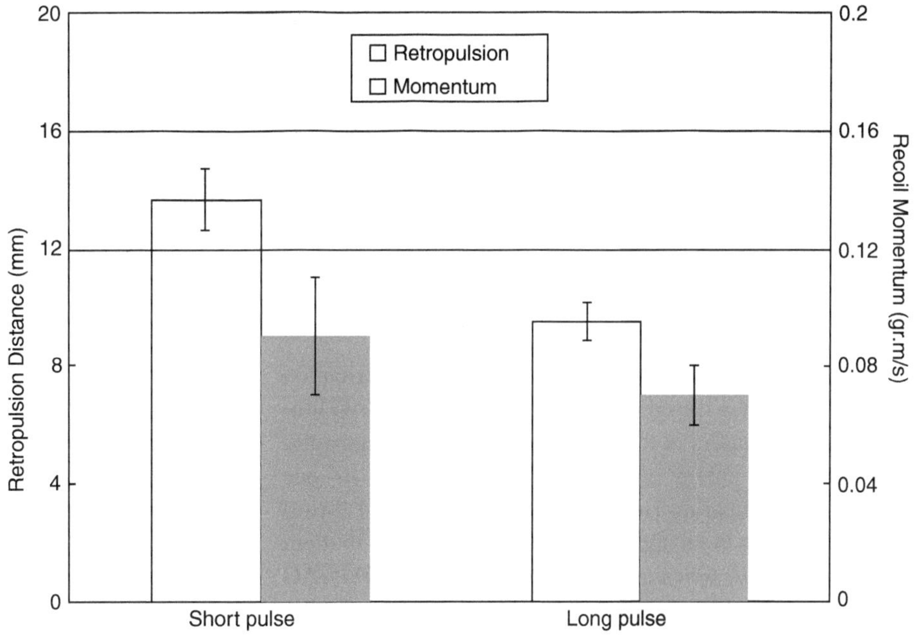

Fig. 39.7 Comparison of stone retropulsion distance (mm, left vertical axis) and corresponding recoil momentum (g·m/s, right vertical axis) between short pulse (~170 μs at FWHM) and long pulse (~320 μs at FWHM). Fiber diameter 550 μm, pulse energy 1 J, and single pulse on stone phantom

high energy output may cause fiber tip damage and irregular beam output [49]. Erbium and holmium lasers were also compared in vitro [35]. Both were controlled for focal length, energy density, and beam width and profile. Pulse energies varied between 0.2 and 1 J for each. For a single laser pulse, crater volumes were five times greater for all stone types with Er:YAG lasers than Ho:YAG lasers [50]. Clinical use of erbium lasers is limited most importantly by the lack of clini cally useful laser fibers [44]. The relatively inexpensive and reusable low OH silica fibers used with holmium lasers do not transmit laser light from an erbium laser adequately. This is due to energy absorption at the input end of the laser, which can lead to thermal degradation and damage to the fiber and laser. Fluoride fibers are another option for laser fiber material and do transmit Er:YAG irradiation successfully, but tend to be brittle, and have a hygroscopic structure. Single crystal sapphire fibers present another option, but their cost is prohibitive, they only transmit energy adequately up to 200 mJ if a diameter of 425 μm is chosen, and they risk damage at their output ends due to high peak power levels. Fibers still being considered include compound fibers of germanium oxide with silica tips and hollow waveguides (cylindrical tubes that transmit infrared energy). While compound fibers are still under investigation, hollow waveguide fibers have been tested experimentally. Some initial studies showed good flexibility and strength, with energy transmission sufficient to fragment calculi. However, problems remain, including the generation of hot spots and irregular ablation craters [51, 52].

Another promising approach is to use diode lasers emitting at 1.9 μm. A diode emits laser energy in a top-hat

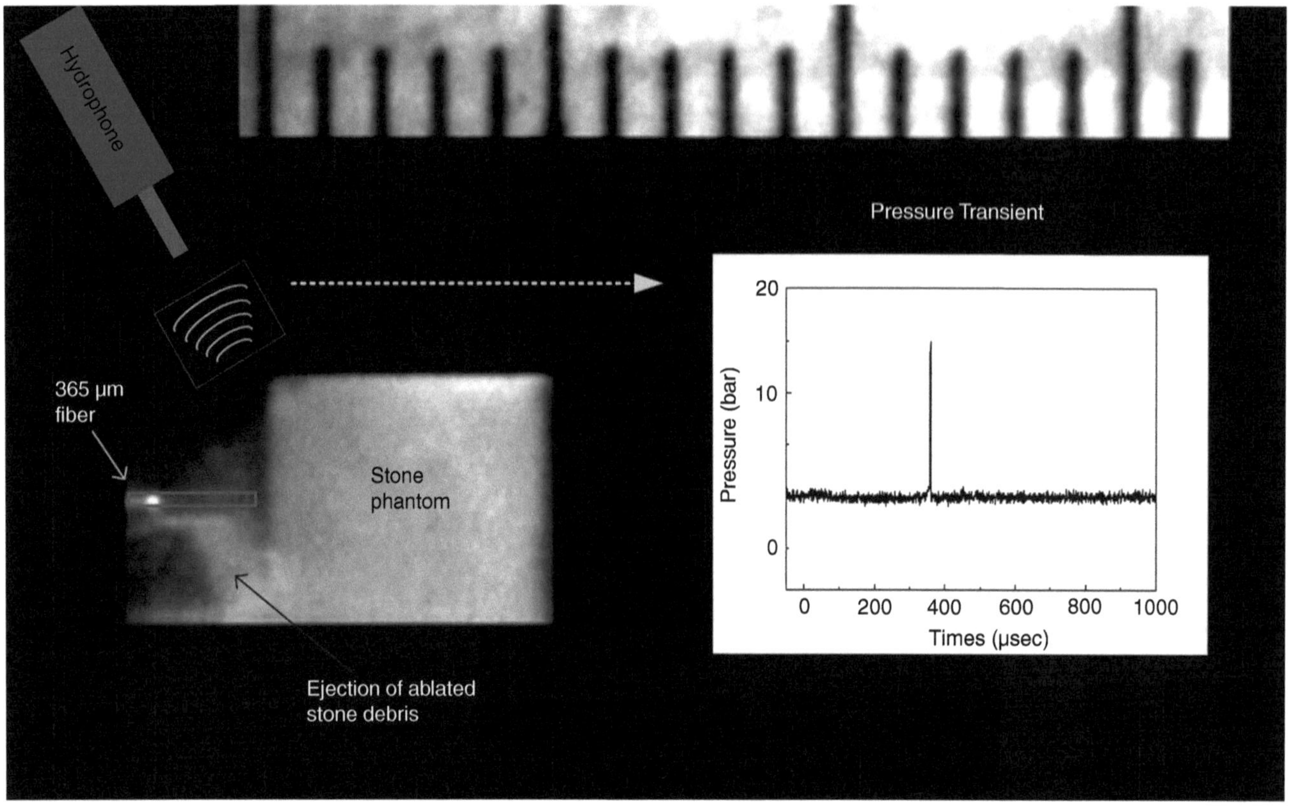

Fig. 39.8 Image of debris ejection during short-pulse (~150 μs at FWHM) irradiation with contact laser lithotripsy (fiber diameter 365 μm, pulse energy 800 mJ, and single pulse). Pressure transient was measured by a PVDF needle hydrophone during laser-stone fragmentation (~15 bars at short pulse versus ~5 bars at long pulse of ~280 μs at FWHM)

configuration compared to the nearly Gaussian distribution of photons seen in doped laser crystals such as Ho:YAG lithotripsy. Diode lasers in theory can achieve more fragmentation per unit energy compared with Ho:YAG. In one experiment comparing Ho:YAG and thulium fiber (1.9-μm) laser lithotripsy in an apples-to-apples comparison, thulium fragmented 5–10 times as much stone material as Ho:YAG for the same total energy applied [53]. Current power limitations and cost of current diode lasers preclude clinical utility. An obvious potential advantage of this technology is the ability to provide an effective laser lithotripsy tool in a small, portable laser fiber package that a urologist could carry from operating room to operating room. The laser fiber would "plug" into an electrical wall outlet, and the distal end of the laser fiber would be inserted as a trunk fiber into a distal fiber cap. A tapered fiber may reduce wear and tear ("burnback") of thulium fiber tip during lithotripsy [54].

Optical Fibers

Basic fiber design consists of an inner circular core surrounded by two to three layers of cladding and a surrounding jacket. Both glasses and polymers can be used as core materials. Among the glasses, silica (amorphous silicon dioxide SiO_2) is the dominant material. The first lasers used clinically in urology used silica fibers. These are ideal laser fibers as they transmit laser energy well with minimal attenuation, are relatively inexpensive, and are small and flexible enough to be used in endoscopic instruments. Ho:YAG lasers use low OH silica fibers since the hydroxyl groups absorb light readily at 2,100 nm, thus reducing transmission of light and potentially causing fiber damage [10]. A high OH concentration is better for UV transmission. Cladding types can also differ. Cladding constructed of fluorine-doped silica has better laser light confinement and a smaller bending radius than fluoroacrylate cladding, which can generate light leakage and damage with lasers of 2-μm wavelength [55]. Most fibers also have a third layer of cladding, called a buffer layer. The buffer often consists of ethylene tetrafluoroethylene (ETFE, Tefzel), which protects the fiber from external mechanical damage.

The laser-fiber interface is usually composed of a protective connector that holds the proximal end of the laser fiber in the proper orientation to receive energy from the laser itself. The subminiature version A connector (SMA) is the industry standard connector, allowing different lasers to accept multiple laser fiber sizes and brands (Fig. 39.9). It consists of a central reinforced housing surrounded by a con-

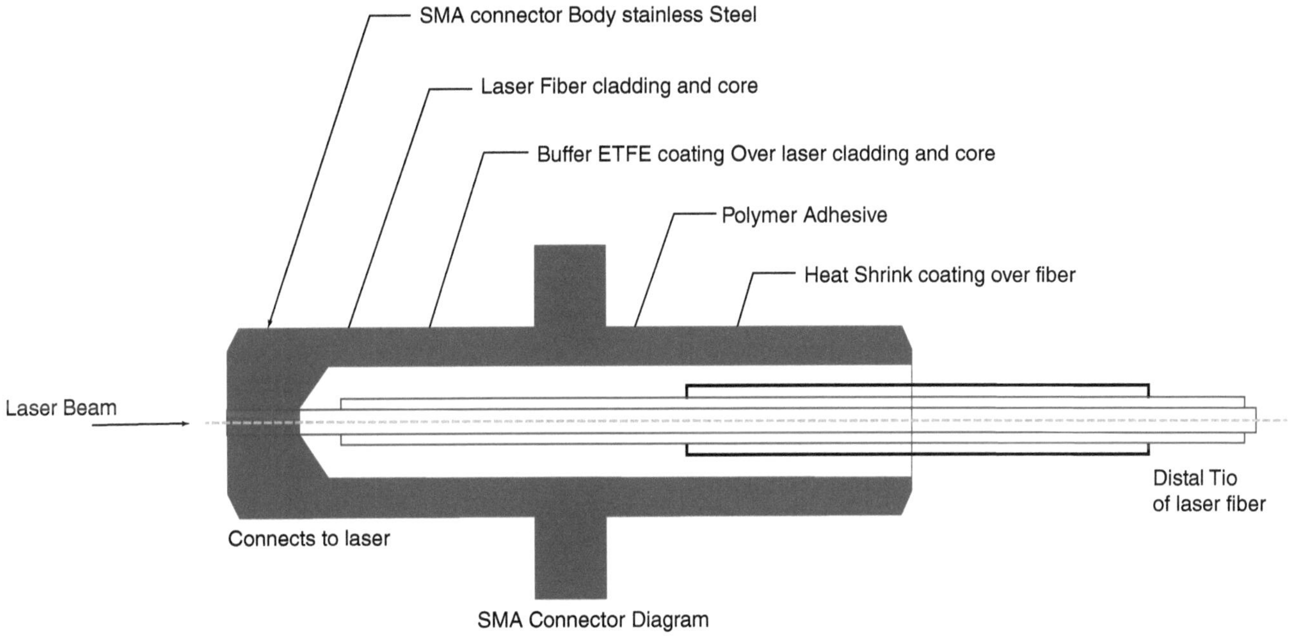

Fig. 39.9 Typical SMA connector. Connector interfaces between laser and laser fiber. Heat shrink-wrap overlaps laser fiber as it enters connector, providing stiffness and decreased mechanical stress at junction. Polymer adhesive envelops laser fiber inside connector (Reprinted with permission from Nazif et al. [55]. Review. Copyright Mary Ann Liebert 2004)

nector shell. The housing is often a polymer material, and the shell is usually composed of steel. The end of the laser fiber exiting the shell is shrink-wrapped in a plastic coating to guard against mechanical damage. With regular use, there will be some misalignment of the laser and the proximal fiber end, which can result in higher-order rays, attenuation, or fiber breakdown. At the input end, stray laser light can be absorbed by the steel shell, which can then vaporize. The condensation of the vapor coats the outer surface of the laser, disrupting its optics and leading to failure. Manufacturers use various mechanisms and engineering to couple the laser to the proximal fiber connector. There are advantages and disadvantages to each design, and a more detailed explanation may be found in Nazif et al. [50].

Urologists may confuse the collimated laser emission generated from ideal lasers as the output from laser fibers. The fiber designs used currently lead to non-collimated output. The collimated laser beam is focused through a lens, so that a convergent beam is delivered from the lens to the proximal fiber tip and the beam launches as a divergent beam down the fiber [50]. If the energy is not launched with a "bull's-eye" strike down the center of the fiber, off-axis rays are increased and proximal fiber failure risk is increased [56]. In order to conduct laser light without having excessive losses or thermal damage, most of the light must be reflected within the fiber to the very distal tip, where it is discharged. This principle, referred to as total internal reflection, is utilized in laser fiber technology. Photons bounce off the cladding and reflect back down the core fiber, where they bounce off the opposite wall cladding, like billiard balls bouncing off the side of a pool table. When light strikes a surface, a portion of it is reflected and a portion may be refracted, depending on the refractive index of both the environment and the material. The refractive index of a material describes how quickly it allows light to pass through it. When light coming from a denser environment strikes a less dense substance, the angle to the normal at which it refracts, or bends, is larger than the incident angle of incoming light. As the incident angle to normal becomes wider, the refracted light in the less dense substance will eventually travel at a 90-degree angle to the normal, or parallel to the surface of the substance. In other words, light will not penetrate into the less dense substance. At this angle of incident light, there is total internal reflection, and laser light is not absorbed by the cladding at all and reflects entirely inside the core fiber. In contrast, if laser approaches the cladding at a more normal incidence, the light refracts and may not reflect. As an example, a pebble can be skipped along the surface of water with a wide incident angle, whereas dropping the pebble at the water surface (narrow incident angle) causes the pebble to fall into the water. The implications for fiber transmission is significant: A laser that launches light with too divergent a beam risks refraction into the cladding, whereas a laser that launches light with a narrowly divergent beam has less risk of refraction into the cladding. The limit of beam divergence a fiber can safely transmit is characterized by the numerical aperture (NA). NA provides a description of what maximum acceptance angle of laser light will provide total internal reflection for a certain fiber. The NA of Ho:YAG lasers ranges from 0.2 to 0.22. An NA of 0.21 corresponds to a maximum acceptance angle of 12°. Despite total internal reflection, some light will partially penetrate the cladding. These penetrating light waves, known as evanescent waves, can damage cladding if they are strong enough. They are accentuated by bending of the fiber.

Bending of the laser fiber can also affect the reflection of light. The high number of bends, or amount of bending, produces a greater number of internal reflections. If the reflected angles produced are smaller than the critical angle, some energy will transmit through the cladding. This is especially damaging in the case of near-infrared lasers such as Ho:YAG, as their wavelengths are well absorbed by plastics. This problem is occasionally encountered during retrograde ureteronephroscopy for lower pole renal calculi, where the flexible ureteroscope is maximally deflected to orient the fiber to the lower pole stone. Laser energy refracts into the cladding at the site of maximal deflection and causes fiber and ureteroscope destruction and possible patient injury [42, 57]. Thulium fiber laser lithotripsy may be advantageous with a "top-hat" beam profile less at risk of photons refracting into the cladding compared to Ho:YAG lithotripsy [47].

The positioning of the fiber during laser lithotripsy is also an important factor to consider. Since an important difference between short-pulse and long-pulse lasers for lithotripsy is that with short pulse duration lasers (<1 μs) where photomechanical lithotripsy occurs, a separation distance of 1 mm between the fiber tip and the stone surface yields maximal fragmentation due to the importance of maximal bubble expansion and collapse-induced pressure transients [12, 14]. In contrast, long-pulse Ho:YAG and Er:YAG lasers (250–350 μs) achieve maximal lithotripsy efficiency in contact mode, as the energy is absorbed efficiently by water [13, 16, 30, 31]. To minimize the amount of Ho:YAG or Er:YAG lost to vaporize a water channel ("Moses effect"), the laser fiber should be placed in contact with the stone surface.

However, the interaction between optical fiber tip and the stone surface during Ho:YAG lithotripsy may lead to fiber tip degradation with irregular laser output and reduced fragmentation efficiency. This "burnback" may reflect the quality of the fiber materials, the stone compositions, and the pulse energy used. Limited data implies that "burnback" is increased with higher pulse energies, but this assertion awaits more testing.

Conclusion

An understanding of the physics of laser design and function will allow the urologist to make informed decisions regarding the clinical application of laser technology in their practice. Central to the clinical application of lasers in urology is basic knowledge of the interaction of lasers with biological tissues and their environments. The physics of laser lithotripsy is one of the most studied applications of lasers in urology, and its understanding is important clinically and also relevant in the advent of new and better laser technology. Lastly, the optical delivery of laser energy is an important component of laser technology with implications for the types of lasers that can be used, how they can be used, and for urological instruments and equipment. In this chapter, we have summarized key points regarding laser physics, which should prove useful to the urologist as it applies to stone disease. As investigators gain further insight into the physics of lasers in urology, further advancements will make lasers in urology safer and more efficient.

References

1. Teichman JMH, et al. Chapter 6a. Lasers. In: Smith AD, Badlani GH, Bagley DH, editors. Smith's textbook of endourology. 2nd ed. Hamilton: BC Decker; 2007. p. 37–40. ISBN: 1-55009-365-7.
2. Maiman TH. Stimulated optical radiation in ruby. Nature. 1960;187:493–4.
3. Patel CK, Mc Farlane RA, Faust WL. Selective excitation through vibrational energy transfer and optical maser action in N_2–CO_2. Physiol Rev. 1964;13:617–9.
4. Rosemberg SK. Carbon dioxide laser treatment of external genital lesions. Urology. 1985;25:555–8.
5. Rosemberg SK. Lasers and squamous cell carcinoma of external genitalia. Urology. 1986;27:430–3.
6. Greenbaum SS, Glogau R, Stegman SJ, et al. Carbon dioxide laser treatment of erythroplasia of Queyrat. J Dermatol Surg Oncol. 1989;15:747–50.
7. Sorokin PP, Lankard JR. Stimulated emission observed from an organic dye, chloroaluminium phthalocyanine. IBM J Res Dev. 1966;10:162.
8. Dretler SP, Watson G, Parrish JA, Murray S. Pulsed dye laser fragmentation of ureteral calculi: initial clinical experience. J Urol. 1987;137:386–9.
9. Bhatta KM, Nishioka NS. Effect of pulse duration on microsecond-domain laser lithotripsy. Lasers Surg Med. 1989;9:454–7.
10. Teichmann HO, Herrmann TR, Bach T. Technical aspects of lasers in urology. World J Urol. 2007;25:221–5. Epub (2007) May 30.
11. Jacques SL. Laser-tissue interactions. Photochemical, photothermal, and photomechanical. Surg Clin North Am. 1992;72(3): 531–58.
12. Berlien H-P, Muller G. Applied laser medicine. Berlin: Springer; 2003.
13. Rink K, Delacrétaz G, Salathé RP. Fragmentation process of current laser lithotriptors. Lasers Surg Med. 1995;16:134–46.
14. Chan KF, Pfefer TJ, Teichman JMH, Welch AJ. A perspective on laser lithotripsy: the fragmentation processes. J Endourol. 2001;15:257–73.
15. Zhong P, Tong HL, Cocks FH, Pearle MS, Preminger GM. Transient cavitation and acoustic emission produced by different laser lithotripters. J Endourol. 1998;12:371–8.
16. Kang HW, Lee H, Teichman JM, Oh J, Kim J, Welch AJ. Dependence of calculus retropulsion on pulse duration during Ho: YAG laser lithotripsy. Lasers Surg Med. 2006;38:762–72.
17. Qiu JZ, Teichman JMH, Wang TY, Neev J, Glickman RD, Chan KF, Milner TE. Femtosecond laser lithotripsy: feasibility and ablation mechanism. J Biomed Opt. 2010;15:028001 (Apr 14, 2010).

18. Chan KF, Hammer DX, Choi B, Teichman JMH, McGuff HS, Pratisto H, Jansen ED, Welch AJ. Free electron laser lithotripsy: threshold radiant exposures. J Endourol. 2000;14:161–7.
19. Teichman JM, Vassar GJ, Bishoff JT, Bellman GC. Holmium:YAG lithotripsy yields smaller fragments than lithoclast, pulsed dye laser or electrohydraulic lithotripsy. J Urol. 1998;159(1):17–23.
20. Dretler SP. An evaluation of ureteral laser lithotripsy: 225 consecutive patients. J Urol. 1990;143:267–72.
21. Fradin D, Bass M. Electron avalanche breakdown induced by ruby laser light. Appl Phys Lett. 1973;22(5):206–8.
22. Doukas AG, Zweig AD, Frisoli JK, Birngruber R, Deutsch TF. Non-invasive determination of shock wave pressure generated by optical breakdown. Appl Phys B. 1991;53:237–45.
23. Denstedt JD, Chun SS, Miller MD, Eberwein PM. Intracorporeal lithotripsy with the Alexandrite laser. Lasers Surg Med. 1997; 20:433–6.
24. Pearle MS, Sech SM, Cobb CG, Riley JR, Clark PJ, Preminger GM, Drach GW, Roehrborn CG. Safety and efficacy of the Alexandrite laser for the treatment of renal and ureteral calculi. Urology. 1998; 51:33–8.
25. Denstedt JD, et al. Intracorporeal lithotripsy with the alexandrite laser. Lasers Surg Med. 1997;20:433–6.
26. Tschepe J, Gundlach P, Leege N, Hopf J, Müller G, Scherer H. The endoscopic laser lithotripsy of salivary gland calculi and the problem of fiber wear. In: Optical fibers in medicine VII, SPIE vol 1649. 1992, p. 254–63. Los Angeles, CA.
27. Helfmann J. Untersuchung der physikalischen Phanomene bei der Zertrummerung von Korperkonkrementen durch laserinduzierte Plasmen. In: Advances in laser medicine. Landsberg/Zurich: Ecomed; 1992.
28. Helfmann J, Muller G. Laser lithotripsy: process overview. Med Laser Appl. 2001;16:30–7.
29. Tischer CF, Koort H, Bazo A, Rasch R, Thiede C. Clinical experiences with a new frequency-doubled double-pulse Nd:YAG Laser (FREDDY) for the treatment of urolithiasis. In: Lasers in Surgery: Advanced Characterization, Therapeutics, and Systems XII, SPIE, vol 4609. 2002. San Jose CA.
30. Schafhauser W, Zorcher W, et al. Erste klinische Erfahrungen mit neuem frequenzverdoppeltem Doppelpuls Neodym:YAG Laser in der Therapie der Urolithiasis. In: Poster presentation at the DGU, Hamburg, 2000.
31. Stark L, Carl P, Zauner R. A new technique for Laser-Lithotripsy: FREDDY, the partially frequency-doubled double-Pulse Nd:YAG Laser. In: Poster presentation at the 1st international consultation on stone disease, Paris, 2001.
32. Dubosq F, Pasqui F, Girard F, Beley S, Lesaux N, Gattengno B, Thibault P, Traxer O. Endoscopic lithotripsy and the FREDDY laser: initial experience. J Endourol. 2006;20:296–9.
33. Stark L, Car P. First clinical experiences of laser lithotripsy using the partially frequency-doubled double-pulse neodymium:YAG laser ("FREDDY") (abstract). J Urol. 2001;165:362A.
34. Vassar GJ, Chan KF, Teichman JM, Glickman RD, Weintraub ST, Pfefer TJ, Welch AJ. Holmium: YAG lithotripsy: photothermal mechanism. J Endourol. 1999;13:181–90.
35. Jansen ED, Asshauer T, Frenz M, Motamedi M, Delacretaz G, Welch AJ. Effect of pulse duration on bubble formation and laser-induced pressure waves during holmium laser ablation. Lasers Surg Med. 1996;18:278–93.
36. Schmidlin FR, Beghuin D, Delacretaz GP, Venzi G, Jichlinksi P, Rink K, Leisinger H-J, Graber P. Laser lithotripsy with the Ho:YAG laser: fragmentation process revealed by time-resolved imaging. In: Lasers in Surgery: Advanced Characterization, Therapeutics, and Systems VIII, SPIE, vol 3245. 1998. p. 123–26. San Jose CA.
37. Chan KF, Vassar GJ, Pfefer TJ, Teichman JMH, Glickman RD, Weintraub ST, Welch AJ. Holmium:YAG laser lithotripsy: a dominant photothermal ablative mechanism with chemical decomposition of urinary calculi. Lasers Surg Med. 1999;25:22–37.
38. Freiha GS, Glickman RD, Teichman JM. Holmium:YAG laser-induced damage to guidewires: experimental study. J Endourol. 1997;11:331–6.
39. Teichman JM, Rogenes VJ, McIver BJ, Harris JM. Holmium:yttrium-aluminum-garnet laser cystolithotripsy of large bladder calculi. Urology. 1997;50:44–8.
40. Teichman JM, Rao RD, Glickman RD, Harris JM. Holmium:YAG percutaneous nephrolithotomy: the laser incident angle matters. J Urol. 1998;159:690–4.
41. Teichman JM, Rao RD, Rogenes VJ, Harris JM. Ureteroscopic management of ureteral calculi: electrohydraulic versus holmium:YAG lithotripsy. J Urol. 1997;158:1357–61.
42. Spore SS, Teichman JM, Corbin NS, Champion PC, Williamson EA, Glickman RD. Holmium: YAG lithotripsy: optimal power settings. J Endourol. 1999;13:559–66.
43. Lee H, Ryan RT, Teichman JM, Kim J, Choi B, Arakeri NV, Welch AJ. Stone retropulsion during holmium:YAG lithotripsy. J Urol. 2003;169(3):881–5.
44. Finley DS, Petersen J, Abdelshehid C, Ahlering M, Chou D, Borin J, Eichel L, McDougall E, Clayman RV. Effect of holmium:YAG laser pulse width on lithotripsy retropulsion in vitro. J Endourol. 2005;19:1041–4.
45. Wezel F, Häcker A, Gross AJ, Michel MS, Bach T. Effect of pulse energy, frequency and length on holmium:yttrium-aluminum-garnet laser fragmentation efficiency in non-floating artificial urinary calculi. J Endourol. 2010;24:1135–40.
46. Sea J, Jonat LM, Chew BH, Qiu J, Wang B, Hoopman J, Milner T, Teichman JMH. Optimal power settings for holmium:YAG lithotripsy. J Urol. 2012;187:914–9.
47. Chan KF, Lee H, Teichman JMH, Kamerer A, McGuV HS, Welch AJ. Erbium:YAG laser lithotripsy. J Urol. 2002;168:436–41.
48. Lee H, Kang HW, Teichman JM, Oh J, Welch AJ. Urinary calculus fragmentation during Ho: YAG and Er:YAG lithotripsy. Lasers Surg Med. 2006;38:39–51.
49. Lee H, Ryan RT, Teichman JM, Landman J, Clayman RV, Milner TE, Welch AJ. Effect of lithotripsy on holmium:YAG optical beam profile. J Endourol. 2003;17:63–7.
50. Teichman JM, Chan KF, Cecconi PP, Corbin NS, Kamerer AD, Glickman RD, Welch AJ. Erbium: YAG versus holmium:YAG lithotripsy. J Urol. 2001;165:876–9.
51. Iwai K, Shi Y, Matsuura Y, Miyagi M. Rugged hollow fiber for the infrared and its use in laser lithotripsy. In: Optics in Health Care and Biomedical Optics: Diagnostics and Treatment, SPIE, vol 4916. 2002. p. 115–9. Shanghai China.
52. Teichman JMH, Kang W, Glickman RD, Welch AJ. Update on Erbium:YAG lithotripsy. In: AIP conference proceedings 2007, vol 900. IOP Institute of Physics Publishing Ltd. p. 216–27. Indianapolis, Indiana.
53. Blackmon RL, Irby PB, Fried NM. Holmium:YAG (lambda = 2,120 nm) versus thulium fiber (lambda = 1,908 nm) laser lithotripsy. Lasers Surg Med. 2010;42:232–6.
54. Blackmon RL, Irby PB, Fried NM. Thulium fiber laser lithotripsy using tapered fibers. Lasers Surg Med. 2010;42:45–50.
55. Nazif OA, Teichman JMH, Glickman RD, Welch AJ. Review of laser fibers: a practical guide for urologists. J Endourol. 2004;18: 818–29.
56. Marks AJ, Mues AC, Knudsen BE, Teichman JMH. Holmium:yttrium-aluminum-garnet lithotripsy proximal fiber failures from laser and fiber mismatch. Urology. 2008;71:1049–51.
57. Knudsen BE, Glickman RD, Stallman KJ, Maswadi S, Chew BH, Beiko DT, Denstedt JD, Teichman JMH. Performance and safety of holmium: YAG laser optical fibers. J Endourol. 2005;19: 1092–7.

Bioeffects of Shock Wave Lithotripsy

40

Ehud Gnessin and James E. Lingeman

Abstract

Injudicious use of shock wave lithotripsy can lead to unwanted effects. The acute bioeffects of shock waves such as renal hemorrhage can be reduced by a number of measures, which include pretreatment with shockwaves, slowing the firing rate, and reducing the total number of shock waves delivered and the power of the shock. Improving the coupling between the patient and machine also improves effectiveness and reduces harm. Long-term effects include renal scarring and new-onset hypertension. This chapter explores the mechanisms by which these bioeffects are produced.

Keywords

Shock wave lithotripsy • Renal stones • Renal hematoma • Renal parenchymal scarring • PCNL • Acoustic coupling • Firing rate • New-onset hypertension • Cavitation bubble • Diabetes • Pretreatment • Acute adverse effects • Long-term adverse effects

Introduction

Shock wave lithotripsy (SWL) was introduced as a clinical treatment during the early 1980s by Chaussy and colleagues [1, 2]. Since the introduction of the first clinical lithotripter, the Dornier HM3 (Dornier MedTech America, Kennesaw, GA, USA), to the United States [3] and worldwide, SWL has been accepted as the primary noninvasive treatment for renal and ureteral stones.

At the time of its introduction, SWL was applied to a wide range of upper tract calculi. SWL soon found application in even complex cases such as multiple stones, bilateral stones, and staghorn calculi [4]. However, as experience with lithotripsy grew, urologists began to recognize its limitations. Some stone types (e.g., calcium oxalate monohydrate, brushite, and cystine stones) could be resistant to SWL. Also, renal anatomic issues (lower pole calyx, acute infundibulopelvic angle, calyceal diverticula, ureteropelvic junction obstruction) could pose a barrier to the clearance of stone fragments [5]. The effectiveness of lithotripsy is also affected by body mass index; studies indicate poorer outcomes when skin-to-stone distance is greater than about 10 cm [6]. In addition, the relatively limited capacity of the ureter to discharge stone fragments restricted SWL treatment to a stone burden of less than about 2 cm.

With growing experience, it became apparent that SWL can cause unexpected and sometimes serious adverse effects [7–12]. Research with experimental animals during the last decade has allowed us to better characterize the structural and functional consequences of SWL [8, 13–15].

Lithotripsy Acute Adverse Effects

It is well established that unwanted renal and extrarenal side effects can occur as a consequence of SWL [8, 9, 13–15]. Shock waves can commonly cause parenchymal bleeding and occasionally mild to severe subcapsular hematomas. Detailed work with animal models has shown that injury can be affected by a variety of risk factors, such as age, the size

E. Gnessin, M.D. (✉) • J.E. Lingeman, M.D.
Department of Urology, Indiana University Health,
1801 North Senate Blvd., Suite 220, Indianapolis, IN 46202, USA
e-mail: egnessin@iupui.edu; jlingeman@iuhealth.org

J.J. Talati et al. (eds.), *Urolithiasis*,
DOI 10.1007/978-1-4471-4387-1_40, © Springer-Verlag London 2012

of the kidney, and the presence of renal disease. Renal damage is also dependent on the number of shock waves, the shock wave firing rate, and the power setting of the lithotripter. For example, measurements of lesion size in the acute (4 h posttreatment) juvenile pig SWL injury model have shown that treatment with a conservative dose of shock waves using the Dornier HM3 lithotripter (1,000 shock waves, 24 kV, 120 shock waves/min) produced a hemorrhagic lesion measuring approximately 0.3 % of the renal parenchyma (functional renal volume, FRV) [13]. Doubling the dose (2,000 shock waves) increased the lesion 20-fold (~6 % FRV), and raising the dose to 8,000 shock waves further doubled the lesion (~14 % FRV) [14]. In the same animal model, but with a dose of 2,000 shock waves, lesion size was observed to be dependent on the power setting of the lithotripter, increasing from approximately 0.3 % FRV at 12 kV to approximately 2.25 % FRV at 18 kV and 6 % FRV at 24 kV [15]. Thus, the severity of acute renal injury in SWL is dose dependent and is affected by the parameters of shock wave delivery.

Although there remains a paucity of data on the precise physical mechanism responsible for tissue injury in SWL, a variety of studies suggest that cavitation (bubble formation and collapse) is involved, but other mechanisms may be at play as well [16–18]. Evidence that cavitation is involved includes the observation of increased hemorrhage when microbubbles are injected into the circulation during SWL [19]. Methods to suppress cavitation such as phase-reverse waveform or tandem delayed SWs to interrupt bubble growth reduce tissue damage [20, 21]. A number of clinical studies report that slowing the firing rate of the lithotripter to 60 shock waves/min not only gives better stone fragmentation but also decreases vascular injury [12]. One possible explanation for the benefits of slow rate may be its effect on the negative pressure wave of the shock wave. Cavitation bubbles generated by the passage of the shock wave grow, collapse, and produce microbubbles that can persist between pulses acting to seed more cavitation initiated by subsequent shock waves [22]. The shorter the interval between shock waves, the more cavitation nuclei survive. The leading positive pressure phase of the shock pulse is unaffected by the very small persistent cavitation bubbles, but the trailing tensile phase of the shock wave is reduced [22, 23]. In vitro studies using high-speed imaging show a reduction in bubble interactions with stone phantoms at fast rate (120 shock waves/min) compared to a slower shock wave rate (60 shock waves/min) [24]. This may begin to explain why stone breakage is less efficient as the firing rate increases.

Although cavitation is a likely mechanism for SW injury, shear forces may be involved as well. In vitro studies have shown that when isolated cells are held under static pressure greater than the threshold for cavitation, SWs cause more cell lysis than in untreated controls [25]. This suggests that cell injury occurs in the absence of cavitation. In an in vivo study, pigs were treated with SWs from a lithotripter (Dornier HM3) fitted with a reflector insert that suppressed cavitation without significantly changing SW peak pressures. This significantly reduced vascular injury compared to animals treated with the standard reflector, but these animals still showed a modest degree of bleeding involving the vessels of the renal papilla [20]. These data demonstrate that cavitation has a prominent role in SWL trauma, but shear forces may be involved as well, creating further SW damage.

Long-Term Adverse Effects of Lithotripsy

The long-term consequences of SWL injury are not nearly as well understood as the acute effects, but there is solid evidence to show that acute SWL injury initiates an inflammatory response with progression to scar formation and permanent loss of functional renal mass [26]. Renal scar formation was demonstrated in patients using single-photon emission computed tomography (SPECT) to measure exclusion of Technicium-99 label from areas of poor perfusion [27]. Patients scanned before and 30 days following SWL showed a loss of marker uptake, and scars that developed measured larger than the focal zone of the lithotripter that was used. Dose-dependent parenchymal fibrosis has also been observed in dogs [28] and in rabbits [29]. In this latter study, a dose-dependent increase in scar formation was observed after treatment with clinical doses of SWs. Scar volume 1 month posttreatment increased nearly tenfold with treatment at 2,000 SWs compared to 1,000 SWs.

Although these manifestations of chronic injury have been identified, it seems likely that the full spectrum of long-term injury has yet to be determined. A number of potential chronic consequences of SWL are emerging. These include rise in systemic blood pressure, increased incidence of diabetes mellitus, an increase in the rate of stone recurrence, and the induction of calcium phosphate and brushite stone disease.

New-onset hypertension is a potential consequence of SWL, and evidence suggests that blood pressure changes following lithotripsy may be dose dependent [7]. Lingeman and associates [30] reported that 8.2 % of 243 patients who were normotensive at the time of SWL developed blood pressure changes requiring antihypertensive medication. Mean follow-up was 1.5 years, giving an annualized incidence of hypertension of 5.5 %. A large study from the same group involving almost 1,000 patients [31] has found a small but statistically significant change in diastolic blood pressure associated with SWL therapy. The observed effect of SWL on diastolic pressure change persisted even after controlling statistically for other variables that might be associated with variation in blood pressure, such as age, sex, pretreatment baseline blood pressure, and number of treatment sessions. A recent, retrospective case-control study from the Mayo Clinic evaluated the long-term effects of SWL on 288 patients with renal and proximal ureteral stones treated with SWL using the HM3 lithotripter in 1985 [32]. Patients were matched with regard to age, gender, and year of presentation to a group of urolithiasis patients treated conservatively who were continuing active follow-up. With a mean follow-up of 19 years, the study found an increased risk of developing hypertension (OR 1.47, 95 % CI 1.03–2.1, $p=0.034$). The development of hypertension was also associated with bilateral SWL treatments ($p=0.033$).

An additional concerning finding in the Mayo Clinic study was that patients treated with SWL were more likely to develop diabetes mellitus compared to controls at long-term follow-up. This risk persisted in multivariate analysis controlling for other factors such as presence of obesity and change in body mass index over 19 years. In addition, the occurrence of diabetes mellitus in these patients was related to the total number of shock waves they received and the power setting of the lithotripter. The significance of the Mayo Clinic study is limited by its retrospective nature and the fact that the control patients in the study represented a different study population. Further, the average stone size of the control group was smaller and may represent less severe stone disease. Nevertheless, this study represents sound data supporting the association between SWL and the onset of diabetes mellitus and hypertension. Two recent retrospective trials have found no association between SWL and the development of diabetes mellitus and hypertension [33, 34], but their limited design leaves these questions unanswered. Until further studies become available, the current data should be considered as a warning of possible long-term association of SWL with diabetes mellitus and hypertension.

There is some evidence to suggest that higher recurrence rates are associated with SWL therapy, mainly due to residual stone debris that may serve as a nidus to further stone formation [35]. Carr et al. [36] studied new stone formation in 298 consecutive patients who initially were determined to be stone-free after SWL and compared those findings with those of 62 patients treated by percutaneous nephrolithotomy (PCNL). They have shown a significant increase in the rate of new stone formation within 1 year of SWL treatment compared with PCNL. The authors concluded that fine sand debris generated from SWL remained in the kidney and may have served as a nidus in the calyceal system for new stone formation.

Multiple lithotripsy procedures have been implicated as a risk factor in the exacerbation of stone disease [37, 38]. That is, patients who had received multiple SWL treatment sessions showed a greater tendency over time for transformation from calcium oxalate stone disease to a calcium phosphate or brushite phenotype. In Parks' work, the calcium phosphate stone formers had received a significantly higher number of procedures than did the idiopathic calcium oxalate stone formers when rates were adjusted for number of stones and duration of stone disease. Furthermore, the brushite stone formers had received a significantly greater number of SWL treatments than had the calcium phosphate stone formers.

Pretreatment with Shock Waves Protects Against Subsequent SWL Injury

Certain treatment or "priming" protocols have been shown to decrease shock wave-induced renal tissue injury in the pig model [39]. Using the HM3 lithotripter, a standard clinical dose of 2,000 shock waves at 24 kV (120 shock waves/min) created a lesion measuring approximately 6 % of the FRV. The lesion size was reduced to 0.3 % of the FRV by simply pretreating the kidney with as few as 100 shock waves at 12 kV before completion of the dose with the higher amplitude pulses. Further studies have suggested that it is not the low-volume priming dose that is protective but rather the interruption of shock wave delivery [40]. In this study, the renal lesion was the same size when the priming dose was delivered at 12, 18, and 24 kV. However, only when a 3- to 4-min pause was instituted following the priming dose before resuming the clinical shock wave treatment was renal protection observed. The physiologic mechanism for this response was not assessed in the study, but work has begun in this area, suggesting that the pretreatment protocol induces renal vasoconstriction during the period of SW application, resulting in a reduction in tissue injury [41].

Shock Wave Rate

It has recently been shown that shock wave rate has a significant effect on the efficiency of stone breakage and limitation of renal vascular injury, with a slower rate being better. Recent studies with pigs indicate that choice of shock wave rate in the clinical range (30–120 shock waves/min) can affect lesion size and slowing the firing rate to 30–60 SWs/min delivers a significant reduction in renal injury [42, 43]. Several prospective clinical trials [44–46] and recently an independent meta-analysis [47] have also reported a significant improvement in stone-breakage outcomes when patients are treated at 60 shock waves/min compared with 120 shock waves/min. This strongly suggests a stone-breakage advantage in reducing the firing rate of the lithotripter. Lengthening treatment time has the potential to create administrative obstacles for high-volume centers, and many urologists would likely find it difficult to treat their patients at the extremely slow rate of 30 shock waves/min that has been shown to be protective. Therefore, a recent study in the pig model has shown that injury is also reduced at 60 shock waves/min compared with 120 shock waves/min (Fig. 40.1) [43]. Thus, there are solid laboratory data to show that injury is reduced when a slower shock wave rate is used, and this finding is complemented by clinical studies reporting improved outcomes at reduced shock wave rate. On the basis of these data, it seems reasonable to suggest that slowing the firing rate of the lithotripter improves both the safety and the efficacy of SW.

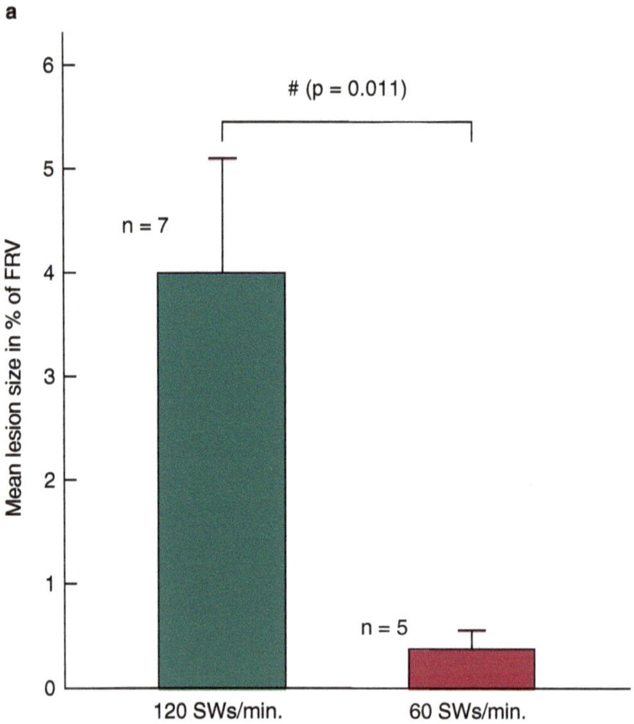

Fig. 40.1 Effect of 2,000 SWs at 120 or 60 SWs/min with an unmodified Dornier HM3 lithotripter on renal hemorrhagic lesion size (% FRV). Slowing the treatment rate demonstrates a decrease in the size of the hemorrhagic lesion

Acoustic Coupling

Coupling of the patient's skin to the lithotripter interface is essential in the propagation of shock waves to the targeted stone. The water bath of the HM3 was an almost perfect means of coupling but was cumbersome, requiring a large surgical facility. Acoustic coupling with modern dry-head lithotripters is not as efficient as when a water bath is used, although these lithotripters eliminated the large space requirements and made lithotripters transportable and readily available to every urologist. Acoustic coupling with modern dry-head lithotripters is more difficult than, and not as efficient as, a water bath. Defects (air pockets) at the coupling interface arise when coupling is first established and worsen if the patient moves or is repositioned. In vitro studies have demonstrated that a 20–40 % reduction in stone breakage can be observed if only 2 % of the coupling interface is covered by air pockets (Fig. 40.2) [49]. Currently there is no way to assess the quality of coupling. However, in vitro work has suggested a few simple measures that can be taken to improve dry-head device coupling [50]. In this study, coupling was enhanced if the gel was applied as a large bolus to the lithotripter cushion directly from the stock jug and not a tube or squeeze bottle. Squeezing the gel from the tube introduced more air bubbles. Spreading the gel over the cushion also introduced air bubbles, and the investigators found that better results were observed if the gel was placed as a large bolus over the treatment head and allowed to spread upon contact between the treatment head and the patient skin. Also, employing the inflation feature of the treatment head to smooth out the gel can significantly improve coupling [50].

Conclusion

SWL is a safe and appropriate treatment option for most urinary tract calculi when appropriately employed. Shock waves have the potential to cause tissue damage, and acute injury may lead to long-term adverse effects. It is likely that the large majority of the patients that are treated with a typical dose of SWs sustain some degree of acute renal injury. It is currently not known whether such injury from a single treatment session will eventually lead to a long-term adverse effect. Treatment protocols have demonstrated potential tissue protective effects, specifically when a 3- to 4-min pause is instituted. By slowing the shock wave rate, treatment efficacy is increased while limiting renal tissue injury. The poor quality and variability of acoustic coupling is an additional challenge that needs to be addressed. Every attempt at maximal coupling should be made to ensure efficient shock wave delivery. By appropriate patient selection and by attention to technique, patient safety can be ensured and limit retreatment rates.

Fig. 40.2 Effects of lithotripter coupling on stone breakage. Stone breakage is reduced as air pockets cover a greater percentage of the coupling interface (Modified from Krambeck and Lingeman [48])

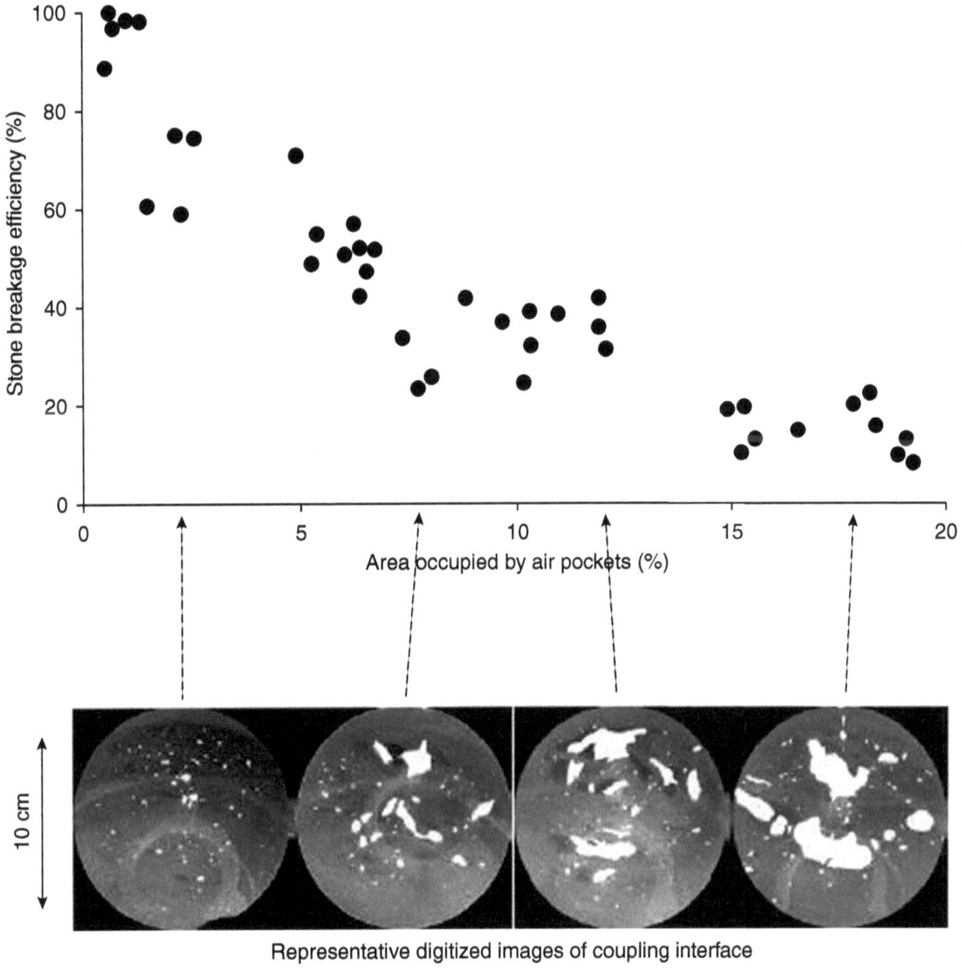

References

1. Chaussy C, Schmiedt E, Jocham D, Brendel W, Forssmann B, Walther V. First clinical experience with extracorporeally induced destruction of kidney stones by shock waves. J Urol. 1982;127(3): 417–20.
2. Chaussy C, Eisenberger F, Forssmann B. Extracorporeal shock-wave lithotripsy (ESWL): a chronology. J Endourol. 2007;21: 1249.
3. Lingeman JE, Newman D, Mertz JH, Mosbaugh PG, Steele RE, Kahnoski RJ, et al. Extracorporeal shock wave lithotripsy: the Methodist Hospital of Indiana experience. J Urol. 1986;135(6): 1134–7.
4. Chaussy CG, Fuchs J. Current state and future developments of noninvasive treatment of human urinary stones with extracorporeal shock wave lithotripsy. J Urol. 1989;141:782–9.
5. Lingeman JE, Matlaga BR, Evan AP. In: Wein AJ, Kavoussi LR, Novick AC, Partin AW, Peters CA, editors. Campbell-Walsh urology. Philadelphia: W. B. Saunders; 2007. p. 1431–507.
6. Pareek G, Hedican SP, Lee Jr FT, et al. Shock wave lithotripsy success determined by skin-to-stone distance on computed tomography. Urology. 2005;66:941.
7. Evan AP, Willis LR. Extracorporeal shock wave lithotripsy: complications. In: Smith AD, Badlani GH, Bagley DH, Clayman RV, Docimo SG, Jordan GH, et al., editors. Smith's textbook on endourology. Hamilton: BC Decker, Inc; 2007. p. 353–65.
8. Evan AP, McAteer JA. Q-effects of shock wave lithotripsy. In: Coe FL, Favus MJ, Pak CYC, Parks JH, Preminger GM, editors. Kidney stones: medical and surgical management. Philadelphia: Lippincott-Raven; 2006. p. 549–70.
9. McAteer JA, Evan AP. The acute and long-term adverse effects of shock wave lithotripsy. Semin Nephrol. 2008;28:200–13.
10. McAteer JA, Evan AP, Willis LR, et al. Shock wave injury to the kidney in SWL: review and perspective. In: Evan AP, Lingeman JE, Williams JC, editors. Renal stone disease: proceedings of the 1st international urolithiasis research symposium. American Institute of Physics conference proceedings, Melville, 2007, vol. 900, p. 287–301.
11. Lingeman JE, Matlaga B, Evan AP. Surgical management of urinary lithiasis. In: Walsh PC, Retik AB, Vaughan ED, Wein J, editors. Campbell-Walsh urology. Philadelphia: W.B. Saunders; 2006. p. 1431–507. Chapter 44.
12. McAteer JA, Evan AP, Williams Jr JC, Lingeman JE. Treatment protocols to reduce renal injury during shock wave lithotripsy. Curr Opin Urol. 2009;19(2):192–5.
13. Connors BA, Evan AP, Blomgren PM, et al. Reducing shock number dramatically decreases lesion size in a juvenile kidney model. J Endourol. 2006;20:607–11.

14. Willis LR, Evan AP, Connors BA, et al. Shock-wave lithotripsy: dose-related effects on renal structure, hemodynamics and tubular function. J Endourol. 2005;19:90–101.
15. Connors BA, Evan AP, Willis LR, et al. The effect of discharge voltage on renal injury and impairment caused by lithotripsy in the pig. J Am Soc Nephrol. 2000;11:310–8.
16. Lingeman JE, Delius M, Evan A, et al. Bioeffects and physical mechanisms of SW effects in SWL. In: Segura JW, Conort P, Khory S, et al., editors. Stone disease: first international consultation on stone disease. Paris: Health Publications; 2003. p. 251–86.
17. Zhong P, Cioanta J, Zhu S, et al. Effects of tissue constraint on shock wave-induced bubble expansion in vivo. J Acoust Soc Am. 1998;104:3126.
18. Zhong P, Zhou Y, Zhu S. Dynamics of bubble oscillation in constrained media and mechanisms of vessel rupture in SWL. Ultrasound Med Biol. 2001;27:119.
19. Matlaga BR, McAteer JA, Connors BA, et al. Potential for cavitation-mediated tissue damage in shockwave lithotripsy. J Endourol. 2008;22:121.
20. Evan AP, Willis LR, McAteer JA, et al. Kidney damage and renal functional changes are minimized by waveform control that suppresses cavitation in shock wave lithotripsy. J Urol. 2002;168: 1556.
21. Zhong P, Zhou Y. Suppression of large intraluminal bubble expansion in shock wave lithotripsy without compromising stone comminution: methodology and in vitro experiments. J Acoust Soc Am. 2001;110:3283.
22. Pishchalnikov YA, McAteer JA, Williams Jr JC, Pishchalnikova IV, Vonderhaar RJ. Why stones break better at slow shockwave rates than at fast rates: in vitro study with a research electrohydraulic lithotripter. J Endourol. 2006;20(8):537–41.
23. Pishchalnikov YA, Sapozhnikov OA, Bailey MR, Pishchalnikova IV, Williams JC, McAteer JA. Cavitation selectively reduces the negative-pressure phase of lithotripter shock pulses. Acoust Res Lett Online. 2005;6(4):280–6.
24. Pishchalnikov YA, Kaehr MM, McAteer JA. Influence of pulse repetition rate on cavitation on the surface of an object targeted by lithotripter shock wave. In: Proceedings of IMECE, Seattle, November 11–15, 2007; 41387.
25. Williams Jr JC, Woodward JF, Stonehill MA, et al. Cell damage by lithotripter shock waves at high pressure to preclude cavitation. Ultrasound Med Biol. 1999;25:1445.
26. Evan AP, Willis LR, Lingeman JE, McAteer JA. Renal trauma and the risk of long-term complications in shock wave lithotripsy. Nephron. 1998;78:1–8.
27. Lechevallier E, Siles S, Ortega MC, et al. Comparison by SPECT of renal scars after extracorporeal shock wave lithotripsy and percutaneous nephrolithotomy. J Endourol. 1993;7:465.
28. Newman R, Hackett R, Senior D, et al. Pathological effects of ESWL on canine renal tissue. Urology. 1987;29:194.
29. Morris JA, Husmann DA, Wilson WT, Preminger GM. Temporal effects of shock wave lithotripsy. J Urol. 1991;145:881–3.
30. Lingeman JE, Kulb TB, Newman DM, et al. Hypertension following ESWL. J Urol. 1987;137(Suppl):142.
31. Lingeman JE, Woods JR, Toth PD. Blood pressure changes following extracorporeal shock wave lithotripsy and other forms of treatment for nephrolithiasis. JAMA. 1990;263:1789–94.
32. Krambeck AE, Gettman MT, Rohlinger AL, et al. Diabetes mellitus and hypertension associated with shock wave lithotripsy of renal and proximal ureteral stones at 19 years of follow-up. J Urol. 2006;175:1742.
33. Sato Y, Tanda H, Kato S, et al. Shock wave lithotripsy for renal stones is not associated with hypertension and diabetes mellitus. Urology. 2008;71:586.
34. Makhlouf AA, Thorner D, Ugarte R, et al. Shock wave lithotripsy not associated with development of diabetes mellitus at 6 years of follow-up. Urology. 2009;73:4.
35. Raman JD, Bagrodia A, Bensalah K, Pearle MS, Lotan Y. Residual fragments after percutaneous nephrolithotomy: cost comparison of immediate second look flexible nephroscopy versus expectant management. J Urol. 2010;183(1):188–93.
36. Carr LK, D'A Honey J, Jewett MA, et al. New stone formation: a comparison of extracorporeal shock wave lithotripsy and percutaneous nephrolithotomy. J Urol. 1996;155:1565–7.
37. Parks JH, Worcester EM, Coe FL, et al. Clinical implications of abundant calcium phosphate in routinely analyzed kidney stones. Kidney Int. 2004;66:777–85.
38. Mandel N, Mandel I, Fryjoff K, et al. Conversion of calcium oxalate to calcium phosphate with recurrent stone episodes. J Urol. 2003; 169:2026–9.
39. Willis LR, Evan AP, Connors BA, et al. Prevention of lithotripsy-induced renal injury by pretreating kidneys with low-energy shock waves. J Am Soc Nephrol. 2006;17:663–73.
40. Connors BA, Evan AP, Blomgren PM, Handa RK, Willis LR, Gao S. Effect of initial shock wave voltage on shock wave lithotripsy-induced lesion size during step-wise voltage ramping. BJU Int. 2009;103(1):104–7.
41. Handa RK, Bailey MR, Paun M, Gao S, Connors BA, Willis LR, Evan AP. Pretreatment with low-energy shock waves induces renal vasoconstriction during standard shock wave lithotripsy (SWL): a treatment protocol known to reduce SWL-induced renal injury. BJU Int. 2009;103(9):1270–4.
42. Evan AP, McAteer JA, Connors BA, et al. Renal injury in SWL is significantly reduced by slowing the rate of shock wave delivery. BJU Int. 2007;100:624–7.
43. Connors BA, Evan AP, Blomgren PM, Handa RK, Willis LR, Gao S, et al. Extracorporeal shock wave lithotripsy at 60 shock waves/ min reduces renal injury in a porcine model. BJU Int. 2009;104:1004–8.
44. Pace KT, Ghiculete D, Harju M, Honey RJD'A. Shock wave lithotripsy at 60 or 120 shocks per minute: a randomized, double-blind trial. J Urol. 2005;174:595–9.
45. Madbouly K, El-Tiraifi AM, Seida M, et al. Slow versus fast shock wave lithotripsy rate for urolithiasis: a prospective randomized study. J Urol. 2005;173:127–30.
46. Yilmaz E, Batislam E, Basar M, et al. Optimal frequency in extracorporeal shock wave lithotripsy: prospective randomized study. Urology. 2005;66:1160–4.
47. Semins MJ, Trock BJ, Matlaga BR. The effect of shock wave rate on the outcome of shock wave lithotripsy: a meta-analysis. J Urol. 2008;179:194–7.
48. Krambeck AE, Lingeman JE. Shockwave lithotripsy: indications and technique. In: Pearle MS, Nakada SY, editors. Urolithiasis, medical and surgical management. London: Informa Health Care UK; 2009. p. 144.
49. Pishchalnikov YA, Neucks JS, VonDerHaar RJ, et al. Air pockets trapped during routine coupling in dry-head lithotripsy can significantly reduce the delivery of shock wave energy. J Urol. 2006;176:2706–10.
50. Neucks JS, Pishchalnikov YA, Zancanaro AJ, et al. Improved acoustic coupling for shock wave lithotripsy. Urol Res. 2008;36: 61–6.

41

History and Development of the Ureteroscope: What Does the Future Hold?

Demetrius H. Bagley and Kelly A. Healy

Abstract

Ureteroscopy has grown from isolated incidental procedures to become a standard portion of urologic endoscopy, both for diagnosis and treatment. The development of fiber optics accelerated the development of the ureteroscope. Initially ureteroscopy was limited by the lack of irrigation, deflection, and working instruments. A major step in ureteroscopy came with distal ureteroscopy using rigid instruments. As the utility of these procedures became evident, there was a rapid development of more endoscopes and associated working instruments, specifically designed for the ureter. One of the major applications has been for urinary calculi. This has been assisted by the development of appropriate intraluminal lithotriptors. The limitations of rigid endoscopes became evident and a great deal of effort was put into developing functional, flexible ureteroscopes with channels adequate for irrigation and working instruments and deflection capabilities which increased access to the lower pole of the kidney. The main limitation is the cross-sectional size of the ureteroscope. The ureter does not accept large instruments easily. The ideal ureteroscope has yet to be made.

Keywords

Ureter • Ureteroscope • Ureteroscopy • Endoscope • Intracorporeal lithotripsy • Laser

Introduction

Ureteroscopy has a long history of stepwise advancement. The isolated initial steps later coalesced into an effort to gain endoscopic access to the ureter. Initially, only visualization was possible. Combined developments of endoscopes and working instruments resulted in very practical devices, which can access the entire upper collecting system for visualization and for functional procedures. Overall, the progress has been dependent on the materials and the instrument designs available at each step.

In 1912, Hugh Hampton Young performed the first ureteroscopy when he unintentionally introduced a pediatric cystoscope into a severely dilated ureter of a pediatric patient with posterior urethral valves. However, Young's experience was not reported until 1929 as part of a larger review article on congenital urethral valves [1]. For the next 30 years, advances in ureteroscopy remained quiescent. During this time, fiber-optic technology was being integrated into medical instrumentation. Later, rigid instruments were developed for practical urologic endoscopes before fiber optics were introduced into the urologic field.

The foundation for contemporary fiber optics began as early as the 1840s with the work of Daniel Colladon at the University of Geneva. In 1841, he disproved the belief that light only traveled in a straight line and introduced the concept of internal reflection and "light guiding," or fiber optics [2]. That same year, Babinet demonstrated this concept of light guided along bent glass rods. Tyndall subsequently

D.H. Bagley, M.D., FACS (✉) • K.A. Healy, M.D.
Department of Urology, Jefferson Medical College,
Thomas Jefferson University,
1025 Walnut Street, Suite 1112 College Building,
Philadelphia, PA 19107, USA
e-mail: demetrius.bagley@jefferson.edu; kelly.healy@jefferson.edu

J.J. Talati et al. (eds.), *Urolithiasis*,
DOI 10.1007/978-1-4471-4387-1_41, © Springer-Verlag London 2012

performed an extravagant demonstration of light guiding at the Royal Institution of Great Britain in 1854. Baird and Hansell obtained patents on fiber bundles providing image transmission through internal reflection in 1927 and 1930, respectively [3]. However, fiber bundles were first applied clinically in the early 1950s in the field of gastroenterology by Hirschowitz, a gastroenterologist, and Curtiss, a physicist [4]. In 1957, Curtiss developed glass cladding, which dramatically improved light propagation. In the same year, Hirschowtiz used fiber optics with glass cladding to develop and test the first flexible gastroscope on himself. The development of the fiberscope spawned interest in endoscopy among other specialties, including urology.

The first flexible ureteroscopy was performed by Marshall in 1960 using a 9 F flexible fiberscope without deflection or a channel. During an open procedure, a ureterotomy was made and the fiberscope was inserted to inspect for renal calculi. In 1962, the first transurethral flexible ureteroscopy was done by McGovern and Walzak and reported by Marshall [5]. During this procedure, the 9 F fiberscope was inserted through a 26 F McCarthy endoscope into the left ureter to visualize a ureteral calculus.

The first determined efforts to develop flexible fiber-optic access to the upper tract were reported by Takagi et al. in 1968 [6]. They described visualization of the renal pelvis and papillae using a newly developed 70-cm 8 F fiber-optic endoscope in both cadavers and patients. The scope was also used to visualize the spinal canal and biliary tract. In these efforts, the authors noted difficulty manipulating the tip within the biliary tract and, thus, recognized the need for a deflectable tip. They also identified difficulty in inserting the flexible endoscope through the bladder into the ureter. They initially used the cystoscope sheath and later developed a flexible introducer sheath [7]. Lack of irrigation was a problem and they attempted to irrigate through the sheath to distend the lumen for visualization. The limitations at this point were one of size. Adding an irrigation channel to the ureteroscope and a deflecting mechanism can significantly increase the overall diameter of the ureteroscope.

Interestingly, the introduction of flexible ureteroscopy preceded rigid ureteroscopy by nearly a decade. However, it was hampered by its limitation as a purely visualizing diagnostic procedure. In the late 1970s, interest developed in two groups who independently accessed the distal ureter with rigid endoscopes. Initially, pediatric cystoscopes were used in female patients and later juvenile endoscopes were used before the development of specific rigid endoscopes. In 1977, Goodman et al. reported rigid ureteroscopy using an 11 F pediatric cystoscope to manage three cases with ureteral abnormalities [8]. Lyon et al. reported transurethral ureteroscopy in women using pediatric instruments and then, in 1979, reported the use of longer endoscopes to reach the ureter, both in males and females [9, 10].

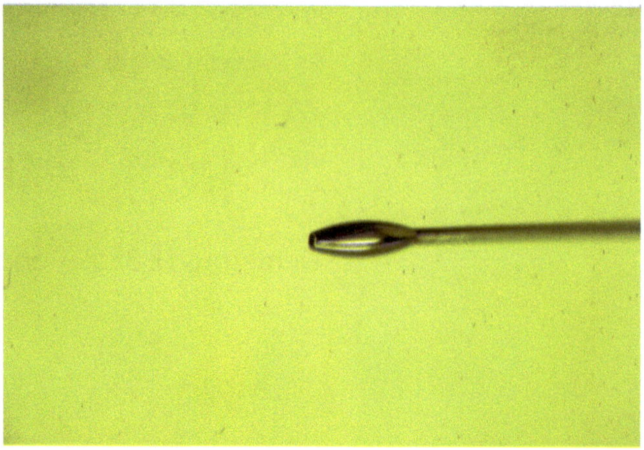

Fig. 41.1 A wire-guided bougie dilation of the distal ureter. Previously, unguided devices had been used with higher risk of perforation

They also described dilation of the ureter to accept the larger (13 F) endoscopes (Fig. 41.1). These contributions stimulated interest in rigid ureteroscopy and then flexible endoscopy, which has continued without cessation to the present.

It is impossible to separate the development of ureteroscopes from the development of working ancillary instruments. Procedures can be done with these ancillary instruments while the ureteroscope provides access and visualization.

The first developments with rigid ureteroscopy dramatically changed the management of ureteral calculi. Until the 1980s, the standard treatment for ureteral calculi was either blind endoscopic manipulation or open ureterolithotomy. However, in 1981 Das reported the first transurethral ureteroscopy with stone basketing under direct vision [11]. Despite this success, the initial widespread adoption of ureteroscopy was thwarted by concerns regarding morbidity, particularly regarding the size of the ureteroscope. Again, the key to practical use of the ureteroscope was the development of smaller functional instruments. The rigid ureteroscopes were somewhat downsized, and by using the rod lens system, excellent visualization was achieved. As noted, Lyon et al. had reported the first application of the 23-cm 13 F specific ureteroscope in men.

Subsequently in 1982, Huffman et al. reported use of this device for treatment of 16 distal ureteral calculi with a relatively high success rate of 69 % [12]. However, its value was limited to the distal ureter because of its length.

Perez-Castro and Martinez-Piniero in 1980 reported a new longer ureteroscope from Karl Storz endoscopy with a length of 41 cm [13]. It was rigid but could often be passed proximally to reach the renal pelvis (Fig. 41.2). This innovation fostered additional advancements in the area of rigid ureteroscopy, including development of endoscopes of various lengths and diameters as well as interchangeable lenses. These early ureteroscopes also incorporated 4–5 F working

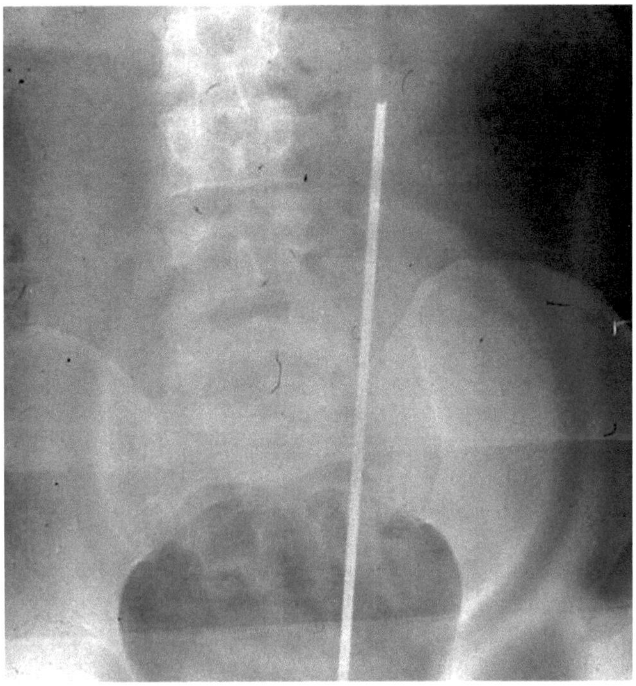

Fig. 41.2 The long 40+ cm rigid ureteroscope can often be passed to the proximal ureter even into the renal pelvis

channels, which allowed for use of working instruments, including stone baskets, biopsy forceps, and wires.

In 1983 Huffman et al. validated the safety of the new longer rigid ureteroscopes in their early clinical experience [14]. They also reported the first ureteroscopic ultrasonic lithotripsy of large renal pelvic calculi. This was also dependent upon emerging technical developments. Ultrasonic lithotripsy was based on the availability of a long ultrasonic probe 2.5 mm in diameter, which can be used through a long ureteroscope with interchangeable telescope. By this technique, the calculus was visualized. It was then trapped within a basket and the telescope was removed. The ultrasound probe was then placed. In a "tactile technique," the tip could be felt impinging upon the stone. The ultrasound was then activated and a portion of the stone was removed. The operator would hold the basket in one hand and the probe in the other and feel if the basket was actually touching the stone. It was then necessary to replace the telescope, reposition the stone, and repeat the procedure. In this way, the stone was gradually fragmented (Fig. 41.3), and although this was a time-consuming and demanding procedure, the authors found that "any stone that can be visualized can be extracted using a combination of stone basket or forceps and the ultrasonic transducer."

The next step in ultrasonic lithotripsy was based on two instrument changes. The ureteroscope itself was designed with an angled eyepiece so that there remained a straight channel through the ureteroscope. Thus, the newly developed 4 F ultrasound probe could pass directly through the ureteroscope while being observed through the offset optical system. There was also a channel for a basket to engage the stone and hold it (Fig. 41.4) while the ultrasound could work. With this combination, only tiny fragments could be removed through the probe, but the stone could be treated effectively and slowly. The electrohydraulic lithotriptor (EHL) offered another modality for endoscopic lithotripsy. It had been used successfully in the bladder with probes as large as 7 and 9 F to break bladder stones. An earlier attempt at blind ureteral lithotripsy by placing the probe into the ureter to the level of the stone resulted in ureteral damage and stricture [15]. The development of the 3 F probe along with a ureteroscope with a working channel allowed it to be placed directly under vision of the calculus for fragmentation. Several series demonstrated the safety of this technique [16–18]. The electrohydraulic also had the advantage that it utilized a flexible probe and could be used with flexible ureteroscopes as they became available. Later progress occurred with downsizing of the EHL probe to 2.5, 1.9, and 1.7 F (Fig. 41.5).

This growing experience with rigid ureteroscopy, including access to the renal pelvis, pointed out the glaring need for visualization and access to the entire intrarenal collecting system. This would be possible with a deflectable, flexible ureteroscope. There were attempts to use passively deflectable, flexible ureteroscopes that really could not access selected portions of the intrarenal collecting system. Bagley et al. [19] combined the rigid and flexible ureteroscopes through the sheath of a rigid ureteroscope. Again, irrigation and function were severely limited.

In the 1980s, interest and momentum continued and the flexible ureteroscope was further refined. Several designs were introduced that could be inserted over a wire and used to visualize the renal pelvis without a stabilizing sheath. Access to the often difficult lower pole was achieved with the use of active primary and secondary passive deflection of the tip. Based on the analysis of radiographs of 30 patients, it was recommended that a flexible ureteroscope should deflect 175° to reach the lower pole [20]. However, in practice, this often did not occur with the endoscope designed with those specifications. Deflection may be limited by working instruments in the channel and even by the collecting system itself (Fig. 41.6). Therefore, active deflection has continued to increase up to 230°.

Grasso et al. described a 7.5/8.2 F flexible ureteroscope, which had 2-way active deflection of 170 and 120° as well as secondary passive deflection [21]. This ureteroscope featured a 3.6 F working channel that could accommodate a variety of instruments including stone baskets, flexible probes, and laser fibers. More recently, ureteroscopes have been designed with either active secondary deflection, which allows further deflection in the lower pole, or with continuous control deflection, which allows the tip to advance into the lower pole. Thus, it became clear that the versatility of flexible ureteroscopy had dramatically expanded (Fig. 41.7a, b).

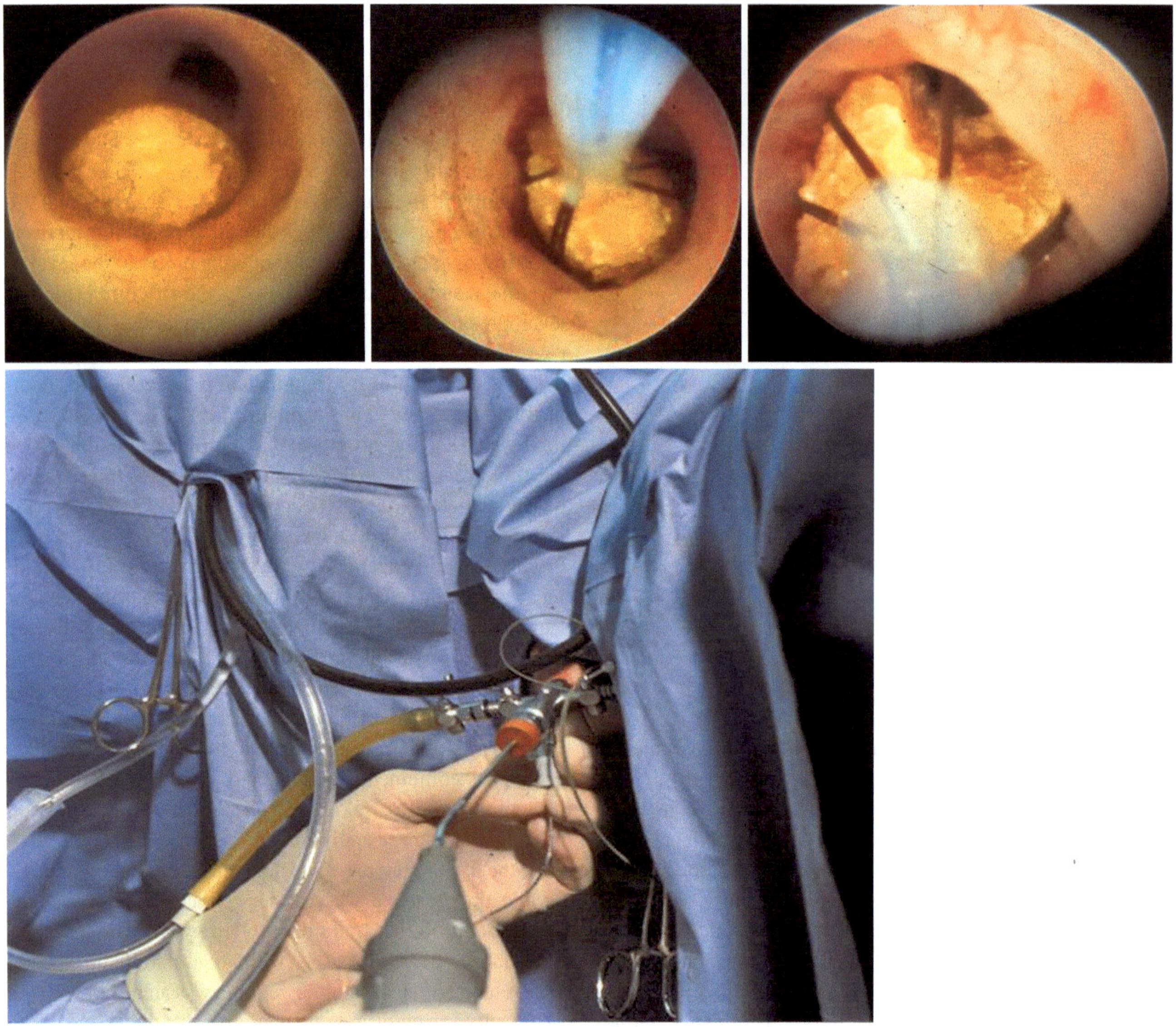

Fig. 41.3 The visualized calculus is grasped with the basket and withdrawn to the tip of the ureteroscope. After removing the telescope, the ultrasound probe was passed to touch the stone. As it cut a groove in the stone and moved beyond, the operator could feel the movement and then reposition the stone

Flexible ureteroscopes are noted for their fragility with a high repair rate. At one time there was considerable interest in developing disposable flexible ureteroscopes because of the high cost and repair rate with standard designs. In each of the designs that became products, the tip itself was disposable while the handle containing the optics was reusable. Vantec produced the first practical disposable ureteroscope. They had flexible tips of 7 or 8.5 F with a working channel. There was also a small rigid scope at 7 F and a tip used in general surgery in the shape of a Bake's dilator. While these were available, there were remarkable changes in the optics and the mechanics. The project was discontinued when the company was taken over by Boston Scientific.

Bard also had a flexible ureteroscope that had a similar design with a flexible tip but with deflection. It was over 8 F. The deflecting mechanism was a turn knob and was both slow and awkward (Fig. 41.8a,b). In the production models, the image was upside down and backward apparently due to a missing lens, and the endoscope was not clinically useful. More recently, a semi-reusable flexible ureteroscope has been introduced. It also is 8 F. In the authors' experience, it was not torque stable so that it was impossible to control rotation within the ureter but had acceptable deflection.

During this period, rigid ureteroscopy continued to evolve with the development of smaller scopes. These became possible with the use of fiber-optic imaging bundles rather than rod lens systems. The first "semirigid" ureteroscope was reported by Dretler in 1988 [22]. It featured two working channels, each 2.3 F and a tapered tip (distal end 7.2 F, proximal end 11.9 F), which allowed for distal ureteral insertion

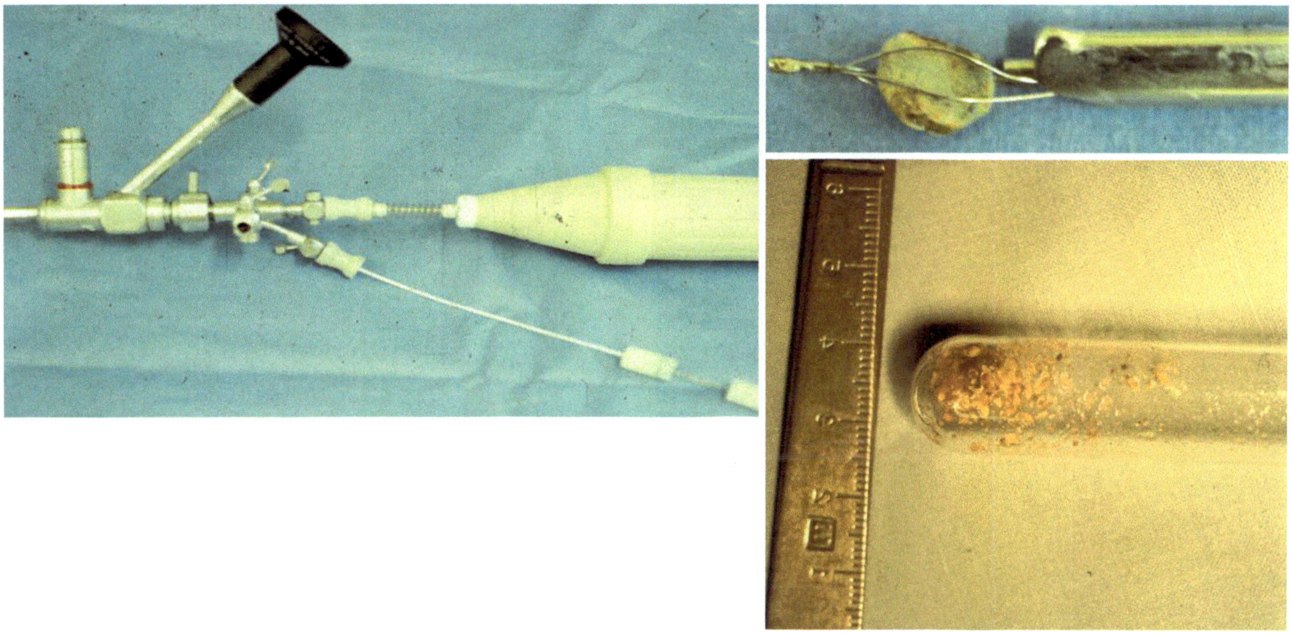

Fig. 41.4 The offset ureteroscope allows direct ultrasonic lithotripsy under vision. The probe is placed onto the stone and activated to fragment it. Although the probe is small, tiny fragments could be removed

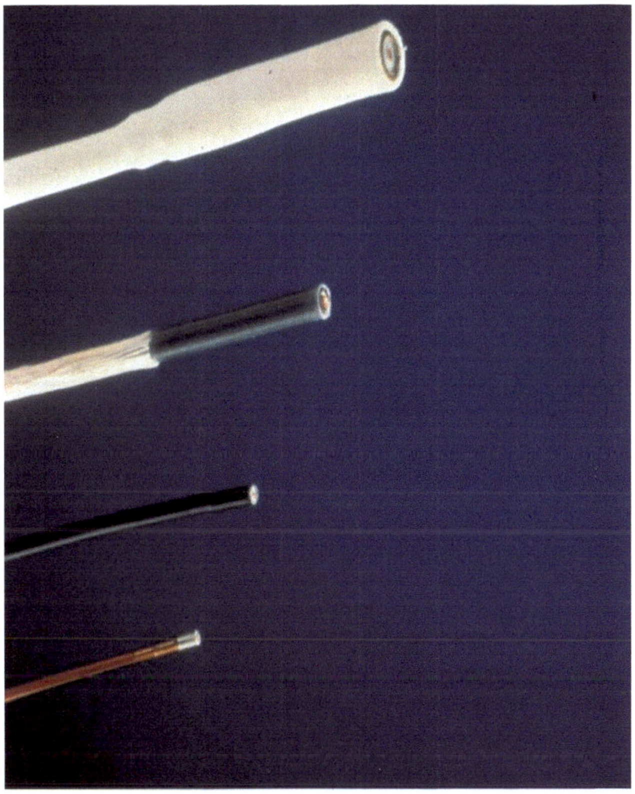

Fig. 41.5 Electrohydraulic probes are available in sizes as small as 1.7 F

without dilation. The instrument was designed specifically to be used with the pulsed dye laser as the channels were adequate for delivery of the fiber. Other improvements continued, and when a similar sized endoscope with a 3.4 F channel became available, it markedly expanded the options for use [23] (Fig. 41.9).

Much of the progress in ureteroscope design was paralleled by developments of intracorporeal lithotripsy, beginning with ultrasonic lithotripsy. In 1952, Mulvaney et al. performed ultrasonic lithotripsy using an 0.8-kHz device [24]. Coates partially fragmented both urinary and biliary calculi using a 15-kHz device in 1955 [25]. In that same year, the first electrohydraulic (EHL) lithotripsy was attempted by Yutkin of Kiev [26]. Higher success rates were reported both for bladder stones and for ureteral stones, but there remains concern regarding the safety of electrohydraulic lithotripsy in the ureter despite evidence to the contrary.

Direct impact, or "ballistic," methods were initially used in 1832 for lithotripsy of bladder calculi. Based on these principles, Languetin et al. introduced the Swiss LithoClast in 1990 for management of ureteral calculi [27]. There are no thermal or cavitation effects with this device, and therefore, the risk of inadvertent ureteral injury is minimal. It provided excellent fragmentation but without removal of fragments. There are now several pneumatic devices available, all with similar high success rates of fragmentation [28]. The impact devices and ultrasound suffer from a heavy transducer, which mounts awkwardly on the ureteroscope, and are limited to a rigid endoscope.

An excellent combination for stone treatment is a small endoscope that can accept a small effective lithotrite. It has largely been achieved with a combination of ureteroscopes and laser fibers as the laser has become practical in urologic

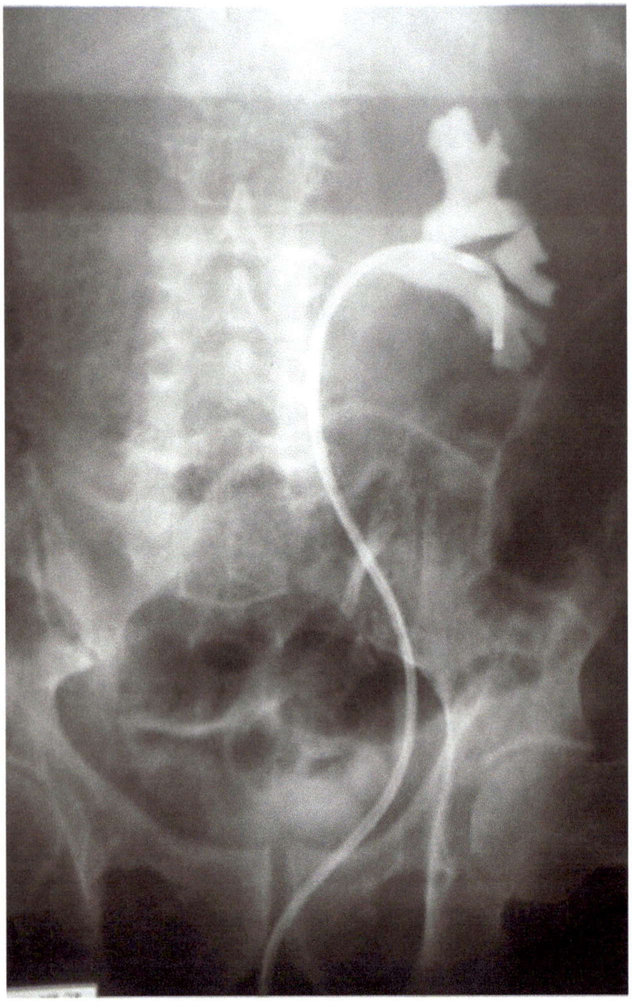

Fig. 41.6 A fully deflectable, flexible ureteroscope is essential to reach the entire intrarenal collecting system

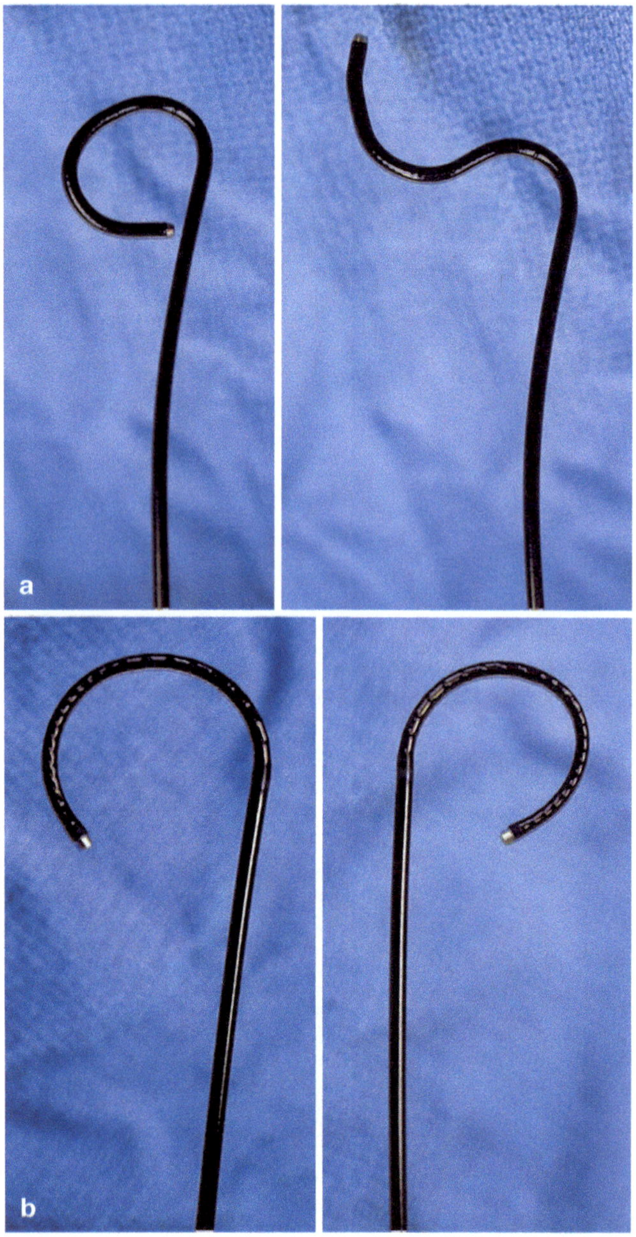

Fig. 41.7 Modifications in deflection of flexible ureteroscopes were made to try to reach the lower pole. It has taken two forms: (**a**) active secondary deflection and (**b**) continuous controlled deflection. The latter has become the standard for use

applications. As early as 1968, the laser beam was described in the urological literature by Mulvaney et al. who tried to treat a bladder calculus using a ruby laser, which is a solid-state laser (λ[lambda] 694 nm) that uses a synthetic ruby crystal as its medium [29]. However, there have been improvements since then. The Q-switched neodymium:YAG laser (λ[lambda] 1,064 nm) was utilized for ureteral calculi in 1989 [30]. The pulsed dye laser, which used coumarin green as the medium, was very successful and popular for endoscopic lithotripsy. It did not damage tissue and the only thing it could do was break stones. The first version at 60 mJ was poorly successful against the harder stone, such as calcium oxalate monohydrate [31]. Only as the power was increased to 140 mJ [32] and then 200 mJ could it treat all stones and become a very successful lithotrite.

The next step in laser lithotripsy development was the holmium:YAG laser (Ho:YAG). Johnson et al. in 1992 and 1993 [33, 34] reported on this laser including successful ureteroscopic lithotripsy. It also increases the versatility as well as safety. For example, it is effective for all stone compositions. It can also cut and ablate tissue. It can accomplish all of these functions with the same device depending on the energy level used and the position of the fiber. It could be very selectively applied. The fibers used with these lasers range from 100 to 1,000 μm. Thus, they can be delivered through flexible ureteroscopes with very little loss of deflection and applied even to lower pole calculi [35].

There remains a challenge to access the ureter and to deliver visualizing mechanisms and working devices to the appropriate location, although this is limited by the size of

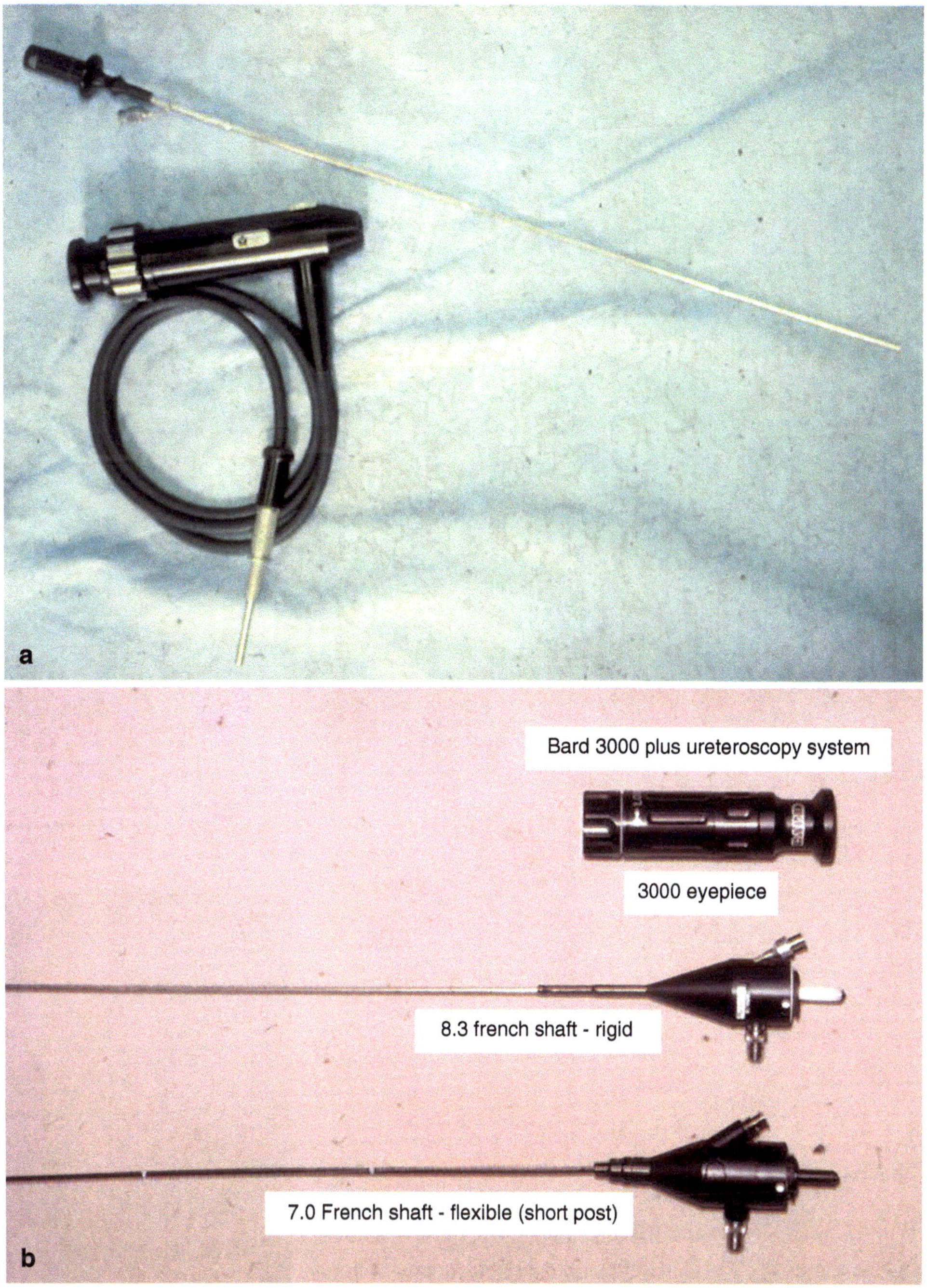

Fig. 41.8 Disposable ureteroscopes were designed with a reusable optical head and interchangeable tips, both rigid and flexible. (**a**) Vantec and (**b**) Bard

the ureter. As Lyon had noted, portions of it can be actively dilated. It can also be dilated by pre-placing a stent, but that alters the endoluminal anatomy and appearance and requires a second procedure. It is best to use an endoscope that can enter the ureter without additional prior manipulation. In evaluating, for example, a flexible ureteroscope, it is important to know the true size. French size or Charriere is defined as 3 × the diameter of the endoscope in mm (Table 41.1). For non-round endoscopes, the equivalent F size can be calculated from the circumference. Often, the instruments are advertised as having a 6+ French tip. They may, in fact, have a tip that size but 2–5 mm proximally on the shaft, it may be 7 or possibly 8+ French. The shaft is the important figure for passing into the ureter (Fig. 41.10). In the series comparing the passing of ureteroscopes, it was noted that a 7.4 F instrument failed to pass in only 1 out of 99, while at 9.0 it was 11 of 30 [36] (Table 41.2). The newer video scopes can provide an excellent image but at a cost of increased size of the ureteroscope. Other video scopes, which will be less than 8 F, are now in preparation.

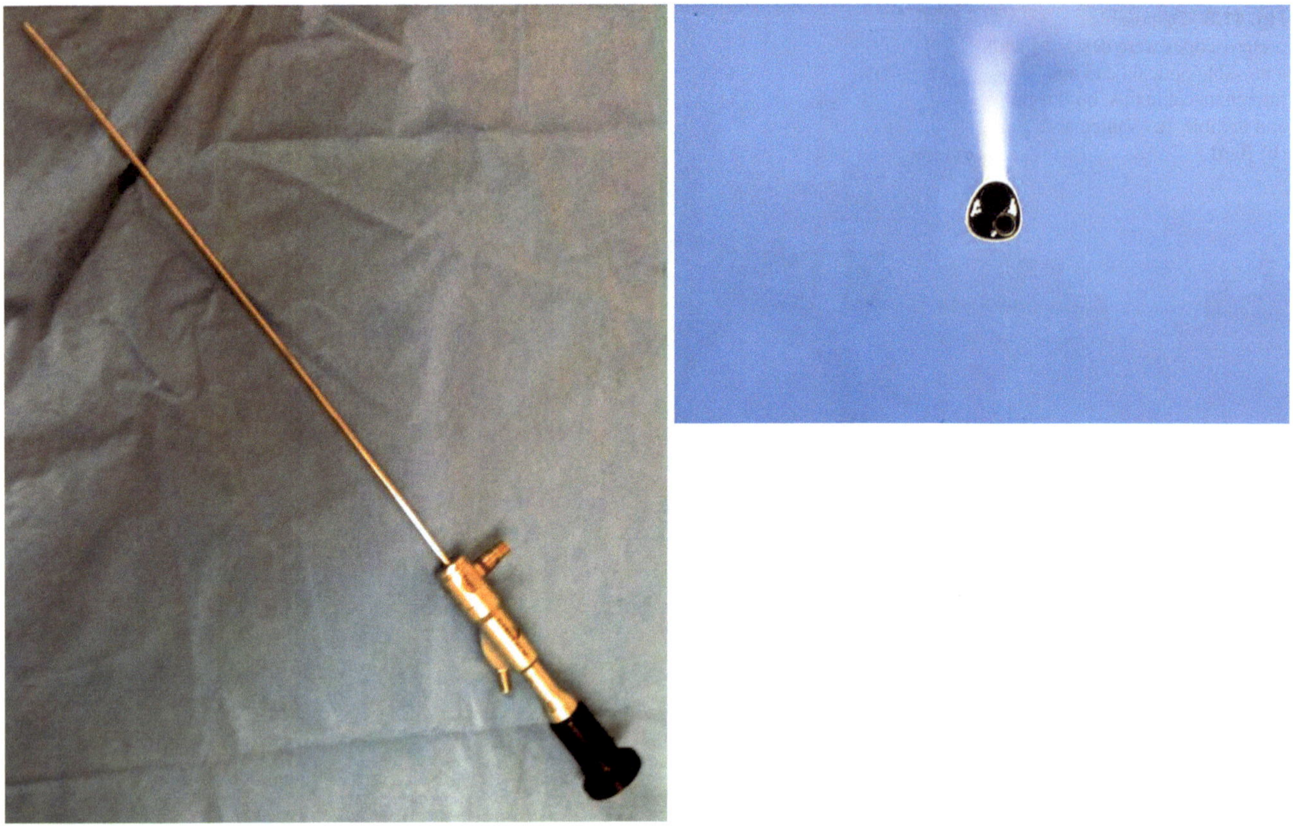

Fig. 41.9 The small rigid ureteroscope with two channels has adequate illumination with fiber bundles packed into the space between the fiber-optic imaging bundle and the working channels

Table 41.1 Sizing of urologic instruments

French (F) or Charriere (Ch) size = Circumference in mm, which is calculated from the diameter [diameter × π] or 3 × circumference
π

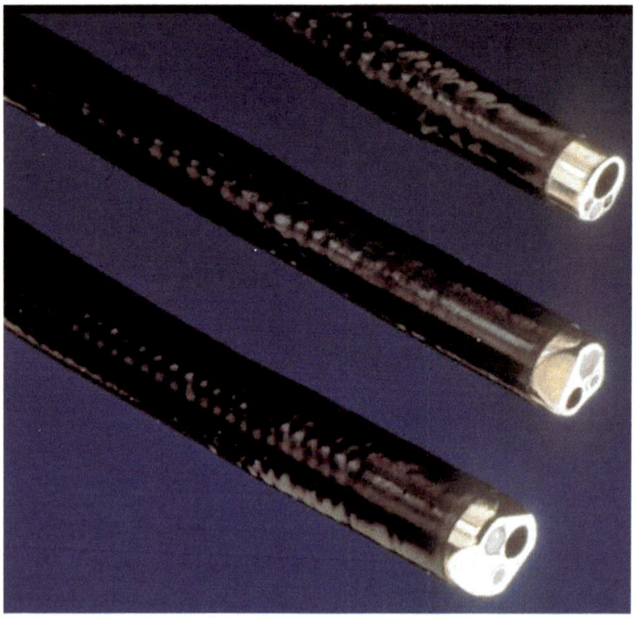

Fig. 41.10 Different-size ureteroscopes are obvious to inspection, feel, and the ureter. Upper 7.6 F, mid 8.3 F, and lower 9.9 F

The Ideal Scope

There is great promise for the development of more effective and anatomically correct deflectable ureteroscopes. There are several factors that can be combined to make something closer to the ideal instrument. For example, the size of the shaft should not be more than 7.5 F for the portion that is inserted into the ureter and 7 F would be preferable. The 7 F endoscope could enter almost any ureter throughout its length, while the 7.5 F would be too large for only a few. This size, of course, limits the imaging capabilities. As video chips become available and become smaller, that problem should also be solved. The best image available today is a video chip design. Endoscopes made with these chips can also theoretically be more durable. The present size of the chip necessitates a flexible ureteroscope that is actually too large for routine use in the ureter.

The ideal technique for flexible ureteroscopy would be to pass the ureteroscope transurethrally into the bladder and directly into the ureter. Many of the present-day endoscopes

Table 41.2 Passing flexible ureteroscopes [36]

Effect of size				
Size	9.0	8.6	8.4	7.4
Failed	11	4	2	1
Total	30	27	38	95
%	36.7	14.8	5.2	1.1

Table 41.3 Ideal flexible ureteroscope

Small diameter, 7 F or less
Excellent imaging
Durable
Relatively rigid
Handle ergonomically designed
Pressure monitoring
Robotic control

are too flexible to allow that maneuver. Therefore, the ideal scope would either be relatively more rigid or incorporate a mechanism to cause rigidity for insertion into the ureter and then allow flexibility after that point. Irrigation will remain necessary to distend or at least open the ureter and the intrarenal collecting system for full inspection and access. An ideal system would be to have constant pressure monitoring in the inflow and measurement of pressure of the outflow within the pelvis since they are not directly related until the pelvis is full and distended.

Since the urologist will not be looking directly through the endoscope, the handle of the endoscope can be altered to make it more ergonomically functional. Early work with a robotic ureteroscope demonstrated the ease of teaching and performing the rotate and deflect maneuvers as necessary to inspect the upper collecting system [37]. Again, this instrument in its present form is much too large for the normal ureter. Therefore, most of the changes needed to provide an ideal ureteroscope are related to the size. Appropriate imaging must become available. Delivery by altering the stiffness of the shaft should be relatively easily achieved. Handle changes should be considered as soon as possible while more irrigation and robotic designs can be expected further into the future (Table 41.3).

Conclusion

Ureteroscopes have developed in steps which have been dependent upon the available technology and materials. The first device was flexible and dependent upon the early fiber optic imaging available. However, the lack of deflection and working channels rendered these instruments only marginally useful for inspection alone. The emphasis changed strongly to rigid ureteroscopy with applications both for stones and tumors, initially in the distal ureter. The development of longer scopes and suitable-size working devices changed the range of ureteroscopy throughout most of the ureter. As the limitations of the rigid scope were evident, flexible ureteroscopes allowed endoscopic access to the intrarenal collecting system. Further refinements including extended deflection and smaller more flexible working instruments, including lasers and small flexible fibers, extended therapeutic procedures throughout the collecting system, including the lower pole. The ideal ureteroscope has yet to be produced. Newer designs in the prototype stage appear to come closer to the ideal designs than endoscopes presently available.

References

1. Young HH, McKay RW. Congenital valvular obstruction of the prostatic urethra. Surg Gynecol Obstet. 1929;48:509.
2. Colladon D. On the reflections of a ray of light inside a parabolic liquid stream. Compt Rend. 1842;15:800.
3. Hecht J. City of lights: the story of fiber optics. New York: Oxford University Press; 1999. p. 13–27.
4. Hirschowitz BI, Curtiss LE, Peters CW, Pollard HM. Gastroenterology. 1958;35:50; Barlow DE. Fiberoptic instrument technology. In: Small animal endoscopy. St. Louis: C.V. Mosby; 1990. p. 1.
5. Marshall VF. Fiber optics in urology. J Urol. 1964;91:110.
6. Takagi T, Go T, Takayasu H, Aso Y. A small-caliber fiberscope for visualization of the urinary tract, biliary tract, and spinal canal. Surgery. 1968;64:1033.
7. Takayasu H, Aso Y. Recent development for pyeloureteroscopy: guide tube method for its introduction into the ureter. J Urol. 1974;112:176.
8. Goodman TM. Ureteroscopy with pediatric cystoscope in adults. Urology. 1977;9(4):394.
9. Lyon ES, Kyker KS, Shoenberg HW. Transurethral ureteroscopy in women: a ready addition to the urological armamentarium. J Urol. 1978;119:35.
10. Lyon ES, Banno JJ, Shoenberg HW. Transurethral ureteroscopy in men using juvenile cystoscopy equipment. J Urol. 1979;122:152.
11. Das S. Transurethral ureteroscopy and stone manipulation under direct vision. J Urol. 1981;125:112.
12. Huffman JL, Bagley DH, Lyon ES. Treatment of distal ureteral calculi using rigid ureteroscope. Urology. 1982;20(6):574.
13. Perez-Castro EE, Martinez-Piniero JA. Transurethral ureteroscopy-a current urologicalprocedure. Arch Esp Urol. 1980;33(5):445–60.
14. Huffman JL, Bagley DH, Schoenberg HW, Lyon ES. Transurethral removal of large ureteral and renal pelvic calculi using ureteroscopic ultrasonic lithotripsy. J Urol. 1983;130:31–4.
15. Raney AM. Electrohydraulic ureterolithotripsy-preliminary report. Urology. 1978;12:284–5.
16. Green DF, Lytton B. Early experience with direct vision electrohydraulic lithotripsy of ureteral calculi. J Urol. 1985;133:767.
17. Begun FP, Jacobs SC, Lawson T. Use of a prototype 3F electrohydraulic electrode with ureteroscopy for treatment of ureteral calculus disease. J Urol. 1988;139:1188–91.
18. Willscher MK, Conway JF, Babayan RK, Morisseau P, Sant GR, Bertagnall A. Safety and efficacy of electrohydraulic lithotripsy by ureteroscopy. J Urol. 1988;140:957–8.
19. Bagley DH, Huffman JL, Lyon ES. Combined rigid and flexible ureteropyeloscopy. J Urol. 1983;130:243–4.

20. Bagley DH, Rittenberg MH. Intrarenal dimensions: guidelines for flexible ureteropyeloscopes. J Surg Endosc Ultrasound Interv Tech. 1987;1:119–21.
21. Grasso M, Bagley DH. A 7.5F actively deflectable, flexible ureteroscope: a New device in both diagnostic and therapeutic upper urinary tract endoscopy. Urology. 1994;43(4):435–41.
22. Dretler SP. An evaluation of ureteral laser lithotripsy: 225 consecutive patients. J Urol. 1990;143:267–72.
23. Abdel-Razzak OM, Bagley DH. The 6.9F semi-rigid ureteroscope in clinical use. Urology. 1993;41(1):45–8.
24. Mulvaney WD. Attempted disintegration of calculi by ultrasonic vibrations. J Urol. 1953;70:704–7.
25. Coats EC. The application of ultrasonic energy to urinary and biliary calculi. J Urol. 1956;75:856–74.
26. Rouvalis P. Electronic lithotripsy for vesical calculus with "Urat-1". an experience of 100 cases and an experimental application of the method to stones in the upper urinary tract. Br J Urol. 1970;42:486.
27. Languetin JM, Jichlinski P, Farre R, van Niederhausern W. The Swiss lithoclast. J Urol. 1990;143:179A.
28. Chew BH, Arsovska O, Lange D, et al. The Canadian StoneBreaker trial: a randomized, multicenter trial comparing the LMA StoneBreaker™ and the Swiss LithoClast® during percutaneous nephrolithotripsy. J Endourol. 2011;25(9):1415–9.
29. Mulvaney WP, Beck CW. The laser beam in urology. J Urol. 1968;99:112–5.
30. Hofmann R, Hartung R, Schmidt-Kloiber H, Reichel E. First clinical experience with a Q-switched neodymium: YAG laser for urinary calculi. J Urol. 1989;141:275–9.
31. Dretler SP, Watson G, Parrish JA, Murray S. Pulsed dye laser fragmentation of ureteral calculi. Initial clinical experience. J Urol. 1987;137:386–99.
32. Bagley DH, Grasso M, Shalaby M, Abass El-Akkad M. Ureteral laser lithotripsy using the pulsolith. J Endourol. 1989;3(1):91–8.
33. Johnson PE, Crameens DM, Price RE. Use of the holmium:YAG laser in urology. Lasers Surg Med. 1992;12:353–63.
34. Webb DR, Kocklburgh R, Johnson WF. The versapulse holmium:YAG laser in clinical urology: a pilot study. Minim Invas Ther. 1993;2:23–6.
35. Erhard M, Bagley DH. Urologic applications of the holmium laser: preliminary experience. J Endourol. 1995;9(5):383–6.
36. Hudson RG, Conlin MJ, Bagley DH. Ureteric access with flexible ureteroscopes: effect of the size of the ureteroscope. BJU Int. 2005;95(7):1043–4.
37. Desai MM, Aron M, Gill IS, et al. Flexible robotic retrograde renoscopy: description of novel robotic device and preliminary laboratory experience. Urology. 2008;72(1):42–6.

The Operating Room Technicians' and Nurses' Roles in Urologic Surgery

42

Mohammad Iqbal and Khurram Mutahir Siddiqui

Abstract

Successful completion of an operative procedure requires careful planning and coordination on the part of operating room staff. This chapter outlines the behind-the-scene preparations that support safe and successful surgery.

Keywords

Operating room • Percutaneous nephrolithotomy (PCNL) • Ureteroscopy (URS) • Instrument care • C-arm image intensifier • Role of circulator • Role of scrub nurse

Introduction

The role of the operating room support staff in the efficient functioning of the operating list is very demanding. The advancements in the surgical techniques and the use of a wide array of armamentarium to surgically treat stones have put extra demands on the entire support system. We now need to maintain a larger inventory, as minimal access surgery relies heavily on the efficiency of the instruments used. We strive to provide the best patient care in the operating room. In order to ensure a safe environment, we have systematically assigned roles at different stages of patient care.

The Day Before: In the Operating Room

The operating list is generated a day prior to the schedule list. We check the procedures accordingly in order to look for any special requirements and to keep updated equipment for the aforementioned list.

M. Iqbal
Department of Nursing, Aga Khan University,
Stadium Road, P.O. Box 3500, Karachi 74800, Pakistan
e-mail: mohammad.iqbal@aku.edu

K.M. Siddiqui, FCPS, FRCS (UK), FEBU (✉)
Department of Nursing, Section of Urology, The Aga Khan University,
Stadium Road, Karachi 74800, Pakistan
e-mail: khurram.siddiqui@aku.edu

Procedure Day

When the patient arrives in the operating room, we are involved with "time-out" procedures that ensure the right identity of the patient, confirm the details of the procedure, and ensure equipment availability, marking of the side of the operation, availability of radiologist/C-arm/ultrasound, and patient position. We also confirm the availability of previous radiological investigations of the patient before taking the patient into the operating room. We check the availability of equipment; because of the high cost of these gadgets, they are often used by multiple specialties (i.e., C-arm). We ensure that a radiolucent operating table is available if fluoroscopy is to be used. When the surgical procedure starts, the operating room nurse takes either the role of a "scrub person" or "the circulator."

Role of Circulator

At the start of the day, the circulator checks the overall preparation of the operating room. He is responsible for assembling and disassembling equipment and for checking that all equipment is in working order. Equipment required for the potential ancillary procedure is also kept ready so that it is available on short request; for example, for a cystolitholapaxy, there might be a need for dilatation or an optical urethrotomy.

J.J. Talati et al. (eds.), *Urolithiasis*,
DOI 10.1007/978-1-4471-4387-1_42,

The circulator nurse checks the operating table and prepares lithotomy poles, the camera monitor trolley, light source, lithoclast machine, ultrasound machine, and computer recording system. In our institute, we take snaps of endourological procedures and provide them with the discharge note.

Role of Scrub Nurse

The scrub nurse prepares the surgical trolley. He/she again checks the operating instruments on trolley and assembles, checks, and then disassembles the instruments.

Some of the practices in our unit for common procedures are elaborated in the following sections.

Preparation for Ureterorenoscopy

The operating room (OR) nurse prepares two sizes of ureteroscopes (URS) (6.4-mm Olympus URS and 8-Fr Wolf URS) and sets the lithoclast handpiece with 0.8-Fr or 1-mm lithoclast probe according to the stone size and URS. In the first step, he/she prepares the cystoscope and, after placement of the guide wire, hands over the ureteric dilators to be used under guidance of fluoroscopy. The OR nurse keeps instruments ready for retrograde pyelography. If the ureter is difficult to negotiate, we use 6.4 Fr URS. However, this size only allows for diagnostic ureteroscopy or for treatment of small stones for which the urologist uses a 0.8-mm lithoclast probe to break stones. Retrieval forceps are weak and difficult to use. The standard 8 Fr URS is used for routine URS; it allows for the use of 1-mm probe of the lithoclast and is good for breaking stones into small pieces. A 7.5 Fr Wolf flexible URS is also useful in narrow ureters where rigid URS difficult to use. Holmium laser would be use according to size and classification of stone. Holmium laser setting vary according to stone but not exceed to 20 watt in ureter with 200 micron laser fiber.

For irrigation we use sodium chloride 0.9 %, and the circulator nurse ensures that an adequate supply of pre-warmed packs is available.

We have multi-length double-J stents of six various sizes and provide them to the urologist when required.

Preparation for Cystolitholapaxy

The scrub nurse prepares his/her trolley with cystoscopy instruments, stone punch, lithoclast, and Ellik evacuator.

After cystoscopy the urologist decides, according to stone size, whether to use the stone punch or Cystolithoclast or Holmium laser. A 2-mm lithoclast probe is used for treatment of bladder stones. We use it with a 24 Fr Wolf cystolitholapaxy instrument with built-in channel for scope. An Ellik evacuator is used to remove stone fragments from the bladder, and we usually have a set available on the table.

Preparation of Percutaneous Nephrolithotomy (PCNL)

The circulator nurse prepares patients in the lithotomy position and is responsible with the anesthesiologist and surgery team for the change of position under anesthesia to a prone position, after insertion of retrograde catheter. We also check that the patient is stabilized with the help of belts and tapes if required. We also ensure that the pressure points are supported with gel pads.

The scrub nurse makes available all the instruments and hands them over to the surgeon when requested. Puncture needle, guide wire, facial dilator, Ellik dilators, and Amplatz sheaths of various sizes are available. Nephroscope, lithoclast, ultrasound, Holmium laser machine with 365 micron laser probe, flexible scope for narrow calyx, C-arm, camera monitor, light source, and so on are also essential equipment and are placed on the table for use, if required.

Postprocedure Instrument Care

After the procedure it is the responsibility of the scrub nurse to wash/clean all instruments. We emphasize the use of personal protective equipment (PPE) for endoscopy instrument washing (Fig. 42.1). We use tap water to wash endoscopy instruments. The channels are also brush cleaned (Fig. 42.2). After drying with dry air, they are lubricated (Fig. 42.3) and stored in the safe place and use appropriate boxes for sterilization (Fig. 42.4).

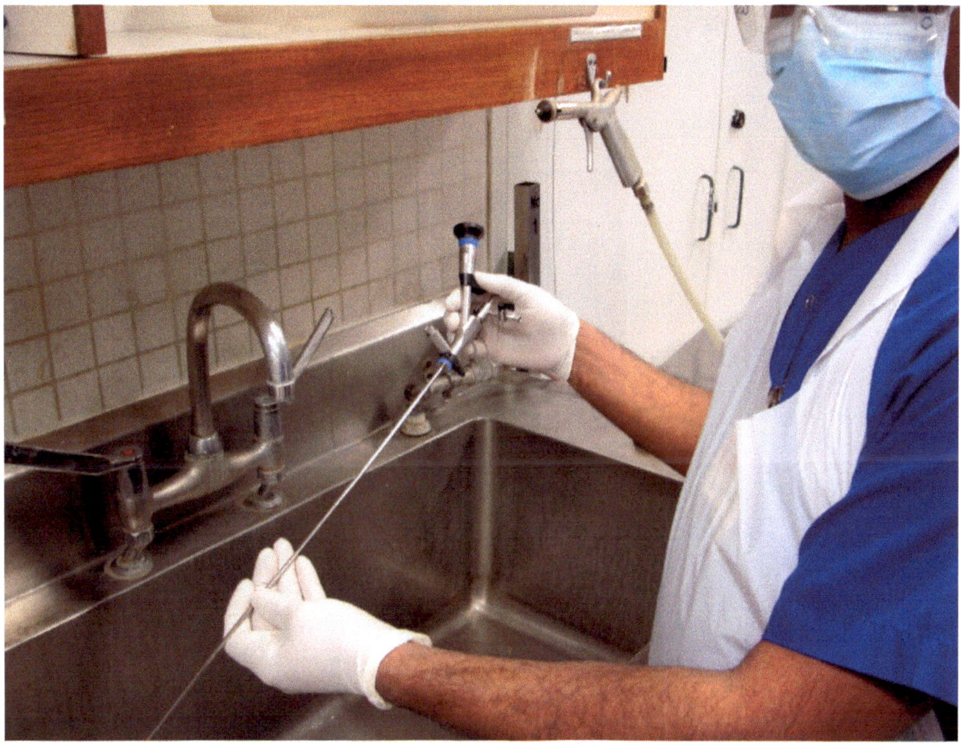

Fig. 42.1 Scrub nurse washing the endoscope while wearing the personal protective equipment

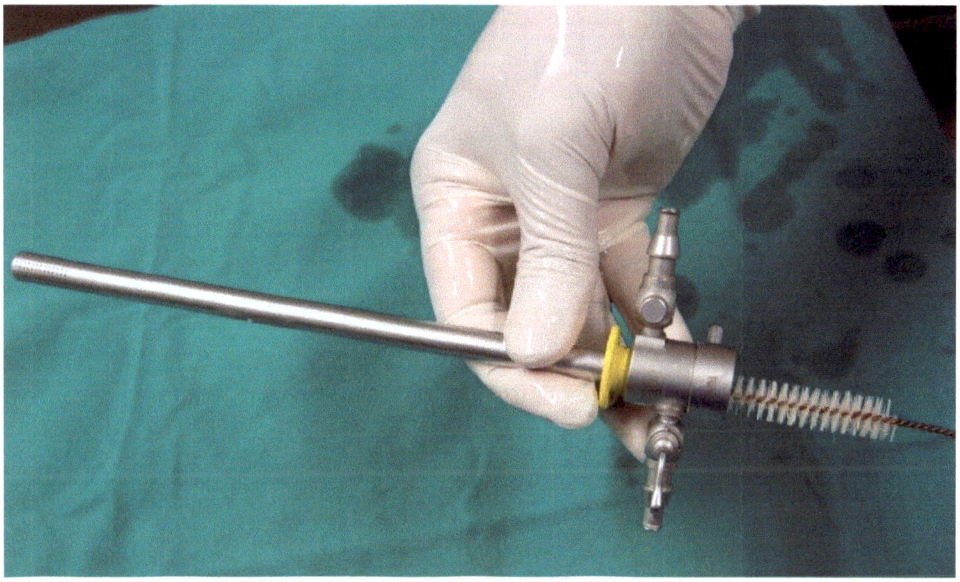

Fig. 42.2 Use of brush to clean the endoscope channel

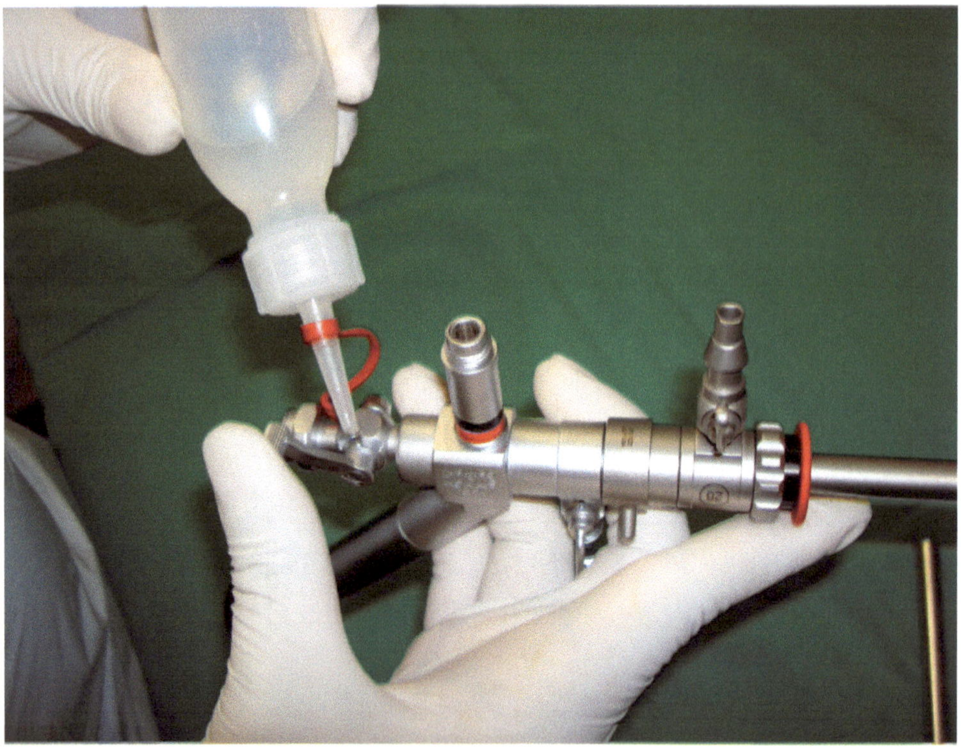

Fig. 42.3 Equipment being lubricated

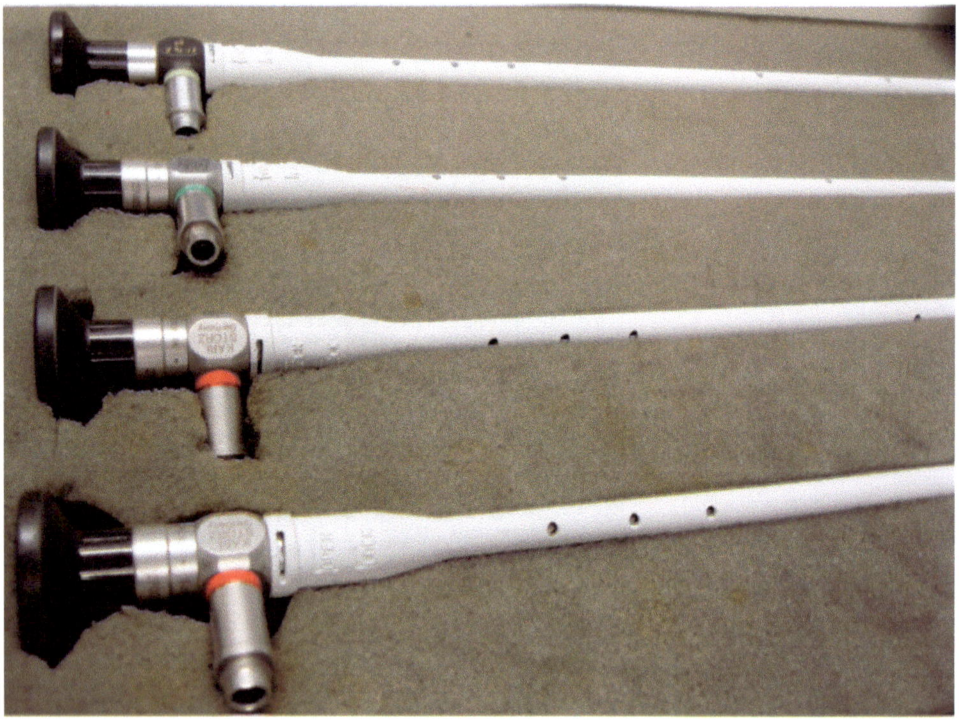

Fig. 42.4 Proper storage of lens

Conclusion

Close coordination between resident staff, consultants, and operating staff leads to an apparently effortless conduct of an operation. A significant amount of preparation, organization, role assignment, and postprocedure instrument care is required to achieve efficiency and safety in the operating room.

Innovation in Stone Disease

43

Brian H. Eisner and Stephen P. Dretler

Abstract

Stone disease has been a part of medical practice since the birth of medicine, mentioned by Hippocrates in the Hippocratic Oath. For hundreds of years, open surgery was the treatment for stones from the kidney to the bladder. Innovation has changed the field dramatically—since the late 1970s, the advent of shock wave lithotripsy, ureteroscopy, and percutaneous nephrolithotomy has completely altered the treatment of nephrolithiasis. This would not have been possible without the creativity and foresight of innovators in treatment of kidney stones. We identified key innovators whose work forever changed the treatment of kidney stones and asked for their thoughts and opinions on innovation in stone disease in a Web-based survey.

Keywords

Innovation • Shock wave lithotripsy • Ureteroscopy • Percutaneous nephrolithotomy Minimally invasive • Creativity • Innovation

Introduction

The Merriam-Webster dictionary defines *innovation* as "the introduction of something new" and *innovator* as a person who "makes changes" or [does] "something in a new way." With this definition in mind, certainly the treatment of kidney stone disease has undergone a number of field-changing innovations since the late 1970s. Specifically, the surgical treatment of kidney stones has changed from open surgery to one of the most minimally invasive fields in urology and perhaps in all of surgery. This is underscored by reports of the near "extinction" of open stone surgery in many centers over the past three to four decades.

To truly understand the effects that innovation has had on the surgical treatment of kidney stones, one must consider a body of recent literature that attests to the declining use of open surgery to treat urolithiasis. One study noted that open surgery accounted for only 1.6 % of all stone surgeries among a large United States-based cohort in 1998, while shock wave lithotripsy (SWL) and ureteroscopy comprised 54 and 41 % of surgical procedures among the same group [1]. A recent study from the United Kingdom noted an 83 % reduction in open stone surgery within the last decade alone [2]. The 1997 and 2007 published guidelines for the treatment of ureteral calculi note that open stone surgery "may well be appropriate for non-standard cases" [3] and that open stone surgery might "rarely be considered" in extreme cases or in cases of "simultaneous open surgery for another purpose" [4]. Similarly, the American Urological Association Guideline on the Management of Staghorn Calculi (2005) noted that open surgery "should not be used for most patients" with large branched renal stones [5].

The three major innovations in the treatment of kidney stones—shock wave lithotripsy, ureteroscopy, and percutaneous nephrolithotomy (PCNL)—were all born in the late 1970s and early 1980s [6–9]. Clearly urologists and their colleagues who pioneered these procedures were true innovators—their forward thinking, creativity, and perseverance

B.H. Eisner, M.D. (✉) • S.P. Dretler, M.D.
Department of Urology, Massachusetts General Hospital, Harvard Medical School, Boston, MA, USA
e-mail: beisner@partners.org; sdretler@partners.org

J.J. Talati et al. (eds.), *Urolithiasis*,
DOI 10.1007/978-1-4471-4387-1_43, © Springer-Verlag London 2012

changed the treatment of kidney stone disease in their own lifetimes and laid the foundation for progress to come. We performed a survey of several early thought leaders in minimally invasive treatment of stone disease in order to gain a better understanding of innovation as it relates to their accomplishments and to modern kidney stone treatment.

Steps to Innovation

B. J. Fogg, an expert on changing human behavior at Stanford University, recently posted his ideas on the key steps to innovation. His ideas, along with those of other similar writers, laid the groundwork for our survey to innovators in stone disease. Fogg's key steps to innovation, first written to a graduate student in 2003, are as follows:

1. Identify an institutional need that intersects with your passion.
2. Get a clear vision of your goal.
3. Enlist support from others and seek feedback.
4. Create value—at first this means working on your own time without compensation or recognition.
5. Document and share your success/progress.
6. Work to institutionalize your product/service/vision.
7. Persist despite setbacks.

> The steps come in the order above, but you also need to return to previous steps. It's iterative. For example, at certain points, you'll need to refocus your vision, you'll need to continue to create value, etc. By doing these seven steps you have the best chance to succeed…. [10]

Survey Format

A Web-based survey was sent to key thought leaders in kidney stone disease over the past four decades. The survey was sent to the urologists who were the early innovators and champions of minimally invasive treatment of stone disease. Respondents were given 3 months to respond to the survey. The following are the questions that comprised the survey. The remainder of this chapter is a compilation of the survey responses and how they relate to innovation in kidney stone disease. All quotations or references to survey responses are included with the permission from the survey respondents.

- When did you first conceive of your innovation (i.e., your "aha" moment)?
- How long did it take from this moment for your innovation to become a reality?
- What "unmet need" did your innovation address?
- Was there an inspiring event or person?
- What other people were instrumental in your innovation?
- What were the barriers or obstacles to getting your innovation accepted and how were they overcome?
- Was your innovation accepted at the outset or did you meet resistance?
- Was your innovation rejected from publications and meetings?
- Were there times you wanted to give up? What brought you back?
- Have others built on your innovation?
- What impact will your innovation have on the future of stone disease?
- Can you name others who you consider innovators in the treatment of nephrolithiasis?
- What innovators do you draw inspiration from (not limited to medical field)?

Respondents to our survey are pioneers in the field of minimally invasive stone treatment and endourology. They were central to the adoption of SWL, ureteroscopy, and percutaneous nephrolithotomy—the three most common treatments for stone disease. They were also central in the development of key concepts in stone treatment, which include stone fragility, multi-access PCNL, ultrasound-guided PCNL, and expanding the use of flexible ureteroscopy to treat lesions of the renal collecting system and ureter.

Inspiration and Building on the Work of Others

> If I have seen further, it is only by standing on the shoulders of giants.
> Sir Isaac Newton

In the preceding quotation, Sir Isaac Newton, arguably one of history's greatest innovators, recognizes that his work would not have been possible without those who came before him and laid the foundations for future innovation. Innovation in stone disease clearly invokes this theme as well. Respondents to our survey noted that their own work built upon that of their predecessors and without which they may not have succeeded:

> Arthur Smith and Ralph Clayman supported the concept of creating new words for new ideas and [allowed me to publish this work] in the *Journal of Endourology*. – Survey respondent
> I adopted [the technique] of percutaneous nephrolithotomy after seeing Peter Alkin present [his] lecture at the SIU meeting in 1982 in San Francisco. – Survey respondent

Other respondents of our survey noted inspiring patients and other influences on their early work:

> The first endourology book was dedicated to my wife and [patient name]. [He] had difficult stone disease and allowed us to perform multiple procedures percutaneously to approach his stones…He was far braver than I and deserves the credit for our getting into the various endoscopic areas of PCNL. – Survey respondent
> [I was inspired by] patients presenting with difficult problems. – Survey respondent

Respondents also noted their own "inspiring innovators"—figures within and outside the field of medicine. These include the following:

- *Nonphysicians*: Isaac Newton, Galileo, Albert Einstein, Thomas Edison
- *Physicians*: Joseph Segura, Inderbir Gill, Stephen Dretler, Peter Alken, Christian Chaussy, Arthur Smith, Jim Lingeman, Ralph Clayman, Margaret Pearle, Demetrius Bagley, Ed Lyon, Glenn Preminger, Dean Assimos

Goals, Unmet Needs, and Enlisting Help and Support

The perceived needs of the patients and of the urological community to treat them provided the motivation and inspiration for innovation. Innovators cited the following goals that were crucial to their innovations: "surgical cure without or with less morbidity," "[improving treatment] safety," "to teach visiting urologists whom to treat and whom not to treat," "[the desire to be] minimally invasive," and "to extend endourologic access" as their goals at the outset of their work.

The help of others (in the urologic community, collaborators, etc.) was done largely through "teaching and training," and survey respondents repeatedly cited "stepwise demonstration of the use of [their innovation]" and "repetition" of their findings and ideas as key steps to enlisting the help of others. Several respondents also noted that support of and collaboration with industry (i.e., technological advancements in machinery, endoscopy, and disposables) as well as colleagues in other fields such as diagnostic and interventional radiology were important aspects of their success.

Failure, Rejection, and Persistence

> If at first you don't succeed, try, try, try again.
> William E. Hickson

B. J. Fogg, cited previously, notes that the final key step to innovation is to *persist despite setbacks*. This appears to have been one of the most valuable concepts for the innovators from our survey. Their stories demonstrate perseverance, without which they may have failed. Respondents noted the time for their innovation to become accepted once they brought it to the eye of the general urologic community. From percutaneous stone extraction (months) to ureteroscopy and shock wave lithotripsy (years), each of these key innovations was not accepted "overnight." Furthermore, innovators in shock wave lithotripsy, ureteroscopy, and percutaneous nephrolithotomy all noted that they "met resistance" at the onset of their innovation. The earliest attempts at publication and meeting presentation were in many cases rejected from journals and meetings, including concepts of clinical use of shock wave lithotripsy, the initial paper on rapid dilation of the nephrostomy tract, percutaneous nephrolithotomy, and the concept of stone fragility. One respondent stated that "a high level of resistance proved that the concept was new—the more resistance, the more innovative the concept." Respondents noted that the scientific community demanded "proper scientific evidence, especially complications and long-term results [of PCNL]," and "scientific proof was demanded [even when concepts appeared to be common sense]." Several other respondents noted that others were slow to adopt their innovations because they "challenged standard accepted techniques" and also that people were uncomfortable trying new techniques such as trying to "pass a flexible ureteroscope."

Shock wave lithotripsy, currently the most common treatment modality for all stone disease [1], provides a particular resonant example of persistence and success—the first patient to be treated with SWL was in February 1980. Subsequent to that, *The Lancet* published the first clinical results of SWL. Nonetheless, that year the presentation was rejected by the American Urological Association (AUA) annual meeting. The following year, the clinical data was accepted for presentation at the AUA annual meeting. The first paper on SWL in the United States did not appear until 2 years after the first lithotripters were used in America. Ten years after the first patient was treated with SWL in Munich, the authors (Chaussy, Eisenberger, and Schmiedt) were presented with the Distinguished Contribution Award by the AUA [11].

The "Aha" Moment

Aha moment (noun): "a moment of sudden insight or discovery"[1]

Aha moment (noun): "an instant at which the solution to a problem becomes clear" [2]

Innovators became aware of solutions to problems that led to their innovations at various times and in various places. Inspirations for the "aha moment" included patients, colleagues, and concepts.

> I had a patient with a leak from reimplantation of the ureter. When I could not [place a ureteral] stent from below, I did a percutaneous nephrostomy, passed a tube down the ureter, and fixed the stent to that tube, then pulled it up the ureter. After that, I realized that the percutaneous access was the gateway to the upper tract. – Survey respondent
> The use of ultrasound in urology [gave me the concept of ultrasound and percutaneous nephrolithotomy]. – Survey respondent

[1] www.oxforddictionaries.com

[2] www.dictionary.com

While teaching physicians how to use the [shock wave] lithotripter, they would ask "How many shocks will it take to break this stone…." All of a sudden I realized that stones looked different on X-ray and that I could predict the fragmentability of the stone by predicting its fragility… – Survey respondent

Other respondents noted that they developed their ideas "as instruments became available," "[when they were presented with] patients with difficult problems," or as a result of "questions and challenges from [their] residents and trainees."

Their Legacy

Survey respondents were asked what their lasting contribution to stone disease would be and what they will be remembered for. Their responses are as follows:

The end of open stone surgery…In 25 years I have not done a single open stone procedure. I believe the same is true of many other urologists….
Choosing the right procedure based on stone size, location, and stone fragility.
[PCNL allows for] preservation of renal function with reduced morbidity [in treatment of large stones].
Change to the approach treatment of calculi [with popularization of ureteroscopy].
Open surgery for stone disease will cease to take place.
Development of the technique of percutaneous stone extraction.
Today there are more than 5,000 lithotriptors in use worldwide, and the more than a million treatments per year show the method's global acceptance [11].

Conclusion

Since the late 1970s, significant changes in the treatment of nephrolithiasis have completely changed this field. Open stone surgery has become obsolete, and it is used with extreme rarity in most centers. The urological community owes a debt of gratitude to those who were creative, bold, and perseverant enough to innovate and change the face of kidney stone treatment. Their words of wisdom, contained within this chapter, should inspire urologists of future generations to continue to create new and innovative methods for stone treatment.

Acknowledgements The authors are indebted to the innovators in stone disease who responded to our survey and made this chapter possible.

References

1. Pearle MS, Calhoun EA, Curhan GC, Urologic Diseases of America Project. Urologic diseases in America project: urolithiasis. J Urol. 2005;173(3):848–57.
2. Turney BW, Reynard JM, Noble JG, Keoghane SR. Trends in urological stone disease. BJU Int. 2012;109(7):1082–7. Epub 2011 Aug 26.
3. Segura JW, Preminger GM, Assimos DG, Dretler SP, Kahn RI, Lingeman JE, et al. Ureteral stones clinical guidelines panel summary report on the management of ureteral calculi. The American Urological Association. J Urol. 1997;158(5):1915–21.
4. Preminger GM, Tiselius HG, Assimos DG, Alken P, Buck C, Gallucci M, et al. 2007 guideline for the management of ureteral calculi. J Urol. 2007;178(6):2418–34.
5. Preminger GM, Assimos DG, Lingeman JE, Nakada SY, Pearle MS, Wolf Jr JS, et al. Chapter 1: AUA guideline on management of staghorn calculi: diagnosis and treatment recommendations. J Urol. 2005;173(6):1991–2000.
6. Chaussy C, Schmiedt E, Jocham D, Brendel W, Forssmann B, Walther V. First clinical experience with extracorporeally induced destruction of kidney stones by shock waves. J Urol. 1982; 127(3):417–20.
7. Alken P, Hutschenreiter G, Gunther R, Marberger M. Percutaneous stone manipulation. J Urol. 1981;125(4):463–6.
8. Wickham JE, Kellet MJ. Percutaneous nephrolithotomy. Br Med J (Clin Res Ed). 1981;283(6306):1571–2.
9. Conlin MJ, Marberger M, Bagley DH. Ureteroscopy. Development and instrumentation. Urol Clin North Am. 1997;24(1):25–42.
10. Fogg BJ. BJ Fogg's steps to innovation. Available at: http://bjfogg.com/innovation.htm. Accessed July 2, 2003.
11. Chaussy C, Eisenberger F, Forssmann B. Extracorporeal shock-wave lithotripsy (ESWL): a chronology. J Endourol. 2007;21(11): 1249–53.

Part V

Management Strategies

The Management of a Patient with an Acute Stone Problem

44

Ahmed S. El-Hefnawy, Ahmed Abed, and Ahmed A. Shokeir

Abstract

Objectives: Pain management is a critical component of high-quality patient care. Renal colic (RC) is the most bothersome presentation of urolithiasis. In this chapter, we aim to present different management modalities involved in care of patients presented with RC resulting from urolithiasis. In addition guidelines for treatment are provided with critical review of the most recent advances in this field.

Materials and Methods: Database of PubMed and the Cochrane Database were searched through March 2011 without time limit. The following keywords were used: renal pain, renal colic, management, nonsteroidal anti-inflammatory drugs, opioids, alpha blockers, renal obstruction, and medical expulsive therapy. A total of 1,021 publications were retrieved. Articles of evidence-based levels of I and II were included together with publication of level III that contain large number of patients.

Results: RC is the ultimate result of obstruction of the ureter or renal collecting system. It represents one of the most frequent presentations in the emergency room (ER). Most of randomized controlled trials (RCT) have documented the efficacy of nonsteroidal anti-inflammatory drugs (NSAIDs) as pharmacological agent of choice in initial management of RC. Diclofenac sodium is recommended to reduce the recurrent episodes. Opioids can be used as a second line; recent studies reported better efficacy when combined with NSAIDs without added adverse effects, while alpha blockers and calcium channel blockers are recommended for medical expulsive therapy (MET). Tamsulosin is the most studied agent with proven safety and efficacy in many RCT. Combination protocols between alpha blockers and corticosteroids might provide better results. In patients with obstructed kidneys, drainage with nephrostomy tubes or stenting should be attempted first before definitive intervention.

Conclusions: The current trends recommended NSAIDs for pain relief and alpha blockers for MET. Combination protocols are gaining more acceptance; however, dose standardization is warranted.

A.S. El-Hefnawy, M.D. • A. Abed, M.D., M.S.
Department of Urology, Urology and Nephrology Center, Mansoura University, Mansoura, Egypt
e-mail: a_s_elhefnawy@yahoo.com

A.A. Shokeir, M.D., Ph.D., FEBU (✉)
Department of Urology, Urology and Nephrology Center, Mansoura University, Mansoura, Egypt
e-mail: ahmed.shokeir@hotmail.com

J.J. Talati et al. (eds.), *Urolithiasis*,
DOI 10.1007/978-1-4471-4387-1_44, © Springer-Verlag London 2012

Keywords
Renal pain • Renal colic • Management • Nonsteroidal anti-inflammatory drugs • Opioids • Alpha blockers • Renal obstruction • Medical expulsive therapy

Introduction

Acute renal colic (RC) is one of the most severe forms of pain in humans. Patients with acute renal colic are often seen and evaluated by emergency physicians at the beginning before referral for definitive management. However, physician perspectives are not limited only on pain management. After establishment of diagnosis, the ultimate goals of the attending physician are to relieve renal pain, expulsion of the stone, and protection of the kidney from any further damage caused by obstructive effects of stones. In order to achieve such goals, the treating doctor should have a good knowledge of a wide spectrum of pharmacological and surgical modalities that can be used in each specific situation.

In this chapter we present different management modalities involved in care of patients who present with RC secondary to urolithiasis. In addition, guidelines for treatment are provided with a critical review of the most recent advances in management of patients with acute stone problems.

Epidemiology and Economic Burden

Renal colic (RC) due to obstruction by urolithiasis represents one of the most frequent presentations in emergency departments (ED). Renal colic affects approximately 1.2 million people each year and accounts for 1 % of all emergency department visits [1] and 1 % of hospital admissions [2]. The peak onset of symptomatic nephrolithiasis occurs in the third and fourth decades of life with an estimated male-to-female ratio of 3:1 [3]. There are concrete data reporting higher incidence of admissions due to RC in hotter climates and in the summer [4] with a high likelihood of stone formation as a result of dehydration and increased concentration, crystallization, and acidification of urine.

According to anecdotal evidence, people are more at risk of RC during the night. However, recent data suggested a circadian variability for the occurrence of RC, with a pattern characterized by a morning peak [5, 6]. Urine production and renal excretion rates of solutes rise during daytime and reach minimum values at night. Also, the glomerular filtration rate (GFR) exhibits a circadian rhythm peaking in the morning [7]. Studies on healthy people and people who have had kidney stones showed a higher risk of calcium oxalate crystallization in the morning [8].

In a study that included 574 patients, mean total hospital cost in patients admitted to the ED due to RC was calculated to be 55.77 €. The greatest contribution to the total cost was made by radiological investigations in the ED (40.5 %) followed by treatment costs (19.7 %) [9]. Annual cost of urinary calculi was estimated to exceed US $2 billion annually [10]. According to the best of our knowledge, no available studies estimated the indirect cost as a result of disability associated with RC, although association between recurrent renal colic and both anxiety and depression has been suggested [11]. Both psychological problems are largely responsible for physical limitations, loss of functional roles and workdays, as well as the frequent use of health services in various countries on different continents [12, 13].

Pathophysiology

Understanding the pathophysiology of RC, involved neurotransmitters, and subsequent molecular events after renal obstruction is important in development of therapeutic pharmaceuticals as well as in determination of management strategies.

The resulting increase in the intraluminal pressure from ureteric obstruction leads to stretching and stimulation of nerve endings in the lamina propria. In addition, expansion of the renal capsule and collecting system is followed by hyperperistalsis of the ureter because the smooth muscle in the wall of the ureter contracts as it tries to move the stone. If the stone becomes lodged and unable to move, these muscles go into spasm [14]. Activation of adrenergic and muscarinic receptors increases the amplitude of ureteric contraction [15]. A prolonged isotonic contraction leads to increased production of lactic acid, which irritates both slow-type A (myelinated and fast conducting; 12–30 m/s, responsible for sharp and stabbing pain) and fast-type C fibers (nonmyelinated, slow conducting; 1 m/s, responsible for dull continuous pain) [16]. Afferent impulses are generated and travel to the posterior horn of the spinal cord at the T11–L1 levels with subsequent projections to higher levels of the central nervous system (CNS). This pain can also be perceived in any organ sharing the urinary tract innervations such as the gastrointestinal organs and other components of the genitourinary system [14].

Because of the pathophysiological complexity, it is not surprising that animal experiments are in mostly small and not well-controlled studies [17]. Moody and colleagues in experimental study have shown that renal pelvic pressure and renal blood flow (RBF) pass into triphasic change following total unilateral ureteral obstruction. In the initial 1.5 h, pressure and flow increase, and then, over the next 4 h, renal pelvic pressure remains high but renal blood flow starts to decline. After this time there is a decline in both renal pelvic pressure and renal blood flow [18]. The initial increase in renal blood flow is due to preglomerular vasodilatation and is mediated by prostaglandins, which cause a diuresis that further increases renal pelvic pressure. The role of nitric oxide in reducing preglomerular vascular resistance has also been suggested [19].

The subsequent decrease in renal blood flow is due to an increase in intrarenal resistance caused by preglomerular vasoconstriction. Consensus does not exist on the mediators of vasoconstriction; among these are angiotensin II, thromboxane A2, antidiuretic hormone, and endothelin [20]. The decline in ureteric pressure is due to a decrease in glomerular filtration rate and an increase in the venous and lymphatic reabsorption of urine. Such decrease is considered as a defense mechanism against parenchymal atrophy and may provide possible explanation for spontaneous improvement in severity of renal colic a few hours after its onset in most patients [14]. The reduction in glomerular filtration rate is due to a decrease in the net hydraulic pressure gradient across the glomerular capillaries and to an increase in the tubular pressure caused by the increase in ureteric pressure.

In a recent review on molecular pain, compelling evidence has been presented for the role of purinergic mechanosensory transduction where adenosine triphosphate (ATP), released from epithelial cells lining the ureter, acts on P2X3 and/or P2X2/3 receptors on subepithelial sensory nerve terminals to relay nociceptive messages via sensory ganglia and spinal cord to pain centers in the CNS [21]. With increasing interest in the role of expulsive therapy for treatment of ureteral stones, attention has been focused to address the various modulators that affect ureteric contraction. The purinergic system is found to be important not only in sensory but also in motor functions. ATP is an important non-adrenergic non-cholinergic (NANC) agent causing contraction. Serotonin causes contraction, while nitric oxide (NO) is a major inhibitory NANC neurotransmitter causing relaxation. Prostaglandin F2 alpha contracts whereas prostaglandin E1/E2 relaxes the ureter. Phosphodiesterases (PDE) and the Rho-kinase pathway have recently been identified in the human ureter [15].

Lines of Management of Patients with Acute Stone Problem

The primary goal of management of acute stone problems is relief of pain. Several treatment modalities have been employed including pharmacological and nonpharmacological therapies.

Pharmacological Treatment for Pain Relief

Pain relief still remains as the most urgent step in patients with an acute stone episode. Several pharmaceutical drugs have been involved in management of acute attacks of renal colic including nonsteroidal anti-inflammatory drugs (NSAIDs), opiate analgesics, and antimuscarinics, and more recently use of desmopressin has been reported.

NSAIDs

NSAIDs block prostaglandin-induced effects, such as afferent arteriolar vasodilatation, which causes an increase in diuresis and consequently raises pelvic pressure. They also reduce local edema and inflammation and inhibit the stimulation of ureteric smooth muscle, which is responsible for increased peristalsis and subsequently increased ureteric pressure [14]. NSAIDs are used in the treatment of renal colic using a variety of routes including intramuscular, intravenous (IV), oral, rectal, and sublingual, with the former route having the best analgesic effect.

Several NSAIDs have been described for management of RC including diclofenac, indomethacin, ibuprofen, and ketorolac. In a systemic review of 20 studies conducted by Cochrane Renal Group and involving 1,613 patients, NSAIDs were found to have better analgesic effect compared with opioids; 10 out of 13 studies reported lower pain scores in patients receiving NDAIDs [22]. More recent studies support the effectiveness of NSAIDs [16, 23–26]. Diclofenac has been recommended as the first drug of choice in RC (grade A) according to the European Association of Urology (EAU) guidelines [23]. In a prospective double-blinded randomized study, ketorolac and diclofenac were equal with respect to pain level over time, the number of patients requiring rescue medicine, and the level of adverse effects [27].

Recently, it has been demonstrated that ureteral obstruction is associated with increased cyclooxygenase (COX)-2 expression and that selective COX-2 inhibitors provide potent analgesia with fewer side effects in patients with ureteral stones. Moreover, selective COX-2 inhibitors have been shown to decrease in vitro contractility of the human ureter [28, 29]. However, in a recent RCT, celecoxib was not superior to placebo for management of RC and does not facilitate stone passage or decrease narcotic requirements in patients with RC [30].

Although NSAIDs reduce pain associated with renal colic, they may potentially interfere with the kidney's autoregulatory response to obstruction with marked reduction of renal blood flow [31]. Moreover, some NSAIDs were shown to decrease the tubular damage and interstitial fibrosis [32] caused by ureteric obstruction. In healthy individuals, these effects are well tolerated [33], although the diagnostic accuracy of resistive index may be affected. In a recent experimental study on rats, administration of diclofenac sodium during a relatively long period of unilateral ureteric obstruction, similar to its use in the management of ureteric colic, appears to ameliorate the alterations in the hemodynamic glomerular functions including the GFR and the RBF at least 2 weeks following the reversal of obstruction [34].

In patients with preexisting renal disease, however, administration of NSAIDs can induce renal failure [35, 36]. This potentially toxic renal effect of NSAIDs was also supported by the clinical observation of renal function deterioration in some individuals such as elderly patients [37, 38]. NSAIDs can also have serious gastrointestinal side effects. Cyclooxygenase-2 inhibitors had been developed to reduce gastrointestinal effects, but they also inhibit renal vasoactive substances and are contraindicated in patients with renal insufficiency [14].

Opiate Analgesics

Opioids have been the traditional first-line therapy for patients suffering from acute renal colic. The two most common opioids studied are morphine and meperidine. A randomized controlled trial (RCT) comparing 10 mg of IV morphine with 100 mg of IV meperidine found they were equally effective [39]. However, because of meperidine's greater abuse potential and increased side effect profile, morphine is recommended over meperidine [40]. Narcotic analgesics can induce adverse effects such as sedation, respiratory depression, constipation, addiction, nausea, and vomiting.

Papaverine hydrochloride (HCl) is a nonaddictive opium-derived agent, extracted from the poppy plant genus *Papaver*. It interferes with the phosphodiesterase enzyme, resulting in an increase in cyclic adenosine monophosphate, which ultimately causes smooth muscle relaxation [41]. This specific effect makes it a potent vasodilator in the vascular system. It has been used in patients with renal colic as a part of systemic treatment [42] with reported high efficacy in patients unresponsive to commonly used conventional agents [43].

Tramadol, a centrally acting analgesic structurally related to codeine and morphine, consists of two enantiomers, both of which contribute to analgesic activity via different mechanisms [44], with fewer opioid-type side effects and less potential for dependence [45]. In a prospective study involving 300 patients with RC, continuous intravenous drip was proven to be effective and safe [46].

Combination Therapy

A Cochrane Database review from 2004 suggested that nonsteroidal anti-inflammatory drugs are superior single agents compared with opiates for the treatment of renal colic [10]. However, a more recent study by Safdar et al. reported that combination therapy with ketorolac and morphine may result in more effective analgesia and a reduced need for rescue medications versus nonsteroidal anti-inflammatory drugs or opiates alone [47]. In another study, ketorolac and meperidine were randomly compared for analgesia in acute RC. Results showed the combination of both drugs resulted in better pain control than meperidine alone. Interestingly, ketorolac alone was found to have equal efficacy as the combination group in pain relief [48].

Nonopiate Analgesics

Paracetamol (acetaminophen) is a safe and effective analgesic administered orally or rectally. At therapeutic doses, it is associated with fewer adverse effects than either opioids or nonsteroidal anti-inflammatory drugs [49]. Safety and efficacy of intravenous paracetamol has been reported in a randomized, double-blind, placebo-controlled clinical trial in which single intravenous doses of paracetamol (1 g) were compared with morphine (0.1 mg/kg) and placebo (normal saline solution) [50].

Metamizol is an effective, non-opioid analgesic, which was originally introduced to the therapy in the year 1922. Metamizol has proved to be a very effective analgesic. When administered in equipotent doses, its effects are comparable to various opioid analgesics [51], and it has been used effectively in RC [52].

Parasympatholytics

N-butyl scopolamine is a parasympatholytic that has been historically used in RC. It acts in the distal ureter parasympathetic innervation. A very high dose should be administrated in order to achieve an effect on the smooth muscles of the distal ureter, which inevitably results in side effects such as tachycardia and intestinal obstruction.

In a study that compared effect of hyoscine *N*-butylbromide with placebo for patients with stone related renal colic, Holdgate et al. demonstrated that hyoscine *N*-butylbromide does not reduce opioid requirements or the need for ongoing opioid analgesia [53]. Currently, anticholinergics are no longer mentioned in guidelines of RC management; however, some textbooks still state that *N*-butyl scopolamine (Buscopan®) has a beneficial effect in RC. This, however, could be applied on Buscopan compositum®, which is an effective combination product that contains metamizol [17].

Desmopressin

Desmopressin is a vasopressin analogue with a potent antidiuretic activity and less pressor effects in comparison with vasopressin. Several studies have showed that desmopressin can reduce pain in patients with acute renal colic, and the response to the desmopressin is not a placebo effect [54–56]. In a prospective randomized study, the effect of intranasal desmopressin and intramuscular hyoscine *N*-butylbromide combination was compared with intramuscular hyoscine *N*-butylbromide alone. Results showed that desmopressin in combination with hyoscine *N*-butylbromide appears to be a promising alternative or adjunct to analgesic medications in patients with acute renal colic, especially in patients in whom narcotics cannot be used [57].

The mechanism of analgesic action of desmopressin in RC is uncertain. At the peripheral level, desmopressin may alleviate pain through its potent antidiuretic effect or by relaxing renal pelvic and ureteral smooth muscles. The central analgesic effect of desmopressin by stimulating the release of the hypothalamic β(beta)-endorphin is also proposed [14].

Nonpharmacological Treatment of Renal Pain

Sterile Water and Forced Hydration

Intracutaneous injection of sterile water has been reported as an efficient pain relief therapy in cases of RC [58, 59]. The possible mechanisms include endorfinergic action and stimulation of pain regulatory centers because of painful stimuli.

Although the usefulness of hydration is well established in the prevention of stone formation, the use of forced hydration to promote stone expulsion has recently become controversial. Forced intravenous hydration in the ED setting (2 L normal saline) did not impact narcotic use, pain scores, or stone passage rates [60].

Acupuncture

Acupuncture is another method for the treatment of RC that is common in China. A possible mechanism may be related to increased endogenous endorphins in cerebrospinal fluids [61]. A recent study has proven meridian electrical conductance in patients with renal colic, which may provide better results for acupuncture in the future [62].

Heat Therapy

A few reports speculated that renal colic pain can be treated effectively with warming the low back [63]. Heat therapy might have a suppressive effect on the sympathetic hyperactivity [63, 64] seen during RC.

Standardization of Pain Management Protocol

Despite a huge number of publications on management of RC (the vast majority are well-designed controlled trials), lack of standard of care for patients presented with RC in ED is acknowledged. A recent study evaluating current practice patterns in United States emergency rooms for the diagnosis, treatment, and counseling of patients with ureteral calculi showed that only 13 % of evaluated ERs have guidelines for the management of ureteral calculi [2]. Wessie and coworkers conducted an experimental design using medical vignettes to evaluate if patient gender and race affects decisions about pain management [65]. In that study, a convenience sample of 11 primary care physicians was asked to treat three hypothetical patients with pain (kidney stone, back pain) or a control condition (sinusitis). Interestingly, gender and racial differences were evident when the role of physician gender was examined, suggesting that many male and female physicians react differently to gender and/or racial cues. With the application of standardized pain management protocol involving treatment of patients with ketorolac, 30 mg IV, and morphine, 0.05–0.1 mg/kg IV, Steinberg and colleagues have succeeded in gaining marked improvement in quality of care as evidenced by a 49 % reduction in time to effective analgesia [24].

Based on the last American Urological Association (AUA) and EAU guidelines (Chicago 2010 and Vienna 2011) for management of pain in RC, the following steps are recommended:

> NSAIDs should be used as a first-line management. Diclofenac sodium could be used also to counteract recurrent pain after an episode of ureteral colic. Hydromorphine or Tramadol could be used as a second line while spasmolytics (e.g., metamizole sodium) may be given when a nonnarcotic agent is mandatory. If pain relief cannot be achieved by medical means, drainage or stone removal should be carried out.

Despite the AUA and EAU annually publishing guidelines for management of pain in urolithiasis, however, on reality basis, the aforementioned studies may underscore the importance of development of collaborative practice guidelines between urology and emergency medicine associations. In addition, educational programs in urinary stone emergencies for primary care providers are warranted.

Drainage of Obstructed Infected Kidneys

Obstructed infected kidneys secondary to stone with subsequent septicemia represent a true life-threatening emergency. A recent systematic review [66] found that only two randomized control trials [67, 68] investigated the optimum method for drainage. A little evidence supports the superiority of percutaneous nephrostomy over retrograde stenting. El-Hefnawy et al. reported that direct bilateral same-session ureteroscopy is safe and effective in distal ureteric stones even in patients with anuria, but not recommended in presence of signs of infection [69].

Medical Expulsive Therapy (MET)

In this section, medical expulsive therapy (MET) is discussed only briefly since it is beyond the focus of this chapter.

According to evidence-based guidelines, the most promising drugs studied for MET are alpha blockers and calcium channel blockers [23, 70, 71]. Several other modalities have been reported, but none of them have succeeded in gaining wide acceptance, including high fluid intake [72], NSAIDs [30], and anticholinergic *N*-butylscopolamine [22]. Use of corticosteroids has been reported to facilitate stone expulsion [73] due to its anti-inflammatory action. However, such ability is a matter of question if it is used as a monotherapy. Recently, the ureteral smooth muscle relaxing effects of phosphodiesterase (PDE) type 4 inhibitor (PDE4-I) and PDE type 5 inhibitor (PDE5-I) in vitro have been reported. Results were similar to those reported for tamsulosin, suggesting the potential for using PDE inhibitors in the treatment of ureteral colic [74]; however, their potential role in expulsion therapy has to be assessed in controlled studies.

The calcium channel blockers nifedipine and verapamil inhibit endogenous prostaglandin synthesis and calcium influx, reducing spontaneous rhythmic contractions of the human ureter [75]. Similarly, α(alpha)-blockers inhibit contractions of ureteral musculature, reduce basal tone, and decrease peristaltic frequency and colic pain, possibly facilitating ureteral stone expulsion and suggesting a beneficial effect for MET [76]. A recent systematic review involved 47 randomized control trials on medical expulsion therapy showed that MET with α(alpha)-blockers or calcium channel blockers augments stone expulsion rates, reduces the time to stone expulsion, and lowers analgesia requirements for ureteral stones with and without extracorporeal shock wave lithotripsy (ESWL) for stones $\leq$10 mm. There is some evidence that a combination of α(alpha)-blockers and corticosteroids might be more effective than treatment with α(alpha)-blockers alone [70].

Conservative management is not appropriate in patients with risk factors for urosepsis, such as prolonged obstruction, persisting pain, or associated infection. Moreover, there is an absolute indication for actively removing urinary stones in some subcategories of patients, such as pilots or sailors [45]. MET in children cannot be recommended due to the limited data. Patients who elect for MET should have well-controlled pain, no clinical evidence of sepsis, and adequate renal function reserve [23].

Acute Stone Problems in Special Patients

Pregnancy

The incidence of symptomatic nephrolithiasis during pregnancy varies between 1 in 244 and 1 in 2,000 pregnancies [77, 78]. The treatment of such patients requires a multidisciplinary team approach involving the urologist, obstetrician, and radiologist [79]. Pharmacotherapy has a restricted role because most drugs in RC are contraindicated during pregnancy. Opiates are the first-line choice during pregnancy as NSAIDs because of concern about oligohydramnios, early spontaneous abortion, and cardiac malformations [80]. There is no data available for drugs used in MET during pregnancy [81].

Indication of invasive interventions is largely based on individual patient factors including uncontrolled pain, sepsis, bilateral obstruction, solitary kidney obstruction, obstetric complications (preeclampsia), and poor access to urology care/equipment [82]. Temporary percutaneous nephrolithotomy (PCNL) is indicated, especially in the case of sepsis, where excessive ureteral manipulation is not recommended. It is also possible to insert a retrograde ureteral stent under local anesthesia and ultrasound guidance. When necessary, ureteroscopy with holmium:YAG laser lithotripsy is likely to be the safest and most effective management choice [79].

Stones in Children

Pediatric urolithiasis occurs in three epidemiological patterns: (1) endemic stones seen in Middle and Far East, (2) infection-related stones occurring most commonly in Great Britain, and (3) metabolic stones encountered most frequently in the United States and Scandinavian countries [36].

Shokeir and coworkers have reported that percutaneous nephrolithotomy is better than shock wave lithotripsy for treatment of 1–2-cm renal stones in children, yielding higher stone-free and lower re-treatment rates [83]. In recent era, the management of ureteral stones in children is becoming more similar to that in adults [84]. However, limited data of MET prevents wide popularity of such a line of management. ESWL has become the primary line of treatment particularly in proximal ureteral stones in children [85]. Ureteroscopic lithotripsy is safe [86] and considered the first line of therapy in symptomatic distal and mid-ureteral calculi [84]. There is growing evidence that both lines are equally effective and safe [84]; the choice between either modality for ureteral stones in children must be tailored according to the clinical situation [36].

Prolonged Stone Impaction and Renal Function

Although no doubt that any renal obstruction secondary to urolithiasis should be managed once diagnosed, however, in many clinical situations, patients may present after a lagging time sufficient for functional deterioration of the involved renal unit. In another case scenario, partial or complete ureteric obstruction by small gravels might happen after ESWL that could be managed with MET but may take several weeks. Under such circumstances, solutions should be searched for possible recoverability of lost function or at least minimizing the hazards of obstruction.

Unilateral ureteral obstruction is associated with histopathological changes, including interstitial fibrosis, tubular atrophy, apoptosis, and macrophage infiltration [87]. All these changes contribute to renal parenchymal damage leading to sustained decrease in renal function. One of the promising drugs is losartan, an angiotensin receptor blocker. In an experimental prospective study, losartan decreased the deterioration of renal function in pelviureteral obstruction and enhanced recoverability of renal function after relief of obstruction [88]. MG 132 and lactocystine are proven to inhibit in vitro transforming growth factor-β(beta), which is involved in renal tubulointerstitial fibrosis [89]. These promising results on experimental basis will encourage its application on humans in the near future as these open wider insights for management of obstruction secondary to urolithiasis.

Conclusion

Unless contraindicated, NSAIDs represent the first line of pain relief in cases with RC. Better efficacy and proven safety of combination protocols with opioids has been provided; however, a standard regimen protocol in ERs is still lacking. For septic patients with obstructing stones, kidneys must be urgently drained using either PCN or ureteral stenting. Alpha blockers in combination with corticosteroid may increase stone expulsion compared with alpha blockers alone. New management modalities enhance recoverability of renal function after obstructions by urolithiasis are warranted.

References

1. Brown J. Diagnostic and treatment patterns for renal colic in US emergency departments. Int Urol Nephrol. 2006;38(1):87–92.
2. Phillips E, Kieley S, Johnson EB, Monga M. Emergency room management of ureteral calculi: current practices. J Endourol. 2009;23(6):1021–4.
3. Serinken M, Karcioglu O, Turkcuer I, Ozkan HI, Keysan MK, Bukiran A. Analysis of clinical and demographic characteristics of patients presenting with renal colic in the emergency department. BMC Res Notes. 2008;1:79.
4. Manthey DE, Teichman J. Nephrolithiasis. Emerg Med Clin North Am. 2001;19(3):633–54, viii.
5. Manfredini R, Gallerani M, Cecilia O, Boari B, Fersini C, Portaluppi F. Circadian pattern in occurrence of renal colic in an emergency department: analysis of patients' notes. BMJ. 2002;324(7340):767.
6. Boari B, Manfredini R. Circadian rhythm and renal colic. Recenti Prog Med. 2003;94(5):191–3.
7. Koopman MG, Koomen GC, Krediet RT, de Moor EA, Hoek FJ, Arisz L. Circadian rhythm of glomerular filtration rate in normal individuals. Clin Sci (Lond). 1989;77(1):105–11.
8. Singh RK, Bansal A, Bansal SK, Singh AK, Mahdi AA. Circadian periodicity of urinary inhibitor of calcium oxalate crystallization in healthy Indians and renal stone formers. Eur Urol. 1993;24(3): 387–92.
9. Turkcuer I, Serinken M, Karcioglu O, Zencir M, Keysan MK. Hospital cost analysis of management of patients with renal colic in the emergency department. Urol Res. 2010;38(1):29–33.
10. Pearle MS, Calhoun E, Curhan GC. Urolithiasis. In: Litwin MS, Saigal CS, editors. Urologic diseases in America. US Department of Health and Human Services, Public Health Service, National Institutes of Health, National Institute of Diabetes and Digestive and Kidney Diseases. Washington, D.C.: US Government Printing Office; 2007. p. 283–317. NIH Publication No. 07–5512.
11. Diniz DH, Blay SL, Schor N. Anxiety and depression symptoms in recurrent painful renal lithiasis colic. Braz J Med Biol Res. 2007;40(7):949–55.
12. Greenberg PE, Leong SA, Birnbaum HG, Robinson RL. The economic burden of depression with painful symptoms. J Clin Psychiatry. 2003;64 Suppl 7:17–23.
13. Herrman H, Patrick DL, Diehr P, Martin ML, Fleck M, Simon GE, et al. Longitudinal investigation of depression outcomes in primary care in six countries: the LIDO study. Functional status, health service use and treatment of people with depressive symptoms. Psychol Med. 2002;32(5):889–902.
14. Shokeir AA. Renal colic: new concepts related to pathophysiology, diagnosis and treatment. Curr Opin Urol. 2002;12(4):263–9.
15. Canda AE, Turna B, Cinar GM, Nazli O. Physiology and pharmacology of the human ureter: basis for current and future treatments. Urol Int. 2007;78(4):289–98.
16. Forster TH, Bonkat G, Wyler S, Ruszat R, Ebinger N, Gasser TC, et al. Diagnosis and therapy of acute ureteral colic. Wien Klin Wochenschr. 2008;120(11–12):325–34.
17. Hess B. Medical management of acute renal colic – there is more than hydration and Buscopan®.... Praxis (Bern 1994). 2011;100(5): 293–7.
18. Moody TE, Vaughn Jr ED, Gillenwater JY. Relationship between renal blood flow and ureteral pressure during 18 hours of total unilateral ureteral occlusion. Implications for changing sites of increased renal resistance. Invest Urol. 1975;13(3):246–51.
19. Lanzone JA, Gulmi FA, Chou SY, Mooppan UM, Kim H. Renal hemodynamics in acute unilateral ureteral obstruction: contribution of endothelium-derived relaxing factor. J Urol. 1995;153(6): 2055–9.
20. Reyes AA, Klahr S. Renal function after release of ureteral obstruction: role of endothelin and the renal artery endothelium. Kidney Int. 1992;42(3):632–8.
21. Burnstock G. Purinergic mechanosensory transduction and visceral pain. Mol Pain. 2009;5:69.
22. Holdgate A, Pollock T. Nonsteroidal anti-inflammatory drugs (NSAIDs) versus opioids for acute renal colic. Cochrane Database Syst Rev. 2004;(1):CD004137. Review. Update in: Cochrane Database Syst Rev. 2005;(2):CD004137.
23. Türk C, Knoll T, Petrik A, Sarica K, Straub M, Seitz C. Guidelines on urolithiasis. Arnhem: European Association of Urology; 2011, Chapter 11, section 1.
24. Steinberg PL, Nangia AK, Curtis K. A standardized pain management protocol improves timeliness of analgesia among emergency department patients with renal colic. Qual Manag Health Care. 2011;20(1):30–6.
25. Wen CC, Coyle TL, Jerde TJ, Nakada SY. Ketorolac effectively inhibits ureteral contractility in vitro. J Endourol. 2008;22(4): 739–42.
26. Duquenne S, Hellel M, Godinas L, De Leval J. Spasmolytics indication in renal colic. a literature review. Rev Med Liege. 2009;64(1):45–8.
27. Cohen E, Hafner R, Rotenberg Z, Fadilla M, Garty M. Comparison of ketorolac and diclofenac in the treatment of renal colic. Eur J Clin Pharmacol. 1998;54(6):455–8.
28. Lee SY, Lee MY, Park SH, Kim TH, Moon YT, Han JH, et al. NS-398 (a selective cyclooxygenase-2 inhibitor) decreases agonist-induced contraction of the human ureter via calcium channel inhibition. J Endourol. 2010;24(11):1863–8.

29. Nakada SY, Jerde TJ, Bjorling DE, Saban R. Selective cyclooxygenase-2 inhibitors reduce ureteral contraction in vitro: a better alternative for renal colic. J Urol. 2000;163:607–12.
30. Phillips E, Hinck B, Pedro R, Makhlouf A, Kriedberg C, Hendlin K, et al. Celecoxib in the management of acute renal colic: a randomized controlled clinical trial. Urology. 2009;74(5):994–9.
31. Perlmutter A, Miller L, Trimble LA, Marion DN, Vaughan Jr ED, Felsen D. Toradol, an NSAID used for renal colic, decreases renal perfusion and ureteral pressure in a canine model of unilateral ureteral obstruction. J Urol. 1993;149(4):926–30.
32. Miyajima A, Ito K, Asano T, Seta K, Ueda A, Hayakawa M. Does cyclooxygenase-2 inhibitor prevent renal tissue damage in unilateral ureteral obstruction? J Urol. 2001;166(3):1124–9.
33. Shokeir AA, Abdulmaaboud M, Farage Y, Mutabagani H. Resistive index in renal colic: the effect of nonsteroidal anti-inflammatory drugs. BJU Int. 1999;84(3):249–51.
34. Hammad FT, Lubbad L. The effect of diclofenac sodium on renal function in reversible unilateral ureteric obstruction. Urol Res. 2010;39(5):351–6. PubMed PMID: 21190019.
35. Brater DC. Effects of nonsteroidal anti-inflammatory drugs on renal function: focus on cyclooxygenase-2-selective inhibition. Am J Med. 1999;107(6A):65S–70; discussion 70 S–71 S.
36. Shokeir AA. Renal colic: pathophysiology, diagnosis and treatment. Eur Urol. 2001;39:241–9.
37. Schneider V, Lévesque LE, Zhang B, Hutchinson T, Brophy JM. Association of selective and conventional nonsteroidal antiinflammatory drugs with acute renal failure: a population-based, nested case–control analysis. Am J Epidemiol. 2006;164(9):881–9.
38. Swan SK, Rudy DW, Lasseter KC, Ryan CF, Buechel KL, Lambrecht LJ, et al. Effect of cyclooxygenase-2 inhibition on renal function in elderly persons receiving a low-salt diet. A randomized, controlled trial. Ann Intern Med. 2000;133(1):1–9.
39. O'Connor A, Schug SA, Cardwell H. A comparison of the efficacy and safety of morphine and pethidine as analgesia for suspected renal colic in the emergency setting. J Accid Emerg Med. 2000;17(4):261–4.
40. Ghuman J, Vadera R. Ketorolac and morphine for analgesia in acute renal colic: is this combination more effective than monotherapy? CJEM. 2008;10(1):66–8.
41. Becker AJ, Stief CG, Meyer M, Truss MC, Forssmann WG, Jonas U. The effect of the specific phosphodiesterase-IV-inhibitor rolipram on the ureteral peristalsis of the rabbit in vitro and in vivo. J Urol. 1998;160(3 Pt 1):920–5.
42. Jönsson PE, Olsson AM, Petersson BA, Johansson K. Intravenous indomethacin and oxycone-papaverine in the treatment of acute renal colic. A double-blind study. Br J Urol. 1987;59(5):396–400.
43. Yencilek F, Aktas C, Goktas C, Yilmaz C, Yilmaz U, Sarica K. Role of papaverine hydrochloride administration in patients with intractable renal colic: randomized prospective trial. Urology. 2008;72(5):987–90.
44. Grond S, Sablotzki A. Clinical pharmacology of tramadol. Clin Pharmacokinet. 2004;43(13):879–923.
45. Osorio L, Lima E, Autorino R, Marcelo F. Emergency management of ureteral stones: recent advances. Indian J Urol. 2008;24(4):461–6.
46. Mortelmans LJ, Desruelles D, Baert JA, Hente KR, Tailly GG. Use of tramadol drip in controlling renal colic pain. J Endourol. 2006;20(12):1010–5.
47. Safdar B, Degutis LC, Landry K, Vedere SR, Moscovitz HC, D'Onofrio G. Intravenous morphine plus ketorolac is superior to either drug alone for treatment of acute renal colic. Ann Emerg Med. 2006;48(2):173–81.
48. Cordell WH, Wright SW, Wolfson AB, Timerding BL, Maneatis TJ, Lewis RH, et al. Comparison of intravenous ketorolac, meperidine, and both (balanced analgesia) for renal colic. Ann Emerg Med. 1996;28(2):151–8.
49. Hyllested M, Jones S, Pedersen JL, Kehlet H. Comparative effect of paracetamol, NSAIDs or their combination in postoperative pain management: a qualitative review. Br J Anaesth. 2002;88(2):199–214.
50. Bektas F, Eken C, Karadeniz O, Goksu E, Cubuk M, Cete Y. Intravenous paracetamol or morphine for the treatment of renal colic: a randomized, placebo-controlled trial. Ann Emerg Med. 2009;54(4):568–74.
51. Fendrich Z. Metamizol – a new effective analgesic with a long history. Overview of its pharmacology and clinical use. Cas Lek Cesk. 2000;139(14):440–4.
52. Pavlik I, Suchy J, Pacík D, Bokr R, Sust M, Villoria J, Abadías M, Evaluation of Cizolirtine Citrate to Treat Renal Colic Pain Study Group. Comparison of cizolirtine citrate and metamizol sodium in the treatment of adult acute renal colic: a randomized, double-blind, clinical pilot study. Clin Ther. 2004;26(7):1061–72.
53. Holdgate A, Oh CM. Is there a role for antimuscarinics in renal colic. A randomized controlled trial? J Urol. 2005;174(2):572–5; discussion 575.
54. el-Sherif AE, Salem M, Yahia H, al-Sharkawy WA, al-Sayrafi M. Treatment of renal colic by desmopressin intranasal spray and diclofenac sodium. J Urol. 1995;153(5):1395–8.
55. Lopes T, Dias JS, Marcelino J, Varela J, Ribeiro S, Dias J. An assessment of the clinical efficacy of intranasal desmopressin spray in the treatment of renal colic. BJU Int. 2001;87(4):322–5.
56. Roshani A, Falahatkar S, Khosropanah I, Atrkar Roshan Z, Zarkami T, Palizkar M, et al. Assessment of clinical efficacy of intranasal desmopressin spray and diclofenac sodium suppository in treatment of renal colic versus diclofenac sodium alone. Urology. 2010;75(3):540–2.
57. Kheirollahi AR, Tehrani M, Bashashati M. A comparison of the effect of intranasal desmopressin and intramuscular hyoscine N-butyl bromide combination with intramuscular hyoscine N-butyl bromide alone in acute renal colic. J Res Med Sci. 2010;15(4):214–8.
58. Bengtsson J, Worning AM, Gertz J, Struckmann J, Bonnesen T, Palludan H, et al. Pain due to urolithiasis treated by intracutaneous injection of sterile water. A clinically controlled double-blind study. Ugeskr Laeger. 1981;143(51):3463–5.
59. Ahmadnia H, Younesi Rostami M. Treatment of renal colic using intracutaneous injection of sterile water. Urol J. 2004;1(3):200–3.
60. Springhart WP, Marguet CG, Sur RL, Norris RD, Delvecchio FC, Young MD, et al. Forced versus minimal intravenous hydration in the management of acute renal colic: a randomized trial. J Endourol. 2006;20(10):713–6.
61. Lee YH, Lee WC, Chen MT, Huang JK, Chung C, Chang LS. Acupuncture in the treatment of renal colic. J Urol. 1992;147(1):16–8.
62. Lee CT, Chang YH, Lin WY, Xu JM, Chen HY, Chou PL, et al. Applications of meridian electrical conductance for renal colic: a prospective study. J Altern Complement Med. 2010;16(8):861–6.
63. Kober A, Dobrovits M, Djavan B, Marberger M, Barker R, Bertalanffy P, et al. Local active warming: an effective treatment for pain, anxiety and nausea caused by renal colic. J Urol. 2003;170(3):741–4.
64. Kaymak B, Ozçakar L, Aksoy S. Urinary colic during low-back treatment: out of the frying pan into the fire? Pain Med. 2009;10(4):771–3.
65. Weisse CS, Sorum PC, Sanders KN, Syat BL. Do gender and race affect decisions about pain management? J Gen Intern Med. 2001;16(4):211–7.
66. Ramsey S, Robertson A, Ablett MJ, Meddings RN, Hollins GW, Little B. Evidence-based drainage of infected hydronephrosis secondary to ureteric calculi. J Endourol. 2010;24(2):185–9.
67. Pearle MS, Pierce HL, Miller GL, Summa JA, Mutz JM, Petty BA, et al. Optimal method of urgent decompression of the collecting

system for obstruction and infection due to ureteral calculi. J Urol. 1998;160(4):1260–4.

68. Mokhmalji H, Braun PM, Martinez Portillo FJ, Siegsmund M, Alken P, Köhrmann KU. Percutaneous nephrostomy versus ureteral stents for diversion of hydronephrosis caused by stones: a prospective, randomized clinical trial. J Urol. 2001;165(4):1088–92.
69. El-Hefnawy AS, El-Nahas AR, El-Tabey NA, Shoma AM, El-Assmy AM, El-Kenawy MR, et al. Bilateral same-session ureteroscopy for treatment of ureteral calculi: critical analysis of risk factors. Scand J Urol Nephrol. 2011;45(2):97–101.
70. Seitz C, Pliatsikas E, Porpiglia F, Tiselius HG, Zwergel U. Medical therapy to facilitate the passage of stones: what is the evidence? Eur Urol. 2009;56(3):455–71.
71. Tzortzis V, Mamoulakis C, Rioja J, Gravas S, Michel MC, de la Rosette JJ. Medical expulsive therapy for distal ureteral stones. Drugs. 2009;69(6):677–92. doi:10.2165/00003495-200969060-00003.
72. Worster A, Richards C. Fluids and diuretics for acute ureteric colic. Cochrane Database Syst Rev. 2005;20(3):CD004926.
73. Mikkelsen AL, Meyhoff HH, Lindahl F, Christensen J. The effect of hydroxyprogesterone on ureteral stones. Int Urol Nephrol. 1988;20(3):257–60.
74. Gratzke C, Uckert S, Kedia G, Reich O, Schlenker B, Seitz M, et al. In vitro effects of PDE5 inhibitors sildenafil, vardenafil and tadalafil on isolated human ureteral smooth muscle: a basic research approach. Urol Res. 2007;35(1):49–54.
75. Sahin A, Erdemli I, Bakkaloglu M, Ergen A, Basar I, Remzi D. The effect of nifedipine and verapamil on rhythmic contractions of human isolated ureter. Arch Int Physiol Biochim Biophys. 1993;101(5):245–7.
76. Al-Ansari A, Al-Naimi A, Alobaidy A, Assadiq K, Azmi MD, Shokeir AA. Efficacy of tamsulosin in the management of lower ureteral stones: a randomized double-blind placebo-controlled study of 100 patients. Urology. 2010;75(1):4–7.
77. Lewis DF, Robichaux 3rd AG, Jaekle RK, Marcum NG, Stedman CM. Urolithiasis in pregnancy. Diagnosis, management and pregnancy outcome. J Reprod Med. 2003;48(1):28–32.
78. Swartz MA, Lydon-Rochelle MT, Simon D, Wright JL, Porter MP. Admission for nephrolithiasis in pregnancy and risk of adverse birth outcomes. Obstet Gynecol. 2007;109(5):1099–104.
79. Srirangam SJ, Hickerton B, Van Cleynenbreugel B. Management of urinary calculi in pregnancy: a review. J Endourol. 2008;22(5):867–75.
80. Briggs GG. Medication use during the perinatal period. J Am Pharm Assoc (Wash). 1998;38(6):717–26; quiz 726–7.
81. Singh A, Alter HJ, Littlepage A. A systematic review of medical therapy to facilitate passage of ureteral calculi. Ann Emerg Med. 2007;50(5):552–63.
82. Biyani CS, Joyce AD. Urolithiasis in pregnancy. II: management. BJU Int. 2002;89(8):819–23.
83. Shokeir AA, Sheir KZ, El-Nahas AR, El-Assmy AM, Eassa W, El-Kappany HA. Treatment of renal stones in children: a comparison between percutaneous nephrolithotomy and shock wave lithotripsy. J Urol. 2006;176(2):706–10.
84. Minevich E. Management of ureteric stone in pediatric patients. Indian J Urol. 2010;26(4):564–7.
85. Landau EH, Shenfeld OZ, Pode D, Shapiro A, Meretyk S, Katz G, et al. Extracorporeal shock wave lithotripsy in prepubertal children: 22-year experience at a single institution with a single lithotriptor. J Urol. 2009;182(4 Suppl):1835–9.
86. El-Assmy A, Hafez AT, Eraky I, El-Nahas AR, El-Kappany HA. Safety and outcome of rigid ureteroscopy for management of ureteral calculi in children. J Endourol. 2006;20(4):252–5.
87. Chevalier RL. Obstructive nephropathy: towards biomarker discovery and gene therapy. Nat Clin Pract Nephrol. 2006;2(3):157–68.
88. Soliman SA, Shokeir AA, Mosbah A, Abol-Enein H, Barakat N, Abou-Bieh E, et al. Recoverability of renal function after relief of chronic partial unilateral ureteral obstruction: study of the effect of angiotensin receptor blocker (losartan). Urology. 2010;75(4):848–52.
89. Sakairi T, Hiromura K, Takahashi S, Hamatani H, Takeuchi S, Tomioka M, et al. Effects of proteasome inhibitors on rat renal fibrosis in vitro and in vivo. Nephrology (Carlton). 2011;16(1):76–86. doi:10.1111/j.1440-1797.2010.01367.x.

Open Surgery: Current Status and Techniques

45

Nagaraja P. Rao

Abstract

The introduction and widespread use of minimally invasive techniques such as extracorporeal shock wave lithotripsy (ESWL), percutaneous nephrolithotomy (PCNL), ureteroscopy (URS), and retrograde intrarenal surgery (RIRS) using fine fiber-optic scopes have drastically reduced the need and indications for open surgery for renal and ureteric stones. However, in a small minority of cases such as those with large and complex staghorn stones that are not amenable for minimally invasive surgery or in some of those with recurrent stone disease, open surgery is still required. Since open surgery is rarely performed, the issue of training is important and needs to be addressed. Although in the not-too-distant future, if as it seems likely that the laparoscopic approach will take over the need for conventional open operations, centralization of complex stone surgery will become inevitable in the future.

Keywords

Complex stones • Open surgery • Staghorn calculi • Anatrophic nephrolithotomy • Stone-free rates • Renal stones • Urinary stones • Open surgery • Nephrolithotomy • Pyelo-nephrolithotomy • Ileal replacement of ureter • Bench surgery • Treatment

Introduction

Until the introduction of minimally invasive techniques in the early 1980s, most of the stones in the urinary tract, except small stones in the pelvic part of the ureter, were removed by open surgery. The arrival of extracorporeal shock wave lithotripsy (ESWL), percutaneous nephrolithotomy (PCNL), ure teroscopy (URS), and, more recently, retrograde intrarenal surgery (RIRS) has completely reversed the process, so much so that only a minority of cases are now treated by open surgery. For example, a report in 1989 from Wake Forest University Baptist Hospital, Winston-Salem in USA, showed that during the early months after the institution of a lithotripter, 4.1 % of 893 stone procedures were performed by open surgery [1]. In the same hospital, between January 1998 and May 2001, of the 986 procedures for stones, only 0.7 % was by open surgery, [2] as a result of further developments in endourological techniques. Bichler et al. [3] and Kane et al. [4] also reported a similar decline in open surgery. This rapid decline in open surgery is not limited to developed countries as Ather et al. [5] reported a reduction in the number of open operations performed in their hospital in Pakistan from 26 % between 1987 and 1995 to 8 % between 1996 and 1998. With the introduction of flexible ureteroscopes and holmium laser for fragmentation of stones, the need for open surgery has

N.P. Rao, M.B.B.S., ChM, FRCS Ed
Formerly Director of Total Stone Management Centre, University Hospital of South Manchester, Manchester, UK

NTR University of Health Sciences, Vijayawada, Andhra Pradesh, India, 66760, Pegeia, Paphos 8592, Cyprus
e-mail: pnagaraja.rao@googlemail.com

J.J. Talati et al. (eds.), *Urolithiasis*,
DOI 10.1007/978-1-4471-4387-1_45,

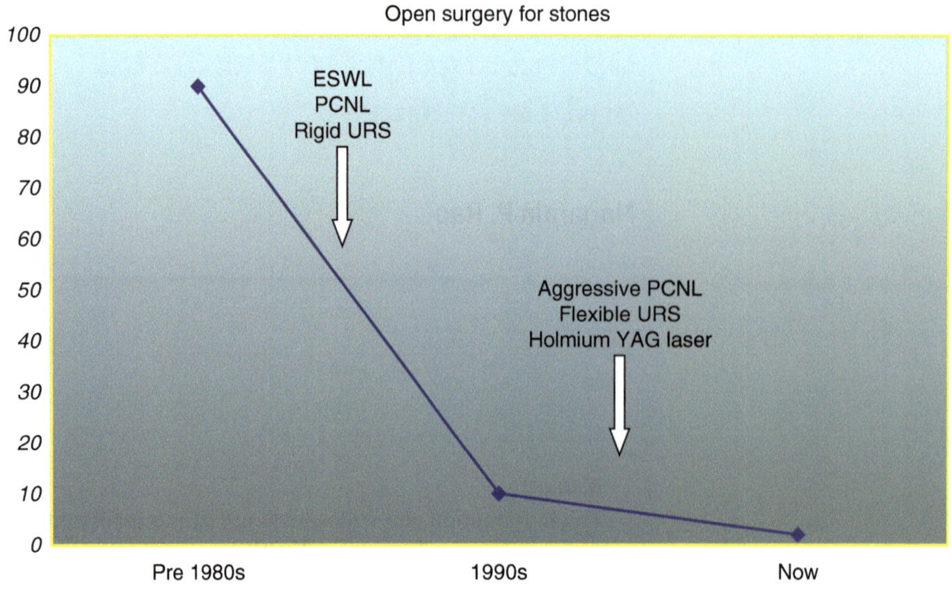

Fig. 45.1 Decline in open surgery for stones (from various sources)

declined even further. In my own practice, between 2003 and 2007, open surgery was necessary only in 0.2 % of cases (Fig. 45.1).

The attractions of minimally invasive surgery (MIS) are reduced postoperative pain, hospitalization, and recuperation time before going back to work. Yet questions have been asked (but often ignored) about the efficacy of MIS particularly in respect of renal stones. These center mainly around stone-free rates (after all, the object of stone surgery is to make the patient stone-free). Do minimally invasive techniques offer better stone-free rates?

Another issue that may be of importance, particularly in health-care systems where patients have no state or private insurance and have to pay for the treatment, is the reoperation rate. There is some evidence to suggest that open surgery offers a better stone-free rate than minimally invasive procedures and is probably cheaper. Al-Kohlan et al. [6], in a randomized study of open surgery versus PCNL for staghorn stones, found a stone-free rate at discharge of 66 % for open surgery and 49 % after PCNL.

Therefore, open surgery still has an important role to play and a case can be made to reduce the threshold for MIS. This raises the question of training and by whom and where open surgery should be performed. One option is management of complex cases in one center [7]. Laparoscopic surgery in urology is advancing very rapidly and some recent reports suggest that this may replace conventional open surgery (see section "The Future").

In this chapter, the indications, preoperative investigations, surgical techniques, complications, postoperative management, and the management of residual calculi after open surgery are reviewed.

Indications for Open Surgery

All the reports have emphasized that open surgery should be considered when MIS has failed, in very obese patients, and in anatomically abnormal kidneys in patients, or if open surgery is necessary for other indications. The 2011 European Association of Urologists (EAU) guidelines on urolithiasis [8] give a comprehensive list of indications for open surgery (Table 45.1).

The other indications for open surgery are nonavailability of equipment for MIS due to economic or other reasons, limited experience of the surgeon, or the patient's preference for financial or other reasons (as a single procedure may be cheaper than multiple procedures). The first indication on the list (i.e., "complex stone burden") is somewhat vague as it can depend on the experience of the surgeon. Nobody, however, disputes that the best procedure for a very large staghorn stone with predomi-

Table 45.1 EAU guidelines on indications for open surgery

Complex stone burden
Treatment failure of ESWL, PCNL, and/or ureteroscopy
Intrarenal anatomical abnormalities (e.g., infundibular stenosis, stone in calyceal diverticulum—especially anterior diverticulum, stone + UPJ obstruction)
Morbid obesity
Skeletal deformity, contractures, and fixed deformities of hips and legs
Comorbid medical disease
Concomitant open surgery
Nonfunctioning lower pole (partial nephrectomy), nonfunctioning kidney (nephrectomy)
Patient choice—the patient may prefer a single procedure
Stone in an ectopic kidney where PCNL and/or ESWL may be difficult or impossible

nantly peripheral stone burden with multiple calyceal stones and especially with infundibular stenosis is open surgery. The other indications for open surgery are ileal replacement of ureter to facilitate easy passage of stones in recurrent stone formers and cases of severe stenosis and scarring of the upper ureter.

Preoperative Investigations

As with any surgical procedure, good preoperative planning and investigations are important for a successful outcome. It is important that the planned procedure is discussed in detail with the patient. The patient should understand the risks, complications, and alternative management options. In addition to assessing the overall medical condition and comorbidities and clinical examination and routine blood tests to assess hemoglobin (Hb) and serum urea, electrolytes, and creatinine, the following investigations are recommended to assess the anatomy of the kidney(s): stone size, shape, location, and burden; renal function; and presence or absence of urinary infection.

Urine Culture

At least 3 weeks before surgery, urine culture should be performed to allow time for the results to come through and allow adequate time for antibiotic treatment. If infection is shown, it should be treated with appropriate antibiotics and the urine culture repeated a week later to check for sterility. In case of "infection stones," it may not be possible to eliminate bacteria in urine completely. In this case, the antibiotic treatment should continue until after surgery. Even if the urine is sterile, it is wiser to perform surgery under antibiotic cover. The author's preference is gentamicin and a cephalosporin at appropriate dosage starting 24 h prior to surgery.

Plain X-Ray of Abdomen and IVU

Plain X-ray is useful as it gives a general idea of the size and location of stone(s) if they are radiopaque. The preoperative X-ray can also be compared with postoperative films. Intravenous urogram (IVU) is optional as currently the imaging modality of choice is a computed tomography (CT) urogram.

Computed Tomography

A helical CT is strongly recommended prior to surgery. It should include both non-contrast and post-contrast phases. CT gives valuable information regarding the thickness of parenchyma, presence or absence of hydronephrosis, and the size, shape, and location of stone(s). If necessary, a three-dimensional (3D) view of the stone can be reconstructed. CT is particularly useful in the assessment of radiolucent stones such as cystine and uric acid stones.

Isotope Renogram

The main purpose of isotope renogram is to assess split renal function and compare the preoperative results to those in the follow-up after surgery.

Surgical Techniques

The need for simple pyelolithotomy by open method is now extremely rare. If indeed, a pyelolithotomy is indicated, it can be performed laparoscopically, thus avoiding the need for open incision.

Surgical Approach

A loin or flank incision gives the best exposure. A subcostal incision (even if the scar of a previous operation is below the ribs) is not recommended. It should be at least above the 12th rib or higher, depending on the size and location of the stone(s), patient's size, and whether the patient had previous operations on the kidney. The pleura should be identified and protected. It may be necessary to gently release it off the rib below the incision. It is not uncommon for the pleura to tear when the wound is retracted, especially when a self-retaining retractor is used. Care should be exercised in this respect. The Gerota's fascia is incised over the posterolateral aspect of the kidney. It is important to identify the peritoneum and not incise it by mistake—hence the reason for incising the fascia on the posterior aspect of the kidney. Once the Gerota's fascia is incised, the kidney with the perinephric fat and the retroperitoneal space are exposed. If there is minimal perinephric fat, it is possible to identify the ureter at this stage, but often it may be necessary to clear the fat off the lower pole of the kidney. The ureter is isolated and placed in a vascular sling. All the perinephric fat is then cleared, exposing the whole kidney and the renal pelvis. The vascular pedicle is identified and cleanly exposed after removing the fat surrounding it. It is recommended to expose the main trunks of both the vein and the artery.

Extended Pyelolithotomy of Gil-Vernet

First described by Gil-Vernet in 1965 [9], the technique is used to remove a simple staghorn stone without extensive calyceal extensions or combined with radial nephrotomy incisions for a complex staghorn stone. After mobilizing the kidney as described previously, the fatty tissue covering the renal pelvis is cleared completely and the space between the renal pelvis and parenchyma exploited on the posterior aspect by lifting the latter gently by blunt dissection to expose the calyceal necks (Fig. 45.2). This dissection should be gentle (to reduce bleeding from the small sinus veins) and is achieved by using blunt scissors and/or "peanut" gauze swabs. Sometimes, a small branch of the posterior renal artery crosses the renal sinus area [10]. It should be carefully preserved. The renal parenchyma is then retracted with small sinus retractors. The retraction should be gentle to prevent a tear in renal parenchyma. A U-shaped incision is made over the renal pelvis extending up to the calyceal necks (see Fig. 45.2). This exposes the pelvic part of the stone. The stone may sometimes be adherent to the mucosa. If an attempt is made to remove the stone, it may produce superficial tears of the mucosa and this may cause bleeding. It is therefore necessary to separate the stone from the mucosa with the help of a flat McDonald type of a dissector. The pelvic part of the stone is then extracted (Fig. 45.3). If the calyceal neck is wide, it should be possible to extract the stone along with the calyceal extensions. Sometimes, the calyceal extension(s) may break off and remain in the calyces. It is therefore important to inspect the extracted stone for the tell-tale signs that one or more of the calyceal part of the stone has become detached or not. If they have, then they can be extracted through the opening in the pelvis, although in some cases additional nephrotomy incisions may have to be made to remove the fragment(s) in the calyces. The collecting system is flushed out with saline and may be inspected with a flexible nephroscope for any residual fragments. Small- to medium-sized fragments can be extracted with a zero-tip basket.

It is important to ensure that all the stone is removed as any residual stones can grow very quickly, particularly if the stone is of "infection type." A 12F nephrostomy tube of Malecot type is brought into the renal pelvis through the parenchyma, and the incision in the pelvis is closed with absorbable suture such as 4-0 Vicryl® (Ethicon Inc). The nephrostomy tube is brought out through a separate stab incision. A 20F drainage tube should be left in to drain the perinephric space and is brought out through another stab incision. If at all possible, the kidney should be placed inside the perinephric fat, in case further open surgery is required in the future.

The drain may be removed 48–72 h after the operation if there is no urinary drainage from the tube. The nephrostomy tube is left draining for 7 days when a plain X-ray of the kidney and bladder area, and a nephrostogram is performed. If there are no ureteric stone fragments or extravasation, the tube is clamped for 24 h and then removed. For management of ureteric stone fragments, see section "Management of Residual Stones."

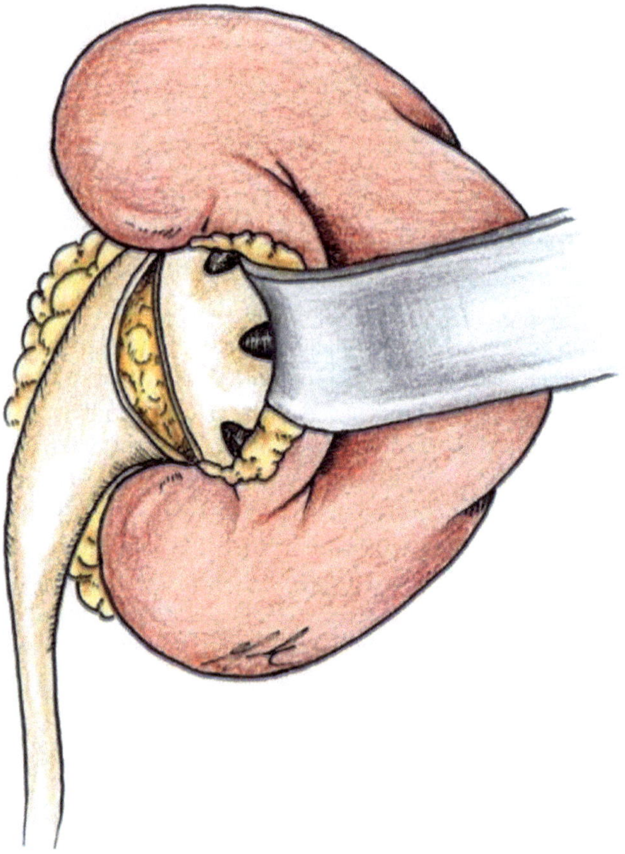

Fig. 45.2 Extended pyelolithotomy, showing retraction of parenchyma and incision over renal pelvis (Reproduced from Wendt-Nordahl et al. [31]. By kind permission of Springer-Verlag)

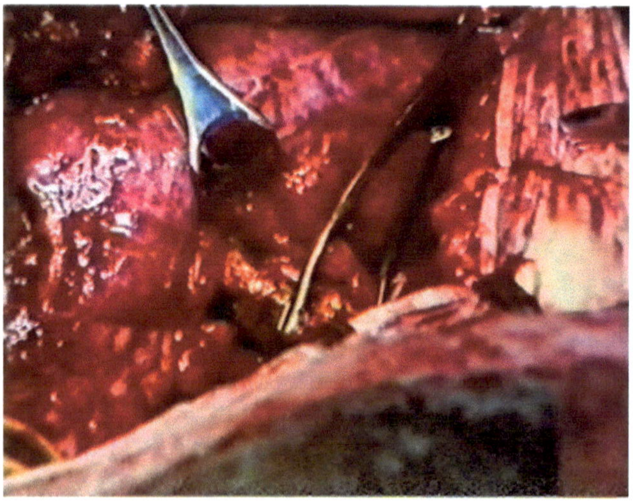

Fig. 45.3 Extraction of stone by extended pyelolithotomy

Renal Ischemia

Clamping of the renal artery may be necessary during open pyelo-nephrolithotomy. The resulting renal ischemia may produce renal damage. Many studies have shown that warm ischemia of more than 30 min produces some permanent reduction in renal function and the kidney can withstand cold ischemia for at least 2 h without incurring any permanent damage [11–14]. Removal of a solitary calyceal stone can easily be achieved during warm ischemia, but for complex staghorn stones (Fig. 45.4), the kidney should be protected from ischemic damage. Intravenous or intrarenal arterial injection of inosine, verapamil, and angiotensin-converting enzyme inhibitors has been reported to offer protection to the kidney [15–17]. However, by far, the safest way to preserve renal function is by renal hypothermia or removal of the stone without clamping the renal artery.

It has been well recognized that it is adequate to cool the parenchyma to between 15 and 20 °C [11, 14]. Renal hypothermia may be achieved by three methods: (1) using cooling coils as described by Wickham [10], (2) infusion of cold saline into renal artery after occluding the artery with double-lumen balloon catheter [18], and (3) the well-accepted method of packing the space round the kidney with slush ice.

Infusion of cold saline into the renal artery produces uniform and controlled cooling of the whole of the parenchyma. The procedure is more complicated and invasive. A double-lumen balloon catheter is passed through the ipsilateral femoral artery and placed in the main renal artery in the radiology department. The patient is then transferred into the operating theater. Prior to any incisions into the parenchyma, the balloon is inflated and cold saline is slowly infused into the kidney for 10–15 min. Thereafter, the renal artery is clamped and nephrolithotomy is carried out. This technique produces a more controlled and uniform reduction of temperature of the parenchyma, and it is not too difficult to produce re-cooling should that become necessary. Its main disadvantage is that it is very invasive and may produce additional complications such as damage to the renal artery.

It is therefore not surprising that the most popular technique is packing the space round the kidney with slush ice. It has the advantage of simplicity and cost effectiveness. It does, however, add to the work load of the theater personnel. In the author's practice, saline bags are deep frozen, and under sterile conditions, the ice is crushed. Several small (no bigger than 10 cm^3) packets are made in polythene bags. At the appropriate time, these are packed around the kidney for at least 15 min after clamping the renal artery.

It is difficult to operate with the ice still present in the wound, and therefore, the ice packs are removed before proceeding with removal of the stone. The biggest dilemma is when to re-cool the kidney. Removal of a complex stone is time consuming, and there is a constant worry in the mind of the surgeon that the kidney may be reheating. The temptation to release the clamp to reperfuse the kidney should be avoided as this may produce reperfusion injury. It is better to leave the renal artery clamped and re-cool the kidney once every 30 min or so. In this situation, a temperature probe monitoring the intrarenal temperature would be extremely useful.

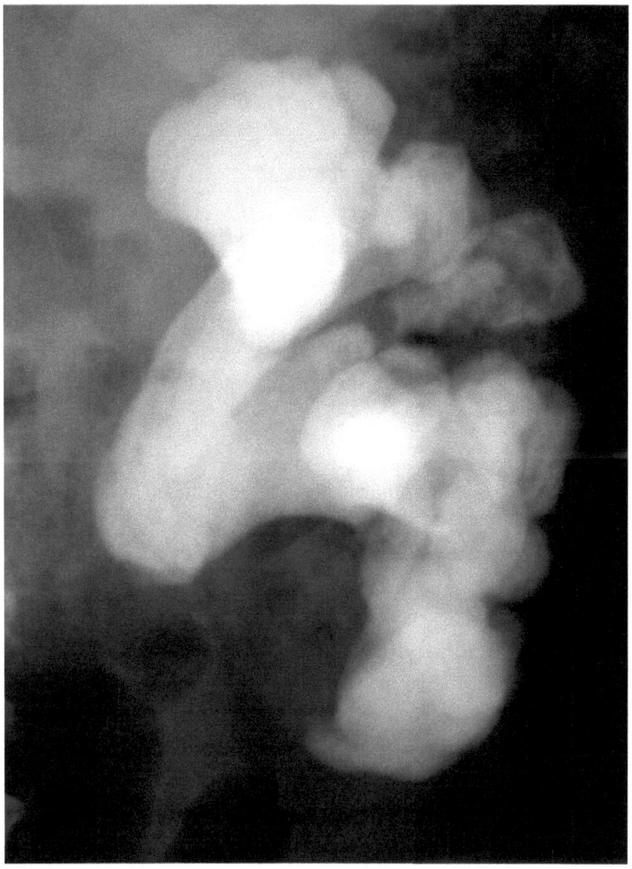

Fig. 45.4 A complex staghorn stone suitable for open pyelo-nephrolithotomy

Anatrophic Pyelo-Nephrolithotomy

Brödel in the early twentieth century suggested that there is a relatively avascular plane below the posterior aspect of the convex border of the kidney [19]. This has been widely recognized as "the bloodless line of Brödel." The keyword here is "relative" as incising through the Brödel's line does produce some (but not heavy) bleeding.

Boyce has exploited this anatomical phenomenon and has developed the technique of anatrophic nephrolithotomy [20]. The line is identified by clamping the posterior branch of the renal artery and injecting 20 ml of methylene blue intravenously. Part of the posterior aspect of the kidney turns blue and the rest remains pink (Fig. 45.5). The next step is to mark the segmental boundary. There are two ways to do this. One is to place a few interrupted sutures along the line just going deeper than the capsule. The other is to make a superficial incision, again just beyond the capsule with a diathermy needle. The latter is preferable as it is definitive and the incision in that area has to be made eventually anyway.

The main renal artery is clamped with a small bulldog arterial clamp (the type of clamp shown in Fig. 45.5), and the perirenal space is packed with slush ice as described

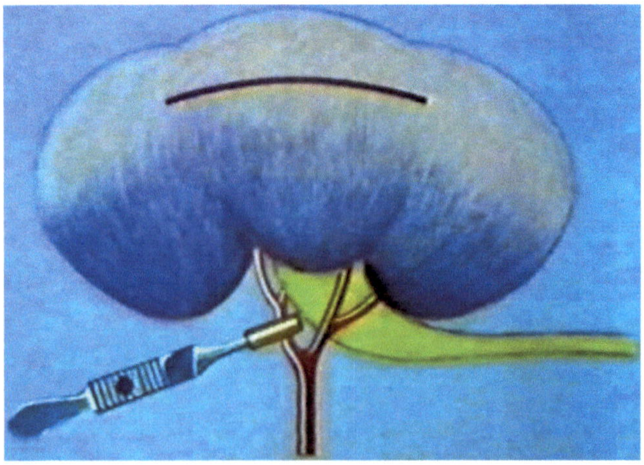

Fig. 45.5 Showing the "the bloodless line of Brödel" after clamping the posterior branch of the renal artery and injecting Methylene *blue* intravenously

previously. Once hypothermia is established, the parenchyma is dissected bluntly down the incision already made. This prevents tearing of small vessels, which can be identified and dealt with by gentle diathermy. Occasionally, they may need to be tied with 5-0 Vicryl and divided. The dissection is continued down toward the renal pelvis (Fig. 45.6). The location of the stone will determine which calyces are to be opened. The pelvic part and the calyceal extensions of the stone are then removed. Sometimes, it is possible to remove the stone *en bloc*. After removing the stone, if a stricture of the infundibulum of any of the calyces is noted, calioraphy may be performed by suturing the base of the calyx to the renal pelvis. Once complete stone removal is achieved, the collecting system is flushed with saline using high-pressure irrigation. A Malecot type of nephrostomy tube is left in situ and is brought out through the parenchyma. This technique may not be appropriate for a very complex staghorn stone with multiple calyceal extensions. In these cases, it is better to combine Gil-Vernet pyelolithotomy with multiple radial nephrotomies.

The nephrostomy and drain tubes are managed as described earlier.

Radial Nephrotomy Using Doppler Ultrasound

Although anatrophic nephrolithotomy is a very good option for some staghorn stones, in the author's experience, it may not be suitable for very extensive stones. It has also been suggested that it may produce renal damage and reduce renal function [21]. An alternative is extended pyelolithotomy to remove a large portion of the stone through the renal pelvis and deal with the peripheral stones through multiple radially placed nephrotomies.

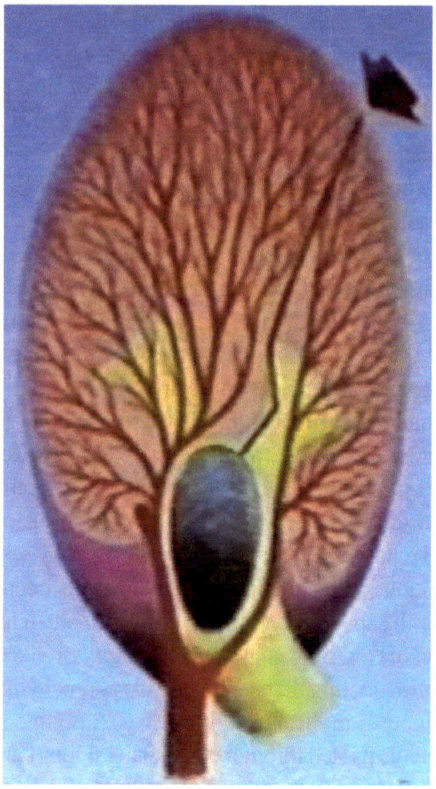

Fig. 45.6 Line of dissection (shown by the *arrow*) during anatrophic pyelo-nephrolithotomy

The kidney is mobilized and the vascular pedicle exposed as described previously. Next, an extended pyelolithotomy is performed. Often it may be necessary to break the large pelvic part off the calyceal extensions if they are too large to be negotiated through a narrow infundibulum. After removing as much stone as possible through the pelvic route, the kidney is placed in an elastic net, the other end of which is clamped or tied to the retractor. This allows the kidney to be stretched without the need for the surgeon's hand in the wound in preparation for contact X-ray. A few randomly placed metal vascular clips placed over the net helps to identify the location of the stones (Fig. 45.7). It is better to wait until the X-rays are developed before proceeding (in case the X-ray may need to be repeated).

The main renal artery is clamped and renal hypothermia induced. The next step is to locate the calyceal stones. This may be achieved in two ways. One is by simple needle probing. The grating sensation felt when the needle comes into contact with the stone is unmistakable. The other is by real-time ultrasound scanning by placing the probe over the surface of the kidney [22].

The concept of radial nephrotomies was originally described by Wickham [23]. Because the small regional vessels run radially from the hilum to the periphery of the kidney (see Fig. 45.6), placing radial nephrotomies parallel to the

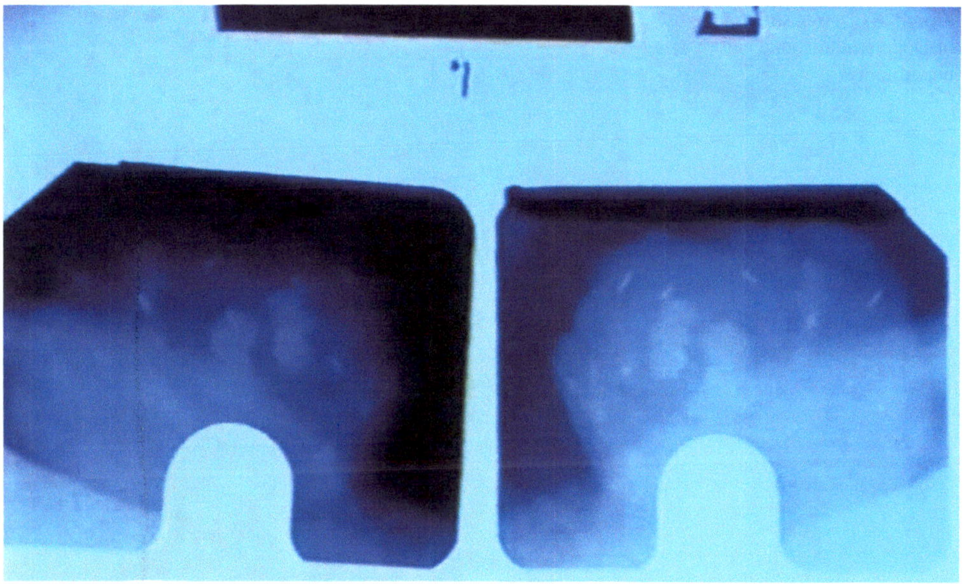

Fig. 45.7 Contact X-ray (this X-ray was in fact taken after removal of few calyceal stones)

vessels on the posterior aspect of the kidney produces minimal bleeding. While this may be true in theory, in practice radial nephrotomy still produces a fair amount of bleeding. Radial nephrotomy with Doppler assistance reduces blood loss considerably.

After locating the calyceal stone, Doppler probe is placed over the calyx (Fig. 45.8). A silent area (indicating that there are no significant sized vessels underneath) is located and radial nephrotomy is placed over that area. The incision is deepened to the level of the stone, which is gently eased out with the help of a flat dissector and stone forceps (Fig. 45.9). It is important not to extend the incision by "tearing" the parenchyma.

After removing all the stones confirmed by either contact X-ray (Fig. 45.10) or by ultrasound scanning, all the calyces are flushed out with saline by passing a catheter through each of the nephrotomy incisions. The renal pelvis is also flushed. A Malecot type of nephrostomy tube is placed in the renal pelvis and the end brought out through one of the nephrotomy incisions. The renal pelvis is closed with 3 or 4-0 Vicryl. The renal capsule over the nephrotomy incisions is closed with 4-0 Vicryl. The wound is closed leaving a drain, which is brought out through a stab incision. Similarly, the nephrostomy tube is also brought out through a separate stab incision.

The nephrostomy and drain tubes are managed as described earlier.

Ileal Replacement of Ureter

There are many indications for replacing the ureter with ileum such as extensive ureteric stricture, which cannot be managed endoscopically or by other open procedures. The main indication for this procedure in stone disease is recurrent stone formation, resulting in repeated hospital admissions for stone episodes and multiple interventions to remove the stones. The most usual categories are cystine stone formers and renal tubular acidosis. Idiopathic calcium oxalate stone formers rarely require this procedure. In uric acid stone formers, recurrence can easily be reduced or prevented with a combination of high fluid intake, alkalinization of urine, and allopurinol.

Preoperative Preparation

As with all procedures for stones in the urinary tract, it is important to treat any urinary tract infection prior to surgery. Even if the urine is sterile, antibiotic prophylaxis covering the perioperative period is recommended. Bowel preparation with sodium picosulfate (Picolax® Ferring Pharmaceuticals, UK) is recommended the day before surgery. The patient should be informed during the consent process that although only a short segment of ileum is isolated, in rare cases some patients may suffer from increase in bowel movements after surgery. The patient should also be warned that the bowel produces mucous and sometimes the mucous may produce difficulties in urination. In the author's experience, the amount of mucous produced by the ileal segment decreases with time and is negligible after 2–3 years. Additionally, the patients should be assured that when large stones drop into the bladder requiring a cystoscopy to remove the stone, it is far better and safer than procedures to remove stones in the upper urinary tract. Some recommend insertion of a percutaneous nephrostomy tube prior to surgery [24]. The author's practice is to insert a nephrostomy tube during surgery.

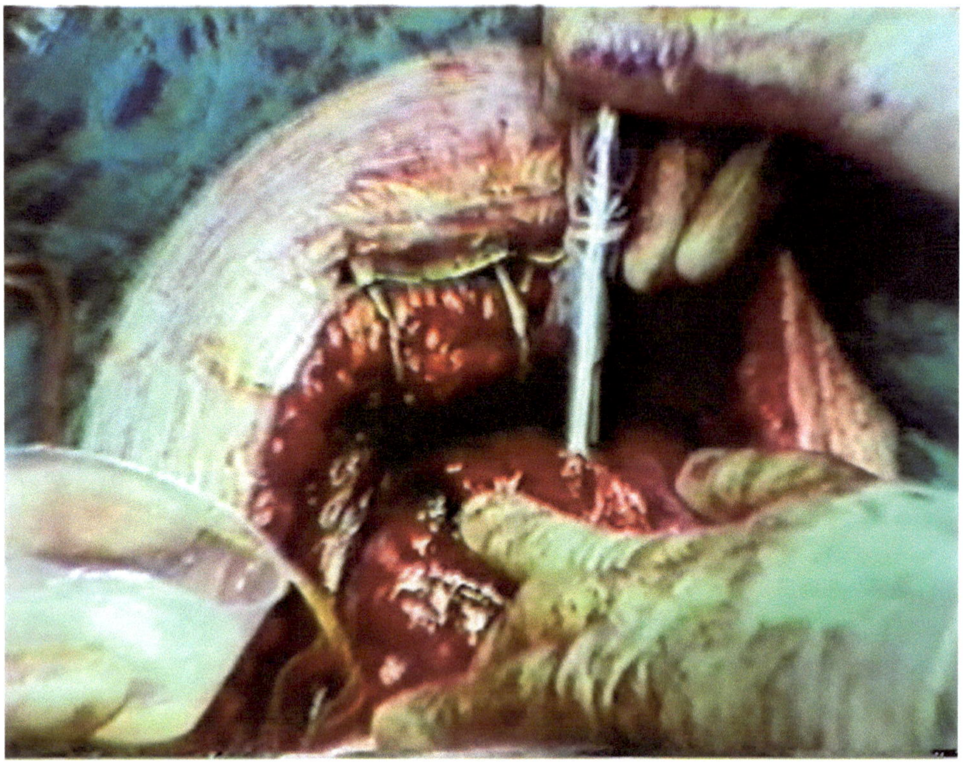

Fig. 45.8 Demonstrating the use of Doppler ultrasound before a nephrotomy

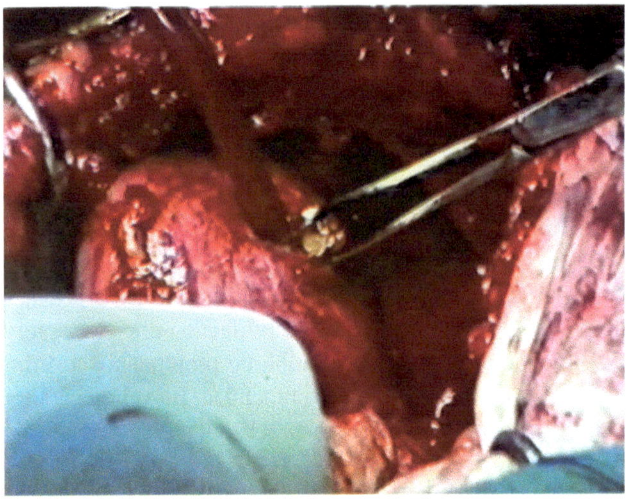

Fig. 45.9 Demonstrating extraction of stone through a nephrotomy

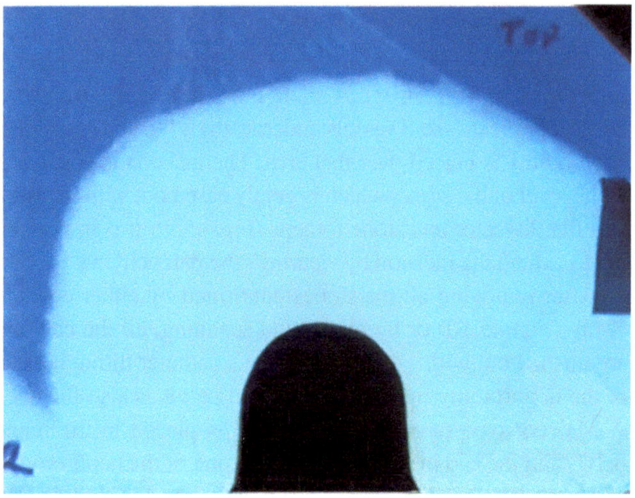

Fig. 45.10 Contact X-ray showing complete stone clearance

Technique

A 22F Simplastic® catheter (Rüsch, UK) is inserted into the bladder. This would not only allow urinary drainage but also facilitate washing out of mucous in the postoperative period. A midline incision from the pubic symphysis to midway between the umbilicus and xiphisternum gives good access. One advantage of this incision is, if needed, it can be extended upward and in extremely rare situations (in the obese) even subcostally. Initially, the small bowel is packed away to expose the ipsilateral colon, which is mobilized. The kidney is then mobilized. Usually, it is only necessary to mobilize the lower half of the kidney, the renal pelvis, and the proximal 2–3 cm of the ureter. A segment of distal ileum 15–20 cm from the ileocecal junction is isolated on its own mesentery. It is important to divide the mesentery as close to the base as possible (without damaging the main mesenteric artery) to allow the ileal segment to be brought to the renal pelvis without any tension on the mesentery (Fig. 45.11). The length of the ileal segment should be long enough to bridge the gap between the renal pelvis and the bladder. It is important to remember that it is the length of the mesentery that

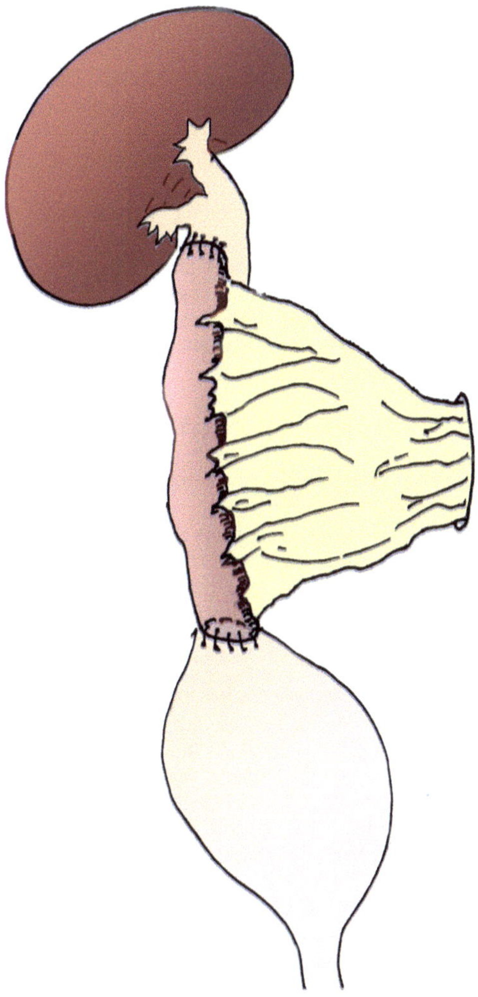

Fig. 45.11 Ileal replacement of ureter (Reproduced from Zuckerman and Assimos [24]. By kind permission of Springer-Verlag)

determines how the proximal part of the ileal segment will stretch toward the renal pelvis and not how long the segment is. The distal end of the isolated ileal segment is marked with a stitch to ensure orientation. The continuity of the main ileum is established by either a stapling technique (the author's choice) or by suture. The ileal segment is then thoroughly washed out with saline (without contaminating the peritoneal cavity).

An opening is made (as posteriorly as possible) in an avascular area of the colonic mesentery, as close to the renal pelvis as possible. The ureter is ligated just below the pelvi-ureteric junction and a longitudinal incision is made in the renal pelvis long enough to match the diameter of the ileal segment, which is anastomosed to the renal pelvis with 3 0 Vicryl. The posterior lips of ileum and renal pelvis are anastomosed first. Prior to performing the anastomosis, a 10-French Malecot-type nephrostomy tube is placed in the renal pelvis and the end brought out of the parenchyma. If part of the pelvis is intrarenal, the space between the pelvis and the parenchyma is exploited (as per extended pyelolithotomy). If the renal pelvis is completely intrarenal, a partial lower pole nephrectomy may be necessary to allow anastomosis between the ileum and renal pelvis and lower pole calyx. The opening in the mesentery is closed.

Some recommend a psoas hitch on the ipsilateral side but this maneuver is not essential. The peritoneum over the dome of the bladder is separated from the bladder. An incision is made in the bladder to match the diameter of the ileum the lower end of which is brought through an incision in the peritoneum. The lower end of ileum is anastomosed to the bladder using 3-0 Vicryl. No attempt should be made to use antireflux techniques or narrowing or "tailoring" the distal end of the ileal segment. Two tube drains are placed draining each anastomotic point and brought out through separate stab incisions. Placement of a ureteric stent is not recommended as it is of no value.

Postoperatively, the drains may be removed after 5 days (usually anastomotic leaks occur around the fourth postoperative day) if there is no urinary drainage. The nephrostomy is kept open until the seventh day when a nephrostogram is performed. If that shows no leaks, the nephrostomy tube is closed and removed after 24 h. The bladder catheter is removed on the tenth day.

Bench Surgery and Autotransplantation

There have been many reports on extracorporeal bench surgery to remove the stones followed by autotransplantation into the iliac fossa and pyelocystostomy to facilitate passage of stones directly into the bladder [25, 26]. Nephrectomy is performed as per donor nephrectomy for renal transplantation either by open or laparoscopic method. The kidney is made hypothermic by placing it in ice packs and/or perfusing it through the renal artery with a cold lactated Ringer solution at 5 °C. Open bench surgery to remove the stone is performed by any of the methods described earlier. The kidney is X-rayed to ensure complete stone clearance. Methylene blue solution can be injected into the renal artery to detect major arterial leaks. If any are found, they are ligated or underrun with absorbable sutures. The kidney is transplanted into the right iliac fossa using the same technique as for conventional renal transplantation except that the renal pelvis is directly anastomosed to the bladder.

The indications for this procedure are the same as for ileal replacement. However, this operation is rarely performed because the group of patients who need bench surgery and autotransplantation often may have had multiple procedures on the kidney to remove stones in the past. This makes dissection of the kidney and the vessels difficult. Therefore, it is far easier to perform an ileal replacement. Furthermore, there is nearly 5 % chance of loss of the kidney after bench surgery and autotransplantation [26].

Management of Residual Stones

If nephrostogram reveals stone fragment(s) in the ureter, the nephrostomy tube is left open for at least 2 weeks when a ureteroscopy is performed to deal with the stone(s). After successful fine fragmentation of the stone or removal of the fragments, a ureteric stent is left in situ. The nephrostomy tube is clamped for 24 h and removed. The ureteric stent is removed under local anesthesia with a flexible cystoscope 2 weeks later.

Ideally, there should not be any residual stones in the kidney. Should some be discovered, attempts at using the existing nephrostomy tract to remove the stones should be avoided as the tract is always tortuous and long. At least a month after the original procedure, the residual stones are managed in the conventional manner by ESWL, ureteroscopy, or PCNL, depending on the stone size, burden, and location.

The Future

In the author's opinion, the future is laparoscopic stone surgery where currently open surgery is performed. The safety and efficacy of laparoscopic pyelolithotomy is well established, although most of the stones in the renal pelvis will be dealt with by PCNL and the laparoscopic approach will be limited to those cases where reconstruction of the upper urinary tract (such as pyeloplasty) is required [27]. For larger branched calculi, reports of successful laparoscopic anatrophic nephrolithotomy have started appearing [28–30]. Although these series are small in numbers, successful stone removal was achieved with warm ischemia times of 32, 31, and 26 min, respectively. It is therefore likely that the future would see publication of larger series from highly centralized stone service units.

Conclusion

Despite great advances in endoscopic surgery and extracorporeal shock wave lithotripsy to remove renal stones, there is still the need for open surgery in a very small selected group of patients. The main procedures are extended pyelolithotomy, anatrophic nephrolithotomy, and nephrolithotomy by radial nephrotomy incisions with or without the aid of Doppler ultrasound. Expertise for open surgery is rapidly declining in developed countries because so few cases are performed every year even in large-volume centers. This argues for a centralized delivery of open stone surgery. In the future, it is highly likely that all operations that are now performed by open method will be performed laparoscopically, again in centralized units.

References

1. Assimos DG, Boyce WH, Harrison LH, McCullough DL, Kroovand RL, Sweat KR. The role of open surgery since extracorporeal shock wave lithotripsy. J Urol. 1989;142:263–7.
2. Matlaga BR, Assimos DG. Changing indications of open surgery. J Urol. 2002;59:493–4.
3. Bichler KH, Lahme S, Strohmaier WL. Indications for open stone removal of urinary calculi. Urol Int. 1997;59:102–8.
4. Kane CJ, Bolton DM, Stoller ML. Current indications for open surgery in an endourology center. Urology. 1995;45:218–21.
5. Ather MH, Paryani J, Menon A, Sulaiman MN. A 10 year experience of managing ureteric calculi: changing trends towards endourological intervention – is there a role for open surgery? BJU Int. 2001;88:173–7.
6. Al-Kohlan KM, Shokeir AA, Mosbaha A, et al. Treatment of complete stag horn stones: a prospective randomised comparison of open surgery versus percutaneousnephrolithotomy. J Urol. 2005; 173(2):469–73.
7. Buchholz NP, Hitchings A, Albanis S. The (soon forgotten) art of open surgery: to train or not to train. Ann R Coll Surg Engl. 2006;88:214–7.
8. Tűrk C, Knoll T, Petrick A, Sarica K, Seitz C, Straub M. European Association of Urology guidelines. 2011 edition. ISBN-13: 978-90-79754-60-1.
9. Gil-Vernet J. New surgical concepts in removing renal calculi. Urol Int. 1965;20:255–88.
10. Wickham JEA. The surgical treatment of renal lithiasis. In: Wickham JEA, editor. Urinary calculus disease. Edinburgh: Churchill Livingstone; 1979. p. 145–98.
11. Petersen HK, Moller BB, Iversen HG. Regional hypothermia in renal surgery for severe lithiasis. Scand J Urol Nephrol. 1977; 11(1):27–34.
12. Thompson RH, Frank I, Lohse CM, et al. The impact of ischemia time during open nephron sparing surgery on solitary kidneys: a multi-institutional study. J Urol. 2007;177:471–6.
13. Becker F, Van Poppel H, Hakenberg OW, et al. Assessing the impact of ischaemia time during partial nephrectomy. Eur Urol. 2009; 56:625–35.
14. Novic AC. Renal hypothermia: in vivo and ex vivo. Urol Clin North Am. 1983;10(4):637–44.
15. Wickham JE, Fernando AR, Hendry WF, et al. Inosine: clinical results of ischaemic renal surgery. Br J Urol. 1978;50(7): 465–8.
16. Aganović D, Kulovac B, Prcić A, Hadziosmanović O. Using verapamil as protective factor in renal ischemia reperfusion injury doing anatrophic nephrolithotomy. Bosn J Basic Med Sci. 2007;7(3): 235–8.
17. Krishnan P, Sharma A, Singh M. Effect of angiotensin converting enzyme inhibitors in ischaemia-reperfusion-induced renal injury in rats. Pharmacol Res. 1998;37:23–9.
18. Marberger M, Georgi M, Guenther R, Hohenfellner R. Simultaneous balloon occlusion of the renal artery and hypothermic perfusion in situ surgery of the kidney. J Urol. 1978;119(4):463–7.
19. Brödel M. The intrinsic blood vessels of the kidney and their significance in nephrotomy. Bull Johns Hopkins Hosp. 1911;12: 10–3.
20. Boyce WH. The surgical treatment of renal lithiasis (quoting his publications of 1967, 1972, 1975). In: Wickham JEA, editor. Urinary calculous disease. Edinburgh: Churchill Livingstone; 1979. p. 171–3.
21. Gough DC, Baillie CT. Paediatric anatrophic nephrolithotomy; stone clearance – at what price? BJU Int. 2000;85(7):874–8.

22. Thuroff JW, Alken P, Riedmiller H, Hohenfellner R. Doppler and real-time ultrasound renal surgery. Eur Urol. 1982;8(5): 298–303.
23. Wickham JEA, Gower R, Sleight MW. Demonstration: radial nephrotomy for nephrolithotomy. Baus annual meeting, 1978.
24. Zuckerman JM, Assimos DG. Autotransplantation and ureteric replacement: in whom and how? In: Rao NP, Preminger GM, Kavanagh JP, editors. Urinary tract stone disease. London: Springer; 2011.
25. Pettersson S, Bryner H, Henriksson C, et al. Autologous renal transplantation with direct pyelocystostomy in the treatment of recurrent calculi. BJU. 1983;55(2):154–61.
26. Bondevik H, Albrechtsen D, Sodal G, et al. Extracorporeal surgery and autotransplantation for complicated renal calculous disease in 108 kidneys. Scand J Urol Nephrol. 1990;24(4):301–6.
27. Badalato GM, Hemal AK, Menon M, et al. Current role of robot-assisted pyelolithotomy for the management of large renal calculi: a contemporary analysis. J Endourol. 2009;23(10):1719–22.
28. Simforoosh N, Aminsharifi A, Tabibi A, et al. Laparoscopic anatrophic nephrolithotomy for managing large stag horn calculi. BJU Int. 2008;101(10):1293–6.
29. Zhou L, Xuan Q, Wu B, et al. Retroperitoneal laparoscopic anatrophic nephrolithotomy for large stag horn calculi. Int J Urol. 2011;18(2):126–9.
30. Nouralizadeh A, Simforosh N, Masoudi P, et al. Bilateral laparoscopic anatrophic nephrolithotomy for managing renal calculi. Urol J. 2010;7:133–5. www.uj.unrc.ir.
31. Wendt-Nordahl G, Knoll T, Alken P. Open surgery to remove stones: when and how? In: Rao NP, Preminger GM, Kavanagh JP, editors. Urinary tract stone disease. London: Springer; 2011.

Shock Wave Lithotripsy: Present Indications and Future Prospects

46

Michael E. Lipkin and Glenn M. Preminger

Abstract

This chapter describes the fundamentals of shock wave lithotripsy (SWL), the instrumentation for SWL, shock wave generation, rate of delivery and focusing, coupling of the shock wave, and stone localization. The process of fragmentation through spallation, cavitation, and comminution is described. The contemporary indications and contraindications to SWL for renal and ureteral calculi, large and staghorn calculi, and calculi in calyceal diverticula are discussed. Lithotripsy advances in the form of changes to the lithotripter, modifications to treatment strategy, and adjuncts that improve SWL safety and efficacy are described. Future technological advances are explored.

Keywords

Shock wave lithotripsy • Instrumentation • Shock wave generation • Shock wave focusing • Coupling • Stone localization • Indications and contraindications to SWL • Renal calculi • Ureteral calculi • Staghorn calculi • Calculi in calyceal diverticula • Advances • Modifications to treatment strategy • Adjuncts that improve SWL safety and efficacy

Introduction

Shock wave lithotripsy (SWL) was introduced clinically in 1980. Since its inception, SWL technology has advanced rapidly in terms of shock wave generation, focusing, patient coupling, and stone localization. The indications for SWL continue to evolve as well. SWL can be considered a first-line therapy for the treatment of most intrarenal stones and many ureteral stones.

This chapter reviews the fundamental physics and instrumentation for SWL. Current indications and contraindications of SWL are discussed. Finally, advances in lithotripsy technology and adjuncts to improve the efficacy of SWL are presented.

Fundamentals of SWL

Shock waves are high-energy amplitudes of pressure generated in the air or water by an abrupt release of energy in a small space. They consist of an initial sharp peak in positive pressure followed by a prolonged negative pressure wave. While they travel unimpeded through substances of similar densities, when a shock wave encounters a boundary between substances of differing acoustic impedance, such as water and stone, compressive stresses are generated along the initial surface, which may overcome the tensile strength of that object. As a shock wave crosses the trailing edge of the stone, part of the energy is reflected, creating tensile stress and fragmentation along the trailing edge (spallation) [1]. These stresses lead to a dynamic fracture process consisting of nucleation, coalescence, and growth of micro-fractures in the

M.E. Lipkin, M.D. (✉)
Division of Urologic Surgery, Department of Surgery, Duke University Medical Center, DUMC 3167, Durham, NC 27710, USA
e-mail: michael.lipkin@duke.edu

G.M. Preminger, M.D.
Department of Urologic Surgery, Duke University Medical Center, RM 1573 White Zone, Duke South, DUMC 3167, Durham, NC, 27710, USA
e-mail: glenn.preminger@duke.edu; premi001@mc.duke.edu

J.J. Talati et al. (eds.), *Urolithiasis*,
DOI 10.1007/978-1-4471-4387-1_46, © Springer-Verlag London 2012

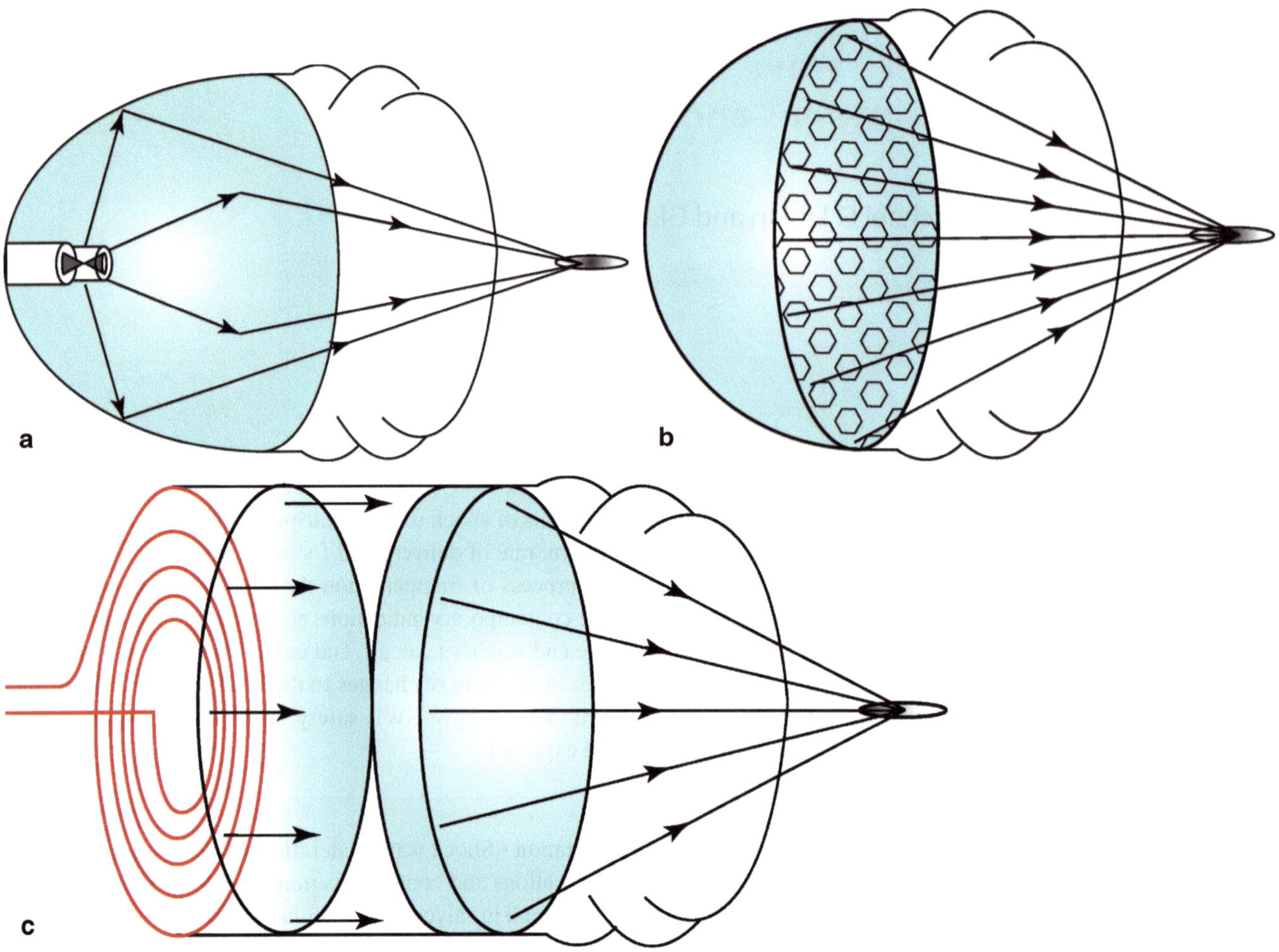

Fig. 46.1 Shock wave sources. The schematics demonstrate shock wave generation and focusing: (**a**) electrohydraulic generator, (**b**) electromagnetic generator, and (**c**) piezoelectric generator

stone leading to fragmentation [2]. Cavitation also plays a major role in stone comminution. As a shock wave passes through fluid, bubbles form and grow at the stone surface during the negative/tensile pressure component of the wave. When the next shock wave arrives, the positive pressure causes these bubbles to violently collapse releasing a microjet of energy directed toward the stone. These forces act in conjunction to ultimately fragment a stone in vivo [3, 4].

While clinical experience has shown that SWL is safe and effective, animal and human studies have demonstrated acute and chronic side effects to SWL. Recent basic science has demonstrated that SWL-induced chronic renal injury is primarily a vascular event [5]. SWL induces vasoconstriction that results in ischemia [6, 7]. In addition, cavitation bubble expansion in small blood vessels during SWL causes rupture [8]. High-speed photography has demonstrated that cavitation bubbles generated during SWL can cause vessel distension and vessel invagination, and this distension and invagination along with liquid jets causes vascular rupture during SWL [9]. Accumulation of shear forces during repeated shock applications can also lead to vessel damage [10]. This damage to blood vessels leads to localized ischemia and may result in free-radical formation as the final pathway of tissue injury [11, 12]. The focus of investigators has not only been to optimize the shock wave for stone fragmentation but to also make it safer.

Instrumentation for Shock Wave Lithotripsy

Shock Wave Generation and Focusing

There are four features common to all shock wave lithotripters: (1) an energy source to generate the shock wave, (2) a focusing device to direct the shock wave at a focal point, (3) a coupling medium, and (4) a stone localization system [1]. There are three common mechanisms utilized by lithotripters for generating shock waves: electrohydraulic, piezoelectric, and electromagnetic generators (Fig. 46.1a–c). The electrohydraulic generator, exemplified by the original Dornier HM3 lithotripter, produces shock waves by an electrical spark gap at the base of a water bath located in an ellipsoidal reflector. The high-voltage discharge causes the rapid vaporization of water at the tip of the electrodes (F1), and this produces a shock wave. The acoustic shock wave is focused at a second focal point (F2) by the ellipsoidal reflector. The potential advantage of electrohydraulic lithotripters is their efficacy in fragmenting stones; however, a disadvantage is the relatively short life of the electrode [5].

Piezoelectric shock waves are generated by the sudden expansion of ceramic elements excited by a high-frequency, high-voltage energy pulse. The sudden expansion generates an ultrasonic wave. The elements are placed in a spherical dish that allows for the convergence of the ultrasonic waves generated from each of the ceramic elements. This produces a single, high-energy shock wave directed at the focal point, which is the center of the sphere [13]. The spherical focusing mechanism allows for a wide area of skin for shock wave energy, which minimizes patient discomfort. This also produces a relatively narrow focal point [14]. Advantages of piezoelectric lithotripters include longer service life, better focusing, and the possibility to perform SWL without anesthesia [5, 14]. The major disadvantage is the decreased power it delivers compared to other lithotripter types [5].

Shock waves generated by electromagnetic devices are produced when an electrical impulse moves a thin, circular metallic membrane that is housed within a "shock tube." The resulting shock wave passes through the water-filled shock tube and is then directed at the focal point by an acoustic lens [15]. Electromagnetic lithotripters introduce the shock wave into the patient's body over a large surface area, reducing the need for anesthesia while maintaining a high amount of energy at the focus [5]. The relatively small focus with high energy produced by electromagnetic lithotripters may increase the risk of subcapsular hematomas [5].

Coupling of the Shock Wave

The original Dornier HM3 utilized a 1,000-l water bath for coupling shock waves to the patient. In an attempt to minimize space requirements and the physiological and functional disadvantages of a large water bath, second- and third-generation lithotripters were developed with several different couplings. Water cushions with ultrasound gel are commonly used [16]. The quality of the coupling media can have a significant impact on the efficacy of SWL. It is important to minimize the amount of air bubbles trapped in the coupling media as these bubbles can reduce the efficiency of the shock waves [17, 18].

Stone Localization

Localization of calculi during lithotripsy is accomplished with either fluoroscopy or ultrasonography. Fluoroscopy has the advantage of being more familiar to the urologist as well as increased ability to localize ureteral stones. The major disadvantages of fluoroscopy are increased risks of ionizing radiation exposure to the patient and to the surgical team and inability to identify radiolucent stones. Automated fluoroscopic localization has been shown to decrease radiation exposure [16]. However, many newer lithotripters utilize ultrasonographic technology for stone localization. Ultrasound offers the advantages of stone localization with real-time monitoring and effective identification of radiolucent stones while eliminating the radiation exposure inherent to fluoroscopy. Ultrasound has been shown to be effective in localizing stone fragments as small as 2–3 mm and may even be superior to routine kidney-ureter-bladder (KUB) imaging in assessing residual stone fragments following lithotripsy [13]. However, localization of stones is hampered when located in the middle ureter.

Contemporary Indications and Contraindications to SWL

The 2007 American Urologic Association/European Urologic Association clinical guidelines for the management of ureteral calculi state that SWL is an acceptable first-line therapy for the treatment of ureteral stones [19]. SWL is also considered first-line treatment for renal stones less than 2 cm, though as stone burden increases stone-free rates for SWL decrease [5]. Relative contraindications to SWL include stone size greater than 2 cm, cystine or calcium oxalate monohydrate stones (due to their relative resistance to fragmentation by SWL), active infection, proximate calcified abdominal aortic or renal artery aneurysms, distal obstruction, pregnancy, bleeding diathesis, and poorly informed patients [5]. Obesity can be a relative contraindication to SWL. Increasing skin-to-stone distance decreases the efficacy of SWL [20, 21]. A skin-to-stone distance greater than 110 mm has been proposed as a cutoff that best predicts failure of SWL [21].

Renal Calculi

Shock wave lithotripsy has been shown to be effective at treating intrarenal stones. However, there are three factors that need to be accounted for when deciding whether SWL is the appropriate treatment modality for a stone: (1) size, (2) location, and (3) composition. As stone burden increases, the stone-free rates achieved with SWL decrease [22–24]. Stone size less than 10 mm has been shown to be a significant predictor of stone-free rate after SWL [23]. The stone-free rates reported for renal stones less than 10 mm are approximately 80 % [23, 25]. Shock wave lithotripsy is not recommended as first-line treatment for stones greater than 2 cm due to poor stone-free rates [5, 24, 26]. For stones larger than 2 cm, percutaneous nephrolithotomy (PCNL) should be considered first-line treatment [5, 26].

Stone location also plays a role in determining the efficacy of SWL. In general, SWL is effective for renal pelvic, upper calyx, and middle calyx stones less than 2 cm [27]. For stones located in the lower pole, SWL is not as effective. In a randomized, prospective trial comparing SWL to PNL for the treatment of lower pole stones, SWL had a 37 % stone-free rate compared to a 95 % stone-free rate for PCNL [28]. Percutaneous nephrolithotomy outperformed SWL even when stratified by stone size. If SWL is to be used to treat lower pole stones, it should be done on stones less than 10 mm.

Certain stone compositions are less amenable to SWL. Cystine, calcium oxalate monohydrate, and brushite stones are all resistant to fragmentation with SWL [29]. Cystine stones are resistant to SWL due to the fact that they are ductile, meaning they are better able to absorb energy from shock waves by plastic deformation [29]. Brushite and calcium oxalate monohydrate stones are hard. They are resistant to deformation from shock waves, fracture propagation, and cavitation microjet impact [29]. Resistance to fragmentation can be predicted by measuring Hounsfield units on preoperative computed tomography. Stones with a density greater than 900 Hounsfield units have been shown to be more resistant to fragmentation with SWL [21]. Stone composition can be accurately determined using dual-energy computed tomography [30, 31]. This technology can differentiate between numerous stone types allowing for better preoperative planning for treatment.

Ureteral Calculi

Shock wave lithotripsy is still considered a first-line treatment for ureteral stones less than 10 mm [19]. Similar to the treatment of renal stones, location, size, and stone composition continue to dictate the utility of SWL for the management of ureteral stones. The same limitations for treating cystine, calcium oxalate monohydrate, and brushite stones apply to ureteral stones. Stone location and size play a major role in determining the efficacy of SWL for the treatment of ureteral stones. The stone-free rate for proximal ureteral stones treated with SWL is approximately 82 % [19]. This is comparable to stone-free rates achieved with flexible ureteroscopy. The majority of patients with ureteral stones treated with SWL clear their fragments within 1–3 days, with a mean of 4.6 days to stone-free status [32]. Routine ureteral stenting is not recommended prior to SWL of ureteral stones [19]. Medical expulsive therapy with alpha-adrenergic blockers and calcium channel blockers has been shown to improve stone clearance after SWL for ureteral stones [33, 34].

For stones in the distal and mid-ureter, the stone-free rate decreases to 74 and 73 %, respectively [19]. In these cases, ureteroscopy has a clear advantage in terms of stone-free rates. The reported stone-free rate for mid-ureteral stones treated with ureteroscopy is 86 % and for distal ureteral stones is 94 % [19]. A potential advantage of SWL over ureteroscopy is the ability to perform the procedure with intravenous sedation or minimal anesthesia. Several investigators have promoted the use of shock wave lithotripsy for the treatment of distal and juxtavesical stones with the patient in a prone or modified sitting position. Studies have demonstrated >85 % stone-free rate with one treatment on the HM3 lithotripter, with patients positioned in the prone position [35–37]. With improvements in endoscopic technology including digital ureteroscopes, high-powered holmium lasers, nitinol baskets, and anti-retropulsion devices, the efficacy of ureteroscopy in the treatment of ureteral stones is likely to increase and supplant SWL as the primary treatment of ureteral stones.

Large Calculi/Staghorn Calculi

Percutaneous nephrolithotomy is considered first-line treatment for staghorn or partial staghorn calculi [26]. There may be a role for SWL as an adjunct to PCNL for these larger stones. If SWL is to be used in conjunction with PCNL for the treatment of staghorn calculi, it is recommended that SWL precede PCNL [26]. Alternatively, SWL can be effective at treating small post-PCNL residual fragments. In selected patients with smaller staghorn stones and normal collecting system anatomy, SWL can be attempted with renal drainage via either a ureteral stent of nephrostomy tube [26].

Calyceal Diverticular Calculi

Calyceal diverticula are urine-filled cavities connected to the normal collecting system by a narrow isthmus. The most common indication for treatment of calyceal diverticular calculi is ipsilateral flank pain; others include recurrent infection or persistent gross hematuria. The goal of treatment for calyceal diverticular stones includes removal of the stones and eradication of the diverticulum [5, 38]. Treatment options for calculi within calyceal diverticula are numerous, ranging from SWL to PCNL to URS; however, SWL cannot be used to obliterate the diverticulum [38]. The stone-free rates reported for the treatment of calyceal diverticular stones with SWL average 21 % [39]. A majority of patients will have resolution of their symptoms after SWL treatment for calyceal diverticular stones; however, many of these patients will have recurrence of symptoms when followed for longer periods of time [40]. The preferred treatment for calyceal diverticular stones is endoscopic management with either PNL or ureteroscopy [38].

Lithotripsy Advances

Based on our current understanding of cavitation in stone fragmentation as well as the role of cavitation, vasoconstriction, and free-radical formation in SWL-induced tissue injury, several groups are investigating ways to improve the clinical safety and efficacy of SWL. This increased knowledge of the mechanisms of stone fragmentation and tissue injury has led to advances in lithotripter designs, improvement in treatment strategies, and the medical adjuncts to improve SWL safety and efficacy.

Changes to the Lithotripter

A reflector insert has been designed that can be integrated with the original Dornier HM3 reflector to create a second shock wave immediately after the original shock wave. This second shock wave partially cancels the negative tensile component of the original wave, preventing cavitation bubbles from overexpanding in blood vessels, reducing their chance of rupture. This combination resulted in improved stone comminution of stones implanted in swine kidneys and decreased renal parenchymal injury compared to the unmodified HM3 [41]. Importantly, these modifications can be applied to other lithotripters, to reduce tissue injury while preserving the impact of cavitation on stone comminution.

Electrohydraulic lithotripters generate a second direct wave from the source in addition to the focused shock wave. This direct wave can induce cavitation prior to the arrival of the focused wave, which may interfere with the cavitation activity of the focused wave. A device has been constructed that can suppress the direct wave. The cavitation activity from the direct wave can be suppressed by installing a direct wave suppressor close to the spark source [42].

Modifications have been made to electromagnetic and piezoelectric lithotripters as well. The Storz Modulith SLX-F2 (Storz-Medical, Kreuzlingen, Switzerland) has a dual focus system that allows the operator to change the focal size depending on the clinical situation [43]. It accomplishes this by modifying the pulse duration from the electromagnetic source [16]. The PiezoLith 3000 (Richard Wolf, Knittlingen, Germany) utilizes a double-layer design to increase shock wave energy [16].

Another way in which investigators have attempted to modify the shock wave is by delivering a shock wave from two lithotripters to the same focal point, F2. This can be accomplished by placing the shock sources at a 90° angle from one another [44]. This dual-pulse lithotripsy has been shown to increase comminution at the focus without increasing tissue injury in animal studies [45]. In clinical trials, patients treated with the dual-head device showed minimal morphological changes to the renal parenchyma despite delivering twice as many shocks [46]. These results appear to confirm the relative safety of dual-pulse lithotripsy in a patient population, although the long-term effects have not been assessed.

Modifications to Treatment Strategy

Investigators have evaluated ways in which treatment strategy can be modified to improve the efficacy and safety of SWL. The two variables that have been most extensively evaluated are the rate of shock wave delivery and the energy. A randomized controlled trial comparing a rate of 60 shocks/min versus 120 shocks/min demonstrated a significantly higher stone-free rate in the group treated with the slower rate [47]. The stone-free rate for patients treated with 60 shocks/min was 60 versus 28 % in patients treated with the faster rate. Patients treated with the slower rate required fewer total shocks, but the procedure did take longer. Other studies have confirmed improved stone-free rates in patients treated with a slower shock wave rate [48, 49]. A recent meta-analysis looking at randomized controlled trials comparing 60 shocks/min versus 120 shocks/min confirmed the findings of improved treatment success with 60 shocks/min [50]. The utilization of slower shock rates during SWL leads to fewer additional procedures and improved cost-effectiveness when compared to faster rates [49].

A number of studies have demonstrated improved stone comminution and decreased renal tissue injury with a treatment strategy that begins with a low energy and gradually increases energy. An in vitro study comparing a gradual increase in energy versus a gradual decrease in energy found improved fragmentation efficiency with the increasing energy strategy [51]. These findings were confirmed in an in vivo study performed in a porcine model [52]. In this study, stones treated with an increasing strategy of 18, 20 and 22 kV for 600, 800, and 800 shocks, respectively, had better fragmentation efficiency than those treated with a decreasing strategy of 22, 20, and 18 kV for 800, 600, and 600 shocks, respectively. A recent randomized controlled trial demonstrated improved stone-free rates in patients treated with an escalating voltage strategy versus those treated with a fixed voltage [53]. Pretreatment with low-energy shock waves has also been shown to reduce renal damage [54, 55]. The low energy shock waves induce vasoconstriction during SWL whereas standard protocols lead to vasoconstriction after SWL [55]. This vasoconstriction early on during treatment likely prevents vascular injury from high-energy shock waves.

Adjuncts to Improve SWL Safety and Efficacy

A large body of evidence suggests that free radicals play a role in SWL-mediated tissue injury. Several studies have investigated the role of antioxidants in protecting the renal parenchyma against free-radical injury [56–58]. Patients pretreated with mannitol, a known free-radical scavenger, have been shown to have reduced urinary β(beta) 2-microglobulin compared to a control group [56]. Urinary β(beta)2-microglobulin is a sign of renal cell damage. Other investigators have demonstrated that both pretreatment and posttreatment with antioxidants reduce signs of renal cellular damage in patients undergoing SWL [58]. Vitamin E and citrate have also been shown to reduce shock wave-induced increase in free radicals in an in vitro model [57]. Patients at high risk of renal damage during SWL may benefit from use of peri-procedure antioxidants and free-radical scavengers.

Medical expulsive therapy has been shown to improve stone passage after SWL. Two large meta-analyses evaluating the use of medical expulsive therapy with either calcium channel blockers or alpha-adrenergic blockers after SWL demonstrated significantly higher stone-free rates with the use of medical expulsive therapy [33, 34]. The calcium channel blocker nifedipine increased the success rate of SWL treatment of ureteral stones in a randomized prospective study [59]. Tamsulosin, an alpha-adrenergic blocker, has also been shown to improve stone-free rates after SWL in a randomized prospective study [60]. Potassium citrate has also been shown to improve residual fragment clearance after SWL [61].

Another way to enhance the efficacy of SWL is to improve patient selection. Preoperative evaluation of patients with computed tomography (CT) is helpful in this regard. Advances in CT have allowed better determination of internal stone architecture [62]. As a consequence, a few studies have demonstrated that determining the Hounsfield units (i.e., density unit of material on CT) of renal stones on pretreatment, non-contrasted CT could predict stone-free rates of patients treated with SWL [21, 63]. More recently, the use of multi-detector CT has been shown to very accurately predict different stone compositions in vivo [31]. Therefore, stone compositions that are "SWL resistant" such as calcium oxalate monohydrate or cystine stones can be identified, and those patients can be treated with endoscopic modalities, thereby avoiding additional procedures in these patients. Preoperative CT is also useful in determining skin-to-stone distance. A number of studies have shown decreased efficacy of SWL as skin-to-stone distance increases [20, 21, 63].

Conclusion

Upon its introduction, SWL revolutionized the treatment of urolithiasis. It provided a minimally invasive technique to treat both renal and ureteral stones. Though the technology for SWL continues to evolve, the fundamental principles of delivering a shock wave to fragment a stone have not. Increasing experience with SWL has allowed better patient and stone selection to improve both safety and efficacy. Modifications have treatment strategies and medical adjuncts, such as antioxidants and medical expulsive therapy that have further improved the safety and efficacy of SWL. Future research will be dedicated to modifying lithotripters' design to improve the delivery of shock waves, coupling of shock waves to patients, and stone localization.

References

1. Zhong P, Preminger G. Physics of shock wave lithotripsy. In: Coe FL, Favus MJ, Pak CY, Parks JH, Preminger G, editors. Kidney stones: medical and surgical management. Philadelphia: Lippincott-Raven Publishers; 1996. p. 529–48.
2. Lokhandwalla M, Sturtevant B. Fracture mechanics model of stone comminution in ESWL and implications for tissue damage. Phys Med Biol. 2000;45(7):1923–40.
3. Zhu S, Cocks FH, Preminger GM, Zhong P. The role of stress waves and cavitation in stone comminution in shock wave lithotripsy. Ultrasound Med Biol. 2002;28(5):661–71.
4. Coleman AJ, Saunders JE, Crum LA, Dyson M. Acoustic cavitation generated by an extracorporeal shockwave lithotripter. Ultrasound Med Biol. 1987;13(2):69–76.
5. Lingeman JE, Matlaga BR, Evan AP. Surgical management of urinary lithiasis. In: Wein AJ, Kavoussi LR, Novick AC, Partin AW, Peters CA, editors. Campbell's-Walsh urology, vol. 3. 9th ed. Philadelphia: Saunders; 2007. p. 1431–507.
6. Willis LR, Evan AP, Connors BA, Reed G, Fineberg NS, Lingeman JA. Effects of extracorporeal shock wave lithotripsy to one kidney on bilateral glomerular filtration rate and PAH clearance in minipigs. J Urol. 1996;156(4):1502–6.
7. Willis LR, Evan AP, Connors BA, Fineberg NS, Lingeman JE. Effects of SWL on glomerular filtration rate and renal plasma flow in uninephrectomized minipigs. J Endourol. 1997;11(1):27–32.
8. Zhu S, Dreyer T, Liebler M, Riedlinger R, Preminger GM, Zhong P. Reduction of tissue injury in shock-wave lithotripsy by using an acoustic diode. Ultrasound Med Biol. 2004;30(5):675–82.
9. Chen H, Brayman AA, Bailey MR, Matula TJ. Blood vessel rupture by cavitation. Urol Res. 2010;38(4):321–6.
10. Freund JB, Colonius T, Evan AP. A cumulative shear mechanism for tissue damage initiation in shock-wave lithotripsy. Ultrasound Med Biol. 2007;33(9):1495–503.
11. Delvecchio F, Auge BK, Munver R, et al. Shock wave lithotripsy causes ipsilateral renal injury remote from the focal point: the role of regional vasoconstriction. J Urol. 2003;169(4):1526–9.
12. Munver R, Delvecchio FC, Kuo RL, Brown SA, Zhong P, Preminger GM. In vivo assessment of free radical activity during shock wave lithotripsy using a microdialysis system: the renoprotective action of allopurinol. J Urol. 2002;167(1):327–34.
13. Abernathy BB, Morris JS, Wilson WT, Miller GL, Preminger GM. Evaluation of residual stone fragments following lithotripsy: sonography versus KUB. In: Lingeman JE, Newman DM, editors. Shock wave lithotripsy II. New York: Plenum Press; 1989. p. 247–54.
14. Preminger GM. Sonographic piezoelectric lithotripsy: more bang for your buck. J Endourol. 1989;3:321–7.
15. Rassweiler J, Kohrmann U, Heine G, Back W, Wess O, Alken P. Modulith SL 10/20 – experimental introduction and first clinical

experience with a new interdisciplinary lithotriptor. Eur Urol. 1990;18(4):237–41.

16. Rassweiler JJ, Knoll T, Kohrmann KU, et al. Shock wave technology and application: an update. Eur Urol. 2011;59(5):784–96.
17. Pishchalnikov YA, Neucks JS, VonDerHaar RJ, Pishchalnikova IV, Williams Jr JC, McAteer JA. Air pockets trapped during routine coupling in dry head lithotripsy can significantly decrease the delivery of shock wave energy. J Urol. 2006;176(6 Pt 1):2706–10.
18. Jain A, Shah TK. Effect of air bubbles in the coupling medium on efficacy of extracorporeal shock wave lithotripsy. Eur Urol. 2007;51(6):1680–6; discussion 1686–1687.
19. Preminger GM, Tiselius HG, Assimos DG, et al. 2007 Guideline for the management of ureteral calculi. J Urol. 2007;178(6):2418–34.
20. Patel T, Kozakowski K, Hruby G, Gupta M. Skin to stone distance is an independent predictor of stone-free status following shockwave lithotripsy. J Endourol. 2009;23(9):1383–5.
21. Wiesenthal JD, Ghiculete D, D'A Honey RJ, Pace KT. Evaluating the importance of mean stone density and skin-to-stone distance in predicting successful shock wave lithotripsy of renal and ureteric calculi. Urol Res. 2010;38(4):307–13.
22. el-Damanhoury H, Scharfe T, Ruth J, Roos S, Hohenfellner R. Extracorporeal shock wave lithotripsy of urinary calculi: experience in treatment of 3,278 patients using the Siemens Lithostar and Lithostar Plus. J Urol. 1991;145(3):484–8.
23. Elkoushy MA, Hassan JA, Morehouse DD, Anidjar M, Andonian S. Factors determining stone-free rate in shock wave lithotripsy using standard focus of Storz Modulith SLX-F2 lithotripter. Urology. 2011;78(4):759–63.
24. Logarakis NF, Jewett MA, Luymes J, Honey RJ. Variation in clinical outcome following shock wave lithotripsy. J Urol. 2000;163(3): 721–5.
25. Clayman RV, McClennan BL, Garvin TJ, Denstedt JD, Andriole GL. Lithostar: an electromagnetic acoustic shock wave unit for extracorporeal lithotripsy. J Endourol. 1989;3:307–13.
26. Preminger GM, Assimos DG, Lingeman JE, Nakada SY, Pearle MS, Wolf Jr JS. Chapter 1: AUA guideline on management of staghorn calculi: diagnosis and treatment recommendations. J Urol. 2005;173(6):1991–2000.
27. Wen CC, Nakada SY. Treatment selection and outcomes: renal calculi. Urol Clin North Am. 2007;34(3):409–19.
28. Albala DM, Assimos DG, Clayman RV, et al. Lower pole I: a prospective randomized trial of extracorporeal shock wave lithotripsy and percutaneous nephrostolithotomy for lower pole nephrolithiasis-initial results. J Urol. 2001;166(6):2072–80.
29. Zhong P, Preminger GM. Mechanisms of differing stone fragility in extracorporeal shockwave lithotripsy. J Endourol. 1994;8(4): 263–8.
30. Ferrandino MN, Pierre SA, Simmons WN, Paulson EK, Albala DM, Preminger GM. Dual-energy computed tomography with advanced postimage acquisition data processing: improved determination of urinary stone composition. J Endourol. 2010;24(3): 347–54.
31. Zilberman DE, Ferrandino MN, Preminger GM, Paulson EK, Lipkin ME, Boll DT. In vivo determination of urinary stone composition using dual energy computerized tomography with advanced post-acquisition processing. J Urol. 2010;184(6):2354–9.
32. Resit-Goren M, Dirim A, Ilteris-Tekin M, Ozkardes H. Time to stone clearance for ureteral stones treated with extracorporeal shock wave lithotripsy. Urology. 2011;78(1):26–30.
33. Schuler TD, Shahani R, Honey RJ, Pace KT. Medical expulsive therapy as an adjunct to improve shockwave lithotripsy outcomes: a systematic review and meta-analysis. J Endourol. 2009;23(3): 387–93.
34. Seitz C, Liatsikos E, Porpiglia F, Tiselius HG, Zwergel U. Medical therapy to facilitate the passage of stones: what is the evidence? Eur Urol. 2009;56(3):455–71.
35. Turk TM, Jenkins AD. A comparison of ureteroscopy to in situ extracorporeal shock wave lithotripsy for the treatment of distal ureteral calculi. J Urol. 1999;161(1):45–6; discussion 46–47.
36. Becht E, Moll V, Neisius D, Ziegler M. Treatment of prevesical ureteral calculi by extracorporeal shock wave lithotripsy. J Urol. 1988;139(5):916–8.
37. Rodrigues Netto Junior N, Lemos GC, Claro JF. In situ extracorporeal shock wave lithotripsy for ureteral calculi. J Urol. 1990;144(2 Pt 1):253–4.
38. Cohen TD, Preminger GM. Management of calyceal calculi. Urol Clin North Am. 1997;24(1):81–96.
39. Renner C, Rassweiler J. Treatment of renal stones by extracorporeal shock wave lithotripsy. Nephron. 1999;81 Suppl 1:71–81.
40. Jones JA, Lingeman JE, Steidle CP. The roles of extracorporeal shock wave lithotripsy and percutaneous nephrostolithotomy in the management of pyelocaliceal diverticula. J Urol. 1991;146(3): 724–7.
41. Marguet CG, Young MD, Maloney M, et al. Improved stone comminution and simultaneously reduced tissue injury with an upgraded electrohydraulic lithotripter: in vivo studies. Paper presented at American Urological Association Annual Meeting, San Francisco, 2004.
42. Matula TJ, Hilmo PR, Bailey MR. A suppressor to prevent direct wave-induced cavitation in shock wave therapy devices. J Acoust Soc Am. 2005;118(1):178–85.
43. De Sio M, Autorino R, Quarto G, et al. A new transportable shockwave lithotripsy machine for managing urinary stones: a single-centre experience with a dual-focus lithotripter. BJU Int. 2007; 100(5):1137–41.
44. Sheir KZ, Zabihi N, Lee D, et al. Evaluation of synchronous twin pulse technique for shock wave lithotripsy: determination of optimal parameters for in vitro stone fragmentation. J Urol. 2003;170(6 Pt 1):2190–4.
45. Sheir KZ, Lee D, Humphrey PA, Morrissey K, Sundaram CP, Clayman RV. Evaluation of synchronous twin pulse technique for shock wave lithotripsy: in vivo tissue effects. Urology. 2003;62(5):964–7.
46. Sheir KZ, El-Diasty TA, Ismail AM. Evaluation of a synchronous twin-pulse technique for shock wave lithotripsy: the first prospective clinical study. BJU Int. 2005;95(3):389–93.
47. Pace KT, Ghiculete D, Harju M, Honey RJ. Shock wave lithotripsy at 60 or 120 shocks per minute: a randomized, double-blind trial. J Urol. 2005;174(2):595–9.
48. Chacko J, Moore M, Sankey N, Chandhoke PS. Does a slower treatment rate impact the efficacy of extracorporeal shock wave lithotripsy for solitary kidney or ureteral stones? J Urol. 2006;175(4): 1370–3; discussion 1373–4.
49. Koo V, Beattie I, Young M. Improved cost-effectiveness and efficiency with a slower shockwave delivery rate. BJU Int. 2010;105(5):692–6.
50. Semins MJ, Trock BJ, Matlaga BR. The effect of shock wave rate on the outcome of shock wave lithotripsy: a meta-analysis. J Urol. 2008;179(1):194–7; discussion 197.
51. Zhou Y, Cocks FH, Preminger GM, Zhong P. The effect of treatment strategy on stone comminution efficiency in shock wave lithotripsy. J Urol. 2004;172(1):349–54.
52. Maloney ME, Marguet CG, Zhou Y, et al. Progressive increase of lithotripter output produces better in-vivo stone comminution. J Endourol. 2006;20(9):603–6.
53. Lambert EH, Walsh R, Moreno MW, Gupta M. Effect of escalating versus fixed voltage treatment on stone comminution and renal injury during extracorporeal shock wave lithotripsy: a prospective randomized trial. J Urol. 2010;183(2):580–4.
54. Willis LR, Evan AP, Connors BA, Handa RK, Blomgren PM, Lingeman JE. Prevention of lithotripsy-induced renal injury by

pretreating kidneys with low-energy shock waves. J Am Soc Nephrol. 2006;17(3):663–73.
55. Handa RK, Bailey MR, Paun M, et al. Pretreatment with low-energy shock waves induces renal vasoconstriction during standard shock wave lithotripsy (SWL): a treatment protocol known to reduce SWL-induced renal injury. BJU Int. 2009;103(9):1270–4.
56. Ogiste JS, Nejat RJ, Rashid HH, Greene T, Gupta M. The role of mannitol in alleviating renal injury during extracorporeal shock wave lithotripsy. J Urol. 2003;169(3):875–7.
57. Delvecchio FC, Brizuela RM, Khan SR, et al. Citrate and vitamin E blunt the shock wave-induced free radical surge in an in vitro cell culture model. Urol Res. 2005;33(6):448–52.
58. Al-Awadi KA, Kehinde EO, Loutfi I, et al. Treatment of renal calculi by lithotripsy: minimizing short-term shock wave induced renal damage by using antioxidants. Urol Res. 2008;36(1):51–60.
59. Porpiglia F, Destefanis P, Fiori C, Scarpa RM, Fontana D. Role of adjunctive medical therapy with nifedipine and deflazacort after extracorporeal shock wave lithotripsy of ureteral stones. Urology. 2002;59(6):835–8.
60. Agarwal MM, Naja V, Singh SK, et al. Is there an adjunctive role of tamsulosin to extracorporeal shockwave lithotripsy for upper ureteric stones: results of an open label randomized nonplacebo controlled study. Urology. 2009;74(5):989–92.
61. Cicerello E, Merlo F, Gambaro G, et al. Effect of alkaline citrate therapy on clearance of residual renal stone fragments after extracorporeal shock wave lithotripsy in sterile calcium and infection nephrolithiasis patients. J Urol. 1994;151(1):5–9.
62. Williams Jr JC, Kim SC, Zarse CA, McAteer JA, Lingeman JE. Progress in the use of helical CT for imaging urinary calculi. J Endourol. 2004;18(10):937–41.
63. Perks AE, Schuler TD, Lee J, et al. Stone attenuation and skin-to-stone distance on computed tomography predicts for stone fragmentation by shock wave lithotripsy. Urology. 2008;72(4):765–9.

What You Should Know About Extracorporeal Shock Wave Lithotripsy and How You Can Improve Your Performance

47

Christian G. Chaussy and Hans-Göran Tiselius

Abstract
Shock wave lithotripsy still remains the only noninvasive treatment modality for urolithiasis besides conservative stone management. Overall it has high efficacy, comfortable application without the need of general anesthesia, low rate of side effects, and high patient acceptance. To obtain the best results, careful attention has to be paid to choice of lithotripter, coupling issues, power and spacing of shocks, post-ESWL care, and case selection.

Keywords
Improved performance • ESWL • Renal stones • Ureteric stones • Newer technical developments • Lower caliceal stones • Asymptomatic small caliceal stones • Obesity • Renal anomalies • Caliceal diverticula • Pregnancy • Stone composition • Brushite • Cystine • Pediatric urolithiasis • Contraindications • Good clinical practice • Disintegration efficiency • Target stability • Analgesia • Optimal coupling • Reduction of tissue trauma • Low-energy shock waves • Tissue injury • Percussion • Inversion • Diuresis therapy • Clinically insignificant residual fragment • Ancillary drug therapy • Coupling • Stenting • Patient positioning • Radiation

Introduction

In 1980, shock wave lithotripsy (SWL) found its way into clinical practice [1]. This marked a milestone and tremendous change in the therapy of kidney stones [2]. First therapy studies proved the efficacy of this noninvasive treatment modality and resulted in excellent stone-free rates of 90 % [3, 4]. Studies with subsequent second- and third-generation lithotripters displayed inferior outcomes compared to the unmodified Dornier HM3.

Due to these changes, the leading role of SWL in stone therapy has come under discussion. The treatment results of new devices showed an enormous variability between different systems and even with the same lithotripter.

An optimization of SWL due to efficacy and side effects has to focus on two main topics: lithotripter technology and the modalities of shock wave application. For this purpose it is essential to analyze the reasons why the Dornier HM3—of which the last model was built in 1986—is still regarded as the most effective lithotripter:

1. The electrohydraulic shock wave source was characterized by a wide focal area and provided high shock wave energy with moderate energy flux density.
2. The patient was immersed completely in water; therefore, a perfect coupling without loss of shock wave energy was guaranteed.
3. The treatment was performed using general or spinal anesthesia; therefore, only minimal movements of the stone occurred during the treatment procedure.
4. The administration of shock waves.

C.G. Chaussy, M.D. (✉)
Department of Urology, Caritas Medical Center St. Josef, University of Regensburg, Landshuter Strasses 65, 93053 Regensburg, Germany
e-mail: cgchaussy@gmail.com

H.-G. Tiselius, M.D., Ph.D.
Division of Urology, Department of Clinical Science, Intervention and Technology, Karolinska Institutet, Stockholm, SE-141 86, Sweden
e-mail: hans-goran.tiselius@telia.com; hans-goran.tiselius@ki.se

J.J. Talati et al. (eds.), *Urolithiasis*,
DOI 10.1007/978-1-4471-4387-1_47, © Springer-Verlag London 2012

5. There were restricted indications for SWL treatment.
6. The treatment was performed by urologists with ample experience in shock wave therapy.

Stone-free rate in SWL depends not just on the lithotripsy device that is used but also on stone characteristics such as localization, size, and composition. The patient's body habitus, the anatomy of the urinary tract system, and, last but extremely essential, the expertise of the performing urologist have substantial impact on the treatment results [5, 6].

Technical Developments

New developments in lithotripsy technology are mainly focused on the increase of disintegrative power to disprove the reproach that newer lithotripters are less effective than the unmodified Dornier HM3. Therefore, the manufacturers introduced shock wave systems with wider focal geometry, selectable focus size, or dual shock wave systems to deliver higher shock wave energy. Further progress was made in stone targeting. Dual imaging with simultaneous use of ultrasound and fluoroscopy in some lithotripters and computer-assisted stone localization (autopositioning) enable a more reliable stone tracking during treatment. Finally, modern lithotripters have a modular design, offer more flexibility in positioning of the shock wave source, and are designed for multifunctional use (SWL and endourology) [7].

Basically, lithotripsy systems are very simple in regard to their main components, which are:

1. Shock wave source
2. Localization system (fluoroscopy/ultrasound)
3. Energy coupling and patient positioning

Each of the above components has the potential for improvement.

The Shock Wave Source

The shock wave generator is the most important component of a lithotripsy device, and all manufacturers modify their energy sources to combine a maximum of disintegration efficacy with a minimum of tissue traumatization. Further aspects are a long lifespan of the system with low running costs, a moderate pain level, and an adequate penetration depth. Electromagnetic and piezoelectric systems are characterized by relatively small focal areas in comparison to the unmodified electrohydraulic shock wave system of the Dornier HM3. This enables anesthesia-free and comfortable treatment, and the long lifespan of the shock wave system guarantees low running costs. Therefore, most manufacturers of high-end lithotripters favor electromagnetic shock wave generators despite the criticism that these units may be less effective than the electrohydraulic lithotripters. Shock wave energy is the most important parameter for stone disintegration, and energy flux density is an important factor for renal tissue damage. Based on these facts, the manufacturers introduced changes in the systems involving focal geometry, focus size, or dual shock wave systems to deliver higher shock wave energies. A wider focal area allows the application of high shock wave energy without increase of the energy flux density. Another important advantage of a wide focal area is the partial compensation of stone movements caused by respiration and pain induced by patient's motion. Thus, the fraction of shock waves, hitting the stone, is much higher with the consequence of a better disintegration.

The Localization System

A powerful shock wave system alone is not a guarantee for efficient stone fragmentation. Precise and reliable stone localization represents another key issue. Fluoroscopy is the preferred option for most users because it is easy to use and allows the localization of all radio-opaque stones (kidney and ureter), but it is associated with some disadvantages. Radiological stone targeting exposes the patient to radiation, allows no continuous visualization of the stone position, and needs additional measures for radiolucent stones (i.v. contrast dye or placement of a ureteral catheter). Fluoroscopy is normally realized with an isocentric C-arm, rotating in longitudinal or lateral (orbital) direction. For a three-dimensional localization, the stone must be targeted in two X-ray projections.

Ultrasound is a radiation-free modality and visualizes stones of any composition (radio-opaque and radiolucent) and allows real-time monitoring of the localization and stone disintegration. However, it is limited to renal and proximal/lower ureteral stones. Furthermore, it depends much more on the experience of the user and needs a longer training period for reliable use. Modern lithotripters normally offer fluoroscopy and ultrasound in some machine designs simultaneously, combining the benefits of both imaging modalities.

The precision of stone localization with ultrasound is mainly dependent on the localization principle. Sound waves are deflected in the body tissue at interfaces with changing impedance and lead to a deviation of the visualized target in regard to the focal spot. Offline localization with a flexible scanner, fixed at an isocentric probe holder, is very convenient for the user but can lead to a lateral deviation up to 6 mm in some situations (obese patients). Coaxial or inline localization can compensate this deviation because diagnostic ultrasound and shock waves have the same propagation path and are deflected in the same direction. For this reason, inline localization (fluoroscopy and ultrasound) provides the most precise localization modality [8].

Energy Coupling and Patient Positioning

The delivery of shock wave energy is very sensitive to any obstacles in the shock wave propagation path. A "dry" coupling with a water cushion and ultrasound gel presents the preferred method for shock wave coupling in most lithotripsy systems. This contact area between a patient's skin and coupling bellows acts as an acoustic interface, and air pockets in this area are able to attenuate the quantity of transferred shock wave energy considerably, resulting in a reduced treatment efficacy [9–12]. Unfortunately, the coupling area is not visible and the user has no opportunity to check directly whether this area is free of any structures interfering with the transmission of shock waves. An inline ultrasound enables the user to inspect the shock wave propagation path for any obstacles (like air pockets) on the coupling surface. Unfortunately, this tool is not available in every lithotripter.

A comfortable and stable positioning of the patient is an important topic to avoid movements during the SWL procedure. Therefore, new lithotripsy devices use a flat table design with table cutouts for the positioning of the shock wave source. Additionally, these tables possess a radiolucent area and rails for the fixation of accessories (e.g., leg holders). They allow endoscopic measures like auxiliary procedures before SWL without repositioning the patient. Movable shock wave systems, which are mounted on an isocentric C-arm, allow a rotation around the patient without losing the focal spot. Thus, all localizations of the urinary tract system are accessible, and the option of SWL treatment with the shock wave source in over-table position avoids the necessity to treat patients in prone position (prone position is always associated with compromised patient comfort and hampered respiration of a patient under analgosedation). A further advantage is the selection of a suitable shock wave propagation path that is free of any obstacles such as bones or bowel gas.

Children and morbidly obese patients represent special situations in SWL. Some manufacturers provide special pediatric positioning equipment to fit the table to the smaller anatomical conditions of children. For an efficient treatment of obese patients, new lithotripsy devices provide table weight limits beyond 200 kg and shock wave sources with a penetration depth of 16 and more centimeters.

Indications for Shock Wave Treatment

The uncritical use for all stones deteriorated the treatment results in comparison to the unmodified Dornier HM3. Newer generation lithotripters made all areas of the urinary tract system accessible for SWL; however, the correct indication is an important factor to guarantee a favorable treatment outcome.

Without any doubt, SWL is the preferred treatment modality for patients with renal stones located in the upper/middle calix and renal pelvis up to a size of 2 cm and normal renal anatomy [13]. The lower caliceal stone was always a target of controversial debates. The lower pole study I, published in 2001, reported a reduced efficacy of SWL for calculi in this localization [14].

Endoscopic stone removal of ureter stones has gained increasing importance because of the higher primary success rate and the decreasing complication rates. Nevertheless, SWL is a noninvasive treatment option with no need for general anesthesia and with a low potential for complications and should therefore be considered as first choice therapy for ureteric stones, as stated by Lindquist [15] in the comparative study "SWL versus ureteroscopy."

Renal Calculi

Lingeman pronounced in 2007 that most (80–85 %) simple renal calculi can be treated successfully with shock wave lithotripsy [16]. There is no doubt that SWL is the first choice treatment option for renal calculi until 2 cm in size and normal anatomy of the urinary tract system. This statement is incorporated in the "Guidelines on Urolithiasis" of the European Urological Association (EAU) and the American Urological Association (AUA).

Preoperative Stenting

Several randomized trials indicate that preoperative stenting provides no advantage over in situ shock wave lithotripsy regarding stone clearance or complication rate [17, 18]. Furthermore, the stent itself is associated with side effects such as dysuria or infection. Therefore, routine stenting for patients with stones less than 2 cm prior to SWL is not necessary. Ureteral stenting should be considered for patients with high stone burden, bilateral obstruction, or obstruction in a solitary kidney and is obligatory for patients with infected hydronephrosis or intractable colicky pain.

Lower Caliceal Stones

Lower caliceal stones remain a subject of controversial debates, because many studies display a worse treatment outcome for SWL in comparison to other localizations of the urinary tract system. In the treatment for lower pole stones, Albala et al. found in their prospective analysis of SWL and percutaneous nephrostolithotomy (PNL) a cumulative stone-free rate of 37 % for SWL versus 95 % for PNL [14]. Numerous studies suggested that the unfavorable spatial anatomy of the lower pole collecting system may be a reason for the complicated discharge of stone debris. Sampaio et al. described already in 1992 that anatomical characteristics of the lower pole collecting system as an acute lower pole infundibulopelvic angle, a tight infundibular width, and a long infundibular length may predict a decreased stone-free rate [19]. Danuser et al. could not find significant influence of the collecting system anatomy on the clearance of disintegrated material from the lower calyx [20]. Different methods of measuring anatomical parameters and inter- and intra-observer variability might be an explanation for these diverse findings.

Obek and Riedler found a cumulative stone-free rate of 63 and 65.5 % for lower pole calculi, treated with second- and third-generation lithotripters [21, 22]. Obek could not find significant differences in treatment outcome regarding stone localization in lower, middle, or upper calix. Robert et al. achieved a stone-free rate of 84 % for lower caliceal stones between 5 and 15 mm with piezoelectric ESWL [23]. The use of electromagnetic or piezoelectric lithotripsy systems and the acceptance of a higher re-treatment rate result in smaller stone fragments and achieve treatment results that are superior to the 37 % stone-free rate reported in the lower pole study [14].

These studies show that the anatomy of the lower pole collecting system does play a certain role, but it remains unclear which parameter can serve as a predictor for treatment success. Stone size seems to be the most important factor influencing treatment outcome [14, 21–23].

SWL remains the treatment of choice for lower pole stones until 10 mm. Pearle et al. compared SWL and ureteroscopic lithotripsy (URS) for the treatment of small lower pole stones in a randomized multicenter study and could not find a significant difference in stone-free rate. SWL, however, was associated with greater patient acceptance and shorter convalescence [24]. For lower pole stones between 11 and 20 mm, treatment outcome for SWL is inferior to endoscopic stone removal, but SWL might be the treatment of choice due to its noninvasive nature and low potential of complications.

Asymptomatic Small Caliceal Stones

Asymptomatic small caliceal stones are the second issue of controversy. There is no consensus whether these stones should be treated or actively monitored. Glowacki et al. analyzed the records of 107 patients with asymptomatic calculi and found that 32 % of these patients became symptomatic during a mean 31.6-month follow-up; spontaneous passage only occurred in 15 %. They concluded that the risk for symptomatic episodes was 10 % per year, and within a 5-year interval, nearly 50 % of the patients became symptomatic [25]. If active stone treatment is required, SWL represents a good option for these patients.

Ureteral Calculi

Newer lithotripsy systems with flat table and flexible shock wave head positioning eliminated the disadvantages of the Dornier HM3, which was only capable to treat proximal ureter stones. These new devices enable the treatment of mid- and distal ureter stones with SWL. Tiselius et al. reported in a review of approximately 20,000 patients treated for ureteral calculi with SWL that 81 % became stone-free with a re-treatment rate of 12 % [26]. A more detailed analysis is given in Table 47.1. The results of this meta-analysis display that URS—except in proximal ureteral stones smaller 10 mm—yields a better stone-free rate with a single procedure, while SWL is characterized by its noninvasive nature, no requirement for general anesthesia, and the low potential of significant complications. Finally, SWL outcome—in comparison to URS—is less dependent on the expertise of the performing urologist, and an eventually needed re-treatment can be performed without bigger efforts [27]. Therefore, both SWL and URS should be considered as first choice treatments for patients requiring ureteral stone removal.

In an analysis of 598 consecutive patients with ureteral stones, Tiselius reported that the consistent use of SWL with an average of 1.3 sessions facilitated a stone-free rate of

Table 47.1 AUA/EAU ureteral stones guideline panel and EAU guideline on urolithiasis (update March 2008)

Stone-free rate: primary treatments or first treatment				
	Shock wave lithotripsy		Ureterorenoscopy	
	n	SF rate (med/95 % CI)	*n*	SF rate (med/95 % CI)
Distal ureter	6.981	74 % (73–75 %)	5.952	94 % (93–95 %)
<10 mm	1.684	86 % (80–91 %)	1.622	97 % (96–98 %)
>10 mm	966	74 % (57–87 %)	412	93 % (88–96 %)
Mid-ureter	1.607	73 % (66–79 %)	1.024	86 % (81–89 %)
<10 mm	44	84 % (65–95 %)	80	91 % (81–96 %)
>10 mm	15	76 % (36–97 %)	73	78 % (61–90 %)
Proximal ureter	6.428	82 % (79–85 %)	2.242	81 % (77–85 %)
<10 mm	886	90 % (85–93 %)	243	80 % (73–85 %)
>10 mm	293	68 % (55–79 %)	230	79 % (71–87 %)

more than 97 %, which is comparable to the outcome of endoscopic stone removal [28].

Special Situations

Obesity

Obesity is becoming an epidemic problem in industrialized countries and is meanwhile identified as an important risk factor for the formation of urinary stones. SWL in morbidly obese patients is challenging due to the inferior stone visualization and the difficulties to center the stone in the shock wave focus. Therefore, some authors consider obesity as a contraindication for SWL with reference to the low stone-free rates that have been reported. Pareek et al. analyzed the skin-to-stone distance (SSD) of 64 patients with lower pole stones, treated with SWL, and concluded that an SSD longer than 10 cm will predict a treatment failure [29]. In contrast to these findings, Munoz et al. reported a 72 % 3-month stone-free rate for obese stone patients undergoing SWL and concluded that lithotripter characteristics and operator experience are the clue for a reasonable treatment outcome [30]. Mezentsev et al. achieved an overall 3-month stone-free rate of 73 % in SWL of morbidly obese patients (BMI>40 kg/m^2) [31].

In experienced hands, SWL is a reasonable therapy option for obese patients with stones <2 cm, though the coincidence of obesity, large stone size, and hard stone composition is bound to result in poor stone clearance.

Renal Anomalies

Renal anomalies such as renal ectopia, malrotation, renal duplication, or fusion abnormality (horseshoe kidney) are often associated with an impaired drainage of urine due to a stenosis of the ureteropelvic junction and a reduced clearance of stone debris.

The treatment procedure should be chosen individually under consideration of kidney function and location, stone size, availability of equipment, and expertise of the performing urologist. SWL represents an effective treatment option for stones smaller than 2 cm, when an obstruction of the urinary tract system is excluded prior to treatment. Sheir et al. reported in their review of 11-year experience with SWL in anomalous kidneys a 72.2 % stone-free rate after 3 months [32].

Stones in *caliceal diverticula* are an indication for treatment when the calculi become symptomatic or increase in size. Turna et al. concluded in a retrospective analysis of the management of caliceal diverticular stones that SWL is suitable to render most patients symptom-free with minimal complications despite a low stone-free rate of 21 % [33].

Pregnancy

Pregnancy is still one of few absolute contraindications for SWL because of the danger of spontaneous abortion and premature contractions as well as ruptures of the fetal vessels [34].

Stone Composition

Stone composition and internal stone structure present important characteristics that define the hardness of urinary calculi and therefore the responsiveness to shock waves.

Ringden and Tiselius calculated a "hardness factor" for different stone compositions using the treatment records of 2,100 SWL patients (Table 47.2) [35]. Shock wave energy, number of shock waves, and number of re-treatments required for a satisfactory stone disintegration were assumed to reflect the hardness.

Brushite and cystine calculi possess the "highest hardness factor" but are not a contraindication for SWL when the stone burden is small and the patient favors a noninvasive therapy. The treating urologist has to keep in mind that these stones may need repetitive treatments for a sufficient disintegration and may only achieve inferior treatment results. Matrix calculi respond only poorly to shock waves despite their very soft composition and should not be treated with SWL.

Some authors suggest the measurement of stone density (Hounsfield unit) in non-contrast computed tomography (NCCT), to estimate the treatment outcome in SWL. However, there is no consensus which HU values will predict SWL failure. Zarse et al. investigated the Hounsfield unit values and internal structure of calcium oxalate monohydrate stones and stated that stone morphology (heterogeneity) rather than stone density (HU values) correlates with stone fragility in SWL [36].

Table 47.2 Hardness factor according to Ringden and Tiselius

Stone composition	Hardness factor
Calcium oxalate dihydrate	1.0
Calcium oxalate monohydrate	1.3
Hydroxyapatite	1.1
Brushite	*2.2*
Uric acid/urate	1.0
Cystine	*2.4*
Carbonate apatite	1.3
Magnesium ammonium phosphate	1.0

> In general, radiological homogenous, sleek-surfaced, strongly radio-opaque, or glass-like looking stones are normally very hard and require high shock wave energy to be disintegrated.

Pediatric Urolithiasis

Pediatric urolithiasis is a rare but challenging condition. SWL is effective and safe and remains the treatment of choice for pediatric patients. Despite the small dimension of the pediatric anatomy, the ureter has a high transport capacity for stone debris. Therefore, the reported stone-free rates for children were superior to that in adult patients, and children did become stone-free more rapidly [37]. Though some concerns have been raised regarding safety, there is no evidence that SWL causes irreversible short- or long-term functional or morphological changes.

However, treatment of children needs to be modified according to their smaller anatomic dimensions. Therefore, the following recommendations may be helpful:

- Pediatric positioning aid
- Lung protection for children (e.g., polystyrene between chest and coupling bellows)
- Minimizing radiation exposure (preferably ultrasound localization)
- Reduced shockwave parameters (see also device-specific suggestions)

Contraindications for Extracorporeal Shock Wave Lithotripsy

Worldwide accepted absolute contraindications for SWL are pregnancy, untreated urinary tract infection, untreated obstruction distal to stone, and patients with uncorrected bleeding diathesis (hemophilia, low platelets) or under medical anticoagulation therapy (coumarin, heparin, platelet aggregation inhibitors).

For SWL, anticoagulation therapy must be stopped and treatment can be performed after the coagulation parameters have returned to normal. Medication with platelet aggregation inhibitors such as salicylates should be suspended 10 days prior to treatment. Flexible ureterorenoscopy is a suitable treatment option if a withdrawal of medication is not possible.

Suggestions for Good Clinical Practice

Compared with endoscopic stone therapy, many doctors see SWL as a "simple procedure that can be learned easily with a short learning curve and may also be delegated to nonmedical personal." In fact, SWL represents a delicate procedure with a complex physical background. All urologists performing SWL should have a basic understanding of the underlying physical process of stone comminution and tissue injury and the correct selection of shock wave parameters. Furthermore, a detailed knowledge of the characteristics of the shock wave generator and the available lithotripter features in combination with a "patient-adapted" application of shock waves enables an improved stone comminution with simultaneous reduction of tissue traumatization.

As stated before,

> Shock wave lithotripsy is a complex technology and requires comprehensive knowledge of the underlying physics and treatment strategies, to improve stone disintegration and to minimize tissue injury.

Increase of Disintegration Efficacy

Only shock waves directed to the stone will result in a fragmentation of the calculus. Inadequate setting of shock wave parameters, absorption of shock wave energy along the blast path, and stone movements are the main causes for disappointing treatment results.

Target Stability

Stone movements, induced by patient's respiration or pain, reduce the number of effective shock waves significantly. Therefore, a stable patient position and flat respiration are the keys for good disintegration results and also for lithotripters with a wide focal area. Cormack et al. compared high-frequency jet ventilation, which causes only minimal stone movements, with spontaneous ventilation and found a significant lower need of shock waves for the patients with high-frequency jet ventilation [38]. Honey et al. used an abdominal compression belt for SWL and achieved a 32 % reduction of stone movements. The increase of pressure in the abdominal cavity caused by the compression belt in combination with sufficient i.v. analgesia can reduce diaphragmatic excursion and therefore stone movements [6, 39].

To achieve the utmost stability of the target, the following measures should be considered.

Adequate Analgesia

ESWL can be a painful therapy. Insufficient analgesia may cause a reduction in hit rate and efficacy. At the same time increasing blood pressure caused by pain can increase the risk for kidney hematoma.

We found the following i.v. analgesia schedule useful for clinical routine:

- Intravenous analgesia with alfentanil under monitoring (ECG, O_2 saturation, RR)
- 2 l O_2/min through a nasal tube

- 0.5 mg alfentanil initially, immediately before treatment
- 0.5 mg alfentanil repetitive, on patient's demand

Fixation of the Patient with a Compression Belt

Patient fixation and abdominal compression reduce the respiration-induced stone movement and increase efficacy of the SWL treatment. The use of abdominal compression is recommended.

Please note: It is important to attach the belt on the abdomen—not the thorax!

Optimized Coupling

Air bubbles in the coupling area between patient and coupling bellows reduce the efficacy of the shockwaves significantly (e.g., an air bubble of 2 cm diameter cuts the efficacy of the SWL treatment by half). Application of large quantity (approximately 50 cc) of low viscous ultrasound gel on the coupling bellows, shaving of the patient's skin at the shock wave entry, the use of a proper inflation of the coupling bellows, and application of new gel after loss of coupling are important precautions to achieve optimal coupling conditions. Inline ultrasound is a helpful tool to check the quality of coupling:

- Remove hair at the shockwave entry area.
- Store the gel bottle head down and do not shake it before use.
- Apply sufficient amount (approximately 30–50 ml) of low viscous ultrasound gel on the coupling bellows.
- During the coupling procedure, slip your hand between the coupling bellows and the patient (smooth out air bubbles).
- Control the coupling area by inline ultrasound.

Bypassing Disturbing Structures (Bones, Intestinal Gas)

Osseous structures and intestinal gas in the shockwave path reflect and absorb shockwave energy. This results in less efficacy and more pain during treatment. Furthermore, gas in the shockwave path is a potential risk for damage of the intestine.

Selection of Shock Wave Parameters

Three different shock wave parameters can be modified in SWL. The users normally adjust the total number of shock wave impulses and the power level but neglect the shock wave administration rate (SW/min) because most new lithotripters enable an ECG-ungated treatment with a fixed frequency of 90 or 120 SW/min. This is in contrast to the HM3, which needed ECG triggering and, consequently, resulted in most cases in a lower shockwave administration rate (which may be an additional reason for higher stone disintegration efficacy of the HM3). In vitro and animal studies showed that stones disintegrate better at a slower rate because of a reduction of cavitation in the shock wave propagation path. Semins et al. found in their meta-analysis of four randomized clinical trials that patients treated at a rate of 60 shocks per minute had a significantly greater likelihood of a successful treatment outcome than patients treated at a rate of 120 shocks/min [40].

A further aspect is the strategy of how to adjust the power level. Protocols with gradual increase of shock wave energy (ramping) produced superior stone fragmentation in comparison with constant or decreasing shock wave energy [41]. Most users performing SWL with i.v. analgesia perform SWL anyway with stepwise increase of energy to adapt the patient to the shock waves. Operators who apply SWL under full anesthesia and start immediately with high-power shock wave level should change their strategy to a gradual energy increase in favor of better results.

Summary

The aim of SWL is to disintegrate the stone in fragments that can pass the urinary tract system spontaneously by simultaneous reduction of shock wave-induced injury of renal parenchyma. Shock waves induce vasoconstriction of the renal vasculature. The reduced renal blood flow decreases the risk of hematomas in the kidney. The tensile wave of the shock wave produces transient cavitation bubbles in the coupling bellows and along the shock wave propagation path of the patient, which reduces the efficacy of the following shock wave. Thus, the reduction of the shock wave frequency increases the efficacy of the SWL therapy. The reason for this phenomenon is that the bubbles will be resolved when the interval between the single shock waves is longer.

Note: The chosen energy level and number of shock wave pulses have to be adapted to the patient's and stone's characteristics.
The treatment should be applied with 60 or 90 shock waves/minute
The first 100 shock waves should be applied at a minimal energy level.

Treatment Parameters

Energy levels and shock wave numbers vary and depend on the following factors:

- Stone composition (important aspect)
- Stone size/stone localization
- Patient's characteristics (obesity, children, anomalies)

Reduction of Tissue Trauma

Cavitation and shear stress do have a destructive impact not only on stone material but also on body tissue—mainly as vascular lesions—clinically noticeable as functional and morphological changes of renal parenchyma (release of tubular enzymes, hematuria) and rarely as renal hematoma. Unfortunately, there is no diagnostic tool to detect tissue damage early during treatment, apart from ultrasound examination for the diagnosis of renal hemorrhage. But some easy precautions can be useful to reduce the risk of tissue injury.

Patient Monitoring

Uncontrolled arterial hypertension or excessive rise of blood pressure induced by pain during treatment seems to be an important risk factor for the development of renal hemorrhage [42]. Therefore, all patients should be monitored during procedure, including ECG, oxygen saturation, and blood pressure to eliminate this unnecessary risk.

Important: The safety of the patient is always first priority. Therefore, patients with additional risk factors, as listed below, should be treated with low shock wave parameters:

- Untreated hypertension
- Diabetes mellitus
- Age > 65 years
- Impaired renal function, hydronephrosis

Pretreatment with Low Shock Wave Energy

Animal studies have shown that shock waves reduce the glomerular filtration rate and the renal plasma flow in the shock wave-exposed and even contralateral kidney due to an induction of vasoconstriction. Willis et al. explored this phenomenon and reported an easy measure to protect renal tissue from shock wave-induced injury. A pretreatment (100–500 SW) at low energy levels prior to the SWL reduces the risk of hemorrhagic lesions in the kidney significantly [43].

Prevention of Tissue Injury

Tissue injury in SWL is dose dependent. This had been proven by Delius et al. already in 1988 [44]. Consequently, treatment should be performed with the lowest number of shock wave pulses required for stone fragmentation. Until today, there is no reliable instrument to judge stone breakage during treatment accurately, and therefore most patients are "overtreated" and subjected to unnecessary tissue damage.

Tissue protection can easily be obtained by reducing the rate of SW delivery. A significant protective effect on the integrity of the kidney's vasculature can be achieved by reducing the rate of SW delivery to 30 SW/min. A slow rate of shock waves appears to improve both safety and efficacy of SWL [45].

Summary

The strategy for kidney protection implies:

- Monitoring of blood pressure during SWL
- Pretreatment with low shock wave energy,
- Shock wave application with a rate of 60 SW/min (or less)

Supportive Measures for Fragment Passage

SWL disintegrates stones into small pieces, which should pass the urinary tract system spontaneously. The likelihood for the passage of stone debris depends on the anatomy of the patient's urinary tract system, the patient's behavior, as well as additional physical and medical measures taken to facilitate the discharge of the debris.

Mechanical *p*ercussion, *i*nversion therapy, and *d*iuresis (the so-called PDI therapy) is useful to assist the passage, especially of lower pole stone fragments after SWL [46, 47]. In a randomized prospective study, Chiong et al. reported a significant higher stone-free rate for patients with a combination of SWL and PDI in comparison to SWL therapy alone (62.5 vs. 35.4 % stone-free rate) [47]. In reality, the physical measures are mostly limited to recommendations for the patient to increase the daily fluid intake and to take more exercise.

Despite all auxiliary medical therapy, patience is the most important virtue to improve SWL outcome. The so-called clinically insignificant residual fragments (CIRF) show remarkable dynamics. Rassweiler et al. found in an analysis of the literature, including more than 14,000 patients, that CIRF will pass continuous up to 24 months after shock wave therapy [48]. Thus, the stone-free rate after 3 months will not display the definite treatment outcome, and follow-up should

Table 47.3 Possible schedule for medical expulsive therapy (MET)

Patients after SWL of a ureteral stone	
Diclofenac	100 mg 1-0-0 for 5 days
Omeprazole	20 mg 1-0-1 for 5 days
Tamsulosin	0.4 mg 0-0-1 for 14 days
Patients after SWL of a kidney stone	
Tamsulosin	0.4 mg 0-0-1 for 14 days

be extended. Oman et al. evaluated patients with a mean follow-up time of 4.9 years who had been treated with SWL and released with CIRF. In 78.6 %, CIRF cleared spontaneously and did not reappear [49].

Drugs

Medical expulsive therapy (MET) represents an effective measure to facilitate the passage of small ureteral calculi. A meta-analysis, conducted by Losek et al., evaluated the efficacy of tamsulosin combined with SWL and suggested that adjunctive tamsulosin therapy is safe and effective in enhancing stone clearance in patients with renal stones 10–24 mm in diameter. Evidence regarding ureteral stone clearance is inconclusive, although adjunctive tamsulosin has been reported to reduce painful episodes [50] (Table 47.3).

Potassium citrate as metaphylaxis for calcium oxalate stone formers is beneficial to improve stone-free rates in patients with residual fragments and to reduce stone recurrence after SWL [51]. In patients stone-free after SWL and receiving medical treatment, the stone recurrence rate was 0 %, whereas untreated patients showed a 28.5 % recurrence rate after 12 months. Similarly, in the residual fragment group, the medically treated patients had a significantly greater remission rate than the untreated patients (44.5 vs. 12.5 %).

Patient Behavior and Physical Therapy

Mechanical percussion and inversion therapy (PDI) is a safe and effective treatment option to promote the discharge of residual lower caliceal stone fragments after SWL [46]. Due to the expenditure of PDI, in everyday practice, patients are only advised to ensure an adequate daily fluid intake and to take more physical exercises.

Physical Measures
- Increasing the daily fluid intake (>2.5 l/day)
- Physical exercise
- Vibro trainer

Acute and Long-Term Side Effects

Acute tissue injury induced by shock waves is normally mild and well tolerated by the patient. But it remains a controversial topic whether SWL has the potential to induce long-term side effects like the development of arterial hypertension or diabetes mellitus. Krambeck et al. found in a retrospective case–control study with 19-year follow-up that patients treated with SWL were significantly more likely to develop hypertension or diabetes mellitus than conservatively treated patients [52]. In contrast, neither Sato et al. nor Eassa et al. found any evidence that SWL is linked to the new onset of hypertension [53, 54]. Strohmaier et al. compared different types of stone treatment (conservative, SWL, PNL) and found significant higher blood pressure after 24 months independent from treatment modality. They concluded that stone disease itself, rather than the type of treatment, seemed to increase the systolic and diastolic blood pressure during a follow-up period of 24 months [55].

Only few data are available regarding shock wave-induced pancreatic tissue damage. The only prospective evaluation of acute endocrine pancreatic injury by SWL was performed by Wendt-Nordahl et al. in 2007. Neither the variables indicating islet cell damage nor those indicating damage of exocrine pancreatic cells changed significantly within the observation time. Therefore, the hypothesis that SWL leads to pancreatic trauma with consecutive development of diabetes mellitus seems to be unlikely [56].

More recently, Krambeck et al. reported that there were no significant differences in the long-term development of renal insufficiency, hypertension, or diabetes mellitus in patients treated with SWL, percutaneous nephrolithotomy, or under conservative management. Most likely the previously described changes were attributable to the general metabolic situation of stone formers than to the effects of SWL or other treatment [57].

Many efforts have been made within the last years to maximize stone comminution and to reduce shock wave-related traumatization. As it has been shown here, only minor modifications in shock wave application and treatment strategy are necessary to achieve this goal.

Conclusion

In spite of all newly arisen discussions, SWL still remains the only noninvasive treatment modality for urolithiasis besides conservative stone management, and it plays a major role in stone therapy due to its efficacy, low rate of side effects, comfortable application without the need of general anesthesia, and last but not least patient's acceptance.

References

1. Chaussy C, Eisenberger F, Forssmann B. Extracorporeal shock wave lithotripsy (ESWL): a chronology. J Endourol. 2007;21(11):1249–53.
2. Chaussy C, Brendel W, Schmiedt E. Extracorporeally induced destruction of kidney stones by shock waves. Lancet. 1980; 2(8207):1265–8.
3. Chaussy C, Schmiedt E, Jocham D, Brendel D, Forssmann B, Walther V. First clinical experience with extracorporeally induced destruction of kidney stones by shock waves. J Urol. 1982;127(3):417–20.
4. Schmiedt E, Chaussy C. Extracorporeal shock-wave lithotripsy of kidney and ureteric stones. Urol Int. 1984;39(4):193–8.
5. Bergsdorf T, Chaussy C. New trends in shock wave application regarding technology and treatment strategy. In: Loske A, editor. New trends in shock wave application to medicine and biotechnology. Trivandrum: Research Signpost; 2009. p. 1–19.
6. Bergsdorf T, Thueroff S, Chaussy C. Extracorporeal shock wave lithotripsy. In: Chaussy C, Haupt G, Jocham D, Koehrmann KU, editors. Therapeutic energy applications in urology II. Stuttgart: Thieme; 2010. p. 8–16.
7. Rassweiler JJ, Knoll T, Köhrmann KU, et al. Shock wave technology and application: an update. Eur Urol. 2011;59(5):784–96.
8. Folberth W, Hassler D. Value of in-line and out-off-line ultrasound targeting in extracorporeal shock wave lithotripsy. Eur Urol. 1990;18(3):215–21.
9. Pishchalnikov YA, Neucks JS, VonDerHaar RJ, et al. Air pockets trapped during routine coupling in dry head lithotripsy can significantly decrease the delivery of shock wave energy. J Urol. 2006;176(6Pt1):2706–10.
10. Jain A, Shah TK. Effect of air bubbles in the coupling medium on efficacy of extracorporeal shock wave lithotripsy. Eur Urol. 2007;51(6):1680–6.
11. Bergsdorf T, Chaussy C, Thueroff S. Energy coupling in extracorporeal shock wave lithotripsy – the impact of coupling quality on disintegration efficacy. J Endourol. 2008;22(Suppl1):A161.
12. Bergsdorf T, Chaussy C, Thueroff S. The significance of accurate shock wave coupling in extracorporeal shock wave lithotripsy. J Endourol. 2009;23:1042.
13. Rassweiler JJ, Grenacher G, Haupt S, et al. The management of caliceal calculi: consensus report. In: Chaussy C, Eisenberger F, Jocham D, Wilbert D, editors. High energy shock waves in medicine. Stuttgart: Thieme; 1997. p. 44–51.
14. Albala DM, Assimos DG, Clayman RV, et al. Lower pole I: a prospective randomized trial of extracorporeal shock wave lithotripsy and percutaneous nephrostolithotomy for lower pole nephrolithiasis-initial results. J Urol. 2001;166(6):2072–80.
15. Lindqvist K, Holmberg G, Peeker R, et al. Extracorporeal shock wave lithotripsy or ureteroscopy as primary treatment for ureteric stones. A retrospective study comparing two different treatment strategies. Scand J Urol Nephrol. 2006;40(2):113–8.
16. Miller N, Lingeman JE. Management of kidney stones. BMJ. 2007;334:468–72.
17. Pryor JL, Jenkins AD. Use of double-pigtail stents in extracorporeal shock wave lithotripsy. J Urol. 1990;143(3):475–8.
18. El-Assmy A, El-Nahas AR, Sheir KZ. Is pre-shock wave lithotripsy stenting necessary for ureteral stones with moderate or severe hydronephrosis? J Urol. 2006;176(5):2059–62.
19. Sampaio FJ, Aragao AH. Inferior pole collecting system anatomy: it's probable role in extracorporeal shock wave lithotripsy. J Urol. 1992;147(2):322–4.
20. Danuser H, Müller R, Descoeudres B, et al. Extracorporeal shock wave lithotripsy of lower calyx calculi: how much is treatment outcome influenced by the anatomy of the collecting system? Eur Urol. 2007;52:539–46.
21. Obek C, Onal B, Kantay K, et al. The efficacy of extracorporeal shock wave lithotripsy for isolated lower pole calculi compared with isolated middle and upper caliceal calculi. J Urol. 2001;166(6):2081–4.
22. Riedler I, Trummer H, Hebel P, et al. Outcome and safety of extracorporeal shock wave lithotripsy as first-line therapy of lower pole nephrolithiasis. Urol Int. 2003;71(4):350–4.
23. Robert M, Marotta M, Rakotomalala E, et al. Piezoelectric extracorporeal shock-wave lithotripsy of lower pole nephrolithiasis. Eur Urol. 1997;32(3):301–4.
24. Pearle MS, Lingeman JE, Leveillee R, et al. Prospective randomized trial comparing shock wave lithotripsy and ureteroscopy for lower pole caliceal calculi 1 cm or less. J Urol. 2005;173(6):2005–9.
25. Glowacki LS, Beecroft ML, Cook RJ, et al. The natural history of asymptomatic urolithiasis. J Urol. 1992;147:319–21.
26. Tiselius HG, Ackermann D, Alken P, et al. Guidelines on urolithiasis. Eur Urol. 2001;40:362–71.
27. Thueroff S, Chaussy C. Ureteral calculi. In situ ESWL treatment with booster technique. Urologe A. 1997;36(3):209–16.
28. Tiselius HG. How efficient is extracorporeal shockwave lithotripsy with modern lithotripters for removal of ureteral stones? J Endourol. 2008;22(2):249–55.
29. Pareek G, Hedican SP, Lee FT, et al. Shock wave lithotripsy success determined by skin-to-stone distance on computed tomography. Urology. 2005;66(5):9141–4.
30. Munoz RD, Tirolien PP, Belhamou S, et al. Treatment of reno-ureteral lithiasis with ESWL in obese patients. Apropos of 150 patients. Arch Esp Urol. 2003;56(8):933–8.
31. Mezentsev VA. Extracorporeal shock wave lithotripsy in the treatment of renal pelvicalyceal stones in morbidly obese patients. Int Braz J Urol. 2005;31(2):105–10.
32. Sheir KZ, Madbouly K, Esobky E, et al. Extracorporeal shock wave lithotripsy in anomalous kidneys: 11 year experience with two second generation lithotripters. Urology. 2003;62(1):10–5.
33. Turna B, Raza A, Moussa S, et al. Management of calyceal diverticular stones with extracorporeal shock wave lithotripsy and percutaneous nephrolithotomy: long term outcome. BJU Int. 2007; 100(1):151–6.
34. Chaussy GC, Fuchs GJ. Current state and future developments of non-invasive treatment of human urinary stones with ESWL. J Urol. 1989;141:782.
35. Ringden I, Tiselius HG. Composition and clinically determined hardness of urinary tract stones. Scand J Urol Nephrol. 2007;41(4): 316–23.
36. Zarse CA, Hameed TA, Jackson ME, et al. CT visible internal stone structure, but not Hounsfield unit value, of calcium oxalate monohydrate (COM) calculi predicts lithotripsy fragility in vitro. Urol Res. 2007;35(4):201–6.
37. Gofrit ON, Pode D, Meretyk S, et al. Is the pediatric ureter as efficient as the adult ureter in transporting fragments following extracorporeal shock wave lithotripsy for renal calculi larger than 10 mm? J Urol. 2001;166(6):1862–4.
38. Cormack JR, Hui R, Olive D, et al. Comparison of two ventilation techniques during general anesthesia for extracorporeal shock wave lithotripsy: high-frequency jet ventilation versus spontaneous ventilation with a laryngeal mask airway. Urology. 2007;70(1):7–10.
39. Honey RJ, Healy M, Yeung M, et al. The use of an abdominal compression belt to reduce stone movement during extracorporeal shock wave lithotripsy. J Urol. 1992;148(3):1034–5.
40. Semins MJ, Trock BF, Matlaga BR. The effect of shock wave rate on the outcome of shock wave lithotripsy: a meta-analysis. J Urol. 2008;179(1):194–7.
41. Maloney ME, Marguet CG, Zhou Y, et al. Progressive increase of lithotripter output produce better in-vivo stone comminution. J Endourol. 2006;20(9):603–6.
42. Collado Serra A, Huguet Perez J, Monreal Garcia de Vicuna F. Renal hematoma as a complication of extracorporeal shock wave lithotripsy. Scand J Urol Nephrol. 1999;33(3):171–5.

43. Willis LR, Evan AP, Connors BA, et al. Preventing of lithotripsy-induced renal injury by pretreating kidneys with low-energy shock waves. Am Soc Nephrol. 2006;17(3):663–73.
44. Delius M, Enders G, Xuan ZR, et al. Biological effects of shock waves: kidney damage by shock waves in dogs – dose dependence. Ultrasound Med Biol. 1988;14(2):117–22.
45. Evan AP, McAteer JA, Conners BA, et al. Renal injury in SWL is significantly reduced by slowing down the rate of shock wave delivery. BJU Int. 2007;100:624–7.
46. Pace KT, Tariq N, Dyer SJ, et al. Mechanical percussion, inversion and diuresis for residual lower pole fragments after shock wave lithotripsy: a prospective, single blind, randomized controlled trial. J Urol. 2001;166(6):2065–71.
47. Chiong E, Hwee ST, Kay LM, et al. Randomized controlled study of mechanical percussion, dieresis, and inversion therapy to assist passage of lower pole renal calculi after shock wave lithotripsy. Urology. 2005;65(6):1070–4.
48. Rassweiler JJ, Renner C, Chaussy C, et al. Treatment of renal stones by extracorporeal shockwave lithotripsy: an update. Eur Urol. 2001; 39(2):187–99.
49. Osman MM, Alfano Y, Kamp S. 5-year-follow-up of patients with clinically insignificant residual fragments after extracorporeal shock wave lithotripsy. Eur Urol. 2005;47(6):860–4.
50. Losek RL, Mauro LS. Efficacy of tamsulosin with extracorporeal shock wave lithotripsy for passage of renal and ureteral calculi. Ann Pharmacother. 2008;42(5):692–7.
51. Soyguer T, Akbay A, Kuepeli S. Effect of potassium citrate therapy on stone recurrence and residual fragments after shockwave lithotripsy in lower caliceal calcium oxalate urolithiasis: a randomized controlled trial. J Endourol. 2002;16(3):149–52.
52. Krambeck AE, Gettmann MT, Rohlinger AL, et al. Diabetes mellitus and hypertension associated with shock wave lithotripsy of renal and proximal ureteral stones at 19 years of followup. J Urol. 2006;175(5):1742–7.
53. Sato Y, Tanda H, Kato S, Ohnishi S, et al. Shock wave lithotripsy for renal stones is not associated with hypertension and diabetes mellitus. Urology. 2008;71(4):586–91.
54. Eassa WA, Sheir KZ, Gad HM, et al. Prospective study of the long-tem effects of shock wave lithotripsy on renal function and blood pressure. J Urol. 2008;179(3):964–8.
55. Strohmaier WL, Schmidt J, Lahme S, et al. Arterial blood pressure following different types of urinary stone therapy. Eur Urol. 2000;38(6):753–7.
56. Wendt-Nordahl G, Krombach P, Hannak D, et al. Prospective evaluation of acute endocrine pancreatic injury as collateral damage of shock-wave lithotripsy for upper urinary tract stones. BJU Int. 2007;100(6):1339–43.
57. Krambeck AE, LeRoy AJ, Patterson DE, Gettman MT. Long-term outcomes of percutaneous nephrolithotomy compared to shock wave lithotripsy and conservative management. J Urol. 2008; 179(60):2233–7.

Examples of Clinical Problems that Might Be Encountered in Patients Treated with Extracorporeal Shock Wave Lithotripsy

48

Hans-Göran Tiselius and Christian G. Chaussy

Abstract

A number of considerations are necessary for an optimal result of extracorporeal shock wave lithotripsy. In this chapter, we present some examples of patients that pose specific problems that need to be identified and appropriately dealt with in order to achieve the desirable result of a satisfactory disintegration without serious complications. It is emphasized that the precise solution to some clinical stone problems requires proper understanding of the relationship between the shock wave path, the anatomy, and the position and composition of the stone.

Keywords

Ureteral stone • Kidney stone • Extracorporeal shock wave lithotripsy (ESWL) • Percutaneous surgery • Intestinal gas • Treatment position • Chemolysis • Salicylates • Bacteriuria

Introduction

During the past decades, extracorporeal shock wave lithotripsy (ESWL) has become established as a standard procedure for active removal of stones from the kidneys and ureters. This matter has been extensively discussed in a previous chapter. The result of ESWL, however, varies considerably from one center to another, and many urologists have experienced and realized that successful stone disintegration does not come automatically. A number of considerations are necessary for an optimal result. In this chapter, we present some examples of patients that pose specific problems that need to be identified and appropriately dealt with in order to achieve the desirable result of a satisfactory disintegration without serious complications.

Although different lithotripters do not have the same geometrical properties, the aspects and considerations that will be presented are generally applicable. It needs to be emphasized, however, that the precise solution to some problems requires proper understanding of the relationship between the shock wave path, the anatomy, and the position of the stone.

Case 1

A 72-year-old woman presented with right-sided pain. She was in a relatively poor medical condition suffering from both diabetes and hypertension. Her list of medications included salicylates. The plain radiograph depicted in Fig. 48.1a shows a multilayered stone obviously located in the right renal pelvis. The size of the stone measured 27 × 15 mm. Calculation of the stone surface area with the formula

H.-G. Tiselius, M.D., Ph.D. (✉)
Division of Urology, Department of Clinical Science, Intervention and Technology, Karolinska Institutet, Stockholm SE-141 86, Sweden
e-mail: hans-goran.tiselius@telia.com; hans-goran.tiselius@ki.se

C.G. Chaussy, M.D.
Department of Urology, Caritas Medical Center St. Josef, University of Regensburg, Landshuter Strasses 65, Regensburg, Oberpfalz 93053, Germany
e-mail: cgchaussy@gmail.com

J.J. Talati et al. (eds.), *Urolithiasis*,
DOI 10.1007/978-1-4471-4387-1_48, © Springer-Verlag London 2012

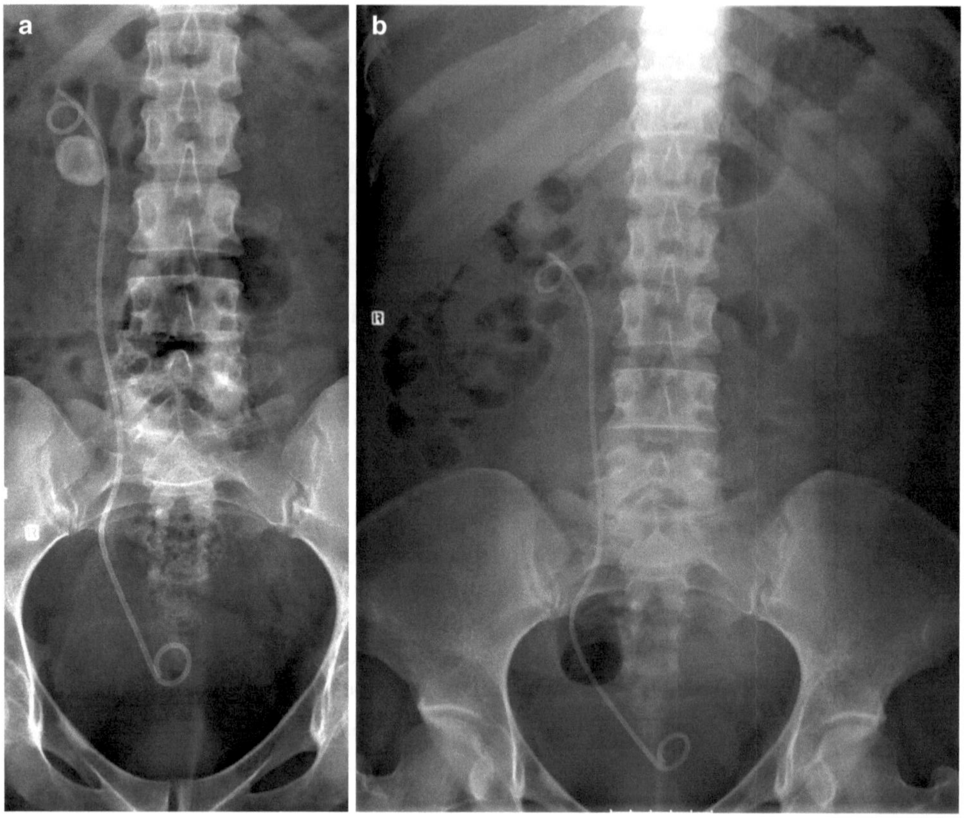

Fig. 48.1 Large (27 × 15 mm) stone in the right renal pelvis with an internal stent in place, before (**a**) and after (**b**) ESWL

$$0.25 \times \text{length} \times \text{width} \times \pi\ (\text{pi})$$

gives a value of 318 mm^2.

The method for stone removal in this particular patient can be discussed because the largest stone diameter exceeds 20 mm and the surface area is greater than 300 mm^2. According to the recommendations in recent guideline documents, the first-line treatment for stones of that size should be percutaneous lithotripsy (PNL) or retrograde intrarenal surgery (RIRS). In this patient, a gentle and maximally low-invasive procedure was preferable. The major reason for that was the medical condition of the patient. Another reason was that the image indicated that the stone might be brittle and easy to disintegrate. Accordingly, ESWL was chosen as the primary procedure.

Before proceeding to ESWL, there are some essential considerations that need to be made.

The multilayered morphology is typical for a stone that has developed as a result of urinary tract infections (urease-producing microorganisms) and also with a negative test for bacteriuria—a test that should be carried out in all patients before ESWL—a pretreatment antibiotic should be given. If a previous urine culture is available, an antibiotic should be selected according to the resistance pattern. Otherwise, aminoglycosides—e.g., gentamycin (120 mg) or ceftazidim (1–2 g)—are suggested alternatives that should be given intravenously *1 hour* before the procedure.

The patient who is normally taking salicylates had stopped that treatment 10 days before the planned procedure. To make sure that no tablet has been taken by mistake, it is wise to measure the bleeding time that was found to be 4.5 min, and accordingly, there was no pharmacological hindrance for ESWL.

The blood pressure was well treated 150/85.

The size of the stone demands an internal stent to avoid a Steinstrasse and to counteract the risk of ureteral obstruction. For a patient with a renal pelvic stone that can be expected to contain bacteria, it might be worthwhile to consider an internal stent also for a smaller stone volume than was the case in this patient.

Both hypertension and diabetes increase the risk of bleeding from capsular and renal arteries. The shock wave energy should be slowly increased, and the lowest energy level at which disintegration is observed should be chosen for the rest of the treatment. Recommended shock wave frequency for patients with the listed risk factors is 60/min (1 Hz).

The geometrical conditions are favorable. There are no skeletal structures that to any significant extent will interfere with the shock wave propagation, irrespective if the shock wave enters the body from a lateral side or directly from the back.

This woman was treated with one shock wave session. A good disintegration was recorded, and she became stone-free as the result of the treatment (Fig. 48.1b). Both ESWL and insertion of the internal stent were carried out with surface anesthesia, analgesics, and sedation only.

No complications were recorded. Stone analysis disclosed a mixture of magnesium ammonium phosphate, carbonate

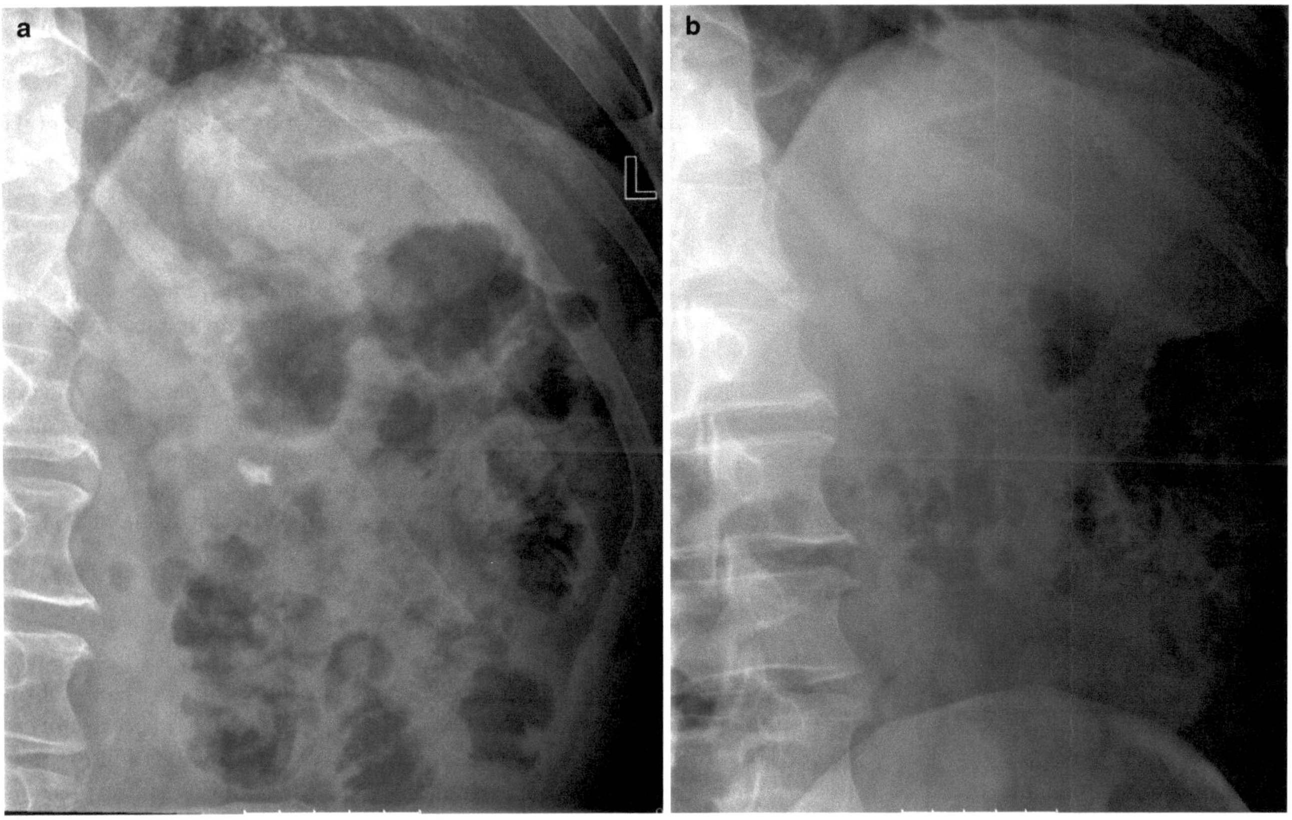

Fig. 48.2 Stone measuring 6 × 4 mm located in the left kidney just below the 12th rib. The situation is shown before (**a**) and after treatment (**b**)

apatite, hydroxyapatite, and a small fraction of calcium oxalate. A urine culture showed *Proteus mirabilis*, and the patient was subsequently treated with a 3-month course of low-dose antibiotics. Ammonium chloride was given as long-term treatment with 1g three times one day each week.

Case 2

A small 6 × 4 mm stone was discovered in a 30-year-old woman who had suffered from intermittent left-sided pain since several months.

It is obvious from the plain X-ray film (Fig. 48.2a) that the stone projects directly over the 12th rib. Although ESWL is the preferred method for this patient, the anatomy is unfavorable for shock waves delivered from the side or from the back. The shock wave power will be reduced by the rib, and, moreover, a shock wave that hits the rib is known to be extremely painful.

Two options are available, and which one to choose depends on the type of lithotripter that is used. Either an attempt can be made to tilt the patient to the left so that the shock wave path does not interfere with the skeleton or the patient is placed in prone position (or in a position that allows passage of shock waves from the abdominal side).

A problem that might be encountered when delivering shock waves through the abdominal cavity is interference with intestinal gas. If gas covers the stone, do not proceed with ESWL, but either try to remove the gas or postpone the ESWL session.

Gas in the left colon can be eliminated with an enema. Pretreatment preparation with dimethicone during a few days before the ESWL session can be of value for a patient in whom it can be anticipated that shock wave administration from in front might be necessary. A plain film taken just before the planned ESWL session, helpful for identification, is helpful not only for showing the stone location but also for demonstration of the intestinal gas situation.

The treatment outcome is shown in Fig. 48.2b.

Case 3

This 38-year-old male patient was medically evaluated because of a few episodes of macroscopic hematuria and dull ache in the right flank. The radiographic examination showed a large renal stone (Fig. 48.3).

There is a stone that has a very large size (26 × 24 mm, surface area 490 mm^2) and a high density. Measurement of Hounsfield units (HU) on non-contrast computed tomography (CT) examinations gives a clue to the stone composition. With a density of approximately 1,200 HU, it can be concluded that the composition is either calcium oxalate monohydrate or brushite.

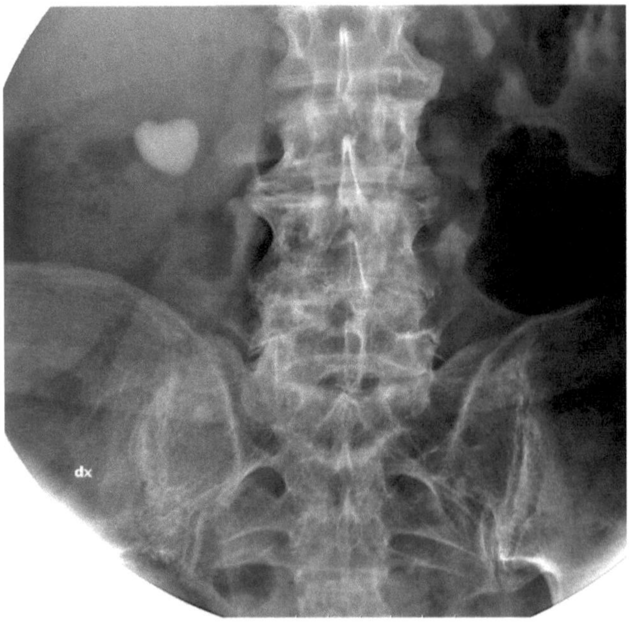

Fig. 48.3 A large (26 × 24 mm) and solid stone in the right kidney. Because of the stone appearance, this patient was referred to percutaneous stone removal

Although stones built up of any of these constituents can be treated with ESWL provided the stone volume is reasonably small, this large stone is unlikely to be eliminated unless a more invasive approach is applied. Percutaneous disintegration is suggested, but in this particular patient, a laparoscopic technique also might be an option.

Following percutaneous stone removal, there were some small collections of residual fragments in the kidney. Stone analysis disclosed brushite, and it is of note that brushite (as well as other calcium phosphate salts) is soluble in Renacidin® (hemiacidrin). When the patient still has a nephrostomy tube in the kidney, it is a good alternative to proceed with chemolytic treatment with the aim of dissolving the residual fragments. This is particularly important in view of the high recurrence rate of brushite stones. Chemolysis is a less invasive alternative than a second-look PNL or RIRS and is likely to get a better stone-free rate than an auxiliary ESWL session.

For a safe chemolytic treatment, a second percutaneous nephrostomy catheter should be inserted, and it is also recommended to have an internal stent in place during the chemolytic procedure.

Case 4

Figure 48.4a shows a stone located in the left ureter just above the sacroiliac joint. This is an example of a mid-ureteral stone. The mid-ureter covers the ureteral section from the upper pelvic brim down to a few centimeters below the sacroiliac joint.

Although the stone seems to be projected free from the adjacent skeletal structures, there is no doubt that the shock wave will interfere with the skeleton. The loss of energy will be greater, the longer the distance is from the body surface to the stone.

Stones in the mid-ureter should always be treated with shock waves directed from in front (through the abdomen). The requirement for a successful disintegration is, however, that there is no intestinal gas in front of the stone. If this condition cannot be met, URS is another alternative, but if steps are taken so that there is a good shock wave hit on the stone, mid-ureteral stones generally can be successfully treated with ESWL.

The result after successful ESWL is shown in Fig. 48.4b.

Case 5

A typical example of a patient with a distal ureteral stone is shown in Fig. 48.5a. At this level, the stone successfully can be treated with either ESWL or ureteroscopy (URS). Both methods have been shown to give acceptable results. The retreatment rate that is statistically higher for ESWL than for URS can be explained either by insufficient care to allow for an optimal effect of the shock wave or by the difficulty associated with an impacted stone that usually only disintegrates at the surface area during a first ESWL session.

ESWL in a patient like this can be carried out with shock waves from the gluteal or abdominal side. In the first case, it is essential to establish a free passage for the shock wave path between the sacrum and the lateral skeleton. In the second case, it is essential to make sure that there is no intestinal gas that extinguishes the shock wave power. It is necessary to use the abdominal direction of the shock wave if a free path cannot be achieved from the back.

For both left- and right-sided distal ureteral stones, gas is often present in the sigmoid colon and rectum, and accordingly, an enema might be helpful to clear the field from gas.

Figure 48.5b shows the result of ESWL.

Case 6

In this patient, a 7 × 6 mm stone was demonstrated in the proximal right ureter (Fig. 48.6a). The stone is located close to a transverse process.

In this situation, it is extremely important to make sure that the transverse process of the spine does not protect the stone from adequate shock wave hits. The majority of these patients

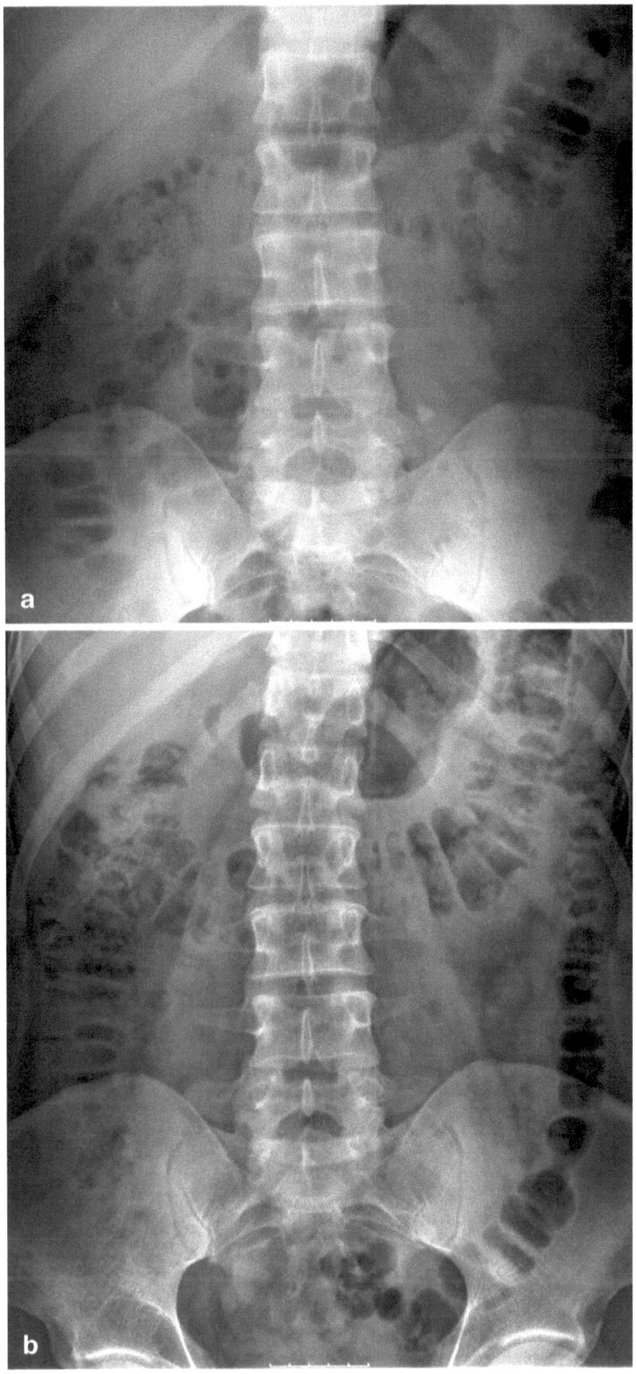

Fig. 48.4 Mid-ureteral stone on the left side at a level just below the pelvic brim, before (**a**) and after (**b**) ESWL

can be adequately treated with shock waves directed from the back. Tilting the patient to the right might be necessary to get a free shock wave path.

If the circumstances do not appropriately assure a free passage from the back, it is recommended to administer the shock waves abdominally.

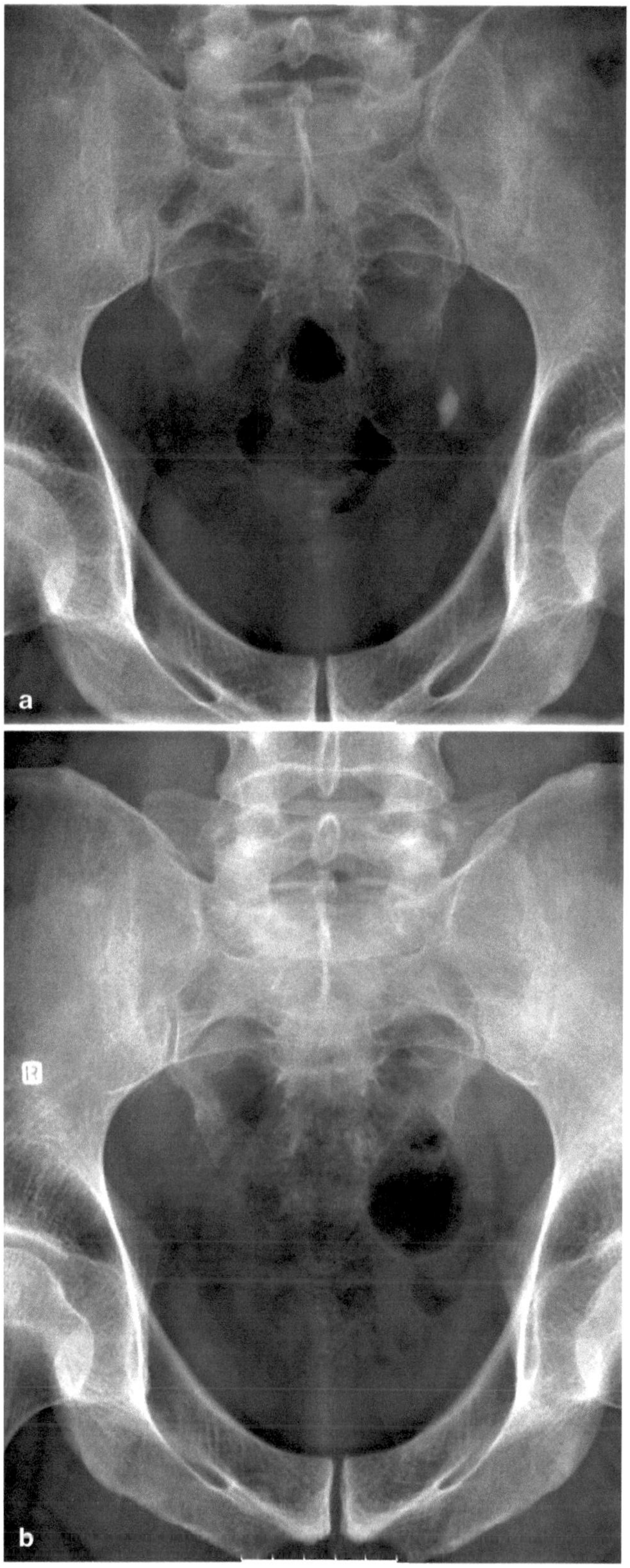

Fig. 48.5 A stone in the left distal ureter before (**a**) and after (**b**) ESWL

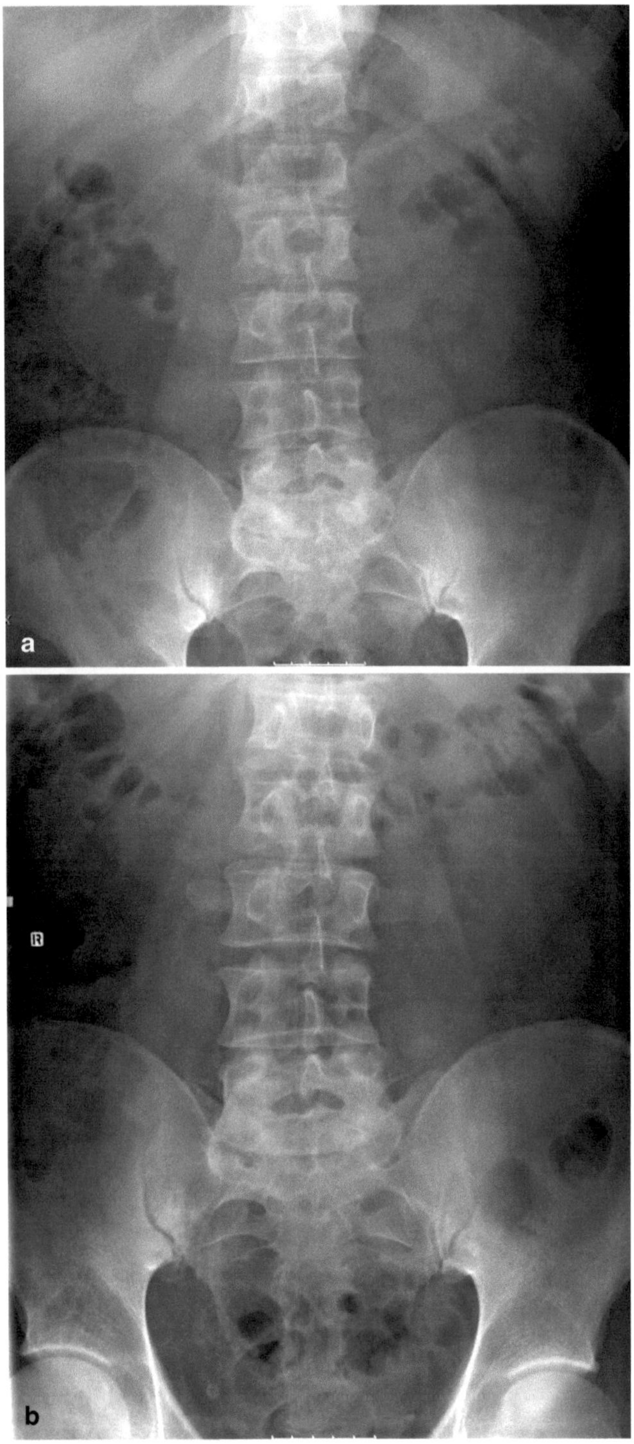

Fig. 48.6 A stone (7 × 6 mm) located in the proximal right ureter. The situation is shown before (**a**) and after (**b**) ESWL

The patient was successfully rendered stone-free with one ESWL procedure (Fig. 48.6b).

Conclusion

The bottom line of the various aspects and recommendations discussed previously is that the anatomical, medical, and transmission conditions for a specific stone situation require an individualized approach for an optimal result. ESWL cannot be carried out in a standardized routine way without carefully observing a number of factors that can or will interfere with transmission of the shock wave power. It is also necessary to take a careful medical history in order to avoid every risk of negative side effects that might occur immediately or in the follow-up period.

SWL of Renal and Ureteral Stones: The Chinese Experience

49

Xizhao Sun, Xiaoming Cong, and Luming Shen

Abstract

The purpose of this chapter is to outline the history of the development of shock wave lithotripsy (SWL) of renal and ureteral stones in China and to present our experiences. The technological aspects and clinical use of Chinese lithotripters are further described. Most lithotripters used for SWL in China are indigenously produced. Lithotripter fabrication began relatively early in China; consequently, our lithotripters have developed distinctive technical characteristics that result in an advantageous cost-benefit ratio, shock waves of lower peak pressure and broader focal zone, and a greater opportunity for anesthesia-/analgesia-free and sedation-free SWL. A single ultrasound is the predominant mode for imaging. Today, SWL has become the first-line modality for renal and ureteral stones across China. Our recommended indications for SWL are similar to the European Association of Urology (EAU) and American Urological Association (AUA) guidelines on urolithiasis. In practice, patients often prefer and select SWL in preference to other modes of treatment due to the aforementioned characteristics. The reported results of SWL in China show comparable or even higher stone-free rates at 3 months; however, there is a higher re-treatment rate compared to Western countries' reported literature. Auxiliary procedures are less used in SWL in China. In our experiences, the most frequent and commonly seen complication post-SWL was temporary hematuria. Other complications were infrequent, and serious complications were rarely reported. In recent years in China, SWL has also been widely used to treat children with renal and ureteral stones. For such cases, serious complications rarely occurred, and the few long-term studies have yet to show any evidence of negative effects of SWL on children's renal morphology and function.

SWL with indigenous lithotripters has been widely used in China as an effective and safe first-line modality for adult and pediatric patients with renal and ureteral stones.

Keywords

Shock wave lithotripsy • China • Chinese lithotripters • Broad focal zone • Pediatric urolithiasis • Re-treatment rates • Complications • Hematuria

X. Sun, M.D. (✉) • X. Cong, Ph.D. • L. Shen, Ph.D.
Department of Urology, Nanjing Drum Tower Hospital
The Affiliated Nanjing Drum Tower Hospital
of Nanjing University Medical School,
321 Zhongshan Road, Nanjing, Jiangsu 210008, China
e-mail: sunxizhaonj@163.com;
oneon2n@163.com; shenluming2008@163.com

J.J. Talati et al. (eds.), *Urolithiasis*,
DOI 10.1007/978-1-4471-4387-1_49, © Springer-Verlag London 2012

Introduction

The Dornier prototype lithotripter (HM1) was first used on humans in 1980. Ever since shock wave lithotripsy (SWL) has revolutionized the treatment of renal and ureteral stones and rapidly gained worldwide acceptance. In China, the first SWL machine ET8410 was produced in Beijing in 1984, as the first human trial with the device followed a year later. In 1987, the Western-produced EDAP-01 and HM3 devices were imported into China. Since then, an increasing number of domestic manufacturers began developing the distinctive features of Chinese lithotripters.

At a rough estimate, >6,000 Chinese lithotripters have been operational in clinical practice compared to <200 imported Western lithotripters. The primary reason for this discrepancy is the advantageous cost-benefit ratio of domestic lithotripters. Their sale price varies between 10,000 and 100,000 US dollars, far less than that of Western lithotripters in China. Consequently, domestically produced lithotripters have been widely used for SWL in China, even in county-level cities in remote areas.

SWL has become the first-line modality for the majority of renal and ureteral stones in China. Financial considerations still influence this treatment choice to a great degree. The average cost of SWL is about 100–200 US dollars, while the cost of re-SWL is roughly 20 US dollars, far less than the 1,200–3,000 US dollars required for percutaneous nephrolithotomy (PCNL) or ureteroscopic stone removal. Therefore, patients frequently opt for the choice of SWL. With the recent progression of endourological technology and the current socioeconomic development in China, the use of PCNL and ureteroscopic stone removal are rapidly on the rise, especially in the more economically developed cities. Still however, SWL is the most preferred among stone management options and plays an irreplaceable role in treatment of urinary stones in China.

The Technology of Chinese Lithotripters

Shock Wave Generation

Electrohydraulic and electromagnetic shock wave generators are currently used in Chinese lithotripters; piezoelectric shock wave generators are unavailable. The initial shock wave generators installed in Chinese lithotripters were electrohydraulic shock wave generators. Beginning in the mid-1990s, electromagnetic shock wave generators started to be installed in Chinese lithotripters, of which there are of three types: electromagnetic flat coil, electromagnetic cylinder, and electromagnetic self-focusing element.

The lifespan of shock wave generators is an important factor for consideration when choosing the types of shock wave generators in China. The lifespan of an electrode is about 3,000–5,000 impulses, and the lifespan of the electromagnetic system is roughly 300,000 impulses. This disadvantage of electrodes may cause inconvenience during operations as well as higher maintenance costs. As a consequence, domestic clients are inclined to purchase electromagnetic lithotripters.

Imaging Systems

The imaging systems used in Chinese lithotripters tend to be fluoroscopy, ultrasound, or both. In the case of fluoroscopic modality, a digitized X-ray imaging source mounted on a mobile C-arm with integrated shock wave source is most frequently used. Whereas for the other modality, an ultrasound imaging system fixed on a lateral articulated arm is exclusively utilized.

Due to a significant cost difference between the two systems, the single ultrasound imaging is much more common than the X-ray or combination system in Chinese lithotripters. Compared with Western machines, the resolution of the X-ray image of the fluoroscopy system is relatively lower in Chinese lithotripters.

Other Technological Characteristics

After an extensive period of research and development, the Chinese lithotripter industry not only came to produce higher quality machines but also created distinctive technological characteristics in its products. Table 49.1 lists the technical data of most lithotripters produced in China. The parts of a typical Chinese lithotripter are shown in Figs. 49.1, 49.2, and 49.3, respectively.

The Low-Moderate Pressure and Broad Focal Zone

A main feature that distinguishes one lithotripter from another is its acoustic output, that is, the amplitude and spatial distribution of acoustic energy delivered to the focal zone. Different from Western lithotripters, most Chinese lithotripters inherently have low-moderate pressure (20–50 MPa) and wide focal zone (16–20 mm). These design characteristics were influenced by the first-generation lithotripter Dornier HM3 and the technical capability of Chinese manufacturers; the Dornier HM3 was considered a gold standard device, a wide focal zone was easier to develop, and it also more easily targeted stones in practice. Interestingly, recent in vitro studies have demonstrated the advantages of a wide focal zone in SWL in several ways [1, 2].

The Low Voltage and High Capacitance in the Circuit

In most circuits, it is necessary to store electrical energy using capacitors. The ability of the capacitor to hold a charge

Table 49.1 A list of the technical data of electrohydraulic and electromagnetic lithotripters made in China

Company	Machine	Focal distance (mm)	Maximum pressure (MPa)	Focal zone ($w \times h$, mm)	Discharge voltage (kV)	Capacitance (μF)	Localization system (F,U)
Electrohydraulic							
Sody	9600 C	120	45	18×70	9–13	0.50	U
Sody	9600D	120	45	18×70	9–13	0.50	U
Sody	9600-FXB[a]	128	50	20×70	NA	0.50	F and U
Hyde	HD-ESWL-Vm[b]	130	50	15×25	5–11	0.40	F and U
Huikang	HK-SWL-V[b]	130	50	18×60	5–10	0.40	F and U
Huikang	HK-SWL-108A	130	50	18×60	5–10	0.40	U
Jiaoda	JDPN-IV	132	50	16×60	15–18	0.32	U
Jiaoda	JDPN-VB	132	50	16×60	15–18	0.32	F
Houyuan	YC9200	120	30	17×60	NA	0.50	U
Keda	NE-3	110	40	20×60	NA	1.00	U
Keda	NE-4	110	40	20×60	NA	1.00	U
XiXin	CS-2000MP	135	30	20×30	4–7	1.00	U
Haibin	HB-SWL-VB	110	NA	17×65	3–9	0.40	F and U
Haibin	HB-SWL-108A	110	NA	17×65	3–9	0.40	U
Jianan	KDE-2001	120	40	NA	6–16	NA	F
Jianan	KDE-2002	120	40	NA	6–16	NA	U
Jianzhong	ESWL-3/ZM[c]	127.5	50	17.5×60	9–18	NA	F and U
Jianzhong	JZS-600[c]	127.5	50	17.5×60	9–18	NA	F and U
Changfa	YS-A[c]	130	50	NA	8–18	0.32	F
Boke	Superman 2000[c]	125	65	18×65	10–20	0.60	F and U
Zhonglian	ZL-502[c]	124	50	17×50	8–20	0.40	F
Songhai	XT03-C[c]	137	40	18×50	8–13	0.60	F
Weida	WD-SWL91[c]	118	NA	17×70	8–12	0.80	U
Weida	WD-SWL98[c]	118	NA	17×70	8–12	0.80	Not available
Yizhou	BD-8828[c]	118	NA	17×70	4–10	1.00	U
Yinxing	153-B	108	NA	17×60	8–12	0.40	F
Xihang	NS-15-1[c]	135	50	NA	12–17	0.66	F
Xihang	NS-15-2[c]	135	50	NA	12–17	0.66	F
Xihang	NS-15-3[c]	135	50	NA	12–17	0.66	F and U
Tiansai	TS-SWL538[c]	130	NA	17×60	NA	NA	F
Aishen	DESUNT-6030[c]	135	65	18×60	10–20	NA	F
Electromagnetic							
Keda	NE-5B	110	NA	20×70	17–22	1.00	U
Keda	NE-5 C	110	NA	20×70	17–22	1.00	F and U
Huikang	HK-SWL-V[b]	135	50	18×60	15–20	0.40	F and U
Huikang	HK-SWL-VI[b]	130	50	18×60	9–16	0.60	F and U
Hyde	HD-ESWL-Vm[b]	130	50	18×60	5–11	0.64	F and U
Hyde	HD-ESWL-109	130	50	15×25	12–18	0.64	U
XiXin	CS-2012MP	145	33.9	NA	12	NA	U
Zhongjia	ZDE-2000	130	50	14×20	8–14	NA	U
Zhongjia	ZDE-2000A	130	50	14×20	8–14	NA	U

The data was excerpted from a study of Sun et al. [9], except for the lithotripters HD-ESWL-Vm, HD-ESWL-109, ZDE-2000, and ZDE-2000A
F fluoroscopy, *U* ultrasound
[a]Lithotripter equipped with tandem-pulse shock wave technology
[b]Shock wave's source could be either electrohydraulic or electromagnetic
[c]Not to be manufactured

(and hence the electric potential energy stored) is termed capacitance. Compared with Western lithotripters, the capacitance of the capacitor (measured in farads) in Chinese lithotripters is often significantly high ranging from 0.3 to 1.2 μF. By the equation of primary energy

$$E = \frac{1}{2}CV^2 \quad (C \sim \text{capacitance}, V \sim \text{voltage}),$$

with an equivalent output of primary energy, the discharge voltage in Chinese lithotripters is accordingly lower.

However, this lower value of discharge voltage does not mean lower energy in Chinese lithotripters. In addition, this circuit feature may affect the shock wave characteristics to some degree, by rising the time of pressure pulse, width of pressure pulse, etc.

SWL Sans Analgesia or Sedation

Patients treated by most Chinese lithotripters do not require or ask for analgesia or sedation. In these cases, pain-free treatment was not achieved by a widening of the aperture, as in most Western lithotripters—for example, the aperture of XX-ES is only 120 mm. Rather, the pain-free lithotripsy could be because the shock waves are delivered at relatively low pressures. Additionally, the larger capacitance of the capacitors mostly used in Chinese lithotripters might influence the characteristics of the shock wave waveform and consequently the amount of pain felt.

New-Generation Lithotripters

Tandem-Pulse Shock Wave Lithotripters

In 1999, the first tandem-pulse shock wave technology in the world was developed in China [3]. With this technology, the SD9600-FXB (Sody Medical Equipment Co. Ltd., Beijing) (see Fig. 49.1) and HB-ESWL-VG (Haibin Medical Equipment Co. Ltd., Zhanjiang) have been put into clinical use for many years [4]. Different from recently reported approaches that utilize an auxiliary shock wave source to generate a second shock wave, the Chinese tandem-pulse shock wave technology used a modified emission-control system to emit tandem-pulse shock waves from a single shock wave source.

Low-Pressure and Wide-Focus Lithotripter

Eisenmenger initially discussed the principal potentials of a wide-focus concept in SWL in 1988 [5]. In 2002, an electromagnetic lithotripter, the ES-XX CS-2012 (see Fig. 49.2) produced by XiXin Medical Instruments Co. Ltd. (Suzhou, China) in cooperation with Eisenmenger, was used to treat patients at a very slow SW rate (27 SWs/min) [6]. The device has an exceptionally wide focus (18 mm) and a relative low pressure (<20 MPa) and has successfully attracted wide interest worldwide.

Real-Time Tracking Lithotripter

Secondary to respiratory movement, stone movement affects the efficacy and safety of SWL. Several targeting systems have been developed to track stones during treatment. Of them, a lithotripter LM-9200 ELMA, which is equipped with an ultrasound-based real-time tracking system (LiteMed Co., Taiwan), is currently in clinical practice [7].

Clinical Use of SWL in China

Selection of Patients for SWL

Stone size and location are the most common indicators used to determine the appropriate treatment choice for stone cases in China. According to the Chinese Urological Association (CUA) guidelines on urolithiasis [8], SWL should be the first-choice procedure for renal stones ≤ 20 mm in diameter and could be used as a secondary procedure for residual stones after PCNL for patients with renal stones > 20 mm in diameter and staghorn calculi. For ureteral stones, SWL should be the first-choice procedure for stones ≤ 10 mm in diameter in upper ureter. Compared with criteria of the European Association of Urology (EAU) or the American Urological Association (AUA), the indications for SWL recommended by the CUA remain relatively inclusive.

In practice, the chosen modality is affected by many factors such as patient and stone characteristics, experience of the urologist, patient preference, and technological factors. These factors often vary across different regions considering the diverse geographical conditions and wide range of socioeconomic conditions in China. The practical selection of patients for SWL may therefore have very distinctive differences across China. In general, Chinese patients with renal and ureteral stones often prefer SWL because of the lower cost, noninvasive nature, and freedom from anesthesia.

Operative Technique of SWL

Nearly all SWL in China are carried out on an outpatient basis. Patients routinely undergo history, physical, and laboratory examination to exclude contraindications. Patients with definite urinary tract infections need specific antimicrobials until their urine culture turns negative. Auxiliary procedures such as retrograde mobilization, stent placement, and nephrostomy are less commonly used prior to treatment. Most cases are carried out as in situ SWL. During SWL procedures, practical steps such as slowing shock wave rate, stepwise power ramping, and proper gel handling have been widely disseminated and used in practice. Post-SWL, patients are encouraged to drink adequate amounts of water and exercise. Chinese herbal medicines for easy passage of calculi fragments are also frequently administrated.

Almost all patients are treated without analgesia or sedation. Being treated "free of analgesia or sedation" does not imply the procedure is free of pain, but rather that the pain is tolerable. Eisenmenger et al. [6] and Sun et al. [9] reported detailed information on pain level in their studies; in the former report, most patients felt mild pain, but only 3 of 297 patients needed sedation during SWL.

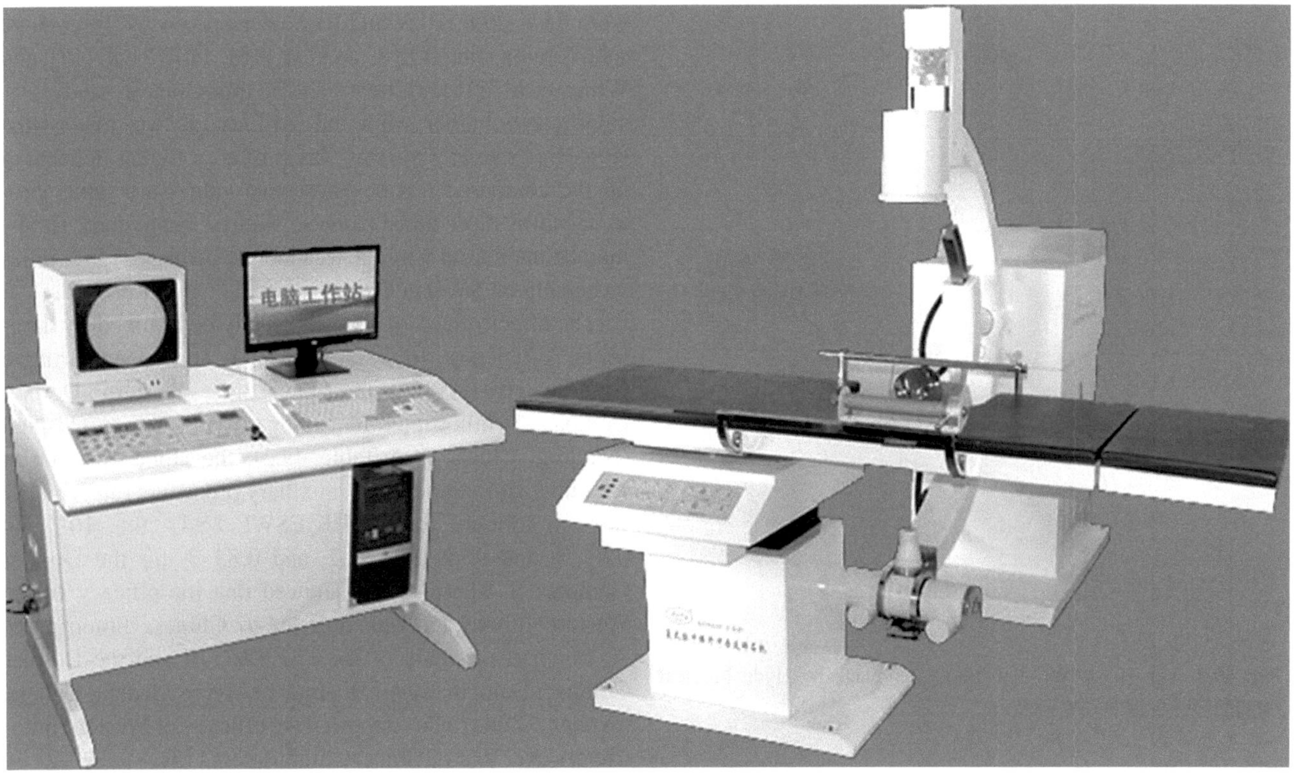

Fig. 49.1 The 9600-FXB lithotripter with the tandem-pulse shock wave technology made by Sody Medical Equipment Co. Ltd., Beijing

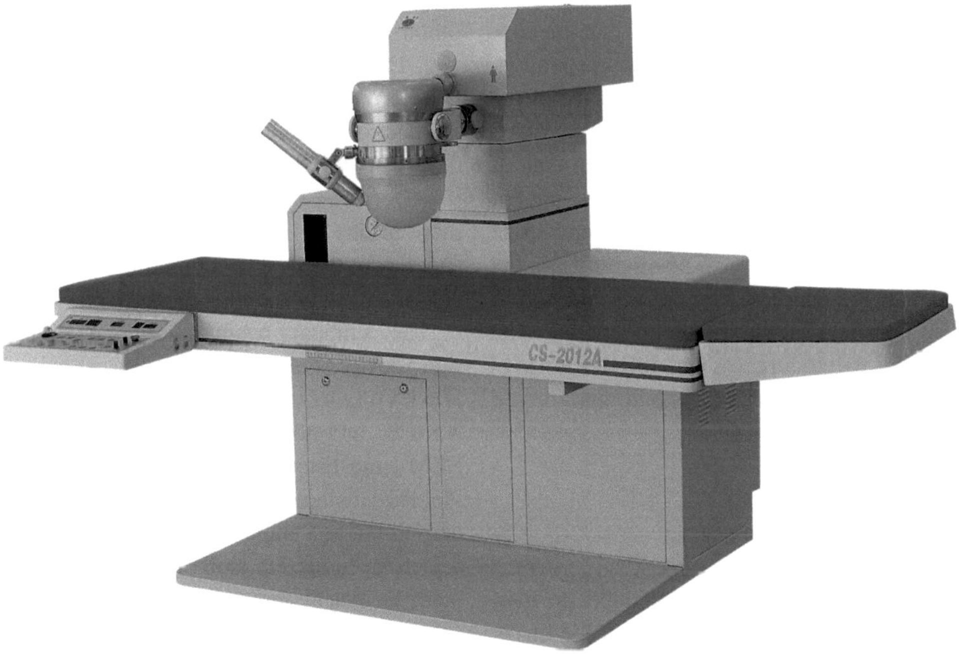

Fig. 49.2 The "low pressure and wide-focus" lithotripter XX-ES made by XiXin Medical Instruments Co. Ltd., Suzhou

Whether or not a stone can be localized successfully will largely determine both the safety and efficacy of a given SWL. In contrast with Western lithotripters, a single ultrasound system is used in a large proportion of Chinese lithotripters. Such imaging equipment has been criticized to pose difficulties in localizing calculi in middle ureter. However, in our experience, the successful localization often depends on whether sufficient urine has filled the bladder. The distended bladder

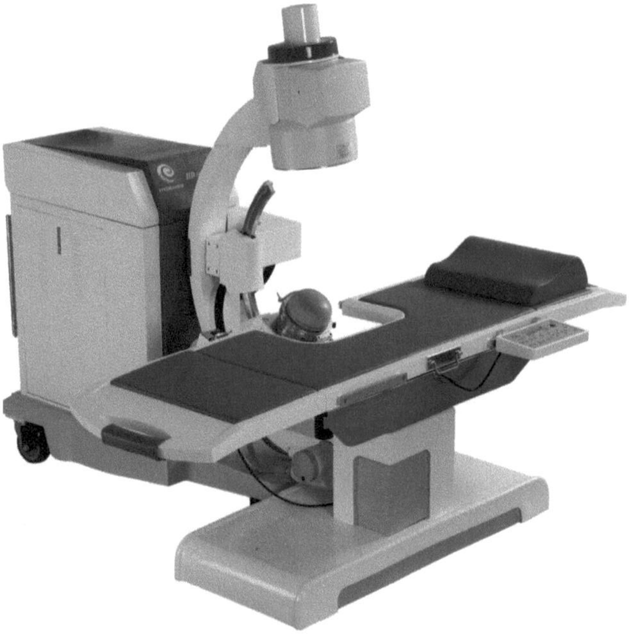

Fig. 49.3 The HD-ESWL-Vm lithotripter made by Hyde Medical Equipment Co. Ltd., Shenzhen

provides a medium through which the ultrasound can be transmitted [10]. As middle ureteral stones lie over the bony pelvis, it can also be difficult to localize these calculi via fluoroscopic imaging. Sun et al. have proposed that the continuously mobile images of stone caused by the respiration, seen against the background of the immobile images of the bony pelvis, can assist the localization of stones [11].

The supine position is generally used for the treatment of stones in the kidneys and upper ureters, whereas the patient is often positioned prone for middle and lower ureter stone procedures. Sun et al. support a prone positioning for the treatment of stones in the middle ureter for two merits: to partly displace the intestines on the ipsilateral side onto the contralateral side (so as to interfere less with the shock wave) and to decrease the distance between the stones and the top of the shock wave generator [11].

Efficacy of SWL

SWL has been shown to be an effective modality to treat both renal stones and ureteral stones. A review of the literature [11–15] showed stone-free rates (at 3 months) of 55–100 %, re-treatment rates of 13.7–42.9 %, and auxiliary treatment rates of 0–10.2 %. In a study of 4,830 patients at an academic institution using a common Chinese lithotripter (Table 49.2), the stone-free rate at 3 months, re-treatment rate, auxiliary procedure rate, and efficiency quotient (EQ) were 85.1, 29.6, 10.2, and 0.61 %, respectively. In contrast with foreign studies by Cass et al. [16], Tailly et al. [17], and White et al. [18], re-treatment in this Chinese study was significantly higher, while the auxiliary rate was lower—the stone-free rate at 3 months was similar or higher depending on the compared report. These two values are rather pronounced in most other Chinese studies; such study results may be the reason why the treatment of urinary stones relies so heavily on SWL in China.

The effectiveness of SWL is greatly determined by lithotripter efficiency. In a large sample study comparing a Chinese HK-ESWL lithotripter to a Western Dornier Compact S lithotripter in Nanjing Drum Tower Hospital (Nanjing, China) (see Table 49.2), the stone-free rate at 3 months, re-treatment rate, auxiliary procedure rate, and EQ were as follows: for the HK-ESWL 85.1, 29.6, 10.2 and 0.61 % and 95.9, 13.4, 2.2, and 0.83 % for the Dornier Compact S. These results showed that the efficacy of the Western lithotripter was superior to Chinese lithotripters. A comparison study of the JT-ESWL-III and the Dornier Compact Delta in Tongji Hospital of Tongji Medical College (Wuhan, China) also supported the efficacy of Western lithotripters over that of Chinese lithotripters [13].

Because stones in the lower ureter are of a relatively similar size and less affected by respiration, Sun et al. considered these stones a suitable model for comparing the efficacy of different lithotripters [11]. In their comparison study of four lithotripters, viz., EDAP-01 (piezoelectric), JDPN-IV (electrohydraulic), HK-ESWL-V (electromagnetic), and Dornier Compact S (electromagnetic), the EQ was noted to be 0.69 (for EDAP-01), 0.74 (for JDPN-IV), 0.80 (for HK-ESWL-V), and 0.81 (for Dornier Compact S). In terms of stone fragmentation, these results showed that the electromagnetic lithotripter was superior to the other two types of lithotripters and the piezoelectric was worst among the three types of lithotripters.

The clinical results of three Chinese new-generation devices—the tandem-pulse shock wave lithotripter HB-ESWL-VG, the pressure and wide-focus lithotripter XX-ES, and the real-time tracking lithotripter LM-9200 ELM—are listed in Table 49.2. Each of these lithotripters yielded satisfactory outcomes. The studies were not, however, carried out at a single institution, so the variability in patient selection, follow-up methodology, definition of success, etc. made an exact comparison of these lithotripters difficult.

Safety of SWL

The safe practice of SWL is a crucial issue in China as SWL is the most widely used stone treatment and, further, because a large number of distinct Chinese lithotripters are available.

Table 49.2 A clinical comparison of typical lithotripters used in China

	Chinese lithotripters				
	A single center study				
	Dornier compact S (n = 9,124)	HK-ESWL-V (n = 4,830)	HB-ESWL-V (n = 769)	XX-ES (n = 389)	LM-9200 (n = 1,332)
Stone size					
£10 mm %	65	57	–	41.6	59.5
10–20 mm %	30	37	–	55.2	23.2
>20 mm %	5	6	0	3.2	17.3
Stone site %					
Upper+middle calyx %	8.1	9.6	26.5	32	45
Lower calyx %	15.8	19.2	28.9	–	40.6
Pelvis %	11.2	12.9	9.8	7	14.4
Upper ureter %	37.3	39.5	34.8	21.5	0
Middle ureter %	4.8	2.8		5.5	
Lower ureter %	22.8	16		30	
Bladder %	0	0	0	4	
Treatment data					
Anesthesia	Yes	No	No	No	No
Localization	F and U	F and U	F and U	U	F and U
Rate SWs/min	70	60	–	27	90
Shock waves per session	2,106	2,482	2,300	1,532	1,716
Results					
SFR at 3 months %	95.9	85.1	89.5	86.2	80
Re-treatment rate %	13.4	29.6	11.2	33	15.7
Auxiliary procedure rate %	2.2	10.2	–	0	3.5
EQ	0.83	0.61	–	0.65	0.67

The results of HB-ESWL-V, XX-ES, and LM-9200 were extracted from the studies of Zhang et al. [4], Eisenmenger et al. [6], and Chen et al. [7], respectively. The results of Dornier Compact S and HK-ESWL-V are extracted from an unpublished study in Nanjing Drum Tower Hospital, the affiliated hospital of Nanjing University Medical School, Nanjing, China

SFR stone-free rate, *EQ* efficiency quotient = stone-free percentage/(100 % + re-treatment percentage + auxiliary procedures percentage) × 100 %

Our review of the literature [9–15] showed hematuria to be the most common short-term complication, occurring in 80–100 % of patients after SWL. However, it was almost always temporary and did not require special management. Renal colic and urinary tract infection (UTI) were minor complications occurring in 1–10 % of patients; serious complications such as perirenal hematoma, hematochezia, hemoptysis, and ureteral injury were rarely reported. The incidence of perirenal hematoma is estimated at about 0.05 % and is often associated with too brief a time interval between treatment sessions. In terms of long-term safety of SWL, there is no report of studies on the effects of the treatment on hypertension, diabetes mellitus, or reproductive function in long-term follow-up.

Almost all Chinese lithotripters have a wide focal zone in terms of acoustic output. Some might think that a wider focal zone would expose a larger region of tissue to potentially damaging shock waves; in our opinion, however, a wide focal zone is not less safe than a narrower focal zone lithotripter. Using a theoretical analysis, Cleveland suggested that wide focal zone lithotripters have the potential to adequately fracture stones with a lower risk of side effects [19]. Leistner et al., also using ex vivo data, showed that renal vascular injury was independent of focal size at an identical number of shock waves [20]. In a prospective study that compared a Chinese lithotripter with Western lithotripter, the HK-ESWL and Dornier Compact S had similar rates of complications; yet, use of the HK-ESWL caused a significantly higher occurrence of skin injury [21].

SWL has been shown to cause acute but reversible decreases in function of the treated and contralateral kidneys [22]. The mechanism of this effect of SWL on kidney function is supposed at least to be correlated with free radical production and a change of renal hemodynamics. A number of clinical studies in China showed that the drugs such as verapamil, nifedipine, and mannitol used during operation have a significantly protective role on decrease of acute renal function in SWL of renal calculi and vitamin E could eliminate free radicals but had a less protective role [23–25]. These findings provided some possible methods of protecting patients from short-term renal injury caused by SWL.

SWL in the Management of Pediatric Urolithiasis

Urinary calculi incidence among children has been reported to be from 0.1 to 5 %. Speculation continues regarding the perceived increase in pediatric urolithiasis in recent years. SWL has been used in children for ~20 years; however, there has been limited attention to pediatric SWL until recently. The US Food and Drug Administration has yet to give approval for use of SWL in pediatric populations, but SWL has been widely used to treat renal and ureteral stones in children in China. The choice for this treatment modality and the technique of SWL do not differ between adult and pediatric patients.

A review of the literature [26–32] shows that stone-free rates at 3 months range from 75 to 100 % and re-treatment rates range from 16 to 35.5 %, while auxiliary procedure rates are often not reported in Chinese studies. In a large sample study, He et al. [31] treated 311 children with the Dornier Compact S, 196 of whom had renal stones and 115 had ureteral stones. The total stone-free rates of renal and ureteral stones at 3 months were 95.8–94.8 % with an EQ of 0.84 and 0.80, respectively. The results also showed that treatments of renal and ureteral calculi in children have comparable efficiency, except that the EQ is lower for stones in lower calyces and the middle ureter compared to those at other sites.

The side effect of SWL is a question of common interest because of the smaller and potentially more fragile kidney in children. In a number of reported datasets [26–33], hematuria occurred in 55.6–91.7 % of patients, colic in 2.6–22.0 %, UTI or fever in 2.6–6.9 %, skin petechiae in 4.2–37 %, and a Steinstrasse in 1–11.9 %, while other serious complications rarely occurred. In general, these complications were significantly reduced in more recent studies. The reduction in morbidity is possibly related with the advancement of shock wave lithotripsy and increased experience of the practicing urologists. In a study of the long-term safety of SWL [32], 16 of 54 pediatric patients were followed up for 24–91 months (average 56.5 months). The results showed blood pressure, renal function, as well as renal form to be normal in all 16 patients.

The prone position is widely used in SWL for distal ureteral stones. However, in a study by Sun et al. [33], the prone position was thought to inhibit the movement of the thorax and possibly lead to decreased total lung capacity. Additionally, it made observation of children's countenance difficult. Rather, distal ureteral stones in young children were treated in the supine position with the path of shock wave through the greater and lesser ischial foramina (Fig. 49.4). A total of 22 young children with distal urinary calculi were treated using the Dornier Compact S lithotripter; stone size ranged from 5 to 16 mm (mean 6.8). Stone-free rate at 2 weeks after lithotripsy was 77.3 %, which increased to 100 % at 3 months after a single lithotripsy session. No serious side effects were observed. The results showed that SWL in the supine position with the path of shock wave through the greater and lesser ischial foramina treats distal ureteral stones in young children with an excellent success rate and few side effects.

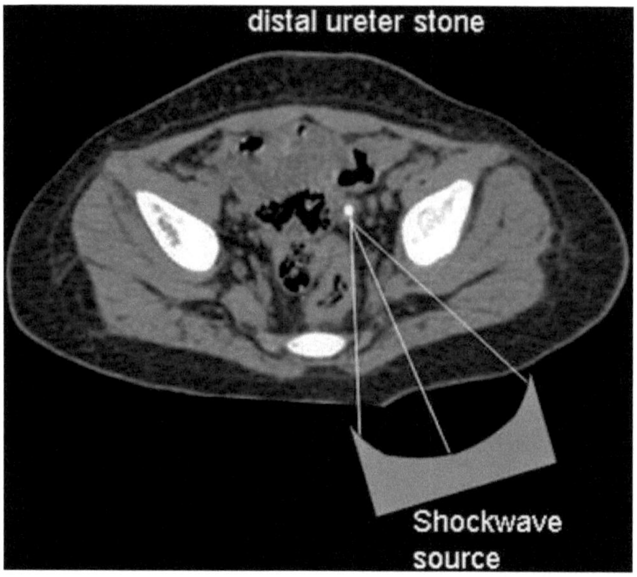

Fig. 49.4 Approach of shock wave treating distal ureteral stone in supine position in children

> **Conclusion**
>
> Most lithotripters used in China are indigenously made and affordably priced and have shock waves of low peak pressure and broad focal zone, which differs from the Western alternatives. As an inexpensive, noninvasive, and free-of-analgesia procedure, SWL has been widely used as the first-line modality for adult and pediatric patients with renal and ureteral stones in China. Usually following SWL, the stone-free rates are satisfactory and high, the re-treatment rates are relatively high, and the auxiliary rates are low. The occurrence of SWL complications is often low with the exception of temporary hematuria; serious complications have been rarely observed in the treatment.

References

1. Sapozhnikov OA, Maxwell AD, Macconaghy B, Bailey MR. A mechanistic analysis of stone fracture in lithotripsy. J Acoustic Soc Am. 2007;121:1190–2.
2. Eisenmenger W. The mechanisms of stone fragmentation in ESWL. Ultrasound Med Biol. 2001;27:683–93.
3. Zhou Y, Sun XZ. Experimental research and investigation of binary repetitive pulsed power technology. Adv Technol Electrical Eng Energy. 2002;21:67–9.

4. Zhang Z, Li X, Xia MY, Tang FL, Long T, Chen GZ, et al. Treatment of renal and ureteral calculi with duplex pulse low-energy ESWL (report of 717 cases). Chin J Urol. 2004;25:448–9.
5. Eisenmenger W. Physikalisch-medizinische Aspekte selbstfokussierender elektromagnetisch erzeugter stosswellen. Verh Ber Dtsch Ges Urol. 1988;34:69–70.
6. Eisenmenger W, Du XX, Tang C, Zhao S, Wang Y, Rong F, et al. The first clinical results of "wide-focus and low-pressure" ESWL. Ultrasound Med Biol. 2002;28:769–74.
7. Chen CJ, Hsu HC, Chung WS, Yu HJ. Clinical experience with ultrasound-based real-time tracking lithotripsy in the single renal stone treatment. J Endourol. 2009;23:1811–5.
8. Ye ZQ. Guidelines for urolithiasis. In: Na YQ, editor. CUA guidelines, vol. I. Beijing: People's Medical Publishing House; 2008. p. 231–41, Chap. 7.
9. Sun XZ, Zhang ZW. Shockwave lithotripsy: instrumentation and status in China. J Endourol. 2005;19:774–9.
10. Fu HX, Li HY, Wu WH, Liang PY. B-ultrasound guided treatment of ureteral calculi with extracorporeal shock wave lithotripsy. J Hainan Med Coll. 2007;15:780–2.
11. Sun XZ, Wang Y, Yu HB, Sun ZY, Chen CZ. Extraeorporeal shock wave lithotripsy in situ for middle ureteral stones. Chin J Urol. 1999;37:438–9.
12. Wu ZX. Treatment of upper urinary calculi with duplex pulse low-energy ESWL. Chin J Clin Ration Drug Use. 2009;2:18–9.
13. Zhou XC, Ye ZQ, Zeng XY, Zhu J, Xia K. In situ ESWL of ureteral stones: comparsion between an electrohydraulic and an electromagnetic SW-source. J Clin Urol. 2004;19:385–7.
14. Liu XG, Deng SZ, Peng SP, Xiong LS, Wang DR, Xie P, et al. Therapeutical effect of ESWL on renal calyceal stones. J Clin Urol. 2000;15:205–6.
15. Han H, Dong C, Li X, Zhong HG, Wu ZJ. The curative effect of ureteral stone: comparison between ESWL and URL. J Clin Urol. 2006;21:296–8.
16. Cass AS. Comparison of first generation (Dornier HM3) and second generation (Medstone STS) lithotripters: treatment results with 1,3864 renal and ureteral calculi. J Urol. 1995;153:588–92.
17. Tailly GG. Consecutive experience with four Dornier lithotripters: HM4, MPL 9000, compact, and U/50. J Endourol. 1999;13: 329–38.
18. White W, Klein F. Five-year clinical experience with the Dornier delta lithotripter. Urology. 2006;68:28–32.
19. Cleveland RO. The advantage of a broad focal zone in SWL. In: Evan AP, Lingeman JE, McAteer JA, Williams Jr JC, editors. Renal stone disease 2. 2nd international urolithiasis research symposium. Melville: American Institution of Physics; 2008. p. 219–5.
20. Leistner R, Wendt-Nordahl G, Grobholz R, Michel MS, Marlinghaus E, Kohrmann KU, et al. A new electromagnetic shock-wave generator "SLX-F2" with user-selectable dual focus size: ex vivo evaluation of renal injury. Urol Res. 2007;35:165–71.
21. Lian HB, Guo HQ, Wang Y, Sun XZ, Sun ZY. Comparison of China- and Germany-made electromagnetic lithotripters for upper urinary tract calculi: preliminary report of perspective study. Chin J Min Invasive Surg. 2008;8:311–3.
22. Delvecchio F, Auge BK, Munver R, Brown SA, Brizuela R, Zhong P, et al. Shock wave lithotripsy causes ipsilateral renal injury remote from the focal point: the role of regional vasoconstriction. J Urol. 2003;169:1526–9.
23. Jiang HM, Guo M, Zhang CY, Li CG, Zhang DT. Experimental study on protective effect of verapamil on ESWL induced renal damage. J Liaoning Med Univ. 2009;30:405–6.
24. Xu YM, Gao WZ, Xu CX. The protective nifedipine for acute renal function impairment caused by ESWL. China J Urol. 2001;22: 601–3.
25. Li ZW, Zheng BZ, Xu ZH, Zhou ZL, He WJ. The protective role mannitol and vitamin E on renal function in SWL and the study of their mechanisms. Shangdong Med Drug. 2000;40:23–4.
26. Wu TC, Huang YD, Liu TJ, Yang N, Cheng ZY, Gou YF, et al. ESWL for the treatment of upper urinary tract stone in children. Chin J Urol. 1991;12:186–7.
27. Liu XY, Zheng WX, Xiao DM. Treatment of renal stones in 42 children. Chin J Urol. 2001;22:361.
28. Zheng XQ, Chen XY, Li YT. Study of the safety and efficacy of extracorporeal shock lithotripsy (ESWL) as a treatment for urolithiasis in children. J Materal Child Health Care. 2005;20:1627–8.
29. Jia JY, Ye M, Chen F, Xu MS, Xie H, Geng HQ. Low-energy extracorporeal shock wave lithotripsy for children with urinary calculi. Chin J Pediatr Surg. 2005;26:239–41.
30. Lin W, Huang HP, Huang H, Meng DL, He JQ. Renal calculi treated with extracorporeal shock wave lithotripsy in children: a report of 27 cases. Chin J Gen Pract. 2010;9:280–2.
31. He L, Sun X, Lu J, Cong X, Zhu H, Shen L, Wang Y. Comparison of efficacy and safety of shock wave lithotripsy for upper urinary tract stones of different locations in children: a study of 311 cases. World J Urol. 2011;29(6):713–7.
32. Wang Q, Chen CZ, Xiong XM. Clinical effects and long-term of extracorporeal shock wave lithotripsy in children. J Clin Urol. 1997;12:330–2.
33. Sun X, He L, Lu J, Cong X, Shen L, Wang Y, Zhu H. Greater and lesser ischiadic foramina as path of shock wave lithotripsy for distal ureteral stone in children. J Urol. 2010;184:665–8.

Retrograde Intrarenal Surgery (RIRS)

50

Andreas J. Gross and Christopher Netsch

Abstract

Technological progress has evolved retrograde intrarenal surgery (RIRS) into a safe and efficacious modality for the treatment of the upper urinary tract and has expanded its potential indications to intrarenal large stones (>25 mm), shock wave lithotripsy (SWL) failure, infundibular stenosis, morbid obesity, renoureteral malformations, musculoskeletal deformities, and bleeding diathesis. The development of flexible ureteroscopes and accessory instrumentation like guidewires, ureteral access sheaths, intracorporeal lithotriptors, and stone retrieval baskets has facilitated RIRS and has given more safety to the procedure. Although neither European Association of Urology (EAU) nor American Urological Association (AUA) guidelines recommend RIRS as first-line treatment for intrarenal stones, RIRS has, however, progressed to be a real alternative to shock wave lithotripsy and percutaneous nephrolithotomy (PCNL) for treating renal calculi—offering the low morbidity of SWL combined with stone-free rates comparable with PCNL for small- to moderate-sized renal calculi. Safety and efficacy of RIRS has also been confirmed in children. Thus, RIRS potentially may become first-line treatment for intrarenal stones. We give a description of the technical aspects and the latest developments of flexible ureteroscopes and accessory instrumentation for RIRS. Potential indications of RIRS, the procedure itself, and its complications are described and were reviewed with the current literature.

Keywords

Retrograde intrarenal surgery (RIRS) • URS • Ureteroscopy • Guidewires • Nitinol • Ureteral access sheath • Ho:YAG laser • Lithotripsy • Stone retrieval devices • Laser lithotripsy Ureteral stenting

Introduction

Technological progress of ureterorenoscopes (URS) and endoscopic instrumentation has evolved retrograde intrarenal surgery (RIRS) into a safe and efficacious modality for the treatment of the upper urinary tract. These improvements in technology have expanded the potential indications of RIRS to intrarenal large stones (>25 mm), shock wave lithotripsy (SWL) failure, infundibular stenosis, morbid obesity, renoureteral malformations, musculoskeletal deformities, and bleeding diathesis [1–7]. RIRS can be considered for multiple or large intrarenal calculi with a high stone-free rate and low morbidity, albeit neither European Association of Urology (EAU) nor American Urological Association (AUA) guidelines recommend RIRS as the treatment of choice for intrarenal stones at this time [1, 2, 8–10]. However, safety and efficacy of RIRS is predominantly influenced by choosing the adequate instrumentation.

A.J. Gross, M.D. (✉) • C. Netsch, M.D.
Department of Urology, Asklepios Hospital Barmbek, Ruebenkamp 220, Hamburg 22291, Germany
e-mail: an.gross@asklepios.com

J.J. Talati et al. (eds.), *Urolithiasis*,
DOI 10.1007/978-1-4471-4387-1_50, © Springer-Verlag London 2012

Instrumentation

Guidewire

The placement of a safety wire facilitates and maintains access to the upper urinary tract. However, the necessity of a guidewire remains controversial as successful wireless RIRS is currently being shown in the literature [11]. Ideally, a guidewire will require little force to flex in response to resistance encountered along a tortuous path and will contrarily require a large force to perforate tissue. Manifold guidewires are on the market: in an in vitro examination, the lubricous, soft-tip nitinol demonstrated to be the safest wire for initial access to the ureter; it is less likely to perforate and more likely to bend when a point of obstruction is encountered [12]. Hybrid wires have been developed to combine various advantageous features: a smooth, hydrophilic distal tip, a kink-resistant nitinol body, and a flexible proximal tip. The clinical application of these wires is limited due to their greater cost compared to the standard alternatives. At the same time, it is possible that a hybrid wire may decrease the need to open a second guidewire if a standard wire fails to pass a point of obstruction [13].

Ureteral Access Sheath

Ureteral access sheaths facilitate the insertion and straight alignment of the URS into the upper urinary tract during multiple stone fragment extractions, decrease operative time and cost, minimize patient morbidity, and optimize overall success with RIRS [14]. The access sheath also allows efflux of irrigant fluid through the sheath and around the URS, maintaining intrapelvic pressures below 20 cm H_2O with irrigant fluid pressurized up to 200 cm H_2O [15]. The reliance on axial dilating force of current ureteral access sheaths, however, exposes the urothelium to the potential risk of an abrasive shearing force. A new balloon-based ureteral access sheath combines radial balloon dilation and access sheath placement in a single step, which may reduce both the axial force and urothelial disruption [16].

Ureteral Balloon Dilator/Catheters

Ureteral balloon dilation may be utilized in approximately 5 % of cases when the ureteral access sheath will not advance to the site of pathology due to ureteral stricture, spasm, or a tight ureteral orifice [13].

Irrigation

Adequate irrigation flow is necessary to maintain visibility. Flexible URS have either two separate channels (one working channel for an instrument and the second for irrigation) or one common channel for both irrigation and working instruments. Irrigation can be provided by gravity, a pressure bag, or a variety of hand or foot pumps. It should be emphasized that manual hand irrigation has been shown to produce pressures greater than 100 mmHg in the kidney [17], which may lead to bacteremia or sepsis due to increased fluid absorption.

Flexible Ureteroscope

Advancements in flexible URS design and functionality have led to improved lower pole caliceal access and instrument longevity. URS differ in terms of working channel, optical resolution, accessing all calices, and the durability of the scopes. The newer, actively deflecting flexible URS offer increased lower pole access compared to older passively deflecting scopes [13]. It has been demonstrated that the ideal outer diameter of a flexible ureteroscope, defined in terms of the ease of introduction without the need for ureteral dilation, was 7.4 F [18]. Another critical consideration regards the durability of flexible URS: Traxer et al. demonstrated deterioration of maximal dorsal/ventral deflection from 270 to 133° and 270–208° after 50 consecutive RIRS with the same scope [19]. It was suggested that scopes returned from major repairs have less than 25 % of the life expectancy of a new scope and that it may be more cost-effective to replace the device than repair it [20].

Intracorporeal Lithotriptors

Intracorporeal lithotripsy is used for large stone fragmentation. Holmium (Ho):YAG laser lithotripsy has been shown to fragment all compositions of urinary calculi, as well as produce smaller stone fragments than pneumatic or electrohydraulic lithotripsy [21, 22]. In addition, the Ho:YAG laser energy is absorbed efficiently in a fluid medium, minimizing the risk of urothelial injury compared to the electrohydraulic lithotrite. Retropulsion of the stone is also less likely than with a pneumatic lithotrite. However, using the Ho:YAG laser with a deflected flexible URS does elevate the risk of collateral damage to instrumentation, including the flexible URS [23].

Stone Retrieval Devices

Since Dormia presented a spiral basket for stone retrieval [24], basket design has improved with regard to wires (number, material, shape), shaft (size, material), and configuration (spherical, helical, paired wire, tipless) [25, 26]. The previously used stainless steel gave way to the soft "memory metal" nitinol, a flexible and kink-resistant alloy of nickel and titanium; nitinol is also less rigid than stainless steel and imposes less limitation on URS deflection [25]. Important properties of these devices include visibility during stone manipulation, sufficient radial force to open in the ureter, and the ability to capture, retain, or if necessary disengage a stone. Compared to alligator or rat tooth forceps, tipless nitinol-based basket designs are more versatile and atraumatic in stone retrieval; this is due both to the unique pliability of the wires, as well as the flexibility that allows full lower pole deflection of a flexible URS in the majority of cases [27, 28].

The RIRS Procedure

Preparation of the Patient

Preparation of the patient includes informed consent and explanation of the potential complications, as well as the possible of insertion of a ureteral stent if necessary [29]. General anesthesia is favored; however, neuroleptic anesthesia is also feasible.

Antibiotic Prophylaxis

The rate of urinary tract infection following ureteroscopy ranges from 4 to 25 %, even when prophylactic antibiotics are administered. Therefore, the use of preoperative antibiotic prophylaxis is still controversial [30]. Patients at risk with a preoperative ureteral stent, catheter, or nephrostomy tube should be treated with antibiotic prophylaxis; additionally, so should patients with heart valves and murmurs at risk of bacterial endocarditis, immunocompromised patients, and those with drug or radiation induced immunosuppression [30, 31].

Positioning of the Patient

Ureteroscopy has been described in the supine, prone, and flank position; the flank position has, however, only been demonstrated with flexible instruments [32]. We prefer the dorsal lithotomy position in routine URS.

Cystoscopy

Depending on the urologist's training and available equipment, flexible or rigid cystoscopes can be used for initial guidewire placement into the ureter. Cystoscopes and URS should be combined with a video monitoring system as it is ergonomically beneficial, ideal for teaching trainees, and useful for documentation purposes. Rigid cystoscopy is the preferred modality for retrograde pyelography, although it may cause more ureteral trauma, particularly in males [29].

Safety Guidewire

Fluoroscopy is used to confirm the position of the guidewire as it is advanced. The wire acts as a safety wire. A general principle of RIRS is always to have a safety wire present intraoperatively [29].

Ureteroscope Insertion

When a safety wire is in place, a second working wire must be inserted in order to backload the endoscope, allowing the wire to act as a guide for the advancement of the instrument into the ureter or kidney under fluoroscopic guidance [33]. For this purpose, manifold ways are described to establish the second wire.

Ureteral Stenting Following Ureteroscopy

Placement of a ureteral catheter or internal ureteral stent has been the standard of care following RIRS to prevent renal colic by obstructing stone fragments or ureteral edema after surgery [29]. However, routine stenting might add morbidity to the procedure by infection, dysuria, flank pain, hematuria, or stent migration. In a randomized controlled trial, patients assigned to ureteral stents following ureteroscopy had increased pain compared with non-stented patients; yet, incidence of emergency room visits, urosepsis, and hospitalization, as well as stone-free rates, did not differ between the two groups [34, 35]. The authors advise against routine stent placement in the ureter if the stone burden is small, if the ureter has not been balloon dilated, or if the Ho:YAG laser has been used without ureteral trauma [35]. Although these series analyzed the usefulness of stenting post-ureteral stone extraction, these principles can also be applied to RIRS. Strict indications for stent insertions include ureteral perforation, ureteral dilation greater than 10 F, ureteral edema due to stone treatment/size, failure to advance the RIRS procedure due to narrow ureter or ureteral orifice, infected urinary system with an obstructing system, large stone burden with many fragments remaining to pass, and solitary kidney [29].

Postoperative Care

If a stent is left indwelling, it is typically removed 3–10 days after the procedure. Postoperative radiographs are obtained within 1–2 weeks to determine the success of the procedure [29]. Small stone fragments (<4 mm) normally pass after the stent has been removed due to the passive ureteral dilation that occurs from stenting [36]. Postoperative imaging has been recommended to examine for residual calculi or silent obstruction [29, 37]. Secondary silent obstruction may occur from ureteral edema, trauma, or stricture and can result in renal failure if it remains undetected. Despite this, some working groups do not recommend routine imaging as long as there is no history of preexisting ureteral stricture, perforation, or significant stone impaction at the time of surgery [38].

RIRS for the Treatment of Kidney Stones

RIRS has progressed to become an alternative to SWL and PCNL for the treatment of renal calculi, offering the low morbidity of SWL combined with similar stone-free rates as PCNL for small- to moderate-sized renal calculi [39]. Significant lower pole stone burden is the limiting factor for success. Even with new flexible URS, the lower pole calyces can only be accessed in 93 % of cases [5]. Fabrizio et al. reported a 77 % (50 %) stone-free rate for renal stones <10 mm (>16 mm) with a complication rate of 3 % [40]. For single intrarenal stones>20 mm [4] and 30 mm [2], the stone-free rates were 93.3–90.9 % after an average of 2.4 and 1.8 procedures, respectively. There are a few published series regarding RIRS for multiple unilateral, intrarenal stones [5, 7, 9, 10, 40, 41]. Breda et al. reported overall stone-free rates after one and two procedures of 64.7–92.2 % for multiple unilateral, intrarenal stones and a complication rate of 13.6 % [9]. Herrera et al. presented the largest series on RIRS for multiple renal stones to date. They reported an overall stone-free rate after one procedure of 74.4 % for multiple unilateral, intrarenal stones and a complication rate of 5.6 % [10]. To conclude, this series supports the usefulness of RIRS throughout the renal collecting system with a high success and low complication rate [9, 10, 40, 42–45].

Ureteroscopy in Children

Since Shepherd et al. [46] and Ritchey et al. [47] have published their experiences, ureteroscopy has gained widespread acceptance among pediatric urologists. The safety and efficacy of ureteroscopy in children has been confirmed [48–52], although these series differ in terms of instruments, techniques, and calculi location. The access to the upper urinary tract remains controversial due to the risk of ureteral trauma and/or bleeding. Shepherd et al. have shown that dilation of the ureter up to 12 F did not result in the development of vesicoureteral reflux (VUR) postoperatively [46]. In addition, VUR resolved spontaneously with conservative management in most children [53]. Some authors believe that stent preplacement provides a safe and effective alternative in achieving access to the child's ureter, resulting in higher overall stone-free rates, as shown in adults [54]. Antegrade ureteral access may be considered in children who have a percutaneous nephrostomy in place and a completely obstructed ureter [53, 55]. Ureteroscopic disintegration of ureteral calculi has also gained acceptance [48–53]. The outcomes in prepubertal children were comparable with those in adults [56]. Nerli et al. have recently reported an overall stone-free rate after one RIRS procedure (with Ho:YAG lithotripsy) of 90 % for ureteral calculi [52]. They concluded that complete stone clearance after one procedure is possible if the stone is small (<10 mm), solitary, and below the level of the pelviureteral junction [52].

Complications of RIRS

Urosepsis

Manipulation of a stone in the presence of an infection is likely to result in bacteremia and possible urosepsis. In patients who present with an infected collected system and an obstructing stone, urinary decompression should be the initial modality followed by culture sensitive antibiotic treatment. Postoperative bacteremia and sepsis should be treated with culture-sensitive intravenous antibiotics, followed by oral antibiotics when the patient has defervesced [29].

Ureteral Avulsion

Ureteral avulsion is an uncommon but serious complication of ureteroscopy. Avulsion typically occurs during basket extraction of a stone fragment that is too large and becomes caught in the ureteral mucosa, telescoping and avulsing the ureter as the stone is extracted. To avoid these catastrophic complications, a safety wire should be always used. And, the stones should also be broken small enough for ureteral passage [29].

Ureteral Stricture

The ureteral perforation rate has decreased concurrently with the ureteral stricture rate over the past 20 years to 1.7–0.1 % in a large contemporary series of semirigid URS, respectively [57]. Risk factors for ureteral perforation included operation time, stone location, use of electrohydraulic lithotripsy, and surgeon experience [29].

Conclusion

Technological progress has evolved RIRS into a safe and efficacious modality for the treatment of the upper urinary tract and has expanded its potential indications. The development of flexible ureteroscopes and accessory instrumentation has facilitated RIRS and has additionally given more safety to the procedure. RIRS has progressed to be a real alternative to SWL and PCNL for renal calculi treatment and offers the low morbidity of SWL as well as stone-free rates comparable with PCNL for small- to moderate-sized renal calculi. Thus, RIRS may potentially become a first-line treatment for intrarenal stones.

References

1. Preminger GM, Tiselius HG, Assimos DG, et al. Guideline for the management of ureteral calculi. J Urol. 2007;178:2418–34.
2. Riley JM, Stearman L, Troxel S. Retrograde ureteroscopy for renal stones larger than 2.5 cm. J Endourol. 2009;23:1395–8.
3. Yinghao S, Yang B, Gao X. The management of renal caliceal calculi with a newly designed ureteroscope: a rigid ureteroscope with a deflectable tip. J Endourol. 2010;24:23–6.
4. Breda A, Ogunyemi O, Leppert JT, et al. Flexible ureteroscopy and laser lithotripsy for single intrarenal stones 2 cm or greater – is this the new frontier? J Urol. 2008;179:981–4.
5. Grasso M. Ureteropyeloscopic treatment of ureteral and intrarenal calculi. Urol Clin North Am. 2000;27:623–31.
6. Grasso M, Bagley D. In discussion of: small diameter, actively deflectable, flexible ureteropyeloscopy. J Urol. 1998;160:1648–53.
7. Wen CC, Nakada SY. Treatment selection and outcomes: renal calculi. Urol Clin North Am. 2007;34:409–19.
8. Tiselius HG, Ackermann D, Alken P, et al. Guidelines on urolithiasis. Eur Urol. 2001;40:362–71.
9. Breda A, Ogunyemi O, Leppert JT, et al. Flexible ureteroscopy and laser lithotripsy for multiple unilateral intrarenal stones. Eur Urol. 2009;55:1190–7.
10. Herrera-Gonzalez G, Netsch C, Oberhagemann K, et al. Effectiveness of single flexible ureteroscopy for multiple renal calculi. J Endourol. 2011;25:431–5.
11. Dickstein RJ, Kreshover JE, Babayan RK, et al. Is a safety wire necessary during routine flexible ureteroscopy? J Endourol. 2010; 24:1589–92.
12. Clayman M, Uribe CA, Eichel L, et al. Comparison of guide wires in urology. Which, when and why? J Urol. 2004;171:2146–50.
13. Holden T, Pedro RN, Hendlin K, et al. Evidence-based instrumentation for flexible ureteroscopy: a review. J Endourol. 2008;22:1423–6.
14. Kourambas J, Byme RR, Preminger GM. Does a ureteral access sheath facilitate ureteroscopy? J Urol. 2001;165:789–93.
15. Rehman J, Monga M, Landman J, et al. Characterization of intrapelvic pressure during ureteropyeloscopy with ureteral access sheaths. Urology. 2003;61:713–8.
16. Harper JD, Ebrahimi KY, Auge BK, et al. Comparison of a novel radially dilating balloon ureteral access sheath to a conventional sheath in the porcine model. J Urol. 2008;179:2042–5.
17. Auge BK, Pietrow PK, Lallas CD, et al. Ureteral access sheath provides protection against elevated renal pressures during routine flexible ureteroscopic stone manipulation. J Endourol. 2004;18:33–6.
18. Hudson RG, Conlin M, Bagley D. Ureteric access with flexible ureteroscopes: effect of the size of the ureteroscope. BJU Int. 2005;95:1043–4.
19. Traxer O, Dubosq F, Jamali K, et al. New-generation flexible ureterorenoscopes are more durable than previous ones. Urology. 2006;68:276–9.
20. Carey RI, Gomez CS, Maurici G, et al. Frequency of ureteroscope damage seen at a tertiary care center. J Urol. 2006;176:607–10.
21. Chan KF, Vassar GJ, Pfefer TJ, et al. Holmium:YAG laser lithotripsy: a dominant photothermal ablative mechanism with chemical decomposition of urinary calculi. Lasers Surg Med. 1999;25:22–37.
22. Teichman JM, Vassar GJ, Bishoff JT, et al. Holmium:YAG lithotripsy yields smaller fragments than lithoclast, pulsed dye laser or electrohydraulic lithotripsy. J Urol. 1998;159:17–23.
23. Vassar GJ, Teichman JM, Glickman RD. Holmium:YAG lithotripsy efficiency varies with energy density. J Urol. 1998;160:471–6.
24. Dormia E. Dormia basket: standard technique, observations, and general concepts. Urology. 1982;20:437.
25. Zeltser IS, Bagley DH. Basket design as a factor in retention and release of calculi in vitro. J Endourol. 2007;21:337–42.
26. Monga M, Hendlin K, Lee C, et al. Systematic evaluation of stone basket dimensions. Urology. 2004;63:1042–4.
27. Bagley D, Ramsay K, Zeltser I. An update on ureteroscopic instrumentation for the treatment of urolithiasis. Curr Opin Urol. 2004;14:99–106.
28. Honey RJ. Assessment of a new tipless nitinol stone basket and comparison with an existing flat-wire basket. J Endourol. 1998; 12:529–31.
29. Chew BH, Denstedt JD. Chapter 45: Ureteroscopy and retrograde ureteral access. In: Campbell MF, Walsh PC, editors. Urology. 9th edn, Vol. II. Philadelphia: Saunders; 2007. p. 1508–25.
30. Grabe M. Controversies in antibiotic prophylaxis in urology. Int J Antimicrob Agents. 2004;23 Suppl 1:S17–23.
31. Amin M. Antibacterial prophylaxis in urology: a review. Am J Med. 1992;92:114S–7.
32. Herrell SD, Buchanan MG. Flank position ureterorenoscopy: new positional approach to aid in retrograde caliceal stone treatment. J Endourol. 2002;16:15–8.
33. Afane JS, Olweny EO, Bercowsky E, et al. Flexible ureteroscopes: a single center evaluation of the durability and function of the new endoscopes smaller than 9Fr. J Urol. 2000;164:1164–8.
34. Borboroglu PG, Amling CL, Schenkman NS, et al. Ureteral stenting after ureteroscopy for distal ureteral calculi: a multi-institutional prospective randomized controlled study assessing pain, outcomes and complications. J Urol. 2001;166:1651–7.
35. Denstedt JD, Wollin TA, Sofer M, et al. A prospective randomized controlled trial comparing nonstented versus stented ureteroscopic lithotripsy. J Urol. 2001;165:1419–22.
36. Deliveliotis C, Giannakopoulos S, Louras G, et al. A double-pigtail stents for distal ureteral calculi: an alternative form of definitive treatment. Urol Int. 1996;57:224–6.
37. Harmon WJ, Sershon PD, Blute ML, et al. Ureteroscopy: current practice and long-term complications. J Urol. 1997;157:28–32.
38. Bugg Jr CE, El-Galley R, Kenney PJ, et al. Follow-up functional radiographic studies are not mandatory for all patients after ureteroscopy. Urology. 2002;59:662–7.
39. Galvin DJ, Pearle MS. The contemporary management of renal and ureteric calculi. BJU Int. 2006;98:1283–8.
40. Fabrizio MD, Behari A, Bagley DH. Ureteroscopic management of intrarenal calculi. J Urol. 1998;159:1139–43.
41. Preminger GM, Assimos DG, Lingeman JE, et al. Chapter 1: AUA guideline on management of staghorn calculi: diagnosis and treatment recommendations. J Urol. 2005;173:1991–2000.
42. Gupta PK. Is the holmium:YAG laser the best intracorporeal lithotripter for the ureter? A 3-year retrospective study. J Endourol. 2007;21:305–9.
43. Grasso M, Beaghler M, Loisides P. The case for primary endoscopic management of upper urinary tract calculi: II. Cost and outcome assessment of 112 primary ureteral calculi. Urology. 1995; 45:372–6.
44. Grasso M. Experience with the holmium laser as an endoscopic lithotrite. Urology. 1996;48:199–206.
45. Stav K, Cooper A, Zisman A, et al. Retrograde intrarenal lithotripsy outcome after failure of shock wave lithotripsy. J Urol. 2003;170: 2198–201.
46. Shepherd P, Thomas R, Harmon EP. Urolithiasis in children: innovations in management. J Urol. 1988;140:790–2.

47. Ritchey M, Patterson DE, Kelalis PP, et al. A case of pediatric ureteroscopic lasertripsy. J Urol. 1988;139:1272–4.
48. Koura AC, Ravish IR, Amarkhed S, et al. Ureteroscopic stone management in prepubertal children. Pediatr Surg Int. 2007;23:1123–6.
49. Smaldone M, Cannon Jr GM, Wu HY, et al. Is ureteroscopy first line treatment for pediatric stone disease? J Urol. 2007;178:2128–31.
50. Satar N, Zeren S, Bayazit Y, et al. Rigid ureteroscopy for the treatment of ureteral calculi in children. J Urol. 2004;172:298–300.
51. Tan AH, Al-Omar M, Denstedt JD, et al. Ureteroscopy for pediatric urolithiasis: an evolving first-line therapy. Urology. 2005;65:153–6.
52. Nerli RB, Patil SM, Guntaka AK, et al. Flexible ureteroscopy for upper ureteral calculi in children. J Endourol. 2011;25:579–82.
53. Reddy PP. Pediatric ureteroscopy. Urol Clin North Am. 2004; 31:145–56.
54. Rubenstein RA, Zhao LC, Loeb S, et al. Prestenting improves ureteroscopic stone-free rates. J Endourol. 2007;21:1277–80.
55. Gupta R, Manohar T, Desai MR. Antegrade flexible ureteroscopy in supine position for impacted multiple ureteric calculi. Indian J Urol. 2006;22:139–41.
56. Reddy PP, Nishinaka K, DeFoor W. Ureteroscopy is safe and effective in prepubertal children. J Endourol. 2003;17:A212.
57. Geavlete P, Georgescu D, Niţă G, Mirciulescu V, Cauni V. Complications of 2735 retrograde semirigid ureteroscopy procedures: a single-center experience. J Endourol. 2006;20:179–85.

Percutaneous Nephrolithotomy (PCNL)

51

Mahesh R. Desai and Arvind P. Ganpule

Abstract

The techniques and technology for management of stones has evolved rapidly over the past 30 years. Percutaneous nephrolithotomy (PCNL) is the preferred modality for kidney stone management; the usual indications for PCNL include stones larger than 20 mm^2, staghorn, partial staghorn calculi, and stones in patients with chronic kidney disease. Various modifications of the procedure such as "miniperc," "multiperc," and tubeless PCNL have been described. In this chapter, we review the technique of PCNL and also allude to the various modifications.

The method of access and tract dilatation is a matter of the operator's preference. If safety measures are followed, the complications can be minimized and even prevented. Special situations such as PCNL in pediatric cases or anomalous kidneys should be handled by surgeons with adequate experience. Training in a surgical skills laboratory is useful for honing the skills of percutaneous surgery.

Keywords

Percutaneous nephrolithotomy (PCNL) • PCNL training • Pediatric PCNL • PCNL complications • Ectopic kidney PCNL • PCNL anomalous kidney

Introduction

Goodwin and colleagues were the first to describe percutaneous renal access; interestingly, their drainage tube was placed without imaging [1]. The first percutaneous renal surgery was performed by Fernstorm and Johnson in 1976. The patient was noted to have a stone in the nephrostomy tract, which was successfully removed [2]. Since the description of this percutaneous procedure, the specialty of endourology has grown by leaps and bounds.

The techniques and technology for stone management has evolved rapidly over the past 30 years. Percutaneous nephrolithotomy (PCNL) is the preferred option for managing stones in the kidney [3]. Various modifications of the procedure such as "miniperc," [4] "multiperc," [5] and tubeless [6] PCNL have been described. This chapter reviews the technique of PCNL and also alludes to the various modifications.

Indications

Technically, most renal stones can be managed with a percutaneous nephrolithotomy. However, the usual indications for PCNL are stones larger than 20 mm^2, staghorn, partial staghorn calculi, and stones in patients with chronic kidney disease [7].

Since the landmark publication by Blandy and Singh in 1976 [8], wherein they emphasize the need for an aggressive approach for the management of staghorn calculi, percutaneous nephrolithotomy has become the treatment of choice

M.R. Desai, M.S., FRCS (✉) • A.P. Ganpule, M.S., DNB, MNAMS
Department of Urology, Muljibhai Patel Urological Hospital,
Dr. Virendra Desai Road, Nadiad, Gujarat 387001, India
e-mail: mrdesai@mpuh.org; doctorarvind1@gmail.com

J.J. Talati et al. (eds.), *Urolithiasis*,
DOI 10.1007/978-1-4471-4387-1_51, © Springer-Verlag London 2012

for such stones. These findings have been further ratified by others [9], while the American Urological Association (AUA) guidelines now recommend percutaneous surgery in this group of patients [3].

Preoperative Evaluation

The preoperative evaluation routinely includes appropriate blood investigations such as complete blood count, coagulation profile, and serum creatinine. In addition, urine microscopy and culture sensitivity are regularly performed. All PCNL patients receive the appropriate culture-sensitive antibiotics prior to the procedure and are evaluated for comorbidities such as diabetes, hypertension, infection, and renal insufficiency. Any concomitant anemia is evaluated and corrected prior to surgical intervention.

Preoperative Imaging

The access in PCNL can be planned with intravenous urography (IVU), renal ultrasound, and three-dimensional (3D) contrast-enhanced computed tomography (CT) with reconstruction. A standard X-ray of the kidneys-ureters-bladder (KUB) is the first imaging modality for the diagnosis of stone disease. Ultrasound examination, if done by the surgeon preoperatively, offers a wealth of information. The degree of hydronephrosis, the cortical thickness, and the location of stone can be ascertained. If an ultrasound-guided puncture is being contemplated for the procedure, the surgeon can decide the line and path of puncture preoperatively. Excretory urography has been the gold standard in the workup for urolithiasis and is very helpful in planning the number and location of punctures. Contrast-enhanced CT has been described as a modality for preoperative imaging; the maximum intensity projection images and VR images improvably help to map the pelvicalyceal system (Fig. 51.1). In addition, 3DCT also captures images of the adjacent abdominal organs, which can help predict potential hazards [10, 11].

The Procedure

Positioning

Proper positioning is crucial for obtaining the correct percutaneous access. The anesthetist and the surgeon are responsible for preventing slippage of the endotracheal tube and cushioning the patient's pressure points (Fig. 51.2). The patient's arms supported both at the elbow and the neck; however, the placement of the supporting bolsters may differ from one surgeon to another. Few surgeons opt not to use a support bolster, while others position one under the abdomen. The bolsters should be firm and may be made up of towels, particularly for pediatric patients. At our center, we prefer to place the bolsters below the iliac crest and the lower chest, which allows the abdominal pannus to droop down and help avoid possible bowel injury (see Fig. 51.2).

Retrograde Ureteric Access

Prior to percutaneous access, a retrograde ureteric catheter, preferably a 5 or 6 Fr, is inserted periurethrally (Fig. 51.3). Placing a ureteric catheter serves the following purposes:

1. It acts as a conduit for opacification of the pelvicalyceal system for retrograde contrast instillation.
2. It facilitates continuous saline administration, which helps distend the pelvicalyceal system; this is particularly helpful if an ultrasound-guided puncture is contemplated. The egress of clear fluid assures the proper positioning of the dilators during the procedure.
3. It aids the passage of retrograde or antegrade double-J stents, intraoperatively or postoperatively.
4. The ureteric catheter also acts as guide beyond which dilatation should not proceed.
5. If a double-J stent is not placed during the procedure, a ureteric catheter can be placed alone for 48 h.
6. If an occlusion or ureteric catheter is placed retrograde, it can help prevent the migration of fragmented stones into the upper ureter.

Selection of Calyx for Access

The method of access is a matter of surgeon preference, which largely depends on his or her training and the equipment available. The basic tenet to achieve a perfect percutaneous access is having a tract/puncture that is short and straight, with the minimal possible distance from the skin to the concerned calyx. The location of the stone, the burden, and the anatomy will dictate the site of puncture. A solitary stone within a calyx may necessitate a stone-bearing calyx puncture. The case objective should be to clear the maximum stone bulk with a minimum number of tracts.

The access needles and guidewires are the "key" instruments needed for optimal access. The access needles can be 18 or 21 gauge and can be either two part or three part. The 18-gauge needle helps to admit a 0.035- and 0.038-in. guide- or glidewire. The stiffness of the shaft is responsible for the "echoreflective" property of the needle; this property is of great importance when gaining ultrasound-guided access. An available "echotip" needle has enhanced echoreflective

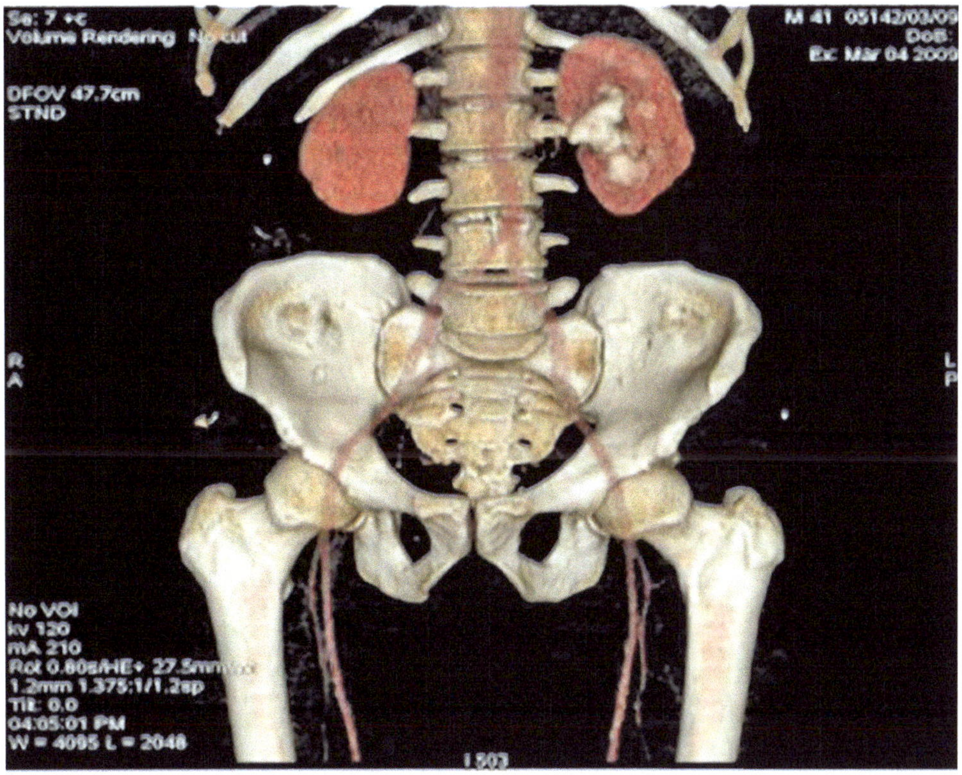

Left kidney staghorn calculus - volume rendered image

Fig. 51.1 Three-dimensional contrast-enhanced computed tomography scan helps to assess preoperatively the pelvicalyceal anatomy

property, making it easily observable on ultrasound. The 21-gauge needle, on the other hand, solely admits a 0.038 guidewire. A three-part needle helps to instill contrast without removing the stylet.

Percutaneous Renal Access

Access can be gained with either ultrasound or fluoroscopic guidance. Occasionally, the access can be gained with retrograde access devices as well.

Ultrasound-Guided Access

The ultrasound-guided access has the distinct advantage of minimizing radiation and allowing visualization of the intervening structures. The key to a successful ultrasound-guided puncture is the visualization of the needle along the path. Once the calyx to be punctured is identified, the ultrasound scan commences at the posterior axillary line; the first calyx sighted is the posterior calyx; clear urine indicates a proper puncture (Fig. 51.4). This method can be technically demanding, and the path may, at times, be ascertained by "jiggling" the needle along the access route.

The application of ultrasound guidance as the modality for access has been applied in pediatric PCNL and even in ectopic kidney PCNL [12].

Fluoroscopy-Guided Access

Under this methodology, the targeted calyx is identified via fluoroscopy, and an 18-gauge needle is directed into the calyx. A mediolateral adjustment of the needle will show the point of entrance to the calyx, while cephalad or caudal adjustments of the needle show the depth of penetration. The C-arm should be rotated obliquely as much as possible relative to the needle axis. It remains crucial that the orientation of the needle is maintained in both the planes; an aspiration of clear urine aids in affirming the proper position of the needle.

Retrograde Renal Access

Such can be gained using ureteroscopic guidance or retrograde access devices.

Ureteroscopically Assisted Percutaneous Access

Under direct vision, a flexible ureteroscope can be advanced to select the exact calyx of interest. A fluoroscopically guided percutaneous puncture is performed using the distal end of the ureteroscope as a landmark, and an antegrade guidewire is both advanced and withdrawn through the urethra. With this through and through, guidewire access is gained.

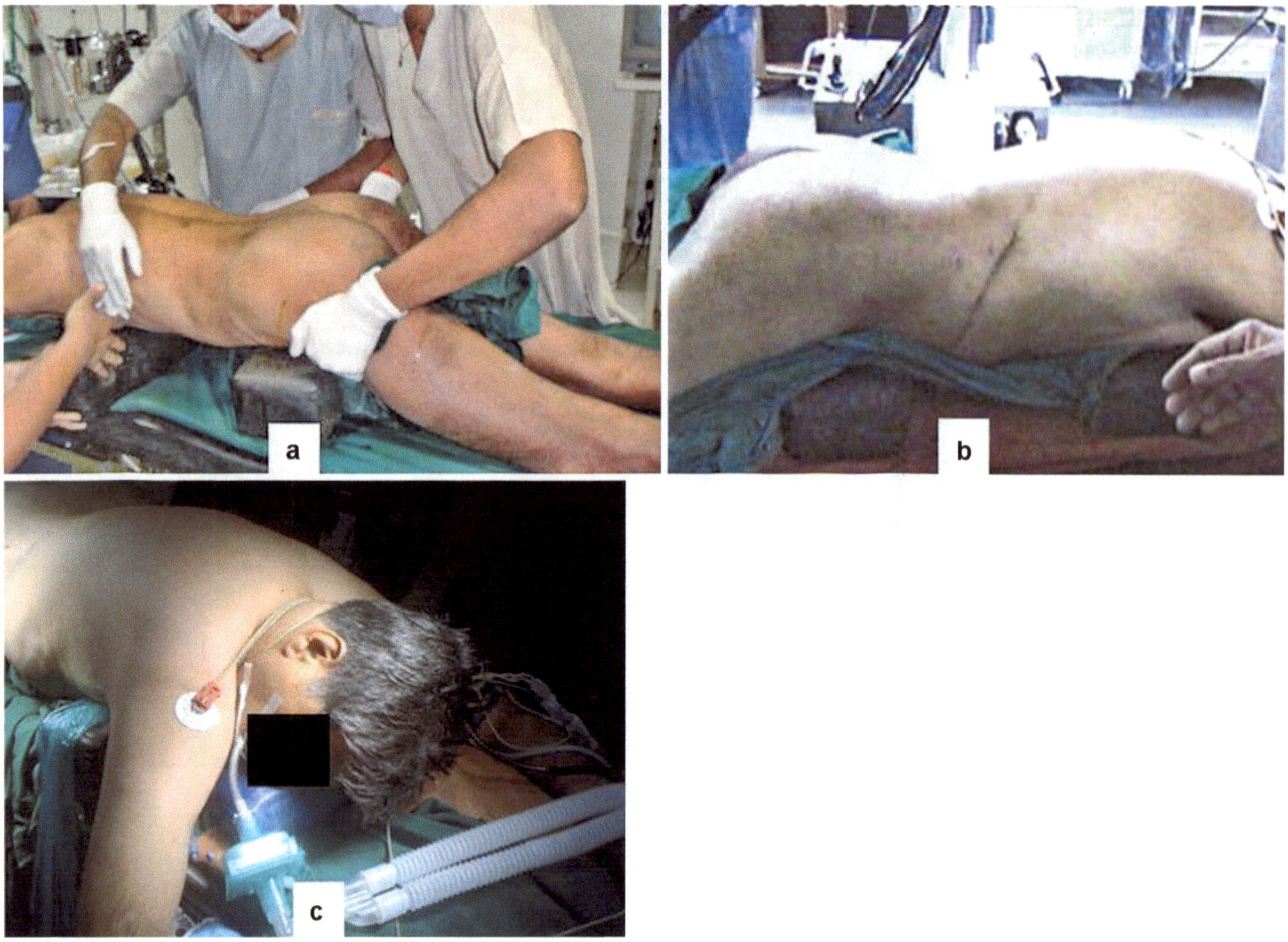

Fig. 51.2 (**a**) An adequate number of assistants should be available for proper positioning of the patient. (**b**) The chapter authors prefer to place a bolster below the hip and the chest during PCNL. (**c**) The endotracheal tube and the pressure points should be padded

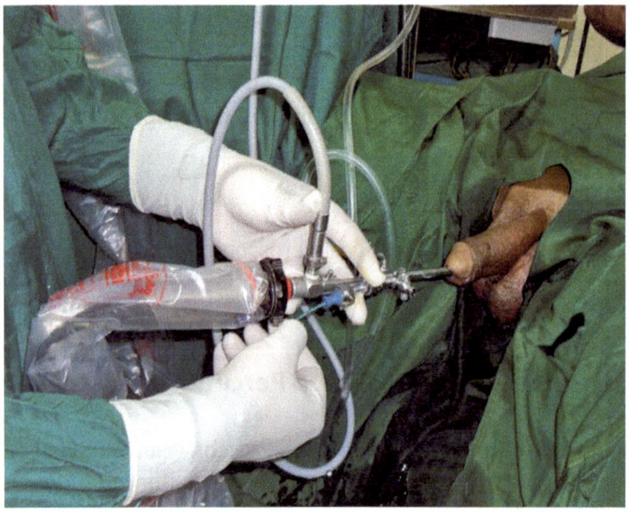

Fig. 51.3 The ureteric catheter is mandatory prior to gaining access

Retrograde Percutaneous Access

Retrograde percutaneous access to the kidney can be obtained using the Lawson retrograde nephrostomy wire puncture set (Cook Urological; Spencer, IN). Retrograde contrast study is performed, and a floppy-tip 0.038-in. guidewire is then advanced into the collecting system. Following, a 7.5-Fr Torcon deflectable catheter is passed over the guidewire, which is then removed through the skin. A posterior calyx is the calyx that is selected by these preceding steps [13].

Optical Puncture System

Recently, an "all see through" optical puncture needle has been described for percutaneous renal access. The assembly consists of microptics, with an integrated light lead inserted

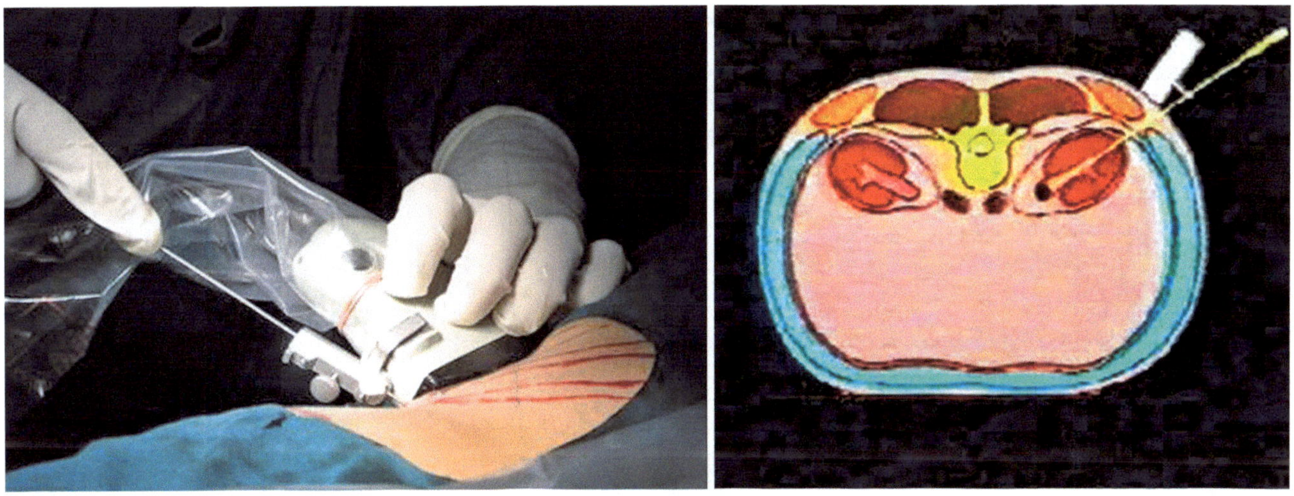

Fig. 51.4 The needle housed in the needle attachment helps in accurate access. (**a**) The needle housed in the needle attachment helps in accurate access. (**b**) The ultrasound guided access helps in gaining a straight tract from the skin to the calyx

through the sheath of the puncture needle, and an incorporated irrigation system for vision. Although still investigational, the authors concluded that optical puncture needle appears helpful for confirming optimal percutaneous access prior to dilatation of the tract [14].

Insertion of Safety Wire

Once there is egress of clear urine (Fig. 51.5), a hydrophilic guidewire is passed preferably into the ureter or a distal calyx. Once the guidewire is in position, the authors prefer to dilate the tract with single-step screw dilator. If a guidewire is utilized here, care should be taken to prevent kinking of the wire. Once the tract is dilated, a safety guidewire can be placed using a telescopic metallic two-part needle. Through this coaxial needle, a second guidewire is passed—this acts as a safety guidewire. The primary guidewire acts as a conduit over which the tract can be dilated using variety of dilator instruments. On basic principle, the axis of the tract should be maintained while one is dilating; the ureteric catheter inserted at the commencement of the procedure acts as a guide beyond which the dilators should not move. The central rod (in the case of metallic dilators) or the Teflon catheter (in the case of Amplatz dilators) should be held in position to avoid this problem.

Tract Dilatation

Available methods of dilatation include serial fascial dilators, Amplatz renal dilator sets, metal coaxial dilators (Alkens dilators), and high-pressure balloon systems. Each of which has its own advantages and disadvantages.

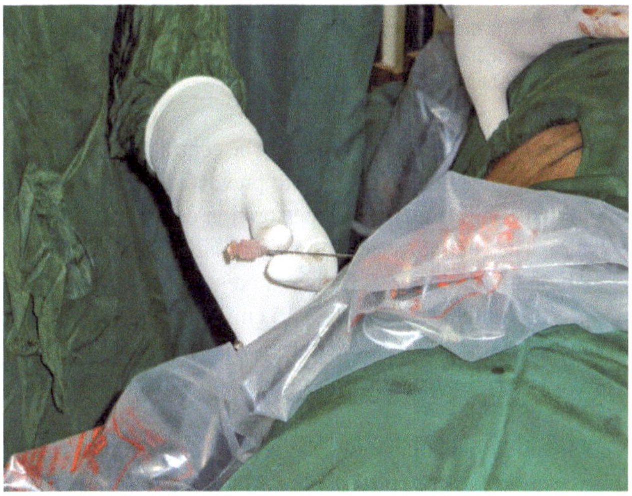

Fig. 51.5 A proper puncture is confirmed with return of clear fluid

The fascial dilators are inexpensive and, however, require multiple insertions and run the risk of kinking and buckling the guide-/glidewires. Theoretically, this practice seems difficult for dilating in obese patients. In our opinion, these dilators are associated with more oozing.

The telescopic metal dilators (Alkens dilators) are available with an 8-Fr central rod, which is passed over a guidewire; the serial dilators vary in size. The tract can be dilated up to 26 Fr (Fig. 51.6). The metallic "nob" at the center of the central rod helps to prevent under or over dilatation, as the stiffness and rigidity of the system help to dilate the tract

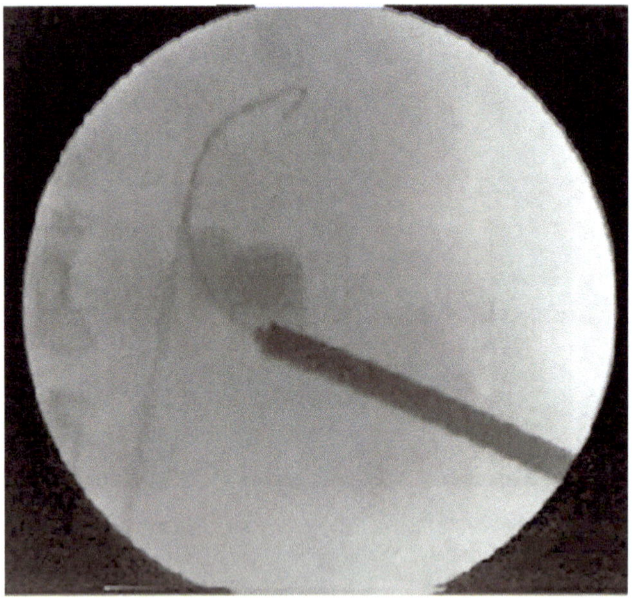

Fig. 51.6 The metallic telescopic dilator has a knob at the tip, as seen in the figure, that prevents over dilatation. The guidewire is seen safely coiled in a distant calyx

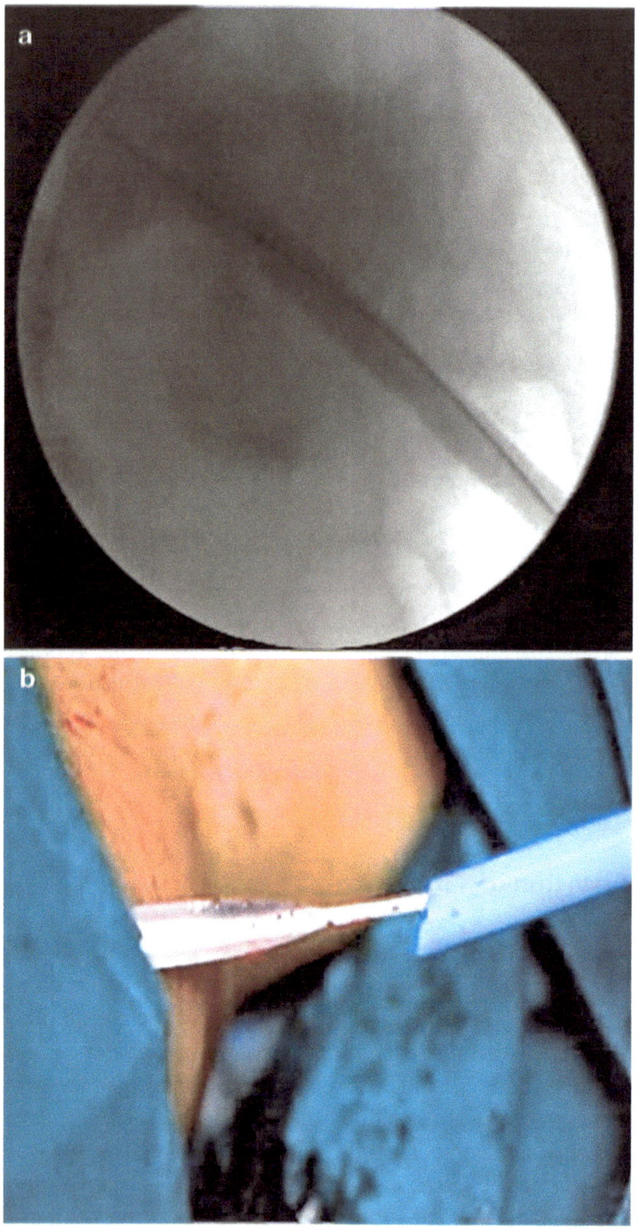

Fig. 51.7 The balloon dilator produces a pressure of 30 atm and is a one-step dilator. (**a**) The balloon dilator produces a pressure of 30 atm and is a one-step dilator. (**b**) The Amplatz sheath is inserted over the balloon dilator

even in dense perinephric scarring. The central rod does, however, need to be held in position to prevent inadvertent movement that could cause medial perforation of the pelvicalyceal system. The central rod additionally stabilizes the guidewire.

The balloon dilators produce a pressure of up to 30 atm (Fig. 51.7) and have a length of 15 cm. The advantage of balloon dilators is that they are easy to use and they generate a lateral rather than angular force. The disadvantages being that they are not effective in dilating tough tissues and may require additional dilatation with rigid dilators in some cases. Furthermore, these instruments are the most expensive among the available dilator options.

The Amplatz dilator set has an 8-Fr coaxial dilator, which is inserted over a guidewire. This assembly prevents buckling of the guidewire and has a maximum size of 30 Fr. An additional advantage is the availability of a wide range of sheaths that are compatible with the set's variety of dilators (Fig. 51.8).

Stone Fragmentation

Stones as small as 10 mm in size can be extracted intact through an appropriate-sized working sheath. However, most of the stones treated today will require some amount of fragmentation. The stone can be fragmented with a variety of energy sources available that include holmium laser, pneumatic lithotripsy, and a combination of ultrasonic and pneumatic energy. Laser fragmentation is slow and can be used for soft, small stones. Pneumatic energy is useful for breaking harder stones into large fragments.

The combination of ultrasound and pneumatic lithotripsy will facilitate quick fragmentation, particularly in hard stones. The stones should not be fragmented into small fragments, as these tend to migrate into distant calyces and become difficult to remove. The stones can be removed with triflange or biflange forceps, or alternatively, with a dormia basket.

In the event of migration of stones into a distant calyx, the options available are the use of a flexible nephroscope, creation of an additional tract and direct extraction of the stone, and/or use of a saline or puncture wash. The use of a suction

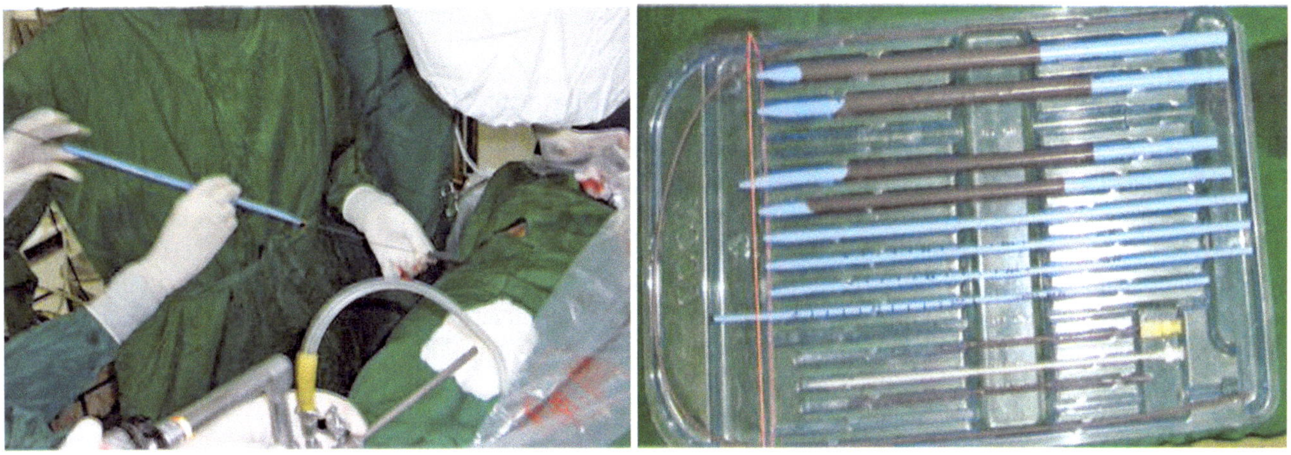

Fig. 51.8 The Amplatz dilator is advanced over a coaxial catheter. It is available as a set of dilators

channel in these stones helps in faster evacuation of fragments.

Postoperative Drainage

The decision to place a nephrostomy tube or otherwise is at the discretion of the surgeon and often depends on the location and size of the stone, as well as intraoperative findings.

At our center, the policy is to insert a nephrostomy if the procedure is done for a calyceal stone or an unimpacted pelvic stone. We prefer to place a 20-Fr Nelaton; the nephrostomy remains clamped for 6 h. The current literature is mutually supportive of and against the placement of nephrostomy. The advantage of the modality is adequate renal drainage, tamponade of renal tract, and the allowance of mature tract for a second-look procedure. The advantages of a tubeless PCNL are less pain and discomfort and a shorter hospital stay. The downside of tubeless PCNL is its feasibility only in a selected population; additionally, there is a possibility of missed residual stone fragment (4–5 mm, invisible on initial postoperative fluoroscopy) that later becomes apparent, and the tubeless operation precludes a "second-look" procedure [15].

A recent meta-analysis has suggested that tubeless PCNL should be carried out only for a select few cases. Those suitable cases are characterized by stone burden of <3 cm, single-tract access, no significant residual stones, no perforation, minimal bleeding, and no requirement for a secondary procedure [15].

Management of Complications

Complications occur both during and after percutaneous nephrolithotomy. Proper case selection, preparation, and application of technique are important. The reported incidence of major complications following PCNL is 0.9–4.7 % for septicemia, 0.6–14 % for renal hemorrhage, 2.3–3.1 % for pleural injury, and 0.2–0.8 % for colonic injury [16]. Similarly, a large multicenter analysis of 96 sites with more than 5,000 patients showed a complication rate of 7.8 % for bleeding, among those more than 5 % required blood transfusions [17].

Prevention of Complications

Measures that can prevent complications are as follows:

1. Manipulation of the pelvicalyceal system should be done under endoscopic or fluoroscopic control.
2. Reduce the amount of fluid absorption by restricting the nephroscopy time.
3. Use of an open system such as an Amplatz sheath should theoretically help keep the pelvic pressure low and decrease the incidence and amount of absorption.
4. In case of major perforations, the procedure should be terminated. In such cases, a nephrostomy tube should be placed.
5. The collecting system should be punctured in the posterior calyx.
6. The dilatation should proceed to the tip of the calyx.
7. In the event that bleeding hampers vision, the tract can be tamponaded temporarily before restarting the procedure. If the bleeding is persistent, the procedure can be staged.
8. In cases where severe postoperative bleeding causes hemodynamic instability, an angioembolization ought to be considered.
9. Documenting sterile urine prior to intervention is mandatory.
10. On occasions where purulent urine is seen after the initial puncture, the collecting system should be drained with a nephrostomy [18, 19].

Special Considerations

PCNL in Horseshoe Kidneys

Stones in horseshoe kidney can be tackled by PCNL effectively. The access to these kidneys can be gained via ultrasound or fluoroscopy guidance. Horseshoe kidneys are low placed; hence, upper calyx access in these cases does not often require supracostal access, which lends to the avoidance of attendant complications. At times, specialized equipment such as long nephroscopes may be necessary. At our center, we prefer to employ multiple tracts and use flexible nephroscopy for stones in inaccessible calyces. Although novel and not commonly used, the laparoscopic approach for tackling horseshoe stones is described for pyelolithotomy and guiding percutaneous renal access [20]. Maheshwari et al. described a case wherein a preoperative CT scan was suggestive of an unfavorable vascular and pelvicalyceal anatomy for a routine renal access; the patient was offered laparoscopic-guided access, and the stone was in the dilated isthmic calyx of the kidney [21].

PCNL in Ectopic and Fused Kidneys

Percutaneous renal access can be gained either with laparoscopic assistance or sonography guidance. The approach depends on the surgeon's expertise and the available equipment.

Ultrasound-Guided PCNL in Ectopic Kidney

This procedure is usually done under general anesthesia. After a retrograde catheterization, the pelvicalyceal system is opacified. The patient will be placed in a supine oblique position with a bolster under the ipsilateral hemipelvis. Pressure on the ultrasound probe is used to displace the bowel away from the puncture line. The dilatation is performed with telescopic dilators, and contrast study follows at the end of the procedure. In a study by Desai et al., none of the patients had any bowel injury, while all had complete clearance on follow-up. The average hemoglobin drop was 0.9/dL, and the average hospital stay was 5.2 days [12].

Laparoscopy Guidance for Access

This approach for stone management in ectopic kidneys has gained acceptance and is now commonly practiced. The procedure is performed with the patient in a Trendelenburg position after a ureteric catheter has been inserted. Once pneumoperitoneum is established, a 10-mm port and two 5-mm ports are placed in the umbilicus, the midclavicular line at level of the umbilicus, and the iliac fossa, respectively. The puncture needle is introduced under laparoscopic and fluoroscopic guidance; once clear fluid is aspirated, the rest of the procedure is performed as in standard PCNL [22].

Supine or Prone PCNL

Traditionally, PCNL has been performed in the prone position, first described by Valdevia et al. [23]. The stated advantages of the prone position are easy access to the posterior calyx, minimal chance of bowel injury, and wide surface area for the manipulation and creation of tract. A major disadvantage of the prone position is that it causes respiratory compromise and cannot be always performed in obese patients or those with poor cardiorespiratory function.

Positioning in a supine or modified supine position is less demanding, time consuming, and is more anesthesia-friendly (Fig. 51.9). A simultaneous ureteroscopic access can also be offered. Theoretically, as the tracts are inclined downward, the intrapelvic pressures are kept low. The surgeon may also perform the procedure while sitting for more comfort. The limitations of supine PCNL are limited space for manipulation and difficulty accessing the upper calyx [24].

Pediatric PCNL

PCNL in the pediatric age group with large complex stones poses a challenge for the surgeon. Pediatric PCNL has been performed in children as young as 19 months old [25]. PCNL offers good clearance rates in experienced hands, even for complex and complete staghorn stones, as described in the literature.

The special considerations in these young patients are:

1. The preoperative evaluation should be done with both an intravenous and CT urogram in cases with anomalous anatomy.
2. In these young patients, we employ ultrasound guidance to gain initial access. This reduces the risk to adjacent organs, particularly the spleen and liver.
3. The smaller the tract size, the better. The authors prefer to use an Amplatz sheath smaller than 20 Fr. Recently, tract size has further reduced to 14 Fr with the addition of a 14-Fr nephroscope in our armamentarium.
4. The combination of ultrasonic and pneumatic lithotripsy or laser lithotripsy helps in faster fragmentation and clearance of stones.

Miniperc

Miniperc PCNL was first described by Jackman et al. with a peel-away sheath, as opposed to its use for larger stones.

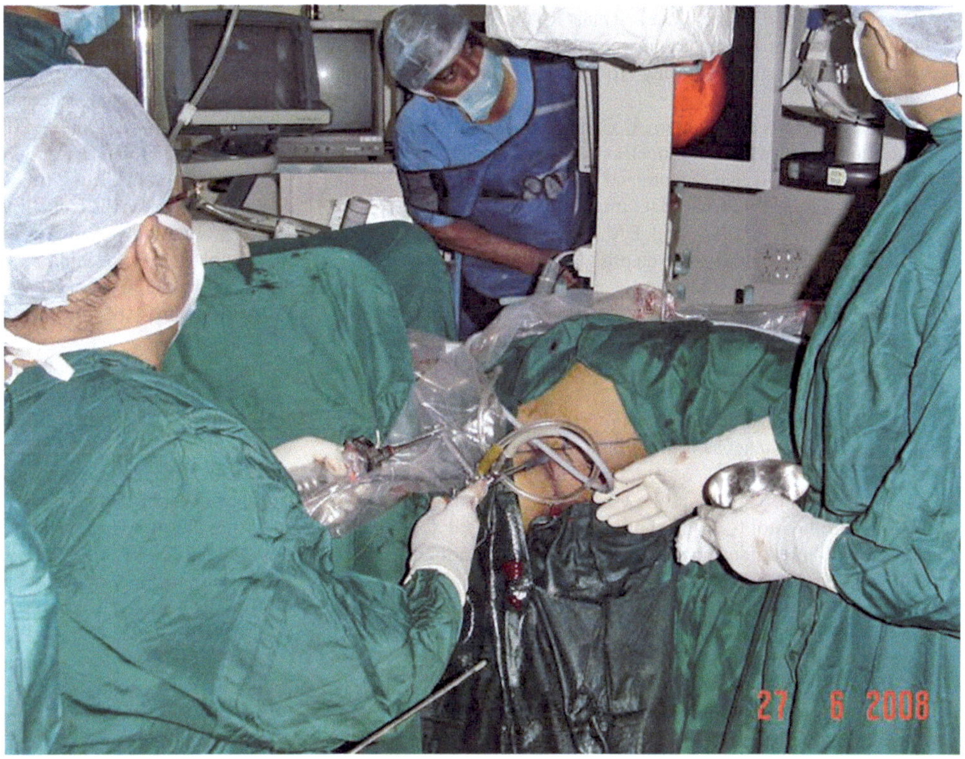

Fig. 51.9 The supine PCNL: positioning of the operator and the patient

With more experience, this technique has become useful for stones smaller than 2 cm. Although the definition of tract size varies, this term generally describes tracts smaller than 20 Fr. In a recently published study comparing mini-perc PCNL with standard PCNL, the mean tract size was 18.2 and 26 Fr, respectively. The authors found that the miniperc procedures had advantages of reduced bleeding and shorter hospital stay when compared to the standard PCNL group. The stone-free rates and complications were comparable in both [4].

PCNL Training

As with any other procedure, a novice needs to be trained in gaining percutaneous renal access prior to performing the procedure on the patient. A variety of training models have been described, which include both bench models and virtual reality simulators. The drawback of bench models is that the trainee is without tactile sensation. Hammond and coworkers have utilized a porcine kidney with pebbles (to simulate renal stones) within a chicken carcass as a training model [26]. On the other hand, virtual reality simulators do provide a real feel, are interactive, and provide a risk-free environment [27]. The Perc Mentor (Simbionix, Israel) is such a simulator that provides a tactile feedback to the trainee. A study by Mishra et al. compared PCNL training on porcine models to the Perc Mentor and showed that the Perc Mentor was superior for repetitive tasking and setup feasibility, while the porcine models were more realistic [28].

Conclusion

PCNL is the treatment of choice for large-volume renal calculi. The method of access and tract dilatation is a matter of surgeon preference. If safety measures are followed, complications are minimized and even can be prevented altogether. Special cases such as pediatric PCNL and anomalous kidneys should be done by surgeons with adequate experience. Training in a surgical skills laboratory is useful for honing the necessary skills for the procedure.

References

1. Goodwin JE, Casey WC, Woolf W. Percutaneous trocar (needle) nephrostomy in hydronephrosis. J Am Med Assoc. 1955; 157(11):891–4.
2. Fernström I, Johansson B. Percutaneous pyelolithotomy. A new extraction technique. Scand J Urol Nephrol. 1976;10(3):257–9.
3. Preminger GM, Assimos DG, Lingeman JE, et al. Nephrolithiasis guideline panel chapter 1 AUA guideline on management of staghorn calculi: diagnosis and treatment recommendation. J Urol. 2005;173:1991–2000.
4. Mishra S, Sharma R, Garg C, Kurien A, Sabnis R, Desai M. Prospective comparative study of miniperсs and standard PCNL for treatment of 1 to 2 cm size renal stone. BJU Int. 2011;108(6):896–9.

5. Desai M, Jain P, Ganpule A, Sabnis R, Patel S, Shrivastav P. Developments in technique and technology: effect on the results of percutaneous nephrolithotomy for staghorn calculi. BJU Int. 2009;104:542–8.
6. Mishra S, Sabnis RB, Kurien A, Ganpule A, Muthu V, Desai M. Questioning the wisdom of tubeless percutaneous nephrolithotomy (PCNL): a prospective randomized controlled study of early tube removal vs tubeless PCNL. BJU Int. 2010;106(7):1045–8.
7. Turk C, Knoll T, Petrik A, et al. EAU guidelines on urolithiasis. Eur Assoc Urol. 2010. www.uroweb.org/gls/pdf/18_Urolithiasis.pdf.
8. Blandy JP, Singh M. The case for a more aggressive approach to staghorn stones. J Urol. 1976;115(5):505–6.
9. Tiechman JM, Long RD, Hulbert JC. Long term renal fate and prognosis after staghorn calculus management. J Urol. 1995;153: 1403.
10. Aga P, Bansal R. Is intravenous urogram no longer an imaging of choice for percutaneous nephrolithotomy. Indian J Urol. 2010;26: 303–4.
11. Thiruchevallam N, Mostafid H, Ubhaykar G. Planning percutaneous nephrolithotomy using multidetector computed tomography urography, multiplanar reconstruction and 3D reformatting. BJU Int. 2005;95:1280–4.
12. Desai MR, Jasani A. Percutaneous nephrolithotripsy in ectopic kidneys. J Endourol. 2000;14(3):289–92.
13. Smith AD. Percutaneous management of the upper urinary tract, chapter 46. In: Gupta M, Ost MC, Shah JB, McDougall Wein EM, editors. Campbell-Walsh urology. 9th ed. Philadelphia: W.B. Saunders; 2007.
14. Bader MJ, Gratzke C, Seitz M, Sharma R, Stief CG, Desai M. The all-seeing needle: initial results of an optical puncture system confirming access in percutaneous nephrolithotomy. Eur Urol. 2011;59(6):1054–9.
15. Agrawal MS, Agrawal M. Tubeless percutaneous nephrolithotomy. Indian J Urol. 2010;26:16–24 (cited 2011 Apr 22).
16. Skolarikos A, De la Rossette J. Prevention and treatment of complications following percutaneous nephrolithotomy. Curr Opin Urol. 2008;18:229–34.
17. la Rossette D, Assimos D, Desai M, Gutierrez J, Lingeman J, Scarpa R, et al. The Clinical Research Office of the Endourological Society percutaneous nephrolithotomy global study: indications, complications, and outcomes in 5803 patients; CROES PCNL Study Group. J Endourol. 2011;25(1):11–7.
18. Michel SS, Trojan L, Rassweiler JJ. Complications in percutaneous nephrolithotomy. Eur Urol. 2007;51:899–906.
19. Lee WJ, Smith AD, Cubelli V, et al. Complications of percutaneous nephrolithotomy. AJR Am J Roentgenol. 1987;148:177–80.
20. Nambirajan T, Jeschke S, Albqami N, Abukora F, Leeb K, Janetschek G. Role of laparoscopy in management of renal stones: single centre experience and review of literature. J Endourol. 2005; 19:353–9.
21. Maheshwari PN, Bhandarkar DS, Shah RS, Andankar MG, Saple AL. Laparoscopic assisted transperitoneal percutaneous nephrolithotomy for recurrent calculus in isthmic calyx of horseshoe kidney. J Endourol. 2004;18:858–61.
22. Goel R, Yadav R, Gupta NP, Aron M. Laparoscopic assisted percutaneous nephrolithotomy (PCNL) in ectopic kidneys: two different techniques. Int Urol Nephrol. 2006;38(1):75–8.
23. Valdevia JG, Valle J, Lopez JA, et al. Technique and complications of percutaneous nephroscopy: experience with 557 patients in supine position. J Urol. 1998;160:1975–8.
24. De la Rosette JJ, Tsakiris P, Ferrandino MN, Elsakka AM, Rioja J, Preminger GM. Beyond prone position in percutaneous nephrolithotomy: a comprehensive review. Eur Urol. 2008;54:1262–9.
25. Callaway TW, Lingardh G, Basata S, Sylven M. Percutaneous nephrolithotomy in children. J Urol. 1992;148:1067–8.
26. Hammond L, Ketchum J, Schwartz BF. A new approach to urology training: a laboratory model for percutaneous nephrolithotomy. J Urol. 2004;172:1950–2.
27. Stern J, Zelster IS, Pearle MS. Percutaneous renal access simulators. J Endourol. 2007;21(3):270–3.
28. Mishra S, Kurein A, Ganpule A, Muthu V, Sabnis R, Desai M. Percutaneous renal access training: content validation comparison between a live porcine and a virtual reality(VR) simulation model. BJU Int. 2010;106:1753–6.

Tubeless Percutaneous Nephrolithotomy

52

Chong H. Choe, James O. L'Esperance, Suzanne R. Gudeman, and Brian K. Auge

Abstract

Tubeless percutaneous nephrolithotomy (PCNL) is a viable option and is actually preferred over the standard technique of nephrostomy tube placement by many surgeons. This chapter suggests modifications in the technique that allow tubeless PCNL to be performed safely.

Tubeless PCNL reduces postoperative pain, need for analgesics, hospital stay, and postoperative urinary leakage. "Totally" tubeless PCNL (in which even a ureteral stent is avoided) may be safely performed in select patients with similar advantages of tubeless PCNL. Tubeless PCNL is facilitated by the use of hemostatic agents—liquid products and flowable or gelatin matrix products. Matrix agents require a bleeding source for fibrinogen, whereas the fibrin sealants do not. Fibrin sealants have both hemostatic and adhesive properties. Since hemostasis and collecting system sealing of a fresh, unsutured percutaneous nephrostomy tract are desired, the use of the liquid sealants may prove to be better suited than the gelatin matrix substances for tubeless PCNL. Diathermal techniques may have a role in enhancing the tubeless PCNL technique, thereby obviating the need for additional hemostatic biomaterials.

Keywords

Percutaneous nephrolithotomy (PCNL) • Tubeless • Hemostatic agents • Risk • Hemorrhage • Flowable or gelatin matrix products • Fibrin sealants • Electrocautery

Introduction

The practice of placing a nephrostomy tube after percutaneous renal surgery was thought to aid in healing of the nephrostomy tract, promote tract hemostasis, drain urine and prevent extravasation, drain purulent material, and allow reentry into the kidney for future adjunct procedures [1]. Nephrostomy tubes of various sizes (5–32 F) and types have been used for this purpose [2–4]. In recent years, attempts have been made to modify the standard PCNL technique with a growing realization that substantial postoperative pain and morbidity after PCNL were caused by the presence of the nephrostomy tubes [1]. New experiences in the technique of tubeless PCNL have suggested that only a few indications still remain for the standard technique PCNL. Those include significant collecting system injury, excessive hemorrhage with poor visualization for placement of an antegrade stent, pyonephrosis necessitating reliable external drainage, or need for second-look procedure. Otherwise, tubeless PCNL is a viable option and is actually preferred over the standard technique of nephrostomy tube placement by many surgeons [5, 6].

C.H. Choe, M.D. (✉) • J.O. L'Esperance, M.D.
S.R. Gudeman, M.D.
Department of Urology, Naval Medical Center,
34800 Bob Wilson Drive, San Diego, CA 92134, USA
e-mail: chong.choe@med.navy.mil;
james.lesperance@med.navy.mil;
suzanne.gudeman@med.navy.mil

B.K. Auge, M.D.
Mountain States Urology,
510 N 2nd Street, Boise, ID 83702, USA
e-mail: brianauge@me.com

J.J. Talati et al. (eds.), *Urolithiasis*,
DOI 10.1007/978-1-4471-4387-1_52, © Springer-Verlag London 2012

The presence of a typical-sized nephrostomy tube (14–18 F) inserted following the standard PCNL technique causes the patient not only discomfort and pain, but it also causes increased hospital stay and increased analgesic use and is associated with increased incidence of urinary leakage around the nephrostomy tube site. Agrawal and associates performed a randomized comparison of a total of 202 patients of tubeless PCNL versus standard PCNL from 2002 to 2005. Their study demonstrated that the tubeless PCNL technique reduced postoperative urinary leakage and local pain related to the drainage tube. They also found tubeless PCNL minimized the patients' hospital stay [7]. Similarly, Al-Ba'adani and associates performed tubeless PCNL in 121 patients between 2004 and 2006 and, when compared to standard PCNL, concluded tubeless PCNL was a good option with the advantages of reduced hospital stay, lower overall postoperative pain, and decreased need for postoperative analgesia [8].

Investigators have further suggested that "totally" tubeless PCNL may be safely performed in select patients with similar advantages of tubeless PCNL [9–12]. "Totally" tubeless refers to the technique in which ureteral stents are not used unlike in other cases of tubeless PCNL in which ureteral stents were placed antegrade at the conclusion of the procedure. Karami and colleagues performed 30 totally tubeless PCNL and compared their results with those of a control group of 30 patients who underwent standard PCNL. They concluded the totally tubeless PCNL in select patients was safe and was associated with significantly reduced postoperative discomfort, length of hospitalization, and analgesic requirements [10]. Crook, et al. analyzed 100 totally tubeless PCNL in a 10-year period from 1996 to 2006 and concluded this technique was safe and well tolerated in select patients [11]. A prospective randomized trial of a total of 90 patients was then completed by Istanbulluoglu in 2007 which compared the totally tubeless PCNL to the standard PCNL group. Similar to others previously reporting on the totally tubeless technique, they concurred that this modification to the procedure was a safe method and reduced hospitalization time and analgesic requirements [12].

Hemostatic Agents

The United States Food and Drug Administration (FDA) defines hemostatic agents as substances intended to produce hemostasis by accelerating the clotting process of blood. With the surge in the advances in percutaneous endoscopic surgery and in the era of "minimally invasive" surgery, several adjunctive hemostatic agents have been proposed in order to achieve optimal intraoperative hemostasis. The most commonly used hemostatic agents in percutaneous stone surgery are the liquid products and the flowable or gelatin matrix products (Table 52.1). Both flowable and liquid products aid in augmenting the clotting cascade: the liquid products typically contain all the components necessary to produce a fibrin clot independent of the patient-derived factors, while the flowable gelatin materials provide a matrix for platelet adhesion and aggregation and aid in the formation of a clot when mixed with thrombin. The gelatin materials do not contain fibrinogen, therefore relies upon the patient's natural fibrinogen to undergo enzymatic activation by the thrombin provided in the matrix in order to form the fibrin clot. Moreover, the gelatin material will swell within the tract to 19–400 % greater than the applied volume, thereby theoretically adding to hemostasis by means of a compressive effect.

Fibrin Sealants

Fibrin sealants have been used in a wide range of surgical specialties since the 1970s. The first surgical liquid fibrin sealant to be approved in the United States was Tisseel® (Baxter Healthcare, Westlake Village, CA), which is utilized for hemostasis in cardiac surgery, splenic trauma, and liver surgery and for sealing colonic anastomosis (Figs. 52.1a, b). Since its initial approval in 1998, its use in multiple urologic procedures has been reported in the literature. There is a rise in trend in the use of fibrin sealants to obtain hemostasis in laparoscopic partial nephrectomy as well as in newer off-label use in urinary tract reconstruction and in percutaneous tract closure after tubeless PCNL [13] (Fig. 52.2).

The fibrin sealants have both hemostatic and adhesive properties. The mechanical strength of the fibrin matrix is ultimately determined by the relative concentration of fibrinogen versus thrombin, plus possibly factor XIII and/or *an* antifibrinolytic agent such as bovine aprotinin or tranexamic acid. A high thrombin concentration forms a more rapid meshwork, while a higher fibrinogen concentration induces a stronger meshwork but in a slower time period.

Tisseel is a four-component product consisting of vapor heat-treated human pooled plasma thrombin and fibrinogen along with a synthetic antifibrinolytic aprotinin and calcium chloride (Fig. 52.3). It is manufactured with aprotinin because it is not a plasminogen-free material and requires a stabilizer [14]. Baxter Corporation recently modified Tisseel to remove the bovine aprotinin to prevent sensitivity reactions such as skin rash, coagulopathy, anaphylaxis, and even death from preformed antibodies. Tisseel is applied by dripping the solutions onto the area of interest via applicator supplied within the package (see Fig. 52.3). This allows for immediate mixing of the components to form the clot. Once mixed, the solutions or applicator cannot be reused.

Evicel™ (Johnson & Johnson, Somerville, NJ) is a second-generation plasminogen-free pooled human plasma

Table 52.1 Comparison of commonly used hemostatic agents

	Agent	Components	Action	Prep time
Liquid agents	Tisseel (Baxter)	Fibrinogen Thrombin Synthetic aprotinin Calcium chloride	Clot formation Hemostasis Tissue sealing	20 min, requires mixing in Fibrinotherm machine
	Evicel (Johnson & Johnson)	Fibrinogen Thrombin	Clot formation Hemostasis Tissue sealing	<1 min
	Thrombin (several companies available)	Thrombin	Convert fibrinogen to fibrin for clot formation	30 s
Flowable agents	FloSeal (Baxter)	Flowable gelatin (bovine)	Provides matrix for platelet aggregation	1–2 min
		Thrombin (human)	Added thrombin aids in clot formation	
	Surgiflo (Johnson & Johnson)	Flowable gelatin (porcine)	Provides matrix for platelet aggregation	30 s
		Thrombin or saline	Added thrombin aids in clot formation	
	CoSeal (Baxter)	Synthetic hemostatic sealing agent	Mechanically seals areas of small vessel leakage	1–2 min

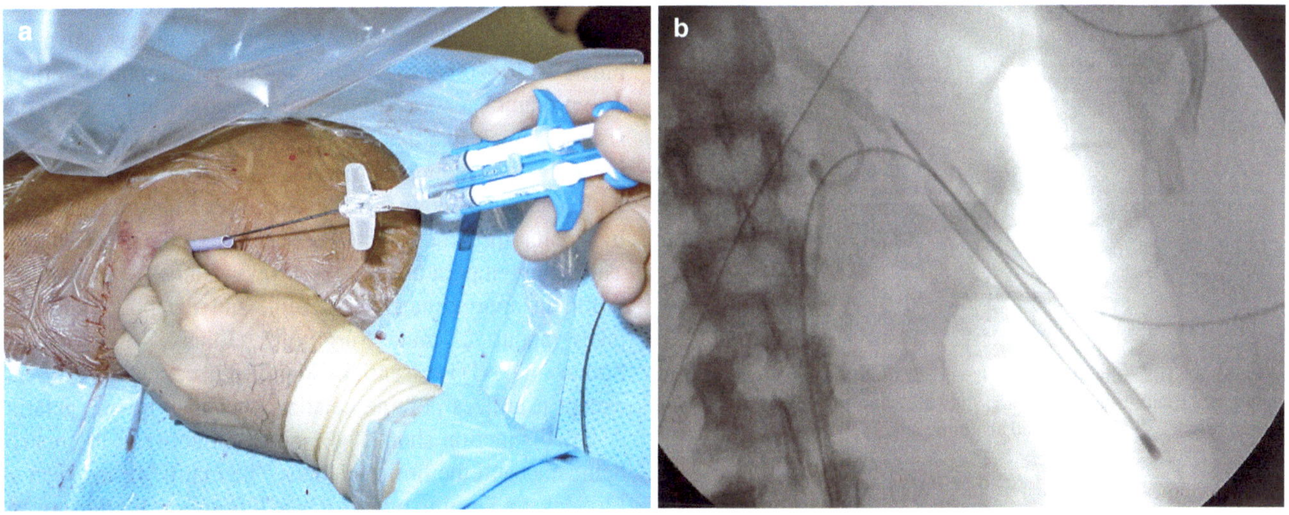

Fig. 52.1 (**a**) Application of fibrin sealant through the nephrostomy tract. (**b**) Fluoroscopic guidance is utilized to ensure proper positioning of the needle or applicator tip within the renal parenchymal defect

product (Fig. 52.4). The terms first generation and second generation refer to the presence or absence of animal products. Therefore, Evicel is an all-human plasma-derived fibrin sealant commercially available in the USA. However, as with all human pooled products, the potential for viral disease transmission exists. Although no unequivocally confirmed reports of viral disease transmission have been reported in approximately six million uses of this material, there are some scattered reports of possible hepatitis transmission associated with its use [15]. Evicel can also be dripped onto the area requiring hemostasis or can be sprayed on using a pressurized spray device. The applicator is a three-channeled device which prevents mixing of the components until they reach their intended target (Fig. 52.5).

The reconstitution of Baxter's Tisseel *does not* require thawing since it no longer requires refrigeration. However, it still requires the mixing steps that are done with the company-provided mechanical mixer. With the second-generation Evicel, it is possible to use the product more rapidly since preparation takes a matter of seconds, and the components can be refrigerated for up to a period of 30 days so they can be ready for more immediate use [16]. The components of unopened vials are stable at room temperature for 24 h.

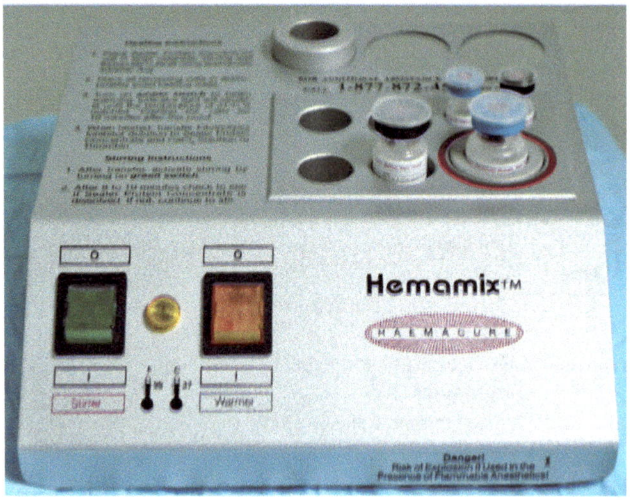

Fig. 52.2 Example of mechanical mixer required in the preparation of Tisseel

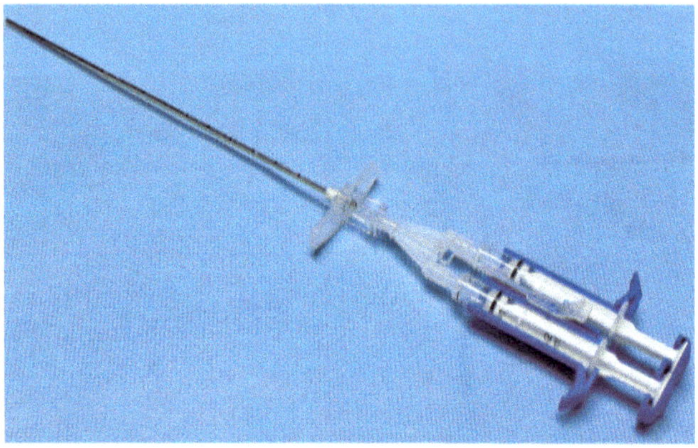

Fig. 52.3 The components of Tisseel are drawn up into two syringes and placed within the applicator, thus allowing for immediate mixing when dripped onto the desired anatomic site

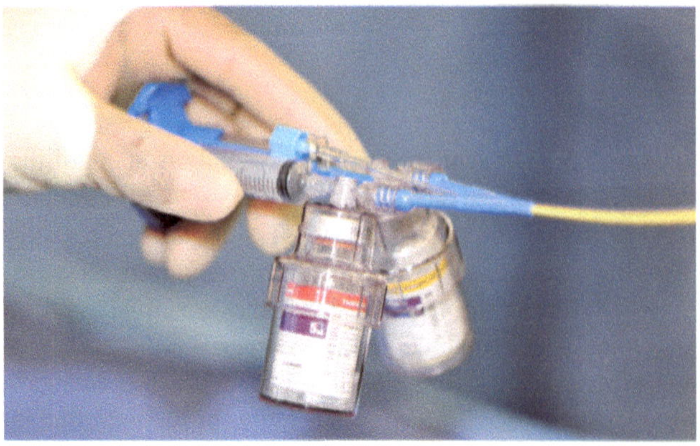

Fig. 52.4 Evicel (Johnson & Johnson, Somerville, NJ) is a second-generation fibrin sealant. The solutions (thrombin and fibrinogen) are premixed within separate vials allowing for easy preparation into the applicator syringes

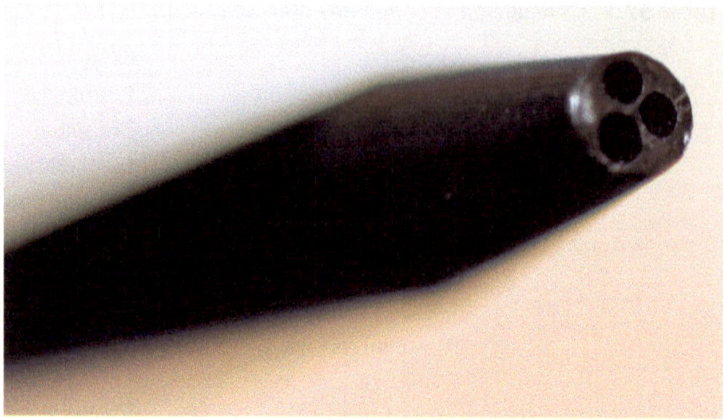

Fig. 52.5 The Evicel applicator contains three separate channels: one for thrombin, one for fibrinogen, and one capable of attaching to compressed air to allow for spray application. If spray is not desired, then the two solutions can alternatively be dripped onto the structure, thereby immediately mixing the solutions on contact to form the fibrin clot

Flowable Products

FloSeal® (Baxter Healthcare, Westlake Village, CA) is a matrix hemostat comprised of bovine gelatin protein and pooled human thrombin. The thrombin is mixed before use, and upon contact with blood, the matrix may swell by as much as 20–400 % providing additional tamponade effect. The product is expressed through the applicator with a consistency much like that of cream of wheat. Once applied to the actively bleeding source, it can be manually compressed with a surgical sponge, which increases the surface contact by forcing the product into the crevices of the tissue planes. The room temperature storage allows relatively rapid preparation in approximately 1–2 min, and the polymerization takes about 2 min. Surgiflo™ (Johnson & Johnson, Somerville, NJ) is essentially identical in concept to FloSeal, except it utilizes porcine gelatin rather than bovine gelatin. A key distinction should be mentioned between the matrix hemostats and the fibrin sealants. The matrix agents such as FloSeal and Surgiflo require a bleeding source for fibrinogen, whereas the fibrin sealants do not. Therefore, the matrix sealants are best suited for obtaining adjunctive hemostasis rather than for tissue adhesion and sealing. CoSeal™ (Baxter Healthcare, Westlake Village, CA) is a synthetic hemostatic sealing agent made of two polyethylene glycols (PEGs) primarily used to seal leaks around sutures (surgical stitches), staples, or other mechanical closure devices in natural or artificial blood vessels. To our knowledge, it has not been utilized in percutaneous renal procedures.

Electrocauterization/Diathermal Methods of Tract Closure

Diathermal techniques, such as those commonly performed during open or laparoscopic surgery (monopolar or bipolar cautery), have been utilized for nephrostomy tract bleeding during PCNL [17]. Jou et al. performed 249 consecutive PCNLs from 2001 to 2003 in which they used electrocauterization of bleeding points with an elongated electrode probe at the end of their tubeless procedure [18]. An 8 F elongated electrode probe which fits through the working channel of a nephroscope was used to provide spot electrocoagulation of various bleeding points along their nephrostomy tract. Their results demonstrated a statistically significant difference in the need for transfusion between the electrocauterized group (3/249 or 1.2 %) and the non-electrocauterized group (6/92 or 6.5 %). There were no differences in the operative time, hospital stay, or infections between the two groups. They concluded that the use of electrocoagulation of various bleeding points was safe and effective and significantly lowered the transfusion rate. The use of a rollerball electrode to electrocauterize the nephrostomy tract using a 26 F resectoscope at the end of the procedure has been effectively performed to control bleeding from the nephrostomy tract following tubeless PCNL [19].

Due to the limited data on the use of diathermal techniques for hemostasis following PCNL, we cannot conclude that it is without merit. In fact, the use of electrical energy to reduce hemorrhage may obviate the need for hemostatic agents, thereby reducing the potential for infectious complications, allergic reactions, and additional procedural costs. Conceptually, the destruction of tissue and the radiating effects of heat on the healing tissue could pose potential long-term problems with tract healing. Although spot electrocauterization of bleeding may provide some immediate benefit, the use of adjunctive hemostatic agents seems to provide not only hemostatic control but also a framework on which the tissues could heal and acute sealing of the urinary collecting system if applied properly.

Discussion

Concerns regarding the tubeless PCNL technique include inability for a "second look," inability to adequately drain an infected system, and the inability to monitor significant collecting system injury and excessive hemorrhage. For these reasons, the current literature which advocates tubeless PCNL stipulates it is a good option and preferable to standard PCNL in "select" cases.

Multiple randomized trials and cohort studies evaluating the safety and efficacy of fibrin sealants for its hemostatic and sealant properties in tubeless PCNL are present in the literature. Noller et al. assessed the usefulness and ability of fibrin sealants (Tisseel) to facilitate tubeless PCNL in select patients by demonstrating stable hematocrit in the early postoperative period and lack of hematoma or urinary extravasation on contrast-enhanced CT scan [20]. Mikhail and colleagues performed a retrospective review of 20 consecutive patients who underwent tubeless PCNL with 2–3-mL injection of Tisseel through the nephrostomy tract compared to a control group of 23 consecutive patients who underwent tubeless PCNL without Tisseel. The results were equivocal in that it did not show a statistically significant difference in hematocrit changes or in the amount of analgesia use between the Tisseel and non-Tisseel groups [21]. Shah and colleagues performed a prospective randomized trial in 2005 with a total of 32 patients who underwent Tisseel tubeless PCNL and compared them with a control group of 31 patients who underwent tubeless PCNL without Tisseel. They found there were no differences in the hematocrit changes or the need for blood transfusions in the two groups. However, they did note that the Tisseel tubeless PCNL group experienced less postoperative pain and required less analgesia [22].

Reports of other types of adjunctive hemostatic agents used to augment tubeless PCNL are present in the literature. However, agents such as the gelatin matrix hemostats and oxidized cellulose do not act as sealants and therefore bear little additional lattice or mesh-like strength to the renal parenchymal defect [23]. Surgicel (Johnson & Johnson Wound Management, Somerville, NJ) was placed in the nephrostomy tract after tubeless PCNL in ten randomized patients by Aghamir and associates, and when compared to the control group of ten patients whose tracts were unsealed, they did not notice any statistically significant difference in bleeding or extravasation from the tract. [24] Concerns for collecting system obstruction stem from reports by Clayman et al. demonstrating the inability for hemostatic agents to dissolve in human urine in vitro. They witnessed that FloSeal formed a fine suspension of particles in contact with urine, but other substances, such as the fibrin sealant Tisseel, created a thicker mucoid material which failed to dissolve after 5 days. [25] This potentially persistent material could settle within the ureteropelvic junction causing acute or subacute obstruction with subsequent morbidity related to that obstruction. Borin et al. reported on a technique for applying FloSeal into the tubeless PCNL nephrostomy tract utilizing a 7 F, 11.5-mm occlusion balloon catheter passed retrograde to the level of entry of the 30 F Amplatz sheath [26]. This occlusion balloon therefore would prevent the passage of gelatin matrix particles into the collecting system and prevent subsequent obstruction. It should be noted, however, that there are no current case reports or studies which implicate that the hemostatic agents have lithogenic properties. The use of gelatin matrix hemostats and liquid sealants in other urological procedures such as laparoscopic partial nephrectomy is established, yet again there is a paucity of evidence implicating lithogenic properties in gelatin matrix hemostats and liquid sealants. Since hemostasis and collecting system sealing of a fresh, unsutured percutaneous nephrostomy tract are desired, the use of the liquid sealants may prove to be better suited than the gelatin matrix substances for tubeless PCNL.

Conclusion

The trend in literature and its data support the technique of tubeless PCNL in select cases. To allay the fears of nephrostomy tract bleeding and extravasation of urine into the retroperitoneum with resultant morbidity, multiple authors advocate the use of adjunctive hemostatic agents. Primarily, the fibrin sealants have been used as the adjunctive hemostatic agent of choice due to its known properties of hemostatic and adhesive/sealing properties. Surprisingly, we discovered that fibrin sealant administration into the nephrostomy tract at the conclusion of the tubeless PCNL did not consistently result in significant decrease in postoperative bleeding or the need for blood transfusion. However, the patients in whom the hemostatic agents were used seemed to experience less postoperative pain. Flowable gelatin matrix agents may prove beneficial for procedures where robust bleeding is encountered if applied cautiously to avoid administration into the collecting system. Unfortunately, they have not been successful in providing collecting system sealing and, therefore, may not be as effective as a primary agent for routine uncomplicated procedures. Finally, diathermal techniques may have a role in enhancing the tubeless PCNL technique, thereby obviating the need for additional hemostatic biomaterials.

Randomized studies comparing fibrin sealants, flowable gelatin matrix materials, electrocautery, and no adjuncts should be conducted to assess the superior technique when performing tubeless PCNL. Furthermore, totally tubeless versus tubeless with a stent requires additional investigation.

Acknowledgement The views expressed in this article are those of the authors and do not reflect the official policy or position of the Department of the Navy, Department of Defense, or the United States government.

References

1. Pietrow PK, Auge BK, Lassas CD, Santa-Cruz RW, Newman GE, Albala DM, et al. Pain after percutaneous nephrolithotomy: impact of nephrostomy tube size. J Endourol. 2003;17:411–4.
2. Maheshwari PN, Andankar MG, Bansal M. Nephrostomy tube after percutaneous nephrolithotomy: large-bore versus pigtail catheter? J Endourol. 2000;14:735–8.
3. Desai MR, Kukreja RA, Desai MM, Mhaskar SS, Wani KA, Patel SH, et al. A prospective randomized comparison of type of nephrostomy drainage following percutaneous nephrostolithotomy: large bore versus small bore versus tubeless. J Urol. 2004;172:565–7.
4. Paul EM, Marcovich R, Lee BR, Smith AD. Choosing the ideal nephrostomy tube. BJU Int. 2003;92:672–7.
5. Bellman GC, Davidoff R, Candela J, Gerspach J, Kurtz S, Stout L. Tubeless percutaneous renal surgery. J Urol. 1997;157:1578–82.
6. Tefekli A, Altunrende F, Tepeler K, Tas A, Aydin S, Muslumanoglu AY. Tubeless percutaneous nephrolithotomy in selected patients: a prospective randomized comparison. Int Urol Nephrol. 2007;39:57–63.
7. Agrawal MS, Agrawal M, Gupta A, Bansal S, Yadav A, Goyal J, et al. A randomized comparison of tubeless and standard percutaneous nephrolithotomy. J Endourol. 2008;22:439–42.
8. Al-Ba'adani TH, Al-Kohlany KM, Al-Adimi A, Al-Towaity M, Al-Baadani T, Alwan M. Tubeless percutaneous nephrolithotomy: the new gold standard. Int Urol Nephrol. 2007;40:603–8.
9. Aghamir SM, Hosseini SR, Gooran S. Totally tubeless percutaneous nephrolithotomy. J Endourol. 2004;18:647–8.
10. Karami H, Gholamrezaie HR. Totally tubeless percutaneous nephrolithotomy in selected patients. J Endourol. 2004;18:475–6.
11. Crook TJ, Lockyer CR, Keoghane SR, Walmsley BH. Totally tubeless percutaneous nephrolithotomy. J Endourol. 2008;22:267–71.
12. Istanbulluoglu MO, Ozturk B, Gonen M, Cicek T, Ozkardes H. Effectiveness of totally tubeless percutaneous nephrolithotomy in selected patients: a prospective randomized study. Int Urol Nephrol. 2009;41(3):541–5.
13. Hong YM, Loughlin KR. The use of hemostatic agents and sealants in urology. J Urol. 2006;176:2367–74.
14. Pipan CM, Glasheen WP, Matthew TL, Gonias SL, Hwang LJ, Jane JA, et al. Effects of antifibrinolytic agents on the life span of fibrin sealant. J Surg Res. 1992;53:402–7.
15. Makris M, Garson JA, Ring CJ, Tuke PW, Tedder RS, Preston FE. Hepatitic C viral RNA in clotting factor concentrates and the development of hepatitis in recipients. Blood. 1993;81:1898–902.
16. Spotnitz WD. Active and mechanical hemostatic agents. Surg. 2007;142:34–8.
17. Jou YC, Cheng MC, Sheen JH, Lin CT, Chen PC. Cauterization of access tract for nephrostomy tube-free percutaneous nephrolithotomy. J Endourol. 2004;18(6):547–9.
18. Jou YC, Cheng MC, Sheen JH, Lin CT, Chen PC. Electrocauterization of bleeding points for percutaneous nephrolithotomy. Urology. 2004;64(3):443–6, discussion 446–7.
19. Mouracade P, Spie R, Lang H, Jacqmin D, Saussine C. "Tubeless" percutaneous nephrolithotomy: a series of 37 cases. Prog Urol. 2007;17(7):1351–4.
20. Noller M, Baughman S, Morey A, Auge B. Fibrin sealant enables tubeless percutaneous stone surgery. J Urol. 2004;172:166.
21. Mikhail A, Kaptein J, Bellman G. Use of fibrin glue in percutaneous nephrolithotomy. Urology. 2003;61:910.
22. Shah HN, Hedge S, Shah JN, Mohile PD, Yuvaraja TB, Bansal MB. A prospective, randomized trial evaluating the safety and efficacy of fibrin sealant in tubeless percutaneous nephrolithotomy. J Urol. 2006;176:2488–92.
23. L'Esperance J, Sung J, Marguet C, Maloney M, Springhar W, Preminger G, et al. Controlled survival study of the effects of Tisseel or a combination of FloSeal and Tisseel on major vascular injury and major collecting-system injury during partial nephrectomy in a porcine model. J Endourol. 2005;19:1114.
24. Aghamir SM, Khazaeli MH, Meisami A. Use of surgicel for sealing nephrostomy tract after totally tubeless percutaneous nephrolithotomy. J Endourol. 2006;20:293–6.
25. Uribe CA, Eichel L, Khonsari S, Finley DS, Basillote J, Park HK, et al. What happens to hemostatic agents in contact with urine? an in vitro study. J Endourol. 2005;19:312–7.
26. Borin JF, Sala LG, Eichel L, McDougall EM, Clayman RV. Tubeless percutaneous nephrolithotomy using hemostatic gelatin matrix. J Endourol. 2005;19:614–7.

Minimally Invasive Percutaneous Nephrolithotomy: The Chinese Approach

53

Guohua Zeng, Wen Zhong, and Zhaohui He

Abstract

The Chinese approach of minimally invasive percutaneous nephrolithotomy (Chinese MPCNL) is mostly similar to standard percutaneous nephrolithotomy, but there are some differences. The first difference is tract size and dilator; only 14–18-Fr percutaneous working tracts were used during the procedure. We also modified fascial dilators, a dilator with marks on the lateral view to indicate how deeply it had been introduced, without the use of fluoroscopy, thus decreasing the X-ray exposure for both the operators and patients. The second difference is that endoscope, semirigid ureteroscope, and pediatric nephroscope replaced the rigid nephroscope; with the small sheath, it is normally possible to inspect the renal pelvis, upper and lower calyx, and proximal ureter up to L4, which decreased the risk of bleeding and increased the stone-free rate. The third difference is the irrigation pump, which we had modified. A specially designed endoscopic pump could provide an impulse wave pressurized irrigation to facilitate flushing out of stone fragments, which could shorten operative time. Over the past 19 years, 10,452 patients with all kinds of upper tract urinary calculi were treated with Chinese MPCNL, which has a high stone-free rate and lower complications. It was proved to be effective and safe.

Keywords

Percutaneous nephrolithotomy • Minimally invasive • PCNL • Chinese MPCNL

Introduction

The first case of percutaneous nephrolithotomy (PCNL) in China was performed in 1984 in this Minimally Invasive Surgery Center, of the First Affiliated Hospital of Guangzhou Medical College [1, 2]. Based on the belief that a smaller percutaneous tract would bring less trauma to the renal parenchyma than the standard PCNL, we modified the traditional technique of standard PCNL in an attempt to decrease the morbidity. We have been using an 8/9.8-Fr rigid ureteroscope, via a 14–18-Fr percutaneous working tract provided by fascial dilators and peel-away sheath since 1992. We termed this procedure minimally invasive percutaneous nephrolithotomy (MPCNL) [2, 3].

PCNL using a small tract for stone removal was first reported in 1997 by Helal and his colleagues [4]. They used a 15-Fr Hickman peel-away sheath as the working sheath with a 10-Fr pediatric cystoscope and forceps to remove three stones of 5–7 mm in a 2-year-old child weighing 10 kg. In same year, Jackman et al. [5], paralleling their work in the pediatric population in 11 children, introduced the mini-percutaneous nephrolithotomy (mini-perc) technique, in which they carried out the percutaneous procedure through an 11-Fr Amplatz sheath. Since then, several small case series were reported, and various terms were used to describe the procedure. Monga and Oglevie [6] performed it with a 20-Fr tract

G. Zeng, M.D., Ph.D.(✉) • W. Zhong, Ph.D. • Z. He, M.D.
Department of Urology, Minimally Invasive Surgery Center, Guangdong Key Laboratory of Urology, The First Affiliated Hospital of Guangzhou Medical College, Kangda Road 1#, Haizhu District, Guangzhou, Guangdong 510230, China
e-mail: gzgyzgh@vip.tom.com

J.J. Talati et al. (eds.), *Urolithiasis*,
DOI 10.1007/978-1-4471-4387-1_53, © Springer-Verlag London 2012

and called the procedure "mini-PCNL." In 2001, Lahme and colleagues [7] used a specially designed rigid nephroscope of 12 Fr through a 15-Fr Amplatz sheath to treat 1–2-cm renal calculi in 19 patients and termed this procedure minimally invasive PCNL, or MPCNL. Despite the use of various sheath sizes and instruments and the different terms for the procedure, all the authors believe that a small tract has the potential advantage of decreased bleeding and trauma to renal parenchyma. However, because of lack of proper endoscopes and special equipment, they found it difficult to maintain a good endoscopic view and even more difficult to remove the stone fragments via the smaller tract. Since the smaller-sized percutaneous tract would result, potentially, in a longer time to dislodge stones than for standard PCNL, the indication for MPCNL, in their studies, was limited to (1) those cases with a stone burden of less than 2 cm in diameter for pediatric upper urinary tract stones and (2) situations where a secondary tract for inaccessible or residual fragments was required to supplement standard PCNL.

During the evolution of practice of Chinese MPCNL, we designed appropriate equipment and modified the traditional PCNL technique (discussed later). The innovations of equipment and modifications of traditional PCNL technique together provided the assurance for a high effectiveness of Chinese MPCNL in treating upper urinary tract stones. In this center, Chinese MPCNL is now routinely performed on upper tract stones of all sizes, including staghorn stones, stones in transplanted kidneys, upper ureteric stones, and stones in a solitary kidney [8–10].

All procedures were performed under continual epidural anesthesia or general anesthesia. After retrograde ureteric catheterization with a 5–6-Fr open-ended ureteric catheter (Boston Scientific Corporation, Miami Technology Center, USA), all other procedures were performed in the prone position. Fluoroscopy-guided percutaneous punctures were made by the urologists, followed by passage of an 18-gauge coaxial needle (Cook Incorporated, Bloomington, IN) into the designed calyx after retrograde injection of contrast medium. A flexible 0.035-in. Zebra™ guide wire (Boston Scientific Corporation, Miami Technology Center, USA) was then inserted into renal collecting system or down the ureter through the needle sheath under fluoroscopic guidance. Fluoroscopy was used to guide the puncture; the line of the puncture holder was directed toward the calyx. If the puncture holder was unavailable, the pathway of the puncture needle was identified under ultrasonic imaging. Then under the real-time ultrasonic monitor, the needle can be seen to reach the targeted calyx. The tract was dilated to 14–18 Fr by fascial dilators. A matched peel-away sheath (Cook Incorporated, Bloomington, IN) was then inserted. The renal stone was fragmented by pneumatic lithotripter or holmium:yttrium-aluminum-garnet laser (Ho:YAG) or a combination, using an 8/9.8-Fr rigid ureteroscope (Richard Wolf GmbH, German). The small fragments can be flushed out by the forceful pulsed flow, which was produced by a special perfusion pump (Jielun Medvice Ltd, Guangzhou, China) (Fig. 53.1). At the end of the procedure, a 5-Fr double-J stent and a 14–18-Fr Silastic nephrostomy tube were fixed in place.

The choice of correct equipment is the key to efficient MPCNL. Lack of suitable equipment for this procedure is often lamented by many urologists. We solved this problem by standardizing the equipment used and simplifying surgical technique. The optimal equipment for solution of all problems in MPCNL includes a Zebra guide wire as the only type of guide wire used, a set of fascial dilators and peel-away sheath, a semirigid Wolf ureteroscope, ballistic lithotripter, and stone removal by irrigation supplemented as necessary by a rigid 5-Fr forceps. These equipment are readily available in all units providing a stone treatment service. We had specially modified the pump (see Fig. 53.1a) to provide a pressurized intermittent irrigation to flush out stone fragments. Additionally the fascial dilators (see Fig. 53.1b) were marked on the side to indicate the depth to which it had been introduced, without the use of fluoroscopy, thus decreasing the X-ray exposure for both the operators and patients.

A combination of sonography guidance and X-ray fluoroscopy is used to guide the puncture (Fig. 53.2). This approach resulted from our increasing awareness of the effects of exposure to irradiation from X-rays. The classical role of fluoroscopy is to confirm the puncture, monitor the passage of a guide wire, or guide a puncture into a specific calyx in difficult cases, and also to detect the remained stones. The preoperative imaging of intravenous urogram (IVU) or computed tomography (CT) was reviewed prior to puncture. Retrograde pyelography via ureteral catheter is most useful for obtaining an initial impression of the spacial distribution of calyceal structures, which helps determine where and how to puncture. After distension of the system by injection of normal saline via the ureteric catheter, the puncture was performed with an 18-gauge needle. As the target is achieved, there will be a feel as if one is piercing through into a cavity, or one will feel a grinding sensation when the needle hits the stone. A Zebra guide wire was preferred by our department, as it is soft enough to be passed down the ureter or coiled up in a dilated calyx. The tract was dilated to 14–18 Fr with fascial dilators under fluoroscopic guidance, and the initial guide wire was left in place through the sheath as a safety guide wire at the start of lithotripsy. It is removed later to facilitate the removing of stone fragments.

We prefer the middle calyceal puncture rather than lower pole puncture under the prone position. The preferred puncture site was a supracostal approach puncture at the 11th intercostal space, bounded laterally by the posterior

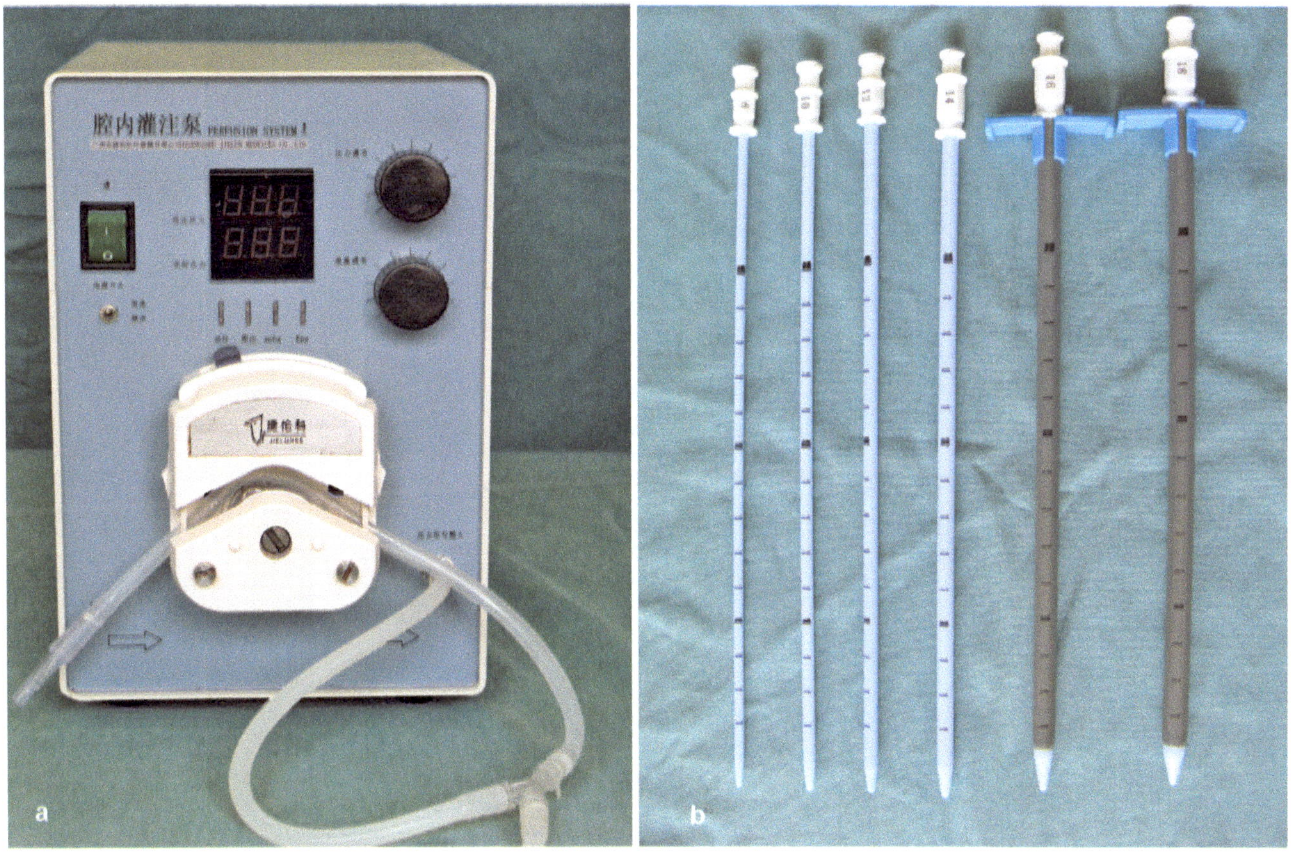

Fig. 53.1 (**a**) A specially designed endoscopic pump that can generate intermittent pressures of up to 350 mmHg for about 3 s, then stop for 2 s, and then repeat the cycle. (**b**) Dilators with markings

axillary line and medially by a line projected from the tip of the scapula [1, 11]. This puncture site has the advantage of hitting the middle calyx without resorting to an oblique tract while having minimal risk of injury to surrounding organs. This also contributed significantly to the subsequent improved maneuverability of the endoscope as there is minimal impingement of endoscope movement by the abdominal wall. The tract should take the shortest route through the renal parenchyma to the stone or the destination calyx. As stated, this is usually the middle calyx, but the actual selected calyx is tailored to the stone location and calyceal configuration. Maximal intrarenal access can be achieved via the "neutral position" of the midcalyceal puncture as the endoscope can swing a full arc [11, 12]. With the small sheath and miniaturized endoscope, it is normally possible to inspect the renal pelvis, upper and lower calyx, and proximal ureter up to L4 in Chinese MPCNL, which would be impossible using the large rigid renoscope as it will bring severe torque on the tissue, risking parenchymal tear. These instruments and maneuvers increase the possibility of clearing the stones through a single percutaneous tract [9].

The strategy of stone fragments removal by irrigant flushing is an important concept. It avoids the tedious process of picking up every fragment by forceps. The process of stone fragment removal occurs concurrently with stone fragmentation and saves time, explaining why operative time in our described (Chinese) technique for MPCNL has been significantly shortened [12]. Intraoperatively the small size of the ureteroscope, together with a straight short tract through the abdominal wall, allows access to most calyces and upper ureter as far down as the L4 level. This improves the clearance rate. Only a parallel calyx with an acute angle to the puncture calyx may be inaccessible, in which case, an additional tract can be inserted as required.

There is concern about the safety of the use of this pressurized irrigation. High renal pelvic pressure could risk systemic absorption of irrigation fluid containing bacteria or endotoxin, which can lead to postoperative fever. Renal pelvic pressure (RPP) during Chinese MPCNL was evaluated between July 2005 and December 2007 [13]; 80 patients who were candidates for MPCNL were selected for RPP measurement by a baroceptor that connected to the open-ended ureteric catheter introduced retrogradely into the renal pelvis. A computer recorded the RPP each second, and all the data were evaluated statistically with SPSS 12.0 software. During MPCNL with 14-Fr, 16-Fr, 18-Fr, and double-16-Fr percutaneous tracts, the mean RPP was 24.55, 16.49, 11.22, and 6.64 mmHg, respectively. Logistical analysis

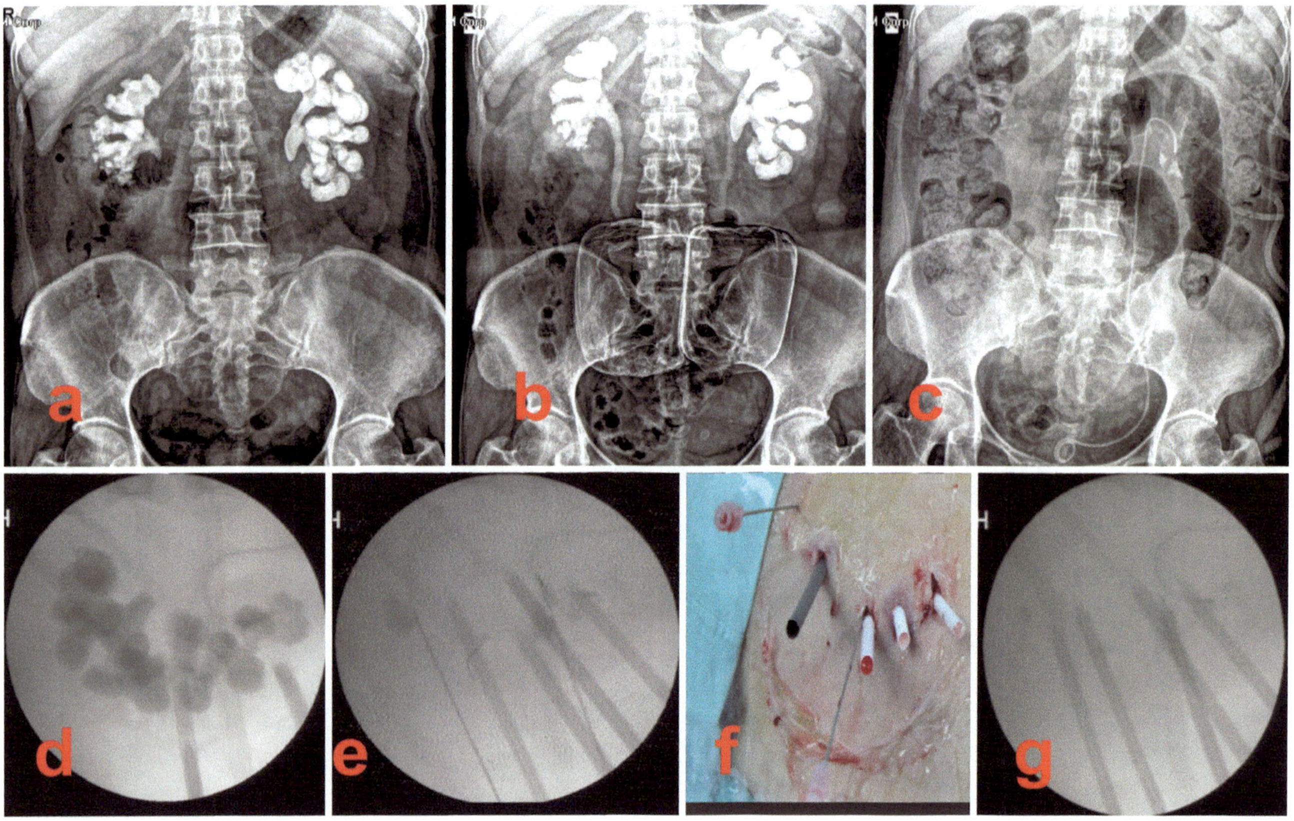

Fig. 53.2 Fluoroscopic view and external view of MPCNL procedures of the same case (**a**) X-rays of kidneys-ureters-bladder (*KUB*), (**b**) intravenous urogram (*IVU*), (**c**) postoperative KUB (**d–g**)

suggested that postoperative fever did not correlate to sex ($P=0.195$), age ($P=0.641$), urinary tract infection (UTI; $P=0.663$), postoperative white blood cell count $\geq 8 \times 10^9$/L ($P=0.751$), or a single occurrence of a renal pelvic pressure reading of ≥30 mmHg during the operation ($P=0.662$). In contrast, infection calculi ($P=0.000$), mean RPP ($P=0.036$), mean RPP ≥ 20 mmHg ($P=0.013$), accumulative time of RPP ≥ 30 mmHg ($P=0.010$), and RPP ≥ 30 mmHg for longer than 50 s ($P=0.024$) may contribute to postoperative fever. In our study, renal pelvic pressure generally remains lower than the 30-mmHg pressure level, which allows backflow (30 mmHg), during Chinese MPCNL via 14–18-Fr percutaneous tract. Any factor that impacted drainage would result in a temporal elevation of RPP to >30 mmHg. Episodes of high pressure had a cumulative effect, with additional risk of enough backflow to bring about bacteremia or postoperative fever. Thus, we concluded that pressurized continuous irrigation through the working channel of an 8/9.8-Fr ureteroscope was safe. Clinically, we did not notice a high sepsis rate in our study.

Modern instrumentation and technical improvement have revitalized Chinese MPCNL. The previous difficulty in stone fragmentation and stone removal has been resolved. Now, Chinese MPCNL has a much wider application. Our experience has shown that it may be applied to large stone loads, including staghorn calculi, with operating time, clinical stone clearance rate, and complication comparable to standard PCNL [1, 12, 14, 15]. In the recently published paper from our department [10], we reported on the use of MPCNL to treat staghorn calculi via multiple mini (16-Fr) tracts in a single session and compared the morbidity with that of standard PCNL procedures in a prospective randomized trial. Chinese MPCNL was associated with higher clearance rate (89.7 vs. 68 %, $P=0.049$), less chance to the need for adjunctive procedure of shock wave lithotripsy (SWL) or second-look PCNL (24.1 vs. 60 %, $P=0.007$), and a similar complication rate (37.9 vs. 52 %, P=0.300).

Conclusion

We recently audited our results (not yet published) of Chinese MPCNL over the past 19 years. These results speak for themselves: 11,801 procedures were performed on 10,876 renal units (5,493 left and 5,383 right) in 10,452 patients. There were 10,102 first-stage procedures, 1,604 s-look procedures, 86 third procedures, and 9 fourth procedures. There were 4,097 (39.2 %) cases of bilateral calculi, 4,600 (44.10 %) cases of calculi in multiple calyces, 1,900 (18.18 %) staghorn calculi, 395 (3.78 %) simple pelvic stone, 645 (6.17 %) lower caliceal stone, 358 (3.43 %) cases of solitary renal stone, 430 (4.11 %) cases of simple ureteral stone, 236 (2.26 %) cases of Steinstrasse after extracorporeal shock wave lithotripsy (ESWL), and 269 (2.57 %) cases of residual stone after open surgery. A total of 956 (9.23 %) renal units were managed with multiple tracts, which included 846 (7.78 %) units that required 2 tracts, 85 (0.78 %) units that required 3 tracts, 18 (0.17 %) units that required 4 tracts, and 7 (0.06 %) units that required 5 tracts. In those 10,876 renal units, a total of 11,830 tracts were established, and 1,207 (10.20 %), 9,174 (77.55 %), and 1,449 (12.25 %) tracts were targeted to upper, middle, or lower renal calyx, respectively. A total of 762 (6.93 %) cases needed ESWL to clear the stone after Chinese MPCNL. The mean stone burden was 777.44 ± 740.34 (20–4,080) mm^2, and the average operative time was 101.3 ± 44.23 (10–240) minutes for each patient including several sessions in together. The stone-free rate was 89.9 %, which increased to 93 % with adjunctive ESWL. Significant complications were noted on 273 (3.05 %) cases, including the need for blood transfusion in 294 patients. Fifty-three cases needed superselective renal arterial embolization for hemorrhage, 9 cases developed a pneumothorax, 12 cases had sepsis, 2 cases had a colon injury, and 2 cases died—one from disseminated intravascular coagulation and one from a myocardial infarction.

Chinese MPCNL has established itself as an effective and safe endourological procedure.

References

1. Li X, He Z, Wu K, et al. Chinese minimally invasive percutaneous nephrolithotomy: the Guangzhou experience. J Endourol. 2009;23: 1693–7.
2. Li X, Zeng GH, Yuan J, et al. Treatment of upper urinary calculi with the PCNL technique(experience of 20 years). Beijing Da Xue Xue Bao. 2004;36:124–6 (article in Chinese).
3. Wu K, Li X, Yuan J, et al. Mini nephrostomy with ureteroscopic lithotripsy for staghorn stones. Acad J Guangzhou Med Coll. 1993;2:13–4 (article in Chinese).
4. Helal M, Black T, Lockhart J, et al. The Hickman peel-away sheath: alternative for pediatric percutaneous nephrolithotomy. J Endourol. 1997;11:171–2.
5. Jackman SV, Docimo SG, Cadeddu JA, et al. The "mini-perc" technique: a less invasive alternative to percutaneous nephrolithotomy. World J Urol. 1998;16:371–4.
6. Monga M, Oglevie S. Minipercutaneous nephrolithotomy. J Endourol. 2000;14:419–21.
7. Lahme S, Bichler KH, Strohmaier WL, et al. Minimally invasive PCNL in patients with renal pelvic and calyceal stones. Eur Urol. 2001;40:619–24.
8. He Z, Li X, Chen L, et al. Minimally invasive percutaneous nephrolithotomy for upper urinary tract calculi in transplanted kidneys. BJU Int. 2007;99:1467–71.
9. Guohua Z, Zhong W, Li X, et al. Minimally invasive percutaneous nephrolithotomy for staghorn calculi: a novel single session approach via multiple 14–18Fr tracts. Surg Laparosc Endosc Percutan Tech. 2007;17:124–8.
10. Zhong W, Zeng G, Wu W, et al. Minimally invasive percutaneous nephrolithotomy with multiple mini tracts in a single session in treating staghorn calculi. Urol Res. 2011;39:117–22.
11. Li X, Zeng G, Liu J, et al. Minimally invasive percutaneous nephrolithotomy in the management of complex urinary calculi: a middle calyx puncture approach. J Chin Urol. 2005;20:147–9 (article in Chinese).
12. Li SK, Tai D, Chau L, et al. Minimally invasive percutaneous nephrolithotomy (MPCNL) according to the Chinese method. In: Baba S, Ono Y, editors. Recent advances in endourology. New York: Springer; 2006. p. 41–63.
13. Zhong W, Zeng G, Wu K, et al. Does a smaller tract in percutaneous nephrolithotomy contribute to high renal pelvic pressure and postoperative fever? J Endourol. 2008;22:2147–51.
14. Deane LA, Clayman RV. Advances in percutaneous nephrostolithotomy. Urol Clin North Am. 2007;34:383–95.
15. Aron M, Yadav R, Goel R, et al. Multi-tract percutaneous nephrolithotomy for large complete staghorn calculi. Urol Int. 2005;75:327–32.

Percutaneous Nephrostomy, Antegrade Stent Placement, and Radiological Control of Post-PCNL Bleeding

54

Tanveer ul Haq and Basit Salam

Abstract

Percutaneous nephrostomy is a well-established technique for relief of obstruction of the renal outflow tract. The technique can be extended into nephrolithotomy for stone removal, nephroscopy, ureteroscopy, and antegrade ureteral stent placement. Serious vascular complication can be avoided by entering the pelvicalyceal system from relatively avascular area under radiological guidance.

The puncture site can be from the lower pole, interpolar region, or upper pole, depending on the indication for which nephrostomy is being performed. Appropriate entry requires proper visualization of the collecting system, which is optimum whenever there is hydronephrosis.

Puncturing a nondilated system is difficult and associated with a higher complication rate.

Transient hematuria, which is mostly managed conservatively, occurs in virtually every patient after percutaneous nephrostomy; however, severe bleeding that may require transfusion or intervention is uncommon. Other complications that may be seen include urosepsis, which can be avoided by minimal manipulation and protective antibiotic cover.

Knowledge of basic technique of nephrostomy and its complications is therefore very important; it allows the operator to extend the technique with safety, whenever required.

Keywords

Percutaneous nephrostomy • Stenoses • Drainage • Antegrade nephrostomy • Ureteral stent • Percutaneous nephrolithotomy • Hemorrhagic complication • Embolization

Percutaneous Nephrostomy

Percutaneous nephrostomy (PCN) has been in clinical practice for urinary diversion in patients presenting with obstructive uropathy for more than 40 years. Fernstrom and Johannson reported the first percutaneous nephrostomy in 1976 [1]. The principles applied to percutaneous puncture for nephrostomy apply equally well to percutaneous nephrolithotomy (PCNL), which has now become an established technique for renal stone removal [2]. A similar percutaneous approach can also be used for placement of antegrade double-J stent (DJS) in patients for whom the retrograde insertion is difficult or has failed. The major indications for percutaneous nephrostomy include urinary diversion in obstructed system, urinary leak or fistula management, renal stones, urosepsis, antegrade DJS placement, and nephrostogram examination [2].

T.ul. Haq, M.B.B.S., FCPS, FRCR (✉) • B. Salam, M.B.B.S., FCPS
Department of Radiology, Aga Khan University Hospital,
Stadium Road, Karachi, Sindh 74800, Pakistan
e-mail: tanveer.haq@aku.edu; basit.salam@aku.edu

J.J. Talati et al. (eds.), *Urolithiasis*,
DOI 10.1007/978-1-4471-4387-1_54, © Springer-Verlag London 2012

Anatomy

Precise understanding of perirenal anatomy is essential prior to performing PCN to avoid injury to other organs. Kidneys are retroperitoneal and are surrounded by perirenal fat and Gerota's fascia. A clear understanding of the renal vascular anatomy also allows the operator to avoid vascular complication associated with percutaneous nephrostomy. The renal artery divides into major anterior and posterior branches, which creates a zone of relative avascularity between the divisions (known as *the Brödel's bloodless line of incision*) that lies just posterior to the lateral convex border of the kidney. The optimal entry plane lies posterolaterally, at the junction of the anterior two-thirds and posterior one-third of the kidney [3, 4]. The renal artery and the renal vein are fortunately situated anterior to the renal pelvis; however, the posterior branch supply for the dorsal segment runs behind the renal pelvis.

A percutaneous nephrostomy tract that enters the pelvis through a calyx has the least possibility of causing arterial injury. It is important to realize that puncturing directly into the renal pelvis is to be avoided, as the risk of hemorrhagic complication increases by this approach. It is recommended to puncture the posterior calyx, which can be identified easily on ultrasound (US) and computed tomography (CT) scan. However, if the approach is under fluoroscopy after intravenous/retrograde contrast injection, the calices that appear end on are posterior [5]. Other structures and their relationship with the kidney are important to recognize for safe and uneventful percutaneous nephrostomy placement. Use of Doppler ultrasound can provide additional information; however, it is not mandatory particularly for experienced operator.

While gaining percutaneous access for nephrostomy, an important consideration is the pleural space that extends posteriorly down to T_{12} vertebral body level. On the left side, the descending colon is anterior in relation with the left kidney, but in approximately 1 % of patients, it may be present behind the kidney [5]. This may result in a serious complication, of colonic injury, particularly in PCNL, if access is under fluoroscopic guidance alone. Ultrasound helps in recognizing the presence of retrorenal colon.

Techniques

Patient Preparation

Before starting this procedure, the patient must be screened and, if required, treated for coagulopathy. A review of the patient's complete medical record will help in planning the nephrostomy approach and in identifying any variant anatomy. Prophylactic antibiotics should be administered before the procedure and continued according to the patient's condition [6, 7].

Informed consent must always be obtained and should follow on a discussion prior to the procedure, which explains the indications for doing the procedure, use of anesthesia, and potential complications that can be encountered [2, 6].

The patient is then placed in a prone position on the fluoroscopy table with rotating C-arm facility, along with ultrasound scanner. Some interventionists prefer placing a 45° foam pad to elevate the side where the nephrostomy is to be done [2, 5]. Under US guidance and local anesthesia, the puncturing needle (21–18 gauge), depending on operator experience and preference, is advanced into the dilated collecting system (using Seldinger technique). After this the procedure is done under fluoroscopic guidance. The contrast is injected to outline the collecting system followed by placement of a guide wire (0.018–0.035 in.). Various guide wires may be used in different situations (Fig. 54.1), *Amplatz Super Stiff wire* (short, straight tip with stiff wire), *Bentson Starter wire* (tapered floppy tip forms a J when advanced, but can also be advanced through stenoses in straight format), glide wire (hydrophilic-coated nitinol with polyurethane coating, excellent tortuous tracking), and *Lunderquist Extra Stiff wire* (malleable tip with stiff wire). Some of these are used for vascular access as well.

Serial dilatation over the guide is achieved, and a nephrostomy catheter is then passed over the guide wire and placed ideally in the renal pelvis. The guide wire is then removed, taking care not to displace the catheter. The external surface of the nephrostomy catheter is secured to the skin with sutures, and then a sterile dressing is applied. It may sometimes be necessary to make the initial puncture under CT scan guidance (Fig. 54.2) when there are technical difficulties, especially when the patient is obese or has severe scoliosis, making the procedure difficult and risky under ultrasound or fluoroscopy [5].

Post-placement care of the nephrostomy catheter is important (Fig. 54.3a, b). The catheter is normally left for temporary drainage; however, whenever it is to be kept for longer duration, it should be exchanged every 3–6 months (over a guide wire) to avoid encrustation and occlusion [2].

Complications of percutaneous nephrostomy can be characterized as minor or major. Minor complications requiring no treatment occur in 15–25 % of procedures and include minor bleeding that gradually resolves [3, 4, 8, 9]. The mortality for percutaneous nephrostomy that has been reported in the literature is 0.46–0.3 % [4, 9, 10]. Transient hematuria is frequently seen and requires conservative management. However, incidence of major hematuria is 1–3 % [10].

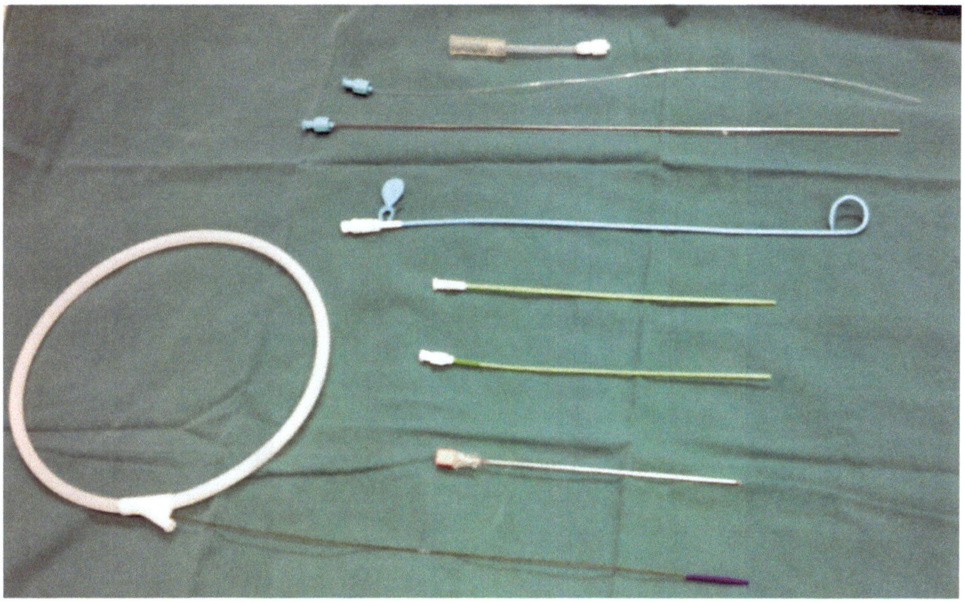

Fig. 54.1 PCN set with 0.038 guide wire, puncture needle (18 G), dilators 6 and 8 Fr, 8-Fr locking nephrostomy catheter, stiffeners, and connector

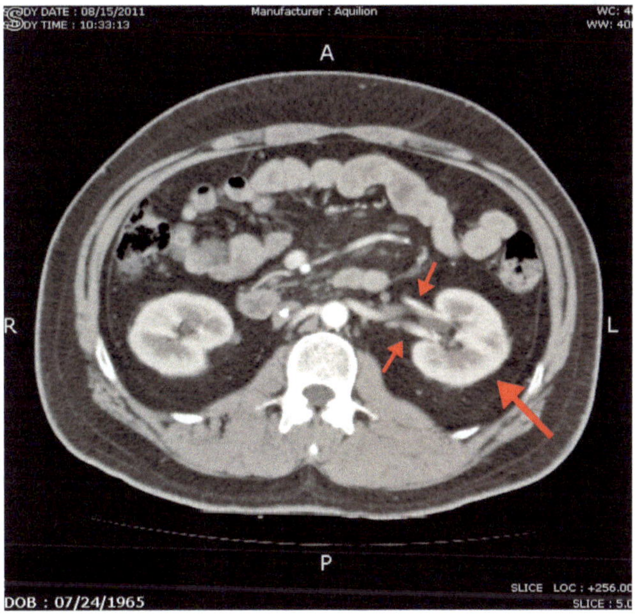

Fig. 54.2 CT scan image showing the left renal artery dividing into anterior and posterior branches marked by the *smaller arrows*. The *larger arrow* signifies relative avascular area

Antegrade Ureteral Stent Placement

Percutaneous nephrostomy can be extended into antegrade ureteral stent placement. It is reserved for those cases in which either the retrograde attempt had fail or was not feasible [2].

Ideally, the decision for antegrade stent placement should be made at the time of percutaneous nephrostomy, as the puncture site should be at the interpolar or upper polar region [2], which will have an impact on renal pelvis access and provides a straighter course for antegrade ureteral stent placement.

Techniques

The technique for antegrade ureteral stent placement is the same as described in the section for nephrostomy, keeping in mind the entry into the dilated collecting system via the interpolar or upper pole calyx. After puncture and placement of guide wire, a vascular access sheath is placed (usually of size 7 Fr), which will facilitate catheter and guide wire exchange, as well as the contrast injection required during the procedure.

Through the sheath a simple curved catheter (5-Fr C1 catheter, Cordis) is introduced along with hydrophilic guide wire (Terumo). The catheter is advanced to the site of stricture, which is then manipulated with the help of hydrophilic wire. The anatomy is initially outlined by injecting contrast via the sheath. The stricture is usually successfully negotiated by this technique; however, if the stricture is not crossed after multiple attempts, it can be reattempted after a 5–7-day interval of external drainage, which allows mucosal edema and ureter redundancy to resolve [5].

After negotiating the stricture, the guide wire is advanced into the bladder, followed by advancing the catheter into the bladder, over which the exchange wire (Amplatz Super Stiff) is also placed into the bladder. The stricture may need to be dilated with an angioplasty balloon—usually a 3–4-mm

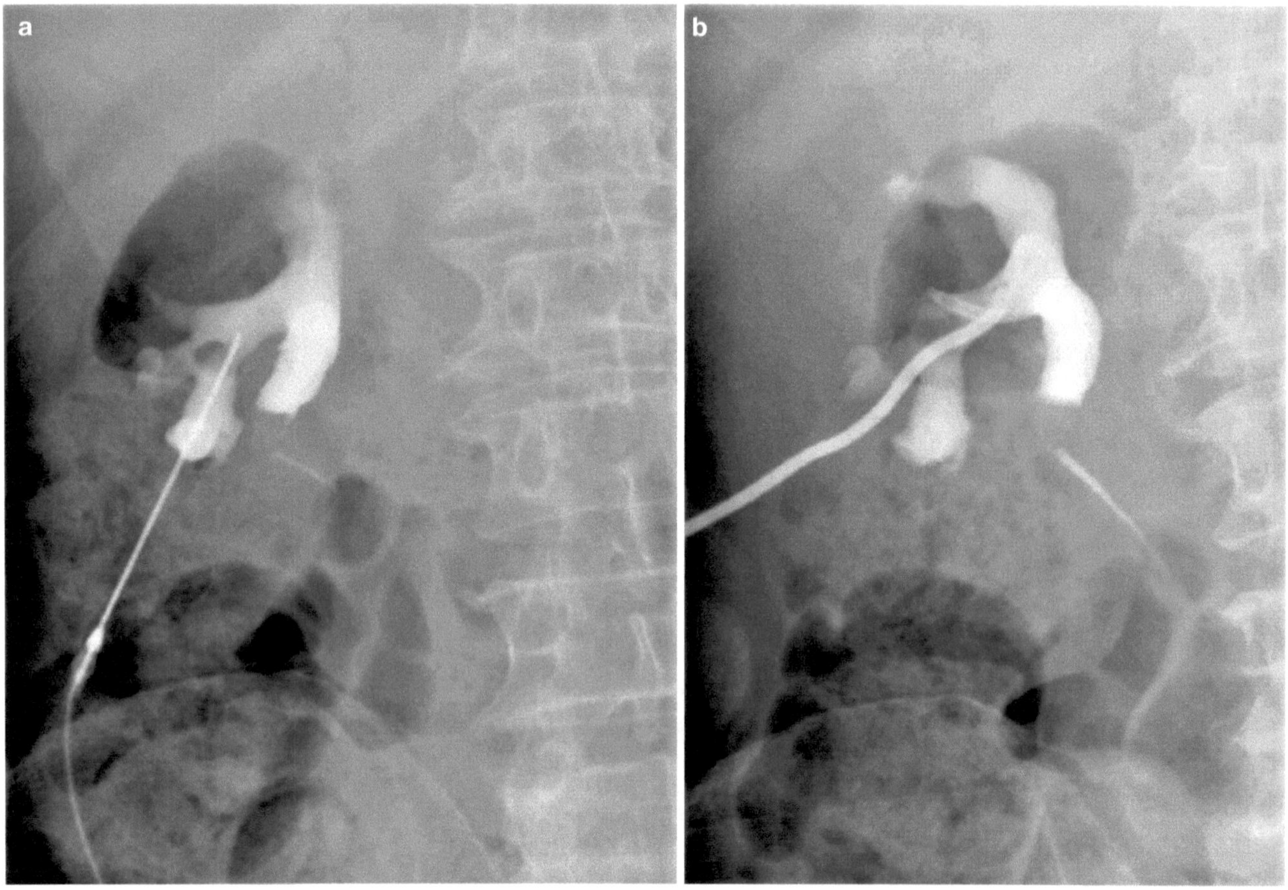

Fig. 54.3 (**a**) Fluoroscopic image showing needle in place while doing (**b**) percutaneous nephrostomy and subsequent nephrostomy catheter placement. Note the collecting system is opacified by contrast

angioplasty balloon is required for this purpose [5]. After the balloon dilatation has been done over the super stiff wire, the stent is deployed with the help of the pushing catheter. Usually 22–24-cm-length stents are suitable in majority of these patients. The distal loop of the catheter should be carefully deployed inside the bladder and should not be excessively advanced, as such may cause bladder irritation [2]. The guide wire is gradually and carefully withdrawn. The proximal end is then advanced with another catheter (the "pusher") to form a coil in the renal pelvis. Sometimes it may be required to slightly withdraw the sheath to make a coil of proximal loop of the stent. For safety, temporary nephrostomy drainage is instituted. The guide wire is reintroduced and coiled into the renal pelvis; a nephrostomy catheter is then advanced over the guide wire. The external drainage can be clamped after 24 h followed by nephrostogram to document stent patency. On confirmation of the patency, the nephrostomy catheter can be removed [2].

Ureteral stents have few complications, among which stent occlusion is the most frequently seen due to encrustation. Long-term patency can be achieved by encouraging the patient to maintain high fluid intake. Stent patency varies from 2 to 18 months [5]. Trimonthly evaluation of these patients is recommended; if stent occlusion is suspected, either ultrasound or cystogram examination should be ordered. The stent is to be exchanged at 6 months.

Other complications described include improper position of stent, ureteral perforation, stent migration, stent fracture, ureteric wall ischemia, urinary tract infection, and bladder irritation.

Hemorrhagic Complication of PCNL

Transient hematuria occurs in virtually every patient after PCNL and is managed conservatively. Significant hemorrhage requiring transfusion occurs in 1–3 % of the cases [2]. Major arterial injury is seen in about 0.5 % cases [5]. This should be suspected whenever gross hematuria persists for 3–5 days, with new clots demonstrated in the collecting system upon a follow-up nephrostogram, and when an accompanying drop in hematocrit is observed. These patients should be evaluated by angiography with embolization whenever possible. While performing angiography, renal

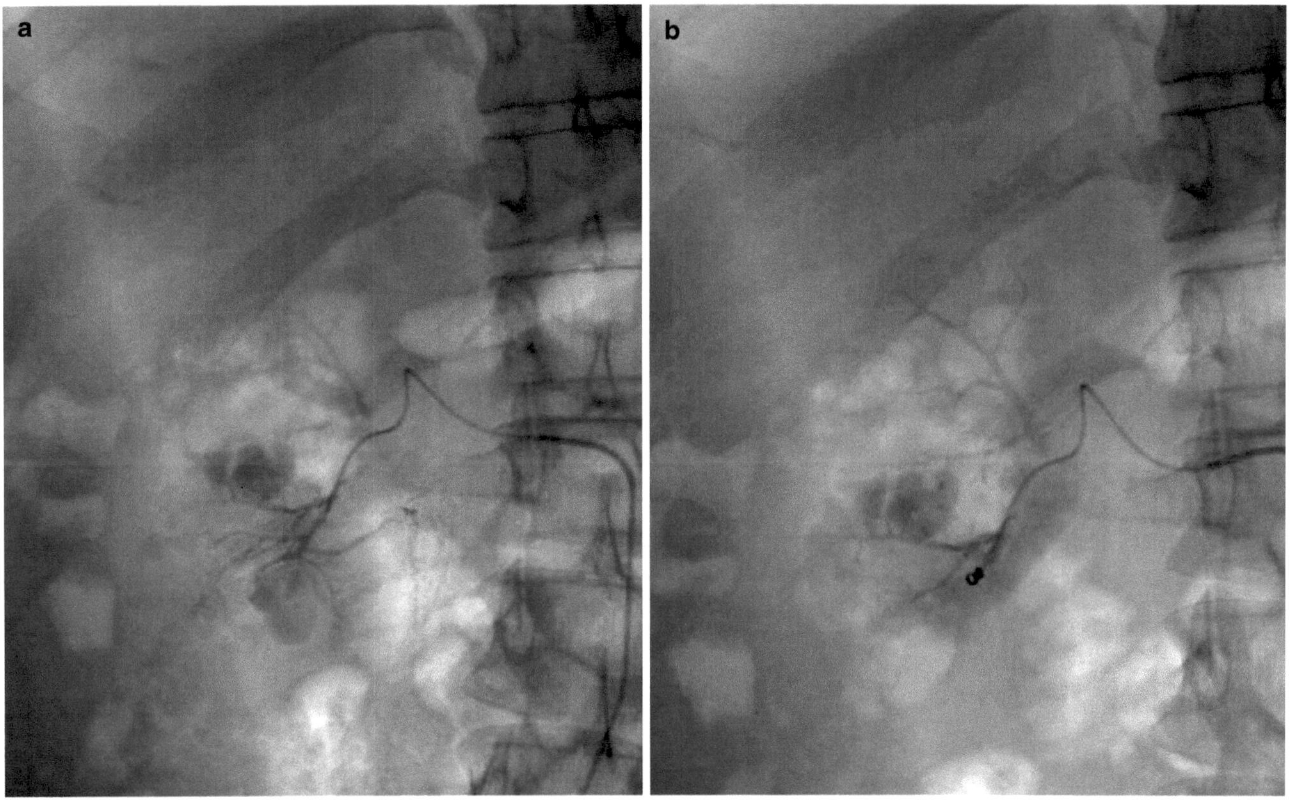

Fig. 54.4 (**a**, **b**) Pseudoaneurysm after PCNL, which was superselectively cannulated and embolized with microcoil

arteriovenous fistula, pseudoaneurysm, and/or vessel laceration are the major vascular complications that can be detected and subsequently embolized [2].

After doing a selective angiogram of the main renal artery, the region where intervention was done should be evaluated carefully with microcatheter technique. A microcatheter is introduced via a coaxial approach, and the abnormal vessel is identified by superselective cannulation and subsequently treated with embolization with coils [11–14] (Fig. 54.4a, b).

Conclusion

Minimally invasive radiological techniques have been established as safe and reliable treatment options in patients with obstructive nephropathy. The technique can be utilized in the primary management of these patients with excellent outcome. Simple nephrostomy can be extended for placement of antegrade ureteral stent in patients for whom retrograde stent placement was unsuccessful. It can further be extended into percutaneous nephrolithotomy.

The role of radiological intervention has also been well established in the management of vascular complication of PCNL; these urological emergencies have been dealt with reliably via minimally invasive radiological intervention.

References

1. Fernstrom I, Johannson B. Percutaneous pyelolithotomy. A new extraction technique. Scand J Urol Nephrol. 1976;10(3):257–9.
2. Dyer RB, Regan JD, Kavanagh PV, Khatod EG, Chen MY, Zagoria RJ. Percutaneous nephrostomy with extensions of the technique: step by step. Radiographics. 2002;22:503–25.
3. Cochran ST, Barbaric ZL, Lee JJ, Kashfian P. Percutaneous nephrostomy tube placement. An outpatient procedure? Radiology. 1991;179:843–7.
4. Lang EK. Percutaneous nephrostolithotomy and lithotripsy: a multi-institutional survey of complications. Radiology. 1987;162:25–30.
5. Valji K. Vascular and interventional radiology. Philadelphia: W.B. Saunders Company; 1999. p. 448–9.
6. LeRoy AJ, May GR, Bender CE, Williams Jr HJ, McGough PF, Segura JW, et al. Percutaneous nephrostomy for stone removal. Radiology. 1984;151:607–12.
7. Patel U, Hussain FF. Percutaneous nephrostomy of nondilated renal collecting systems with fluoroscopic guidance: technique and results. Radiology. 2004;233:226–33.
8. Hogan MJ, Coley BD, Jayanthi VR, Shiels WE, Koff SE. Percutaneous Nephrostomy in Children and Adolescents: Outpatient Management. Radiology. 2001;218:207–10.
9. Lee WJ, Smith AD, Cubelli V, Badlani GH, Lewin B, Vernace F, et al. Complications of percutaneous nephrolithotomy. AJR. 1987; 148:177–80.
10. Ramchandani P, Cardella JF, Grassi CJ, Roberts AC, Sacks D, Schwartzberg MS, et al. Quality improvement guidelines for percutaneous nephrostomy. J Vasc Interv Radiol. 2003;14:S277–81.
11. Chazen MD, Miller KS. Intrarenal pseudoaneurysm presenting 15 years after penetrating renal injury. Urology. 1997;49:774–6.

12. Mavili E, Dönmez H, Ozcan N, Sipahioğlu M, Demirtaş A. Transarterial embolization for renal arterial bleeding. Diagn Interv Radiol. 2009;15(2):143–7.
13. Yamakado K, Nakatsuka A, Tanaka N, Takano K, Matsumara K, Takeda K. Transcatheter arterial embolization of ruptured pseudoaneurysms with coils and n-butyl cyanoacrylate. J Vasc Interv Radiol. 2000;11:66–72.
14. Parildar M, Oran I, Memis A. Embolization of visceral pseudoaneurysms with platinum coils and N-butyl cyanoacrylate. Abdom Imaging. 2003;28:36–40.

Management Strategies for Staghorn Stones

55

Markus Margreiter and Michael Marberger

Abstract

Staghorn stones represent most advanced renal stone disease and, if not treated adequately, will result in loss of the kidney. PCNL is usually the treatment of choice, but the surgical technique has to be adapted to the individual situation. It provides stone clearance rates equal to those obtained with open surgery, but at significant lower overall morbidity. Nevertheless, it is challenging and requires significant expertise and frequently staged procedures. Even with complete stone removal, the risk of recurrent stone formation is inherently high. Eliminating underlying reasons for stone formation, close long-term follow-up and aggressive treatment of recurrent stones are therefore essential for successful management. The following chapter provides a detailed review of the current management strategies for staghorn stones.

Keywords

Staghorn stones • Staghorn calculi • Complex stones • Urolithiasis • Percutaneous nephrolithotripsy • PCNL • Ureteroscopy • Shock wave lithotripsy • Nephrolithotomy

Definition of Staghorn Stones

Staghorn stones are regarded as the combination of a large stone mass filling much or all of the renal collecting system [1–3]. Irrespective of the number of calices involved, the term is often applied to any branched stone occupying a significant portion of the collecting system [1–3]. Early attempts to categorize staghorn stones failed to gain clinical acceptance, rendering comparison of clinical studies unreliable [4, 5]. In general staghorn stones are today only subclassified into "partial" and "complete" staghorn stones; whereas "partial" staghorn stones fill only parts of the collecting system, "complete" staghorn stones occupy all calices and the renal pelvis [1–3]. In contrast the term "complex" stone is utilized to define situations difficult to treat not only because of stone burden but also because of other aggravating factors such as abnormal anatomy of the collecting system, multiplicity of stones, abnormal renal function, concomitant urinary tract infection, or special metabolic situations [6]. Although most staghorn stones are considered complex stones, lower-volume stones in abnormal collecting systems and in horseshoe, pelvic, or transplant kidneys may result in clinically more challenging scenarios [6]. Stone mass per se is therefore not the decisive factor defining the clinical problem in a specific situation [7]. The exception from this is if shock wave lithotripsy (SWL) is to be used for treatment as its success clearly depends on the stone mass to be expelled. A surface area of 300 mm^2 or a diameter >2.0 cm is the upper limit where this approach should be used [1–3].

Prevalence

Approximately 5–10 % of the population in Europe and North America are affected by urinary calculi needing therapy [8], but the proportion of these being staghorn stones at

M. Margreiter, M.D., FEBU (✉) • M. Marberger, M.D., FRCS (ed)
Department of Urology, Medical University of Vienna, Waehringer Guertel 18-20, A-1090 Vienna, Austria
e-mail: markus.margreiter@meduniwien.ac.at; michael.marberger@al.net

J.J. Talati et al. (eds.), *Urolithiasis*,
DOI 10.1007/978-1-4471-4387-1_55, © Springer-Verlag London 2012

the time of diagnosis and therapy seems to mainly be determined by access to modern stone treatment. With the availability of less invasive, non-incisional therapy, early removal of upper tract stones has become the rule, and the prevalence of large-volume stones has dropped dramatically. At the author's institution, renal stones with a diameter >2.5 cm have decreased from 12.4 % of all upper tract stones removed from 1,175 reno-ureteral units in 1998 stones to 4.5 % in 882 kidneys in 2008. This could, of course, also reflect a changing referral pattern at a tertiary care stone center. Austria has a healthcare system covering the entire population, and its database precisely reflects the type of renal stones being treated: In 2007 of the 11,690 patients coming for surgical therapy for upper tract stones in all of Austria, 49 % had SWL, 46 % ureteroscopy, 4.8 % percutaneous nephrolithotripsy, and only 0.2 % incisional surgery [9]. As staghorn stones are mainly managed by percutaneous nephrolithotripsy today, their actual prevalence has obviously become very low. True staghorn stones were removed from only 131 renal units at this institution from 1997 to 2007, in spite of ~900 patients with stones being treated annually, as compared to ~60 staghorn stones treated by the author annually before 1985. Most staghorn stones clearly need a long time to develop, and with aggressive early management of upper urinary tract urolithiasis, "the pond is rapidly overfished."

Although staghorn stones still accumulate at tertiary care centers in Europe and North America, large series are today almost only reported from countries with expanding medical systems. The Clinical Research Office of the Endourological Society (CROES) Percutaneous Nephrolithotomy (PCNL) Global Study is a prospective patient registry to assess the current indications, perioperative morbidity, and stone-free outcomes for percutaneous nephrolithotomy (PCNL) conducted at 96 centers worldwide with 5,803 patients enrolled so far. Seventy percent of these patients were registered from centers in Europe and North America, and 1,466 (27.5 %) patients had staghorn stones [10]. In one of the largest recent series on the treatment of upper tract stones from India, 1,466 of 5,335 patients (i.e., 27.5 %) had staghorn stones. Up to 67 % of kidney stones coming to treatment at centers in Thailand were classified as staghorn stones. The median age of patients was 51.0 with 51.8 % being male and 48.2 % female [11]. This development is even more pronounced for staghorn stones in children: Staghorn stones are rarely seen in children in Europe and the United States, whereas Kumar et al. treated 33 children with complex renal stones by percutaneous nephrolithotripsy in a 3-year period [12].

Etiology of Staghorn Stones

The etiology of staghorn stones is variable, but the combination of a calculus too large to be passed, ongoing supersaturation, crystallization, sludge formation, and impaired urinary drainage are the compounding factors for ongoing growth. As this process can develop with any metabolic imbalance, staghorn stones can show a wide spectrum of stone compositions, but magnesium ammonium phosphate (struvite), calcium carbonate apatite (brushite), cystine, or/and uric acid are dominant (Figs. 55.1a, b, c) [13]. Only calcium oxalate stones rarely grow to become branched stones [13]. Apart from obvious significant metabolic imbalances, abnormal urinary drainage and urinary infection are promoting factors for growth, with the vicious cycle of the more impact, the bigger the stone. Impaired urinary drainage may be congenital, such as with horseshoe kidneys, or a result of previous surgery. Urinary tract infection with urease-splitting bacteria that result in high local concentrations of ammonium and an alkaline urinary environment, with crystallization of magnesium ammonium phosphate (struvite), is the single most important factor for rapid stone growth. Because of the multifactorial etiology of most staghorn stones, successful therapy requires complete removal of all calculous material, elimination of urinary infection, normalization of urinary drainage, and correction of obvious metabolic imbalances.

Natural History of Untreated Staghorn Stones

Staghorn stones in general do not cause acute obstruction, and patients therefore rarely present with the acute pain problems typical for most stone episodes. Symptoms tend to be dominated by concomitant urinary infection, hematuria, chronic obstruction, and/or ultimately renal failure. The paucity of symptoms in many of the patients and also the often fairly slow progression of the disease may render patients reluctant to seek invasive therapy, especially if they are elderly and feeble. In the past a conservative approach with surgical intervention only with acute problems has clearly demonstrated that staghorn stones are always a progressive condition that when left untreated ultimately lead to loss of the affected kidney [14]. Koga et al. reported long-term follow-up data of 167 patients with staghorn calculi, including 61 patients that were treated conservatively. Following conservative treatment, 36.1 % of patients developed chronic renal failure, and 11.5 % died from uremia compared to only 6.0 % of patients developing chronic renal failure and no one dying following nephrolithotomy [15].

Today there is a general agreement that all staghorn stones have to be removed as soon as possible [1–3]. A delay in therapy only aggravates the situation and increases the risk for the patient. The only exceptions from this rule are rare situations of very advanced disease with threatening end-stage renal failure, where complete stone removal may cause too much renal trauma even with modern minimally invasive procedures. Selective removal of obstructing stone segments may then be the preferred approach to minimize renal trauma (Fig. 55.2).

Treatment Strategy

In the management of staghorn stones, the treating urologists face two major challenges:

- Removal of complex stones is technically demanding and prone to complications.
- The high risk of recurrent stone formation necessitates long-term follow-up and/or treatment.

Key to successful treatment of staghorn stones is an individualized treatment strategy with complete removal of all stone burden at lowest possible morbidity and correction of the underlying reasons for stone formation [16].

Pre-therapeutic Evaluation

Precise evaluation of the situation before treatment is essential for success. This requires comprehensive understanding of the medical condition, detailed knowledge of the individual anatomical situation and the location of the stone within the collecting system, and the recognition of potential risk factors and elimination of these wherever possible before the intervention. A complete medical history with precise information on previous surgery of the urological tract is essential. If the patient has a history of stone formation, previous stone analyses should be obtained. Obvious indicators for metabolic disorders such as a family history of stone disease, recurrent stone formation at early age and at short intervals, significant weight loss within a short period of time, highly abnormal dietary habits, and signs of urinary infection should be recognized.

Urinalysis (including a semiquantitative nitroprusside test or quantitative cystine analysis), a urine culture, and, if positive, an antibiotic resistance profile are mandatory diagnostic steps. Any proven urinary infection must be treated with an appropriate antibiotic agent prior to therapy, albeit urinary infection can frequently not be eliminated before the stone is removed. Renal function is usually adequately assessed by serum creatinine and eGFR. Where split renal function between the affected and contralateral kidney impacts clinical decisions, this is evaluated by split Tc-99m MAG3 scintigraphy, if necessary supplemented with furosemide diuresis.

Four-phase, multiparameter computerized tomography, ideally with three-dimensional reconstruction, usually depicts the stone, its shape and location within the collecting system, and its correlation to the renal parenchyma in the perfect manner [17, 18]. Renal ultrasonography,

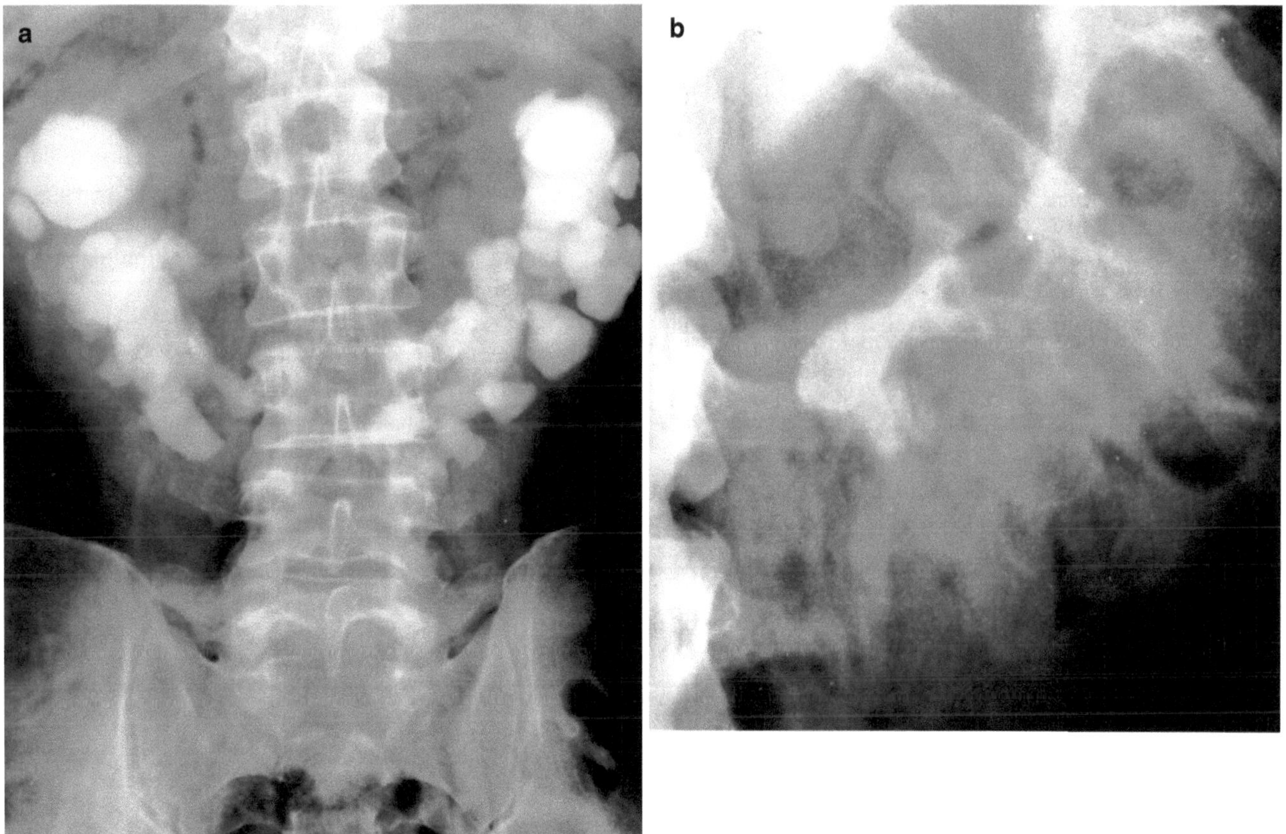

Fig. 55.1 (a) Bilateral sterile apatite staghorn stone in horseshoe kidney. (b) Struvite stone in solitary left kidney of a 39-year-old female with recurrent urinary tract infections. (c) Brushite staghorn stone in pediatric patient

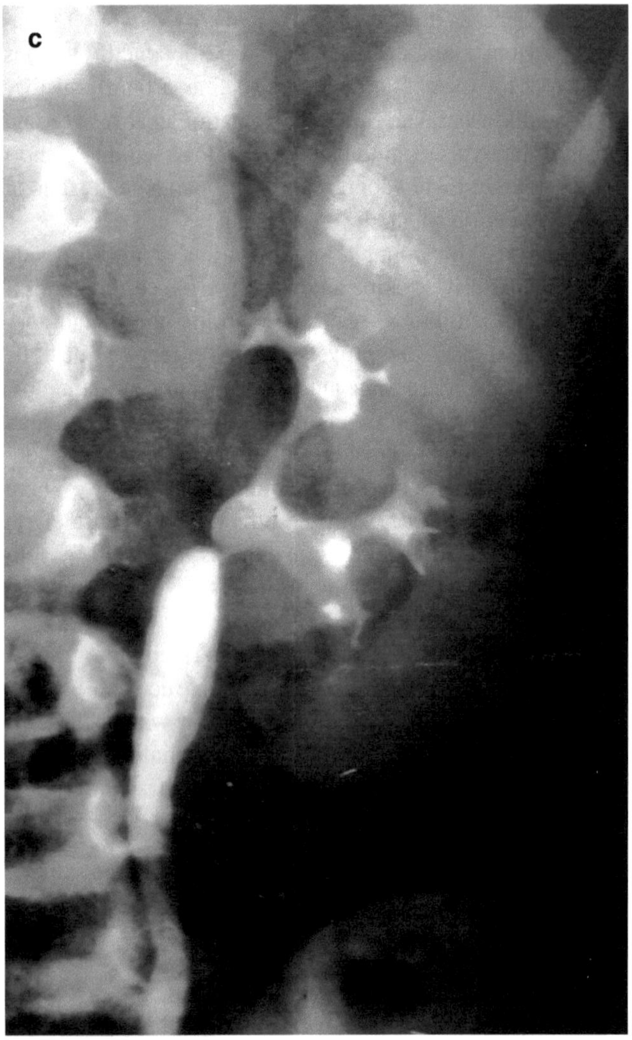

Fig. 55.1 (continued)

preferably by or in the presence of the surgeon, will clarify the last remaining questions such as the choice of the access route for percutaneous nephrolithotripsy. KUB and intravenous urography, even when supplemented with tomography and at various angles, clearly provide less information [16]. Calculous material is not depicted adequately at magnetic resonance tomography. As some staghorn stones cause significant obstruction, it may occasionally be difficult to clarify ureteral anatomy adequately even with state-of-the-art CT imaging. In this situation retrograde ureterography at the time of definitive surgery is still a reliable mainstay.

Detailed explanation of the therapeutic approach, of potential complications that may occur, and especially the potential need for staged interventions are essential for informed consent.

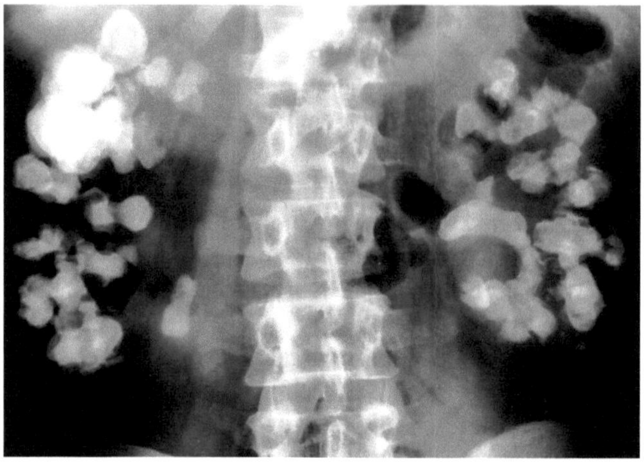

Fig. 55.2 Advanced stone disease with threatening end-stage renal failure

Selection of the Individual Therapeutic Approach

Open surgery using extended pyelolithotomy and/or nephron-sparing anatrophic nephrolithomy techniques, if needed in renal ischemia and regional hypothermia, achieve complete stone clearance rates with complete staghorn stones of up to 90 % [16, 19]. Percutaneous nephrolithotomy (PCNL) has been proven equally effective at lower morbidity [20, 21]. Staghorn stones have a high recurrence rate regardless of the surgical approach, even with complete stone removal [22]. Incisional redo surgery for stones is complex and limited in how often it can be performed. In contrast, redo endourological procedures are not aggravated by previous surgery. As a result, they have become the "gold standard" for the treatment of staghorn stones today and have eliminated open surgery for this indication [1–3, 23, 24].

Open surgery has occasionally been advocated to simultaneously correct a concomitant urinary drainage problem with stone removal. The last 20 years of endourological stone removal has shown that there rarely is a true need to correct apparent obstruction at the ureteropelvic junction, a horseshoe kidney, or segmental obstruction of the collecting system at the time of stone removal. In the rare case where this is indeed needed, laparoscopic surgery has also replaced open surgery today [25].

Percutaneous Nephrolithotripsy (PCNL)

Percutaneous nephrolithotripsy is not limited by the stone mass to be removed and the drainage situation and therefore has become the standard approach for managing staghorn stones. The surgical technique is detailed in Chap. 51. As staghorn stones present the most daunting challenge in stone therapy, PCNL has to be adapted to the individual situation [22]:

- We routinely insert a ureteric catheter as the first step. This permits administration of contrast dye at any time of the procedure, helps identify the ureteropelvic junction during endoscopic manipulation, and prevents dislocation of stone fragments into the ureter.
- PCNL can be performed either in the supine or prone position. The decision mainly depends on the surgeon's experience, and systematic data analyses have shown neither approach to offer significant advantages over the other [10, 26]. With patients at higher risk of cardiopulmonary complications, we usually select the supine position for anesthesiological considerations, whereas with severe obesity, with very large stone mass, or if bilateral PCNL in the same session is an option, we always prefer the prone position. If PCNL is to be combined with retrograde ureteroscopy, a modified supine semioblique position with the legs slightly extended and flexed permits performing both procedures simultaneously without having to change the patient's position [27].
- Fluoroscopy in two planes must be available throughout the procedure without having to change the patient's position. This is best achieved with a modern C-arm unit, which permits fluoroscopy at multiple angles and hardcopy radiographs where needed for documentation. In addition we routinely use intraoperative ultrasonography with 3.5–6 MHz for establishing the nephrostomy tract, as it simultaneously depicts the stone, the calyx to be punctured, and the overlying parenchyma.
- Key to successful PCNL is correct percutaneous access to reach all calculous material. In staghorn stones this has to be selected individually, mainly depending on the location of the stone within the collecting system. In general a first nephrostomy tract is placed into the calyx, which permits access to the largest stone mass, and additional tracts are placed to reach calyces that cannot be reached from the first tract. Posterior lower pole calyces are easiest to puncture, but it may be difficult to reach middle calyces or even lower pole anterior calyces from this point of entry. An upper pole posterior calyx may provide better access to more of the collecting system (Fig. 55.3), but this frequently requires a supracostal approach with a higher potential for complications [28].
- In the last years, with availability of better flexible nephroscopes, miniaturized nephroscopes, holmium-Nd:YAG stone fragmentation, and the option of simultaneous retrograde ureteroscopy, we have changed our PCNL strategy for staghorn stones. Supracostal puncture, multiple nephrostomy tracts, larger caliber tracts, and long intrarenal surgery are driving factors for a higher complication rate, especially from hemorrhage, and we try to avoid them as much as possible [23, 29, 30]. A first tract is placed into an easy-to-puncture calyx from which the bulk of the stone can be accessed. This tract is then used for removing the remaining stone with the flexible nephroscope wherever possible. Calculous material that cannot be reached is then approached with additional tracts, but with smaller caliber nephroscopes (15–21-F tracts) [31]. The procedure usually becomes more difficult after step one, removal of the bulk of the stone, as bleeding at this time often obscures vision and flexible and small-caliber rigid endoscopes become more difficult to use. Stone removal is therefore staged: Easy-to-remove stone material is removed in a first session, and the difficult-to-reach residuals in a second procedure within 24–48 h. The primary nephrostomy tract remains intubated with a 14–16-F nephrostomy tube during this period. When bleeding clears, the residual stone situation can be reassessed radiologically if necessary, and the second phase of the procedure can be performed under optimum endoscopic conditions. In 131 kidneys with complete staghorn stones treated at our institution from 1997 to 2009, complete stone removal was achieved in 54 % after the first session and 89 % after the second session, with major complications (requiring a reintervention) in 3.8 % and a mean time of hospitalization of 6.1 days.
- Combining PCNL at the second session with retrograde ureteroscopy for stone removal from upper and middle anterior calyces improves stone clearance in difficult situations [27]. The advent of true mini-nephroscopes which can be introduced through the needle used to establish the tract promises further reduction of complications [32].
- Drainage after PCNL with only an internal ureteric stent ("tubeless" PCNL) has been advocated to reduce treatment morbidity. With staghorn stones this is hazardous, as unnoticed residual stones, bleeding, and urinary extravasation are more common than with standard PCNL and a percutaneous access may again be needed. Moreover, many staghorn stones are infected at the time of surgery in spite of antibiotic pretreatment, and postoperative infectious problems are more common. Large-caliber tubes to tamponade the tract are unneeded and even hazardous; one 12–14-F nephrostomy tube left in place provides secure drainage and access to the collecting system if needed [33]. After the redo-procedure complete stone removal and free ureteric drainage are again controlled radiologically, the tube can then be removed within 24 h.

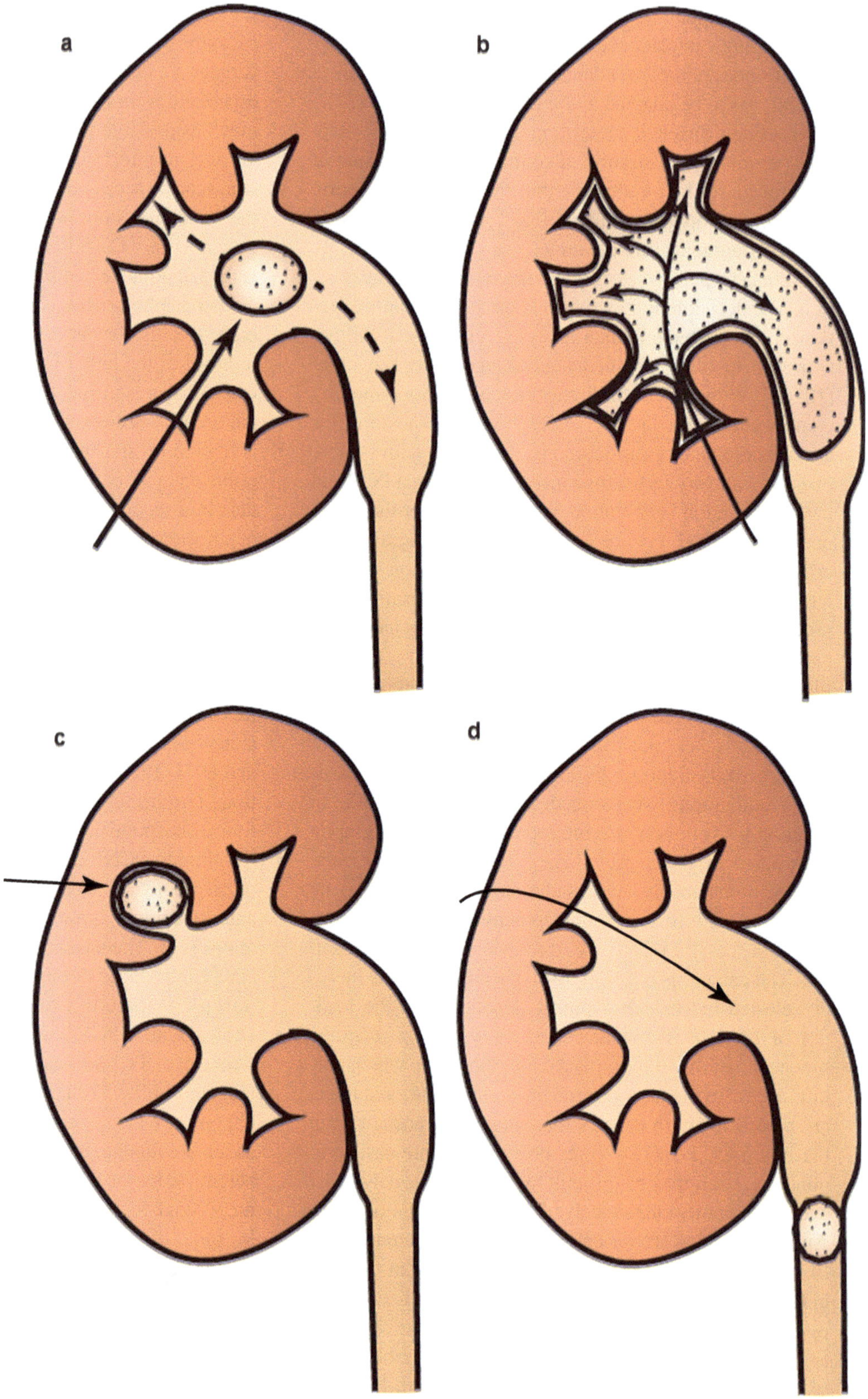

Fig. 55.3 Percutaneous access depending on stone location. (**a**) Pelviceal stone. (**b**) Branched stone. (**c**) Diverticulum stone. (**d**) Stone in the upper ureter

- Residual stone material is the single most important reason for recurrent stone formation, especially in struvite stones [20]. Complete stone removal is therefore essential. If residual stones are detected even after the second PCNL, we today tend to do another endoscopic redo procedure (PCNL/URS), preferably again within 24–48 h. We have abandoned all attempts of dissolving residual calculous material by percutaneous irrigation only [2]. Adjuvant SWL is very rarely used any more; in our series mentioned above, 8 % of the patients had adjuvant SWL, and this dropped to <2 % in the last 5 years.

With bilateral staghorn stones, bilateral PCNL is feasible in the same session and, if performed prudently, results in equal stone-free rates at lower overall complication rates than when each side is treated separately [34]. After inserting ureteral catheters on both sides, the patient is brought into the prone position. The stone on the side technically simpler to remove, or with significant obstruction the more threatened side, is treated first. PCNL follows the previously outlined approach, i.e., with vision becoming obscured by bleeding, the procedure on this side is terminated, good nephrostomy drainage is established, and the more tedious removal of difficult-to-reach stone segments is delayed for an early second procedure. If no major problems were encountered at this point, the contralateral side is now to be approached in an identical manner. The second intervention 24–48 h later can then be used to complete stone clearance at both sides.

Staghorn stones in children can be treated by PCNL along the same principles, but with the use of adequately miniaturized instruments [35]. With tract over-dilatation renal parenchyma may fragment in a radial direction from the tract, potentially resulting in significant renal trauma and bleeding. A 28-F tract in a kidney with a length of 12 cm corresponds in trauma to a 56-F tract in a kidney of 6-cm length. Pediatric nephroscopes 12–18 F in diameter, corresponding small-caliber sheaths, and adequate small-caliber ultrasonic, pneumatic, or laser lithotrites must be available. As SWL is far more effective for branched stones in children than in adults, we tend to treat these stones by primary SWL [1].

Retrograde Ureteroscopic Intrarenal Stone Removal

Approaches via natural orifices with their inherent low morbidity represent an attractive alternative to PCNL with its perforating trauma. The development of better flexible ureteroscopes and reliable disintegration techniques through small working ports today permits effective, albeit tedious, removal of renal stones of up to 35 mm in diameter [1, 36, 37].

With staghorn stones, which by definition have a large stone mass and complex stone location, an all-natural orifice approach is rarely feasible, but it may become a future option. Combining PCNL and retrograde ureteroscopy to reach upper pole calyces to avoid supracostal nephrostomy tracts is already being used today [27].

Shock Wave Lithotripsy (SWL)

Large stone mass renders this a very unsatisfactory approach, and early attempts to use staged SWL in conjunction with internal stenting of the ureter have largely been abandoned because of the need of multiple treatments, the long time needed to reach stone-free status, and the high rate of adjuvant procedures. In a prospective, randomized, single center study, Meretyk et al. compared the use of extracorporeal shock wave lithotripsy to the combination of SWL and PCNL in 50 patients with complete staghorn calculi. Stone-free rate was significantly higher with the latter technique (74 vs. 22 %, respectively), and septic complications were 1.5-fold higher after SWL [24]. All guidelines today recommend limiting SWL as first-line treatment for stones with a diameter <20 mm respective to a stone cross section <300 mm^2 [1–3].

The situation differs with staghorn stones in children. Apparently as a result of less interference with energy transmission by the thinner abdominal wall, softer stones and a better capability of the ureter to expand more readily with obstruction for fragment expulsion children achieve complete stone clearance after SWL considerably faster and at higher rates than adults [38]. SWL is therefore the first choice of treatment for larger stones up to 20 mm in diameter or 300-mm^2 surface area, in particular for children <6 years of age [1]. Of course the renal trauma generated by shock waves, radiation exposure, and the amount of stone debris generated per session has to be minimized. This requires a modern, small-focus lithotripter with ultrasound-based targeting of the stone and staged SWL treating stone segments in the renal pelvis and upper calices first. Because of the excellent fragment expulsion in children, we do not use ureteric stents in children. Where lithotripters suitable for children are not available, staghorn stones can be removed by PCNL, albeit at somewhat higher morbidity than with SWL [35].

With proven uric acid stones, oral dissolution is possible even for large-volume stones. As dissolution is more effective with larger surface of stone material to be dissolved, SWL prior to dissolution increases stone surface multifold and hence improves dissolution. In patients with staghorn stones and a high likelihood of having uric acid stones (previous analysis-proven uric acid stones, constant urine pH < 5.2, radiolucent stone on KUB), this approach can be considered, especially with a fairly delicate, low-volume staghorn stone. Fragments may rapidly block the ureter, and this cannot be discerned on a KUB. The ureter must therefore be stented. Close urologic surveillance is essential. Any fragment passed must be analyzed to confirm the composition of uric acid. As even stone formers with proven recurrent uric acid stones may suddenly form stones with a calcium oxalate or urate component which prevents dissolution, failure to document a reduction of stone mass or signs of increasing obstruction should trigger the decision for endoscopic removal. In view of the long treatment time involved with the SWL/oral dissolution approach, we today favor immediate PCNL also for larger, more complex uric acid stones.

Treatment and Follow-Up After Complete Stone Removal

Staghorn stones in general have a higher recurrence rate than uncomplicated stones [39]. Identifying the reason for stone formation and eliminating causative factors therefore become an essential part of therapy. The essential first steps are the precise analysis of the stone composition by radio diffractometry or spectrometry and metabolic evaluation (as detailed in Chap. 85). Any risk factor for recurrent stone formation is corrected by adequate behavioral and medical measures. The patient must remain under close urologic surveillance to monitor both the elimination of risk factors and compliance. Urinary infection is a common etiological factor, especially in patients after urinary diversion or after reconstructive procedures of the urinary tract. If appropriate medical therapy cannot eliminate infection in these situations, secondary surgical correction of any underlying problem may be become necessary. Any recurrent stone should be detected and treated aggressively as early as possible. The main problem of stones comes from stone mass, and this is almost always a result of treatment being initiated too late.

Conclusion

Staghorn stones represent most advanced renal stone disease and, if not treated adequately, will result in loss of the kidney. PCNL is usually the treatment of choice, but the surgical technique has to be adapted to the individual situation. It provides stone clearance rates equal to those obtained with open surgery, but at significant lower overall morbidity. Nevertheless, it is challenging and requires significant expertise and frequently staged procedures. Even with complete stone removal, the risk of recurrent stone formation is inherently high. Eliminating underlying reasons for stone formation, close long-term follow-up and aggressive treatment of recurrent stones are therefore essential for successful management.

References

1. EAU Guidelines on Urolithiasis. www.uroweb.org. Accessed 10 Sept 2011.
2. AUA Guideline on managment of staghorn calculi: diagnosis and treatment recommendations. www.auanet.org. Accessed 10 Sept 2011.
3. ICUD Guidelines on Stone Disease. www.icud.info. Accessed 10 Sept 2011.
4. Wickham JEA. The surgical treatment of renal lithiasis. In: Urinary calculous disease. Edinburgh: Churchill Livingstone; 1979.
5. Rocco F, Mandressi A, Larcher P. Surgical classification of renal calculi. Eur Urol. 1984;10:121–3.
6. Rassweiler JJ, Renner C, Eisenberger F. The management of complex renal stones. BJU Int. 2000;86:919–28.
7. Lam HS, Lingeman JE, Russo R, Chua GT. Stone surface area determination techniques: a unifying concept of staghorn stone burden assessment. J Urol. 1992;148:1026–9.
8. Pak CY, Resnick MI, Preminger GM. Ethnic and geographic diversity of stone disease. Urology. 1997;50:504–7.
9. Statistik Austria. www.statistik.at. Accessed 11 Sept 2011.
10. de la Rosette J, Assimos D, Desai M, Gutierrez J, Lingeman J, Scarpa R, et al. The clinical research office of the endourological society percutaneous nephrolithotomy global study: indications, complications, and outcomes in 5803 patients. J Endourol. 2011; 25:11–7.
11. Desai M, De Lisa A, Turna B, Rioja J, Walfridsson H, D'Addessi A, et al. The clinical research office of the endourological society percutaneous nephrolithotomy global study: staghorn versus nonstaghorn stones. J Endourol. 2011;25(8):1263–8. Epub 2011 Jul 20.
12. Kumar R, Anand A, Saxena V, Seth A, Dogra PN, Gupta NP. Safety and efficacy of PCNL for management of staghorn calculi in pediatric patients. J Pediatr Urol. 2011;7:248–51.
13. Tiselius HG. Epidemiology and medical management of stone disease. BJU Int. 2003;91:758–67.
14. Blandy JP, Singh M. The case for a more aggressive approach to staghorn stones. J Urol. 1976;115:505–56.
15. Koga S, Arakaki Y, Matsuoka M, Ohyama C. Staghorn calculi – long-term results of management. Br J Urol. 1991;68:122–4.
16. Marberger M, Fitzpatrick JM. A guide to treatment selection. In: Marberger M, Fitzpatrick JM, Jenkins AD, Pak CYC, editors. Stone surgery. Edinburgh: Churchill Livingstone; 1991. p. 233–57.
17. Hubert J, Blum A, Cormier L, Claudon M, Regent D, Mangin P. Three-dimensional CT-scan reconstruction of renal calculi. A new tool for mapping-out staghorn calculi and follow-up of radiolucent stones. Eur Urol. 1997;31:297–301.
18. Patel U, Walkden RM, Ghani KR, Anson K. Three-dimensional CT pyelography for planning of percutaneous nephrostolithotomy: accuracy of stone measurement, stone depiction and pelvicalyceal reconstruction. Eur Radiol. 2009;19:1280–8.
19. Boyce WH, Elkins IB. Reconstructive renal surgery following anatrophic nephrolithotomy: followup of 100 consecutive cases. J Urol. 1974;111:307–12.
20. Marberger M. Percutaneous stone manipulation. In: Marberger M, Fitzpatrick JM, Jenkins AD, Pak CYC, editors. Stone surgery. Edinburgh: Churchill Livingstone; 1991. p. 49–115.
21. Al-Kohlany KM, Shokeir AA, Mosbah A, Mohsen T, Shoma AM, Eraky I, et al. Treatment of complete staghorn stones: a prospective randomized comparison of open surgery versus percutaneous nephrolithotomy. J Urol. 2005;173:469–73.
22. Michael M, Fitzpatrick JM, Jenkins AD. Stone surgery. Edinburgh: Churchill Livingstone; 1991.
23. Desai M, Jain P, Ganpule A, Sabnis R, Patel S, Shrivastav P. Developments in technique and technology: the effect on the results of percutaneous nephrolithotomy for staghorn calculi. BJU Int. 2009;104:542–8, discussion 8.
24. Meretyk S, Gofrit ON, Gafni O, Pode D, Shapiro A, Verstandig A, et al. Complete staghorn calculi: random prospective comparison between extracorporeal shock wave lithotripsy monotherapy and combined with percutaneous nephrostolithotomy. J Urol. 1997;157: 780–6.
25. Simforoosh N, Aminsharifi A, Tabibi A, Noor-Alizadeh A, Zand S, Radfar MH, et al. Laparoscopic anatrophic nephrolithotomy for managing large staghorn calculi. BJU Int. 2008;101: 1293–6.
26. de la Rosette JJ, Tsakiris P, Ferrandino MN, Elsakka AM, Rioja J, Preminger GM. Beyond prone position in percutaneous nephrolithotomy: a comprehensive review. Eur Urol. 2008;54: 1262–9.

27. Scoffone CM, Cracco CM, Cossu M, Grande S, Poggio M, Scarpa RM. Endoscopic combined intrarenal surgery in Galdakao-modified supine Valdivia position: a new standard for percutaneous nephrolithotomy? Eur Urol. 2008;54:1393–403.
28. Lojanapiwat B, Prasopsuk S. Upper-pole access for percutaneous nephrolithotomy: comparison of supracostal and infracostal approaches. J Endourol. 2006;20:491–4.
29. Yamaguchi A, Skolarikos A, Buchholz NP, Chomón GB, Grasso M, Saba P, et al. Operating times and bleeding complications in percutaneous nephrolithotomy: a comparison of tract dilation methods in 5,537 patients in the Clinical Research Office of the Endourological Society Percutaneous Nephrolithotomy Global Study. J Endourol. 2011;25:933–9.
30. Ganpule AP, Mishra S, Desai MR. Multiperc versus single perc with flexible instrumentation for staghorn calculi. J Endourol. 2009;23:1675–8.
31. Kukreja R, Desai M, Patel S, Bapat S. Factors affecting blood loss during percutaneous nephrolithotomy: prospective study. J Endourol. 2004;18:715–22.
32. Desai MR, Sharma R, Mishra S, Sabnis RB, Stief C, Bader M. Single-step percutaneous nephrolithotomy (microperc): the initial clinical report. J Urol. 2011;186:140–5.
33. Marcovich R, Jacobson AI, Singh J, Shah D, El-Hakim A, Lee BR, et al. No panacea for drainage after percutaneous nephrolithotomy. J Endourol. 2004;18:743–7.
34. Holman E, Salah MA, Toth C. Comparison of 150 simultaneous bilateral and 300 unilateral percutaneous nephrolithotomies. J Endourol. 2002;16:33–6.
35. Desai MR, Kukreja RA, Patel SH, Bapat SD. Percutaneous nephrolithotomy for complex pediatric renal calculus disease. J Endourol. 2004;18:23–7.
36. Prabhakar M. Retrograde ureteroscopic intrarenal surgery for large (1.6-3.5 cm) upper ureteric/renal calculus. Indian J Urol. 2010;26:46–9.
37. Ricchiuti DJ, Smaldone MC, Jacobs BL, Smaldone AM, Jackman SV, Averch TD. Staged retrograde endoscopic lithotripsy as alternative to PCNL in select patients with large renal calculi. J Endourol. 2007;21:1421–4.
38. D'Addessi A, Bongiovanni L, Sasso F, Gulino G, Falabella R, Bassi P. Extracorporeal shockwave lithotripsy in pediatrics. J Endourol. 2008;22:1–12.
39. El-Nahas AR, Eraky I, Shokeir AA, Shoma AM, El-Assmy AM, El-Tabey NA, et al. Long-term results of percutaneous nephrolithotomy for treatment of staghorn stones. BJU Int. 2011;108:750–4.

Ureteral Stone Management: An Overview

56

Sutchin R. Patel and Stephen Y. Nakada

Abstract

Technologic changes in the field of endourology and the introduction of medical expulsive therapy have led to changes in the treatment of ureteral calculi. Non-contrast computed tomography pre-procedure parameters such as stone size, stone attenuation (Hounsfield units), and skin-to-stone distance can allow selection of the treatment modality with the highest success rate. Medical expulsive therapy with periodic evaluation may be used for <10-mm ureteral stones in a patient whose symptoms are controlled and who is not infected. Both shock wave lithotripsy and ureteroscopy with laser lithotripsy are acceptable first-line treatments for ureteral stones. Other treatment options such as percutaneous antegrade ureteroscopy or laparoscopic/open ureterolithotomy may be considered in rare cases when ureteroscopy or shock wave lithotripsy has failed.

Keywords

Ureteral stone management • Medical expulsive therapy • Shock wave lithotripsy • Ureteroscopy • Hounsfield units • Skin-to-stone distance • Non-contrast computed tomography

Introduction

The treatment of ureteral calculi has evolved over the years with the technologic changes in endourology and the recognition of medications to aid in stone expulsion. The American Urological Association (AUA) and European Association of Urology (EAU) guidelines for the management of ureteral calculi assert that stone size and location are two of the most important factors in determining the appropriate intervention [1]. Thus, accurate quantification of stone burden is an important factor in the selection of the appropriate treatment modality. Non-contrast computed tomography (NCCT) has been the imaging modality of choice for evaluating stone burden due to its high sensitivity (95–100 %) and specificity (94–96 %) in detecting urolithiasis [2–4]. Due to concerns regarding the radiation dose associated with computed tomography, newer low-dose CT protocols (with radiation dose reductions to the level of a KUB [kidney-ureter-bladder]) are available and have been shown to have a high sensitivity, specificity, and accuracy in evaluating urolithiasis [5, 6].

Whether it be for preoperative or postoperative evaluation, it is important for urologists to understand the limitations and errors associated with the common imaging modalities used to quantify stones. Despite the relatively low cost and radiation dose of a plain abdominal X-ray, KUB is associated with a magnification error of approximately 20 % [7]. The sensitivity and specificity for KUB in the detection of ureteral calculi are 45–59 % and 71–77 %, respectively [8]. Ultrasound (US), which has no associated radiation exposure, can be used to measure stone dimensions in any plane, but reproducibility of size measurements can be

S.R. Patel, M.D. • S.Y. Nakada, M.D. (✉)
Department of Urology, University of Wisconsin School of Medicine and Public Health, 1685 Highland Ave, Madison, WI 53705, USA
e-mail: sutchin_patel@yahoo.com; nakada@urology.wisc.edu

J.J. Talati et al. (eds.), *Urolithiasis*,
DOI 10.1007/978-1-4471-4387-1_56, © Springer-Verlag London 2012

difficult as US does not have fixed planes as does KUB or NCCT. US has also been shown to overestimate stone size by ≤50 % when compared to NCCT for smaller stones (≤5 mm) [9]. US may also have difficulty localizing mid-ureteral calculi. Yilmaz et al. found US to have poor sensitivity in the detection of ureteral calculi (sensitivity: 19 %, specificity: 97 %) [10]. Heterogeneity exists in the literature regarding the imaging modality used both pre- and post-procedure (for SWL and ureteroscopy); thus, it is important for urologists to be aware of the limitations of different radiographic tests in the evaluation of ureteral stone burden [11, 12].

Observation and Medical Expulsive Therapy

It has long been noted that many ureteral calculi pass spontaneously. Knowledge regarding how long a patient should expect to wait prior to stone passage and which factors predict spontaneous passage are important in determining which patients can be observed. Though observation is the least invasive treatment option, it is important to be cognizant of the pain expectations of the patient, how it may affect the patient in regard to time off from work, and the potential risk of renal injury. Miller and Kane analyzed the impact of clinical factors such as patient age, gender, stone size, location, pain medication requirements, and interval to stone passage [13].

Multivariate analysis revealed that patient sex, age, and degree of pain were unrelated to the time for stone passage and that together stone size, location, and side were statistically related to stone passage interval ($p=0.012$). The mean time for stone passage for ≤2, 2–4, and ≥4 mm was 8.2, 12.2, and 22 days, respectively. For 95 % of stones ≤6 mm to pass spontaneously, 30–40 days were required. The likelihood of intervention for stones >4 mm was 50 %. Hubner et al. evaluated 100 patients managed with observation and found that stone passage rates based on stone location were 12, 22, and 45 % for proximal, middle, and distal ureteral stones [14]. Stone passage rates based on stone size in the same cohort of patients were 57, 35, and 8 % for <4-mm, 4- to 6-mm, and >6-mm stones. They also found that complications increased significantly with time, with 20 % of complications occurring after 4 weeks compared to only 7 % of complications occurring prior to 4 weeks of observation.

Though pain management and antiemetic therapy allow for patient comfort during a trial of observation, a number of other pharmacologic agents can also be used to help increase the rate of stone passage and reduce the chance of surgical intervention. Patients who elect to undergo an attempt at spontaneous stone passage or medical expulsive therapy should have well-controlled pain, no clinical evidence of sepsis, and adequate renal function reserve [1]. Nonsteroidal anti-inflammatory drugs (NSAIDs) have been shown to inhibit ureteral contractions as well as block the local release of pain-mediating prostaglandins [15, 16]. Though NSAIDs are used for pain control in patients with renal colic, they have not been shown to increase the rate of stone passage [17]. Corticosteroids, such as deflazacort and prednisone, have been shown to inhibit stretch-induced ureteral contractility in the porcine model as well as stabilize neutrophil lysosomes, thereby decreasing inflammation and edema related to mechanical irritation [18, 19]. In a study of patients treated with tamsulosin, the addition of deflazacort reduced mean expulsion time from 139.2 to 103.3 h ($p=0.04$) and also slightly increased stone expulsion rates (90.0 vs. 96.7 %) [20]. Thus, corticosteroids may be beneficial in reducing the time to stone expulsion.

The two best studied pharmacologic agents used in medical expulsive therapy are the calcium channel blocker, nifedipine, and alpha-receptor antagonists. The panel for the 2007 AUA/EAU guidelines on the management of ureteral calculi performed a meta-analysis of available randomized controlled trials that compared either nifedipine or alpha blockers to control therapies [1]. They found that nifedipine showed an absolute increase of 9 % in stone passage rates, which was not statistically significant. A meta-analysis of alpha blocker therapy versus control showed an absolute increase of 29 % in the stone passage rate, which was statistically significant. Porpiglia et al. performed the first randomized controlled trial comparing the efficacy of tamsulosin versus nifedipine for stone passage [21]. Eighty-six patients with stones <10 mm in the distal ureter were randomly divided into three groups: (1) 30 mg/day nifedipine + 30 mg/day deflazacort, (2) 0.4 mg/day tamsulosin + 30 mg/day deflazacort, and (3) no medication (control group). There was a statistically significant difference in the time to stone passage when comparing groups 1 and 2 to group 3 (control), but there was no statistically significant difference in time to stone passage when comparing the nifedipine + deflazacort group (group 1) to the tamsulosin + deflazacort group (group 2). Dellabella et al. performed a large randomized controlled trial of 210 patients with distal ureteral calculi >4 mm that were randomized to 1 of 3 groups: (1) tamsulosin, (2) nifedipine, and (3) phloroglucinol, and each group was given a corticosteroid drug [22]. The stone expulsion rate was significantly higher in the tamsulosin group (97 %) when compared to the nifedipine (77 %) and phloroglucinol (64 %) groups. The time to stone passage was also significantly shorter for the tamsulosin group compared to the nifedipine and phloroglucinol groups (Table 56.1). Yilmaz et al. studied the efficacy of three different alpha blockers (tamsulosin, terazosin, and doxazosin) in the passage of distal ureteral stones and found similar stone expulsion rates (79, 79, and 76 % for tamsulosin, terazosin, and doxazosin respectively compared to 54 % for a control group) among the three medications [23]. Hollingsworth et al. performed a meta-analysis

Table 56.1 Tamsulosin versus nifedipine trials

Study	Stone size studied (no patients)	Treatment	Stone passage rate (%)	Time to stone passage (days)
Porpiglia et al. [21]	<10 mm (n=86)	Nifedipine + deflazacort	80	9.3
		Tamsulosin + deflazacort	85	7.9
		Observation	43	12
Dellabella et al. [22]	>4 mm (n=210)	Tamsulosin	97	3
		Nifedipine	77	5
		Phloroglucinol	64	5

of randomized controlled trials to assess the efficacy of medical therapy in facilitating spontaneous passage of ureteral stones. Their study showed that patients given calcium channel blockers or alpha blockers had a 65 % greater likelihood of stone passage than those not given such treatment [24].

Though both calcium channel blockers and alpha-adrenergic agents have been shown to increase the rate of stone passage and shorten stone expulsion times, it is important to be aware of and counsel patients regarding the side effects of these medications. The AUA/EAU guideline panel considers it a standard that not only should patients be counseled on the attendant risks of medical expulsive therapy including associated drug side effects but that they should also be informed that it is administered for an "off-label" use [1]. There has been growing literature on intraoperative floppy iris syndrome (IFIS) in patients taking tamsulosin and undergoing phacoemulsification cataract surgery [25]. Other alpha-antagonists (doxazosin, terazosin, alfuzosin) have also been associated with IFIS, and thus, urologists need to be aware of this potential side effect in order to counsel patients and recommend that patients discuss the use of alpha blockers with their ophthalmologist and consider stopping the use of alpha blockers in patients that may undergo cataract surgery [26]. Once a patient has been placed on a trial of observation or medical expulsive therapy, they should be monitored with periodic imaging studies to monitor stone position and to assess for hydronephrosis. Miller and Kane found that 50 % of patients with stones >4 mm ultimately fail conservative management. Patients considering observation need to allow from 2 to 4 weeks in order to give an adequate trial of observation or medical expulsive therapy. Indications for intervention include poor pain control, failure of stone progression on serial imaging, the presence of increasing or unremitting renal colic, or development of a urinary tract infection (AUA/EAU panel consensus, level IV evidence) [1].

Shock Wave Lithotripsy

Since its first scientific and clinical description by Chaussy, extracorporeal shock wave lithotripsy (SWL) has provided a noninvasive surgical treatment modality for urinary tract calculi [27, 28]. As the technology has developed over the years, different types of lithotripters have been developed, and the science behind stone fragmentation via shock wave lithotripsy has begun to be better understood. As with any surgical intervention, it is important to understand the contraindications for the procedure as well as the technical limitations in order to select the patients that will have the highest success rate via SWL. Absolute contraindications to SWL include pregnancy, acute pyelonephritis, urinary sepsis, coagulopathy, implanted cardiac devices containing an abdominal crystalline component, and calcified vascular aneurysms located within 5 cm of the target stone (or measuring greater than 2 and 5 cm in absolute diameter for renal and aortic aneurysms). There have also been concerns regarding the use of SWL to treat distal ureteral calculi in women of childbearing age because of the theoretical possibility of damage to the ovaries and/or unfertilized eggs. Though there has been no objective evidence regarding this concern, many centers require women that are of childbearing age to be fully informed of the possibility and give their consent before treatment with SWL [1, 29, 30].

It is also important to be aware of the technical limitations of SWL as certain situations may limit the effectiveness of SWL such as morbid obesity, stone composition, and distal urinary tract obstruction. Stone compositions that are relatively resistant to SWL include matrix calculi, cystine stones, pure calcium oxalate monohydrate, and calcium phosphate stones [31–34]. Radiographic parameters on non-contrast computed tomography (NCCT) can be used to help predict SWL success. Hounsfield unit measurement on NCCT has been shown to help predict the difference between calcium oxalate and uric acid stones [35]. Stone attenuation on computed tomography can thus be used to predict stone fragmentation via SWL [36]. Kacker et al. performed a retrospective case-control study to determine radiographic parameters that predict SWL success and found that mean stone attenuation cutoff of less than 1,000 Hounsfield units could be used to predict SWL success for solitary 6- to 10-mm stones [37]. Several factors may also limit SWL in the obese patients. Patients may exceed the weight limit of the machine (which can be as high as 400 lbs, equivalent to 181 kg, approximately). The increased amount of intervening adipose tissue may both dampen the peak shock wave focal pressure and may hinder stone localization and targeting. The focal length, maximum skin-to-stone distance, may be too short for some obese patients. On NCCT, skin-to-stone distances (SSD) greater than 10 cm have been shown to predict treatment failure via SWL when compared to SSD < 10 cm for lower pole renal calculi [38]. Skin-to-stone distance has not been found to be a predictive parameter for ureteral calculi (SSD: 127.0 vs. 138.6 for SWL success and failure respectively for ureteral calculi), but studies have not compared obese to nonobese populations [18]. SWL success requires adequate fragmentation and spontaneous passage of stone fragments; thus, SWL monotherapy in the setting of distal urinary tract obstruction is not recommended unless a simultaneous procedure to correct the obstruction, such as ureteral stent placement, is planned.

The panel of the AUA/EUA ureteral stone guidelines performed a meta-analysis analyzing stone-free rates for ureteral calculi. The SWL stone-free rates were 82 % in the proximal ureter (41 studies, 6,428 patients), 73 % in the mid-ureter (31 studies, 1,607 patients), and 74 % in the distal ureter (50 studies, 6,981 patients) (Table 56.2) [1]. The procedure counts that include primary procedures (the number of times the intended procedure was performed), secondary procedures (the number of times an alternative stone removal procedure was performed), and adjunctive procedures (procedures related to the primary/secondary procedures such as stent removals) were also analyzed. The numbers of primary/secondary/adjunctive procedures for SWL based on ureteral stone location were the following: distal ureter = 1.22, 0.12, and 0.03; mid ureter = 1.11, 0.18, and 0.23; and proximal ureter = 1.31, 0.07, and 0.24. SWL complication rates for ureteral calculi that were reported in the studies analyzed were the following: 3–5 % sepsis, 4–8 % Steinstrasse, 0–2 % stricture, 1–2 % ureteral injury, and 1–4 % urinary tract infection [1]. Krambeck et al. reported that SWL for renal and proximal ureteral stones using an HM-3 lithotripter was associated with the development of hypertension and diabetes at 19 years follow-up [39]. Barbosa et al. found a small (prevalence of 37.8 % in SWL population vs. 32.5 % in controls; $p = 0.0009$) but significant increase in the risk of hypertension after SWL at a median follow-up of 6 years using a third-generation electrohydraulic lithotripter [40]. Studies by Sato et al. and Chew et al., with a median follow-up of 17 and 20 years, respectively, did not report an association between SWL for renal and proximal ureteral stones with hypertension or diabetes mellitus [41, 42]. The role of SWL used to treat ureteral stones in the development of hypertension and diabetes mellitus remains unclear. The AUA/EUA guideline panel recommends that both SWL and ureteroscopy are acceptable first-line treatments for patients requiring stone removal. Routine stenting as a part of SWL was not recommended as there is no improved fragmentation with stenting and ureteral stents are associated with frequent symptoms [1, 43–46].

Table 56.2 Stone-free rates for SWL and ureteroscopy for ureteral calculi (AUA/EAU ureteral stone guideline panel) [1]

Stone location	SWL SFR (95 % CI)	URS SFR (95 % CI)
Distal ureter	*74 % (73–75 %)*	*94 % (93–95 %)*
Distal ureter < 10 mm	86 % (80–91 %)	97 % (96–98 %)
Distal ureter > 10 mm	74 % (57–87 %)	93 % (88–96 %)
Mid-ureter	*73 % (66–79 %)*	*86 % (81–89 %)*
Mid-ureter < 10 mm	84 % (66–95 %)	91 % (81–96 %)
Mid-ureter > 10 mm	76 % (36–97 %)	78 % (61–90 %)
Proximal ureter	*82 % (79–85 %)*	*81 % (77–85 %)*
Proximal ureter < 10 mm	90 % (85–93 %)	80 % (73–85 %)
Proximal ureter > 10 mm	68 % (55–79 %)	79 % (71–87 %)

Ureteroscopy

With the technologic advances, including smaller caliber flexible and semirigid ureteroscopes and the introduction of the holmium: YAG laser, ureteroscopy has become a mainstay in the treatment of ureteral stones. The improvements in instrumentation have led to a safer and more efficacious modality to treat urolithiasis in all locations in the ureter [1, 47]. Currently available flexible ureteroscopes have a tip diameter of 5.3–8.7 Fr and a midshaft diameter of 7.5–9.3 Fr, allowing them to be passed into the ureter often without active dilation [48]. Complication rates have decreased to less than 5 %, and long-term complications such as stricture formation occur less than 2 % [49]. Overall stone-free rates for ureteral stones range from 81 to 94 % depending on stone location (see Table 56.2).

Treatment of stones in the distal ureter by ureteroscopy is associated with a high success rate. The overall stone-free rate using semirigid or rigid ureteroscopy was 94 %, with similar stone-free rates for both large and small distal ureteral stones (<10 mm = 97 % SFR, >10 mm = 93 % SFR) [1]. The middle ureter can be accessed with either the semirigid ureteroscope or via flexible ureteroscopy. SWL for middle ureteral stones may be problematic due to the underlying bone. The location over the iliac vessels may occasionally hinder access via a semirigid ureteroscope, but ureteroscopic management still yields a high stone-free rate (86 %) [1]. It should be noted that stone-free rates for larger stones are much less than those for smaller stones (>10 mm = 78 % SFR; <10 mm = 91 %).

The 1997 AUA nephrolithiasis clinical guideline panel recommended SWL for <1-cm stones in the proximal ureter and either SWL or URS for >1-cm proximal ureteral stones [43]. The current technology and instrumentation allows for much easier access to the proximal ureter leading to improved efficacy and low morbidity of flexible ureteroscopic treatment of proximal ureteral stones. Stone-free rate of ureteroscopy for proximal ureteral stones is 81 % with similar stone-free rates for both large and small stones (<10 mm = 80 % SFR; >10 mm = 79 % SFR). El-Nahas et al. performed a multivariate analysis of semirigid ureteroscopy for ureteral stones and found that factors predisposing to unfavorable results included proximal ureteral stones, ureteroscopy performed by surgeons that were not experienced endourologists, stone impaction, and stone width [50]. This further confirmed that semirigid ureteroscopy is best used for the treatment of mid- and distal ureteral stones. Best and Nakada studied outcomes of flexible ureteroscopy for the treatment of proximal ureteral stones in the obese and nonobese patient population and found similar stone-free rates between both groups [51]. With the increase in obesity in the general population, ureteroscopy may play an even larger role in the treatment of urolithiasis as SWL may be limited by the difficulty in visualizing and targeting the stone as well as the longer skin-to-stone distance in this patient population. In regard to post-ureteroscopy stenting, a number of randomized trials have shown that for uncomplicated ureteroscopy, the ureter may be left unstented without an increase in the risk of obstruction or colic [52–54].

Comparison of SWL and Ureteroscopy for Ureteral Stones

Though randomized controlled trials comparing SWL and ureteroscopy (URS) for ureteral stones are lacking, the meta-analysis performed by the 2007 AUA/EUA panel allows us to compare the stone-free rates between SWL and ureteroscopy for ureteral calculi. A multicenter prospective randomized trial by Pearle et al. compared SWL and ureteroscopy for the management of distal ureteral calculi <15 mm in size in 64 patients [55]. Follow-up KUB was performed at 21–24 days post-procedure in 91 % of the patients and showed resolution of the target stone in all cases. The minor complication rates were 9 % and 25 % for SWL and URS, respectively. SWL required less operating room time (72 vs. 97 min) and showed a trend toward less flank pain and quicker convalescence. The meta-analysis from the 2007 AUA/EUA guidelines found that stone-free rates for ureteroscopy were significantly better than SWL rates for both small (<10 mm) and large (>10 mm) distal ureteral calculi (see Table 56.2). Regarding stone-free rates for mid-ureteral calculi, though ureteroscopy appears to be superior (ureteroscopy = 86 % SFR; SWL = 73 % SFR), no statistically significant difference was found between ureteroscopy and SWL, possibly due to the small number of patients [1].

Lee et al. performed a prospective randomized trial comparing the efficiency quotient and cost-effectiveness index of SWL and ureteroscopic lithotripsy for the treatment of large (>15 mm) upper third ureteral stones [56]. The efficiency quotient (EQ) takes into account the need for retreatment and auxiliary procedures:

EQ = % stone-free/(100% [1 treatment] + % requiring retreatment + % requiring auxillary procedure) x 100%.

The efficiency quotients of SWL and ureteroscopy were 0.61 and 0.63, respectively. The authors, however, did note that the degree of hydronephrosis significantly influenced the success rate of SWL. Thus, the authors concluded that SWL should not be recommended as the first-line treatment option for the management of upper third ureteral stones larger than 1.5 cm with severe hydronephrosis. The cost-effectiveness index, treatment time, pain score, and hospital stay were greater in the ureteroscopy group. In the 1997 AUA nephrolithiasis clinical guidelines, the panel recommended SWL for <1-cm stones in the proximal ureter and either SWL or URS for >1-cm proximal ureteral stones [1, 43]. With the improved efficacy of ureteroscopic management for proximal ureteral stones, the 2007 AUA/EUA guidelines deemed ureteroscopy or SWL the appropriate treatment modality for proximal ureteral stones. However, proximal ureteral stones <10 mm treated with SWL were noted to have a higher stone-free rate than those treated with ureteroscopy (SWL = 90 % SFR; ureteroscopy = 80 % SFR). Conversely, proximal ureteral stones >10 mm treated with ureteroscopy were noted to have a higher stone-free rate than those treated with SWL (ureteroscopy = 79 % SFR; SWL = 68 % SFR) [1]. We have developed an algorithm that can be used alongside the AUA/EUA ureteral stone guidelines to help determine which patients should undergo medical expulsive therapy, SWL, or ureteroscopy (Fig. 56.1).

Other Procedures for Ureteral Calculi

Percutaneous antegrade ureteroscopy with laser lithotripsy and stone removal can be considered in the treatment of large (>15 mm) impacted proximal ureteral stones [57]. Stone-free rates in these cases range from 85 to 100 % [58, 59]. Percutaneous antegrade ureteroscopy for the treatment of ureteral stones can be an alternative when SWL has failed and in cases where retrograde ureteroscopy may not be amenable (patients with urinary diversion or renal transplants) [60–62].

SWL, ureteroscopy, and percutaneous antegrade ureteroscopy can successfully treat almost all ureteral calculi. In rare cases, such as very large impacted ureteral calculi, in which SWL or ureteroscopy have failed, can one consider laparoscopic or open ureterolithotomy [63, 64]. Laparoscopic ureterolithotomy is preferred if the surgeon has expertise in laparoscopy as it is less invasive and has a shorter recovery time compared to open ureterolithotomy. Laparoscopic or open ureterolithotomy, though highly effective, is thus not a first-line treatment for the treatment of ureteral calculi [1].

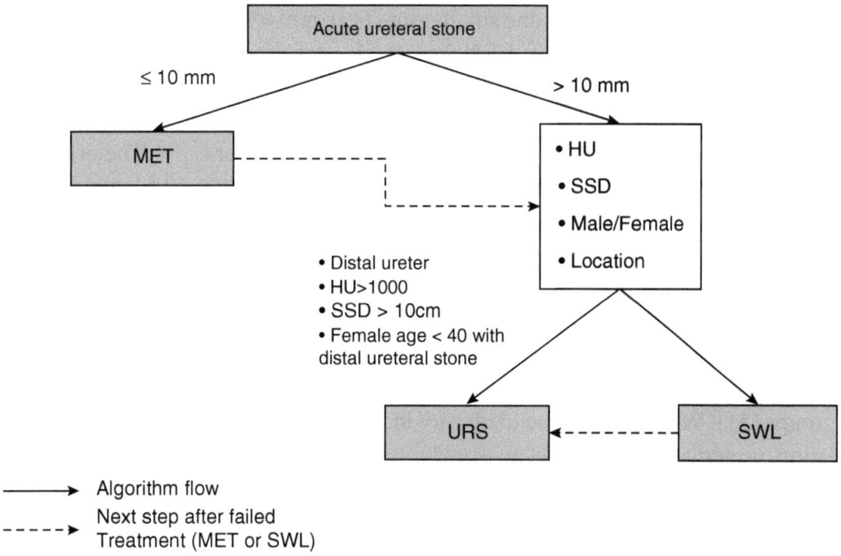

Fig. 56.1 An algorithm to help determine which patients should undergo medical expulsive therapy, *SWL*, or ureteroscopy. *HU* Hounsfield unit stone attenuation on NCCT, *SSD* skin-to-stone distance, *MET* medical expulsive therapy, *URS* ureteroscopy, *SWL* shock wave lithotripsy

Conclusion

The changes that have occurred from the 1997 to the 2007 ureteral stone guidelines have illustrated the changes in technology and instrumentation available to urologists [1, 43].

The AUA/EUA 2007 guidelines form the basis of the treatment of ureteral calculi today [1]. For ureteral stones <10 mm in a patient whose symptoms are controlled and who is not infected, observation with medical expulsive therapy is an option for initial treatment as long as the patient undergoes periodic evaluation. All patients who are started on medical expulsive therapy should be counseled regarding the associated drug side effects and that it is administered for an "off-label" use. The guidelines state that both SWL and ureteroscopy are acceptable first-line treatments for patients with ureteral stones. Ureteroscopy has been shown to have a higher stone-free rate than SWL for distal ureteral stones of all sizes as well as for large (>10 mm) proximal stones. SWL has been shown to have a higher stone-free rate for small (<10 mm) proximal ureteral calculi. Routine stenting is not recommended as part of SWL, and stenting following uncomplicated ureteroscopy is optional. Other treatment modalities such as percutaneous antegrade ureteroscopy are acceptable first-line treatments in select cases (large impacted stones in the proximal ureter). Laparoscopic or open surgical stone removal may be considered in rare cases when SWL, ureteroscopy, and percutaneous ureteroscopy fail or are unlikely to succeed.

References

1. Preminger GM, Tiselius HG, Assimos DG, Alken P, Buck C, Gallucci M, et al. 2007 guideline for the management of ureteral calculi. J Urol. 2007;178:2418–34.
2. Vieweg J, Teh C, Freed K, Leder RA, Smith RH, Nelson RH, et al. Unenhanced helical computerized tomography for the evaluation of patients with acute flank pain. J Urol. 1998;160:679–84.
3. Dalrymple NC, Verga M, Anderson KR, Bove P, Covey AM, Rosenfield AT, et al. The value of unenhanced helical computerized tomography in the management of acute flank pain. J Urol. 1998; 159:735–40.
4. Boulay I, Holtz P, Foley WD, White B, Begun FP. Ureteral calculi: diagnostic efficacy of helical CT and implications for treatment of patients. AJR Am J Roentgenol. 1999;172:1485–90.
5. Ferrandino MN, Bagrodia A, Pierre SA, Scales Jr CD, Rampersaud E, Pearle MS, et al. Radiation exposure in the acute and short-term management of urolithiasis at 2 academic centers. J Urol. 2009;181: 668–73.
6. Liu W, Esler SJ, Kenny BJ, Goh RH, Rainbow AJ, Stevenson GW. Low-dose nonenhanced helical CT of renal colic: assessment of ureteric stone detection and measurement of effective dose equivalent. Radiology. 2000;215:51–4.
7. Olcott EW, Sommer FG, Napel S. Accuracy of detection and measurement of renal calculi: in vitro comparison of three-dimensional spiral CT, radiography and nephrotomography. Radiology. 1997; 204:19–25.
8. Levine JA, Neitlich J, Verga M, Dalrymple N, Smith RC. Ureteral calculi in patients with flank pain: correlation of plain radiography with unenhanced helical CT. Radiology. 1997;204:27–31.
9. Ray AA, Ghiculete PKT, Honey RJ. Limitations to ultrasound in the detection and measurement of urinary tract calculi. Urology. 2010;76:295–300.
10. Yilmaz S, Sindel T, Arslan G, Ozkaynak C, Karaali K, Kabaalioglu A, et al. Renal colic: comparison of spiral CT, US and IVU in the detection of ureteral calculi. Eur Radiol. 1998;8:212–7.
11. Patel SR, Nakada SY. Quantification of preoperative stone burden for ureteroscopy and shock wave lithotripsy: current state and future recommendations. Urology. 2011;78(2):282–5.
12. Hyams ES, Bruhn A, Lipkin M, Shah O. Heterogeneity in the reporting of disease characteristics and treatment outcomes in studies evaluating treatments for nephrolithiasis. J Endourol. 2010;24: 1411–4.
13. Miller OF, Kane CJ. Time to stone passage for observed ureteral calculi: a guide for patient education. J Urol. 1999;162:688–91.
14. Hubner WA, Irby P, Stoller ML. Natural history and current concepts for the treatment of small ureteral calculi. Eur Urol. 1993; 24:172–6.

15. Sterret SP, Nakada SY. Medical expulsive therapy. Semin Nephrol. 2008;28:192–9.
16. Wen CC, Coyle TL, Jerde TJ, Nakada SY. Ketorolac effectively inhibits ureteral contractility in vitro. J Endourol. 2008;22:739–42.
17. Laerum E, Ommundsen OE, Gronseth JE, Christiansen A, Fagertun HE. Oral diclofenac in the prophylactic treatment of recurrent renal colic: a double-blind comparison with placebo. Eur Urol. 1995;28:108–11.
18. Bandi G, Wilkinson EA, Cary-Coyle TL, Jerde TJ, Nakada SY. Third prize: effect of hydrocortisone on porcine ureteral contractility in vitro. J Endourol. 2008;22:1169–73.
19. Cooper J, Stack G, Cooper T. Intensive medical management of ureteral calculi. Urology. 2000;56:575–8.
20. Dellabella M, Milanese G, Muzzonigro G. Medical-expulsive therapy for distal ureterolithiasis: randomized prospective study on role of corticosteroids used in combination with tamsulosin-simplified treatment regimen and health-related quality of life. Urology. 2005;66:712–5.
21. Porpiglia F, Ghigone G, Fiori C, Fontana D, Scarpa RM. Nifedipine versus tamsulosin for the management of lower ureteral stones. J Urol. 2004;172:568–71.
22. Dellabella M, Milanese G, Muzzonigro G. Randomized trial of the efficacy of tamsulosin, nifedipine and phloroglucinol in medical expulsive therapy for distal ureteral calculi. J Urol. 2005;174:167–72.
23. Yilmaz E, Batislam E, Basar MM, Tuglu D, Ferhat M, Basar H. The comparison and efficacy of 3 different α1-adrenergic blockers for distal ureteral stones. J Urol. 2005;173:2010–2.
24. Hollingsworth JM, Rogers MA, Kaufman R, Bradford TJ, Saint S, Wei JT, Hollenbeck BK. Medical therapy to facilitate urinary stone passage: a meta-analysis. Lancet. 2006;368:1171–9.
25. Kayes O, McLoughlin J. Tamsulosin and intraoperative "floppy iris" syndrome – keeping an eye on the problem. BJU Int. 2010;368:2–3.
26. Chatziralli IP, Sergentanis TN. Risk factors for intraoperative floppy iris syndrome: a meta-analysis. Ophthalmology. 2011;118:730–5.
27. Eisenberger F, Chaussy C. Contact-free renal stone fragmentation with shock waves. Urol Res. 1978;6:111.
28. Chaussy C, Schmiedt E, Jocham D, Brendel W, Forssmann B, Walther V. First clinical experience with extracorporeally induced destruction of kidney stones by shock waves. J Urol. 1982;127:417–20.
29. Carol PR, Shi RY. Genetic toxicity of high energy shock-waves: assessment using the induction of mutations or micronuclei in Chinese hamster ovary. J Urol. 1986;135:292a.
30. Erturk E, Herrman E, Cockett AT. Extracorporeal shock wave lithotripsy for distal ureteral stones. J Urol. 1993;149:1425–6.
31. Stoller ML, Gupta M, Bolton D, Irby 3rd PB. Clinical correlates of the gross, radiographic and histologic features of urinary matrix calculi. J Endourol. 1994;8:335–40.
32. Preminger GM, Zhong P. Mechanisms of differing stone fragility in extracorporeal shockwave lithotripsy. J Endourol. 1994;8:263–8.
33. Kim SC, Burns EK, Lingeman JE, Paterson RF, McAteer JA, Williams Jr JC. Cystine calculi: correlation of CT-visible structure, CT number, and stone morphology with fragmentation by shock wave lithotripsy. Urol Res. 2007;35:319–24.
34. Krambeck AE, Handa SE, Evan AP, Lingeman JE. Brushite stone disease as a consequence of lithotripsy? Urol Res. 2010;38:293–9.
35. Nakada SY, Hoff DG, Attai S, Heisey D, Blankenbaker D, Pozniak M. Determination of stone composition by noncontrast spiral computed tomography in the clinical setting. Urology. 2000;55:816–9.
36. Perks AE, Schuler TD, Lee J, Ghiculete D, Chung DG, D'A Honey RJ, et al. Stone attenuation and skin-to-stone distance on computed tomography predicts for stone fragmentation by shock wave lithotripsy. Urology. 2008;72:765–9.
37. Kacker R, Zhao L, Macejko A, Thaxton CS, Stern J, Liu JJ, et al. Radiographic parameters on noncontrast computerized tomography predictive of shock wave lithotripsy success. J Urol. 2008;179:1866–71.
38. Pareek G, Hedican SP, Lee FT, Nakada SY. Shock wave lithotripsy success determined by skin-to-stone distance on computed tomography. Urology. 2005;66:941–4.
39. Krambeck AE, Gettman MT, Rohlinger AL, Lohse CM, Patterson DE, Segura JW. Diabetes mellitus and hypertension associated with shock wave lithotripsy of renal and proximal ureteral stones at 19 years of followup. J Urol. 2006;175:1742–7.
40. Barbosa PV, Makhlouf AA, Thorner D, Ugarte R, Monga M. Shock wave lithotripsy associated with greater prevalence of hypertension. Urology. 2011;78(1):22–5.
41. Sato Y, Tanda H, Kato S, Ohnishi S, Nakajima H, Nanbu A, et al. Shock wave lithotripsy for renal stones is not associated with hypertension and diabetes mellitus. Urology. 2008;71:586–91.
42. Chew BH, Zavaglia B, Sutton C, Masson RK, Chan SH, Hamidizadeh R, et al. Twenty-year prevalence of diabetes mellitus and hypertension in patients receiving shock-wave lithotripsy for urolithiasis. BJU Int. 2012;109(3):444–9.
43. Segura JW, Preminger GM, Assimos DG, Dretler SP, Khan RI, Lingeman JE, et al. Ureteral stones clinical guidelines panel summary report on the management of ureteral calculi. The American Urological Association. J Urol. 1997;158:1915–21.
44. Pryor JL, Jenkins AD. Use of double-pigtail stents in extracorporeal shock wave lithotripsy. J Urol. 1990;143:475–8.
45. Preminger GM, Kettelhut MC, Elkins SL, Seger J, Fetner CD. Ureteral stenting during extracorporeal shock wave lithotripsy: help or hindrance? J Urol. 1989;142:32–6.
46. Low RK, Stoller ML, Irby P, Keeler L, Elhilali M. Outcome assessment of double-J stents during extracorporeal shock wave lithotripsy of small solitary renal calculi. J Endourol. 1996;10:341–3.
47. Francesca F, Scattoni V, Nava L, Pompa P, Grasso M, Rigatti P. Failures and complications of transurethral ureteroscopy in 297 cases: conventional rigid instrumentation vs. small caliber semi-rigid ureteroscopes. Eur Urol. 1995;28:112–5.
48. Buscarini M, Conlin M. Update on flexible ureteroscopy. Urol Int. 2008;80:1–7.
49. Johnson DB, Pearle MS. Complications of ureteroscopy. Urol Clin North Am. 2004;31:157–71.
50. El-Nahas AR, El-Tabey NA, Eraky I, Shoma AM, El-Hefnawy AS, El-Assmy AM, et al. Semirigid ureteroscopy for ureteral stones: a multivariate analysis of unfavorable results. J Urol. 2009;181:1158–62.
51. Best SL, Nakada SY. Flexible ureteroscopy is effective for proximal ureteral stones in both obese and nonobese patients: a two year, single surgeon experience. Urology. 2011;77:36–9.
52. Byrne RR, Auge BK, Kourambas J, Munver R, Delvecchio F, Preminger GM. Routine ureteral stenting is not necessary after ureteroscopy and ureteropyeloscopy: a randomized trial. J Endourol. 2002;16:9–13.
53. Chen YT, Chen J, Wong WY, Yang SS, Hsieh CH, Wang CC. Is ureteral stenting necessary after uncomplicated ureteroscopic lithotripsy? A prospective, randomized controlled trial. J Urol. 2002;167:1977–80.
54. Borboroglu PG, Amling CL, Schenkman NS, Monga M, Ward JF, Piper NY, et al. Ureteral stenting after ureteroscopy for distal ureteral calculi: a multi-institutional prospective randomized controlled study assessing pain, outcomes and complications. J Urol. 2001;166:1651–7.
55. Pearle MS, Nadler R, Bercowsky E, Chen C, Dunn M, Figenshau RS, et al. Prospective randomized trial comparing shock wave lithotripsy and ureteroscopy for management of distal ureteral calculi. J Urol. 2001;166:1255–60.

56. Lee YH, Tsai JY, Jiann BP, Wu T, Yu CC. Prospective randomized trial comparing shock wave lithotripsy and ureteroscopic lithotripsy for management of large upper third ureteral stones. Urology. 2006; 67:480–4.
57. Goel R, Aron M, Kesarwani PK, Dogra PN, Hemal AK, Gupta NP. Percutaneous antegrade removal of impacted upper-ureteral calculi: still the treatment of choice in developing countries. J Endourol. 2005;19:54–7.
58. Karami H, Arbab AH, Hosseini SJ, Razzaghi MR, Simaei NR. Impacted upper-ureteral calculi >1 cm: blind access and totally tubeless percutaneous antegrade removal or retrograde approach? J Endourol. 2006;20:616–9.
59. Maheshwari PN, Oswal AT, Andankar M, Nanjappa KM, Bansal M. Is antegrade ureteroscopy better than retrograde ureteroscopy for impacted large upper ureteral calculi? J Endourol. 1999; 13:441–4.
60. El-Assmy A, El-Nahas AR, Mohsen T, Eraky I, El-Kenaway MR, Shaban AA, et al. Extracorporeal shock wave lithotripsy of upper urinary tract calculi in patients with cystectomy and urinary diversion. Urology. 2005;66:510–3.
61. Rhee BK, Bretan PN, Stoller ML. Urolithiasis in renal and combined pancreas/renal transplant recipients. J Urol. 1999;161: 1458–62.
62. El-Nahas AR, Eraky I, El-Assmy AM, Shoma AM, El-Kenaey MR, Abdel-Latif M, et al. Percutaneous treatment of large upper tract stones after urinary diversion. Urology. 2006;68:500–4.
63. Kane CJ, Bolton DM, Stoller ML. Current indications for open stone surgery in an endourology center. Urology. 1995;45:218–21.
64. Huri E, Basok EK, Ugulu O, Gurbuz C, Akgul T, Ozgok Y, et al. Experience in laparoscopic removal of upper ureteral stones: multicenter analysis of cases, based on TurkUroLap Group. J Endourol. 2010;24:1279–82.

Ureteroscopy for Ureteric Stones

57

Gerhard J. Fuchs and Steven G. Koopman

Abstract

Endoscopic stone treatment technique and the use of extracorporeal shock wave lithotripsy have revolutionized the interventional management of ureteric stones. While extracorporeal shock wave lithotripsy is truly noninvasive in nature, complete freedom of stone and resolution of symptoms in one treatment session are not predictable; therefore, the minimally invasive endoscopic surgical approach—over time—has become more attractive to many urologic surgeons. In particular, the downsizing of the ureteroscopes and the development of flexible ureteroscopes have facilitated access to the entire course of the ureter. In addition, with the advent of the holmium laser technology, stone fragmentation and vaporization can be achieved in practically all cases. Newer data approximate the success in terms of freedom of stones and resolution of symptoms to almost 100 % over the entire course of the ureter. These techniques have proven safe, efficient, and reproducible and with adherence to detail complications can be kept to a minimum. In this chapter, we provide a comprehensive review of present techniques for interventional management of ureteric stones with detailed description of safe endoscopic treatment techniques.

Keywords

Ureteric stone diagnosis • Differential treatment of ureteric stones • Energy sources for ureteric stone fragmentation • Success rates of ureteric stone treatment • Complications of ureteric stone treatment

Introduction

Ureteroscopy for the management of ureteral stones in the entire course of the ureter is a well-established, minimally invasive, highly effective, outpatient procedure. In addition to stone treatment, ureteroscopy is employed for the diagnostic evaluation of unilateral upper tract bleeding, for further evaluation of radiological filling defects, as well as for management of ureteral and ureteropelvic junction strictures, urothelial tumors, and removal of migrated and encrusted stents [1–4]. Ureteroscopic surgery (URS) is safe and efficacious when performed on the appropriate patient, using the appropriate instrumentation with the appropriate technique.

In this chapter, we will give a step-by-step description of the technical aspects of successful ureteroscopic surgery for stone treatment in the ureter using rigid and flexible instrumentation and present a short review of the results, and management of complications.

G.J. Fuchs, M.D., FACS (✉) • S.G. Koopman, M.D.
Department of Surgery, Minimally Invasive Urology Institute, Cedars-Sinai Medical Center, 8635 West Third Street, Suite 1070, Los Angeles, CA, 90048, USA
e-mail: gerhard.fuchs@cshs.org

J.J. Talati et al. (eds.), *Urolithiasis*,
DOI 10.1007/978-1-4471-4387-1_57, © Springer-Verlag London 2012

Indications

Ureteroscopic surgery can access the entire ureter. When rigid and flexible ureteroscopy are combined, a complete and thorough evaluation and treatment of the entire ureter and, if necessary, the kidney(s) can be achieved with minimal invasiveness [1–4]. The most common indication for ureteroscopic surgery is the treatment of stones in the course of the ureter with low likelihood for spontaneous passage. Alternative treatment such as extracorporeal shock wave lithotripsy (ESWL) and respective results are well covered in the literature [5]. Ureteroscopic stone surgery is safe, effective, and reliable for the treatment of ureteral stones and therefore in many institutions the first choice for most ureteral stones. The indications for ureteroscopy are listed in Table 57.1.

Ureteroscopic surgery can render the ureter stone-free in greater than 90 % of cases, regardless of stone size, stone composition, and stone location (Tables 57.2 and 57.3) [6–12, 15–20, 23]. Stone-free rates with ESWL on the contrary are highly variable, and individual outcomes can vary significantly as ESWL results are highly dependent on patient selection (body habitus, patient mobility) and stone characteristics (size, hardness, location, degree of impaction), choice of lithotripter (first vs. later generations), and selection of the time to intervene (stone embedded in edema) (see Tables 57.2 and 57.3) [8, 10, 11, 13–16, 21–23]. Acceptable results with SWL (greater than 80 % stone free, one treatment session) can be achieved for smaller stones (less than 7 mm) of calcium-dihydrate composition in the distal third of the ureter and short duration of stone location in the stone bed (lesser amount of edema) [13, 15, 16, 21–23]. Stone-free rates with calcium oxalate monohydrate and larger stones have significantly lower stone-free rates—especially when located in the proximal ureter—and higher rates of complications requiring secondary sessions and auxiliary procedures [5, 23, 24]. Both procedures are usually performed in an outpatient setting with anesthesia requirements ranging from oral pain management (piezoelectric lithotripter) over intravenous sedation (both) to general or epidural anesthesia (first-generation lithotripter, complex URS, proximal ureteral URS). Postoperative morbidity and energy-related injury for both procedures are low [5, 23–25]. After uretero-

Table 57.1 Indications for ureteroscopic surgery (URS)

Stone disease
Primary treatment for all stones below crossing with iliac vessels
Failed ESWL procedures (especially proximal ureter)
Obstructive radiolucent stones (after failed medical therapy)
Concomitant ureteral and renal stones (when renal stone <1.0 cm)
Encrusted/calcified retained ureteral stents
Stones and urinary diversion (conduit)
Morbidly obese patients with ureteral stones
Patients with ureteral stones and coagulopathy
Aviation pilots (need to be free of stones)
Strictures
Strictures of ureter (shorter than 1 cm)
Strictures of ureteropelvic junction (with mild/moderate hydronephrosis)
Strictures of uretero-enteric anastomosis (ileum conduit)
Tumors
Tissue diagnosis and removal of select ureteral TCC (low grade, papillary)

Table 57.2 Results of URS versus ESWL for proximal ureteral stones

	Number of patients	Stone size mean (mm)	Stone-free rate (%)
Ureteroscopic treatment of proximal ureteral calculi <1 cm			
Fong et al. [6]	51	9.0	90
Krambeck et al. [7]	237	5.9	87
Salem [8]	59	6.8	100
Best and Nakada [9]	55	9.1	86
Ureteroscopic treatment of proximal ureteral calculi >1 cm			
Wu et al. [10]	39	15.1	92
Lee et al. [11]	20	18.5	35
Mugiya et al. [12]	54	20.4	87
Salem [8]	48	12.2	88
ESWL treatment of proximal ureteral calculi			
Wu et al. [10]	51	12.1	35
	68	6.9	85
Lee et al. [11]	21	18.5	64
Tiselius [13]	580	4.2	73
Ziaee et al. [14]	126	10–15	78
Salem [8]	42	12.5	60
	58	6.2	80

Table 57.3 Results of URS versus ESWL for distal ureteral stones

	Number of patients	Stone size mean (mm)	Stone-free rate (%)
Ureteroscopic treatment of distal ureteral calculi <1 cm			
Pearle et al. [15]	32	6.4	91
Zeng et al. [16]	180	6–20	93
Aghamir et al. [17]	247	<10	96
Sozen et al. [18]	464	8.8	95
Krambeck et al. [7]	342	5.9	94
Ureteroscopic treatment of distal ureteral calculi >1 cm			
Sofer et al. [19]	348	10.3	99
Zeng et al. [16]	180	6–20	93
Elashry et al. [20]	3,542	10.9	97
ESWL treatment of distal ureteral calculi			
Pearle et al. [15]	32	7.4	91
Zeng et al. [16]	210	5–21	78
Hochreiter et al. [22]	518	9	91
Tiselius [13]	580	4.2	83

scopic surgery patient discomfort is related to the commonly used indwelling ureteral stent, and in the ESWL patients the episodes of obstruction with stone colic and need for secondary procedures are rather common problems [5, 23].

Contraindications

Ureteroscopic surgery for ureteral stone is absolutely contraindicated in the presence of an active urinary tract infection (UTI). Even if the urine cultures from the bladder are negatives, the appearance of purulent urine from above the stone should be an indication to abort the procedure with placement of a ureteral stent; otherwise, septic complications are likely. After drainage and appropriate antibiotic treatment, a second-stage URS procedure can be performed once sterile urine has been confirmed. URS may be relatively contraindicated in pregnancy and anticoagulation, with complex anatomical variations, and in patients with poor medical status. In these patients, the use of URS, on a case-by-case selection, can be successful without increasing the risk of complications. The use of URS with lithotripsy has been shown to be safe and efficacious during pregnancy [26, 27], but its use has not gained wide acceptance and therefore has remained listed as a relative contraindication (Table 57.4). Likewise, URS with a direct contact laser energy source (holmium or thulium laser) can be performed safely and successfully on the anticoagulated patient, whereas the risk of bleeding increases when other energy sources such as ultrasound or the pneumatic lithoclast are employed. By optimizing the patient's medical condition and lowering anesthesia risk (IV sedation, local anesthesia), patients who have poor performance and medical status may be treated safely with ureteroscopic surgery techniques (see Table 57.4) [28].

Table 57.4 Contraindications for ureteroscopic surgery (URS)

Infection of urinary tract:
Absolute: Untreated urinary tract infection (UTI)
Treat according to C&S with antibiotics for 10 days
If obstruction, start antibiotic and manage obstruction with ureteral stent or PCN tube
Caution: Infection stone or history of UTIs
Pretreat with broad-spectrum abx for 10 days even if culture negative
Pregnancy: Anesthesia and obstetric monitoring, radiation exposure
Coagulopathy and anticoagulation:
Relative: Preferred management to correct coagulopathy if medically safe
Relative: Untreated coagulopathy
Cautious treatment with direct contact laser (holmium, thulium)
Use access sheath to reduce bleeding (prostate, frequent passage up/down ureter)

Instrumentation

The success of ureteroscopic surgery depends on the surgeon's skill and the availability of ureteroscopes, working instruments, accessories, and energy sources. Instrument manufacturers have developed their own ureteroscope design and offer endoscopic camera systems and various accessories [29]. Endoscopic camera systems are now routinely used to facilitate surgery (ergonomic and safety aspects for surgeon, increased team involvement through visualization). Basically, all scopes are similar in design and well suited for ureteroscopic surgery. The differences lie in the outer diameter, length, eyepiece position, and the number and size of working channels. Most ureteroscopes come in two different lengths. The shorter scopes (31–34 cm) are ideal for distal pathology that is below the iliac vessels; above this point we prefer to use the longer scopes (41–43 cm), which reach the proximal ureter and commonly the renal pelvis as well. Both lengths of the semirigid scopes and a flexible ureteroscope should be available at the time of surgery.

Different wires, stone retrieval devices, ureteral catheters, and stents are essential when planning URS. Wires for urologic procedures vary in diameter, length, and composition. Diameter varies from 0.025 in. (0.64 mm) to 0.038 in. (0.97 mm). Lengths are available ranging from 80 to 260 cm. The usual length for ureteroscopic work is 145–150 cm. The outer coating can be Teflon, polytetrafluoroethylene (PTFE), or hydrophilic polymer. Most wires have a soft tip with an angled, J-shaped, or straight tip. We prefer Teflon-coated, straight tip, 0.038 wires with a length of about 150 cm. These wires are atraumatic yet fairly inexpensive and sturdy (floppy tip and stiff body), and do not readily slip out of the ureter. When a tight stricture (narrow stone bed) or a tortuous ureter is encountered and the regular Teflon wire cannot negotiate its way past, a hydrophilic-coated wire, like a glidewire, may be helpful to bypass those areas. As soon as access to the kidney is achieved with a hydrophilic-type wire, it should be exchanged for a regular Teflon-coated wire. By advancing the angiographic catheter above the obstruction first, it is assured that the wire will be in the correct position. If this maneuver is omitted, wire slippage out of the ureter may occur, thus losing an already established difficult access to the ureter and kidney.

Ureteral dilators for sequential, coaxial, or balloon dilation are frequently used to facilitate access for URS to the upper tract [30]. Ureteral dilation should always be performed over a second guidewire to avoid losing the safety wire in an already tenuous situation. Overaggressive dilation against resistance may result in ureteral tears and subsequent submucosal passage of a "blindly" placed guidewire with the risk of more severe ureteral damage if an instrument is advanced over such a wire; it is advisable to use a coaxial access sheath for placement of a second wire (assures correct position) and then dilate over the second wire. Serial Teflon or coaxial Teflon dilators (inexpensive) or balloon dilators (expensive) may be used to facilitate access in difficult situations [5, 30]. Hydrophilic ureteral access sheaths, cobra catheters, coaxial introductory sheets, and Zebra or Amplatz super stiff wires are all important and useful tools to gain access to the ureter, but in our experience this is rarely needed.

Technique of Rigid Ureteroscopy

Rigid ureteroscopy of the upper urinary tract is a well-established procedure. With adherence to proper guidelines and following a step-by-step approach, access to the upper tract and successful treatment can be accomplished in the vast majority of patients with minimal morbidity and very few complications.

Preoperative Preparation

Immediate preoperative preparation includes confirmation of a sterile urine sample within 5 days of surgery, start of intravenous hydration in the preoperative area, and administration of perioperative antibiotic coverage (e.g., 1 dose of ampicillin and gentamicin). If the treatment is for stone disease or the patient has an indwelling stent, immediate preoperative imaging with a plain abdominal X-ray or fluoroscopy will confirm the patient's status. The patient then undergoes anesthesia (Table 57.5).

Anesthesia for URS

The choice of anesthesia may vary with the location of the stone, the patient's sex, and general medical condition. While general or epidural anesthesia is frequently the anesthesia of choice, intravenous sedation may well suffice for a distal ureteral stone, or in a female patient, or when dictated by the patient's medical status. Occasionally, a small retained stone in a stented patient can be removed in the office setting with topical anesthesia (Xylocaine jelly) to the urethra only.

Table 57.5 Patient preparation for ureteroscopic surgery (URS)

Patient selection (see Tables 57.1 and 57.2) and informed consent
Medical clearance for anesthesia and optimization of comorbidity
Sterile urine (negative C&S)
Preoperative PO antibiotics, if positive C&S or history of UTIs
IV hydration (>100 cc/h)
IV perioperative antibiotics (e.g., ampicillin + gentamicin)
KUB (for stones <1.0 cm to r/o spontaneous passage)
General anesthesia (regional, IV sedation, or local optional)

The patient is positioned in the low lithotomy position (cave: proper padding of pressure point areas). Modifications of positioning such as ipsilateral leg extension or patient rotation are not necessary or helpful in a patient with normal body habitus.

Access to the Ureter

The first procedural step is a cystoscopy (21 Fr. rigid or 15 Fr. flexible [in males, when IV sedation is used]) with inspection of the bladder and a retrograde pyelogram under fluoroscopic control (5-Fr. straight angiocatheter and floppy-tipped 0.038 Bentson guidewire) to assess the technical complexity of the case by delineating the course of the ureter [31]. Then, the Bentson wire is advanced up the ureter and into the kidney to serve as a safety wire. Placement of a safety wire is one of the essential steps for assuring success and reducing the risks of iatrogenic damage of ureteroscopic instrumentation. Once the safety wire has been advanced past the obstructing ureteral stone and into the kidney, the patient receives 20 mg of furosemide (weight adjusted; 0.25 mg/kg) to induce diuresis and reduce the risk of pyelorenal reflux and infectious complications (Table 57.6). Technical difficulty with safety wire placement can be encountered at the level of the intramural ureter (impacted stone, stricture, ureterocele, reimplanted ureter, tumor, large prostate middle lobe, female bladder descensus), or the level of an impacted stone, or by ureteral tortuosity. Iatrogenic damage of the ureteral mucosa in the intramural ureter should be consistently avoided with the use of a floppy-tipped Bentson wire and the angiographic catheter. If the guidewire cannot negotiate the intramural ureter, the next step is the use of a hydrophilic glidewire (straight or angled), which often will allow advancement well into the ureter. Before further manipulation is undertaken, one needs to confirm that the wire is correctly positioned in the ureter by advancing the angiographic catheter beyond the narrow segment, removing the wire, and observing for obstructive urine drip from the angiographic catheter; a small amount of dilute contrast is helpful to delineate the course of the ureter and confirm the correct position when no urine is seen. Note that if there is any indication of infected urine draining from the previously obstructed upper tract, the treatment should be terminated with placement of an indwelling stent, the urine sampled and cultured, and treatment of the ureteral pathology postponed until confirmation of sterile urine.

Provided the correct position of the angiocatheter is confirmed and there is no sign for infected urine from the obstructed upper tract, a regular Bentson wire is placed and advanced to the kidney (mind that the glidewire is a specialty wire and is only used for overcoming difficulty in access; it is best replaced as soon as proper access is established, for otherwise the risk of loss of access is likely). If a glidewire

Table 57.6 Essential procedural steps of ureteroscopic surgery (URS)

Steps	Goal	Execution	Equipment used
1	Evaluate bladder	Cystoscopy	Fluoroscopy X-ray table
	Assess upper tract anatomy for treatment planning	Retrograde pyelogram under fluoroscopic control	19- to 21-Fr. cystoscope
	Place safety guidewire		5-Fr. straight angiocatheter
			0.038 Bentson guidewire
2	Establish access to ureter	Optical dilation of ureter (working and safety wire in 6 and 12 o'clock position)	9.5-Fr. semirigid ureteroscope
			Second guidewire
3	Treat stone	Stone fragmentation and stone retrieval	Holmium/thulium laser
			Stone baskets/graspers
			Access sheath (optional)
4A	Treat stone (special situations)	Consider hydrophilic glidewire for safe passage of safety wire	Hydrophilic glidewire (straight and angle tip)
	Impacted stone	If wire cannot bypass stone, cautiously fragment stone until enough space created for guidewire passage	
		Exchange glidewire as soon as stone has been bypassed	
4B	Treat stone (special situations)	Advance the fulcrum; use angiographic catheter and guide- or glidewire to negotiate tortuosity	5-Fr. angiographic catheter
	Tortuous ureter below or above stone		5-Fr. angle-tip catheter
			Hydrophilic wire
4C	Treat stone (special situations)	Establish safety wire, see 4A, 4B	Holmium/thulium laser (possible ESWL combo)
	Steinstrasse	Consider use of energy source to fragment or dislodge impacted stone gravel	Hydrophilic glidewire
			Zero-tip nitinol basket
5	Safe exit from upper tract	Place indwelling ureteral drainage stent over safety wire	6/7-Fr. ureteral double pigtail stent

through the stabilizing angiocatheter will not advance, then the 9.5-Fr. semirigid ureteroscope is cautiously advanced into the intramural ureter. Under direct endoscopic control a guide- or glidewire can then often be successfully placed. In the very few cases where this may not be feasible (<2 %, authors' experience), careful fragmentation of an intramural stone until such time that a safety wire can be placed may be attempted. If this does not allow access or is deemed too dangerous, placement of a percutaneous drainage tube and subsequent percutaneous antegrade surgery is preferred. If the safety wire passes through the intramural ureter but cannot be advanced past a higher ureteral pathology, the first salvage step is the use of the angiocatheter to provide fulcrum for better wire manipulation. The angiocatheter is advanced to within 1/2 in. of the obstacle and then wire manipulation is again attempted. This being successful, the same procedural steps as previously described are followed to confirm correct position of the wire. If the regular wire does not negotiate the obstacle, a specialty glidewire (straight or angled) is utilized. Ureteroscopy up to the obstacle and manipulation of a wire under direct endoscopic control (but without the benefit of a safety wire) obviously is more risky but in experienced hands often successful and avoids the next level of invasiveness—the placement of a percutaneous access. If ureteral tortuosity is encountered, the combination of an angiographic catheter (advancing the fulcrum) and guide/glidewire will usually allow successful negotiation of the obstacle and placement of a safety wire. Advancing the angiographic catheter over the guidewire all the way up to the kidney oftentimes will straighten out the ureter. For placement of a working wire, a coaxial sheath (7 and 11 Fr.) or a dual guidewire introductory catheter is best used to assure correct position. If an impacted stone is located within a ureteral kink or right above a ureteral kink, safe manipulation of a guidewire may not be possible. In such rare cases, placement of a percutaneous drainage tube will drain the obstructed kidney and straighten the course of the ureter in a matter of 10 days. Then, retrograde ureteroscopic surgery will be most likely feasible; otherwise, percutaneous antegrade ureteroscopy can be performed after dilating the percutaneous access.

Once a safety wire is placed into the kidney, ureteroscopic access to the ureter is the next procedural step. Ureteroscopic access to the ureter using the ureteroscope as "optical dilator" with a 9.5-Fr. instrument is technically feasible in 97 % of cases (author's experience) without additional formal dilation of the intramural ureter or higher ureteral segments. In a female patient, the instrument often can be directly advanced alongside the safety wire. In the male patient, the use of a second wire (working wire) through the work channel of the instrument will allow proper access. It is helpful to turn the scope clockwise and counterclockwise until the working wire (resting against the base of the orifice in the 6 o'clock position) and the safety wire (against the roof of the orifice in the 12 o'clock position) form an inverted V. This alignment of the guidewires will then allow the gradual advancement of the scope through the intramural and into the pelvic ureter. Note that the "real" narrowing is the junction from the intramural to the pelvic ureter not the orifice per se. In select complex cases where advancement of the scope is not possible (pelvic surgery, radiation, extrinsic compression, young muscular males, large prostate middle lobes, large cystoceles), placement of an indwelling stent is preferable over dilation of the orifice for it will allow easier and safe instrumentation in the entire ureter usually after 10–14 days. Scopes with smaller distal tip designs (6–7.5 Fr.) are of no advantage over the 9.5-Fr. bevel type instrument design. As a matter of fact, the square distal tip of many of these scopes is potentially more dangerous, and these instruments are best used over a guidewire. If the surgeon decides on dilating the ureteral orifice (or higher ureteral segments), a variety of methods are available. Natural caveats are not to dilate adjacent to a stone (risk of intramural or ureteral perforation) and to use a separate working wire and not the safety wire for placement of serial dilators or a balloon dilator. The intramural ureter "tolerates" dilation up to 30 Fr., which in reality will rarely be necessary since 12- to 15-Fr. dilation or "optical dilation" usually suffices.

Advancement of the scope should always be done under continuous visualization of the ureter. If difficulty is encountered (edema, tortuosity, relative narrowing), the use of a working wire is helpful. If visualization is impaired and safe advancement therefore not possible, placement of an indwelling stent and return to surgery in 10–14 days will avoid risks of iatrogenic damage and greatly facilitate the procedure and usually result in successful completion. Hydration pumps or other means of raising the pressure of irrigant are usually not helpful in negotiating the difficult ureter. On the contrary, there is increased risk of fluid overload, forniceal rupture with extravasation, and infectious complications (pyelorenal reflux).

Treatment of Ureteral Stone(s)

The goal of ureteroscopic surgery for the management of ureteral stone(s) is to render the ureter free of stone in a minimally invasive fashion in one outpatient treatment session. Once the stone is endoscopically approached, the next step is the choice of the appropriate means for stone removal, i.e., for intact removal with a basket or grasper or for fragmentation with an energy source (laser, pneumatic, ultrasound, electrohydraulic) [32, 33]. Stone size, degree of impaction, and ureteral anatomy will determine the mode of stone removal. Stones that can be positioned into a wide enough ureteral segment to be grasped with a 2-prong rigid 4.7-Fr. forceps can either be removed intact (usually size less than 4 mm, e.g., Steinstrasse or residual gravel in patients with previous ureteral stent) or mechanically fragmented using the forceps (calcium oxalate dihydrate) and then removed. Although nitinol baskets are most commonly used for ureteral stone retrieval, the use of the rigid forceps has several advantages in that it can cheaply fragment stones (calcium oxalate dihydrate, struvite, uric acid) as no energy source is needed. The grasper will avoid getting "stuck" with the stone above a narrow ureteral segment as might happen when a stone is trapped in a basket, and it is reusable (no extra cost). The rigid forceps necessitate the use of an ureteroscope with an offset lens and straight work channel of appropriate sizes (9.5 Fr. with 5-Fr. work channel).

If the stone is too large for intact removal, fragmentation with any of the energy sources is performed. Holmium laser energy is most popular for its efficient stone fragmentation regardless of stone composition and stone debulking capabilities (vaporization). Alternative, less expensive energy sources such as the pneumatic lithotrites, electrohydraulic energy, and ultrasound energy are not only less effective but also require somewhat more technical skills to overcome their inherent technical limitations (insufficient breakage of stone, upward migration of the stone, mild bleeding from energy delivery). Before fragmenting an impacted stone, it is always advisable to obtain a contrast imaging study to assess the degree of surrounding edema and to be forewarned if there is ureteral tortuosity involving the stone bed (increased risk of ureteral damage and perforation). If the ureter is dilated above the stone (which is usually the case) and the stone is not impacted (no significant narrowing and edema at the stone site), it is helpful to carefully dislodge the stone from the stone bed into the dilated portion of the ureter for there it can be handled easier (fragmentation and use of the rigid forceps). Using Holmium laser energy (5–10 W), any stone (regardless of composition) is readily fragmented and vaporized. The resultant gravel (any pieces larger than 2 mm as compared to the 1-mm size of the safety wire) is removed from the ureter using either a rigid forceps or any of the baskets. In male patients, we usually deposit the gravel in the bladder so as to avoid numerous passages through the urethra. With the use of baskets, one needs to be careful not to take larger stone pieces since negotiating a stone out of the basket in the ureter is technically difficult and may not be feasible, resulting in a "stuck" basket. If a basket gets "stuck" above a narrow ureteral segment (e.g., iliac vessel crossing, intramural ureter), no attempt should be made to pull forcefully (due to risk of ureteral avulsion).

The instrument should be withdrawn leaving the basket in place. If the stone gets "stuck" in the distal third of the ureter, the scope can be withdrawn and positioned outside the patient while leaving the basket intact. A second scope is then advanced into the ureter, and the stone is fragmented with careful avoidance of damaging/cutting the wires (pneumatic or ultrasound energy are safe; Holmium and electrohydraulic lithotripter [EHL] may cut the wires). Once the stone is fragmented sufficiently, the basket and stone gravel are removed from the ureter; provided the basket withstood the salvage maneuver, it can be used for the remainder of the case. If the basket is "stuck" higher up in the ureter, it has to be dismantled or cut to allow complete withdrawal of the ureteroscope. The same salvage maneuver is utilized, albeit at the expense of needing an additional basket to complete stone retrieval. Upward migration of a stone or stone pieces is not considered a complication unless the surgeon is not prepared to retrieve the pieces from the upper ureter or renal collecting system by having the appropriate instrumentation available (flexible ureteroscope) for retrograde intrarenal surgery.

Steinstrasse

Steinstrasse after ESWL is a complex ureteral stone scenario (ureter packed with stone gravel, encased in edema) and one of the challenges of ureteroscopic surgery. In these cases, even the passage of a safety wire may become a formidable task. For placement of a safety wire, the same maneuver for advancing the fulcrum—angiocatheter and guide- or glidewire—is successful as in the manipulation of a ureteral tortuosity. Length of the Steinstrasse and degree of stone impaction and surrounding edema will determine the complexity of the ureteroscopic procedure. A ureteral stent when already in place should not be removed before a safety wire is well established in the renal collecting system. When the ureter is tightly packed with stone gravel, it may not be possible to safely engage pieces with a basket or grasper. In those instances, the impacted gravel can be loosened using a direct contact energy source (holmium, ultrasound, or pneumatic). The cautious use of a direct contact energy source can fragment larger pieces and separate impacted gravel; EHL is not recommended in this setting because of the stone bed usually being edematous, and release of EHL energy will result in mild bleeding making the procedure technically more challenging with increased risk of ureteral injury. For removal of the dislodged pieces, the use of a 4-wire tipless basket (nitinol) is helpful. The basket is used like a parachute with the wires left open to separate the gravel until safe engagement of pieces small enough for retrieval can be ascertained. If stone impaction is very tight with copious edema and no stent is present, placement of an indwelling ureteral stent for 2 weeks will drain the kidney and passively dilate the ureter thus greatly facilitating the task of successful stone retrieval.

For the management of extensive Steinstrasse, use of a ureteral access sheath is often helpful, especially for proximal ureteral involvement. An access sheath placed below the level of the stone impaction in conjunction with a flexible ureteroscope and a holmium laser may expeditiously clear such a ureter. Also, with large amounts of gravel in the proximal ureter and additional renal stone burden, a combined retrograde/antegrade (percutaneous) approach should be considered in the interest of expeditious resolution of the situation.

Ureteroscopic Surgery in Patients with Skeletal Abnormalities

Patients with severe skeletal abnormalities may not be physically able to be positioned in low lithotomy position, the traditional position for URS. In most cases, ureteroscopic surgery can be successfully performed with the use of flexible scopes and occasionally using ultrasound instead of X-ray for stent position verification.

Ureteroscopic Surgery in Patients with Upper Tract Reconstruction

Patients with upper urinary tract reconstruction or urinary diversion may develop stones secondary to chronic UTI and/or reflux of infected urine. The conduit or neobladder reconstruction can usually be navigated with a flexible cystoscope for identification of the ureteral anastomosis and guidewire access. Initially all mucous should be evacuated from the conduit or continent pouch. Fluoroscopic evaluation with injection of contrast and use of a guidewire (contained in a 5-Fr. angiocatheter for advancing the fulcrum) can both be helpful when the bowel reservoir is tortuous. If the ureterointestinal anastomoses are of the refluxing type, fluoroscopy with contrast injection usually allows identification of the anastomoses (unless the anastomosis is obstructed by a stone or stricture). It is often helpful to have some knowledge of the implantation method that was used (Wallace type vs. single ureter anastomosis) and the topographical location of the anastomoses. When fluoroscopy with contrast does not identify the location of the anastomoses, we carefully search for sessile well-circumscribed areas in the reservoir/conduit wall, using a floppy-tipped guidewire to gently probe these areas. Administration of IV methylene blue can also be useful in directing the endoscopist to the area of upper tract access. Once identified, the ureteral orifice should be cannulated with a safety wire preloaded in a 5-Fr. angiocatheter. The wire should then be advanced under fluoroscopic control and coiled in the kidney prior to advancing the angiocatheter up the ureter. Contrast is then injected to define the upper tract anatomy. The hydrophilic glidewire is then exchanged for a regular Bentson type wire, and a coaxial access catheter set should then be used to place a second (working) wire. An access sheath will facilitate reaccess to the upper tract and reduce the risk of losing access in a tenuous situation. URS treatment of ureter stones should follow the principles previously described in this chapter. Frequently, a hydroureter is encountered, and upward migration of ureteral stone into the kidney is more common than in a regular ureter. Since most URS instrumentation in these patients is by use of flexible ureterorenoscopes, access to the kidney and treatment of those stones should not unduly complicate the treatment.

Ureteral Healing

Diagnostic ureteroscopy and ureteroscopic surgery are minimally invasive procedures. Patients undergoing a diagnostic procedure with a flexible instrument do well without stenting, while patients undergoing ureteral surgery usually do better with an indwelling stent [4, 34].

Although new controversy surrounds the routine use of stenting after uncomplicated ureteroscopic surgery for stone removal without the need for dilation of the orifice, we believe that most patients treated at a tertiary center for more complex stone scenarios fare better with an indwelling stent [4, 37]. After treatment of ureteral stones with uncomplicated access to the ureter, a small stone burden, without significant edema at the stone bed, and without gross hydronephrosis, a stent does not necessarily need to be placed. However, in our experience, we mostly encounter patients with larger stones, impacted stones, patients after failed previous treatment attempts, and with other complicating factors, and we therefore advocate the use of an indwelling stent for such patients. An indwelling time of 3–14 days (depending on the amount of edema) will invariably result in resolution of edema and hydronephrosis and after stent removal morbidity is minimal.

Postoperative Care

After surgery, the patient is recovered in the outpatient area. The Foley catheter is removed, and the patient discharged as soon as fully recovered from anesthesia and tolerating oral fluids and, if necessary, oral pain medication. Discharge medications are usually pyridium 100 mg TID for 5 days and Darvocet N-100 PRN; if a stent remains indwelling, we also prescribe Flomax 0.4 mg qhs during the indwelling time. Antibiotics are not routinely given. If treatment is performed on what appears to be an infection-induced stone, urine and stone is sampled for culture and sensitivity testing at the conclusion of the procedure, and oral antibiotics are given for 5 days. Patients return to clinic for a physical examination after between 3 and 14 days depending on the determination of the length of ureteral stenting. A physical examination is performed, and once a renal ultrasound confirms a normal kidney without residual hydronephrosis, the indwelling stent is removed under topical urethral anesthesia.

Complications of Ureteroscopic Surgery

Prevention

Complications of ureteroscopic surgery overall are exceedingly rare with strict adherence to safe surgery guidelines. Medically, urinary tract infection with symptoms ranging from mild postoperative temperature elevation to full septic complications (very rare) can be encountered. Potential surgical complications of ureteroscopic surgery include damage to the ureteral orifice, upper urinary tract perforation, and postoperative ureteral stricture.

Awareness of preoperative positive urine culture results with appropriate antibiotic treatment, the use of perioperative antimicrobial agents, and maintaining low pressures within the upper urinary tract during URS will help to reduce infectious complications to a minimum. As described earlier in this chapter, the routine use of a loop diuretic and avoidance of pressurized fluid flow will help to keep upper tract pressure low. Furthermore, use of a ureteral access sheath—especially for prolonged cases of stones in the proximal ureter—will also help to reduce intraoperative renal pelvis pressure and the risk of infectious complications.

Damage to the urinary tract can best be prevented by always visualizing the action of the ureteroscope, accessory instruments, and energy sources—avoiding blunt damage to the ureter, either by the scope itself or by the sharp tips of instruments and accessories (guidewires, baskets, and graspers) passed through the scope working channel. In addition, lithotripsy energy sources should never be activated unless the stone, the fiber/probe, and the ureteral wall are directly visualized. Always maintaining a safety wire access to the kidney will help in the management of URS complications; should one occur.

Table 57.7 Technical complications of ureteroscopic surgery and management

Complications (medical)	Prevention and management
Acute urinary retention	Avoid overdistention of bladder intraoperatively
	Voiding trial for male patients with large prostates
Infection	
Bacteremia, sepsis	Sterile urine preoperative, perioperative, IV antibiotics sterile technique, drainage (stent or PCN)
Urethritis, prostatitis, cystitis	Antibiotics and symptomatic (antispasmodic)
Periureteral fluid collection (extravasation)	
Hematoma (sterile/infected)	Observe (sterile); PCN – drain (infected)
Irrigation fluid	Observe (sterile); PCN – drain (infected)
Positional	
Nerve damage	Proper positioning and cushioning
	Evaluate, physical therapy
DVT (deep vein thrombosis)	Proper positioning and cushioning, pulsatile stockings
	Medical treatment

Table 57.8 Medical complications of ureteroscopic surgery and management

Complications (technical)	Management
Ureteral injury	
Mucosal tear with/without extravasation	Drainage (1. stent; 2. stent+Foley 3. stent+Foley+PCN)
False passage (guidewire)	Endoscopically correct guidewire placement and stent for 2 weeks
Perforation (with extravasation), false passage	Drainage with stent (safety wire!!), check with US/CT, PCN drainage of urinoma/hematoma
Ureteral bleeding (from scope or energy source)	Observe, mostly will cease unless perforation or damage of large, adjacent vessel
Ureteral intussusception/avulsion	Laparoscopic or open surgery required
Damage to adjacent structures (vessels, bowel)	Open surgery likely required

Management of Complications of Ureteroscopic Surgery

Sepsis complications can be severe, especially after treatment of infectious stones. If patients exhibit signs or symptoms of sepsis (high temperature, elevated white count, tachycardia, hypotension), they should be closely monitored and treated with broad-spectrum antimicrobial agents. Appropriate intravenous access should be in place, as blood pressure support and intensive care management may be required.

If bleeding from the use of an energy source or instrumentation occurs and vision is impaired, termination of the procedure with placement of an indwelling ureteral stent is the best course of action. Occasionally, a discreet bleeder can be identified and coagulated with the holmium (defocused beam) or Nd:YAG laser, but more commonly bleeding is more of a generalized oozing nature involving edema in the stone bed and will self-terminate in short order after placement of an indwelling stent. A second look for completion of the procedure can usually be safely performed within 7–10 days. Breech of the integrity of the ureteral wall (perforation) rarely occurs. In such instances, the area of perforation should be examined either with fluoroscopy and contrast injection of endoscopically.

In most situations, placement of an indwelling ureteral stent will allow the injury to heal, and the urologist can return at a later date to reassess the damaged area and complete the surgery. Severe injury, such as a circumferential ureteral tear, may require urgent operative intervention (Tables 57.7 and 57.8) [35–37].

Conclusion

In general, all stones in the ureter can be removed endoscopically regardless of size, composition, or complicating anatomical factors. Even in the setting of a tertiary care referral center, less than 4 % of patients need a second session, and less than 4 % need a combination with percutaneous antegrade techniques to achieve stone-free status. In more than 3,500 consecutive cases, there has been no incident of ureteral stricture or iatrogenic ureteral damage necessitating further action (authors' experience).
Ureteroscopic surgery with rigid and flexible instrumentation is a highly successful, minimally invasive treatment modality for patients with a variety of ureteral pathology. The indications are well established in particular for patients with stones in the entire course of the ureter. With the evolution of the ureteroscopic surgical technique and advances in instrumentation over the past 30 years as well as the advances in flexible ureteroscopy as an adjunct to the semirigid instruments, ureteroscopic surgery has become one of the essential surgical skills for any successful urologist. The surgical techniques can be easily learned, and the results are reproducible with a low rate of intra- and perioperative surgical complications.

References

1. Kumon H, et al. Ureteroscopy: indication for surgical intervention, chapter 28. In: Smith AD, Badlani GH, Bagley DH, editors. Smith's textbook of endourology. St. Louis: Quality Medical Publishing; 1996. p. 397–411.
2. Gerber GS, Lyon ES, et al. Treatment of ureteral stones, chapter 33. In: Smith AD, Badlani GH, Bagley DH, editors. Smith's textbook of endourology. 1996th ed. St. Louis: Quality Medical Publishing; 1996. p. 455–63.

3. Tawfiek ER. Management of upper urinary tract calculi with ureteroscopic techniques. Urology. 1999;53:25–31.
4. Colon I, Fuchs G. Rigid ureteroscopy. AUA Update Ser. 2005; vol. 24, lesson 17:127–9.
5. Segura JW, Preminger GM, Assimos DG, Dretler SP, Kahn RI, Lingeman JE, et al. Ureteral Stones Clinical Guidelines Panel summary report on the management of ureteral calculi. J Urol. 1997;158:1915–21.
6. Fong YK, Ho SH, Peh OH, Ng FC, Lim PH, Quek PL, et al. Extracorporeal shockwave lithotripsy and intracorporeal lithotripsy for proximal ureteric calculi – a comparative assessment of efficacy and safety. Ann Acad Med Singapore. 2004;33:80–3.
7. Krambeck A, Murat FJ, Gettman MT, Chow GK, Patterson DE, Segura JW. The evolution of ureteroscopy: a modern single-institution series. Mayo Clin Proc. 2006;81(4):468–73.
8. Salem HA. A prospective randomized study comparing shock wave lithotripsy and semirigid ureteroscopy for the management of proximal ureteral calculi. Urology. 2009;74:1216–22.
9. Best SL, Nakada SY. Flexible ureteroscopy is effective for proximal ureteral stones in both obese and nonobese patients: a two-year, single-surgeon experience. Urology. 2011;77:36–9.
10. Wu CF, Chen CS, Lin WY, Shee JJ, Lin CL, Chen Y, et al. Therapeutic options for proximal ureter stone: extracorporeal shock wave lithotripsy versus semirigid ureterorenoscope with holmium: yttrium-aluminum-garnet laser lithotripsy. Urology. 2005;65:1075–9.
11. Lee YH, Tsai JY, Jiaan BP, Wu T, Yu CC. Prospective randomized trial comparing shock wave lithotripsy and ureteroscopic lithotripsy for management of large upper third ureteral stones. Urology. 2006;67:480–4.
12. Mugiya S, Ozono S, Nagata M, Takayama T, Nagae H. Retrograde endoscopic management of ureteral stones more than 2 cm in size. Urology. 2006;67:1164–8.
13. Tiselius H. How efficient is extracorporeal shockwave lithotripsy with modern lithotripters for removal of ureteral stones? J Endourol. 2008;22(2):249–56.
14. Ziaee SA, Halimiasl P, Aminsharifi A, Shafi H, Beigi FM, Basiri A. Management of 10–15-mm proximal ureteral stones: ureteroscopy or extracorporeal shockwave lithotripsy. Urology. 2008;71:28–31.
15. Pearle MS, Nadler R, Bercowsky E, Chen C, Dunn M, Figenshau RS, et al. Prospective randomized trial comparing shock wave lithotripsy and ureteroscopy for management of distal ureteral calculi. J Urol. 2001;166:1255–60.
16. Zeng GQ, Zhong WD, Cai YB, Dai QS, Hu JB, Wei HA. Extracorporeal shock wave versus pneumatic ureteroscopic lithotripsy in treatment of lower ureteral calculi. Asian J Androl. 2002;4(4):303–5.
17. Aghamir SK, Mohseni MG, Ardestani A. Treatment of ureteral calculi with ballistic lithotripsy. J Endourol. 2003;17:887–90.
18. Sozen S, Kupeli B, Tunc L, Senocak C, Alkibay T, Karaoğlan U, et al. Management of ureteral stones with pneumatic lithotripsy: report of 500 patients. J Endourol. 2003;17(9):721–4.
19. Sofer M, Denstedt J. Flexible ureteroscopy and lithotripsy with the holmium:YAG laser. Can J Urol. 2000;7:952–6.
20. Elashry O, Elgamasy AK, Sabaa MA, Abo-Elenien M, Omar MA, Eltatawy HH, et al. Ureteroscopic management of lower ureteric calculi: a 15-year single-centre experience. Br J Urol. 2008;102:1010–7.
21. Coz F, Orvieto M, Bustos M, Lyng R, Stein C, Hinrichs A, San Francisco I. Extracorporeal shockwave lithotripsy of 2000 urinary calculi with the Modulith SL-s20: success and failure according to size and location of stones. J Endourol. 2000;14(5):239–46.
22. Hochreiter W, Danuser H, Perrig M, Studer UE. Extracorporeal shock wave lithotripsy for distal ureteral calculi: what a powerful machine can achieve. J Urol. 2003;169:878–80.
23. Preminger GM, Tiselius HG, Assimos DG. Guidelines for management of ureteral calculi. European Urology. 2007;52:1610–31.
24. Kim HH, Lee JH, Park MS, Lee SE, Kim SW. In situ extracorporeal shockwave lithotripsy for ureteral calculi: investigation of factors influencing stone fragmentation and appropriate number of sessions for changing treatment modality. J Endourol. 1996;10:501–5.
25. Pace KT, Weir MJ, Tariq N, Honey RJ. Low success rate of repeat shock wave lithotripsy for ureteral stones after failed initial treatment. J Urol. 2000;164:1905–7.
26. Ulvik NM, Bakke A, Hoisaeter PA. Ureteroscopy in pregnancy. J Urol. 1995;154:1660–3.
27. Scarpa RM, De Lisa A, Usai E. Diagnosis and treatment of ureteral calculi during pregnancy with rigid ureteroscopes. J Urol. 1996;155:875–7.
28. Hosking DH, Bard RJ. Ureteroscopy with intravenous sedation for treatment of distal ureteral calculi: a safe and effective alternative to shock wave lithotripsy. J Urol. 1996;156:899–901.
29. Conlin MJ, Marberger M, Bagley DH. Ureteroscopy. Development and instrumentation. Urol Clin North Am. 1997;24:25–42.
30. Perez-Castro E, Iglesias JI, et al. Ureteral dilation: indications and techniques, chapter 29. In: Smith AD, Badlani GH, Bagley DH, editors. Smith's textbook of endourology. St. Louis: Quality Medical Publishing; 1996. p. 411–20.
31. Chew BH, Denstedt JD. Ureteroscopy and retrograde ureteral access, chapter 45. In: Wein AJ, Kavoussi LR, Novick AC, Partin AW, Peters CA, editors. Campbell Walsh-urology, vol. 2. 9th ed. Philadelphia: Saunders Elsevier; 2007, sect XI.
32. Pattaras JG, O'Keefe SC. Ureteroscopic lithotripsy. AUA Update Ser. 2003; vol. XXII, lesson 19:195–8.
33. Knudsen BE, Denstedt JD. Intracorporeal lithotripters, chapter 5. In: Smith AD, Badlani GH, Bagley DH, Clayman RV, Docimo SG, editors. Smith's textbook of endourology. 2nd ed. Hamilton: BC Decker Inc; 2007.
34. Netto AR, Ikonomidis J, Zillo C. Routine ureteral stenting after ureteroscopy for ureteral lithiasis: is it really necessary? J Urol. 2001;166:1252.
35. Smith AD. Management of iatrogenic ureteral strictures after urological procedures. J Urol. 1988;140:1372.
36. Semins MJ, Matlaga BR. Complications of ureteroscopy. AUA Update Ser. 2008; vol. 27, lesson 27:258–63.
37. Kau EL, Ng CS, Fuchs GJ. Complications of ureteroscopic surgery. In: Taneja SS, Smith RB, Ehrlich RM, editors. Complications of urologic surgery. Philadelphia: Saunders; 2009. p. 303–17.

Tricks for Successful Ureteroscopy

58

Zhong Wu and Chen-Chen Feng

Abstract

Ureteral calculus is a common condition in urological practice. Ureteroscopic laser lithotripsy is currently widely used as the first-line therapy for stones reaching indicated size. Successful lithotripsy needs not only adept maneuver techniques but swift decision making as well. In this chapter, the author shares his experience with some of the tricks that could help fresh practitioners manage ureteroscopy faster and with fewer complications. As choice of correct equipment is crucial, this chapter lists the various ureteroscopes, guidewires, and ureteral access sheaths that are helpful in difficult cases. Then, the tips for gaining access into the ureteral orifice with a semirigid ureteroscope are delineated, as these are maneuvers to guarantee safe practice whenever resistance is encountered during passage of the ureteroscope. Lithotripsy is then described in detail to ensure maximum clearance at the first attempt. Furthermore, step-by-step maneuvers of flexible ureteroscopy are described, as these instruments are increasingly used in the minimally invasive therapy for stones in the renal pelvis and calyx. Finally, decisions on stent placement are discussed based on experience of the author's, as well as other, institutes.

Keywords

Ureteroscopy • Ureteroscope • Ureteral calculi • Renal calculi • Lithotripsy • Laser • Stone occlusion • Stone retropulsion • Guidewire • Ureteral stent

Introduction

Approximately 26 % of all admissions of urologic diseases [1] are for urolithiasis, especially upper urinary tract calculi. Extensive experience has broadened the indications of ureteroscopic lithotripsy with only a few contraindications, such as intolerance of the surgery, severe coagulant disorders, and some congenital urinary tract deformations. In China, the utilization of ureteroscopy is presently extensive. Almost all hospitals and clinics above the county level are equipped with more than one semirigid ureteroscope. Treating a large population with urolithiasis, urologists in China have encountered various complicated situations from time to time. This has enriched their clinical experience with a variety of difficult cases. Previously contraindicated scenarios like huge incarcerated stones (≥2 cm), pyonephrosis, and post-renal acute renal failure (ARF) are now commonly being treated effectively with ureteroscopy [2].

Z. Wu, M.D., Ph.D. (✉) • C.-C. Feng, M.D.
Department of Urology, Huashan Hospital, Fudan University, 12 Central Urumqi Rd, Shanghai 200040, People's Republic of China
e-mail: hmgsh188@126.com

Electronic supplementary materialThe online version of this chapter (doi:10.1007/978-1-4471-4387-1_58) contains supplementary material, which is available to authorized users.

J.J. Talati et al. (eds.), *Urolithiasis*,
DOI 10.1007/978-1-4471-4387-1_58, © Springer-Verlag London 2012

Instrumentation

Current ureteroscopes are either semirigid or flexible devices. The semirigid instrument may accommodate to a certain degree of bend and have a tapering tip as wide as 6.75–9 Fr. Some of the currently available semirigid ureteroscopes are summarized in Table 58.1. The flexible ureteroscopes are characterized as active or passive deflections with a smaller tip calibration. The degree of deflection currently available [3, 4] allows access to the entire urinary system including the lower pole of the kidney (Fig. 58.1). In the author's department, the flexible ureteroscope is most frequently used as an intraoperative supplement when the semirigid device is unable to reach and fragment migrating calculi [5]. Table 58.2 lists certain types of currently used flexible ureteroscopes.

Ancillary equipment is of critical importance for successful ureteroscopy. A complete video tower set with virtual monitoring and continuous irrigation is prerequisite. Guidewires are crucial for ureteral passage of the ureteroscope and can be classified as polytetrafluoroethylene (PTFE) coated, hydrophilic, extra-stiff, combination wires, double

Table 58.1 Characteristics of some of the current semirigid ureteroscopes

Manufacturer	Model	Working length (cm)	Tip (F)	Proximal shaft (F)	Channel caliber (F)
Wolf	8703/8705/8708/8709/8719	31/31.5/42.5/43	8	9.8	1×5.0/2×3.0
Wolf	8702	31.5/43	6	7.5	1×4.0/2×2.4
Wolf	8708	31.5/43	6.5	8.5	1×4.0/2×2.2
Gyrus ACMI	Bagley MR-6/MR-6LA	33/43	6.9	10.2	3.4/2.3
Gyrus ACMI	MR0-742A	42	7.0	11.2	5.4
Olympus	Endoeye	43	8.5	9.9	4.2
Storz	27001K/L	34/43	7.0	8.0	5.0
Storz	27002K/L	34/43	8.0	–	5.5
Stryker	SRU-6	33/43	6.9	–	3.4/2.5

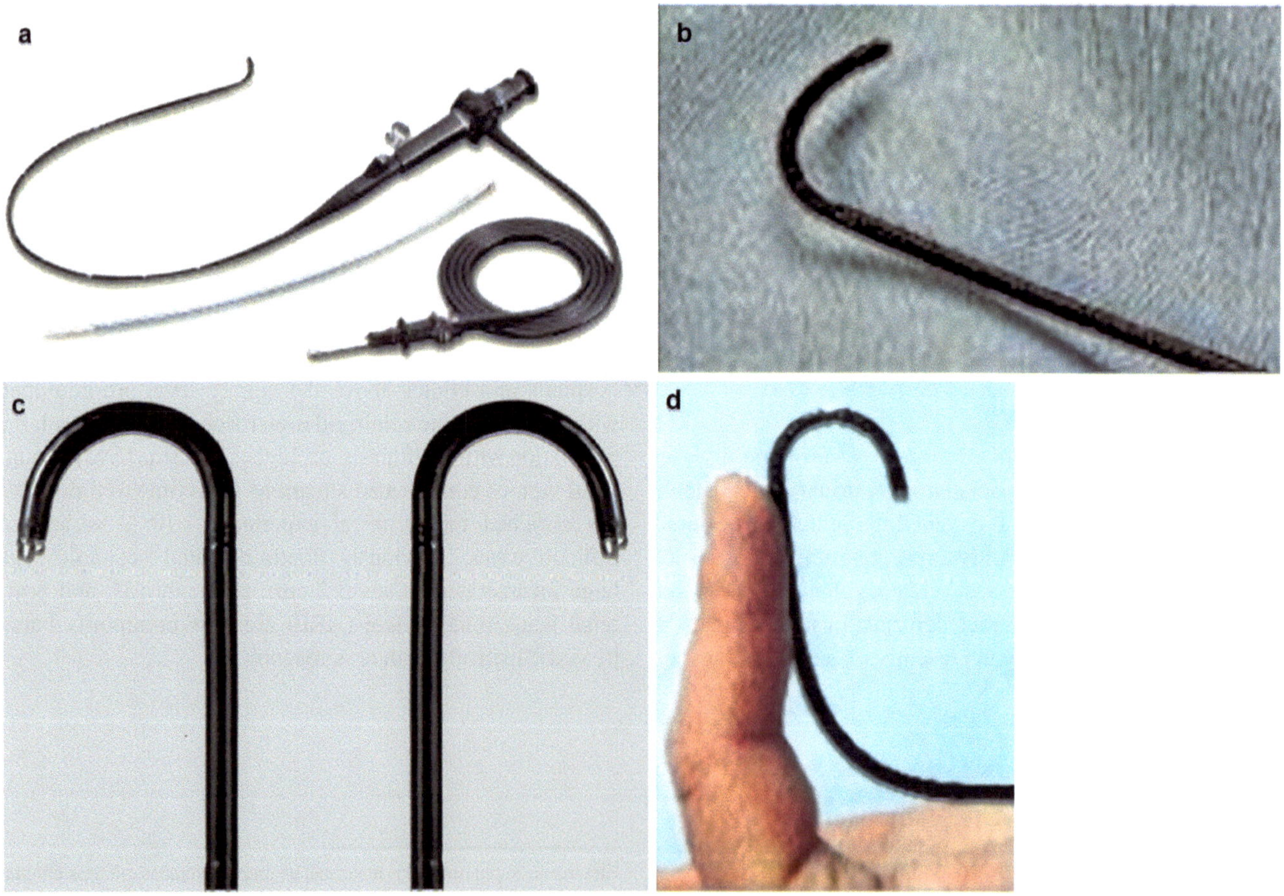

Fig. 58.1 (**a**) Whole vision of a flexible ureteroscope. (**b**) Deflections reaching 180–270°. (**c**) Active deflection. (**d**) Passive deflection

Table 58.2 Characteristics of some of the current flexible ureteroscopes

Manufacturer and model	Tip size (F)	Shaft size (F)	Working length (cm)	Active tip deflection	Active deflection
ACMI DUR 8 Elite	6.75	8.7–10.1	64	180/170–130 dual	Primary and secondary
Storz flex-X (11278A)	7.5	8.4	67.5	270/270 dual	Primary and secondary
Wolf 7325.172 7.5 F	7.5	8.0–9.0	70	160/130	Primary
Olympus URF-P3	6.9	8.4	70	180/180	Primary

floppy tip, and exchange wires, among which the PTEF and hydrophilic wires are the most commonly used [6].

Intracorporeal lithotriptors utilized currently are mainly characterized as ballistic, electrohydraulic (EHL), and laser mediated. The advent of holmium: YAG has made laser lithotripsy the gold standard for ureteral calculi treatment. Unlike its predecessor, the neodymium:YAG laser (which is incapable of fragmenting calcium oxalate monohydrate and brushite calculi), the holmium laser can fragment stones of any composition and can be conducted by a fiber that can be passed through both semirigid and flexible ureteroscopes [7, 8].

Tips and Tricks

Preoperative Preparation

A single dose of prophylactic antibiotic is used to prevent postoperative infection. Any patients with hydronephrosis and confirmed infection are to be cleared of infection before surgery. Appropriate antibiotics should be prescribed on the basis of urine culture reports, and endoscopic ureteral drainage should be provided using a JJ stent. Percutaneous nephrostomy (PCN) should be performed if the stent placement fails. Ureteroscopy should not be attempted until infection is controlled. Either epidural or general anesthesia is utilized for the procedure.

Step-by-Step Maneuver of the Semirigid Ureteroscope

Retrograde Passage

The patient is placed in lithotomy position and the semirigid ureteroscope is inserted into the bladder according to standard protocol. Once the ureteral orifice is detected, a guidewire with a floppy tip should be introduced, as it is less traumatic to the ureteral mucosa. In case the ureteral orifice cannot be identified, or the guidewire cannot negotiate the orifice, the operator should:

1. Locate the contralateral orifice and slowly rotate the scope, searching along the ureteral crest to the corresponding ipsilateral region, and then introduce a guidewire with a floppier tip. If this fails, then
2. Catheterize the patient with a fine Nelaton catheter to empty the bladder and attempt to identify the orifice, observing carefully with the ureteroscope. If this fails, then
3. Use a rigid or flexible cystoscope (more applicable in male patients) to insert the guidewire. The cystoscope provides a much larger field of view with an angle of 70°, which facilitates the detection of an occult ureteral orifice (while the ureteroscope is usually only 5–10°). If this fails, then
4. Give the patient an intravenous injection of furosemide and swiftly insert the guidewire while urine is spurting through the orifice. Keep the guidewire indwelling and insert ureteroscope over the guidewire.

In the process of advancing through the ureteral orifice and the very distal ureter, the operator may experience resistance. This could be due to either obstruction caused by the anterior wall of the orifice over the terminal ureter or stenosis of the distal ureter. Solutions to this include:

1. Rotate the ureteroscope through an arc of 90–180° clockwise at the orifice to enlarge the opening by the passive stretch. If the advancement is impeded despite this maneuver, then
2. Dilate the ureteral orifice and distal part of the ureter. The current, most widely used semirigid ureteroscope seldom necessitates a dilator as they have a small diameter (6–9.8 Fr), which allows easy access to the ureter. In the case of difficulty, however, a balloon or coaxial dilator should be introduced. The balloon dilator is more commonly utilized as it is less traumatic. The balloon caliber ranges from 3 to 8 Fr. If dilation fails, then
3. Change over to a ureteroscope with a more tapering tip, example 6/7.5 Fr, which can usually negotiate the distal ureter. If changing the ureteroscope still fails, then
4. Terminate the operation and place a JJ stent in retrograde fashion. This will allow passive dilation over time and facilitate entry at a second attempt a week later. The second maneuver has substantially better chances of success (refer to Fig. 58.2).

When the ureteroscope has been successfully inserted and is being advanced through the ureter, the guidewire tip should not be advanced too far ahead to prevent pushing the calculus back into the kidney (especially for those in the upper ureter and those below the ureteropelvic junction). The irrigation pressure should be adjusted by syringe or pump to give a clear field of vision; excessive pressure

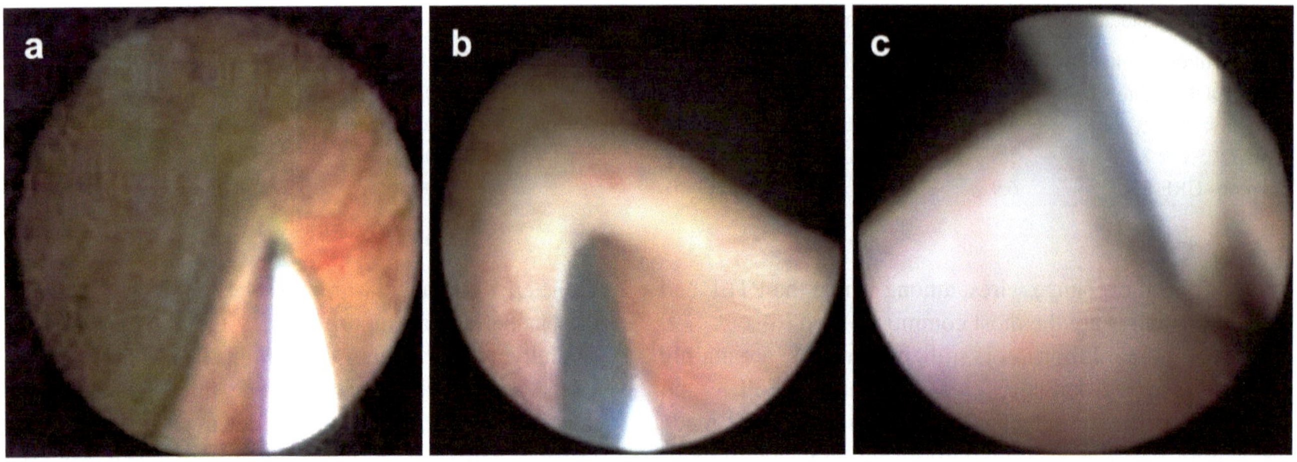

Fig. 58.2 Tips on successful entering the ureteral orifice: (**a**) introduction of a zebra guidewire into the ureteral orifice, (**b**) approaching the orifice with the ureteroscope, and (**c**) a 180° clockwise rotation of the ureteroscope to cause a stretch of the guidewire, enlarging the orifice and facilitating the passage

should be avoided to prevent retropulsion, bacteremia, and compromised renal function. During the procedure, the lumen should always be kept in view. In those cases where the ureteroscope or guidewire cannot be easily advanced in the ureter because of significant kinking or stenosis from previous surgery, the maneuvers should be very gentle to best avoid perforation.

Difficulty during ureteroscopic passage in the ureter can be resolved by performing the following sequential steps:

1. Switching to a guidewire with a floppier tip, as stiff wires like zebra guidewire have a higher chance of submucosal tunneling. If one encounters extreme tortuosity of the ureter, one should switch to hydrophilic guidewires, and gently advance the ureteroscope through the stenosis. If this fails, then
2. A second guidewire can be introduced and may bypass the obstruction easily, by minimizing the angulation. If this fails, then
3. The staff urologist should elevate the patient's flank, compress the abdomen, or place the patient in a head down Trendelenburg position to straighten the ureter as much as possible. If this fails, then
4. Introduce onto the guidewire a 5-Fr ureteral catheter to reinforce the tension of the guidewire. If this fails, then
5. Try the balloon dilator as mentioned previously. Alternatively a short, <2-cm stenosis can be incised by holmium:YAG laser to facilitate the passage [9] of the instrument. If this fails, then
6. Inject contrast via the 5-Fr catheter and perform an intraoperative pyelography to examine the anatomic abnormality (kinks or tortuosity) at the site of obstruction. From the author's experience, incarcerated calculi located just beyond the torsion or kinking appear to provide the most difficult condition to overcome. Such ureters are usually inflamed and edematous and present with polyps and mucosal erosion. Violent passage with either the guidewire or the ureteroscope will lead to perforation. If the intraoperative retrograde pyelography exhibits contrast extravasations implying perforation, the urologist should attempt to advance the catheter into the renal pelvis and thereby terminate the operation, or, alternatively, the surgeon should complete the lithotripsy as quickly as possible. A JJ stent then should be left in place. In case it is difficult to advance the catheter into the collecting system, a percutaneous nephrostomy (PCN) should be used in antegrade fashion to drain the kidney.

In a straightforward case, lithotripsy is performed once the calculus is seen. The guidewire is advanced lateral to the stone and into the upper collecting system; this serves to provide a safety wire to guide stent placement in case perforation occurs and sustains a correct working channel prior to the introduction of intracorporeal lithotriptors (such as laser, ballistic device, or ultrasound).

Retropulsion

Retropulsion remains a major problem for mid- and upper ureteral calculi or stones located in the renal pelvis. Possible preventive measures include:

1. Adjust the patient into reverse Trendelenburg position, or
2. Reduce irrigation pressure or apply intermittent irrigation, or
3. Down-switch the lithotriptor energy to 0.5–0.8 J/5–6 Hz, or
4. In the case of incarcerated calculi, initiate lithotripsy from the margin of the stone and advance the guidewire as soon as a gap is created. Alternatively,

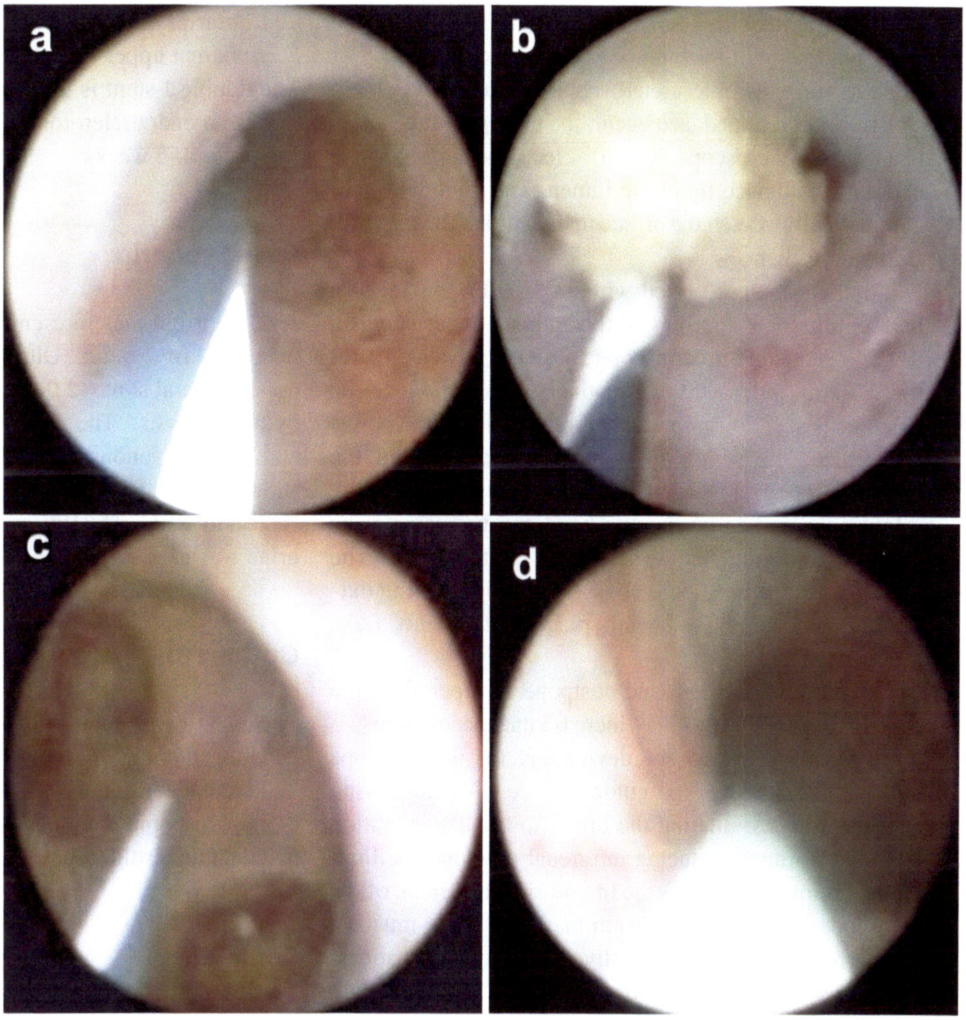

Fig. 58.3 Lithotriptic tips for semirigid ureteroscope: (**a**) Slow passage in guidance of a guidewire always with lumen in vision. (**b**) Advance the guidewire to the collecting system laterally once the stone is met, followed by lithotripsy. (**c**) Do routine examination of the renal pelvis and calyx to ensure there are no large residual fragments remaining after lithotripsy. (**d**) After lithotripsy the guidewire should be kept indwelling for stent implanting under visual monitoring

5. Start the lithotripsy from the margin of the stone leaving the portion where the adhesion of the stone to the ureteral mucosa is the most severe to the last part of fragmentation.
6. Lithotripsy should be delivered step-by-step in a "worm-encroach" pattern and not be started from the central part nor multiple lateral spots of the stone. This reduces the frontal impact of shock waves on the stone.
7. Use occlusive instruments if available, such as Ntrap, Innovex, Stone Cone, or Lidocaine gel (all of which can significantly deter retropulsion), to increase success and stone-free rates [10] (refer to Fig. 58.3 for details).

Antegrade Passage

Should the retrograde ureteroscopy fail or prove extremely difficult due to a complicated anatomical situation at the distal ureter, an antegrade approach via PCN channel may be considered. The passage provides equal options for maneuvers such as pyelography, guidewire passage, and lithotripsy to the corresponding retrograde pathway.

Step-by-Step Maneuver of the Flexible Ureteroscope

Cystoscopic or semirigid ureteroscopic placement of a first working guidewire is a prerequisite. A second safety guidewire is subsequently introduced through the ureteral access sheath (UAS) or double-conduit catheter. The safety guidewire is left in the ureter throughout the procedure to prevent loss of direction and to facilitate JJ stent placement in case of perforation. Nonetheless, Dickstein et al. [11] recommended that the safety guidewire should be introduced in case of concomitant obstruction, associated encrusted ureteral stent, or difficult access secondary to a large stone burden (Steinstrasse or staghorn) or aberrant anatomy.

On entering the ureteral orifice with guidance by the working guidewire, it may not be necessary to use a UAS or dilators, as most flexible ureteroscopes are narrow enough (<7.5 Fr). Should impedance occur, the urologist may:

1. Rotate the ureteroscope 90–180° clockwise at the orifice and aim the device tip at the lumen. The guidewire will automatically stretch the orifice and facilitate the passage. If this fails, then
2. Dilation can be performed with an 8/10 Fr coaxial or a balloon dilator. According to the author's experience, an 8/9.8 Fr semirigid ureteroscope is usually advanced after the working guidewire is effectively in place. Once the calculus is seen, or in the case of renal calculi, the pelvis is reached, the semirigid scope is extracted, and the flexible scope is advanced. Such a maneuver benefits by dilating the orifice on the one hand and previewing the ureteral condition below the stone on the other. The working guidewire should always be left indwelling during the procedure for sheath placement. If this fails, then
3. Implant a double J stent and postpone the operation to a date 1 week later—this may increase the success rate.

When a UAS is utilized, the device and the ureteroscope should be advanced via the guidewire. A UAS may bring various advantages: dilating the ureter to modify irrigation and visual clearance, reducing intrarenal pressure, facilitating stone removal, as well as the in-and-out movement of the ureteroscope. However, the sheath may also cause mucosal injury, perforation, and postoperative stenosis. Thus, patients should be carefully selected for UAS and a 9/11-Fr sheath should typically be utilized. The whole procedure should be conducted under video monitoring. If any impedance is noted during the passage, the procedure should be carried out under X-ray imaging to avoid false passage or perforation. Once the stone is located, the safety guidewire should be kept indwelling while the working guidewire is extracted. The tip of the ureteroscope should be controlled at 0° as an optic fiber of 200–400 μm is introduced through the working channel for lithotripsy. In the case of renal calculi, each calyx should be examined in order to avoid missing any stone.

It remains controversial whether a double J stent should be placed postoperatively. According to the author's experience, a stent is necessary when:

1. Ureteral injury or perforation is encountered.
2. The ureteral mucosa is edematous and hemorrhagic.
3. An incarcerated stone is larger than 1 cm.
4. A polyp is noted.
5. Ureteral stricture is associated with/without endoureterotomy or dilation.
6. A heavy fragment load is left following treatment of a large stone
7. Lithotripsy is insufficient or fails.
8. Apparent upper urinary infection is detected.

The double J stent is usually left indwelling for 1–2 weeks, unless an endoureterotomy is performed, in which case it is left in for 4–6 weeks.

Case Scenario

A 41-year-old male presented with left flank pain occurring over the last 2 years. Ultrasonograms revealed a large left upper ureteral stone (2.0 cm × 0.9 cm in size) associated with hydronephrosis. The kidney-ureter-bladder (KUB) X-ray and the intravenous pyelogram exhibited similar results as shown in Fig. 58.4. Urine analysis demonstrated WBC, 12/HPF and RBC, 15/HPF, and the culture-sensitivity test of urine was negative.

Options for Treatment

1. Shock wave lithotripsy (SWL)
2. Ureteroscopic lithotripsy (URSL)
3. Percutaneous nephrolithotomy (PCNL)
4. Laparoscopic ureterolithotomy
5. Open ureterolithotomy

Comments

The patient suffers from left hydronephrosis and dilation of upper ureter secondary to the ureteral stone. Immediate intervention should be carried out to remove the occlusion and minimize further compromise of renal function, utilizing the least invasive approach. As the course of disease has lasted for more than 2 years, it is quite probable that the stone is incarcerated, and the mucosa edematous, with polyps encapsulating the stone. The size and the dense nature of the stone predicted from the X-ray appearance indicates a relatively unsatisfactory result from shockwave lithotripsy. The SWL has a lower single procedure stone-free rate and is unable to promptly remove the occlusion. The second SWL intervention should preferably be prescribed after an interval of 14 days. SWL therefore appears inappropriate especially as it will not help procure early recovery of renal function. Thus, SWL is not an optimal treatment option.

PCNL, despite its capability of successful single lithotripsy and creation of a free conduit, will inevitably cause some nephron injury. Clayman et al. [12] has reported a 1–2 % of permanent nephron impairment in each PCNL channel. In this patient, PCNL can be considered, yet is not the optimal technique.

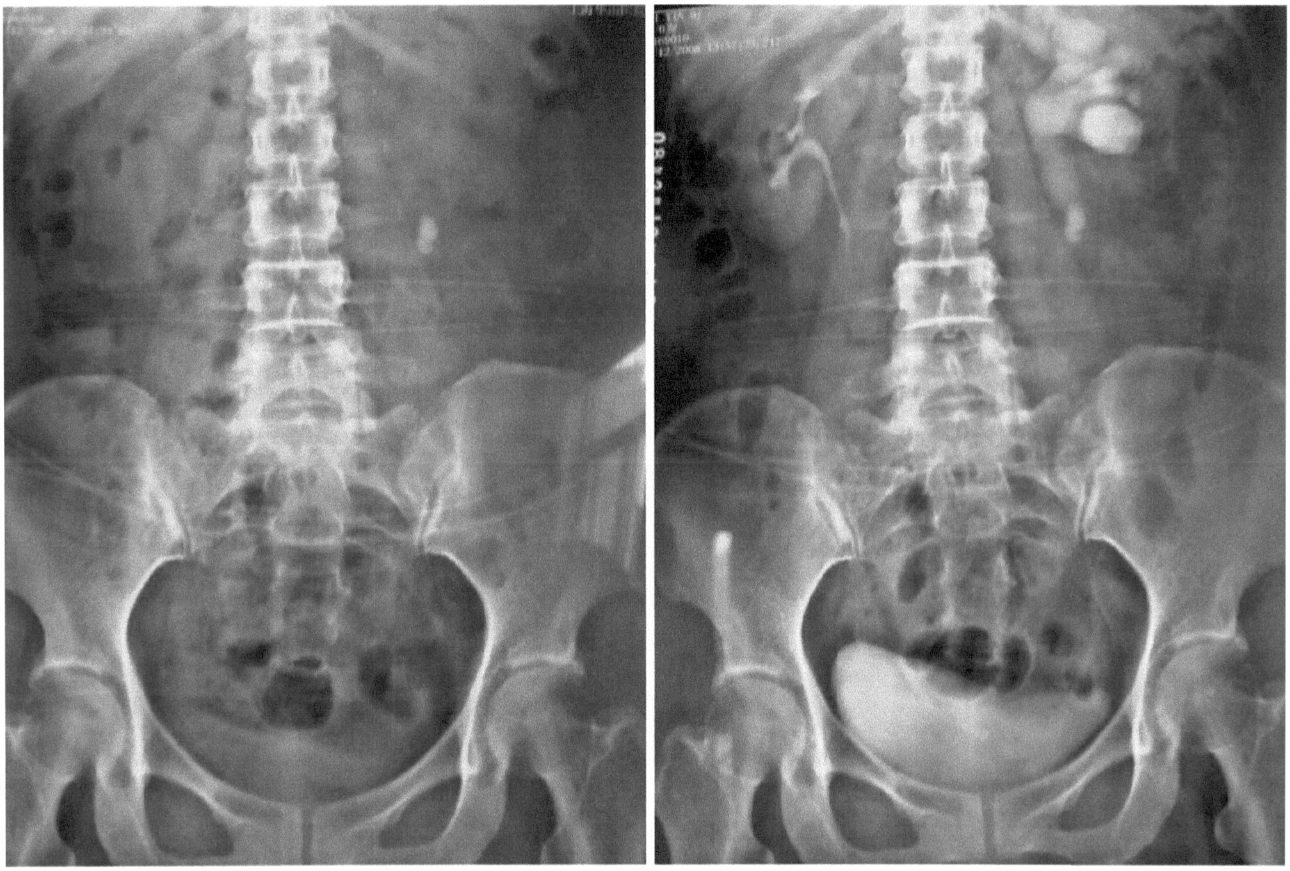

Fig. 58.4 Preoperative KUB (*left*) and intravenous pyelography (IVP) (*right*) showing left upper ureteral calculi with ureteral dilation and hydronephrosis

Laparoscopic ureterolithotomy avoids the long cutaneous incision of an ureterolithotomy, yet requires opening and suturing of the ureter, which causes the same trauma to the ureter as a corresponding open surgery. As the procedure is comparatively more traumatic and conceives higher rate of complications like stricture and urine leakage, it is difficult to consider it the optimal technique.

Ureteroscopic lithotripsy (URSL) accesses the stone through a natural orifice and requires no skin incision. In association with novel intracorporeal lithotriptors like holmium:YAG laser, the URSL is capable of fragmenting any stone without compromising the nephrons. The procedure is prompt and highly effective and leads to a swift salvage of renal function. In this patient, therefore, URSL is the optimal choice.

However, several difficulties may be encountered and one needs to be cautious while performing lithotripsy. The stone is incarcerated in the upper ureter and below the ureteropelvic junction (UPJ) where the collective system is severely dilated, conditions conducive to retropulsion. The precautions are listed in the preceding sections of this chapter and include change of position, reduce irrigation pressure, and especially the use of occlusive devices.

How We Did It

We optioned semirigid ureteroscope (Wolf 8/9.8 F) associated with holmium:YAG laser lithotripsy. The ureteroscope was advanced with the aid of a guidewire and was arrested well below the UPJ because of significant kinking of the ureter. We introduced another guidewire with a curved tip, associated with position change and elevation of the ipsilateral flank, to advance over the torsion and locate the stone, which was incarcerated and encapsulated with polyps. As the lumen was completely occluded, the guidewire could not be further advanced. The lithotripsy started from one side of the stone margin, taking care to avoid impacting multiple spots of the stone margin or its central part, which maneuvers are both more disposed to retropulsion. Then, when a gap was created between the calculus and mucosa, an Ntrap was immediately advanced and opened to prevent upward migration of stone or fragments. Lithotripsy was then continued at 1.5 J/15–20 Hz, the aim being to produce stone particles no larger than 0.2 cm. The procedure was completed and the pelvis examined for stone fragments. A double J stent was placed. There was no intraoperative hemorrhage or perforation. The patient

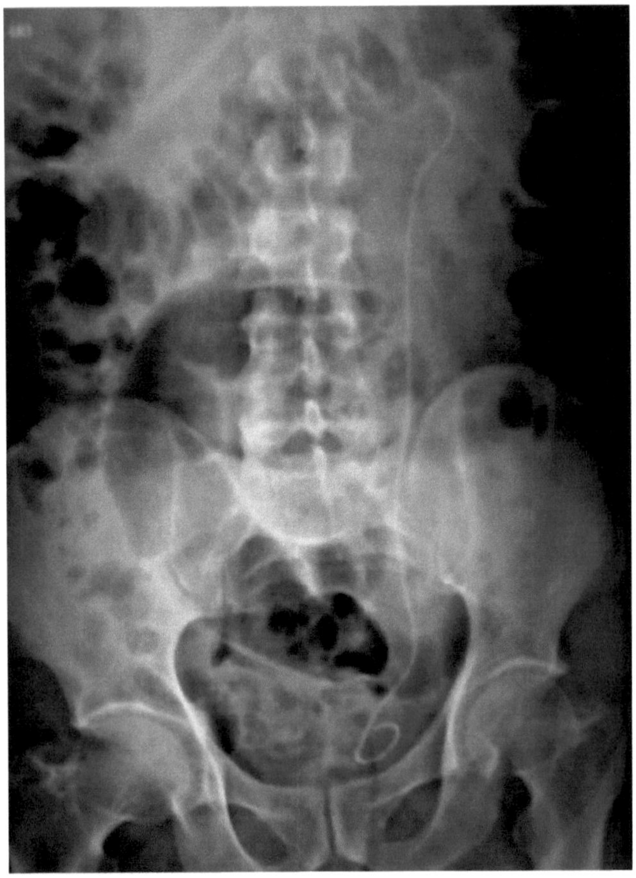

Fig. 58.5 KUB on postoperative day 7 exhibiting complete stone clearance

was discharged on postoperative day 1, and follow-up was conducted in a week with KUB and ultrasonograms, showing complete stone clearance (Fig. 58.5).

Conclusion

Choosing the correct instrument and ancillary equipment can lead to excellent results with laser lithotripsy. Commonly encountered difficulties can be overcome by simple maneuvers. Experience gradually enlarges the skills of the surgeon to cope with a wide range of difficult cases, so that ultimately the most difficult stones can also be fragmented effectively.

References

1. Wu JP. Wujieping urology. 1st ed. Jinan: Shandong Science and Technology Press; 2004. p. 743.
2. Jiang H, Wu Z, Ding Q. Ureteroscopy and holmium: YAG laser lithotripsy as emergency treatment for acute renal failure caused by impacted ureteral calculi. Urology. 2008;72(3):504–7.
3. Shvarts O, Perry KT, Goff B, Schulam PG. Improved functional deflection with a dual-deflection flexible ureteroscope. J Endourol. 2004;18(2):141–4.
4. Ankem MK, Lowry PS, Slovick RW, Munoz del Rio A, Nakada SY. Clinical utility of dual active deflection flexible ureteroscope during upper tract ureteropyeloscopy. Urology. 2004;64(3):430–4.
5. Jiang H, Wu Z, Ding Q, Zhang Y. Ureteroscopic treatment of ureteral calculi with holmium: YAG laser lithotripsy. J Endourol. 2007;21(2):151–4.
6. Feng C, Ding Q, Jiang H, Gao P, Wen H, Gu B, et al. Use of NTrap during ureteroscopic holmium: YAG laser lithotripsy of upper ureteral calculi. Minim Invasive Ther Allied Technol. 2012;21(2):78–82.
7. Binbay M, Tepeler A, Singh A, Akman T, Tekinaslan E, Sarilar O, et al. Evaluation of pneumatic versus holmium: YAG laser lithotripsy for impacted ureteral stones. Int Urol Nephrol. 2011;43(4):989–95.
8. Denstedt JD, Zheng W. Intracorporeal lithotripsy. Update on technology. Urol Clin North Am. 2000;27:301–13.
9. Wu Z, Feng C, Ding Q, Jiang H, Zhang Y. Ureteroscopic holmium: YAG laser endopyelotomy is effective in distinctive ureteropelvic junction obstructions. Videosurg Other Miniinvasive Tech. 2011;6(3):144–9. doi:10.5114/wiitm.2011.24692.
10. Farahat YA, Elbahnasy AE, Elashry OM. A randomized prospective controlled study for assessment of different ureteral occlusion devices in prevention of stone migration during pneumatic lithotripsy. Urology. 2011;77(1):30–5.
11. Dickstein RJ, Kreshover JE, Babayan RK, Wang DS. Is a safety wire necessary during routine flexible ureteroscopy? J Endourol. 2010;24(10):1589–92.
12. Clayman RV, Elbers J, Miller RP, Williamson J, McKeel D, Wassynger W. Percutaneous nephrostomy: assessment of renal damage associated with semi-rigid (24 F) and balloon (36 F) dilation. J Urol. 1987;138(1):203–6.

Lasers in Stone Disease

59

Anne Sophie Knipper and Andreas J. Gross

Abstract

Ho: YAG represents the most widely used and most efficacious lithotripter in endourology. While combining the laser fibers with smaller caliber ureterorenoscopes, semirigid and flexible, literally every urinary calculus can be treated. And even though technical developments are still ongoing, modern laser and fiber technology has already shifted ureteroscopy from a diagnostic to a serious therapeutic option in urolithiasis.

Keywords

History • Physics • Instrumentation and devices • Fibers • Laser systems • Photoacoustic lasers • Pulsed-dye laser • FREDDY laser • Photothermal lasers • Erbium:yttrium aluminum garnet (Er:YAG) laser • Ability to fragment stones • Plasma formation • Collapse of the bubble • Collateral damage • Tissue safety

Introduction

History

It is well-known that Albert Einstein was the first to introduce the theory of "stimulated emission." During this process, photons with the correct amount of energy can disturb an excited atom and cause it to drop to a lower energy level, in turn leading to the creation of another identical photon. The original photon interacting with the atom, as well as the photon subsequently released, will be discharged simultaneously and will therefore have the identical wavelength and direction of propagation [1].

The concept of stimulated emission was the foundation on which subsequent laser development would be undertaken.

A.S. Knipper, M.D. (✉) • A.J. Gross, M.D.
Department of Urology, Asklepios Hospital Barmbek, Ruebenkamp 220, Hamburg 22291, Germany
e-mail: an.gross@asklepios.com

J.J. Talati et al. (eds.), *Urolithiasis*,
DOI 10.1007/978-1-4471-4387-1_59, © Springer-Verlag London 2012

Physics

It is the active medium in a laser (acronym for light amplification by stimulated emission of radiation) that determines the wavelength (and therefore color) and frequency of the light that it emits. The wavelength and frequency are inversely proportional to one another.

The design of a laser is basically that of a laser medium placed within an optical resonator, which is defined by two mirrors. Light at the characteristic laser wavelength receives amplification whenever it passes through the excited laser medium. The reflective surfaces of the optical resonator ensure multiple passes of the light beam through the medium, leading to repetitive amplification. Excitation energy is required for this amplification process and can be derived from an electrical current. A fraction of the amplified light inside the optical resonator escapes as a beam of light out of one or both mirrors.

A classification of laser output of particular practical importance in urology is that of pulsed wave (PW) versus continuous wave (CW). During CW operation, the output of the laser is continuous and of constant amplitude. The clinical effect is a more controlled interaction with the tissue. PW operation on the other hand delivers forceful bursts of laser energy, which is useful for stone fragmentation [2].

Lasers for the treatment of kidney and bladder stones have been one of the earliest uses of lasers in medicine. Mulvaney Beck attempted to fragment urinary calculi in vitro in 1968, using a ruby and a carbon dioxide laser [3]. Energy applied was up to 300 J or 50 W output. Already at this early stage of laser lithotripsy, it was recognized that the effect was dependent on stone composition, fragmenting compact stones with more difficulty. It took another 20 years before the first commercially available lasers for lithotripsy were introduced, which use 504 nm of light delivered through optical quartz fibers. This was a nonthermal safe laser that produced plasma between the tip of the fiber and the calculus, fragmenting stones with a photoacoustic effect. The small flexible probes were complimentary to both the semirigid and flexible ureteroscopes and could fragment most urinary calculi, including cystine [4]. Limiting factors to this kind of lithotripsy were high initial costs, expensive disposables such as coumarin dye, as well as trouble with fragmentation of hard stones composed of calcium oxalate monohydrate [5].

Instruments and Devices

Today various laser types have been introduced for stone treatment. In addition, the technical development of instruments in endourology is still ongoing. All manufacturers offer a variety of cutting-edge semirigid and flexible instruments enabling the surgeon to perform lithotripsy in almost any location of the upper urinary tract. Simultaneously, an endless selection of devices such as wires, baskets, and access sheaths (internal and external) has been created to achieve a higher success rate and more safety during ureteroscopic procedures. To successfully treat calculi, there are two main characteristics of the instruments that need to be fulfilled. To begin with, the energy source (laser) should fragment urinary stones efficiently but with the lowest possible risk of damaging the surrounding tissue. Additionally, high demands on the delivery system (laser fibers) are made. They should transfer the energy to the expected location within the collecting system. To achieve this, without affecting the function of the instrument, it requires that fibers are as small and as flexible as possible so as to be able to reach any calculus within the urinary tract. The laser fibers are an important tool for disintegration of the stone, but can impact on the durability of the expensive ureteroscope.

Fibers

Laser fibers are built with an inner circular optical core and up to three concentric layers. The laser radiation is delivered through the core, while the next layer confines the radiation inside the core by total reflection. The outer layers provide mechanical stability. Mostly low-OH silica fibers with an optical cladding of fluorine doped silica are used, since they allow smaller bending radius and provide a very focused beam, both important essentials during flexible ureterorenoscopy. Alternatively, fibers with fluoroacrylate cladding exist but are much more rigid. Also, radiation may leak through these fibers and can consequently damage the working channel and integrity of the scope.

Laser Systems

Several laser types for stone treatment are available. They can vary in terms of emitted wavelength, used fiber diameter, and pulse duration, with consequent different mechanisms of stone fragmentation. The laser systems can be divided into photoacoustic and photothermal lasers. Photoacoustic lasers operate in the blue-green portion of the spectrum, whereas photothermal lasers are in the mid-infrared portion. Photoacoustic effects are produced in lasers with short pulse durations, typically <1 μs. Well-known lasers of the photoacoustic group are the FREDDY laser (frequency-doubled double pulse ND:YAG laser) and the pulsed-dye laser. Photothermal effects are produced in lasers with long pulse durations, normally >10 μs. Typical examples of the photothermal group are the Ho:YAG (holmium:YAG) and the erbium:YAG laser. Whereas photothermal lasers need to be in contact with the stone to disintegrate it, photoacoustic lasers do not. During this contact, energy is absorbed in the surface of the stone within 0.4 mm [6]. Consequently, photothermal lasers produce smaller fragments than photoacoustic lasers. On the other hand, the latter causes less collateral damage in the ureter, because they do not perforate or coagulate the ureter as easily as the photothermal lasers. It has been shown that two pulses with a Ho:YAG laser may perforate the ureter, whereas 2,000 pulses with the FREDDY laser failed to do so [7]. At the same time, hard stones present a challenge to the photoacoustic lasers since they do not work well in stones that are not dark or colored. In conclusion, the FREDDY lasers achieved success in some 50 % of stones only and therefore did not stay the test of time. At the price of a higher chance of collateral damage, photothermal lasers may fragment all types of calculi. The two best known photothermal lasers are the Ho:YAG and the erbium:YAG laser. There is no doubt, that nowadays Ho:YAG lasers are the energy source of choice in the endoscopical treatment of urolithiasis. But even though erbium lasers have shown a five times more efficient stone fragmentation in vitro, the use of this laser is limited for endourological procedures, because up to date there is a lack of suitable fiber [8].

Photoacoustic Lasers

Photoacoustic lasers emit laser energy at a wavelength in the blue-green portion of the spectrum where it is absorbed by hemoglobin. Examples for those kinds of lasers used in endourological procedures are the FREDDY laser (wavelength at 532 nm) and the pulsed-dye laser (504 nm). Another laser in this category is the Alexandrite laser with a wavelength at 755 nm. These photoacoustic lasers provide a high safety margin due to the absorption of their energy in hemoglobin [9]. If laser energy accidentally hits surrounding tissue, it will be absorbed and carried away by the blood flow. In this case, hemoglobin can be regarded as a cooling element for the laser energy [10].

When the energy of photo acoustic lasers is transferred to water or stones, it creates a vapor bubble. The collapse of the vapor bubble leads to a pressure effect on the calculi, which results in fragmentation of the stone [11]. The fiber needs to be positioned in front of the stone, with a little distance though, to allow best bubble expansion in order to achieve maximum fragmentation efficacy. Since the photoacoustic effect spreads circumferentially, the laser fiber can be positioned aside of the stone and fragmentation of the stone can be achieved equally. Nevertheless, photoacoustic lasers have deficiencies in the ability of fragmenting cystine as well as calcium oxalate monohydrate calculi [12].

Pulsed-Dye Laser

One of the first lasers to be utilized in the treatment of urinary calculi was the pulsed-dye laser. Initial reports on the use of it for stone fragmentation appeared in 1987 [4]. The pulsed-dye laser has an emission wavelength of 504 nm. It employs a short pulse duration of approximately 1 ps that allows effective stone fragmentation. The energy is not absorbed in water, revealing a diminished risk of thermal damage to the urothelium during stone workup. Therefore, the use of a pulsed-dye laser reduces the reliance on direct visualization. But as mentioned above, calcium oxalate monohydrate, brushite, and cystine stones cannot be fragmented efficiently with this laser, since these types of stones present with a low optical absorption of the laser energy. This characteristic pushed the pulsed-dye laser out of the endourological routine [13].

FREDDY Laser

The FREDDY laser was created by placing a KTP crystal into the resonator of an Nd:YAG laser. Therefore, it produces pulses with two possible wavelengths simultaneously: a 20 % green light component at 532 nm and an 80 % infrared component at a wavelength of 1,064 nm. The high pulse intensity, which can be reached by this laser, permits stone fragmentation. In contrast to the pulsed-dye laser, the FREDDY laser generates a plasma bubble instead of steam in front of the fiber tip. While the pulse at 532 nm initiates plasma formation at the surface of the stone, the laser radiation at a wavelength of 1,064 nm heats the plasma bubble, leading first to its expansion and then inducing the collapse of the bubble. After these steps the mechanism can be compared with physical characteristics of the pulsed-dye laser. By the collapse of the plasma bubble, a mechanical shock wave is provoked. This leads to the stone fragmentation. Regular pulse durations of FREDDY lasers lie within 0.3 and 1.5 μs [14]. In comparison to the Ho:YAG laser, the FREDDY laser has a low risk of collateral damage, and the clinical results from the use of the FREDDY laser are promising. Stone-free rates of up to 95 % after ureteral stone treatment are reported. However, like the pulsed-dye laser, the FREDDY laser fails to fragment hard urinary calculi like calcium oxalate monohydrate, cystine, and brushite stones [15]. On the other hand, because of its intrinsic safety to soft tissues and the low cost, the FREDDY laser is still an alternative in the treatment of calcium phosphate stones. It is particularly useful in clinical situations where visualization is limited or a close tissue contact is inevitable, for example, during the fragmentation of impacted stones [13].

Photothermal Lasers

Photothermal lasers emit energy in the mid-infrared portion of the light spectrum. At these wavelengths laser energy is absorbed by water. Prominent examples are the holmium:YAG or the erbium:YAG laser. Laser types releasing photothermal effects show a relatively long pulse duration of approximately 300 μs. This leads to a slow energy transfer in water that lets the vapor bubble appear torpedo-shaped in the Er:YAG laser and pear-shaped in the Ho:YAG laser, reducing cavitation and insignificant acoustic pressure waves. In contrast to photoacoustic lasers, photothermal lasers are contact lasers. Here, the fiber needs to be positioned in contact to the stone surface due to the fact that the energy is absorbed within the first 0.4 mm^3. Compared to photoacoustic lasers, photothermal stone fragmentation produces smaller fragments. On the other hand, photothermal lasers have a lower safety margin than photoacoustic lasers and can actually coagulate or even perforate the ureter [7]. On the positive side, these laser types permit the fragmentation of all types of calculi.

Holmium:Yttrium Aluminum Garnet (Ho:YAG) Laser

The Ho:YAG laser is currently the most commonly used laser in urology. It releases energy at a wavelength of 2,140 nm and at a pulse duration of 350 μs. Because of these features, the radiation of holmium lasers is efficiently absorbed by water. Therefore, a high safety profile can be emphasized for an aqueous surrounding like the urinary tract. With the incident laser pulse water is vaporized immediately in front of the stone, with a cavitation bubble forming at the tip of the optical fiber [16]. The energy of the holmium laser is then transmitted through this "vapor window" to the stone. When laser radiation is transferred to a urinary stone, some of the energy is absorbed by the stone, and this causes stone fragmentation by forming a pressure wave inside the stone [17]. In addition, by the implosion of the vapor bubble, a shock wave is caused and then transmitted to the stone leading to fragmentation. In terms of effectiveness, by decreasing the laser pulse duration at a given energy, a more effective stone fragmentation can be achieved since the peak of the pulse power will increase. In combination with flexible silica fibers, this characteristic is used in calculi fragmentation. The holmium laser permits the fragmentation of all types of stones; even cystine stones are fragmented efficiently. By that, with the holmium laser, the need for percutaneous procedures in cystine stone patients is considerably reduced. Laser settings are particularly important in the use of the holmium laser since the efficacy of stone fragmentation is largely influenced by settings like used energy, frequency, and fiber diameter. It has been shown that laser settings for small caliber fibers are optimal below 1.0 J and at 5–10 Hz [18].

The Ho:YAG lithotripsy has another important advantage. By now, laser fibers with a very small optical core have been developed (200 μ), allowing the holmium laser lithotripsy to be used during flexible ureterorenoscopic procedures. However, a diminished deflection capacity of the scope caused by the stiffness of the laser fiber still needs to be considered [19].

Multiple clinical studies could already show the efficacy of stone treatment using the holmium laser. For the treatment of urinary calculi, stone-free rates around 95 % have been published [20].

Potential limitations of the use of holmium lasers are the risks of collateral tissue damage that requires optimal visualization during the procedure.

Erbium:Yttrium Aluminum Garnet (Er:YAG) Laser

The erbium:YAG laser has already been used in dentistry and ophthalmology, while the employment in urology is still experimental. The possibly valuable potential of the Er:YAG laser for stone treatment is based on known energy absorption of urinary calculi. Maximum energy absorption appears to be near 2.9 μm. In theory, the Er:YAG laser (wavelength 29–2.94 μm, pulse duration 275 μs) should then be the optimal energy source. As stated above, the mechanism of stone fragmentation is also photothermal and thereby comparable to that of the Ho:YAG laser. It has been shown in vitro that stone fragmentation with the Er:YAG laser seems to be up to 3–5 times more efficient than with holmium lasers [8]. This is why this laser is thought to have the potential to become a valuable substitute to the holmium laser.

Nevertheless, for an application in endourology, up to date there is a lack of suitable fibers. This excludes this promising implement from clinical use in urology.

Conclusion

In summary, various laser systems are currently available for urologists. Today, the Ho:YAG represents the most widely used and most efficacious lithotripter in endourology. While combining the laser fibers with smaller caliber ureterorenoscopes, semirigid and flexible, literally every urinary calculi can be treated. And even though technical developments are still ongoing, modern laser and fiber technology has already shifted ureteroscopy from a diagnostic to a serious therapeutic option in urolithiasis [21].

References

1. Einstein A. Zur Quantentheorie der Strahlung. Phys Z. 1917; 18:121–8.
2. Gordon JP, Zeiger HJ, Townes CH. Molecular microwave oscillator and new hyperfine structure in the microwave spectrum of NH_3. Phys Rev. 1954;95:282–4.
3. Mulvaney WP, Beck CW. The laser beam in urology. J Urol. 1968; 99:112–25.
4. Dretler SP, Watson G, Parrish JA, Murray S. Pulsed dye laser fragmentation of ureteral calculi: initial clinical experience. J Urol. 1987;137:386–9.
5. Floratos DL, de la Rosette JJ. Lasers in urology. BJU Int. 1999; 84(2):204–11.
6. Freiha GS, Glickmann RD, Teichman JM. Holmium:YAG laser induced damage to guidewires: an experimental study. J Endourol. 1997;11:331–6.
7. Santa Cruz RW, Leveillee RJ, Krongrad A. Ex vivo comparison of four lithotripters commonly used in the ureter: what does it take to perforate? J Endourol. 1998;12:417–22.
8. Teichman JM, Chan KF, Cecconi PP, Corbin NS, Kamerer AD, Glickman RD, et al. Erbium:YAG versus Ho:YAG. J Urol. 2001; 165:876–9.
9. Nishioka NS, Kelsey PB, Kibbi AG, Delmonico F, Parrish JA, Anderson RR. Laser lithotripsy: animal studies of safety and efficacy. Lasers Surg Med. 1988;8(4):357–62.
10. Teichmann JM. Lasers. In: Smith AD, Badlani GH, Bagley DH, Clayman RV, Docimo SG, editors. Smith's textbook of endourology. Hamilton: BC Decker; 2006.

11. Rink K, Delacrétaz G, Salathé RP. Fragmentation process of current laser lithotriptors. Lasers Surg Med. 1995;16(2):134–46.
12. Denstedt JD, Chun SS, Miller MD, Eberwein PM. Intracorporeal lithotripsy with the Alexandrite laser. Lasers Surg Med. 1997; 20(4):433–6.
13. Marks AJ, Teichman JMH. Lasers in clinical urology: state of the art and new horizons. World J Urol. 2007;25:227–33.
14. Helfmann J, Muller G. Laser lithotripsy: process overview. Med Laser Appl. 2001;16:30–7.
15. Dubosq F, Pasqui F, Girard F, Beley S, Lesaux N, Gattegno B, et al. Endoscopic lithotripsy and the FREDDY laser: initial experience. J Endourol. 2006;20(5):296–9.
16. Cinman NM, Andonian S, Smith AD. Lasers in percutaneous renal procedures. World J Urol. 2010;28(2):135–42.
17. Teichmann HO, Herrmann TR, Bach T. Technical aspects of lasers in urology. World J Urol. 2007;25(3):221–5.
18. Kuo RL, Aslan P, Zhong P, Preminger GM. Impact of holmium laser settings and fiber diameter on stone fragmentation and endoscope deflection. J Endourol. 1998;12(6):523–7.
19. Bach T, Geavlete B, Herrmann TR, Gross AJ. Working tools in flexible ureterorenoscopy – influence on flow and deflection: what does matter? J Endourol. 2008;22(8):1639–43.
20. Wu CF, Shee JJ, Lin WY, Lin CL, Chen CS. Comparison between extracorporeal shock wave lithotripsy and semirigid ureterorenoscope with holmium:YAG laser lithotripsy for treating large proximal ureteral stones. J Urol. 2004;172:1899–902.
21. Bagley DH. Ureteroscopic surgery: changing times and perspectives. Urol Clin North Am. 2004 Feb;31(1):1–4, vii.

Ureteric Stents: Their Use and Abuse

60

Stuart J. Graham and Simon Choong

Abstract

Ureteric stents are used to prevent or treat obstruction of the urine flow from the kidney or to allow appropriate healing after a procedure on the renal pelvis or ureter. Placement of stents is in most circumstances a simple procedure if care is taken to follow a few principles. They can be inserted retrogradely up the ureter or percutaneously down the ureter. Stents are made of soft, synthetic material with memory molecules that uncurl to facilitate insertion, but remain coiled in the human body after placement. Stents have a limited life when inserted into the human body. They are prone to encrustation and upward migration and can easily be forgotten unless there is a tracking system to record and remind patients of the due date of removal.

Keywords

Bladder • Biofilm • Catheter • Encrustation • Hydrophilic • Guidewire • Percutaneous • Ureteroscope • Ureteric stent • Urine • History

Introduction

A ureteric or ureteral stent is a thin prosthetic device, often tubular, inserted into the ureter to prevent or treat obstruction of the urine flow from the kidney or to allow appropriate healing after a procedure on the renal pelvis or ureter. Often considered a necessary evil, these very necessary devices can cause significant morbidity, which needs to be clearly understood when counseling a patient prior to their insertion.

The classic ureteric stent most commonly in use today is the "double pigtail" design that involves a long and narrow central portion, normally hollow to allow easy placement, with a complete curl at either end (Fig. 60.1). As the stent is made usually of a soft, plastic type biomaterial (Fig. 60.2), these end pieces completely uncurl to facilitate insertion, but remain coiled inside the human body after placement, to hold the stent in place. The lower curl stops upward migration into the kidney, making retrieval from the bladder easier, and the upper curl stops the stent from falling out.

Not all stents are such hollow tubes. Several companies make solid stents that may be placed in conditions that cause significant ureteric obstruction such as in compression due to intra-abdominal tumors (Fig. 60.3). The basis for their use is that they tend to be incompressible, and small grooves in the stent wall allow urine passage. They are technically more difficult to place, however.

Another type of device used in compressive ureteric disease is the Memokath® stent (Fig. 60.4a–c). This is a metal coil placed permanently within the ureter that holds the wall fully open. They may also be difficult to pass and require a section of normal ureter below the stent.

Much of the development of stents in recent years has focused on increasing the in vivo life of the device using novel biomaterials to resist encrustation and infection, and

S.J. Graham, B.Sc., M.B.B.S., FRCSEd, FRCS (Urol) (✉)
Department of Urology,
Whipps Cross Hospital, Barts Health NHS Trust,
Whipps Cross Road, Leytonstone, London F11 INR, UK
e-mail: stuart@stuartgraham.com

S. Choong, M.B.B.S. (Lon), FRCS (Eng), FRCSEd, MS, FRCS (Urol)
The Stone Unit, University College London Hospital,
London, UK
e-mail: schoong@aol.com

J.J. Talati et al. (eds.), *Urolithiasis*,
DOI 10.1007/978-1-4471-4387-1_60, © Springer-Verlag London 2012

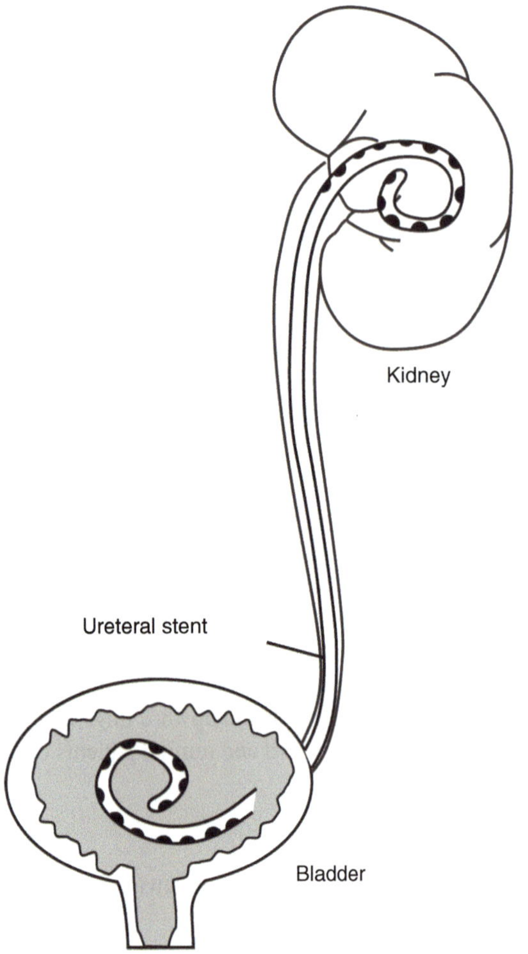

Fig. 60.1 Left side of the urinary tract containing a ureteric stent

increasing the patient comfort, by altering the lower end and shaft of the stent and by softening at body temperature.

The History of the Ureteric Stent

The first ureteric stents were used to aid alignment of the cut ends in ureteric anastomotic surgery. The first described case is by Gustav Simon in the nineteenth century [1]. True endoscopic placement had to wait until the development of cystoscopy in 1876 by Nietze [2].

Initially, ureteric catheters were made from materials such as varnish-coated fabric (Fig. 60.5). Plastic replaced this, which was easier to place and more robust. The catheters would run through the bladder and out to an external drainage bag. However, the rate of infections and therefore encrustation and blocking was very high. In 1952, Tulloch [3] used polythene tubing to repair a ureter. In 1967, Zimskind et al. [4] described the use of a silicone device and introduced it cystoscopically.

These devices all had the problem that, being straight tubes, they migrated easily out of the ureter, into the bladder,

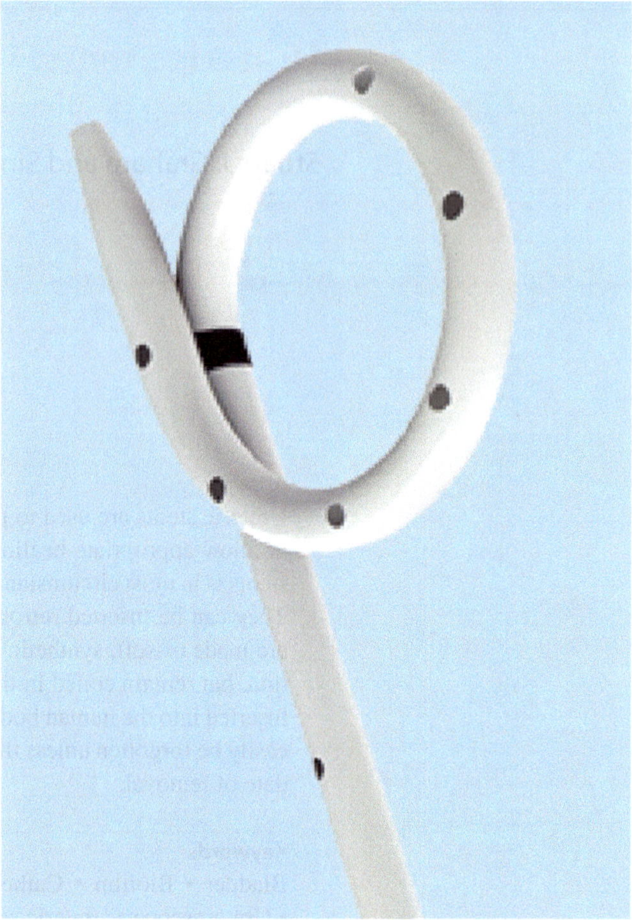

Fig. 60.2 The upper curl of a typical JJ stent. Note the tapered end, the black mark that shows the start of the coiled portion and the multiple side holes

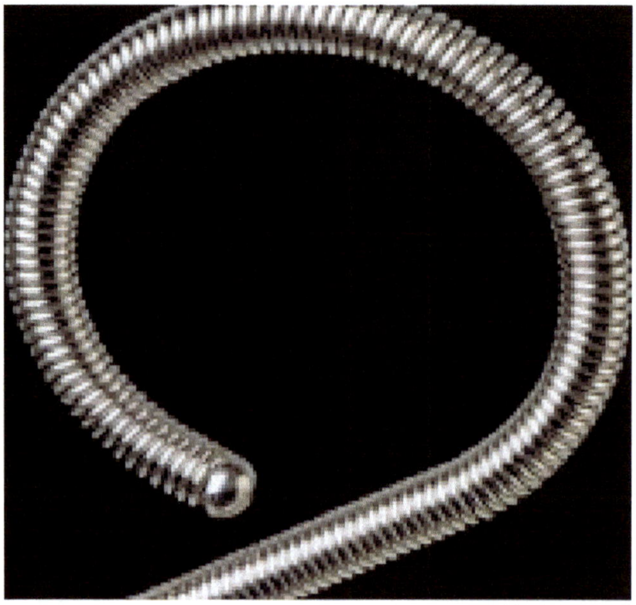

Fig. 60.3 A solid metal coil stent. Note the coiled groove running round the side of the stent (Permission for use granted by Cook Medical Incorporated, Bloomington, IA)

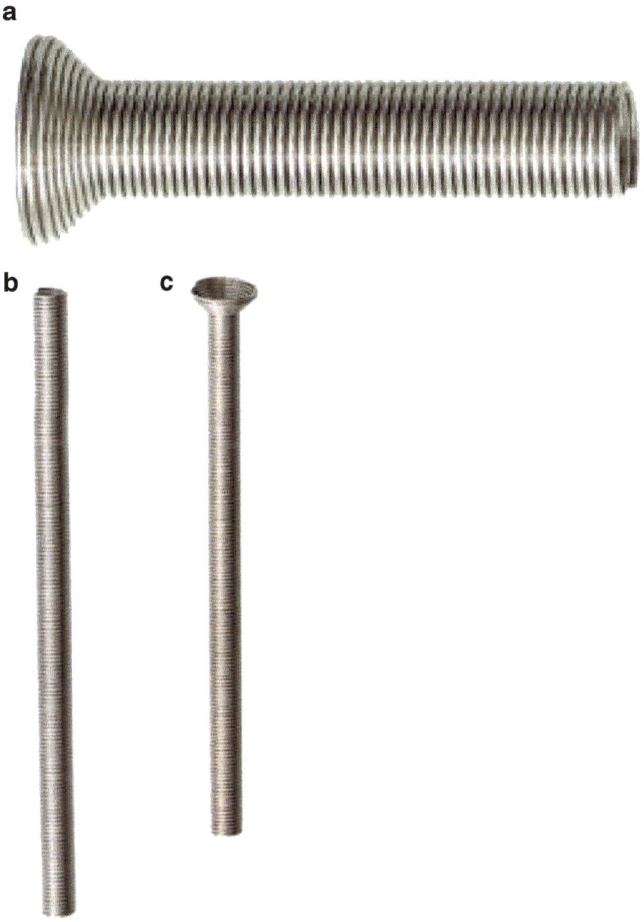

Fig. 60.4 (**a**) A Memokath stent, in the flange-ended configuration. A Memokath stent (**b**) before and (**c**) after thermal expansion

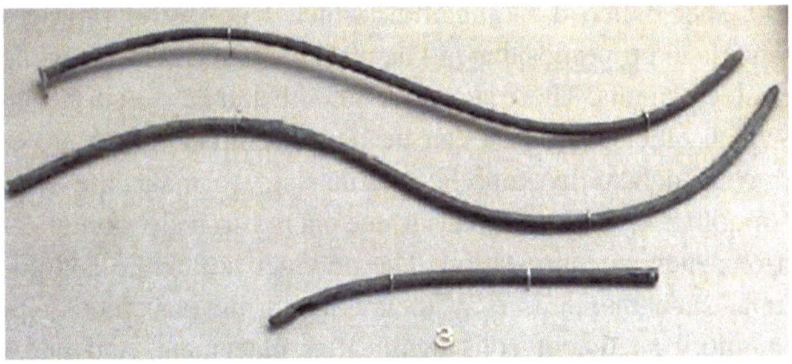

Fig. 60.5 Ancient lead catheters (Courtesy of British Museum)

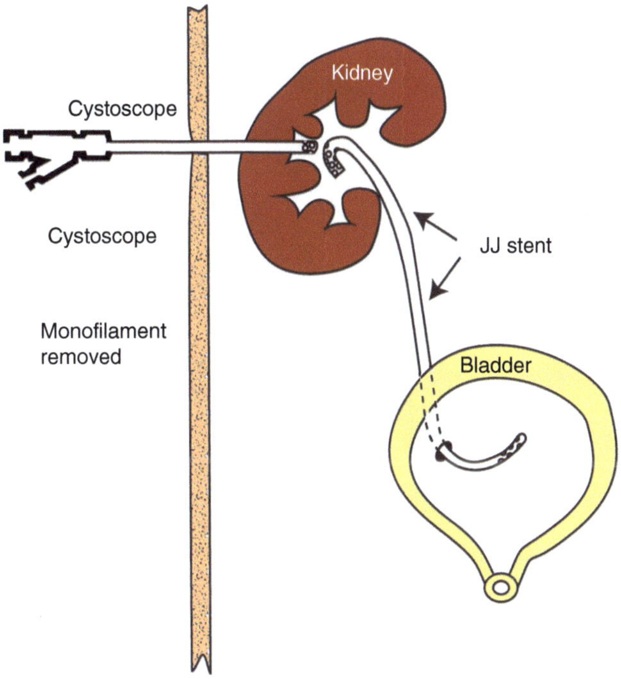

Fig. 60.6 Description of placing the Finney JJ stent (Adapted [7])

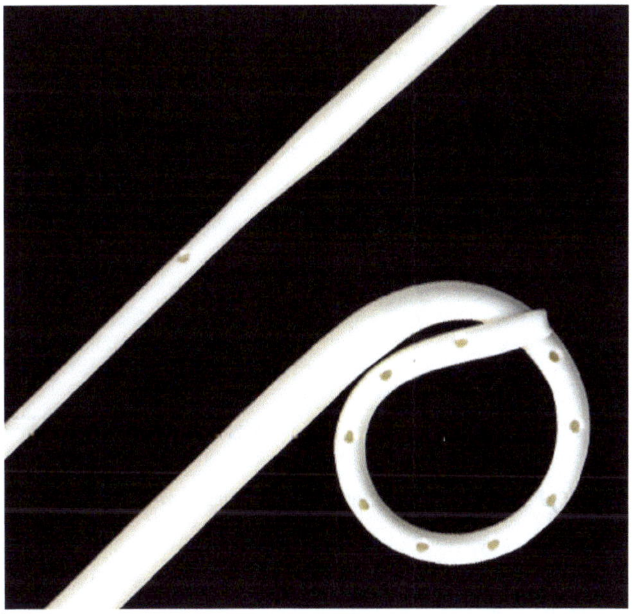

Fig. 60.7 Endopyelotomy stent. Note the change in diameter to allow a widened ureteric caliber during healing

thus losing their function. The modern stent derives its shape and characteristics from strategies developed to overcome movement. Gibbons et al. [5] devised a catheter with molded barbs, which reduced the rate of expulsion. The barbs increased the external diameter, making placement tricky, as did later attempts to address this problem, using a distal flange.

Hepperlen and Mardis [6] described the first design with a curled or "J" tip in 1978. This device had a curl at the top end that was placed into the kidney, but no provision was made to prevent proximal movement of the device.

Finney [7] described the first "double-J" stent in 1978 (Fig. 60.6). It had a constant diameter and, being hollow, could be mounted on a wire, straightening the curl at the leading end to facilitate placement, and placed via a cystoscope. The stent thus created was used primarily to bypass

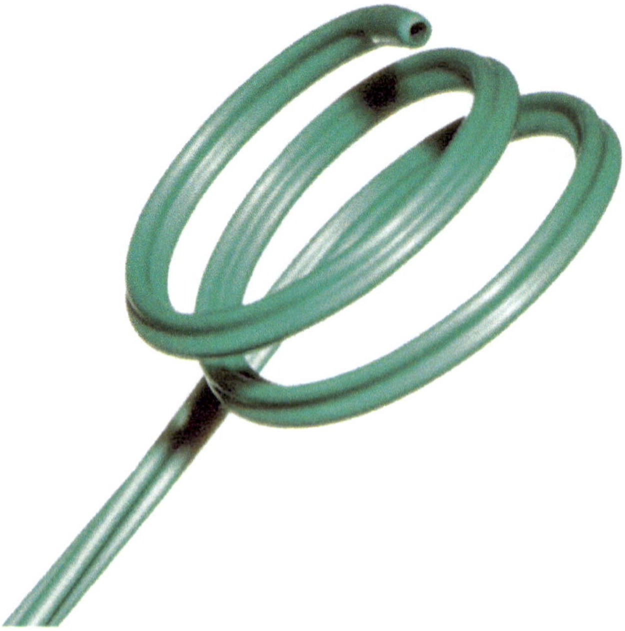

Fig. 60.8 Grooved tower stent

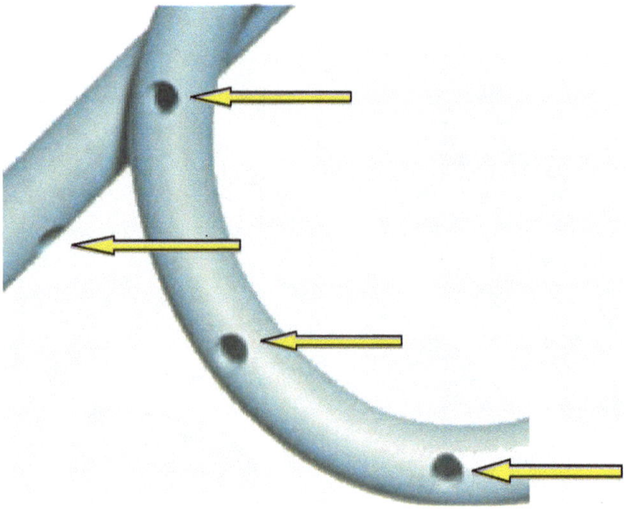

Fig. 60.9 Close up of stent showing side holes (*arrows*)

malignant obstruction, but over time, its use has expanded to protective and other treatment roles.

Each step in the design process has modified the stent to a more "ideal" state. The ideal appliance will give benefits both to the surgeon placing it and the patient, in whom it is being placed. For the surgeon, the stent needs to be easy to handle, easy to place, easy to remove, but not migratory while in place. From the patient's perspective, the stent must be comfortable, with as few side effects as possible. It needs ideally to be placed and removed or replaced with the minimum of time and effort.

To that end the modern double-J stent is hollow, usually of constant diameter (Fig. 60.7), made of a polymer, with or without a coating, and with or without holes along its length possibly to facilitate drainage. The stent is also radiopaque to facilitate its positioning by fluoroscopy.

Stent designers have tried other strategies for anchoring the device in place. Single and multicoil devices have been used. As one might expect, single coil stents tended to migrate more, and there are reports of multicoil stents knotting, requiring percutaneous removal. Stent variations abound, including the use of grooves (Fig. 60.8) and helical screws.

Side holes are a regular feature of stents (Fig. 60.9), although their original purpose is difficult to ascertain. Certainly some researchers feel that they have a detrimental effect on peristaltic function, and some do not use them in their design at all. This assertion has been questioned in animal studies that show the main determinant on reducing peristaltic function is stent diameter. There is, however, some evidence that the presence of side holes may be useful. In one study, a stent containing no holes, the Tower stent, was compared to other stents with side holes. The holeless stent performed badly with regard to drainage properties.

The usefulness of the stent as a hollow tube has been described previously. However, it does not necessarily mean it is the best shape from a consideration of fluid dynamics. Little work has been done on the flow dynamics of the ureter containing a solid stent. There are, however, some devices that used a solid portion of stent for part of their length. However, the inability to use a guidewire for its placement has meant that it has not found favor with most surgeons.

Materials Used in Ureteric Stents

The modern ureteric stent is usually made of a synthetic polymer called a biomaterial, which has several physicochemical properties that aid its placement and comfort while inside patients. These stents are smooth and have a surface to which other chemicals can be bonded, either to aid placement, such as hydrophilic coatings, or to make the stent smoother or have a lower surface energy to resist complications such as encrustation. The polymer is flexible and pliable such that it is easy to uncoil during placement, has memory so that it coils again after placement, and has a degree of elasticity so that it resists fracturing of continued patient movement and during removal.

However, polymers are not the only material used to make stents. The Memokath stent is a metallic coil made of a nickel titanium alloy (nitinol) and has a wide lumen that resists compression. It can be used when ureters are compressed by external malignant tumors or in benign strictures. This material has specific memory properties such that it exists in two states based on the temperature of fluid passing over it. This allows the surgeon to place the stents and pass warm saline to expand the proximal end of the stent to keep the stent in place. The Memokath stents have no proximal or distal coils and do not usually cause stent symptoms. They are ideal for

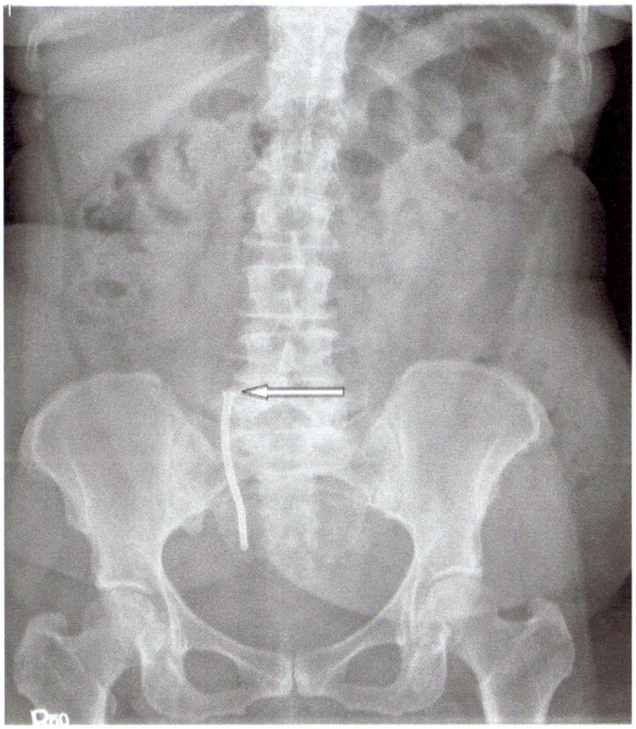

Fig. 60.10 A Memokath stent in situ. Note the expanded upper end holding it in place (*arrow*)

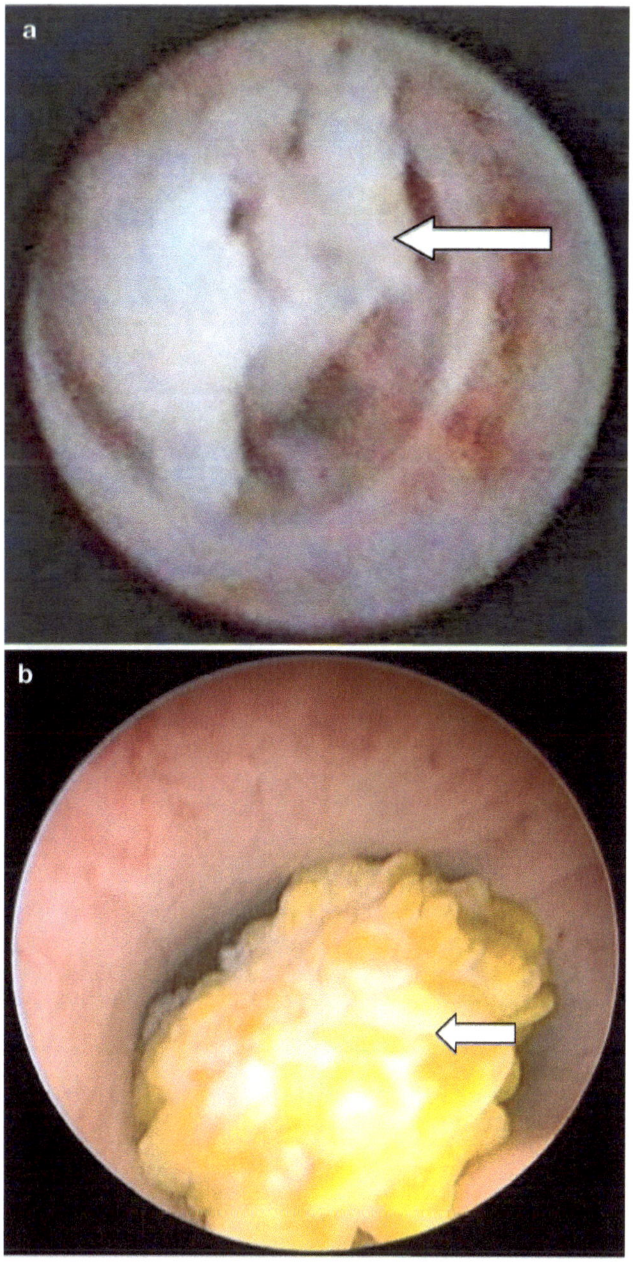

Fig. 60.11 (**a**) Endoscopic view of a ureteric tumor (*arrow*). (**b**) Endoscopic view of a ureteric stone (*arrow*)

malignant compression and can usually last for 1–2 years or longer (Fig. 60.10). If used in benign cases, regular 6-month checks are required to ensure the stent remains in a good position and no blockage has occurred.

Other metallic devices are available and also made of nitinol that do not change shape at different temperatures. These devices are designed for longer term use. They do not rust or corrode, and tend to resist encrustation well, so are suited for long-term use. They tend to be uncomfortable, however; are more expensive; and are more difficult to place.

Conditions Suited to Ureteric Stent Insertion

The ureteric stent is used for three main purposes:

1. The relief of renal obstruction
2. To facilitate later passage of endoscopic equipment to the upper urinary tract in an unsafe ureter
3. To allow safe healing in a damaged ureter, either accidentally or deliberately

The Relief of Renal Obstruction

An obstructed kidney will cease to function as a filtering and detoxification unit within hours of an obstruction happening. Long-term obstruction may end in the destruction of the renal unit involved, and short-term obstruction associated with infection may become rapidly fatal.

Relief of such obstruction therefore is important in all but the most transient of causes. This may be best done by percutaneous drainage of the kidney (nephrostomy, antegrade stenting) or via a transurethral method (retrograde stenting). One must not overlook the lower tract as a cause of dilatation; an obstructing prostate or a failing bladder may lead to renal obstruction, which is best treated with a catheter. Also, kidneys may be dilated without obstruction, and as such in a situation of doubt, isotopic renography may be helpful.

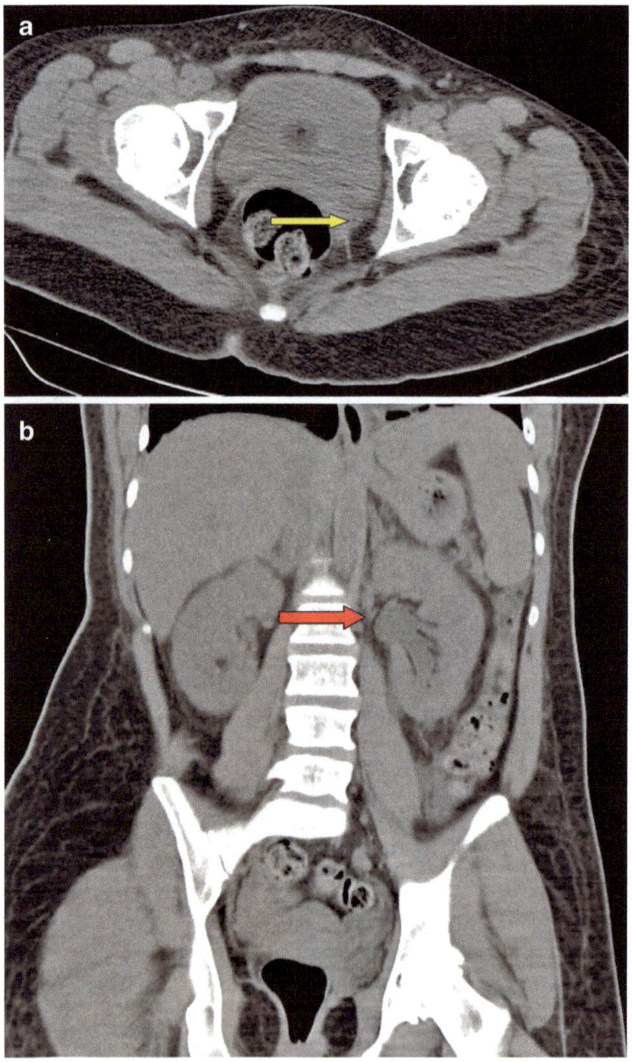

Fig. 60.12 Plain CT KUB showing (**a**) sloughed renal papilla (*yellow arrow*) leading to (**b**) pyonephrosis (*red arrow*)

Renal obstruction may be intraluminal, luminal, or extra-luminal:

1. Intraluminal
   (a) Stone (Fig. 60.11a, b)
   (b) Sloughed renal papilla (Fig. 60.12a, b)
   (c) Papillary transitional cell carcinoma (TCC) (Fig. 60.13)
2. Luminal
   (a) Stricture
   (b) Annular TCC
   (c) Pelviureteric junction (PUJ) obstruction (Fig. 60.14)
3. Extra-luminal
   (a) Tumor
   (b) Iatrogenic (clip or a stitch)
   (c) Procidentia, causing fish-hooking of the ureters

The commonest of these is the obstructing stone; one in ten men in the UK will develop a stone over their lifetimes, and these may be excruciatingly painful. Placement of a stent may aid pain relief and allow effective treatment of a stone at a later date while preserving renal function in the meantime.

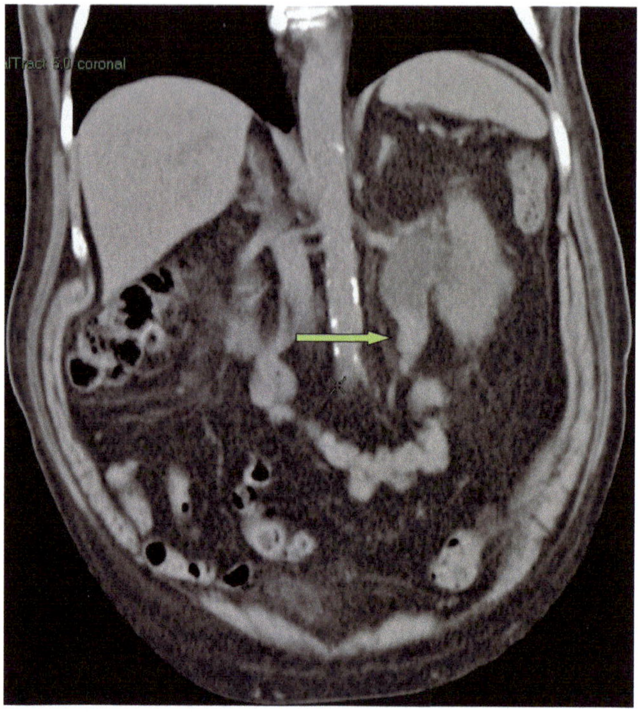

Fig. 60.13 Ureteric tumor (*green arrow*) causing obstruction of the left kidney on CT KUB

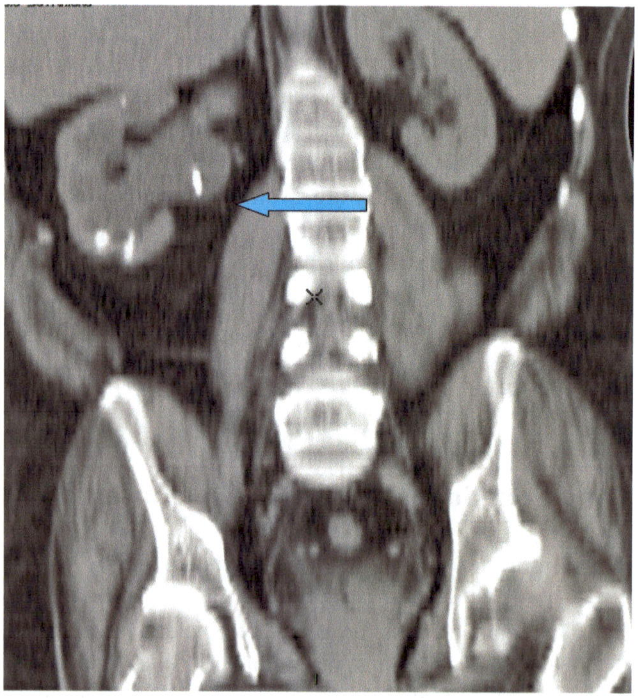

Fig. 60.14 PUJ obstruction (*blue arrow*) leading to renal obstruction and stone formation

To Facilitate Later Passage of Endoscopic Equipment to the Upper Urinary Tract in an Unsafe Ureter

Many centers especially treating stone disease find that patients will often need obstruction relieving in an acute setting, often in the late evening or middle of the night. It may be that specialist equipment or expertise is not available at this time or that it is simply not possible to treat the obstruction in one go. A stone may often have developed a significant tissue reaction, leading to a friable edematous ureter below it that bleeds easily. In these cases, a ureter may be "rested" for a number of weeks with a stent prior to a second look, which is often a technically easier exercise.

To Allow Safe Healing in a Damaged or Operated Ureter

Injured tubular structure tends to heal with scarring, and as this contracts, strictures may form. Repairing a ureter over a stent allows a more patent ureter as the stent acts like a scaffold, holding the ureter open as it heals. Ureteric and renal surgeons will often leave a stent after endoscopic surgery to allow easy passage of debris, and promote patent healing of the ureter.

Placing a Ureteric Stent

Basic Technique

Placing a ureteric stent can take a few minutes to perform. Likewise, it can also take several hours in a difficult ureter with an impacted stone, poor visibility, and a challenging lower tract. The key message is to assume the worst. There is no such situation as "just a ureteric stent"!

Two main methods will be discussed: placing a stent via a cystoscope and freehand stenting.

Cystoscopic Stenting Method

1. In a correctly prepared, consented, and draped patient in extended lithotomy position, introduce a cystoscope into the bladder (Fig. 60.15). Find the appropriate ureteric orifice (UO). The authors prefer to have both live fluoroscopy available and the most recent static images available in theater to check the appropriate side.
2. Cannulate the UO using the floppy tip of a guidewire (Fig. 60.16). It must be remembered that the wire will tend to exit the scope in a slight downward direction and the scope may need to be turned 90° away from the UO to facilitate passage. If the wire exits the scope unkindly so that it cannot be seen, pull the scope back to the bladder neck and reposition the wire. Occasionally taking the scope partly apart may help. If the wire does not sit in a comfortable viewing position, pass a ureteric catheter over the top to leave a few millimeters of the wire showing. The ureteric catheter will stiffen the wire allowing a better viewing position. It may also be used for retrograde pyelography if desired.
3. Run the guidewire up to the renal pelvis using image intensification. It is the authors' contention that placing the wire under continuous X-ray screening holds no benefit over static pictures and increases the radiological load to the patient. Inexperienced operators will often obtain a "road map" by obtaining a retrograde pyelogram first (Fig. 60.17). More experienced operators tend to use a mixture of tactile feedback from placing the guidewire, pattern recognition as to where the top of the wire is coiling, and judicious use of contrast when the wire or ureter are not behaving in the appropriate way or difficulty is encountered.
4. Slide the stent over the wire into the ureter, over the guidewire, through the cystoscope. Several maneuvers facilitate this. Ask an assistant to help slide the stent over the wire and then ask them to fix their end of the guidewire at a point, such as the patient's leg, so that it does not move as the stent moves. Many stents have one crosscut end and one tapered end. Make sure that the stent is introduced tapered end first into the cystoscope. Hold the scope close to the UO and watch it enter. It will usually go only slightly into the ureter as most of its length will lie within the scope (Fig. 60.18a, b). The authors will perform two exercises prior to inserting the stent: they remove the attached thread from the stent (which is used to remove the stent under local anesthetic in certain conditions) and will note the last mark on the stent before the lower pigtail to be placed.

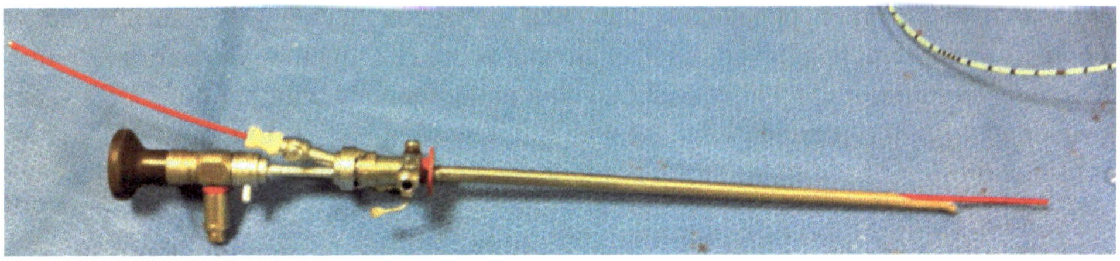

Fig. 60.15 Pusher through a cystoscope. This will allow the surgeon to thread the guidewire through the scope if it has been left at the end of a procedure for stent insertion

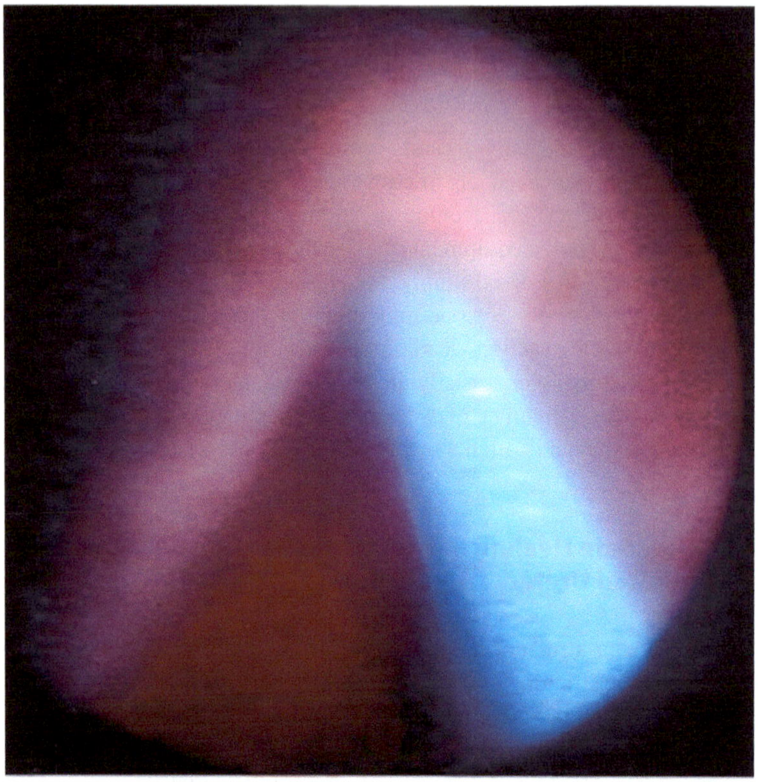

Fig. 60.16 Cannulation of the right ureteric orifice (UO) with a PTFE-coated guidewire

5. Slide the pusher over the guidewire. The wire should be fixed as in point 4 above. The authors tend to keep close to the UO until the noted mark is seen and then use X-ray to check the top end of the stent. Sometimes withdrawing the guidewire partially back facilitates the curling of the stent in the renal pelvis. With the top end of the stent correctly placed, the cystoscope is withdrawn to the bladder neck and the pusher gently advanced until its tip is seen (Fig. 60.19a, b). The guidewire is withdrawn until the stent can be seen to curl in the bladder.

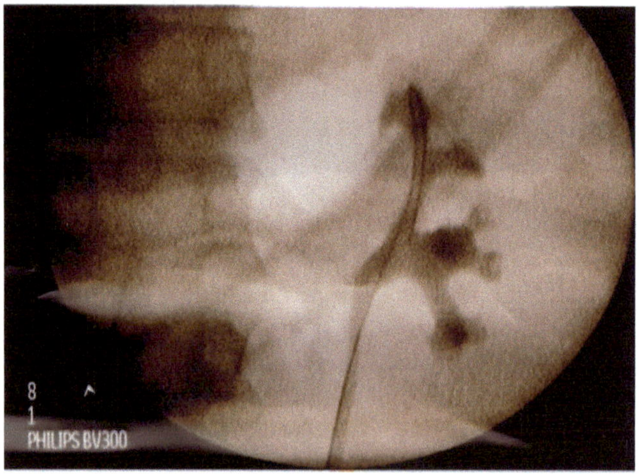

Fig. 60.17 Guidewire within the upper pole and renal pelvis on single shot X-ray. Retrograde study used to demonstrate anatomy

Freehand Stent Placement Method

This is a more advanced technique and the authors would recommend being comfortable with the cystoscopic method before attempting a freehand stent placement (Fig. 60.20). We will usually place a stent through a cystoscope if we happen to be in this position when the stent needs to be placed or in a very difficult ureter with one precious wire that must not lose its position.

With a wire correctly placed into the renal pelvis on fluoroscopy, the stent is slid over the top of the wire as before. The authors prefer to use a stent pusher with a radiopaque marker at its tip. It is paramount that the wire is fixed so that it cannot move with the stent. This tends to leave a coil of wire in the bladder that will stop the stent entering the UO or even the wire to fall out.

The stent is then positioned within the renal pelvis via the pusher, and the wire withdrawn into the upper ureter under fluoroscopy to assess correct coiling. The image intensifier is then placed over the bladder so that the pubic symphysis is seen, along with the bladder. The guidewire is then withdrawn under live screening until it can be seen within the bony pelvis, and the lower portion of the stent starts to move from a predominantly vertical lie to a more horizontal one. At this point, as the wire is withdrawn further, the pusher is pushed further into the bladder, tenting the stent up above the symphysis. It then springs off the

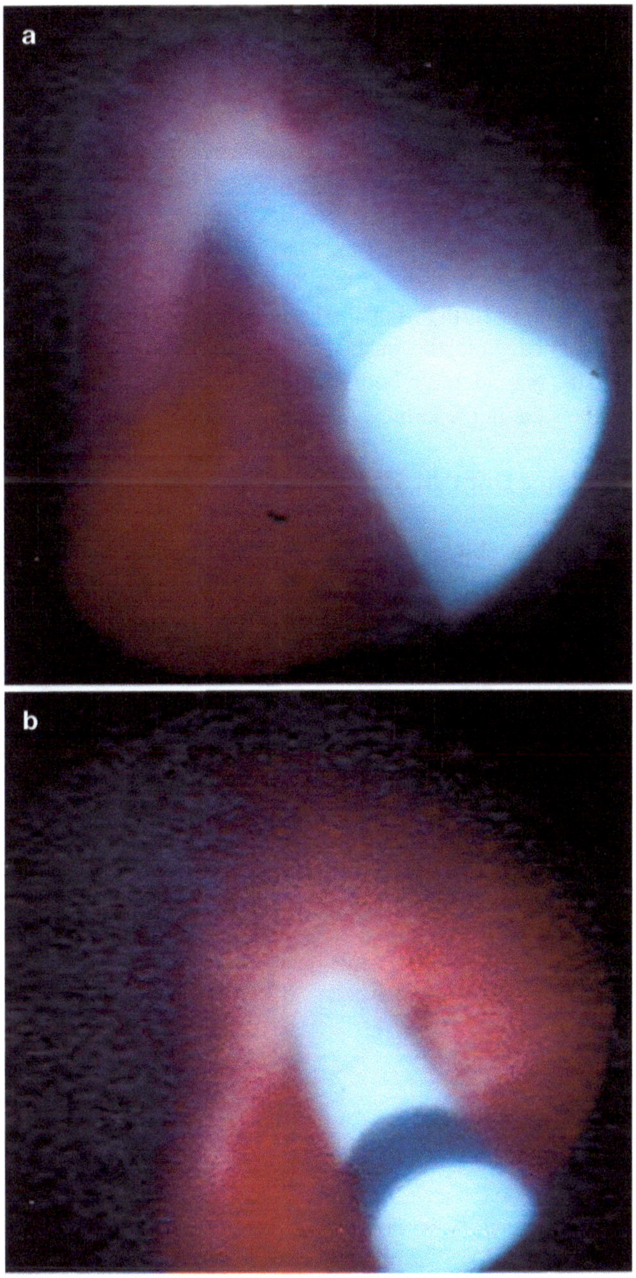

Fig. 60.18 (**a**) Stent seen sliding over guidewire toward OU and (**b**) then partially within the UO. Note the black distance marker

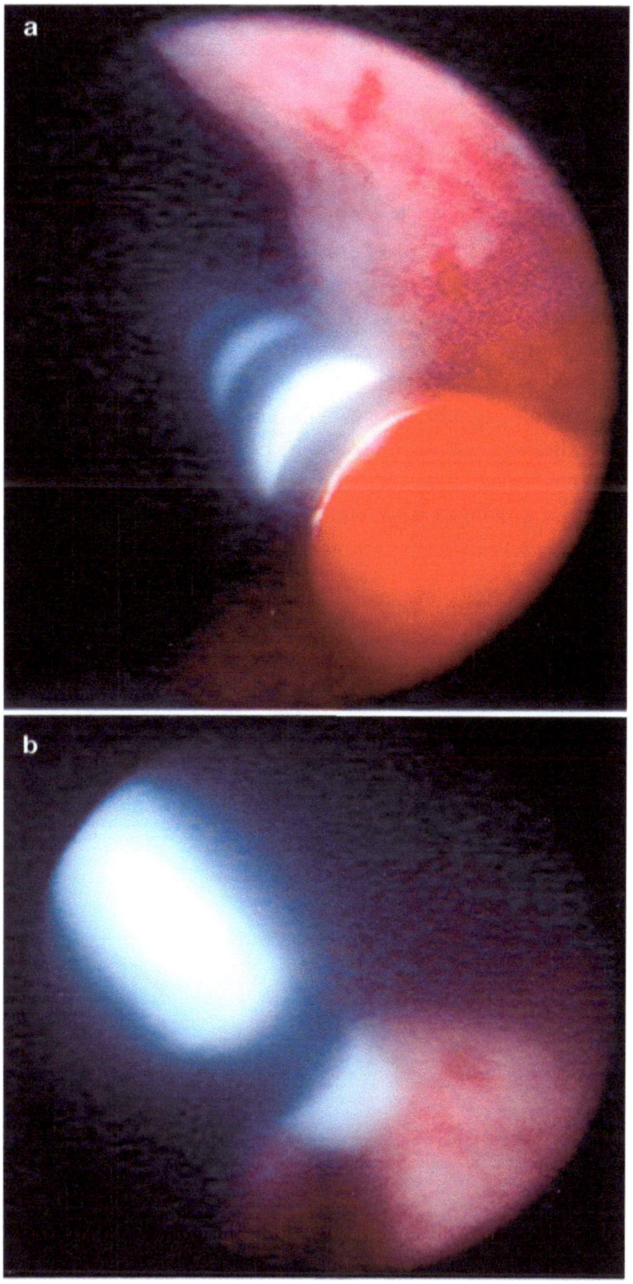

Fig. 60.19 (**a**) Pusher seen at end of stent over guide wire and (**b**) after withdrawal of pusher and wire

pusher as the wire is fully withdrawn, leaving the lower curl visible on fluoroscopy.

Antegrade Stent Placement

This may be performed by a radiologist but is a useful technique to be able to perform, especially for surgeons undertaking percutaneous nephrolithotomy. With a renal puncture performed, and a guidewire placed such that a large proportion sits coiled in the bladder, the stent is placed in an antegrade fashion so that the lower end crosses the midline on fluoroscopy. The wire is withdrawn with a holding pusher on the antegrade end of the stent to stop it from being pulled back out. Position is confirmed via fluoroscopy.

Troubleshooting

Several key factors may make an easy stent placement difficult. There are also several useful points that may make a difficult stent insertion easier.

Keeping an Easy Stent Insertion Easy

Several important points will aid in the insertion of a ureteric stent and promote success:

1. Keep the wire straight—wires coiled in the bladder will not accept a stent. It is best to check position using image intensification and pull back on the wire until it is straight and begin again rather than struggle with a curled wire.
2. Discard a bent wire—if you force a wire and it bends, it is better to begin again or perform a guidewire exchange (see later) than struggle on (Fig. 60.21). Wires work by transmitting the forward force applied at their base in a straight line, and this advantage is lost in a bent wire. Also, it is difficult to pass a bent wire through a cystoscope and very difficult to pass a stent over the bent portion of a wire.
3. Keep the wire fixed—if the wire is held such that it cannot move as the stent, pusher, or ureteric catheter is advanced, the overlying tube will move into position. If the wire is allowed to move, it has the opportunity to move sideways, resulting in coiling.
4. Use X-ray to check position—Think of X-ray as a car rearview mirror. This is used to check that what one has done is correct or if a difficulty has occurred.
5. Check the end marker before the stent is inserted and stay close to the UO—this will allow the operator confidence to insert the stent until the mark is reached.
6. If the stent is in the kidney and it is difficult to push the pusher in further, but the endpoint marker has not been reached, hold the pusher and withdraw the wire 5 cm. This may increase both the room for and the pliability of the stent in the kidney, making it easier to insert.

Making a Difficult Stent Insertion Easier

1. Assume difficulty—it is far better to enter a stent insertion expecting the worst. Keep to basic principles, be

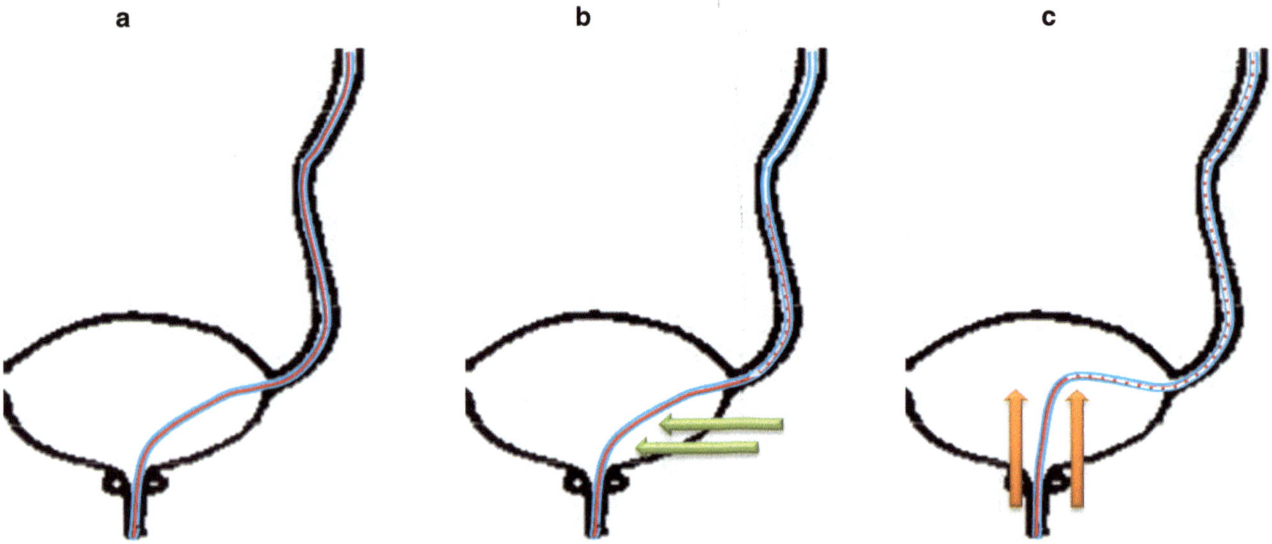

Fig. 60.20 Diagram showing the steps involved in hand stenting. (**a**) The stent (*blue*) contains the guidewire (*red*). As the wire is screened down the lower ureter, the stent moves from a relatively vertical to a more horizontal position (*green arrows*) (**b**). (**c**) At the same time the pusher pushes the stent into the bladder (*orange arrows*), and the wire is withdrawn further until the stent coils as normal within the bladder

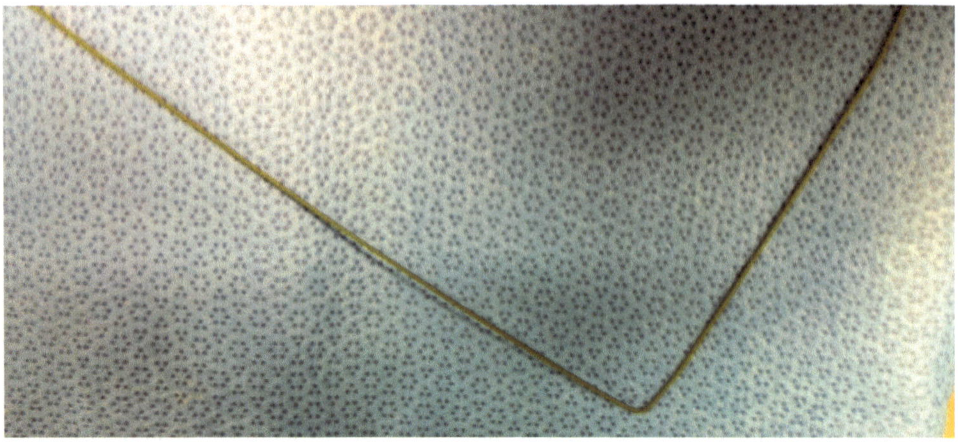

Fig. 60.21 A bent guidewire. Throw it away

aware of complications, and be prepared to stop and consider alternatives such as a nephrostomy.

2. The wire will not go up the ureter—there are a number of reasons this may happen:
   (a) Something (i.e., the stone) is in the way.
   (b) The ureter is tortuous and dilated.
   (c) The wire is bent or coiled (see previous).

In the first two situations, it is worth the operator being wary. It is very easy to lose a precious wire that is partway placed or push a wire either through a suburothelial tunnel in the ureter or outside the ureter and make a difficult situation much worse.

The first maneuver to try is to use a hydrophilic floppy wire. These must be made wet before use and are difficult to handle. In placing them through a cystoscope, it is often useful to grasp them with a gauze swab. It is extremely easy to lose position with them or for them to fall out. Judicious use of fluoroscopy aids in checking position. The authors feel that it is unwise to place a stent over one of these wires, and as such, when correct position has been obtained, the wire should be exchanged with a standard guidewire. This can be achieved by passing a ureteric catheter over the top of the hydrophilic wire, removing the wire and placing a standard wire, or using a dual lumen catheter, preloaded with the standard wire.

In tortuous and dilated systems, a hydrophilic wire again may be helpful. Generally two factors help stent placement: having as much wire beyond a problem point so that it will not slip out and rotating the wire so that the ureter straightens. Occasionally, live screening may help this maneuver. It cannot be emphasized enough that a straight wire will always allow an easier stent insertion than a curved one. If the wire will not straighten, introduce a ureteric catheter over the top of the wire to stiffen it and keep it straight. This allows more accurate work at points of difficulty. If this is unhelpful, it may be necessary to pass a ureteroscope.

With a difficult obstruction, such as impacted stone, it may be useful if a hydrophilic wire will not pass, to look under direct vision using a small ureteroscope. While the authors will often manage a ureteric stone with a primary ureteroscopy, it is not often possible in all cases, especially if infection is suspected or present. Nevertheless, if a stent will not pass an obstruction, it is better to introduce a small ureteroscope and visually try to pass a wire past the obstruction using fluoroscopy to confirm position. If a wire has been passed out of the ureter or into a suburothelial tunnel, leave it in place and return with a ureteroscope and a fresh wire and try in a different position. The first wire will occlude the hole made and reduce extravasation. Extreme care needs to be taken in ureteroscopic techniques; the ureter may be extremely friable and may avulse very easily. If all techniques fail, it is by far safer to pull out and insert a nephrostomy, with subsequent antegrade stent insertion than to pursue a difficult and worsening situation in a retrograde fashion.

The Lost Stent

It is very possible, especially by an inexperienced freehand stent inserter to lose the stent into the lower ureter. In this situation, a ureteroscope should be passed into the lower ureter and ureteroscopic graspers or baskets used to manipulate the stent back into the bladder. If this fails, a percutaneous antegrade approach may be needed first to temporize the situation and to subsequently remove the stent.

Encrustation

Basic Concepts

Encrustation is a multifactorial process that occurs on a great many surfaces. Its effects are significant not only for medicine in general, and for urology in particular, but also in the fermentation industry, in gas turbines, and in many other industrial processes. In the medical sphere, encrustation or sludging can happen in respect to other stents, such as those used in coronary arteries and the biliary tree, and may also affect other implants, such as orthopedic prostheses, intraocular implants, and ventricular shunts. Encrustation often necessitates changing or altering the device in some way, involving operations or further procedures for the patient, which have attendant risks of mortality and morbidity.

Dental plaque is a common form of crusting that is thought to be deposited in a similar way to urological encrustation. Both processes involve the position of a basic conditioning film, which may or may not be followed by bacterial events, but eventually salts and other compounds are deposited on the surface forming a crust. In dentistry such a crust is called plaque and is removed by brushing or by a visit to a dental practitioner. In urological practice, encrustation may affect any device that lies in contact with urine, i.e., at least in part above the bladder outflow sphincter, and this usually necessitates removing the device and replacing it with a new one.

Bacterial Biofilm and Its Role in Encrustation

Overview

There is much debate in microbiological, industrial, medical, and surface science circles as to the contribution that bacteria give to encrustation. It is certainly true that bacteria are not essential to cause encrustation on a ureteric stent. However, most, if not all, stents had associated bacteria on the surface after removal. These bacteria are not in the standard "planktonic" or free form. They have properties that would promote encrustation, such as causing changes of pH to their microenvironment and their ability to secrete extracellular polymeric substances.

The association between urinary infection and stone formation was first recognized by Horton Smith in 1897 [8] and Brown in 1901 [9]. However at this time, the pathogenesis of stone formation and calculus structure was not understood, and the role of urease-producing organisms was also not appreciated.

Putative Steps in Biofilm Formation and Encrustation

A number of steps have been proposed:

1. Absorption of proteins and other urinary constituents onto the device surface to form a conditioning film due to interaction between electrostatic forces of these urinary constituents and the device itself.
2. Weak attachment of planktonic bacteria to the device surface by a similar process of electrostatic attraction. This process is promoted by the presence of the conditioning film.
3. Genetic upregulation in the bacteria leading to ultrastructural changes.
4. Strong attachment of the bacteria to the device.
5. Production of extracellular polymeric substances (EPS).
6. Bacteria-community interactions, communication, and turnover, as explained later. This includes production of enzymes such as urease.
7. Splitting of urea by urease causing an increased local pH, leading to salting out of calcium and magnesium salts from solution. These salts are then deposited onto the device surface as a layer of encrustation.

Bacterial Activity and Its Role in Encrustation

The bacterial composition associated with ureteric stents is usually a monoculture; this will usually take the form of *Proteus mirabilis*. *Proteus mirabilis* produces the enzyme urease that causes the hydrolysis of urea. The resultant reaction yields NH_4^+ and OH^- ions.

The urine pH rises and the newly generated NH_4^+ ions are available for the formation of struvite crystals. The alkaline environment also increases the formation of CO_3^{2-} ions from CO_2, which are available for calcium carbonate crystal formation. In addition, a high pH increases the formation of PO_4^{3-} and HPO_4^{2-}, which are able to generate calcium phosphate crystals. Urine is supersaturated with many of these ions, and the extra crystal load is readily deposited on the device surface.

Strategies to Combat Biofilm

Antibiotics are commonly given up to the time of surgical implantation. The evidence for their usefulness is, however, not convincing. In one study, 12,000 times the dose of gentamicin was required to kill the biofilm on a device in vitro compared to that required for free bacteria. This resistance is thought to be due to the conformational changes that occur during genetic upregulation. Changes in protein coats of the bacterial cell wall are thought to inhibit penetration and render standard antibiotic modalities ineffective.

There has been some effort to bind antibiotics onto devices. One major problem is that antibiotics bound to a device's surface tend to release their load rapidly so that only for a short time the effective concentration is reached. One of the aims of this thesis is to examine the timing of biofilm formation and to see whether antibiotics would have a role in preventing encrustation.

The next modality of prevention of device-related infection is the modification of biopolymers. Much work done in this area has been at the instigation of device manufacturers. Various chemical or physical modifications intended to change properties such as surface free energy charge and surface roughness have been devised, but none has yet been of clinical benefit. One of the major problems is that surfaces are coated by conditioning films rapidly and this tends to obliterate many modified surfaces.

Metal coatings, especially silver, have been used extensively. Results tend to be good in vitro but animal and clinical studies do not support the findings. Coatings including silver tend to have two main problems: the first is that the glycoproteins in the conditioning film tend to interact with the coating, and secondly, once in contact with urine, the metal ions are rapidly eluted. There is some evidence that impregnation of the polymer matrix with physicochemically compatible antimicrobials rather than layering them on the surface may yield promising results.

Health Economics of Urinary Encrustation

The most common devices placed within the urinary tract are urethral catheters and ureteric stents. It has been estimated that 28 % of all patients in chronic care facilities require indwelling urinary catheters. Fifty percent of patients with a long-term indwelling catheter suffer regular encrustation and catheter blockage. The great majority of patients with a catheter in situ are elderly and accounts for 4 % of the community nursing caseload. It is impossible to predict which patients will suffer from catheter blockage, and an individual patient may at some time experience catheter blockage and at other times will not.

Encrustation and catheter blockage can be extremely distressing and often lead to an episode in accident and emergency, which can be costly for the National Health System (NHS) and also very inconvenient to the patient. It has been estimated that the district nurse commitment to urethral catheters is about 500 h/month or 1,000 visits per year in a district with a total population of 500,000. Furthermore, changing a male urethral catheter requires a skill that requires training and is not necessarily a prerequisite for district nursing.

Catheter Blockage Symptoms

When a catheter blocks, it ceases to function as a drainage device (Fig. 60.22). The bladder will fill to a maximum amount, causing pain. As the bladder reaches its elastic limit, and as encrustation irritates the bladder wall, strong, often painful, bladder contractions force urine around the sides of the catheter. This is known as bypassing and leaves the patient wet and uncomfortable.

As the encrustation rubs on the bladder wall, it may also cause bleeding. Symptoms are often considered to be caused by infection, but this is not always the case. Bacteria associated with the device surface, a biofilm, are not necessarily susceptible to antibiotics and do not cause a conventional cystitis. Device removal and placement of a new catheter is the best form of treatment. Another problem is that a piece of encrustation may fall off into the bladder and become a nidus for bladder stone formation.

On occasions, patients may need hospitalization, with its attendant risks of morbidity and mortality. Changing the catheter increases the risk of infection and septicemia, due to trauma and introduction of urinary pathogens into the bloodstream.

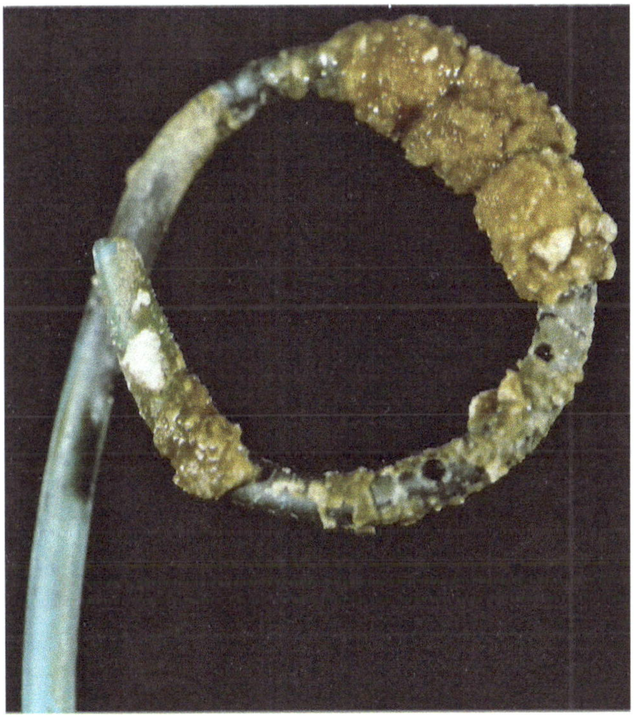

Fig. 60.22 An encrusted and blocked catheter

Ureteric Stents

Ureteric stents suffer from similar problems. While many stents are placed for the short term, severe encrustation and stone formation has been reported, but there are instances of neglected stents that have not encrusted. It is impossible to predict who will have problems with encrustation and who will not. However, encrustation will limit the useful lifespan of a ureteric stent. At present, all stents are licensed for a maximum of 6 months within a patient, but some devices may soon gain licenses for a year. The important point is that a stent that can be left in a patient for a longer time reduces the number of replacement sessions, thus lowering morbidity and mortality associated with operative events, as well as reducing bed usage and hospital time.

It has been estimated that an improved urological device, able to remain within the body for 12 months rather than 6, by reducing encrustation and urinary tract infection, would save approximately €1 billion annually in health care spending in the European Union and a similar amount in North America. It remains clear that finding a solution to this problem is important.

The Lost or Neglected Stent

Stents can become, from time to time, lost (Fig. 60.23). Various methods have been employed to avoid this difficult situation, but all methods (stent registers, email alerts, on the day booking of removal, etc.) have their limitations. Some patients default follow-up for various reasons, and

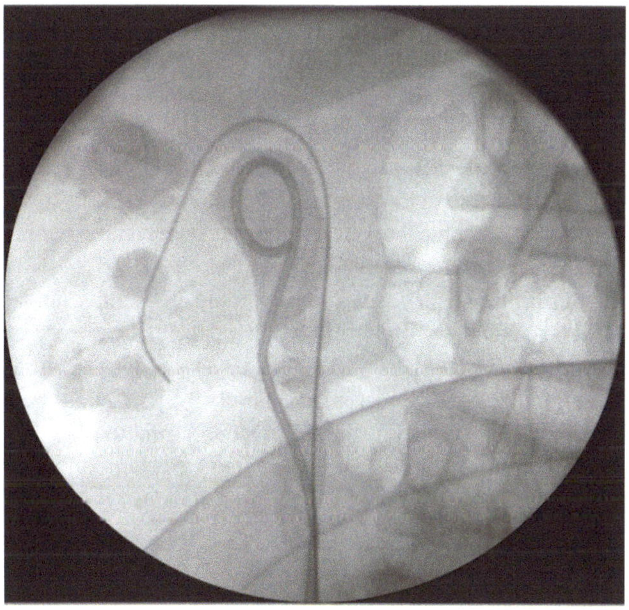

Fig. 60.23 Intraoperative pictures showing the upper coil and associated encrustation on a stent lost for 2 years

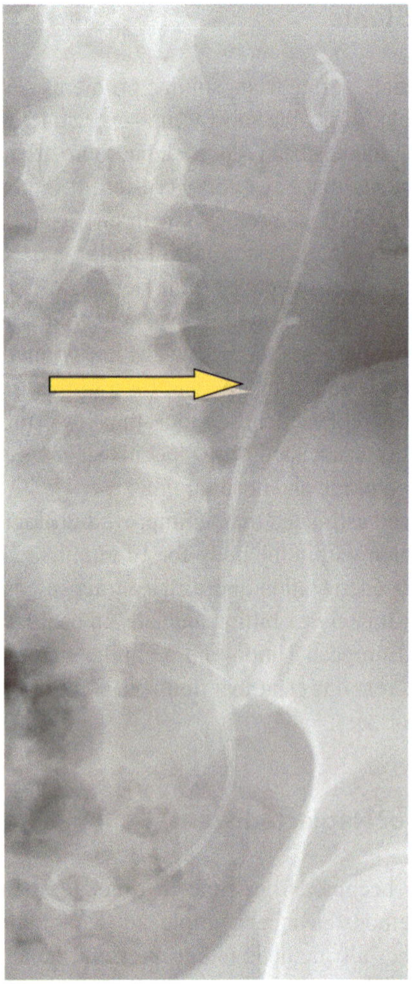

Fig. 60.24 Close up of a system containing a ureteric stent and a broken portion of a stent (*orange arrow*)

booking follow-up can be missed. Four scenarios can be encountered:

1. The pristine stent—this is rare and should be treated with suspicion. Stents immersed in urine for long periods of time become brittle (see scenario 2), and encrustation may not be so evident on a plain radiograph. Such stents should be screened out in theater under fluoroscopic guidance.
2. The brittle stent—again, these should be remove under live screening, with a full complement of ureteroscopes, wires, and baskets available if the stent fractures (Fig. 60.24). All pieces of a broken stent should be removed as they form a nidus of stone formation.
3. The encrusted stent—encrusted stents may uncoil when screened out, but may well not. The standard practice is to attempt to pass a ureteroscope alongside the stent and remove encrustation using a laser or a lithoclast. If this fails, percutaneous treatment is needed. Careful consideration is needed to decide on replacing the stent.

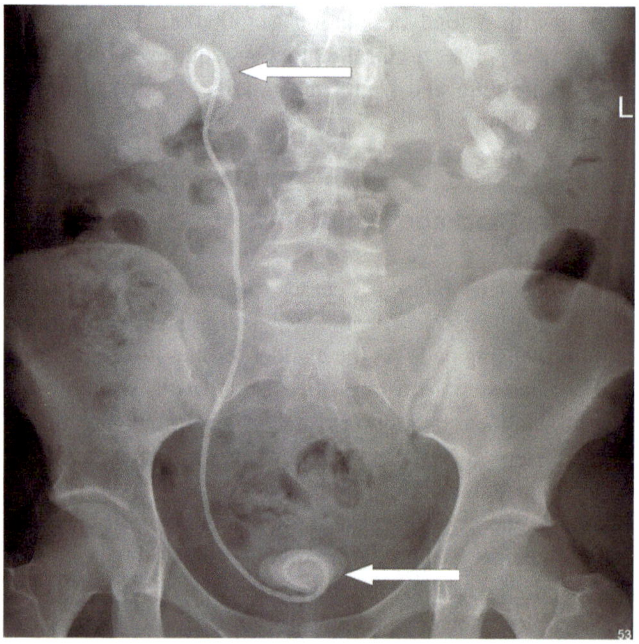

Fig. 60.25 Plain KUB demonstrating bilateral stones and a neglected stent with significant encrustation affecting the upper and lower coils (*arrows*)

4. The heavily encrusted stent—these are often too difficult to be treated in a retrograde pattern and need percutaneous management (Fig. 60.25).

Knotted Stents

Stents can catch their upper coil within itself (Fig. 60.26), and this may stop the stent from being removed. If a wire can be passed through the middle of the stent, then this will uncurl it and the stent can be screened out. If this is not possible, the authors tend to pass a ureteroscope to help uncurl the stent. By pinning the end of the stent, it may be possible to allow it to unravel. If this fails, percutaneous management is needed.

Conclusion

The Ideal Ureteric Stent

The ideal stent has not yet been discovered, but we have a fair idea of what it should be like. It should be easy to place, should be comfortable for the patient, can be inserted or replaced using the minimum of anesthesia and analgesia, can resist encrustation and loss of elasticity, and should allow excellent flow in an antegrade fashion, while resisting flow in a retrograde fashion. We are not there yet, but advances continue to be made toward this ideal.

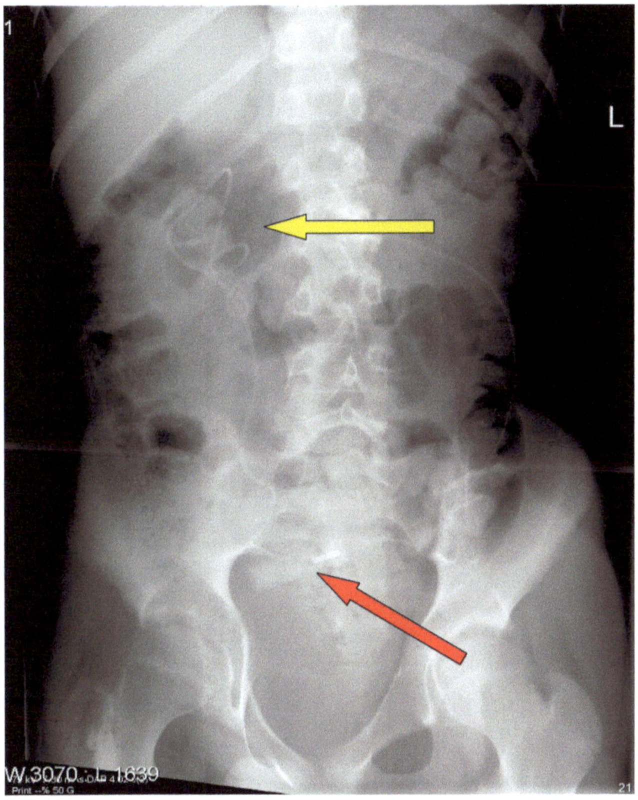

Fig. 60.26 A knotted stent. Note the large amount of coil in the kidney (*yellow arrow*) and the lower end has retracted into the ureter (*red arrow*)

References

1. Lewis B. History of urology, vol. 1. Baltimore: Williams and Wilkins; 1988. p. 70–5.
2. Nietze M. Lehrbuch de kystosskopie: Ihre lechnik und klinische bedeutung. Berlin: JE Bergman; 1907.
3. Tulloch RB. Restoration of the continuity of the ureter by means of polythene tubing. Br J Urol. 1952;24:42–5.
4. Zimskind PD, Fetter TR, Wilkerson JL. Clinical use of long term indwelling silicone rubber ureteral splints injected cystoscopically. J Urol. 1967;97:840–4.
5. Gibbons RP, Mason JT, Correwa RJ. Experience with indwelling rubber silicone ureteral catheters. J Urol. 1974;111:594.
6. Hepperlen TK, Mardis HK. Pigtail stent, termed means of ureteral surgery. Trends Clin Urol. 1978;1:405.
7. Finney RP. Experience with a new "double J" ureteral catheter stent. J Urol. 1978;120:678–81.
8. Horton-Smith P. On bacillus *Proteus* urinae: A new variety of the *Proteus* group, discovered in the urine of a patient suffering from cystitis. J Pathol. 1897;4:210–5.
9. Brown TR. On the relation between the variety of microorganisms and the composition of stone in calculous pyelonephritis. JAMA. 1901;36:1395–7.

Ureteric Stenting: Tips and Tricks

61

Syed Muhammad Nazim, Ali Akbar Zehri,
and Khurram Mutahir Siddiqui

Abstract

Ureteric stents are indispensable tools in urology, especially endourology. Technical difficulties can arise during their placement and removal. It is therefore important that stent procedures should not be regarded as "minor." This chapter describes the basic protocol for stent placement and describes some "tricks of the trade" to combat the technical difficulties. The tips, approaches, and instruments that are needed to deal with these problems are also described.

Keywords

Ureteric stent • Techniques • Tips • Difficulties • Endourology • Stent placement

Introduction

Ureteric stents are placed for various indications by both retrograde and antegrade approaches. The learning curve is not steep, and residents rapidly develop the expertise in stent placement. However, this seemingly easy "5-minute case" should not be considered a minor procedure, as it can result in significant frustration and anxiety [1]. This chapter is written with the intention of showing how to make the task easy and what to do in difficult situations.

S.M. Nazim, M.B.B.S., MCPS, MRCS (Glasgow), FCPS (Urology) (✉)
Section of Urology,
The Aga Khan University,
Stadium Road, Karachi, Sindh 74800, Pakistan
e-mail: Muhammad.nazim@aku.edu

A.A. Zehri, M.B.B.S., FCPS (Urology)
Section of Urology,
The Aga Khan Hospital, Dar Es Salaam,
Tanzania

K.M. Siddiqui, FCPS, FRCS (UK), FEBU
Department of Nursing, Section of Urology,
The Aga Khan University,
Stadium Road, Karachi, Sindh 74800, Pakistan
e-mail: khurram.siddiqui@aku.edu

J.J. Talati et al. (eds.), *Urolithiasis*,
DOI 10.1007/978-1-4471-4387-1_61,

The first step of retrograde placement is cystoscopy and localization of the ureteric orifice (UO). The UO is then cannulated with a guidewire or open-ended ureteric catheter that is then passed up to the kidney under fluoroscopy guidance. A retrograde pyelogram can be obtained, if necessary, by exchanging the guidewire with a 5-Fr ureteric catheter to outline the collecting system. The self-retaining stent can be inserted and pushed into the ureter under vision via a cystoscope sheath, or in case a guidewire is in place, using only fluoroscopy with a radiopaque stent pusher to guide its proper positioning in the kidney and bladder. Table 61.1 lists the protocol for routine stent placement.

Calculating the Length of Stent Required

Nowadays, multi-length ureteric stents are available and used in a majority of cases; however, calculation of appropriate length may be necessary if a fixed-length stent is to be placed. The appropriate stent length can be determined by three different methods:

1. For a patient's height <1.78 m, the appropriate stent length would be 22 cm; for patients 1.78–1.93 m tall, 24 cm; and for patients 1.93 m, 26 cm [2].

Table 61.1 Protocol for the routine stent placement

Radiolucent table
General/regional/sedo-analgesia
Dorsal lithotomy position
Flexible/rigid cystoscope
Image intensifier/fluoroscope
Guidewire of appropriate length and size
Ureteral catheter and radiopaque contrast media
Ureteric stent of appropriate length and size

2. Direct perioperative measurement (from renal pelvis to ureteric orifices) during open surgery using guidewire or open-ended ureteric catheter.
3. Measuring the distance from the ureteropelvic junction (UPJ) to ureteral-vesical junction (UVJ) (on intravenous urography [IVU] or retrograde pyelogram [RPG]) [2, 3].

Tips and Tricks

The most critical step in uneventful completion of the procedure is the cannulation of the ureteric orifice. Care must be taken to ensure a very gentle and atraumatic entry.

- If a false passage is created, a retrograde study can be obtained by gently instilling contrast under continuous fluoroscopy. Often, one is able to see the distal ureter; however, if resistance is encountered and only extravasation of contrast is seen, then it is best not to pursue any further.
- If the guidewire gets arrested in a false passage, a smaller caliber ureteroscope can be introduced as far as easily possible; while withdrawing the scope, use irrigation under pressure and have the guidewire ready, positioned in the channel. On withdrawing the scope, you can sometimes see the opening of the ureter and quickly cannulate it. Once access is gained, the procedure is completed as per plan, and an indwelling stent is placed.
- If the stent is not sliding over the guidewire, the beak of the cystoscope should be kept close to ureteric orifices with the ureteric orifice at the bull's eye. This allows more efficient transfer of force.
- If it is still not sliding into the ureter, then use a smaller caliber stent.
- The guidewire should be held tight by the assistant to avoid looping in the bladder, and the bladder should not be overdistended (Fig. 61.1a, b).
- Sometimes the ureteric orifice is located at a difficult location. Use of an Albarran lever attached to the cystoscope channel may be useful to direct the guidewire/ureteral catheter.
- A narrowed/stenotic ureteric orifice can be managed by balloon dilatation or graduated metallic dilators.
- When a guidewire or stent cannot get pass a Steinstrasse or stone impacted in the distal ureter, a ureteroscope can be used to fragment or dis-impact the stone, or flush it with saline (introduced through its irrigation channel). The guidewire can then be passed between the stone and the mucosa under vision (Fig. 61.2).
- A tortuous or kinked ureter may pose a challenge. Difficulty in retrograde access may result in false passage or even perforation with bacteremia and urinary extravasation [4]. These tortuosities/kinks can sometimes be negotiated by placing the patient in a steep Trendelenburg position.
- Mertz maneuver [4] is a useful trick that involves pushing the kidney upwards and medially, using a closed fist on the flank beneath the costal margin, to straighten the ureter.
- Another useful trick is to pass a guidewire halfway up to the kink; then advance an open-ended ureteric catheter over it and pull both as a unit in order to straighten it by traction. Keeping the open-ended catheter at this position, now the guidewire is pushed in. This traction maneuver can perhaps be done better with the help of a balloon catheter inflated and pulled just below the kink.
- Passing a slippery hydrophilic (glide) wire that glides through the kink can also be used.
- The ureteroscope can be used to bypass the kink under direct vision and maneuver the guidewire through its working channel.
- If available, a specialized (angled) ureteric catheter—e.g., Cobra catheter—can be used in combination with hydrophilic guidewire under fluoroscopic guidance.
- A conventional guidewire can cause trauma to the mucosa and is more likely to kink or bend rather than curl against the obstruction [5]. Issa et al. described a glide wire loop technique by using a hydrophilic-coated floppy-tipped guidewire that binds water to create a well-lubricated coating, which diminishes friction [6]. This is passed under fluoroscopic control to form a wedge between the stone and the wall of the ureter. It is further manipulated to form a curl that then forces the walls of the ureter to stretch at the site of impaction, resulting in the entry of this loop into the renal pelvis. The ureteric catheter is then passed over the guidewire into the pelvis. The wire is pulled back and redirected to curl in the renal pelvis, over which the stent can be advanced.

Stent Placement in Extrinsic Compression/ Stricture

At times a stone lies above the strictured segment of ureter. Retrograde passage can be a problem in extrinsic obstruction and stricture. The success rate in extrinsic ureteric obstruction varies from 40 to 60 % [7]. Under such circumstances, a hydrophilic guidewire is preferred because it has a greater chance of traversing through the stricture. A balloon dilatation

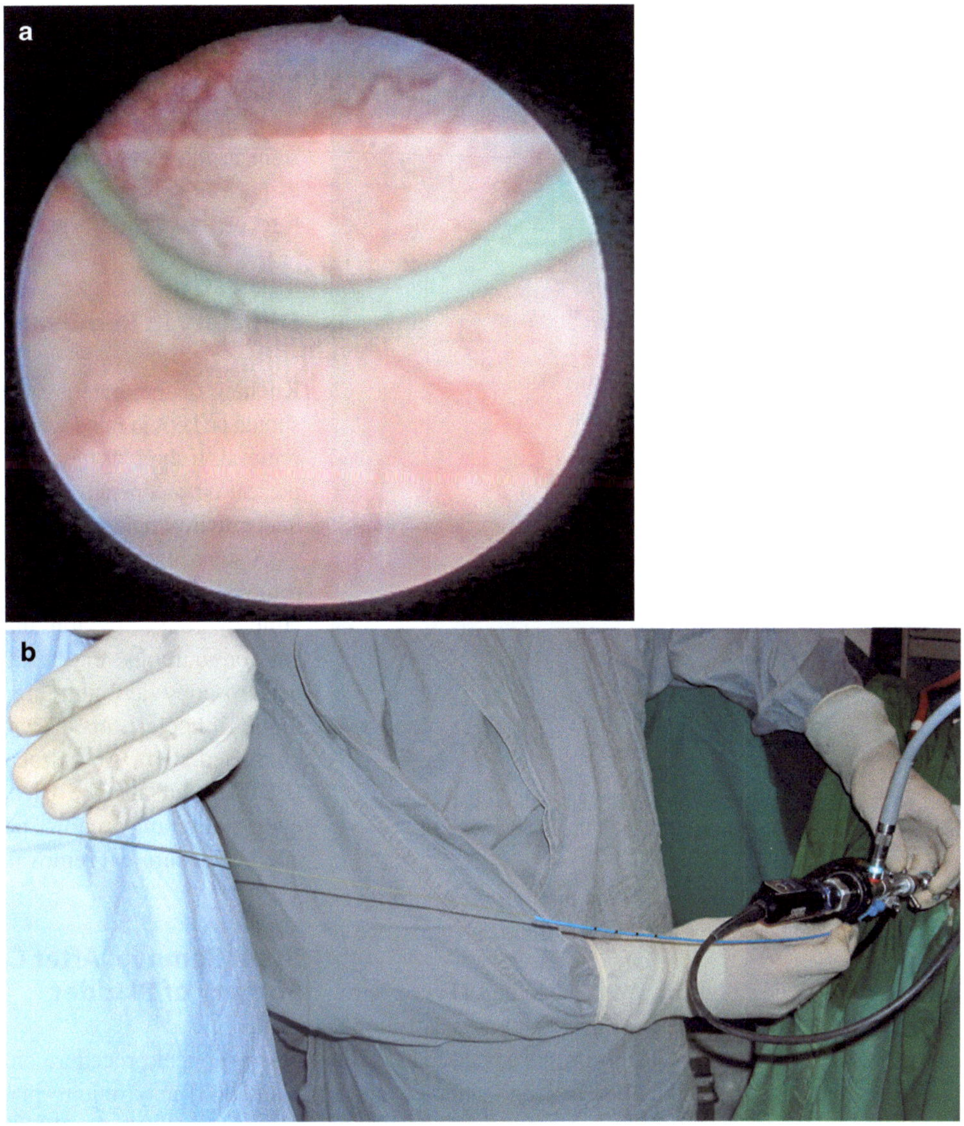

Fig. 61.1 (**a**) Cystoscopic picture showing looping of guidewire in the urinary bladder. (**b**) The assistant is holding the guidewire taut in the line of ureter, while the surgeon is pushing the double J stent

under fluoroscopy might be needed prior to this approach. The placement of two ipsilateral parallel ureteric stents (size 4.7 Fr) or a specialized metallic ureteric stent helps avoid stent failure [8, 9].

Changing/Exchanging the Ureteric Stent

In patients who require long-standing stent placement (e.g., due to stricture), replacement may be problematic. This may be because of extensive bullous reaction/edema around the ureteric orifice. An attempt to pass another guidewire next to/parallel to the stent should be made once the stent is removed because it will be difficult to re-localize the UO. Alternatively, the distal tip of the stent can be pulled out of the urethra while the guidewire is passed through its lumen under fluoroscopic guidance. There is, however, a possibility that the internal lumen of the stent might be occluded with stone debris.

Stent Placement in Open Surgical Procedures

In open surgical procedures like pyelolithotomy/pyeloplasty or ureterolithotomy, the confirmation of lower curl of stent in the bladder can be perioperatively done by filling the bladder with 50–100 cc of diluted methylene blue and then looking for oozing dye from multiple holes in the stent as it reaches the bladder. This obviates the need for intraoperative fluoroscopy or postoperative radiology [10].

Stent Placement Through Urinary Diversion

Retrograde stent placement is difficult in patients who have had urinary diversion procedures because of intrinsic peristalsis, the presence of intestinal mucosal folds, and the redundancy of the bowel loop. The guidewire and catheter can also coil in the diversion. After an intravenous injection of up to 20 mg/5 ml

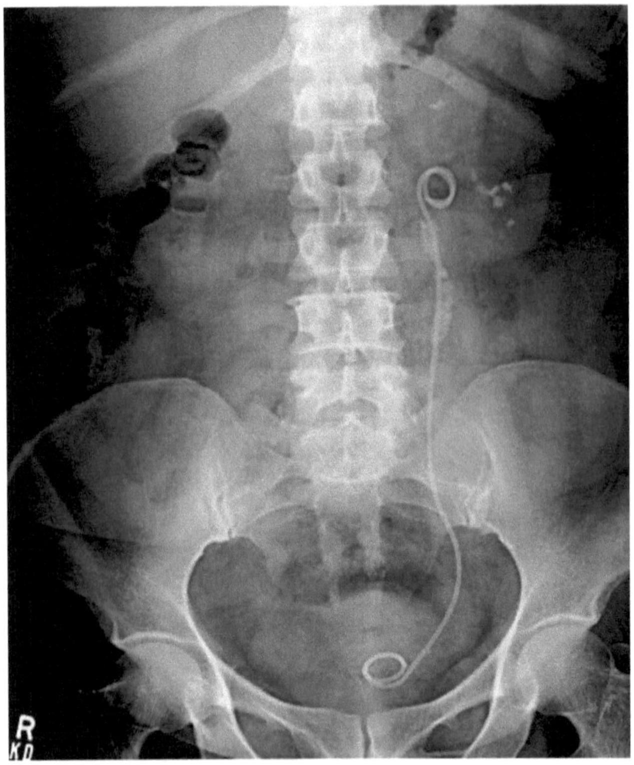

Fig. 61.2 Steinstrasse in the proximal ureter following ESWL. It was successfully negotiated with a JJ stent

indigo carmine, efflux of blue urine through ureteric orifices can be localized by using a flexible cystoscope/ureteroscope.

A technique described by Wah and Kellett [11] to retrogradely catheterize the ureter via ileal conduit is as follows: A 16-Fr Foley's catheter is cut at its tip and advanced as far up the ileal conduit as is possible. The balloon is inflated, and a loopogram is obtained, which allows contrast to reflux up both the ureters. Using the Foley's catheter as a fulcrum, an angiographic Cobra catheter is maneuvered, so an angled wire can be advanced up to the ureter under fluoroscopic guidance.

Removal of Stents

A stent should be removed as soon as it has served its purpose. The authors prefer to remove the stent under local anesthesia using a flexible cystoscope with the help of grasper forceps. It can also be removed under general anesthesia, by snares or Dormia basket.

Stent and PCN

When a kidney has both a percutaneous nephrostomy (PCN) and a JJ stent in place, there is always a chance that the loop of the JJ stent will curl in between the loop of PCN, creating trouble in the removal of either due to the pulling of one tube on the other. To avoid such a complication, a guidewire should be passed through the tube to be removed, which will straighten it and prevent it from pulling on the other tube. A migrated stent in the distal ureter can be pulled back in the bladder using a ureteroscope and various instruments like grasping forceps, stone baskets and snares, and Fogarty catheters.

Difficulty in Removal of Stent

Knotting of the ureteric stent is an unusual complication but should be kept in mind when difficulty or resistance is felt in its removal. If three or more coils of proximal end of JJ stent are present on preoperative imaging, the stent should be removed under fluoroscopic guidance to avoid irreversible knotting [12].

A stent placed for a long time may cause difficulty in its removal due to encrustations. If stent removal is not possible by gentle traction and radiology shows minimal linear or bulbous encrustation with low stone burden, ureteroscopy and intracorporeal lithotripsy (with pneumatic lithoclast or laser) can successfully remove the encrusted stent. An extracorporeal shock wave lithotripsy (ESWL) can also be tried [13]. Larger stone burden or encrustation may require percutaneous nephrolithotomy or even open surgical removal.

Stent Removal After Cases of Open Surgery of Bladder

Open surgical procedure on the bladder (e.g., ureteric reimplantation) may require placement of a stent. A JJ stent is placed and attached to the suprapubic catheter within the urinary bladder with a nonabsorbable suture. This method prevents the need for a second hospital admission because by simply pulling the supra pubic catheter out later on, it brings the removal of the attached JJ stent with it [14].

Forgotten and Retained Stents

Forgotten stents pose a significant management dilemma for physicians. They can give rise to serious and fatal complications like urosepsis or renal failure. There should be some effective system to ensure timely removal. To reduce the incidence of retained stents, a variety of solutions have been published including manual and computerized systems [15, 16]. Using only the logbook system, Thomas et al. reported delayed removal of up to 6 % of stents [15]. Ather et al. reported a reduction in the incidence of forgotten stent from 12.5 to 1.2 % in their series after the inception of computer generated program [16].

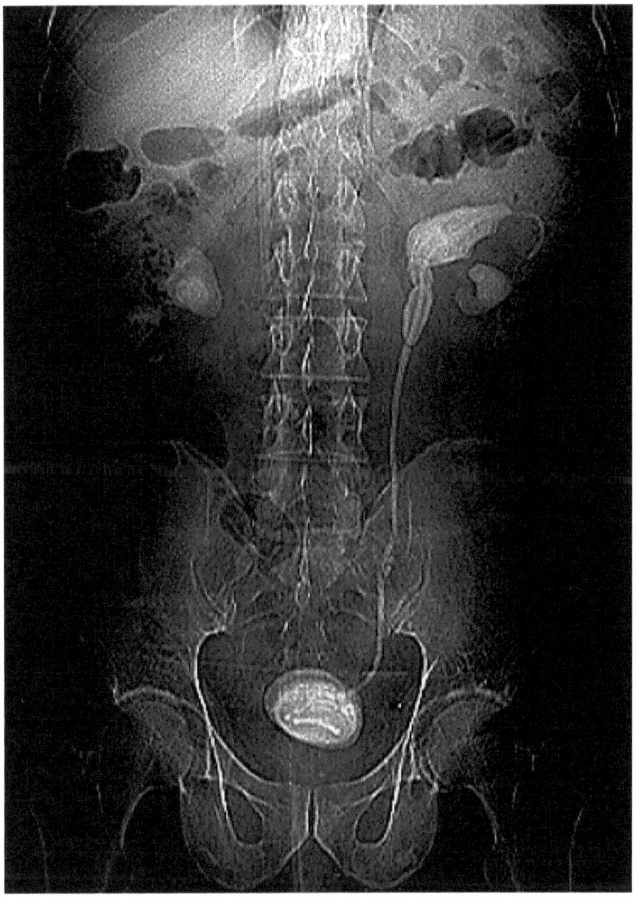

Fig. 61.3 X-ray of kidneys-ureters-bladder (KUB) showing overdue stent on left side with severe encrustation along with bladder stone and partial staghorn calculus on right side

The Resultant of Forgotten Stents: A Case Scenario

A 45-year-old gentleman with history of left pyelolithotomy and JJ stent placement presented with bilateral flank pain and lower urinary tract symptoms along with UTI 7 years after pyelolithotomy. A non-contrast computed tomography scan showed an overdue JJ stent on the left side with severe encrustation and a cast along its length, as well as the development of a large laminated calculus in the left kidney and urinary bladder around the encrusted stent. There was a partial staghorn calculus in the right kidney (Fig. 61.3).

Conclusion

Urologists should be familiar with the technical innovations to cope with the difficult situations to increase their efficiency of ureteric stenting. This involves following a logical sequence and both knowing and using various instruments like glide wire, ureteroscopes, balloon dilators, and forceps, along with various "tricks of the trade."

References

1. Eiley DM, McDougall EM, Smith AD. Techniques for stenting the normal and obstructed ureter. J Endourol. 1997;11(6):419–29.
2. Pilcher JM, Patel U. Choosing the correct length of ureteric stent: a formula based on the patient's height compared with direct ureteric measurement. Clin Radiol. 2002;57(1):59–62.
3. Paick SH, Park HK, Byun SS, Oh SJ, Kim HH. Direct ureteric length measurement from intravenous pyelography: does height represent ureteric length? Urol Res. 2005;33(3):199–202.
4. Schwalb DM, Eshghi M. Techniques to negotiate the tortuous ureter. J Urol. 1994;151(4):939–42.
5. Leveillee RJ, Bird V. A new tool to aid the urologist in the placement of stents for impacted ureteral stones or strictures: the glide catheter. Urology. 2000;55(6):944–6.
6. Issa MM, Pruthi RS, McNamara DE. New technique of ureteral stent placement for impacted ureteral calculus: the glidewire loop technique. Urology. 1997;49(4):614–7
7. Kouba E, Wallen EM, Pruthi RS. Management of ureteral obstruction due to advanced malignancy: optimizing therapeutic and palliative outcomes. J Urol. 2008;180(2):444–50.
8. Kilciler M, Erdemir F, Bedir S, Coban H, Erten K, Ors O, et al. Using two ipsilateral double J ureteral stents for extrinsic ureteral obstruction due to colon carcinoma. Urol Int. 2005;75(4):319–21.
9. Al Aown A, Iason K, Panagiotis K, Liatsikos EN. Clinical experience with ureteral metal stents. Indian J Urol. 2010;26(4):474–9.
10. Singh KM, Goel A, Shankhwar SN, Dalela D. Confirmation of the correct placement of lower end of DJ stent during open surgery: point of technique. Int Urol Nephrol. 2004;36(3):335–6.
11. Wah TM, Kellett MJ. Ureteric catheterization via an ileal conduit: technique and retrieval of a JJ stent. Clin Radiol. 2004;59(11):1041–3.
12. Ho CH, Chung SD, Huang KH, Yu HJ. Retrieval of a misplaced double-J ureteral stent in the renal pelvis: a novel technique. Surg Laparosc Endosc Percutan Tech. 2009;19(1):e24–5.
13. Polat F, Ye il S, Kiraç M, Tan MO, Biri H, Bozkirli I. An uncommon application of shock wave lithotripsy: encrusted double pigtail ureteral stent. Int Urol Nephrol. 2005;37(2):231–3.
14. Barbour KW, Arunachalam P, King PA, McAndrew HF. The use of ureteral stents and suprapubic catheter in vesicoureteric reflux surgery. Pediatr Surg Int. 2004;20(5):387–8.
15. Thomas AZ, Casey RG, Grainger R, McDermott T, Flynn R, Thornhill JA. The forgotten ureteric JJ stent and its prevention: a prospective audit of the value of a ureteric stent logbook. Ir J Med Sci. 2007;176(2):117–9.
16. Ather MH, Talati J, Biyabani R. Physician responsibility for removal of implants: the case for a computerized program for tracking overdue double-J stents. Tech Urol. 2000;6:189–92.

Transperitoneal Laparoscopic and Retroperitoneoscopic Stone Treatment

62

Marcel Hruza and Jens J. Rassweiler

Abstract

Objectives: This chapter focuses on the role of laparoscopic and retroperitoneoscopic stone surgery, especially in Europe and Northern America, where endourology and shock wave lithotripsy have replaced open stone surgery almost completely but also in developing and emerging nations.

Indications: There are no absolute indications for laparoscopic or retroperitoneoscopic stone surgery. Relative indications are residual stones after failure of other treatment modalities, very large or hard stones, stones in patients with anatomic variations of kidney and ureter, stones in patients who have to be safely treated within one treatment session, and stones in patients with other pathologies requiring surgical interventions.

Preparation and Techniques: Proper imaging and planning are mandatory in every single case. The access to the ureter and kidney (laparoscopic transperitoneal or retroperitoneoscopic) depends on the anatomy, on the localization of the stone, and on the skills and preferences of the surgeon. We propose that an organ bag should be used for removal of the stone from the body to prevent loss of a stone.

Discussion: We prefer inserting a double-J stent before starting surgery, if possible. However, there is an ongoing discussion whether to stent the ureter or not. The use of thermal energy for opening of the ureter may lead to higher rates of stricture formation; however, this is not verified yet. After removal of the stone, we do an intracorporeal suture to close the ureter and leave a drain as most authors do. Other groups negate suturing of the ureter to prevent stricture formation from too tight sutures. Laparoscopic and retroperitoneoscopic stone removal can be carried out with high stone-free rates and low complication rates in experienced hands. Less postoperative pain, shorter hospital stay, and time to convalescence and better cosmetic results are advantages compared to open surgery; however, operating room times are longer. In Europe and Northern America, retroperitoneoscopic and laparoscopic stone surgery is rarely performed because endourological techniques and shock wave lithotripsy are widespread. However, in developing and emerging nations, there is a large potential for these minimally invasive surgical methods for stone removal in replacing open surgery.

Conclusions: Despite the advances in endourology and shock wave lithotripsy, open stone surgery is still used in special stone situations. Laparoscopic and retroperitoneoscopic stone removal can be a good alternative to open surgery in most of these cases.

M. Hruza, M.D. (✉)
Department of Urology, SLK-Kliniken GmbH,
Am Gesundbrunnen 20-26, 74078 Heilbronn, Germany
e-mail: marcel.hruza@gmail.com

J.J. Rassweiler, M.D.
Department of Urology,
SLK-Kliniken GmbH, University of Heidelberg,
Am Gesundbrunnen 20-24, D 74078 Heilbronn, Germany
e-mail: jens.rassweiler@slk-kliniken.de

J.J. Talati et al. (eds.), *Urolithiasis*,
DOI 10.1007/978-1-4471-4387-1_62, © Springer-Verlag London 2012

Keywords
Stone surgery • Laparoscopy • Retroperitoneoscopy • Transperitoneal laparoscopic stone removal • Retroperitoneoscopic stone removal • Endourology

Introduction

For many centuries, open surgery has been the only possibility for active removal of renal and ureteral calculi all over the world. With the development of ureteroscopy (URS), percutaneous renoscopy, and extracorporeal shock wave lithotripsy (ESWL), new possibilities for stone treatment have emerged and, especially in Europe and Northern America, replaced open surgery in most cases. The increased use of laparoscopy and, more recently, robotic-assisted laparoscopic surgery also provide new possibilities for stone treatment. This chapter focuses on indications and techniques of transperitoneal laparoscopic and retroperitoneoscopic stone surgery today.

Indications

There are no absolute indications for laparoscopic or retroperitoneoscopic stone surgery. Relative indications are all cases of failure of shock wave lithotripsy and endourological techniques. This might be due to very hard, very large, or impacted stones or due to an awkward position of the stone within the renal calices. Symptomatic calculi within an anterior diverticulum of a calyx, for example, might not be reached by ureterorenoscopic instruments; the fragments after shock wave lithotripsy might not be able to pass the narrow orifice of the diverticulum, and it might not be possible to perform a percutaneous procedure because of the anterior location of the diverticulum. In cases of cicatrization of the renal pelvis, after previous stone treatment procedures or infections, stones might also be unreachable using endoscopic techniques.

Another relative indication for laparoscopic or retroperitoneoscopic procedures are renal or ureteral stones in patients with anatomic variations in location or shape of the kidney, for example, pelvic kidney, horseshoe kidney, malrotated kidney, or transplant kidney. It has to be checked properly in every single case which technique of stone treatment might be the best.

If definite removal of calculi within one treatment session is important due to comorbidity, incompliance of the patient, or social or economic necessities, retroperitoneoscopic or laparoscopic stone surgery may be more favorable than endourological techniques or shock wave lithotripsy.

In morbidly obese patients, laparoscopy or retroperitoneoscopy causes less wound-healing complications compared to open stone surgery in complicated stone situations.

One of the most frequent indications for laparoscopic or retroperitoneoscopic stone surgery is the coincidence of urolithiasis and other pathologies of kidney or ureter that need surgical intervention, for example, renal stones in a kidney with ureteropelvic junction (UPJ) obstruction.

Preparation

As laparoscopic or retroperitoneoscopic stone management is mostly used in complicated stone situations, a proper planning of the procedure is mandatory. Preoperatively, ultrasound and X-rays as well as a computed tomography (CT) should be used to check the anatomy of the kidneys and ureters and the precise location of the stones. In difficult cases, an additional magnetic resonance imaging (MRI), combined with a urography, may be useful to define the optimal treatment strategy.

Ultrasound probes that can be passed through a trocar for intracorporeal sonography can be very useful to identify the stone during the procedure.

Before starting the laparoscopic procedure, a ureteral stent (double-J stent) should be inserted transurethrally if possible. In most cases, this is much easier than laparoscopic intraoperative antegrade stenting of the ureter.

Technique

Retroperitoneal Access to Kidney and Ureter

After placement of the patient in flank position, a 15-mm incision is made in the lumbar triangle between the twelfth rib and the iliac crest, bounded by the lateral edges of the latissimus dorsi and external oblique muscles (Petit triangle). First, a tunnel to the retroperitoneal space is created using overholt forceps for blunt dissection. Then, the tunnel is dilated with the index finger pushing the peritoneum forward. Afterward, a balloon trocar system can be used to widen the cavity. Two secondary trocars (10 and 5 mm) are placed under palpation with the index finger introduced through the primary incision. Then, the primary incision is closed around a camera port to prevent the leakage of gas. A pneumoretroperitoneum can be established using a maximum carbon dioxide pressure of 12 mmHg and a flow of 3.5 l/min. A fourth trocar may be used if needed. The psoas muscle is the most important landmark to expose the ureter, the spermatic/ovarian vein, and the kidney. The Gerota fascia has to be incised completely.

Transperitoneal Access to Kidney and Ureter

The patient is positioned in a lateral 45° decubitus position. To establish a pneumoperitoneum, a Veress needle is used. The camera port is then inserted paraumbilically. After inspection of the peritoneal cavity, two other trocars are placed under endoscopic vision to avoid injuries of the bowel. To reach the retroperitoneal space, the ascending or descending colon has to be mobilized. The peritoneum is incised laterocolically along the white line of Toldt. When the colon is free to fall medially, additional trocars may be inserted into the exposed retroperitoneum. The psoas muscle and the ureter are identified and followed cranially toward the renal hilum. Gerota's fascia is inserted.

Laparoscopic and Retroperitoneoscopic Removal of Kidney Stones

In most cases, the renal pelvis can be reached sufficiently from the retroperitoneoscopic access. However, in cases of malrotated kidneys or horseshoe kidneys, the renal pelvis may point ventrally and can be reached via the transperitoneal route more easily. In case of pelvic kidneys or after prior retroperitoneal surgery, we also recommend a transperitoneal access. Proper preoperative imaging and planning of the procedure is therefore essential.

Stones within the renal pelvis are exposed by performing a longitudinal incision of the renal pelvis. Sometimes, however, the stone or a part of it slips into a calyx, which can make both identification and removal more difficult. Intracorporeal ultrasound may be used in these cases to find the stone. Irrigation can be used to bring the calculus into sight. For stone removal, different types of laparoscopic forceps and graspers are available and should be chosen depending on the size and shape of the stone (Fig. 62.1). We recommend the use of an organ bag to prevent the loss of a stone during extraction from the body (Fig. 62.2). After stone removal, the renal pelvis is closed with an intracorporeal running suture.

Some authors describe the use of a flexible endoscope introduced through one of the trocars to find and remove stones that cannot be reached using laparoscopic instruments [1]. However, this technique is complex, time-consuming, and not always successful.

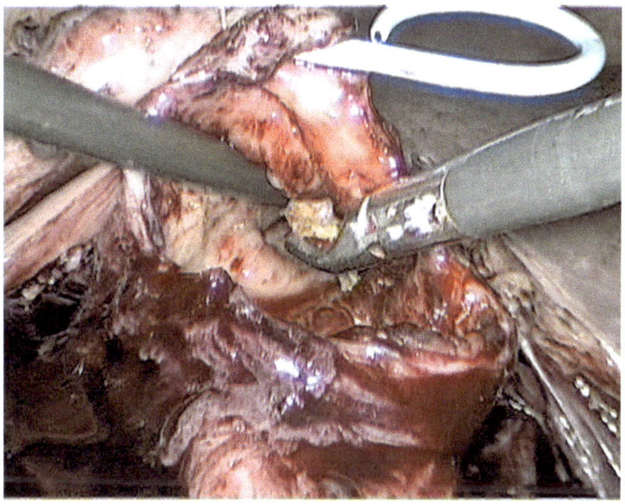

Fig. 62.1 The size and shape of the stone should determine the type of forceps and graspers used for laparoscopic stone removal

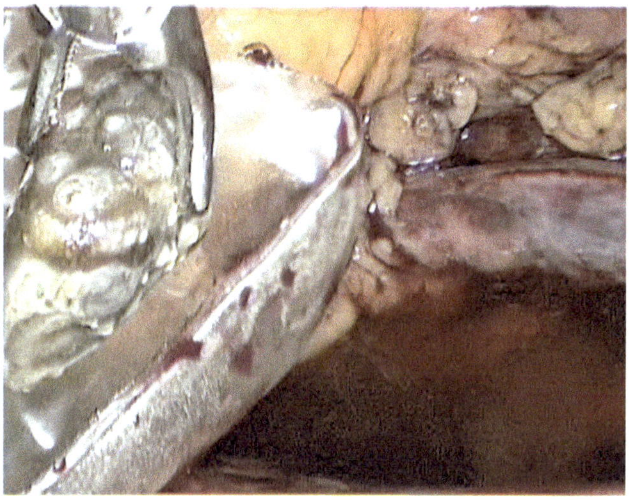

Fig. 62.2 A stone is placed into a bag to prevent its loss during extraction from the body

In cases with a calculus within a diverticulum of a calyx, the diverticulum itself is incised to remove the stone. In some cases, with the diverticulum bulging out over the contour of the kidney, the identification may be easy. In other cases, intracorporeal ultrasound should be used. After stone removal, the gap should be filled with fatty tissue, Gerota's fascia, or synthetic glue to prevent the formation of new stones.

In pelvic kidneys and horseshoe kidneys, a technique of laparoscopic-assisted percutaneous stone removal has been described: The percutaneous puncture of the renal pelvis is performed with a needle under laparoscopic guidance to prevent injuries of other structures in difficult anatomic situations. The removal of the stone is then performed via nephroscope in the conventional technique of percutaneous nephrolithotripsy (PNL) [2].

Laparoscopic Ureterolithotomy

A proximal ureteral stone usually can be reached using a retroperitoneal access, while distal stones should be removed via transperitoneal route. The psoas muscle and the gonadal veins are important landmarks during identification of the ureter. While large stones can often be localized easily because they buckle the ureter, smaller stones have sometimes to be found using intraoperative intracorporeal ultrasound. The ureter is longitudinally incised over the stone to remove it using forceps (Fig. 62.3). Again, especially in cases with more than one stone, we suggest the use of an endobag to bring the stones out of the body to prevent the loss of a stone. After stone removal, we close the ureter using an intracorporeal running suture over a double-J stent. A drain is inserted through one of the incisions to prevent the formation of an urinoma.

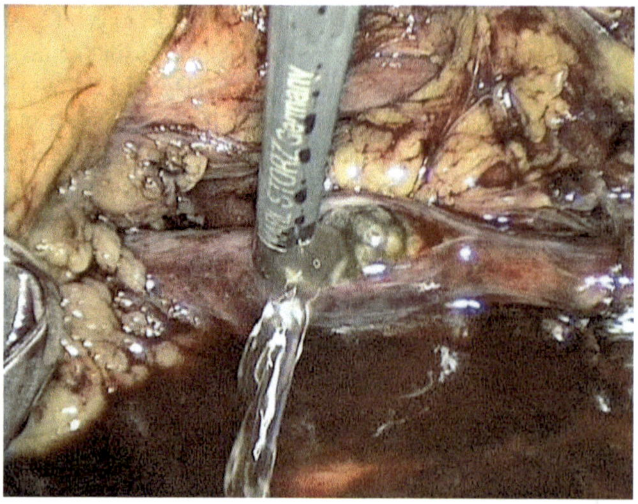

Fig. 62.3 A longitudinal incision allows the use of forceps to remove a stone

Discussion

The question of whether a laparoscopic procedure for removal of a renal or ureteral stone should be performed via transperitoneal or retroperitoneal access route has to be answered in every single case depending not only on the localization of the stone but also on the preference of the surgeon. The transperitoneal route may be favored because it provides a more familiar overview of the anatomic landmarks and a larger working space. The advantages of the retroperitoneoscopic operation are less complication may be a better wording than less complication related to the bowel and the prevention of an extravasation of urine into the peritoneal cavity. After previous retroperitoneoscopy, however, a second operation via the same access should be avoided because adhesions can make the development of the retroperitoneal working space extremely difficult in these cases.

The stricture rate after laparoscopic ureterolithotomy is about 3 % [3]. The impact of different patho-mechanisms on stricture formation remains unclear: An inflammation of the ureteric wall due to the impacted stone, thermal energy used to incise the ureter, too tight sutures for closing the ureter, or a fibrosis of the tissue surrounding the ureter caused by an extravasation of urine may play a role.

There is no consensus on the right instrumentation for incision of the ureter: Nouira and coworkers reported a higher rate of ureteral strictures when using a diathermal hook compared to a cold knife [4]. Other authors, however, found no strictures after the use of thermal energy on the ureter [5]. We usually incise the ureter or pyelon with a cold knife to prevent stricture formation.

We always recommend double-J stenting of the ureter for 3–4 weeks after laparoscopic stone removal, although there is no consensus on this subject in literature; some authors have abandoned the use of a double-J stent. They just left in a drain for some days to prevent the formation of a urinoma and reported few cases with secondary necessity of double-J stenting due to persisting extravasation of urine [6–8]. Other groups proposed to use a double-J stent and a retroperitoneal drain, but to leave to ureter without suture [9, 10] or just with a few adapting sutures [4] to prevent stricture formation from too tight sutures. In contrary, Mitchinson and Bird recommended a watertight suture of the ureter to prevent fibrosis of the surrounding tissue due to an extravasation of urine [11].

To date, few studies have been published on stone-free rates after laparoscopic stone surgery. Many case reports on this intervention for difficult stone situations can be found; some small series have also been published. However, there are no randomized controlled trials comparing laparoscopic stone therapy to open surgery or endourological treatment options. This may be due to low numbers of laparoscopic procedures for this indication even in centers of laparoscopic excellence. There are two non-randomized comparative studies by Goel and Hemal [12] and Skrepetis et al. [13] comparing laparoscopic versus open surgical ureterolithotomy: They found a shorter hospital stay, a lower demand for analgesics, and a shorter time to convalescence as benefits of laparoscopic treatment. Operating room times were significantly longer in the laparoscopic group. However, stone-free and complication rates showed no significant differences. In 2011, Falahatkar et al. presented a non-randomized comparison between transurethral lithotripsy, laparoscopic ureterolithotomy, and open ureterolithotomy including 60 patients with residual ureteral calculi >10 mm after shock wave lithotripsy [14]. Operative time showed significant differences between all three groups with a maximum in the laparoscopic group. Mean time of hospital stay was equal after open and laparoscopic surgery, but significantly lower after ureteroscopy. Mean time to return to full activity was longest after open surgery (21.7 days) compared to 14.6 days after laparoscopy and 8.9 days after transurethral lithotripsy. Stone-free rates were 100 % after open surgery, 95 % after laparoscopy, and 90 % after the transurethral procedure. Blood transfusions were necessary only after open surgery (15 %). No major complications occurred; minor complications (pain, fever, ileus, bleeding, pulmonary edema) were lower after laparoscopic ureterolithotomy (45 %) compared to open surgery (70 %). Transurethral lithotripsy showed the lowest complication rate (25 %). No ureteral strictures were found in the three groups; however, the follow-up time was short (7–21 months).

In Europe and North America, the importance of surgery for ureteral and renal stones has decreased in daily clinical practice due to the widespread availability of transurethral and percutaneous endoscopic treatment options and shock wave lithotripsy [15]. Today, technical advancements in the endourological instrumentation have made it possible to treat almost every stone, independent from size and localization. However, there are still special situations making surgical procedures necessary, especially after failure of endoscopic treatment. Most of these cases can be managed laparoscopically today. Robot-assisted pyelolithotomies have also been reported in some cases.

The rarity of open stone surgery in Europe and North America causes a major problem, especially for younger urologists trained in the era of endourologic stone treatment: Their experience in stone surgery is low, cases to train these procedures are rare, and the cases recommending surgery are difficult due to the size of the stone or anatomic variations. The question how young urologists can be sufficiently trained for these procedures remains unanswered to date.

In developing countries and even in emerging nations, however, the situation is completely different. When poor financial resources and medical infrastructure meet a higher incidence of large calculi compared to the industrial countries, open stone surgery still plays an important role. The instruments needed are simple, inexpensive, low maintenance, and available; surgeons are often only trained in open surgery, and patients benefit from removal of the stone within one single procedure because every visit to a medical doctor and every day in hospital is expensive for people having no adequate health insurance. In this context, Kijvikai and Patcharatrakul from Thailand reported that an increasing number of surgeons in their country use the advantages of laparoscopy to combine the benefits of open surgery (removal of the most stones within one treatment session) with the benefits of minimally invasive treatment (low consumption of analgesics, short hospital stay, and time to convalescence) [7]. An important difference between the acquisition of endourological and laparoscopic equipment in these countries is the possibility to use the laparoscopic instruments for a variety of different surgical procedures, not only for stone therapy.

Conclusion

Laparoscopic transperitoneal and retroperitoneoscopic stone treatment can be an alternative to open surgery, when endourologic treatment options and shock wave lithotripsy fail or are not feasible, for example, due to anatomical variations of kidney or ureter. Both, laparoscopic/retroperitoneoscopic and open stone surgery, are rarely performed in Europe and North America today. The access route and the use of special techniques as intracorporeal ultrasound depend on the localization and size of the stones. Accurate treatment planning and sufficient preoperative imaging are mandatory. In experienced hands, laparoscopic and retroperitoneoscopic stone surgery can be carried out with high stone-free rates, low complication rates, and all benefits of minimally invasive surgery. However, operating room times may be longer compared to open surgery. Training of young urologists for these interventions is necessary because laparoscopic and retroperitoneoscopic stone surgery is mostly used in difficult stone situations. However, it remains unclear how training can be arranged for an intervention that is so rarely performed. In developing countries and emerging nations, the importance of laparoscopic/retroperitoneoscopic stone surgery may increase because it provides advantages of minimally invasive treatment when endourological equipment is not available.

References

1. Kramer BA, Hammond L, Schwartz BF. Laparoscopic pyelolithotomy: indications and technique. J Endourol. 2007;21:860–1.
2. El-Kappany HA, El-Nahas AR, Shoma AM, El-Tabey NA, Eraky I, El-Kenawy MR. Combination of laparoscopy and nephroscopy for treatment of stones in pelvic ectopic kidneys. J Endourol. 2007; 21:1131–6.
3. Wolf Jr JS. Treatment selection and outcomes: ureteral calculi. Urol Clin North Am. 2007;34:421–30.
4. Nouira Y, Kallel Y, Binous MY, Dahmoul H, Horchani A. Laparoscopic retroperitoneal ureterolithotomy: initial experience and review of literature. J Endourol. 2004;18:557–61.
5. Harewood LM, Webb DR, Pope AJ. Laparoscopic ureterolithotomy: the results of an initial series, and an evaluation of its role in the management of ureteric calculi. Br J Urol. 1994;74:170–6.
6. Demerici D, Gulmez I, Ekmekcioglu O, Karacagil M. Retroperitoneoscopic ureterolithotomy for the treatment on ureteral calculi. Urol Int. 2004;73:234–7.

7. Kijvikai K, Patcharatrakul S. Laparoscopic ureterolithotomy: its role and some controversial technical considerations. Int J Urol. 2006;13:206–10.
8. Hemal AK, Goel A, Goel R. Minimally invasive retroperitoneoscopic ureterolithotomy. J Urol. 2003;169:480–2.
9. Gaur DD, Agarwal DK, Purohit KC, Darshane AS. Retroperitoneal laparoscopic pyelolithotomy. J Urol. 1994;151:927–9.
10. Keeley FX, Gialas I, Pillai M, Chrisofos M, Tolley DA. Laparoscopic ureterolithotomy: the Edinburgh experience. BJU Int. 1999;84:765–9.
11. Mitchson MJ, Bird DR. Urinary leakage and retroperitoneal fibrosis. J Urol. 1971;105:56–8.
12. Goel A, Hemal AK. Upper and mid-ureteric stones: a prospective unrandomized comparison of retroperitoneoscopic and open ureterolithotomy. BJU Int. 2001;88:679–82.
13. Skrepetis K, Doumas K, Saifakas I, Lykourinas M. Laparoscopic versus open ureterolithotomy. Eur Urol. 2001;40:32–7.
14. Falahatkar S, Khosropanah I, Allakbar A, Jafari A. Open surgery, laparoscopic surgery, or transurethral lithotripsy – which method? Comparison of ureteral stone management outcomes. J Endourol. 2011;25:31–4.
15. Hruza M, Schulze M, Teber D, Gözen AS, Rassweiler JJ. Laparoscopic techniques for removal of renal and ureteral calculi. J Endourol. 2009;23:1713–8.

Role of Robotic-Assisted Surgery in the Management of Urolithiasis

63

Tyler Luthringer, Khurram Mutahir Siddiqui, and David Mois Albala

Abstract

The means by which urolithiasis is managed continues to evolve with innovative surgical technology. Recently, the da Vinci® robotic system has been utilized for the treatment of certain stone disease indications, notably simultaneous pyeloplasty-pyelolithotomy, as well as stone extractions that have been difficult with established techniques. The efficacy of new adjuncts to the robotic system for ureterorenoscopy and laser lithotripsy is also being investigated. While increased operative time for joint stone procedures has been reported, successful outcomes of this application have been published in the literature. Pertinent indications for the robotic management of urinary tract calculi are continuously being documented. The field of urology would greatly benefit from large, multi-institutional studies that evaluate the effective advantages of the robotic approach against well-established methodologies in the treatment of stone disease.

Keywords

Urolithiasis • Robotic • Robotic-assisted • Pyeloplasty-pyelolithotomy

Introduction

At this juncture in the era of modern medicine, laparoscopic alternatives have been established for almost all invasive surgical procedures. Advancements in endoscopic equipment as well as improvements in techniques of percutaneous access have left relatively few indications for open surgery in contemporary urologic operating suites. While prevailing minimally invasive techniques have nearly monopolized the management of urolithiasis, not all cases of stone disease can yet be handled endoscopically. Despite the progression, the wide variation of human genitourinary anatomy continues to puzzle physicians and demands further innovative methods to effectively treat the most technical cases of urolithiasis [1].

While the learning curve for pure laparoscopic reconstruction is steep due to the requirement of suturing, the need to consistently reproduce excellent results has been greatly facilitated by the da Vinci® robotic system. Already well validated for numerous urologic surgical procedures, the robotic platform has recently been applied to surgically manage urolithiasis in select scenarios (large impacted ureteral stone, stones resistant to extracorporeal shock wave lithotripsy [ESWL] and/or laser therapy, stones associated with pelviureteric junction obstruction, etc.). Unlike ablative procedures, it is almost always necessary to reconstruct the collecting system following stone removal. The role of robotic-assisted surgery continues to expand in this arena, especially for cases in which a more complex reconstruction is required. Although one may argue that the reconstruction can be performed by pure laparoscopic technique

T. Luthringer, B.A. • D.M. Albala, M.D. (✉)
Division of Urology, Associated Medical Professionals,
1226, East Water Street, Syracuse, NY 13104, USA
e-mail: tluthringer@ampofny.com;
dalbala@ampofny.com

K.M. Siddiqui, FCPS, FRCS (UK), FEBU
Department of Nursing, Section of Urology,
The Aga Khan University, Stadium Road, Karachi 74800, Pakistan
e-mail: khurram.siddiqui@aku.edu

J.J. Talati et al. (eds.), *Urolithiasis*,
DOI 10.1007/978-1-4471-4387-1_63, © Springer-Verlag London 2012

in the majority of cases, the known advantages of the robot-assisted approach—enhanced optics, dexterity, wristed instrumentation, and ergonomics—can facilitate a complex reconstruction of the collecting system for surgeons who may find intracorporeal suturing challenging. Beyond suturing and intracorporeal reconstruction, the robotic interface also improves upon the limits of tissue dissection and stone extraction during laparoscopy. The robotic advantage offers the potential for the improvement of patient outcomes in complex stone cases and for a flatter learning curve in surgeons with little laparoscopic experience.

Development of the Surgical Robot

The challenge of laparoscopic reconstructive surgery within difficult anatomical confines and the need to enhance surgeon capabilities in such areas greatly fueled the enthusiasm for the development of the robotic surgical system. The initial application of robot assistance in a urological case occurred in 1988 when the Probot was employed to perform prostatic surgery. The modern surgical robot that is used in clinical practice today was introduced by Intuitive Surgical Inc. (Sunnyvale, CA) as the da Vinci® Surgical System—first approved by the US Food and Drug Administration (FDA) for general laparoscopic surgery in the year 2000.

During robotic-assisted procedures, the surgical instruments are controlled by the surgeon from a remote console that functions as a "telemanipulator" to execute operative tasks at bedside via computer assistance. That is, the physician makes his or her surgical movements by manipulating hardware controls at the console station; those movements are instantaneously reproduced by the electromechanical arms at the operating table in a scaled-down, micro-fashion, permitting superhuman surgical precision. The platform also detects and filters out any tremors in the surgeon's hand movements, so such inaccuracies are not duplicated robotically within the patient.

The da Vinci Surgical System is comprised of three main components: the surgeon console, the patient-side robotic cart with four (or fewer, depending on the da Vinci model) arms (one camera and up to three surgical instruments), and a high-definition 3D vision system. Task specific instruments may be connected to the robotic cart and introduced via cannula in the patient as required by the surgeon during a given procedure. The camera used in the system provides a true stereoscopic picture transmitted to the surgeon's console.

Since the release of the original da Vinci device, numerous attachment upgrades and updated models have been brought to market by Intuitive Surgical Inc. The da Vinci *S* and da Vinci *Si* are currently the latest surgical robots commercially available to healthcare institutions. The latter of these two is now compatible with a single-entry port adaptation, a second console for training purposes, and further specialized arms to enhance case-specific surgical competency.

Future Robotic Systems

Although the progression of the surgical robotic system has greatly augmented our capabilities in the operating room, the platform is not without flaw. What is likely the most frequently reported shortcoming of the current da Vinci robot is the lack of force feedback offered to the surgeon; the superior visual acuity has, however, been said to sufficiently compensate for the absence of this tactile sensation. The future of robotic surgery may be revolutionized by a new robot, Titan Medical Inc.'s Amadeus® (Toronto, ON), or by new adjuncts for the da Vinci system, which may offer robotic surgeons haptic feedback for the first time.

Clinical Application of Robotic Surgery for Urolithiasis

The benefits of robotic-assisted laparoscopic pyeloplasty (RALP) have already been demonstrated by a number of reviews [2–5]. In a 4-year retrospective case control study, Lee et al. found that pediatric RALP offers advantages of shorter hospital stay and decreased need for pain medication compared to the open procedure [2]. Other research has shown that this procedure is advantageous for patients beyond the hospital setting; RALP has been described as financially and cosmetically favorable for patients over the open alternative [3, 4]. More recently, the robotic approach has been implemented for genitourinary stone removal in a variety of operations. One of the indications for which robotic-assisted surgery has shown a clear advantage is simultaneous pyeloplasty-pyelolithotomy [6–9]. While the aforementioned joint procedure is a relatively young methodology for robotic practice, its application has shown positive results in a few small studies.

Hemal et al. published a case series of 50 robotic-assisted laparoscopies (RAL) for upper tract stones that included 29 cases of joint pyeloplasty-pyelolithotomy, those of which had a mean operative time of 105 min and a range of 86–135 min [6]. This combined procedure (pyeloplasty-pyelolithotomy) is similar in time to performing a laparoscopic pyelolithotomy. In their study, Hemal et al. also reported five cases of successful tailoring of the ureter and ureteroneocystostomy with additional ureteric calculi removal; they concluded that RAL is a safe and efficacious treatment approach for upper tract urolithiasis.

As expected, additionally removing calculi in the midst of a distinct procedure has been shown to increase operative time; yet doing so has not been shown to compromise the benefits of a robotic-assisted reconstruction. Atuq et al. described 55 concomitant procedures and reported an average increase in operative time of roughly 60 min for cases requiring stone removal [7]. In their study series, no conversions to open surgery were necessary, all patients were confirmed stone-free by imaging, and there were no intraoperative or delayed complications during a mean follow-up of 12.3 months. Both of these aforementioned studies concluded that robotic assistance can be advantageous in cases of simultaneous reconstruction, while neither documented any major perioperative issues nor considerable incidence of failed stone extraction [6, 7].

Abnormally located and anomalous renal units (e.g., horseshoe kidneys) pose a technical challenge for stone removal and treatment of pelviureteric junction obstruction (PUJO). Authors have reported success in the management of these conditions with assistance of the da Vinci robotic system [9, 10]. Despite these promising results, the application of the robotic technique for such difficult operations remains to be validated by a large sample study. Similarly, in their contemporary analysis of the role of robot-assisted pyelolithotomy for large renal calculi, Badalato et al. concluded that a longitudinal, multi-institutional study was necessary to validate the early encouraging results of this application [11]. Such investigations could greatly benefit the field of urology in the near future.

From Henry Ford Hospital in Detroit, Michigan, Badani et al. reported 13 cases of robotic-assisted extended pyelolithotomy for staghorn calculi without open or laparoscopic conversion; the mean operative time was 158 min while the average time console time averaged 108 min. The authors describe this modality as an alternative to PCNL in appropriately selected cases, excluding those patients with complete staghorn stones [12]. In an alternative evaluation, Lee et al. retrospectively reviewed their experiences of five adolescent robotic-assisted laparoscopic pyelolithotomies; four patients had cystine staghorn stones, while the fifth had calcium oxalate calculi concurrent with PUJO [13]. Open conversion was necessary for the removal of one staghorn calculus, while 75 % of the pure robotic cases left patients completely stone-free (one of four concluded with a residual 6-mm lower pole stone).

In what may be the first documented clinical assessment of remote robotic ureterorenoscopy and laser lithotripsy for renal calculi, Desai et al. yielded encouraging results with a novel flexible robotic system [14]. The surgeons manually placed a robotic catheter system into the renal collecting cavity via guidewire and fluoroscopic control prior to executing all stone fragmentation and relocation from the robotic console. Of the 18 subjects with an average stone diameter of 11.9 mm, only one required a secondary percutaneous nephrolithotomy. With continued technological innovation and increasingly complex adjuncts to the robotic platform, the robotic management of stone disease may have a promising future.

Conclusion

A current literature search on the use of robotic surgery for urolithiasis extracts considerably few articles. On top of the immature nature of this application, the small number of published reports regarding robotic management of urolithiasis may be due to a lower prevalence of large stones within the catchment area of major academic robotic programs. As the availability of the robotic system and new stone-specific adjuncts expands, this application may as well. The early, yet promising, efforts of robotic-assisted stone management ought to be compared against other minimally invasive techniques in similar stone cases to effectively determine the benefits of each approach. Perhaps such research will lead to the next major breakthrough in stone treatment and prove advantageous for physicians, patients, and healthcare institutions alike.

References

1. Gross AJ, Fisher M. Management of stones in patients with anomalously sited kidneys. Curr Opin Urol. 2006;16(2):100–5.
2. Lee RS, Retik AB, Borer JG, Peters CA. Pediatric robot assisted laparoscopic dismembered pyeloplasty: comparison with a cohort of open surgery. J Urol. 2006;175(2):683–7.
3. Behan JW, Kim SS, Dorey F, De Filippo RE, Chang AY, Hardy BE, et al. Human capital gains associated with robotic assisted laparoscopic pyeloplasty in children compared to open pyeloplasty. J Urol. 2011;186(4Suppl):1663–7.
4. Freilich DA, Penna FJ, Nelson CP, Retik AB, Nguyen HT. Parental satisfaction after open versus robot assisted laparoscopic pyeloplasty: results from modified Glasgow Children's Benefit Inventory Survey. J Urol. 2010;183(2):704–8.
5. Singh I, Hemal AK. Robot-assisted pyeloplasty: review of the current literature, technique and outcome. Can J Urol. 2010;17(2):5099–108.
6. Hemal AK, Nayyar R, Gupta NP, Dorairajan LN. Experience with robotic assisted laparoscopic surgery in upper tract urolithiasis. Can J Urol. 2010;17(4):5299–305.
7. Atug F, Castle EP, Burgess SV, Thomas R. Concomitant management of renal calculi and pelvi-ureteric junction obstruction with robotic laparoscopic surgery. BJU Int. 2005;96(9):1365–8.
8. Ilbeigi P, Lovallo GG, Bhalla RS, Sawczuk IS, Munver R. Robotic-assisted laparoscopic pyeloplasty with concomitant laparo-endoscopic pyelolithotomy of calyceal calculi. J Endourol. 2005;19(Suppl):270.
9. Nayyar R, Singh P, Gupta NP. Robot-assisted laparoscopic pyeloplasty with stone removal in an ectopic pelvic kidney. JSLS. 2010;14(1):130–2.
10. Chammas Jr M, Feuillu B, Coissard A, Hubert J. Laparoscopic robotic-assisted management of pelvi-ureteric junction obstruction

in patients with horseshoe kidneys: technique and 1-year follow-up. BJU Int. 2006;97(3):579–83.

11. Badalato GM, Hemal AK, Menon M, Badani KK. Current role of robot-assisted pyelolithotomy for the management of large renal calculi: a contemporary analysis. J Endourol. 2009;23(10):1719–22.
12. Badani KK, Hemal AK, Fumo M, Kaul S, Shrivastava A, Rajendram AK, et al. Robotic extended pyelolithotomy for treatment of renal calculi: a feasibility study. World J Urol. 2006;24(2):198–201. Epub 2006 May 16.
13. Lee RS, Passerotti CC, Cendron M, Estrada CR, Borer JG, Peters CA. Early results of robotic assisted laparoscopic lithotomy in adolescents. J Urol. 2007;177(6):2306–9.
14. Desai MM, Grover R, Aron M, Ganpule A, Joshi SS, Desai MR, Gill IS. Robotic flexible ureteroscopy for renal calculi: initial clinical experience. J Urol. 2011;186(2):563–8.

Management of Urinary Bladder Calculi

64

Jai Pal Paryani and Syed Raziuddin Biyabani

Abstract

The most common cause of bladder stones in the adult is bladder outlet obstruction from mechanical or neurogenic causes. Pediatric bladder stones, on the other hand, are likely due to nutritional factors. Open surgery for bladder stones has almost completely been replaced by endoscopic methods. Yet, it remains an effective modality of treatment in low-resource countries.

Keywords

Bladder stone • Bladder outlet obstruction • Neurogenic bladder • Laser • Electrohydraulic Cystolitholapaxy • Cystolithotripsy • Suprapubic cystolithotripsy • Suprapubic cystolitholapaxy • Cystolithotomy • Shock wave lithotripsy

Introduction

The reported incidence of vesical calculi is 5 % in the Western world. The majority of them are reported in men older than 50 years and are associated with bladder outlet obstruction [1]. However, in the developing world, urinary bladder calculi are more common in children. Asper et al. demonstrated an association of bladder calculi with socioeconomic conditions [2]—more than 40 % of all stones in countries with poor socioeconomic conditions were vesical as compared to <10 % in countries with high socioeconomic conditions.

Due to lack of documentation, the exact incidence of bladder calculi in underdeveloped countries is not known. In high-volume urology centers in public and private sectors, bladder calculi still form a substantial part of the workload of urolithiasis management. However, the incidence is decreasing in recent years in urban centers. Hussain et al., reporting from a large urology center in lower Sindh, noted that the numbers of patients treated for bladder stone are decreasing—cystolitholapaxy formed 6.4 % of the treatment provided for urolithiasis prior to 1996. This has now declined to 2.5 % in the recent times [3].

Historical Background

Archeologists in the early twentieth century found the oldest bladder stones in mummies of Egypt. These stones were about 6,800 years old [4]. The first literary reference to bladder stone was quoted in Hippocrates's oath, "I will not cut for stone, even for the patients in where the disease is manifest; I will leave this operation to be performed by practitioners." He warned the future lithotomists about this lethal disease [5]. A number of famous personalities, including Napoleon Bonaparte, Peter the Great, Benjamin Franklin, scientist Isaac Newton, and physician Harvey, developed vesical calculi.

Accounts of open operation to remove bladder stone can be found in the accounts of the Hindu surgeon Susruta who wrote about perineal lithotomy. Apart from him, other Greek, Roman, and Arab surgeons also described this procedure.

J.P. Paryani, M.B.B.S., FCPS, FEBU (✉)
Department of Urology,
Liaquat University of Medical and Health Sciences,
Jamshoro, Sindh 75500, Pakistan
e-mail: jpsindh@yahoo.com

S.R. Biyabani, M.B.B.S., FCPS (Urol), FEBU
Section of Urology, Department of Surgery, The Aga Khan University,
Stadium Road, P.O. Box 3500, Karachi, Sindh 74800, Pakistan
e-mail: raziuddin.biyabani@aku.edu

J.J. Talati et al. (eds.), *Urolithiasis*,
DOI 10.1007/978-1-4471-4387-1_64, © Springer-Verlag London 2012

Suprapubic litholapaxy was performed by Pierro Franco in 1500 CE, while in 1600 CE Fere Jacques introduced the lateral approach to perineal vesicolithotomy [6]. In 1800 CE, Egyptian surgeons suggested avoiding incision by using large wooden or cartilage cannula via urethra to manually aspirate the stone from bladder.

Another technique in which a long nail was passed though the urethra and then struck with a blacksmith's hammer, fragmenting the stone, became popular in the 1700s. Then, in the nineteenth century, a significant technological advancement occurred with the advent of a device used to grasp and fragment the stone in order to allow removal of smaller pieces via suction into a glass bottle. Sir Philip Crampon was the pioneer who developed litholapaxy in 1834, which was popularized in 1878 by Henry J. Bigelow, a professor of surgery at Harvard.

Over the last four decades, robust development of technology has greatly refined the treatment of bladder stone and has made the treatment safer and quicker [7].

Etiology

The most common causes of bladder stones in the adult is bladder outlet obstruction. Conditions like prostatic enlargement, high bladder neck, urethral strictures, and neurogenic bladder cause stasis of urine, which allows crystal aggregation, nucleation, and ultimately stone formation. Chronic urinary tract infection and foreign bodies like catheters, stents, sutures, and staples also are sources of bladder calculi formation. In one study, 36 % of patients with spinal cord injuries developed bladder calculi. Chronic bladder irritation and inflammation secondary to radiotherapy and schistosomiasis can also predispose to bladder stones. Congenital or acquired diverticuli of the urinary bladder may serve as a reservoir of stagnating urine and hence lead to stone formation. There are other risk factors that can lead to urinary bladder stone formation including procedures like bladder augmentation and repair of cloacal abnormalities [8].

There are various studies published in developing countries that mention the formation of primary bladder stones in children is due to low-protein and high-carbohydrate diet and chronic dehydration from diarrheal disease, all of which predispose to endemic stone.

Pathophysiology

The majority of bladder stones are formed within the bladder, but some may have initially formed in the upper tracts and then passed down to the bladder where additional crystal deposition allows the stone to grow in size. However, most renal stones that are small enough to pass from kidney and ureter are also small enough to pass from bladder and urethra. The majority of bladder stones in adults are struvite and uric acid, but calcium oxalate stones are also commonly encountered [9]. Other less frequently encountered stones are composed of calcium phosphate, cystine, etc. Patients with uric acid calculi are not always hyperuricemic, and the core and surface component of the calculi may be different.

Stones in children are mainly made of ammonium urate followed by calcium oxalate or a mixture. An association has been shown in endemic areas with breast-feeding and consumption of polished rice. These foods are low in phosphorus leading to high ammonia excretion.

Bladder stones could be single, multiple, and vary in size. Their consistency ranges from soft to extremely hard, while they may appear rounded, with smooth or jagged spiculated surfaces. Most of the bladder stones are mobile, but some may be fixed on sutures, stents, or papillary growths [10].

Clinical Presentation

Bladder calculi are often found incidentally at the time of evaluation of patients presenting with obstructive or irritative lower urinary tract symptoms. Recurrent infection is also one of the common presentations and a known risk factor for vesical stone. Smaller calculi may be voided spontaneously, while larger calculi may present with acute urinary retention. Other symptoms such as suprapubic pain, dysuria, intermittency, frequency, hesitancy, or nocturia also occur. Sudden interruption of stream while voiding due to impaction of stone at the bladder neck or prostatic urethra is also a common feature and change of position may alleviate the symptoms as the stone rolls back into the bladder. Parents of children may notice their child rubbing the penile tip or may notice priapism or enuresis. On physical examination, common findings include suprapubic tenderness, fullness, and a palpable bladder when patient is in urinary retention. Other findings like cystocele in women, stomal stenosis in urinary diversion, and neurological deficit in patients with neurogenic bladder may indicate their etiology [10].

Diagnosis

Historically, vesical stones were diagnosed through passage of van Buren sounds transurethrally. The contact of this instrument with stone causes transmission of a clicking noise or vibration that confirmed the presence of stone. With the availability of bladder imaging modalities, this maneuver is rarely used [11].

Laboratory Investigations

Urinalysis

A urine dipstick can be a cheap and rapidly performed investigation for a quick evaluation. The dipstick test in bladder calculi may reveal positive nitrites, leukocyte esterase, and blood. Specific gravity may be increased as patients decrease their fluid intake in fear of dysuria and urinary retention. In patients with uric acid calculi, the pH may be acidic, while on microscopic examination red blood cells (RBCs) and white blood cells (WBCs) may be present. Microscopic crystals, when found, are usually consistent with composition of bladder stone.

Urine Culture and Sensitivity

This test is important to document the infection and initiate and direct appropriate treatment.

Other Tests

The white blood cell count may be elevated with neutrophilia when associated with infection.

The serum creatinine level may be raised in cases of obstructive uropathy or urosepsis.

Imaging Modalities

The initial imaging study of choice is a plain X-ray of kidneys, ureters, and bladder (KUB), as it is inexpensive, readily available everywhere, and can diagnose the radiopaque stones easily. In radiolucent stones, an outer layer of calcification may be faintly visible on the X-ray [11].

Ultrasonography is now being used extensively because of its widespread availability and high sensitivity for vesical calculi. Bladder calculi can be seen as moving hyperechoic object with posterior acoustic shadowing. Ultrasound can detect both radiopaque as well as radiolucent stones [12].

When X-ray KUB remains inconclusive, cystography and intravenous urography can be used. Bladder calculi may be visible as a filling defect moving with change of posture. At times, the stone is adherent to mucosa or tumor, or situated in a diverticulum, in which case it will be seen as a nonmobile filling defect. Intravenous urography is also useful in identifying associated abnormalities such as upper tract stone, enlarged prostate, diverticulum, cystocele, and urethrocele.

An unenhanced non-contrast computed tomography (NCCT) scan of the abdomen is not freely available in developing countries but is superior to other methods for detection of bladder calculi. It can detect small stones with accuracy. A contrast-enhanced CT scan, on the other hand, can obscure bladder calculi.

Diagnostic Procedures

Cystoscopy is the most common and reliable method to confirm the bladder stone and plan treatment. Cystoscopy can identify the stones, their number, size, and position. Apart from this, it helps in identifying other problems such as urethral stricture, enlarged prostate, bladder diverticulum, or tumors.

Treatment

Medical Therapy

Oral potassium citrate has been used to produce urinary alkalinization to dissolve uric acid calculi. Other agents like Suby G or M solution are now rarely used. Irrigation of bladder or continent diversion has been done to prevent debris collection and stone formation and ensure adequate drainage in patients with neurogenic bladder [7].

Surgical Treatment

Surgical management of bladder calculi has changed with the passage of time and technological advancement. The modality of treatment chosen depends upon the size, composition of stone, previous stone treatment, etiology, the presence of risk factor for stone formation, recurrence, previous lower urinary tract surgery, age, comorbid conditions, as well as equipment availability and the level of the surgeon's expertise.

Cystolitholapaxy

Cystolitholapaxy is the most commonly performed procedure in adults [1]. Initially, cystoscopy is performed to visualize the stone. Cystolitholapaxy is performed with a stone-crushing forceps, a stone punch, or an optical lithotrite. During the procedure, the bladder should be filled with at least 150 ml of fluid. Care should be taken to ensure that the bladder mucosa has not been caught by the grasping jaws. This can be done by rotating the instrument, which should occur freely if the grip is mucosa-free. The stone is then crushed manually, and the procedure repeated on the fragments until they are comminuted to a size that allows their evacuation through the sheath. An Ellick evacuator is used to evacuate the small fragments from the bladder expeditiously [13].

Contraindications to this procedure include a small capacity bladder, a stone larger than 3 cm (which is difficult to engage in the punch or forceps), a very hard stone, and a vesical stone in some children, where the inadequate urethral size will not allow the introduction of these instruments.

Complications have been reported in 9–25 % of patients [14]. Rizvi et al. have reported simultaneous cystolitholapaxy and transurethral resection of the prostate (TURP). They did not find any difference in the complication rate of cystolitholapaxy as monotherapy or combined procedure [15]. However, some authors reported a complication rate of up to 21 % for the combined procedures and suggested simultaneous therapy should be avoided.

Transurethral Cystolithotripsy

This procedure is useful in larger and relatively harder stones that are not easy to grasp or crush manually. Various energy sources such as electrohydraulic, ultrasonic, or pneumatic lithotripter are used. Pneumatic lithotripsy remains successful most of the time for fragmenting the stone into smaller pieces. It is an easy, safe, and effective procedure with a success rate of 85 % and minimal complications. It has been found to be more effective than ultrasonic and electrohydraulic lithotripsy [15]. This is also an effective and safe procedure for children with bladder stones. In the past, electrohydraulic lithotripsy has been used by many authors. They found that in very hard stones it takes a longer time with incomplete fragmentations, while in relatively softer stones it is a good modality with a reported success rate of 92 % [16]. Ultrasonic lithotripsy: In one series, a success rate of 88 % was reported in medium-sized stones with minimal complications [15]. Laser lithotripsy: Holmium:YAG laser has been used for the treatment of large and hard bladder stones with safety and efficacy. Teichman and Gould reported 100 % success rate in using this modality [17].

Procedure Details

Anesthesia

Patients are given general or spinal anesthesia depending upon the patient's comorbidities and choice of anesthetist.

Position

Patients are placed in a dorsal lithotomy position. A supine position can be used when procedure is performed with a flexible cystoscopy or percutaneous suprapubic access is used. A cystoscope with adult-size sheath is used through which energy sources are used. If a Lithoclast is being used, its probe should be advanced 1 cm away from the lens. This probe should also be at a safe distance from bladder mucosa to avoid bladder injury and perforation. The probe is postured over the middle part of the stone, and stone fragmentation proceeds under direct vision—pressing the stone against the wall of the bladder may reduce the time of procedure. Fragmentation should be continued until the pieces are small enough to pass through the sheath. Manual suction with an Ellick evacuator is commonly used to remove the stones.

Suprapubic Cystolitholapaxy and Cystolithotripsy

In these procedures, percutaneous access is obtained as in percutaneous renal surgery. An Amplatz sheath or trocar sheath is left in place. The instrument for manual crushing or a cystolithotripsy is introduced through the sheath and the procedure performed—in the case of litholapaxy, by manual crushing.

Percutaneous cystolithotripsy has now become the treatment of choice in children and in patients with inadequate urethra. Through the Amplatz sheath inserted as previously described, an adequately sized rigid nephroscope is passed, through which an electrohydraulic lithotriptor (EHL) probe or a pneumatic lithoclast is then used to fragment the stone. A grasper is used to retrieve the stone fragments. Contraindications to this procedure include prior lower abdominal or pelvic surgery and small capacity noncomplaint bladder.

Maheshwari and associates have reported a 100 % success rate for appropriately selected patients [18]. Isen et al. have shown that a rigid ureteroscope with holmium laser lithotripsy can be used to treat bladder stones in young patients with smaller urethras [19].

Postoperative Details

At the end of the procedure, the bladder is drained with a urethral catheter for 24 h in all patients. A single perioperative antibiotic dose is sufficient in patients with previously documented sterile urine.

Open Cystolithotomy

Open cystolithotomy has been used with high success rates, but now it is less commonly used in the developed world [20–22].

Indications

Indications for open surgery include large, hard stones refractory to an endoscopic approach, abnormal anatomy not allowing safe access, or concomitant open prostatectomy and open bladder diverticulectomy. In such instances, open surgery is the procedure of choice. This is a good procedure in terms of stone clearance, but it is associated with longer hospital stay and bladder drainage.

Preparation on the Operating Table

The patient is placed in the supine position with slight hyperextension of the lumbar spine. A Foley catheter is inserted transurethrally and filled with 200–300 ml of normal saline.

Surgical Procedure

A transverse Pfannenstiel, Czerny, or vertical lower midline incision is made. The linea alba is incised, and the retropubic space is a created with blunt dissection. The bladder is identified, and peritoneum is reflected upward. Aspiration of urine through a 23-G needle inserted into the bladder further confirms that indeed the structure to be incised is the bladder (and not any other viscus). The bladder is then opened between two stay sutures of 2.0 chromic catgut placed in the bladder wall. When removing large stones, it is useful to place two additional sutures at the end of the wound, to prevent further tearing of the bladder as the large stone is removed. The stone is removed by a stone-holding forceps. The bladder is closed in two layers with fine Vicryl. A drain may be placed in the retropubic area. It is never brought out through the main incision; rather, it is pulled out through a separate stab. The peritoneum is replaced in the previous position. The rectus abdominis muscle is approximated with Vicryl 2.0. The rectus sheath is then closed with Vicryl 1.0. The skin wound edges are then approximated with Prolene 2.0. The catheter is kept indwelling for 5 days. The drain is removed after 1–2 days.

Surgical Complications

Intraoperatively, occasionally bleeding and injury to the peritoneum or gut has been seen. Postoperatively, urinary leakage, extravasation, wound infection, and urinary tract infections may occur.

Extracorporeal Shock Wave Lithotripsy (ESWL)

The first reported series of treating bladder calculi with extracorporeal shock waves was from Vandeurson and Baert in 1990 [23]. The experience from our center with 29 patients over a 2-year period showed that 75 % stones were cleared with a single session of ESWL [24]. The patients with bladder outflow obstruction secondary to enlarged prostate can be treated on the next day. Al-Ansari et al. reported ESWL monotherapy for the treatment of urethraland bladder stones presenting with urinary retention [25].

Indications

The use of EWSL for bladder stones has been reported for stones less than 2 cm in the greatest diameter. Other potential indications are presence of a penile prosthesis or artificial urinary sphincter and orthotopic urinary diversion. In all of these situations, prolonged urethral instrumentation may be risky [26].

In cases where there is associated bladder outlet obstruction secondary to enlarged prostate or urethral stricture, the endoscopic treatment might be preferable, as stone and prostate can be dealt with in the same sitting.

Method

The procedure is done under sedoanalgesia. In children or patients with poor pain threshold, general anesthesia may be required. The urethral stone can be pushed back into the bladder. The urinary bladder needs to be full in order to localize the stone with an ultrasound. The number of recommended shock waves per session is an average of 3,400 (1,000–5,000) [24]. The limit of shock waves per session and the interval between sessions remain to be defined.

Complications

The potential complications include hematuria, retention from retained fragments, and infection. In cases where prostate surgery is contemplated, the procedure is performed prior to the TURP so that the fragments can be evacuated endoscopically.

Case Scenario

This case highlights the extent of adult urinary bladder stone disease encounters in rural areas in Pakistan. A 65-year-old female presented with a long-standing history of lower urinary

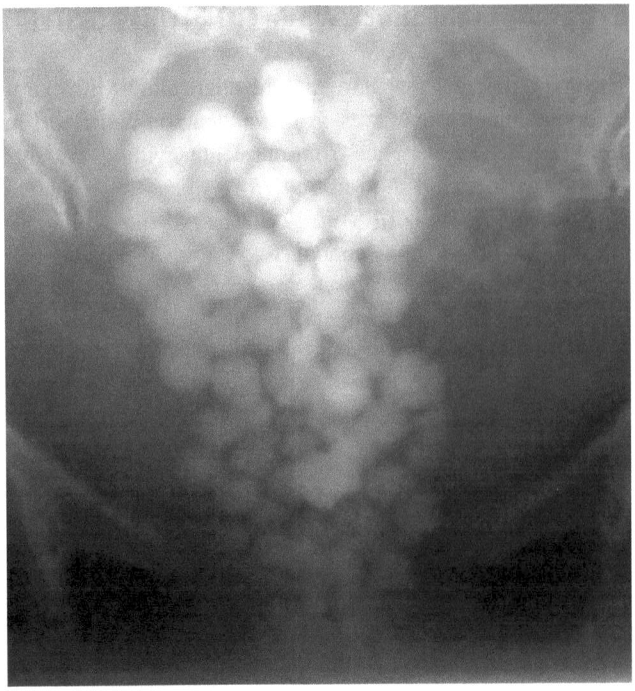

Fig. 64.1 KUB X-rays showing bladder calculi

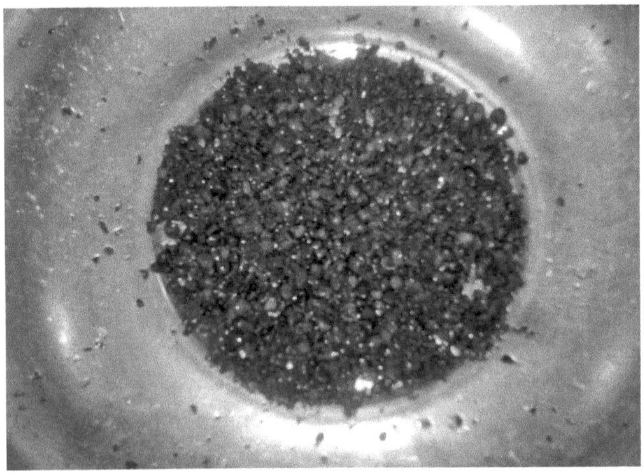

Fig. 64.2 Stone fragments retrieved at cystolitholapaxy

tract symptoms, urinary tract infections, and something coming out from the vagina. Examination showed suprapubic fullness and a cystocele. The serum creatinine was 8.9 mg/dl (0.8–1.3). X-ray KUB (Fig. 64.1) showed multiple relatively smaller stones in the urinary bladder. She was managed by hemodialysis followed by cystolitholapaxy (Fig. 64.2). Following recovery, she was referred for management of cystocele (case by Dr. Jai Pal Paryani).

Conclusion

Multiple options are available for treating vesical calculi. Open surgery is reserved for situations in which instrumentation for alternative methods is not available. Endoscopic approaches are now the gold standard. In addition to the stone, coexisting diverticula and mechanical or neurogenic outflow obstruction should also be appropriately dealt with.

References

1. Athansios GP, Iaonnis V, Athaniosis D, Charlambos D. Bladder lithiasis: from open surgery to lithotripsy. Urol Res. 2006;34:163–7.
2. Asper R. Epidemiology and socioeconomic aspect of urolithiasis. Urol Res. 1984;12:1–5.
3. Hussain M, Rizvi SAH, Askari H, et al. Management of stone disease: 17 year experience of a stone clinic in a developing country. J Pak Med Assoc. 2009;59(12):843–6.
4. Shattock SG. A prehistoric or pedynastic Egyptian calculus. Trans Pathol Soc Lond. 1905;56:275.
5. Ellis H. A history of bladder stone. Oxford: Blackwell; 1969. p. 3.
6. Ganem JP, Carson CC. Frere Jacques Beaulieu. From rogue lithotomist to nursery rhymes characters. J Urol. 1999;161:1061–9.
7. Huffman JL, Ginsberg DA. Calculi in the bladder and urinary diversions. In: Coe FL, Favus MJ, Pak CY, Parks JH, Premingers GM, editors. Kidney stones: medical and surgical management. Philadelphia: Lippincott-Raven; 1996. p. 1025–34.
8. Drach GW. Urinary lithiasis. Etiology, diagnosis and medical management. In: Walsh PC, Retik AB, Stamey TA, Vaughn ED, editors. Campbell's urology. 6th ed. Philadelphia: W.B Saunders; 1992. p. 2140.
9. Hammad FT, Kaya M, Kazim E. Bladder calculi. Did the clinical picture change? Urology. 2006;67:1154–6.
10. Bakane BC, Nagtilak SB, Patil B. Urolitiasis! A tribal scenario. Indian J Paediatr. 1999;66:863.
11. Ho K, Segura J. Lower urinary tract calculi. In: Wein A, Kavousi L, Novick A, Partin A, Pters C, editors. Campbell-Walsh urology. 9th ed. Philadelphia: Saunders Elsevier; 2007. p. 2663–7.
12. Haung WC, Yang JM. Sonographic appearance of bladder calculus secondary to a suture from a bladder neck suspension. J Ultrasound Med. 2002;21:1303.
13. Bapat SS. Endoscopic removal of bladder stones in adults. Br J Urol. 1977;49:527–30.
14. Bhatia V, Biyani CS. Vesical lithiasis. Open surgery vs cystolithotripsy vs ESWL. J Urol. 1996;151:660.
15. Rizvi HA, Song TY, Denstedt JD. Management of vesical calculus. Comparison of lithotripsy devices. J Endourol. 1996;10:559.
16. Bülow H, Frohmüller HG. Electrohydraulic lithotripsy with aspiration of the fragments under vision – 304 consecutive cases. J Urol. 1981;126(4):454–6.
17. Teichman JMH, Rogenes VJ, McIver BJ. Holmium YAG: laser cystolithotripsy of large bladder calculi. Urology. 1997;50:44.
18. Maheshwari PN, Oswal AT, Bansal M. Percutaneous suprapubic cystolithotripsy for vesical calculi: a better approach. Tech Urol. 1999;5:40–2 www.ncbi.nlm.nih.gov/pubmed/10374793.
19. Ise K, Em S, Kilic V, Utku V, Bogatelium S. Management of bladder stone with pneumatic lithotripsy using ureteroscope in children. J Endourol. 2008;22:1037.
20. Rizvi SA, Sultan S, Ijaz H, Mirza ZN, Ahmed B, Saulat S, et al. Open surgical management of pediatric urolithiasis: a developing country perspective. Indian J Urol. 2010;26:573.
21. Al-Mahroon MS, Sarhan OM, Awad BA, Helmy T, Ghali A, Dawaba MS. Comparison of endourological and open cystolithotomy in the management of bladder stones in adults. J Urol. 2009;181:2684–7.
22. Mahran MR, Dwaba MS. Cystolitholapaxy versus cystolithotomy in children. J Endourol. 2000;14:423–5.

23. Vandeursen H, Baert L. Extracorporeal shock wave lithotripsy monotherapy for bladder stones with the second generation lithotriptors. J Urol. 1990;143(2):252–6.
24. Hotiana MZ, Khan LA, Talati J. Extracorporeal shock wave lithotripsy for bladder stones. Br J Urol. 1993;71(6):692–4.
25. Al-Ansari A, Shamsodini A, Younis N, Jaleel OA, Al-Rubaiai A, Shokeir AA. Extracorporeal shock wave lithotripsy monotherapy for treatment of patients with urethral and bladder stones presenting with acute urinary retention. Urology. 2005;66(6):1169–71.
26. Bosco PJ, Nieh PT. Extracorporeal shock wave lithotripsy in combination with transurethral surgery for management of large bladder calculi and moderate outlet obstruction. J Urol. 1991;145(1):34–6.

Current Status of Medical Expulsion Therapy for Urinary Calculi

65

Zhangqun Ye and Huan Yang

Abstract

The current, predominant therapies to remove urinary calculi include the minimally invasive treatments of extracorporeal shock wave lithotripsy (ESWL), percutaneous nephrolithotomy (PCNL), ureteroscopy (URS), and laparoscopy. Conservative medical expulsion therapy is certainly a desirable option for urinary stone removal. This chapter summarizes the application of noninvasive medical expulsion therapy utilized in previous clinical experiments. Related drugs include α1-receptor blockers, calcium channel antagonists, nonsteroidal anti-inflammation drugs and prostaglandin synthesis inhibitors, gonadal hormones, glucocorticoids, potassium sodium hydrogen citrate, and even some traditional Chinese medicines. Although medical expulsion therapy of urinary calculi has yielded encouraging results, further double-blind, placebo-controlled studies ought to be performed to better evaluate the current medicines and to develop other treatments.

Keywords

Medical expulsion therapy • Urinary calculi • α1-receptor blocker • Calcium channel antagonist • Nonsteroidal anti-inflammation drugs • Prostaglandin synthesis inhibitors Gonadal hormones • Glucocorticoid • Potassium sodium hydrogen citrate

Introduction

Currently, the majority of urinary calculi are treated via minimally invasive surgery (MIS), which reduces the metabolic response to surgical trauma while maintaining a success rate similar to that achieved by the traditional open approach. Available minimally invasive treatments for patients with urinary tract stones include extracorporeal shock wave lithotripsy (ESWL), percutaneous nephrolithotomy (PNL), ureteroscopy (URS), and laparoscopy. However, the advantages of MIS, which include risk reduction and minimal surgical trauma, are offset by the fact that minimally invasive treatment remains expensive and still exposes the patient to potential, albeit small risk [1, 2].

Small calculi that can be expected to pass spontaneously, and calculi in patients where there are no clear indications for MIS, can be treated with a more conservative strategy. It will be advantageous to include medical expulsion therapy (MET) in the treatment plan of such patients, as an effective, safe, and noninvasive approach for outpatient use. The search for an ideal MET agent has become a focus of basic and clinical research over recent decades [3]. Such a treatment option may be perfect for those patients who wish to have their minimally or asymptomatic stones removed nonsurgically.

Z. Ye, M.D., Ph.D. (✉) • H. Yang, M.D., Ph.D.
Division of Urology, Tongji Hospital, Tongji Medical College, Huazhong University of Science and Technology, Wuhan, China
e-mail: zhangqun_ye@yahoo.com.cn

J.J. Talati et al. (eds.), *Urolithiasis*,
DOI 10.1007/978-1-4471-4387-1_65, © Springer-Verlag London 2012

Factors That Influence Stone Expulsion

The factors influencing expulsion of calculi are twofold: (1) pathological factors of urinary tract infection, edema, and convolutions and (2) calculus-related factors such as stone size, shape, and location. Of these, the location of the calculus and its size are the most important factors at play [4]. A previous study indicated that 29–98 % of proximal ureteral calculi with diameters of less than 5 mm could be spontaneously expelled without medical intervention. In contrast, 71–98 % of distal ureteral calculi were spontaneously passed. For 4- to 6-mm calculi or those larger than 6 mm, the spontaneous expulsion rates were only 59 and 21 %, respectively [5]. As a conservative approach, the effectiveness of spontaneous expulsion is rather unpredictable. Pharmacological expulsion therapy, on the other hand, provides an effective supplementary strategy. Based on the hypothesis that ureteral edema affects calculi expulsion rates, the following agents have come into common use for medical expulsion therapy: α1-receptor blockers, calcium antagonists (calcium channel blockers), nonsteroidal anti-inflammatory drugs, prostaglandin synthesis inhibitors, gonadal hormones, and glucocorticoids.

Alpha 1-Receptor Blocking Agents

Previous studies have shown that there are α and β adrenergic receptors, as well as muscarinic receptors in the ureteral smooth muscle. Generally, α1-receptors have a much higher spatial density than β and muscarinic receptors [6]. The α1-receptor density in the distal segment is the greatest compared to other ureteral regions; the distribution characteristic of α1-receptor subtypes in the distal, middle, and proximal ureteral segments is, however, still similar (i.e., α1D>α1A>α 1B) [7]. Of the known subtypes, α1D-receptors have the strongest effect on the distal ureter and detrusor muscle, especially for the wall segment of the ureter, and therefore play an important role in the lower ureteral region. Alpha1-receptor blocking agents can relax the ureteral smooth muscles, reduce peristaltic frequency and amplitude, decrease the pressure of the intra-wall segment of the ureter, enhance the transporting capacity of the urine boluses, and increase the pressure above the stone. In effect, these agents may establish a pressure around the stone, relax the smooth muscles of the bladder neck and urethra, and finally initiate a thrust to expel the stone. Alpha1-receptor blockers can also affect the C-type fast fibers of the spinal cord and sympathetic postganglionic neurons, blocking the pain transmission pathway to the central nervous system and reducing renal colic during calculi expulsion [8]. Alpha1A-receptors mainly exist in the proximal ureteral segment, the prostatic urethra, and the bladder neck, while α1D-receptors mainly reside the in the distal segment of the ureter, ureteral smooth muscles, and bladder detrusor [9]. Alpha-receptor blockers affect the prostate and bladder neck and, therefore, are recommended for the treatment of lower urinary tract symptoms. Among these agents, tamsulosin selectively affects α1A- and α1D-receptors and is commonly used in the management of prostate diseases [10].

Over the past 10 years, extensive clinical randomized control experiments have testified that α1-receptor blocking agents promote the expulsion of ureteral calculi and control renal colic. In 1999, Ukhal et al. first found that doxazosin could promote expulsion of distal ureteral calculi [11]. In 2002, Cervenakov et al. performed the first randomized double-blind study investigating the effect of tamsulosin in 104 cases of distal ureter calculi. Their results proved tamsulosin advantageous over the control group in terms of expulsion rate, time to expulsion, and recurrent colic [12]. In a 2004 study of 86 distal ureteral calculi of less than 1 cm, Porpiglia et al. randomized three groups to receive tamsulosin, nifedipine, or control. Tamsulosin and nifedipine enhanced calculi expulsion rate and reduced the need of pain killers, but compared to each other, tamsulosin was more effective in reducing time to expulsion [13]. Yilmaz et al. later compared three α1A-receptor blockers (tamsulosin, terazosin, and doxazosin) in 114 patients with lower ureteral calculi in 2005; they concluded that all three drugs increased the expulsion rate of distal calculi with equal effect [14]. In 2007, Sakip et al. compared the expulsive effect of tamsulosin and tolterodine on distal calculi and found that tamsulosin promoted calculi expulsion, while tolterodine did not [15].

Sefa utilized tamsulosin in 67 cases of lower ureter calculi formed post-renal ESWL. He found that tamsulosin administered together with regular conservative therapy was helpful in reducing the frequency and extent of renal colic after ESWL [16]. In 2005, Gravina et al. performed a randomized prospective study of 130 cases of renal stone fragments after ESWL. The experimental group was treated with self-defined standard medication plus 0.4 mg of tamsulosin daily for a 12-week maximum duration, while the control group was treated only with self-defined standard medication. The results indicated that the 3-month rates of stone absence were 78.5 and 60 % for the experimental and control groups, respectively. The success rate in the experimental group was much higher for stones with a diameter less than 1 cm. Additionally, the renal colic rates were 76.9 and 26.1 % for the control and experimental groups, respectively. The authors concluded that ESWL with tamsulosin was safer and more effective than ESWL alone in treating renal calculi larger than 1 cm and that tamsulosin could reduce the usage of pain medication [17]. In 2007, Micali et al. [18] analyzed the expulsive effect of either tamsulosin or nifedipine combined with ketoprofen after ESWL treatment in 113 cases of ureteral calculi. Nifedipine was prescribed for upper and middle ureteral calculi, while tamsulosin was prescribed for lower ureteral calculi. Of the 113 patients, 37 had upper, 27 had middle, and 49 had lower ureteral calculi. Thirty-five patients received 30 mg of nifedipine daily and 28 received 0.4 mg of tamsulosin daily. In the control groups, there were 29 and 21 cases, respectively. In the nifedipine and tamsulosin groups, the stone-free rates were 85.7 and 82.1%, respectively. And the stone-free rates in the control groups were 51.7 and 57.1 %, respectively. Post-ESWL medical expulsive therapy can facilitate passage of ureteral calculi, increase the stone-free rate at 1 and 2 months, and reduce the need of re-treatment.

In 2009, Seitz et al. [19] performed a meta-analysis of the randomized control experiments in which calcium or α-receptor blockers had been used, including studies with combined application of ESWL. The information was collected from the databases of MEDLINE, EMBASE, the Cochrane Central Register of Controlled Trials, and the Cochrane Database of Systematic Reviews. The authors found that α-receptor blockers could promote stone expulsion from the distal ureter and reduce the need of analgesic treatment of renal colic, as well as hospitalization time. The same results were recorded regardless of whether the patients had been treated with ESWL or not.

Ye et al. [20] compared the effectiveness of tamsulosin and nifedipine in the management of distal ureteral stones in a prospective randomized trial of 3,189 outpatients from 10 centers in China. The spontaneous stone expulsion rates in groups treated with tamsulosin and nifedipine were 95.9 and 73.5 %, respectively. The average time to stone expulsion for the tamsulosin and nifedipine groups was 78 and 138 h, respectively. The mean necessary consumption of diclofenac for episodes of renal colic was less in the tamsulosin group (52.35 mg) than in the nifedipine group (109.33 mg). Administration of tamsulosin and nifedipine as MET for ureteral stones with renal colic was concluded to be both safe and effective. However, tamsulosin was significantly better than nifedipine in relieving renal colic and facilitating ureteral stone expulsion [20].

Calcium Channel Antagonists

The basic functional unit of the ureter, the smooth muscle cell, reacts to changes in calcium concentration, exhibiting contraction when calcium concentrations rise and relaxation when calcium concentrations decrease. Ureteral calculi can induce ureter convulsion and thereby inhibit calculi expulsion. Ideal anticonvulsive agents should prevent incongruous contraction without influencing slow peristaltic activity. Previous studies have shown that calcium antagonists can inhibit the fast contraction phase of the animal and human ureter (i.e., convulsion) without effect on tonic activities [21, 22]. As a result, this type of drug was considered for use as a stone-passing facilitator. Nifedipine is a calcium channel antagonist with fewer reported adverse effects; this agent has therefore been the first-line choice for clinical investigation.

In 1994, Borghi et al. performed a randomized double-blind experiment in 86 patients with ureteral calculi smaller than 15 mm. The authors either used nifedipine with methylprednisolone or nifedipine with placebo. The results indicated that nifedipine with methylprednisolone increased the stone expulsion rate (nifedipine with methylprednisolone 86 % vs. nifedipine with placebo 65 %) and reduced expulsion duration (nifedipine with methylprednisolone 11.2±7.5 days vs. nifedipine with placebo 16.4±11.0 days) [23].

In 2007, Michael et al. administered tamsulosin post-ESWL to patients treated for upper and mid-ureteric stones and nifedipine post-ESWL for those treated with lower ureteric stones. Both treatments were effective in obtaining a greater stone clearance than in respective control arms of the study and reducing the need for a second session to attain stone-free status [18].

In the meta-analysis by Seitz et al. previously discussed, the same conclusion was reached; that is, calcium channel antagonists can promote expulsion of distal ureteral calculi, and reduce the need of analgesic treatment, the intensity of renal colic, and period of hospitalization [19].

Nonsteroidal Anti-inflammatory Drugs and Prostaglandin Synthesis Inhibitors

Ureteral calculi tend to cause obstruction, which is frequently worsened by accompanying ureteral inflammation. Such ureteral obstruction may increase pressure in the urine collection system and promote the secretion of prostaglandins. Prostaglandins can dilate the afferent arterioles and result in a series of responses including increased renal blood flow, subsequent pressure increase in the pelvis and ureter, as well as inflammation and further edema. These changes may result in renal colic and increase the sensitivity of nociceptors to chemical and mechanical stimuli, which in turn aggravates the pain. Experiments have documented that nonsteroidal anti-inflammatory agents can inhibit the synthesis of prostaglandins, reduce blood vessel dilation and inflammation, and decrease the glomerular filtration rate and consequently the intrarenal pressure [24]. At the same time, it has been proved that COX-2 inhibitors can inhibit release of prostaglandins and ureteral contraction [25], effects that help facilitate stone expulsion.

Although diclofenac and celecoxib did not promote stone expulsion in one randomized double-blind test, the two drugs did significantly prevent renal colic and hospitalization stays [26, 27]. The use of nonsteroidal anti-inflammatory drugs is still common in stone treatment and used with other pharmacological agents for stone expulsion.

Gonadal Hormones

Several types of gonadal hormones can affect the tension of the urinary tract. Estrogen affects α-receptors to increase the contraction of renal collecting system, bladder, and ureter, while progesterone affects β-receptors to reduce the tension of urinary tract, bladder, and ureter [28]. Progesterone acts by relaxing smooth muscles and inhibiting sympathetic nerve activity, thus reducing the pain impulses of sympathetic afferent fibers that innervate the kidneys and ureters. These effects of progesterone can produce analgesia and large volume diuresis, which aids calculi expulsion. By this effect, progesterone could theoretically be used as a calculi expulsion facilitator.

Despite this, studies on progesterone are rare. In 1988, Mikkelsen et al. [29] treated patients with ureteral calculi with 250 mg of hydroxyprogesterone for 8–10 days and recorded an effectiveness of 66 %. For patients with symptoms less than 3 weeks, the effectiveness was 75 %. Although there was no control group, the effectiveness rate was significantly higher than the spontaneous expulsion rate in the literature. The role of progesterone in stone expulsion remains to be demonstrated in further studies.

Glucocorticoids

As previously mentioned, edema is a noteworthy counteractive factor of stone expulsion. For this reason, glucocorticoids have been used as a pharmacological agent to reduce ureteral edema and promote stone expulsion. Glucocorticoids inhibit the release of prostaglandins, thus preventing or reducing stone-induced edema as well as the inflammatory response and ureteral convulsion. Clinical studies have indicated that glucocorticoids combined with α1-receptor blockers or calcium antagonists effectively promote calculi expulsion [30, 31]. Alone, however, glucocorticoids were not found to enhance the stone expulsion rate [32].

Traditional Chinese Medicine

Lysimachia christinae is a traditional Chinese medicine important for the removal of urinary stones by the following effects: diuresis, increased pressure in the renal pelvis and ureter, promotion of peristalsis in the ureter, inhibition of calcium oxalate crystal growth, nucleation and aggregation, and the lowering of urate concentration in serum. All of these effects might facilitate stone passage and counteract recurrent stone formation. Moreover, *Lysimachia christinae* also has protective properties against kidney damage [33].

Conclusion

In summary, pharmacological expulsive therapy used for appropriate patients can effectively increase stone expulsion rate and reduce both time to expulsion, as well as complications faced. This therapeutic approach may also reduce medical costs and periods of hospitalization. Statistical evidence has shown that α1-receptor blockers and calcium channel antagonists have a satisfactory effect in this regard. In combination with nonsteroidal anti-inflammatory drugs or prostaglandin synthetase inhibitors, glucocorticoids might prove beneficial to stone passage. Although medical expulsive therapy of urinary calculi has encouraging results, additional studies must be performed to further evaluate the role of current pharmacological agents and to develop new treatment approaches.

References

1. Lotan Y, Gettman MT, Roehrborn CG, Cadeddu JA, Pearle MS. Management of ureteral calculi: a cost comparison and decision making analysis. J Urol. 2002;167(4):1621–9.
2. Preminger GM, Tiselius HG, Assimos DG, Alken P, Buck C, Gallucci M, et al. 2007 guideline for the management of ureteral calculi. Eur Urol. 2007;52(6):1610–31.
3. John MH, Mary AMR, Samuel RK. Medical therapy to facilitate urinary stone passage:a meta-analysis. Lancet. 2006;368: 1171–9.
4. Segura JW, Preminger GM, Assimos DG, Dretler SP, Kahn RI, Lingeman JE, et al. Ureteral stones clinical guidelines panel summary report on the management of ureteral calculi. J Urol. 1997;158: 1915–21.
5. Ueno A, Kawamura T, Ogawa A, Takayasu H. Relation of spontaneous passage of ureteral calculi to size. Urology. 1977;10(6): 544–6.
6. Morita T, Ando M, Kihara K, Oshima H. Function and distribution of autonomic receptors in canine ureteral smooth muscle. Neurourol Urodyn. 1994;13:315–21.
7. Obara K, Takeda M, Shimura H, Kanai T, Tsutsui T, Komeyama T, et al. Alpha-1 adrenoreceptors subtypes in the human ureter. Characterization by RT-PCR and in situ hybridization. J Urol. 1996;155[Suppl]:472A.
8. Kinnman E, Nygards EB, Hansson P. Peripheral alpha-adrenoreceptors are involved in the development of capsaicin induced ongoing and stimulus evoked pain in humans. Pain. 1997;69(1–2): 79–85.
9. Dellabella M, Milanese G, Muzzonigro G. Randomized trial of the efficacy of tamsulosin, nifedipine and phloroglucinol in medical expulsive therapy for distal ureteral calculi. J Urol. 2005;174(1): 167–72.

10. Yasuda K, Yamanishi T, Tojo M, Nagashima K, Akimoto S, Shimazaki J. Effect of naftopidil on urethral obstruction in benign prostatic hyperplasia: assessment by urodynamic studies. Prostate. 1994;25:46–52.
11. Ukhal M, Malomuzh O, Strashny VV. Administration of doxazosin for speedy elimination of stones from lower section of ureter. Eur Urol. 1999;35 Suppl 2:4–6.
12. Cervenakov I, Fillo J, Mardiak J, Kopecny' M, Smirala J, Lepies P. Speedy elimination of ureterolithiasis in lower part of ureters with the alpha 1-blocker – tamsulosin. Int Urol Nephrol. 2002;34: 25–9.
13. Porpiglia F, Ghignone G, Fiori C, Fontana D, Scarpa RM. Nifedipine versus tamsulosin for the management of lower ureteral stones. J Urol. 2004;172(2):568–71.
14. Yilmaz E, Batislam E, Basar MM, Tuglu D, Ferhat M, Basar H. The comparison and efficacy of 3 different α1-adrenergic blockers for distal ureteral stones. J Urol. 2005;173:2010–2.
15. Erturhan S, Erbagci A, Yagci F, Celik M, Solakhan M, Sarica K. Comparative evaluation of efficacy of use of tamsulosin and/or tolterodine for medical treatment of distal ureteral stones. Urology. 2007;69(4):633–6.
16. Resim S, Ekerbicer H, Ciftci A. Role of tamsulosin in treatment of patients with steinstrasse developing after extracorporeal shock wave lithotripsy. Urology. 2005;5:945–94.
17. Gravina GL, Costa AM, Ronchi P, Galatioto GP, Angelucci A, Castellani D, et al. Tamsulosin treatment increases clinical success rate of single extracorporeal shock wave lithotripsy of renal stones. Urology. 2005;66:24–8.
18. Michael S, Grande M, Sighinolfi MC, De Stefani S, Bianchi G. Efficacy of expulsive therapy using nifedipine or tamsulosin, both associated with ketoprofene, after shock wave lithotripsy of ureteral stones. Urol Res. 2007;35:133–7.
19. Seitz C, Liatsikos E, Porpiglia F, Tiselius HG, Zwergel U. Medical therapy to facilitate the passage of stones: what is the evidence? Eur Urol. 2009;56:455–71.
20. Ye Z, Yang H, Li H, Zhang X, Deng Y, Zeng G, et al. A multicentre, prospective, randomized trial: comparative efficacy of tamsulosin and nifedipine in medical expulsive therapy for distal ureteric stones with renal colic. BJU Int. 2011;108(2):276–9.
21. Andersson KE, Forman A. Effects of calcium channels blockers on urinary tract smooth muscle. Acta Pharmacol Toxicol. 1986;58 Suppl 2:193–200.
22. Hannappel J, Rohrmann D, Lutzeyer W. Pharmacologic modifications of ureteral activity. Urologe A. 1986;25:246–51.
23. Borghi L, Meschi T, Amato F, Novarini A, Giannini A, Quarantelli C, et al. Nifedipine and methylprednisolone in facilitating ureteral stone passage: a randomized, double-blind, placebo-controlled study. J Urol. 1994;152(4):1099–100.
24. Ahmad M, Chaughtai MN, Kahn FA. Role of prostaglandin synthesis inhibitors in the passage of ureteric calculus. J Pak Med Assoc. 1991;41:268–70.
25. Jerde TJ, Calamon-Dixon JL, Bjorling DE, Nakada SY. Celecoxib inhibits ureteral contractility and prostanoid release. Urology. 2005;65:185–90.
26. Laerum E, Ommundsen OE, Gronseth JE, Christiansen A, Fagertun HE. Oral diclofenac in the prophylactic treatment of recurrent renal colic: a double-blind comparison with placebo. Eur Urol. 1995;28:108–11.
27. Phillips E, Hinck B, Pedro R, Makhlouf A, Kriedberg C, Hendlin K, et al. Celecoxib in the management of acute renal colic: a randomized controlled clinical trial. Urology. 2009;74:994–9.
28. Miodrag A, Castleden CM, Vallance TR. Sex hormones and the female urinary tract. Drugs. 1988;36(4):491–504.
29. Mikkelsen AL, Meyhoff HH, Lindahl F, Christensen J. The effect of hydroxyprogesterone on ureteral stones. Int Urol Nephrol. 1988;20(3):257–60.
30. Salehi M, Fouladi Mehr M, Shiery H, et al. Does methylprednisolone acetate increase the success rate of medical therapy for passing distal ureteral stones? Eur Urol Suppl. 2005;4(3):25.
31. Porpiglia F, Destefanis P, Fioric C, Fontana D. Effectiveness of nifedipine and deflazacort in the management of distal ureter stones. Urology. 2000;56(4):579–82.
32. Porpiglia F, Vaccino D, Billia M, Renard J, Cracco C, Ghignone G, et al. Corticosteroids and tamsulosin in the medical expulsive therapy for symptomatic distal ureter stones: single drug or association? Eur Urol. 2006;50:339–44.
33. Hua-fang C. Effects and mechanisms of *Lysimachia christinae* on urolithus treatment. Natl Med Front China. 2010;5(12):7–8.

Dissolution of Stones by Oral and Irrigative Therapy

66

Ruslan Korets, Joseph A. Graversen, and Mantu Gupta

Abstract

Advancement in percutaneous and endoscopic techniques has revolutionized surgical treatment options for upper and lower urinary tract calculi. However, while the use of oral and irrigative therapies for stone dissolution has declined over the last decades, these therapies continue to serve as a safe alternative to surgery, especially in patients with significant comorbidities. This chapter examines principles of chemolysis for component-specific stone dissolution including pH manipulation, cation chelation, and mixed disulfide bond formation, as well as setup and deployment of percutaneous irrigation systems.

Keywords

Chemolysis • Stone dissolution • Urinary alkalinization • Irrigation system • Uric acid Struvite • Cystine • Potassium citrate • Hemiacidrin • Acetohydroxamic acid • THAM Alpha-mercaptopropionylglycine • D-penicillamine

Introduction

With the development of minimally invasive procedures such as shock wave lithotripsy (SWL), ureteroscopy, and percutaneous nephrolithotomy (PNL), treatment of urolithiasis has changed dramatically. While open renal surgery for urinary calculi is now rarely employed, chemolysis with systemic or irrigative therapy may still play a role in the management of urinary calculi. There are several factors that determine whether dissolution therapy can be performed. The first is the chemical composition and molecular structure of the stone. More amorphous minerals such as struvite will enter the solution much faster than will highly crystalline salts such as calcium oxalate [1]. Additionally, the surface area exposed to the chemolytic agent affects the time to complete dissolution. For example, large single stones (with a smaller exposed surface area/volume) will dissolve slower than multiple smaller stones with a similar combined volume (because of the greater exposed surface area). Chemolysis involves increasing dissolution kinetics of the stone and can be achieved through a variety of means including pH manipulation, chelation, and disulfide rearrangement.

Oral Chemolytic Therapy

Uric Acid Stones

Uric acid is a weak organic acid with a pK_a of 5.4 that precipitates to form uric acid crystals in an acidic renal environment. When in solution, it is present in two forms: as an undissociated acid and as urate anion. Alkalinization shifts the equilibrium from undissociated acid to urate, which is significantly more soluble. As a result, a urinary pH change from 5.0 to 6.5 makes uric acid 11 times more soluble and therefore more

R. Korets, M.D. • J.A. Graversen, M.D.
Department of Urology, Columbia University College of Physicians and Surgeons, New York Presbyterian Hospital Kidney Stone Center, New York, NY, USA
e-mail: rk317@columbia.edu

M. Gupta, M.D. (✉)
Director of Endourology, Columbia University and NYPH Kidney Stone Center,
New York, NY, USA
e-mail: mg392@columbia.edu

J.J. Talati et al. (eds.), *Urolithiasis*,
DOI 10.1007/978-1-4471-4387-1_66, © Springer-Verlag London 2012

Table 66.1 Oral pharmacotherapy for urinary calculi chemolysis

Drug	Mechanism of action	Stone type	Dose
Potassium citrate	Alkalinization of urine/decreases urinary calcium supersaturation	Uric acid, calcium oxalate	10 mEq TID
Sodium bicarbonate	Increases uric acid solubility by raising urinary pH	Uric acid	650–1,950 mg PO q4h
AHA (acetohydroxamic acid)	Inhibits urease production by urea-splitting bacteria/decreases ammonium production in urine	Struvite	250 mg TID
D-penicillamine	Forms a mixed disulfide bond with cystine, promoting cystine dissolution	Cystine	250–500 mg QID
Alpha-mercaptopropionylglycine (α-MPG)		Cystine	200–400 mg TID

likely to remain suspended in solution [1]. Urinary alkalization to a pH above 6.5 can be accomplished by the oral administration of sodium bicarbonate or potassium citrate. Of the two, potassium citrate is preferable to that of sodium bicarbonate. The increased sodium load associated with $NaHCO_3$ can cause increased urinary calcium excretion and thereby calcium stone formation. Contrarily, potassium citrate gets metabolized to bicarbonate, thus raising urinary pH levels without an associated sodium load. Furthermore, citrate has the additional benefit of decreasing urinary calcium supersaturation by combining with calcium ions to form a complex that is more soluble than calcium oxalate [2, 3].

Several studies have reported on symptomatic stone recurrences, with highest recurrence rates reported following SWL therapy (36.5 %) [4] compared to symptomatic events following ureteroscopy (19.6 %) [5] and PNL (26.3 %) [6]. Because of inherent morbidity and higher healthcare costs associated with secondary surgical interventions [7], oral chemolytic therapy administered in an adjuvant setting may be helpful in preventing symptomatic stone recurrence (Table 66.1). Two randomized-control studies have shown that patients with residual fragments receiving potassium citrate after SWL had higher clearance rates (80–100 %) compared to controls (66–72 %) [8, 9]. Similarly, Kang et al. found decreased stone formation rates in patients receiving medical therapy after undergoing PNL, independent of whether they had residual fragments or were stone-free at the end of the case [10]. Medical therapy consisted of potassium citrate for patients with hypocitraturia or renal tubular acidosis, thiazide diuretics in patients with hypercalciuria, or allopurinol in patients with hyperuricosuria. In summary, adjuvant medical therapy following surgical intervention may be an effective strategy to decrease residual stone burden and prevent new stone growth.

Struvite Stones

Struvite stones account for 10–15 % of all urinary calculi. Struvite stones typically form in urine infected with urea-splitting bacteria and are composed of magnesium ammonium phosphate and carbonate apatite. These bacteria catalyze hydrolysis of urea into ammonium, bicarbonate, and hydroxyl equivalents. Ammonium combines with trivalent phosphates that are excreted by the renal tubules resulting in struvite crystal formation.

The most commonly used oral agent, acetohydroxamic acid (AHA), irreversibly inhibits urease production by bacteria. This causes inhibition of urea hydrolysis leading to reduced ammonium production in the urine. However, reversing the chemical conditions that permit struvite and carbonate apatite to form usually rarely causes dissolution of existing stones, though it does inhibit new stone growth. In a study by Griffith et al., 17 % of patients receiving AHA experienced stone growth, compared to 46 % receiving placebo [11].

Side effects of AHA administration include gastrointestinal upset, headaches, weakness, hemolytic anemia, and neuropathy. A dose reduction is indicated for patients with mild renal impairment and is contraindicated in severe renal insufficiency (CrCl < 20) and pregnancy.

Cystine Stones

Cystine stones are rare, accounting for less than 1 % of all renal calculi. However, oral dissolution of cystine stones can be challenging and requires a high degree of patient compliance. The main objective of treatment for cystinuria is to lower urinary cystine concentration below its solubility point (<250 mg/L). First-line treatment involves increasing fluid intake to maintain urine output of 2.5 L or more, along with the administration of an oral alkali, such as potassium citrate, to raise urinary pH to 6.5–7.0. If conservative therapy fails, cystine chelators such as D-penicillamine or alpha-mercaptopropionylglycine (α[alpha]-MPG) can be added [12]. These agents form a thiol-cystine mixed disulfide bond, which is up to 50 times more soluble than the pure disulfide bonds of cystine stones. In more than 60 % of patients, oral thiol administration has been associated with side effects that include dermatitis, pancytopenia, arthralgia, nephritic syndrome, as well as significant gastrointestinal side effects (abdominal pain, nausea, vomiting, and diarrhea). And while α-MPG is better tolerated than D-penicillamine, about one-third of patients in one study were still unable to tolerate α-MPG therapy [13].

Despite its side effects, several studies have reported on the effectiveness of urinary alkalization coupled with thiol therapy for cystine stone dissolution [14, 15]. In the study by Pareek et al., surgical intervention rates were compared between cystinuria patients who were compliant with a strict oral dissolution regimen and a second group of noncompliant patients [16]. Medical therapy consisted of urinary alkalization with potassium citrate and a cystine chelator, with the goal of decreasing in urinary cystine to levels below 300 mg/L. After a mean follow-up of 43 months, patients that adhered to medical therapy were four times less likely to undergo a surgical intervention compared to noncompliant patients.

Calcium Oxalate

Calcium oxalate stones are the most common type of stone in industrialized countries. Unfortunately, the need for extreme pH changes to resuspend precipitated crystals also makes CaOx stones the least amenable to oral dissolution. Use of a chelating agent, ethylenediaminetetraacetic acid (EDTA), for calcium calculi dissolution has been reported by several groups, with success rates ranging from 30 to 66 % [17–20]. The deleterious effects of EDTA on urothelial mucosa, however, limit its applicability [21]. As a result, other modalities should be considered when dealing with these calculi.

Irrigative Therapy

With the advent of flexible nephroscopy, irrigative dissolution techniques are now utilized less often; some of the solutions that are discussed in this section may no longer be available. Stone dissolution by direct irrigation was first reported by Crowell in 1924 [22]. Two decades later, Howard Suby and Fuller Albright described using intermittent instillation of Suby G solution for dissolution of calcium phosphate calculi [23]. In 1959, Mulvany made further modifications to the Suby solution with the addition of citric, malonic, and gluconic acids as well as magnesium hydrocarbonate to create hemiacidrin solution [24]. Both hemiacidrin and Suby G solutions form complexes with calcium and phosphate in the stone, promoting dissolution. Furthermore, the relatively low pH of these solutions is advantageous in struvite dissolution.

Calculi can be dissolved in vitro by manipulation of the chemistry of the bathing solution.

However, for an effective solution to be used in vivo, the irrigant must (1) be compatible with biological tissue, (2) not cause significant precipitation of other minerals, (3) dissolve stones in a timely fashion, and (4) there must not be systemic absorption of any substance that may be toxic. The irrigation system must maintain low renal pelvic pressures, so as to preclude pyelovenous backflow and risk of bacteremia [25]. As long as the renal pelvic pressure is maintained below 25 cm H_2O, pyelovenous backflow is unlikely to occur.

The basic irrigation system involves a method of washing the stone in the chemolytic agent, a pressure "pop-off" valve, and a simple tolerability test. A three-way valve on the irrigation catheter with a vent approximately 25 cm above the renal pelvis ensures low intrarenal pressures [26]. After waiting 24 h to allow the skin to seal around the tube, infusion of normal saline at 30 mL/h is started. The patient is monitored for any signs of discomfort and to ensure that the system is functioning properly. The infusion rate is then slowly increased up to 125 mL/h as long as the patient remains pain free, and the intrarenal pressure does not exceed 25 cm of H_2O. To ensure that the infused irrigant reaches the stone, patient positioning and catheter manipulation may be necessary. For example, a seated position may be helpful to maximize dissolution of lower pole stones, while having the patient lie supine or in mild Trendelenburg position may assist in dissolution of upper pole calculi [27].

Uric Acid Dissolution

Urinary alkalization with oral therapy is the preferred method for uric acid dissolution. However, in certain instances where the patient cannot tolerate the dose necessary to alkalize their urine or is noncompliant with oral therapy, irrigative therapy can be employed. The three most commonly used alkalinizing irrigants are sodium bicarbonate (pH 7.0–8.0), tromethamine (THAM, pH 8.6), and THAM-E (pH 10.5) [28]. Due to an increased risk of calcium and phosphate precipitation with bicarbonate use, and the potential for urothelial toxicity from the high pH associated with THAM-E use [29], THAM is the preferred agent of choice for uric acid dissolution.

Cystine Stones

Irrigative chemolysis of cystine stones poses a significant challenge due to the relatively high pH and lengthy periods of irrigative therapy that are required for dissolution. As a result, there is no consensus as to the best agent for cystine stone dissolution. Several publications have reported on successful dissolution of cystine with THAM-E alone [30], 0.3-M solution of *N*-acetylcysteine in THAM-E [31], penicillamine [32], and α(alpha)-MPG [21], with some therapies taking as long as 6 months. It has been estimated that 9 days of irrigative therapy are necessary to dissolve a 1-cm stone. As a result, irrigative dissolution of cystine stones should be performed for small stone burden or as an adjunct to PNL or SWL therapy.

Struvite Stones

Irrigative therapy for struvite dissolution is significantly more effective than oral therapy. Struvite stones will dissolve in an acidic environment; however, this process can take weeks to months with oral therapy alone. Stronger acids hasten the process, but cannot be taken orally. Contrarily, hemiacidrin and Suby G solution have a pH of approximately 4.0, and renal pelvis irrigation rapidly lowers the pH to allow for struvite dissolution.

The successful use of hemiacidrin irrigation as primary therapy has been reported by Dretler and Pfister [33]. However, modern endourological technology and techniques have relegated irrigative therapy to an adjuvant role. In this setting, irrigation ensures stone-free status, shorter treatment durations, and decreased urothelial irritation that is often seen with more intense therapy [34].

Due to the presence of bacteria in these stones, it is of paramount importance that patients be monitored to ensure that the system has adequate drainage and the intrapelvic pressure does not exceed 25 cm of water. Preoperative antibiotics may be of benefit, but unfortunately bladder cultures are known to have poor correlation with stone and renal pelvis cultures [35]. If flank pain or fever develops, irrigation must be immediately stopped. Patients with renal insufficiency undergoing hemiacidrin irrigation should be monitored for signs of hypermagnesemia (respiratory depression, hyporeflexia, and mental status changes) [36].

Conclusion

Effective primary oral dissolution therapy is limited to the alkalinization of urine for the treatment of uric acid stones. Oral alkalinization with potassium citrate also has a preventive role for the treatment stones. The use of chemolytic irrigative modalities has been demonstrated to be both well tolerated and efficacious; however, modern techniques have relegated irrigation to more of an adjuvant role. The benefits of adjuvant irrigation include improved stone-free rates, shorter therapy times, and less urothelial irritation from the chemolytic agent.

References

1. Rodman JS, Williams JJ, Peterson CM. Dissolution of uric acid calculi. J Urol. 1984;131(6):1039–44.
2. Meyer JL, Smith LH. Growth of calcium oxalate crystals. II. Inhibition by natural urinary crystal growth inhibitors. Invest Urol. 1975;13(1):36–9.
3. Tiselius HG, Fornander AM, Nilsson MA. The effects of citrate and urine on calcium oxalate crystal aggregation. Urol Res. 1993;21(5):363–6.
4. Krambeck AE, LeRoy AJ, Patterson DE, Gettman MT. Long-term outcomes of percutaneous nephrolithotomy compared to shock wave lithotripsy and conservative management. J Urol. 2008;179(6):2233–7.
5. Rebuck DA, Macejko A, Bhalani V, Ramos P, Nadler RB. The natural history of renal stone fragments following ureteroscopy. Urology. 2011;77(3):564–8.
6. Altunrende F, Tefekli A, Stein RJ, Autorino R, Yuruk E, Laydner H, et al. Clinically insignificant residual fragments after percutaneous nephrolithotomy: medium-term follow-up. J Endourol. 2011;25(6):941–5.
7. Raman JD, Bagrodia A, Bensalah K, Pearle MS, Lotan Y. Residual fragments after percutaneous nephrolithotomy: cost comparison of immediate second look flexible nephroscopy versus expectant management. J Urol. 2009;183(1):188–93.
8. Cicerello E, Merlo F, Gambaro G, Maccatrozzo L, Fandella A, Baggio B, et al. Effect of alkaline citrate therapy on clearance of residual renal stone fragments after extracorporeal shock wave lithotripsy in sterile calcium and infection nephrolithiasis patients. J Urol. 1994;151(1):5–9.
9. Soygur T, Akbay A, Kupeli S. Effect of potassium citrate therapy on stone recurrence and residual fragments after shockwave lithotripsy in lower caliceal calcium oxalate urolithiasis: a randomized controlled trial. J Endourol. 2002;16(3):149–52.
10. Kang DE, Maloney MM, Haleblian GE, Springhart WP, Honeycutt EF, Eisenstein EL, et al. Effect of medical management on recurrent stone formation following percutaneous nephrolithotomy. J Urol. 2007;177(5):1785–8; discussion 1788–9.
11. Griffith DP, Gleeson MJ, Lee H, Longuet R, Deman E, Earle N. Randomized, double-blind trial of Lithostat (acetohydroxamic acid) in the palliative treatment of infection-induced urinary calculi. Eur Urol. 1991;20(3):243–7.
12. Gupta M, Bolton DM, Stoller ML. Etiology and management of cystine lithiasis. Urology. 1995;45(2):344–55.
13. Pak CY, Fuller C, Sakhaee K, Zerwekh JE, Adams BV. Management of cystine nephrolithiasis with alpha-mercaptopropionylglycine. J Urol. 1986;136(5):1003–8.
14. Barbey F, Joly D, Rieu P, Mejean A, Daudon M, Jungers P. Medical treatment of cystinuria: critical reappraisal of long-term results. J Urol. 2000;163(5):1419–23.
15. Pietrow PK, Auge BK, Weizer AZ, Delvecchio FC, Silverstein AD, Mathias B, et al. Durability of the medical management of cystinuria. J Urol. 2003;169(1):68–70.
16. Pareek G, Steele TH, Nakada SY. Urological intervention in patients with cystinuria is decreased with medical compliance. J Urol. 2005;174(6):2250–2. discussion 2.
17. Burns JR, Cargill 3rd JG. Kinetics of dissolution of calcium oxalate calculi with calcium-chelating irrigating solutions. J Urol. 1987;137(3):530–3.
18. Heap GJ, Perrin DD, Cliff WJ. Dissolving urinary stones with a chelating agent. Med J Aust. 1976;1(19):714–5.
19. Timmermann A, Kallistratos G. Modern aspects of chemical dissolution of human renal calculi by irrigation. J Urol. 1966;95(4):469–75.
20. Timmermann A, Kallistratos G. Chemotherapy in nephrolithiasis. Isr J Med Sci. 1971;7(5):689–95.
21. Kane MH, Rodman JS, Horten B, Reckler J, Marion D, Vaughan Jr ED. Urothelial injury from ethylenediaminetetraacetic acid used as an irrigant in the urinary tract. J Urol. 1989;142(5):1359–60.
22. Crowell A. Cystine nephrolithiasis report of ease with roentgenographic demonstration of disintigration of stone by alkanizaiton. Surg Gynecol Obstet. 1924;38:87.
23. Suby HI, Albright F. Dissolution of phosphatic urinary calculi by the retrograde introduction of a citrate solution containing magnesium. N Engl J Med. 1943;228(3):81–91.

24. Mulvaney WP. A new solvent for certain urinary calculi: a preliminary report. J Urol. 1959;82:546–8.
25. Dretler SP, Pfister RC. Percutaneous dissolution of renal calculi. Annu Rev Med. 1983;34:359–66.
26. Rodman JS, Williams JJ. Adjunctive therapy for struvite stone management. Infect Surg. 1985;4:867–74.
27. Rodman JS, Reckler JM, Israel AR. Hemiacidrin irrigations to dissolve stone remnants after nephrolithotomy. Problems with solution flow. Urology. 1981;18(2):127–30.
28. Sadi MV, Saltzman N, Feria G, Gittes RF. Experimental observations on dissolution of uric acid calculi. J Urol. 1985;134(3): 575–9.
29. Chernesky CE, Rodman JS, Reckler J, Rotterdam H, Marion D, Boolbol J, et al. Urothelial injury to the rabbit bladder from alkaline irrigants useful in the treatment of uric acid stones. J Urol. 1987;138(4):893–4.
30. Singer A, Das S. Cystinuria: a review of the pathophysiology and management. J Urol. 1989;142(3):669–73.
31. Saltzman N, Gittes RF. Chemolysis of cystine calculi. J Urol. 1986;136(4):846–9.
32. Stark H, Savir A. Dissolution of cystine calculi by pelviocaliceal irrigation with D-penicillamine. J Urol. 1980;124(6):895–8.
33. Dretler SP, Pfister RC. Primary dissolution therapy of struvite calculi. J Urol. 1984;131(5):861–3.
34. Reckler J, Rodman JS, Jacobs D, Rotterdam H, Marion D, Vaughan Jr ED. Urothelial injury to the rabbit bladder from various alkaline and acidic solutions used to dissolve kidney stones. J Urol. 1986;136(1):181–3.
35. Korets R, Graversen J, Kates M, Mues A, Gupta M. Post-PCNL systemic inflammatory response: a prospective analysis of preoperative urine, renal pelvic urine, and stone cultures. J Urol. 2011;186:1899–903.
36. Cato AR, Tulloch AG. Hypermagnesemia in a uremic patient during renal pelvis irrigation with renacidin. J Urol. 1974;111(3): 313–4.

Traditional Chinese Medicine for Treatment of Urinary Stones

67

Xiao He

Abstract

This chapter describes the use of traditional Chinese medicine in treatment of patients with urinary stones. The diagnosis and treatment of urinary stone disease has a long history in China. The disease is classified into six types by Liqiang. The chapter describes the pharmacological mechanism of *Lysimachia christina* and some commonly used clinical medicines.

Keywords

Traditional Chinese medicine • Urolithiasis • *Shi Lin* • *Lysimachia christinae* • *Desmodium styracifolium* (Osh.) Merr. • *Glechoma longituba* (Nakai) Kupr. • Niao Shitong • Pai Shi • *Spora lygodii* • Semen plantaginis • *Folium pyrroslae* • Talcum • *Chingma abutilon* seed flavonoids • Triterpenoids

Introduction

The diagnosis and treatment of urinary stone disease has a long history in China, recorded in ancient Chinese medical literature. In the Canon of Internal Medicine, urolithiasis, especially the condition associated with irritant symptoms from the bladder caused by bladder stones, was called *Lin* [1, 2]. In the Han Dynasty, Hua Tuo (the author of *Zhong Zang Jing*) termed the condition where fine particulate matter ("sand") and stones were discharged through the urethra as *Sha Lin*, and he described in detail the symptoms as well as the size and color of different stones. The mechanism of stone formation was considered similar to that when salt is boiled in water—stones were formed at high (environmental) temperatures when urinary volumes decreased—similar to the current view of crystallization in supersaturated solutions. In the Sui Dynasty, Chao Yuanfang (the author of *General Treatise on the Causes and Syndromes of Disease*) concluded that stones were caused by kidney failure and bladder heat. In the Ming Dynasty, Yu Tuan (the author of *Yixue Zhengchuan*) for the first time presented the relationship between diet (food of damp and heat, such as fat meat and fine grain, liquor, and roast) and *Shi Lin*, which is the same as the international view on the etiological role of sugar, alcoholic drink, and meat.

X. He, MB
Department of Urology, Peking Union Medical College Hospital, No 1, Shuaifuyuan Wangfujing, Beijing, 100730, China
e-mail: pumchxiaohe@hotmail.com

Etiology and Pathogenesis

In Chinese traditional medicine, urolithiasis is thought to be mainly caused by kidney *qi* deficiency, impaired kidney *yang*, damp-heat retention and fumigation in lower *Jiao*, and *qi* stagnation and blood stasis. Among these factors, kidney deficiency, damp and heat, *qi* stagnation, and stasis are considered crucial. Stone disease accordingly is classified into six types by Li Qiang [3]:

- *Qi stagnation and damp-heat type*: treated by clearing of heat, regulation of *qi*, dissipation of dampness, induction of diuresis, and removal of stones
- *Qi stagnation and blood stasis type:* treated by promotion of *qi* and removal of stasis, relief of stranguria and removal of the stones, as well as dissipation of dampness and heat

J.J. Talati et al. (eds.), *Urolithiasis*,
DOI 10.1007/978-1-4471-4387-1_67, © Springer-Verlag London 2012

- *Spleen-kidney deficiency and damp-heat retention type*: treated by strengthening of spleen and kidney functions and by clearance and relief of stranguria
- *Kidney yin deficiency type*: treated by nourishing the *yin* and kidney, by induction of diuresis, relief of stranguria, and removal of dampness and heat
- *Kidney yang deficiency type*: treated by tonifying spleen and kidney and by inducing diuresis and relieving stranguria
- *Spleen-kidney deficiency type*: treated by enforcing the spleen and nourishing the kidney, relieving stranguria, removing the stones, and regulating *qi*

Traditional Chinese Medicines

Herbs capable of clearing heat and promoting diuresis, relieving stranguria, and removing the stones—such as *Herba lysimachiae*, *Spora lygodii*, semen *Plantaginis*, folium *Pyrrosia*, talcum, and chingma *Abutilon* seed—were commonly used for treatment of urinary stones by doctors even in the past dynasties. Attributable to the identified effects, *Herba lysimachiae* became the first choice for treating patients with urinary stones, and this agent has achieved a reputation as a "stone decomposition miracle."

Herba lysimachiae—a commonly used herb for treating patients with urinary stones—has many varieties. According to the origin and function, this agent can be classified into *Lysimachia christinae Hance*, *Desmodium styracifolium* (Osh.) Merr., and *Glechoma longituba* (Nakai) Kupr. *Herba lysimachiae* mainly contains flavonoids, amino acids, choline, tannin, sterols, potassium chloride, and lactones. Among them, flavonoids are the main component of *Herba lysimachiae*.

Pharmacological Mechanism of Action of *Lysimachia christina*

This herb preparation has the following properties:

1. Increased ureteral peristalsis and urine output: After intravenous injection of a decoction or an extract of *Lysimachia christina* or following its experimental introduction into the duodenum of anesthetized dogs, increased ureteral peristalsis is seen. Additionally, the urine flow increases to a level similar to that obtained following administration of hydrochlorothiazide.
2. Inhibition of the crystallization process: The polysaccharide component of *Lysimachia christina* has an inhibitory effect on calcium oxalate monohydrate crystal growth. In the absence of seed crystals, the polysaccharide component of *Lysimachia christina* can delay the nucleation of calcium oxalate monohydrate. The prolongation of the crystallization induction period is directly proportional to the concentration of the administered drug.
3. Changes in urine pH: *Lysimachia christina* can help to make blood and urine acidic and dissolve those urinary stones that form and exist in an alkaline environment. The preparation can also decrease crystal growth rate and reduce the degree of crystal aggregation. In addition, *Lysimachia christina* also has an anti-inflammatory, analgesic, antibacterial, and antioxidant effects. Lipid peroxidation in the liver is counteracted.

Wang Yongquan et al. carried out an inhibition experiment in kidneys with calcium oxalate stones [4]. They injected decoctions or extracts of *Lysimachia christina* and, using transmission electron microscopy, showed that *Lysimachia christina* reduced ethylene glycol-induced renal tubular cell disintegration and necrosis. Furthermore, it reduced the debris in the renal tubular cavity. The oxalate and calcium concentration in kidney tissue was 1.40 ± 0.86 mg/g (15.6 μmol/g) and 3.99 ± 1.28 μmol/g, respectively, in the injection group and 5.67 ± 0.70 mg/g (63.0 μmol/g) and 8.62 ± 1.44 μmol/g, respectively, in the extract group. All values were significantly lower than those recorded in the untreated stone group ($p < 0.05$). Polarizing microscopy showed that the number of calcium oxalate crystals in the treated groups was significantly smaller than that in the untreated renal stone-forming group. Therefore, *Lysimachia christina* was considered to have a significant inhibitory effect on the formation of calcium oxalate crystals.

Wang Ping and coworkers studied the effect of extracts of *Lysimachia christinae* on calcium oxalate crystal growth in urine from healthy subjects. The gained crystals were characterized by scanning electron microscopy (SEM), Fourier transform infrared spectroscopy (FT-R), and X-ray diffraction analysis (XRD). The result indicated that different crystal phases appeared in urine from healthy subjects, such as calcium oxalate monohydrate (COM) and calcium oxalate dihydrate (COD). When the extract of *Lysimachia christinae* was added to healthy urine, COM crystals disappeared completely, the shape of COD crystals changed, and their size apparently was reduced when the concentration of *Lysimachia christinae* extract increased in urine. These results suggested that extracts of *Lysimachia christinae* might prohibit the formation of urinary stones.

Lysimachia christinae with its remarkable clinical efficacy has been the preferred medicine for urinary stones. At present in the clinical practice, the conventional daily dosage of *Lysimachia christinae* is 15–30 g, but many masters use even larger doses in the treatment of patients with urinary stones.

Through the proven long-term clinical efficacy and practical experience predominantly of *Lysimachia christinae*, several other Chinese traditional medical preparations have been developed. The following clinical medicines are commonly used: Niao Shitong soluble granules, Pai Shi granules, etc.

Niao Shitong Soluble Granules

This medicine is mainly composed of *Lysimachia christinae*, *Spora lygodii*, endothelium corneum gigeriae galli, radix *Paeoniae rubra*, radix *Angelicae sinensis*, and radix astragali [5]. An Gang reports on 200 cases of urinary stone patients undergoing shock wave lithotripsy divided randomly into 2 groups—a treatment group and a control group [6]. All patients in the treatment group were given Niao Shitong soluble granules after extracorporeal shock wave lithotripsy. The clinical outcome was much better in the treatment group than in the control group, and the difference was statistically significant ($p<0.05$).

Pai Shi Granules

The most important components of this medicine are *Lysimachia christinae*, *Spora lygodii*, herba dianthi, *Chingma abutilon* seed, talcum, *Folium pyrroslae*, endothelium corneum gigeriae galli, amber, radix curcumae, spica prunellae, processed carapax trionycis, and herba plantaginis. Pai Shi granules were used by Su Peiyan in the treatment of urinary stones in 122 cases of small ureteral stones (<0.8 cm) diagnosed by ultrasound [7]. In 113 of these patients the treatment was successful (92.6 %), in 3 patients the condition was improved (2.5 %), and in 6 cases the treatment failed (4.9 %). The total effective rate was thus 95.1 %.

Research continues into the mechanisms of action of extracts of traditional Chinese medicines [8–10]. Two examples are given as follows.

Hirayama et al. noted that a triterpenoid (Ds-t) extracted from *Desmodium styracifolium* (Osbeck) Merr. has an inhibitory effect on the formation of ethylene glycol-vitamin 1 alpha D3 (EO-D3) induced calcium oxalate renal stones [9]. Eighty-one percent of the control group (who received only EO-D3) developed renal stones, while only 29 % of those treated with Ds-t in addition to EO-D3 formed stones. Hirayama noted that Ds-t increased urinary volume, decreased the excretion of calcium, and increased the urinary excretion of citrate and concluded that Ds-t may be useful in preventing the recurrence of urinary Ca oxalate stones in the clinical setting.

Sheng, using a decoction of six drugs containing rhizoma *Rehmanniae preparata* and supplements of other traditional Chinese medicinal herbs, proved that they exerted a protective effect against renal injury induced by shock waves in rabbits [10]. They noted a much smaller increase in post-ESWL plasma nitric oxide (NO), endothelin-1 (ET-1), malondialdehyde (MDA), and serum tumor necrosis factor-- α(alpha) (TNF-α) in the medicated group as compared to controls ($p<0.05$).

Conclusion

Chinese traditional medicines have beneficial effects in the treatment of patients with urinary stones, with the advantages of good efficacy, low price, and absence of side effects. These medicines may also have a potential additional role in the treatment of stones. When combined with Western methods of treatment (such as SWL), their renoprotective effects, increase of ureteric peristalsis, the induced dieresis, and change of pH may all combine to enhance the safety and effectiveness of such treatments, reducing renal damage and increasing stone-free rates [11]. Such combination therapies might provide an effective way to improve the effectiveness of therapeutic measures for urolithiasis.

References

1. Wu X, Zeng B, Shu Y. Prescription after syndrome differentiation for treatment of urinary stone disease. New Chin Tradit Med. 1998;30(5):32–3.
2. Wang K, Guo J. Development of traditional Chinese medicine in treatment of urinary stones. Med Recapitulate. 2009;15(11):1716–8.
3. Li Q, Lu Y, Liu L. Professor Lai Zhentian's clinical experience for treatment of urinary stones disease. New Chin Tradit Med. 2002; 33(7):9–10.
4. Wang Y, Zhu B, An R, Qi Y, Li C. Inhibitory effect of *Desmodium styracifolium* (Ds) injection on calcium oxalate renal stone formation. Chinese J Urol. 1999;20(11):689–91.
5. Peng H. Niao Shitong soluble granules for treatment of 76 cases of urinary stone disease. Pract Tradit Chin Med. 2011;27(8):526.
6. An G. Clinical observation of Niao Shitong soluble granules in patients with urinary stones after lithotripsy. Health Digest. 2008; 5(9):49–50.
7. Su P, Sheng Z, Zhang H. Pai Shi granules for treatment of 122 cases of ureteral stones. State Medical Forum. 2007;5:38.
8. He Z, Cao L. The prevention and treatment of urolithiasis of flavored eight from the changes of surface zeta potential of calcium oxalate crystals. Chinese J Urol. 1991;12(1):51–3.
9. Hirayama H, Wang Z, Nishi K, Ogawa A, Ishimatu T, Ueda S, et al. Effect of *Desmodium styracifolium*-triterpenoid on calcium oxalate renal stones. Br J Urol. 1993;71(2):143–7.
10. Sheng B, He D, Zhao J, Chen X, Nan X. The protective effects of the traditional Chinese herbs against renal damage induced by extracorporeal shock wave lithotripsy: a clinical study. Urol Res. 2011;39(2):89–97. Epub 2010 Jul 6.
11. Yu Z, Que D, Xiaocheng J, et al. Holmium laser lithotripsy with traditional Chinese medicine for treatment of ureteral and bladder stones in 60 patients. Tradit Chin Med He Bei Province. 2007; 9(12):1084–5.

Patient Safety and the Importance of Informed Consent

68

Robyna Irshad Khan

Abstract

Safety of the patients in health care is a subject that has received significant attention over the last decade. This attention stemmed from the realization that human beings are bound to make errors. However, these errors can be considerably decreased if systems are changed appropriately. Multiple factors have been identified for reducing errors and improving safe practices in clinical care. One of these factors is procurement of well-understood informed consent, especially from patients having language barriers or low health literacy. In order to achieve this objective, various methods have been suggested. "Teach-back" is one such method, where patients or family members are requested to teach the health-care providers, in their own words, what they have understood during the consent process. This and other measures used to procure a well-understood informed consent have shown a significant decrease in the incidence of medical errors, leading to safer health care for patients and providers. There might be logistic problems in obtaining consent from some of the patients, but for the delivery of safe health care, a well-understood informed consent is mandatory.

Keywords

Well-understood informed consent • Patient safety • Respect for person • Clinical care • Teach-back • Medical errors • Protection from harm • Low health literacy • Language barriers • Communication

Introduction

In ethics, informed consent is a process whereby a patient or research participant is given sufficient information to be able to understand the potential benefits, risks, and alternatives of the offered treatment or research project. The principle of informed consent is "respect for person," as human beings have an intrinsic value, and this value makes them worthy of being respected. It is presumed that to be respectful is to let the patients/participants of research decide what is being done to them and obtain their voluntary permission. Though immense significance has been awarded to informed consent in biomedical research, it must be appreciated that there is considerable difference between the application of informed consent in research and clinical settings. The objective of informed consent in research is to protect human beings from harm, while science is looking for answers to questions, important from the perspective of the health of the human race. Contrarily, the objective of informed consent in clinical care is to devise a treatment plan for the patient, with an aim to cure disease, improve health, and alleviate suffering. Unfortunately, well-understood informed consent is a rarity in health care [1, 2]. This chapter will explore the relationship of well-understood informed consent with safety of the patient in health-care settings.

R.I. Khan, FCPS (anaesthesiology), M.B.B.S., MHSc (bioethics)
Department of Anesthesia and Intensive Care,
Aga Khan University, 3500 Stadium Road,
Karachi, Sindh 74800, Pakistan
e-mail: robyna.khan@aku.edu

J.J. Talati et al. (eds.), *Urolithiasis*,
DOI 10.1007/978-1-4471-4387-1_68,

Concept of Safe Practices

Patient safety is a new health-care discipline that emphasizes the reporting, analysis, and prevention of medical errors that often leads to adverse health-care events [3]. Linda Emanual states that, "Patient safety is an attribute of health care systems; it minimizes the incidence and impact of, and maximizes recovery from, adverse events" [4]. The incident of preventable adverse patient events was not well known until the 1990s, when several countries reported an increased morbidity and mortality as a result of medical errors. One of the important outcomes of this realization has been the development of an interest in patient safety across the world. In October 2004, the World Health Organization (WHO) launched a patient safety program in response to a World Health Assembly Resolution (2002) urging WHO and member states to pay the closest possible attention to the problem of patient safety. The aim was to "coordinate, disseminate and accelerate improvements in patient safety worldwide" while recognizing patient safety as a global health-care issue.

Medical Errors and Informed Consent

Medical errors are often described as human errors in health care [5]. They are errors or mistakes committed by health professionals that result in harm to the patient. They include errors in diagnosis, in the administration of drugs and other medications, in the performance of surgical procedures, in the use of other types of therapy, in the use of equipment, and in the interpretation of laboratory findings. Medical errors are differentiated from malpractice in that the former are regarded as honest mistakes or accidents, while the latter is the result of negligence, reprehensible ignorance, or criminal intent [6].

When patients do not understand what is to be done to them, medical errors can result, e.g., incorrect medication prescriptions, drug interactions, wrong-site surgery, or severe or life-threatening reactions. Well-understood informed consent has a potential of making health care safer. In 2000, a report published by the Institute of Medicine (IOM) in the United States titled "To Err Is Human: Building a Safer Health System" received considerable attention [7].

Similarly, in order to reduce the number of surgical deaths across the world, WHO started an initiative titled "Safe Surgery Saves Lives" in 2008 that led to the implementation of surgical checklist in the operating rooms. In this checklist, the operating team is understood to comprise of the surgeons, anesthesiologists, nurses, technicians, and other operating room personnel involved in surgery [8]. This checklist is enforced when the patient is awake. Recently, in a patient undergoing left-sided radical nephrectomy, the mark was placed on the right side of the patient. During the checklist, the patient, who was a banker, said out loud that "it is my left and not the right kidney that will be operated upon." After a moment's stunned silence, everyone recovered, thanked the patient, and realized that the on-call resident has given the wrong-site booking to the operating list clerk. There is sufficient evidence now that involving patients in their care have decreased the incidence of mortality and morbidity in health care [9].

In May 2003, the National Quality Forum (NQF) published Safe Practices for Better Healthcare, a report specifying 30 evidence-based practices that would substantially reduce the risk of health-care errors. Among these 30 practices, Safe Practice 10 that calls for improved communication in the informed consent process stood out due to its importance to patients who are being exposed to medical errors as a result of insufficient communication.

Safe Practice 10: Teach-Back

Safe Practice 10 [10] states that all health-care professionals should ask patients to repeat or "teach-back" what they have been told during the informed consent process. The objective for Safe Practice 10 is to ensure that patients or legal surrogates understand the proposed treatment and its potential complications. Asking patients to "teach-back" helps assess how well they understand. Patients are asked to explain, in their own words, their diagnosis, health problem for which they need care, name and nature of treatment or procedure they will undergo, and the risks, benefits, and alternatives to the treatment. Patients should be able to show they have understood and not just be asked to repeat what they have been told. There is sufficient evidence that this is an effective way of communicating, especially with patients having limited literacy because it increases information retention and actively involves patients in their own health-care decisions [11–13].

NQF carried out a project to identify key lessons learned by the three hospitals that have already implemented Safe Practice 10 [14]. In this project, specified benefits of this practice are:

- It ensured medication safety
- Corrected misperceptions and promoted informed decision making
- Prevented surgical errors
- Promoted a culture of quality, safety, and patient-centeredness
- Saved cost

Some of the examples of the benefits of using "teach-back" cited in the report are:

- Since "teach-back" was used as part of the preoperative process, one of the patients had an additional opportunity to state the specific medications he was taking, allowing anesthesiologists to change the planned course of anesthesia that otherwise may have been fatal.

- A Spanish-speaking woman refused the surgery when she understood that the procedure planned for her, tubal ligation, was a permanent sterilization technique and not a temporary method of birth control.

Neil Baum, a practicing urologist in the United States, who writes a regular blog promoting meaningful informed consent as a major tool to prevent medical errors, delivered a paper entitled "Automating Informed Consent: Are You Overlooking a Safety Opportunity?" at the 2006 HIMSS Conference. In this, he described automated informed consent as an adjunct to "teach-back." He writes, "An automated informed consent offers providers access to a comprehensive library of detailed, procedure-specific forms that include explanations of risks, benefits, and alternatives written in a style that is easy to understand. This opportunity for enhanced communication, coupled with the availability of easy-to-understand documentation, is critical to a patient being able to comprehend and 'teach back' basic information about his or her procedure" [15].

Toward a Well-Understood Informed Consent

It is evident that communication gap between health-care teams and patients can lead to medical errors. This gap is wider where patients and families are disadvantaged by language barriers, poverty, educational limitations, and illiteracy. Treating these patients without ensuring that they have understood what is to be done to them can result in treatments/procedures that are either not required, not anticipated by the patients, or with side effects/adverse reactions that are not acceptable for the patients. To be able to achieve a solution for all these problems, improvement in communication strategies leading to a well-understood informed consent is mandatory. Fay A. Rozovsky, a past president of the American Society for Healthcare Risk Management who has worked on the topic of informed consent in clinical care for more than 30 years, says "Informed consent process is more than a legal tool, it is a patient safety tool. It is more than a piece of paper. At its core, this communication process is the most powerful, inexpensive patient safety tool that you have in your armamentarium" [16].

Right Actions for the Right Reasons

Despite the significance awarded to informed consent in medical literature, its meaningful procurement is not at par. The reasons are multifactorial and vary from place to place [17]. Informed consent for clinical care is driven more for protection from litigation and self-defense of health systems rather than an honest respect for human beings. The word medicine is derived from the Latin *ars medicina*, meaning the art of healing. The true meaning of "medicine" is service. This service is provided to human beings who are sick and suffering. The relationship between patients and health-care providers will always be an unequal one. Health-care providers have knowledge of the disease and a power to cure it, while patients are suffering. No matter what measures are taken to make this an equal relationship, patients will always be in a position of vulnerability. Respect for person entails that human beings are respected in this interaction not only in word but by correct actions. Taking a well-understood informed consent is one of the ways of expressing this respect and protecting them from harm.

Conclusion

Respect for person demands that human beings are treated with dignity, especially when they are sick and vulnerable. Clinical medicine places health-care providers in a unique position where they have to provide care and cure to these human beings while keeping them safe from harm. If patients are not aware of what is being done to them, some of the decisions made for their health care or the consequences of these decisions can result in medical errors. To be able to prevent medical errors and avoid increased morbidity and mortality resulting from them, it is imperative that extra measures are taken to make the informed consent process a truly meaningful one, a well-understood informed consent. This has been recognized as one of the major factors correlating with patient safety in health care.

References

1. Saw KC, Wood AM, Murphy K, et al. Informed consent: an evaluation of patients' understanding and opinion (with respect to the operation of transurethral resection of prostate). J R Soc Med. 1994; 87(3):143–4.
2. Bergler JH, Pennington AC, Metcalfe M, et al. Informed consent: how much does the patient understand? Clin Pharmacol Ther. 1980;27(4):435–40.
3. Definition of patient safety. From Wikipedia, the free encyclopedia. http://en.wikipedia.org/wiki/Patient_safety. Accessed on 14 July 2011.
4. Emanuel L, Berwick D, Conway J, et al. What exactly is patient safety? Advances in Patient Safety: New Directions and Alternative Approaches. AHRQ Publication Nos. 08-0034 Volume 1, July 2008. http://www.ahrq.gov/qual/advances2. Accessed in May 2011.
5. Zhang J, Patel VL, Johnson TR. Medical error: is the solution medical or cognitive? J Am Med Inform Assoc. 2008;6 Suppl 1:75–7. doi:10.1197/jamia.M1232.
6. Reference.MD. Definition of medical errors. http://www.reference.md/files/D019/mD019300.html. Accessed on 10 Sepi 2011.

7. Institute of Medicine, Kohn LT, Corrigan JM, Donaldson MS, editors. To err is human: building a safer health system. Washington D.C.: National Academy Press; 2000.
8. Implementation manual – surgical safety checklist. http://www.who.int/patientsafety/safesurgery/tools_resources/SSSL_Manual_finalJun08.pdf. Accessed on June 2011.
9. Haynes AB, Weiser TG, Berry WR, et al. A surgical safety checklist to reduce morbidity and mortality in a global population. N Engl J Med. 2009;360:491–9.
10. National Quality Forum. Implementing a national voluntary consensus standard for informed consent – A user's guide for healthcare professionals. 2005. Washington D.C.: Author. www.qualityforum.org/publications.html. Accessed in May 2011 at URL http://www.qualityforum.org/Publications/2005/09/Implementing_a_National_Voluntary_Consensus_Standard_for_Informed_Consent__A_User%E2%80%99s_Guide_for_Healthcare_Professionals.aspx.
11. Doak CC, Doak LG, Root JH. Teaching patients with low literacy skills. 2nd ed. Philadelphia: JB Lippincott Company; 1996. 24.
12. Schillinger D, Piette J, Grumbach K, et al. Physician communication with diabetic patients who have low health literacy. Arch Intern Med. 2003;163(1):83–90.
13. The National Work Group on Literacy and Health. Communicating with patients who have limited literacy skills: report of the National Work Group on Literacy and Health. J Fam Pract. 1998;46(2):168–76.
14. National Quality Forum. Improving patient safety through informed consent for patients with limited health literacy an implementation report. 2005. Washington D.C.: Author. www.qualityforum.org/publications.html. Accessed in July 2011 at URL http://www.qualityforum.org/Publications/2005/09/Improving_Patient_Safety_Through_Informed_Consent_for_Patients_with_Limited_Health_Literacy.aspx
15. Baum N. Comprehension is the key: the challenge hospitals face is that many patients do not understand the fundamental information regarding their treatment plans. http://www.psqh.com/mayjun06/informed.html Accessed on Aug 2011.
16. Mcdonagh C. Informed consent, part two: how to enhance the physician-patient dialogue. http://www.aao.org/publications/eyenet/201001/practice_perf.cfm. Accessed on 10 Sept 2011.
17. Khan RI. Informed consent and some of its problems in Pakistan. J Pak Med Assoc. 2008;58:82–4.

Anesthesia and Pain Relief for Procedures Performed to Manage Urolithiasis

69

Gauhar Afshan and Aliya Ahmed

Abstract

Anesthetic considerations for extracorporeal shock wave lithotripsy (ESWL), percutaneous nephrolithotomy (PCNL), and concepts of pain management are discussed in this chapter. The pain associated with ESWL has cutaneous, somatic, and visceral origins. General anesthesia, regional anesthesia, and several others miscellaneous techniques (e.g., monitored anesthesia care [MAC]) have been used successfully. The continuous monitoring of hemodynamics and oxygenation is of paramount importance in patients undergoing ESWL regardless of anesthesia technique. Currently the patient undergoing lithotripsy with a new-generation device usually requires MAC with conscious sedation only.

For patients undergoing PCNL, general anesthesia is a preferred technique. Hemodynamic parameters in prone patients need to be closely monitored as pressure on vena cava and iliac veins may cause impaired venous return and decreased cardiac preload. A multimodal analgesia and combined spinal-epidural anesthesia are alternative techniques to general anesthesia. No matter what anesthesia technique is used, the anesthetist must plan the postoperative pain management for PCNL.

Effective postoperative pain management is essential for early rehabilitation, improved recovery, and better patient satisfaction. Regular pain assessment is essential for effective pain management. Several scales have been defined for this purpose, for example, verbal rating scale, visual analogue scale, and numeric rating scale. It is essential to have a basic knowledge of the pharmacology of the commonly used analgesic medications to use them safely and effectively.

An individualized approach to management is important for effective postoperative pain management. A multimodal pain management regime should be employed whenever possible since it helps to increase efficacy while minimizing adverse effects. Analgesics should be given on demand after extracorporeal shock wave lithotripsy, and analgesics with a spasmolytic effect may be useful. Postoperative pain associated with percutaneous nephrolithotomy is much worse and requires stronger analgesics. Titration of the opioid dose is important to achieve effective analgesia. Patient-controlled analgesia may improve patient satisfaction. Epidural analgesia provides superior postoperative analgesia and has been shown to reduce pulmonary complications.

G. Afshan, FCPS (Pakistan)(✉) • A. Ahmed, FFARCS (Ireland)
Department of Anaesthesia, Aga Khan University,
Stadium Road, P.O. Box 3500, Karachi 74800, Pakistan
e-mail: gauhar.afshan@aku.edu; aliya.ahmed@aku.edu

J.J. Talati et al. (eds.), *Urolithiasis*,
DOI 10.1007/978-1-4471-4387-1_69, © Springer-Verlag London 2012

Keywords
Extracorporeal shock wave lithotripsy (ESWL) • Percutaneous nephrolithotomy (PCNL) • Patient-controlled analgesia • Monitored anesthesia care (MAC) • Epidural anesthesia • General anesthesia • Analgesics • Multimodal pain management

Introduction

Surgical management options and minimally invasive therapies for patients with renal stones present unique challenges to anesthetists. These conditions most often require anesthetic management, but at times only pain relief is required. We believe that a holistic and rational approach toward preoperative, intraoperative, and postoperative care leads to improved surgical outcomes, and therefore these are considered a vital part of the anesthesia care for surgical patients with renal stones. Basic anesthetic considerations for extracorporeal shock wave lithotripsy (ESWL) and percutaneous nephrolithotomy (PCNL) and the concept of pain management are discussed in this chapter. The same principles apply to anesthesia for open, laparoscopic, and all endoscopic surgery for stone disease.

Preoperative Anesthesia Evaluation

Preoperative anesthesia evaluation lays the clinical foundation for perioperative management of the surgical patient. It can potentially reduce operative morbidity and enhance patient outcome. During the preoperative visit, anesthetists perform focused clinical examination and determine the need for relevant laboratory tests and diagnostic studies. They develop an anesthesia plan according to surgical requirements, patient preference, and presence of any medical disease. This preoperative visit reduces the patient's and family's anxiety and also provides an opportunity for the patient to discuss with the anesthetist the overall perioperative care, potential anesthesia risks, and options for postoperative pain control.

Anesthetic Choices for ESWL

Extracorporeal shock wave lithotripsy has become the treatment of choice for disintegration of stones in the kidney and upper part of the ureter. The pain associated with ESWL has cutaneous, somatic, and visceral origins [1]. It has been attributed to shock wave-induced and cavitation-mediated irritation of the renal capsule, lumbar muscles, periosteum of the rib, vertebrae, or skin at the coupling site [2, 3]. Numerous anesthetic techniques have been used successfully to address the discomfort associated with ESWL treatments. These include:

- General anesthesia
- Regional anesthesia, for example, epidural anesthesia and spinal anesthesia
- Miscellaneous technique, for example, flank infiltration with or without intercostal nerve blocks and monitored anesthesia care (MAC) or conscious sedation

Currently, general or regional anesthesia is used with first-generation lithotripters (water bath immersion) and MAC, or conscious sedation is used with second- or third-generation (i.e., non-water bath) lithotripters [4].

General Anesthesia (GA)

General anesthesia (GA) provides a rapid onset and adequately controls patient movements. Diaphragmatic movement with spontaneous ventilation can produce a downward displacement of renal stones in excess of 12 mm [4]. This stone excursion may increase treatment times and expose tissues into the injurious shock waves. Sedation of spontaneously breathing patients diminishes tidal breathing volumes by 25 % and can decrease stone movement to about 5 mm. Application of an abdominal binder also was shown to decrease stone movement by an average of 32 % during spontaneous ventilation [4].

Stone excursions are exaggerated and can exceed 60 mm when patients undergo ESWL with general anesthesia and conventional mechanical ventilation. High-frequency jet ventilation has been advocated as one strategy to reduce the mean stone movement from 30.6 mm during conventional mechanical ventilation to 2.2 mm [4]. Despite many advantages of GA, one should be careful about positional injury and difficulty in transporting an anesthetized patient to other locations if some other adjunctive procedure is also planned.

Regional Anesthesia

Both techniques of regional anesthesia—either epidural or spinal anesthesia—offer the advantage of keeping the patient awake, which can help with the transfers and so may reduce the likelihood of positional injuries. For epidural anesthesia, it is better to use saline (rather than air) for loss of resistance technique to identify the epidural space. Air in the epidural space provides an interface and causes dissipation of shock wave energy and local tissue injury [5]. In animal experiments, epidural tissue damage after injection of air and exposure to shock waves has been seen; however, no neurologic injury has been reported in human subjects worldwide [6]. Spinal anesthesia offers a reasonable alternative with its rapid onset compared to epidural anesthesia. However, the main disadvantage of spinal anesthesia is hypotension, which often requires treatment.

Miscellaneous Techniques

Attempts by manufacturers to decrease pain associated with ESWL have resulted in lithotripters designed to use a lower working voltage, which generally cause less pain than lithotripters using other energy sources [7]. These enable most patients to undergo ESWL without regional or general anesthesia; however, these so-called anesthesia-free systems continue to provoke sufficient cutaneous and deep discomfort, and many patients still require supplemental sedative and analgesic agents. Local anesthetic infiltration of the flank with or without intercostal blocks provides adequate comfort level when combined with intravenous sedation. Intravenous combined analgesia using patient-controlled analgesia (PCA) and sedation has been used successfully for ESWL as a daycare procedure [8].

An alternative method for achieving cutaneous anesthesia is topically applied lidocaine-prilocaine mixture (EMLA cream) to the area of skin at the treatment site. Studies have shown that although EMLA decreases pain during ESWL and seem to be similar in efficacy to local skin infiltration at low-energy settings, it does not eliminate the need for supplemental analgesia when ESWL energy is increased [9]. A spectrum of analgesic and sedative agents such as pethidine and rectal diclofenac, intravenous pethidine with intramuscular promethazine, intravenous midazolam with alfentanil, fentanyl, or ketamine has been used effectively. Oral lorazepam alone has also been used successfully for ESWL [4].

Physiological Effects of Immersion (Water Bath) Lithotripsy Under General Anesthesia

Placing a patient into the water bath during lithotripsy produces a number of physiological alterations including increase central venous pressure (CVP), capillary wedge pressure, and increased work of breathing [4]. The continuous monitoring of hemodynamic and respiratory system including oxygenation is of paramount importance in patients undergoing ESWL immersed in a water bath.

Intraoperative ECG Monitoring for Cardiac Arrhythmias

Cardiac arrhythmias can be seen in 80 % of patients undergoing ESWL with first-generation lithotripters. The most likely mechanism of inducing arrhythmias is 10–20 kV discharge (preceding each shock), which results in premature electrical stimulation of the atria. The mechanical irritation of the shock wave itself also has been identified as the initiating event for reentrant atrial tachycardia [4]. Most lithotripters synchronize SWL with the EKG, initiating the shock at the least vulnerable moment, namely, the R wave.

The most recent lithotripters may offer an incorporated cardiac simulator to improve ESWL treatment times. The simulator produces an externally generated cardiac rhythm and drives the lithotripter to increase the shocks delivered per minute. Use of the simulator precludes use of intrinsic electrocardiogram (ECG) gating and results in a 20 % incidence of induced arrhythmias. Deactivating the simulator and returning to an ECG-triggered mode of operation eliminate the arrhythmias [10].

Anesthetic Complications

Complications have been reported with all types of anesthesia including general and regional anesthesia techniques. However, monitored anesthesia care (MAC) associated with conscious sedation technique using narcotic and sedative agents can be tricky. Currently, the patient undergoing lithotripsy with a new-generation device usually requires conscious sedation only. The usual complications associated with this anesthesia technique include hypoventilation with desaturation and nausea and vomiting, which are treated conservatively. For hypoventilation, supplemental oxygen is usually sufficient; however, assisted mask ventilation or intubation may sometimes be needed. For narcotic induced nausea and vomiting, intravenous antiemetic is recommended for symptomatic management.

Anesthesia Options for Percutaneous Nephrolithotomy (PCNL)

Percutaneous nephrolithotomy (PCNL) is a preferred surgical treatment for larger stones (size more than 25 mm). General anesthesia with endotracheal intubation is recommended for the patients undergoing PCNL [4]. Achieving and maintaining adequate ventilation in the prone position is one of the most important steps in the overall management. Care must be taken in achieving prone position by maintaining the head in a neutral position relative to the body. One should remember that both positions of head, flexion or extension, could result in the dislodgment or displacement of the endotracheal tube. To ensure that the endotracheal tube does not dislodge, ventilation of the lungs should be confirmed with bilateral auscultation of chest after final prone positioning of the patient.

The anesthetist must ensure that there is no pressure on testicles or nipples or face, including eyes, lips, nose, and ears. All joints and limbs must also be protected. Limbs generally are placed in positions approximately halfway between extremes of joint movements. Final positioning should avoid angles at the joints more than 90° from neutral in any plane.

Hemodynamic parameters in prone patients under general anesthesia should be closely monitored as pressure on vena cava and iliac veins may cause decreased cardiac preload and impaired venous return. Sometimes extreme obesity, restriction of the diaphragm, and lung excursions by abdominal contents may complicate ventilation. With careful positioning, clinically significant cardiovascular or ventilatory consequences can be avoided.

Intraoperatively the anesthetist must be aware of the possibility of increased airway pressure and desaturation and hypercarbia. Periodical bilateral auscultation of both the lungs is recommended. A close working relationship between the anesthetist and the surgeon allows the coordination of the percutaneous access puncture with deflation of the lung and ventilator standstill to minimize pleural injury.

Recently the possibility of performing PCNL under a multimodal analgesia regime using paracetamol, a COX(2) inhibitor, epidural morphine, and infiltration of the surgical field with *local* anesthetics has been evaluated and found a well-tolerated and safe alternative to general or regional anesthesia [11]. The combined spinal-epidural anesthesia has also been evaluated for efficacy and safety with good results as an alternative to general anesthesia [12].

Some patients are unfit to receive general anesthesia or regional anesthesia due to severe comorbidities specially associated with morbid obesity. In obese patients this procedure has also been performed under IV sedation with local anesthetic infiltration at surgical site in order to avoid obesity-related anesthetic complications specially the cardiorespiratory compromise in the prone position [13, 14].

No matter what anesthesia technique is used, the anesthetist must plan the postoperative pain management for PCNL.

Complications and Special Considerations

Anesthesia during PCNL for big stones like staghorn stones is a challenge because of the possibility of fluid absorption, dilutional anemia, hypothermia, or significant blood loss [4]. Repeat hemoglobin measurement should be considered during the perioperative period [15]. The most common complications of PCNL are pain, fever, urinary infection, septicemia, and bleeding sufficient to require transfusion [15]. The other possible complications include organ injury, for example, pneumothorax and hydrothorax. A chest X-ray in the recovery room is recommended after every PCNL [15]. In spite of identifiable anesthesia-related side effects, PCNL has been successfully performed in high-risk patients [16]. Prolongation of postanesthesia recovery has been reported with mild intraoperative hypothermia in this high-risk population.

Postoperative Pain Management

Effective postoperative pain management is an essential component of the perioperative management of a surgical patient as it has the potential to lead to early rehabilitation, increased patient satisfaction, and a reduced chance of progression to chronic pain [17]. Inadequately treated postoperative pain may have physiological, psychological, economic, and social adverse effects on the patients and also increases the burden on their families [17, 18]. In order to improve the quality of pain relief, it is important to streamline and standardize the method of pain assessment and to enhance the standard of the different strategies available for pain management.

Pain Assessment

Pain is a subjective sensation and therefore difficult to measure. Reliable assessment of pain is one of the most important aspects of effective pain management. When addressing postoperative pain, careful determination of the location and intensity of pain is essential not only for adequate pain management but also for evaluating the effectiveness of the pain management strategies employed. For this purpose, several pain assessment scales have been defined [19], for example, verbal rating scale (VRS), visual analogue scale (VAS), and numeric rating scale (NRS) (Fig. 69.1). These scales are not equally sensitive and reliable [20]. A standardized pain assessment method should be used throughout the hospital by both the medical and nursing staff to avoid miscommunication between teams and to allow a smooth multiteam approach to pain management. The pain scale used should be simple and easy to understand. For this purpose, the NRS has been found to be very practical [19]. It uses numbers from 0 to 10; zero meaning no pain and 10 representing the worst imaginable pain. The patient denotes a number from 0 to 10 to represent the severity of his/her pain. It can even be used to determine the intensity of pain accurately on the telephone after a patient's discharge.

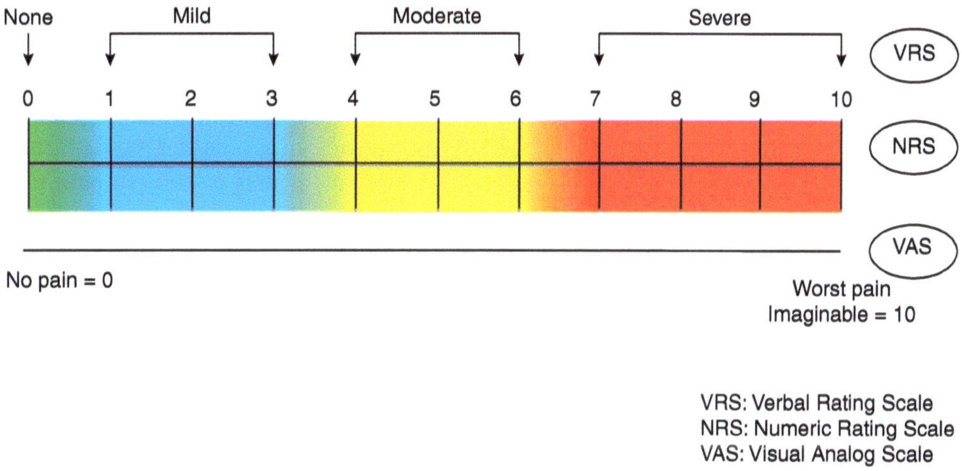

Fig. 69.1 Commonly used pain assessment scales

As pain is a subjective experience, pain assessment becomes very challenging when the patients have difficulty in communication, for example, those with cognitive impairment or young children. For children less than 3 years of age, the faces pain scale, with happy and unhappy faces, has been well validated [21]. In patients having communication problems, observation of physical behavior like restlessness, tense muscles, frowning, grimacing, and groaning helps in making an estimation of the severity of pain [22]. The method of pain assessment must be explained to the patients before surgery, preferably at the preoperative anesthetic evaluation. It is essential to assess the pain both at rest and on movement (dynamic pain)—that is, during coughing, changing position, etc.—and to manage the pain accordingly [19, 22]. Effective relief of dynamic pain helps in improved physiotherapy and early mobilization and reduces the risk of cardiorespiratory and thromboembolic complications and therefore has the potential to improve long-term outcome after surgery [23]. Pain should be assessed at regular intervals after moderate to major surgery, at least for the first 24–72 h. In addition to the assessment of the pain score, the presence of side effects related to pain management should also be assessed at regular intervals and managed as required.

Pain Management

Postoperative pain should be treated adequately to avoid postoperative cardiopulmonary complications and the development of chronic pain and to enhance patient comfort and allow early rehabilitation and discharge [24]. An individualized approach to management is an important step toward improvement in postoperative pain management. One must take into account the patient's age, gender, personality, weight, and comorbidities, in addition to the surgical procedure, when planning the postoperative pain management. A multimodal pain management regime should be employed whenever possible since it helps to increase efficacy while minimizing adverse effects [17, 25].

Analgesics should be given on demand after extracorporeal shock wave lithotripsy because not all patients need pain relief. Analgesics with a spasmolytic effect (e.g., hyoscine-*N*-butylbromide [Buscopan]) may be required after ESWL [26]. However, nonsteroidal anti-inflammatory drugs (NSAIDs) are often sufficient. If possible, opioids should be avoided for outpatients. For postoperative pain control in outpatients, multimodal analgesia with a combination of NSAIDs and paracetamol with infiltration of local anesthetics is usually adequate [27]. Postoperative pain associated with percutaneous nephrolithotomy is much worse and requires stronger analgesics. Multimodal analgesia with a combination of opioid, NSAIDs, and paracetamol should be able to control the immediate postoperative pain [12]. Regular assessment of pain and titration of the opioid dose is important to achieve effective analgesia. NSAIDs decrease the need for opioids [22, 28] and are often sufficiently effective in mild to moderate pain. Similarly, paracetamol can be very useful for postoperative pain management as it also reduces the consumption of opioids [22]. It can alleviate mild postoperative pain as a single therapy without major adverse effects.

The most effective method for systemic administration of opioids is patient-controlled analgesia (PCA), which has been shown to improve patient satisfaction [29]. It is usually employed as the main component of a multimodal analgesic regime. Patient-controlled analgesia can be used safely in children more than 6 years old [30]. Locoregional techniques such as wound infiltration, nerve blocks, and caudal and epidural analgesia are also used successfully. Epidural analgesia provides superior postoperative analgesia and has been shown to reduce pulmonary complications [31]. When the PCNL procedure is conducted under an epidural anesthetic technique, the epidural should be continued postoperatively for the provision of analgesia for 24–48 h.

Nurses play a major role in postoperative pain management of the drugs prescribed by the physicians [32]. Hence, teaching and training of nurses should be an integral part of strategies to improve postoperative pain management. Formal guidelines must be available for safe and effective management of patients receiving regional analgesia or opioids in the surgical wards. It is also important to have a basic knowledge of the pharmacology of the commonly used analgesic medications if they are to be used safely and effectively.

Pharmacology of Analgesic Agents Commonly Used in the Postoperative Period

Opioid Agents

Opioid agents produce their effects by acting on the opioid receptors, which are found in the brain, spinal cord, and various sites outside the central nervous system [33]. The main receptors are mu, delta, and kappa. The pharmacological effects of a given opioid are the result of its receptor specificity, affinity, and intrinsic activity at various receptors [33]. According to their intrinsic activity, opioid drugs are classified as agonists (stimulate opioid receptors and are capable of producing a maximal response), antagonists (bind to but do not stimulate receptors), partial agonists (stimulate receptors but produce a submaximal response with a ceiling effect), and agonist-antagonists (agonist at one type of receptor and antagonist at another). The effective range of blood concentration of a given opioid varies widely between patients [6]. The amount of opioid required also varies with the severity of pain. Thus, management must be individualized with titration of the opioid dose to achieve effective analgesia with minimal side effects. The more common side effects of opioids include nausea and vomiting, sedation, respiratory depression, constipation, and urinary retention [22, 33].

Non-opioid Analgesics

The pharmacology of the most commonly used non-opioid analgesics is outlined in the ensuing paragraphs:

Nonsteroidal Anti-inflammatory Drugs (NSAIDs)

Nonsteroidal anti-inflammatory drugs (NSAIDs) have analgesic, anti-inflammatory, antipyretic, and antiplatelet actions [34]. Their mechanism of action involves a reduction in prostaglandin synthesis by inhibition of the enzyme cyclooxygenase (COX). All NSAIDs are characterized by a high degree of protein binding and small volumes of distribution [34]. Differences in clearance of these drugs account for the variability in half-life among these drugs. The majority are metabolized by the liver through a variety of pathways and excreted by the kidney. Their use may lead to a considerable reduction in the requirement of opioid agents to achieve pain relief [26, 35]. These agents have kinetic properties of good absorption after oral administration and strong binding to plasma protein. Most drugs of this class predispose to the development of peptic ulcer disease. In addition, due to the inhibitory effects on thromboxane biosynthesis, prolonged use of most of these drugs results in decreased blood clotting, which can lead to serious bleeding problems in certain situations. They should also be avoided in patients with renal impairment and in asthmatics.

Selective COX-2 (an isoform of cyclooxygenase) inhibitors are available and can be used for postoperative pain, especially as a component of multimodal analgesia [27, 35]. These drugs do not impair platelet function and do not have similar deleterious effects on the gastrointestinal mucosa as do the nonselective NSAIDs [35].

Paracetamol

Paracetamol is an analgesic and antipyretic agent and, despite its long history of use, there is uncertainty about its mechanism of action. Currently, a central effect is believed to be the mode of action for its analgesic and antipyretic actions [36]. Paracetamol is usually given orally or rectally and now an intravenous preparation is also available, which makes its perioperative use simpler. Intravenous administration results in higher concentration of the drug in the central nervous system with better analgesia than the oral and rectal routes. An opioid-sparing effect has been reported with the addition of paracetamol to opioid analgesic regimens [26]. A dose limit of 4 g in 24 h has been suggested, and this dose is well tolerated and has minimal adverse effects. A big overdose can lead to massive liver damage. It undergoes glucuronide and sulfate conjugation in the liver and is excreted by the kidney [22]. Paracetamol can be used alone for mild to moderate pain and is a useful component of multimodal analgesia for moderate to severe pain [26, 27].

Local Anesthetic Agents

Local anesthetic agents (LA) block sodium channels in the cell membrane, thereby preventing the influx of sodium into the cell. This action blocks the generation of action potential and the conduction of nerve impulses [37]. Thus, these agents produce analgesia by blocking nerve conduction at sensory fibers, although they do not have specific analgesic effects of their own. The lipid solubility of LA agents mainly determines the efficacy of these agents [37].

The adverse effects caused by local anesthetic agents can be caused by the physiological effects of blocking of certain nerves, local toxicity, or systemic toxicity [22, 37]. Local neurotoxicity could be caused by the LA itself or result from the preservatives added to the solution. Inadvertent intravascular injection or systemic absorption can lead to signs and symptoms of systemic toxicity due to the effects of local anesthetic agents on CNS and cardiovascular system. These signs and symptoms include circumoral numbness, tinnitus, drowsiness, convulsions, coma, cardiovascular depression, and respiratory arrest [37].

Conclusion

In conclusion, careful conduct of preoperative assessment and anesthetic management of patients undergoing procedures for urolithiasis is essential for a good outcome. Effective pain relief is also very important for further improving the postoperative outcome. In order to manage pain effectively, one must have a good understanding of the pharmacology of pain medications and make a special effort to assess pain regularly and manage it accordingly.

References

1. Irwin MG, Campbell RCH, SiuLun T, et al. Patient maintained alfentanil target-controlled infusion for analgesia during extracorporeal shock wave lithotripsy. Can J Anaesth. 1996;43:919–24.
2. Schelling G, Weber W, Mendl G, et al. Patient-controlled analgesia for shock wave lithotripsy: the effect of self-administered alfentanil on pain intensity and drug requirement. J Urol. 1996;155:43–7.
3. Tiselius H. Cutaneous anesthesia with lidocaine-prilocaine cream: a useful adjunct during shock wave lithotripsy with analgesic sedation. J Urol. 1993;149:8–11.
4. Dietrich Gravenstein MD. Extracorporeal shock wave lithotripsy and percutaneous nephrolithotomy. Anesthesiol Clin North America. 2000;18(4):953–71.
5. Saberski LR, Kondamuri S, Osinubi OY. Identification of the epidural space: is loss of resistance to air a safe technique? Reg Anesth. 1997;22:3–15.
6. Terai T, Yukioka H, Fujimori M. A double-blind comparison of lidocaine and mepivacaine during epidural anesthesia. Acta Anaesthesiol Scand. 1993;37:607–10.
7. Lingeman JE. Extracorporeal shock wave lithotripsy: development, instrumentation, and current status. Urol Clin North Am. 1997;24:185–211.
8. Tailly GG, Marcelo JB, Schneider IA, et al. Patient-controlled analgesia during SWL treatments. J Endourol. 2001;15:465–71.
9. Ganapathy S, Razvi H, Moote C, et al. Eutectic mixture of local anaesthetics is not effective for extracorporeal shock wave lithotripsy. Can J Anaesth. 1996;43:1030–4.
10. Ganem JP, Carson CC. Cardiac arrhythmias with external fixed rate signal generators in shock wave lithotripsy with the Medstone lithotripter. Urology. 1998;51:548–52.
11. Aravantinos E, Kalogeras N, Stamatiou G, Theodorou E, Moutzouris G, Karatzas A, et al. Percutaneous nephrolithotomy under a multimodal analgesia regime. J Endourol. 2009;23(5):853–6.
12. Kuzgunbay B, Turunc T, Akin S, Ergenoglu P, Aribogan A, Ozkardes H. Percutaneous nephrolithotomy under general versus combined spinal-epidural anesthesia. J Endourol. 2009;23(11):1835–8.
13. Kanaroglou A, Razvi H. Percutaneous nephrolithotomy under conscious sedation in morbidly obese patients. Can J Urol. 2006;13(3):3153–5.
14. Aravantinos E, Karatzas A, Gravas S, Tzortzis V, Melekos M. Feasibility of percutaneous nephrolithotomy under assisted local anaesthesia: a prospective study on selected patients with upper urinary tract obstruction. Eur Urol. 2007;51(1):224–7; discussion 8. Epub 2006 Jun 30.
15. Vasevold R, Endrez N, Andrei S, Leonard M, Noris G, Yosef K, Natan W. Anesthetic consideration during percutaneous nephrolithotomy. J Clin Anesth. 2007;19:351–5.
16. Patel SR, Haleblian GE, Pareek G. Percutaneous nephrolithotomy can be safely performed in the high-risk patient. Urology. 2010;75(1):51–5. Epub 2009 Sep 25.
17. White PF, Kehlet H. Improving postoperative pain management: what are the unresolved issues? Anesthesiology. 2010;112:220–5.
18. Apfelbaum JL, Chen C, Mehta SS, Gan TH. Postoperative pain experience: results from a national survey suggest postoperative pain continues to be undermanaged. Anesth Analg. 2003;97:534–40.
19. Brevik H, Borchgrevink PC, Allen SM, et al. Assessment of pain. Br J Anaesth. 2008;101:17–24.
20. Cork RC, Isaac I, Elsharydah A, et al. A comparison of the verbal rating scale and the visual analog scale for pain assessment. Internet J Anesthesiol. 2004;8. Website: http://www.ispub.com/ostia/index.php?xmlFilePath=journals/ija/vol8n1/vrs.xml. Accessed on 18 Apr 2011.
21. Hicks CL, von Baeyer CL, Spafford PA, et al. The faces pain scale revised: toward a common metric in paediatric pain measurement. Pain. 2001;93:173–83.
22. Macintyre PE, Schug SA, editors. Acute pain management: a practical guide. Edinburgh: Elsevier Health Sciences; 2007.
23. Stubhaug A, Breivik H. Prevention and treatment of hyperalgesia and persistent pain after surgery. In: Breivik H, Shipley M, editors. Pain best practice and research compendium. London: Elsevier; 2007. p. 281–8.
24. White PF, Kehlet H, Neal M, et al. Role of the anesthesiologist in fast track surgery: from multimodal analgesia to perioperative medical care. Anesth Analg. 2007;104:1380–96.
25. White PF. Multimodal analgesia: its role in preventing postoperative pain. Curr Opin Investig Drugs. 2008;9:76–82.
26. Bader P, Echtle D, Fonteyne V, et al. Guidelines on pain management in urology. 2010. http://www.uroweb.org/gls/pockets/english/Pain%20Management%20in%20Urology%202010.pdf. (Text update April). Accessed on 09 May 2011.
27. Elvir-Lazo OL, White PF. The role of multimodal analgesia in pain management after ambulatory surgery. Curr Opin Anaesthesiol. 2010;23:697–703.
28. Jin F, Chung F. Multimodal analgesia for postoperative pain control. J Clin Anesth. 2001;13:524–39.
29. Hudcova J, McNicol ED, Quah CS, Lau J, Carr DB. Patient controlled opioid analgesia versus conventional opioid analgesia for postoperative pain. Cochrane Database Syst Rev. 2006;4: CD003348. doi: 10.1002/14651858.CD003348.pub2. http://www.cochrane.org/reviews/en/ab003348.html. Accessed on 09 May 2011.
30. Grandinetti CA, Buck ML. Patient controlled analgesia: guidelines for use in children. Pediatr Pharmacother. 2000;6. http://www.healthsystem.virginia.edu/alive/pediatrics/PharmNews/20011.pdf. Accessed on 09 May 2011.
31. Nimmo SM. Benefit and outcome after epidural analgesia. Contin Educ Anaesth Crit Care Pain. 2004;4:44–7.
32. Rawal N. Acute pain services revisited: good from far, far from good? Reg Anesth Pain Med. 2002;27:117–21.
33. Trescot AM, Datta S, Lee M, Hansen H. Opioid pharmacology. Pain Physician. 2008;11:S133–53.
34. Brater DC. Clinical pharmacology of NSAIDs. J Clin Pharmacol. 1988;28:518–23.

35. White PF. The role of non-opioid analgesic techniques in the management of pain after ambulatory surgery. Anesth Analg. 2002;94: 577–85.
36. Graham GG, Scott KF. Mechanism of action of paracetamol. Am J Ther. 2005;12:46–55.
37. Becker DE, Reed KL. Essentials of local anaesthetics pharmacology. Anesth Prog. 2006;53:98–109.

Part VI

Management of Stones Under Special Circumstances

Shock Wave Lithotripsy, Endourological Intervention, and Hemostatic Defects

70

Bushra Moiz and Syed Raziuddin Biyabani

Abstract

Extracorporeal shock wave lithotripsy and minimally invasive procedures for the management of urolithiasis are currently considered safe and effective. Yet, treatment-related hemorrhagic complications are common and at times dreadful. The risk of such complications is increased by the widely prevalent use of antiplatelet and anticoagulant medications as well as when operating on patients having inherited or acquired bleeding disorders. This chapter describes the perioperative management of these situations and depicts real-life scenarios of management of such cases.

Keywords

Hemostatic defects • Coagulation disorders • Antiplatelet medication • Hematological considerations

Introduction

Experience of more than two decades has reflected a high safety profile for extracorporeal shock wave lithotripsy (ESWL). Its minimally invasive nature coupled with its effectiveness renders it an ideal tool for the treatment of urinary tract calculi. In skilled hands, this technology has minimally associated complications. However, acute renal and perirenal hemorrhages are recognized as the two most common and devastating clinical consequences with a reported frequency of 1–30 % [1, 2]. Indeed, deaths subsequent to ESWL are exceptional events but can result from hemorrhagic complications [3, 4]. This risk of bleeding is increased several folds by the intake of oral anticoagulants (vitamin K antagonists, e.g., warfarin) or antiplatelet drugs (aspirin, clopidogrel, etc.). Similarly, patients with bleeding diathesis are at increased risk of blood loss during the procedure. Correction of hemostatic defects has allowed safe ESWL in various hematological disorders, which therefore should not be considered as contraindications for the treatment. Unfortunately, despite the extensive use of antithrombotic drugs in the general population and the significant prevalence of inherited and acquired bleeding disorders, our current knowledge is limited to few case reports and small series. This chapter underscores the perioperative management of these high-risk patients.

Managing Patients Treated with Vitamin K Antagonists

The presently available oral anticoagulants are vitamin K antagonists (VKAs). They inhibit hepatic synthesis of vitamin K-dependent clotting factors (II, VII, IX, and X). Based on the half-lives of these factors, VKAs usually take five days to establish their full anticoagulant effects. Patients who are taking oral anticoagulants and require ESWL present a

B. Moiz, M.B.B.S., MCPS (Path), FCPS (Haem) (✉)
Section of Hematology, Department of Pathology and Microbiology, The Aga Khan University, Stadium Road, Karachi, Sindh 74800, Pakistan
e-mail: bushra.moiz@aku.edu

S.R. Biyabani, M.B.B.S., FCPS (Urol), FEBU
Section of Urology, Department of Surgery, The Aga Khan University, Stadium Road, 3500, Karachi, Sindh 74800, Pakistan

J.J. Talati et al. (eds.), *Urolithiasis*,
DOI 10.1007/978-1-4471-4387-1_70, © Springer-Verlag London 2012

therapeutic dilemma. The risk of bleeding during reinitiation of VKAs should be precisely balanced with the thromboembolic risk during their interruption. Alternatively, flexible ureterorenoscopy and Holmium:YAG lithotripsy can be safely and efficaciously utilized in these patients without discontinuing anticoagulation [5].

Practical Considerations

Fatal hemorrhage following ESWL was reported as a complication of warfarin therapy [6]. In contrast, when fourteen elderly patients taking warfarin due to previous cardiac surgery and atrial fibrillation were converted to low-molecular-weight heparin (LMWH) before intervention, treatment with ESWL was performed safely in all the patients [7]. This highlights the significance of appropriate handling of anticoagulants during and after surgery. The American College of Chest Physicians has laid down evidence-based clinical practice guidelines for perioperative management of patients on antithrombotic therapy [8]. They stratified surgeries based on hemorrhagic risk, but ESWL was not mentioned. Since the kidney is enclosed in Gerota's fascia and perirenal hematomas can cause mass effect, ESWL is considered as a high hemorrhagic risk procedure [9].

The management protocol described here [8] is based on these guidelines considering that there is high risk of bleeding associated with ESWL which necessitates interruption of warfarin therapy at least 5 days before the procedure. Patients at low thromboembolic risk do not require bridging anticoagulation during temporary cessation of warfarin therapy. However, high thromboembolic risks such as mechanical cardiac valves, atrial fibrillation, recent arterial or venous thromboembolism, and inherited thrombophilias (Protein C, S, or antithrombin III deficiency, factor V Leiden, antiphospholipid syndrome) demand bridging anticoagulation through IV unfractionated heparin (UFH) or low-molecular-weight heparin (LMWH). UFH should be monitored through APTT, while LMWH requires lab monitoring only in obesity and renal failure through anti-Xa assay. UFH/LMWH should be discontinued 4 or 24 h respectively prior to surgery. International normalized ratio (INR) measured at this time should be normal or less than 1.5. Failing to achieve this should prompt administration of low-dose (1 mg) oral vitamin K. Warfarin can be resumed on the evening of surgery or next day, provided adequate hemostasis has been achieved. Similarly therapeutic-dose LMWH/UFH can be started 24–48 h after surgery. INR and complete blood counts (CBC) should be done on third postoperative day. While INR indicates the effective anticoagulation, CBC is important in monitoring hemoglobin and platelet count which may respectively fall secondary to bleeding or heparin-induced thrombocytopenia. The bridging anticoagulation should be discontinued if therapeutic INR has been achieved. This usually takes 3–5 days after ESWL depending on the time when warfarin was resumed.

An emergency ESWL for a patient taking oral anticoagulants demands rapid reversal of coagulopathy. This can be achieved by administering intravenous, oral, or subcutaneous vitamin K and/or fresh frozen plasma (10–15 mL/kg) prior to intervention [8]. It must be emphasized that peri-ESWL management of patients at high risk of thromboembolism requires team work with cooperation as well as understanding between hematologist, anesthetist, and urologist.

Managing Patients with Antiplatelet Therapy

Today, the two most commonly used antiplatelet drugs are aspirin and clopidogrel. Aspirin irreversibly binds with COX-1 in the platelets and therefore blocks the synthesis of thromboxane-A_2. The latter is an effective agonist for platelets' activation during primary hemostasis. Platelets lack the capability to resynthesize new cyclooxygenase enzyme; therefore, the action of aspirin lasts for 7–10 days equivalent to the life span of platelets. Clopidogrel irreversibly binds to a cysteine residue of the platelet PY_{12}ADP receptor. It usually takes 8–11 days to demonstrate its full antiplatelet effects.

Practical Considerations

Life-threatening hemorrhage following ESWL had been described in patients taking aspirin or clopidogrel [10–12]. Therefore, antiplatelet agents should be discontinued at least 7–14 days prior to ESWL. However, great caution should be exercised, as even when discontinued up to 2 weeks before treatment, these drugs have been linked to hematoma formation [2]. Platelet aggregometry [13] and flow cytometry [14] are helpful laboratory tools in evaluating the restoration of platelet functions before proceeding with the intervention. Unfortunately, there are no standard guidelines for patients requiring antiplatelet agents and ESWL. Zanetti and his colleagues stratified such patients into two groups depending on their risk for thromboembolism [15]. Accordingly, antiplatelet therapy was suspended 8 days prior to elective ESWL in all patients and was resumed 10–14 days post-ESWL. Those having a low risk of thromboembolism (e.g., myocardial infarction in last 1 year) did not receive any bridging anticoagulation. In contrast, patients with high thromboembolic risk (e.g., coronary bypass surgery, atrial fibrillation, cerebrovascular disease, peripheral occlusive disease) received bridging anticoagulation with 5,000 U UFH at 8 h intervals which was continued for another 10–14 days after surgery. All the patients had an uneventful postoperative course.

The patients with drug-eluting stents in their coronary arteries are even more challenging. There is an increasing threat of stent thrombosis during the first year post insertion if antiplatelet therapy is discontinued. It is recommended that all elective surgical procedures should be postponed during this period [16]. For those requiring emergency surgery, management protocols have been defined [16]. Recently, a guideline has been proposed by Din Minno et al. for managing patients on antiplatelets requiring surgical procedures based on thromboembolic risk of underlying disease [17].

Patients requiring emergency ESWL require brisk reversal of platelet dysfunction through intravenous injection of de-amino D arginine vasopressin (DDAVP)/prohemostatic drugs and/or platelet transfusions prior to surgery [8]. DDAVP, a vasopressin analogue, induces release of endothelial cell-associated Weibel-Palade bodies including von Willebrand factor. DDAVP causes a marked rise of von Willebrand factor and associated factor VIII and by a yet unexplained pathway; it causes a marked augmentation of primary hemostasis [18]. A dose of 4–6 units of whole blood-derived platelets or one unit of apheresis platelets (single donor platelets) may suffice. Repeat transfusions may be required.

Managing Patients with Bleeding Diathesis

Normal hemostasis aims at preventing bleeding from an injured vessel. It results from a complex interaction of the vessel wall with the platelets and clotting factors. An adequate number of functioning platelets is responsible for primary hemostasis by initially adhering to the traumatized vessel followed by their aggregation. Secondary hemostasis results in formation of a stable clot when elements of extrinsic and intrinsic pathways are stimulated. Patients with bleeding disorders are at increased risk of hematoma following ESWL, but this is not an absolute contraindication.

Assessment of Bleeding Disorders and Their Severity

A thorough, detailed clinical history along with local and physical examinations is mandatory. These steps assist in differentiating inherited from acquired disorders and platelet-type bleeding from clotting insufficiency. A mild bleeding disorder is usually the most difficult to assess as patient might present later in life subsequent to hemostatic challenges. Primary or screening tests include complete blood count with peripheral film examination, prothrombin time (PT), activated partial thromboplastin time (APTT), bleeding time (BT), and urea clot assay. Based on the results of these tests, more specialized tests should be requested for a definitive diagnosis. For example, platelets function test is required in suspected platelet dysfunction. Similarly, factor VIII assay is required for diagnosing a patient with hemophilia A. Factor XIII assay is indicated if the clot dissolves in urea. A consultation with hematologist is very essential at this point to ensure proper diagnosis and hence management of the patient.

Management of Perioperative Hemorrhage in Bleeding Diathesis

Streem et al. in 1990 treated five patients with ESWL known to have bleeding diathesis such as liver disease and von Willebrand disease. They concluded that ESWL can be performed in such patients, provided specific therapy is instituted to reverse coagulopathy before intervention [19]. Similarly, ESWL has been safely performed in liver disease and cirrhosis after administration of vitamin K or FFP transfusions, and no excessive bleeding was observed when an INR of <1.5 was maintained [20]. Recombinant factor VII can be used to control intractable bleeding in the perioperative period [21]. Glanzmann's thrombasthenia is a rare inherited qualitative platelet defect. ESWL was uneventful in four such cases receiving platelet transfusions without any severe hemorrhagic complications [22, 23]. Immunosuppressive treatment and/or splenectomy were successfully used in 23 patients with immune-mediated thrombocytopenia (ITP) allowing safe SWL treatment [20].

The uneventful postoperative course following ESWL was described in hemophiliacs receiving substitution therapy [24, 25]. In the largest series of 11 patients with hemophilia, 25 ESWL sessions were performed [26]. Substitution therapy was started on the day of treatment, and a factor level of 80–100 % was maintained in the perioperative period. Replacement therapy was withdrawn based on clinical status and absence of bleeding. No hemorrhagic complications were observed. In developing countries where clotting factors are not available, alternative sources include fresh whole blood, fresh frozen plasma (FFP), cryoprecipitate (CP), and cryosupernatant. A dose of 10–15 mL/kg of FFP or 1 unit of CP/10 kg body weight is required in hemophilia A. The treatment should be given twice daily and must be continued until satisfactory hemostasis is achieved. Literature search did not reveal any report of ESWL treatment in acquired hemophilia A. However, such a patient would require administration of factor VIII, steroids, immunosuppressive therapy, and/or plasmapheresis to control bleeding and suppress synthesis of autoantibodies prior to any urgent intervention.

There is evidence that ESWL can be safely used in patients with various hemostatic defects, provided coagulopathy is fully reversed prior to intervention. Careful clinical evaluation, laboratory monitoring, and discussion with a hematologist are key elements of successful treatment.

Some Clinical Scenarios

Case 1

A 75-year-old male presented with urinary retention following an episode of hyponatremia-associated altered consciousness. Comorbidities included a long-standing history of lower urinary tract symptoms, diabetes, and hypertension. His neurological examination was normal, while digital rectal examination revealed a grossly enlarged prostate gland. Additionally, ultrasonography showed a vesical calculus. The serum creatinine was within reference range and urine culture showed no bacterial growth.

An initial trial with alpha-blocking drug administration without catheterization failed to relieve his symptoms. This prompted planning for the transurethral resection of prostate (TURP) and cystolitholapaxy (CLL). Preoperative cardiac risk assessment with perfusion scanning indicated myocardial ischemia for which angioplasty with a nondrug-eluting stent was performed. Aspirin and clopidogrel were initiated as antithrombotic management while TURP was temporarily postponed for 4 weeks. Subsequently, clopidogrel was discontinued without interrupting aspirin therapy. The patient had a smooth recovery following CLL and TURP under spinal anesthesia. The clopidogrel was resumed 2 weeks later.

The case underscores the temporary interruption of clopidogrel well ahead of elective surgical procedures which can safely be resumed once postsurgical hemostasis is achieved.

Case 2

A 99-year-old male presented with chronic urinary retention with progressive deterioration of urinary stream. Comorbidities included hypertension and ischemic heart disease. Surgical history revealed TURP, right herniorrhaphy, right hydrocelectomy, and coronary angioplasty. Examination revealed a suprapubic catheter, while investigations revealed bladder neck stenosis associated with urethral stricture and right ureteric calculus. He was scheduled to undergo an optical urethrotomy and bladder neck incision along with right ureteroscopy for the ureteric stone.

Preoperative workup showed a low platelet count of 63×10^9/L (reference range: 150–400). The counts were reassessed and the hematological team was involved. The patient did not have any past or family history of a bleeding disorder. Moreover, the patient had not shown any significant bleeding in the previous hemostatic challenges. Peripheral blood film showed large platelets with clumping. A repeat count in citrated sample was suggested which showed a platelet count of 88×10^9/L. Subsequent counts were normal. No perioperative hemostatic care was advised. The surgical and postsurgical courses of the patient were uneventful without any significant bleeding.

This is the classical example of pseudothrombocytopenia commonly resulting from platelet clumping. Such cases demand repeating platelet count with peripheral film examination. The surgical procedures can safely be performed with a platelet count of $50–100 \times 10^9$/L.

Case 3

A 45-year-old female was referred from a local urology/nephrology center for management of a right staghorn renal calculus measuring 3 cm. The patient was warfarinized since 8 years for aortic valve replacement. Her cardiac function was stable with no arrhythmias or heart failure. An isotope renal scan showed outflow stasis with 30 % right split renal function.

Prior to elective surgery, the warfarin treatment was interrupted and anticoagulation was achieved through low-molecular-weight heparin (LMWH), which was also stopped the night before surgery. She underwent a routine PCNL with internal ureteral stent placement. Postoperatively, she had cardiogenic hypotensive episodes and hematuria requiring blood transfusions and inotropic support. The patient gradually recovered in the next 3 days. The patient received LMWH in immediate postoperative period while warfarin was reinitiated. The ureteral stent was removed after 8 weeks.

This case highlights the significance of interrupting warfarin therapy before planned surgical procedures and its reinitiation following achievement of surgical hemostasis. The bridging treatment with LMWH is essential to prevent thrombotic risk during period of warfarin cessation.

Conclusion

There is evidence that ESWL and minimally invasive endourological procedures for urolithiasis can be safely used in patients with various hemostatic defects, provided coagulopathy is fully reversed prior to intervention. Careful clinical evaluation, appropriate laboratory monitoring, and timely consultation with hematologists are key elements for the successful management of such patients.

References

1. Dhar NB, Thornton J, Karafa MT, Streem SB. A multivariate analysis of risk factors associated with subcapsular hematoma formation following electromagnetic shock wave lithotripsy. J Urol. 2004; 172:2271–4.

2. Silberstein J, Lakin CM, Parsons JK. Shock wave lithotripsy and renal hemorrhage. Rev Urol. 2008;10:236–41.
3. Toro K, Kardos M. Fatal renal hemorrhage after extracorporeal shock wave lithotripsy. J Forensic Sci. 2008;53:1191–3.
4. Uemura K, Takahashi S, Shintani-Ishida K, Nakajima M, Saka K, Yoshida K. A death due to perirenal hematoma complicating extracorporeal shockwave lithotripsy. J Forensic Sci. 2008;53:469–71.
5. Turna B, Stein RJ, Smaldone MC, Santos BR, Kefer JC, Jackman SV, et al. Safety and efficacy of flexible ureterorenoscopy and holmium:Yag lithotripsy for intrarenal stones in anticoagulated cases. J Urol. 2008;179:1415–9.
6. Inoue H, Kamphausen T, Bajanowski T, Trubner K. Massive retroperitoneal haemorrhage after extracorporeal shock wave lithotripsy (ESWL). Int J Legal Med. 2011;125:75–9.
7. Sighinolfi MC, Micali S, Grande M, Mofferdin A, De Stefani S, Bianchi G. Extracorporeal shock wave lithotripsy in an elderly population: how to prevent complications and make the treatment safe and effective. J Endourol. 2008;22:2223–6.
8. Douketis JD, Berger PB, Dunn AS, Jaffer AK, Spyropoulos AC, Becker RC, et al. The perioperative management of antithrombotic therapy: American College of Chest Physicians evidence-based clinical practice guidelines (8th edition). Chest. 2008;133:299S–339.
9. Alsaikhan BAS. Shock wave lithotripsy in patients requiring anticoagulation or antiplatelet agents. Can Urol Assoc J. 2011;5:53–7.
10. Ruiz H, Saltzman B. Aspirin-induced bilateral renal hemorrhage after extracorporeal shock wave lithotripsy therapy: implications and conclusions. J Urol. 1990;143:791–2.
11. Sare GM, Lloyd FR, Stower MJ. Life-threatening haemorrhage after extracorporeal shockwave lithotripsy in a patient taking clopidogrel. BJU Int. 2002;90:469.
12. Bahceci M, Tuzcu A, Akay F, Agil C, Akay H. Serious clopidogrel associated renal hematoma in a type 2 diabetic patient with primary hyperparathyroidism after extracorporeal shock wave lithotripsy. Saudi Med J. 2005;26:1007–9.
13. Weber AA, Braun M, Hohlfeld T, Schwippert B, Tschope D, Schror K. Recovery of platelet function after discontinuation of clopidogrel treatment in healthy volunteers. Br J Clin Pharmacol. 2001; 52:333–6.
14. Zisman E, Erport A, Kohanovsky E, Ballagulah M, Cassel A, Quitt M, et al. Platelet function recovery after cessation of aspirin: preliminary study of volunteers and surgical patients. Eur J Anaesthesiol. 2010;27:617–23.
15. Zanetti G, Kartalas-Goumas I, Montanari E, Federici AB, Trinchieri A, Rovera F, et al. Extracorporeal shockwave lithotripsy in patients treated with antithrombotic agents. J Endourol. 2001; 15:237–41.
16. Grines CL, Bonow RO, Casey Jr DE, Gardner TJ, Lockhart PB, Moliterno DJ, et al. Prevention of premature discontinuation of dual antiplatelet therapy in patients with coronary artery stents: a science advisory from the American Heart Association, American College of Cardiology, Society for Cardiovascular Angiography and Interventions, American College of Surgeons, and American Dental Association, with representation from the American College of Physicians. J Am Coll Cardiol. 2007;49:734–9.
17. Di Minno MN, Prisco D, Ruocco AL, Mastronardi P, Massa S, Di Minno G. Perioperative handling of patients on antiplatelet therapy with need for surgery. Intern Emerg Med. 2009;4:279–88.
18. Levi M, Vink R, de Jonge E. Prevention and treatment of bleeding by pro-hemostatic treatment strategies. WMW Wiener Medizinische Woechenshrift 19/20/2003. http://www.springerlink.com/content/n1118t1183k31391. Accessed on September 5, 2011.
19. Streem SB, Yost A. Extracorporeal shock wave lithotripsy in patients with bleeding diatheses. J Urol. 1990;144:1347–8.
20. Tse GH, Qazi HA, Halsall AK, Nalagatla SR. Shockwave lithotripsy: arterial aneurysms and vascular complications. J Endourol. 2011;25:403–11.
21. Franchini M. The use of recombinant activated factor vii in platelet disorders: a critical review of the literature. Blood Transfus. 2009;7:24–8.
22. Onishi T, Shibahara T, Kise H, Okuno T, Hayashi N, Arima K, et al. Extracorporeal shock wave lithotripsy in patients with coagulopathies: report of three cases. Hinyokika Kiyo. 1998;44:657–60.
23. Montanari E, Zanetti G, Guarneri A, Trinchieri A, Seveso M, et al. Extracorporeal lithotripsy in patients with acquired or congenital coagulopathies. Prog Urol. 1995;5:706–10.
24. Becopoulos T, Karayannis A, Mandalaki T, Karafoulidou A, Markakis C. Extracorporeal lithotripsy in patients with hemophilia. Eur Urol. 1988;14:343–5.
25. Christensen JG, McCullough DL, Cline Sr WA. Extracorporeal shock-wave lithotripsy in hemophiliac patient. Urology. 1989;33: 424–6.
26. Czaplicki M, Jakubczyk T, Judycki J, Borkowski A, Jaskowiak W, Ziemski JM, et al. ESWL in hemophiliac patients. Eur Urol. 2000;38:302–5.

Cardiac Rhythm Management Devices

71

Azam Shafquat

Abstract

This chapter describes the concepts behind cardiac rhythm management devices and the practical measures that improve patient safety when operating on patients with such devices.

Keywords

Pacemakers • Internal cardiac defibrillators • Cardiac resynchronization therapy devices • Sensing • Pacing • Electrocautery • Shock wave lithotripsy • Surgery

Introduction

Cardiac rhythm management devices such as pacemakers, internal cardiac defibrillators (ICD), and cardiac resynchronization therapy (CRT) devices are implanted for the management of patients with bradycardia (pacemakers), for prevention of sudden death due to ventricular arrhythmias (ICDs), or for treatment of severe heart failure (CRTs). These devices assess the heart rhythm continuously—they "sense" the electrical activity of the heart and provide an appropriate response. This chapter will review management of patients with different types of cardiac rhythm devices who may need to undergo urologic procedures.

Basic Concepts

Cardiac pacemakers are electronic devices that consist of a pulse generator and leads that connects it to the heart. Pacemakers stimulate the heart at a set time interval to prevent the heart rate from falling below a lower rate limit. For this to be achieved, the pacemaker needs to be able to recognize the intrinsic activity of the heart. Each time the myocardium depolarizes, there is electrical activity in the heart that is "sensed" by the pacemaker via the lead. When the pacemaker "senses" the heart's own activity, it is "inhibited" and does not deliver a pacing stimulus. On the other hand, if the pacemaker does not sense any electrical activity within the set time interval, it will deliver a pacing stimulus. This electrical stimulus initiates cardiac depolarization and contraction. For example, a pacemaker set at 60/min will wait for an interval of 1 second before delivering a pacemaker stimulus. If there is a sensed event within this time, the interval will be reset and will again wait for 1 s before delivering the next stimulus. Application of a magnet on top of the pacemaker can turn the sensing function off. In this situation when the pacemaker can no longer "see" the intrinsic activity, it will pace continuously.

Many pacemakers have a *rate responsive* (R) mode that senses physical activity and increases the heart rate. The most common type of rate responsive sensor is set to detect motion and increases the heart rate with increased movement.

A single chamber pacemaker has a lead in either the right atrium or the right ventricle. A dual chamber pacemaker has leads in both the chambers. Dual chamber pacemakers pace at the lower rate when there is no intrinsic activity. If the intrinsic atrial rate is faster than the set lower rate, the pacemaker senses each atrial depolarization and "triggers" a pacing stimulus to be delivered in the ventricle.

A. Shafquat, M.B.B.S., FHRS
Department of Cardiology,
King Faisal Specialist Hospital and Research Center,
Takhassusi Road, MBC 16, 3354, Riyadh 11211, Saudi Arabia
e-mail: azamshafquat@gmail.com

J.J. Talati et al. (eds.), *Urolithiasis*,
DOI 10.1007/978-1-4471-4387-1_71, © Springer-Verlag London 2012

Pacemakers are often referred to by their North American Society of Pacing and Electrophysiology/British Pacing and Electrophysiology Group (NASPE/BPEG) code, which describes the chamber paced, the chamber sensed, and the response to the sensed event [1]. For example, a VVI pacemaker will pace the ventricle, sense electrical activity of the ventricle, and if it senses ventricular activity its response will be to inhibit the delivery of a pacing stimulus. Addition of the letter R in the fourth position in this code (e.g. VVIR) indicates that the pacing rate will increase with activity.

A major concern with pacemakers is unwanted inhibition by electrical signals originating outside the heart. The pacemaker may sense extrinsic electrical activity, for example, from electrocautery, and be inappropriately inhibited and fail to pace. This phenomenon is called *electromagnetic interference* (EMI).

Having the electrocautery device or its pad close to the pacemaker can cause other problems besides EMI. It may cause failure to deliver pacing, changes in pacing behavior, or inadvertent electrical reset to backup pacing modes [2].

Extracorporeally delivered shockwave lithotripsy (SWL) poses some special issues. SWL shocks can induce ventricular ectopy, and to prevent it, the shocks delivered by the lithotripter are synchronized to the R wave on the electrocardiograph (ECG). During ECG gating, atrial spikes can be inappropriately sensed as R waves resulting in inappropriately timed shocks. Pacemaker rates have been known to increase during shocks if rate response is on. Shocks have also been known to inhibit pacing. Moreover, components of the pacemaker may be damaged if the beam is focused on the pacemaker [3].

Preoperative Assessment of Patients with Pacemakers

Prior to surgery, the pacemaker needs to be assessed and the procedure evaluated in terms of risk of EMI.

The type of pacemaker including the manufacturer, model and programmed mode, and lower rate should be determined. Often the patient will have a card detailing these. At this stage in an elective situation, it is best to have the patient seen by a heart rhythm specialist or a representative of the pacemaker manufacturer to have the device interrogated and assessed.

The cardiologist should be made aware of the procedure being contemplated and its details. It should be documented if the patient is completely dependent on the device or if there is an underlying stable rhythm present.

A 12-lead ECG with and without a magnet application should be performed in all patients. This can help in determining the type of pacemaker and if there is appropriate atrial or ventricular "capture" following each pacing stimulus.

The possibility of EMI during the procedure being contemplated has to be assessed. If the patient is dependent on the pacemaker and there is a chance that EMI may inhibit pacing, then it would be appropriate to reprogram the pacemaker to a nonsensing mode, that is, VOO or DOO mode. By doing this the pacemaker will be unable to sense any electrical activity and will not get inappropriately inhibited. Arrangements for this to be done at the time of surgery need to be preplanned during a preoperative visit.

Management of Patients with Pacemakers During Surgical Procedures

It should be ensured that the heart can be monitored during the procedure. ECG monitors develop artifacts when electrocautery is applied, obliterating the underlying ECG. Application of a pulse oximeter that shows heart rate or physically palpating the pulse during electrocautery can demonstrate if the pacemaker is being inappropriately inhibited.

In patients who are pacemaker dependant and undergoing a procedure with EMI, the device should be programmed to a nonsensing mode (VOO or DOO) with rate response turned off. Alternatively, sensing can be transiently suppressed by application of a magnet.

Management of EMI associated with electrocautery includes (1) assuring that the cautery tool and current return pad are positioned so that the current pathway does not pass through or near the pulse generator and leads; (2) avoiding proximity of the cautery's electrical field to the pulse generator or leads (>6 cm Medtronic advisory); (3) using short, intermittent, and irregular bursts at the lowest feasible energy levels; and (4) using a bipolar electrocautery system or an ultrasonic (harmonic) scalpel, if possible [4].

During SWL there are suggestions that the shocks may be safe if they are focused 6 cm away from the pacemaker [3]. Rate response should be turned off as the pacemaker rate may increase on sensing vibrations. Recommendation from at least one of the manufacturers [5] suggests that devices 18 cm from the lithotripsy focal point need only be monitored. Those between 5 and 18 cm may have oversensing and can be programmed to a nonsensing mode. While those less than 5 cm away can have both oversensing and device damage and should be programmed in a nonsensing mode, and device should be interrogated postprocedure to ensure there is no damage. Lithotripsy shocks are often timed with the ECG "R" wave, because inappropriately timed shocks may cause arrhythmias. Hence it should be ensured that the lithotripter does not sense the pacing spike as an R wave. Dual chamber pacemakers which may have two pacing spikes in addition to the R wave may be programmed to a single chamber mode and the lithotripter amplifier adjusted to synchronize on the R wave [5].

During surgery it is imperative that there be provision for emergency cardioversion and insertion of temporary pacemaker, should the need arise [4].

Postoperative Management

After surgery the patient should be monitored until the device is interrogated again as programming changes and resets can occur with EMI. It needs to be ensured that the device is reprogrammed to its original settings if any temporary changes were made for the surgery.

Internal Cardiac Defibrillator (ICD)

An internal cardiac defibrillator (ICD) is a device that can be implanted similar to a pacemaker. In addition to working as pacemakers, ICDs can detect ventricular arrhythmias and treat them automatically either by overdrive pacing or by delivering a direct current shock. The ICD detects tachyarrhythmias when it senses rapid ventricular activity. The ICD may consider EMI as ventricular arrhythmias, thereby causing inappropriate shocks to be delivered.

All the precautions previously mentioned for pacemakers should also be applied to the ICD. Additionally, immediately prior to surgery all sensing should be deactivated to prevent inappropriate shocks [4]. It is imperative that the patient be under constant ECG monitoring with standby external defibrillator while ICD sensing is off. Postprocedure ICD should be interrogated and previous settings restored by competent staff.

Cardiac Resynchronization Devices (CRT)

Some patients with severe heart failure also have conduction abnormalities such as bundle branch blocks. This results in slight delay in the contraction of some parts of the heart, resulting in intraventricular dyssynchrony. CRT-P (cardiac resynchronization device pacemakers) and CRT-D (CRT with defibrillator) devices have leads in right atrium and right ventricle and through the coronary sinus onto the epicardial surface of the left ventricle (LV). Near simultaneous contraction of the lateral wall and the septum results in synchrony being reestablished, with the majority of patients experiencing marked improvement in symptoms.

Since these patients often do not have a bradycardic indication for their devices, they may not be pacemaker dependant. If interrogation reveals them to be not dependant, the devices may not need to be reprogrammed to an asynchronous mode. As with other patients at the end of the procedure, the device should be assessed and, if necessary, reprogrammed.

Conclusion

With proper planning it is safe to have urological procedures done in patients who have cardiac rhythm management devices. Electromagnetic interference should be minimized as far as possible. The device can be programmed to an asynchronous mode. During surgery, heart rate and rhythm should be monitored continuously, if needed by palpating the pulse or using a pulse oximeter. At end of surgery, the device should be reinterrogated and appropriately reprogrammed. Special precautions need to be taken when SWL is being considered.

References

1. Bernstein AD, Daubert JC, Fletcher RD, Hayes DL, Lüderitz B, Reynolds DW, et al. The revised NASPE/BPEG generic code for antibradycardia, adaptive-rate, and multisite pacing. North American society of pacing and electrophysiology/British pacing and electrophysiology group. Pacing Clin Electrophysiol. 2002;25(2):260–4.
2. Stone ME, Apinis A. Current perioperative management of the patient with a cardiac rhythm management device. Semin Cardiothorac Vasc Anesth. 2009;13(1):31–43.
3. Ellenbogen KA, Kay GN, Lau CP, Wilkoff BL. Clinical cardiac pacing, defibrillation and resynchronization therapy. 3rd ed. Philadelphia: WB Saunders; 2006.
4. American Society of Anesthesiologists. Practice advisory for the perioperative management of patients with cardiac implantable electronic devices: pacemakers and implantable cardioverter-defibrillators. Anesthesiology. 2011;114(2):247–61.
5. Medtronic. Lithotripsy considerations, Rev. A2. 18-JUL-2008. http://cacgas.com/uploads/Medtronic___ESWL.pdf. Accessed 2 Jan 2012.

Stone Disease in Pregnancy

72

Ahmed Mohamed Elshal and Ahmed A. Shokeir

Abstract

With increasing burden of urolithiasis among the daily urologic practice, it is no longer rare to see urolithiasis in a pregnant woman. Consequently, the practicing obstetrician has to master the diagnostic approach available for its diagnosis and know how to manage the associated risks. Diagnosis of urolithiasis during pregnancy can be a challenge due to the physiological changes of pregnancy and the need to limit exposure to ionizing radiation. Conservative management is the first treatment option for noncomplicated urolithiasis in pregnancy. If spontaneous passage of the stone does not occur or if complications develop, urologic consultation should be obtained. Urologist effort should be paid to relieve obstructed kidney to prevent obstetric complications and sepsis. A place for active endoscopic treatment procedures is still present after proper patient counseling with minimal obstetric sequelae.

Keywords

Urolithiasis • Pregnancy • Ureteroscopy • PNL • Multiparous • Hydronephrosis of pregnancy • Gestational hypercalciuria

Introduction

Although urolithiasis during pregnancy is not a common daily urologic practice, nevertheless, it can pose many risks to both the pregnant mother and the unborn fetus. Nowadays, symptomatic urolithiasis has been reported to affect from 1 in 200 to 1 in 1,500 pregnant women [1–4]. Urolithiasis in pregnancy may be more common in multiparous women during the second and third trimesters. Both kidneys have been reported to be affected equally [5, 6].

The question about the role of pregnancy in pathogenesis of urolithiasis is controversial. Despite the physiological processes that favor stone formation during pregnancy, urine stasis and the elevated concentration of urinary calcium, most studies have reported no difference in the incidence of kidney stones between pregnant and nonpregnant women [7]. It appears that in addition to alterations that may increase stone formation, there are also changes that may have an inhibitory influence. The increased glomerular filtration rate (GFR) as well increases the urinary excretion of citrate, glycoproteins, and magnesium, and it has been well documented that these substances can inhibit stone formation both in vivo and in vitro [6]. Thus, it seems likely that these positive and negative effects on stone formation counterbalance each other.

Anatomical and Physiological Changes in Pregnancy

Pregnancy results in numerous normal anatomic and physiological changes in the urinary tract, which may be correlated to the pathogenesis of urolithiasis. Urinary stasis is

A.M. Elshal, M.Sc., FEBU
Department of Urology, Mansoura Urology and Nephrology Center, Mansoura University, Elgomhoria Street, 35516 Mansoura, Egypt
e-mail: elshalam@hotmail.com

A.A. Shokeir, M.D., Ph.D., FEBU (✉)
Department of Urology, Urology and Nephrology Center, Mansoura University, Mansoura, Egypt
e-mail: ahmed.shokeir@hotmail.com

J.J. Talati et al. (eds.), *Urolithiasis*,
DOI 10.1007/978-1-4471-4387-1_72, © Springer-Verlag London 2012

typically described as hydronephrosis of pregnancy. It is usually attributed to mechanical compression of the collecting system by the growing uterus and hormonal "physiological dilation" secondary to elevated progesterone levels. The latter leads to a relaxation of ureteral smooth muscle and decreased peristalsis [4]. Urinary stasis facilitates aggregation of crystals in the urine.

Another change associated with pregnancy is a 30–50 % increase in the glomerular filtration rate due to increase in cardiac output in combination with a decrease in renal vascular resistance [6]. This results in a higher filtration rate of calcium and uric acid by the kidneys which are typical stone promoters and also the increased urinary excretion of citrate, glycoproteins, and magnesium which are typical stone inhibitors.

The elevated concentration of urinary calcium "gestational hypercalciuria" is further amplified by the higher serum concentration of placental-derived 1, 25-dihydroxyvitamin D that increases the intestinal absorption of calcium. The increased intestinal calcium absorption in response to increased fetal needs ultimately leads to increased urinary calcium levels [4]. This promotes nucleation of calcium crystals. The pregnancy-related urinary stasis then provides an adequate time for the crystals to aggregate and form stones.

Scope of the Problem

Pregnant women with nephrolithiasis have a greater risk of preterm delivery compared to women without stones. Lewis et al. reviewed more than 21,000 deliveries in their database and found that among the 86 patients diagnosed with a stone disease during pregnancy, there was an increased risk of premature rupture of membranes (2.9 % in non-stone patients versus 7 % in stone patients) [8]. Premature rupture of membranes is associated with an increased risk of neonatal morbidity and mortality. However, a population-based study from Hungary (from 1980 through 1996) did not find a higher risk of preterm birth in pregnant women with nephrolithiasis [9]. Interestingly, the source data for this study was obtained from patient questionnaires, with different compliance rates between the study and control groups. Therefore, nephrolithiasis during pregnancy remains a real concern.

Diagnostic Challenge

Clinical Presentation

The pregnant patient with nephrolithiasis might represent a diagnostic dilemma, both clinical and radiological (Fig. 72.1) present an algorithm to assist decisions when managing pregnant patients with urolithiasis. The presenting symptom of flank pain can be atypical in a pregnant lady, leading to further confusion. In fact, up to 28 % of pregnant patients with renal colic and urinary calculi are misdiagnosed with medical conditions like appendicitis, cholecystitis, pyelonephritis, or hydronephrosis of pregnancy [3]. Past history of stone disease might be a clue for diagnosis in a high percentage of pregnant women with flank pain with or without other urinary symptoms. Laboratory studies may have a role in diagnosis of urolithiasis during pregnancy, as microscopic hematuria occurs in more than 75 % of patients [10]. The presence of two out of the following—recurrent urinary tract symptoms, microscopic hematuria, or a sterile pyuria—significantly raises the suspicion of urinary stones in most of pregnant females [11].

Conventional X-Ray

Although urinary tract plain X-ray combined with intravenous urography is the cornerstone for diagnosis of stone disease in nonpregnant women, there is a need to minimize radiation exposure especially in the first trimester of pregnancy. However, the American College of Obstetricians and Gynecologists recommends that "Women should be counseled that the X-ray exposure from a single diagnostic procedure does not result in harmful effects"—specifically exposure to less than 50 mGy, which is not associated with an increase in fetal anomalies or pregnancy [12].

Grayscale Ultrasound (US)

Although conventional ultrasound is considered a safe, bed site, and obstetrician friendly assessment tool, it misses up to 20 % of patients with complete obstruction because they are thought to have "physiological hydronephrosis" of pregnancy [13]. However, ureteral dilatation usually is not present distal to pelvic brim. Thus, a dilated ureter beyond the iliac artery is suggestive for a distal ureteral obstruction [14]. Additionally, a vaginal ultrasound evaluation may facilitate the diagnosis of distal ureteral stones and should be considered [15, 16].

Doppler US

Using Doppler US may add to the sensitivity and specificity of US in diagnosis of acute obstruction; Delta resistive index (Δ(Delta) RI) is a sensitive and specific test for diagnosis of acute unilateral ureteric obstruction in pregnant women with cutoff value of more than 0.04 [17]. In addition, ureteric

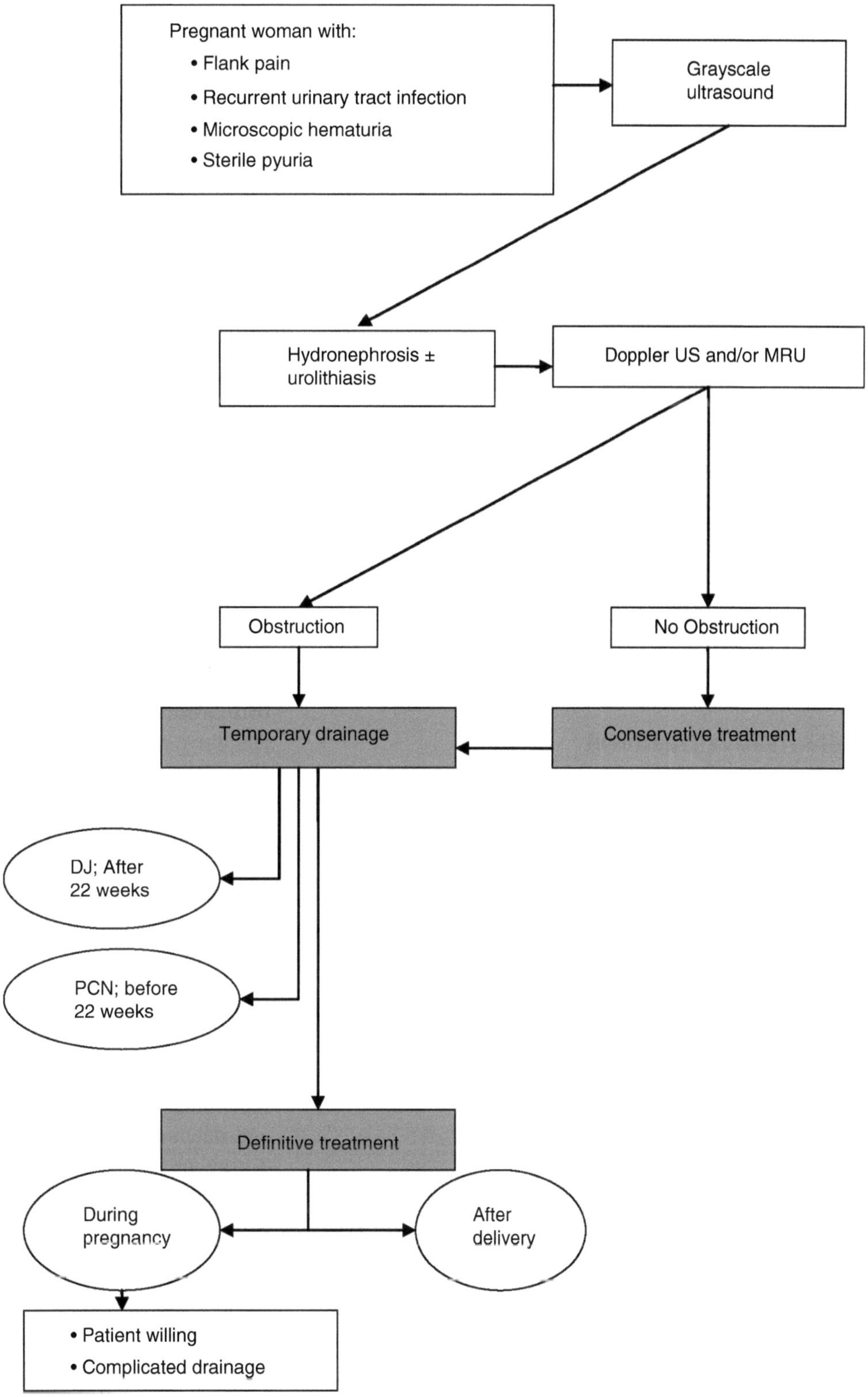

Fig. 72.1 Algorithm for management of urolithiasis during pregnancy. *US* ultrasound, *MRU* magnetic resonance urography, *PCN* percutaneous nephrostomy, *DJ* double J stent

jets assessment is useful only for unilateral obstruction. The symptomatic side is compared to the normal side for 10–15 min after good hydration. Complete obstruction is diagnosed if no jets were detected [18].

Magnetic Resonance Urography (MRU)

Although ultrasound should be used as the first-line imaging modality in patients with suspected urolithiasis, MRU possesses the potential for problem solving because it enables a distinction to be made between the physiological and pathologic bases of ureter obstructions. Furthermore, the MRU can be used to detect the size of signal void urinary calculi and its exact site, which are important factors in defining management [19].

Treatment Approach

In the era of evidence-based medicine, by the end of the year 2010, there was no single high-level evidence report on the treatment of urolithiasis during pregnancy either in the urologic or the obstetric literature. With many case series reporting on various algorithms for treatment, successful conservative therapy was reported in most of the cases. Urine diversion procedures come to the second line in the urologic armamentarium for such group of patients in terms of either internal ureteral stenting or percutaneous nephrostomy drainage. Eventually, the door is opened to the stone-freeing procedures, as many urologists as well obstetricians coined the phrase "expectant therapy for the expectant mother" [11].

Conservative Treatment

Pain management, hydration-rehydration regimen, and suppressive antimicrobial therapy are the corner stones in conservative management strategy. While alpha-adrenoceptor blockers and calcium channel blockers enhance spontaneous stone passage, safety of these medications in pregnancy is not well established. The routine use of medical expulsive therapy cannot be recommended [20]. However, 64–84 % spontaneous stone passage rate with conservative therapy was reported [8, 21].

Temporary Drainage Procedures

The two main urine diversion procedures available are ureteral stent placement and percutaneous nephrostomy (PCN). Ureteral stents are placed under cystoscopic guidance under local or regional anesthesia [22] with the assistance of pulsed fluoroscopy or ultrasound guidance. Although stents facilitate drainage of urine around the stone and sometimes assist in passage of smaller stones, they have disadvantages of obstruction with encrustation, which is secondary to the triad of gestational hypercalciuria, hyperuricosuria, and infection. US-guided PCN allows safe and effective drainage of the obstructed kidney. However, the external tube may be bothersome to the gravid woman as frequent dislodgment and obstruction of the tube might be a nightmare. Table 72.1 provides a comparison between the advantages and disadvantages of external and internal urine drainage procedures in pregnant women with urolithiasis.

Extracorporeal Shockwave Lithotripsy (ESWL)

ESWL is contraindicated in pregnancy because of the potential hazardous effects of the shockwave on the fetus [26]. However, there have been reports of SWL treatment in young women with unrecognized early pregnancies, who went on to have uncomplicated pregnancies and healthy babies [27, 28]. Mandatory termination of pregnancy in such situations is not recommended [24].

Endoscopic Stone Treatment

It is important to minimize ionizing radiation exposure to the pregnant patient during endoscopic procedures by the use of a below-table X-ray source and to shield the fetus with a lead apron placed below the patient.

Indications

Definitive management of the stone is usually delayed until after delivery. However, for ureteral stones or obstructing renal pelvis stones in patients who either refuse or suffer complicated temporary drainage procedures, endoscopic stone removal might be an option especially when the stone presents early in pregnancy with an expected long delay. Clear written consent explaining all possible risks should be signed by the patient and the husband.

Lithotripsy

Mechanical stone extraction with or without disintegration is utilized. The optimal method for stone disintegration is Holmium-YAG laser lithotripter. Ultrasonic lithotripters and pneumatic lithotripters are not recommended for use during pregnancy as they produce high-intensity sound waves. They have a theoretical risk for damaging fetal auditory system [29].

Ureteroscopy (URS)

With many reports for successful ureteroscopy for lower ureteral stones during pregnancy and with advancement in the technology of flexible ureteroscopy and Holmium-YAG laser, access to the upper ureteral stones could be feasible. Also, management of ureteral stones in the third trimester with flexible URS allows manipulation of tortuous ureter. Table 72.2 shows the results of URS in treatment of ureteral stones in pregnant women in the current literature [10, 30–38].

Table 72.1 Percutaneous nephrostomy versus internal stent for drainage of obstructed kidney

	PCN	Internal stent
Advantages	Minimally invasive	No external device
	Immediate and effective decompression of the obstructed system	Rarely dislodged once properly placed
	Local anesthesia without ionizing radiation	May be fixed retrograde or antegrade via PCN
	Urine collection for culture and sensitivities	May allow passage of small stones
	No ureteral manipulation	
	Access for future PNL	
	Minimal LUTs	
	Easy exchange	
	Cost-effective	
Disadvantages	Risk of bleeding during insertion	Irritative LUTs
	Bacterial colonization	Stent related pain
	Dislodgement	Possible trauma to the ureter
	Tube blockage; encrustation	Risk of ascending UTIs
	External device burden	Stent blockage; encrustation
Recommendations [4, 25]	Before 22 weeks of pregnancy	Later on in pregnancy to avoid frequent exchange

Modified after [23, 24]
LUTs lower urinary tract symptoms, *UTIs* urinary tract infections

Table 72.2 Different series of endoscopic stone treatment during pregnancy

Series	Procedure	Patients (number)	Fluoroscopy	Lithotripsy	Trimester	Complications	Stone-free
Juan et al. [30]	URS	3	No	No	3	No	3/3
Alkpinar et al. [31]	URS	7	No	Hol-YAG	1, 2, 3	No	6/7
Khoo et al. [32]	URS	2	?	?	3	No	2/2
Yang et al. [33]	URS	3	No	EHL	1, 2	No	3/3
Lemos et al. [34]	URS	14	1/14	USL	2, 3	No	13/13
Lifshitz and Lingeman [35]	URS	6	Yes	No	2, 3	No	4/4
Watterson et al. [36]	URS	8	Yes	Hol-YAG	1, 2, 3	No	7/9
Butler et al. [10]	URS	2	?	?	?	No	2/2
Shokeir and Mutabagani [37]	URS	10	No	USL	?	No	5/8
Scarpa et al. [38]	URS	15	No	Pulsed dye and Hol-YAG	2, 3	No	10/13
Hosseini et al. [39]	PNL	1	No	No	2	No	1/1
Csaba et al. [40]	PNL	1	No	No	1	No	1/1
Shah et al. [41]	PNL	1	Yes	No	2	No	1/1

PNL percutaneous nephrolithotomy, *URS* ureteroscopy, *Hol-YAG* holmium-YAG, *USL* ultrasound lithotripsy, *EHL* electrohydraulic lithotripsy

Percutaneous Nephrolithotomy (PNL)

Patients with an indwelling nephrostomy tube may proceed to PNL after delivery, but the indications of PNL during pregnancy are questionable. The necessity for general anesthesia, the need for fluoroscopy, and prone position of the patient make it a hazardous procedure. However, there have been a few case reports describing successful PNL in pregnancy (Table 72.2) [39–41]. Prone position can be adopted only early in pregnancy. However, with establishment of the experience of PNL in supine position in many centers, PNL in supine position may be utilized in late pregnancy. Under total ultrasonic guidance, needle puncture of the collecting system with insertion of a guide-wire and sequential tract dilatation till Amplatz sheath insertion are performed.

Outcome

The postoperative stone control status assessment is done by renal US both early postoperatively and 2 weeks after discharge following endoscopic lithotripsy. Assessment of the fetal parameters in the postoperative period after any

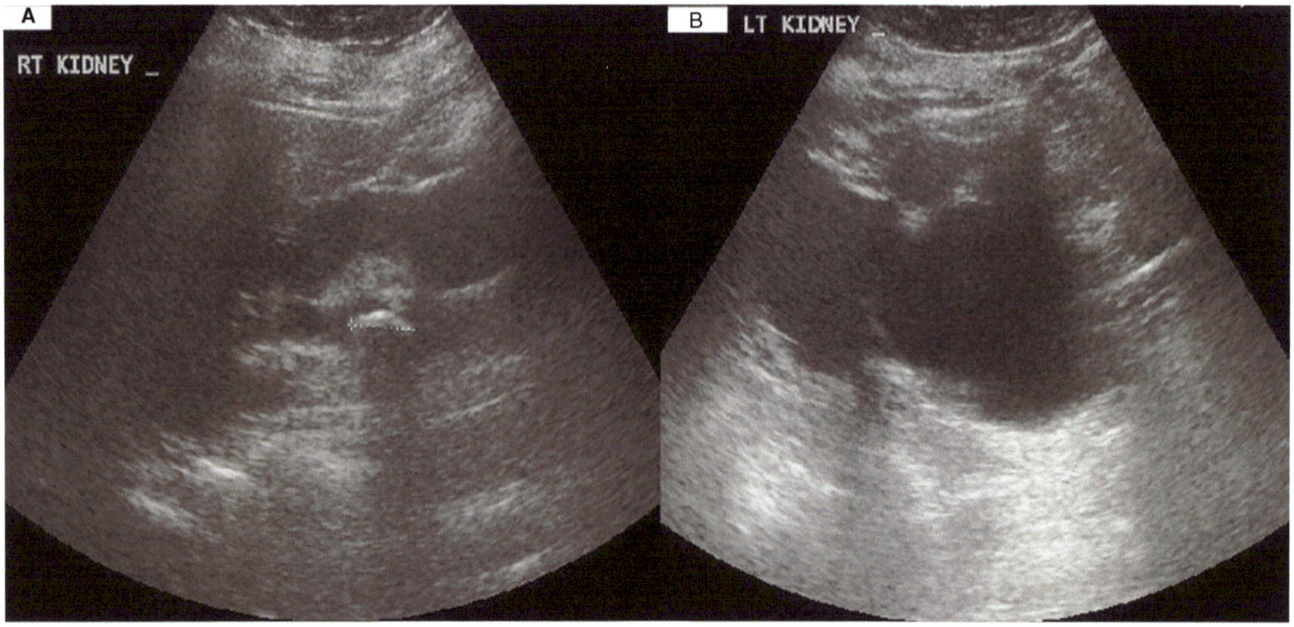

Fig. 72.2 Grayscale ultrasound. (**a**) Mild hydronephrosis of the right kidney with stone renal pelvis of 2 cm in diameter. (**b**) Marked hydronephrosis of the left kidney with thinned parenchyma with non-dilated ureter

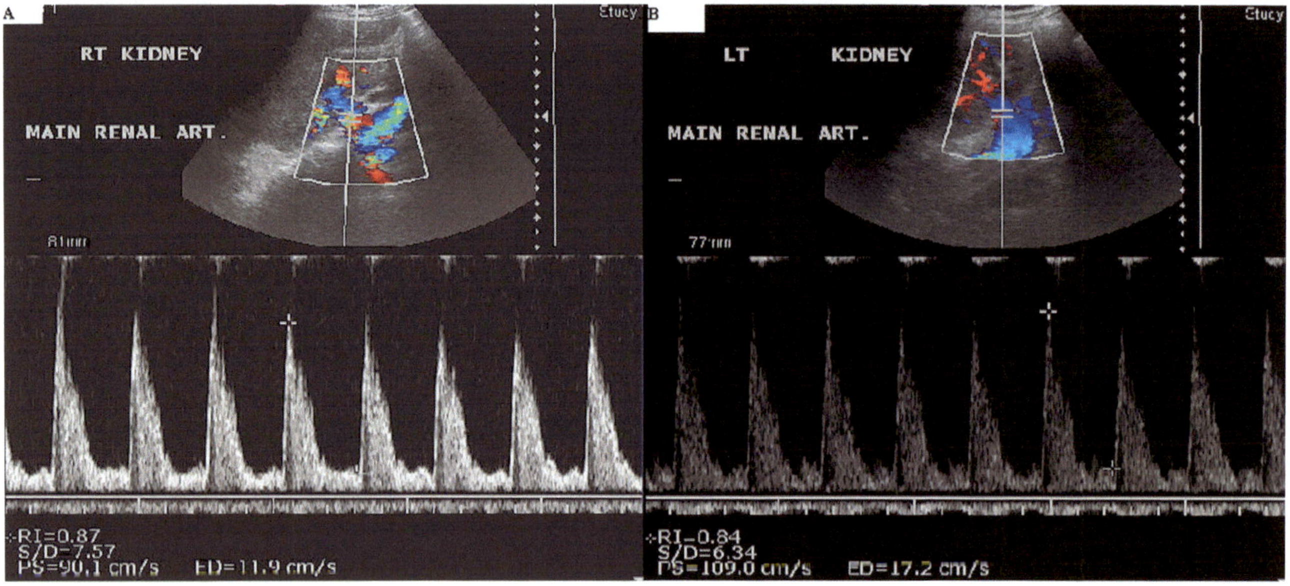

Fig. 72.3 Color Doppler ultrasound. (**a**) RI of the right kidney 0.87 (suggestive of obstruction). (**b**) RI of the left kidney 0.84 (suggestive of obstruction)

endoscopic management is mandatory. No adverse effects for the baby were reported in any of the published series for endoscopic lithotripsy in pregnancy [10, 30–41].

Open Surgery

Open surgery is rarely indicated in management of stone disease; in rare instances, it has been used when endourology expertise or equipments are not available [42].

Case Scenario

A 25-year-old female, 2nd gravida (26th week of gestation) and primipara, with a history of left PNL 4 years previously, complained of recurrent attacks of fever and bilateral flank pain mainly on the left side during the previous 2 months. Her obstetrician advised a high fluid intake, oral antimicrobial medications, and antipyretics with minimal symptom

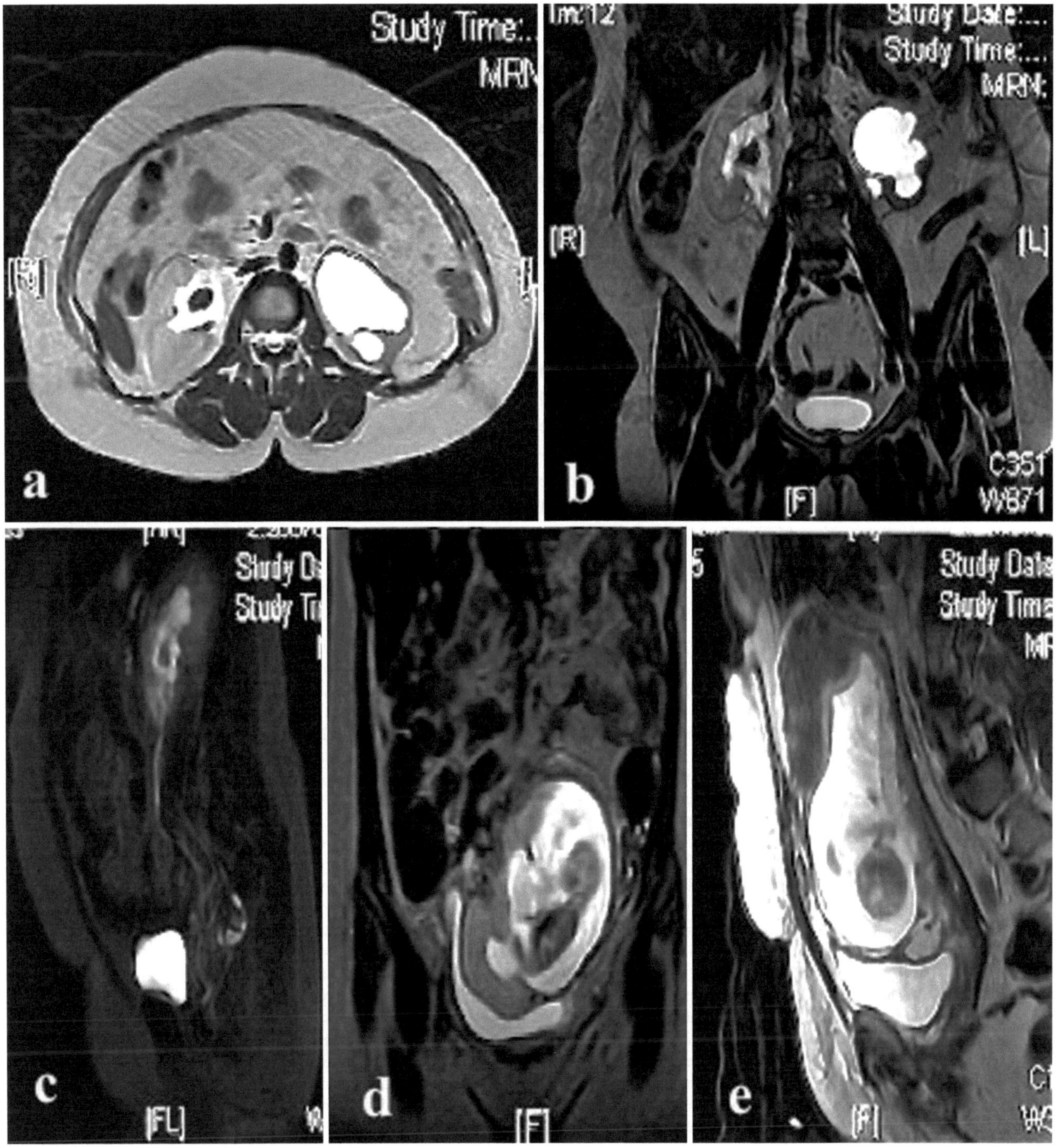

Fig. 72.4 MRI-MRU. (**a**) Coronal section T2 image showing signal void stone in the right kidney and picture of left pelviureteric junction obstruction (PUJO). (**b**) Axial section T2 image showing signal void stone in the right kidney with marked left hydronephrosis. (**c**) Sagittal one shot MRU showing signal void stone in the right kidney with non-dilated ureter. (**d**) Coronal section T2 image showing gravid uterus. (**e**) Sagittal section T2 image showing gravid uterus

control. She presented to a urologist with a 39 °C fever, urine analysis findings of microscopic hematuria and pyuria, and grayscale US findings of bilateral hydronephrosis and stone in the right renal pelvis (Fig. 72.2).

While awaiting the results of urine culture and sensitivity test, she was initially managed by intravenous empirical antimicrobial medications, intravenous fluids, and antipyretics.

Doppler US was requested with assessment of delta resistive index. Bilateral renal obstruction was suggested (Fig. 72.3), and MRU was performed for an accurate assessment of the cause and degree of obstruction on both sides (Fig. 72.4). Minimal hydronephrosis with stone in right renal pelvis was depicted as well-marked hydronephrosis with thinned parenchyma on the left side with no stones and picture suggestive of pelviureteric junction obstruction. A urine culture and sensitivity test revealed heavy growth of *E. coli* with high sensitivity to ceftriaxone. Five days of intravenous ceftriaxone and left side double J (DJ) stent were sufficient to control symptoms without urologic or obstetric complications until delivery of a full-term healthy baby. Three months later, right PNL was performed. As the right kidney was obstructed and had better function than the left, the right kidney was managed first.

Conclusion

It is imperative that practicing obstetricians possess knowledge about current diagnostic modalities and management protocols of urolithiasis in pregnant women. Fortunately enough, a conservative treatment policy will succeed in most cases; however, a high index of suspicion is required for a prompt urologic intervention. Improvements in the technology allowed both safe temporary drainage procedures and definitive treatment in some cases. Ureteroscopic access to stones at any location in the collecting system of the pregnant patient is feasible safely nowadays.

References

1. Rodriguez PN, Klein AS. Management of urolithiasis during pregnancy. Surg Gynecol Obstet. 1988;166:103–6.
2. Meria P, Anidjar M, Hermieu JF, Boccon-Gibod L. Urinary lithiasis and pregnancy. Prog Urol. 1993;3:937–43.
3. Cheriachan D, Arianayagam M, Rashid P. Symptomatic urinary stone disease in pregnancy. Aust N Z J Obstet Gynaecol. 2008;48:34–9.
4. McAleer SJ, Loughlin KR. Nephrolithiasis and pregnancy. Curr Opin Urol. 2004;14:123–7.
5. Maikranz P, Coe FL, Parks JH, Lindheimer MD. Nephrolithiasis and gestation. Baillieres Clin Obstet Gynaecol. 1987;1:909–19.
6. Maikranz P, Lindheimer M, Coe F. Nephrolithiasis in pregnancy. Baillieres Clin Obstet Gynaecol. 1994;8:375–86.
7. Drago JR, Rohner TJ, Chez RA. Management of urinary calculi in pregnancy. Urology. 1982;20:578–81.
8. Lewis DF, Robichaux 3rd AG, Jaekle RK, Marcum NG, Stedman CM. Urolithiasis in pregnancy: diagnosis, management and pregnancy outcome. J Reprod Med. 2003;48:28–32.
9. Banhidy F, Acs N, Puho EH, Czeizel AE. Maternal kidney stones during pregnancy and adverse birth outcomes, particularly congenital abnormalities in the of spring. Arch Gynecol Obstet. 2007;275:481–7.
10. Butler EL, Cox SM, Eberts EG, et al. Symptomatic nephrolithiasis complicating pregnancy. Obstet Gynecol. 2000;96:753–6.
11. Horowitz E, Schmidt JD. Renal calculi in pregnancy. Clin Obstet Gynecol. 1985;28:324–38.
12. American College of Obstetricians and Gynecologists Committee on Obstetric Practice. Guidelines for diagnostic imaging during pregnancy. ACOG Committee opinion no 158. Washington DC: ACOG; 1995.
13. Laing FC, Jeffrey Jr RB, Wing VW. Ultrasound versus excretory urography in evaluating acute flank pain. Radiology. 1985;154:613–6.
14. MacNeily AE, Goldenberg SL, Allen GJ, et al. Sonographic visualization of the ureter in pregnancy. J Urol. 1991;146:298–301.
15. Laing FC, Benson CB, DiSalvo DN, et al. Distal ureteral calculi: detection with vaginal US. Radiology. 1994;192:545–8.
16. Loughlin KR. Management of urologic problems during pregnancy. Urology. 1994;44:159–69.
17. Shokeir AA, Mahran MR, Abdulmaaboud M. Renal colic in pregnant women: role of renal resistive index. Urology. 2000;55(3):344–7.
18. Shokeir AA. The diagnosis of upper urinary tract obstruction. BJU Int. 1999;83(8):893–900.
19. Spencer JA, Chahal R, Kelly A, et al. Evaluation of painful hydronephrosis in pregnancy: magnetic resonance urographic patterns in physiological dilatation versus calculous obstruction. J Urol. 2004; 171:256–60.
20. Porpiglia F, Vaccino D, Billia M, et al. Corticosteroids and tamsulosin in the medical expulsive therapy for symptomatic distal ureter stones: single drug or association? Eur Urol. 2006;50:339–44.
21. Parulkar BG, Hopkins TB, Wollin MR, Howard Jr PJ, Lal A. Renal colic during pregnancy: a case for conservative treatment. J Urol. 1998;159:365–8.
22. Delakas D, Karyotis I, Loumbakis P, et al. Ureteral drainage by double-J catheters during pregnancy. Clin Exp Obstet Gynecol. 2000;27:200–2.
23. Pearle MS, Pierce HL, Miller GL, et al. Optimal method of urgent decompression of the collecting system for obstruction and infection due to ureteral calculi. J Urol. 1998;160:1260–4.
24. Shalom J, Srirangam B, Hickerton B, Van Cleynenbreugel B. Management of urinary calculi in pregnancy: a review. J Endourol. 2008;22(5):865–75.
25. Denstedt JD, Razvi H. Management of urinary calculi during pregnancy. J Urol. 1992;148:1072–5.
26. Streem SB. Contemporary clinical practice of shockwave lithotripsy: a reevaluation of contraindications. J Urol. 1997;157: 1197–203.
27. Asgari MA, Safarinejad MR, Hosseini SJ, Dadkhah F. Extracorporeal shock wave lithotripsy of renal calculi during early pregnancy. BJU Int. 1999;84:615–7.
28. Deliveliotis CH, Argyropoulus B, Chrisofos M, Dimopoulos CA. Shockwave lithotripsy in unrecognized pregnancy: interruption or continuation? J Endourol. 2001;15:787–8.
29. Menon M, Resnick MI. Stones in pregnant women. In: Walsh PC, Retik AB, Vaugh ED, editors. Campbell's urology. 8th ed. Philadelphia: WB Saunders; 2002. p. 3292–3.
30. Juan YS, Wu WJ, Chuang SM, Wang CJ, Shen JT, Long CY, Huang CH. Management of symptomatic urolithiasis during pregnancy. Kaohsiung J Med Sci. 2007;23:241–6.
31. Akpinar H, Tüfek I, Alici B, Kural AR. Ureteroscopy and holmium laser lithotripsy in pregnancy: stents must be used postoperatively. J Endourol. 2006;20:107–10.
32. Khoo L, Anson K, Patel U. Success and short-term complication rates of percutaneous nephrostomy during pregnancy. J Vasc Interv Radiol. 2004;15:1469–73.
33. Yang CH, Chan PH, La SK, Chang HC, Chiu B, Lin HM, Sheu MH. Urolithiasis in pregnancy. J Chin Med Assoc. 2004;67:625–8.
34. Lemos GC, El Hayek OR, Apezzato M. Rigid ureteroscopy for diagnosis and treatment of ureteral calculi during pregnancy. Int Braz J Urol. 2002;28:311–6.
35. Lifshitz DA, Lingeman JE. Ureteroscopy as a first-line intervention for ureteral calculi in pregnancy. J Endourol. 2002;16:19–22.
36. Watterson JD, Girvan AE, Beiko DT, Nott L, Wollin TA, Razvi H, Denstedt JD. Ureteroscopy and holmium:YAG laser lithotripsy: an emerging definitive management strategy for symptomatic ureteral calculi in pregnancy. Urology. 2002;60:383–7.
37. Shokeir AA, Mutabagani H. Rigid ureteroscopy in pregnant women. Br J Urol. 1998;81:678–81.
38. Scarpa RM, De Lisa A, Usai E. Diagnosis and treatment of ureteral calculi during pregnancy with rigid ureteroscopes. J Urol. 1996;155: 875–7.
39. Hosseini MM, Aminsharifi AR, Mostafavi M. S188 Radiation-free percutaneous nephrolithotomy (PCNL) in pregnancy. Eur Urol. 2010;9(6):604.
40. Csaba T, Gyorgy T, Attila V, Tibor F, Morshed AS. Percutaneous nephrolithotomy in early pregnancy. Int Urol Nephrol. 2005;37:1–3.
41. Shah A, Chandak P, Tiptaft R, Glass J, Dasgupta P. Percutaneous nephrolithotomy in early pregnancy. Int J Clin Pract. 2004;58(8):809–10.
42. Meares EM. Urologic surgery during pregnancy. Clin Obstet Gynecol. 1978;21:907–20.

73 Minimally Invasive Treatment of Calculi in Renal Anomalies

Ahmed R. El-Nahas and Ahmed A. Shokeir

Abstract

Treatment of calculi in patients with congenital renal anomalies (such as horseshoe, ectopic, autosomal dominant polycystic kidneys, and duplex systems) requires special considerations. These kidneys had abnormal vascular, altered calyceal orientation, and variable anatomical relations with the surrounding viscera. Nowadays, minimally invasive techniques (such as extracorporeal shock wave lithotripsy [SWL], flexible ureterorenoscopy [F-URS], percutaneous nephrolithotomy [PNL] and laparoscopic pyelolithotomy) are the most frequently used modalities for treatment of calculi in both normal and anomalous kidneys. They offer high stone-free rates with minimal morbidity and improved recovery. However, there are many challenges in utilization of these modalities in patients with renal anomalies.

In this chapter, we describe indications, techniques, and results of minimally invasive treatments for calculi in anomalous kidneys.

Keywords

Renal calculi • Congenital anomalies • Ectopic • Horseshoe • Duplex • Malrotated • Shock wave lithotripsy • Percutaneous nephrolithotomy • Flexible ureteroscopy • Laparoscopy

Introduction

Calculi in kidneys with anomalous anatomy pose a particular challenge for the urologist. These kidneys vary significantly in terms of position, calyceal orientation, relations of the calices to the renal pelvis, renal vasculature, relations with other intra-abdominal organs, and abnormal ureteral insertion [1]. These factors must be considered before making a treatment decision. However, the principle treatment guidelines remain the same as those for normal kidneys to achieve stone-free status with minimal number of procedures, treat concomitant obstruction to prevent stone recurrence, and use minimally invasive techniques whenever feasible.

Historically, most of those patients were treated with open surgery. Currently, and after the marked improvements in technology and availability of wide variety of instruments, minimally invasive modalities (such as extracorporeal shock wave lithotripsy [SWL], flexible ureterorenoscopy [F-URS], percutaneous nephrolithotomy [PNL], and laparoscopic pyelolithotomy) have almost replaced open surgery.

In this chapter, we will describe minimally invasive treatment modalities that have been employed in managing calculus disease in patients with congenital renal anomalies. The focus will be on indications, techniques, results, and the criteria for judging which approach is likely to be successful without undue morbidity in this challenging patient population.

A.R. El-Nahas, M.D. • A.A. Shokeir, M.D., Ph.D., FEBU (✉)
Department of Urology, Urology and Nephrology Center, Mansoura University, Mansoura, Egypt
e-mail: ar_el_nahas@yahoo.com; ahmed.shokeir@hotmail.com

J.J. Talati et al. (eds.), *Urolithiasis*,
DOI 10.1007/978-1-4471-4387-1_73,

Extracorporeal Shock Waves Lithotripsy (SWL)

Indications of SWL in Anomalous Kidneys

In the past 25 years, SWL had become the most widely performed procedure for treatment of urolithiasis including stones in anomalous kidneys [2]. It is indicated for treatment of stones smaller than 20 mm without distal obstruction. It was recommended by some authors as the first choice of treatment for calculi in kidneys with congenital anomalies being the least invasive modality [3, 4]. When anatomic obstruction requires surgical correction, SWL is no longer the therapeutic modality of choice [5]. The indications for SWL treatment in patients with autosomal dominant polycystic kidneys disease (ADPKD) are renal calculi less than 2 cm. Larger or branched calculi are treated with PNL and residual stones were treated with secondary nephroscopy and SWL [6].

Technique of SWL in Anomalous Kidneys

All patients can be treated on an outpatient basis using sedoanalgesia, except for children who require general anesthesia. Pretreatment simulation is important for stones that are too anterior or those obscured by the spine. Ultrasound localization is needed for lucent stones. Retrograde urography can be used in some patients to visualize a lucent stone. In cases of ectopic kidneys, the water cushion must be applied to the anterior abdominal wall to avoid hitting the iliac bone by the shock waves if it passed through a posterior site. Therefore, the patients must be in prone position in some machines when the water cushion cannot be moved to anterior position.

Results of SWL in Anomalous Kidneys

Results of SWL in Ectopic Kidneys

Good fragmentation could be obtained with SWL for stones in pelvic ectopic kidneys [7]. The resultant fragments did not clear easily because these kidneys have an inadequate urinary drainage. Therefore, the stone-free rates ranged from 25 to 100 % (Table 73.1). Multiple sessions are often required before patients become stone-free when using SWL in these patients compared to one to two sessions when PNL or ureteroscopy is used [4]. Residual fragments may lead to regrowth of symptomatic stones in 50–86 % of patients. These levels indicate a high risk of stone recurrence in patients with abnormal kidneys. In 2001, Gallucci et al. recommended that these patients should be considered at high risk for recurrence and they need to be followed up carefully [16].

Results of SWL in Horseshoe Kidneys

Stone-free rates after ESWL for horseshoe kidneys vary widely, ranging from 28 to 80 % [3, 17, 18] (Table 73.2). In 1996, Kirkali et al. reported 78 % fragmentation rate, but only 28 % of patients became stone-free at the end of follow-up [17]. Urinary drainage from the dependent lower calyces of horseshoe kidney may impair the passage of stone fragments. In 2004, Tunc et al. reported SWL for 45 horseshoe kidneys; the stone-free rate was 66 % and with an additional 22 % sufficient fragmentation rate and overall success of 88 % [8].

Results of SWL in ADPKD

Table 73.3 summarizes the results of SWL for treatment of calculi in autosomal dominant polycystic kidney disease (ADPKD). Delakas et al. in 1997 reported their experience with SWL for 16 renal units of ADPKD [26]. Ten renal units had complete fragmentation with one session; three units had successful complete fragmentation after a second SWL session, and three units had no fragmentation and needed other procedures. In 2002, Deliveliotis et al. reported SWL for treatment of four patients with calyceal stones in ADPKD [29]. The mean stone diameter was 1 cm. Although stone fragmentation was successful in all patients, only one patient (25 %) became stone-free. In 1995, Cass published a study of 13 patients with renal cysts who were treated for urolithiasis using SWL (included 4 patients with ADPKD) [25]. In spite of the fragmentation of stones in the four patients, only two of them (50 %) were stone-free at 3 months.

Results of SWL in Duplex and Malrotated Kidney

The stone-free rate after SWL for stones in duplex systems ranges from 55 to 86 % (Table 73.4). Tunc et al. considered SWL to be the preferred therapeutic option for duplex kidneys [8]. The stone-free rate after SWL for stones in malrotated kidneys ranged from 50 to 69 % (Table 73.5).

Factors Affecting Stone-Free Rate After SWL for Anomalous Kidneys

In 2003, Sheir et al. published a large series of patients (198) who were treated for urolithiasis in anomalous kidneys using ESWL [3]. Stone-free rates vary with stone size and location. In patients with stones of 1.5 cm or less, a stone-free rate of 79 % was achieved, compared with 53.3 % for calculi larger than 1.5 cm. The minimum success rate was obtained in patients with multiple calyceal stones (20 %). Comparisons of the stone-free rate among the types of anomalies showed that the type of renal anomaly had no statistical impact on the stone-free rate.

Tunc et al., in 2004, published a study on 150 patients with stones in anomalous kidneys, which were treated by ESWL [8]. The minimum success rate was obtained in

Table 73.1 Results of minimally invasive treatment of renal stones in ectopic kidney

References, year	*N*	Treatment Method	Stone-free rate (%)
Kupeli et al. (1999) [2]	13	SWL	54
Tunc et al. (2004) [8]	14[a]	SWL	57
	4[b]		25
Al-Tawheed et al. 2006 [4]	10	SWL	100
Weizer et al. (2005) [9]	4	Flexible URS	75
Fayad (2008) [10]	4	Flexible URS	75
Desai and Jasani (2000) [11]	9	PNL	100
Holman and Tóth (1998) [12]	15	Lap-assisted PNL	100
Maheshwari et al. (2004) [13]	3	Lap-assisted PNL	100
Matlaga et al. (2006) [14]	8	Lap-assisted PNL: 6	100
		PNL: 2	100
El-kappany et al. (2007) [15]	11	Lap. pyelolithotomy: 6	100
		Lap-assisted PNL: 5	80

N number of renal units
[a]Simple ectopia
[b]Crossed fused ectopic

Table 73.2 Results of different treatment methods of renal stones in horseshoe kidneys

References, year	*N*	Treatment method	Stone-free rate (%)
Kirkali et al. (1996) [17]	18	SWL	28
Semerci et al. (1997) [19]	18	SWL	60
Sheir et al. (2003) [3]	49	SWL	71.4
Tunc et al. (2004) [8]	45	SWL	66
Al-Tawheed et al. (2006) [4]	9	SWL	76.9
Weizer et al. (2005) [9]	4	Flexible URS	75
Janetschek and Kunzel (1988) [20]	8	PNL	89
Lampel et al. (1996) [18]	41	SWL: 37	76
		PNL: 4	75
Shokeir et al. (2004) [21]	45	PNL	82
Mosavi-Bahar et al. (2007) [22]	7	PNL	71
Razvi and Zaidi (2007) [23]	19	PNL	93
Gupta et al. (2009) [24]	37	PNL	100

Table 73.3 Results of different methods for treatment of renal stones in ADPKD

References, year	*N*	Treatment method	Stone-free rate (%)
Cass (1995) [25]	4	SWL	50
Delakas et al. (1997) [26]	16	SWL	81
Ng et al. (2000) [6]	8	SWL: 6	100
		PNL+ESWL: 2	100
Al-Kandari et al. (2009) [27]	20	PNL	89.4
Umbreit et al. (2010) [28]	11	PNL	82

patients with lower-calyceal stones (50 %), followed by middle-calyceal (60 %) calculi. Success was size dependent. In patients with stones larger than 3 cm, only 34 % became stone-free, compared with 92 % for calculi smaller than 1 cm. In 2006, Al-Tawheed et al. observed better clearance for calculi in the renal pelvis or upper pole [4].

Table 73.4 Results of different methods for treatment of renal stones in duplex kidneys

References, year	*N*	Treatment method	Stone-free rate (%)
Semerci et al. (1997) [19]	27	SWL	60
Gallucci et al. (2001) [16]	34	SWL	55
Sheir et al. (2003) [3]	29	SWL	86.2
Tunc et al. (2004) [8]	57	SWL	80
Rana and Bhojwani (2009) [1]	12	PNL	91.6

In ADPKD, the combination of anatomical complexity and cyst calcifications may compromise precise SWL stone localization [28]. In patients with nephrolithiasis in cystic kidneys, renal cysts may interfere with the passage of stone fragments due to urinary stasis from the stretching and distortion of the calyces by the renal cysts. Therefore, the rates of stone clearance were lesser compared with the non-ADPKD kidneys. The stone-free rate was 25 % in ADPKD compared with 83 % in solitary renal cyst [29].

Table 73.5 Results of different methods for treatment of renal stones in malrotated kidneys

References, year	*N*	Treatment method	Stone-free rate (%)
Sheir et al. (2003) [3]	120	SWL	69
Al-Tawheed et al. (2006) [4]	4	SWL	50
Mosavi-Bahar et al. (2007) [22]	5	PNL	80
Rana and Bhojwani (2009) [1]	14	PNL	92.8
Binbay et al. (2011) [30]	44	PNL	77.4

In duplex kidneys, insufficient spontaneous passage of fragments after SWL may be due to ectopic ureteral insertion or kinking and narrowing at the junction of two ureters [8].

Complications of ESWL in Anomalous Kidneys

Tunc et al. reported renal colic in 26.6 % of patients, acute pyelonephritis in 5.3 % of cases, and Steinstrasse formation in 4 % [8]. Sheir et al. observed Steinstrasse in 3.5 % of patients, but no perirenal hematoma or fluid collection was detected by regular follow-up ultrasonography [3]. Acute pyelonephritis was treated with appropriate antibiotics and Steinstrasse were treated with ureteral stent or ureteroscopic stone extraction.

Cass [25] and Deliveliotis et al. [29] reported no significant changes in blood pressure during or after SWL for patients with cystic kidneys. No hemorrhage, rupture, or infections within the cysts were reported immediately or after 1 month after the procedure. They concluded that SWL is the primary treatment for small calculi in cystic kidneys. In 1987, Rubin et al. performed computed tomography (CT) scans for 50 patients with ADPKD after SWL to study the effect of shock waves on the renal parenchyma and cysts [31]. Post-SWL scans demonstrated asymptomatic subcapsular hematomas in eight (15 %) patients (two large, six small) and intrarenal hematomas in two (4 %) patients. In three (6 %) patients, small subcapsular fluid collections of uncertain cause were seen. The effect of the shock waves on the renal cysts of normal kidneys was evaluated by different authors. In 1985, Kaude et al. documented hemorrhage into renal cyst in two of three kidneys examined by magnetic resonance imaging after SWL [32]. In 1990, Williamson et al. detected hemorrhage into the cyst in one of three kidneys after SWL with computerized tomography [33]. The patient with hemorrhage had thrombocytopenia, which probably predisposed him to bleeding.

Flexible Ureterorenoscopy (F-URS)

Indications of F-URS in Anomalous Kidneys

F-URS have been recommended as an alternative procedure to SWL in patients with large renal calculi, stones in dependent or obstructed portions of the renal collecting system, and unfavorable stone composition (calcium oxalate monohydrate, brushite, cystine). It is also indicated when some patient characteristics such as obesity and body habitus deformities can limit the efficacy of SWL. In addition, there are circumstances under which SWL and PNL are not clinically or medically feasible for managing patients with renal calculi in ectopic kidneys [34].

In recent years, new developments in endourological techniques have allowed retrograde intrarenal surgery (RIRS) of stone therapy to gain more and more influence. Virtually the whole collecting system can be inspected using small actively deflectable flexible ureteroscopes. Holmium laser lithotripsy has provided an effective method to fragment stones [35]. Therefore, some groups prefer primary endoscopic treatment for stones in anomalously sited kidneys [9].

Technique of F-URS

A flexible or rigid cystoscope is used to insert a 0.035-in. polytetrafluoroethylene-coated guide wire into the ureter under fluoroscopic guidance until it is coiled in the kidney. A second "working" hydrophilic-coated wire must be inserted to backload the endoscope, allowing the wire to act as a guide for the instrument to be advanced into the ureter or kidney under fluoroscopic guidance.

Alternatively, a ureteral access sheath (UAS) can be used to allow access to the renal pelvis. The access sheath has many benefits. It allows free drainage of the irrigation from the kidney, thus improving vision and prevents potentially harmful elevations in intrarenal pressure. It has the potential to improve stone-free rates by allowing passive or active retrieval of fragments as the F-URS can be introduced many times in short time through the sheath. On the other hand, UAS can lead to ischemia of the ureter. Therefore, it is advised to use a suitable size of the UAS and to hydrate its outer surface adequately. UAS should also be introduced gently under fluoroscopic guidance, and if it does not pass upward, a ureteral stent can be left for a few days for passive dilatation of the ureter [36].

Flexible URS is performed with a 7.5–9.5 F actively deflecting tip ureteroscope. Holmium laser is essential for stone fragmentation. Tipless nitinol graspers or baskets are used in repositioning of the renal calculi from the lower pole into an upper pole calyx, in which intracorporeal lithotripsy can be performed more effectively [37] and they are used for extraction of fragments. A ureteral stent is placed at the completion of the procedure [9]. Figure 73.1 shows a case of F-URS for treatment of renal stones in crossed ectopic kidney.

Results of F-URS in Anomalous Kidneys

Many patients with renal calculi in orthotropically positioned kidneys are successfully treated by a retrograde approach

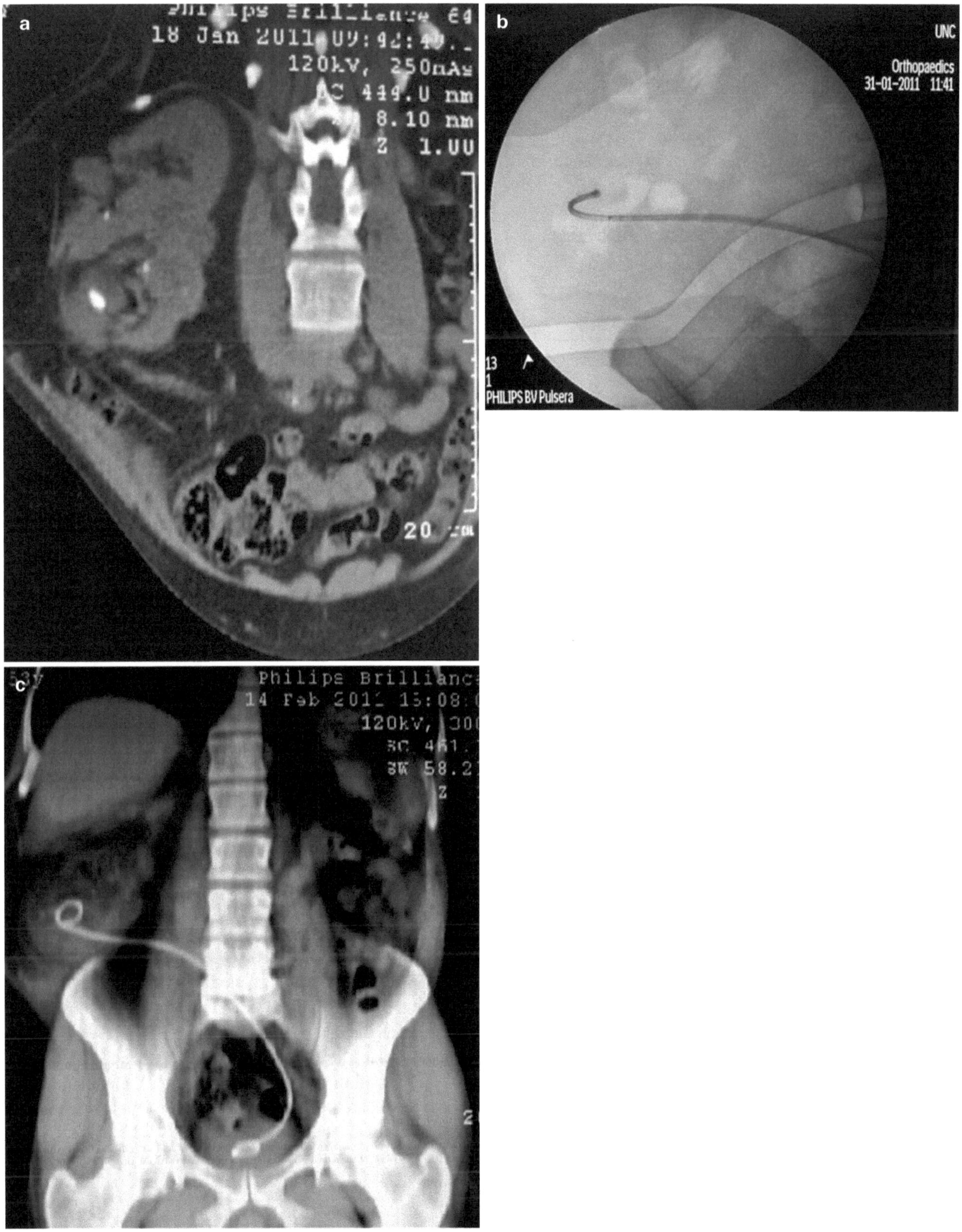

Fig. 73.1 (**a**) Preoperative noncontrast computed tomography (*NCCT*), coronal-oblique view showing a stone in the renal pelvis of crossed fused ectopic left kidney in the *right* iliac region. (**b**) Intraoperative fluoroscopy showing the flexible URS passing from *left* to *right* to reach the stone in the crossed ectopic kidney. (**c**) Postoperative NCCT, coronal view showing no residual stones and the double-J stent

with excellent stone-free rates. To date, only individual cases of retrograde management of patients with renal calculi in pelvic kidneys have been reported. The stone-free rate for treatment of intrarenal calculi in pelvic kidneys treated with URS is 75 % [9, 10] (see Table 73.1). In horseshoe kidneys, the stone-free rate was also 75 % with no reported intraoperative or postoperative complications [9] (see Table 73.2).

Percutaneous Nephrolithotomy (PNL)

Indications of PNL in Anomalous Kidneys

PNL is an established modality of stone management. In anomalous kidneys, PNL can be used for treatment of complex, branched, and large calculi of 2.5 cm or more or in patients with failed SWL.

Techniques of PNL in Anomalous Kidneys

Technique of PNL in Ectopic Kidneys

PNL has been applied to ectopic kidneys occasionally—fear of injury to abdominal viscera makes it a technically challenging procedure [11]. The procedure is done under general anesthesia. A supine oblique position with a pack under the ipsilateral hemi-pelvis is utilized. After retrograde fixation of a ureteral catheter, the pelvicalyceal system is opacified. Then side-to-side mobility of the kidney is assessed, and ability to displace the kidney close to the abdominal wall by contralateral pressure is determined. The desired calyx of entry is localized using ultrasound guidance. Pressure on the ultrasound probe itself is utilized to displace any intervening loops of bowel away from the puncture line to the targeted calyx.

Dilatation is performed under fluoroscopic control followed by fixation of an Amplatz sheath. Ultrasound lithotripsy is used for stone fragmentation through a rigid nephroscope. When using flexible nephroscope, laser disintegration is utilized [24]. In all cases, after stone clearance, an on-table ultrasound study and a contrast study through the Amplatz sheath are done. Then a double-J stent is inserted. The contrast study is repeated prior to nephrostomy tube removal [11].

Technique of PNL in Horseshoe Kidneys

In horseshoe kidneys, two main factors differ from the normal renal anatomy, namely, blood supply and the orientation of the collecting system. In an anatomic and radiologic study, Janetschek and Kunzel have shown that all blood vessels enter the kidney from its ventromedial aspect, except for some to the isthmus [20]. Therefore, percutaneous access must be obtained on the opposite—far from the major arteries. The dorsal arteries to the isthmus are protected by the spine and are situated away from the nephrostomy tract. The risk of arterial bleeding is not greater than in a normal kidney. In a horseshoe kidney, most of the calyces point either dorsomedial or dorsolateral. The calyces of the isthmus lie within a coronal plane and point medially. The anatomic situation results in a lower and more medial position of the nephrostomy tract, whose orientation is more or less dorsoventral [20].

Upper pole access is preferred because it allows access to the upper pole calices, renal pelvis, lower pole calices, pelvi-ureteral junction, and proximal ureter. Access to the calices in the isthmus is gained across the pelvis [20]. Furthermore, upper pole access can decrease blood loss, because the long axis of the nephroscope is aligned with the long axis of the kidney, thereby minimizing nephroscope torque on renal tissue during manipulation [38]. Figure 73.2 shows upper pole access for PNL in horseshoe kidney. However, upper pole access will result in an unusually long tract, and the instruments may not reach the lower and medial calices. This problem is exacerbated in obese patients, but it can be overcome using long nephroscopes [39]. In horseshoe kidney, upper pole percutaneous access is often essential and is relatively safe owing to the inferior displacement of the kidneys away from the pleura. Violation of the pleural cavity is decreased because a supracostal approach is less likely [38].

Technique of PNL in ADPKD

In ADPKD, calyceal distortion is common because of the large, multiple renal cysts. Simple cyst aspiration may facilitate calyceal localization and percutaneous access and more than one access tract may be needed [28]. A prone position is suitable with fluoroscopic guidance after retrograde ureteral catheterization. Choosing the proper calyx for puncture depends on the stone location and the width of the target calyx. To avoid dilating the cysts, the contrast material is mixed with methylthioninium chloride; thus, only when blue dye comes from the puncture, the next steps are undertaken. Dilatation is performed using sequential facial dilators or balloons. A polytetrafluoroethylene (PTFE)-coated guide wire with a J-tip is initially used to negotiate the target calyx and to reach the renal pelvis. The use of flexible nephroscope is encouraged for retrieval of distant fragments [27].

At completion of the PNL procedures, nephrostogram is done to evaluate the collecting system for injury, extravasation, or residual stone fragments. An 18–22-Fr nephrostomy tube and a 6-Fr ureteral catheter are inserted [28]. Figure 73.3 shows PNL in ADPKD.

Technique of PNL in Duplex Kidney

PNL in duplex kidney is relatively straightforward. The most important requirements are to create perfect calyceal punctures and to maintain the accessibility of the PNL tract with a guidewire throughout the procedure [1].

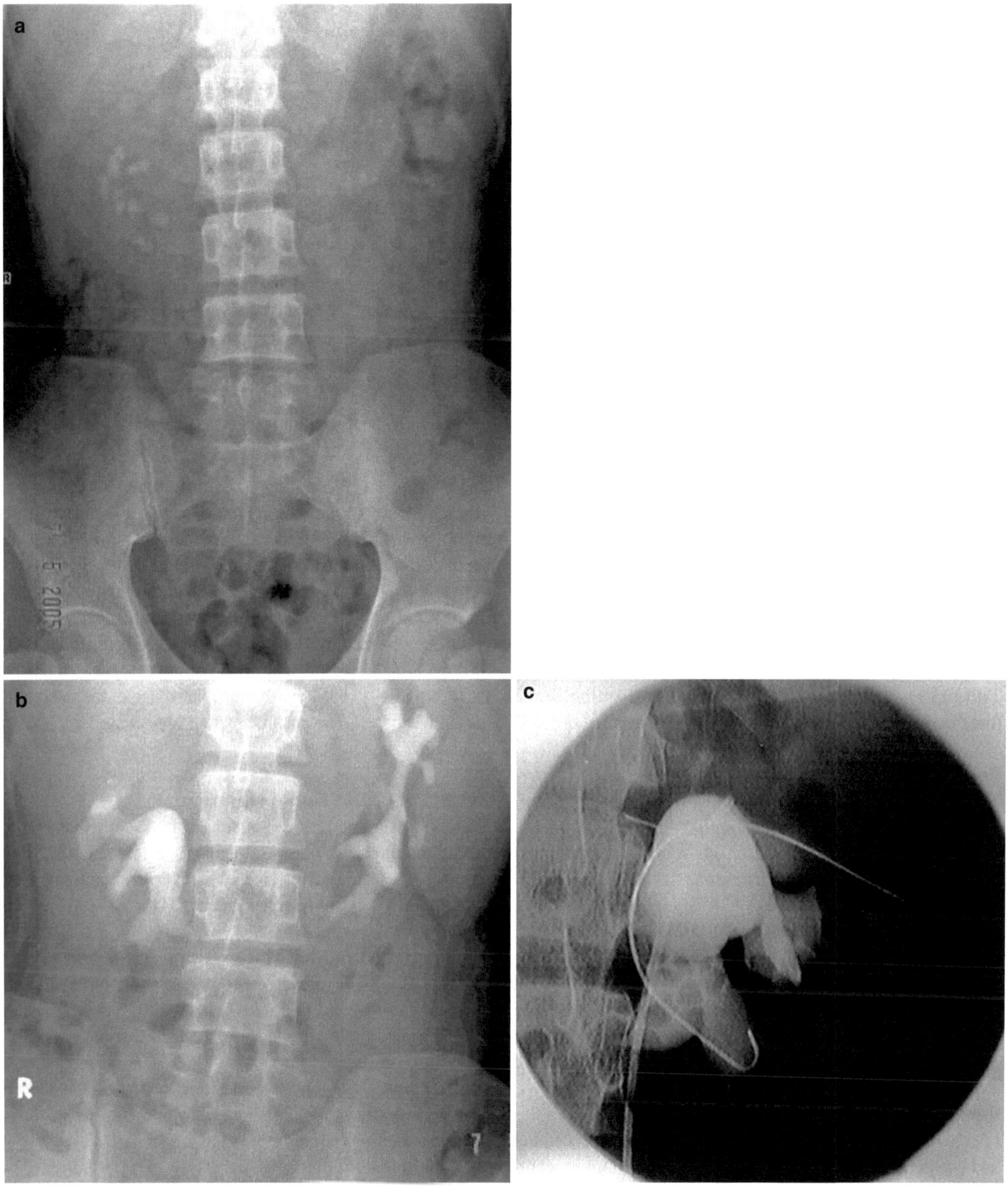

Fig. 73.2 (**a**) Kidneys-ureters-bladder (*KUB*) X-ray showing multiple radio-opaque shadows in the right kidney region. (**b**) Intravenous urogram (*IVU*) showing that these multiple stones are present in a horseshoe kidney. (**c**) Intraoperative fluoroscopy showing the ureteral catheter and the guide wire passed through the upper pole calyx

Technique of PNL in Malrotated Kidney

Although it was thought that it is not always easy to achieve optimal access in malrotated kidneys due to altered calyceal position, Binbay et al. in 2011 described the technique of PNL for calculi in patients with simple renal malrotation [30]. They found that most calices face posterior while the renal pelvis is anterior. Therefore, percutaneous renal access using fluoroscopy seems to be easier than normal kidneys.

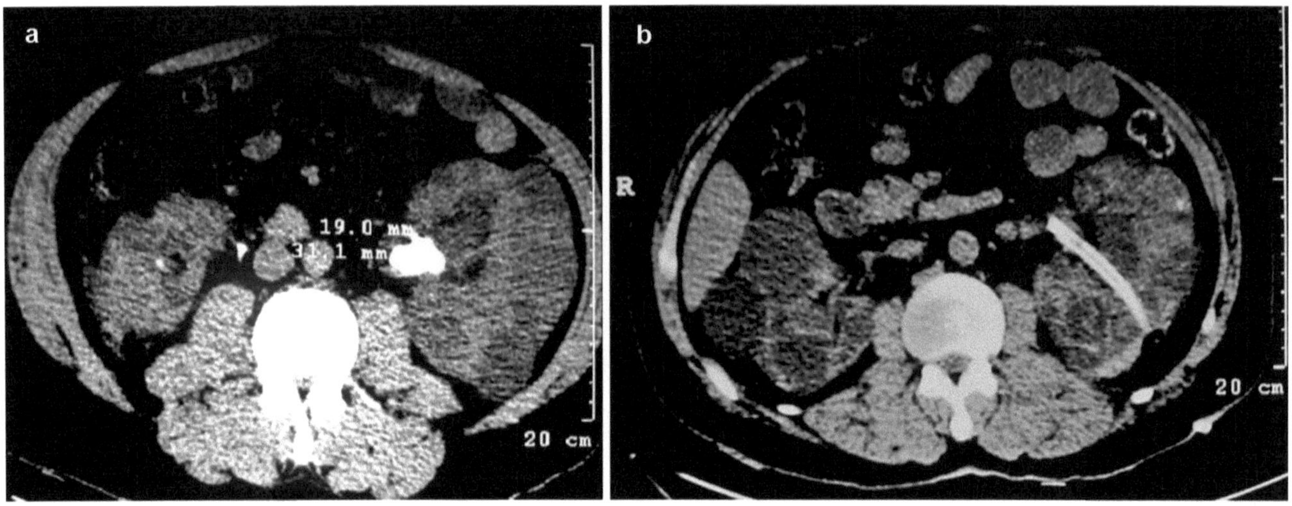

Fig. 73.3 (**a**) Preoperative noncontrast computed tomography (*NCCT*), axial scan showing hyperdense stone in the renal pelvis of the left polycystic kidney. (**b**) Postoperative NCCT, axial scan showing left nephrostomy tube and no residual stones

Results of PNL in Anomalous Kidneys

Results of PNL in Ectopic Kidneys

In 2000, Desai and Jasani published a study of nine patients with stones in ectopic kidneys who were treated by PNL [11]. The mean hospital stay was 5.2 days (range 3–8 days), complete stone clearance was achieved in all cases (see Table 73.1). Six cases were cleared in a single sitting, while three cases required a second-look nephroscopy.

Results of PNL in Horseshoe Kidney

Table 73.2 summarizes the results of PNL for treatment of calculi in horseshoe kidneys. Shokeir et al., in 2004, reported a single-center experience of PNL in 34 patients (45 renal units) with horseshoe kidneys [21]. The stone-free rate was 82.2 % and the mean hospital stay was 4 ± 1.9 days (range 3–12 days). Auxiliary procedures were required in (35.3 %) of patients, including ureteroscopy, second-look PNL, and ESWL to fragment residual calyceal stones. In 2009, Gupta et al. published a study of 31 patients (37 renal units) with stones in horseshoe kidneys who were treated by PNL [24]. The overall stone-free rate was 100 % and the mean hospital stay was 3.2 days (range 1–8 days). The criteria for considering a second-look PNL were postoperative plain X-ray showing residual stones, intraoperative bleeding causing nonprogression of the procedure, and a large stone burden requiring longer than 90 min for completion of the procedure.

Results of PNL in ADPKD

Table 73.3 summarizes the results of PNL for treatment of calculi in ADPKD. In 2010, Umbreit et al. reported their experience of PNL in 11 renal units with ADPKD [28]. The average stone burden was 2.5 cm (range 1.6–3.6). Overall, four patients required repeat percutaneous procedures to become stone-free and the mean hospital stay was 3.1 days (range 2–6 days). Al-Kandari et al. in 2009 reported on PNL in 20 renal units with ADPKD [27]. The proper puncture could not be achieved in one patient. Second-look PNL through the already present nephrostomy tract was required in three patients (15 %) with multiple stones in the renal pelvis and calyces. The mean hospital stay was 3 ± 1.2 days (range 2–5 days).

Results of PNL in Duplex Kidneys

Table 73.4 summarizes the results of PNL for treatment of calculi in duplex kidneys. Rana and Bhojwani, in 2009, reported 92 % stone-free rates after PNL for treatment of 12 patients with stones in duplex kidneys [1].

Results of PNL in Malrotated Kidneys

The results of PNL for treatment of stones in malrotated kidneys are summarized in Table 73.5. In 2007, Mosavi-Bahar et al. reported their experience of PNL in five patients [22]. In a single-stage single-tract operation, 80 % of the patients became stone-free, and second-look procedure produced 100 % stone-free rate. The mean hospital stay was 3 days and mean hemoglobin drop was 0.8 mg/dl.

A multicenter comparative study was reported in 2011 by Binbay et al. for PNL treatment of stones in malrotated and normal kidneys [30]. They observed comparable stone-free rates (77 % for malrotated and 79 % for normal kidneys). The mean operative time, number of access tracts, and rate of blood transfusion were also comparable.

Complications of PNL in Anomalous Kidney

Rana and Bhojwani, in 2009, reported their experience with PNL in 48 patients with various types of renal anomalies [1]. No major complications were observed. The reported complications included blood transfusion in three patients (6 %), postoperative pyrexia >38 °C in three patients, perinephric collection in two patients, and one patient developed intraperitoneal urine leak after laparoscopic-assisted PNL.

Ectopic Kidney

In ectopic kidneys, intraperitoneal spill of contrast on nephrostogram and persistent leak from the nephrostomy site were observed in 22.2 % of patients [11].

Horseshoe Kidney

In horseshoe kidneys, Shokeir et al., in 2004, reported complications in 13.3 % of patients [21]. They included significant hematuria requiring blood transfusion, septicemia, ureteral obstruction by stone fragments, and colonic injury. Angio-embolization was necessary to control bleeding in 0.02 % of patients. Raj et al., in 2003, reported pneumothorax in one out of 15 patients with an upper pole nephrostomy tract in a horseshoe kidney [38]. However, all other series with large number of patients did not observe pleural injury [21, 24].

Colonic perforation during PNL of horseshoe kidneys was encountered in 3 of 51 procedures (5.9 %). It may produce dangerous morbidity in the form of septicemia, peritonitis, abscess formation, and nephrocolic or colocutaneous fistula. Advanced age and horseshoe kidneys were found to be independent risk factors for colonic perforation during PNL. Early diagnosis and proper treatment are keys to minimize patient morbidity and avoid serious complications [40]. Some investigators recommend CT with contrast before PNL in patients with horseshoe kidneys to avoid colonic injury [41].

ADPKD

In ADPKD, minor complications were seen in 15 % of patients. They included low-grade fever (10 %), mild hematuria with no need for a blood transfusion (5 %), and bleeding via the nephrostomy tube (5 %). The mean decrease in the hemoglobin level was 1.2 ± 1.1 g. Bleeding during or after the procedure is a risk in patients with ADPKD as they have varying degrees of chronic renal impairment, which is commonly associated with a coagulation defect [27].

Malrotated Kidney

In malrotated kidneys, Binbay et al., in 2011, had found that complications of PNL in malrotated kidneys were comparable to non-malrotated kidneys [30]. They included transient fever, urinary tract infection (UTI), and urine leakage through the nephrostomy tube.

Laparoscopic Pyelolithotomy

Indications of Laparoscopic Pyelolithotomy in Anomalous Kidneys

In 1985, Esghi et al. were the first to report laparoscopic stone removal in a pelvic kidney [42]. The indications for treatment of patients with stones in ectopic kidneys by laparoscopic pyelolithotomy are stones larger than 3 cm or branched renal-pelvic stones or multiple pelvic and caliceal stones [15]. Laparoscopic pyelolithotomy seems to be ideal treatment for large renal-pelvic stones in ectopic kidneys because it has the advantage of avoiding renal parenchymal puncture in addition to the advantages of minimally invasive procedures. It is a well-tolerated and feasible technique for treatment of stones in ectopic kidneys with better visualization, avoiding iatrogenic injuries of concomitant vascular abnormalities [43].

Technique of Laparoscopic Pyelolithotomy

After administration of general anesthesia, the patient is placed in the dorsal lithotomy position and the procedure starts with cystoscopic insertion of an open-end ureteral catheter under fluoroscopic guidance. The patient is then placed in the Trendelenburg position with slight lateral elevation of the side to be operated on to help the bowel to fall away from the operative field. The primary surgeon stands on the side opposite the affected kidney and the assistant on the same side.

Three or four transperitoneal ports are placed in a fan-shaped distribution (Fig. 73.4): an umbilical port for the laparoscope, two pararectal ports for the primary surgeon, and one port in the iliac fossa for the assistant. The intestinal loops are dislodged away from the anterior surface of the kidney, the posterior peritoneum is incised in the right side, and the mesocolon is incised on the left side to expose the kidney surface [15].

The renal pelvis is identified with fluoroscopy: by viewing of the large pelvic stone or with the aid of retrograde ureteropyelography to localize the renal pelvis accurately. The renal pelvis is exposed by dissection of the peripelvic fatty tissue then incised with a laparoscopic scalpel or endoscissors. The pelvic stone is retrieved with an endograsper, entrapped in the cutoff finger of a surgical glove, and removed

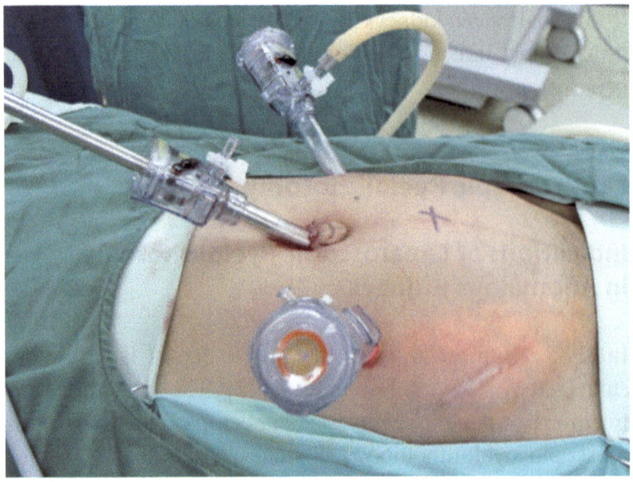

Fig. 73.4 Intraoperative picture showing ports distribution for laparoscopic pyelolithotomy of a stone in a pelvic kidney

through a 10-mm port site at the end of the procedure. In patients with an additional large calyceal stone, a nephroscope is passed through one of the 10-mm ports and then through the pyelotomy, where the stone is broken up, and the fragments are retrieved.

After removal of all stones as confirmed with fluoroscopy, the pyelotomy is closed with 4/0 polyglactin sutures. The incision in the peritoneum or mesocolon is closed, and a 20 F transperitoneal perinephric tube drain is left. The ureteral catheter is removed after 3 days, followed by removal of the tube drain the next morning [15].

Results of Laparoscopic Pyelolithotomy in Ectopic Kidneys

Table 73.1 summarizes the results of laparoscopic pyelolithotomy for treatment of calculi in ectopic kidneys. The patient benefits by avoiding the morbidity of an abdominal incision. Pyeloplasty can be performed simultaneously. El-Kappany et al. in 2007 published a study of five patients with stones in ectopic kidneys who were treated by laparoscopic pyelolithotomy [15]. The mean hospital stay was 3.8 ± 0.4 days and the stone-free rate was 100 % with no reported cases of conversion to open surgery. There are some case reports of laparoscopic pyelolithotomy in pelvic kidneys [43–47].

Laparoscopic-Assisted PNL

Indications of Laparoscopic-Assisted PNL

The indications for laparoscopic-assisted PNL for treatment of stones in ectopic kidneys are large calyceal stones and failed ESWL. The combination of laparoscopic and percutaneous approaches is an attempt to avoid the risk of injury to surrounding abdominal viscera and blood vessels by the establishment of a percutaneous tract into the kidney safely under direct vision [15]. The general consensus is that laparoscopic guidance is important for percutaneous renal access because adhesions between the bowel and the peritoneal surface of the kidney were found in 13–27 % of patients [12, 15]. Therefore, laparoscopic dissection of these adhesions was performed prior to the establishment of the percutaneous tract. This method also provides the opportunity for safe access to the pelvicalyceal system and stone clearance in a single session [13].

Technique of Laparoscopic-Assisted PNL

The type of anesthesia, patient placement, insertion of the ureteral catheter, and port placement are similar to laparoscopic pyelolithotomy. The primary surgeon stands on the side of the affected kidney and the assistant on the opposite side. Intestinal loops are dislodged away from the anterior surface of the kidney.

Retrograde pyelography is performed, and percutaneous renal access to the targeted calyx is established through a separate skin puncture under both laparoscopic vision and fluoroscopic guidance (C-arm). A stiff guide wire with a floppy J-tip is passed to coil in the upper calyx (in cases of lower-calyceal puncture) or negotiated into the ureter (in cases of upper-calyceal puncture). The tract is dilated and an Amplatz sheath is fixed (Fig. 73.5). Through the rigid nephroscope, large stones are broken up with a pneumatic lithotripter, and small stones are removed with forceps.

At the end of the procedure, the Amplatz sheath is removed; a nephrostomy tube and a transperitoneal tube drain are left. A control plain film is performed after 24 h. The nephrostomy tube is removed after 48 h, followed 6 h later by the ureteral catheter. The tube drain is removed the next morning, and the patient is discharged home [15].

Results of Laparoscopic-Assisted PNL in Ectopic Kidneys

The results of laparoscopic-assisted PNL for treatment of calculi in ectopic kidneys are summarized in Table 73.1. Holman and Tóth, in 1998, published their experience with 15 cases; all the stones could be removed successfully [12]. The only complication was delayed urine leakage through the abdominal drain in one patient. The average operating time was 55 min (range 40–85); the average hospital stay was 4.8 days (range 4–11). El-Kappany et al. in 2007 performed the same technique for five patients; one patient had

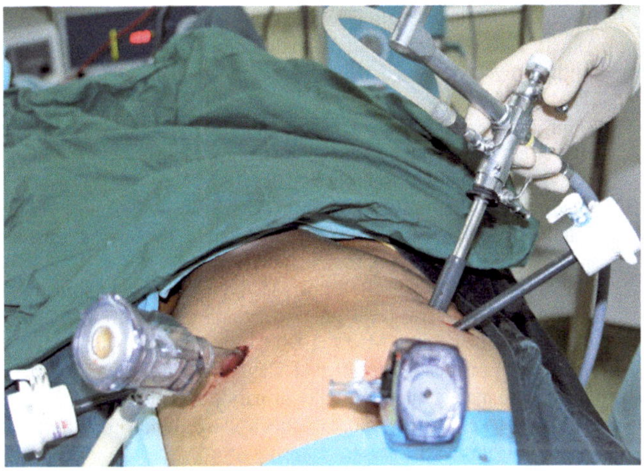

Fig. 73.5 Intraoperative picture showing ports distribution and Amplatz site for laparoscopic-assisted PNL in right pelvic kidney

a residual calyceal fragment that was treated with ESWL, and a hemostatic suture was needed to control brisk parenchymal bleeding beside the nephrostomy tube [15]. In 2006, Matlaga et al. reported on six patients who were treated for stones in ectopic kidneys using laparoscopic-assisted PNL [14]. The stone-free rate was 100 % with no reported cases of conversion to open surgery. Various authors had reported case reports with complete stone clearance without intraoperative or postoperative morbidity [48, 49].

Conclusion

For minimally invasive treatments of calculi in anomalous kidneys, SWL is recommended only for small stones (<2 cm) and when urinary drainage is not hindered while PNL is the treatment of choice for large and complex stones. The role of F-URS is not completely defined because of the limited number of published data. However, F-URS can be more frequently utilized in treatment of these patients.

- *In ectopic kidneys*, failed SWL can be considered for F-URS and holmium laser lithotripsy. Laparoscopic-assisted PNL and laparoscopic pyelolithotomy are the choice for large and complex stones as they avoid complications caused by anatomical abnormalities. Laparoscopic approach is also helpful in patients with associated UPJO because pyeloplasty can be done simultaneously.
- *In horseshoe kidneys*, stones that have failed SWL or that are larger than 2 cm are best managed by F-URS or PNL. However, PNL was associated with less residual stones and more complications.
- *In ADPKD*, therapeutic planning for calculus disease must consider the anatomical kidney distortion and patient's medical complexity. PNL is a safe and efficacious approach. It has a satisfactory stone-free rate and accepted morbidity. The outcome and complications are comparable to the already published results of PNL in the kidneys with normal anatomy.
- *In duplex kidney*, upper tract urinary stasis is common; the lower pole of the duplex system is dependent and may have impaired clearance of fragments after SWL. F-URS and PNL in duplex kidney are relatively straightforward procedures.
- *In malrotated kidneys*, most calices face posterior while the renal pelvis is anterior. Therefore, percutaneous renal access seems to be easier than normal kidneys.

Finally, the choice of treatment of calculi in patients with congenital renal anomalies requires strategic planning after studying all preoperative laboratory and radiological investigations. It is important to discuss with the patients the options of treatment and the reported outcomes of each. The decision is usually individualized in each case depending on many factors such as the patient's general condition, renal function, stone burden, surgeon experience, and available instruments.

References

1. Rana AM, Bhojwani JP. Percutaneous nephrolithotomy in renal anomalies of fusion, ectopia, rotation, hypoplasia, and pelvicalyceal aberration: uniformity in heterogeneity. J Endourol. 2009;23: 609–14.
2. Küpeli B, Isen K, Biri H, Sinik Z, Alkibay T, Karaoğlan U, et al. Extracorporeal shockwave lithotripsy in anomalous kidneys. J Endourol. 1999;13:349–52.
3. Sheir KZ, Gad HM. Prospective study of the effects of shock wave lithotripsy on renal function: role of post-shock wave lithotripsy obstruction. Urology. 2003;61(6):1102–6. discussion 1106.
4. Al-Tawheed AR, Al-Awadi KA, Kehinde EO, Abdul-Halim H, Hanafi AM, Ali Y. Treatment of calculi in kidneys with congenital anomalies: an assessment of the efficacy of lithotripsy. Urol Res. 2006;34:291–8.
5. Grossa AJ, Fisher M. Management of stones in patients with anomalously sited kidneys. Curr Opin Urol. 2006;16:100–5.
6. Ng CS, Yost A, Streem SB. Nephrolithiasis associated with autosomal dominant polycystic kidney disease: contemporary urological management. J Urol. 2000;163:726–9.
7. Bhatia V, Biyani CS. Urolithiasis with congenital upper tract anomalies: a 4-year experience with extracorporeal shock wave lithotripsy. J Endourol. 1994;8:5–8.
8. Tunc L, Tokgoz H, Tan MO, Kupeli B, Karaoglan U, Bozkirli I. Stones in anomalous kidneys: results of treatment by shock wave lithotripsy in 150 patients. Int J Urol. 2004;11(10):831–6.
9. Weizer AZ, Springhart WP, Ekeruo WO, Matlaga BR, Tan YH, Assimos DG, et al. Ureteroscopic management of renal calculi in anomalous kidneys. Urology. 2005;65:265–9.
10. Fayad AS. Retrograde holmium:YAG laser disintegration of stones in pelvic ectopic kidneys: would it minimize the risk of surgery? J Endourol. 2008;22:919–22.
11. Desai MR, Jasani A. Percutaneous nephrolithotripsy in ectopic kidneys. J Endourol. 2000;14:289–92.

12. Holman E, Tóth C. Laparoscopically assisted percutaneous transperitoneal nephrolithotomy in pelvic dystopic kidneys: experience in 15 successful cases. J Laparoendosc Adv Surg Tech A. 1998; 8:431–5.
13. Maheshwari PN, Bhandarkar DS, Andankar MG, Shah RS. Laparoscopically guided transperitoneal percutaneous nephrolithotomy for calculi in pelvic ectopic kidneys. Surg Endosc. 2004; 18:1151.
14. Matlaga BR, Kim SC, Watkins SL, Kuo RL, Munch LC, Lingeman JE. Percutaneous nephrolithotomy for ectopic kidneys: over, around, or through. Urology. 2006;67:513–7.
15. El-Kappany HA, El-Nahas AR, Shoma AM, El-Tabey NA, Eraky I, El-Kenawy MR. Combination of laparoscopy and nephroscopy for treatment of stones in pelvic ectopic kidneys. J Endourol. 2007; 10:1131–6.
16. Gallucci M, Vincenzoni A, Schettini M, Fortunato P, Cassanelli A, Zaccara A. Extracorporeal shock wave lithotripsy in ureteral and kidney malformations. Urol Int. 2001;66:61–5.
17. Kirkali Z, Esen AA, Mungan MU. Effectiveness of extracorporeal shockwave lithotripsy in the management of stone-bearing horseshoe kidneys. J Endourol. 1996;10:13–5.
18. Lampel A, Hohenfellner M, Schultz-Lampel D, Lazica M, Bohnen K, Thürof JW. Urolithiasis in horseshoe kidneys: therapeutic management. Urology. 1996;47:182–6.
19. Semerci B, Verit A, Nazlı O, Ilbey O, Ozyurt C, Cikili N. The role of ESWL in the treatment of calculi with anomalous kidneys. Eur Urol. 1997;31:302–4.
20. Janetschek G, Kunzel KH. Percutaneous nephrolithotomy in horseshoe kidneys: applied anatomy and clinical experience. Br J Urol. 1988;62:117–22.
21. Shokeir AA, EL-Nahas AR, Shoma AM, Eraki I, El-Kenawy M, Mokhtar A, et al. Percutaneous nephrolithotomy in treatment of large stones within horseshoe kidneys. Urology. 2004;64:426–9.
22. Mosavi-Bahar SH, Amirzargar MA, Rahnavardi M, Moghaddam SM, Babbolhavaeji H, Amirhasani S. Percutaneous nephrolithotomy in patients with kidney malformations. J Endourol. 2007;21: 520–4.
23. Razvi S, Zaidi Z. Percutaneous nephrolithotomy (PNL) in horse shoe kidneys. J Pak Med Assoc. 2007;57:222–5.
24. Gupta NP, Mishra S, Seth A, Anand A. Percutaneous nephrolithotomy in abnormal kidneys: single-center experience. Urology. 2009;73:710–5.
25. Cass AS. Extracorporeal shock wave lithotripsy for renal stones with renal cysts present. J Urol. 1995;153:599–601.
26. Delakas D, Daskalopoulos G, Cranidis A. Extracorporeal shock wave lithotripsy for urinary calculi in autosomal dominant polycystic kidney disease. J Endourol. 1997;11:167–70.
27. Al-Kandari AM, Shoma AM, Eraky I, El-Kenawy MR, Al-Eezi H, El-Kappany HA. Percutaneous nephrolithotomy for management of upper urinary tract calculi in patients with autosomal dominant polycystic kidney disease. J Urol. 2009;2:273–7.
28. Umbreit EC, Childs MA, Patterson DE, Torres VE, LeRoy AJ, Gettman MT. Percutaneous nephrolithotomy for large or multiple upper tract calculi and autosomal dominant polycystic kidney disease. J Urol. 2010;183:183–7.
29. Deliveliotis C, Argiropoulos V, Varkarakis J. Extracorporeal shock wave lithotripsy produces a lower stone-free rate in patients with stones and renal cysts. Int J Urol. 2002;9:11–4.
30. Binbay M, Istanbulluoglu O, Sofikerim M, Beytur A, Skolarikos A, Akman T, et al. Effect of simple malrotation on percutaneous nephrolithotomy: a matched pair multicenter analysis. J Urol. 2011; 185:1737–41.
31. Rubin JI, Arger PH, Pollack HM, Banner MP, Coleman BG, Mintz MC, et al. Kidney changes after extracorporeal shock wave lithotripsy: CT evaluation. Radiology. 1987;162:21–4.
32. Kaude JV, Williams CM, Millner MR, Scott KN, Finlayson B. Renal morphology and function immediately after extracorporeal shock-wave lithotripsy. AJR. 1985;145:305–13.
33. Williamson BR, Paling MR, Lippert MC, Jenkins AD. Computerized tomographic appearance of renal cysts after extracorporeal shock wave lithotripsy. South Med J. 1990;83:287–9.
34. Grasso M, Loisides P, Beaghler M, Bagley D. The case for primary endoscopic management of upper urinary tract calculi: I. A critical review of 121 extracorporeal shock-wave lithotripsy failures. Urology. 1995;45:363–71.
35. Kuo RL, Aslan P, Zhong P, Preminger GM. Impact of holmium laser settings and fiber diameter on stone fragmentation and endoscope deflection. J Endourol. 1998;12:523–7.
36. Stern JM, Yiee J, Park S. Safety and efficacy of ureteral access sheaths. J Endourol. 2007;21:119–23.
37. Kourambas J, Delvecchio FC, Munver R, Preminger GM. Nitinol stone retrieval-assisted ureteroscopic management of lower pole renal calculi. Urology. 2000;56:935–9.
38. Raj GV, Auge BK, Weizer AZ, Denstedt JD, Watterson JD, Beiko DJ, et al. Percutaneous management of calculi within horse shoe kidneys. J Urol. 2003;170:48–51.
39. Munver R, Delvecchio FC, Newman GE, Preminger GM. Critical analysis of supracostal access for percutaneous renal surgery. J Urol. 2001;166:1242–6.
40. El-Nahas AR, Shokeir AA, El-Assmy AM, Shoma AM, Eraky I, El-Kenawy M, et al. Colonic perforation during percutaneous nephrolithotomy: study of risk factors. Urology. 2006;67:937–41.
41. Skoog SJ, Reed MD, Gaudier Jr FA, Dunn NP. The posterolateral and the retrorenal colon: implication in percutaneous stone extraction. J Urol. 1985;134:110–2.
42. Esghi AM, Roth JS, Smith AD. Percutaneous transperitoneal approach to a pelvic kidney for endourological removal of a staghorn calculus. J Urol. 1985;134:525.
43. Kamat N, Khandelwal P. Laparoscopic pyelolithotomy: a technique for the management of stones in the ectopic pelvic kidney. Int J Urol. 2004;11:581–4.
44. Chang TD, Dretler SP. Laparoscopic pyelolithotomy in an ectopic kidney. J Urol. 1996;156:1753.
45. Harmon WJ, Kleer E, Segura JW. Laparoscopic pyelolithotomy for calculus removal in a pelvic kidney. J Urol. 1996;155:2019.
46. Hoenig DM, Shalhav AL, Elbahnasy AM, McDougall EM, Clayman RV. Laparoscopic pyelolithotomy in a pelvic kidney: a case report and review of the literature. JSLS. 1997;1:163–5.
47. Gupta N, Yadav R, Singh A. Laparoscopic transmesocolic pyelolithotomy in an ectopic pelvic kidney. JSLS. 2007;11:258–60.
48. Dos Santos AR, Rocha Filho DC, Tajra LC. Management of lithiasis in pelvic kidney through laparoscopy-guided percutaneous transperitoneal nephrolithotripsy. Int Braz J Urol. 2004;30:32–4.
49. Troxel SA, Low RK, Das S. Extraperitoneal laparoscopy-assisted percutaneous nephrolithotomy in a left pelvic kidney. J Endourol. 2002;16:655–7.

Kidney Stones and Chronic Kidney Disease

74

Absar Ali, Quratulain Khan, and Tazeen H. Jafar

Abstract

Chronic kidney disease has become a global public health problem with serious social and economic effects from premature morbidity and deaths. Kidney stone formers are at increased risk for chronic kidney disease (CKD)—both early and advanced stages—with the stone acting either as the initiating or a contributing factor. Recent data indicates that prevalence and incidence of kidney stone are increasing worldwide. Individuals with kidney stones should be screened for the presence of underlying CKD. This chapter reviews the burden of CKD, the risk of kidney stone formation, and the association of CKD with kidney stones and underscores the need for screening and preventive strategies for CKD in individuals with kidney stones.

Keywords

Chronic kidney disease • Kidney stone • End-stage kidney disease • Nephrolithiasis

Introduction

Chronic kidney disease (CKD) has become a global public health problem with serious economic implications not only from the cost of renal replacement therapy but also in terms of premature morbidity and deaths from cardiovascular risk at young age [1]. This problem is magnified in developing countries with large populations, and epidemiologic studies have shown that the incidence of kidney diseases is higher in these countries than in developed world [2].

In the United States, where reliable data are available, the number of patients enrolled in the end-stage renal disease (ESRD) Medicare-funded program has increased from approximately 10,000 beneficiaries in 1973–86,354 in 1983 and to 547,982 as of December 31, 2008 [3]. Reliable data from most low- and middle-income countries are not available due to lack of registries despite the urgent need, albeit renal replacement therapy remains prohibitively expensive [4, 5].

A. Ali, M.D., FACP • Q. Khan, M.B.B.S • T.H. Jafar, M.D., MPH (✉)
Department of Medicine, Aga Khan University,
Stadium Road, 3500, Karachi, Sindh 74800, Pakistan
e-mail: tazeen.jafar@aku.edu

The prevalence of earlier stages of CKD is even higher. CKD is defined by the presence of persistent (3 months or greater) albuminuria (30 mg/day or more) or a reduction in glomerular filtration rate and classified into five stages on the basis of glomerular filtration rate (GFR): more than 90 mL/min/1.73 m^2 (stage 1), 60–89 mL/min/1.73 m^2 (stage 2), 30–59 mL/min/1.73 m^2 (stage 3), 15–29 mL/min/1.73 m^2 (stage 4), and less than 15 mL/min/1.73 m^2 (stage 5). In the United States, the prevalence of CKD (stage 1 or higher) rose from 10 to 12 % from 1999 to 2006 [6].

Epidemiologic studies provide robust evidence that the risk of premature deaths from cardiovascular disease is also significantly increased in individuals with earlier stages of CKD [7]. Unfortunately, the burden of CKD is increasing in transitioning and developing countries, with an overall prevalence of about 6 % in Saudi Arabia, 12–18 % in Iran, and 17 % in Thailand [8–10].

Kidney stone formers are at increased risk for chronic kidney disease (CKD), both early and advanced stages, with the stone acting either as the initiating or a contributing factor. It is challenging to determine the precise etiology of renal injury in stone-forming individuals with CKD. However, the risk for CKD has been reported to be about 50 % higher in

J.J. Talati et al. (eds.), *Urolithiasis*,
DOI 10.1007/978-1-4471-4387-1_74, © Springer-Verlag London 2012

symptomatic kidney stone formers as compared to control population in large cohort in the United States [11].

The identification of individuals with kidney stones and associated risk factors is important from CKD perspective in terms of prevention of stone and also for early institution of strategies for detection and prevention of CKD. In this chapter, we will review the evidence linking kidney stones with CKD.

Prevalence of Kidney Stones

There is scarcity of nationally representative data on the global prevalence of kidney stones. An accurate estimation will require imaging studies on population-based samples to account for asymptomatic kidney stones, in addition to reported prevalence relying solely on symptoms of acute pain. However, the former endeavors are laborious and resource-intensive, and most available prevalence estimates rely on symptomatic kidney stones. The prevalence of kidney stones varies by age, sex, and race [12]. In the United States, up to 12 % of men and 6 % of women will have one symptomatic episode of urinary stone by the age of 70 years and recurrence rate reaches 50 % [13]. If untreated, reported recurrence rate is around 30–40 % in 5 years [14, 15].

In the nationally representative Third National Health and Nutrition Examination Survey (NHANES III) conducted during the period 1988–1994 in the United States, the prevalence of symptomatic kidney stones increased with age until age 70, then declined, and was higher in men than women and in whites than blacks. Ethnic variation was observed in the prevalence of kidney stones with Hispanic and Asian men having an intermediate burden compared to whites and blacks. Regional variability was also observed among US whites; the age-adjusted prevalence increased from north to south and from west to east [16].

Geographic differences in the overall probability of forming kidney stones have been reported in various parts of the world (see chapters in Part I). In the United Kingdom, about 8 % of men and 4 % of women will form at least one renal stone by the age of 60. The lifetime risk for stone formation is about 5–9 % in Europe, 13 % in North America, and 20 % in oil-rich Arabian Gulf countries [17–19]. However, recent data indicate that prevalence and incidence of kidney stone are increasing worldwide and that global warming may be a contributing factor [20–22].

Prevalence of Kidney Stones Associated with CKD

Overall, of all patients with ESRD who start maintenance hemodialysis, about 3.2 % are directly attributed to kidney stones [23]. In addition, kidney stones could be a contributing factor in the development of CKD and its progression even when the underlying etiology for ESRD is different. For example, black patients on maintenance hemodialysis regardless of etiology of ESRD were three times more likely to be stone formers than age, sex, and race adjusted counterparts in the general population [24]. In addition, reduced kidney function is well documented in overweight individuals with history of kidney stones [25]. These data suggest a significant association between kidney stone formation and loss of kidney function.

Moreover, there has been variation in reported prevalence of kidney stones associated with ESRD with estimates of up to 10 % in Sri Lanka and Sudan [26, 27]. Studies from Thailand indicate nephrolithiasis is very common in patients with CKD [28]. In Iran and Pakistan, obstructive uropathy mainly from kidney stones was noted in 12 % of CKD patients [29–32]. Well-conducted studies from less-developed countries are needed to provide more insight into the potential contribution of kidney stones to CKD.

Risk Factors for Kidney Stones

Kidney stones are usually associated with an anatomic or metabolic abnormality or occur in the presence of an environmental or genetic determinant. Some of the anatomic abnormalities associated with kidney stones are listed in Table 74.1 and illustrated in Fig. 74.1a, b.

The metabolic factors, including hypercalciuria, hyperphosphaturia, hyperoxaluria, hypocitraturia, hyperuricosuria, cystinuria, a low urinary volume, and a defect of urinary acidification, enhance the susceptibility to kidney stone formation [33–35]. The presence of complex gene-environment interaction further catalyzes this process [36, 37].

The environmental determinants of kidney stones include high dietary intake of salt, protein, calcium, and other nutrients; low fluid intake; urinary tract infections; low socioeconomic status of the individual; and tropical climate [38, 39].

Table 74.1 Anatomic and urodynamic abnormalities associated with stone formation

Abnormalities associated with stone formation
Medullary sponge kidney
Ureteropelvic junction obstruction
Calyceal diverticulum, calyceal cyst
Ureteral stricture
Vesico-uretero-renal reflux
Horseshoe kidney
Ureterocele
Urinary diversion (via enteric hyperoxaluria)
Neurogenic bladder dysfunction

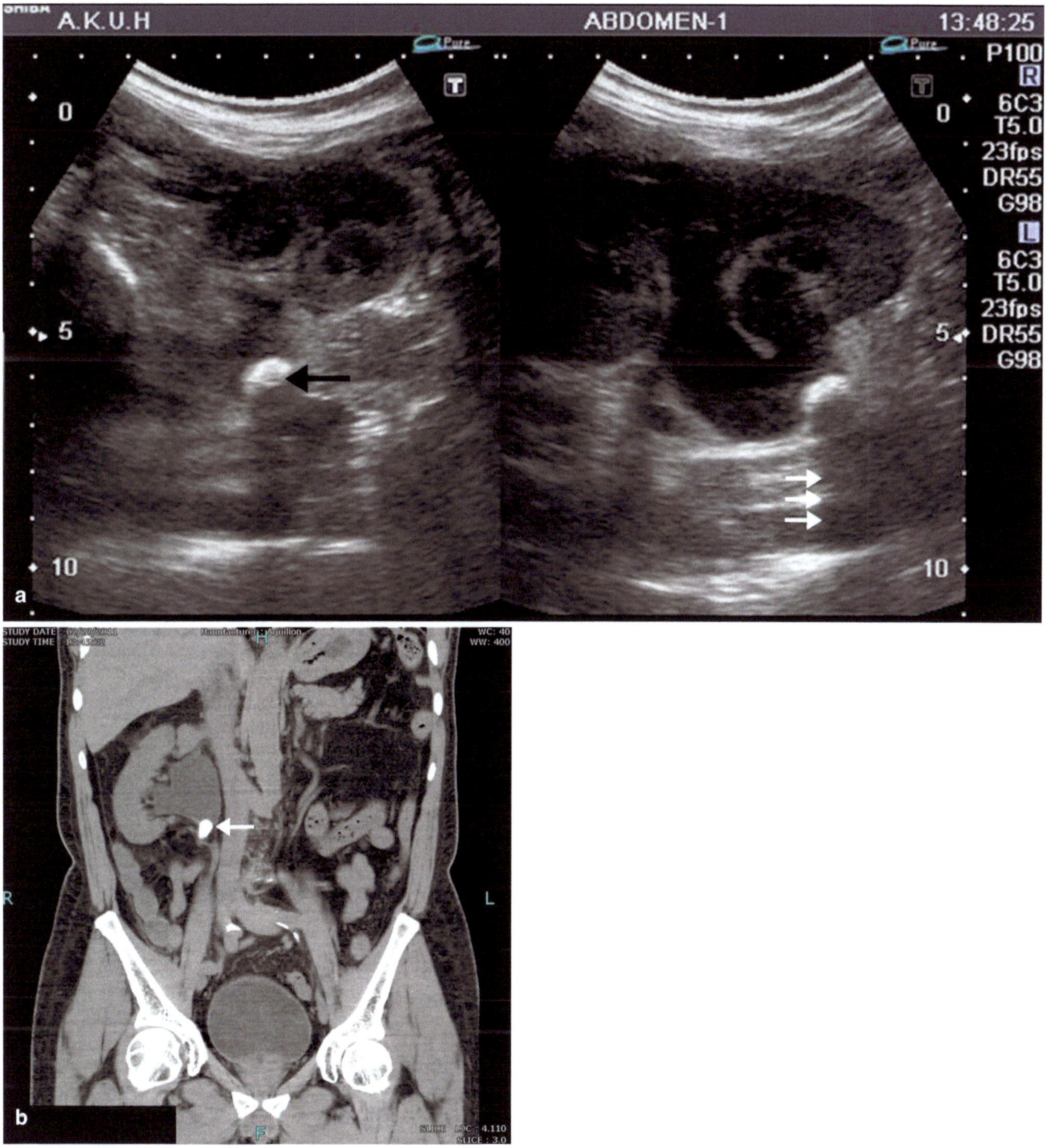

Fig. 74.1 (**a**) Ultrasound of the kidney showing a calculus impacted at the pelvi-ureteric junction (*black arrow*) with posterior echoic shadowing (*white arrows*) with resultant hydronephrosis. (**b**) Coronal reformatted computed tomography (*CT*) scan showing a calculus (*white arrow*) impacted at the pelvi-ureteric junction (*PUJ*) with resultant hydronephrosis (Courtesy of Dr. Zafar Sajjad, MRCP(UK), FRCR, The Abdul Mahomed Noormahomed Sherrif Chair and Associate Professor, Department of Radiology, Aga Khan University, Karachi, Pakistan)

A few drugs are known to increase the risk of stone formation by impairing the urine composition and crystallizing in urine by their active compounds (Table 74.2).

Studies have also shown that ambient temperature and sunlight levels are important risk factors for stones and that difference in exposure to temperature and sunlight and beverages may contribute to the geographic variability in the prevalence of kidney stones. It is postulated that global warming will lead to a marked increase in the prevalence of kidney stones [40, 41].

The genetic determinants may confer a strong risk of kidney stones as well. Studies have shown that 55 % of those with recurrent kidney stones have a positive family history of this condition [42, 43]. Evidence also suggests that the familial risk of forming kidney stones remained high even when potentially modifiable factors such as calcium consumption and other urinary metabolite excretion were adjusted for; thus, this risk is mediated only in part by an abnormal metabolic profile or cultural and familial habitual diets. Genetic studies suggest that stone formation may be the result of a polygenic defect with partial penetrance [16, 38, 42, 43].

Table 74.2 Drugs associated with stone formation

Active compounds crystallizing in urine	Substances impairing urine composition
Allopurinol and oxypurinol	Acetazolamide
Amoxicillin and ampicillin	Allopurinol
Ceftriaxone	Aluminum magnesium hydroxide
Ciprofloxacin	Ascorbic acid
Ephedrine	Calcium
Indinavir	Furosemide
Magnesium trisilicate	Laxatives
Sulfonamide	Methoxyflurane
Triamterene	Vitamins

Pathophysiology and Factors Associated with Kidney Stones and CKD

The pathogenesis of CKD due to kidney stones is not entirely clear and may be multifactorial; thus, causality per se remains to be established, albeit association between the two is well documented [11, 25].

Pathophysiologically, obstructive nephropathy is characterized by an inflammatory state in the kidney, that is, promoted by cytokines and growth factors produced by damaged tubular cells, infiltrated macrophages, reactive myofibroblasts, and other chronic inflammatory cells. This inflammatory state leads to tubular atrophy and interstitial fibrosis. Tubular thyroidization (thyroid-like appearance due to formation of pink colloid casts of Tamm-Horsfall glycoprotein in dilated renal tubules) is not diagnostic but is a common finding in obstructive nephropathy secondary to renal calculi. Renal blood flow progressively falls with continued obstruction, resulting in ischemia and incremental nephron loss. Recovery of renal function depends on the duration and level of obstruction, pre-obstruction blood flow, and coexisting medical illness or infection [16, 44–46]. Some of the typical pathological findings are illustrated in Fig. 74.2a, b, c.

Although back pressure from the blockage may be the initiating event, other factors, such as chronic infection from

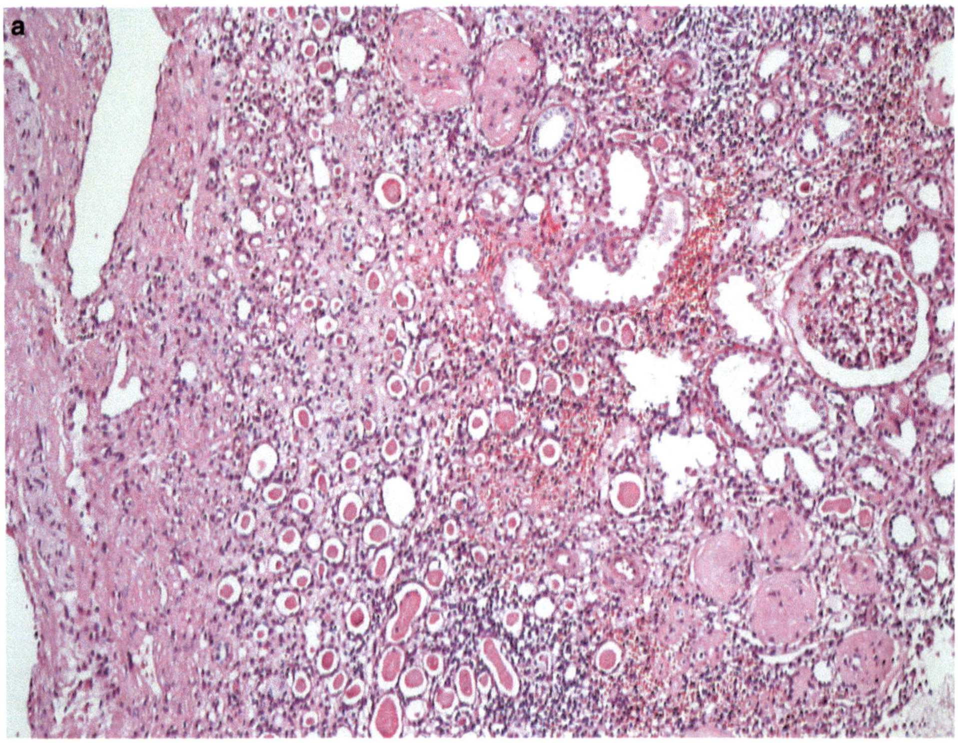

Fig. 74.2 (**a**) Tubular thyroidization with a viable glomeruli at the periphery (10×). (**b**) Reactive fibroblasts, chronic inflammatory cells, and occasional tubules with thyroidization (20×). (**c**) Transitional lining of pelvis with thyrodized tubules and interstitial inflammation (10×) (Courtesy of Dr. Saira Fatima, Senior Instructor, and Dr. Romana Idrees, Assistant Professor, Department of Pathology and Microbiology, Aga Khan University Hospital, Karachi, Pakistan)

Fig. 74.2 (continued)

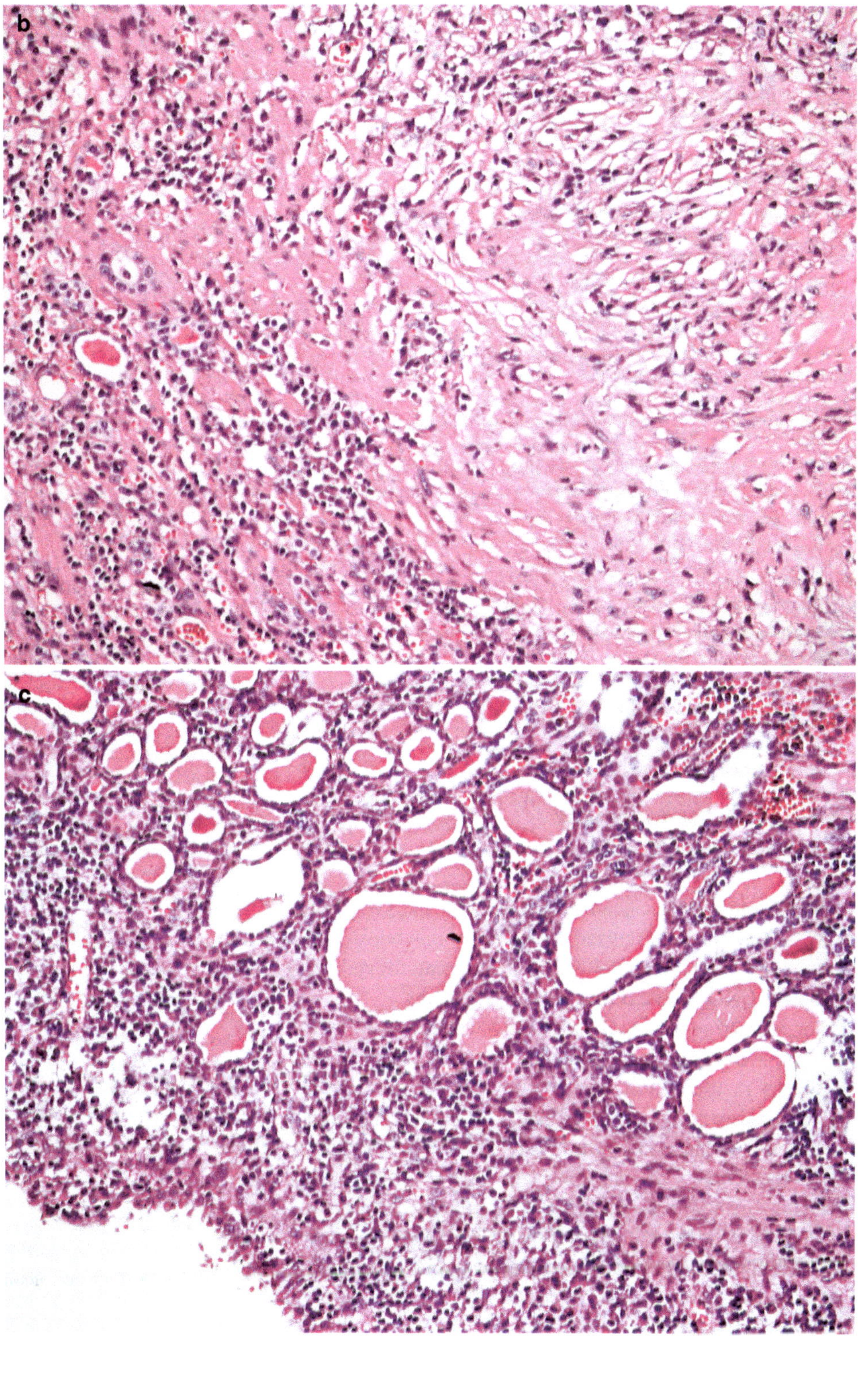

urinary stasis, use of medications to treat pain or infection, and treatment of the stone itself, are equally important in potentially perpetuating the damage leading to the progression to ESRD [45]. The factors that have been associated with ESRD in stone formers include hereditary stone disease, struvite stones, urinary tract infections, frequent stone episodes, obstructive uropathy, and urinary tract anomalies (Table 74.3) [23].

Table 74.3 Factors associated with obstructive uropathy leading to kidney damage

Initiating factor
Back pressure from the blockage is the initiating event
Perpetuating factors
Chronic infection
Prolonged use of nonsteroidal anti-inflammatory drugs
Extracorporeal shock wave lithotripsy
Use of antibiotics (see Table 74.2)

Table 74.4 General preventive measures

Fluid intake 2.5–3 L/day
Circadian drinking
Neutral pH beverages
Diuresis: 2.0–2.5 L/day
Specific gravity of urine: <1.010
Balanced diet rich in vegetable and fiber
Normal calcium content: 1,000–1,200 mg/day
Limited sodium chloride content: 4–5 g/day
Limited animal protein content: 0.8–1.0 g/kg/day
Lifestyle advice to normalize general risk factor
Body mass index: 18–25 kg/m^2 for adults
Stress limitation measures
Adequate physical activity
Balancing of excessive fluid loss

Conclusion: Management and Prevention of CKD

In addition to the management of relief of acute symptoms from kidney stones (discussed elsewhere in this book), prevention of recurrent kidney stones and screening for and prevention of CKD should be key therapeutic goals.

For prevention of recurrence of kidney stones, the majority of stone formers can be managed with education on modest dietary restrictions and advised to increase fluid intake. Table 74.4 lists the general guidelines for evaluation of individuals with kidney stones and lifestyle modification to prevent recurrence. For the recurrent stone former with metabolically active stone disease, it is probably best to individually tailor medical therapy to treat the specific urinary chemical abnormality to halt the disease process. Research is needed to determine the precise contribution of these factors in different populations [47–58].

Due to the high risk of CKD, patients with kidney stones should be screened for subclinical CKD. This would include measurement of serum creatinine for estimated glomerular filtration rate and urine albumin excretion. If detected to have CKD, patients should be initiated on therapy to slow down the progression of CKD including blood pressure control and blockers of the renin-angiotensin system and screened for presence of cardiovascular disease [59, 60]. In addition, aggressive measures to prevent stone recurrence are likely to prevent CKD as well. Timely referral to nephrologist is important for optimal patient outcomes.

References

1. Hemmelgarn BR, Manns BJ, Lloyd A, James MT, Klarenbach S, Quinn RR, et al. Alberta kidney disease network. Relation between kidney function, proteinuria, and adverse outcomes. JAMA. 2010; 303(5):423–9.
2. Remuzzi G. A research program for COMGAN. ISN News. July 2001:1–6.
3. Collins AJ, Foley RN, Herzog C, Chavers B, Gilbertson D, Ishani A. US renal data system 2010 annual data report. Am J Kidney Dis. 2011;57(1 Suppl 1):A8, e1–526.
4. Jafar TH. The growing burden of chronic kidney disease in Pakistan. N Engl J Med. 2006;354:995–7.
5. Barsoum RS. Chronic kidney disease in the developing world. N Engl J Med. 2006;354:997–9.
6. Levey AS, Coresh J. Chronic kidney disease. Lancet. 2012; 379(9811):165–80.
7. Sarnak MJ, Levey AS, Schoolwerth AC, Coresh J, Culleton B, Hamm LL, et al. Kidney disease as a risk factor for development of cardiovascular disease. A statement from the American Heart Association Councils on kidney in cardiovascular disease, high blood pressure research, clinical cardiology, and epidemiology and prevention. Circulation. 2003;108:2154–69.
8. Alsuwaida AO, Farag YM, Al Sayyari AA, Alhejaili F, AlHarbi A, Houswi A. Epidemiology of chronic kidney disease in the Kingdom of Saudi Arabia (Seek Saudi Investigators). Saudi J Kidney Dis Transpl. 2010;21:1066–72.
9. Husseinpanah F, Kasraei F, Nassiri AA, Azizi F. High prevalence of kidney disease in Iran: a large population based study. BMC Public Health. 2009;9:44.
10. Ingsathit A, Thakkiinstian A, Chaipraset A, Sangthawan P, Sangthawan P, Gojaseni P, et al. Prevalence and risk factors for chronic kidney disease in the Thai adult population: Thai SEEK study. Nephrol Dial Transplant. 2010;25:1567–75.
11. Rule A, Krambeck AE, Lieske JC. Chronic kidney disease in kidney stone formers. Clin J Am Soc Nephrol. 2011;6:2069–75.
12. Curhan GC. Epidemiology of stone disease. Urol Clin North Am. 2007;34:287–93.
13. Stamatelou KK, Francis ME, Jones CA, Nyberg LM, Curhan GC. Time trends in reported prevalence of kidney stones in the United States: 1976–1994. Kidney Int. 2003;63:1817–23.
14. Johnson CN, Wilson DM, O'Fallen WM, Malek RS, Kurland RT. Renal stone epidemiology: a 25 years study in Rochester Minnesota. Kidney Int. 1979;16:624–31.
15. Lieske JC, de la Pena Vega LS, Slezak JM, Bergstralh EJ, Leibson CL, Ho KI, et al. Renal stone epidemiology in Rochester, Minnesota. An update. Kidney Int. 2006;69:760–4.
16. Soucie JM, Thun MJ, Coates RJ, McClellan W, Austin H. Demographic and geographic variability of kidney stones in the United States. Kidney Int. 1994;46:893–9.
17. Robertson WG. Epidemiology of urinary stone disease. Urol Res. 1990;18 Suppl 1:S3–8.
18. Johri N, Jaeger P, Robertson W, Choong S, Unwin R. Renal stone disease. Medicine. 2011;39(7):371–7.
19. Ramello A, Vitale C, Marangella M. Epidemiology of nephrolithiasis. J Nephrol. 2000;13 Suppl 3:S45–50.
20. Romero V, Akpinar H, Assimos DG. Kidney stone: a global picture of prevalence, incidence, and associated risk factors. Rev Urol. 2010;12:e86–96.

21. Yoshida O, Okada Y. Epidemiology of urolithiasis in Japan: a chronological and geographical study. Urol Int. 1990;45(2):104–11.
22. Yanagaw M, Kawamura J, Onishi T, Soga N, Kameda K, Sriboonlue V, et al. Incidence of urolithiasis in northeast Thailand. Int J Urol. 1997;4(6):537–40.
23. Jungers P, Joly D, Barbey F, Choukroun G, Daudon M. ESRD caused by nephrolithiasis: prevalence, mechanism, and prevention. Am J Kidney Dis. 2004;44:799–805.
24. Stankus N, Hammes M, Gillen D, Worcester E. African American ESRD patients have a high pre-dialysis prevalence of kidney stones compared to NHANES III. Urol Res. 2007;35(2):83–7. Epub 2007 Feb 20.
25. Gillen DL, Worcester EM, Coe FL. Decreased renal function among adults with a history of nephrolithiasis: a study of NHANES III. Kidney Int. 2005;67(2):685–90.
26. Gooneratne IK, Ranaweera AK, Liyanarachchi NP, Gunawardane N, Lanerolle RD. Epidemiology of chronic kidney disease in Sri Lankan population. Int J Diabetes Dev Ctries. 2008;28:60–4.
27. Abboud OL, Osman EM, Musa AR. The etiology of chronic renal failure in adult Sudanese patients. Ann Trop Med Parasitol. 1989;83:411–4.
28. Sitiprija V. Nephrology in south east Asia: fact and concept. Kidney Int. 2003;63(S83):s128–30.
29. Afshar R, Sanavi S, Salimi J. Epidemiology of chronic renal failure in Iran: a four year single center experience. Saudi J Kidney Dis Transplant. 2007;18:191–4.
30. Daudon M. Epidemiology of nephrolithiasis in France. Ann Urol (Paris). 2005;39:209–31.
31. Safaraninejad MR. Adult urolithiasis in a population bases study in Iran: prevalence, incidence, and associated risk factors. Urol Res. 2007;35:73–82.
32. Rizvi SAH, Manzoor K. Causes of chronic renal failure in Pakistan: a single large center experience. Saudi J Kidney Dis Transplant. 2002;13:376–9.
33. Frick KK, Bushinsky DA. Molecular mechanisms of primary hypercalciuria. J Am Soc Nephrol. 2003;14:1082–95.
34. Scheinman SJ. Nephrolithiasis. Semin Nephrol. 1999;19:381–8.
35. Robertson WG, Peacock M, Marshall RW, Speed R, Nordin BE. Seasonal variations in the composition of urine in relation to calcium stone-formation. Clin Sci Mol Med. 1975;49:597–602.
36. Moe OW, Bonny O. Genetic hypercalciuria. J Am Soc Nephrol. 2005;16:729–45.
37. Parry ES, Lister IS. Sunlight and hypercalciuria. Lancet. 1975;1:1063–5.
38. Curhan GC, Willett WC, Rimm EB, Stampfer MJ. Family history and risk of kidney stones. J Am Soc Nephrol. 1997;8:1568–73.
39. Curhan GC, Willett WC, Rimm EB, Stampfer MJ. A prospective study of dietary calcium and other nutrients and the risk of symptomatic kidney stones. N Engl J Med. 1993;328:833–8.
40. Serio A, Fraioli A. Epidemiology of nephrolithiasis. Nephron. 1999;81 suppl 1:26–30.
41. Fakheri RJ, Goldfarb DS. Ambient temperature as a contributor to kidney stone formation: implications of global warming. Kidney Int. 2011;79(11):1178–85.
42. Resnick M, Pridgen DB, Goodman HO. Genetic predisposition to formation of calcium oxalate renal calculi. N Eng J Med. 1968;278:1313–8.
43. Ljunghall S, Danielson BG, Fellström B, Holmgren K, Johansson G. Family history of renal stones in recurrent stone patients. Br J Urol. 1985;57(4):370–4.
44. Pishchalnikov YA, McAteer JA, Williams Jr JC, et al. Why stones break better at slow shockwave rates than at fast rates: in vitro study with a research electrohydraulic lithotripter. J Endourol. 2006;20(8):537–41.
45. Connors BA, Evan AP, Blomgren PM, et al. Extracorporeal shock wave lithotripsy at 60 shock waves/min reduces renal injury in a porcine model. BJU Int. 2009;104(7):1004–8.
46. Bander SJ, Buerkert JE, Martin D, Klahr S. Long-term effects of 24-h unilateral ureteral obstruction on renal function in the rat. Kidney Int. 1985;28:614.
47. Borghi L, Meschi T, Amato F, et al. Urinary volume, water and recurrences in idiopathic calcium nephrolithiasis: a 5-year randomized prospective study. J Urol. 1996;155(3):839–43.
48. Curhan GC, Willett WC, Speizer FE, et al. Beverage use and risk for kidney stones in women. Ann Intern Med. 1998;128(7):534–40.
49. Siener R, Ebert D, Nicolay C, et al. Dietary risk factors for hyperoxaluria in calcium oxalate stone formers. Kidney Int. 2003;63(3):1037–43.
50. Borghi L, Schianchi T, Meschi T, et al. Comparison of two diets for the prevention of recurrent stones in idiopathic hypercalciuria. N Engl J Med. 2002;346(2):77–84.
51. Fink HA, Akornor JW, Garimella PS, et al. Diet, fluid, or supplements for secondary prevention of nephrolithiasis: a systematic review and meta-analysis of randomized trials. Eur Urol. 2009;56(1):72–80.
52. Hesse AT, Tiselius H-G, Siener R, Hoppe B, editors. Urinary stones, diagnosis, treatment and prevention of recurrence. 3rd ed. Basel: S Karger AG; 2009.
53. Stitchantrakul W, Sopassathit W, Prapaipanich S, et al. Effects of calcium supplements on the risk of renal stone formation in a population with low oxalate intake. Southeast Asian J Trop Med Public Health. 2004;35(4):1028–33.
54. von Unruh GE, Voss S, Sauerbruch T, et al. Dependence of oxalate absorption on the daily calcium intake. J Am Soc Nephrol. 2004;15(6):1567–73.
55. Coe FL. Hyperuricosuric calcium oxalate nephrolithiasis. Adv Exp Med Biol. 1980;128:439–50.
56. Sarig S. The hyperuricosuric calcium oxalate stone former. Miner Electrolyte Metab. 1987;13(4):251–6.
57. Ettinger B. Hyperuricosuric calcium stone disease. In: Coe FL, Favus MJ, Pak CYC, Parks JH, Preminger GM, editors. Kidney stones: medical and surgical management. Philadelphia: Lippincott-Raven; 1996. p. 851–8.
58. Constanzo LS, Windhager EE. Calcium and sodium transport by the distal convoluted tubule of the rat. Am J Physiol. 1978;235(5):F492–506.
59. Jafar TH, Schmid CH, Landa M, Giatras I, Toto R, Remuzzi G, et al. Angiotensin-converting enzyme inhibitors and progression of nondiabetic renal disease: a meta-analysis of patient-level data. Ann Intern Med. 2001;135:73–87.
60. Jafar TH, Paul C, Stark PC, Schmid CH, Landa M, Maschio G, et al. Progression of chronic kidney disease: the role of blood pressure control, proteinuria, and angiotensin-converting enzyme inhibition: a patient-level meta-analysis. Ann Intern Med. 2003;139:244–52.

Calculus Renal Failure in Pakistan

75

Saiyid Jaffar Ali Naqvi

Abstract

The proportion of patients presenting with anuria or requiring support for end-stage renal disease (ESRD) is higher in Pakistan than in industrialized nations. This chapter draws attention to the relationship between stone and renal failure, the proportion of end-stage renal disease due to stone, and the changing proportions of renal failure from stone disease, glomerulonephritis, and diabetes and hypertension, due to increasing longevity and probably lifestyle.

Keywords

Calculi • Calculus renal failure • Urinary tract obstruction • Anuria • End-stage renal failure • Dialysis • Transplant

Introduction

There are marked differences between the rates of renal failure in calculus-plagued patients in advanced societies and underdeveloped nations. The key cause for the higher rate of renal failure in countries such as Pakistan is the unfortunate fact that health care has not received the attention it deserves. A healthy individual in industry or agriculture can galvanize the economy of any country. Without health, nations remain impoverished. The resulting national poverty restricts the introduction of health-promoting measures perpetrating a vicious cycle.

The situation is compounded by the fact that education receives just 2.1 % of the gross domestic product (GDP) [1]. In contrast, the public sector spending on education in Vietnam is 5.3, Iran 5.2, Malaysia 4.7, Thailand 4.5, Nepal 3.2, and India 3.3 %. The result is that the major part of society remains uneducated (in fact, illiterate) and consequently unaware about the important aspects of maintaining health.

Pakistan is a signatory to the Alma-Ata Declaration of 1976 where the nation committed to provide for all health needs for its people by the year 2000. It is already 12 years past that deadline, and Pakistan's expense on health is only 0.6 % of the gross national production (GNP). The nation's health budget is a meager PKR 60 billion/annum, i.e., Rs. just 353/person/annum [2].

Health care, which should be the responsibility of the state, becomes a burden on the shoulders of the patient, who may be earning a meager PKR 170 (US $2)/day [3]. Pakistan appears to be one of the leading countries in the world as far as philanthropic support is concerned, but philanthropy cannot provide for all the needs. It is laudable that schools and hospitals built by the community are being looked after by philanthropists. However, in addition to money, there is the question of organizing a national health system. Philanthropic support can supplement national efforts, but cannot take on the responsibility for total provision of health care.

As far as the health scenario is concerned, communicable diseases like tuberculosis, small pox, hepatitis, gastrointestinal disorders, polio, typhoid, and malaria have rightly taken the priority among health providers. Efforts are being made for hepatitis, polio, and tuberculosis in the extended

S.J.A. Naqvi, F.R.C.P.
Department of Nephrology, The Kidney Foundation, National Institute of Kidney & Urological Diseases (NIKUD), University of Karachi, Gate No.4, Haque Nawaz Jhangvi Road, Karachi, Pakistan
e-mail: exceldia@cyber.net.pk

J.J. Talati et al. (eds.), *Urolithiasis*,
DOI 10.1007/978-1-4471-4387-1_75, © Springer-Verlag London 2012

prevention program. Stone disease does not qualify for the same level of attention, but it is important that it receives appropriate attention. This is because it is one additional cause of renal damage.

As a consequence of the disease prevention strategies, people are living progressively longer lives, and we as physicians are facing problems of noncommunicable diseases (NCD). According to the National Survey of Pakistan Medical Council [4], high blood pressure (BP) is present in 17.9 % of adults and only 3 % have controlled blood pressure. The second important noncommunicable disease is diabetes [5], which affects 9.1 % of the population, but according to the National Health Survey, less than 3 % have controlled diabetes. Chronic kidney disease (CKD) is present in about 7 % of those 40–49 years old; its incidence increases with age and rises to 17 % in the age group of 59 years in urban area and 13 % in rural area. Less than 2 % of females have laboratory evidence of chronic kidney disease. It is possible that women die early because of other complication of BP and diabetes and do not survive to have kidney diseases [6].

That is the background scenario in which urinary tract calculi occur. In this vast landscape of unattended disease, it does not attract attention. In such settings, data is inadequately documented and infrequently published.

The Kidney Foundation of Pakistan started publishing a Dialysis Registry in 2002. The available data are based upon the voluntary participation of institutions who agreed to share their experience. In 2002, only 105 centers in Pakistan shared their experience. The number of patients at that time was 2,387. The causes of end-stage renal disease (ESRD) needing dialysis, at that time, included chronic nephritis in 29.1 %, diabetes in 26.6 %, hypertension (HPT) in 10.3 %, urinary stone disease in 4.5 %, polycystic kidney disease in 0.7 %, and unknown in 28.6 %. As participation increased, data was available from 224 centers and for 6,127 patients [7] (Fig. 75.1).

It is interesting that the etiology of renal failure has completely changed over the years. The leading cause of ESRD in Pakistan now is diabetes (seen in 42.6 % of all ESRD patients), high blood pressure (29.46 %), chronic nephritis (now only 10.45 %), stone diseases (8.05 %), and unknown causes now contribute only 5.54 % (Table 75.1). The probable reason is the availability of diagnostic tools such as ultrasound, biochemical tests, kidney biopsies, urological tests, etc. The increased incidence of diabetes and hypertension as the etiology of ESRD is due to a poor control of 3 % of each, according to National Survey of Pakistan Research Council.

According to the Dialysis Registry of Pakistan, stone disease does not appear to be a leading cause of ESRD requiring renal replacement therapy. The maximum percentage available in recent registry of 2010 is 8 %, which is almost similar to 7.2 % mentioned by other centers [8]. But as mentioned in Chap. 3, up to 8 % of stones may be asymptomatic, thus possibly continuing to contribute to the pool of renal failure patients in adulthood. An untold number of children unable to access care might be dying from bilateral urinary tract obstruction from stones.

Treatment of end-stage renal diseases (ESRD) requiring renal replacement therapy in the form of dialysis and transplantation is expensive. The cost of renal replacement therapy in Pakistan is about PKR 200,000 (USD 2,383)/patient/year. As mentioned previously, neither the government nor the patients are able to support this treatment, and philanthropy has a limited outreach. As a result, the majority of patients have no access to the treatment.

It is all the more important to institute appropriate treatment of stone disease at the earliest to forestall destruction of the kidney. It is even more important in Pakistan where the state, which is responsible for care, spends a paltry 0.6 % on health, leaving the individual who earns USD 2/day to face an unfortunate situation: death from kidney failure and death by default.

The cost of renal replacement therapy (RRT) forced the medical profession all over the world to adopt a rational approach. All over the world, the emphasis is now to find out the causes of ESRD, which should be amenable to preventive measures. The Dialysis Registry of Pakistan gives the causes. Diabetes and high blood pressure only requires Rs. 5/day (angiotensin-converting enzyme [ACE] inhibitors + metformin). Unfortunately, the detection and management of stone disease is very expensive.

Stones and Renal Failure

The prevalence of kidney stone has risen over the past 30 years in the USA. Eleven percent of men and 5.6 % of women will have kidney stone symptoms [9]. Stone is not a minor problem. In Pakistan, 52 % of patients attending the busy nephrourology outpatient department at Jinnah Post-Medical Centre-Karachi have stone disease symptoms.[1]

The availability of lithotripsy and other urological measures to break the stones has completely changed the management from operative procedure to minor procedures like breaking stone in the bladder and ureteroscopy (URS) for the stones in the midthird of the ureter. These procedures have done away with some of the fears associated with open surgery and saved the kidneys from total damage leading to ESRD.

[1] Personal unpublished data

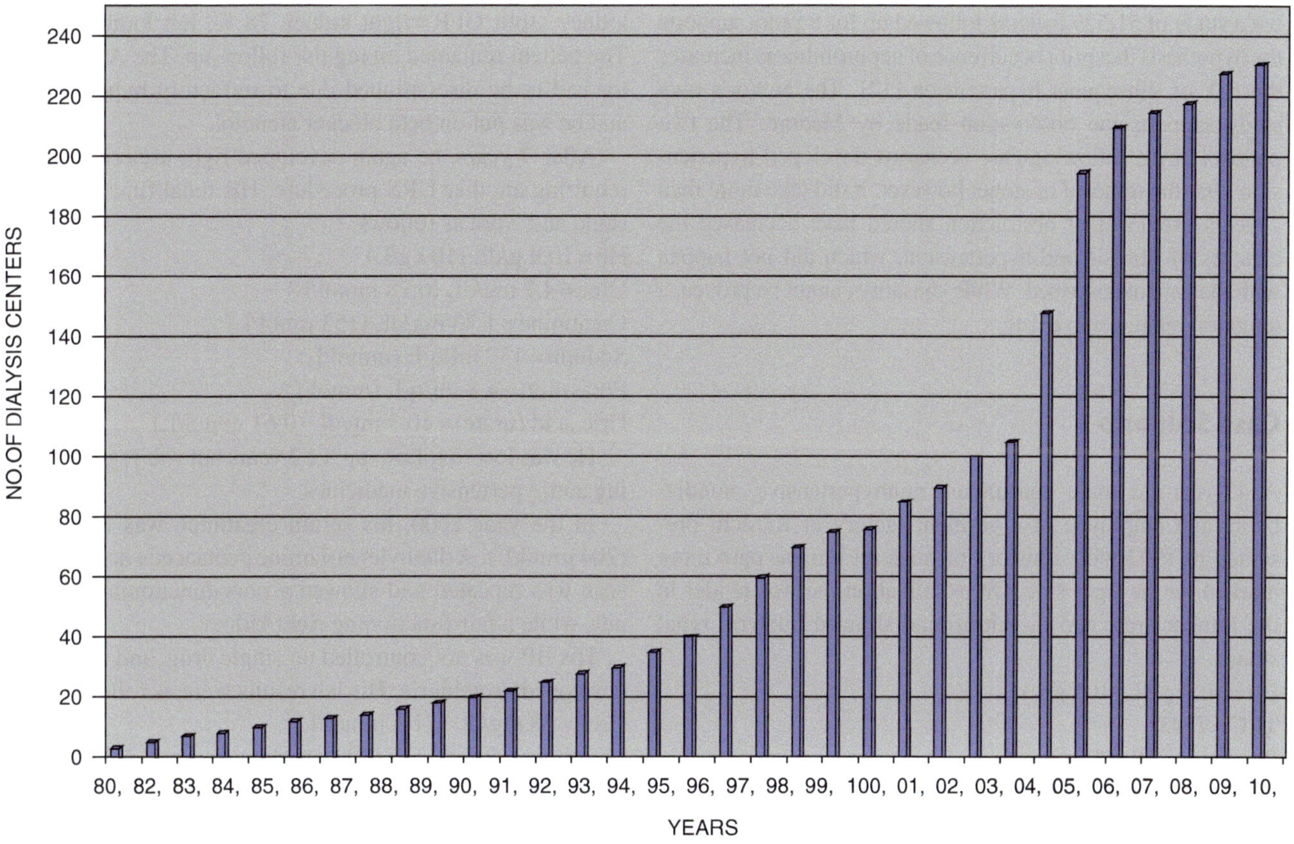

Fig. 75.1 The number of dialysis centers in Pakistan has steadily increased since 1980

Table 75.1 The causes of end-stage kidney disease

Diagnosis available	No. of patients	%
Diabetic nephropathy	2,282	42.60
Hypertensive renal failure	1,578	29.46
Chronic glomerulonephritis	560	10.45
Calculus disease	431	8.05
ADPKD	200	3.73
Other/unknown	297	5.54

If we take the recent figures of 8 % of ESRD patients due to stone diseases needing dialysis (which translates to the 431 patients on Dialysis Registry 2010), the cost of these patients will be PKR 86.2 million/year, i.e., 14 % of the government's health budget. It is a fact that patients in our country come very late, and they have already been treated with unscientific remedies, which delays the treatment and damages the kidneys.

Obstructive nephropathy [10] has bimodal distribution, and it is common in children. It declines with age until late childhood. During the years 1989–1993, 4,869 patients with obstruction were treated for ESRD in the USA, 7 % of whom were younger than 20 years, 36 % were within 20–64 years, and 57 % were older than 64 years. Males constituted 74 % of the patients; 81 % were white, 16 % African-American, 2 % Asians, and 1 % Native Americans.

Stones leading to obstruction can cause changes in the tubulointerstitial compartment of the kidney. This leads to fibrosis, with the glomeruli becoming involved later [11]. Interstitial damage plays the major role in destroying the kidney [10]. The tubulointerstitium comprises approximately 80 % of total renal volume. The interstitium is surrounded by vascular and tubular compartment. Its communication with the glomerular and extraglomerular mesangium makes it especially vulnerable to pathological events in these neighboring areas. There is an accumulation of matrix protein in the interstitium. This accumulation of protein leads to tubular atrophy, infiltration of the macrophages, and an increased number of fibroblasts. These tubular changes appear to be responsible for glomerular damage leading to a decrease in glomerular filtration rate (GFR). It is now certain that obstructive uropathy characterized by primary tubulointerstitial changes leads to involvement of glomerular structures.

The Association of Stones and Hypertension

The association of stone diseases with hypertension (according to *American Journal of Hypertension*) remains controversial, but a study of 51,529 patients followed up for 8 years supports the hypothesis that prior occurrence of nephrolithiasis increases the risk of subsequent hypertension [12]. The author's own study supports the observation made by Madore. The two patients in the following case scenarios developed hypertension after the removal of stone; however, it did take more than 2 years. Removal of obstruction should have decreased the chances of fibrosis and hypertension, which did not happen with the patient described. While causality cannot be proven, a temporal relationship exists.

Case Scenario 1

A 42-year-old male nonsmoker, nonhypertensive, nondiabetic, and employee of a garment factory at Karachi presented in 1992 with a history of bilateral lumbar pain more marked on the right side. On examination, he was tender in the lumbar area, and his ultrasound showed bilateral renal stones.

Hb = 10.5 g/dL (105 g/L)
TLC = 7,400
Platelets = 210,000
Urea = 29 mg/dL (4.83 mmol/L)
Creatinine = 1.3 mg/dL (115 μmol/L)
Sodium = 139 mEq/L (mmol/L)
Potassium = 4.7 mEq/L (mmol/L)
Uric acid (urate) = 6.7 mg/dL (0.40 mmol/L)

Two sessions of ESWL were performed. After the second session of ESWL, he developed fever, burning maturation, and decreased urine output. He was hospitalized in Karachi. His investigations were as follows:

Hb = 10.9 g/dL (109 g/L)
TLC = 17,000
Urea = 4.7 mg/dL (0.78 mmol/L)
Creatinine = 1.8 mg/dL (159 μmol/L)
Sodium = 140 mEq/L (mmol/L)
Potassium = 4.7 mEq/L (mmol/L)

He had a urinary tract infection (UTI) with pseudomonas. An ultrasound of kidneys-ureters-bladder (KUB) revealed bilateral hydronephrosis. He was started on intravenous antibiotics, and bilateral percutaneous nephrostomies were inserted. Unfortunately, his urine output gradually decreased and renal functions deteriorated as well. Hemodialysis started with a temporary jugular catheter. Five sessions of hemodialysis were performed. During a hospital stay, right pyelolithotomy and left-sided URS were performed. The patient improved gradually. On discharge, the patient remained hypertensive and was put on ACE inhibitor. His renal functions were mildly deranged with serum creatinine levels of 1.5 mg/dL (133 μmol/L). A radioisotope scan revealed a poor-functioning left kidney and well-functioning right kidney (split GFR = right kidney 78 %, left kidney 22 %). The patient remained on regular follow-up. The ACE inhibitor had to be discontinued due to refractory hyperkalemia, and he was put on beta blocker atenolol.

After 7 years, he again developed right ureteric calculus requiring another URS procedure. His renal functions were static and were as follows:

Hb = 10.9 g/dL (109 g/L)
Urea = 4.7 mg/dL (0.78 mmol/L)
Creatinine = 1.73 mg/dL (153 μmol/L)
Sodium = 139 mEq/L (mmol/L)
Potassium = 4.8 mEq/L (mmol/L)
Uric acid (urate) = 10.3 mg/dL (0.61 mmol/L)

He was lost to follow-up for 2 years but was regularly taking antihypertensive medicines.

In the year 2000, his serum creatinine was 2.3 mg/dL (204 μmol/L). A diethylenetriamine pentaacetic acid (DTPA) scan was repeated and showed a poor-functioning left kidney, while a fair-functioning right kidney.

His BP was not controlled on single drug, and the patient developed proteinuria. His lab results were as follows:

Urea = 68 mg/dL (11.3 mmol/L)
Creatinine = 2.3 mg/dL (204 μmol/L)
Sodium = 139 mEq/L (mmol/L)
Potassium = 5.5 mEq/L (mmol/L)
Bicarbonate = 18 mEq/L (mmol/L)
Urine protein = 3 g in 24 h

A calcium channel blocker was added, and his blood pressure was controlled with disappearance of proteinuria. Angiotensin receptor blocker (ARB) was started, but he did not tolerate that medication, and ARB administration was discontinued due to hyperkalemia.

Creatinine = 2.6 mg/dL (230 μmol/L)
Potassium = 6.32 mEq/L (mmol/L)

During the course of his illness, he had multiple attacks of gouty arthritis, for which he was given colchicines and steroids. He was also given allopurinol, initially 300 mg and after a month 150 mg daily.

He was on regular follow-up and continued his treatment. His blood pressure required multiple drugs including atenolol, prazosin, and hydralazine. His renal functions slowly deteriorated.

Hb = 10.4 g/dL (104 g/L)
Urea = 160 mg/dL (26.7 mmol/L)
Creatinine = 8.7 mg/dL (770 μmol/L)
Sodium = 137 mEq/L (mmol/L)
Potassium = 5.3 mEq/L (mmol/L)
Platelets = 241,000

In May 2010, a permanent arteriovenous (AV) fistula was created. He was vaccinated for hepatitis B. In August 2010, maintenance hemodialysis started twice a week, and the patient remains on dialysis as of this writing.

Case Scenario 2

A 62-year-old male was seen 21 years ago with a history of operation on the left kidney for stone in 1983. According to the patient, the kidney functions were normal, and the BP was normal as well before operation. His postoperative recovery was uneventful.

In 1990, he felt unwell, had nausea and vomiting, and was short of breath. He also had chest pain. He was found to have high blood pressure (250/160). His weight was 61 kg. His investigations were as follows:

Hb = 14.3 g/dL (143 g/L)
WBC = 5,400
Polys = 61 %
Lympho = 39 %
Urea = 130 mg/dL (21.7 mmol/L)
Creatinine = 2.4 mg/dL (212 μmol/L)
Sodium = 134 mEq/L (mmol/L)
Potassium = 4.6 mEq/L (mmol/L)
Urine volume = 1 L
Protein = Nil
RBC = Nil
WBC = 152
ALT = 31 units
ALK phosphatase = 299 units: normal
Cholesterol = 180 mg/dL
Triglycerides = 180 mg/dL: normal
Lipid = 870 mg/dL: normal
LE = negative
RA = negative
C3 = 1.4 units
C4 = 0.5 units: normal

He had UTI with *Klebsiella pneumoniae*. His creatinine rose to 4.1 mg/dL (363 μmol/L) with normal electrolytes; his creatinine clearance was 9 mL/min with urine output of 1,650 mL. He was treated with antibiotics. With control of BP and infection, he improved gradually, and in June 1990 his clearance was 24 mL/min with urine output of 2,540 mL. His Hb was 12 g/dL (120 g/L).

He continued to improve: his creatinine clearance with 35 mL/min and by August 1990, 42 mL/min; in 1991, 44 mL/min; in 1992, 57 mL/min; in 1993, 49 mL/min; and in 1995, 47 mL/min.

In August 1995 he had renal colic, his right kidney 9.6 with mild hydronephrosis, left side was normal. His creatinine rose to 3.2 and 4 mg/dL later with UTI; he was treated with antibiotics and drips with improvement of his serum creatinine to 2.8 mg/dL (248 μmol/L). With control of BP and UTI, he gradually improved with creatinine and achieved stable creatinine of 2.1 mg/dL (186 μmol/L).

He developed liver abscess, which was treated, and clearance improved to 33 mL/min, with serum creatinine 2.5 mg/dL (221 μmol/L). His BP was effectively controlled with atenolol.

In 1992, he developed another stone leading to a rise in serum creatinine to 3.4 mg/dL (301 μmol/L) with clearance of 19 mL/min. He was treated with drips and passed the stone. He remained symptom free. In 2006, his clearance was 25 mL/min; in 2007, his serum creatinine was 3.7 g/dL (327 μmol/L) with clearance of 17 mL/min, and Hb 12.1 g/dL (121 g/L). In 2009, his serum creatinine was 3.5 mg/dL (310 μmol/L) with clearance of 19 mL/min.

On his last attendance on April 22, 2011, his serum creatinine was 3.7 mg/dL (327 μmol/L) with creatinine clearance of 18 mL/min, and Hb 12.4 g/dL (124 g/L). He remained symptom free as of this writing.

These two cases with stone diseases did not have hypertension, prior to the development of chronic kidney disease (CKD). The high BP developed after removal of the stone with the passage of more than 2 years.

The patients reported show that hypertension developed late after removal of stones by operative and nonoperative procedures. Repeated attacks of stones might possibly have given rise to the pathological change described previously leading to hypertension.

For case number 1, dialysis started after 12 years. Case number 2 is symptom free and stable with serum creatinine 3.7 mg/dL (327 μmol/L) and clearance of 18 mL/min.

Conclusion

The total contribution of stone disease to the ESRD burden is small and in the order of 8 %. In a country with poor resources and low income, it is an even more imperative that this small proportion of potential ESRD patients is attended aggressively before the start of renal failure. This is now possible through minimally invasive strategies that have transformed the management of urolithiasis, through the selective deployment of a plethora of technology.

References

1. Alam M. Gov't move over universal primary education sought. Daily Dawn. 4 May 2011.
2. http://www.infopak.gov.pk/SALIENT%20FEATURES%20OF%20PAKISTAN%20ECONOMY.pdf. Accessed on 5 Aug 2011.
3. Ali M. Per capita income of Pakistan (2010). http://www.einfopedia.com/per-capita-income-of-pakistan.php. Accessed on 5 Aug 2011.
4. Ahmad K, Jafar TH, Chaturvedi N. Self-rated health in Pakistan: results of a national health survey. BMC Public Health. 2005;5:51.
5. International Diabetes Federation. A call to action on diabetes. 2010. http://www.idf.org/webdata/Call-to-Action-on-Diabetes.pdf. Accessed on 5 Aug 2011.
6. National Health Survey. http://www.measuredhs.com/pubs/pdf/FR200/FR200.pdf. Accessed on 5 Aug 2011.
7. Data from Dialysis Registry of Pakistan. The Kidney Foundation of Pakistan. www.kidneyfoundation.net.pk.

8. Rizvi SAH, Manzoor K. Causes of chronic renal failure in Pakistan: a single large center experience. Saudi J Kidney Dis Transpl. 2002;13(3):376–9.
9. Worcester EM, Coe FL. Calcium kidney stones. N Engl J Med. 2010;363:954–63.
10. Klahr S. Obstructive nephropathy. Kidney Int. 1998;54:286–300.
11. Rastegar A, Kashgarian M. The clinical spectrum of tubulointerstitial nephritis. Kidney Int. 1998;54:313–27.
12. Madore F, Stampfer MJ, Rimm EB, Curhan GC. Nephrolithiasis and risk of hypertension. Am J Hypertens. 1998;11(1 Pt 1):46–53.

Urolithiasis in Renal Transplant Donors and Recipients

76

Ahmed M. Harraz and Ahmed A. Shokeir

Abstract

Allograft nephrolithiasis is an uncommon complication following renal transplantation. Stones may develop de novo in the graft or may be present in the grafted kidney at the time of transplant. A donor with history of stone disease is suitable for donation if he does not have any risk factors that predict recurrent stone formation. If a potential donor has a stone, he is accepted for donation if stone is less than 1.5 cm and if this can be removed during transplantation. Ex vivo removal of graft stone is a viable option, but this adds to the cold ischemia time and has the potential for injuring the pelvicalyceal system. For stones less than 0.5 cm, a watchful waiting strategy is optimal unless there is obstruction. For 0.5–1.5-cm stones, shock wave lithotripsy is feasible, but a percutaneous nephrostomy or double-J stent insertion may be necessary if the outflow tract is obstructed. Percutaneous nephrolithotomy and antegrade ureteroscopy are the management of choice for bigger stone burden with special care to avoid bleeding and bowel injury. Open surgery is restricted to select cases. A multidisciplinary approach is tailored according to stone and graft conditions.

Keywords

Urolithiasis • Renal transplant • Donor • Allograft nephrolithiasis • Amsterdam forum

Introduction

Kidney allograft urolithiasis is an uncommon event after renal transplantation, with incidence ranging from 0.17 to 3 % [1–8]. Allograft calculi, albeit that they are uncommon, are still more common than in the general population [9]. Allograft calculi may be donor gifted or may develop subsequent to transplantation.

Certain considerations need to be borne in mind when transplanting stone-bearing kidneys. Additionally, both the donors and recipients should be counseled about the risk of stone development and the potential impact on graft outcome. The recipients should know that unique factors might predispose the graft to further stone formation and that the symptoms and signs may be quite different because of the characteristics of the allograft and that the management strategies of urolithiasis in allografts are complicated by altered kidney location and ureteral anatomy.

In this chapter, we will discuss urolithiasis in renal transplants from both the donor and recipient perspectives.

Donor Perspectives

Criteria for Accepting Stone-Bearing Kidneys for Transplantation

A report of the Amsterdam Forum on the care of the live kidney donor has suggested that an asymptomatic potential donor with history of a single stone may be suitable for

A.M. Harraz M.D., M.S., MRCS
Department of Urology and Nephrology Center, Mansoura University, Mansoura, Egypt

A.A. Shokeir, M.D., Ph.D., FEBU (✉)
Department of Urology,
Urology and Nephrology Center, Mansoura University, Mansoura, Egypt
e-mail: ahmed.shokeir@hotmail.com

J.J. Talati et al. (eds.), *Urolithiasis*,
DOI 10.1007/978-1-4471-4387-1_76,

kidney donation if there is no known stone-associated metabolic syndrome or urinary tract infection (UTI) and the donor does not have multiple stones or nephrocalcinosis on computed tomography (CT) scan. If the donor has a stone, he should meet the previous criteria, and the stone should be less than 1.5 cm and potentially removable during transplant [10]. In addition, the possibility of further stone formation in the remaining kidney (of the donor) and its morbidity should be discussed clearly and in detail with the potential donors. The presence of stone in the allograft kidney and the implications should be explained to the potential recipient. The need for regular follow-up should be stressed, and access to the nearest center that could offer help in case of a stone-related emergency must be ascertained and the patient so informed [11].

Contraindications of Kidney Donation in Donors with Stone-Bearing Kidneys

Stone-bearing kidneys have been considered an important factor in donor exclusion [12]. The Amsterdam Forum guidelines indicated that in addition to aforementioned criteria, stone formers should not donate if they have bilateral stone disease or a stone type prone to a high recurrence rate. Examples of such stones include cystine stones; struvite stones; stones associated with inherited or systemic disorders such as primary or enteric hyperoxaluria, distal renal tubular acidosis, and sarcoidosis; stones in the setting of inflammatory bowel diseases; and stones that recur while on appropriate therapy [10]. Other criteria for exclusion include stone-forming donors younger than 25 years [13].

Management of Stone Disease in Donors Before Transplantation

Ex Vivo Ureteroscopic Stone Extraction

Ex vivo ureteroscopic stone extraction had been adopted to clear small calculi in transplanted kidneys before transplantation [14]. This procedure was performed for donor stones ranging from 1 to 8 mm (average 5.2).

Technique

The whole procedure is performed while the kidney is embedded in sterile ice-cold solution. Ureteral dilatation may be needed if the caliber is not adequate for passage of ureteroscopy. A 6.9 F semirigid or flexible ureteroscope can be used and the stone can be localized by careful revisiting of the preoperative imaging or with the help of fluoroscopy. Laser or pneumatic energy disintegration of the stone could be accomplished. A ureteral stent is placed while performing the subsequent ureteroneocystostomy [15].

Advantages and Disadvantages

Performing the procedure in this manner has some merit. There are no normal constrictions as would be encountered in the transplanted ureter, and secondly, as the ureter is not fixed, the ureteroscopy can be used at different angles, with resulting better access to all calyces. Done at the time of the transplant, these procedures obviate the need for performing further interventions on the allograft [14, 15]. However, it should be empathized that this manipulation would lead to an increased ischemia time and in addition could possibly damage the kidney owing to instrumentation [13].

Shock Wave Lithotripsy (SWL)

Devasia and associates have performed shock wave lithotripsy (SWL) for a stone in the future graft; the fragments have passed after 3,000 shocks, and the kidney was harvested with a 4-mm fragment that passed spontaneously later [11]. However, a waiting period after lithotripsy should be considered to avoid allograft edema or tissue friability that cannot be assessed accurately by routine clinical testing.

Fate of Donors Who Have Donated Stone-Bearing Kidneys

The incidence of stone recurrence after a single episode of stone disease has been reported to be up to 28 % over a 5–10-year follow-up period [16]. Nevertheless, to date, no reports have assessed the incidence of stone recurrence after donation of a stone-bearing kidney. A long-term follow-up of donors has demonstrated that stone disease developed in 5 (14.7 %) out of 339 donors and all were managed by lithotripsy with no recurrence. The authors have not delineated whether those donors have donated stone-bearing kidneys or not [17]. In another report, stones have developed in 6 (6.9 %) donors, which is not higher than the normal population [18]. Therefore, further studies should be conducted to demonstrate the fate of donors of stone-bearing kidneys.

Recipient Perspectives

Stones in renal transplant recipients may be the one gifted from the donor or one that develops because of metabolic abnormalities and risk factors leading to stone formation.

Donor-Gifted Nephrolithiasis

Urolithiasis in living donors has been considered a relative contraindication for donation. However, as there are no national organ-sharing programs for cadaver transplants in most developing countries and because of the demonstrated safety of therapy in graft lithiasis and the minimal estimated risk of lithiasis recurrence, there is a trend toward accepting stone-bearing kidneys [11, 19]. Donor-gifted nephrolithiasis occurred in the past unknowingly as there were less sensitive imaging techniques for donor selection. Conversely, the current computerized tomography (CT) era for donor screening allows for better donor selection and intentional transplantation with insignificant donor stones [13].

The De Novo Development of Stones in Renal Transplant Recipients

Incidence of New Stone Formation in Allograft Recipients

Although multiple risk factors are involved in stone formation in renal transplant recipients, the risk of stone formation in the transplant is not significantly higher than in the normal population [20]. Different hypotheses have been developed to explain such findings. Dumoulin et al. demonstrated that there is lack of increased urinary calcium oxalate supersaturation in long-term kidney transplant recipients [21]. Rhee et al. demonstrated increase in urinary IL-6 in patients with urolithiasis and its usefulness as a potential marker for stone disease [22], at the same time, suggesting a role of cyclosporine, as an IL-2 inhibitor, in the development of stones. Furthermore, the graft recipients also had lower urinary calcium and uric acid excretion and larger urine volume than the healthy controls, suggesting a combination of these factors in preventing the development of lithiasis [21].

Stone Composition

The reported stone composition in allograft kidneys has included calcium oxalate, calcium phosphate, calcium oxalate with uric acid, uric acid, struvite, and struvite mixed with calcium phosphate stones; however, no certain type has been determined to be the most common [6, 23–28].

Pathogenesis of Stone Development in Renal Transplant Recipients

Calcium Oxalate Stones

The primary determinant of calcium oxalate stone formation is the supersaturation of urine with calcium and oxalate salts. In renal transplant recipients, multiple factors might contribute to hypercalcemia and, subsequently, hypercalciuria. Steroid-induced hypercalciuria secondary to bone resorption is well recognized, and cyclosporine has also been hypothesized to contribute to bone loss and persistent tertiary hyperparathyroidism. In addition, hypocitraturia has been reported in renal transplant recipients [8]. Urinary tract infection, citrate malabsorption, and systemic acidosis (the latter being the most important factor) are the main causes [29–31]. Furthermore, a higher oxaluria has been reported in renal transplant recipients more than their control healthy subjects, favoring the interaction between calcium and oxalate salts and forming calcium oxalate stones [21]. On the other hand, as urinary volume is a primary determinant of urinary calcium oxalate saturation, a significantly higher urinary output in renal recipients clearly decreases the clinical incidence of kidney stone.

Calcium Phosphate Stones

A high urinary pH is a critical risk factor for calcium phosphate precipitation. Excessively alkaline urine associated with the renal tubular acidosis in renal transplant recipients, which also causes hypercalciuria, facilitates calcium phosphate stone formation [20]. The renal tubular acidosis could result from proximal wasting of bicarbonate due to the common persistent hyperparathyroidism in these patients or from distal renal tubular acidosis in some kidney recipients [21].

Uric Acid Stones

Hyperuricosuria, caused by cyclosporine [32] or a purine-rich diet in renal transplant recipients, predisposes to uric acid stone development. This can be treated with chemolysis [8, 32]. In rare instances, the stones may be composed of 2,8-dihydroxyadenine, but such stones would be formed in a renal transplant recipient with a homozygous adenine phosphoribosyltransferase deficiency. In this context, long-term maintenance with allopurinol and a low-purine diet could effectively prevent stone formation and renal failure [33].

Urological Risk Factors

Urological causes included recurrent urinary tract infection with urea-splitting bacteria [34, 35], use of nonabsorbable sutures [36], voiding dysfunction and retained double-J ureteral stent, ureteric stricture, and poor urinary drainage due to changes in anatomical positioning [37–40]. In addition, advances in immunosuppression have extended graft survival and have allowed longer periods for stones to form and become symptomatic.

Diagnosis

Clinical Presentation

Clinical presentation is quite different from normal kidney stones. As the allograft is denervated during procurement, the patient does not experience renal colic. The presenting symptoms are often a urinary tract infection, hematuria, impaired renal function, or obstructive anuria [7, 41]. Furthermore, the presence of a stone can produce a clinical presentation that is frequently mistaken for acute rejection or acute tubular necrosis [37, 40, 42]. In early graft obstruction, hydronephrosis is minimal and is seldom as dramatic in the transplant as in the acutely obstructed native kidney, causing ultrasound to be less diagnostic [43]. In pediatric patients, the first symptoms might be hematuria with or without dysuria, urine retention, or anuria [36].

Imaging Studies

Radiological evaluation for recipient lithiasis does not differ from ordinary imaging modalities for diagnosis of stone disease. Plain X-ray shows radiopaque shadow at the proposed location of the graft at the iliac fossa. However, small stones are missed in plain film, since the transplant kidney overlies iliac bone [44]. Ultrasonography detects the stone in the graft or the hydronephrosis caused by a stone at the graft ureter and can be used for follow-up after diagnosis. On the other hand, the low sensitivity of ultrasound should be considered [11], and in order not to miss any stones, as in other stone patients, a non-contrast CT (NCCT) scan should be done as it continues to be the most sensitive for diagnosing transplant urolithiasis [44]. In addition, apart from the risk associated with the use of iodinated contrast agents in patients with impaired renal function, CT urography has proved to be an important diagnostic tool in the evaluation of urological complications of kidney allografts particularly stone disease, showing a diagnostic accuracy greater than 90 % [45].

The stone disease can also be diagnosed by antegrade pyeloureterography after fixation of a nephrostomy tube for obstructed pelvicalyceal system (please see section "Case Scenario").

Treatment of the Graft and Transplanted Ureter Calculi

Conservative Treatment

The fact that some stones may pass spontaneously through the transplanted ureter may favor the watchful waiting option. Good diuresis and small stones <4mm are more likely to pass [23]. The passage could have resulted from the already high spontaneous rates coupled with increased urine output and possible dislodgement during manipulation of the kidney ex vivo. In addition, it has been speculated that the increased glomerular filtration rate and urine output in a transplanted kidney might prevent future stone formation [13]. Nevertheless, this should not be applied if there were impairment of graft function, and the compliance has to be very good to follow this option and the patient counseled accordingly [11].

Up to date, no definite criteria had been specified for adopting conservative treatment for allograft nephrolithiasis. In the study by Martin and associates, five out of the eight stones have passed spontaneously at follow-up (mean 508 days). Those remaining were two upper-pole stones and one mid-pole stone. In addition, the two patients with remaining stones had a significantly shorter length of follow-up, suggesting the possibility that these stones might pass with more time [13]. Lancina and associates have reported no intervention for one peripheral stone in the kidney, five stones passed spontaneously, and medical treatment for 7 patients who were diagnosed with hyperuricosuria and were treated by urinary alkalinization [6]. Two out of 18 stones had passed spontaneously, as reported by Rifaioglu et al. [40]. In another report, two patients developed stones in a series of 1,523 renal transplants required no interventions [2]. Three stones out of 19 allograft nephrolithiasis passed spontaneously, as reported by Klingler et al. [23]. Similarly, many reports described spontaneous stone passage with no intervention [6, 20, 27, 41].

In summary, transplantation of small (less than 4 mm) asymptomatic stones in situ can be safely performed with adequate follow-up and monitoring for the development of obstructing transplant stones [13].

Shock Wave Lithotripsy (SWL)

Indications and Outcome

Non-obstructing calculi less than 1.5 cm are suitable for shock wave lithotripsy (SWL) disintegration and have satisfactory outcome [4]. Similarly, Klingler et al. recommended SWL under close surveillance for calyceal stones (5–15 mm). They did not perform a percutaneous nephrostomy as a safety measure prior to ESWL [23]. For obstructing calculi, fast relief of the obstruction via nephrostomy tube or insertion of a ureteric double-J stent, followed by one or more sessions of SWL, appeared to be sufficient for stone clearance [4].

No adverse effect of shock wave on allograft function was noted both on short- and long-term follow-up [19], and successful outcome has been reported in many series.

Challacombe and associates reported stone clearance in the 13 cases with one residual fragment that passed spontaneously. This is in concordance with other reports [46]. Similarly, four out of five patients were rendered free after SWL for their graft stones; in the fifth case, fragmentation of the calyceal stone was not achieved after four sessions. The authors recommended SWL for 2-cm stones or less, with or without fixation of double-J stent [47].

Complications

Steinstrasse is a serious complication of SWL that can obstruct the allograft and impair renal function. However, conservative management with close monitoring of the Steinstrasse is highly recommended except when infection and/or oliguria is present, provided the overall stone burden is low [13, 23]. In a series of five patients with six stones, all were rendered stone free apart from one that required percutaneous nephrostomy placement for hydronephrosis secondary to impacted stone gravel. Transient hematuria was reported to always occur either during or after the treatment session [23].

Limitations

Many factors may contribute to reducing the success of SWL in clearing allograft stones—for example, the abnormal pelvic location of transplant kidney in the iliac fossa; its proximity to pelvic bones and alteration in kidney hydrodynamics resulted from malrotation. Clearance of stone fragments may be limited, especially with lower calyceal stones. In addition, residual fragments carry the risk of urinary tract infection and may serve as nidi for new stones [48]. The management of Steinstrasse is difficult because of the altered pain response and abnormal location of ureteral orifice near bladder dome. Rifaioglu et al. reported two transplants underwent percutaneous nephrolithotomy (PNL) after SWL failure [40].

Retrograde Endoscopy

Retrograde access to the transplanted ureter is technically challenging. It is often limited by the domal or posterolateral location of the ureteroneocystostomy and the frequently met tortuous course of the ureter. Nevertheless, in one report, retrograde ureteroscopy was used in 14 renal transplant recipients for different indications including obstructing ureteral stones in 4 patients [49]. Ureteroscopy was successful in removing all the stones without any complications. Three of the stones were 3–4 mm in size and were impacted in the distal third of the ureter; in the fourth patient, a 3-mm calculus was impacted at the ureteral orifice. All stones were removed with the basket without mechanical disintegration. The ureteroscopy was unsuccessful in only one case that required ureteroneocystostomy later. The authors suggested using cobra curved-tip open-ended catheters and a stiff Amplatz wire to afford support to the allograft ureter in much the way that retroperitoneal structures support the native ureter. This support facilitates passage of the ureteroscope and allows examination and treatment of the ureter under direct vision all the way up to the renal pelvis.

Percutaneous Nephrolithotomy (PNL) and Antegrade Ureteroscopy

Fisher and associates described the first report of percutaneous removal of calculi from transplanted kidneys in 1982 [50], and this is now often the treatment of choice when there is a significant stone burden as it has the ability to remove all the stone fragments. It is recommended that PCNL be carried out on larger calculi (>1.5 cm) in specialist centers with a large PCNL experience because of the risks inherent in treating a solitary kidney [4].

Advantages

The superficial location of a renal allograft to the abdominal wall makes PNL an appealing alternative in treating urinary calculi, and it has the advantage of potentially removing all stone fragments at one procedure [38]. In addition, the procedure has been performed in the early postoperative period, with minimal morbidity and preservation of renal function. No adverse effects due to immunosuppression were noted [48].

Technical Aspects and Difficulties

Initially, all patients should have preoperative urine cultures followed by culture-guided antibiotic therapy. Patients with positive cultures should probably be treated for at least 1 week before surgery. The procedure is conducted with patients in supine position under general or occasionally epidural anesthesia [21]. Calyx puncture of the graft is performed with a radiopaque 18-gauge needle guided by ultrasound in combination with fluoroscopy in either interventional radiology setting or in the operative room. Ultrasound guidance is recommended to avoid potential injury to the overlying bowel and to minimize radiation exposure, while fluoroscopy alone may be inconvenient because of the difficulty in opacifying the collecting system using a retrograde approach. For complex anatomy around the transplant, CT guided access might be the safest modality [40]. Unlike PNL in a normal kidney, the anterior calyx is usually preferred for puncture for transplanted kidney [37, 40]. This is a result of the anterior location of the transplanted kidney in the true pelvis, as well as the change in the axis of the kidney. In patients with renal pelvic calculi or a retained stent, an interpolar or lower-pole calyx can be chosen for puncture, while an upper-pole calyx seems suitable for branched calculi [38].

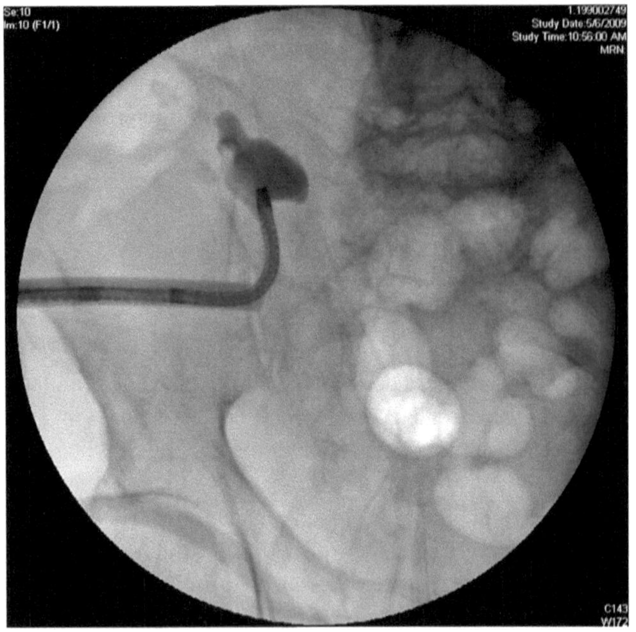

Fig. 76.1 A flexible nephroscope that is used to check for residuals in upper calyx after completion of the procedure with a standard nephroscope

Following guidewire placement, tract dilation is initially performed with radiopaque Amplatz dilators and then a balloon dilator (20 atm), allowing the placement of a 30-Fr Amplatz radiopaque sheath [37]. An expected difficulty is usually anticipated owing to the dense pericapsular scarring. In some cases, the loops of bowel can overlie the transplant, risking injury at the time of establishing renal access. Therefore, scheduling a CT before nephrostomy tube placement seems to be a prudent recommendation [38]. There is also possibility for iliac vessel injury because of the abnormally located pelvic graft.

The procedure can be performed with standard-sized nephroscope, usually 26 F, a 16-F peel-away sheath with an 8.5-F to 11-F nephroscope or a 15-F mini-nephroscope with no increase in complications using the larger scopes [38]. A smaller tract (16 F) is usually preferred to decrease the risk of bleeding and tearing of the renal cortex [24]. A flexible nephroscope or ureteroscope might be beneficial in select cases with a smaller stone burden. Flexible nephroscope can check for any small residuals in every calyx without the need to mobilize the graft, therefore minimizing risk of bleeding (Fig. 76.1). After dilation, PNL is initiated with combined ultrasound, pneumatic lithotripsy, and holmium: YAG laser with forceps extraction of the fragments. A 12.5 F flexible ureteroscope with holmium: YAG laser can be used for disintegration of distal ureteric stones out of reach of the nephroscope. In addition, antegrade ureteroscopy can be used as an adjunct to failed SWL [51]. A gentle manipulation should be conducted not to vigorously change the axis of the graft and predispose to bleeding. The bleeding risk can also be increased by platelet dysfunction in the early transplant period from preexisting renal failure [40]. Following the procedure, a nephrostomy tube is left and is removed after antegrade nephrostogram. An indwelling double-J stent remains an option tailored according to operative details and surgeon preferences.

Postoperative Complications

Minimal postoperative complications have been reported after PNL for stones in allograft kidneys. A urinary fistula developed after PNL for coralliform lithiasis in a patient with trans-ileal Bricker-type ureterostomy. The Bricker ureterointestinal anastomosis was located at the same level as the nephrostomy orifice, which maintained upper urinary high pressures as well as the fistula [52]. Table 76.1 lists criteria and outcome of PNL in renal transplant recipients.

Open Surgery

Open approach is a universally unaccepted alternative for treating allograft calcular disease because of many factors. The extensive fibrosis around the graft limits the chances of successful surgical nephrolithiasis intervention. In addition, the loss of capsular vessels and the use of ischemic drugs may be underlying conditions for the extensive fibrosis [37]. Furthermore, immunosuppressive use increases the potential risk of infection and poor wound healing [24]. Notwithstanding, open approach is typically restricted to large stone burden not suitable for PNL or residual calculi left over after PNL with no reported graft failure [4]. It is recommended that a transplant surgeon and an endourologist be part of the operating team for these open procedures, since intraoperative nephroscopy may be required for removal of residual stone disease [20].

Bladder Calculi

Vesical calculus formation in renal transplant patients is uncommon with different reported causes. Bladder calculus might develop on a polypropylene suture nidus at the site of a ureteroneocystostomy. Therefore, the use of a nonabsorbable suture in the urinary tract is not recommended [53]. El-Mekresh and associates reported vesical stones that developed following reimplantation by the Politano-Leadbetter procedure [51]. In addition, the development of bladder calculi in pancreas/renal transplant recipients might be attributed to the alkaline urine caused by the pancreas allograft, dehydration commonly reported in this population, use of nonabsorbable suture, or exposed staples near the pancreas-bladder anastomosis [20]. Bladder calculi can be treated with cystolitholapaxy with open approach reserved for difficult cases [51].

Impact of Graft Stones on Patient and Graft Survival

Limited data are available about the incidence of stone recurrence and the effect on graft survival. In a report of 16 renal transplants diagnosed with stone disease, a long-term follow-up (mean 69 months) showed 4 patients had lost the real graft (only one case was related to urinary calculi [primary hyperoxaluria]) and 4 patients had recurrent calculi [6]. In another report, 2 out of 12 stone patients have relapsed with no affection of graft function for any of these patients [7]. Cho and colleagues reported, during long-term follow-up, only one patient (out of 9) lost the renal graft 14.5 years after transplantation, primarily from causes unrelated to urinary calculi, and one instance of stone recurrence was noted [28]. It has been postulated that increased urine output on a per nephron basis of the graft might be sufficient to overcome any propensity of the kidney for subsequent stone formation [15].

Case Scenario

A 22-year-old male patient received left iliac renal allotransplantation for primary oxaluria. The patient was maintained on an immunosuppressant regimen with static graft function (creatinine 1.6 mg/dl). Two years later, the patient presented with graft impairment (creatinine 2 mg/dl) with incidentally diagnosed lower calyceal graft stone by ultrasonography (Fig. 76.2). The diagnosis was confirmed by NCCT that delineated hyperdense stone (8×7 mm) at graft lower calyx (Fig. 76.3). The decision was taken for close observation for this stone. One year later, the patient developed marked reduction of urine output with rising of serum creatinine up to 3 mg/dl. Emergent NCCT scan revealed mild graft hydronephrosis down to stone at the lower-end ureter (Fig. 76.4). A graft percutaneous nephrostomy was emergently placed within 24 h of presentation (Fig. 76.5). Twelve days later, creatinine decreased to its nadir level

Table 76.1 Outcome of PNL in renal allograft recipients

Reference	No. of patients	Average stone size (mm)	Average operative time (min)	Complications	Average hospital stay (day)	Stone-free rates no. (%)
Oliveira et al. [37]	7	32.8 (20–50)	102 (75–150)	–	6.9 (4–9)	6 (85.7)
Wyatt et al. [38]	16	–	84 (25–170)	1 (bleeding)	5.1	13 (81)
Rifaioglu et al. [40]	15	13 (6–40)	79	No	–	15(100)
He et al. [24]	7	–	53 (20–100)	No	–	7 (100)
Tanneau et al. [52]	1	–	–	1 (urinary fistula)	–	1 (100)
Challacombe et al. [4]	3	–	–	No	–	3 (100)
Klingler et al. [23]	3	34 (22–47)	–	No	–	3 (100)

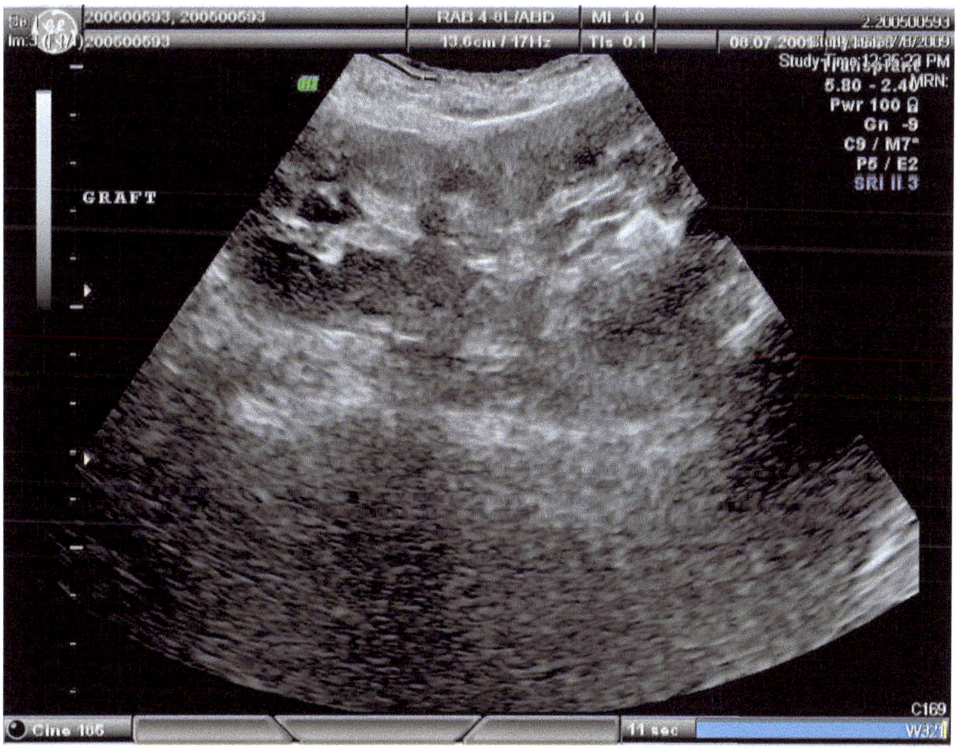

Fig. 76.2 Gray scale ultrasonography shows a hyperechoic stone shadow with acoustic shadow behind a lower calyx

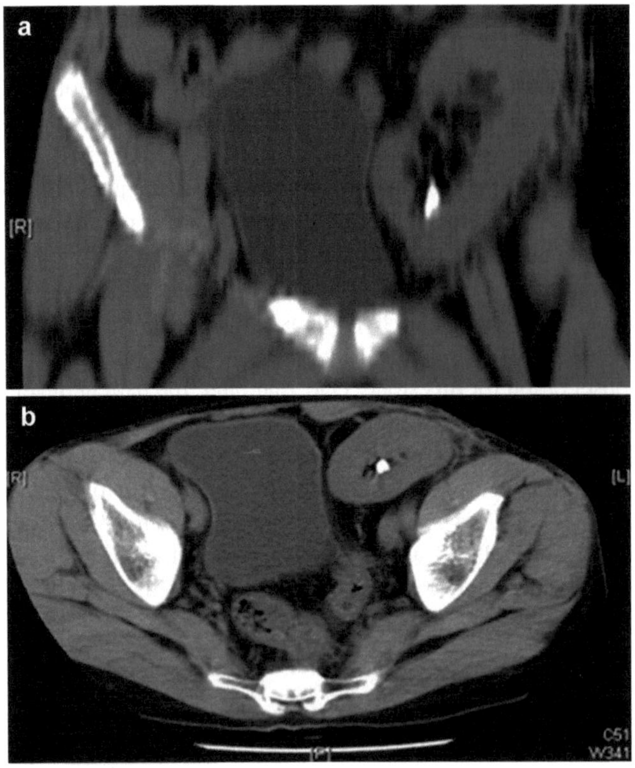

Fig. 76.3 Non-contrast computerized tomography scan showing hyperdense stone in the allograft at the lower calyx, (**a**) sagittal section, (**b**) axial section

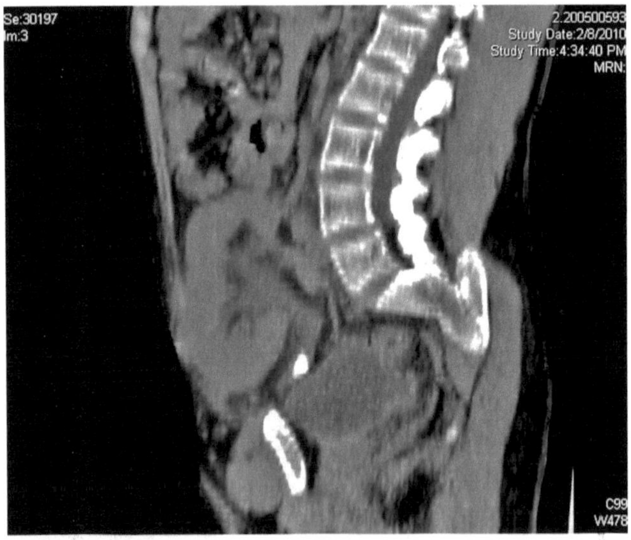

Fig. 76.4 Non-contrast computerized tomography scan showing hyperdense stone in the lower end of the allograft ureter

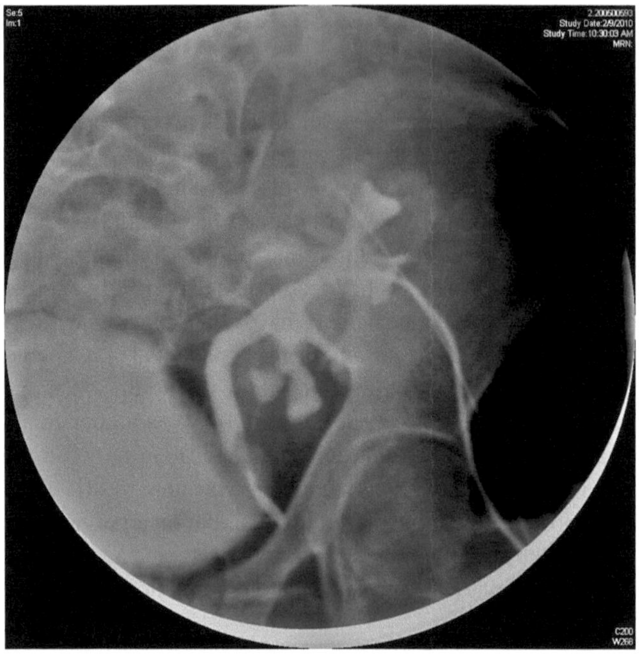

Fig. 76.5 Under biplanar fluoroscopy, fixation of upper calyceal graft percutaneous nephrostomy

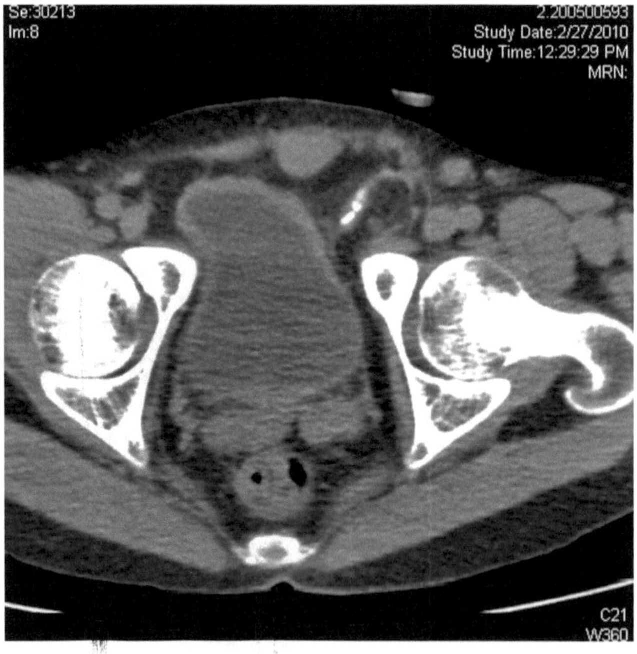

Fig. 76.6 Axial cuts of non-contrast computerized tomography scan showing hyperdense fragments at the lower end of the allograft ureter

(1.6 mg/dl), and the patient was scheduled for SWL. The stone was disintegrated using 3,000 shocks, and the patient experienced free passage of the stone fragments through the urethra (Fig. 76.6). Follow-up NCCT scan revealed complete passage of the stones 1 week later. Antegrade pyeloureterography revealed patent pelvicalyceal system with free passage of dye to the bladder (Fig. 76.7). Intermittent clamping of the PCN was performed with no development of fever or pain, then PCN was removed and

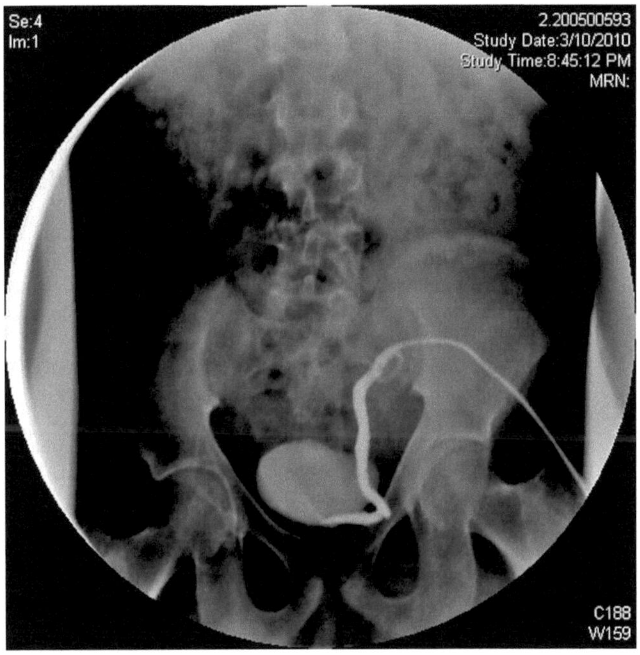

Fig. 76.7 Antegrade pyeloureterography reveals free passage of dye down to the bladder

patient was discharged free of stones and creatinine level 1.6 mg/dl.

Conclusion

Donor-gifted lithiasis is no longer a contraindication for transplantation in select cases. Stones could be managed by SWL and ex vivo extraction before transplantation. Incidence of recipients' nephrolithiasis is quite rare, with available armamentarium for stone retrieval if it becomes complicated and endangering the graft function. Limited data exists about the effect of urolithiasis on long-term graft function.

References

1. Buresley S, Samhan M, Moniri S, Codaj J, Al-Mousawi M. Postrenal transplantation urologic complications. Transplant Proc. 2008;40:2345–6.
2. Dalgic A, Boyvat F, Karakayali H, Moray G, Emiroglu R, Haberal M. Urologic complications in 1523 renal transplantations: the Baskent University experience. Transplant Proc. 2006;38:543–7.
3. Shokeir AA, Osman Y, Ali-El-Dein B, El-Husseini A, El-Mekresh M, Shehab-El-Din AB. Surgical complications in live-donor pediatric and adolescent renal transplantation: study of risk factors. Pediatr Transplant. 2005;9:33–8.
4. Challacombe B, Dasgupta P, Tiptaft R, et al. Multimodal management of urolithiasis in renal transplantation. BJU Int. 2005;96:385–9.
5. Nuininga JE, Feitz WF, van Dael KC, de Gier RP, Cornelissen EA. Urological complications in pediatric renal transplantation. Eur Urol. 2001;39:598–602.
6. Lancina Martin JA, Garcia Buitron JM, Diaz Bermudez J, et al. Urinary lithiasis in transplanted kidney. Arch Esp Urol. 1997; 50:141–50.
7. Benoit G, Blanchet P, Eschwege P, Jardin A, Charpentier B. Occurrence and treatment of kidney graft lithiasis in a series of 1500 patients. Clin Transplant. 1996;10:176–80.
8. Harper JM, Samuell CT, Hallson PC, Wood SM, Mansell MA. Risk factors for calculus formation in patients with renal transplants. Br J Urol. 1994;74:147–50.
9. Abbott KC, Schenkman N, Swanson SJ, Agodoa LY. Hospitalized nephrolithiasis after renal transplantation in the United States. Am J Transplant. 2003;3:465–70.
10. Delmonico F. A report of the Amsterdam forum on the care of the live kidney donor: data and medical guidelines. Transplantation. 2005;79:S53–66.
11. Devasia A, Chacko N, Gnanaraj L, Cherian R, Gopalakrishnan G. Stone-bearing live-donor kidneys for transplantation. BJU Int. 2005;95:394–7.
12. Wafa EW, Donia AF, Ali-El-Dein B, et al. Evaluation and selection of potential live kidney donors. J Urol. 2004;171:1424–7.
13. Martin G, Sundaram CP, Sharfuddin A, Govani M. Asymptomatic urolithiasis in living donor transplant kidneys: initial results. Urology. 2007;70:2–5; discussion -6.
14. Rashid MG, Konnak JW, Wolf Jr JS, et al. Ex vivo ureteroscopic treatment of calculi in donor kidneys at renal transplantation. J Urol. 2004;171:58–60.
15. Trivedi A, Patel S, Devra A, Rizvi J, Goel R, Modi P. Management of calculi in a donor kidney. Transplant Proc. 2007;39:761–2.
16. Trinchieri A, Ostini F, Nespoli R, Rovera F, Montanari E, Zanetti G. A prospective study of recurrence rate and risk factors for recurrence after a first renal stone. J Urol. 1999;162:27–30.
17. El-Agroudy AE, Sabry AA, Wafa EW, et al. Long-term follow-up of living kidney donors: a longitudinal study. BJU Int. 2007; 100:1351–5.
18. Azar SA, Nakhjavani MR, Tarzamni MK, Faragi A, Bahloli A, Badroghli N. Is living kidney donation really safe? Transplant Proc. 2007;39:822–3.
19. Bhadauria RP, Ahlawat R, Kumar RV, Srinadh ES, Banerjee GK, Bhandari M. Donor-gifted allograft lithiasis: extracorporeal shockwave lithotripsy with over table module using the Lithostar Plus. Urol Int. 1995;55:51–5.
20. Rhee BK, Bretan Jr PN, Stoller ML. Urolithiasis in renal and combined pancreas/renal transplant recipients. J Urol. 1999;161:1458–62.
21. Dumoulin G, Hory B, Nguyen NU, et al. Lack of increased urinary calcium oxalate supersaturation in long-term kidney transplant recipients. Kidney Int. 1997;51:804–10.
22. Rhee E, Santiago L, Park E, Lad P, Bellman GC. Urinary IL-6 is elevated in patients with urolithiasis. J Urol. 1998;160:2284–8.
23. Klingler HC, Kramer G, Lodde M, Marberger M. Urolithiasis in allograft kidneys. Urology. 2002;59:344–8.
24. He Z, Li X, Chen L, Zeng G, Yuan J. Minimally invasive percutaneous nephrolithotomy for upper urinary tract calculi in transplanted kidneys. BJU Int. 2007;99:1467–71.
25. Thakar CV, Lara A, Goel M, Nally Jr JV. Staghorn calculus in renal allograft presenting as acute renal failure. Urol Res. 2003;31: 414–6.
26. Jayawardene SA, Goldsmith DJ. Staghorn calculi complicating renal transplantation in patients with persistent post-transplantation hyperparathyroidism. Clin Nephrol. 2003;59:222–4.
27. Kim H, Cheigh JS, Ham HW. Urinary stones following renal transplantation. Korean J Intern Med. 2001;16:118–22.
28. Cho DK, Zackson DA, Cheigh J, Stubenbord WT, Stenzel KH. Urinary calculi in renal transplant recipients. Transplantation. 1988;45:899–902.

29. Menon M, Koul H. Clinical review 32: calcium oxalate nephrolithiasis. J Clin Endocrinol Metab. 1992;74:703–7.
30. Fegan J, Khan R, Poindexter J, Pak CY. Gastrointestinal citrate absorption in nephrolithiasis. J Urol. 1992;147:1212–4.
31. Simpson DP. Citrate excretion: a window on renal metabolism. Am J Physiol. 1983;244:F223–34.
32. Norlen BJ, Hellstrom M, Nisa M, Robertson WG. Uric acid stone formation in a patient after kidney transplantation–metabolic and therapeutic considerations. Scand J Urol Nephrol. 1995;29:335–7.
33. Glicklich D, Gruber HE, Matas AJ, et al. 2,8-Dihydroxyadenine urolithiasis: report of a case first diagnosed after renal transplant. Q J Med. 1988;68:785–93.
34. Hess B, Metzger RM, Ackermann D, Montandon A, Jaeger P. Infection-induced stone formation in a renal allograft. Am J Kidney Dis. 1994;24:868–72.
35. Locke DR, Steinbock G, Salomon DR, et al. Combination extracorporeal shock wave lithotripsy and percutaneous extraction of calculi in a renal allograft. J Urol. 1988;139:575–7.
36. Guest G, Tete MJ, Beurton D, Broyer M. Urinary lithiasis after kidney transplantation. Experience at a pediatric center. Arch Fr Pediatr. 1993;50:15–9.
37. Oliveira M, Branco F, Martins L, Lima E. Percutaneous nephrolithotomy in renal transplants: a safe approach with a high stone-free rate. Int Urol Nephrol. 2011;43(2):329–35.
38. Wyatt J, Kolettis PN, Burns JR. Treatment outcomes for percutaneous nephrolithotomy in renal allografts. J Endourol. 2009;23:1821–4.
39. Strang AM, Lockhart ME, Amling CL, Kolettis PN, Burns JR. Living renal donor allograft lithiasis: a review of stone related morbidity in donors and recipients. J Urol. 2008;179:832–6.
40. Rifaioglu MM, Berger AD, Pengune W, Stoller ML. Percutaneous management of stones in transplanted kidneys. Urology. 2008;72: 508–12.
41. Hayes JM, Streem SB, Graneto D, Hodge EE, Steinmuller DR, Novick AC. Renal transplant calculi. A reevaluation of risks and management. Transplantation. 1989;47:949–52.
42. Greif F, Dreznick Z, Jacob ET. Calculus in 16-year-old cadaveric kidney transplant: a unique case and literature review. Nephron. 1990;55:423–8.
43. Heron SP, O'Brien 3rd DP, Whelchel JD, Neylan JF. Ureteral obstruction due to calculi in the early postoperative period in renal cadaveric transplantation: a case report and discussion of ureteral obstruction in the renal transplant patient. J Urol. 1995;153: 1211–3.
44. Rajiah P, Lim YY, Taylor P. Renal transplant imaging and complications. Abdom Imaging. 2006;31:735–46.
45. Sciascia N, Zompatori M, Di Scioscio V, et al. Multidetector CT-urography in the study of urological complications in renal transplant. Radiol Med. 2002;103:501–10.
46. Wheatley M, Ohl DA, Sonda 3rd LP, Wang SC, Konnak JW. Treatment of renal transplant stones by extracorporeal shock-wave lithotripsy in the prone position. Urology. 1991;37:57–60.
47. Rodrigo Aliaga M, Morera Martinez J, Lopez Alcina E, et al. Lithiasis of the transplanted kidney: therapeutical potential. Arch Esp Urol. 1996;49:1063–70.
48. Lu HF, Shekarriz B, Stoller ML. Donor-gifted allograft urolithiasis: early percutaneous management. Urology. 2002;59:25–7.
49. Del Pizzo JJ, Jacobs SC, Sklar GN. Ureteroscopic evaluation in renal transplant recipients. J Endourol. 1998;12:135–8.
50. Fisher MF, Haaga JR, Persky L, Eckel RE, LiPuma J. Renal stone extraction through a percutaneous nephrostomy in a renal transplant patient. Radiology. 1982;144:95–6.
51. El-Mekresh M, Osman Y, Ali-El-Dein B, El-Diasty T, Ghoneim MA. Urological complications after living-donor renal transplantation. BJU Int. 2001;87:295–306.
52. Tanneau Y, Vidart A, Sibert L, Grise P, Pfister C. Management of coralliform lithiasis on renal allograft with Bricker-type ureterointestinal anastomosis. Transplant Proc. 2005;37:2104–6.
53. Klein FA, Goldman MH. Vesical calculus: an unusual complication of renal transplantation. Clin Transplant. 1997;11:110–2.

Primary Hyperoxaluria: The Role and Timing of Liver and Kidney Transplantation

77

Harshal Rajekar and Shrawan K. Singh

Abstract

Primary hyperoxaluria is an uncommon metabolic defect resulting from the deficiency of the enzyme alanine-glyoxylate aminotransferase in the liver. Deficiency of the enzyme results in overproduction and increased urinary excretion of oxalate, resulting in renal deposition of oxalate, which manifests as recurrent renal stones and nephrocalcinosis, often leading to renal failure early in life.

Renal replacement therapy in the form of dialysis, peritoneal or hemodialysis, is ineffective in clearing oxalate, and the ensuing systemic oxalosis results in the various clinical manifestations of the disease. Several medications like high-dose pyridoxine, orthophosphate, magnesium, glycosaminoglycans, and probiotic oxalobacter and measures to increase urinary output are useful in the management of raised serum oxalate and promoting urinary excretion of oxalate. The isolated kidney transplantation performed for renal failure does not take care of the biochemical defect which lies in the liver, and therefore, overproduction of oxalate and subsequent deposition in tissues continue unabated. Most recent authors advise against isolated kidney transplant for primary hyperoxaluria due to poor graft outcomes and recurrent renal insufficiency. Preemptive isolated liver transplant might be the first option in selected patients before advanced chronic renal failure has occurred, though it is unusual. With the onset of renal disease, combined liver-kidney transplantation serves to correct the metabolic defect as well as the renal failure. Liver-kidney transplant may be performed either simultaneous (immunological benefit) or sequential (biochemical benefit). In the future, advances in gene therapy and increased insight into the pathophysiological course of primary hyperoxaluria raise the hope to change the outlook of this problem with dismal prognosis.

Keywords

Primary hyperoxaluria • Oxalosis • Combined liver-kidney transplantation • Oxalobacter • Nephrocalcinosis • Pyridoxine • Renal failure

H. Rajekar, M.S., MRCS, DNB (✉)
Department of General Surgery,
Post Graduate Institute of Medical Education & Research,
Chandigarh, Chandigarh 160012, India
e-mail: harshal_rajekar@yahoo.co.in

S.K. Singh, M.S., MCh (Urology)
Department of Urology,
Postgraduate Institute of Medical Education & Research,
Sector 12, Chandigarh, Chandigarh 160012, India
e-mail: shrawanksingh2002@yahoo.com

Introduction

Archer and colleagues in 1957 first used the term "primary hyperoxaluria" (PHO) to specifically denote a suspected metabolic origin for the marked hyperoxaluria [1], recurrent urolithiasis, and renal and extrarenal calcium oxalate crystal deposition that characterized affected children. The urine oxalate excretion in affected patients is typically 3–6 times normal with severe clinical consequences. Children with

J.J. Talati et al. (eds.), *Urolithiasis*,
DOI 10.1007/978-1-4471-4387-1_77, © Springer-Verlag London 2012

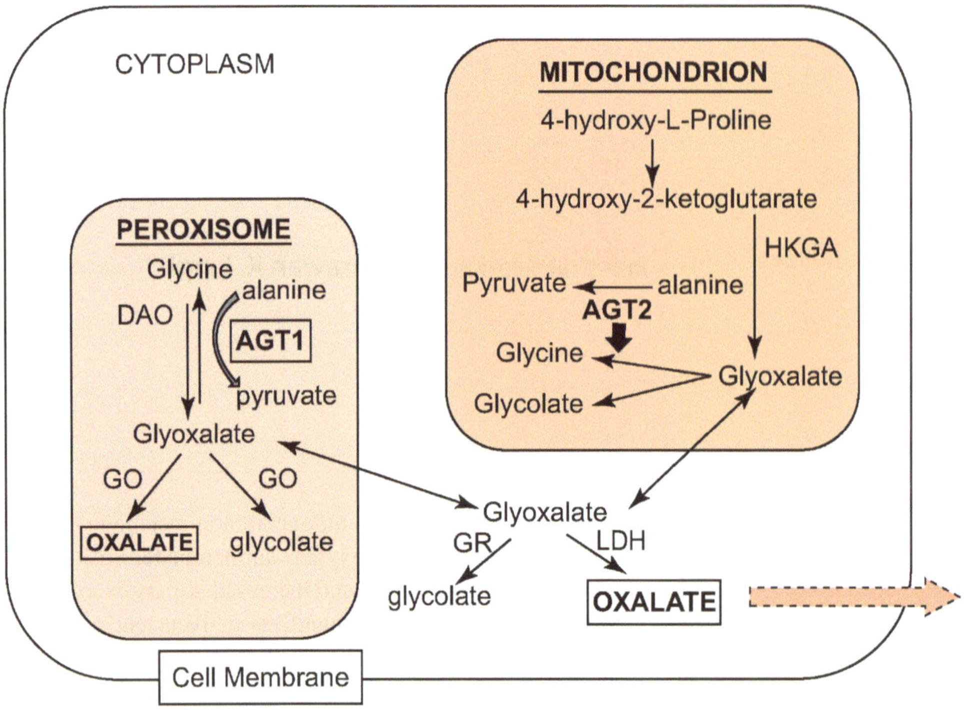

Fig. 77.1 The glyoxylate pathway in the human hepatocyte. *AGT* alanine-glyoxylate aminotransferase, *HKGA* 4-hydroxy-2-ketoglutarate lyase, *GO* glycolate oxidase, *LDH* lactate dehydrogenase, *DAO* D-amino acid oxidase

type I disease and a glomerular filtration rate (GFR) of 15 mL/min/1.73 m^2 excrete high amounts of both oxalate and glycolate. Normal urinary oxalate excretion per 1.73 m^2 body surface area is less than 45 mg/day or 0.5 mmol/day; values as high as 135–270 mg/day can occur in primary hyperoxaluria [2]. Kidney stones and/or calcification of the kidney occurs in childhood or adolescence. Renal injury due to oxalate deposition and consequences of the stones often leads to renal failure. Loss of renal function, if not addressed promptly by transplantation, leads to markedly increased plasma concentrations of oxalate with deposition of calcium oxalate in body tissues.

Deficiency or abnormal targeting of alanine-glyoxylate aminotransferase (AGT) to mitochondria in humans in primary hyperoxaluria type I (PH-1) results in buildup of glyoxylate and increased oxalate production (Fig. 77.1). Deficiency of an enzyme with dual glyoxylate reductase (GR) and hydroxypyruvate reductase (HPR) activities gives rise to increased hydroxypyruvate and glyoxylate, precursors of L-glycerate, and oxalate, respectively, in primary hyperoxaluria type II (PH-2).

Clinical Features

Oxalate is eliminated primarily by renal excretion, and there are no known metabolic pathways for its degradation, and so, marked hyperoxaluria ensues in PHO. Calcium oxalate deposition causing urolithiasis or nephrocalcinosis occurs early in the course of the disease. Symptoms usually appear within the first year of age in 15 % of patients and by 5 years of age in 50 %. The infantile form is characterized by renal insufficiency due to massive parenchymal oxalosis, and these patients often do not develop renal calculi. Older patients usually present with renal calculi or its sequelae such as renal colic, hematuria, or urinary tract infection [3]. Renal failure typically develops later, followed by calcium oxalate deposition in bone, blood vessels, myocardium, and other organs [4].

Other clinical manifestations include cardiac conduction defects and even cardiac arrest, digital gangrene, and difficulties with vascular access for hemodialysis. Bone and joint manifestations are seen in patients who have been on dialysis for more than a year [4]. Bands of increased radiodensity and subperiosteal cortical defects are seen due to calcium oxalate deposition in the bone. Calcium oxalate deposits can be seen in the retina and macula [5].

Diagnosis is often delayed due to the lack of clinical suspicion on account of the rarity of the disease. Even on clinical presentation with nephrocalcinosis and renal stones, suspicion of primary hyperoxaluria is uncommon. Strong clinical suspicion in patients with renal stones or nephrocalcinosis and renal dysfunction may prove useful in the early diagnosis of primary hyperoxaluria. Liver biopsy has been deemed essential for definitive diagnosis of PH-1 by measuring AGT catalytic activity. As an alternative approach, genetic analysis of AGT gene allows the detection of mutations in most of suspected patients.

A slow progressive decline in renal function is seen in most patients with episodes of obstructive uropathy and urinary tract infection. The resulting systemic oxalosis results in significant morbidity and may lead to metabolic bone disease, refractory anemia, cardiomyopathy, cardiac conduction system abnormalities, and ischemic ulcers of the skin. These cause severe morbidity and, ultimately, mortality. Historically, the median age at death is only 36 years. While a smaller number of patients present initially with renal failure, some as early as in infancy, the median age of end-stage renal failure is 25 years. Eighty percent of patients require renal replacement by the third decade [6, 7].

A less common variant, primary hyperoxaluria type II, also characterized by hyperoxaluria and urolithiasis but less frequently by renal failure, is caused by a defect in a different hepatic enzyme (glyoxylate-hydroxypyruvate reductase) [8]. Aside from increased oxalate production, hepatic function remains normal in both these disorders, even in late stages of disease progression. In type I primary hyperoxaluria, extrahepatic manifestations drive the need for orthotopic liver transplantation.

Management

In 1975, the American College of Surgeons and the National Institutes of Health recommended that primary hyperoxaluria was "unsuitable for treatment by renal transplantation" [9]. In 14 transplantations performed in 10 patients, the committee reported 7 deaths. Oxalate deposition in single or multiple allografts resulted in death from uremia in 4 patients, ranging from 49 days to 2.5 years after transplantation. Similarly, disappointing results with isolated renal transplantation caused by disease recurrence and the inefficiency of oxalate removal by standard modes of dialysis were noted by other investigators [10]. With improved understanding of the pathophysiological course of primary hyperoxaluria over the past two decades combined with advances in transplantation, improved outcomes have been obtained in type I hyperoxaluria [11, 12]. Understanding the effects and distribution of oxalate resulted in therapeutic designs to minimize oxalate-related tissue damage. These include initiation of renal replacement therapy earlier in the course of renal failure and specific approaches to the management of hyperoxalemia and hyperoxaluria both before and after transplantation. To minimize the renal calcium oxalate deposition, therapy should begin early with early diagnosis of PHO. The following measures may be tried:

- Maintenance of high urine output (>3 L/1.73 m^2 body surface area) to decrease tubular fluid oxalate concentration and diminish tubular oxalate deposition.
- Avoidance of high oxalate-containing foods.
- A trial of high-dose pyridoxine (3 mg/kg), which is an AGT coenzyme, and may be useful in some homozygous patients by reducing the production and urinary excretion of oxalate. It is more effective in heterozygotes where urinary oxalate excretion may fall by almost 10 % [13].
- Calcium oxalate solubility may be increased by the administration of neutral phosphate (orthophosphate at a dose of 30–40 mg/kg, but higher during periods of growth), potassium citrate (0.15 g/kg), and/or magnesium oxide (500 mg/day/m^2).
- Thiazide diuretics may be tried in an attempt to reduce urinary calcium excretion, whereas loop diuretics should be avoided in these patients as they tend to increase urinary calcium excretion.

Long-term therapy with pyridoxine and orthophosphate should begin early in the course of the disease and probably should be tried in most patients with primary hyperoxaluria [14]. Orthophosphates should be discontinued if the patient progresses to renal failure to prevent phosphate accumulation and genesis of tertiary hyperparathyroidism. Citrate may also be used to stabilize renal function in patients with type I disease, though the role remains uncertain [15]. With the development of renal stones, intervention is required for the management of urinary obstruction and urinary tract infection.

Increasing the colonization of the gut with oxalate-degrading anaerobic microflora *Oxalobacter formigenes* in enteric-coated capsules has been described to significantly decrease the urinary oxalate in patients with PHO [16]. Hoppe et al. recently reported the efficacy and safety of reduction of plasma oxalate levels by oral administration of *Oxalobacter formigenes* in two patients with infantile oxalosis [17].

Renal Transplantation

Renal transplantation was proposed for the management of the renal failure resulting from PHO since the oxalate elimination by current available methods of dialysis is suboptimal and cannot prevent systemic oxalosis and subsequent deposition of oxalate crystals in body tissues [18].

However, the transplant experience has been disappointing in primary hyperoxaluria type I due to the recurrence of oxalosis in the transplanted kidney resulting in graft loss in many patients. Both newly produced oxalate resulting from the metabolic defect and oxalate mobilized from the tissue contribute to the renal deposits [14].

Data from European Dialysis and Transplant Association showed a 3-year survival of only 23 % in living related donor kidneys and 17 % in cadaveric renal transplants [19].

However, many manipulations have been suggested and tried with varying degrees of success in making renal allograft more successful.

Preventive therapy includes:

- Aggressive preoperative dialysis to deplete the systemic oxalate pool [14].
- Consideration of early transplantation when the GFR is just below 20 mL/min to minimize systemic oxalate accumulation [5] and the preferential use of living related transplants to minimize the possibility of posttransplant renal failure that will limit the oxalate accumulation.
- Some physicians avoid nephrotoxic drugs including cyclosporine to maintain adequate GFR.

The degree of hyperoxaluria in type II PHO is lower and the clinical course more favorable than in type I disease. Hence, kidney-alone transplantation is recommended for patients with PH-2 [14].

Combined Liver-Kidney Transplantation

Identification along with isolation of the causative enzyme defect in the liver in the mid-1980s [20] opened up a new avenue of treatment. Simultaneous correction of the hepatic metabolic defect and renal failure by combined liver-kidney transplantation (LKT) for PHO was first tried successfully in 1984 in an adolescent with a failing cadaveric renal allograft secondary to oxalate deposition [21]. Oxalate dynamic studies performed in this patient confirmed correction of the metabolic defect by the orthotopic hepatic allograft [22]. Combined liver-kidney transplantation for the infantile presentation of PH-1 is associated with excellent outcome when the approach includes early diagnosis and early combined transplantation, aggressive pretransplant dialysis, and avoidance of posttransplant renal dysfunction [23].

Although LKT for correction of the metabolic defect and renal failure is now widely adopted for the treatment of PH-1, controversy remains regarding specific indications for and timing of hepatic transplantation. In PH-2, which is characterized by a more benign clinical course and localization of the enzyme defect to organs other than liver [24], experience has been limited to kidney-alone transplantation. To date, published reports of transplant outcomes in PHO are derived predominantly from registry sources. Little information is available with respect to urine oxalate excretion rates, plasma oxalate concentrations, and renal clearance after transplantation.

Bergstralh et al. reported the results of kidney graft survival among 203 patients in the International Primary Hyperoxaluria Registry from 1976 to 2009. They compared kidney alone versus combined liver and kidney as well as early versus recent experience. They concluded that the early diagnosis and determining the type of hyperoxaluria have made a significant difference. The outcomes of transplantation in PHO have improved over time, especially with recent combined liver and kidney transplantation [25].

Strategies for optimum patient as well as renal and liver graft outcomes must take into account the specific pathophysiological characteristics of PHO. Important considerations include patient selection for type of transplantation, appropriate timing of transplantation, and clinical management, both at the time of transplantation and long term. With the development of end-stage renal disease, the waiting list time for receiving a graft should be kept to a minimum to minimize oxalate accumulation.

Preemptive liver transplantation for correction of the metabolic defect and as a mode of preventing end-stage renal disease remains controversial. Supporters of preemptive transplant favor the deterrence of renal failure and avoidance of systemic oxalosis. However, with currently available knowledge, it is not possible to predict the prognosis of an individual patient with type I PHO.

Auxiliary liver as a means of enzyme replacement is not appropriate in PHO as the presence of increased oxalate production rather than decreased catabolism would continue in the remaining native liver tissue.

Careful management specific to PHO involves control of plasma oxalate concentrations with intensive dialysis pretransplantation, maintenance of high-volume diuresis posttransplantation, and, as soon as renal allograft function permits, initiation of neutral phosphate therapy to reduce calcium oxalate crystallization and supersaturation. Close monitoring is recommended to maintain plasma oxalate levels at less than 20–30 mmol/L, with dialysis as needed, and urine oxalate concentration at less than 0.3 mmol/L, with hydration as needed. Attention to the presence of calcium oxalate crystals in urine and stone formation also is important, as is prompt adjustment of doses of cyclosporine A, tacrolimus, and other potentially nephrotoxic agents. It should be kept in mind that not all renal allograft loss in kidney-alone transplantation is caused by oxalate deposition, and renal allografts even in liver-kidney transplant recipients remain at risk for loss caused by recurrent oxalosis until urine oxalate excretion rates approach normal. Pretransplantation, perioperative, and posttransplantation management guidelines are shown in Table 77.1.

Although plasma oxalate concentrations appear to decrease promptly with replacement of renal function, hyperoxaluria may persist for years after hepatic transplantation. This is caused by the length of time required for the mobilization and excretion of tissue oxalate. Gradual resolution of tissue oxalate deposits is achieved over the next 2–3 years. In this situation, increased oxalate excretion may persist as long as 3 years due to mobilization of tissue oxalate. Daily urine output should be maintained above 3 L till hyperoxaluria subsides.

Table 77.1 Management guidelines for patients with primary hyperoxaluria

Objectives	Renal clearance		
	Pretransplantation – <25 mL/min/1.73 m^2	Perioperative variable renal clearance	Posttransplantation – >30 mL/min/1.73 m^2
Stone prevention	Hydration as tolerated by renal function	Goal urine output of 4–7 L/day with fluids, diuretics as needed	Fluid intake to maintain urine output >4 L/24 h
	Pyridoxine	Pyridoxine in kidney-only transplant recipients	Pyridoxine in kidney-only transplant recipient
		Neutral phosphate if serum creatinine >2 mg/dL	Neutral phosphate
			Magnesium or citrate in selected patients
Prevention of systemic oxalosis	Intensive hemodialysis or combined hemodialysis and peritoneal dialysis	Hemodialysis or CVVHD pretransplantation and daily posttransplant until plasma oxalate is <20 μmol/L	Maintain hydration
		Pyridoxine in kidney-only transplant recipient	Minimize nephrotoxic agents
			Pyridoxine in kidney-only transplant recipient
Monitor	Urine volume	Daily urine volume	Renal function
	Urine oxalate excretion rate and concentration	Urine oxalate excretion rate and concentration	Plasma oxalate
	Renal function	CaOx crystalluria	Urine volume
	Plasma oxalate	Daily plasma oxalate and serum phosphorus	Urine oxalate excretion rate and concentration
			CaOx crystalluria
			Renal imaging for stones, nephrocalcinosis

Domino liver transplantation is unsuitable in PHO since the metabolic defect in the liver may lead to renal dysfunction in the recipient with attendant morbidity and mortality.

Indian Perspective

In India, primary hyperoxaluria is rare, and the exact incidence is not known since there may be patients who remain undiagnosed. Across the world, type I PHO occurs in 0.11–0.26/100,000 births and results in severe disease, while there are less than 30 reported cases of the less severe type II PHO [26]. Presently, approximately 3,200 renal transplants are done in India every year, a majority of which are living donor transplants. Barely 5 % of all renal transplants come from cadaveric organ donors. Even with this high number of renal transplants, it is barely enough because the annual requirements for kidney transplants exceed 150,000 [27]. A kidney transplant costs about 6,000 US dollars, with a lifetime monthly postoperative care costing approximately 250 US dollars. At present, deceased organ donation in India amounts to 0.7/million and is woefully inadequate [27] because of lack of health insurance, institutional and financial support, and the absence of a national program for organ transplants in the public sector. Moreover, most patients are unable to bear the costs of renal transplantation in addition to the unavailability of suitable donors.

Kidney-only transplantation is appropriate in patients with pyridoxine-responsive PH-1, in PH-2, and as an interim step preceding cadaveric liver transplantation in patients with pyridoxine-resistant PH-1 when a living donor kidney is available, and waiting time for a living donor liver is expected to be significant.

In the authors' country (India), the prohibitive costs of undergoing transplant surgery preclude a vast majority from getting a transplant. The average cost of liver-kidney transplantation at a private hospital in India could be between 40,000 and 50,000 US dollars. In addition, approximately 300–400 US dollars/month is required for ongoing postoperative health care and medication. The cost of continuous ambulatory peritoneal dialysis (CAPD) is approximately 400 US dollars/month.

At our institute, we have seen five patients with primary hyperoxaluria in the last 10 years, two of whom underwent renal transplantation and one received CAPD. The diagnosis in all our patients was indirect evidence of oxalosis in bone marrow biopsy or in allograft biopsy. None of the patients were diagnosed with PHO before the development of renal failure. The PHO was suspected on the basis of indirect evidence such as younger age with bilateral renal stones and calcified kidneys (Fig. 77.2). There has been one instance when a patient had early allograft dysfunction and required dialysis within a week after transplantation secondary to oxalate deposition in the allograft [28].

Though we are in the process of setting up an organ transplant program in the public sector, it is still in its infancy, and it would be expected to grow only with increasing awareness of brain death. In one of the private sector hospitals in India,

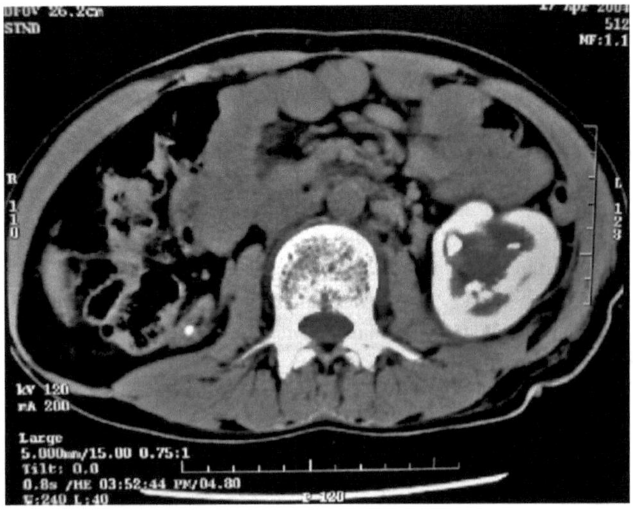

Fig. 77.2 Noncontrast computed tomogram showing stones in both the kidneys and calcified left kidney. The right kidney showed postobstructive atrophy and became nonfunctional before the patient developed renal failure

approximately 150 live donor liver transplants are being performed annually. One of the authors (HR) has experience with two cases of simultaneous liver-kidney transplantation from living donors. That liver transplant center has since then performed eight simultaneous liver-kidney transplants (three of them for oxalosis) of which seven have been successful. Simultaneous liver-kidney transplant is a complex operation with its attendant complications, and when a living donor is involved, the attendant risks to a healthy donor need to be carefully evaluated and communicated to the family.

Conclusion

Primary hyperoxaluria type I is a genetically determined disease and has dismal prognosis due to systemic deposition of oxalate. It is caused by overproduction of oxalate due to deficiency of enzyme AGT in the liver. The lack of early clinical feature and cumbersome screening by liver biopsy are the limitation for establishing an early diagnosis. The conservative and medical measures with high-dose pyridoxine may be beneficial in a sizeable proportion of patients. Among patients with partial or complete pyridoxine responsiveness, an excellent outcome can be expected with kidney-only allograft. Combined living donor kidney and living donor liver transplant may be an alternative in other cases of primary hyperoxaluria type I. PHO type II has a relatively benign course; however, it cannot be reliably distinguished from PHO type I based on plasma oxalate concentrations or other clinical parameters [29]. Moreover, in type II PHO, the deficiency of oxalate reductase is not limited to the liver only, but is more widespread. Therefore, kidney-alone transplantation is recommended in these patients with renal failure since it is not known whether the metabolic defect can be corrected by liver-kidney transplantation. With a better understanding of the pathophysiology of PHO, mechanisms of oxalate-related renal injury and advances in gene therapy will hopefully obviate the need for kidney and orthotopic liver transplant and thus changing the outlook of this problem in the near future.

References

1. Archer HE, Dormer AE, Scowen EF, Watts RW. Primary hyperoxaluria. Lancet. 1957;273(6990):320–2.
2. Watts RW. Primary hyperoxaluria type I. Q J Med. 1994;87:593.
3. Latta K, Brodehl J. Primary hyperoxaluria type I. Eur J Pediatr. 1990;149:518.
4. Morgan SH, Purkiss P, Watts RWE, Mansell MA. Oxalate dynamics in chronic renal failure. Comparison with normal subjects and patients with primary hyperoxaluria. Nephron. 1987;46:253–7.
5. Small KW, Scheinman K, Klintworth GK. A clinicopathological study of ocular involvement in primary hyperoxaluria type I. Br J Ophthalmol. 1992;76:54.
6. Latta K, Brodhel J. Primary hyperoxaluria type I. Eur J Pediatr. 1990;149:518–22.
7. Cochat P, Deloraine A, Rotily M, Olive F, Liponski I, Deries N, et al. Epidemiology of primary hyperoxaluria type I. Nephrol Dial Transplant. 1995;10 suppl 8:S3–7.
8. Giafi CF, Rumsby G. Primary hyperoxaluria type II: enzymology. J Nephrol. 1998;11 suppl 1:S29–31.
9. Wilson RE. Renal transplantation in congenital and metabolic disease. A report from the ACS/NIH renal transplant registry. JAMA. 1975;232:148–53.
10. Monico CG, Milliner DS. Combined liver-kidney and kidney-alone transplantation in primary hyperoxaluria. Liver Transpl. 2001;7(11):954–63.
11. Jamieson NV. The results of combined liver/kidney transplantation for primary hyperoxaluria (PH1) 1984–1997. The European PH1 transplant registry report. J Nephrol. 1998;11 Suppl 1:S36–41.
12. Saborio P, Scheinman JI. Transplantation for primary hyperoxaluria in the United States. Kidney Int. 1999;56:1094–100.
13. Milliner DS, Eickholt JT, Bergstralh EJ, et al. Results of long term treatment with orthophosphate and pyridoxine in patients with primary hyperoxaluria type I. N Engl J Med. 1994;331:1553.
14. Niaudet P. Primary hyperoxaluria. Orphanet Encyclopedia. Mars 2004 http://www.orpha.net/data/patho/GB/uk-oxalos.pdf.
15. Leumann E, Hoppe B, Neuhaus T. Management of primary hyperoxaluria: efficacy of oral citrate administration. Pediatr Nephrol. 1993;7:207.
16. Singh SK, Agarwal MM, Sharma S. Medical therapy for calculus disease. BJU Int. 2011;107:356–68.
17. Hoppe B, Dittlich K, Fehrenbach H, Plum G, Beck BB. Reduction of plasma oxalate levels by oral application of *Oxalobacter formigenes* in 2 patients with infantile oxalosis. Am J Kidney Dis. 2011; 58(3):453–5.
18. Watts RW, Morgan SH, Purkiss P, et al. Timing of renal transplantation in the management of pyridoxine resistant type I primary hyperoxaluria. Transplantation. 1998;45:1143.
19. Broyer M, Brunner FP, Brynger H. Kidney transplantation in primary oxalosis: data from the EDTA registry. Nephrol Dial Transplant. 1990;5:332.
20. Danpure CJ. Peroxisomal alanine: glyoxylate aminotransferase deficiency in primary hyperoxaluria type I. FEBS Lett. 1986; 201:20–4.

21. Watts RWE, Calne RY, Williams R, Mansell MA, Veall N, Purkiss P, et al. Primary hyperoxaluria (type I): attempted treatment by combined hepatic and renal transplantation. Q J Med. 1985;57:697–703.
22. Watts RWE, Rolles K, Morgan SH, Williams R, Calne RY, Danpure CJ, et al. Successful treatment of primary hyperoxaluria type I by combined hepatic and renal transplantation. Lancet. 1987;2:474–5.
23. Millan MT, Berquist WE, So SK, Sarwal MM, Wayman KI, Cox KL, Filler G, Salvatierra Jr O, Esquivel CO. One hundred percent patient and kidney allograft survival with simultaneous liver and kidney transplantation in infants with primary hyperoxaluria: a single-center experience. Transplantation. 2003;76(10):1458–63.
24. Giafi CF, Rumsby G. Kinetic analysis and tissue distribution of human D-glycerate dehydrogenase/glyoxylate reductase and its relevance to the diagnosis of primary hyperoxaluria type II. Ann Clin Biochem. 1998;35:104–9.
25. Bergstralh EJ, Monico CG, Lieske JC, Herges RM, Langman CB, Hoppe B, Milliner DS, IPHR Investigators. Transplantation outcomes in primary hyperoxaluria. Am J Transplant. 2010;10(11):2493–501.
26. Leumann E, Hoppe B. The primary hyperoxaluria. J Am Soc Nephrol. 2001;12:1986–93.
27. http://www.livemint.com/2009/02/20002008/India-ranks-2nd-in-kidney-tran.html. Accessed on 13 Sept 2011.
28. Heer MK, Sharma A, Joshi K, Minz M. Early allograft failure in an unrecognized case of primary hyperoxalosis. Nephrology (Carlton). 2005;10:423–4.
29. Milliner DS, Wilson DM, Smith LH. Phenotypic expression of primary hyperoxaluria: comparative features of types I and II. Kidney Int. 2001;59:31–6.

Part VII

Pediatric Urolithiasis

Metabolic Stone Disease in Children

78

Kemal Sarica

Abstract

When compared with the adult population, which has an overall 1–2 % incidence, urinary stone disease in children is relatively rare but often associated with metabolic abnormalities that can lead to recurrent stone episodes, emphasizing the necessity of full metabolic evaluation after the first stone episode. As a recurrent pathology that may reveal functional as well and morphologic changes in the urinary tract, each child should be evaluated thoroughly on an individual basis.

In children, stone recurrence rates range widely from 3.6 to 67 % and appear to be highest in children with metabolic abnormalities. Without close follow-up and medical management, stone recurrence rates have been reported to be as high as 50 % within 5 or 6 years.

Given the high risk of subsequent calculus formation, it could be argued that all children should undergo some form of evaluation to determine the cause of their kidney stone and to provide a basis for proper management strategies. It is well known that certain groups of children should undergo a full metabolic work-up due to the high risk of recurrence. Through these efforts, future stone formation and/or growth may be controlled in pediatric population, limiting the morbidity of this disease.

Keywords

Pediatric urolithiasis • Incidence • Metabolic abnormalities • Recurrent stone • Pathophysiology • Clinical presentation • Hematuria • Stone composition • Calcium oxalate • Phosphate • Struvite • Cystine • Uric acid • Hypercalciuria • Hyperoxaluria • Hyperuricemia • Cystinuria • Hypocitraturia • Diagnostic evaluation

Introduction

Pediatric urolithiasis is a relatively rare disease in developed countries, and in different series, the prevalence values have been reported to be ranging from 2 to 2.7 % [1, 2]. Although recent studies have shown that the annual incidence is increasing in Western populations [3, 4], stone formation is uncommon in children younger than 2 years of age. In contrast to the marked predominance of male gender in adults, boys seem to be affected slightly higher than girls [5, 6]. While the majority of the calculi (up to 90 %) are located in the upper urinary tract in developed countries [7], lower urinary tract calculi are seen more frequently in developing countries. Calcium-containing stones (calcium oxalate and calcium phosphate) constitute the most common type, and nearly 75 % of all stones have this composition [5, 8]. Several factors predispose children to urolithiasis, of which metabolic abnormalities and genitourinary anomalies are particularly important. These factors are frequently combined with dietary, environmental, and infectious causes where underlying metabolic abnormalities may be present in approximately

K. Sarica, M.D., Ph.D.
Department of Urology, Yeditepe University, Medical School, Ankara Caddesi No: 102/104, Kozyatagi, Istanbul 34752, Turkey
e-mail: kemalsarica@superonline.com; kemal64@hotmail.com; ksarica@yeditepe.edu.tr

J.J. Talati et al. (eds.), *Urolithiasis*,
DOI 10.1007/978-1-4471-4387-1_78, © Springer-Verlag London 2012

50–75 % of patients [5, 8]. Due to the common presence of metabolic abnormalities, stone disease may recur in this specific population more often than in adults. Therefore, children require a thorough anatomic and metabolic evaluation for a proper treatment plan to prevent further stone formation. Remarkable improvements in the understanding of both physicochemical principles and pathophysiology of stone formation have increased the need for a thorough metabolic evaluation. Moreover, medical treatment is crucial in the prevention of the recurrences in these patients.

Pathophysiology

Stone formation is a complex process beginning with crystallization and followed by crystal growth, aggregation, and adherence (Fig. 78.1), among which crystal formation has been defined as an important step for the initiation and growth of urinary stones.

These steps are promoted or inhibited by a number of chemical and environmental factors. Supersaturation is defined as the concentration of a salt that is higher than the solubility for that substance and is necessary for the crystallization process. The saturation depends on the total daily excretion of the substances and urine volume. Although the concentration of solutes is the principal determinant, ionic strength, pH, and promoter and inhibitor factors also play an important role in stone formation. Although urine is often supersaturated with calcium oxalate, calcium phosphate, or sodium urate, concentrations of mineral solutes vary throughout the day. In a large series of patients, the relative risk for stone formation was found to be strongly correlated with urinary calcium concentration [9]. In addition to the supersaturation of the urine, some promoting factors were also found to be necessary to trigger new stone formation. Of these factors, some urinary macromolecules, salt crystals and lipids, which may act as a nuclei or an aggregation factor for crystals, have been evaluated

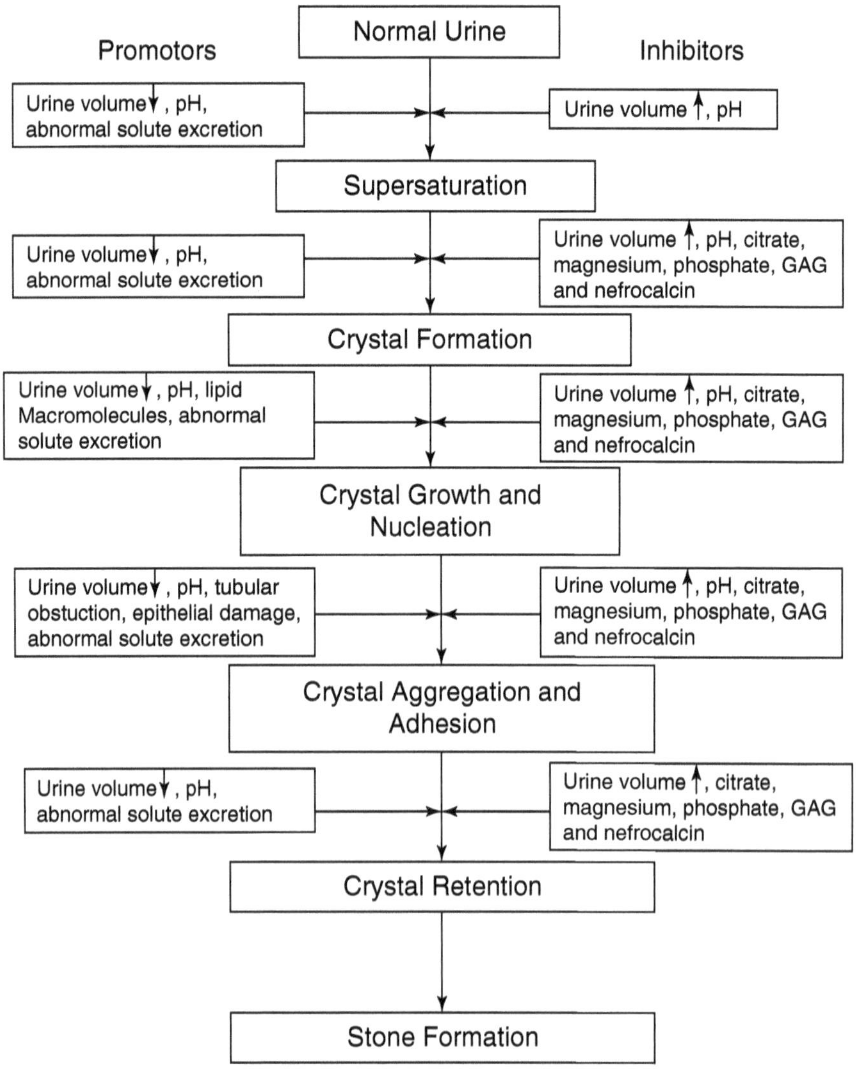

Fig. 78.1 The sequence of events leading to urinary stone formation

in different studies [10–13]. Another important factor for stone formation is urine pH, which may closely affect the solubility of urinary stone-forming risk factors, resulting in an increased risk of crystal formation. While alkaline pH may ease the formation of calcium phosphate-containing stones, an acidic urine lowers the solubility of uric acid and cystine crystals [14]. So, urine pH may act either as a promoting or an inhibiting factor, making this urine variable sometimes important as a therapeutic approach. Inhibitors are the substances that affect the crystal surface, resulting in crystal growth limitation or formation of soluble complexes [15–17]. These natural inhibitors include citrate, magnesium, pyrophosphate, glycosaminoglycans, and nephrocalcin. To form a stone, crystals must reach a sufficient size to obstruct or adhere to a renal tubule. After this step, these crystals may act as nuclei and promote the stone formation. But these steps are very variable, and in the majority of subjects, urinary stones are not formed. Children who form stones usually have underlying predisposing metabolic factors and/or anatomical abnormalities causing higher excretion of solutes, urinary obstruction, or urinary tract infection [18].

Clinical Presentation

In adults, the typical features of nephrolithiasis are flank pain and/or hematuria which are present in more than 90 % of stone patients. In the adolescent period too, approximately 90 % of children present with pain and hematuria, but in children, these typical symptoms are less common. At school age, these symptoms may be present only in 70 % and in those <5 years in only 50 % of patients [5, 19]. Although infants with urinary calculi usually present with colic pain, in younger children, abdominal pain is more common than renal colic.

Hematuria (macroscopic or microscopic) is noted in 14–90 % of the cases in different age groups of children [20–23]. Sometimes hematuria may be present in children with hypercalciuria and hyperuricosuria without any urinary stone [24–27]. Urinary stones may present with urinary infection or sterile pyuria especially in preschool age children. Usually, the diagnosis is made during investigation of a urinary tract infection or sterile pyuria with radiosonographic findings [5]. Dysuria and urinary frequency are manifestations of bladder or urethral stones. The latter are rare in children.

In summary, like the adult cases suffering from urinary stones, the majority of the pediatric cases complain of flank and/or abdominal pain. Although relatively older cases may present with clear symptomatology, such symptoms may not be easily recognized in younger pediatric patients, who are unable to articulate or localize their complaints. Thus, in the light of the increasing incidence of stone disease in children, pediatricians should always keep this pathology in mind when dealing with younger pediatric cases presenting with atypical abdominal pain, which in some cases may be present for a long period of time.

Concerning the location of the calculi, in developed countries, approximately 90 % of urinary stones are found in the upper urinary tract and bladder calculi too, commonly originate in the kidneys. Primary bladder stones on the other hand are usually seen in developing countries and are commonly referred to as endemic bladder stones [28, 29]. These stones are seen in younger children and associated with dietary factors [30, 31]. A diet with whole-grain cereals, oxalate-rich vegetables with low calcium, animal protein, and phosphate increases the risk for bladder stone formation [32, 33]. In Western countries, in contrast, primary bladder stones have usually been found to be related with bladder malformations.

With respect to the stone composition, like the adult population, calcium-containing stones are the most common type of nephrolithiasis in children. Of all the calculi evaluated so far in different series, 40–60 % were composed of calcium oxalate, 15–25 % were calcium phosphate, 10–25 % mixed stones, 17–30 % magnesium ammonium phosphate (struvite), 10 % cystine, and only 2–10 % were composed of uric acid [5, 7, 8, 28, 34–36].

Metabolic Factors

Children with stone disease have at least one predisposing factor, and these factors are identifiable in approximately 75 % of the patients [5, 35–37]. Tekin et al. [23] evaluated the metabolic status of 78 cases with idiopathic calcium stone formation and demonstrated that hypocitruria and hyperoxaluria were 4.3- and 3-fold more common in stone formers than in normal controls, respectively. Depending on the common association of the underlying metabolic disorders, recurrence rates have been found to be higher (65 %) than that in the normal population [5]. In a long-term follow-up study, Noe et al. investigated the recurrence rate in hypercalciuric patients, and they found that 33 % of patients had at least one recurrence in 4–15 years during which period 40 % of the cases did experience multiple recurrences [38]. Children with abnormal urinary tract structure tended to have metabolic abnormalities and chronic infection with incidences of 39 and 29 %, respectively [38]. Certain medical conditions have been shown to be associated with renal lithiasis in children. Calcium oxalate stones have been found to be quite common in malabsorptive states, resulting in enhanced uptake of oxalate and subsequent increased urinary oxalate excretion [39]. Children with cystic fibrosis had significantly elevated oxalate excretion compared to normal healthy children [40]. All these data show that there is tendency for stone recurrence in children with these identifiable risk factors that should be investigated carefully.

The metabolic risk factors for nephrolithiasis in children are the same as in adults: hypercalciuria, hyperoxaluria, cystinuria, hyperuricosuria, and hypocitraturia (Table 78.1).

Table 78.1 Factors associated with urolithiasis

Factors	Pathology	Conditions
Hypercalciuria	Genetic	Idiopathic
		Dent's disease
		Seyberth syndrome
		Williams syndrome
	Dietary	Dietary calcium excess
		Vitamin D excess
		Ketogenic diet
		Phosphate depletion
	Drugs	Corticosteroids
		Loop diuretics
	Endocrine diseases	Hyperthyroidism/hypothyroidism
		Adrenocorticoid excess
		Hyperparathyroidism
	Bone metabolism	Immobilization
		Rickets
		Malignancies
		JRA
	Renal tubular dysfunction	Renal tubular phosphate leak
		Impaired renal tubular calcium absorption
		Type 1 (distal) renal tubular acidosis
		Bartter syndrome
	Others	Prematurity
		Metabolic acidosis
		Increased renal prostaglandin E2 production
	Dietary excess or chronic malabsorption	Primary hyperoxaluria types I and II
Hyperoxaluria	Genetic	Cystinuria
Cystinuria	Genetic	HPRT deficiency
Hyperuricosuria	Dietary	Ketogenic diet
		High-protein diet
	Drugs	Salicylates
		Phenylbutazone
		Sulfinpyrazone
	Other	Malignancies
		Tumor lysis syndrome
		Diabetes
		SIADH
	Tubular dysfunction	Distal RTA
		Hypokalemia
Hypocitraturia	Dietary	Ketogenic diet
	Dietary	Ketogenic diet

Hypercalciuria

Hypercalciuria is defined as a urinary calcium excretion greater than 4 mg/kg/day (0.1 mmol/kg/day) measured in a 24-h urine collection or urinary calcium/creatinine ratio greater than 0.21 while on a normal daily diet [40–42]. During the first 2 years of life, children tend to have higher calcium and lower creatinine excretion. Adolescents, however, may have slightly higher calcium excretion during rapid growth periods. Hypercalciuria is the most common cause of pediatric urolithiasis and can be found in 4 % of the normal population [43, 44]. It is not a single disease or entity, but it is a condition that may be associated with genetic, endocrine, dietary, and renal disorders (see Table 78.1). Children with hypercalciuria generally have normal blood calcium and, in most cases, no underlying pathology and are described as having idiopathic hypercalciuria. Two different types of idiopathic hypercalciuria are described; the first type is associated with excessive gastrointestinal calcium absorption. The urinary calcium-creatinine ratio is normal in fasting condition in these children. The second type is caused by excessive renal excretion, and dietary calcium restriction does not affect the urinary calcium levels [45–47]. Although the pathophysiology of idiopathic hypercalciuria is unclear, some patients with this pathology have an increased number of vitamin D receptors compared with controls [48]. Some of these patients have familial penetrance, but the responsible gene has not been identified so far. The disease appears to be transmitted as an autosomal dominant trait with incomplete penetrance as 40–65 % of patients have a positive family history [49–52]. Hypercalciuria is present in nearly half of the children with urinary stones, and it is often associated with hematuria despite the absence of a stone. In a prospective study, Stapleton et al. found that 27 % of children with unexplained hematuria had hypercalciuria, and when urinary calcium was reduced by treatment, hematuria resolved in the majority of the cases [6]. Hypercalciuria may also cause dysuria, urinary urgency, and perhaps recurrent urinary tract infections [53–56]. In some studies, 4–17 % of patients did develop urinary stones [54–56]. In a prospective study, 8 of 65 patients with hypercalciuria and hematuria developed calculi in a 4-year follow-up period [57]. Garcia et al. revealed that 17 % of patients developed urolithiasis, and the mean period between hematuria and stone formation was 13.1 months. No predictive factor could be identified [55].

Dent's disease is a rare X-linked recessive disorder related to a specific chloride channel (CLCN5), which is located on chromosome Xp11.22. This pathology affects the proximal tubule, loop of Henle, and medullary thick ascending limb and causes hypercalciuria, low-molecular-weight proteinuria, nephrolithiasis, and nephrocalcinosis [58, 59]. The same chloride channel is implicated in four different entities: Dent's disease, X-linked recessive hypophosphatemic rickets, and low-molecular-weight proteinuria with hypercalciuria and nephrocalcinosis [60].

Other causes of hypercalciuria that need to be mentioned are use of corticosteroids and loop diuretics, distal renal tubular acidosis, dietary excess calcium intake, hyperparathyroidism, immobilization, hypo- or hyperthyroidism, osteolytic metastases, idiopathic hypercalcemia of infancy, sarcoidosis, and hypervitaminosis D.

Hyperoxaluria

Hyperoxaluria is found in up to 20 % of children with nephrolithiasis [5, 61]. Oxalate is an end product of normal amino acid metabolism where endogenous oxalate is produced in the liver. Dietary intake of oxalate is also important. Beets, turnips, strawberries, sweet potatoes, wheat bran, tea, cocoa, pepper, chocolate, spinach, dill, nuts, and citrus juices are defined as oxalate-rich foodstuffs. Dietary oxalate normally combines with calcium in the intestine and under normal conditions to form insoluble calcium oxalate, and only 10 % of the totally excreted oxalate is absorbed from the food. In malabsorption syndromes, fatty acids combine with calcium, leaving oxalate free to combine with Mg to form soluble salts, and this leads to excessive oxalate absorption [62, 63].

Renal oxalate excretion reflects the quantum of endogenous and exogenous oxalate load.

Primary hyperoxaluria is a rare autosomal recessive disorder caused by deficiency of hepatic alanine-glyoxylate aminotransferase (AGT) (type 1) or glyoxylate reductase/hydroxypyruvate reductase (type 2). This deficiency leads to a moderate to marked hyperoxaluria [64, 65]. The gene of the enzyme of type 1 disease is located on chromosome band 2q37.3, and type 2 enzyme is located on chromosome 9 [66]. The enzyme deficiency also leads to hyperglyceric aciduria. Type 1 disease is more severe than type 2 disease, and patients with type 2 disease usually do not have any symptoms until the second or third decade of life [67]. Due to moderate to marked hyperoxaluria, recurrent nephrolithiasis occurs during infancy in type 1 disease. Stone disease may progress to end-stage renal failure at early ages. When glomerular filtration rate (GFR) decreases to 30 mL/min/m^2, the blood oxalate level can increase rapidly, resulting in calcium oxalate depositions in multiple organ systems (oxalosis). At this stage, aggressive dialysis is a primary treatment alternative (see Chap. 77).

Pyridoxine is the cofactor for the AGT enzyme, and in cases with type 1 disease, pyridoxine should be a part of treatment regimen. One-third of patients do respond to pyridoxine treatment [68, 69]. Additionally, neutral phosphate administration, alkalinization of urine, and high fluid intake are beneficial measures to prevent urinary supersaturation with calcium oxalate and reduce the stone-forming activity [68]. Diagnosis of hyperoxaluria requires a 24-h urine collection, and hyperoxaluria is defined as urine oxalate levels exceeding 1.0–1.5 mmol/1.73 m^2/24 h. Urine oxalate excretion is higher during infancy [67].

Secondary hyperoxaluria may occur due to malabsorption states, ethylene glycol poisoning, renal tubular acidosis (RTA), pyridoxine deficiency, sarcoidosis, or ingestion of a large amount of vitamin C [70].

Cystinuria

Cystinuria is an autosomal recessive disorder of renal tubular and intestinal reabsorptive transport of cystine and the dibasic amino acids (ornithine, arginine, and lysine) [71]. Mutations of the SLC3A1 gene on chromosome arm 2p and the SLC7A9 gene of chromosome 19 are responsible for the disease [72–74]. Cystine stones account for only 6–8 % of all urinary calculi in children in developed countries. Cystinosis has a wide range of incidence worldwide [75], where the estimated incidence in England is 1/2,000 and in the USA 1/15,000. Large amounts of cystine excreted that cannot be absorbed by the tubules are excreted in urine. It has a low solubility—the soluble concentration of cystine is limited to 1,000 μmol/L (240 mg/L) in normal urine. Cystine crystals form in children with higher excretion levels [76]. Cystine crystals (which have a characteristic flat hexagonal shape) are seen in 25 % of patients [67]. In suspected cases, a positive nitroprusside test indicates excessive excretion of cystine, which needs to be confirmed by quantitive analysis in a 24-h urine collection.

Cystine forms radiopaque stones that generally form during the first decade of life in these children. The majority of cases are asymptomatic until the second or third decade of life. Therefore, a diagnosis of cystinuria often is delayed for several years. Patients with homozygous forms of cystinuria have lifelong recurring stone formation [77]. First-line therapy consists of increased oral fluid intake and a low-salt diet. Alkaline pH increases the solubility of cystine, and alkalinization of the urine is an important part of treatment [76]. If stone formation cannot be controlled, D-penicillamine or tiopronin (a thiol drug) can be added to the therapy.

Hyperuricosuria

As a weak acid, urate is the end product of purine metabolism. Its solubility is mainly dependent on urinary pH and decreases in acidic urine. Idiopathic uricosuria is often familial and asymptomatic where a defect in renal tubular reabsorption or increased secretion may cause the disease [78–80]. Although uric acid crystals may combine with calcium oxalate crystals and act as a nidus, this condition is uncommon in children. Uric acid stones are responsible for 3–4 % of urinary calculi in pediatric patients. Hematuria is a common sign of idiopathic hyperuricosuria [78] and usually accompanies hypercalciuria [5]. These stones may also occur in children in case of urate overproduction. Hereditary disorders associated with overproduction of urate include Lesch-Nyhan syndrome (hypoxanthine-guanine phosphoribosyltransferase deficiency) and type I glycogen storage disease [81]. Increasing cell activity in lymphoproliferative or myeloproliferative disorders and tumor lysis syndrome may also raise the urate levels. Urolithiasis may present as early as the first year of life in patients with Lesch-Nyhan syndrome (an X-linked recessive disorder). Another inborn error of metabolism with hyperuricosuria is hypoxanthine-guanine phosphoribosyltransferase deficiency. The accumulation of phosphoribosylpyrophosphate leads to the overproduction of urate [18]. Pediatric patients who have partial hypoxanthine-guanine phosphoribosyltransferase deficiency also may have gouty arthritis [82].

During the early months of life, urate excretion is relatively high and remains higher than in adults through infancy [81]. However, beginning at 2 years of age, the amount of urate excreted per deciliter of glomerular filtrate does not vary with age [78]. A value of less than 0.56 mg of urate/dL (0.033 mmol/L) of glomerular filtrate may be considered normal after 2 years of age.

Treatment of hyperuricosuria requires a high fluid intake along with the restriction of dietary purines. Alkalinization of urine increases the solubility of urate. In addition to use in the classical clinical cases, allopurinol may also be recommended in an attempt to limit urate excretion in patients with Lesch-Nyhan syndrome or tumor lysis syndrome during chemotherapy [82, 83].

Diagnostic Evaluation

Evaluation of pediatric patients with stone disease includes:

- Patient history (including diet).
- Family history of stone disease and genetic disorders.
- Physical examination.
- Detailed urine analysis (urinalysis, urine culture sensitivity tests). A urinalysis provides greater information than a dipstick test.
- Blood biochemistry including calcium and renal functional parameters (BUN, Cre).
- Radiosonographic imaging.
- 24-h urine collection.
- Stone analysis.

Evaluation of these children should begin with a detailed history specifically asking for a history of prematurity. The patient's age at presentation and signs and symptoms of urinary and other systems may provide clues to an underlying systemic disease. Family history of hematuria, renal failure, urolithiasis, arthritis, and gouty disease is also important. Detailed dietary history including fluid intake, medications, and dietary excesses and deficiencies should be obtained. The physical examination again should include growth evaluation, bone development, body deformities, and blood pressure. Urinalysis is performed for detecting the presence of crystalluria, pyuria, or hematuria. Urinary tract infection should be excluded by urine culture and sensitivity tests. A chemical analysis of the stone is also important to focus on an appropriate metabolic work-up. A 24-h urine collection will be helpful while the patient is healthy, under normal diet, and usual fluid intake without any additional medication (Table 78.2). The excretion rate of urinary stone-forming constituents (calcium, cystine, urate, sodium, oxalate, and citrate) should be measured. Ideally, the urine collection should be obtained at least 6 weeks after the passage of a stone. Abnormal values might be verified with a repeat collection when necessary. But determination of urinary supersaturation with calcium oxalate, calcium phosphate, and uric acid may be helpful if the urine volume is >1 mL/kg/h [84]. The creatinine excretion rate is often used to verify that the total 24-h urine has been collected. An adequate urine collection is gauged from the fact that the majority of the children excrete 15–20 mg/kg/24 h (0.13–0.18 mmol/kg/24 h) of creatinine [18]. Plasma levels of calcium, magnesium, phosphorus, creatinine, bicarbonate, and urate should be investigated. Lastly, intact parathyroid hormone (PTH) levels should be determined in children with hypercalcemia or hypophosphatemia.

Table 78.2 Normal urinary values in school age children: 24-h urine collection [20]

Calcium	<4 mg/kg/day	<0.1 mmol/kg/day
Oxalate	<50 mg/1.73 m^2/day	<0.56 mmol/1.73 m^2/day
Cystine	<60 mg/1.73 m^2/day	<0.25 mmol/1.73 m^2/day
Citrate	>400 mg/g creatinine	>236 mmol/mol creatinine
Urate	<0.56 mg/dL GFR	<0.033 mmol/L GFR
Volume	>20 mL/kg/day	

If a 24-h urine collection cannot be obtained, a random spot urine specimen measuring the solute-to-creatinine ratio can be used. But daily urine volume should be measured. The normal values of solute-to-creatinine ratio are given in Table 78.3.

Radiological imaging is an important part of the diagnostic evaluation of urolithiasis. Most calcium-containing stones are radiopaque on plain films if the size is adequate. While struvite and cystine stones are less radiopaque than calcium stones [5], uric acid and xanthine stones are radiolucent, being diagnosed easily with ultrasonography and computed tomography (CT). Ultrasonography can diagnose all kinds of stones with a false-negative rate of 30 % where small papillary or calyceal stones and ureteral calculi may be missed [85, 86]. Additionally, ultrasonography can outline the

Table 78.3 Normal urinary values in children [20]

	Age	mg/mg	mmol/mmol	mmol/mmol
Calcium/creatinine	0–6 months	<0.8	<2.24	
	6–12 months	<0.6	<1.68	
	2–18 years	<0.2	<0.56	
Oxalate/creatinine	<1 year	<0.3	<0.061	
	1–5 year	<0.15	<0.036	
	5–12 year	<0.1	<0.03	
	>12 year	<0.1	<0.013	
Cystine/creatinine	All ages	<0.02	<0.01	
Citrate/creatinine	All ages	<0.51	*Male*	*Female*
	Infant		<1.9	<0.63
	Child		<0.27	<0.33
Magnesium	>2 year	0.12		
Urate	>3 year	<0.56 mg urate/dL of glomerular filtrate	<0.03 mmol urate/L of glomerular filtrate	

Table 78.4 Selected medications used in the treatment of nephrolithiasis [20]

Chlorothiazide	<6 month – 10–40 mg/kg/day 1–2 doses
	6–12 year – 10–20 mg/kg/day 2 doses
	>12 year – 500–2,000 mg/day in 1–2 doses
Hydrochlorothiazide	<6 month – 3.3 mg/kg/day 2 doses
	6–12 year – 2–2.2 mg/kg/day 2 doses
	>12 year – 25–100 mg/day in 1–2 doses
Urinary alkalinization	Children – 2–3 mEq HCO_3/kg/day 3–4 doses
	Adolescents – 30–60 mEq HCO_3 3–4 times daily
Alkalinizing agents	Potassium citrate – 2 mEq HCO_3/mL
	Sodium citrate/citric acid – 1 mEq HCO_3/mL
	Baking soda – 1 tsp = 42 mEq HCO_3
	Sodium bicarbonate IV solution – 8.4 % = 1 mEq HCO_3/mL
	(given orally) – 4.2 % = 0.5 mEq HCO_3/mL

presence of urinary obstruction or nephrocalcinosis. In a study evaluating the sensitivity for plain film, ultrasonography, and CT, these values were found to be 57, 77, and 100 %, respectively [87, 88]. CT has a high sensitivity and specificity (96–98 %) and does not require any contrast medium [20]. Currently, for the prompt evaluation of acute renal colic, noncontrast CT is the first imaging choice because of its high sensitivity for ureteral stones compared to other modalities [89].

Treatment

Medical Treatment

Because of the high recurrence rate of urolithiasis in children, a medical approach is an important part of the treatment regimen for urolithiasis (Table 78.4). For all kinds of stones, increased fluid intake is the main and essential part of the therapy. A high fluid intake prevents the supersaturation of urine and reduces the concentration of the solutes. Again, the increased urinary flow helps to remove the crystals before they obstruct the renal tubules. However, it is clear that maintenance of the daily urine output over 2 L for an adolescent is usually difficult for a long-term treatment period.

Hypercalciuria

High fluid intake and dietary sodium restriction are the initial steps for the management of hypercalciuria. Also, excessive calcium intake should be restricted to the recommended daily allowance. Children should avoid vitamin C and D supplementation and high protein intake. If the hypercalciuria does not respond to dietary measures, thiazide diuretics may be added to the therapy. Thiazides increase the absorption of calcium in the renal tubule. The effect of thiazide diuretics is increased when combined with salt restriction [90, 91]. Common adverse effects of thiazides are hypokalemia and hyperlipidemia. Hypokalemia, which also causes a decrease in citrate excretion, may require potassium supplementation. Citrate therapy is helpful in patients with hypocitraturia and hypercalciuria. Lastly, amiloride may increase the distal tubular calcium reabsorption and may be useful together with thiazide diuretics. Phosphate is another adjuvant therapy in cases with hypercalciuria [6].

Hyperoxaluria

Initial therapy is similar to hypercalciuria with the recommendation of high fluid and low sodium intake. Additionally, avoidance of oxalate-rich foods is essential. Citrate, magnesium, and phosphate supplements may also help to increase oxalate solubility. In case of accompanying hypercalciuria, thiazides could be given. In primary hyperoxaluria type 1, approximately 30 % of patients respond to pyridoxine medication. Pyridoxine could be given at a dose of 25 mg/day initially and may be increased to 100 mg/day. Calcium intake should not be restricted, but excess calcium intake may be prohibited.

Uric Acid Lithiasis

A high urinary flow rate is essential for the management of hyperuricosuria. Limiting sodium intake may be useful by lowering the urate excretion. If these precautions fail, supplementation with citrate or bicarbonate will be indicated for alkalinization of the urine. In case of failure, allopurinol treatment may be necessary to decrease urate levels. Allopurinol decreases urate synthesis by inhibiting xanthine oxidase and is useful in disorders associated with excessive urate production.

Cystinuria

For cystine stones, treatment aims to increase the urinary flow rate abundantly (1.5 L/m^2) and to increase the urine pH above 7.5. Potassium citrate is the preferred choice for urinary alkalinization. The aim of the fluid therapy is to keep the urinary cystine concentration less than 300 mg/L (1.25 mmol/L). D-penicillamine and *a*-mercaptopropionylglycine can be used as adjunctive therapies if the first-line therapies fail.

Conclusion

The objectives of stone management in children should be complete stone clearance, prevention of stone recurrence and regrowth, preservation of renal functions, control of urinary tract infections (UTIs), correction of anatomic abnormalities, and correction of the underlying metabolic disorders. Long-term postoperative follow-up is mandatory, especially after using newer technical innovations for urinary calculus management during childhood. Regarding the metaphylactic management, there is a great choice of different treatment modalities on which the clinicians have to decide based on metabolic evaluation and stone analysis data, as well as the frequency of stone events.

Because of the multifactorial causes of stones in children (metabolic, anatomic, and/or recurrent UTI), during long-term follow-up, treatment can only be successful when combined with appropriate prophylaxis to prevent recurrence. Numerous treatment regimens for preventing recurrent formation of calcium stones have been designed and published during recent decades. The patients can be treated conservatively by an increased fluid intake with or without dietary manipulations or by administering pharmacological agents. As a pharmacological agent, potassium citrate has been used with acceptable success rates. However, it is really very troublesome to keep the child under a certain preventive measure for a long period of time. Cooperative parents with children at older ages are the cases that may demonstrate acceptable successful outcomes following these measures.

To conclude, we may emphasize that due to the high likelihood of predisposing factors in children with urolithiasis and high recurrence rates, metabolic evaluation of every child with a urinary stone should be undertaken, and medical treatment should be given when necessary. With recent advances in technology, stone management has changed from an open surgical approach to less invasive procedures such as extracorporeal shock wave lithotripsy and endoscopic techniques. The evaluation of metabolic risk factors in children with renal stone disease is the basis of medical treatment aimed at preventing recurrent stone events and the growth of preexisting calculi.

References

1. Vahlensieck EW, Bach D, Hesse A. Incidence, prevalence and mortality of urolithiasis in the German Federal Republic. Urol Res. 1982;10:161–4.
2. Borghi L, Ferretti PP, Elia GF, Amato F, Melloni E, Trapassi MR, et al. Epidemiological study of urinary tract stones in a northern Italian city. Br J Urol. 1990;65:231–5.
3. Tellaloğlu S, Ander H. Stones in children. Turk J Pediatr. 1984;26:51–60.
4. Edvardsson V, Elidottir H, Indridason O, Palsson R. High incidence of kidney stones in Icelandic children. Pediatr Nephrol. 2005;20: 940–4.
5. Milliner DS, Murphy ME. Urolithiasis in pediatric patients. Mayo Clin Proc. 1993;68:241–5.
6. Stapleton FB, Roy S, Noe HN, Jerkins G. Hypercalciuria in children with hematuria. N Engl J Med. 1984;310:1345–8.
7. Gearhart JP, Herzberg GZ, Jeffs RD. Childhood urolithiasis: experiences and advances. Pediatrics. 1991;87:445–50.
8. Stapleton FB, McKay CP, Noe HN. Urolithiasis in children: the role of hypercalciuria. Pediatr Ann. 1987;16:980–92.
9. Curhan GC, Willett WC, Speizer FE, et al. Twenty-four-hour urine chemistries of kidney stones among women and men. Kidney Int. 2001;59(6):2290–8.
10. Khan SR, Glenton PA, Backov R, et al. Presence of lipids in urine, crystals and stones: implication for the formation of kidney stones. Kidney Int. 2002;62:2062–72.
11. Pak CYC, Arnold LH. Heterogeneous nucleation of calcium oxalate by seeds of monosodium urate. Proc Soc Exp Biol Med. 1975; 149:930–2.
12. Fleisch H. Inhibitors and promoters of stone formation. Kidney Int. 1978;13:361–71.
13. Sarica K. Pediatric urolithiasis: etiology, specific pathogenesis and medical treatment. Urol Res. 2006;34:96–101.
14. Pak CYC. Potential etiologic role of brushite in the formation of calcium (renal) stones. J Crystal Growth. 1981;53:202–8.
15. Lingeman JE, Smith LH, Wood JR, et al. Basic considerations of urinary stone formation. In: Moster MB, editor. Urinary calculi. Philadelphia: Lea & Febiger; 1989. p. 51–76.
16. Burdette DC, Thomas WC, Finlayson B. Urinary supersaturation with calcium oxalate before and during orthophosphate therapy. J Urol. 1976;115:418–22.
17. Pak CYC, Fuller C, Sakhaee K, et al. Long-term treatment of calcium nephrolithiasis with potassium citrate. J Urol. 1985;134:11–9.
18. Polinsky MS, Kaiser BA, Baluarte HJ. Urolithiasis in childhood. Pediatr Clin North Am. 1987;34:683–710.
19. Stapleton FB, Roy S, Noe HN. Hypercalciuria in children with hematuria. N Engl J Med. 1984;310:1345–8.
20. Gillespie RS, Stapleton FB. Nephrolithiasis in children. Pediatr Rev. 2004;25(4):131–8.
21. Van Savage JG, Palanca LG, Andersen RD, et al. Treatment of distal ureteral stones in children: similarities to the American Urological Association guidelines in adults. J Urol. 2000;164: 1089–93.

22. Smith SL, Somers JM, Broderick N, Halliday K. The role of the plain radiograph and renal tract ultrasound in the management of children with renal tract calculi. Clin Radiol. 2000;55:708–10.
23. Tekin A, Tekgul S, Atsu N, et al. A study of the etiology of idiopathic calcium urolithiasis in children: hypocitruria is the most important factor. J Urol. 2000;164:162–5.
24. Nijman RJM, Ackaert K, Scholtmeijer RJ, et al. Long-term results of extracorporeal shock wave lithotripsy in children. J Urol. 1989;142:609–12.
25. Payne SR, Ford TF, Wickharnd EA. Endoscopic management of upper urinary stones. Br J Surg. 1985;72:822–5.
26. Smith LH. Stone activity. In: Roth RA, Finlayson B, editors. Stones: clinical management of urolithiasis. Baltimore: Williams & Wilkins; 1983. p. 183–5.
27. Vandeursen H, Devos P, Baert L. Electromagnetic extracorporeal shock wave lithotripsy in children. J Urol. 1991;145:1229–32.
28. Sarkissian A, Baloyan A, Arikyants N, et al. Pediatric urolithiasis in Armenia: a study of 198 patients observed from 1991 to 1999. Pediatr Nephrol. 2001;16:728–32.
29. Milliner DS. Epidemiology of calcium oxalate urolithiasis in man. In: Kahn S, editor. Calcium oxalate in biological systems. Boca Raton: CRC Press; 1995. p. 169–88.
30. Anderson DA. The nutritional significance of primary bladder stones. Br J Urol. 1962;34:160–3.
31. Ashworth M. Endemic bladder stones. BMJ. 1990;301:826–7.
32. Robertson WG. What is the aetiology of urinary calculi? Pediatr Nephrol. 1996;10:763.
33. Milliner DS. Epidemiology of calcium oxalate urolithiasis in man. In: Kahn S, editor. Calcium oxalate in biological systems. Boca Raton: CRC Press; 1995. p. 169–88.
34. Walther PC, Lamm D, Kaplan GW. Pediatric urolithiasis: a 10-year review. Pediatrics. 1980;65:1068–72.
35. Lim DJ, Walker III RD, Ellsworth PI, et al. Treatment of pediatric urolithiasis between 1984 and 1994. J Urol. 1996;156:702–5.
36. Choi H, Snyder HM, Duckett JW. Urolithiasis in childhood: current management. J Pediatr Surg. 1987;22:158–64.
37. Pietrow PK, Pope JC, Adams MC, et al. Clinical outcome of pediatric stone disease. J Urol. 2002;167:670–3.
38. Noe HN. Hypercalciuria and pediatric stone recurrences with and without structural abnormalities. J Urol. 2000;164:1094–6.
39. Faerber GJ. Pediatric urolithiasis. Curr Opin Urol. 2001;11:385–9.
40. Turner MA, Goldwater D, David TJ. Oxalate and calcium excretion in cystic fibrosis. Arch Dis Child. 2000;83:244–7.
41. DeSanto NG, DiLorico B, Capasso G, et al. Population based data on urinary excretion of calcium, oxalate, phosphate and uric acid in children from Cimitile. Pediatr Nephrol. 1992;6:149–57.
42. Hillman LS, Hoff N, Salmon S, et al. Mineral homeostasis in very premature infants: serial evaluation of serum 25 hydroxyvitamin D, serum minerals and bone mineralization. J Pediatr. 1985;106:970–80.
43. Moore ES. Hypercalciuria in children. Contrib Nephrol. 1981;27:20–32.
44. Kruse K, Kracht U, Kruse U. Reference values for urinary calcium excretion and screening for hypercalciuria in children and adolescents. Eur J Pediatr. 1984;143:25–31.
45. Stapleton FB, Noe HN, Jenkins GR, et al. Urinary excretion of calcium following an oral calcium loading test in healthy children. Pediatrics. 1982;69:594–7.
46. Hymes LC, Warshaw BL. Idiopathic hypercalciuria: renal and absorptive subtypes in children. Am J Dis Child. 1984;138:176–80.
47. Pak CYC, Kaplan R, Bone H, et al. A single test for the diagnosis of absorptive, resorptive, and renal hypercalciuria. N Engl J Med. 1975;292:497–500.
48. Favus MJ, Karnauskas AJ, Parks JH, et al. Peripheral blood monocyte vitamin D receptor levels are elevated in patients with idiopathic hypercalciuria. J Clin Endocrinol Metab. 2004;89(10):4937–43.
49. Lerolle N, Coulet F, Lantz B, Paillard F, Houillier P, Soubrier F, et al. No evidence for point mutations of the calcium-sensing receptor in familial idiopathic hypercalciuria. Nephrol Dial Transplant. 2001;16:2317–22.
50. Gillespie RS, Stapleton FB. Nephrolithiasis in children. Pediatr Rev. 2004;25(4):131–9.
51. Mehes K, Szelid Z. Autosomal dominant inheritance of hypercalciuria. Eur J Pediatr. 1980;133:239–42.
52. Coe FL, Parks JH, Moore ES. Familial idiopathic hypercalciuria. N Engl J Med. 1979;300:337–40.
53. Vachvanichsanong P, Malagon M, Moore ES. Urinary tract infection in children associated with idiopathic hypercalciuria. Scand J Urol Nephrol. 2001;35:112–6.
54. Stapleton FB. Idiopathic hypercalciuria: association with isolated hematuria and risk for urolithiasis in children. Kidney Int. 1990;37:807–11.
55. Garcia CD, Miller LA, Stapleton FB. Natural history of hematuria associated with hypercalciuria in children. Am J Dis Child. 1991;145:1204–7.
56. Polito C, La Manna A, Cioce F, et al. Clinical presentation and natural course of idiopathic hypercalciuria in children. Pediatr Nephrol. 2000;15:211–4.
57. Stapleton FB. Idiopathic hypercalciuria: association with isolated hematuria and risk for urolithiasis in children. The Southwest Pediatric Nephrology Study Group. Kidney Int. 1990;37:807–11.
58. Devuyst O, Christie PT, Courtoy PJ, et al. Intra-renal and subcellular distribution of the human chloride channel, CLC-5, reveals a pathophysiological basis for Dent's disease. Hum Mol Genet. 1999;8:247–57.
59. Dent CE, Friedman M. Hypercalciuric rickets associated with renal tubular damage. Arch Dis Child. 1964;39:240–9.
60. Scheinman SJ. X-linked hypercalciuric nephrolithiasis: clinical syndromes and chloride channel mutations. Kidney Int. 1998;53:3–17.
61. Neuhaus TJ, Belzer T, Blau N, et al. Urinary oxalate excretion in urolithiasis and nephrocalcinosis. Arch Dis Child. 2000;82(4):322–6.
62. Hesse A, Schneeberger W, Engfeld S, et al. Intestinal hyperabsorption of oxalate in calcium oxalate stone formers: application of a new test with ($^{13}C_2$) oxalate. J Am Soc Nephrol. 1999;10:329–33.
63. Monico CG, Ford GC, Persson XMT, et al. Potential mechanisms of marked hyperoxaluria not due to primary hyperoxaluria I or II. Kidney Int. 2002;62:392–400.
64. Danpure CJ. Primary hyperoxaluria. In: Schriver CR, Beaudet AL, Sly WS, et al., editors. The metabolic and molecular bases of inherited disease. 8th ed. New York: McGraw-Hill; 2001. p. 3323–67.
65. Giafi CF, Rumsby G. Primary hyperoxaluria type 2: enzymology. J Nephrol. 1998;11:29–31.
66. Cramer SD, Ferree PM, Lin K, et al. The gene encoding hydroxypyruvate reductase (GRHPR) is mutated in patients with primary hyperoxaluria type II. Hum Mol Genet. 1999;8:2063–9.
67. Thomas S, Stapleton FB. Pediatric urolithiasis: diagnosis and management. In: Gonzales E, Bauer SB, editors. Pediatric urology practice. Philadelphia: Lippincott/Raven Press; 1999. p. 607–21.
68. Milliner DS, Eickholt JT, Bergstralh E, et al. Primary hyperoxaluria: results of long-term treatment with orthophosphate and pyridoxine. N Engl J Med. 1994;331:1553–8.
69. Toussaint C. Pyridoxine-responsive PHI: treatment. J Nephrol. 1998;11:49–50.
70. Stapleton FB. Childhood stones. Endocrinol Metab Clin North Am. 2002;31:1001–15.
71. Rosenberg LE, Durant JL, Holland JM. Intestinal absorption and renal extraction of cystine and cysteine in cystinuria. N Engl J Med. 1965;273:1239–45.

72. Purroy J, Bisceglia L, Calonge MJ, et al. Genomic structure and organization of the human rBAT gene (SLC3A1). Genomics. 1996;37:249–52.
73. Chesney RW. Mutational analysis of patients with cystinuria detected by a genetic screening network: powerful tools in understanding the several forms of the disorder. Kidney Int. 1998;54:279–80.
74. Feliubadalo L, Font M, Purroy J, et al. Non-type I cystinuria caused by mutations in SLC7A9, encoding a subunit ($b^{0,+}$ AT) of rBAT. Nat Genet. 1999;23(1):52–7.
75. Rutchik SD, Resnick MI. Cystine calculi: diagnosis and management. Urol Clin North Am. 1997;24:163–71.
76. Dent CE, Senor B. Studies on the treatment of cystinuria. Br J Urol. 1955;27:317–32.
77. Milliner DS. Urolithiasis. In: Avner ED, Harmon WE, Niaudet P, editors. Pediatric nephrology. Philadelphia: Lippincott Williams & Wilkins; 2004. p. 1091–1111.
78. Stapleton FB. Hematuria associated with hypercalciuria and hyperuricosuria: a practical approach. Pediatr Nephrol. 1994;8: 756–61.
79. Baldree LA, Stapleton FD. Uric acid metabolism in children. Pediatr Clin North Am. 1990;2:391–418.
80. Benjamin D, Sperling O, Weinberger A. Familial hypouricemia due to isolated renal tubular defect. Nephron. 1977;18:220–5.
81. Stapleton FB. Renal clearance of uric acid in human neonates. J Pediatr. 1984;14:337–9.
82. Kelley WN. Gout and other disorders of purine metabolism. In: Harrison's principles of internal medicine. 9th ed. New York: McGraw-Hill; 483.
83. Lingeman JE, Smith LH, Wood JR, et al. Medical evaluation and treatment of the stone patient. In: Moster MB, editor. Urinary calculi. Philadelphia: Lea & Febiger; 1989. p. 84–133.
84. Lande MB, Varade W, Erkan E, et al. Role of urinary supersaturation in the evaluation of children with urolithiasis. Pediatr Nephrol. 2005;20:491–4.
85. Diament MJ, Malekzadeh M. Ultrasound and the diagnosis of renal and ureteral calculi. J Pediatr. 1986;109:980–3.
86. Vrtiska TJ, Hattery RR, King BF, et al. Role of ultrasound in medical management of patients with renal stone disease. Urol Radiol. 1992;14:131–8.
87. Nimkin K, Lebowitz RL, Share JC, et al. Urolithiasis in a children's hospital: 1985–1990. Urol Radiol. 1992;14:139–43.
88. Mendelson RM, Arnold-Reed DE, Kuan M, Wedderburn AW, Anderson JE, Sweetman G, et al. Renal colic: a prospective evaluation of non-enhanced spiral CT versus intravenous pyelography. Australas Radiol. 2003;47(1):22–8.
89. Smergel E, Greenberg SB, Crisci KL, et al. CT urograms in pediatric patients with ureteral calculi: do adult criteria work? Pediatr Radiol. 2001;31:720–3.
90. Stapleton FB, Kroovand RL. Stones in childhood. In: Coe FL, Favres MJ, Pak CYC, Parks JH, Preminger GM, editors. Kidney stones: medical and surgical management. Philadelphia: Lippincott-Raven Press; 1996. p. 1065–80.
91. Cohen TD, Ehreth J, King LR, Preminger GM. Pediatric urolithiasis: medical and surgical management. Urology. 1996;47(3):292–305.
92. Greene ML, Fujimoto WY, Seegmiller JE. Urinary xanthine stones: a rare complication of allopurinol therapy. N Engl J Med. 1969;280:426–7.

Pediatric Urinary Stone Disease in China

79

Gang Wang

Abstract

Pediatric urolithiasis is relatively uncommon in China, though still endemic in undeveloped western regions of China. Calcium-containing stone accounts for 67 % and cystine stone accounts for 12 %. The clinical manifestations present with a wide range of uncharacterized symptoms. The principles of treatment are rapid relief of symptoms, complete clearance of stones, preservation of the renal function, and prevention of stone recurrence. To the urologist, it is a specific technical challenge to treat pediatric urolithiasis. Treatment decision should be made according to careful diagnosis and should be individualized. Most patients can be treated conservatively or with shockwave lithotripsy (SWL). Though open surgery is still a treatment option in some places, microinvasive techniques such as ureteroscopy and percutaneous nephrolithotomy (PCNL) are assuming greater importance in recent years.

Keywords

Pediatric urolithiasis • China • Prevalence • Stone composition • Shockwave lithotripsy (SWL) • Ureteroscopy • Laparoscopy • Percutaneous nephrolithotomy (PCNL) • Mini-PCNL (mPCNL) • Cystoscopic lithotripsy

Introduction

Pediatric urolithiasis is a challenging disease in China. It is relatively uncommon and there have been no reports on prospective randomized clinical trials in the management of these calculi in Chinese literature until now. Metabolic, anatomical, infectious, and nutrition-related factors are the main causes of childhood urinary stones. The clinical presentations include a wide range of uncharacterized symptoms. Delayed diagnosis may cause damage to the renal function, thus disturbing the growth and development of the involved child. Great attention should be paid to obtaining an early diagnosis, complete clearance of stones, preservation of renal function, and prevention of recurrence. To the urologist, it is a specific technical challenge to treat pediatric urolithiasis—children are sensitive to radiation and invasive therapies. Microinvasive techniques are now more frequently used in recent years.

This chapter is based on post-2000 literature in Chinese.

Epidemiology

There is no data on true incidence or prevalence of stones in official reports. However, in 2008, several large-scale screening studies on children in different parts of China revealed some information about the prevalence. In southern China, Guangzhou, 22,238 children aged 0–13 years were screened and 347 were found with urinary stones, which accounted for a prevalence of 1.56 % [1]. Meanwhile, among 14,256 children aged 0–17 years in Chongqing (mid-western China) [2] and 7,705 children aged 0–3 years in Xuzhou (eastern China) [3], 82 cases (0.58 %) and 95 cases (1.23 %) of urinary stones were diagnosed, respectively. Altogether, the

G. Wang, M.D., Ph.D.
Department of Urology, Peking University First Hospital, Institute of Urology, Peking University,
8 Xishiku Street, Xicheng District, Beijing, 100034, China
e-mail: gunner.w@263.net

J.J. Talati et al. (eds.), *Urolithiasis*,
DOI 10.1007/978-1-4471-4387-1_79,

urinary stone prevalence is 1.19 % among the 44,199 children in the aforementioned three screening projects. Considering the influence of dietary melamine contamination, the natural prevalence of urolithiasis must be lower than that. In those that claimed to not having been fed with melamine-contaminated milk, the prevalence of urinary stone in children is only 0.32 % [2].

Several data support that pediatric urolithiasis is rare. At the Institute of Urology, Peking University, 4,039 stones were received for analysis from January 2004 to May 2011, 135 of which were from patients under age 18, accounting for 3.34 %.[1] At Children's Hospital, Chongqing Medical University, among 7,024 children admitted with some urinary disease from 1993 to 2007, 187 cases (2.66 %) were diagnosed with urinary stones [4]. In Liuzhou, Guangxi Zhuang Autonomous Region (southern China), among 1,776 inpatients with urinary stone, 53 cases (3.0 %) were under age 20 [5].

The gender distribution of children with urinary stones is similar to that in adults. The large-scale screenings in 2008 in Guangzhou [1] and Chongqing [2] revealed a male-to-female ratio of 2.4:1 and 1.7:1, respectively. In Guangzhou Children's Hospital, 248 cases of pediatric stone disease were treated during 1999–2009; the male-to-female ratio is 2.0:1 [1]. And the ratio is 2.3:1 from the data of Institute of Urology, Peking University, from January 2004 to May 2011.[2] In contrast, most children with lower urinary tract calculi are boys, with a male-to-female ratio of 16:1 [5].

The location of stones in children varies in different reports. Yu and colleagues from Harbin (northeastern China) reported that lower urinary tract stones accounted for 70.9 % of the 117 cases from 1982 to 2003 [15]. Sun et al. reported the ratio 32 % from 1994 to 1996 in Liuzhou, Guangxi Zhaung Autonomous Region [5], while Sun and colleague found the proportion of lower urinary stone was 24.2 % during 1999–2009 [1]. Bladder stone still remains endemic in some of the underdeveloped territories in the vast western regions in China [6] (see also Fig. 6.2 in Chap. 6).

The composition and frequency of urinary stones in children have changed during the past three decades, partly because of the economic development in China. Li et al. reported stone disease accounting for 1.97 % of the inpatients during 1993–1997, and the ratio rose to 2.74 % during 2003–2007 [4]. Zhong and colleagues found the relative proportion of upper urinary stones increased in these years, with the upper/lower urinary stone ratios of 1.48:1 during the 1999–2004 period, 4.75:1 during 2005–2008, and 13.2:1 during 2008–2009 [1].

In summary, the prevalence of pediatric urolithiasis may be around 1 % of the pediatric population in modern China, and there is an increasing trend recently. Calculi in children constitute only 2–3 % of all stone formers in China. The male-to-female ratio is roughly 2:1. The proportion with lower urinary tract stones is greater than that seen in adults, but is showing a decreasing trend with time.

Table 79.1 Stone composition and occurrence in children

Stone composition	Occurrence (%)
Calcium oxalate	32.6
Hydroxyapatite	10.4
Other calcium-containing stones	24.8
Uric acid	9.6
Magnesium ammonium phosphate	10.4
Cystine	12.6

Stone Composition and Etiology

Stone Composition

Results from an analysis of 137 urinary stones in patients under the age of 18 years, at the Institute of Urology, Peking University (January 2004 to May 2011),[3] showed that the most common component of urinary calculi is calcium. Calcium-containing stone makes up nearly 70 % of all stones. Pure calcium oxalate stone accounts for 32.6 %. Hydroxyapatite, uric acid, and magnesium ammonium phosphate stones each contributed approximately 10 %. Cystine stones occurred in 12.6 % of the patients (Table 79.1).

Etiology

Metabolic disorders are of most importance in pediatric stone formers. Liu and colleague [21] found 19 (43.2 %) of the 44 pediatric stone formers had metabolic abnormalities according to a 24-h urine analysis, namely, hyperoxaluria in 6, hypercalciuria in 5, hyperuricosuria in 4, and hypercystinuria in 4. Yang et al. [7] studied 52 children with idiopathic hypercalciuria and found that 12 % of them developed renal stones in 0.6–7 years. Zhuang [8] described 18 children with distal renal tubular acidosis; nephrocalcinosis and multiple renal calculi were found in 50 % of the victims. Interestingly, in the aforementioned stone composition analysis,[4] the cystine stone occurrence is much higher than that in adult stone formers, reminding us that metabolic factors must be more important in children and drawing attention to a possible self-limiting nature of the disease.

The mechanisms of the aforementioned metabolic disorders are described elsewhere in this book.

[1,2,3,4] Unpublished data

Anatomical abnormalities and urinary tract infection, in addition to metabolic disorders, are also important causes of urinary stones in children.

Liu and colleague [21] found that 34.1 % of 44 stone-forming school children (aged 7–14) had different anatomical abnormalities, including ureteropelvic junction obstruction, duplication of the upper urinary tract, renal malrotation, horseshoe kidney, and solitary kidney. Other obstructive disorders such as neurogenic bladder, vesicoureteral reflux, megaureter, and ectopic kidney are also important factors in children calculi formation.

Liu and colleague [21] also found 31.8 % of the children in the same series had concomitant urinary tract infection. Similarly, Yang et al. [22] reported in younger children under age 6 that 42.9 % of the 35 cases had a positive urine culture. *Escherichia coli* was the most common pathogen.

Feeding modality is another important factor in pediatric stone formers. The high carbohydrate diet in western China, such as the Tibet [6] Autonomous Region and the Xinjiang Uygur Autonomous Region, has been suggested as the possible and major cause for the high prevalence of lower urinary tract stones in those regions.

Some drugs may be associated with renal stones. Antimicrobial ceftriaxone [9] and sulfadimidine [10] have been reported to crystalize in urine and cause renal stone.

Clinical Manifestations

Pediatric stone formers may present with different, uncharacterized symptoms depending on age.

Hematuria is common both in infants and children. Wang et al. [23] found hematuria accounted for 58 % of all symptoms in the children presented with urinary stones. And the ratio remained almost the same in different age groups.

Pain is relatively uncommon in child stone formers. Though school-aged children may complain of lumbar aching, small infants cannot express themselves clearly and may present with crying and restlessness.

In case of bilateral upper urinary tract acute obstruction, a child may present with anuria or oliguria. If the obstruction occurs gradually, the child may present with no symptoms in early stage, but in the late stage when chronic renal failure occurs, the child might present with related symptoms and signs such as pallor, nausea, vomiting, decreased appetite, or edema.

Fever and urinary tract infection can also be seen in pediatric stone formers with urinary urgency and frequency and painful urination.

Interrupted urination and sudden dysuria may be the sign of a bladder stone or urethral stone, which is more common in undeveloped areas in China.

A large portion of urinary stones do not present with any clinical symptoms. It is diagnosed incidentally, occasionally, when a radiographic study is done for another reason or for routine examination. For example, in a large-scale screening of asymptomatic children in Chongqing, 0.58 % of all were found with urinary stones [2].

A systematic physical examination should be performed on any child suspected of urolithiasis. During an episode of renal colic, percussion pain may be elicited in the costospinal angle, while there may be little or no abdominal muscular guarding. In a child with huge hydronephrosis, a big mass may be palpable in the abdomen. Signs related with chronic renal failure, such as anemia and edema, can be found. Physical examination is difficult in infants because of difficulties in getting their compliance.

Investigations

The reader is referred to the general comments on investigation of pediatric patients in the following chapter (Chap. 80). The following additional information is provided on the practices in China.

Investigations of a child suspected of urolithiasis should include a history, laboratory tests, and imaging. It is important to inquire of the patient's previous episodes, treatments, and results, as well as family history, feeding or nutritional habits, fluid intake, etc. Aims of laboratory tests are evaluation of metabolic abnormalities, renal function, and urinary infection. Metabolic evaluation in children is relatively more important than that in adults. Imaging is most important to diagnose urinary stone and obtain the patient's anatomical information.

Laboratory Tests

Microscopic hematuria may be found in *routine urine test*. Elevated white blood cell (WBC) count and positive nitrate indicate urinary infection. *Urine culture* is mandatory in stone formers in order to direct antimicrobial drug selection. If the morning urine pH is over 5.8, distal renal tubular acidosis (dRTA) should be considered. Crystals in the urine are helpful in the diagnosis of urinary lithiasis.

Twenty-four-hour urine collection is a relatively simple method to evaluate metabolic status through testing urine calcium, phosphate, magnesium, potassium, uric acid, oxalate, citrate, cystine, and creatinine. Two collections are recommended.

Blood tests may also provide information on metabolic factors including calcium, phosphate, magnesium, uric acid, and oxalate. In case of renal failure, elevated serum creatinine, potassium can be found while total CO_2 in venous blood

(CO_2CP) decreased. When serum calcium ≥2.60 mmol/L, primary hyperparathyroidism should be taken into account and PTH must be tested. In dRTA, blood potassium may be lowered down as chloride and CO_2CP elevated.

Stone analysis is a direct way of metabolic investigation. Any stones should be tested for the composition, no matter if passed spontaneously or after shockwave lithotripsy (SWL) or from operation. Though chemical analysis lacks accuracy, it is used in some hospitals in China. More and more hospitals are using infrared spectroscopy for stone analysis.

Imaging

Because of the uncharacteristic presentations of pediatric stone formers, imaging is pivotal in the diagnosis of urolithiasis. The following modalities are commonly used in China: β(beta)-ultrasound (β-US), plain film of kidneys-ureters-bladder (KUB), intravenous pyelography (IVP), cystourethrogram, helical computerized tomography (CT), magnetic resonance (MR), and nuclear imaging. Imaging helps to establish that a stone is present and indicates its position, size, shape, and multiplicity. Additional information on anatomical configuration of the pelvicalyceal system and some idea of differential renal function can be gauged. Congenital anatomical abnormalities such as ureteropelvic junction obstruction are common in children as well as functional abnormalities such as vesicoureteral reflux and neurogenic bladder, and radiological imaging assists in identifying these conditions.

Several factors may influence the selection of the imaging methods: the potential risk of carcinogenesis from X-ray-related imaging, the lower compliance of younger children during examination, and economic considerations. Generally speaking, B-US and KUB are being used as first-line studies. When diagnosis is not clear or a radiolucent stone is dubiously seen on B-US, IVP or CT can help. CT may provide comprehensive information on anatomy and may evaluate differential kidney function with usage of contrast. Magnetic resonance urography (MRU) is able to provide information on obstruction with no irradiation. Cystourethrogram is used when there are concerns regarding vesicoureteral reflux.

B-Ultrasound (B-US)

Ultrasound is the main imaging in pediatric urology. Its advantages are simple and economic and absence of radiation and anesthesia. Stones, including X-ray lucent uric acid stone, can be easily identified by B-US. US can provide information on anatomy, such as the presence of hydronephrosis; the size of the kidney; the thickness and echo of the parenchyma, which provides a rough estimate of renal function; the dilation of ureter; and presence of ureterocele. US is able to find accompanying renal masses. US can also provide information on urinary system function, such as resistant index for renal obstructive degree, postvoid volume for obstruction of bladder outlet, or neurogenic bladder. The drawbacks of US are difficulty in differentiation between calculus and calcification, invisibility of ureter without dilation, and lack of accuracy in evaluation of differential renal function.

KUB and IVP

About 80–90 % of all urinary stones are radiopaque and thus can be identified by KUB. The stone position, size, and number can be identified with minimum radiation. According to the radiopacity, the stone composition may be estimated. The main disadvantages of KUB are inability to detect radiolucent uric acid stone and lack of information on urinary tract anatomy and function. Multiple radiopaque lesions—such as gall bladder stones, all kinds of calcification, and kidney tuberculosis—cannot be differentiated from urinary stones by KUB. Thus, in some cases KUB is used in combination with IVP. IVP is able to overcome almost all the drawbacks of KUB mentioned. However, IVP has its disadvantages too, mainly because of injection of contrast dye. For patients with creatinine over 200 μ(mu)mol/L and allergy to the contrast dye, IVP is contraindicated. The visualization of urinary tract is depending on the involved renal function. During renal colic episode, IVP may provide false information on function of the involved side.

Computed Tomography (CT)

Computed tomography (CT) is a well-established procedure in diagnosis of pediatric urolithiasis with the highest sensitivity and specificity among all the imaging tools. Though it cannot reflect the renal function, noncontrast helical CT may diagnose stones with accuracy and rapidity without the need of anesthesia or usage of a contrast dye. CT with contrast may provide information about the renal function. By calculation of renal parenchyma integration by CT, glomerular filtration rate (GFR) of both sides may be estimated. Comprehensive information on anatomy obtained by CT scan is helpful in making decision before an operation, such as stone distribution in the kidney and adjacent organ relationship. CT urography (CTU) is a substitute to IVP to some extent though the X-ray exposure is relatively higher.

Magnetic Resonance (MR)

MR urography (MRU) is a T2-weighted image that can demonstrate dilation of the collecting systems and position of stenosis without radiation or usage of a contrast dye. It remains a useful investigation in patients with abnormal renal function and for those who are allergic to contrast dye.

[5] Unpublished data

MRU may also reveal anatomical defects. Role of MRU in stone diagnosis is limited because stones show low signals both on T1- and T2-weighted images. Other drawbacks of MR are relative longer examination time and the need for anesthesia in small children.

Nuclear Imaging

Renogram and dynamic renal imaging are used to demonstrate differential renal function including renal blood supply, excretion, and evacuation, irrespective of renal function. With the injection of diuretics, they may provide information on the nature of obstruction (mechanic or nonmechanic).

Treatment

Treatment of pediatric urolithiasis is challenging to any urologist because the disease is relatively uncommon and a child's body diathesis is different from that of an adult. Before a treatment decision is made, the disease should be diagnosed thoroughly. Any aspect may have influence on treatment results, such as pain degree, stone size, position, possible component, the child's age, renal function, whether accompanying infection or not, whether complicating anatomical abnormalities or not, techniques, and instrument preparation. Treatment should be individualized according to the aforementioned factors. The *principles of treatment* are rapid relief of symptom, complete clearance of stones, preservation of the renal function, and prevention of stone recurrence.

Emergency Management

Though stone colic is common in emergency rooms for adult patients, it is uncommon in children. Sometimes school-aged patients may present with renal colic and can be treated with the same strategy as that used for adults. Drugs for spasmolysis (atropine derivatives) and analgesia (diclofenac sodium, morphine) can be administered, but the dosage should be adjusted according to the child's body weight. Diclofenac sodium is not suitable for patients with renal insufficiency, and opioid drugs are contraindicated for children with asthma. Caution should be taken before giving the drugs to infants. As renal colic may be caused by another reason, such as ureteropelvic junction obstruction, restriction of fluid intake may reduce urine secretion, which is helpful to relieve the pain.

Upper urinary tract stone may be complicated with severe infection, causing pyonephrosis, high fever, and even septicemia. Broad-spectrum antibiotic drugs must be used. If it does not work, percutaneous nephrostomy should be taken. Blood culture or pus culture may find the related bacteria and sensitive drugs.

If the functional kidney(s) are acutely obstructed with resultant anuria, the kidneys must be drained as soon as possible, whether by a ureteric stent or PCN. Usually dialysis is not required.

Conservative and Medical Treatment

The indications for conservative treatment are stones less than 4 mm in diameter without severe symptoms or significant hydronephrosis. Most small stones of 3 mm and less may pass out spontaneously. The role of medical expulsive therapy such as α(alpha)-blockers in children lacks evidence-based support in China. Traditional Chinese medicine containing *Desmodium styracifolium*, *Herba pyrrosiae*, and other herbal drugs has been used for hundreds of years though there are still no randomized controlled trials (RCTs) to support it.

SWL

Shockwave lithotripsy (SWL) has been widely used in China for more than 20 years, and experience has been gained in treating pediatric urolithiasis. For children with renal or ureteral calculi larger than 3 mm in diameter and failed conservative therapy, SWL remains the first-line choice of therapy. SWL can be used to treat bladder stones. Most studies have revealed acceptable results, with the stone-free rates between 70 and 96 % and low rates of complications [11–14]. Contraindications are uncorrected coagulopathy and uncontrolled infection.

The techniques used for SWL in pediatric patients need to be modified because of the special characteristics of children. Because of relative shorter duration of stone formation, relative smaller stone size, and relative thinner body size that cause less attenuation of the shockwave, stones are relatively easier to be fragmented compared to those in adults, and the fragments are relatively easy to pass through the children's ureter because of the ureter compliance. Pu and colleague found 92 % of upper urinary tract stone gained stone-free status after SWL, which was higher than of the lower urinary tract stone-free rate (69 %) [12]. It seems that the lower pole stones in children may gain higher stone-free rates after SWL compared to those in adults.

Repeated SWL is only needed in small group of patients. The average treatment sessions of SWL in the previously cited studies are 1.16–1.35 [12–14]. Few patients need more than two treatment sessions. If two to three sessions of SWL do not work, the child should be converted to other intervention therapies.

Treatment-related complications are neither frequent nor severe. Hematuria is the most common complication.

Steinstrasse occurred in 0.5–2.9 % of the reported group, and some authors recommend double-J stent insertion in patients with large stone burden or with urinary tract infection in advance of SWL [12, 13], but this is controversial. No hematoma happened after SWL in the cited reports. After an average of 6.7 months' follow-up, no renal atrophy was observed.

Generally SWL is performed under general anesthesia, though sedation alone may be satisfactory for teenage patients [12] and even for school-going children [14]. Patient position is the same as that of adults: supine for renal and upper ureteral stones and prone for the mid- and distal ureteral stones. Considering the delicacy of child's body and fragility of stones, lower voltage (5–11 kV) and fewer shocks (2,000) are recommended [12, 13]. With the utility of a twin-pulse lithotripter, 3.5–8-kV voltage and fewer than 2,500 shocks can obtain satisfactory results [14]. The interval recommended for repeated SWL is 2 weeks [11, 13].

It is not clearly defined if shockwaves have side effects on children or not, especially on the ovarian function in girls. Some authors prefer using a grid shield to protect the child's body from irradiation during SWL.

Open Surgery

Nowadays, open surgery is still a treatment option in China for big bladder stones and upper urinary tract stones in children that failed conservative treatment or SWL. Due to the relatively weak diathesis and delicacy of body structure in children, the utilization of endourological techniques in the pediatric department is delayed compared to that in the adult department. In the Department of Urology, Peking Children's Hospital, from 2006 to 2010, 28 cases of urinary stone disease were admitted, 20 were treated conservatively, and 8 were treated with open surgery, including nephrolithotomy, ureterolithotomy, and cystolithotomy.[5] Yu et al. reviewed 117 cases in the past two decades: 92 stones were removed by open surgery, and only 4 cases were treated by endoscopic procedures [15].

Recently the situation is changing gradually. Because of the wide acceptance of microinvasive techniques to treat adult patients and advances in miniaturization of various scopes, the endourological procedures are now being used with increasing frequency in children. However, it appears that open surgery will retain its position in treating large bladder stones and upper urinary tract stones in kidneys with anatomical abnormalities such as UPJ obstruction and for those who failed endo-surgical attempts. Great effort should be taken to preserve the child's kidney even if the GFR of that kidney is lowered down to 10 % of the total combined renal function. Nephrectomy is seldom done in pediatric stone patients.

Laparoscopic and Retroperitoneoscopic Surgery

If it is thought that an open surgical procedure is required, laparoscopic surgery must be considered as an alternative. Large stones 10 mm in diameter or more in the upper ureter are a case in point. Zhou et al. [16] reported 16 cases aged 3–14 years, 12 with upper ureteric and 4 with midureter stones, most of which had failed SWL or ureteroscopic (URS) treatment. They used balloon dilation to create a retroperitoneal cavity, and the operation was done, retroperitoneoscopically, through three trocars. In pediatric patients the pneumoperitoneum pressure is set at 8–12 mmHg, which is a bit lower than that used in adult surgery. Zhou had a 100 % success in their series. Most laparoscopic surgeries on kidney and ureter are done transretroperitoneally in China, though it is also being done transperitoneally, by some other doctors.

Ureteroscopy

Ureteroscopy is gaining wide acceptance in pediatric urology in China. Miniaturization of ureteroscopes made the application of this technique possible in children.

Indications include ureteric stones larger than 4 mm and failed conservative or SWL treatment. It is more suitable for mid- and distal ureter stones. Stone-free rates after ureteroscopy were reported satisfactory with minimal complications. Liu and colleague reported a series of 26 ureter stones, 23 of which were located in mid- and distal ureters [17]. The stone-free rate was 92.3 %. Complications included ureteric perforation in 2 cases, fever in 2 cases, stone migration in 1 case, and conversion to open surgery in 1 case. The 2 patients with perforation were treated conservatively with double-J stent placement without ureter stenosis after 12 months' follow-up. Huang et al. reported similar results in 13 cases (11 were mid- and distal ureter stones) with a stone-free rate 84.6 % [18]; stone migration occurred in 2 cases, and no perforation and stenosis occurred.

Age is not a limit to the procedure. Zeng reported 13 patients who underwent ureteroscopy were less than 6 years old and the youngest child was 8 months [19]. Five cases were successful in the first session. In 7 patients the procedure was taken in a second session after a double-J stent, placed for 1–3 weeks. Only one child converted to open surgery.

The procedure is done under general anesthesia. The caliber of semirigid scopes utilized for child patients in the literature is from F6 to F8.5. Because child body fluid volume is relatively small, caution should be taken to ensure low pressure and low flow of irrigant fluid. Holmium: YAG laser is the preferred lithotripter in ureteroscopic lithotripsy. It is effective and safe with less possibility of stone migration [18, 19].

Percutaneous Nephrolithotomy (PCNL)

Percutaneous nephrolithotomy (PCNL) is an evolving technique in China. It is a regular procedure in most major hospitals today and is used to treat pediatric patients. Indications are large stone burdens in kidney or proximal ureter that failed SWL or URS [20–23]. It is a first choice for staghorn stones. In experienced hands, the stone-free rate is quite high, up to 92 %.

The procedure is performed under general anesthesia, usually in the prone position. The percutaneous access is set up either under fluoroscopy or under ultrasonic guidance. Most urologist use a mini-perc technique (mPCNL). The size of the operating tract is usually F16 and may be adjusted to F14 [20] or F21 [21] according to the child's age, stone size, and degree of hydronephrosis. An F8/9.8 ureteroscope is used as a nephroscope. Most operations are successful in the first session. In case of long fragmentation time, bleeding, and large quantum of residual stones, a second session is needed.

The reported complication rate is low in the literature [20–23]. The most common complication is fever, accounting for 5–29.5 %. Blood transfusion rate is 0–4.5 %. One colon injury was reported in a patient with a horseshoe kidney under X-ray-guided PCNL and cured by conservative therapy [23].

PCNL is safe even in younger children. Yang et al. reported 35 cases aged 14 months to 6 years [22]. They set up a single tract F16 under ultrasound guidance, and the stones were fragmented by a ballistic lithotripter; 92.9 % of their series were rendered stone-free with no transfusion, adjacent organ injuries, or hyponatremia. Holmium laser is a good lithotripter with safety, efficiency, and clear view during operation [21, 23].

Concomitant anatomical abnormalities can be treated simultaneously during PCNL. Liu and colleague treated the ureteropelvic junction stenosis in six cases with a cold knife or holmium laser; only one case needs open surgery during follow-up [21].

Cystoscopic Lithotripsy

Bladder and urethral stones can also be treated endoscopically. Chen et al. reported 22 boys aged 1–12 years with bladder or urethral calculi [24]. The average stone size was 12 mm (range 8–30 mm). They took an F8/9.8 ureteroscope as a cystoscope and fragmented the stones with a pneumatic lithotripter. In 2 patients whose urethras were too narrow for the ureteroscope to pass through, an F16 suprapubic cystotomy was made for the procedure under β(beta)-US guidance. The stone-free rate was 100 % with almost no complications. A decision to use the above endoscopic procedure should be based on the stone burden. If the bladder stone is larger than 3 cm, a longer time is needed for fragmentation, making open surgery a valid alternative.

Conclusion

Pediatric urolithiasis is relatively uncommon in China though still endemic in undeveloped western regions. Calcium-containing stone accounts for 67 % and cystine stone accounts for 12 % of cases. The clinical manifestations present with a wide range of uncharacterized symptoms. The principles of treatment are rapid relief of symptom, complete clearance of stones, preservation of the renal function, and prevention of stone recurrence. To the urologist, it is a specific technical challenge to treat pediatric urolithiasis. Treatment decision should be made according to careful diagnosis and should be individualized. Most patients can be treated with conservation or SWL. Though open surgery is still a treatment option in some places, microinvasive techniques such as ureteroscopy and PCNL have become treating modalities in recent years.

References

1. Fu Z, Yan G, Ying-jie L, et al. Clinical analysis of children urinary stone. Chin J Child Health Care. 2009;17:453–5.
2. Hai-ping Y, Juan L, Cui-cui L, et al. Ultrasound screening of urinary system in 14256 asymptomatic children. J Chongqing Med Univ. 2010;35:926–30.
3. Jun-xia L, Chen D, Li-li G. Status quo analysis of urinary diseases in children under 3 years of age in Xuzhou and its surrounding areas. ACTA Acedemiae Medicinae Xuzhou. 2010;30:247–9.
4. Cui-cui L, Qiu L, Li W, et al. The constituent ratio of urinary system disease had changed among inpatient children in the Children's Hospital Affiliated of Chongqing Medical University during 15 years. J Chongqing Med Univ. 2010;35:938–41.
5. Wei-gui S, Zhi-ren D, Jun Z, et al. The age distribution of urolithiasis patients in Guangxi provice. Chin J Urol. 2001;22:100–2.
6. Yingjun M. Analysis of 91 children lower urinary tract calculi in Gannan Tibetan region. Gansu Sci Technol. 2009;25:150–1.
7. Yi Y, Shaogang W, Zhangqun Y, et al. Clinical features of idiopathic hypercalciuria in 52 children. J Clin Surg. 2005;13:569–71.
8. Jieqiu Z. Diagnosis, treatment and prognosis analysis of primary distal renal tubular acidosis in children. J Wenzhou Med Coll. 2004;34:49–51.
9. Shuhua Z. Ceftriaxone associated renal and gall stones in children, 3 case report. Chin Appl Pediatr J. 2008;23:424.
10. Liming Y. Sulfadimidine associated renal stone in infant, case report. Clin Misdiagnosis Mistherapy. 2006;19:46.
11. Xing-fa C, Xing Z, Naihui L, et al. Extracorporeal shock wave lithotripsy for treatment of urinary tract calculi in children (report of 62 cases). J Clin Urol. 2004;19:338–9.
12. Xiaoyong P, Lilai H, Xinghuan W, et al. Extracorporeal shock wave lithotripsy for ureteral calculi: ten-year experience. Chin J Pediatr Surg. 2006;27:188–90.
13. Zhenfeng L, Yufeng L. Treatment of extracorporeal shock wave lithotripsy in 296 children with urinary calculi. J Appl Clin Pediatr. 2007;22:842–3.
14. Xiaojian G, Lili L, Xianghua Z, et al. Treatment of pediatric upper urinary calculi with twin pulse low-energy ESWL. Xiandai Miniao Waike Zazhi. 2008;13:27–8.

15. You Y, Fu-you H, Qing-bo C, et al. Diagnosis and treatment of pediatric urolithiasis of 1 17 cases. J Harbin Med Univ. 2005;39:379–81.
16. Huixia Z, Xin M, Xu Z, et al. Retroperitoneoscopic ureterolithotomy in children. Chin J Pediatr Surg. 2008;29:227–9.
17. Xingming L, Shengqing R, Xuming W, et al. Treatment of ureteral stone with ureteroscopy in children (report of 26 cases). J Clin Urol. 2006;21:188–9.
18. Yunteng H, Maosheng X, Hongquan G, et al. Ureteroscopic lithotripsy for treatment of ureteral calculi in children: efficacy and safety. Acad J Second Mil Med Univ. 2009;30:1389–92.
19. Guohua Z, Wen Z, Xun L, et al. Ureteroscopy treatment of mid and distal ureteric calculi in preschool children. Clin J Pediatr Surg. 2007;28:240–2.
20. Hongqian G, Xiaogong L, Weidong G, et al. Using of percutaneous nephrolithotomy in pediatric urolithiasis. Chin J Surg. 2006;44: 389–91.
21. Bingqian L, Yudong W, Junfu Y, et al. Percutaneous nephrolithotomy with pneumatic and ultrasonic power for treatment of pediatric calculi. Chin J Urol. 2008;29:681–3.
22. Bo Y, Jianxing L, Xiaobo H, et al. Minimally invasive percutaneous nephrolithotomy in preschool age children. Chin J Pediatr Surg. 2009;30:209–11.
23. Xiang W, Jianming G, Yiqun L, et al. Minimally invasive percutaneous nephrolithotomy for treatment of upper tract calculi in children: a report of 45 cases. Shanghai Med J. 2010;33:246–9.
24. Hequn C, Yiqiang Z, Fan Q, et al. Treatment of lower urinary tract stones in children. J Clin Urol. 2003;18:411–2.

Patient Evaluation and Comparison of Stone-Removing Strategies in Pediatric Patients with Urinary Tract Stones

80

Temuçin Şenkul

Abstract

Urinary stone disease in children is an important health problem worldwide. Presenting signs and symptoms are different from those in adults. Abdominal pain, hematuria, and urinary tract infection are more common in children. Imaging of the pediatric patients is another challenging issue because of potentially harmful effects of ionizing radiation. Children with urinary stone have a high chance of recurrent stone formation; therefore, a complete risk assessment and metabolic evaluation should be performed.

The treatment depends on size and location of the stone. Patient's age and anatomy of the urinary tract are also other important factors that define treatment strategy. In the modern world, extracorporeal shock wave lithotripsy, percutaneous nephrolithotomy, and ureteroscopy are available for pediatric patients, and these procedures have the same level of efficiency and safety as in adults. Today, laparoscopic and robot-assisted laparoscopic stone surgeries are available in advanced health centers. Open surgery has become a historical treatment option in developed countries.

Keywords

Pediatric stone disease • Patient evaluation • Shock wave lithotripsy • Ureteroscopy Percutaneous lithotripsy • Laparoscopic stone surgery • Open surgery

Introduction

Pediatric stone disease is still an important health problem in the world. The disease is different from adult stone disease in terms of its presentation and treatment. In contrast to adults, boys and girls are affected almost equally in the pediatric age group. Most pediatric stones are generally located in the upper urinary tract, but bladder stones are still common in underdeveloped countries. These bladder stones are usually composed of ammonium acid urate and uric acid, strongly related to dietary factors [1]. The incidence of pediatric stones shows a wide geographical variation. In the United States, urinary stones are the reason for 1 out of every 1,000–7,500 pediatric hospital admissions [2]. Although bladder stones are seen in less than 10 % of North American children, they are endemic in other regions such as Turkey, Pakistan, and in some South Asian, African, and South American nations [2, 3]. Anatomic abnormalities such as ureteropelvic junction (UPJ) obstruction or ureterovesical junction (UVJ) obstruction also may be accompanied with stone disease in 11–24 % of children [4]. Infants represent approximately 20 % of pediatric stone cases [5] and tend to have a different history and clinical presentation.

Presenting Symptoms

Although unilateral colic pain is a typical symptom for adults, children with urinary stone disease have varying complaints for different age groups [6]. Pain occurs in 60, 40 and

T. Şenkul, M.D.
Department of Urology, GATA Haydarpasa Training Hospital Üsküdar, Istanbul, 81327, Turkey
e-mail: senkul@ixir.com

J.J. Talati et al. (eds.), *Urolithiasis*,
DOI 10.1007/978-1-4471-4387-1_80,

20 % of adolescents, school-aged children, and children younger than 5 years, respectively [2]. Stone location is another factor that influences pain. Children in the 0–5-year age group are much less likely to have ureteral stones [7]. While ureteral stones tend to be painful, kidney stones are generally asymptomatic and diagnosed incidentally. Pain perception is another important issue, and infants with stone disease generally have nonspecific abdominal pain instead of colicky pain [8].

Hematuria can be the only symptom or occur concomitantly with abdominal pain; 30–55 % of the cases may present with macroscopic hematuria [9, 10].

Irritative symptoms such as urgency or dysuria occur in 10 % of children with stone disease [11]. This is important to consider for the differential diagnosis between stone disease and urinary tract infection. Urinary tract infection may be the etiological agent of stone disease, especially in younger children. Irritative symptoms without urinary infection can be present when vesical or urethral stones are present [12]. In case of recurrent urinary tract infection and nonspecific complaints, all children should undergo renal and bladder ultrasound examination in order to exclude stone disease [4].

In infants, stone(s) impacted in the urethra may be palpable during physical examination, and it is necessary to conduct a detailed examination in younger children with stone disease [13]. In addition, a palpable kidney may be the first sign of polycystic kidney and associated stone disease [10].

Imaging

Plain abdominal radiography has low sensitivity in terms of diagnostic accuracy [14]. Additionally, radiation exposure is another important issue for children which makes renal/bladder ultrasound the imaging modality of choice in the pediatric population. Developments in ultrasound technology and growing experience have dramatically increased the diagnostic accuracy of ultrasonography. Stones located in the kidney and upper ureter are detected perfectly, but this may not be the case for lower ureteral stones. If the suspicion of a stone is high and ultrasonography has not detected any pathology, helical computerized tomography (CT) is indicated with/without contrast [15]. Recently, the authors concluded that CT without contrast has high sensitivity in depicting calculi in a rapid manner and ability to reveal concomitant pathologies. For that reason, like in adults CT plays an important role in the acute evaluation of children with flank pain [16]. The long-term risks of radiation exposure in children are not clear. It has been estimated that a single abdominal CT in a 1-year-old child imparts a 1 in 550 risks of subsequent lethal tumor development [17]. However, with the clinical use of low-dose CT techniques (see Chap. 35), the radiation dose may now be diminished with minimal loss of diagnostic accuracy [18]. The current pediatric guidelines recommended that "if no stone is found but symptoms persist, spiral CT scanning is indicated" [1]. Intravenous pyelography is rarely performed in current practice, but it can be used for detecting radiolucent stones, which cannot be seen on abdominal plain films [14]. Last but not least, endoscopically injected materials (used for treating vesicoureteral reflux) can calcify over time and may be seen as a hyperdense focus on CT [19]. For that reason, the physician should take a detailed medical history.

Urine and Blood Analyses

Complete urine analysis is essential for all children with stone disease. Differentiation of hematuria (glomerular or nonglomerular), presence of leucocytes, and detection of urinary crystals can be made by microscopic examination of urine [10]. The pH and the specific gravity measurements of urine are other important indicators for underlying abnormalities. In case of infection stone disease, urinary pH is almost always alkaline. These (pH) measurements may also be useful to assess children's compliance with oral alkali therapy, and similarly the specific gravity measurements help evaluate the degree of hydration.

Analysis of serum calcium level and spot urine for calcium, urate, and oxalate levels relative to urine creatinine should be the first step in laboratory investigation. Twenty-four-hour urine collection is needed in case of any metabolic abnormality. Hypercalciuria, hyperoxaluria, and hypocitraturia are the most common metabolic factors related to urinary stone disease. If a physician decides to collect the 24-h urine, patients must continue normal dietary habits. Bladder catheterization for 24-h urine collection is not recommended [15].

If urinary obstruction or infection is present, analysis should be deferred. In case of any intervention for stone fragmentation, it is recommended that metabolic investigations on urine should not be done earlier than 1 month after the procedure [20].

Recording of the total volume of urine is essential. Low urine volume (<1 mL/kg/h) may be the most important single factor for stone disease and its relapses [14].

Twenty-four-hour urinary calcium excretion is an important part of the pediatric stone evaluation. In case of hypercalciuria, further evaluation and even medical therapy can be required [1, 15, 21]. Hyperoxaluria is another important pathology in children with stone disease. Detailed analysis should be done by a pediatric specialist. Detailed metabolic evaluation in pediatric stone disease is discussed in Chap. 78.

Analysis of the Stone

Stone analysis is an indispensible part of the evaluation and must be done if the stone or even just a stone fragment is retrieved. Infrared spectroscopy and/or X-ray diffraction are the current methods of value. Chemical stone analysis is no longer recommended [10]. Because stone composition may change over time, recurrent stones should be analyzed.

In summary, evaluation of the pediatric patient with stone disease is different from that in their adult counterparts. Symptomatology is less significant, especially in infants. Radiation exposure is a concern. A full metabolic workup is essential in pediatric stone formers because of frequent metabolic abnormalities and high relapse rates. Every stone should be analyzed.

Management Strategies

Surgical management of pediatric stone disease has changed dramatically in recent years. Nowadays, shock wave lithotripsy (SWL) and ureteroscopic lithotripsy (URS) are equally effective modalities of treatment owing to technological advancements. Miniaturization of the equipment has allowed widespread application of ureteroscopy and percutaneous nephrolithotomy (PNL) in modern centers. The effectiveness and reliability of the management strategies will be discussed in this section.

Shock Wave Lithotripsy

The first SWL treatment for human kidney stone was performed in 1980 [22]. Due to concerns that shock waves might be hazardous for developing kidneys, SWL has not been used for children with urinary stone disease for years. But it has been widely accepted as the gold standard for adult urinary stone disease, and initial trials in pediatric patients were started and the first publications were reported with almost excellent results [23]. Although it has not been approved by the US Food and Drug Administration (FDA) for use in children, it is considered as a first-line minimally invasive treatment alternative for pediatric stone disease [24]. In 2011, the European Association of Urology guidelines recommended that SWL is the first-line treatment option for upper urinary calculi less than 10 mm even located in the lower pole of the kidney [1].

Smaldone showed that when SWL is used for upper urinary system stones, its efficacy varies from 70 to 85 % [25]. Contemporary results of SWL for kidney stones are shown in Table 80.1 [27–31]. In the first study, success of the procedure seemed to be related to stone location and size. But in 2010, He et al. stated that SWL for kidney stone up to 1 cm has excellent results regardless of location [26]. In this study, stone-free status was defined as "no visible fragments on ultrasonography and plain films."

The definition of stone-free status is still not exactly established. When plain radiographs are used to detect residual fragments, stone-free status might be established more easily. But computed tomography scans have higher sensitivity and they may detect very small fragments [32]. On the other hand, ionizing radiation is a concern in the pediatric population, and routine CT evaluation should not be used for detecting stone-free status.

In the literature, there are limited studies that have evaluated SWL for ureteral stones (Table 80.2) [26, 29–31, 33]. Recently, He et al. reported the results of 115 children with ureteral stone. There was no significant difference in stone-free rates between

Table 80.1 Results of SWL for kidney stones

Author	Lithotriptor	Stone-free rate	Mean size (cm)
Raza [27]	Piezolith 2300	53 %	2.6
		76 %	1.3
		84 %	0.7
	Dornier Compact Delta	50 %	2.9
		82 %	1.3
		92 %	0.6
DeFoor [28]	Dornier Compact Delta	68 % after one treatment	0.61
		74 % after two treatment	
Rizvi [29]	EDAP Technomed LT02	84.2	N/A
He [26]	Dornier Compact Sigma	94.3 %	Pelvic 9.7
		98.7 %	Upper and mid calices 9.3
		94.1 %	Lower calices 9.1
Landau [30]	Dornier HM3	80 %	14.9
Slavkovic [31]	Siemens LITHOSTAR	60.2 %	<1
		26.4 %	1.1–2
		44.4 %	2.1–2.5
		40 %	>2.5

Table 80.2 Results of SWL for ureteral stones

Author	Lithotriptor	Stone-free rate (%)	Mean size (cm)
Myers [33]	Siemens LITHOSTAR	91.1	7.3
Rizvi [29]	EDAP Technomed LT02	54.1	N/A
Landau [30]	Dornier HM3	78	9.5
He [26]	Dornier Compact Sigma	98.8	≤1
		85.7	>1
Slavkovic [31]	Siemens LITHOSTAR	94.3	<1
		73.3	1.1–2
		50	2.1–2.5
		100	>2.5

different stone locations [26], but stone size was an important factor in the treatment success. Although ureteral stones are restive and resistant to comminute, they have a shorter distance to pass. Thus, results of SWL for ureteral stones are similar to those of kidney stones.

Although the European Association of Urology (EAU) guidelines indicate that the success rates with SWL are lower for distal ureteral stones [1], He et al. obtained 95.7 % of the stone-free rate at 3 months [26].

Krambeck et al. concluded that SWL increased the risk of diabetes mellitus and hypertension in his study [34]. But there were a couple of debated issues in this study and results of the study have been questioned. Moreover, it has also been shown that SWL has no hazardous effect on pancreatic functions [35].

In the pediatric population, SWL has higher success rates for almost all urinary stones because pediatric stones are more amenable to shock waves and stone clearance is more likely than in adults. But cystine and calcium oxalate monohydrate stones are resistant to SWL, and in the presence of such calculi, other endourologic interventions should be considered [36].

Hydronephrosis, bladder dysfunction, and vesicoureteral reflux are other challenging issues in pediatric stone disease. These abnormalities may alter urinary drainage and stone clearance may be a problem [32]. For that reason, in such situations, SWL may be unsuitable and other endourologic approaches must be chosen.

Stent placement before SWL is still controversial in the pediatric population. Although stent placement did not affect stone-free rates, several studies indicated that stent placement may reduce the complication rates [25, 37]. In a recently reported review, Smaldone concluded that solitary kidney, staghorn calculi, large ureteral calculi, obstruction, and anatomic abnormalities are relative indications for prestenting SWL [25].

SWL for middle or distal ureteral stones is a concern for pediatric ureteral stones. The procedure has not gained wide acceptance because of focusing difficulties and the possibility of injury to immature reproductive systems. In a recent study, He at al. reported that SWL for the middle and distal ureters could be performed with high success rates [26]. Authors suggested that SWL is possible because of the lower density of bony pelvis.

How Shock Wave Lithotripsy in Children Differs from That in Adults

- General anesthesia is almost always required for pediatric SWL. Therefore, in case of SWL failure at first sessions, it may be better to use another treatment modality instead of additional SWL seasons.
- SWL may be more effective in children because pediatric stones are relatively soft, there is less tissue between coupling medium, and stone localization is easier in children.
- Lower power settings and a lower number of shock waves per session are recommended especially in young children.
- Spontaneous stone passage is easier in children after SWL therapy because the pediatric ureter is more compliant than the adult ureter.
- Anatomic or functional urological pathologies such as hydronephrosis, vesicoureteral nephrosis, or neurogenic bladder may accompany stone disease and may affect stone clearance.
- Pulmonary precautions such as shielding the lower chest should be taken particularly when treating small patients with upper pole kidney stone.

In summary, in spite of technological evolution on the other endourologic procedures such as PNL or URS, SWL still remains an effective treatment option in children with urinary stones. Thus, SWL can be considered the first-line treatment for renal pelvic stone less than 20 mm, for lower caliceal stone less than 10 mm, and for upper ureteric stones [1].

Percutaneous Nephrolithotomy (PNL)

PNL has been a safe and efficient treatment modality in adults with large urinary stones. But PNL for pediatric stone disease has not become widespread due to the probability of

Table 80.3 The results of PNL in pediatric patients

Author	Mean size (cm)	Stone-free rate (%)	Complications
Salah [38]	2.25	98.6	Urine leak 8 % Bleeding 0.7 %
Samad [39]	2.72	59.3	Fever 42.8 % Hyponatremia 0.1 % Obstruction 0.1 %
Holman [40]	2.25	98.5	Fever 1.1 % Urine leakage 8 %
Zeren [41]	1.68	86.9	Fever 29.8 % Open conversion 1.6 %
Kumar [42]	Staghorn	91.6	Fever 8.3 % Abdominal collection 8.3 %

damage to developing kidneys and due to the lack of miniaturized devices designed for small kidneys. With the help of the technological advancements and on the basis of accumulated experience so far, PNL has replaced open surgery for the management of pediatric stones larger than 2 cm. In addition, its efficacy and safety are comparable with the results obtained in adults. The results of the modern series are shown in Table 80.3 [38–42].

In the 2011 version of the EAU guidelines, PNL has been stated as the first-line treatment option for staghorn calculi, pelvic stones greater than 2 cm, and lower pole caliceal stones greater than 1 cm [1].

Although acceptable results were reported with adult-sized instruments [38, 41], technological advancements have led to miniaturization of the devices. In 1998, Jackman described a new technique which is called "mini-perc" [43]. But the procedure was not suitable for large stones because of prolonged intervention time and visualization problems from bleeding. In a recently published study, Mishra et al. compared the "mini-perc" with standard PNL. The authors showed that "mini-perc" has significant advantages in terms of diminished bleeding, hospital stay, and analgesic requirements. There were no significant differences in the stone-free rates and complications, but operative time was longer in the "mini-perc" group [44]. Today, technological advancements and increased experience made it possible to carry out PNL in a totally tubeless manner [45] or simultaneously on both kidneys [46] with higher success rates and lower morbidity. Reported stone-free rates of modern series are greater than 90 %.

Concerning the renal scarring and loss of renal function after PNL, Mor et al. investigated the function changes after PNL by radioisotope scans and were able to show no changes in differential function and no evidence of renal scarring [47]. Dawaba showed that PNL has no deleterious effect on kidney; moreover, renal function might improve after PNL [48].

It had been believed that intraoperative hemorrhage is related to the size and number of tracts during PNL. Nowadays, 11–15-Fr access sheaths are available and used successfully for pediatric PNL. Ganpule recommended that tract planning should be done carefully and should enable the endourologist to remove most of the stone, because small fragments can be removed through smaller tracts and the procedure can be completed in a less invasive manner [49]. In a recently reported article, Kumar et al. performed PNL for pediatric staghorn calculi. They used the 24-Fr sheath routinely and 21-Fr adult nephroscope. More than one access were needed in only 2 cases of 12 patients and blood loss was minimal [42]. Although PNL can be performed with adult-sized instruments, miniaturized instruments, holmium: YAG laser, or smaller pneumatic and ultrasound probes must be preferred where available.

SWL can be used for residual fragments but Smaldone recommended that a second-look nephroscopy should be considered before deciding on SWL sandwich therapy [25]. It should be kept in mind that SWL for residual fragments is an additional load in terms of anesthesia and ionizing radiation for children with stone disease. For that reason, every effort should be made to obtain the stone-free status during the initial operation.

The most frequently reported complications of PNL in children are bleeding, postoperative fever or infection, hydrothorax, hypothermia, and persistent urinary leakage. The results of the current series are shown in Table 80.3. Except postoperative fever, other complications have been reported to be very rare. The origin of fever is not thought to be the infection [1].

How PNL in Pediatric Patients Differs from the Procedure in Adults

- Mini-perc technique should be the "technique of choice" especially in smaller children where available. If not, the smallest and least traumatic instruments should be used.
- Balloon dilating technique is more suitable than sequential dilatation especially in smaller children.
- Holmium: YAG laser or smaller pneumatic lithoclast and ultrasound probes must be preferred where available.
- Irrigation solution at body temperature, short anesthetic induction, short operation time, meticulous draping, and

continuous monitoring of body temperature are important because of the risk of hypothermia.

- Low-pressure, isotonic irrigation system should be used to prevent fluid absorption.
- Pediatric cystoscopes sizes 7 and 8 Fr are useful for pediatric PNL.
- Complete stone-free status is very important in children, because stone fragments can be a predisposing factor for infection or stone recurrence.
- Second-look nephroscopy can be considered before deciding on SWL sandwich therapy.
- Staged operation is reasonable option for small patients with complex kidney stone.

Ureteroscopy

In 1988, Ritchey and Shepard first described ureteroscopy for distal ureteral stones in children [50, 51]. Although adult-sized instruments can be used in older children, the ureters in younger children are not suitable for larger instruments. Owing to developing technology, a large number of pediatric-sized instruments are available today; 4.5–8-Fr semirigid ureteroscopes with 2.4–3.5-Fr working channel and 6.9-Fr flexible ureteroscopes with 1.8–3.5-Fr working channel are used with high success [52]. In addition, ureteral access sheaths minimize ureteral trauma and decrease intrarenal pressure [53].

Initially URS has been preferred for middle and distal ureteral calculi or for the proximal ureteral stone which has been refractory to primary SWL [54]. There were some concerns about the de novo formation of vesicoureteral reflux and strictures following the ureteroscopic stone removal. However, Schuster showed that only 2 patients had ureteral strictures and a lower incidence of vesicoureteral reflux in the review of 221 pediatric ureteroscopies [55].

The EAU guidelines recommended that URS should be the first-line treatment option for lower ureteral calculi [1]. Lesani et al. showed that URS for upper urinary tract calculi is also feasible with 100 % stone-free rates [56]. Today URS for upper urinary tract calculi has excellent results with stone-free rates greater than 90 % (Table 80.4) [57–62]. But complex stones may be problematic. Dave et al. had a stone-free rate of only 14 % in 7 children with partial staghorn stones [63]. Additionally, Tanaka et al. stated that most of the upper tract calculi that are greater than 1 cm required multiple interventions to get a stone-free status [64]. In a recently published paper, Nerli et al. stated that complete stone clearance is possible if the stone is single, smaller than 1 cm, and located below the ureteropelvic junction [65]. In other situations, PNL might be a more suitable option.

Antegrade ureteral access is also possible with flexible ureteroscopy in children undergoing percutaneous nephrostomy. Reddy and Gupta reported the antegrade technique in children with complete ureteral obstruction or inability to dilate the ureteral orifice or intramural portion of the ureter [66, 67].

Ureteral stent placement prior to URS is a reasonable method of obtaining passive dilatation in prepubertal children. Reddy recommended the use of 3.7–4.8-Fr stents to get passive dilation of the ureter and found that URS can be done easily after 3–14 days. Additionally, subsequent balloon dilation is rarely needed [68].

The complications of ureteroscopy in children closely match with those reported in adults (see Table 80.4). In experienced hands, URS can be safely done with minimal morbidity. A detailed analysis of this issue is covered elsewhere in this book.

How URS in Pediatric Patients Differs from That in Adults

- General anesthesia is always required for pediatric URS.
- Passive ureteral dilation by placing ureteral JJ stent is a reasonable option when the endourologist encounters difficulty with balloon or coaxial dilators.
- Radiation exposure is a more important issue than adults in the pediatric population, and every effort should be made to decrease the fluoroscopy time.
- Antegrade ureteral access may be considered in children who already have a percutaneous nephrostomy tube and impacted ureteral stone.
- The decision to post-URS stenting should be made on an individual patient basis. The age of the patient, size of the ureter, experience of the surgeon, and degree of ureteral trauma are important factors for decision making.

Table 80.4 The results of the pediatric URS

Author	Location	Stone-free rate	Complications
Bassiri [57]	Ureter	88 %	Pyelonephritis 4 %
De Dominicis [58]	Ureter	94.1 %	None
Koura [59]	Upper ureter 10 % Middle ureter 20 % Lower ureter 70 %	90 % with single season	Pyelonephritis 5 %
Smaldone [60]	Renal 52 % Ureteral 48 %	91 %	Ureteral perforation 4.2 % Ureteral stricture 1 %
Kim [61]	Renal pelvis 60 % Ureter 40 %	97 %	None
Corcoran [62]	Renal 100 %	88 %	Ureteral perforation 9 %

Laparoscopic or Robot-Assisted Laparoscopic Stone Surgery

Laparoscopy and robot-assisted laparoscopy are current treatment modalities for urinary stone disease in adults [69]. Laparoscopic surgery has replaced open surgery, especially in the developed countries. In 2004, Casale et al. performed laparoscopic pyelolithotomy in children with a mean stone size of 2.9 cm. Results were almost excellent and no complications were seen [70]. In 2007, Lee et al. reported early results of robot-assisted laparoscopic pyelolithotomy. Most of the children had cystine stones refractory to PNL and SWL. Conversion to open procedure was required in one case with residual lower pole stone [71]. The early results of the procedures are encouraging but further studies are needed.

Open Surgery

EAU guidelines stated that "good candidates for open stone surgery include very young children with large stones and/or a congenitally obstructed system which also requires surgical correction" [1]. Additionally the children with severe orthopedic deformities or with very large bladder stones may be candidates for open surgery [1]. In developed countries, open surgery is performed for 0.3–5.4 % of children with stone disease [36], but in developing countries, it is used in 14 % of cases [72]. In a recently published report, Rizvi et al. stated that open surgery was still a valid treatment option in 30 % of the pediatric stone patients. Economic constraints and long distance from the center were the main reasons for choosing that modality. The authors concluded that open surgery provides comparable success rates to modern endourologic modalities, and principals of the open surgery should continue to be part of the urologists' armamentarium [73].

Conclusion

Advanced miniaturized instruments and better understanding of the use of laser and SWL have reduced the need for open surgery. As recurrence is frequent in pediatric populations, careful investigation to reveal underlying metabolic, functional, and anatomic abnormalities is mandatory.

References

1. Tekgül S, Riedmiller H, Gerharz E, Hoebeke P, Kocvara R, Nijman R, et al. Urinary stone disease. In: Guidelines on paediatric urology. EAU Guidelines; 2011. p. 53–63
2. Milliner DS, Murphy ME. Urolithiasis in pediatric patients. Mayo Clin Proc. 1993;68:241–8.
3. Nicoletta JA, Lande MB. Medical evaluation and treatment of urolithiasis. Pediatr Clin North Am. 2006;53:479–91.
4. Dursun I, Poyrazoglu HM, Dusunsel R, Gunduz Z, Gurgoze MK, Demirci D, et al. Pediatric urolithiasis: an 8-year experience of single centre. Int Urol Nephrol. 2008;40:3–9.
5. Mohamed J, Riadh M, Abdellatif N. Urolithiasis in infants. Pediatr Surg Int. 2007;23:295–9.
6. Durkee CT, Balcom A. Surgical management of urolithiasis. Pediatr Clin North Am. 2006;53:465–77.
7. Pietrow PK, Pope 4th JC, Adams MC, Shyr Y, Brock 3rd JW. Clinical outcome of pediatric stone disease. J Urol. 2002;167:670–3.
8. Smith RC, Rosenfield AT, Choe KA, Essenmacher KR, Verga M, Glickman MG, Lange RC. Acute flank pain: comparison of non-contrast-enhanced CT and intravenous urography. Radiology. 1995; 194(3):789–94.
9. VanDervoort K, Wiesen J, Frank R, et al. Urolithiasis in pediatric patients: a single center study of incidence, clinical presentation and outcome. J Urol. 2007;177:2300–5.
10. Hoppe B, Kemper MJ. Diagnostic examination of the child with urolithiasis or nephrocalcinosis. Pediatr Nephrol. 2010;25(3):403–13.
11. Sternberg K, Greenfield SP, Williot P, Wan J. Pediatric stone disease: an evolving experience. J Urol. 2005;174:1711–4.
12. Gearhart JP, Herzberg GZ, Jeffs RD. Childhood urolithiasis: experiences and advances. Pediatrics. 1991;87:445–50.
13. Leuman E, Hoppe B. Urolithiasis in childhood. In: Proesmanns W, editor. Therapeutic strategies in children with renal disease, vol. 5. London: Bailliere's Clinical Paediatrics; 1997. p. 655–74.
14. Kokorowski PJ, Hubert K, Nelson CP. Evaluation of pediatric nephrolithiasis. Indian J Urol. 2010;26:531–5.
15. Cilento BG, Mingin GC, Nguyen HT. Urolithiasis. In: Stringer M, Oldham K, Mouriquand P, editors. Pediatric surgery and urology: long-term outcomes. New York: Cambridge University Press; 2006. p. 695–706.
16. Persaud AC, Stevenson MD, McMahon DR, Christopher NC. Pediatric urolithiasis: clinical predictors in the emergency department. Pediatrics. 2009;124:888–94.
17. Brenner D, Elliston C, Hall E, Berdon W. Estimated risks of radiation-induced fatal cancer from pediatric CT. AJR Am J Roentgenol. 2001;176:289–96.
18. Kim BS, Hwang IK, Choi YW, Namkung S, Kim HC, Hwang WC, et al. Low-dose and standard-dose unenhanced helical computed tomography for the assessment of acute renal colic: prospective comparative study. Acta Radiol. 2005;46(7):756–63.
19. Nelson CP, Chow JS. Dextranomer/hyaluronic acid copolymer (Deflux) implants mimicking distal ureteral calculi on CT. Pediatr Radiol. 2008;38:104–6.
20. Beck B, Hoppe B. Pediatric aspects of nephrolithiasis and nephrocalcinosis. In: Chaussy C, Haupt G, Jocham D, Köhrmann KU, Wilbert D, editors. Therapeutic energy applications in urology. Heidelberg: Thieme; 2005. p. 86–91.
21. Duffy PG, Thomas DFM, Flett ME. Stone disease in children. In: Thomas DFM, Duffy PG, Rickwood AMK, editors. Essentials of pediatric urology. 2nd ed. London: Informa; 2008. p. 143–55.
22. Chaussy C, Brendel W, Schmiedt E. Extracorporeally induced destruction of kidney stones by shock waves. Lancet. 1980;2(8207): 1265–8.
23. Sigman M, Laudone VP, Jenkins AD, Howards SS, Riehle Jr R, Keating MA, et al. Initial experience with extracorporeal shock wave lithotripsy in children. J Urol. 1987;138(4):839–41.
24. Muslumanoglu AY, Tefekli A, Sarilar O, Binbay M, Altunrende F, Ozkuvanci U. Extracorporeal shock wave lithotripsy as first line treatment alternative for urinary tract stones in children: a large scale retrospective analysis. J Urol. 2003;170:2405–8.
25. Smaldone MC, Docimo SG, Ost MC. Contemporary surgical management of pediatric urolithiasis. Urol Clin North Am. 2010; 37(2):253–67.
26. He L, Sun X, Lu J, Cong X, Zhu H, Shen L, Wang Y. Comparison of efficacy and safety of shockwave lithotripsy for upper urinary

tract stones of different locations in children: a study of 311 cases. World J Urol. 2011;29(6):713–7. PubMed PMID: 21153828.
27. Raza A, Turna B, Smith G, Moussa S, Tolley D. Pediatric urolithiasis: 15 years of local experience with minimally invasive endourological management of pediatric calculi. J Urol. 2005;174:682–5.
28. DeFoor W, Dharamsi N, Smith P, et al. Use of mobile extracorporeal shock wave lithotripter: experience in a pediatric institution. Urology. 2005;65:778–81.
29. Rizvi SA, Naqvi SA, Hussain Z, Hashmi A, Hussain M, Zafar MN, et al. Management of pediatric urolithiasis in Pakistan: experience with 1,440 children. J Urol. 2003;169(2):634–7.
30. Landau EH, Shenfeld OZ, Pode D, Shapiro A, Meretyk S, Katz G, et al. Extracorporeal shock wave lithotripsy in prepubertal children: 22-year experience at a single institution with a single lithotriptor. J Urol. 2009;182(4 Suppl):1835–9.
31. Slavkovic A, Radovanovic M, Vlajkovic M, Novakovic D, Djordjevic N, Stefanovic V. Extracorporeal shock wave lithotripsy in the management of pediatric urolithiasis. Urol Res. 2006;34(5):315–20.
32. Nelson CP. Extracorporeal shock wave lithotripsy in the pediatric population. Urol Res. 2010;38(4):327–31.
33. Myers DA, Mobley TB, Jenkins JM, Grine WB, Jordan WR. Pediatric low energy lithotripsy with the Lithostar. J Urol. 1995;153(2):453–7.
34. Krambeck AE, Gettman MT, Rohlinger AL, Lohse CM, Petterson DE, Segura JW. Diabetes mellitus and hypertension associated with shock wave lithotripsy of renal and proximal ureteral stones at 19 years of follow-up. J Urol. 2006;75:1742–7.
35. Knoll T, Janitzky V, Michel MS, Alken P, Köhrmann KU. Cystinuria-cystine stones: recommendations for diagnosis, therapy and follow-up. Aktuelle Urol. 2003;34:97–101.
36. Straub M, Gschwend J, Zorn C. Pediatric urolithiasis: the current surgical management. Pediatr Nephrol. 2010;25:1239–44.
37. Al-Busaidy SS, Prem AR, Medhat M. Pediatric staghorn calculi: the role of extracorporeal shock wave lithotripsy monotherapy with special reference to ureteral stenting. J Urol. 2003;169(2):629–33.
38. Salah MA, Tσth C, Khan AM, Holman E. Percutaneous nephrolithotomy in children: experience with 138 cases in a developing country. World J Urol. 2004;22:277–80.
39. Samad L, Aquil S, Zaidi Z. Paediatric percutaneous nephrolithotomy: setting new frontiers. BJU Int. 2006;97(2):359–63.
40. Holman E, Khan AM, Flasko T, et al. Endoscopic management of pediatric urolithiasis in a developing country. Urology. 2004;63(1):159–62.
41. Zeren S, Satar N, Bayazit Y, et al. Percutaneous nephrolithotomy in the management of pediatric renal calculi. J Endourol. 2002;16(2):75–8.
42. Kumar R, Anand A, Saxena V, Seth A, Dogra PN, Gupta NP. Safety and efficacy of PCNL for management of staghorn calculi in pediatric patients. J Pediatr Urol. 2011;7(3):248–51. doi:10.1016/j.jpurol.2011.02.016.
43. Jackman SV, Docimo SG, Cadeddu JA, Bishoff JT, Kavoussi LR, Jarrett TW. The "mini-perc" technique: a less invasive alternative to percutaneous nephrolithotomy. World J Urol. 1998;16(6):371–4.
44. Mishra S, Sharma R, Garg C, Kurien A, Sabnis R, Desai M. Prospective comparative study of Miniperc and standard PNL for treatment of 1 to 2 cm size renal stone. BJU Int. 2011. doi:10.1111/j.1464-410X.2010.09936, 10284.x.
45. Ozturk A, Güven S, Kilinc M, Topba E, Piskin M, Arslan M. Totally tubeless percutaneous nephrolithotomy: is it safe and effective in preschool children? J Endourol. 2010;24(12):1935–9.
46. Guven S, Ozturk A, Arslan M, Istanbulluoglu O, Piskin M, Kilinc M. Simultaneous bilateral percutaneous nephrolithotomy in children: no need to delay. J Endourol. 2011;25(3):437–40.
47. Mor Y, Elmasry YE, Kellett MJ, Duffy PG. The role of percutaneous nephrolithotomy in the management of pediatric renal calculi. J Urol. 1997;158:1319–21.
48. Dawaba MS, Shokeir AA, Hafez AT, Shoma AM, El-Sherbiny MT, Mokhtar A, et al. Percutaneous nephrolithotomy in children: early and late anatomical and functional results. J Urol. 2004;172:1078–81.
49. Ganpule AP, Mishra S, Desai MR. Percutaneous nephrolithotomy for pediatric urolithiasis. Indian J Urol. 2010;26(4):549–54.
50. Ritchey M, Patterson DE, Kelalis PP, Segura JW. A case of pediatric ureteroscopic lasertripsy. J Urol. 1988;139:1272–4.
51. Shepard P, Thomas R, Harmon EP. Urolithiasis in children: innovations in management. J Urol. 1988;140:790–2.
52. Raju GA, Norris RD, Ost MC. Endoscopic stone management in children. Curr Opin Urol. 2010;20(4):309–12.
53. Singh A, Shah G, Young J, Sheridan M, Haas G, Upadhyay J. Ureteral access sheath for the management of pediatric renal and ureteral stones: a single center experience. J Urol. 2006;175:1080–2.
54. Wu HY, Docimo SG. Surgical management of children with urolithiasis. Urol Clin North Am. 2004;31(3):589–94, xi.
55. Schuster TG, Russell KY, Bloom DA, Koo HP, Faerber GJ. Ureteroscopy for the treatment of urolithiasis in children. J Urol. 2002;167(4):1813–5.
56. Lesani OA, Palmer JS. Retrograde proximal rigid ureteroscopy and pyeloscopy in prepubertal children: safe and effective. J Urol. 2006;176:1570–3.
57. Bassiri A, Ahmadnia H, Darabi MR, Yonessi M. Transureteral lithotripsy in pediatric practice. J Endourol. 2002;16:257–60.
58. De Dominicis M, Matarazzo E, Capozza N, Collura G, Caione P. Retrograde ureteroscopy for distal ureteric stone removal in children. BJU Int. 2005;95:1049–52.
59. Koura AC, Ravish IR, Amarkhed S, Nerli RB, Reddy M. Ureteroscopic stone management in prepubertal children. Pediatr Surg Int. 2007;23:1123–6.
60. Smaldone MC, Cannon Jr GM, Wu HY, Bassett J, Polsky EG, Bellinger MF, et al. Is ureteroscopy first line treatment for pediatric stone disease? J Urol. 2007;178:2128–31.
61. Kim SS, Kolon TF, Canter D, White M, Casale P. Pediatric flexible ureteroscopic lithotripsy: the children's hospital of Philadelphia experience. J Urol. 2008;180:2616–9.
62. Corcoran A, Mally D, Smaldone M, Bellinger M, Schneck F, Docimo S. Flexible ureteroscopy for proximal stones in pediatric patients: how complete access simplifies the surgical approach. J Endourol. 2007;21:A84.
63. Dave S, Khoury AE, Braga L, Farhat WA. Single-institutional study on role of ureteroscopy and retrograde intrarenal surgery in treatment of pediatric renal calculi. Urology. 2008;72(5):1018–21.
64. Tanaka ST, Makari JH, Pope 4th JC, Adams MC, Brock 3rd JW, Thomas JC. Pediatric ureteroscopic management of intrarenal calculi. J Urol. 2008;180(5):2150–3.
65. Nerli RB, Patil SM, Guntaka AK, Hiremath MB. Flexible ureteroscopy for upper ureteral calculi in children. J Endourol. 2011;25(4):579–82.
66. Reddy PP. Pediatric ureteroscopy. Urol Clin North Am. 2004;31(1):145–56.
67. Gupta R, Manohar T, Desai MR. Antegrade flexible ureteroscopy in supine position for impacted multiple ureteric calculi. Indian J Urol. 2006;22:139–41.
68. Reddy PP, DeFoor WR. Ureteroscopy: the standard of care in the management of upper tract urolithiasis in children. Indian J Urol. 2010;26:555–63.
69. Nambirajan T, Jeschke S, Albqami N, Abukora F, Leeb K, Janetschek G. Role of laparoscopy in management of renal stones: single-center experience and review of literature. J Endourol. 2005;19(3):353–9.
70. Casale P, Grady RW, Joyner BD, Zeltser IS, Kuo RL, Mitchell ME. Transperitoneal laparoscopic pyelolithotomy after failed percutaneous access in the pediatric patient. J Urol. 2004;172(2):680–3.
71. Lee RS, Passerotti CC, Cendron M, Estrada CR, Borer JG, Peters CA. Early results of robot assisted laparoscopic lithotomy in adolescents. J Urol. 2007;177(6):2306–9.
72. Zargooshi J. Open stone surgery in children: is it justified in the era of minimally invasive therapies? BJU Int. 2001;88(9):928–31.
73. Rizvi SA, Sultan S, Ijaz H, Mirza ZN, Ahmed B, Saulat S, et al. Open surgical management of pediatric urolithiasis: a developing country perspective. Indian J Urol. 2010;26(4):573–6.

Pediatric Vesicle Stone

81

M.S. Ansari, Jatinder Kumar, and Priyadarshi Ranjan

Abstract

Pediatric vesicle calculus is a rare disease in the developed world but still common in developing nations; a large proportion is constituted by endemic vesicle calculus. Diet lacking in animal protein predisposes to this condition and usually affects children less than 10 years of age, with peak incidence at around 3 years of age. The most common type of pediatric vesicle calculus is ammonium acid urate. The diagnosis of this condition mainly depends upon radiological studies, and symptomatology may also help sometimes.

With the advent of newer endoscopic instruments, the treatment options for vesicle calculus are inclining toward percutaneous cystolithotomy for larger stone. Other treatment options include extracorporeal shock wave lithotripsy (ESWL), transurethral cystolitholapaxy, and open cystolithotomy, depending upon the size of stone.

Keywords

Pediatric vesicle calculus • Percutaneous cystolithotomy • Transurethral cystolitholapaxy

Introduction

Vesical calculi refer to the presence of stones or calcified materials in the bladder or bladder substitute that functions as a urinary reservoir. These stones are usually associated with urinary stasis, but they can form in healthy individuals without evidence of anatomic defects, strictures, infections, or foreign bodies. The presence of upper urinary tract calculi is not necessarily a predisposition to the formation of bladder stones.

Bladder stones have been treated both medically and surgically for many centuries. The oldest bladder stone discovered dates back to 4,800 BCE and was found by archeologists in Egypt around the turn of the twentieth century [1]. The first literary references to bladder stones date back to a time as early as, or earlier than, the time of Hippocrates [2].

M.S. Ansari, M.S., MNAMS, MCh, Diplomat National Board (✉)
J. Kumar, M.S. • P. Ranjan, M.S., MCh
Department of Urology and Renal Transplantation,
Sanjay Gandhi Postgraduate Institute of Medical Sciences,
Raebareli Road, Lucknow, Uttar Pradesh, 216014, India
e-mail: ansarimsa@hotmail.com

Although urinary calculi, especially bladder calculi, are a rare entity in children in developed countries, it is a common disease among children in developing countries.

Epidemiology

Urolithiasis in childhood is rare in the developed world; it represents 1–5% of all urinary tract stones, and moreover, urinary bladder stone is very rare [3–5]. At the same time, in the developing countries (such as those in the Middle East, Thailand, and Indonesia), pediatric vesical stones constitute 30% of all urinary tract stones [3, 6].

The incidence of primary bladder calculi in the United States and Western Europe has been steadily and significantly declining since the nineteenth century because of improved diet, nutrition, and infection control. In these countries vesical calculi mainly affects adults, and a steadily declining frequency is noted in children. Bladder calculi remain common in less-developed countries and areas such as Thailand, Burma, Indonesia, the Middle East, and North Africa [7]. Although the prevalence of bladder calculi is declining in

J.J. Talati et al. (eds.), *Urolithiasis*,
DOI 10.1007/978-1-4471-4387-1_81,

these populations, it remains a disease that affects children, being diagnosed far more commonly in boys than in girls [8]. The endemic bladder calculus is still a common disease in childhood.

Etiopathogenesis

Most vesical calculi are formed de novo within the bladder, but some may initially have formed within the kidneys and subsequently passed into the bladder, where additional deposition of crystals causes stone growth. These are termed migrant calculi. Most renal stones that are small enough to pass through the ureter are also small enough to pass through a normally functioning bladder and unobstructed urethra. In children, however, these stones are retained due to small bladder outlet, even though the primary etiology may be related to metabolic factors associated with renal calculi formation, such as hypercalciuria, hyperuricosuria, and hypocitraturia.

Endemic bladder stones form in children in the absence of obstruction, local disease, neurologic lesion, or known primary infection. The incidence has decreased with industrialization and affluence, such that it is a rare pathology in developed countries. However, endemic bladder calculi remain common in infants and children of lower socioeconomic backgrounds in North Africa and the Middle and Far East. They are uncommon in Central and South Africa, Central and South America, and the Pacific Islands. Similarities are seen in the afflicted children of these areas. Stone formation results from dietary and nutritional deficiencies. Children in these areas are dependent on a cereal-based diet that is lacking in animal proteins, especially cow's milk. Cereals commonly used are whole wheat flour, millet, and rice. Less than 25% of the total protein intake is of animal origin. Compared with cow's milk, human breast milk and foods such as polished rice and cereals are low in phosphorus. This dietary phosphate deficiency leads to low urine phosphate excretion and high peaks of ammonia excretion. Chronic dehydration, excessive protein or oxalate consumption, high endogenous oxalate production, and deficiencies in vitamins A, B_1, and B_6 and magnesium have been associated with stone formation [8]. These conditions act to decrease urine production, acidify urine, and increase the concentration of uric acid and calcium oxalate excretion, which in turn lead to precipitation of insoluble salts in the urine.

Children younger than 10 years of age are typically affected, with the peak incidence around 3 years. The cloudy, sandy urine produced by children in endemic areas indicates the early stages of stone formation. Girls are able to pass most of the debris through their short, nontortuous urethra, but boys may retain these potential nidi. This accounts for the male-to-female ratio of 10:1 for endemic bladder calculi.

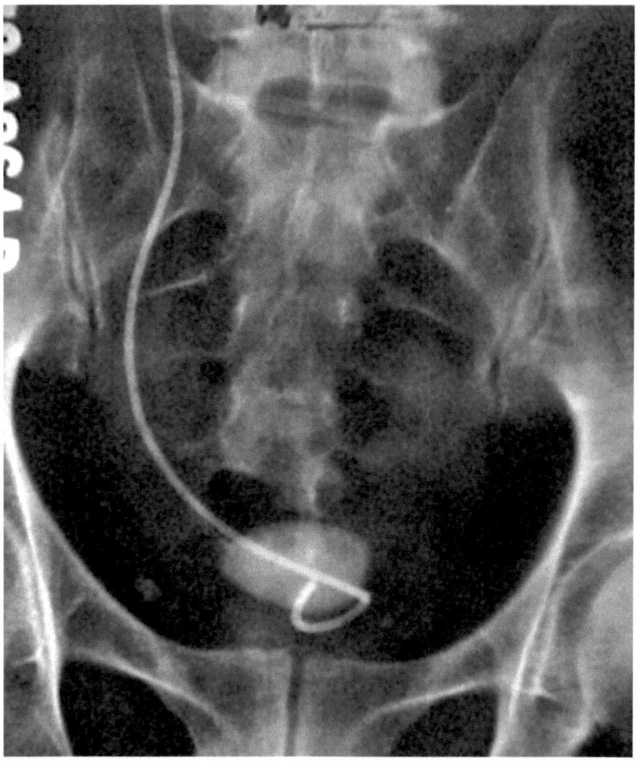

Fig. 81.1 Stone formation in bladder on lower end of JJ stent

Other etiologic factors for bladder stone formation include foreign bodies in the bladder that act as a nidus for stone formation (Fig. 81.1). These are subclassified into iatrogenic and noniatrogenic bodies. The first group includes suture material, shattered Foley catheter balloons, eggshell calcifications that form on a catheter balloon, staples, ureteral stents, and erosions of surgical implants [9–12]. Stones on suture material may have an early presentation if sutures were originally placed within the bladder lumen. A delayed presentation may be caused by erosion through the bladder wall [13]. Noniatrogenic causes include objects placed into the bladder by the patients for recreational and various other reasons [14].

Vesical calculi are also reported in augmented bladders. Mathoera et al. (2000) described risk factors for stone formation in 89 pediatric patients who had undergone bladder augmentation and presented with bladder calculi [15]. Cloacal malformations, vaginal reconstructions, ureteral reimplantations, and bladder neck surgery were all associated with higher risk for stone formation [15]. Risk factors associated with calculi formation include urinary stasis, mucus production, urinary infection with a urea-splitting organism, foreign bodies, and metabolic disturbances. The efficiency of bladder drainage has been implicated as a risk factor for stone formation [16]. This is reflected in the finding that continent diversions had a stone formation rate three times higher than that of orthotopic cystoplasties; those with orthotopic diversions

Table 81.1 Stone composition of bladder calculi in children [16]

Stone type	Patients %
Ammonium acid urate	27.1
Ammonium acid urate+calcium oxalate	29
Ammonium acid urate+uric acid	36.8
Uric acid	3.2
Calcium oxalate	2.6
Struvite+carbonate-apatite	1.3
Total	100

who voided by catheterization through native urethra and/or abdominal stoma had a rate five and ten times higher risks, respectively, than that of those who voided spontaneously.

Pediatric vesical stones in developing countries are composed mainly of ammonium acid urate, calcium oxalate, or an impure mixture of ammonium acid urate and calcium oxalate with calcium phosphate (Table 81.1). Bladder stones in patients with spinal cord injuries are often composed of struvite or calcium phosphate. Contrary to this, in the developed countries, the main component of the rarely existing urinary bladder stone is struvite, while in the developing world, the main component is ammonium acid urate [17, 18]. The common link among endemic areas relates to feeding infants human breast milk and polished rice. This type of diet is low in phosphorus, ultimately leading to high ammonia excretion. These children also usually have a high intake of oxalate-rich vegetables (which increases the risk of oxalate crystalluria) and animal protein (and consequent low urinary citrate).

Vesical calculi may be single or multiple, especially in the presence of bladder diverticula. Vesical calculi can be small or large enough to occupy the entire bladder. Their physical features range from soft to extremely hard and from having smooth-faceted surfaces to jagged spiculated surfaces, the latter termed "jack" stones based on their resemblance to the metal objects in the children's game jacks. In general, most vesical calculi are mobile within the bladder, although some stones are fixed when they form on a suture, on the intravesical portion of a papillary tumor, or on retained stents.

Clinical Presentation

The presentation of vesical calculi varies from completely asymptomatic to symptoms of suprapubic pain, dysuria, intermittency, frequency, hesitancy, nocturia, and urinary retention [19]. Parents of children with vesical calculi may notice priapism and occasional enuresis [20]. Most children may not have any symptoms and are routinely found on radiographic films.

Other common signs include terminal gross hematuria and sudden termination of voiding with some degree of associated pain referred to the tip of the penis, scrotum, perineum, back, or hip. The discomfort may be dull or sharp and is often aggravated by sudden movements and exercise. Assuming a supine, prone, or lateral head-down position may alleviate the pain initiated by the stone impacting the bladder neck by causing it to roll back into the bladder. Less specific signs of vesical calculi include microscopic or gross hematuria, pyuria, bacteriuria, crystalluria, and urine cultures that demonstrate urea-splitting organisms.

A history of prior pelvic surgery should be sought in all patients, especially when synthetic materials were implanted [21]. Common physical examination findings include suprapubic tenderness, fullness, and, occasionally, a palpable distended bladder if the patient is in acute urinary retention.

Diagnosis

Laboratory Studies

Urinalysis

Urinalysis is usually inexpensive and rapid and provides useful information. On the dipstick, bladder calculi can be associated with test results that are positive for nitrite, leukocyte esterase, and blood. Microscopy usually demonstrates red blood cells (RBCs) and pyuria (white blood cells). Microscopic crystals are usually consistent with the composition of the stone.

Urine Culture and Sensitivity

A culture of the urine is integral to help document and direct treatment of associated infections.

Complete Blood Cell Count

In patients with outlet obstruction and infection, the white blood cell (WBC) count may be elevated, with a left shift.

Comprehensive Metabolic Panel

The creatinine level may be elevated in outlet obstruction. Other findings may give a clue to an underlying abnormality.

Imaging Studies

The initial imaging study of choice is plain radiography of the kidneys, ureters, and bladder (KUB) because it is the least expensive and easiest radiologic test to obtain. KUB demonstrates the presence of radiopaque stones (Fig. 81.2). Pure uric acid and ammonium urate stones are radiolucent but are occasionally coated with a layer of opaque calcium sediment. Laminations are common, with the layers stratified according to metabolic and infectious status and the degree of periodic hematuria.

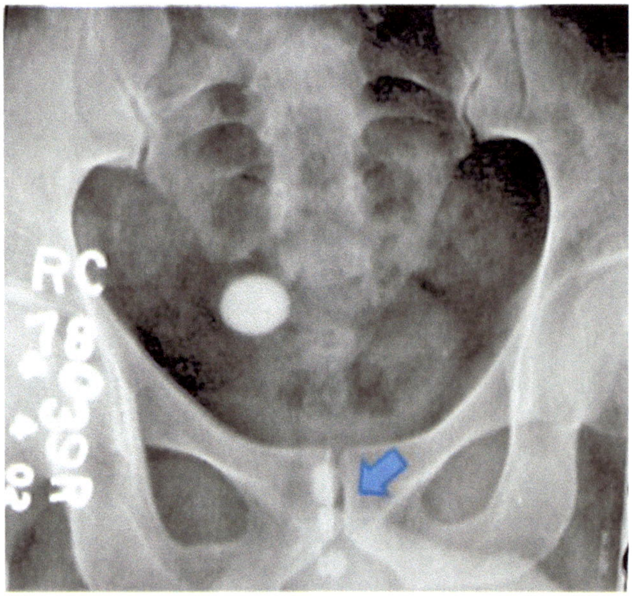

Fig. 81.2 Radiopaque shadows in pelvic region suggestive of bladder and multiple urethral stones

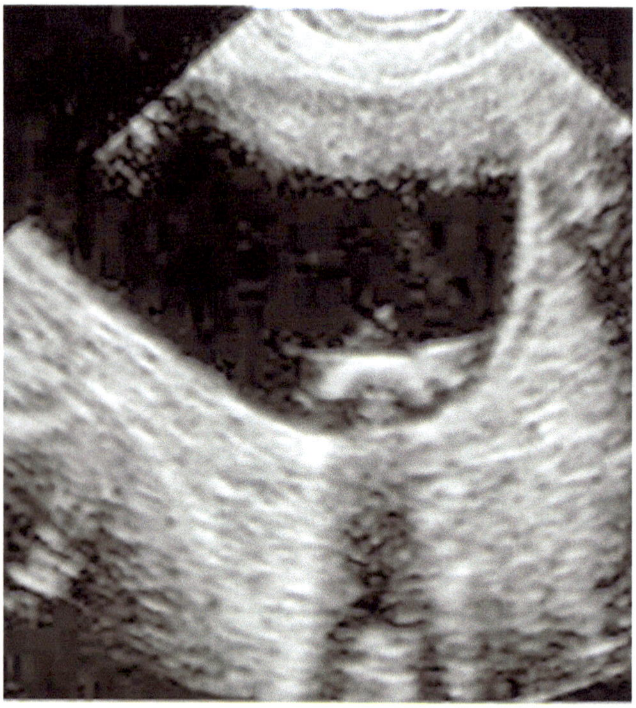

Fig. 81.3 The sonogram showing a classic hyperechoic object in the urinary bladder with posterior shadowing

Before the advent of ultrasonography and spiral computed tomography (CT), if the clinical suspicion was high and the initial KUB revealed no stones, the next step used to be cystography. These tests demonstrate the stone as a filling defect in the bladder [20]. If the filling defect moves when the patient is repositioned, the presence of a stone is highly likely. Nonmobile filling defects could be calculi attached to the bladder wall via a stitch or in a diverticulum. This test is not routinely done these days due to its invasiveness and risk of urinary tract infection.

With the recent widespread availability of ultrasonography, this relatively inexpensive and rapid modality can be more widely used to diagnose bladder calculi. The sonogram, showing a classic hyperechoic object with posterior shadowing, is effective in identifying both radiolucent and radiopaque stones (Fig. 81.3). USG may be limited by bowel gases in the settings of urinary diversion [22].

Noncontrast CT scan (NCCT) is highly sensitive and specific in diagnosing calculi along the urinary tract. Even pure urate calculi can be detected with this method. The stone may be obscured if contrast has been administered. NCCT is more helpful in the settings of lower tract reconstructions [20].

Magnetic resonance imaging (MRI) is an expensive imaging modality that yields poor resolution of calculi. It is not recommended in the evaluation of bladder calculi. If performed, MRI may show an incidental black hole of low water content corresponding to a calculus in an otherwise full bladder. As with MRI, Tc-99m MAG-3 renal scanning is a poor imaging modality in this condition. It may demonstrate the incidental finding of focal photopenia within the bladder resulting from calculus formation [23].

Cystoscopy remains the most commonly used test to confirm the presence of bladder stones and plan treatment. This procedure allows for the visualization of stones and assessment of their number, size, and position. Additionally, examination of the urethra, bladder wall, and ureteral orifices may well allow the identification of strictures, bladder diverticula, and presence of foreign body [20].

Treatment

The majority of bladder calculi are treated endoscopically, but treatment strategies may range from chemolysis to open surgery. The many available management options include shock wave lithotripsy; cystolitholapaxy; cystolithotripsy with mechanical, electrohydraulic, ultrasonic, or laser energy sources; percutaneous cystolithotomy; and open cystolithotomy.

Medical Therapy

The only potentially effective medical treatment for bladder calculi is urinary alkalinization for the dissolution of uric acid stones. Stone dissolution may be possible if the urinary pH can be made greater than or equal to 6.5. However, overly aggressive alkalization may lead to calcium phosphate deposits on the stone surface, making further medical therapy ineffective [20].

Other agents for stone dissolution, such as Suby's G or M solution, are rarely used. Renacidin can be used to dissolve phosphate or struvite calculi, but treatment is slow and invasive because of the use of indwelling irrigating catheters. Patients must also be closely monitored for possible sepsis or hypermagnesemia [7].

When underlying errors of metabolism are discovered during 24-h urine evaluation of stone disease, various treatments are available to prevent further calculus development.

Surgical Treatment

"Cutting for the stone" is a phrase that has been used since the time of Hippocrates. Historically, stones were removed via open operation, either using a suprapubic incision or a perineal incision. In the absence of antibiotic therapy and adequate hemostatic techniques, both operations were associated with high morbidity and mortality rates. Civiale performed the first documented blind transurethral lithotripsy in 1822 [1].

Extracorporeal Shock Wave Lithotripsy (ESWL)

ESWL treatment of bladder stones is a technically easy method; however, its application in children, because of the difficulty in passing the stone fragments, is often questioned [24–26]. To reach a high success rate, one needs more sessions in the cases of large and/or dense stones, but the need for auxiliary procedures and the chance of complications increase as well [24]. The late bioeffects of ESWL in children are still controversial [27, 28]. Another important reason, for not preferring ESWL as the primary modality for management, is the cost of the treatment and possible need for multiple sessions.

Transurethral Cystolitholapaxy

With advancements in instrumentation, the smaller caliber of the pediatric urethra can be accommodated with small-size instruments, allowing these approaches to be applicable in selected children. Cystolitholapaxy is found to be useful in stones sizing up to 2 cm [29, 30].

Following the visualization of the stone(s) at cystoscopy, an energy source is used to fragment the stone and the fragments are removed through the cystoscope (Fig. 81.4). The energy sources available are mechanical, ultrasonic, electrohydraulic, and laser.

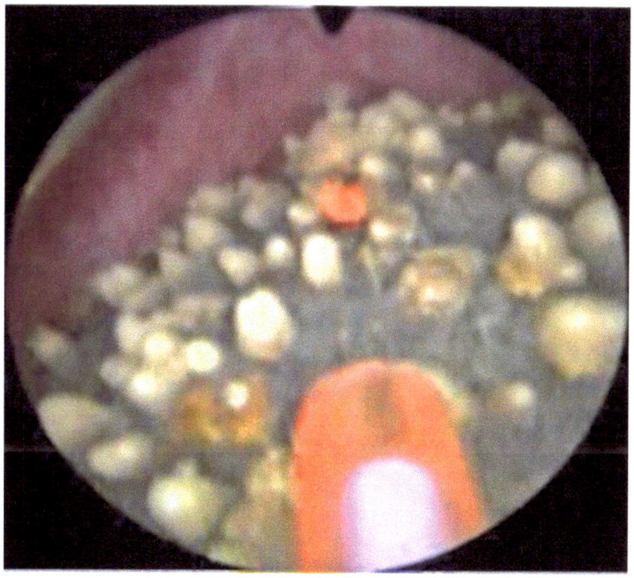

Fig. 81.4 Cystolithotripsy for bladder stone with holmium laser

In boys, because of the size limitations secondary to the small urethra and concerns about iatrogenic urethral stricture, transurethral endoscopic removal may be more difficult and should be approached with great care.

Percutaneous Cystolithotomy (PCCL)

Gopalakrishnan and colleagues were the first to report use of a percutaneous suprapubic approach in managing bladder calculi [31]. The morbidity of percutaneous cystolithotomy (PCCL) is significantly less than that of open cystolithotomy. Using the percutaneous suprapubic approach, a 15-F pediatric nephroscope can be introduced into the bladder without urethral injury (Fig. 81.5) [32–34]. In this manner, the large and hard stones can be disintegrated and removed in large fragments so that the intervention can be performed quickly. In studies, the largest calculus removed was up to 5 cm in diameter [35].

Cystolithotomy

Although rarely used today, open cystolithotomy for the treatment of bladder calculi is associated with a high success rates. Currently cystolithotomy is certainly the preferred alternative for very large and/or hard stones [36]. Other indications are abnormal anatomy precluding safe access, failure of an endoscopic approach, and lastly the need for concomitant procedures like bladder diverticulectomy.

However, it should be kept in mind that open surgery has the inherent problems of a long skin scar, prolonged catheterization, extended hospitalization, and risk of infection [37].

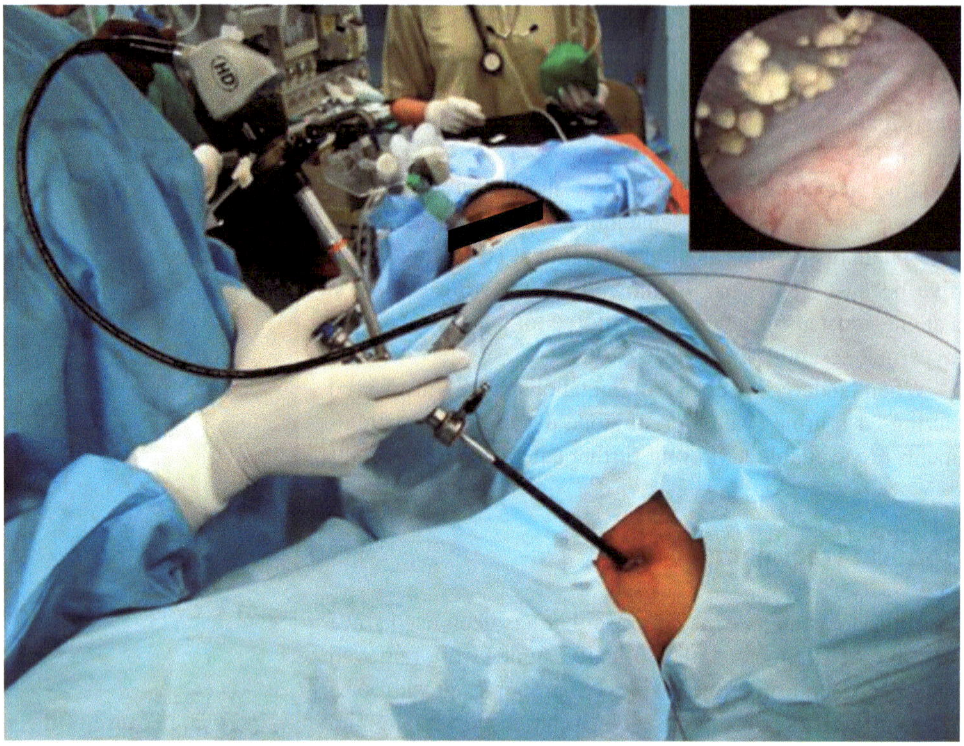

Fig. 81.5 Percutaneous cystolithotomy in a child with a 15-F pediatric nephroscope. Cystoscopic view is shown in *inset*

Conclusion

This relatively common developing world disease with the advent of newer technologies can now be managed safely by minimal invasive procedures.

References

1. Ellis H. A history of bladder stone. Oxford: Blackwell Scientific Publications; 1969.
2. Schwartz BF, Stoller ML. The vesical calculus. Urol Clin North Am. 2000;27(2):333–46.
3. Bichler KH, Strohmaier WL, Korn S. Urolithiasis in childhood. Monatsschr Kinderheilkd. 1985;133:256.
4. Carvajal Busslinger MI, Gygi C, Ackerman D, Kaiser G, Bianchetti M. Urolithiasis in childhood: when to do what? Eur J Pediatr Surg. 1994;4:199.
5. Ansari MS. Pediatric urolithiasis: a challenging problem. Indian J Urol. 2010;26(4):51.
6. Ansari MS, Gupta NP. Impact of socioeconomic status in etiology and management of urinary stone disease. Urol Int. 2003;70(4):255–61.
7. Huffman JL, Ginsberg DA. Calculi in the bladder and urinary diversions. In: Coe FL, Favus MJ, Pak CY, Parks JH, Preminger GM, editors. Kidney stones: medical and surgical management. Philadelphia: Lippincott-Raven; 1996. p. 1025–34.
8. Kancha RK, Anasuya A. Contribution of vitamin A deficiency to calculogenic risk factors of urine: studies in children. Biochem Med Metab Biol. 1992;47:1–9.
9. Rub R, Madeb R, Morgenstern S, Ben-Chaim J, Avidor Y. Development of a large bladder calculus on sutures used for pubic bone closure following extrophy repair. World J Urol. 2001;19(4):261–2.
10. Godbole P, Mackinnon AE. Expanded PTFE bladder neck slings for incontinence in children: the long-term outcome. BJU Int. 2004;93(1):139–41.
11. Eichel L, Allende R, Mevorach RA, et al. Bladder calculus formation and urinary retention secondary to perforation of a normal bladder by a ventriculoperitoneal shunt. Urology. 2002;60(2):344.
12. Hick EJ, Hernandez J, Yordan R, et al. Bladder calculus resulting from the migration of an intrauterine contraceptive device. J Urol. 2004;172(5 Pt 1):1903.
13. Arunkalaivanan AS, Smith AR. Bladder calculus after laparoscopic colposuspension. J Obstet Gynaecol. 2002;22(1):101.
14. Lau S, Zammit P, Bikhchandani J, Buchholz NP. The unbreakable bladder stone-Munchhausen's tale. Urol Int. 2006;77(3):284–5.
15. Mathoera RB, Kok DJ, Nijman RJ. Bladder calculi in augmentation cystoplasty in children. Urology. 2000;56(3):482–7.
16. Zahag H, Yamataka A, Koga H. Bladder stone formation after sigmoidocolocystoplasty: statistical analysis of risk factors. J Pediatr Surg. 2005;40:407.
17. Vanwaeyenbergh J, Vergauwe D, Verbeeck RM. Infrared spectrometric analysis of endemic bladder stones in Niger. Eur Urol. 1995;27:154–9.
18. Salah MA, Holman E, Khan AM, Toth C. Percutaneous cystolithotomy for pediatric endemic bladder stone: experience with 155 cases from 2 developing countries. J Pediatr Surg. 2005;40(10):1628–31.
19. Hammad FT, Kaya M, Kazim E. Bladder calculi: did the clinical picture change? Urology. 2006;67(6):1154–8.
20. Ho K, Segura J. Lower urinary tract calculi. In: Wein A, Kavoussi L, Novick A, Partin A, Peters C, editors. Campbell-Walsh urology, vol. 3. 9th ed. Philadelphia: Saunders Elsevier; 2007. p. 2663–73.
21. Su CM, Lin HY, Li CC, et al. Bladder stone in a woman after cesarean section: a case report. Kaohsiung J Med Sci. 2003;19(1):42–4.
22. Huang WC, Yang JM. Sonographic appearance of a bladder calculus secondary to a suture from a bladder neck suspension. J Ultrasound Med. 2002;21(11):1303–5.
23. Webb M, Fong W. A large bladder calculus and severe vesicoureteric reflux as seen on Tc-99m MAG3 renography. Clin Nucl Med. 2002;27(11):803–4.
24. Husain I, El-Faqih SR, Shamsuddin AB, et al. Primary extracorporeal shockwave lithotripsy in management of large bladder calculi. J Endourol. 1994;8:183–6.

25. Lin CM. Extracorporeal shock wave lithotripsy in children: experience with the multifunctional lithotripter MFL 5000. Chung Hua Min Kuo Hsiao Erh Ko I Hsueh Hui Tsa Chih. 1992;33(5):357–62.
26. Ni YH, Tsau YK, Chen CH, et al. Urolithiasis in children. Chung Hua Min Kuo Hsiao Erh Ko I Hsueh Hui Tsa Chiha. 1991;32(1):9–16.
27. Goel MC, Baserge NS, Babu RVR, et al. Pediatric kidney: functional outcome after extracorporeal shock wave lithotripsy. J Urol. 1996;155:2044–7.
28. Losty P, Surana R, O'Donell B. Limitations of extracorporeal shock wave lithotripsy for urinary tract calculi in young children. J Pediatr Surg. 1993;28:1037–9.
29. Agrawal MS, Aron M, Goyal J, et al. Percutaneous suprapubic cystolithotripsy for vesical calculi in children. J Endourol. 1999;13:173–5.
30. Wollin TA, Singal RK, Whelan T, et al. Percutaneous suprapubic cystolithotripsy for treatment of large bladder calculi. J Endourol. 1999;13:739–44.
31. Gopalakrishnan G, Bhaskar P, Jehangir E. Suprapubic lithotripsy. Br J Urol. 1988;62:389.
32. Salah MA, Holman E, Toth C. Percutaneous suprapubic cystolithotripsy for pediatric bladder stones in a developing country. Eur Urol. 2001;39:466–70.
33. Johnson O. Vesical calculus in Ethiopian children. Ethiop Med J. 1995;33:31–5.
34. Agrawal MS, Aron M, Goyal J, Elhence IP, Asopa HS. Percutaneous suprapubic cystolithotripsy for vesical calculi in children. J Endourol. 1999;13:173–5.
35. Ahmadnia H, Younesi Rostami M, Yarmohammadi AA, Javad Parizadeh SM, Esmaeili M, Movarekh M. Percutaneous treatment of bladder calculi in children: 5 years experience. Urol J. 2006;3(1):20–2.
36. Mohammed S, et al. Comparison of endourological and open cystolithotomy in the management of bladder stones in children. J Urol. 2009;181:2684.
37. Maheshwari PN, Oswal AT, Bansal M. Percutaneous cystolithotomy for vesical calculi: a better approach. Tech Urol. 1999;5:40–2.

Shock Wave Lithotripsy for Renal Stone in Children

82

M. Hammad Ather

Abstract

Interventional management of urolithiasis in children has evolved dramatically over the past 3 decades. Open surgery with its antecedent risks on need for re-treatment has almost completely been replaced by endourological treatment in most centers in the West. The higher incidence of pediatric urolithiasis in the developing world with lack of well-equipped endourological centers still mandates use of knife for stones.

Since its initial reports in the mid-1980s, shock wave lithotripsy (SWL) has become the current standard therapeutic alternative for most of the moderate-sized renal stones. The intrinsic ability of pediatric ureter to transmit relatively large stone fragments encouraged investigators to treat even larger stones as well as staghorn stones with SWL monotherapy in a safe and efficacious manner. Long-term safety of shock wave application on the growing kidneys was a major concern in using SWL in particularly younger children. Although there is lack of quality data on this subject, many contemporary studies have shown long-term safety of SWL even for very young children. Among the major short-term complications, development of obstructive Steinstrasse and urosepsis are two major concerns. Fortunately the overall incidence of major complications is quite low.

In essence, SWL for pediatric renal stone is safe and highly efficacious, and there is lack of evidence that it is associated with any significant long-term consequences. The use of stent is often unnecessary, and relatively larger stones could be treated by SWL compared to adults.

Keywords

Pediatric • Stone • Shock wave lithotripsy • Efficacy • Safety • Stenting • Gated SWL • Use of anesthesia • Clearance rates

Introduction

Interventional treatment of pediatric renal stones has seen a paradigm shift over the past few decades. Although open stone surgery was predominantly used prior to the 1980s [1], clinical introduction of shock wave lithotripsy (SWL) has revolutionized pediatric stone management. Currently, SWL is the gold standard for the minimal invasive management of most upper tract calculi in the developed world. In the Third World, however, open stone surgery is still performed for many reasons [2]. During the same period, development in technology with miniaturization of equipment and refinement of technique of percutaneous surgery led to its application in the pediatric population as well. Percutaneous and endourological access to the entire pediatric urinary tract is now possible. SWL safety and efficacy has been shown in many contemporary series. This chapter provides a focused review of the contemporary literature, on

M.H. Ather, M.B.B.S., FCPS(urol), FEBU
Department of Surgery, Division of Urology,
Aga Khan University, Stadium Road, 3500,
Karachi, Sindh, 74800, Pakistan
e-mail: hammad.ather@aku.edu

J.J. Talati et al. (eds.), *Urolithiasis*,
DOI 10.1007/978-1-4471-4387-1_82, © Springer-Verlag London 2012

recent advances, controversies, and challenges, in the management of pediatric renal stone disease by SWL.

Incidence of Pediatric Renal Stones

There is a lack of quality data on the epidemiology of pediatric renal stone disease. The incidence and characteristics of nephrolithiasis in children reflect a wide geographic variation [3]. Although the disease is uncommon in the western hemisphere, it is considered endemic in developing countries like Turkey, India, Pakistan, and countries in the Far East. In these areas, ammonium acid urate and uric acid stones predominate, strongly implicating dietary factors. The incidence of urinary stones in children has been reported to be from 0.1 to 5 %. In the United States, the prevalence varies from 1 in 1,000 to 1 in 7,600 hospital admissions, depending on the geographic region [4]. In an epidemiological study from Turkey, where urinary stones disease is considered endemic, 17 % of patients with urinary stone disease were noted to be younger than 14 years [5]. The gender distribution among pediatric stone formers varies significantly by age; in the first decade of life, males predominate, whereas in the second decade of life, females predominate [6]. Overall, females in the pediatric population have a greater prevalence of treated stone disease than do males [6]. The reasons for this unique epidemiologic finding are not readily apparent. A smaller study from Central Europe noted an overall male prevalence for hospital admissions for stones [7]. Perhaps the epidemiology differs in Central Europe than in the United States. The possible reasons, put forth by the investigators, for this difference included hormonal changes at puberty, which might be partly responsible for females having a greater likelihood of stone formation than males. Obesity and perhaps sexual activity in adolescent females were the other factors evaluated on this aspect.

Shock Wave Lithotripsy in Children: Efficacy and Safety

Since its initial report in 1986 [8], the emergence of SWL revolutionized the minimally invasive treatment of urolithiasis in children. Many contemporary large series have reported that the rate of complications, safety, and stone-free rates are comparable with those of adults. In a recent report from China, He and colleagues [9] have noted that SWL for both renal stones and ureteral stones in pediatric group have comparable efficacy and safety, except that stones in lower calyxes and middle ureters have a lower efficiency quotient than those in other locations. Ather and Noor [10] noted that stone clearance was not adversely affected by a stone size up to 30 mm; however, lower-pole calyceal stones and stones impacted at the ureteropelvic junction had a relatively poorer clearance in a cohort of 105 children studied younger than 14 years of age. These investigators reported an overall stone-free rate of 95 % after a mean of 1.7 treatments, with 5 % of patients requiring additional procedures as adjuncts to SWL. With a maximum of 30 mm, mean stone size in the treatment success group was 14 mm compared with 16 mm in the treatment failure group. More recently Landau et al. [11] treated 216 children (mean age 6.6 years) with a mean stone size of 14.9 mm by SWL treated on Dornier HM3 lithotripter. They reported a 3-month stone-free rate of 80 %, demonstrating that efficacious stone-free rates can be achieved in appropriate candidates.

Although SWL is well tolerated in children with few complications, stone-free rates following single-session monotherapy occur in less than half of the children [12]. This mandates multiple treatments, often performed under general anesthesia. The impact of multiple treatment sessions is a matter of debate as the effects of shock waves on renal tissue are still not clearly defined. Shock waves result in renal vessel vasoconstriction and that renal tubular injury and subcapsular hematoma from cavitations and shear forces are dependent on the kilo voltage applied [13]. In a large series of 340 adult patients with a mean follow-up of 19 years post SWL, Krambeck and colleagues [14] reported an increased risk of hypertension and diabetes mellitus related to bilateral treatment, number of administered shocks, and treatment intensity. Significant alterations of renal growth in children after SWL were observed in a long-term study, with a mean follow-up of 9 years [15], although the authors could not determine whether alterations were because of the treatment or to some extent underlying conditions intrinsic to pediatric kidneys with urolithiasis. Ather and Noor [10] showed long-term safety with SWL; however, they only assessed serum creatinine and development of de novo hypertension as parameters of long-term safety. The short-term safety has been established in many contemporary series. Aksoy and colleagues [16] noted that a low incidence of major complications such as Steinstrasse (13 cases), urinary tract infection (UTI, 7 cases), urosepsis (1 case), and subcapsular hematoma (1 case) was seen in 22 (8.4 %) patients in a cohort of 263 patients treated over a decade.

Technical Considerations

Preoperative Stent Placement

Stent placement prior to SWL is a controversial issue in children treated by SWL. Most of the indications currently used—such as the size of the stone, the prevention of complications, obstruction, and the management of staghorn calculi—have been borrowed from the adult literature. They have not taken into consideration the unique characteristics of pediatric ureters to transmit stone fragments. There is significant evidence in literature indicating that the fragments pass more easily in children [17] and more easily in younger children than in older children and adults [18]. There is paucity of quality data on the use of stents in children prior to SWL, but review of current data indicates that it should be reserved for a few selected patients. Our current indications of stent placement include patients with obstructing stones and infection or for prevention of posttreatment obstruction, particularly for children residing far from the treatment center.

Use of Anesthesia

The effectiveness of lithotripter to fragment stone largely depends on the power expressed at the focal point. Closely correlated with the power is the pain produced by the shock waves. By reducing the size of the focus, it becomes possible to treat the patient without anesthesia or analgesia. This, however, often results in a higher re-treatment rate. In a nonrandomized study, Raza and Ather [19] noted, in a multivariate analysis, that type of anesthesia/analgesia does not affect the outcome. Older children often tolerate SWL under intravenous sedation, and minimal anesthesia is applicable for most patients treated with second- and third-generation lithotripters. General anesthesia is administered in a majority of smaller children to avoid both patient and stone motion and the need for repeated repositioning.

Gated Versus Ungated SWL

Ungated SWL is not synchronized to the patient's electrocardiogram, in order to have greater freedom in setting the shock wave rate. Ungated SWL is often associated with cardiac arrhythmias in adults; the incidence of arrhythmias in children has not been established [20]. In adults there has been some data indicating that slowing the shock wave rate may result in better clearance; similar work is not yet done in the pediatric age.

Type of Lithotripter

Following initial reports of success on first-generation lithotripters, SWL has become the standard treatment of renal stones. Second- and third-generation lithotripters, which are dry-head lithotripters and equipped with advanced imaging, were subsequently used in children. The impact of SWL machine has been studied by Aksoy and colleagues, who showed that SWL treatment was effective and safe in pediatric urolithiasis using both electrohydraulic (EHL) and electromagnetic (EML) machines [16].

The electromagnetic machine was more effective than the electrohydraulic one for distal ureteral calculi. Additionally, the electromagnetic lithotripter has significant clinical advantages over the electrohydraulic lithotripter in terms of anesthesia requirements, hospitalization duration, and fluoroscopic targeting [16]. In another study comparing the electrohydraulic and electromagnetic lithotripters, Raza and Ather [19] noted that the EHL has a better stone-free rate and efficiency quotient than the EML; however, short-term safety has been found to be marginally better with the EML.

Size and Location of Stones and Clearance Rate

There is no clear definition of stone-free status in children. Earlier works indicate that <4 mm as insignificant residual fragment has been challenged even in adults. Although children are able to clear residual fragments spontaneously better than adults, they are also likely to have an earlier stone recurrence; it is therefore important to document stone clearance.

Earlier work on SWL in children focused on the safety and efficacy profile. More recently there has been significant literature focusing on the anatomical factors, stone-related parameters, and demographic factors of the treated children affecting the stone-free rate. SWL is currently considered the primary treatment for upper tract calculi 15 mm or smaller in children [21], but evidence supporting this stone size cutoff is lacking. Ather and Noor [10] analyzed the correlation between stone size and clearance in 105 children younger than 14 years. These investigators reported an overall stone-free rate of 95 % after a mean of 1.7 treatments, with 5 % of patients requiring additional procedures as adjuncts to SWL. With a maximum of 30 mm, mean stone size in the treatment success group was 14 mm compared with 16 mm in the treatment failure group. In contrast, Elsobky and colleagues [22] reported a 91 stone-free rate versus 75 % stone-free rate for mean stone diameter less than and greater than 10 mm, respectively. Recently, Shouman and colleagues [23] reported a series of 24 children with a mean stone size of 31 mm undergoing SWL with the Dornier DoLi S device. In 53 sessions requiring a mean number of 3,489 shock waves per session, stone-free and complication rates were 83.3 and 25 %, respectively. While it is possible to treat very large stone burdens with SWL, concerns include the necessity of more shock treatments, more frequent re-treatment sessions, and increased risk of postoperative obstruction.

Conclusion

Currently higher stone-free rates can be achieved even for large stones of 20–30 mm in diameter, staghorn stones, and stones located in the lower pole. Staghorn calculi are uncommon in children and represent a management challenge. Although monotherapy success rates are low in adults, acceptable stone-free rates in children have been achieved with SWL. SWL is considered the safest and highly efficacious modality for children with significant stone burden. Current data seem to suggest that systematic preoperative insertion of ureteric stents is unnecessary.

References

1. Wickham J. Current management of urinary calculi. Practitioner. 1989;233(1466):526–9.
2. Rizvi SA, Sultan S, Ijaz H, Mirza ZN, Ahmed B, Saulat S, et al. Open surgical management of pediatric urolithiasis: a developing country perspective. Indian J Urol. 2010;26(4):573–6.
3. Novak TE, Lakshmanan Y, Trock BJ, et al. Sex prevalence of pediatric kidney stone disease in the United States: an epidemiologic investigation. Urology. 2009;74(1):104–7.
4. Kroovand RL. Pediatric urolithiasis. Urol Clin North Am. 1997; 24(1):173–84.
5. Tellaloglu S, Ander H. Stones in children. Turk J Pediatr. 1984; 26(1–4):51–60.
6. Matlaga BR, Schaeffer AJ, Novak TE, Trock BJ. Epidemiologic insights into pediatric kidney stone disease. Urol Res. 2010; 38(6):453–7.
7. Biocic M, Saraga M, Kuzmic AC, et al. Pediatric urolithiasis in Croatia. Coll Antropol. 2003;27:745–52.
8. Newman DM, Coury T, Lingeman JE, et al. Extracorporeal shock wave lithotripsy experience in children. J Urol. 1986;136(1 Pt 2): 238–40.
9. He L, Sun X, Lu J, Cong X, Zhu H, Shen L, Wang Y. Comparison of efficacy and safety of shockwave lithotripsy for upper urinary tract stones of different locations in children: a study of 311 cases. World J Urol. 2011;29(6):713–7.
10. Ather MH, Noor MA. Does size and site matter for renal stones up to 30-mm in size in children treated by extracorporeal lithotripsy? Urology. 2003;61(1):212–5; discussion 215.
11. Landau EH, Shenfeld OZ, Pode D, et al. Extracorporeal shock wave lithotripsy in prepubertal children: 22-year experience at a single institution with a single lithotriptor. J Urol. 2009;182 Suppl 4: 1835–9.
12. Muslumanoglu AY, Tefekli A, Sarilar O, et al. Extracorporeal shock wave lithotripsy as first line treatment alternative for urinary tract stones in children: a large scale retrospective analysis. J Urol. 2003;170(6 Pt 1):2405–8.
13. Lingeman JE, Kim SC, Kuo RL, et al. Shockwave lithotripsy: anecdotes and insights. J Endourol. 2003;17(9):687–93.
14. Krambeck AE, Gettman MT, Rohlinger AL, et al. Diabetes mellitus and hypertension associated with shock wave lithotripsy of renal and proximal ureteral stones at 19 years of followup. J Urol. 2006;175(5):1742–7.
15. Lifshitz DA, Lingeman JE, Zafar FS, Hollensbe DW, Nyhuis AW, Evan AP. Alterations in predicted growth rates of pediatric kidneys treated with extracorporeal shockwave lithotripsy. J Endourol. 1998;12(5):469–75.
16. Aksoy Y, Ziypak T, Yapanoglu T. Comparison of the effectiveness and safety of MPL 9000 and Lithostar Modularis shockwave lithotriptors: treatment results of 263 children. Urol Res. 2009;37(2):111–6.
17. Longo JA, Netto Jr NR. Extracorporeal shock-wave lithotripsy in children. Urology. 1995;46(4):550–2.
18. Myers DA, Mobley TB, Jenkins JM, Grine WB, Jordan WR. Pediatric low energy lithotripsy with the Lithostar. J Urol. 1995; 153(2):453–7.
19. Raza SJ, Ather MH. Does the type of lithotripter affect outcomes in children with upper tract urolithiasis? J Endourol. 2009;23(2):223–7.
20. Palmer JS. Ungated extracorporeal shock wave lithotripsy: safe and effective in the pediatric population. Can J Urol. 2009;16(6):4924–6.
21. Farhat WA, Kropp BP. Surgical treatment of pediatric urinary stones. AUA Update Ser. 2007;26(3):22–7.
22. Elsobky E, Sheir KZ, Madbouly K, et al. Extracorporeal shock wave lithotripsy in children: experience using two second-generation lithotripters. BJU Int. 2000;86(7):851–6.
23. Shouman AM, Ziada AM, Ghoneim IA, et al. Extracorporeal shock wave lithotripsy monotherapy for renal stones >25 mm in children. Urology. 2009;74(1):109–11.

Endourological Approaches to Renal and Ureteric Calculi in Children

83

Zafar Zaidi and Zaheer Alam

Abstract

Pediatric urolithiasis is a management challenge because of the smaller size of the urinary tract and a higher risk of stone recurrence. The standard procedures to treat pediatric urolithiasis do not differ from those used for adults, i.e., extracorporeal shock wave lithotripsy (ESWL), percutaneous nephrolithotomy (PCNL), ureteroscopy (URS), laparoscopy, and open surgery. With improvement in equipment, energy sources, and increasing worldwide experience, open surgery is now limited to few cases requiring anatomical correction also. PCNL and URS can be performed in children with the same efficacy and safety as in adults.

This chapter describes endourological approaches (PCNL and URS) to management of pediatric urolithiasis. PCNL since its first report in the 1970s has undergone much refinement as a procedure, and indications for its use have expanded many folds. This chapter traces the history of PCNL, a very detailed account of step-by-step technique, and discusses PCNL in conditions like bilateral stones and congenital abnormalities. The instruments used, the complications of PCNL, and the effectiveness of this procedure in managing renal stones in children have been described in detail.

Management of ureteric stones with URS in children has been described with a detailed account of the procedure, its complications, and outcomes.

Keywords

Renal calculi in children • ureteric calculi in children • Pediatric PCNL • Pediatric URS • PCNL in special conditions • Effectiveness of PCNL • Ureterorenoscopy in children

Introduction

Pediatric urolithiasis is a management challenge because of the smaller size of the urinary tract and a higher risk of stone recurrence. Due to a longer lifetime risk of stone recurrence, children require complete stone clearance, and residual fragments considered clinically insignificant in adults must be avoided in children. Afshar et al. [1] have shown that 69 % of patients with residual fragments <5 mm after extracorporeal shock wave lithotripsy (ESWL) had symptomatic episodes or an increase in stone size after a mean follow-up of 48 months. As compared with stone-free individuals, children with residual fragments had an increased risk for adverse clinical outcome, with an odds ratio (OR) of 3.9, and this increased to an OR of 11.4 if an underlying metabolic disorder was present.

The standard procedures to treat pediatric urolithiasis do not differ from those used for adults, i.e., SWL, percutaneous nephrolithotomy (PCNL), ureterorenoscopy (URS), laparoscopy, and open surgery. With improvement in equipment, energy sources, and increasing worldwide experience, open surgery for management of renal and ureteric stones is mostly

Z. Zaidi, M.B.B.S., FRCS, FEBU (✉) • Z. Alam, M.B.B.S., MCPS, FCPS Urology
Department of Urology, The Indus Hospital, Korangi Crossing, Karachi, 75190, Pakistan
e-mail: zzaidi@cyber.net.pk; doctorzaheer@yahoo.com

J.J. Talati et al. (eds.), *Urolithiasis*,
DOI 10.1007/978-1-4471-4387-1_83, © Springer-Verlag London 2012

reserved for selected cases, especially those requiring anatomical correction of the urinary tract. PCNL and URS can now be performed in children with the same efficacy and safety as in adults.

Percutaneous Nephrolithotomy (PCNL) in Children

History

The radiologist Fernstorm and Johansson [2] is credited with the first percutaneous renal stone removal in the late 1970s. He dilated the tract to 1 cm, using serial plastic dilators for a radiologically controlled stone extraction. Rusnak and associates [3] added a plastic sheath as a conduit into the urinary tract that later became popular as the Amplatz sheath. The metallic telescoping dilator, the first purpose-built device designed to allow for puncture, dilatation, and endoscopically controlled intrarenal instrumentation in one session, was described by Alken [4]. The balloon dilatation system used for percutaneous transluminal angioplasty was first applied for PCNL access by Clayman and coworkers [5].

In 1985, Woodside [6] and associates rendered seven children (ages 5–18 years) stone-free without complications using adult PCNL equipment. Mor [7] and colleagues treated 25 children using adult equipment. In 1997, Helal et al. [8] reported the use of a 15-Fr Hickman catheter access sheath in a 2-year-old child, where the tract was serially dilated to 16 Fr and a 15-Fr peel-away vascular access sheath was passed into the collecting system for stone extraction. Initially, there was hesitation on the part of urologists to adopt PCNL in children due to concerns regarding use of large instruments in pediatric kidneys resulting in parenchymal damage and the associated effects on renal function and the risk of sepsis and bleeding. Hence, for many years PCNL was considered unsafe in children younger than 5 years and in those with renal impairment or congenital renal abnormalities. In a series of 169 children, the author (Zaidi) [9] showed that PCNL is safe and effective when stratified by patient age (<5 years), anatomy, bilaterality, and renal function and that the stone free outcomes were comparable in all groups.

Indications

There is currently no international consensus on when PCNL is the preferred primary therapy. However, it is a reasonable approach in children with a large upper tract stone burden (>1.5 cm), lower-pole calculi (>1 cm), an impacted stone in the upper ureter, known cystine or struvite stones or where concurrent anatomical abnormality impairs urinary drainage and stone clearance as seen in horseshoe kidneys; ectopic, crossed, or fused kidneys; stone in calyceal diverticulum; transplanted kidney; encrusted foreign objects; or urinary diversions [10–12].

Operative Technique

General Considerations

In order to avoid hypothermia, especially in the very small children, it is important to have a warm operating room, irrigation fluids at body temperature, short operative time, proper draping, and monitoring of body temperature. There is a potential risk of hypothermia from large amounts of irrigation fluid used. This can result in decreased core temperature, shivering, peripheral vasoconstriction, and delayed drug clearance [18]. Effective warming of irrigation fluid may prevent hypothermia even if large volumes are used.

Antibiotic Prophylaxis and Anesthetic Considerations

PCNL is a clean-contaminated procedure in patients with sterile urine documented preoperatively. In a study of 81 patients, Dogan et al. [13] found no significant differences between single-dose and short-term prophylaxis protocols in terms of infectious complications in patients with preoperative sterile urine. Duration of surgery and amount of irrigation fluid are significant risk factors for postoperative fever. Charton et al. [14] found a urinary tract infection (UTI) rate of 35 % and a postoperative fever rate of 10 % without antibiotic prophylaxis, while Clayman and Casteneda-Zuniga [15] reported a 2 % rate of bacteremia after percutaneous surgery performed with antibiotic prophylaxis. Both American Urological Association (AUA) and European Association of Urology (EUA) guidelines recommend antibiotic prophylaxis for all patients undergoing PCNL [16, 17].

All PCNL in children should be performed under general anesthesia. Throughout anesthesia maintenance, the anesthesiologist should auscultate the lungs frequently and should be cognizant of possible airway pressure and $ETCO_2$ elevation and/or decrease in SpO_2. Postoperative fever despite sterile urine and blood cultures may be attributed to an elevated thermostatic set point caused by cytokine response due to postoperative stress [19].

Patient Position

After induction of general anesthesia, the patient is placed in lithotomy position, and retrograde pyelography is performed to outline the collecting system, after which an open-ended ureteral catheter is placed. Children with spinal anomalies like spina bifida can be a challenge for positioning due to contractures and the spinal hardware present [20]. In children, percutaneous access is achieved in complete prone position or with the torso elevated at 30° from the table surface [15]. The authors have always used a completely prone position without any roll below the body or any angulations to torso [21]. PCNL in supine position has been infrequently described in adult patients but none reported in the pediatric age group. This is mainly due the increased chance of colonic perforation when accessing the kidney from lateral side.

Tract Site, Size, and Dilatation

Retrograde pyelography is done using a 4.5-Fr ureteric catheter. Pelviureteric junction (PUJ) occluding balloon catheters have been used, as they stop stone fragment migration into the upper ureter. The authors use a simple ureteric catheter, which successfully prevents migration of stone fragments in the upper ureter and is also cost effective. Radiopaque contrast diluted to 50 % is injected to outline the calyces. After retrograde pyelography, the patient is repositioned for renal access and waterproof drapes applied to avoid hypothermia. The surgeon stands on the side of the kidney to be punctured with the fluoroscopic image intensifier on the opposite side. The alternative use of ultrasound guidance will diminish the risks of radiation exposure to a meaningful extent, but it requires additional expertise.

A thorough evaluation of the collecting system anatomy is mandatory for safe puncture. The most appropriate calyx is selected for puncture. This should allow easy access to stone requiring minimal torque inside the kidney [22]. Lower-pole access is frequently used in most series. However, upper-pole access is useful as it provides visualization of superior calyx, pelvis, lower calyx, PUJ, and upper ureter in selected cases.

Once the calyx to puncture is chosen, an 18-gauge spinal needle is used to puncture the desired calyx. The authors do not use a Chiba needle as length of needle is never an issue in children. We take extra care to follow the "bull's eye" principle. The needle is advanced up to the kidney, and then the C-arm is rotated to 30°. This gives depth perception of how much further the needle needs to be advanced. Additionally by rotating the C-arm away, clear passage of instruments is gained. On removal of the stylet, clear fluid should flow. Further filling of the system with contrast helps visualize parts of the collecting system obstructed by the stone. A 0.035-in. guide wire is passed into the collecting system and preferably directed down the ureter. A J-shaped guide wire should preferentially be used as it turns on contact with the calyceal system wall without the risk of perforation. For cost-effectiveness the authors gently bend the tip of a simple guide wire, and this performs the desired function equally well. The spinal needle is beveled on one side. This side should be directed toward the intended direction of the guide wire. A small incision is made on the skin at the point of entry, and facial dilator 8 Fr in size is passed over the guide wire into the system. Care must be taken to reach exactly the same depth as the needle tip.

The tract can further be dilated using serial dilators or a balloon dilator. Wezel [23] compared metallic telescoping dilatation to balloon dilatation in adults and showed no significant difference in morbidity. The advantages of the metallic telescoping dilatation are maintenance of the original puncture path direction, tamponade of the tract, low cost, and haptic feedback of resistance during dilatation. However, the surgeon needs to be meticulous throughout dilatation with frequent radiological exposures. The balloon dilatation has less risk of forward perforation. The "mini-perc" technique described by Jackman et al. [24] using an 11-Fr peel-away access sheath eliminated the need for sequential dilatation and reduced the size of the tract significantly. They reported an 85 % stone-free rate for 11 procedures in seven children. The limitation of this technique is large stone burden since stone fragments have to be tiny to come out of the small tract. In addition, the small-sized tract does not allow use of standard pediatric nephroscopes; hence, a cystoscope or ureteroscope [25] has to be used, which makes the procedure further less practical. Guisti et al. [26] showed that any advantage gained by a small-diameter tract is far outweighed by poor vision, lengthy operative time, and lower stone-free rates. Bilen et al. [27] compared PCNL results in children after using different sizes of instruments via a 26-, 20-, and 14-Fr tract. They concluded that smaller instruments did not significantly increase operative time and had the same success rates as the adult-sized devices. Nouralizadeh et al. [28] performed 26 PCNLs in patients younger than 5 years old with adult-sized instruments. The mean stone size was 33 mm. Using a single tract, complete stone clearance was achieved in 79.1 % with an overall complication rate of 15.3 %. Only one patient required transfusion. Mahmud and Zaidi [21] performed PCNL in 29 children <5 years old using 17-Fr nephroscope. Only two children required post-procedure transfusion. The authors [9] using a 17-Fr nephroscope via upper-pole access in eight children with congenital renal abnormalities had 90 % stone clearance, and no patient required transfusion.

Nephroscopy and Nephrolithotomy

Once access is obtained, nephroscopy is performed. Successful miniaturizing of endoscopes and lithotripsy tools has allowed use of smaller access tracts. The outer diameter of nephroscopes available for children ranges from 15 to 17 Fr. Adult nephroscopes of 26 Fr have frequently been used. Flexible nephroscope with a 15-Fr outer diameter and 6-Fr working channel is available. Pediatric cystoscopes, semi-rigid ureteroscopes, and flexible ureteroscopes have all been used [29].

For the disintegration of stone, currently available energy sources include electrohydraulic lithotripsy (EHL), ultrasonic lithotripsy, holmium:YAG laser, and pneumatic lithotripsy. The authors prefer pneumatic lithotripsy as this is cost effective.

Renal Drainage After PCNL

At the end of PCNL, a nephrostomy tube is to achieve hemostasis as well as renal drainage left in the tract. Srinivasan et al. [30] reviewed the different techniques of renal drainage after PCNL in adult patients and concluded that the optimal renal drainage method depends on patient characteristics and the operative course which should be individualized accordingly. They grouped patients as routine and problematic based on the increasing complexity of the procedure and its complications. They suggested placement of ureteric stent or a small-bore nephrostomy tube in routine PCNL, while in problematic and complicated procedures, large-bore nephrostomy tube is indicated. The authors use a Foley catheter with its balloon port cut to allow successful removal of Amplatz sheath over it [21]. This is cost-effective drainage. Council tip catheters or Malecot reentry tube (10–16 Fr) have also been used [22].

Tubeless PCNL with a ureteric stent has been described in adult population with less pain, shorter hospitalization, and better patient acceptance [31, 32]. Khairy Salem et al. [33] first evaluated their initial experiences to determine the indications and limitations of tubeless PCNL in children. They reported that tubeless PCNL was less painful and less troublesome and had shorter hospital stay for children. This conclusion is similar to other studies in children comparing tubeless versus conventional PCNL [34]. Totally tubeless PCNL without nephrostomy drainage or ureteric stenting has been described in a small series of eight preschool children by Ozturk et al. [35] to be safe and effective.

Bilateral PCNL

Salah et al. [36] performed simultaneous bilateral PCNL in 13 children with a mean stone size of 2 cm, by using a 26-Fr adult nephroscope, and did not report any complications. The authors [9] in their series of bilateral simultaneous PCNL in 24 renal units used 17-Fr nephroscope in 21 kidneys, and 24-Fr nephroscope in three kidneys have confirmed these encouraging results.

PCNL in Congenital Renal Anomalies

Stone disease is more common with associated congenital anomalies like pelviureteric obstruction and horseshoe or ectopic kidneys. Percutaneous approach facilitates correction of PUJ stenosis along with stone removal [37]. Access in horseshoe kidneys can only be from upper or middle pole, and puncture is more vertical and closer to midline [38, 39] with excellent results, even in children [9]. For ectopic pelvic kidneys, Aquil et al. [40] have performed laparoscopic-assisted PCNL approaching the kidney anteriorly.

Complications of PCNL

Renal Hemorrhage

Renal hemorrhage is one of the most common and worrisome complications of PCNL. When it occurs during operation and hinders visualization, the procedure may need to be abandoned. Desai et al. [41] reported that the number and size of tracts are significantly correlated with the decrease in hemoglobin levels. They reported an average hemoglobin drop of 1.9 g/dl in 116 cases of PCNL with an overall transfusion rate of 14 %. Samad et al. [9] recorded a blood transfusion rate of 4 % during 188 consecutive PCNLs. Mahmud et al. [21] transfused 2 out of 29 preschool-aged children undergoing PCNL. In both series none of the procedures was abandoned or required conversion to open surgery. In 52 children with a mean stone burden of 282 mm^2, Zeren et al. [42] reported a transfusion rate of 24 % and showed an association with operative time, sheath size, and stone burden. While in 135 children with mean stone burden of 507 mm^2, a transfusion rate of only 0.7 % was reported by Salah et al. [43] In the 193 adult PCNLs reviewed by Turna et al. [44], multivariate analysis found that staghorn stones, multiple tracts, presence of diabetes, and large stones are associated with increased renal hemorrhage. Bleeding during PCNL is usually venous in origin and can be managed with the placement of nephrostomy tube or tamponade catheter [45].

Postoperative Fever

Postoperative fever has been reported very frequently with an incidence as high as 30–40 % [9, 41, 45]. The origin of this fever is thought to be cytokine response to stress [19] since it is documented in patients with sterile blood and urine on investigation.

Fluid Absorption During PCNL

Fluid absorption does take place during PCNL and may have clinical significance in patients with impaired renal function or compromised cardiorespiratory status leading to volume overload. Kukreja et al. [46] calculated expired breath ethanol concentration in 148 patients where ethanol was used in the irrigating fluid and found fluid absorption in all patients but no evidence of electrolyte imbalance. They advocated creating a low-pressure system using an Amplatz sheath, reducing the amount of irrigation fluid used, and staging the procedure to reduce the amount of fluid absorbed. In a group of 13 patients with impaired renal function, Samad et al. [9] documented mild electrolyte imbalance in two patients postoperatively with no clinical manifestation.

Urinary Leakage

Postoperative leakage from the tract site is dependent on tract size and internal anatomy of the kidney and is reported in 1.2–8 % cases [41, 43, 47, 48]. It usually settles within 24 h. In grossly hydronephrotic kidneys or those with narrow PUJ, leakage may take longer to stop. Closing the skin wound snugly around the nephrostomy tube when tethering it to the skin is helpful. Prolonged leakage is usually due to a stone fragment obstructing the ureter, and this should be actively investigated when leakage continues beyond 24 h. A secondary procedure with ureteroscopy or insertion of a double-J stent may be required. To avoid prolonged postoperative urinary leakage, it is advisable to insert a double-J ureteric stent if at the end of PCNL there is residual stone fragments likely to obstruct urine passage or a large burden needing a repeat (second look) PCNL or ESWL.

Long-Term Effects on Renal Function

Several animal and clinical studies have revealed that PCNL has no long-term adverse effect on renal function. Dawaba et al. [49] reported an improvement of glomerular filtration rate (GFR) in 65 children after PCNL. They did not detect any renal scarring. Nouralizadeh et al. [50] evaluated the estimated GFR during the first few days after PCNL. In a total of 94 patients, they reported that GFR decreases immediately after PCNL, reaches a nadir 48 h after operation, and then increases slowly. They advise to avoid factors that can bear a negative influence on renal function such as nephrotoxic drugs, contrast agents, ESWL, and redo PCNL during early postoperative period. Mahmud and Zaidi [21] performed ^{99m}Tc-DMSA in 17 children <5 years old 6 weeks after PCNL and did not detect any scarring or loss of renal function. Mor et al. [7] did radioisotope scans in 10 children before and after PCNL and found changes in only 1 child who had undergone three PCNLs within 4 years. On the other hand, Samad et al. [51] demonstrated a 5 % risk of focal damage to renal parenchyma as a direct result of nephrostomy tract formation.

Effectiveness of PCNL

Most large studies demonstrate high success rates after PCNL monotherapy. Stone clearance rates approach 90 % [27, 41, 42] (Table 83.1). In 56 children with mean stone size of 18.4 mm, Desai et al. [41] reported a stone-free rate of 89.8 % with a transfusion rate of 14.3 %. However, 45 % of the cases were treated in a staged manner. Some centers [22] advocate a second-look nephroscopy through the same tract during the same admission. Zeren et al. [42] reported a stone clearance rate of 86.9 % with a transfusion rate of 23.9 % in 55 children with mean stone size of 16.8 mm. In 138 patients with mean stone size of 22.5 mm, Holman et al. [48] had a stone clearance rate of 98.5 %, transfusion rate of 0.4 %, and a urinary leak of 8 %. In patients with large stone burdens, PCNL is often followed by ESWL. In a large series of 188 PCNLs by Samad et al. [9], mean stone size was 27.2 mm; the clearance rate was only 67.4 %. Their transfusion rate was 4 %. However, after follow-up ESWL to residual fragments, the cumulative stone clearance rate improved

Table 83.1 PCNL in children: comparison of outcomes

Study	No. of children/ renal units	Mean age (years)	Mean stone size (mm)	Transfusion (%)	Stone clearance (%)	Combined with ESWL%	Complications and no. of patients
Mahmud and Zaidi [21]	29/30	3.5	26	6	60	40	Ileus 1/29
							Retention 1/29
Zeren et al. [42]	55/62	7.9	16.8	23.9	86.9	1.6	Open conversion 1/55
Desai et al. [41]	56	9.1	18.4	14.3	90	5.4	Urine leak 3/56
Salah et al. [43]	135/138	8.9	22.5	0.7	98.6	0	Urine leak 11/135
Samad et al. [9]	169/188	8.2	27.2	4	67.4	39.6	Ureteric obstruction 1/169
							Hyponatremia 1/169
Shokeir et al. [47]	75/82	6.6	14.4	1.2	95.1	4.8	Urine leak 1/75

to 100 %. In a smaller series of 29 patients of younger age (mean 3.8 years) and large stone burden (mean stone size of 24 mm), Mahmud and Zaidi [21] restricted the PCNL to a single puncture to avoid bleeding, but this resulted in a stone-free rate of 60 %. However, after follow-up on ESWL, the stone-free rate increased to 100 %.

Learning Curve in Pediatric PCNL

De la Rosette [52] and associates studied factors influencing training and maintaining skills in performing PCNL. They observed that obtaining renal access was the most crucial element. The steep learning curve is mainly related to obtaining renal access. They concluded that a resident should perform about 24 PCNL procedures to obtain a good proficiency during residency. Competence at performing PCNL is reached after 60 procedures, and excellence is obtained after performing more than 100 PCNLs.

Ureterorenoscopy in Children

Ureterorenoscopy (URS) in children has been slowly adapted as a means of stone removal and has lagged behind adults due to concerns regarding use of large uretreroscopes in small-caliber ureters. With significant improvements in miniaturization and durability of scopes and use of holmium laser, URS has become an attractive option in children.

History

Hampton Young and McKay [53] performed the first ureteroscopy in 1929 in a 2-week-old infant with posterior urethral valves and massively dilated ureters, using a cystoscope, which advanced easily to the renal pelvis. Ureterorenoscopy and lasertripsy were first described in children by Ritchey et al. [54] in 1988 for ureteric stone. They used rigid URS and successfully removed lower ureteric stone using pulsed dye laser. In the late 1980s, URS started gaining acceptance for stone management in children but was limited to stones below the iliac crest and for upper tract calculi only after ESWL failure [10]. There was reluctance to perform URS in children with proximal and mid-ureteric stones due to concern of iatrogenic ureteral injury, ureteral ischemia, avulsion, perforation, stricture formation, and development of vesicoureteric reflux as a result of excessive dilatation of small-size ureteric orifices. With miniaturizing of endoscopes and wider acceptance of holmium laser, URS has become a more attractive option in children.

Indications of URS

The removal of ureteral stone is indeed the most common indication for URS. Van Savage et al. [55] recommended modification in the American Urological Association (AUA) guidelines to be applied to the pediatric patient and concluded that calculi larger than 4 mm would require surgical management. The joint European Association of Urology (EAU)/AUA Nephrolithiasis Guideline 2010 [56] recommends observation or medical expulsive therapy during observation period for ureteric stone of less than 1 cm. URS is indicated if the stone size is >1 cm or, in the case of smaller stones, if there is persistent obstruction, failure of stone progression, and increasing or unremitting colic. URS also has a role in diagnostic and therapeutic management of renal and ureteral pathologies like renal hemangiomas or arteriovenous malformations, ureteropelvic junction (UPJ) obstruction, ureteral stricture, and ureteral polyps. Diagnostic ureteroscopy is also performed in cases of unexplained hematuria and its lateralization, but, contrary to the adult population, the underlying cause is usually benign lesion like hemangioma or arteriovenous malformation. The incidence of ureteral stricture after upper tract endoscopy has been reported to be 1–11 % [57]. Endoscopic management of UPJ obstruction is now considered a viable alternative to open procedure in pediatric patients [58] with success rates ranging from 55 to 85 % [59].

Contraindication for URS

URS is contraindicated in cases of active urinary tract infection (UTI). In patients with sepsis secondary to an obstructive stone, urgent decompression with percutaneous drainage is indicated, and URS should be deferred until sepsis in resolved. Children with anatomic anomalies that make retrograde access difficult, or with a history of previous endoscopic failures in such, should not be considered for URS.

Procedure

General Considerations

Appropriate prophylactic antibiotics according to the weight of the child are administered before the procedure. Under general anesthesia and caudal block in case of a young child, the patient is placed in lithotomy position with the ipsilateral (same side) leg slightly extended. This position makes surgery easier and faster [60]. Patients <1 year of age can be positioned adequately in an open leg posture. Patients with severe skeletal deformities are a challenge, and antegrade access of the ureter may need to be considered.

Operating room temperature should be adjusted for patient size and age. Normal saline warmed at body temperature should be used, and water should be avoided as it can cause potential intravascular hemolysis and hyponatremia. The anesthesiologist should remember that urethral stimulation can precipitate laryngospasm. Ureteroscopy must be performed with a C-arm image intensifier available in theater.

Ureteric Orifice Dilatation and Ureteroscopy

After complete evaluation of the bladder using a rigid cystoscope appropriate for the size of the child, a working guide wire is placed under fluoroscopic guidance into the ureter and advanced to the renal pelvis or up to/beyond the stone. Most procedures will require some form of ureteral dilatation. Ureteric orifice dilatation remains controversial in pediatric URS. There are several advantages of controlled ureteral dilatation before URS. This can be achieved with 8/10-Fr coaxial dilators or balloon dilators. The wider distal ureter allows larger ureteroscopes to pass, and hence, a bigger working channel is available. There is also increased flow of irrigation fluid around the scope allowing better visibility. There is a belief that controlled dilatation using balloon dilator or gradually dilating catheter may be less traumatic to the ureter than dilatation with a ureteroscope. Shepherd et al. [61] have shown that dilatation up to 12 F did not result in the development of vesicoureteral reflux postoperatively in their patients. Bassiri et al. [62] reviewed 66 prepubertal patients who underwent URS, of whom 25 underwent balloon dilation to allow ureteroscopic access. At 3-month follow-up with intravenous urography, there was no evidence of stenosis or stricture in any patient. Voiding cystourethrogram (VCUG) after URS in children has shown a low-grade and transient vesicoureteric reflux (VUR) to be present in 15 % of the cases resolving spontaneously with conservative management without any symptoms [63–65]. On the basis of reports [66] and the authors' own experience, we do not recommend routine postoperative VCUG to screen for VUR.

Soygur et al. [67] performed URS with a 7.5-Fr rigid ureteroscope in 26 children, obtaining ureteral access with the assistance of a hand irrigation pump without any further active dilation in all cases. Hydrodilation can be achieved most inexpensively by wrapping the irrigation bag with a blood pressure cuff or pressure bag. The limitation of this technique is that it is difficult to control the degree of hydrodilation, potentially resulting in cephalad migration of the stone. Gedik et al. [68] performed semirigid URS in 54 children with a mean age of 8.5 years without ureteral dilatation and found no difficulty in access.

Single-step active dilatation using a ureteral access sheath has been shown to be successful when multiple passages of the ureteroscope are anticipated. The sheath prevents significant trauma to the orifice or the intramural ureter. Various sizes are available ranging from 10 to14 Fr. Initially described in eight children by Singh et al. [69], ureteral access sheaths have been shown to facilitate repetitive upper tract access, reduce intrarenal pressure, decrease operative time, and improve stone-free rates.

Ureteroscopes available for children range from 4.5 Fr rigid, 7.5 Fr semirigid, or 6.9 Fr flexible. Satar et al. [70] found rigid URS to be safe and efficient in every location in children when using rigid 6.9–10-Fr ureteroscope in 35 ureteral units. Tanriverdi et al. [71] compared URS in children using 8-Fr rigid and 6.9-Fr semirigid ureteroscopes and concluded that neither the diameter nor the rigidity of the ureteroscope significantly affects the outcome of the procedure as long as the caliber of the scope is 8 Fr or less. Kim et al. [72] performed flexible ureteroscopy on 167 children with a mean age of 62.4 months and mean stone size of 6.12 mm. Stone clearance was 100 % for stone sizing 10 mm or less and 97 % for burdens greater than 10 mm after a single ureteroscopic procedure. Eighty-six of their patients had stones located in the lower pole making flexible ureteroscopy an excellent modality for managing ureteric calculi as well as small calculi in the lower pole of the kidney. One should bear in mind, however, that currently available flexible ureteroscopes that are smaller than 8 Fr in outer diameter are very delicate instruments.

Passive Ureteral Dilatation

Rubenstein et al. [73] suggested that the use of pre-stenting before ureteroscopy is associated with higher overall stone-free rates in adults. Hubert and Palmer [74] first evaluated the effect of passive dilatation by ureteral stenting before URS, if the ureteral orifice was inaccessible at initial cystoscopic evaluation. Corcoran et al. [75] suggests placing a ureteral stent only if initial attempts at access are unsuccessful for upper tract URS. Passive dilatation of the ureter is used in prepubertal children to minimize the risk of injury to the ureter and possible reflux. A 3.7–4.8-Fr indwelling ureteral stent is placed cystoscopically under general anesthesia and left in place for passive dilatation of the ureter. This is removed after 1–3 weeks, allowing easy passage of a ureteroscope into the ureter. With this staged approach, subsequent balloon dilatation of the ureter for URS is not required; however, an additional procedure under general anesthesia is required.

Stone Fragmentation

The currently available sources of energy for stone fragmentation are holmium:YAG laser, ultrasound lithotripsy, pneumatic lithotripsy, and electrohydraulic lithotripsy (EHL).

The most successful and popular modality is laser as it can be used in flexible ureteroscopes allowing access even to intrarenal calculi [72]. Safwat et al. [76] performed ureteroscopic holmium laser lithotripsy in 15 children successfully on an outpatient basis. Binbay et al. [77] compared pneumatic lithotripsy with holmium:YAG lithotripsy in impacted ureteral stones in adults and found that operating time was diminished, with better stone-free rates of 97.5 % with holmium:YAG laser versus 80 % with pneumatic lithotripsy, making the former more efficient and safe. Pneumatic lithotripsy with a rigid probe is invaluable for lower ureteric stone and can be used successfully for upper ureteric stones in children. Pneumatic lithotripsy remains the authors' choice as it is extremely cost effective and successful in stone fragmentation [78].

Postoperative Stenting

The rationale for postoperative stenting has been potential decrease in stricture formation and pain. However, stents can actually be the cause of significant pain and bothersome lower urinary tract symptoms such as hematuria, dysuria, and pain [79]. Additionally stents can migrate, cause UTI, break, encrust, obstruct, and be forgotten in situ. Some large series [80] advocate routinely leaving a stent postoperatively, while others have found routine stenting after uncomplicated URS to be unnecessary [81]. In our experience, a decision to stent should be made according to situation, and we recommend post URS stenting in case of visible ureteral injury, solitary kidney, renal insufficiency, or a large residual stone burden. If edema at the ureteric orifice is anticipated, the authors would prefer to leave an externally draining ureteric catheter hinged on a Foley catheter for 24 h. This is cost effective and does not require a further procedure for removal.

Complications

The most common complication following pediatric ureteroscopic lithotripsy is hematuria, ureteric colic, and postoperative urosepsis. In a retrospective study [82], the incidences of hematuria and urosepsis were 27 and 8 %, respectively. Reported incidence of ureteral perforation in published studies is 1.4 %, similar to that seen in adult patients [66]. One concern during ureterorenoscopy is fluid absorption, and if water is used, it can lead to severe intravascular hemolysis and hyponatremia resulting in seizure and even death. Cybulski et al. [83] studied fluid absorption during ureteroscopy prospectively. In their series the mean estimated systemic fluid absorption during URS was 54 ml (range 4–137 ml). There were two intraoperative ureteral perforations but no postoperative complications reported.

Outcomes of Ureteroscopy in Children

In terms of overall safety, pediatric ureteroscopy has been validated as a safe modality in contemporary series. Intraoperative complications, defined as ureteral injury (ischemia, perforation, and avulsion), or postoperative complications (mainly ureteral stricture) have shown to be extremely rare. The overall complication rates ranged from 0 to 5.2 % [72, 80, 84]. In a systemic review of the literature encompassing 221 pediatric ureteroscopies, Schuster et al. [66] noted only two ureteral strictures and minimal incidence of VUR.

Stone clearance efficacy of pediatric URS in proximal ureteric stones has been shown to be superior to ESWL. In a prospective randomized study, De Dominicis et al. [85] demonstrated a statistically significant higher success rate of ureteroscopy with intracorporeal lithotripsy (success rate of 94 % with one treatment), compared to ESWL (42 % after one session, 64 % after two sessions). Reddy and DeFoor [86] performed a systematic review of contemporary urological literature on ureteroscopy (URS) looking for all articles published from 1990 to 2009 and indexed in PubMed. A total of 27 papers that met the inclusion criteria for this review were identified and data abstracted. During the past 20 years, the results of 832 pediatric patients (mean age 9.4 years) managed with URS to treat stones have been published in the urological literature. In the same time frame, there were a total of 21 papers published discussing the results with ESWL, including a total of 1,839 patients (mean age 7.9 years). The success rates of URS and ESWL were 93.4 and 80.3 %, respectively. The complication rate associated with the URS procedures is 5.9 % and compares favorably with 8.4 % for ESWL. In a large series of 100 children with a mean stone diameter of 8.3 mm, Smaldone et al. [80] reported a 91 % stone-free rate with 9 % of children undergoing staged procedure. They reported a 4.2 % perforation rate managed with ureteral stenting and one distal ureteric stricture requiring open neocystostomy.

Conclusion

With increasing international experience of endoscopic surgery in children, miniaturizing of instruments, and availability of more effective stone fragmentation devices, PCNL and ureteroscopy in children have become safe and highly effective for stones in children of all ages.

References

1. Afshar K, Mclorie G, Papanikolaou F, Pippi Salle JL, Bagli DJ, Khoury AE. Outcome of small residual stone fragments following shock wave lithotripsy in children. J Urol. 2004;172:1600–3.
2. Fernstorm I, Johansson B. Percutaneous pyelolithotomy. A new extraction technique. Scand J Urol Nephrol. 1976;10:257–9.

3. Rusnak B, Castaneda-Zuniga W, Kotula F, Herrera M, Amplatz K. An improved dilator system for percutaneous nephrostomies. Radiology. 1982;144:174.
4. Alken P. Telescopbougierst zur perkutanen nephrostomie. Akt Urol. 1981;12:216–9.
5. Clayman RV, Castaneda-Zuniga WR, Hunter DW, Miller RP, Lange PH, Amplatz K. Rapid balloon dilatation of nephrostomy track for nephrostolithotomy. Radiology. 1983;147:884–5.
6. Woodside JR, Stevens JF, Strak JL, Borden TA, Ball WS. Percutaneous stone removal in children. J Urol. 1985;134:1166–7.
7. Mor Y, Elmarsy YE, Kellet MJ, Duffy PG. The role of percutaneous nephrolithotomy in the management of pediatric renal calculi. J Urol. 1997;158:1319–21.
8. Helal M, Black T, Lockhart J, Figueroa TE. The Hickman peel-away sheath: alternative for pediatric percutaneous nephrolithotomy. J Endourol. 1997;11:171–2.
9. Samad L, Aquil S, Zaidi Z. Pediatric percutaneous nephrolithotomy: setting new frontiers. BJU Int. 2006;97:353–63.
10. Wu HY, Docimo SG. Surgical management of children with urolithiasis. Urol Clin North Am. 2004;31:589–94.
11. Farhat WA, Kropp BP. Surgical treatment of pediatric urinary stones. AUA Update Ser. 2007;26:22.
12. Mendez Probost CE, Denstedt JD, Razvi H. Preoperative indications for percutaneous nephrolithotomy in 2009. J Endourol. 2009;23:1557–61.
13. Dogan HS, Sahin A, Cetinkaya Y, Akdogan B, Ozden E, Kendi S. Antibiotic prophylaxis in percutaneous nephrolithotomy: prospective study in 81 patients. J Endourol. 2002;16:649–53.
14. Charton M, Vallencien G, Veillon B, et al. Urinary tract infection in percutaneous surgery for renal calculi. J Urol. 1986;135:15–7.
15. Clayman RV, Casteneda-Zuniga WR. Techniques in endourology. A guide to percutaneous removal of renal and ureteral calculi. Chicago: Year Book Medical Publishers; 1984.
16. Wolf Jr JS, Bennet CJ, Dmochowski RR, Hollenbeck BK, Pearle MS, Schaeffer AJ. Urological surgery antimicrobial prophylaxis best practice policy panel. Best practice policy statement on urologic surgery antimicrobial prophylaxis. J Urol. 2008;179:1379–90.
17. Grabe M, Bishop MC, Bjerklund-Johansen TE, Botto H, et al. European Association of Urology. Guidelines on urological infections (updated 2009). European Guidelines office (publ). Web access: www.uroweb.org. Accessed on March 20, 2011.
18. Rozentsveig V, Neulander EZ, Gurevich B, Klein Y, Weksler N. Anesthetic consideration during percutaneous nephrolithotomy. J Clin Anesth. 2007;19:351–5.
19. Frank SM, Kluger MJ, Kunkel SL. Elevated thermostatic setpoint in postoperative patients. Anesthesiology. 2000;93:1426–31.
20. Ost MC, Lee BR. Urolithiasis in patients with spinal cord injuries: risk factors, management and outcomes. Curr Opin Urol. 2006;16:93–9.
21. Mahmud M, Zaidi Z. Percutaneous nephrolithotomy in children before school age: experience of a Pakistani center. BJU Int. 2004;94:1352–4.
22. Schuster TK, Smaldone MC, Averch TD, Ost MC. Percutaneous nephrolithotomy in children. J Endourol. 2009;23:1699–705.
23. Wezel F, Charalampos M, Jorge R, Maurice SM, de la Rosette J, Alken P. Two contemporary series of percutaneous tract dilatation for percutaneous nephrolithotomy. J Endourol. 2009;23:1655–61.
24. Jackman SV, Docimo SG, Cadeddu JA, Bishoff JT, Kavoussi LR, Jarrett TW. The "mini-perc" technique: a less invasive alternative to percutaneous nephrolithotomy. World J Urol. 1998;16:371–4.
25. Sung YM, Choo SW, Jeon SS, Shin SW, Park KB, Do YS. The "mini-perc" technique of percutaneous nephrolithotomy with a 14-Fr peel-away sheath: 3 year results in 72 patients. Korean J Radiol. 2006;7:50–6.
26. Guisiti G, Seveso M, Taverna G, Piccinelli A, Graziotti P. Miniperc ? No thank you. Eur Urol Suppl. 2006;5:110.
27. Bilen CY, Kocak B, Kitirci G. Percutaneous nephrolithotomy in children: lessons learned in 5 years at a single institution. J Urol. 2007;177:1867–71.
28. Nouralizadeh A, Basiri A, Javaherforooshzadeh A, Soltani MH, Tajali F. Experience of percutaneous nephrolithotomy using adult size instruments in children less than 5 years old. J Pediatr Urol. 2009;5:351–4.
29. Smaldone MC, Gayed BA, Ost MC. The evolution of the endourological management of pediatric stone disease. Indian J Urol. 2009;25:302–11.
30. Srinivasan AK, Herati A, Okeke Z, Smith A. Renal drainage after percutaneous nephrolithotomy. J Endourol. 2009;23:1743–9.
31. Limb J, Bellman GC. Tubeless percutaneous renal surgery: review of first 112 patients. Urology. 2002;59:527–31.
32. Yoon GH, Bellman GC. Tubeless percutaneous nephrolithotomy: a new standard in percutaneous renal surgery. J Endourol. 2008;9:1865–9.
33. Khairy Salem H, Morsi HA, Omran A, Daw MA. Tubeless percutaneous nephrolithotomy in children. J Pediatr Urol. 2007;3:235–8.
34. Zaidi Z, Samad L. Tubeless vs tubed PCNL in children. J Pediatr Urol. 2009;5(S1):36–7.
35. Ozturk A, Guven S, Kilinc M, Topbas E, Piskin M, Arslan M. Totally tubeless percutaneous nephrolithotomy: is it safe and effective in preschool children? J Endourol. 2010;24:1935–9.
36. Salah MA, Tallai B, Holman E, Khan MA, Toth G, Toth C. Simultaneous bilateral percutaneous nephrolithotomy in children. BJU Int. 2005;95:137–9.
37. Choong S, Whitfield H, Duffy P. The management of pediatric urolithiasis. BJU Int. 2000;86:857–60.
38. Desai MR, Jasani A. Percutaneous nephrolithotripsy in ectopic kidneys. J Endourol. 2000;14:289–92.
39. Razvi S, Zaidi Z. Percutaneous nephrolithotomy (PCNL) in horseshoe kidneys. J Pak Med Assoc. 2007;57:222–4.
40. Aquil S, Rana AM, Zaidi Z. Laparoscopic assisted percutaneous nephrolithotomy in ectopic pelvic kidney. J Pak Med Assoc. 2006;5:381–3.
41. Desai MR, Kukreja RA, Patel SH. Percutaneous nephrolithotomy for complex pediatric renal calculus disease. J Endourol. 2004;18:23–7.
42. Zaren S, Satar N, Bayazit Y, Bayazit AK, Payasli K, Ozkeceli R. Percutaneous nephrolithotomy in the management of pediatric renal calculi. J Endourol. 2002;16:75–8.
43. Salah MA, Toth C, Khan MA, Holman E. Percutaneous nephrolithotomy in children: experience with 138 cases in a developing country. World J Urol. 2004;22:227–80.
44. Turna B, Nazli O, Demiryoguran S, Mammadov R, Cal C. Percutaneous nephrolithotomy: variables that influence hemorrhage. Urology. 2007;69:603–7.
45. Bogris S, Papatsoris AG. Status quo of percutaneous nephrolithotomy in children. Urol Res. 2010;38:1–5.
46. Kukreja RA, Desai MR, Sabnis RB, Patel SH. Fluid absorption during percutaneous nephrolithotomy: does it matter? J Endourol. 2002;16:221–4.
47. Shokeir AA, Sheir KZ, El-Nahas AR, El-Assmy AM, Eassa W, El-Kappany HA. Treatment of renal stones in children; a comparison between percutaneous nephrolithotomy and shock wave lithotripsy. J Urol. 2006;176:706–10.
48. Holman E, Khan AM, Flasko T, Toth C, Salah MA. Endoscopic management of pediatric urolithiasis in a developing country. Urology. 2004;63:159–62.
49. Dawaba MS, Shokeir AA, Hafez AT, et al. Percutaneous nephrolithotomy in children: early and late anatomical and functional results. J Urol. 2004;172:1078–81.
50. Nouralizadeh A, Sichani MM, Kashi AK. Impact of percutaneous nephrolithotomy on estimated glomerular filtration rate during the first few days after surgery. Urol Res. 2011;39:129–33.

51. Samad L, Qureshi S, Zaidi Z. Does percutaneous nephrolithotomy in children cause significant renal scarring? J Pediatr Urol. 2007;3:36–9.
52. De la Rosette JJMCH, Laguna MP, Rassweiler JJ, Conort P. Training in percutaneous nephrolithotomy – a critical review. Eur Urol. 2008;54:994–1003.
53. Young HM, McKay RW. Congenital valvular obstruction of the prostatic urethra. Surg Gyencol Obstet. 1929;48:509.
54. Ritchey M, Patterson DE, Kelalis PP. A case of pediatric ureteroscopic lasertripsy. J Urol. 1988;139(6):1272–4.
55. Van Savage JG, Palanca LG, Andersen RD, Rao GS, Slaughenhoupt BL. Treatment of distal ureteral stones in children: similarities to American urological association guidelines in adults. J Urol. 2000;164:1089–93.
56. Turk C, Knoll T, Petrik A, Sarcia K, Seitz C, Straub M, Traxer O. Guidelines on urolithiasis. 2010. European Guidelines Office (publ) Web access: www.uroweb.org/guidelines/urolithiasis. Accessed on March 20, 2011.
57. Assimos DG, Patterson LC, Taylor CL. Changing incidence and etiology of iatrogenic ureteral injuries. J Urol. 1994;152:2240.
58. Lam JS, Cooper KL, Green TD, et al. Impact of hydronephrosis and renal function on treatment outcomes: antegrade versus retrograde endopyelotomy. Urology. 2003;61:1107.
59. Reddy PP. Pediatric ureteroscopy. Urol Clin North Am. 2004;31: 145–56.
60. Korkes F, Lopes-Neto AC, Mattos MH, Pompeo AC, Wroclawski ER. Patient position and semirigid ureteroscopy outcomes. Int Braz J Urol. 2009;35:542–50.
61. Shepherd P, Thomas R, Harmon EP. Urolithiasis in children: innovations in management. J Urol. 1988;140:790–2.
62. Bassiri A, Ahmadnia H, Darabi MR, Yonessi M. Transureteral lithotripsy in pediatric practice. J Endourol. 2002;16:257.
63. Caione P, De Gennaro M, Capozza N, et al. Endoscopic manipulation of ureteral calculi in children by rigid operative ureteroscopy. J Urol. 1990;144:484–9.
64. Hill DE, Segura JW, Patterson DE, Kramer SA. Ureteroscopy in children. J Urol. 1990;144:481–3.
65. Thomas R, Ortenberg J, Lee BR, et al. Safety and efficacy of pediatric ureteroscopy for management of calculous disease. J Urol. 1993;149:1082–4.
66. Schuster TG, Russell KY, Bloom DA, Koo HP, Faerber GJ. Ureteroscopy for the treatment of urolithiasis in children. J Urol. 2002;167:1813–6. discussion 1815–6.
67. Soygur T, Zumrutbas AE, Gulpinar O, Suer E, Arikan N. Hydrodilation of the ureteral orifice in children renders ureteroscopic access possible without any further active dilation. J Urol. 2006;176:285–7.
68. Gedik A, Orgen S, Akay AF, Sahin H, Bircan MK. Semirigid ureterorenoscopy in children without ureteral dilation. Int Urol Nephrol. 2008;40:11–4.
69. Singh A, Shah G, Young J, Sheridan M, Haas G, Upadhyay J. Ureteral access sheath for the management of pediatric renal and ureteral stones. A single center experience. J Urol. 2006;175:1080–2.
70. Satar N, Zeren S, Bayazit Y, Aridogan IA, Soyupak B, Tansug Z. Rigid ureteroscopy for treatment of ureteral calculi in children. J Urol. 2004;172:298–300.
71. Tanriverdi O, Silay MS, Kendirci M, Kadihasnoglu M, Aydin M, Horasanli K, et al. Comparison of ureteroscopic procedures with rigid and semirigid ureteroscopes in pediatric population: does the caliber of instrument matter? Pediatr Surg Int. 2010;26:733–8.
72. Kim SS, Kolon TF, Canter D, White M, Casale P. Pediatric flexible ureteroscopic lithotripsy: the Children's hospital of Philadelphia experience. J Urol. 2008;180:2616–9.
73. Rubenstein RA, Zhao LC, Loeb S, Shore DM, Nadler RB. Prestenting improves ureteroscopic stone free rates. J Endourol. 2007;21:1277.
74. Hubert KC, Palmer JS. Passive dilation by ureteral stenting before ureteroscopy: eliminating the need for active dilation. J Urol. 2005;174:1079–81.
75. Corcoran AT, Smaldone MC, Mally D, Ost MC, Bellinger MF, Schneck FX, et al. When is prior ureteral stent placement necessary to access the upper urinary tract in prepubertal children. J Urol. 2008;180:1861–4.
76. Safwat AS, Bissada NK, Kumar U, Taha MI, Abdel-hafez SES, Eltaher AM, et al. Experience with ureteroscopic holmium laser lithotripsy in children. Pediatr Surg Int. 2008;24:579–81.
77. Binbay M, Tepler A, Yuruk E, Sarilar O, Ozkuvanci U, Muslumanoglu AY. Comparative evaluation of pneumatic versus holmium:YAG laser lithotripsy for impacted ureteral stones. In: EAU 5th south eastern European meeting/European urology supplement, 2009, vol. 8, p. 607–55.
78. Fuganti PE, Pires SR, Branco RO, Porto JL. Ballistic ureteroscopic lithotripsy in prepubertal patients: a feasible option for ureteral stones. Int Braz J Urol. 2006;32:322–9.
79. Pryor JL, Langley MJ, Jenkins AD. Comparison of symptoms characteristic of indwelling ureteral catheters. J Urol. 1991;145:719.
80. Smaldone MC, Cannon GM, Wu HY, Basett J, Polsky EG, Bellinger MF, et al. Is ureteroscopy first line treatment for pediatric stone disease? J Urol. 2007;178:2128–31.
81. Byrne RR, Auge BK, Kourambas J, Munver R, Delvecchio F, Preminger GM. Routine ureteral stenting is not necessary after ureteroscopy and ureteropyeloscopy: a randomized trial. J Endourol. 2002;16(1):9–13.
82. Rizvi SA, Naqvi SA, Hussain Z, Hashmi A, Hussain M, Zafar MN, et al. Management of pediatric urolithiasis in Pakistan: experience with 1,440 children. J Urol. 2003;169(2):634–7.
83. Cybulski P, Honey RJ, Pace K. Fluid absorption during ureterorenoscopy. J Endourol. 2004;18(8):739–42.
84. Minevich E, Defoor W, Reddy P, Nishinaka K, Waksman J, Sheldon C, et al. Ureteroscopy is safe and effective in prepubertal children. J Urol. 2005;174:276–9. discussion 279.
85. De Dominicis M, Matarazzo E, Capozza N, Collura G, Caione P. Retrograde ureteroscopy for distal ureteric stone removal in children. BJU Int. 2005;95:1049–52.
86. Reddy PP, DeFoor WR. Ureteroscopy: the standard of care in the management of upper tract urolithiasis in children. Indian J Urol. 2010;26:555–63.

Part VIII

Prevention of Recurrence

Biochemical Risk Evaluation in Patients with Urolithiasis

84

Hans-Göran Tiselius

Abstract

This chapter is an overview of the biochemical evaluation of patients with urinary tract stone disease. The aim is to give practical aspects on how the search for risk factors can be carried out when stone composition is known or unknown. The physical chemistry of stone formation is superficially touched.

Aspects on the importance of the medical history, the radiographic evaluation, and the stone, blood, and urine analysis are discussed. The goal of every metabolic or biochemical evaluation is to provide a basis for a reasonable and effective recurrence prevention. The intention with this chapter is to give information in this regard.

Keywords

Stone analysis • Blood analysis • Urine analysis • Calcium stones • Uric acid stones • Cystine stones • Infection stones • Medical history • Radiography • Preservative of urine • AP(CaOx) index • AP(CaP) index • Protein intake

Introduction

For a rational and effective prevention (metaphylaxis) of recurrent stone formation in the urinary tract, it is necessary to identify relevant risk factors that explain or contribute to the pathology [1]. In view of the fact that almost all patients with uric acid stones, infection stones, and cystine stones and approximately at least 50 % of patients with calcium stones will continue to form new stones, measures aiming at a reduced risk are highly desirable.

It is of note that the introduction of noninvasive or low-invasive methods for active stone removal, undoubtedly, resulted in a rather nihilistic attitude among several urologists who subsequently considered both risk evaluation and recurrence prevention as unnecessary overdoing for their stone patients.

Although a definite explanation for calcium stone formation is lacking, there are several obvious risk factors, the correction of which will result in an arrest or at least a significant reduction in the rate of stone formation. For patients with uric acid, cystine, and infection stone formation, the causes are well recognized and so are the therapeutic tools.

Moreover, it needs to be emphasized that although the procedures for stone removal have become dramatically improved and relatively easy, none of such procedures are entirely without complications and definitely not without cost. Active stone removal—with a slightly increased indication during recent years—is applicable to roughly 30–40 % of the patients [2, 3]. For the remaining patients, stones are expected to pass spontaneously. In most situations, a nonsurgical treatment is superior to all kinds of surgical stone removal in its widest sense. Also for the latter group of patients, it will usually be necessary with medical support and very often repeated visits to an emergency unit. According to several economic analyses, selective recurrence prevention is cost effective [4–10].

H-G. Tiselius, M.D., Ph.D.
Division of Urology, Department of Clinical Science, Intervention and Technology, Karolinska Institutet, Stockholm, SE-141 86, Sweden
e-mail: hans-goran.tiselius@telia.com, hans-goran.tiselius@ki.se

J.J. Talati et al. (eds.), *Urolithiasis*,
DOI 10.1007/978-1-4471-4387-1_84, © Springer-Verlag London 2012

Stone Composition

Search for factors responsible for or contributing to the stone formation requires knowledge of the stone composition. The fundamental step in the evaluation of the disease, therefore, is an appropriate stone analysis. How this analysis technically should be carried out is extensively discussed elsewhere in this book (see Chap. 85). Suffice it here to state that patients always should get instructions to collect passed stones or stone fragments. Analysis of the stone composition is recommended at least once for every patient. Repeated analysis is indicated if it can be assumed that the prerequisites for stone formation for any reason have been changed [4].

With an appropriate stone analysis, we will know whether the patient has produced a calcium stone with calcium oxalate (calcium oxalate monohydrate [COM] and/or calcium oxalate dihydrate [COD]), calcium phosphate (hydroxyapatite [HAP], octacalcium phosphate [OCP], carbonate apatite, whitlockite, or brushite), mixtures of calcium oxalate and calcium phosphate, or a non-calcium stone composed of infection stone material (magnesium ammonium phosphate + carbonate apatite, ammonium urate), uric acid, or cystine. The stone analysis also makes it possible to identify stones composed of less commonly encountered crystal phases such as 2,8-dihydroxyadenine, xanthine, and silicates.

Not unexpectedly a large number of patients never bring a stone to analysis, because the stone material has been lost, passed without any obvious symptoms, or remains in the renal collecting system inaccessible to appropriate analysis. Also in these cases it is desirable to draw reasonable conclusions on the stone composition.

In the absence of a stone analysis, qualified indirect assumptions are necessary [11]. An algorithm for such a procedure is shown in Fig. 84.1.

Today, the stone diagnosis is established by urography; plain radiograph of kidneys, ureters, and bladder (KUB); or non-contrast helical computerized tomography (NCCT). Ideally, when both KUB and NCCT have been carried out, it can be concluded that a stone visible on the NCCT image and not visible on the KUB most likely is composed of uric acid [4, 12]. It should be noted, however, that very large stones composed of uric acid give a weak density also on the KUB.

When only a KUB is available, some features are useful. Infection stones (staghorn or non-staghorn stones) usually, but not always, have a layered morphology. Cystine stones have a radiodensity that is low relative to the size of the stone. Stones with a very compact structure with a high density are usually composed of COM or brushite, whereas stones with burdock (spiky) morphology suggest COD. It is of note that complete staghorn stones can develop with any crystal phase, and the finding of a staghorn stone does not necessarily mean an infection etiology.

When an NCCT examination is available, measurement of Hounsfield units (HU) can be very helpful for the decisions on the stone composition [13]. Unfortunately, there is an overlapping of HU recordings for different stone constituents. The latter problem has recently been addressed by applying dual photon energy technique [14, 15], but such

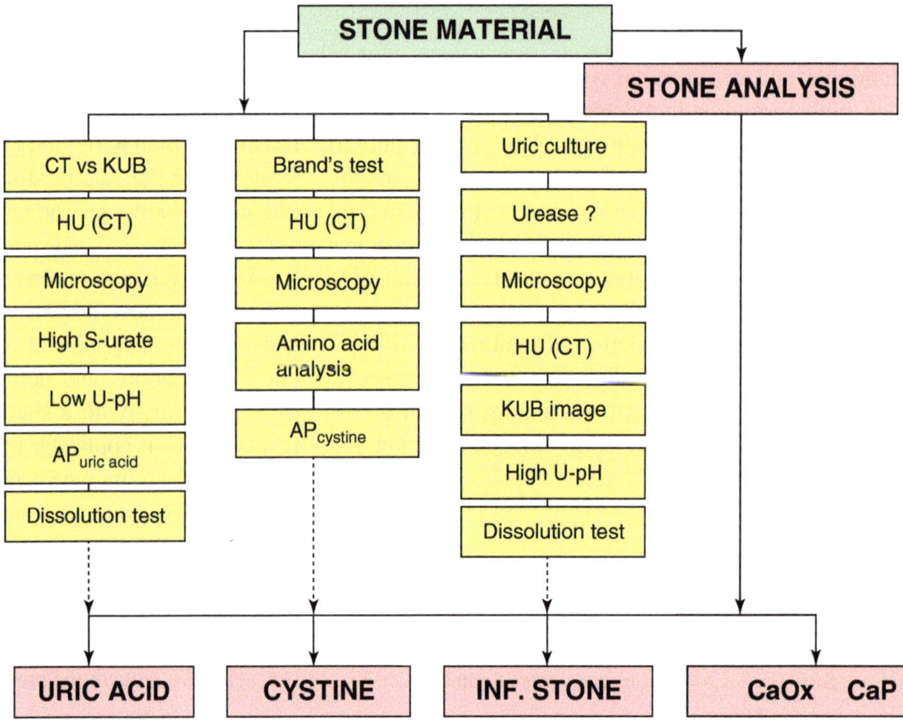

Fig. 84.1 An algorithm for deciding what kind of stone the patient has formed

advanced facilities presently have limited availability. Three HU intervals can roughly be used for practical conclusions on stone composition: high (HU > 1,000), medium (HU = 500–1,000), and low (HU < 500). The low values correspond to stones composed of uric acid, cystine, and struvite (magnesium ammonium phosphate) and the highest for COM and brushite. Stones with intermediate HU values might be composed of COD, HAP, and carbonate apatite. Further support for an appropriate conclusion on stone composition can be made with other tools.

Microscopic identification of typical cystine (hexagonal) or struvite (coffin-shaped) crystals is diagnostic for cystinuria and infection stone disease, respectively [11, 16, 17]. Demonstration of COD crystals might indicate calcium oxalate stone formation, but such crystals are commonly encountered also in urine from non-stone-forming subjects and thus of limited diagnostic value. Urine sediment with brown/red color (from a sample without hematuria) is typically found in association with uric acid stones.

When cystine is a possibility, the sodium nitroprusside test (Brand's test) is a useful qualitative analysis to confirm cystinuria [18].

A low urine pH is associated with uric acid stone formation [19, 20] and a high pH with infection stones and calcium phosphate stones [21]. In the absence of standardized principles for pH measurements, it is usually difficult to use urinary pH for conclusions, unless the pH recordings are extreme. Fasting morning urine samples might be most useful in this regard and also of value for decisions on whether the patient has an acidification defect or not [4, 22–24], but it is not always possible to get such samples.

A high serum or plasma level of urate (in patients with normal renal function) might give further support to uric acid stone formation, provided other observations do not exclude that type of stone.

When still in doubt of the kind of stone disease, measurements of supersaturation levels with uric acid and cystine can give valuable information. This approach is further discussed as follows.

Medical History

Like in most other fields of medicine, a careful medical history can give valuable clues to or a full explanation of the stone disease. There are several medical diseases as well as various forms of pharmacological treatment that are more or less closely associated with an increased risk of abnormalities in urine composition, crystallization, and stone formation. The most important of these factors will be summarized below.

Diseases Associated with Stone Formation

One of the best recognized explanations for calcium stone formation is *hyperparathyroidism* [22, 25–27]. Adenomas or hyperplasia of the parathyroid glands is responsible for an excessive production of parathyroid hormone (PTH). The biochemical consequence that leads to stone formation is hypercalciuria caused by hypercalcemia. The importance of a correct diagnosis is best understood by the fact that a correction of this abnormality usually results in arrest of stone formation.

There are also other conditions with hypercalcemia that result in an increased urinary excretion of calcium and accordingly an increased risk of calcium stone formation. In this regard, *sarcoidosis* and *immobilization* need attention. High urinary calcium levels also are encountered in patients with *hyperthyroidism* [22].

Abnormalities in intestinal function with fat malabsorption, loss of water, and alkali are seen in patients with Crohn's disease, intestinal resection, different forms of bypass procedures used for weight-reducing purposes, pancreatic insufficiency, and other conditions with intestinal malfunction [22, 25–27]. The risk of stone formation is based mainly on high urinary concentrations of oxalate (*enteric hyperoxaluria*), but the small urine volumes together with low pH levels also contribute to a pronounced crystallization propensity. These patients also have low excretion of calcium, but since oxalate is a relatively more powerful determinant of calcium oxalate supersaturation, very high crystallization driving forces are obtained.

Although the majority of patients with intestinal malfunction and diarrhea form calcium oxalate stones, it is of note that uric acid stones commonly are seen in patients with *ileostomy*, because of the very low pH levels encountered as a result of extreme losses of alkali. Similarly in patients with *ulcerative colitis*, both uric acid and calcium oxalate stones might form.

Whereas 24-h oxalate excretion levels in the range of 0.6–1.2 mmol are typical for patients with enteric hyperoxaluria, higher oxalate values might suggest *primary hyperoxaluria* [22]. This rare inborn error of metabolism can present with different degrees of severity. In the most advanced form, it is a life-threatening condition with both excessive calcium oxalate stone formation and calcium oxalate tissue deposits. Primary hyperoxaluria must be excluded when stone formation starts very early in life.

There are some less common disturbances in purine metabolism leading to increased excretion of urate and uric acid stone formation. In *Lesch-Nyhan syndrome*, the treatment with high doses of xanthine oxidase inhibitors might result in precipitation of *xanthine* [22]. Xanthine oxidase is responsible both for the conversion of hypoxanthine to xanthine and of xanthine to urate. Another abnormality in purine metabolism (defect function of adenine phosphoribosyltransferase) is the origin of 2,8-dihydroxyadenine stones [22].

Distal renal tubular acidosis (dRTA) in a complete or partial form causes stone formation by a combination of hypercalciuria and alkaline urine. The acidification defect also leads to hypocitraturia. The condition that is most common in women should be suspected in case of calcium phosphate stone formation [24]. The inability to acidify urine below pH 5.8 is of diagnostic importance [4, 23]. A fasting morning urine pH, analysis of urine pH in repeated collections during the day (pH profile), or analysis of urine after an acid load can be used for diagnostic purposes (discussed later) [24]. Proximal renal tubular acidosis (pRTA) is not associated with stone formation.

Cystinuria is an inborn error of metabolism that explains stone formation in 1–2 % of stone formers. The homozygous form is necessary for cystine concentrations leading to stone formation. The increased excretion of the amino acids lysine, ornithine, and arginine that also are excreted in large quantities is not important for stone formation, and the loss of these amino acids is generally considered to be without important physiological or metabolic consequences.

The increased risk of stone formation in patients with *metabolic syndrome* is well recognized [28, 29], and so is the risk of stone formation in patients with *hypertension* and *diabetes mellitus* [29].

Pharmacological Agents Associated with Stone Formation

There are some forms of pharmacological treatment to which attention should be paid as a possible explanation of stone formation.

Supplements of *calcium* and *vitamin D* commonly used in the treatment of patients with osteoporosis can give rise to hypercalciuria [30]. The intake of these agents together with meals—and not between—should be advised.

Vitamin C in large (orthomolecular) quantities can result in an increased excretion of oxalate. Individual variations most certainly exist, and the allowed amount of vitamin C has remained a matter of debate. It is commonly considered safe if the daily amount of ascorbate does not exceed 2–4 g [31–33].

Thyroid hormone causes hypercalciuria. Acetazolamide increases urine pH while simultaneously reducing urinary citrate in a way similar to that seen with dRTA [34]. These alterations lead to an increased risk of calcium phosphate precipitation and stone formation.

The low solubility of sulfonamides, triamterene, and indinavir might result in precipitation and stone formation with that composition.

Treatment with corticosteroids increases the risk of stone formation by an increased calcium excretion.

Identification of Anatomical and Morphological Abnormalities

Factors causing stagnation of urine or a turbulent flow are probably of great importance in the stone-forming process, and their presence needs to be identified.

Conditions with obstruction of the ureteropelvic junction, ureteral strictures, horseshoe kidneys, and malrotated kidneys are usually associated with hydronephrosis. Crystalline material that develops in retained urine of a dilated collecting system cannot easily be eliminated [35, 36]. In sufficiently supersaturated urine, the crystals grow and aggregate to clinically important stones. Intrarenal obstructions to the urine flow, such as narrow calyx necks and calyx diverticula, are other risk factors of stone formation.

All of the mentioned anatomical abnormalities can usually be detected by NCCT.

Another common clinical entity is tubular ectasia (medullary sponge kidney disease [MSK]). This abnormality might occur in the whole kidney or only in part of the kidney. The best procedure for discovering MSK is probably by a standard urography [37, 38].

With NCCT, the diagnosis can be indirectly suspected from the distribution of calcifications. For correct diagnosis of MSK with NCCT, special image manipulation is necessary, and with the less common use of contrast medium, there is a risk that the diagnosis of MSK often will be overlooked.

It also needs to be emphasized that those patients who have been subjected to invasive surgical procedures might have scar tissue and various iatrogenic intrarenal abnormalities of great importance for stone formation.

Basic Blood Analyses

For all patients with urolithiasis, it is essential to get information on the renal function. Thereby, analysis of *serum(S-) creatinine* is a sufficiently accurate guide.

As mentioned previously, detection of hyperuricemia can give support to an otherwise suspected risk of uric acid stone formation. It is of note, however, that S-*urate* is increased when the renal function is reduced, and a simultaneous *S-creatinine* analysis is necessary for conclusions. Moreover, a normal urate level in no way excludes the possibility of uric acid stone formation. A relationship between hyperuricemia and calcium oxalate stone formation also has been suggested [39]. There are, unfortunately, no recent studies of such a mechanism, and possibly, a high urate level only reflects one of several abnormalities associated with the metabolic syndrome [21, 28, 29].

Inasmuch as most patients form calcium stones, it is important to find those in whom hypercalcemia is an underlying reason. Of conditions with hypercalcemia, it is most essential to identify patients with hyperparathyroidism, because that is in most cases a surgically curable condition. When the serum or plasma calcium exceeds 2.50–2.60 mmol/L, there is good reason to repeat the measurement and to add analysis of *ionized calcium* and *PTH*. Moreover, analysis of *S-phosphate* might be of diagnostic value in these patients.

Another important serum variable is *S-potassium*, since hypokalemia causes hypocitraturia [40, 41] and thereby an increased risk of calcium oxalate and calcium phosphate precipitation, growth, and aggregation [40, 42].

The blood analyses mentioned here are the only ones that I personally find unavoidable in the work-up of patients with stone disease. It is of course important to note that specific circumstances might require other blood analyses, but the variables listed are those that should be considered as a basic set for every stone former.

Solution Chemistry of Uric Acid

Precipitates in which urate is an important constituent are most often composed of uric acid. Although sodium urate theoretically can form stones, that crystal phase is rarely encountered clinically, and the same is true for potassium urate. The most common crystal phase beside uric acid is ammonium urate, but the formation of an ammonium urate precipitate is a result of infection with urease-producing bacteria at sufficiently high concentrations of urinary urate. The latter precipitate therefore should be considered to reflect an infection stone problem (see later) [4].

There are two prerequisites for formation of uric acid stones. Firstly and most important, the pH should be low. Secondly, there must be a reasonably high concentration of urate, either caused by an excessive excretion of urate or by a small urine volume. But it needs to be emphasized that uric acid precipitation can occur also with normal urinary urate concentrations, provided the urine is sufficiently acid. With this basic understanding, the ion-activity product of uric acid $AP_{uric\text{-}acid}$ can be calculated from the following formula [21, 22]:

$$AP_{uric\text{-}acid} = \frac{C_{urate} \cdot 10^{-pH} \cdot 0.53}{(1 + 1.63 \cdot 10^{5} \cdot 10^{-pH})}$$

In this formula, the concentration of urate (C_{urate}) is expressed in mol/L. The formation (FP) and solubility (SP) products of uric acid are approximately $5.0 \cdot 10^{-9}$ (mol/L)^2 and $2.0 \cdot 10^{-9}$ (mol/L)^2, respectively [21].

From a clinical point of view, $AP_{uric\ acid}$ can be derived from analyses of a 24-h urine sample only by measuring urate and pH. It is essential, however, to get a representative measurement of urine pH, and it has been the author's own routine to measure the urine composition in one 16-h and one 8-h urine sample [4, 11]. Even such an approach is not ideal, but in most clinical situations, it gives a rough idea of the supersaturation with uric acid. This analytical step also can be very helpful to confirm or exclude uric acid stone disease. The therapeutic goal in uric acid stone-forming patients should be to decrease $AP_{uric\ acid}$ to a level below $SP_{uric\ acid}$.

Sodium azide (0.3 mmol/L) is an appropriate preservative to add to the collection bottles: 30 mL for a 24-h urine sample, 20 mL for a 16-h sample, and 10 mL for an 8-h sample [11]. Moreover, it needs to be emphasized that the pH should be measured with a glass electrode as soon as possible after completion of the urine collection. That means that the sample should be taken care of within the first few hours after delivery of the sample to the laboratory. It goes without saying that urate cannot be measured in acidified samples!

Corresponding formulas for $AP_{ammonium\ urate}$ and $AP_{sodium\ urate}$ have been derived and can be found elsewhere [21].

The estimate of $AP_{uric\ acid}$ shown previously can be used as part of a risk evaluation, but it is also an excellent tool for follow-up of patients during recurrence prevention or stone dissolution.

Solution Chemistry of Cystine

An estimate of the ion-activity product of cystine ($AP_{cystine}$) is obtained from information on the concentration of cystine in urine and the pH. Although the expression for calculating $AP_{cystine}$ looks complicated, the formula can easily be stored in a computer and only requires information on the concentration of cystine ($C_{cystine}$) and pH in any urine sample [22]:

$$AP_{cystine} = \frac{(10^{-pH})^2 \cdot C_{cystine} \cdot 0.155}{\left[1 + (0.39 \cdot 10^{9} \cdot 10^{-pH}) + ((10^{-pH})^2 \cdot 3.51 \cdot 10^{16})\right]}$$

Roughly and at normal urine pH levels, the risk of forming cystine crystals occurs when the cystine concentration exceeds 1 mmol/L [43]. The solubility of cystine is increased when the pH is increased, and a rule of thumb tells us that approximately 2 mmol/L can be held in solution at pH 7 and 3 mmol/L at pH 8. It is, however, difficult to maintain a urine pH of 8 in a consistent way, and such pH levels can only be expected with powerful pharmacological alkalinizing therapy [43]. Nevertheless, it is important always to include a pH measurement in the biochemical work-up and follow-up of patients with cystinuria.

Similar to what was stated previously for $AP_{uric\ acid}$, $AP_{cystine}$ can be derived from analytical data in 24-h urine, from any other short-term urine collection, or even from a spot urine sample. Sodium azide (3 mmol/L) is an excellent preservative, and 30 mL is recommended for a 24-h sample.

The concentration of cystine should be analyzed with amino acid chromatography, whereby also the concentrations of lysine, ornithine, and arginine are obtained [43]. The latter three amino acids are important for diagnostic purposes, but they are otherwise thought to be without clinical importance. The possible long-term effects of constant loss of all four amino acids, however, have been poorly studied.

The excretion of cystine increases with a high sodium load [44], and if there is a clinical interest in urinary sodium, it should be noted that the collection either has to be made without sodium azide or corrected for the sodium that already is present in the bottle. In a therapeutic and follow-up perspective, it is, of course, necessary to closely look at the urine volumes produced by the patient.

Biochemical Evaluation of Patients with Infection Stone Disease

Although it is possible to get an approximate estimate of the ion-activity product of magnesium ammonium phosphate (AP_{MAP}) [21], the clinical value of such calculations is usually small, partly because of the mixture of crystal phases that comprise the infection stone (struvite, carbonate apatite, and hydroxyapatite) and partly by the fact that infection stones only form and grow in urine with urease-producing microorganisms. The urease activity also brings the pH up to high levels, and it is generally considered that infection stone material does not precipitate unless the pH exceeds 7.5–8 [22]. A standard urine culture in most situations can be used for identification of the microorganism responsible for the stone formation. A specific analysis is required to show whether the microorganism produces urease or not, and the laboratory should be asked to provide that information. Occasionally, infection with *Ureaplasma urealyticum* is the responsible factor, and if no bacterial growth or history of bacterial infection can be demonstrated in patients who apparently have formed infection stones, it is worthwhile to look for that microorganism. Detection of *Ureaplasma urealyticum*, however, requires a special sampling technique with a specific medium [45].

In the work-up of patients with stones and infection, it is essential to distinguish between infection stones and stones with associated infection. The latter group of patients has stones of another composition, usually calcium oxalate, that have been secondarily infected with bacteria not producing urease. Such infection has been associated with originally sterile stones, and it is not unusual that such a development is initiated after invasive stone-removing procedures with or without residual stone material in the kidney.

When urease-producing microorganisms are the cause of secondary infection, it therefore often is necessary to search for risk factors also of calcium stone formation (see below).

Without appropriate recurrence prevention, there is a high risk of rapidly recurring and growing infection stones, and the efficacy of the treatment efforts is better followed with repeated radiographic examinations than with urine analyses. Nevertheless, urine cultures and occasionally pH measurement can be recommended for the long-term recording of these patients.

Biochemical Risk Evaluation of Patients with Calcium Stone Disease

Although our understanding of how calcium stones form in the urinary tract is far from complete, it is undisputable that the composition of urine plays an important role. Hereby, the levels of saturation/supersaturation with calcium oxalate as well as with calcium phosphate [21, 46] together with concentrations of factors that are considered as important modifiers of crystal nucleation, crystal growth, and crystal aggregation are of interest [47]. From a clinical point of view, the available information to a large extent is limited to what we can measure in finally processed and voided urine. This shortcoming becomes particularly obvious when we consider that the initial—and possibly most important—steps in calcium stone formation appear to take place at high nephron levels, where the urine composition is much different from that recorded in caliceal, pelvic, or bladder urine. Nevertheless, it stands to reason that precipitation of calcium oxalate—the major constituent of most stones—obviously in most cases does not take place at levels above the distal part of the collecting ducts [48–51]. Recent evidence, moreover, indicates that the formation of calcium oxalate occurs either at areas of submucosal Randall's plaques exposed to urine by epithelial erosion or as trapped accumulations of calcium phosphate at the opening of the collecting ducts on the tip of the papilla [52–54].

If we disregard changes in urine composition that can be expected to occur during the passage of urine through calices, renal pelvis, ureters, and during storage in the bladder, final urine is likely—at least to some extent—to reflect the biochemical environment in which stone formation takes place.

It is thus logical that the biochemical risk evaluation should comprise analysis of the composition of one or several 24-h urine samples or any other sample of urine collected during a defined period of the day [4]. Although practically convenient, this routine is far from optimal. Urine composition varies considerably during the day as a result of food intake, drinking, and physical activities [55].

The risk of pathological or abnormal crystallization is not a continuous process, but is likely to be associated with peaks of supersaturation with either calcium oxalate or calcium phosphate or with other risk factors of stone formation. Such peaks never can be identified when urine is analyzed in long-term urine collections, in which we only can conclude whether individual urine variables, calculated risk parameters, or levels of saturation seem to be above or below an expected average or not. The ideal risk evaluation accordingly should be carried out by analysis of urine composition in a continuous series of short-term urine samples (e.g., 1, 2, or 4 h) during one or many 24-h periods. Such measurements also have been reported in the literature [55–57], but the extensive number of analyses that such approach requires is a limiting factor in the clinical routine work. Another problem is that there often is an obvious reluctance from patients to handle their own urine, and to accomplish analysis of a large number of correctly collected samples during one or several 24-h periods under normal living conditions, therefore, is less likely to be successful unless in specific cases.

The number of analyses required for useful information might be advantageously reduced by using, for instance, the Bonn Risk Index [58] or direct measurements of the risk of calcium oxalate crystallization [21]. Such procedures, however, cannot be applied without special equipment and analytical expertise that are not commonly available. There are also some test kits aiming at measurement of the crystallization propensity of urine samples, but the experience of such methods is limited [59].

The bottom line is that analysis of composition of 24-h or any urine sample collected during a defined period of the day is useful for the biochemical work-up of patients with calcium stone disease. But it is important to be aware of the limitations outlined previously because they also explain why comparison between normal subjects and stone-forming patients very often only gives discrete differences with a large overlapping of data [60, 61].

Whether one or a series of urine collections are necessary has remained a matter of debate over the years. Most certainly, the likelihood of finding one or several abnormalities increases with the number of collections [23, 59]. The reason for that is that urine composition varies not only from hour to hour but also from day to day and from week to week and is subject to a significant variation during the year. It is not easy to know how such a problem best should be handled from a clinical point of view, but the author's own preference has been that if one urine collection does not give any clues to the individual's risk of stone formation, then a repeated collection appears appropriate [62]. With such a routine, it has been possible to maintain good cooperation with the patients and still to get valuable information as a basis for recurrence preventive measures.

So what should be analyzed? In order to get sufficient information on the saturation levels, relatively accurate ion-activity products of calcium oxalate and various calcium phosphate crystal phases can be obtained by iterative approximation as published in the literature by Robertson and coworkers [63]: EQUIL2 [64], SEQUIL [65], JESS [66], or any other computerized calculation program. A major disadvantage is that all of them require a large set of urine variables.

Based on calculations carried out with the EQUIL program, it was shown that the most important determinants for the ion-activity product of calcium oxalate are the excretion of calcium, oxalate, citrate, magnesium, and the urine volume [21]. For the ion-activity product of calcium phosphate (AP_{CaP}), the corresponding variables are calcium, phosphate, pH, citrate, and urine volume [67]. From these urine constituents, approximate estimates (indices) of the ion-activity products were derived [21]:

$$\text{AP(CaOx) index} = \frac{A \cdot \text{Calcium}^{0.84} \cdot \text{Oxalate}}{\text{Citrate}^{0.22} \cdot \text{Magnesium}^{0.12} \cdot \text{Volume}^{1.03}}$$

$$\text{AP(CaP) index} = \frac{B \cdot \text{Calcium}^{1.07} \cdot \text{Phosphate}^{0.70} \cdot (\text{pH} - 4.5)^{6.8}}{\text{Citrate}^{0.20} \cdot \text{Volume}^{1.31}}$$

These indices, in which the excreted variables during the collection period should be expressed in mmol and the volume in liters, correspond to the ion-activity products as follows:

$$\text{AP(CaOx) index} \sim 10^{8} \cdot AP_{CaOx}$$
$$\text{AP(CaP) index} \sim 10^{13} \cdot AP_{CaP}$$

In the formula for calculating indices, *A* and *B* are numerical factors determined by the duration of the collection periods (Table 84.1). CaP does not represent a specific calcium phosphate crystal phase but reflects the ion-activity products of naturally occurring calcium phosphate crystal phases. Interpretation of $AP_{Brushite}$, AP_{OCP}, and AP_{HAP} in terms of AP(CaP) index has been published elsewhere [67].

Other factors that obviously are of great importance for the risk of abnormal crystal formation are the influence of various small as well as large molecular inhibitors of crystallization [61, 68]. In calculations of AP indices or more accurate ion-activity products, however, no consideration is paid to the influence of urinary macromolecules [47]. Previous studies have shown that by adding an estimate of the inhibition of crystal growth and/or crystal aggregation, an improved distinction can be made between stone-forming patients and normal subjects [61, 68]. Unfortunately, there are so far no generally accepted routine methods for measuring various inhibitory properties.

Table 84.1 Factors *A* and *B* to be used when calculating AP(CaOx) and AP(CaP) index values

Collection period (h)	24	16	12	8	4	2	1
Factor *A*—AP(CaOx) index	1.9	2.3	2.7	3.2	4.5	6.3	8.8
10^3 × Factor *B*—AP(CaP) index	2.7	3.0	3.2	3.6	4.3	5.1	6.1

There is, however, no consensus on whether urinary inhibiting activities exert their most important effect in diluted urine (at high nephron levels) or in whole urine (at a caliceal level). Moreover, although there is an array of large molecules that have an inhibitory or promoting activity, there are no established ways in which they can be therapeutically influenced except by changing pH and by increasing the excretion of citrate and magnesium. Small molecular inhibitors such as citrate and magnesium are already included in the list of important determinants for the ion-activity products of calcium oxalate and calcium phosphate. Therapeutically induced increments in citrate and magnesium might favorably reduce the ion-activity products of calcium oxalate and calcium phosphate and in addition to that increase the inhibition of the crystallization processes of both salts. The clinical importance of other small molecular inhibitors—such as pyrophosphate, phytate, and some metallic ions—has not been definitely established and is therefore not included in the routine risk evaluation suggested later in this chapter.

Analysis of creatinine is of great importance in order to decide whether the urine collection is complete or not. It is common that patients deliver urine samples that do not correspond to the urine produced during the intended collection period. Samples might be too small or too large, but with knowledge of the patient's body weight, the recorded creatinine excretion can be compared with predicted creatinine excretion. For 24-h urine samples, the relationship between body weight and urinary creatinine is shown in Fig. 84.2 [11]. Analysis of urea is useful because the urea level reflects the intake of protein. That value can be obtained from the following formula [11, 24]:

$$\text{Protein intake}\left(\text{g/24 h}\right) = \text{Urea}\left(\text{mmol/24 h}\right)0.18 + 13$$

By comparing the accordingly recorded protein intake with that recommended (0.8–1.0 g/kg body weight), the dietary advice can be facilitated.

It has been suggested that urinary urate concentrations are important for calcium oxalate precipitation. A salting-out effect, as demonstrated experimentally, has been put forward as the reasonable explanation for a relationship between hyperuricosuria and calcium oxalate stone disease [69]. There might be geographical variations of that risk, but it is the author's personal opinion that in most patients, a high urate excretion reflects a diet that also in other ways changes urine composition in a crystallization-promoting direction. Contradictory results also have been reported from allopurinol treatment of patients with calcium oxalate stone disease [39, 70].

Recent as well as earlier reports have indicated that urinary pH is of fundamental importance, not only for calcium phosphate precipitation but also for calcium phosphate dissolution and thereby probably also for calcium oxalate precipitation/nucleation [48]. It is, however, not easy to get a representative measurement of urine pH, which is subject to a considerable variation during the day. What is said previously about the shortcomings of analysis of different urine constituents in 24-h urine is even more relevant for pH. Moreover, pH changes during storage, and if not measured directly after completion of the urine collection, erroneous results can be obtained. Ideally, pH should be recorded as a pH profile with repeated and frequent measurement during the 24-h period [24]. Alternatively, one or several pH measurements in urine collected during well-defined periods are useful and for larger groups of patients, undoubtedly, most practical.

The following variables might be useful to include in the search of risk factors of calcium stone formation [4]:

- Calcium
- Oxalate
- Phosphate
- Citrate
- Magnesium
- pH
- Volume
- Creatinine
- Urate (optional)
- Urea

For the measurement of pH, it has been the author's own preference to collect samples between 22:00 h and 06:00 h, with sodium azide (10mL of a solution with a concentration of 3 mmol/L). Although this is not a fasting urine sample, it comes close to that and in anyway represents urine from a standardized collection period. Inasmuch as the 8-h urine sample suggested does not contain any acidifying agent as preservative, the sample also can be used for analysis of urinary urate. In the latter case, it is also recommended to measure creatinine provided that the total urate excretion, and not only the concentration, is of interest.

The other urine variables should be analyzed in a urine collection to which an acidifying agent has been added. It can be a 24-h sample or any sample collected during another defined period of the day. The author's own routine during recent years has been a 16-h urine sample

Fig. 84.2 Relation between bodyweight and expected 24-h excretion of creatinine in men (*bold*) and women (*thin*) [11]

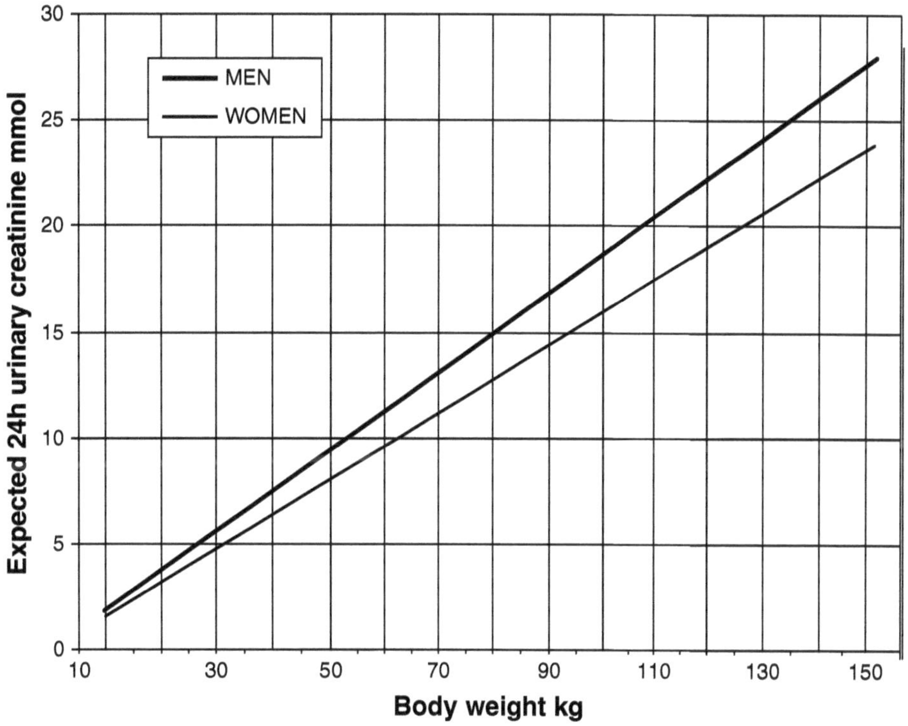

collected between 06:00 h and 22:00 h in a bottle containing 20 mL of 6 mol/L hydrochloric acid. Other acidifiers can be used, but it is essential to keep the pH in the sample sufficiently low (below pH 2) in order to avoid precipitation of calcium oxalate or calcium phosphate in the bottle and to dissolve any crystals that have been excreted with urine. The other—and equally important—role of acidification is to counteract oxidation of ascorbate to oxalate [4]. Insufficiently acidified urine otherwise might result in an overestimation of the excretion of oxalate. In case of large urine volumes, it is recommended to measure pH in the sample upon delivery and if necessary add more hydrochloric acid (or another acidifying agent) to get a pH below 2.0.

There are some points of note before proceeding to analysis of urine for risk factors:

1. After any kind of active stone removal—open surgery, shock wave lithotripsy (SWL), percutaneous nephrolithotomy (PNL), ureteroscopy (URS), retrograde intrarenal surgery (RIRS)—allow 4–8 weeks to pass before collecting urine [4].
2. Wait until there is little or no risk that fragments will be excreted with urine.
3. In case of bacteriuria, ongoing urinary tract infection, or when hematuria is present, discard the sample and wait for a better occasion.
4. Send the sample to the laboratory as soon as possible. If some delay is necessary, the sample can be stored in a refrigerator up to 24–48 h. Otherwise, keep aliquots of urine frozen until analysis.
5. It is important to note that the acidified sample cannot be used for analysis of urate. Although alkalinization is an option, it is better to measure urate in a separate sample that has been collected without acid.
6. Detailed instructions must be given to the patient in oral as well as written form, to make sure that the patient starts and finishes the urine collection in a correct way.
7. Urine collection should be undertaken during conditions that—as far as possible—reflect the normal (average everyday) situation and not that of artificial living conditions with unusual diet and excessive fluid intake.
8. It also is of utmost importance that urine samples are carefully mixed and heated to a temperature of 37 °C before aliquots are drawn for analysis. This might appear unnecessary to emphasize, but I am sure that neglecting these steps explains numerous erroneous results.

Despite careful instructions on how to collect urine, experience has shown that during this procedure, people tend to drink more than they usually do. Standardized estimates of AP(CaOx) index and AP(CaP) index therefore have been developed based on a 24-h urine volume of 1,500 mL (1.5 L in the formula) during 24 h [21]. Inasmuch as the pH cannot be measured in the 16-h sample suggested previously, the standardized AP(CaP) index is derived for a pH of 7.0. These two standardized indices are given the annotations "s": AP(CaOx) $index_s$ and AP(CaP) $index_s$. As mentioned, the factors A and B are determined by the duration of the collection period, and some relevant numbers are given in Table 84.1.

Interpretation of AP(CaOx) and AP(CaP) index values is partly hampered by our incomplete understanding of the calcium stone-forming process. From previous calculations and experiments, the formation of calcium oxalate crystals is less likely to occur at AP_{CaOx} values below 1.5–2.5 · 10^{-8} $(mol/L)^2$ [21]. When a 16-h AP(CaOx) index of 1.5 is recorded, it means that peak values of up to at least 2.5 can have occurred during the collection period. In case of calcium phosphate-induced precipitation caused by dissolution of calcium phosphate, very high local levels of supersaturation with CaOx are likely [48]. Such peak supersaturation levels will never be reflected in AP(CaOx) index levels in samples collected over longer periods of the day.

From a practical point of view, an AP(CaOx) index above 1.5–1.7 might indicate a need for actions to lower the supersaturation. Similarly, an AP(CaP) $index_s$ exceeding 50 indicates an increased risk of calcium phosphate precipitation. In this regard it is of note that AP(CaP) $index_s$ can be assumed to reflect the AP_{CaP} in the distal part of the collecting duct.

With the result obtained from analysis of urine samples as discussed previously, a reasonable basis should be available for conclusions of factors responsible for or contributing to the stone formation. The AP indices give an impression of the concert action exerted by the various urine variables in terms of forming urine critically supersaturated with calcium oxalate and/or calcium phosphate. The individual urine variables subsequently can be used for dietary and drinking advice or for choosing the most appropriate form of pharmacological therapy. Those issues are, however, extensively discussed elsewhere in this book.

When Should Chemical Analysis of Urine Be Carried Out?

If we first look at non-calcium stone-forming patients, it is mandatory to measure the concentration of cystine in patients with cystine stone formation. The supersaturation with cystine ($AP_{cystine}$) should be calculated both as part of the initial risk evaluation as during follow-up during recurrence preventive treatment. For uric acid stone formers, $AP_{uric\ acid}$ might be a helpful estimate in the diagnostic work-up. But recurrence prevention usually can be started and maintained without further analyses. In case of therapeutic failure, it is, however, highly recommended to measure urine urate and pH and calculate $AP_{uric\ acid}$.

Patients with infection stones—like patients with cystine and uric acid stones—always should be given recurrence preventive treatment [71]. The outcome of such a therapy usually is best followed clinically in terms of new stone formation and the presence or absence of bacteriuria. There is thus no absolute need for any further analytical efforts.

In patients with calcium stone disease, there is a great diversity in terms of the severity of stone formation. There is definitely a group of patients in whom a careful analysis of risk factors should be strongly recommended. In others it might be optional, whereas some patients have a mild disease (or what appears to be a mild disease) for whom a complete urine analysis is overdoing. It also is important that the patient is motivated to accept medical advice or treatment based on urinary findings before an extensive risk analysis is undertaken. That is, however, mostly a pedagogic problem.

Several categories of calcium stone formers can be identified [4]. A relatively small group (category Rs) has a frequently recurring stone formation, which by itself calls for effective preventive measures. It is often difficult to get a good estimate of the frequency of stone formation. There is usually insufficient data available, and the patient has only a vague idea when stones have formed. On the other hand, the total number of stones (*N*) that has formed is usually better recorded or known by the patient. With this information, a stone age index (SAI) can be calculated as follows [46]:

$$SAI = \frac{N \cdot 100}{Age}$$

A value above 10 indicates a severe disease (Rs). To that group—irrespective of the previous history of stone formation—should also be added those with specific risk factors such as formation of brushite stones, as well as those with medical diseases, anatomical abnormalities, and pharmacological treatment known to be associated with calcium stone formation. The patients thus referred to category Rs always should be considered for a complete metabolic risk evaluation.

Mild recurrent stone formation (Rm) is defined by longer intervals between stones and SAI usually in a range between 7 and 10. Those patients who do not have any residual stones (Rmo) can probably be left with some general preventive advice. Those with residual stone material (Rmres) might definitely benefit from specific medical advice and/or pharmacological treatment and accordingly that group of patients should be offered a urine examination. The same probably is wise also for first (single) stone formers with residuals (Sres). In contrast, the first-time stone former without residuals (So) can be given general advice, but that is all needed unless the patient highly desires an evaluation in order to find a reason for the stone. Of first-time stone formers, around 75 % remain stone-free during a 10-year period [72].

For the categories (So and Rmo), the evaluation can be restricted to a set of serum (or plasma) analyses including calcium, phosphate, creatinine, potassium, and urate. Spot urine sample can be used to exclude or confirm bacteriuria or leukocyturia, and with a measurement of the pH, no further analyses are necessary.

Acid Load for the Diagnosis of DRTA

An intake of 0.1 g of ammonium chloride per kg body weight together with 150 mL of water is followed by urine collection in five 1-h samples. At each collection, 150 mL of water is taken. The pH should be measured before acidification in each sample. If the pH is reduced to 5.4, the diagnosis of dRTA can be excluded. The distinction between complete and incomplete RTA is made from measurements of pH and bicarbonate in blood. Whereas blood pH and bicarbonate are normal in the incomplete form, low values are seen in patients with complete RTA [24].

Conclusion

Appropriate consideration of relevant aspects of the patient's medical history and radiographic image, together with analyses of stones, blood, and urine, is extremely helpful for identifying risk factors of stone formation. This is a field that unfortunately is neglected by too many urologists, but a lot of problems and expenses can be saved by paying attention to the etiology of stone formation in the individual patient. It is recommended that the principles of risk evaluation are adapted both to the type of stone that the patient has formed (if this is known) and to the severity of the disease. These findings should provide the basis for subsequent recurrence preventive measures.

References

1. Tiselius H-G. Epidemiology and medical management of stone disease. BJU Int. 2003;91:758–67.
2. Straub M, Strohmaier W, Berg W, Beck B, Hoppe B, Laube N, et al. Diagnosis and metaphylaxis of stone disease. Consensus concept of the national working committee on stone disease for the upcoming German urolithiasis guidelines. World J Urol. 2005;23: 309–23.
3. Tiselius HG. Investigation of single and recurrent stone formers. Miner Electrolyte Metab. 1994;20:321–7.
4. Tiselius H-G, Alken P, Buck C, Gallucci M, Knoll T, Sarica K, et al. Guidelines on urolithiasis. European association of urology guidelines. EAU Guideline Office. 2009 edition; 2009.
5. Parks J, Coe F. Evidence for durable kidney stone prevention over several decades. BJU Int. 2009;103:1238–46.
6. Leslie SW. Outpatient metabolic evaluation of patients with recurrent kidney stones. Ohio Med. 1989;85:292–4.
7. Colussi G, De Ferrari ME, Brunati C, Civati G. Medical prevention and treatment of urinary stones. J Nephrol. 2000;13 Suppl 3:S65–70.
8. Robertson WG. The economics and epidemiology of urolithiasis. In: Gohel MDI, Au DWT, editors. Kidney stones: inside and out. Hong Kong: The Hong Kong Technical University; 2004. p. 368–71.
9. Tiselius HG. Routine metabolic evaluation of patients with stone disease – aspects on its cost effectiveness. In: Gohel MDI, Au DWT, editors. Kidney stones: inside and out. Hong Kong: The Hong Kong Polytechnical University; 2004. p. 372–6.
10. Parks JH, Coe FL. The financial effects of kidney stone prevention. Kidney Int. 1996;50:1706–12.
11. Tiselius HG. Medical evaluation of nephrolithiasis. Endocrinol Metab Clin North Am. 2002;31:1031–50.
12. Liebman SE, Taylor JG, Bushinsky DA. Uric acid nephrolithiasis. Curr Rheumatol Rep. 2007;9:251–7.
13. Chevreau G, Troccaz J, Conort P, Renard-Penna R, Mallet A, Daudon M, et al. Estimation of urinary stone composition by automated processing of CT images. Urol Res. 2009;37:241–5.
14. Ferrandino MN, Pierre SA, Simmons WN, Paulson EK, Albala DM, Preminger GM. Dual-energy computed tomography with advanced postimage acquisition data processing: improved determination of urinary stone composition. J Endourol. 2010;24:347–54.
15. Matlaga BR, Kawamoto S, Fishman E. Dual source computed tomography: a novel technique to determine stone composition. Urology. 2008;72:1164–8.
16. Hesse A, Tiselius H, Siener R, Hoppe R. Crystals in the urinary sediment. In: Urinary stones, diagnosis, treatment and prevention of recurrence. Basel: Karger AG; 2009. p. 213–5.
17. Shekarriz B, Stoller ML. Cystinuria and other noncalcareous calculi. Endocrinol Metab Clin North Am. 2002;31:951–77.
18. Brand E, Harris MM, Bildon S. Cystinuria: excretion of a cystine complex which decomposes in the urine with liberation of free cystine. J Biol Chem. 1930;86:315.
19. Marickar YM. Calcium oxalate stone and gout. Urol Res. 2009; 37:345–7.
20. Kenny JE, Goldfarb DS. Update on the pathophysiology and management of uric acid renal stones. Curr Rheumatol Rep. 2010; 12:125–9.
21. Tiselius HG. Solution chemistry of supersaturation. In: Coe FL, Favus MJ, Pak CYC, Parks JH, Preminger GM, editors. Kidney stones: medical and surgical management. Philadelphia: Lippincott-Raven Publishers; 1996. p. 33–64.
22. Tiselius HG. Aetiological factors in stone formation. In: Davison AM, Cameron JS, Grünfeld J-P, Ponticelli C, Ritz E, Winearls CG, van Ypersele C, editors. Oxford textbook of clinical nephrology. New York: Oxford University Press; 2005. p. 1199–223.
23. Hess B, Hasler-Strub U, Ackermann D, Jaeger P. Metabolic evaluation of patients with recurrent idiopathic calcium nephrolithiasis. Nephrol Dial Transplant. 1997;12:1362–8.
24. Hesse A, Tiselius H, Siener R, Hoppe R. Urinary stones: diagnosis, treatment and recurrence prevention. Basel: Karger AG; 2009.
25. Worcester EM. Stones from bowel disease. Endocrinol Metab Clin North Am. 2002;2002:997–9.
26. Asplin JR. Hyperoxaluric calcium nephrolithiasis. Endocrinol Metab Clin North Am. 2002;31:927–49.
27. McConnell N, Campbell S, Gillanders I, Rolton H, Danesh B. Risk factors for developing renal stones in inflammatory bowel disease. BJU Int. 2002;89:835–41.
28. Asplin JR. Obesity and urolithiasis. Adv Chronic Kidney Dis. 2009; 16:11–20.
29. Maalouf NM. Metabolic syndrome and the genesis of uric acid stones. J Ren Nutr. 2011;21:128–31.
30. Domrongkitchaiporn S, Ongphiphadhanakul B, Stitchantrakul W, Piaseu N, Chansirikam S, Puavilai G, et al. Risk of calcium oxalate nephrolithiasis after calcium or combined calcium and calcitriol supplementation in postmenopausal women. Osteoporos Int. 2000; 11:486–92.
31. Taylor EN, Curhan GC. Determinants of 24-h urinary oxalate excretion. Clin J Am Soc Nephrol. 2008;3:1453–60.
32. Auer BL, Auer D, Rodgers AL. Relative hyperoxaluria, crystalluria and haematuria after megadose ingestion of vitamin C. Eur J Clin Invest. 1998;28:695–700.
33. Massey LK, Liebman M, Kynast-Gales SA. Ascorbate increases human oxaluria and kidney stone risk. J Nutr. 2005;135:1673–7.

34. Ahlstrand C, Tiselius HG. Urine composition and stone formation during treatment with acetazolamide. Scand J Urol Nephrol. 1987; 21:225–8.
35. Koul HK, Koul S, Fu S, Santosham V, Seikhon A, Menon M. Oxalate: from crystal formation to crystal retention. J Am Soc Nephrol. 1999;10 suppl 14:S417–21.
36. Khan SR. Renal tubular damage/dysfunction: key to the formation of kidney stones. Urol Res. 2006;34:86–91.
37. Pritchard MJ. Medullary sponge kidney: causes and treatments. Br J Nurs. 2010;12:972–6.
38. Maw AM, Megibow AJ, Grasso M, Goldfarb DS. Diagnosis of medullary sponge kidney by computed tomographic urography. Am J Kidney Dis. 2007;50:146–50.
39. Sorensen CM, Chandhoke PS. Hyperuricosuric calcium nephrolithiasis. Endocrinol Metab Clin North Am. 2002;31:915–25.
40. Caudarella R, Vescini F. Urinary citrate and renal stone disease: the preventive role of alkali citrate treatment. Arch Ital Urol Androl. 2009;81:182–7.
41. Wuermser LA, Reilly C, Poindexter JR, Sakahee K, Pak CY. Potassium magnesium citrate versus potassium chloride in thiazide-induced hypokalemia. Kidney Int. 2000;57:607–12.
42. Tiselius HG, Berg C, Fornander AM, Nilsson MA. Effects of citrate on the different phases of calcium oxalate crystallization. Scanning Microsc. 1993;7:381–90.
43. Tiselius HG. New horizons in the management of patients with cystinuria. Curr Opin Urol. 2010;20:169–73.
44. Goldfarb DS, Coe FL, Asplin JR. Urinary cystine excretion and capacity in patients with cystinuria. Kidney Int. 2006;69:1041–7.
45. Grenabo L, Hedelin H, Pettersson S. Urinary infection stones caused by ureaplasma urealyticum: a review. Scand J Infect Dis. 1988;53(suppl):46–9.
46. Tiselius HG. Factors influencing the course of calcium oxalate stone disease. Eur Urol. 1999;36:363–70.
47. Khan SR, Kok DJ. Modulators of urinary stone formation. Front Biosci. 2004;9:1450–82.
48. Tiselius H, Lindbäck B, Fornander A-M, Nilsson M. Studies on the role of calcium phosphate in the process of calcium oxalate crystal formation. Urol Res. 2009;37:181–92.
49. Luptak J, Bek-Jensen H, Fornander AM, Hojgaard I, Nilsson MA, Tiselius HG. Crystallization of calcium oxalate and calcium phosphate at supersaturation levels corresponding to those in different parts of the nephron. Scanning Microsc. 1994;8:47–62.
50. Kok D, Schell-Feith E. Risk factors for crystallisation in the nephron: the role of renal development. J Am Soc Nephrol. 1999; 10:S364–70.
51. Kok DJ. Crystallization and stone formation inside the nephron. Scanning Microsc. 1996;10:471–86.
52. Evan AP, Lingeman JE, Worcester EM. Role of interstitial apatite plaque in the pathogenesis of common calcium oxalate stone. Semin Nephrol. 2008;28:111–9.
53. Cifuentes Delatte L, Minon Cifuentes J, Medina JA. Randall and his plaque. Urology. 1996;48:343–6.
54. Liu Y, Mo L, Goldfarb DS, Evan A-P, Liang F, Khan SR, Lieske JC. Progressive renal papillary calcification and ureteral stone formation in mice deficient for Tamm-Horsfall protein. Am J Physiol Renal Physiol. 2010;299:F469–78.
55. Vahlensieck EW, Bach D, Hesse A. Circadian rhythm of lithogenic substances in the urine. Urol Res. 1982;10:195–203.
56. Robert M, Roux JO, Bourelly F, Boularan AM, Guiter J, Monnier L. Circadian variations in the risk of urinary calcium oxalate stone formation. Br J Urol. 1994;74:294–7.
57. Ahlstrand C, Larsson L, Tiselius H-G. Variations in urine composition during the day in patients with calcium oxalate stone disease. J Urol. 1984;131(1):77–81.
58. Laube N, Hergarten S, Hoppe B, Schmidt M, Hesse A. Determination of the calcium oxalate crystallization risk from urine samples: the BONN risk index in comparison to other risk formulas. J Urol. 2004;172:355–9.
59. Conte A, Piza P, Garcia-Raja A, Grases F, Csta-Bauza A, Prieto RM. Urinary lithogen risk test: usefulness in the evaluation of renal lithiasis treatment using crystallization inhibitors (citrate and phytate). Arch Esp Urol. 1999;52:305–10.
60. Tiselius HG. Aspects on estimation of the risk of calcium oxalate crystallization in urine. Urol Int. 1991;47:255–9.
61. Tiselius HG, Bek-Jensen H, FA M, Nilsson MA. Crystallization properties in urine from calcium oxalate stone formers. J Urol. 1995;154:940–6.
62. Bek-Jensen H, Tiselius HG. Repeated urine analysis in patients with calcium stone disease. Eur Urol. 1998;33:323–32.
63. Roberston WG, Peacock M, Nordin BEC. Activity products in stone-forming and non-stone-forming urine. Clin Sci. 1968; 34:579–94.
64. Werness PG, Brown CM, Smith LH, Finlayson B. EQUIL2: a basic computer program for calculation of urinary saturation. J Urol. 1985;134:1242–4.
65. Ashby R, Györy AZ. Thermodynamic equilibrium model for calcium salt urolithiasis: clinical application. Exp Nephrol. 1997;5: 246–52.
66. Rodgers A, Allie-Hamdulay S, Jackson G. Therapeutic action of citrate in urolithiasis explained by chemical speciation: increase in pH is the determinant factor. Nephrol Dial Transplant. 2006;21: 361–9.
67. Tiselius HG. A simplified estimate of the ion-activity product of calcium phosphate in urine. Eur Urol. 1984;10:191–5.
68. Roberston WG, Peacock M, Marshall RW, Marshall DH, Nordin B. Saturation inhibition index as a measure of the risk of calcium oxalate stone formation in the urinary tract. N Engl J Med. 1976; 294:249–52.
69. Ryall RL, Grover PK, Marshall VR. Urate and calcium stones-picking up a drop of mercury with one's fingers? Am J Kidney Dis. 1991;17:426–30.
70. Tiselius HG, Larsson L, Hellgren E. Clinical results of allopurinol treatment in prevention of calcium oxalate stone formation. J Urol. 1986;136:5–53.
71. Leusmann DB, Niggemann H, Roth S, von Ahlen H. Recurrence rates and severity of urinary calculi. Scand J Urol Nephrol. 1995;29: 279–83.
72. Ahlstrand C, Tiselius HG. Recurrences during a 10-year follow-up after first renal stone episode. Urol Res. 1990;18:397–9.

Application of Physical Methods to Kidney Stones and Randall's Plaque Characterization

85

Michel Daudon and Dominique C. Bazin

Abstract

Chemical analysis of stones does not identify crystal types, as do physical methods. This chapter describes the principles and application of X-ray energy dispersive spectrometry (EDS), proton-induced X-ray emission (PIXE), Fourier transform infrared spectroscopy (FTIR), X-ray fluorescence (XRF), scanning electron microscopy (SEM), powder neutron diffraction (PND), X-ray absorption spectroscopy (XAS), and FTIR microspectroscopy (FTIRM). Today, fine details regarding the relationship between structural characteristic of kidney stones and the pathology that exists at the macroscopic scale can be obtained at the mesoscopic scale.

Some of the key issues addressed are in addition to chemical composition, the spatial distribution of the different chemical phases inside Randall's plaque, and the nature of the interaction between plaque, stone, and renal epithelium. Details regarding relevant concepts of these different methods used principally in physics and chemistry are not given, as they can be obtained from available excellent reviews and books. Instead, the detailed nature of information that is given by these techniques is discussed, and the link between structural or chemical information and the etiopathogenesis of kidney stones is explored.

Keywords

Randall's plaque • Concretion • Kidney stone • Calcification • Calcium oxalate • Calcium phosphate • Uric acid • Ammonium hydrogen urate • Magnesium ammonium phosphate • Cystine • X-ray energy dispersive spectrometry • Proton-induced X-ray emission • Fourier transform infrared spectroscopy • Nanocrystals • Crystallites • X-ray fluorescence • Scanning electron microscopy • Powder neutron diffraction • Amorphous carbonated calcium phosphate • X-ray absorption spectroscopy • FTIR microspectroscopy

Introduction

From a medical point of view, we may distinguish at least three different families of pathological calcifications. The first is a *concretion* defined as deposition of crystalline material in excretory ducts (kidney stones, gallstones, and salivary stones fall into this category). The second is referred to as ectopic calcification, defined as inappropriate biomineralization occurring in soft tissue (which can be related to severe pathologies like breast or testicular cancer). The third can be associated with physiological calcifications from which a part becomes pathological after a disease. Due to its

M. Daudon, Ph.D. (✉)
Service des Explorations Fonctionnelles,
Tenon Hospital, APHP, 4 Rue de la Chine, Paris 75020, France
e-mail: michel.daudon@tnn.aphp.fr

D. C. Bazin, Ph.D.
Laboratoire de Physique des Solides UMR 8502,
Université Paris Sud, Bât 510, 91405 Orsay Cedex, France

J.J. Talati et al. (eds.), *Urolithiasis*,
DOI 10.1007/978-1-4471-4387-1_85,

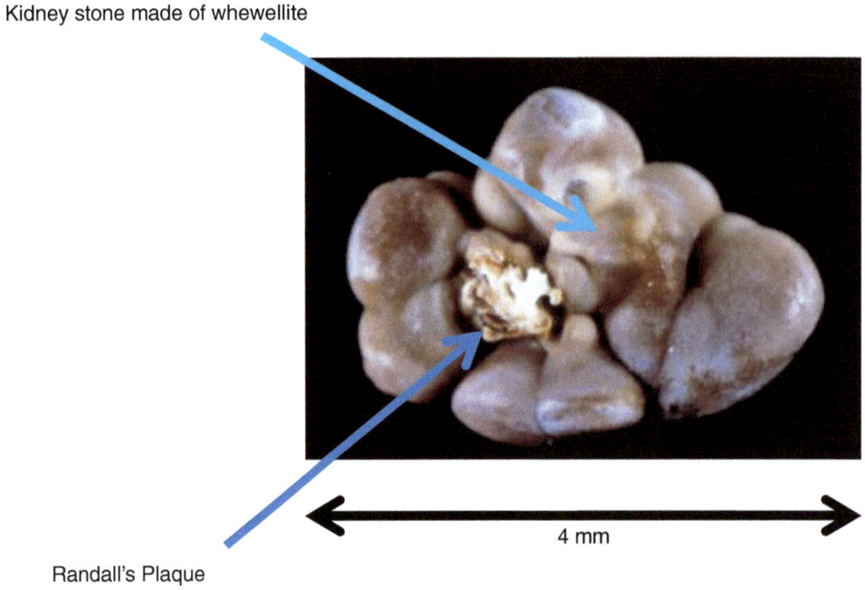

Fig. 85.1 Typical Randall's plaque (*white area*) attached on a calculus made of whewellite

importance, several excellent books have been devoted to this subject [1–4].

As old as mankind, urinary stone disease [5–7] affects an increasing part of the population and thus can be considered as a major health problem [8–11]. In parallel with the increased prevalence of stone disease, a rising prevalence of overweight individuals is noted in the general population, particularly in industrialized countries. Recent epidemiologic studies have emphasized a positive correlation between overweight status or obesity and the risk of kidney stone formation through changes in urine biochemistry [12–16].

The main chemical constituents of stones are calcium oxalate, calcium phosphate, uric acid, ammonium hydrogen urate, and magnesium ammonium phosphate and cystine with differences in their distribution according to the population group being studied. Such diversity in the chemical nature of kidney stone constitutes a mirror of the large set of associated pathologies from alimentary disorder to genetic pathologies [17]. Only a precise description of the macroscopic morphology of the calculus completed with a determination of the spatial distribution from the core to the surface of the kidney stone of the different chemical phases can define the associated disease [18–20].

From a chemistry-based viewpoint, homogeneous and heterogeneous primary nucleation exist in the case of supersaturated urine. It is well accepted that kidney stones may result from homogeneous primary nucleation. However, typical heterogeneous nucleation is commonly observed in the case of calcium oxalate stones developed from a carbapatite Randall's plaque (Fig. 85.1), which is a frequent finding in Western countries.

This ectopic calcification, first described by Alexander Randall in the 1930s, is receiving increasing attention mainly due to its major role in the genesis of calcium oxalate kidney stones [21–23]. Recognized as the origin of renal stones [24, 25], the major increase of its prevalence observed either through ureteroscopy [26] or on the calculus [26] itself has motivated a large number of recent studies. The driving force under this effort is linked to the fact that, as suggested by Kim et al. [27], stone formation is proportional to papillary surface coverage by Randall's plaque (RP).

Although major experimental efforts have led to important general insight in the chemical structure of RP, a satisfactory understanding of the associated biochemical mechanisms is still far from being achieved. Among the key issues to be addressed are the following: (1) their chemical composition, (2) the spatial distribution of the different chemical phases inside the Randall's plaque, and (3) the nature of the interaction between RP and either kidney stone or the epithelium.

In this chapter, the details regarding relevant concepts of these different methods used principally in physics and chemistry are not given, as they can be obtained from available excellent reviews and books [28, 29]. We shall discuss in detail the nature of information that is given by these techniques and will attempt to link structural or chemical information to the etiopathogenesis of kidney stones.

Techniques Used for Routine Analysis

Generalities

In material science, elemental analysis generally constitutes the starting point. To attain this goal, a chemical analysis is usually performed. Physical methods such as X-ray fluorescence spectroscopy can also be used. In that case, fluorescence can be induced by electrons (i.e., X-ray energy dispersive spectrometry

[EDS]), by protons (i.e., proton-induced X-ray emission [PIXE]), or by photons (i.e., X-ray fluorescence spectroscopy). PIXE experimental setup needs an accelerator to obtain a proton beam—the proton energy being around 2.9 MeV. Several excellent papers are based on this technique; most of the measurements used electrons or photons as a probe. All these X-ray fluorescence techniques led to the knowledge of the chemical nature of major as well as trace elements. For some experimental setups, the size of the probe is less than a micrometer, and thus it is possible to map the different elements to different sites.

The next step consists in gathering structural information (i.e., determining the arrangement of atoms in the sample). In the case of kidney stones, Fourier transform infrared (FTIR) spectroscopy and scattering techniques are often used to obtain such structural information. Again, scattering techniques can be based on interaction between matter and electrons, photons, or neutrons. Nevertheless, X-ray scattering is widely used, while very few papers regarding kidney stones deal with neutron or electron scattering. When FTIR and scattering experimental setup use synchrotron radiation as a source, the size of the associated probe can be as low as one micrometer. Moreover, using synchrotron radiation as a source increases the sensitivity of these techniques dramatically. Thus, some basic characteristics of synchrotron radiation will be given in this chapter.

When the chemical phases present in kidney stones are amorphous, some techniques specific to synchrotron radiation, such as X-ray absorption spectroscopy, can be used. This technique describes the local environment of one kind of atom present in the sample. Recently, we used this technique to study the environment of Ca in Randall's plaque as well as the environment of Zn in kidney stones.

Finally, while scattering techniques are used to describe crystals at the nanometer scale, a scanning electron microscope is used to depict the surface of the crystallites at the mesoscopic scale. From a physicochemical point of view, we used the terms "nanocrystals" and "crystallites" according to Van Meerssche and Feneau-Dupont [30] in order to define the structural hierarchy of these mineral concrements. Such three-dimensional (3D) images of the crystallites are of primary importance, and sometimes a relationship can be established between the morphology of crystallites and the pathology involved in stone formation.

Chemical Analysis

Chemical methods for identifying stone components are widely used throughout the world because they are cheap and easy to perform. However, they present a number of major disadvantages: first, they identify ions and not molecules, making difficult the relation to the pathology. They are unable to distinguish between crystalline phases. For example, in the case of calcium oxalate stones, it is not possible to distinguish between whewellite (COM) and weddellite (COD), which have very different etiopathogenic significance. Again, among calcium phosphates, apatite and brushite are not clearly identified, which constitute a major drawback of such an approach. Obviously, the carbonate level of apatite, which may be a fingerprint of infectious process, is not available. Finally, chemical methods fail to identify dihydroxyadenine or drugs or other rare components related to specific pathological conditions. For all these reasons, chemical methods for stone analysis have to be replaced by physical methods.

Infrared Spectroscopy

As recalled by Miller and Dumas [31], FTIR spectroscopy is a technique that probes the vibrational modes of molecules, providing a spectrum that is structure specific. It is well known that vibrational motions associated with chemical bonds lie in the wavelength range of 2.5–25 μm. In fact, for FTIR spectroscopy, a different energy scale is adopted: the reciprocal centimeters ν (in cm^{-1}) $= 10^4/\lambda$ (in μm) (thus, 2.5 μm = 4,000 cm^{-1}; 25 μm = 400 cm^{-1}).

Regarding biological materials made of proteins, lipids, nucleic acids, and carbohydrates, FTIR takes advantage of the fact that these compounds have unique chemical structures and thus distinctive infrared spectra [32]. More precisely, a protein's FTIR spectrum exhibits two prominent features, the amide I (1,600–1,700 cm^{-1}) and amide II (1,500–1,560 cm^{-1}) bands. These two bands come from stretching vibrations of two bonds, namely, C–O and C–N of the peptide backbone. This technique is also sensitive to bonds present in mineral and routinely used to characterize kidney stones as well as Randall's plaques extracted from kidney stones.

At Tenon Hospital, kidney stones are characterized by FTIR using a spectrometer (Vector 22; Bruker Spectrospin, Wissembourg, France) according to an analytical procedure previously defined [33]. Data were collected in the absorption mode between 4,000 and 400 cm^{-1} with a resolution of 4 cm^{-1}. In the case of biopsies, the distribution of calcification may occur at the cell level. When FTIR used synchrotron radiation as a source, it is possible to use a characterization technique that combines high spatial resolution (micrometer scale) with high biochemical (spectral) sensitivity.

In industrialized countries, the main component of urinary calculi is calcium oxalate. However, two crystalline forms exist, namely, calcium oxalate monohydrate (COM) and calcium oxalate dihydrate (COD), which are linked to different etiologies. Even if these two compounds are quite close from a structural point of view, an original method [34]

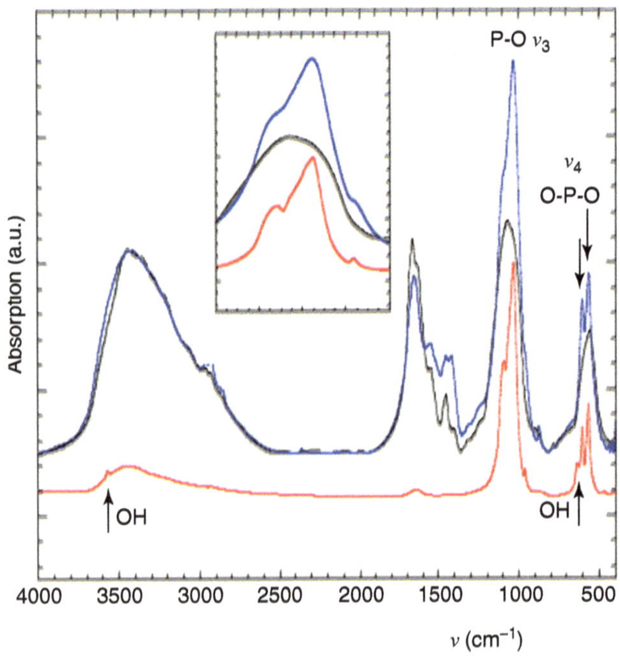

Fig. 85.2 FTIR absorption spectra for the compounds used here as references (*bottom*, hydroxyapatite; *top*, carbapatite; *middle*, amorphous carbonated calcium phosphate)

has been developed to separate the contributions of these two compounds. This method of zero-crossing-point first-derivative spectrophotometry was applied to calcium oxalate species quantitation and revealed to be easy, accurate, precise, and very well adapted to routine laboratories.

In the case of calcium phosphate apatite FTIR spectrum, different absorption bands are well assigned (Fig. 85.2). The (nu) ν_1 and (nu) ν_3 P–O stretching vibration modes are measured at 960–962 cm^{-1} and 1,035–1,045 cm^{-1}, respectively, while the (nu) ν_4 O–P–O bending mode corresponds to the doublet at 602–563 cm^{-1}. The bands at 3,570 and 633 cm^{-1} corresponding to the stretching and vibrational modes of the OH groups are present for the hydroxyapatite (HAP) and almost absent for the biological apatites. Particular attention has to be paid to the presence of a shoulder in the (nu) ν_3 absorption band, which can be used as a fingerprint for the presence of carbapatite. Its disappearance can be considered as a marker for the presence of amorphous carbonated calcium phosphate (ACCP) compound, the (nu) ν_3 P–O peak of which being located at around 1,060 cm^{-1}. From a medical point of view, ACCP is often a fingerprint of a local supersaturation of Ca phosphate in poorly acidic urine. In the case of trioxypurines, uric acid and urates often greatly differ by biochemical conditions involved in their formation. Therefore, stone analysis must be able to distinguish clearly between the various chemical and physical forms of such compounds.

Figures 85.3a–j present the infrared spectra of the main components found in urinary calculi.

Scattering Techniques

In material science, X-ray scattering constitutes a powerful tool [35] giving the spatial arrangement of atoms. More precisely, scattering techniques can be used either to determine the crystal structure [36, 37] or the chemical composition of the samples through the powder diffraction bank data file, which contains more than 64,000 patterns. In the United States, this technique is used routinely to characterize kidney stones, leading to information regarding its chemical composition. We have also used scattering techniques to determine structural characteristics of crystals present in kidney stones.

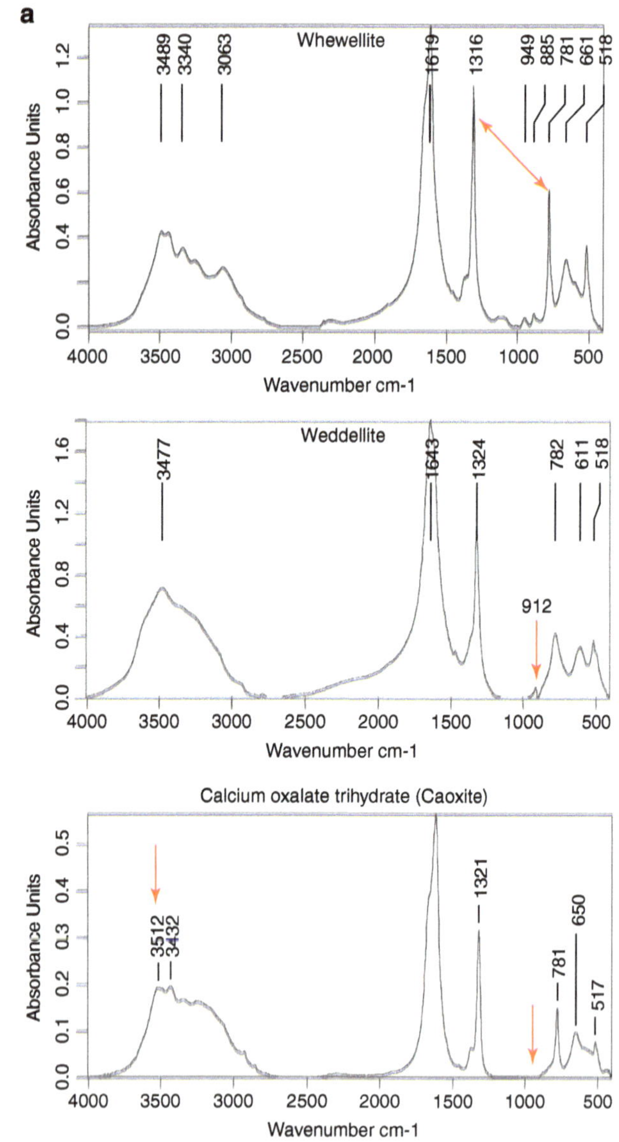

Fig. 85.3 Infrared spectra of urinary calculi: (**a**) calcium oxalates, (**b**) calcium phosphates, (**c**) magnesium phosphates, (**d**) other minerals, (**e**) uric acids, (**f**) urates, (**g**) other purines, (**h**) amino acids, (**i**) proteins and lipids, and (**j**) drugs

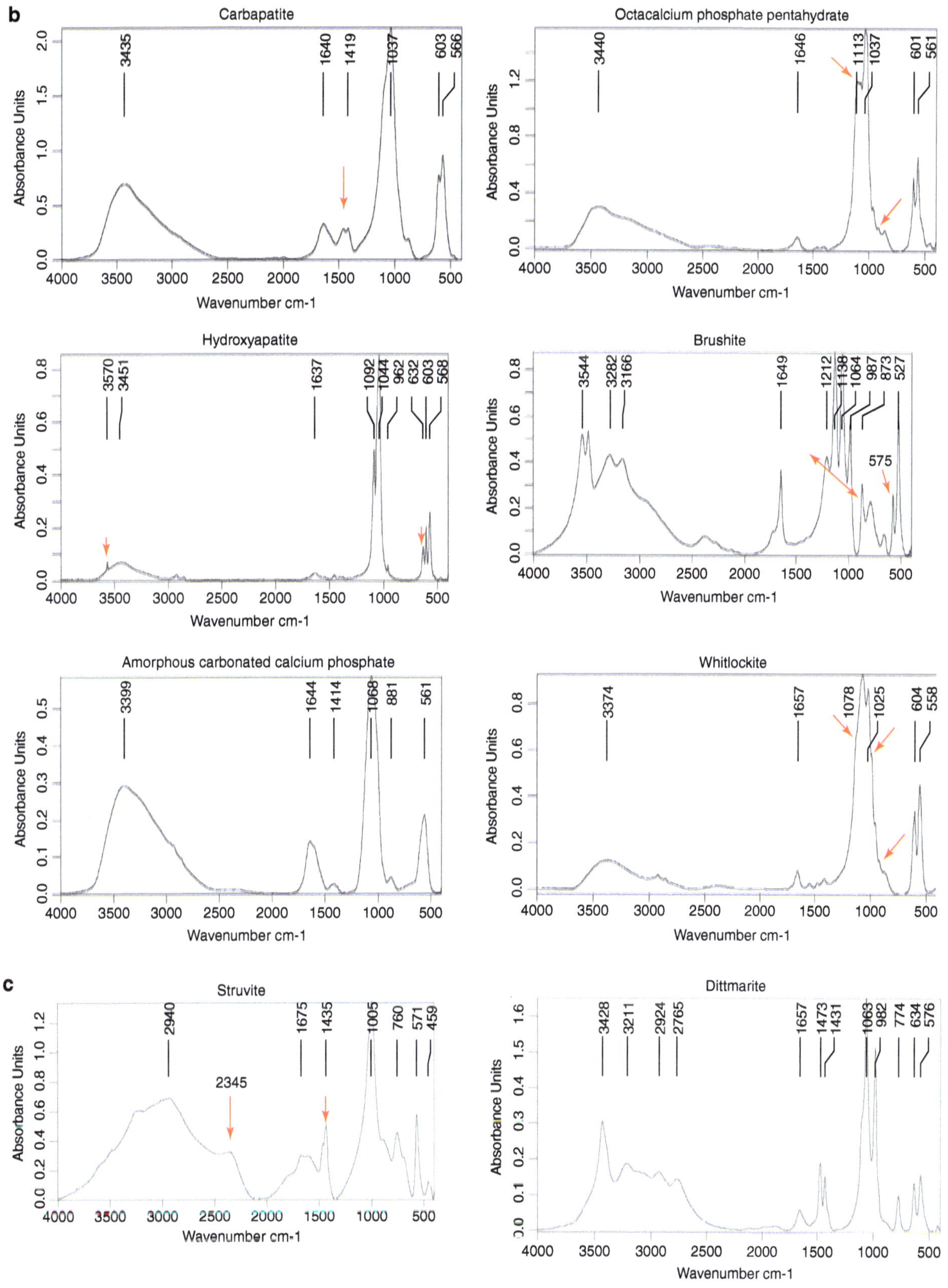

Fig. 85.3 (continued)

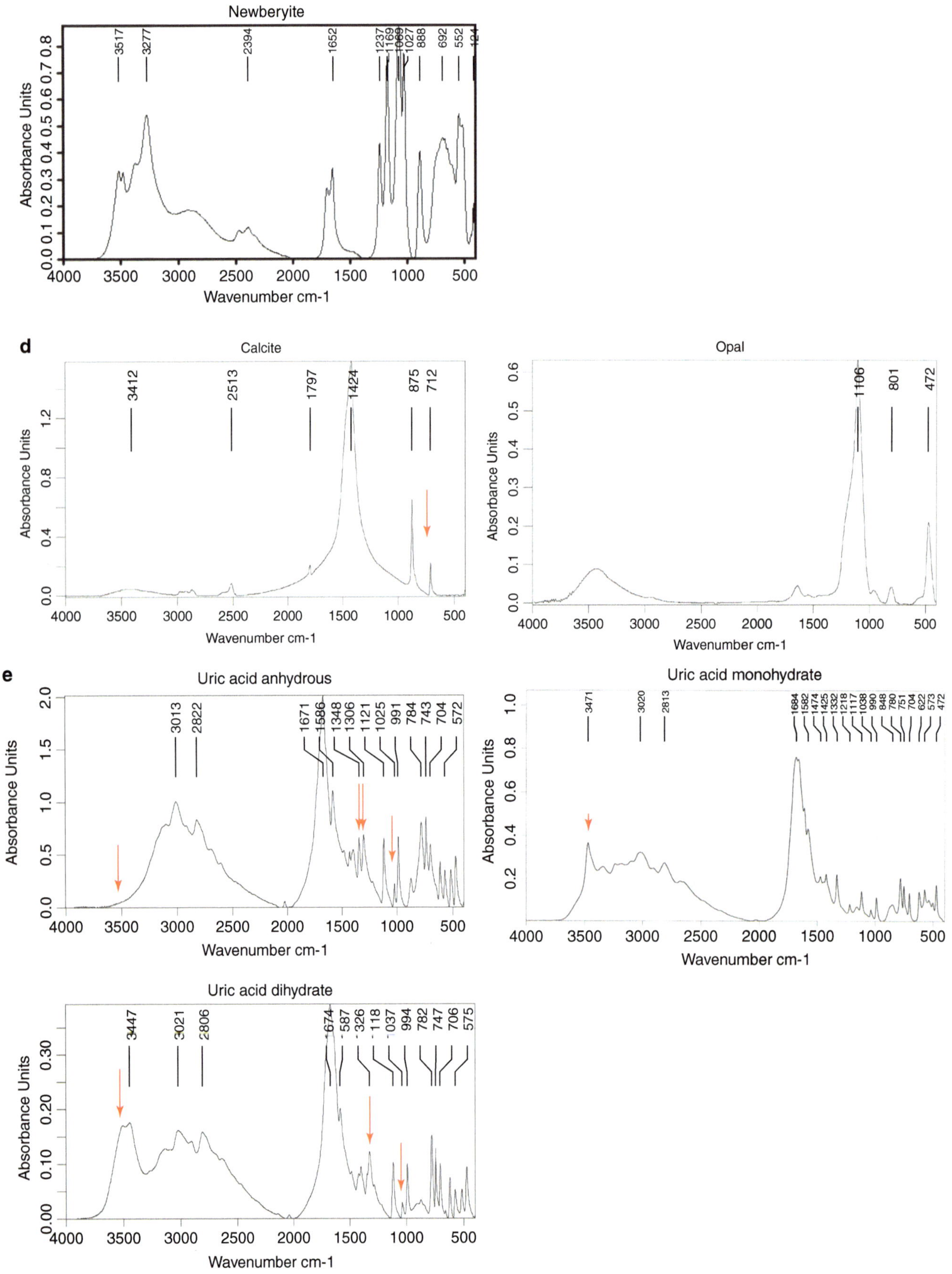

Fig. 85.3 (continued)

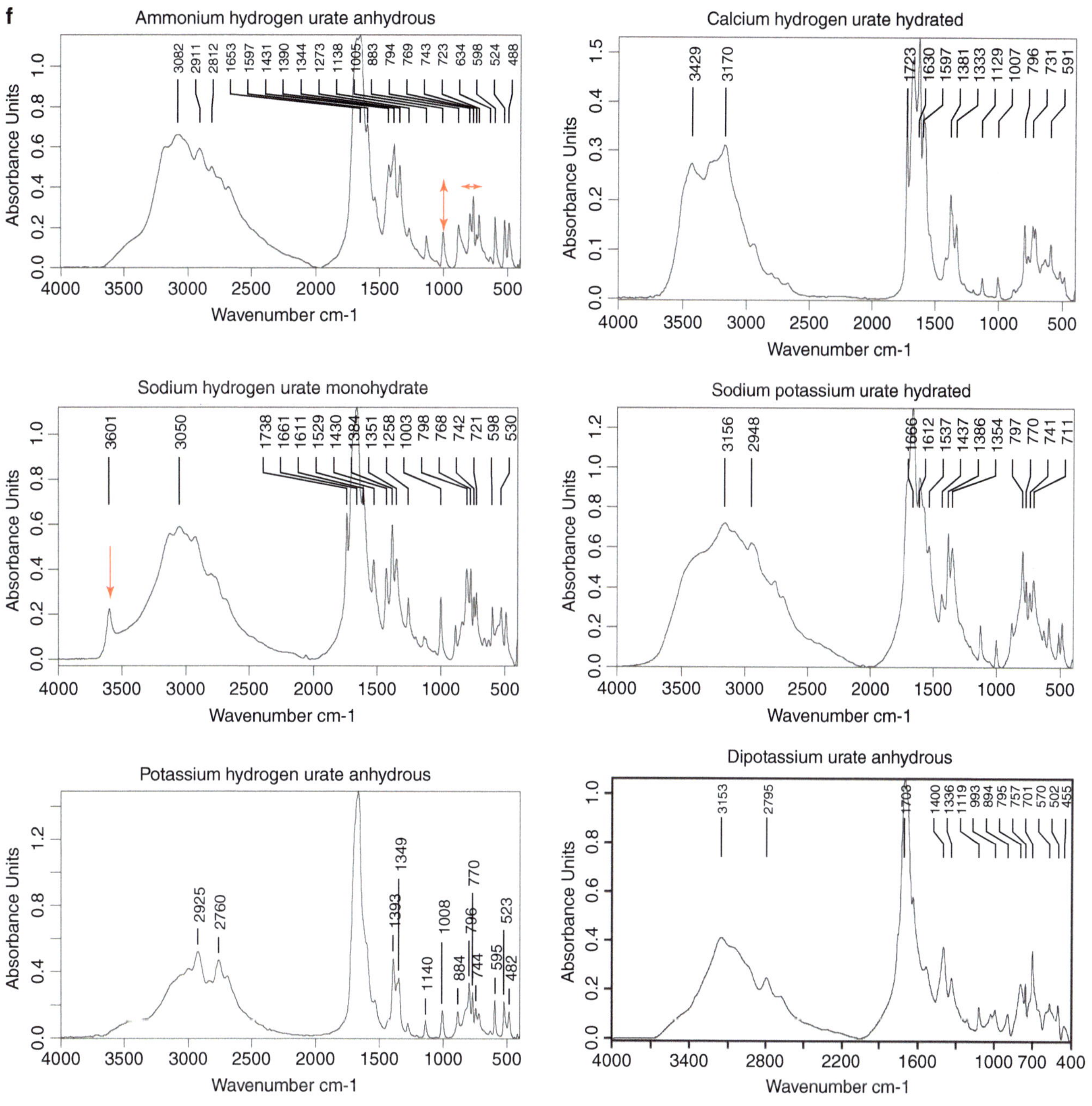

Fig. 85.3 (continued)

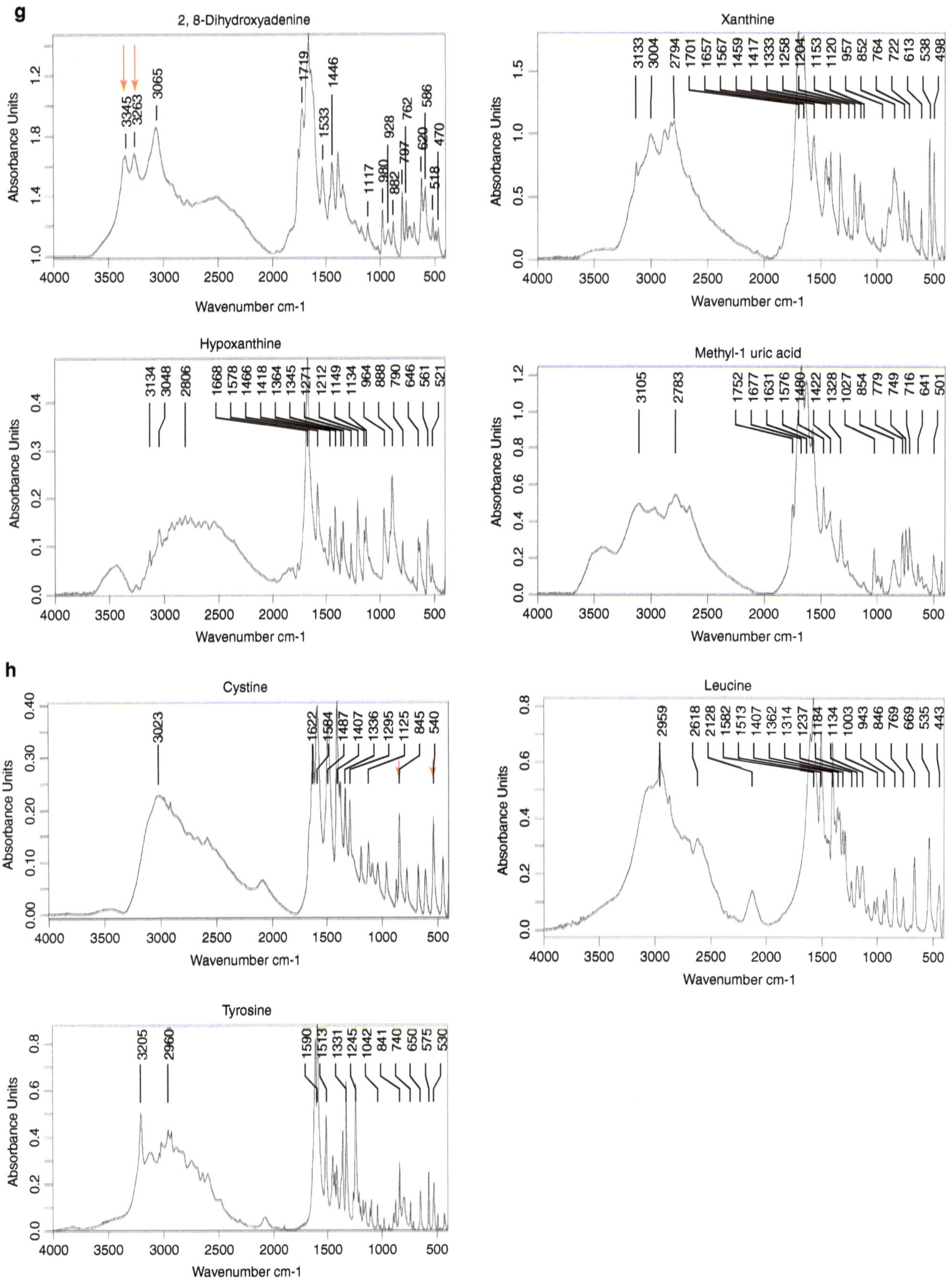

Fig. 85.3 (continued)

i

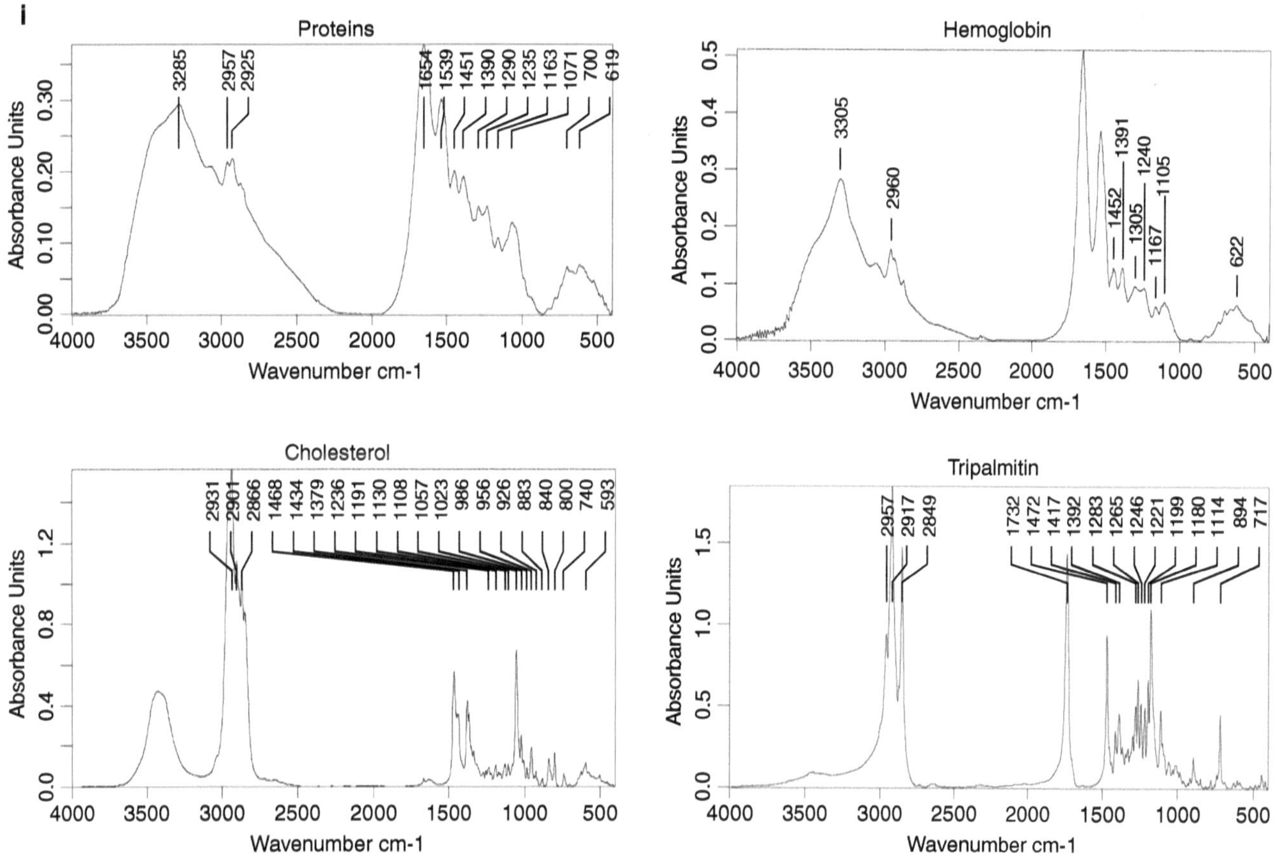

j

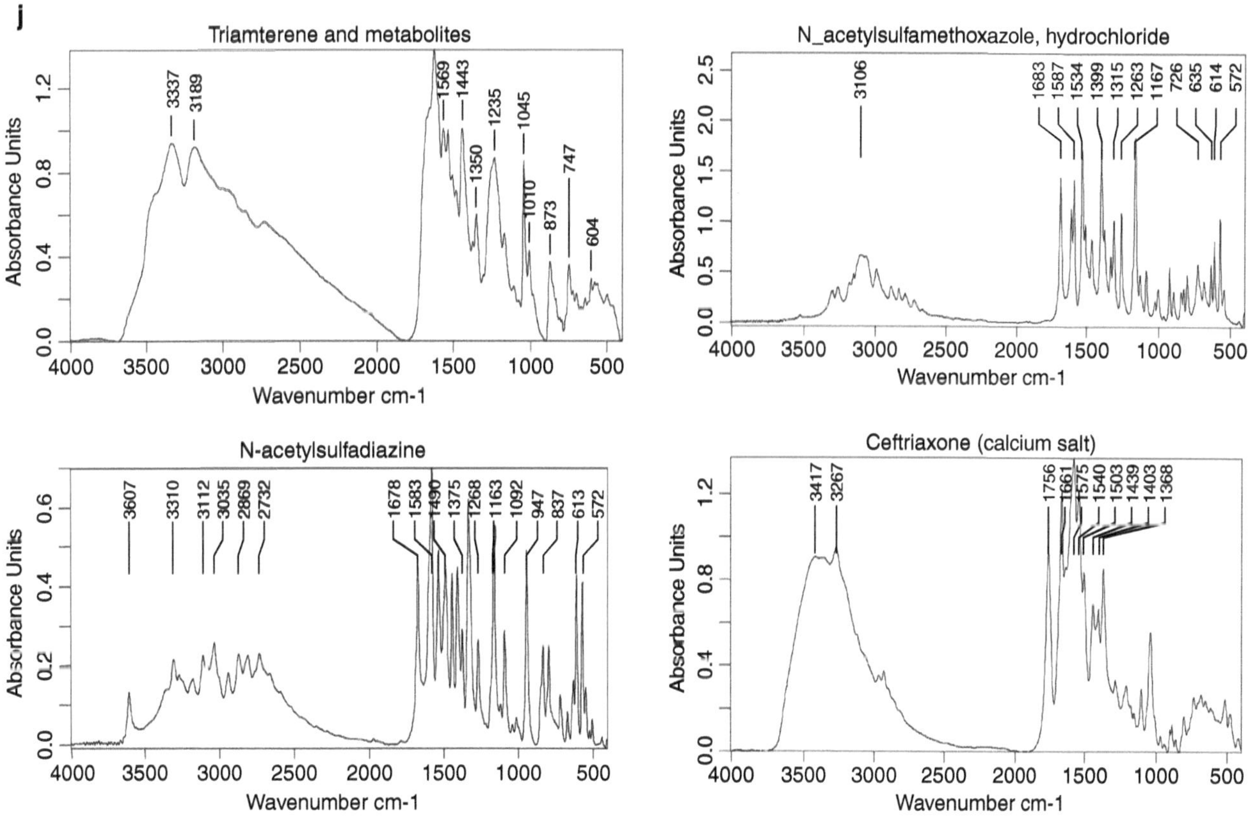

Fig. 85.3 (continued)

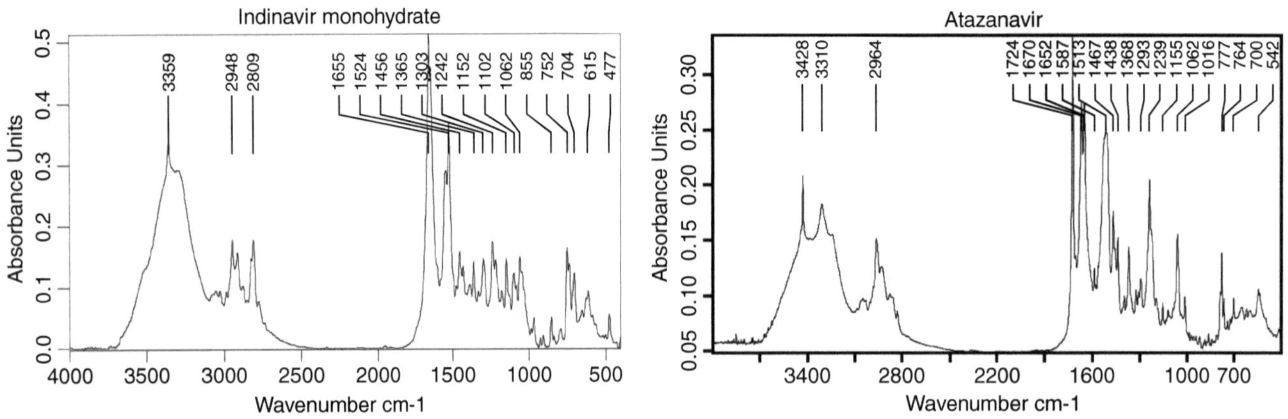

Fig. 85.3 (continued)

Indeed, in our experience, the atomic structure of a new form of calcium tartrate tetrahydrate [$Ca(C_4H_4O_6)$] $4H_2O$ has been identified in rat kidney calculus [38]. The crystal structure has been determined from powder and single-crystal X-ray diffraction.

Basically, at the atomic level, each atom of the sample defines a scattered wave built from an incident beam made either of photons, neutrons, or electrons. The spatial configuration of atoms causes the interference pattern of each wave. From an experimental point of view, this interference pattern is measured through a collection of diffraction peaks, their positions, and their intensities being intimately related to the spatial arrangement of the atoms.

As already underlined, scattering techniques yield some essential information regarding the size, the strain, the morphology, and the orientation of the nanocrystals. Broadening of the diffraction peaks is the result of two physical factors (namely, size and microstrain), and we can evaluate their effect separately [39]. Nanometer scale of crystals yields diffraction peaks that are broadened because the fewer the atomic planes that give rise to Bragg diffraction, the less sharp is the peak. A quantitative analysis based on the Scherrer equation links the broadening of the diffraction peak to the size of the nanocrystals. More precisely, the Scherrer equation (85.1) relates the width of a powder diffraction peak to (beta) β_s, the average (by volume) dimensions of crystallites in a polycrystalline powder:

$$\beta_s\,(2\theta_{hkl}) = \frac{K\lambda}{T\cos(\theta_{hkl})} \qquad 85.1$$

where (beta) β_s is the crystallite size contribution to the peak width (integral or full width at half maximum) in radians, K is a constant near unity, and T is the average thickness of the crystal in a direction normal to the diffracting plane *hkl* [40].

In the case of nanomaterials, the Debye equation (85.2) offers the opportunity to calculate the diffraction intensity:

$$I(q) = \Sigma_{i=1,n}\,\Sigma_{i=1,n} f_i(q) f_j(q)\left[\sin\left(qR_{ij}\right)\right]/\,qR_{ij} \qquad 85.2$$

In this equation, $I(q)$ is the angle-dependent intensity from coherent scattering, the sums over i and j are over all the n atoms, R_{ij} is the distance between the atoms i and j, and fi and f_j are the angle-dependent atomic scattering factors. This atomic factor is related to (rho) $\rho(r)$, the electron density of the atom, where r is the coordinate vector:

$$f_0(q) \;=\; 4\pi\int_0^{\infty} \rho(r)\left[\sin(qr)\right]/\,qr\; r^2 dr \qquad 85.3$$

It is well known that for forward scattering, this parameter tends toward Z plus a relativistic correction in the case of medium and heavy elements. Through these equations, it is thus possible to evaluate the effect of different structural and chemical parameters such as the morphology, the modification of interatomic distance, and partial substitution of Ca^{2+} by other cations such as Zn^{2+} or Sr^{2+}. In the case of size distribution, the Debye function analysis method (simulation done with a linear combination of ab initio calculations of a diffraction diagram) as developed by Vogel et al. [41] can be used; thus, information regarding the size distribution is available.

To obtain X-ray diffraction data on very small samples, several devices have been developed at the Laboratoire de Physique des Solides (LPS) (Fig. 85.4), including a home-built diffractometer using copper Kα (alpha) radiation and a microfocus device. Description of the apparatus has been previously reported [42]. Diffraction patterns can be recorded on photosensitive image plates. Classical (theta) θ/2θ (theta)-diffracted intensity representations were obtained and compared to the diffraction data collected for the reference compounds.

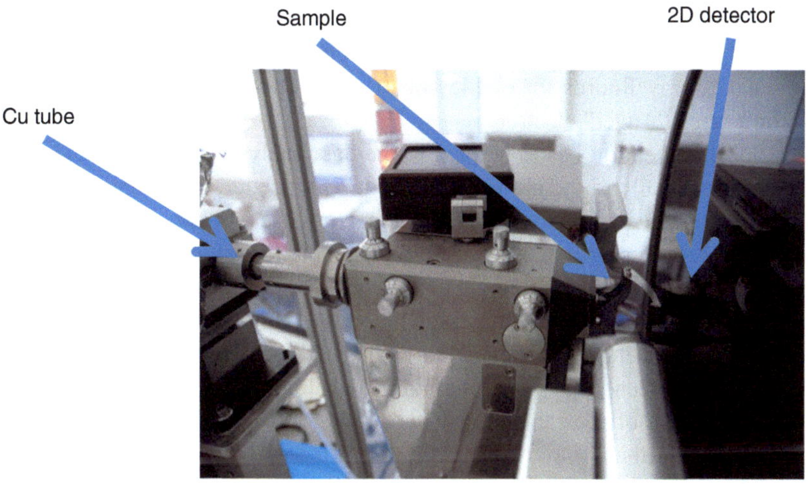

Fig. 85.4 X-ray scattering experimental device on which diagram is collected with a 2D detector

Figure 85.5 shows that the different X-ray diffraction patterns obtained for RP are clearly similar to the one collected on a kidney stone (KS) made of carbapatite (CA), which is used as a reference sample in this study (sample N17105). The selected RP samples are made mostly of nanocrystalline apatite exhibiting the usual anisotropy along the *c* axis. These typical structural characteristics are associated in the X-ray diagram with a relatively fine (002) diffraction peak (at 2(theta)θ=26°) and several poorly resolved lines constituting a broad peak between 2(theta)θ=30° and 2(theta)θ=35°. These structural characteristics are shared by numerous biological apatites [43, 44] associated not only with pathological calcifications but also with physiological ones (bone, dentine).

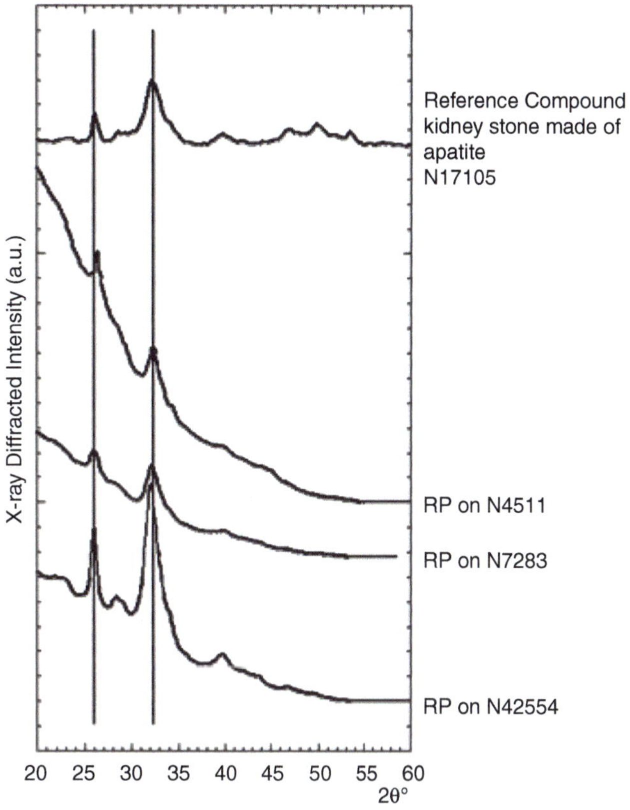

Fig. 85.5 X-ray diffraction diagram collected for a kidney stone and Randall's plaque made of apatite

Physical Methods for Special Investigations

Scientific research performed on kidney stones is based on several techniques that are not used routinely at the hospital—among them X-ray fluorescence spectroscopy. Recently, observations have been performed on field-effect scanning electron microscope, which allows a description at the submicrometer scale of the topology of kidney stones without the conventional deposit of carbon or gold or techniques specific to large-scale instrument such as neutron reactor dedicated to research or synchrotron radiation centers. We present these techniques in the section that follows.

Elemental Analysis Through X-Ray Fluorescence (XRF)

X-ray fluorescence (XRF) is used to determine the elemental composition of a sample by probing the electronic structure of the atoms in the sample, each element having electronic orbitals of characteristic energy. XRF has unique advantages over other analytical methods in that it enables nondestructive, multielemental analysis and does not damage the sample.

The physical process associated with X-ray fluorescence is as follows. When the energy of incident X-ray photon is sufficient, core electrons of atoms are ejected, creating vacancies. These vacancies correspond to an atom in an unstable state. As the atom returns to its stable state, electron transfer from the outer shells to the inner shells is made, and in this transfer, there is a possibility of a photon emission named "X-ray fluorescence" [45] or of an electron emission named "Auger" electron.

Special attention has to be paid to the data analysis and more specifically to the absorption correction procedures in order to obtain quantitative analysis. In fact, *dN*, the number of fluorescence photons, depends both on geometric parameters such as (alpha) α, the angle between the incident beam and the surface, or *D*, the thickness of the sample (Fig. 85.6), as well as more electronic parameters related to the efficiency of the fluorescence process ((sigma) σ^{Fl}_K (epsilon)$\varepsilon(E_K)$) or the absorption of the sample ((mu)μ_0, (mu)μ_{FL}). The equation to use in these corrections is the following (Eq. 85.4), and the integration is performed for $x=0$ to *D*:

$$dN = N_0 \exp(-\mu_0 x / \sin\alpha)\, n\sigma^{Fl}_K\, \varepsilon(E_K) \quad 85.4$$
$$\mathrm{Exp}(-\mu_{FL} x / \sin\beta)\, d\Omega / 4\pi\, dx$$

From an experimental point of view, numerous setups exist. At the LPS, such an experimental device allows the acquisition of a 2D map of elements in biological samples. This experimental device (Fig. 85.7) uses an X-ray tube with a Mo anode followed by a graphite monochromator. It can be operated at a tube voltage of 40 kV and a tube current of 30 mA. Fluorescence photons are collected with a SiLi detector, which allows plotting the number of fluorescence photons versus their energy, leading to a knowledge of the different elements present in the samples. This experimental device has been already used to evaluate the presence of heavy elements such Zn or Pb in different pathological calcifications.

A typical X-ray fluorescence spectrum of a kidney stone made of apatite is shown in Fig. 85.8, where we observe the contributions of different trace elements such as Zn (Kα(alpha) = 8,638 eV, Kβ(beta) = 9,572 eV), Pb (Lα(alpha) = 10,549 eV, Lβ(beta) = 12,613 eV), or Sr (Kα(alpha) = 14,165 eV) and obviously contributions coming from Ca (Kα(alpha) = 3,691 eV, Kβ(beta) = 4,012 eV). In this set of measurements, the highest proportion of the heavy elements was observed for Zn (1,000 ppm), a value in line with those found in previous works.

Scanning Electron Microscopy (SEM)

In order to perform significant research through scanning electron microscopy (SEM), we used two electron microscopes. The first is a FEI/Philips XL40 ESEM equipped with an energy dispersive X-ray spectrometer. Imaging involves a gaseous secondary electron detector, an accelerating voltage of 20 kV, and water pressure 0.4 torr in the chamber. This low pressure is used to keep good spatial resolution for the X-ray analysis by minimizing the scatter of the primary electron beam.

The second is a Zeiss SUPRA55-VP scanning electron microscope (Fig. 85.9). This field-effect "gun" microscope (FE-SEM) operates at 0.5–30 kV. High-resolution observations are obtained by two secondary electron detectors: an

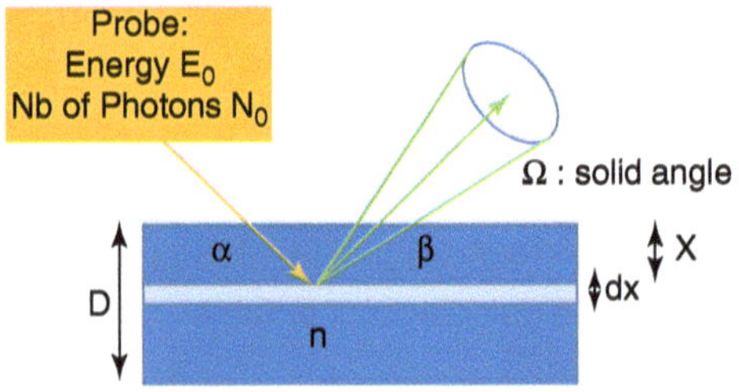

Fig. 85.6 Definition of the geometric parameters which have to be taken into account for performing quantitative analysis of X-ray fluorescence measurements

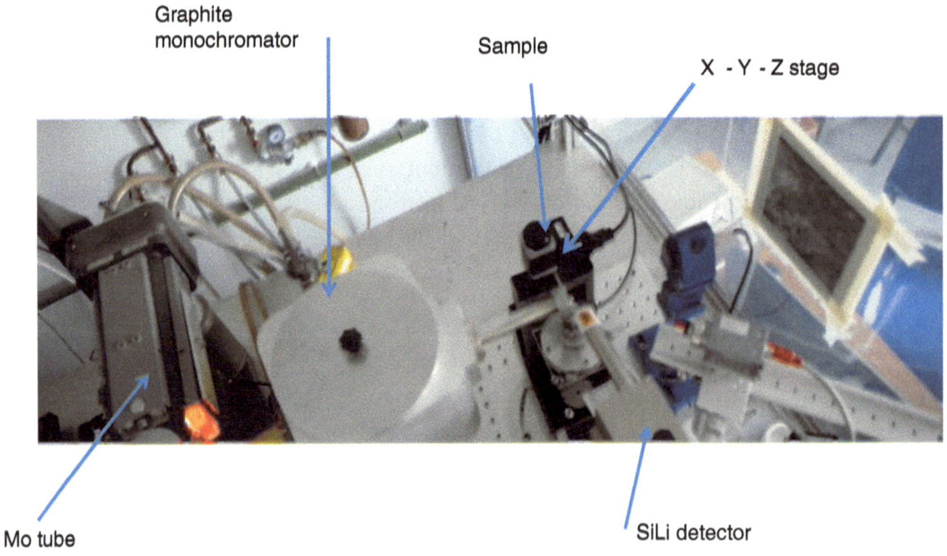

Fig. 85.7 X-ray fluorescence setup implemented in the LPS

in-lens SE detector and an Everhart–Thornley SE detector. To maintain the integrity of the samples, for both scanning electron microscopes, measurements are taken without the usual deposits of carbon at the surface of the sample.

On Fig. 85.10, a SEM image shows clearly the usual spherical morphology of apatite crystallites. For this sample, a homogeneous size distribution is measured. As we can see on Fig. 85.11 collected with a larger magnification, this spherical morphology comes from an agglomeration of smaller entities. This observation is in line with the fact that typical biological apatite crystals display nanometer dimensions.

Numerous structural investigations based on SEM have been already published regarding kidney stones [46–49].

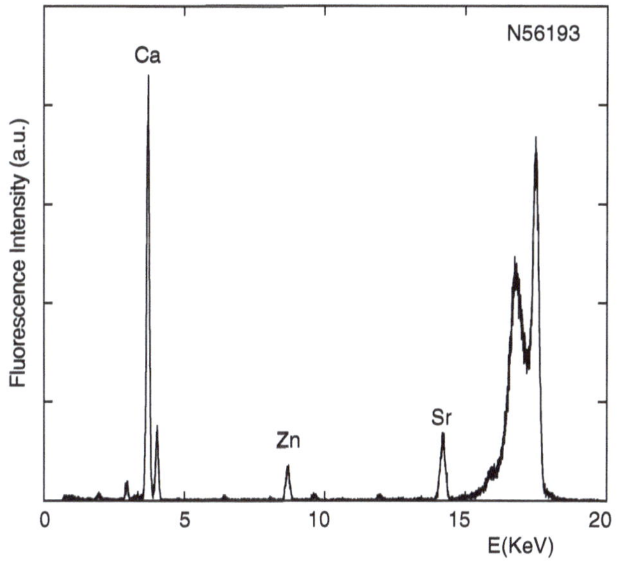

Fig. 85.8 Typical X-ray fluorescence spectrum collected for a biological apatite (kidney stones) linked to a pathological calcification. We can see clearly the contributions of Ca (Kα[alpha] = 3,691 eV, Kβ[beta] = 4,012 eV), Zn (Kα[alpha] = 8,638 eV, Kβ[beta] = 9,572 eV), Pb (Lα[alpha] = 10,549 eV, Lβ[beta] = 12,613 eV), and Sr (Kα[alpha] = 14,165 eV)

Scattering Techniques Using Neutrons as Probe

Powder neutron diffraction (PND) is nondestructive and particularly adapted to nanomaterials made of light elements such as kidney stones. Why neutron diffraction rather than X-ray diffraction? Simply because the average dimension of the nanocrystals is done for the overall sample with the neutrons and not only for the surface of the sample (as X-ray diffraction technique does). Such neutron probe limits possible preferential orientation of the crystals (in our case, X-ray diffraction experimental tests have been performed, but diffraction intensities were significantly affected by such an effect). Also, the result given by the neutron diffraction is more relevant to seek possible correlations between the macroscopic examination and the average nanocrystal dimension.

From an experimental point of view, neutron diffraction diagrams of kidney stones have been collected on the G4.1

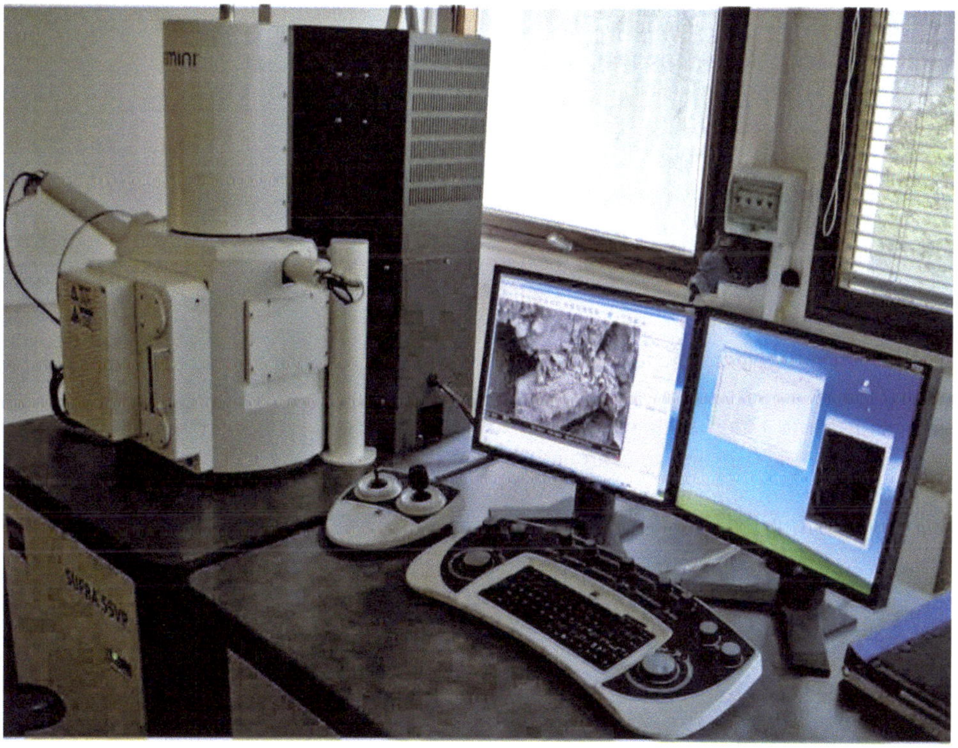

Fig. 85.9 Zeiss SUPRA55-VP scanning electron microscope

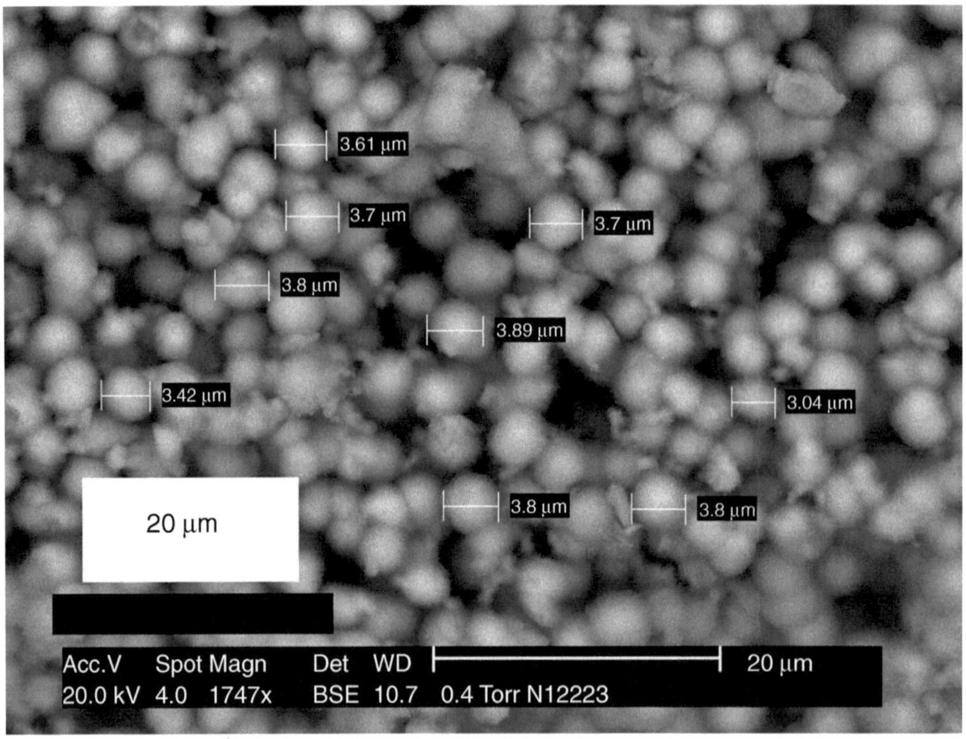

Fig. 85.10 SEM image of a kidney stone made of carbapatite. We can see clearly a spherical morphology for the crystallites

two-axis multidetector powder diffractometer [50] installed at the cold-source beamline of the Orphée reactor (Saclay, France). This beamline (Fig. 85.12) was equipped with a two-axis powder diffractometer with a vertical focusing pyrolytic graphite monochromator and a 800-cell multidetector covering a 80° 2θ (theta) range (step 0.1° between two cells). More precisely, neutron diffraction diagrams have been collected between 7° and 87° using a wavelength of 2.4226 Å, with an acquisition time of about a few hours depending on samples at room temperature. This particular experimental setup offers the opportunity to determine accurately the size of nanocrystals in a range between 5 and 200 nm.

We would like now to show how this technique is sensitive to the nanocrystal size. To attain this goal, we have plotted in Fig. 85.13 the neutron diffraction diagrams of three families of apatites. In the case of high-temperature-calcinated stoichiometric hydroxyapatite, very sharp diffraction peaks are measured, an experimental result in line with the fact that such materials are made of large nanocrystals (their dimension is around 200 nm).

In contrast, diffraction peaks related to nonstoichiometric nanocrystalline apatites synthesized at room temperature are very large. Similar experimental data have been obtained for biological apatites (such as in bones).

For these samples, the size is typically around 10 nm. Moreover, for all these apatites (synthesized at room temperature) and biological ones, the width of a diffraction peak (hkl=002) is smaller than the width of the other diffraction

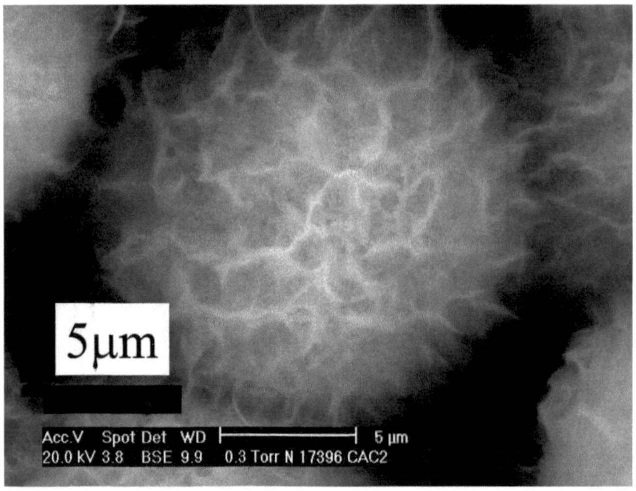

Fig. 85.11 A spherical apatite entity observed at high magnification

peaks, pointing out the anisotropy of the nanocrystals of all these compounds (needle and/or platelet-like morphology).

Synchrotron Radiation Generalities

Across the world, numerous storage rings dedicated to basic and applied research (using synchrotron radiation) exist. More precisely, there are now more than 50 light source facilities around the world, and on each one, dozens

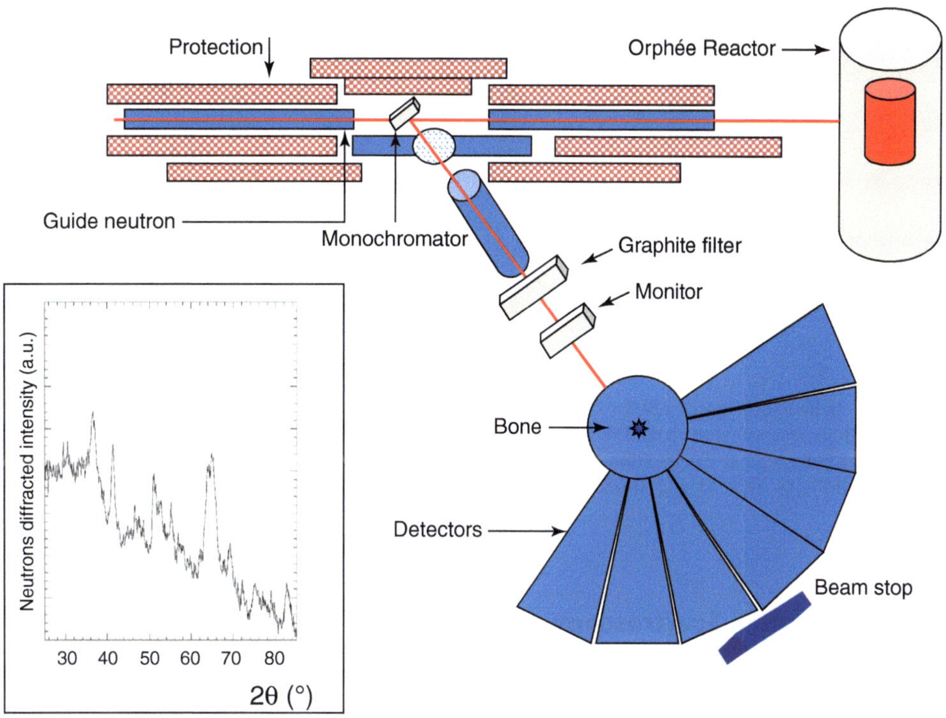

Fig. 85.12 Experimental setup of the beamline G4.1 installed on the Orphée reactor

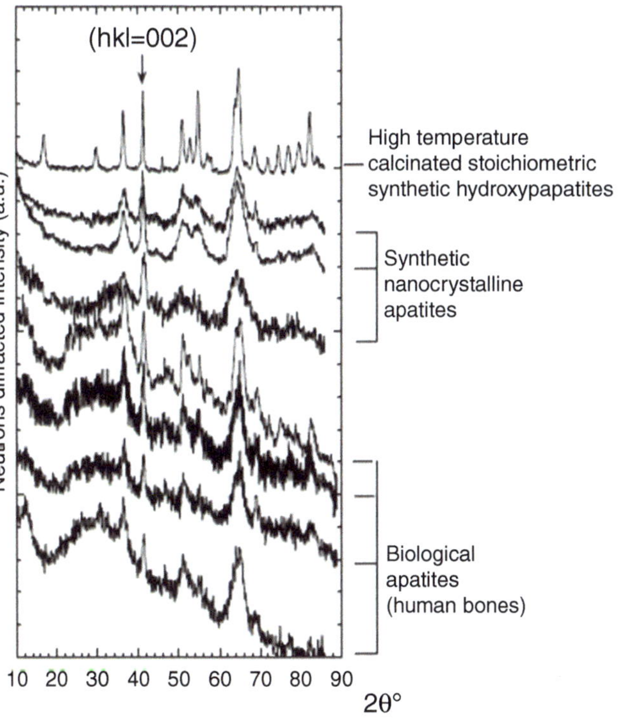

Fig. 85.13 Neutron diffracted intensity of different synthetic and biological apatites

of experiments are implemented, running 24 h a day, seven days a week [51, 52]. Several beamlines in different synchrotron radiation facilities are dedicated to medical research [53–55]. In France, two synchrotron radiation factories exist: ESRF, an acronym for "European Synchrotron Radiation Facility" [56] and SOLEIL [52] for "Source Optimisée de Lumière d'Energie Intermédiaire du LURE." It must be stressed that the first experiments on "a true sample" on SOLEIL were performed on a kidney stone [57].

What the human eye can see—namely, visible light—is only a tiny part of a vast spectrum from radio waves, microwaves, infrared, ultraviolet, and X-rays to gamma rays. Synchrotron radiation can deliver all of this spectrum and be used as a "supermicroscope" to reveal invaluable information from the intimate electronic structure of an atom to the kinetic evolution of the conformation of large proteins.

Due to the relativistic energy of the particles, synchrotron radiation has several specific properties that can be used in medical research. The emitted continuous spectrum is of high intensity. We can use this particularity to study either a very low quantity of sample or a highly diluted element in a matrix [58]. The natural divergence of the radiation is very small [59]. Cartography at the submillimeter scale can be performed [60, 61]. Finally, synchrotron radiation has a time structure, because the particles are stored in pulses. This time structure can be used to investigate time-dependent phenomena like relaxation or diffusion. The time scale ranges from nanoseconds to many hours. We can study the kinetic process of the drug diffusion, for example [62–64]. Several beamlines are of interest for stone analysis, such as DISCO (UV–visible microscopy), SMIS (infrared microscopy), and DIFFABS (X-ray absorption spectroscopy) (Fig. 85.14).

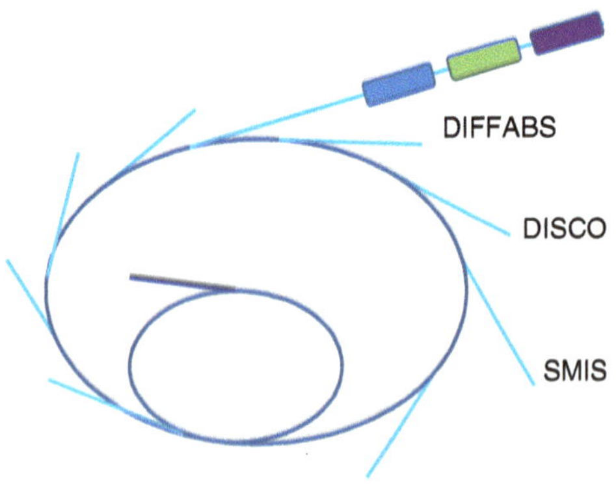

Fig. 85.14 Schematic view of a SOLEIL, a synchrotron radiation factory of third generation. Three beamlines currently used in the characterization of pathological calcifications have been positioned around SOLEIL: DIFFABS, DISCO, and SMIS

X-Ray Absorption Spectroscopy

Modern high brightness synchrotron radiation sources have helped X-ray absorption spectroscopy to become a significant technique for the characterization of low ordered materials [65] or trace elements [66–69].

X-ray absorption spectroscopy is especially useful for characterizing biological calcium phosphates for different valuable reasons. First, calcified deposits are often poorly crystalline and consequently difficult to characterize by classical techniques. Second, the size of the probe is sufficient to establish a mapping of a biological sample for which no specific preparation is necessary. Thus, one main virtue of X-ray absorption spectroscopy (XAS) is that the chemical state of the pathological calcification is preserved.

XAS (Fig. 85.15) includes X-ray absorption near edge structure (XANES) and extended X-ray absorption fine structure (EXAFS). This spectroscopy is able to describe accurately an average of the electronic state, the geometry of the very first neighbors, and finally the first coordination spheres of a selected element. On Fig. 85.15, we collected X-ray absorption spectra after the absorption edge of synchrotron radiation; thus, it is the average local environment of synchrotron radiation that is characterized. The notion of average is quite important, as this technique is insensitive to polydispersity [70].

At the edge of low Z elements, this technique is of great interest since it is highly sensitive to the geometrical environment around the photoabsorbing atom. In the literature, most Ca K edge studies have been devoted to the bones [71].

In EXAFS experiments, a monochromatic X-ray beam is directed at the sample. To extract a monochromatic beam from the white beam coming from the ring, a monochromator

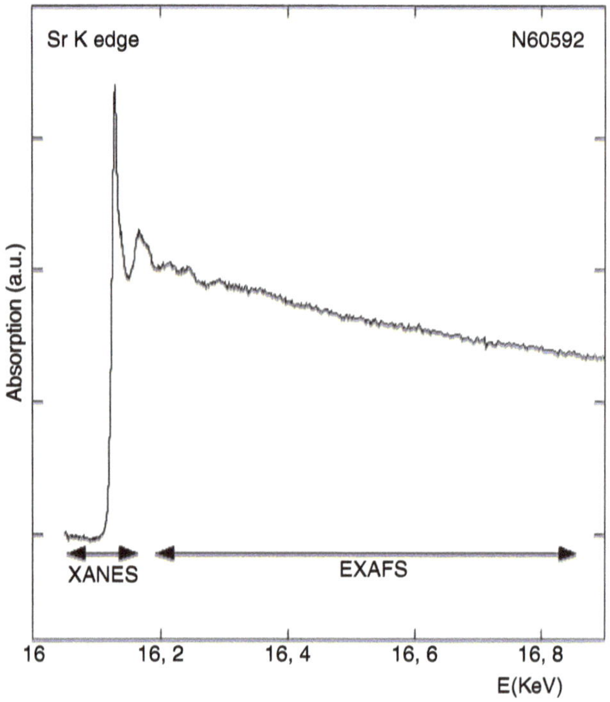

Fig. 85.15 X-ray absorption spectrum (XAS) collected at the Sr K edge

made of two Si crystals is used (see Fig. 85.16). Also, two mirrors are positioned before and after the monochromator in order to obtain a perfect collimated monochromatic beam. The photon energy of the X-rays is gradually increased such that it can excite one of the core electrons. We use thus the possibility to sweep the photon energy. In that case, a large increase in absorption occurs known as the absorption edge. The core electron, now called a photoelectron, is ejected and can be backscattered by the atoms surrounding the emitting atom. The net result is a modulation of the absorption edge that can be used to determine the atomic number, distance, and coordination number of the emitting atoms.

The relation between the modulated part $\chi(k)$ and the structural parameters contained in the absorption spectrum has been established in numerous theoretical studies and can be written as

$$\chi(k) = \sum_j N_j / kR_j^2 f_j(k) \exp(-\Gamma(\text{Gamma})_j R_j/k)$$
$$\exp(-2(\text{sigma})\sigma_j^2 k^2) \sin(2kR_j + (\text{phi})\phi_j(k))$$

where k is the wave vector of the photoelectron and j refers to the different coordination shells around the absorbing atom, each shell containing N_j equivalent atoms. A Debye-Waller factor (sigma) σj takes into account the fact that a spread in distance exists in material, and we assume that this distribution is Gaussian.

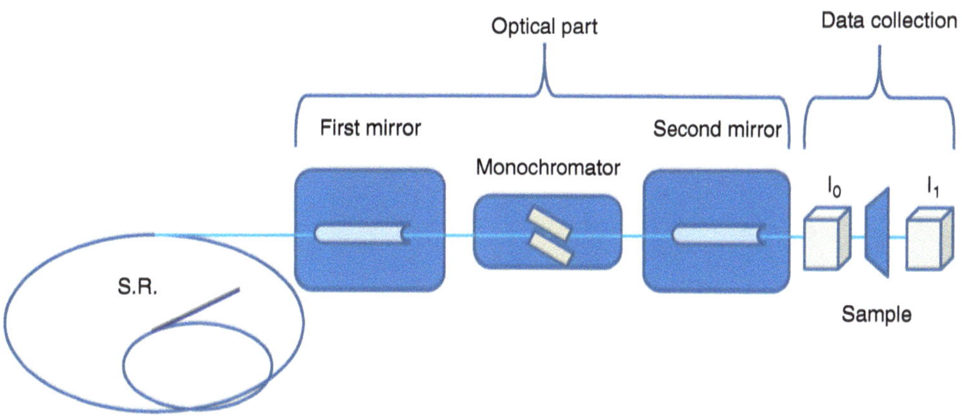

Fig. 85.16 Schematic representation of the DIFFABS beamline

Generally, the electron mean free path (Gamma) Γ_j is introduced in order to reflect the probability that the electron is inelastically scattered.

In the last set of experiments, SOLEIL was running at 2.75 GeV with an average current of 300 mA for our experiments in the new TOP/UP configuration. The monochromatization and horizontal focus is achieved using a double Si (111) crystal monochromator (Fig. 85.16), which offers an energy resolution of (Delta) $\Delta E/E = 10^{-4}$ necessary to resolve the XANES structures [72]. This experimental setup is between two cylindrical vertically focusing (50-nm Rh deposited on Si substrates). At the sample position, the spot size was defined with slits to reach 100 × 250 (mu) μm² (H×V, FWHM).

Either at K or at L edge, XANES contain both electronic and structural information but can be difficult to interpret fully [73]. In fact, similarity between the K and the L edge may point out overlap between cations (4s, 4p, and 3d) and oxygen (2p) orbitals [74].

FTIR Microspectroscopy on Synchrotron

One drawback of FTIR microspectroscopy (FTIRM) is the long wavelength of infrared light, where the diffraction-limited spatial resolution is theoretically predicted to be around 2 (mu) μm in the mid-infrared region (4,000–400 cm^{-1}) [75]. In practice, however, the spatial resolution is often limited by the brightness of the conventional thermal infrared source found in laboratory FTIR spectrometers.

Application of Physical Methods to Stone Characterization

Calcium Oxalate Stones

Regarding calcium oxalate monohydrate (COM) kidney stones, a classification into five main types, namely, Ia, Ib, Ic, Id, and Ie, has been already proposed and confirmed through the analysis of more than 70,000 kidney stones at the Necker Hospital. For example, type Ia stones (the most common), with a dark-brown smooth or mammillary surface, are found in idiopathic stone formers with intermittent hyperoxaluria of dietary origin, while type Ic kidney stones (Fig. 85.17), the surfaces of which have a mulberry-shaped aspect of cream or pale yellow–brown color, are specifically observed in patients with primary hyperoxaluria, a severe inherited metabolic disease.

We have recently used scanning electron microscopy (SEM) to show that the classification of COM kidney stones based on observations at the macroscopic scale exists also at the mesoscopic scale. More precisely, a peculiar morphology for whewellite crystallites exists in stones that exhibit an Ic morphological type associated with primary hyperoxaluria type 1. Such a morphology is significantly distinct from that of the common type of whewellite stones [76, 77].

Finally, the stone morphology as defined by stereomicroscopic examination for 1,270 whewellite calculi first treated by ESWL in clinical practice has been investigated. Among them, 94 were resistant to several (two or more) ESWL sessions and had to be removed by surgical procedures. Among stones that were considered to be successfully treated (i.e., fragmented as small pieces of stone able to be spontaneously passed during the days or weeks following treatment), 98.7 % had a well-organized structure (type Ia or Id), while only 1.3 % were disorganized (type Ib). In contrast, among stones that were resistant to ESWL, 62 (66 %) presented an Ib structure corresponding to large disorganized crystals, and eight exhibited a well-organized structure corresponding to type Ia. Only five stones with type Id morphology were found in the group of unsuccessful ESWL treatment. It is of interest that among 77 stones that exhibited a type Ib morphology, 80.5 % were resistant to ESWL.

Calcium Phosphate Stones

CA stones can be classified according to morphologic criteria, as previously reported. Among the six main types of this classification, type IV includes all calcium and magnesium

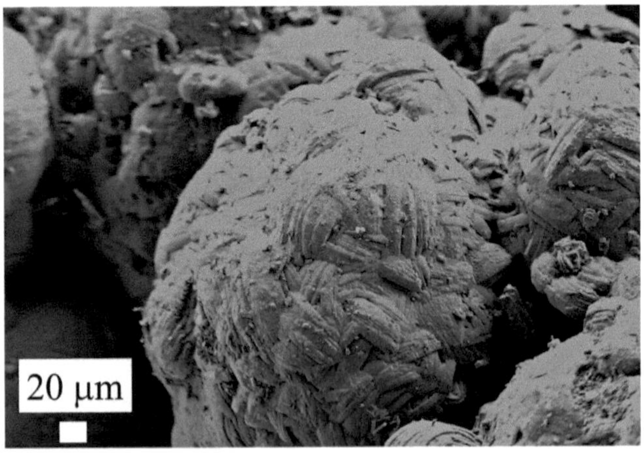

Fig. 85.17 SEM observations of a COM kidney stone type Ic related to primary hyperoxaluria

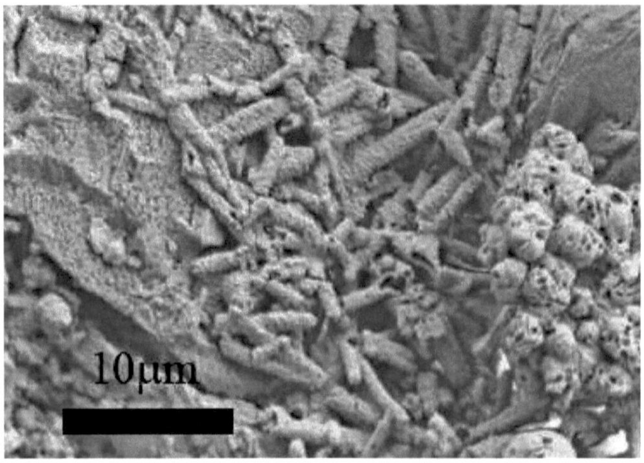

Fig. 85.18 SEM observations of bacterial imprints and calcified bacteriae within a CA kidney stone

phosphate stones, and type II includes stones mainly composed of weddellite. Because CA and weddellite often coexist in stones, especially in patients with hypercalciuria, a mixed type IV + II is frequently observed. According to the morphologic examination findings, three groups could be distinguished in our series of stones: group 1 included 23 stones composed of nearly pure calcium phosphate (type IV), group 2 included 11 stones composed of a mixture of calcium phosphate and weddellite (type IV + II), and group 3 included 5 stones with a complex heterogeneous structure.

The complete set of SEM observations has allowed us to underline a close relationship in group 1 between the presence of bacterial imprints observed through SEM (Fig. 85.18), indicative of past or current urinary tract infection, and both the presence of amorphous carbonated calcium phosphate (ACCP) or whitlockite and a high carbonation rate of CA [78]. Such correlation significantly helps the clinician to define the diagnostic. Thus, SEM may constitute a key technique to establish the existence of infection through the observation of bacterial imprints.

A Classification of Trace Elements Present in Kidney Stones

Usually, the X-ray fluorescence measurements are given in different tables without any kind of comments except on their content. The complete set of X-ray fluorescence data in the 2–18-KeV range we obtained on more than 100 kidney stones leads us to a classification of elements we can find in these concretions. At first, we find calcium or sulfur elements which are elements present in the stoichiometric formulae, for example, calcium in whewellite ($CaC_2O_4 \cdot H_2O$) or weddellite ($CaC_2O_4 \cdot 2H_2O$), which are calcium oxalates or sulfur for the cystine ($[S–CH_2–CH(NH_2)–COOH]_2$). Then, we can find several oligoelements with different origins. For example, the presence of strontium and selenium is pointed out because these elements share the same column in the periodic table as elements present in the stoichiometric formulae, for example, strontium for calcium and selenium for sulfur. In fact, we can add that Sr^{2+} ions follow the Ca^{2+} metabolic pathways. Moreover, from a chemical point of view, Ca^{2+} and Sr^{2+} have similar chemistry (these two elements share the same column in the periodic table) and commonly substitute for one another in minerals [79]. We may also find zinc and copper. These two elements are present in the human body in various metalloproteins. Of note, Zn^{2+} ions can be excreted by the kidney. We may find also iron, probably due to blood at the surface of, or within, kidney stones. Finally, we can find trace elements such as lead or cadmium. In our case, we have noticed the presence of lead, and the quantitative evaluation of this element has been compared to previous study showing a significant decrease in the amount of this element in kidney stones. Other elements used in medicine can be revealed by X-ray fluorescence, such as iodine or platinum, the presence of the first one being noticed in kidney stones.

Application of Physical Methods to Randall's Plaque Characterization

In 1936, Alexander Randall reported on calcium deposits observed at the surface of and beneath the papillary epithelium [21]. Some deposits, also named plaques because some of them partly covered the epithelium, supported small calcium oxalate stones, suggesting these plaques could serve as nucleators for calcium oxalate stone formation. Such observations were confirmed by other authors during the same period [80, 81], and this phenomenon was then forgotten. A renewal of interest in Randall's plaques (RP) more recently resulted from the progress in endoscopic procedures, which now offer the opportunity to see the different parts of the renal cavities and the surface of the papillae with minimally invasive surgery or ureteroscopy. Taking advantage of these new urological procedures, Evan and colleagues obtained papillary biopsies and found that the calcium deposits within the inner medulla initiated in the basement membrane of Henle's loops and spread out in the interstitium around vasa recta and collecting ducts up to the papillary epithelium [82]. Once the epithelium disrupted, calcium phosphate that forms such calcification may be in contact with supersaturated urine, resulting for calcium oxalate deposition on the phosphate and further stone formation [83].

The occurrence of RP in the kidneys of stone formers varies greatly from one country to another. However, epidemiological data highly suggest a significant increase of such RP at the origin of calcium stones in the recent decades in the United States and Western Europe. As suggested by Evan's group and also by other American teams, about 75–80 % of calcium stone formers present with RP in their kidneys [26, 84]. In France, Olivier Traxer, who recommends ureteroscopic procedures as safe and minimally invasive treatment for kidney stones, found that 55–60 % of calcium stone formers present with RP [85] and 27 % of non-stone-former patients who have been explored for other urological problems during the same period. In our experience, based on stone analysis, we found that calcium oxalate stones developed from RP accounted for about 8.9 % at the beginning of the 1980s and dramatically increased to 20.6 % at the beginning of the twenty-first century with a significant decrease in the patient's age [86]. Today, in France, more than 50 % of young calcium oxalate stone formers aged 20–30 years old developed their stone from an RP, the latter being observed at the surface of the stone when examining it under a stereomicroscope.

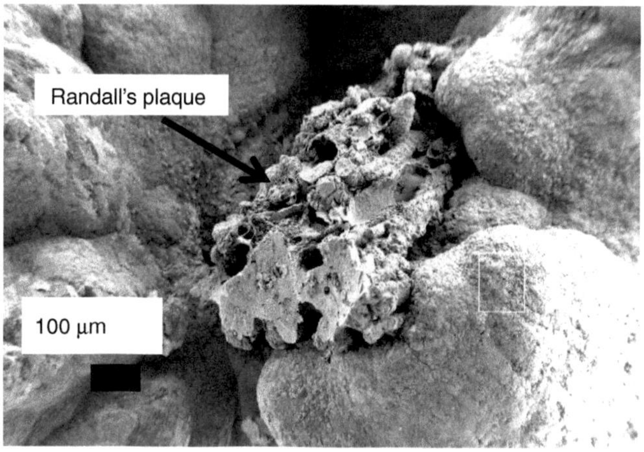

Fig. 85.19 Typical photography at the mesoscopic scale of a Randall's plaque

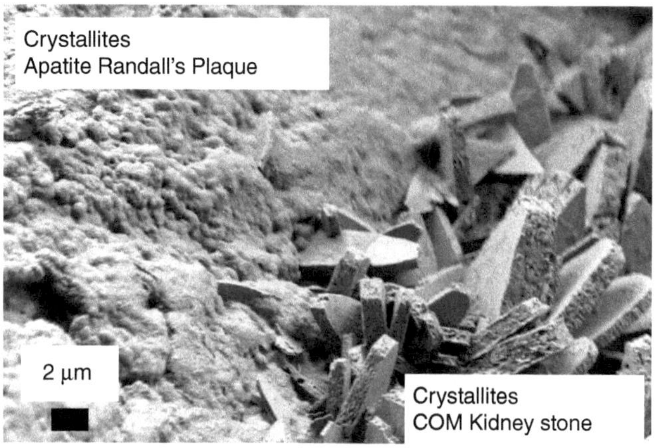

Fig. 85.20 Typical scanning electron micrograph collected at the interface between a Randall's plaque and calcium oxalate monohydrate

Randall's Plaque Described at the Mesoscopic Scale Through SEM

Figure 85.19 illustrates a typical Randall's plaque. As revealed by SEM, its structure is quite complex at the mesoscopic scale. We can see that it is made of an accumulation of calcified tubes that are either full or empty.

The Interface Between RP and Kidney Stones

RP is made of a mixture of spheres of apatite and proteins [84] in which calcium oxalate crystallites are trapped (Fig. 85.20). Such deposits are not allowed on a normal epithelium where different proteins are dedicated to prevent such a process. The fact that this epithelium is now covered with a mixture of mineral and proteins favors the deposit of calcium oxalate monohydrate crystallites. As we can see in the right part of the figure, the building of the kidney stone then results from a simple accumulation of micrometer-sized calcium oxalate crystallites. Such crystallites normally are supposed to be evacuated through urine flowing down to the ureters.

In the following picture (Fig. 85.21), we may understand why it is quite rare to find calcium oxalate dihydrate crystallites. The size of such crystallites can be comparable to the size of the Randall's plaque. It is thus quite difficult to trap such calcium oxalate dihydrate crystallites at the surface of the Randall's plaque. Indeed, from an epidemiologic point of view, the percentage of Randall's plaque present on calcium oxalate dihydrate kidney stones is equal to 12.6 %, while the percentage corresponding to calcium oxalate monohydrate kidney stones is around 49 %.

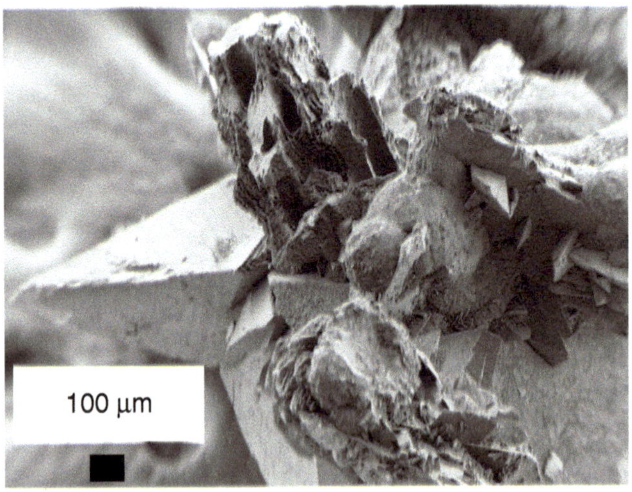

Fig. 85.21 Typical scanning electron micrograph collected at the interface between a Randall's plaque and either calcium oxalate dihydrate crystallites

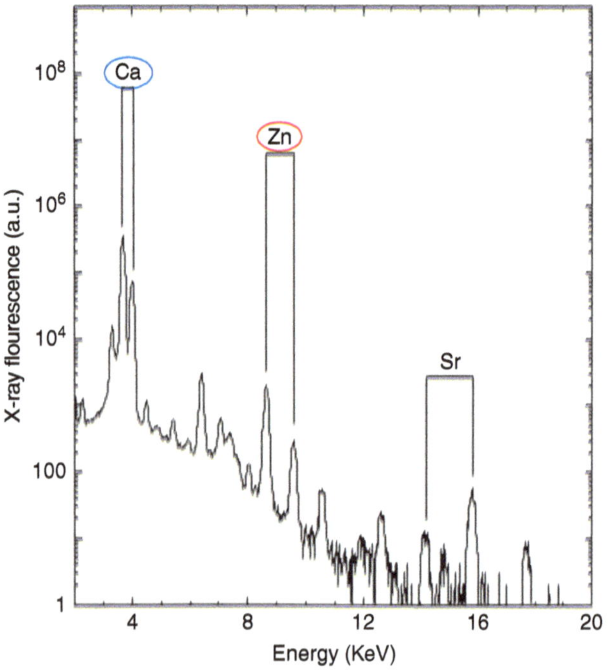

Fig. 85.22 Typical PIXE spectrum collected for a Randall's plaque

Understanding the Role of Oligoelements in the Genesis of Randall's Plaque

Trace elements have been already considered as risk factors regarding kidney stones [87, 88] or from a more chemistry point of view [89]. We have already performed a similar study [90], pointing out the fact that the preponderance of oligoelements such as Zn^{2+} or Sr^{2+}, both bivalent ions, in calcium-containing stones suggests a substitution process of Ca^{2+} by metal ions with similar charge and radius ($R(Ca^{2+})$ = 0.99 Å; $R(Zn^{2+})$ = 0.74 Å; $R(Sr^{2+})$ = 1.12 Å) rather than a contribution of the metals to stone formation.

Here, we consider the investigation of oligoelements as risk factors for the formation of RP as a logical extension of our previous work dedicated to KS. To attain this goal, we consider X-ray fluorescence induced by proton as well as by synchrotron radiation [91]. Particle-induced X-ray emission (PIXE) is a nondestructive, simultaneous trace multielement analytical technique. Depending on the proton energy and sample composition, detection limits may be as low as pg/g.

The spatial distributions of Ca and Zn in Randall's plaque were examined by micro-PIXE. Nuclear microprobe analyses were performed with a 2.8-MeV proton beam at the Pierre Süe Laboratory. The beam was focused down to 3 × 3 µ(mu)m² with an average intensity of 250 pA. X-rays were collected using a 30-mm² silicon SDD detector. Distance from the detector to the sample was fixed to 30 mm, and a 200-µ(mu)m-thick Mylar foil was used to stop backscattered protons.

Figure 85.22 represents a typical PIXE spectra collected for a kidney biopsy. The contributions of the different elements, namely, Ca ($E_{K\alpha}$(alpha) = 3.692 KeV, $E_{K\beta}$(beta) = 4,013 KeV), Zn ($E_{K\alpha}$(alpha) = 8.639 KeV, $E_{K\beta}$(beta) = 9.572 KeV), and Sr ($E_{K\alpha}$(alpha) = 14.17 KeV, $E_{K\beta}$(beta) = 15.84 KeV), are well defined. Elemental maps of Ca and Zn were generated from PIXE spectra. Each element of interest was identified by finding the integrated photopeak area associated with its K_α (alpha) fluorescence emission. Figure 85.22 shows an example of the elemental maps of Ca and Zn obtained at 10-µ(mu)m spatial resolution.

On Figs. 85.23 and 85.24, the cartography for Ca and Zn has been plotted. Some features are particularly interesting. For example, it seems that for the first biopsy (see Fig. 85.23), the spatial repartition of Ca and Zn is clearly very different. Zn is present at the surface of Ca domains. The reverse configuration is observed for the second biopsy (see Fig. 85.24), for which high concentration of Zn domains corresponds to high concentration of Ca.

Such observations suggest a possible inflammatory response of the tissue to the carbapatite deposition in the interstitium, mediated by metalloproteinases. Indeed, we found a very high Zn content in carbapatite RP by comparison to other carbapatite stones developed from tubular lumen or renal cavities [92], which could be a marker of a Zn accumulation in the tissue where calcium phosphate particles are deposited.

First Ex Vivo Experiments on RP

Regarding the chemical composition of RP, even if other phosphate phases such as whitlockite or brushite can be

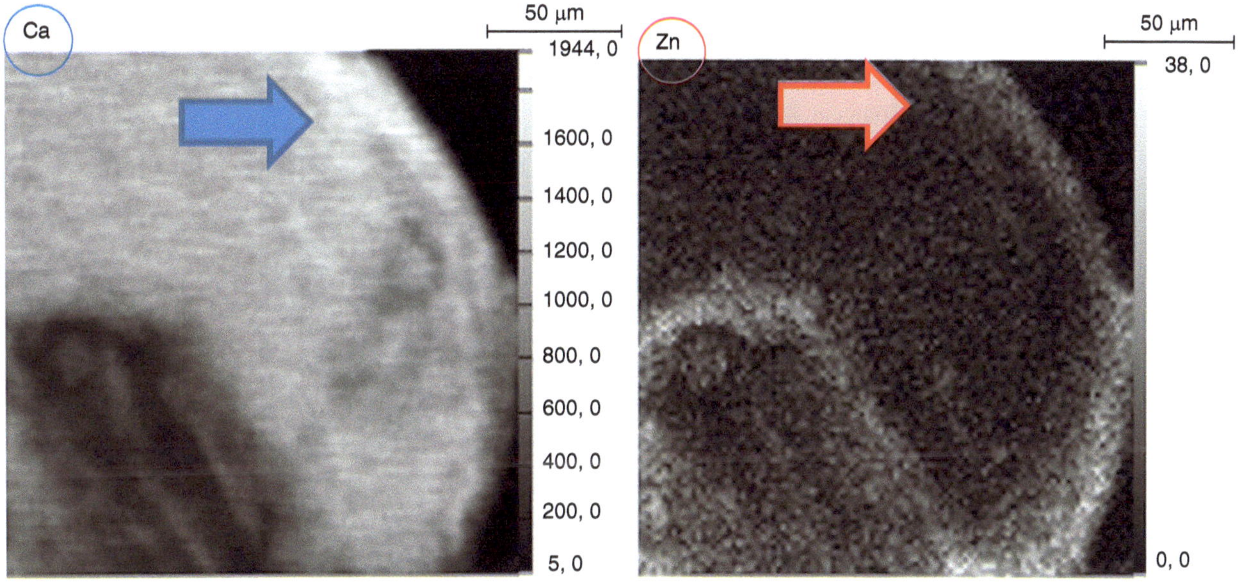

Fig. 85.23 Elemental map of RP for Ca and Zn for a kidney biopsy. Darker regions indicate a lower concentration of the element (scale is 50 µ[mu]m). Total collected beam charge: 0.7 µ(mu)C

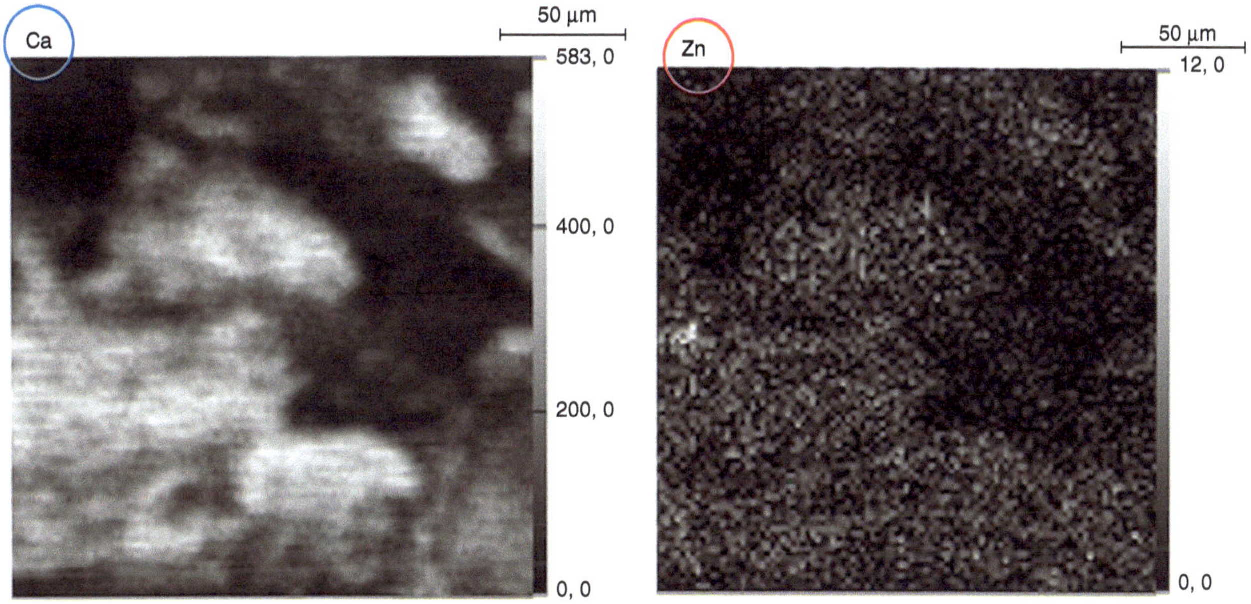

Fig. 85.24 Elemental map of RP for Ca and Zn for another kidney biopsy. Darker regions indicate a lower concentration of the element (scale is 50 µ[mu]m). Total collected beam charge: 0.4 µ(mu)C

found as minor components (less than 5 %), calcium phosphate apatite (CA) and amorphous carbonated calcium phosphate (ACCP) are the major components of most RPs. In fact, at the surface of apatite, an amorphous part (ACCP) can be found. Of note, ACCP can be considered as a precursor for CA, and its chemical stability is controlled by the water content. Thus, it is of primary importance to characterize RP while the sample is hydrated.

X-ray absorption spectroscopy (XAS) is especially useful for characterizing biological calcium phosphates for several reasons. First, calcified deposits and their model compounds may be poorly crystalline or amorphous and consequently difficult to characterize by X-ray powder diffraction. Second, the size of the probe is sufficient to establish a mapping of a biological sample for which no specific preparation is necessary.

The present study is based on the XANES part of the X-ray absorption spectra to evaluate the local environment of Ca atoms. The spectra of possible Ca species, namely, ACCP and calcium phosphate apatite (CA) compounds, in the papilla were measured. Moreover, owing to the submillimeter size of the probe, we will establish a mapping of these compounds from the top of the papilla where the RP is localized to the medulla.

Regarding the reference compounds, the feature labeled A reflects the effective charge and the site symmetry of Ca^{2+} ions (3d0 electron configuration). We consider now that transitions are discrete, with broadening owing to core-hole lifetime and instrumental resolution. Following this simple scheme, this feature A can be attributed to a $1s \rightarrow 3d$ transition or O 2p molecular orbital [93]. This transition is dipole forbidden ($\Delta\lambda$[Delta lambda] = 2) and results from mixing of unoccupied d final states with p-character final states. This structure includes a shoulder-like structure (feature B transition $1s \rightarrow 4s$) and a double peak (features C1 and C2: transition $1s \rightarrow 4p$) whose relative intensities depend on the type of Ca involved (Ca(I) or Ca(II)). At this point, we would like to recall that HAP can be described as a hexagonal stacking of (PO4)3- groups with two kinds of tunnel parallel to the *c* axis. The first one coincides with the ternary axis of the structure and is occupied by Ca^{2+}, noted as Ca(I) ions. The second one is linked by oxygen and other calcium ions, noted Ca(II), and is occupied by OH- ions. Ca(I) and Ca(II) are present in a 2/3 ratio.

While the feature A is quite the same between the three samples HAP, CA, and ACCP, significant variations are measured for the shoulder B as well as for the C1–C2 features (Fig. 85.25). These observations are in line with the work of Eiden-Assmann et al. [94], who have noticed that this shoulder becomes more prominent as the crystallinity of the compounds increases. The XANES part is thus sensitive to the local order around Ca^{2+} cations (i.e., between the samples CA and ACCP). Of note, this type of experimental approach has already been performed on apatitic and non-apatitic calcium phosphates of biological interest [95, 96].

Regarding the experiments that have been performed on the kidney (Fig. 85.26), we have reported the different X-ray absorption spectra collected when we move from the top of the renal papilla to the medulla (Fig. 85.27). The amplitude (la for the spectra a) of the absorption edge (from la to ld in Fig. 85.26) and thus the Ca content decreases rapidly. This is mainly due to the presence of the calcification at the top of the papilla. The feature A that corresponds to the fact that the electronic state of calcium is 2+ is clearly visible. The position of the features B, C1, and C2, which are very sensitive to the crystallinity of the calcification at the edge, has been indicated. Of interest, the morphology of feature B in papilla 1 is close to the morphology of feature B in ACCP

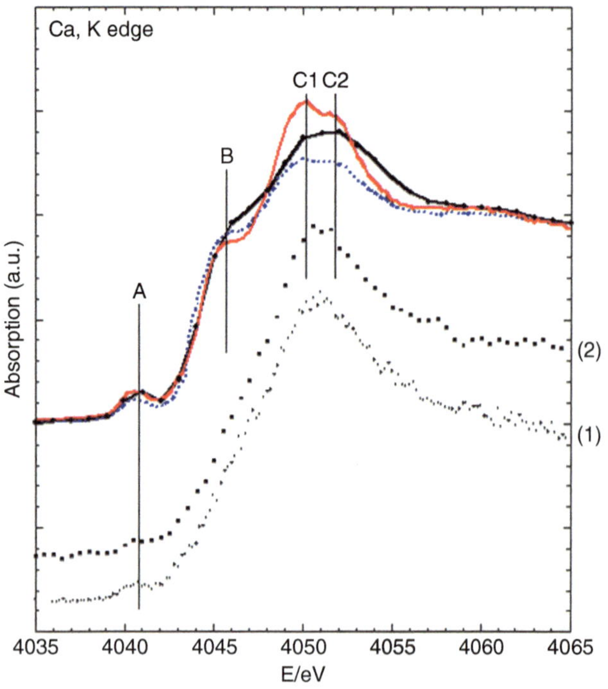

Fig. 85.25 XANES spectra of different compounds. References (in the *upper* part of the figure: around 4050 eV, the first curve corresponds to HAP, well-crystallized synthetic apatite; the second one is ACCP, amorphous biological apatites; the last one is CA, biological apatite) and biopsies (1 and 2 are the X-ray absorption spectra collected when the beam is positioned on the RP). Details regarding the prepeak $A(1s \rightarrow 3d$ transition), the shoulder B (transition $1s \rightarrow 4s$), and the double peaks C1–C2 (transition $1s \rightarrow 4p$ whose relative intensities depend on the type of Ca, namely, Ca(I) or Ca(II), involved in apatite) are visible

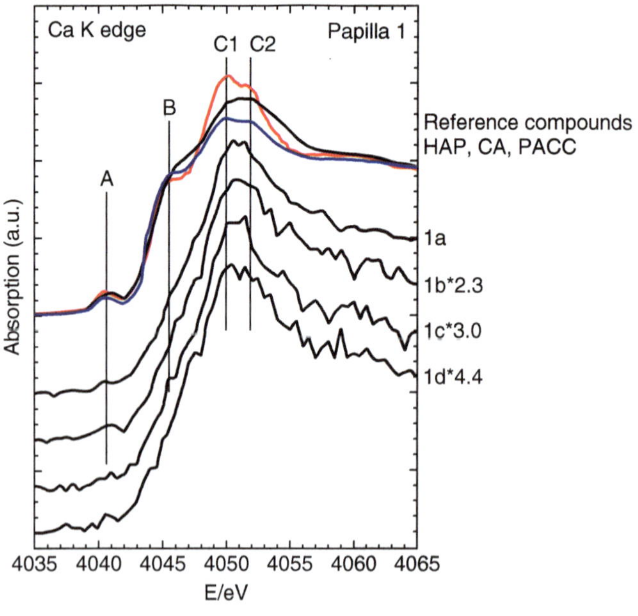

Fig. 85.26 XANES part of the absorption spectra for the papilla 1

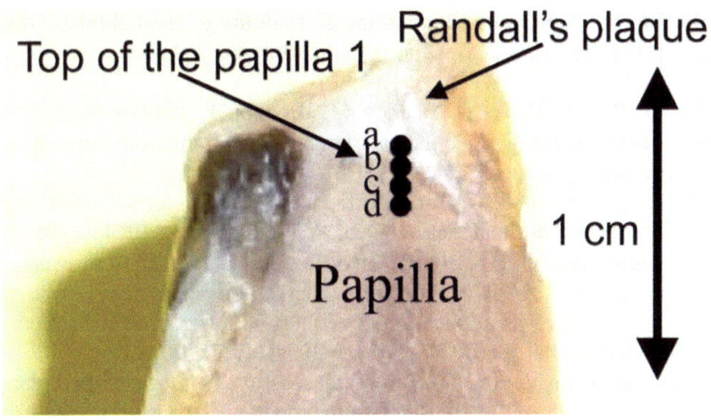

Fig. 85.27 The RP can be clearly seen as the white part at the top of the renal papilla. (**a**), (**b**), (**c**), and (**d**) refer to acquisition points related to X-ray absorption experiments

(see Fig. 85.25). Moreover, the two features C1–C2 are not present at the top of the absorption spectra. These two observations give direct structural evidence that one of the biochemical mechanisms can be described as an agglomeration of ACCP entities in the medulla leading to the formation of RP at the top of the papilla.

We give for the first time direct structural evidence of the significant presence of an amorphous phase similar to ACCP as a major constituent of RP. This set of data shows that this chemical phase can be considered as one precursor in the genesis of RP. Moreover, our measurements suggest that ACCP may be deposited within the tissue and not only at the surface of the papilla.

Conclusion

Stone analysis today should be performed using physical methods. In addition to conventional FTIR spectroscopy or XR scattering methods, techniques usually dedicated to fundamental physics or chemistry offer the opportunity to deeply address major problems in nephrolithiasis. Fine details regarding the relationship between structural characteristic of kidney stones and the pathology that exists at the macroscopic scale can be obtained at the mesoscopic scale. When such description is put in perspective with physiology, the biochemical processes that are associated with the genesis of pathological calcifications can be proposed as, for example, a mechanism for the formation of Randall's plaque when this ectopic calcification is the result of an agglomeration of calcified tubules. These techniques can be used to establish a diagnostic. In the case of hyperoxaluria, SEM images are able to separate the case of intermittent hyperoxaluria of dietary origin to primary hyperoxaluria, which is a severe inherited metabolic disease. Other examples regarding a description of biochemical processes or diagnostic and related to techniques specific to synchrotron radiation such as X-ray absorption have been published. The fact that significant improvements have been obtained in fundamental physics and chemistry will lead to other significant breakthroughs in nephrolithiasis in a close future.

Acknowledgments We wish to thank Dr. I. Brocheriou (Necker Hospital), Dr. X. Carpentier (Nice Hospital), Dr. Ch. Chappard (Lariboisière Hospital), Prof. P. Conort (La Pitié-Salpétrière Hospital), Dr. P. Dorfmüller (La Pitié-Salpétrière Hospital), Prof. D. Hannouche (Lariboisière Hospital), Dr. J. P. Haymann (Tenon Hospital), Prof. P. Jungers (Necker Hospital), Prof. B. Knebelman (Necker Hospital), Dr. E. A. Korn (Lariboisiere Hospital), Dr. E. Letavernier (Tenon Hospital), Prof. F. Lioté (Lariboisière Hospital), Prof. M. Mathonnet (Limoges Hospital), Prof. P. Meria (St. Louis Hospital), Dr. Ch. Nguyen (Lariboisière Hospital), Dr. I. Tostivint (La Pitié-Salpétrière Hospital), Prof. O. Traxer (Tenon Hospital), and Prof. J. C. Williams (Department of Anatomy and Cell Biology, Indiana University School of Medicine, Indianapolis, IN) for providing samples and useful discussions.

Also, regarding the physicochemistry, this research could not have been performed without the scientific advices of Dr. P. A. Albouy (LPS), Dr. G. André (LLB), Dr. A. Bianchi (INSERM-U7561), Dr. P. Chevallier (LURE), Dr. A. Cousson (LLB), Dr. P. Dumas (Soleil Synchrotron), Dr. B. Fayard (LPS), Dr. F. Fayon (CEHMTI), Dr. E. Foy (Laboratoire Pierre Süe), Dr. J. Guicheux (Laboratoire d'Ingénierie Ostéo-Articulaire et dentaire), Dr. J. L. Hazemann (ESRF), Dr. A. Lebail (Laboratoire des fluorures), Dr. Lenaour (INSERM U1004), Dr. O. Mathon (ESRF), Dr. G. Matzen (CEHMTI), Dr. P. Reboul (UMR 7561), Dr. M. Refringiers (Soleil Synchrotron), Dr. S. Reguer (Soleil Synchrotron), Dr. S. Rouzière (LPS), Dr. J. P. Samama (Soleil Synchrotron), Dr. Ch. Sandt (Soleil Synchrotron), Dr. D. Thiaudière (Soleil Synchrotron), Dr. E. Véron (CEHMTI), and Dr. R. Weil (LPS).

This work was supported by the Physics and Chemistry Institutes of CNRS and by contract ANR-09-BLAN-0120-02. The authors are grateful to the SOLEIL SR Facility and the Leon Brillouin laboratory for beam time allocation.

References

1. Mann S. Biomineralisation. Principles and concepts in bioinorganic materials chemistry. Oxford, UK: Oxford University Press, 2001.
2. Bonucci E. Calcification in biological systems. Boca Raton: CRC Press; 1992.
3. Bonucci E. Biological calcification, normal and pathological processes in the early stages. Berlin: Springer Verlag; 2007.
4. Giachelli CM. Ectopic calcification, gathering hard facts about soft tissue mineralization. Am J Pathol. 1999;154:671–5.
5. Jungers P, Daudon M, Leduc A. Lithiase urinaire. Paris: Flammarion Medecine-Sciences; 1989.
6. Conort P, Jungers P, Daudon M. Lithiase rénale, diagnostic et traitement. Flammarion: Medecine-Sciences; 1999.
7. Coe FL, Evan A, Worcester E. Kidney stone disease. J Clin Invest. 2005;115:2598–608.
8. Jungers P, Daudon M. Epidemiology of the kidney stones. Presse Med. 1990;19:1655–7.
9. Jungers P, Joly D, Barbey F, Choukroun G, Daudon M. ESRD caused by nephrolithiasis: prevalence, mechanisms, and prevention. Am J Kidney Dis. 2004;44:799–805.
10. Moe OW. Kidney stones: pathophysiology and medical management. Lancet. 2006;367:333–44.

11. Knoll T. Stone disease. Eur Urol Suppl. 2007;6:717–22.
12. Powell CR, Stoller ML, Schwartz BF, et al. Impact of body weight on urinary electrolytes in urinary stone formers. Urology. 2000;55: 825–30.
13. Sakhaee K, Adams-Huet B, Moe OW, et al. Pathophysiologic basis for normouricosuric uric acid nephrolithiasis. Kidney Int. 2002;62: 971–9.
14. Daudon M. Epidemiology of nephrolithiasis in France. Ann Urol. 2005;39:209–31.
15. Daudon M, Donsimoni R, Hennequin C, et al. Sex- and age-related composition of 10617 calculi analyzed by infrared spectroscopy. Urol Res. 1995;23:319–26.
16. Daudon M, Lacour B, Jungers P. High prevalence of uric acid calculi in diabetic stone formers. Nephrol Dial Transplant. 2005;20:468–9.
17. Joly D, Rieu P, Mejean A, Gagnadoux MF, Daudon M, Jungers P. Treatment of cystinuria. Pediatr Nephrol. 1999;13:945–50.
18. Daudon P, Bader CA, Jungers P. Urinary calculi – review of classification methods and correlations with etiology. Scanning Microsc. 1993;7:1081–106.
19. Daudon M. L'analyse morphoconstitutionnelle des calculs dans le diagnostic étiologique d'une lithiase urinaire de l'enfant. Arch Pediatr. 2000;7:855–65.
20. Daudon M, Jungers P. Clinical value of crystalluria and quantitative morphoconstitutional analysis of urinary calculi. Nephron Physiol. 2004;98:31–6.
21. Randall A. An hypothesis for the origin of renal calculus. N Engl J Med. 1936;214:234–7.
22. Randall A. The origin and growth of renal calculi. Ann Surg. 1937;105:1009–27.
23. Randall A. Papillary pathology as a precursor of primary renal calculus. J Urol. 1940;44:580–9.
24. Ohman S, Larsson L. Evidence for Randall's plaques to be the origin of primary renal stones. Med Hypotheses. 1992;39:360–3.
25. Evan AP, Lingeman JE, Coe FL, et al. Role of interstitial apatite plaque in the pathogenesis of the common calcium oxalate stone. Semin Nephrol. 2008;28:111–9.
26. Low RK, Stoller ML. Endoscopic mapping of renal papillae for Randall's plaques in patients with urinary stone disease. J Urol. 1997;158:2062–4.
27. Kim SC, Coe FL, Tinmouth WW, et al. Stone formation is proportional to papillary surface coverage by Randall's plaque. J Urol. 2005;173:117–9.
28. Guinier A. Théorie et technique de la radiocristallographie. Paris: Dunod; 1964.
29. Materlik G, Sparks CJ, Fisher K, editors. Resonant anomalous X-ray scattering. North-Holland: Amsterdam; 1994.
30. Van Meerssche M, Feneau-Dupont J. Introduction à la cristallographie et à la chimie structurale. Louvain-la-Neuve: Peeters; 1984.
31. Miller LM, Dumas P. From structure to cellular mechanism with infrared microspectroscopy. Curr Opin Struct Biol. 2010;20: 649–56.
32. Miller LM, Dumas P. Chemical imaging of biological tissue with synchrotron infrared light. Biochim Biophys Acta. 2006;1758: 846–57.
33. Estépa L, Daudon M. Contribution of Fourier transform infrared spectroscopy to the identification of urinary stones and kidney crystal deposits. Biospectroscopy. 1997;3:347–69.
34. Maurice-Estepa L, Levillain P, Lacour B, Daudon M. Advantage of zero-crossing-point first-derivative spectrophotometry for the quantification of calcium oxalate crystalline phases by infrared spectrophotometry. Clin Chim Acta. 2000;298:1–11.
35. Warren BE. X-ray diffraction. New York: Dover; 1990.
36. Rietveld HM. A profile refinement method for nuclear and magnetic structure. J Appl Cryst. 1969;2:65–71.
37. Le Bail A, Loüer D. Smoothing and validity of crystallite size distributions from X-ray line profile analysis. J Appl Cryst. 1978; 11:50–5.
38. Le Bail A, Bazin D, Daudon M, Brochot A, Robbez-Masson V, Maisonneuve V. Racemic calcium tartrate tetrahydrate form (II) in rat urinary stones. Acta Cryst B. 2009;65:350–4.
39. Klug H, Alexander L. X-ray diffraction procedures for polycrystalline and amorphous materials. 2nd ed. New York: Wiley; 1974.
40. Burton AW, Ong K, Rea T, Chan IY. On the estimation of average crystallite size of zeolites from the scherrer equation: a critical evaluation of its application to zeolites with one dimensional pore systems. Micropor Mesopor Mat. 2009;117:75–90.
41. Gnutzmann V, Vogel W. Structural sensitivity of the standard platinum/silica catalyst EuroPt-1 to hydrogen and oxygen exposure by in situ X-ray diffraction. J Phys Chem. 1990;94:4991.
42. Chougnet A, Heitz C, Sondergard E, Berquier JM, Albouy PA, Klotz M. Substrates do influence the ordering of mesoporous thin films. J Mater Chem. 2005;15:3340–50.
43. Vallet-Regi M, Gonzalez-Calbet JM. Calcium phosphates as substitution of bone tissues. Progr Solid St Chem. 2004;32:1–31.
44. Drouet C, Bosc F, Banu M, Largeot C, Combes C, Dechambre G, et al. Nanocrystalline apatites: from powders to biomaterials. Powder Technol. 2009;190:118–22.
45. Chevallier P, Wang JX, Brissaud I. S.R. As a tool for X-ray fluorescence analysis of trace elements. Chem Geol. 1988;70: 173–90.
46. McLean RJC, Nickel JC, Noakes VC. An in vitro ultrastructural study of infectious kidney stone genesis. Infect Immun. 1985;2: 805–11.
47. Nickel JC, Reid G, Bruce AW. Ultrastructural microbiology of infected urinary stone. Urology. 1986;28:512–5.
48. Dorian HH, Rez P, Drach GW. Evidence for aggregation in oxalate stone formation: atomic force and low voltage scanning electron microscopy. J Urol. 1996;156:1833–7.
49. Umer S, Sultan S, Zafar M. Composition of renal and bladder calculi in pediatric stone formers. J Pediatr Urol. 2009;5:S32.
50. http://www-llb.cea.fr/spectros/pdf/g41-llb.pdf. Accessed 26 Oct 2011.
51. http://www.lightsources.org/cms/. Accessed 26 Oct 2011.
52. http://www.synchrotron-soleil.fr/. Accessed 26 Oct 2011.
53. Castelli E, Arfelli F, Dreossi D. Clinical mammography at the SYRMEP beam line. NIM A. 2007;572:237–40.
54. http://www.esrf.eu/UsersAndScience/Experiments/Imaging/ID17. Accessed 26 Oct 2011.
55. http://www.synchrotron-soleil.fr/portal/page/portal/Soleil/ToutesActualites/RayonSOLEIL. Accessed 26 Oct 2011.
56. http://www.esrf.eu/. Accessed 26 Oct 2011.
57. Current events. J. Synchroton Radiat 2007;14:297–298.
58. Adam JF, Biston MC, Rousseau J. Heavy element enhanced synchrotron stereotactic radiotherapy as a promising brain tumour treatment. Phys Med. 2008;24:92–7.
59. Chevallier P, Dhez P, Erko A, et al. X-ray microprobes. NIM B. 1996;113:122–32.
60. Grunwaldt JD, Hannemann S, Schroer CG. 2D-Mapping of the catalyst structure inside a catalytic microreactor at work: partial oxidation of methane over Rh/Al2O3. J Phys Chem B. 2006;110: 8674–80.
61. Jamin N, Dumas P, Moncuit J. Highly resolved chemical imaging of living cells by using S.R. Infrared microspectrometry. PNAS. 1998;95:4837–40.
62. Benazeth S, Bazin D, Viosat B, et al. Composé du platine(II) à visée tumorale, dérivés de l'ellepticine et de ses analogues. J Chim Phys. 1989;T86–718:1635–8.
63. Bouvet D, Michalowicz A, Crauste-Manciet S, Curis E, Nicolis I, Olivi L, et al. EXAFS characterization of oxaliplatin anticancer drug and its degradation in chloride media. J Synchroton Radit. 2006;13:477–83.

64. Nicolis I, Deschamps P, Curis E, Bénazeth S. XAS applied to pharmaceuticals: drug administration and bioavailability. J Synchroton Radit. 2001;8:984–6.
65. Bazin D, Sayers D, Rehr J. Comparison between Xas, awaxs, asaxs & dafs applied to nanometer scale metallic clusters. J Phys Chem. 1997;101:11040–7.
66. Chassot E, Oudadesse H, Irigaray J, Curis E, Bénazeth S, Nicolis I. Differentiation of biological hydroxyapatite compounds by infrared spectroscopy, x-ray diffraction and exafs. J Appl Phys. 2001;90: 6440–6.
67. Tang Y, Chappell HF, Dove MT, Reeder RJ, Lee YJ. Zinc incorporation into HAP. Biomaterials. 2009;30:2864–72.
68. Bazin D, Daudon M, Chevallier P, et al. Les techniques de rayonnement synchrotron au service de la caractérisation d'objets biologiques: un exemple d'application, les calculs rénaux. Ann Biol Clin. 2006;64:125–39.
69. Bazin D, Carpentier X, Traxer O, et al. Very first tests on SOLEIL regarding the Zn environment in pathological calcifications made of apatite determined by X-ray absorption spectroscopy. J Synchroton Radit. 2008;15:506–9.
70. Moonen J, Slot J, Lefferts L, Bazin D, Dexpert H. The influence of polydispersity and inhomogeneity on exafs of bimetallic catalysts. Physica B. 1995;208&209:689–90.
71. Harries JE, Hukins DW, Holt C, Hasnain SS. Conversion of amorphous calcium phosphate into hydroxyapatite. J Crystal Growth. 1987;84:563–70.
72. Bazin D, Rehr J. Limits and advantages of xanes for nanometer scale metallic clusters. J Phys Chem B. 2003;107:12398–493.
73. Tew MW, Miller JT, van Bokhoven JA. Particle size effect of hydride formation and surface hydrogen adsorption of nanosized Pd catalysts: L3 edge vs K edge X-ray absorption spectroscopy. J Phys Chem C. 2009;113:15140–7.
74. Bazin D, Rehr J. Soft X-ray absorption spectroscopy at the cutting edge for nanomaterials used in heterogeneous catalysis: the state of the art. Catal Lett. 2003;87:85–90.
75. Dumas P, Sockalingun GD, Sulé-Suso J. Adding synchrotron radiation to infrared microspectroscopy: what's new in biomedical applications? Trends Biotechnol. 2006;25:40–4.
76. Daudon M, Jungers P, Bazin D. Peculiar morphology of stones in primary hyperoxaluria. N Engl J Med. 2008;359:100–2.
77. Daudon M, Jungers P, Bazin D. Stones in primary hyperoxaluria – a clarification. N Engl J Med. 2009;360:100.
78. Carpentier X, Daudon M, Traxer O, et al. Relationship between the carbonate rate of carbapatite, morphological characteristics of calcium phosphate stones and etiology. Urology. 2009;73:968–75.
79. Rokita E, Hermes C, Nolting HF, Rycze K. Substitution of Ca by Sr within selected Ca phosphates. J Crystal Growth. 1993;130:543–52.
80. Rosenow Jr EC. Renal calculi: study of papillary calcification. J Urol. 1940;44:19–23.
81. Vermooten V. The incidence and significance of the deposition of calcium plaques in the renal papilla as observed in the Caucasian and bantu population in South Africa. J Urol. 1941;46:193–6.
82. Evan AP, Lingeman JE, Coe FL, Parks JH, Bledsoe SB, Shao Y, et al. Randall's Plaque of patients with nephrolithiasis begins in basement membranes of thin loops of henle. J Clin Invest. 2003;111: 607–16.
83. Evan AP, Coe FL, Lingeman JE, et al. Mechanism of formation of human calcium oxalate renal stones on Randall's plaque. Anat Rec (Hoboken). 2007;290:1315–23.
84. Matlaga BR, Coe FL, Evan AP, Lingeman JE. The role of Randall's plaques in the pathogenesis of calcium stones. J Urol. 2007; 177:31–8.
85. Daudon M, Traxer O, Williams JC, et al. Randall's plaques. In: Rao N, Khavanagh J, Preminger G, editors. Urinary tract stone disease. New York: Springer; 2011. p. 103–12.
86. Daudon M, Traxer O, Jungers P, Bazin D. Stone morphology suggestive of Randall's plaque. Vol 900. In: Evan AP, Lingeman JE, Williams JC Jr, eds. Renal stone disease. American Institute of Physics Conference Proceedings, Ed. New York: Melville; 2007. p. 26–34.
87. Levinson AA, Nosal M, Davidman M. Trace elements in kidney stones from three areas in the United States. Invest Urol. 1978; 15:270–5.
88. Joost J, Tessadri R. Trace element investigations in kidney stone patients. Eur Urol. 1987;13:264–71.
89. Grases F, Genestar C, Mill A. The influence of some metallic ions and their complexes on the kinetics of crystal growth of calcium oxalate. J Crystal Growth. 1986;94:507–11.
90. Bazin D, Chevallier P, Matzen G, Jungers P, Daudon M. Heavy elements in urinary stones. Urol Res. 2007;35:179–84.
91. Bertsch PM, Hunter DB. Applications of synchrotron-based X-ray microprobes. Chem Rev. 2001;101:1809–42.
92. Carpentier X, Bazin D, Combes C, et al. High Zn content of Randall's plaque: A μ-X-ray fluorescence investigation. J Trace Elem Med Biol. 2011;25:160–5.
93. Rher JJ, Kas JJ, Prange MP, Sorini AP, Takimoto Y, Vila F. *Ab initio* theory and calculations of X-ray spectra. C R Phys. 2009;10:548–59.
94. Eiden-Assmann S, Viertelhaus M. In-situ XANES spectroscopy at the Ca K edge of calcium phosphate compounds. HASYLAB-Jahresbericht 1999, HASYLAB/DESY: Hamburg; 2000.
95. Asokan K, Jan JC, Chiou JW, Pong WF, Tseng PK, Lin IN. X-ray absorption spectroscopy studies of Ba1-xCaxTiO3. J Synchroton Radit. 2001;8:839–41.
96. Eichert D, Salomé M, Banu M, Susini J, Rey C. Preliminary characterization of calcium chemical environment in apatitic and non-apatitic calcium phosphates of biological interest by X-ray absorption spectroscopy. Spectrochim Acta B. 2005;60:850–8.

General and Specific Dietary Advice for the Prevention of Stone Recurrence

86

William G. Robertson

Abstract

This chapter describes the various general and specific dietary regimens that can be used to advise patients on how to prevent the recurrence of their calcium- and uric acid-containing kidney stones. The conclusion is that although there is some general advice that may be useful to most patients, it is more efficacious to screen the patient in order to identify his/her main urinary, metabolic, nutritional, environmental, and lifestyle risk factors for stone formation and then tailor specific advice for that patient on the basis of the findings from these detailed investigations. If the patient can be motivated to adhere strictly over a long time period to this conservative approach to the prophylactic management of their stone problem, then it is possible to prevent their forming further stones. Although this approach to stone management may be relatively expensive in the short term, it is not as expensive as any of the procedures currently available for stone removal or disintegration and in the long term may save health authorities considerable sums within their hospital budgets. It will also be of considerable benefit to the patient not to have to suffer the discomfort and inconvenience of further stone episodes and would save the Exchequer considerable sums in unclaimed sick pay and industry a significant number of days lost from work.

Keywords

Dietary management • Metabolic screening • Urolithiasis • Fluid intake • Calcium intake • Oxalate intake • Animal protein intake • Salt intake • Sugar intake

Introduction

Urolithiasis is a multifactorial disorder involving various genetic, metabolic, nutritional, environmental, demographic, and lifestyle factors that combine in a given individual to produce a urine that has a high potential to form crystals of one or more of the insoluble salts and acids that occur in urinary calculi [1]. The common factor in the formation of all these stone types is that there has to be an imbalance between the supersaturation of a particular urine with respect to one or more of these substances and the factors that decrease (inhibitors) or increase (promoters) the rate of crystallization and/or agglomeration of these substances in that urine. Supersaturation of urine, however, is a *sine qua non* for crystals of all the various stone types to form. In turn, there are several individual urinary risk factors that contribute to differences in these chemical risk factors for stone formation between persons who form stones and those who do not.

Figure 86.1 shows the main factors involved in formation of calcium-containing stones, the most common stone type in most series throughout the world. Analysis of large numbers of urine samples from calcium stone formers and age- and sex-matched normal subjects has shown that there are seven factors in urine that are significantly different between the two groups: a low urine volume; a raised

W.G. Robertson, Ph.D., D.Sc. (✉)
The Physiology Department, Centre for Nephrology,
Royal Free and University College Medical School,
Rowland Hill Street, London, NW3 2PF, UK
e-mail: robertsonwilliam67@gmail.com

J.J. Talati et al. (eds.), *Urolithiasis*,
DOI 10.1007/978-1-4471-4387-1_86,

Fig. 86.1 Model of calcium stone formation

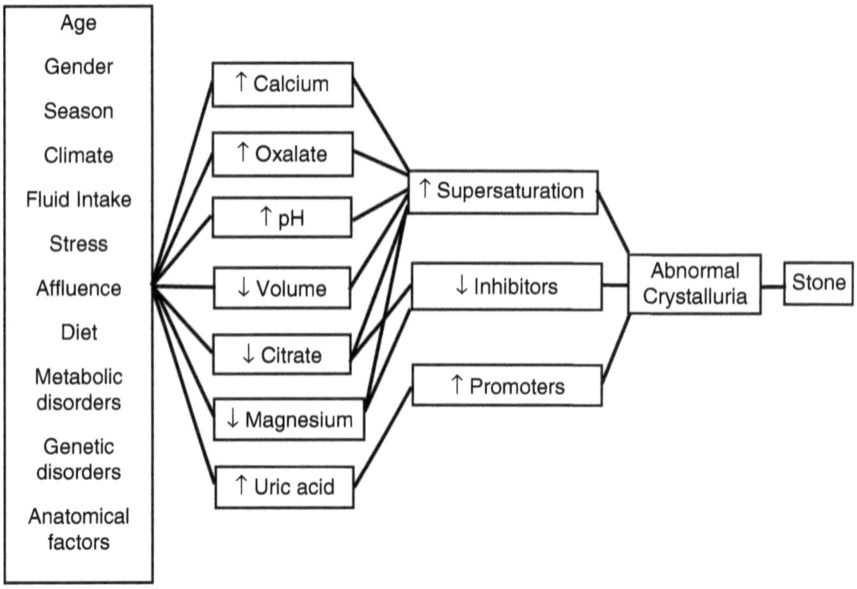

urinary pH; increases in urinary oxalate, calcium, and uric acid; and decreases in urinary citrate and magnesium [2]. Occasionally, only one of these abnormalities is critical for the formation of a stone, but more usually it is a combination of two or more abnormalities that are involved. These abnormalities, sometimes quite small, can be combined into an overall measure of the biochemical risk of forming stones (P_{SF}) of different compositions (pure uric acid, mixed uric acid-calcium oxalate, pure calcium oxalate, mixed calcium oxalate-calcium phosphate, and pure calcium phosphate). The algorithms for calculating the risk of forming these various types of stone based on the analysis of 24-h urine samples have been published elsewhere. P_{SF} brings together the known significant factors that affect supersaturation and the inhibition or promotion of the crystallization of calcium salts in urine. This procedure can also be applied to uric acid stone formation where the main risk factors are a low urinary volume, an acidic urinary pH, and a high urinary excretion of uric acid. P_{SF} is defined on a probability scale from 0 to 1. Fortuitously, untreated stone formers generally have P_{SF} values >0.5 and non-stone formers have P_{SF} values <0.5 on this scale. Moreover, the nearer the P_{SF} value is to 1, the greater is the frequency of stone episodes (i.e., the severity of the disorder) experienced by a given patient.

In turn, there is a multitude of epidemiological risk factors that have been shown to influence the seven urinary risk factors involved in calcium stone formation. These include various genetic, metabolic, nutritional, environmental, demographic, and lifestyle factors that have been widely described in the literature over the past 50 years or so. Similar studies have identified the urinary and epidemiological factors responsible for uric acid stone formation and for other stone types, and these are documented in Fig. 86.2.

Identification of which of these factors are important in a given patient with stones requires a comprehensive screening procedure. The system which I and my various colleagues over the years have developed is called LITHOSCREEN and requires (a) a detailed patient history (patient screen), (b) a metabolic screen based on a blood sample (preferably fasting) and concomitant urine sample (metascreen), (c) completion of a 7-day diet diary by the patient on his/her free home diet (diet screen), and (d) the collection of two 24-h urine samples on the last two days of the diet diary. In addition, (e) quantitative stone analysis is carried out whenever possible (stone screen), and the patients and nursing and medical staff are strongly encouraged to retain any stones or stone fragments for analysis. Quantitative analysis is best carried out by Fourier transform infrared (FTIR) spectroscopy. Full details of the LITHOSCREEN procedure have been published elsewhere [3].

From these various data, a stone profile is constructed of all the factors that contribute to the cause of that particular patient's stones, and suitable prophylactic measures are instituted which are designed to reduce his/her risk of forming further stones by correcting his/her most significant urinary risk factors. As far as possible, this is achieved conservatively through changes in diet and lifestyle. Only if the patient is found to have some metabolic disorder do we resort to drug treatment because, once started, this is likely to be a lifetime process.

It is important to note that dietary treatment is of little value in the management of infection stones and stones that are caused by inborn errors of metabolism such as primary hyperoxaluria, xanthinuria, and 2,8-dihydroxyadeninuria. Nor does dietary treatment affect the formation of iatrogenic stones such as those caused by indinavir, magnesium silicate or calcium-containing antacids, triamterene, and sulfadiazine.

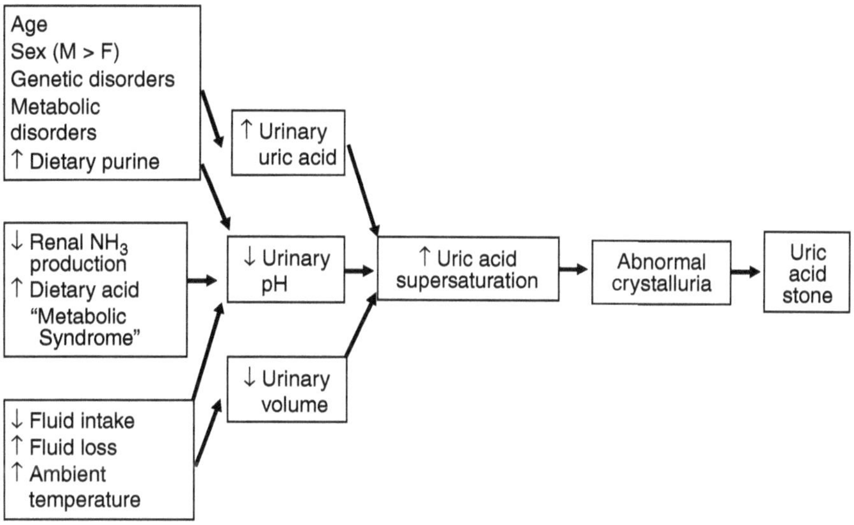

Fig. 86.2 Model of uric acid stone formation

General Principles in the Dietary Management of Stone Risk

There are a few general principles in the dietary management of stone formation.

As may be surmised from the above, the main object in the prevention of stone recurrence must be to reduce the biochemical risk of forming stones. Usually, this involves reducing the supersaturation of urine with respect to the patient's stone type but may also require an increase in the urinary inhibitors of crystallization or a decrease in the urinary promoters of crystallization. In most patients, these goals can be achieved by appropriate manipulation of the patient's diet and lifestyle. Most often, this involves reducing the intake of one or more particular dietary constituents such as oxalate, calcium, sodium, refined sugars, and animal protein or increasing the intake of fluid, potassium, or magnesium. But there are many other possibilities sometimes involving combinations of changes in the intakes of these and other dietary constituents.

It is important to emphasize, however, that one must tailor the treatment regime to the metabolism of the patient concerned, as defined by the risk factors identified by a detailed metabolic, nutritional, and lifestyle screening procedure such as LITHOSCREEN. After all, if you take 100 individuals and feed them all exactly the same foodstuffs for a week and then measure their 24-h urine compositions at the end of the week, these will vary widely from patient to patient. This is because of interindividual variability in the intestinal absorption, metabolism, and renal handling of the various constituents of the diet. Variability in hormonal and vitamin status may also be of importance in this context. Some studies suggest that it is those individuals who are most sensitive to a given dietary, environmental, metabolic, or lifestyle stimulus who frequently end up with the most extreme excretions of the various urinary risk factors mentioned above. These are the individuals who are most likely to form stones.

Specific Dietary Advice for the Preventions of Stone Recurrence

Once the particular urinary risk factors and the reasons for these abnormalities have been identified, it is then possible to treat these either individually or in combination in order to reduce the patient's biochemical risk of forming stones. The following sections describe the specific dietary modalities that are available for achieving this.

High Fluid Intake

Firstly, it is always important to ensure that the patient is passing a diluted urine as possible by means of a high fluid intake as this will reduce the supersaturation of all stone-forming materials and thereby reduce the risk of forming the crystals that appear to trigger off a stone episode [4]. Depending on the patient's other risk factors, our aim is to try and persuade the patient to pass a urine volume of at least 2.0–2.5 l/day under all circumstances. For the average patient living and working in a temperate environment, this will require a total fluid consumption of 2.3–2.8 l/day, but for some (see later) it may require considerably more. Naturally, a high urine volume will reduce the P_{SF} values for the various stone types, the object being to bring all of these values below 0.5 on the probability scale. There are two situations, however, where diluting urine can be counter-productive. The first is in cases where the risk of forming stones is entirely due to a low excretion of the urinary inhibitors of crystallization (citrate and magnesium). Clearly, diluting urine will not help in these patients since it will only serve to dilute further the concentration of these inhibitors and make them even less active than before, thereby increasing the risk of forming further stones. The second situation where diluting urine is not the most efficacious way of reducing stone risk is in cases where the main risk factor is either a very acidic urine (in the case of uric acid-containing stones) or a very alkaline urine (in the case of calcium phosphate-containing stones). The reason for this is that pH is a logarithmic function and urine volume can only be changed linearly by a factor of 2–3 at most. In this situation, even trebling urine volume will have a minimal effect on urinary pH.

Other factors that must be taken into account when recommending a high fluid intake are:

- Does the patient sweat a lot normally or have night sweats?
- Does the patient suffer from stress (when he/she is more likely to lose fluid through anxiety sweating)?
- Does the patient exercise regularly (light, medium, or strenuous) and does he/she sweat a lot when doing so?
- Does the patient travel frequently by air, particularly on long-haul flights (a highly dehydrating situation)?
- Does the patient work in a hot environment or sweat a lot through hard physical work?
- Does the patient travel regularly on business or vacation to countries where the climate is hot?
- Does the patient regularly take high-fiber laxatives, which reduce water absorption in the intestine and cause urine volume to be lower than would be expected from the patient's fluid intake?

In all of these situations, the patients will have to consume considerably more fluid in order to achieve a urine volume of 2.2–2.5 l/day.

There are some situations, however, where a high fluid intake may be difficult or inconvenient for the patient:

- If the patient has any bowel disorder, such as chronic diarrhea, that might make it difficult for them to consume a high fluid diet
- If the patient has had any bowel surgery, such as an ileostomy or a colectomy, which might make it difficult for them to tolerate a high fluid intake
- If the patient has an enlarged prostate and finds it inconvenient to go more frequently to the toilet
- If the patient has an occupation, such as taxi-driving, that makes it difficult to go to the toilet during working hours

These groups of patients are particularly difficult to treat by means of a high fluid intake. I usually encourage them to consume as much as they can without them being inconvenienced or embarrassed and try to find alternative approaches to their stone prevention.

Low Oxalate Intake

Risk factor analysis has shown that after a low urine volume, the next most important risk factor for calcium-containing stones is an increase in urinary oxalate [2, 5]. The average upper limit of normal for urinary oxalate is considered to be around 0.45 mmol/day in most series in the West, although that figure may be much higher in the oil-rich countries of the Arabian Gulf. However, risk factor analysis shows that at a urinary oxalate of 0.45 mmol/day, the risk of forming stones in the average person is already increased by a factor of 1.7. This also underlines the error made by many researchers who rely on so-called upper limits (or lower limits) of normal for defining the abnormalities in the urinary risk factors that lead to stones. It is important to recognize that risk is a continuous function such that the probability of forming stones is already increasing by the time urine reaches the so-called upper (or lower) limit of normal for each of the seven risk factors described previously. It is not a discrete function that suddenly takes off into significance at some arbitrary upper (or lower) limit. Furthermore, risk is generally not a linear function in relation to the urinary excretion of the various risk factors involved in stone formation; it has been shown to increase geometrically or logarithmically with a linear increase (or decrease) in each of the risk factors [2].

If mild hyperoxaluria is important in the formation of calcium-containing stones, then it might be assumed that reducing dietary oxalate might have a major effect on the risk of forming further stones. However, urinary oxalate has at least two components: (a) oxalate derived from exogenously from the diet and (b) oxalate derived endogenously from various normal metabolic pathways in the body. Endogenously produced oxalate comprises at least 50 % (if not more) of urinary oxalate and, at this moment in time, cannot be reduced by any known means. There may also be a third source of oxalate in urine that is derived exogenously from dietary sources other than oxalate itself. These are substances that are absorbed through the intestine and metabolized in the body to produce oxalate as a by-product of metabolism. One example of this phenomenon appears to be animal protein which generally contains more of the amino acids that are partially metabolized to oxalate than protein derived from fruit and vegetables [6]. The most significant of these is hydroxyproline, which is only found in collagen and which, in turn, is only found in meat, fish, and poultry. But other amino acids such as phenylalanine, tyrosine, and tryptophan may also be involved. It has been suggested that some individuals, possibly as a result of polymorphism in alanine-glyoxylate transferase Pro11Leu, may have an increased ability to metabolize one or more of these amino acids to oxalate, thereby possibly accounting for the mixed reports on the effect of a high-animal-protein diet on urinary oxalate [7]. Another exogenous source that has the potential to be metabolized to oxalate in the body is a high dose of vitamin C (>2 g/day). However, researchers still have not agreed on the importance of this [8, 9]. As a precaution, stone patients are usually advised not to take doses of vitamin C greater than 1 g/day.

Another factor that is important in determining the intestinal absorption of oxalate is the bioavailability of oxalate in a given diet [8]. This is due to the fact that oxalate present in a soluble form is more readily absorbed than oxalate present in the form of calcium oxalate (CaOx) crystals. Mixing oxalate-containing foods with dairy products, which have a high content of calcium, can reduce the availability of oxalate for absorption. For example, oxalate is less well absorbed from tea consumed with the addition of a little milk than from tea containing no milk [10], presumably because the calcium in the milk precipitates with the oxalate from the tea and makes it less available for absorption. Similarly, oxalate is less well absorbed from creamed spinach than when it is served without the addition of milk products [11]. Foods with a high fiber content may also affect the bioavailability of oxalate. Thus, sugar beet fiber may reduce the intestinal absorption of oxalate by mechanically binding crystals of CaOx or by chemically binding soluble oxalate and so making the oxalate less available for absorption in the intestine [12].

It is now generally recognized that dietary calcium as a whole exerts a major effect on oxalate absorption. As mentioned previously, at high concentrations of calcium in the intestinal tract, CaOx crystals will precipitate and are unlikely to be redissolved after leaving the stomach unless the ambient calcium concentration becomes very low. Based on this principle, a high calcium intake has been used to reduce the intestinal absorption in patients with enteric hyperoxaluria [13]. It has also been used to normalize urinary oxalate excretion in Saudi stone formers who have marked hyperoxaluria as a result of the high oxalate/calcium ratio in their diet, which is 5–6 times that in the West. This effect of a high intake of calcium was confirmed in a study from Switzerland [14], although providing additional calcium in the form of high Ca-containing mineral water did not reduce urinary oxalate excretion in a study carried out on German stone formers [15].

In general, it is advisable not to consume a diet that is high in oxalate, such as has been found in the Middle East [16, 17]. However, in practice, it is difficult to reduce urinary oxalate by a large amount through a low oxalate diet alone —except in those individuals who are initially consuming a diet with a very high content of oxalate. Table 86.1 contains a list of high-oxalate-containing foods that stone patients should be advised to avoid. A more recent addition to this list are tablets of cranberry juice concentrate. It has been calculated that one 450-mg tablet of cranberry concentrate, which the manufacturers claim is equivalent to 2.88 l of concentrated cranberry juice, contains 2 mmol of oxalate [18]. Therefore, taking the recommended dosage of two tablets per day would add an estimated 4 mmol of oxalate to the diet—two- to threefold increase in the daily intake of oxalate.

Table 86.1 List of high-oxalate-containing food

High-oxalate foods
Rhubarb
Spinach
Beetroot
Okra (ladies' fingers)
Molokhia
Sabanaq
Salaq
Yams
Soya beans and soya products (including tofu)
Nuts (except coconut)
Bran-containing foods
Sesame seeds and sesame seed products (including tahini)
Chocolate
Tea without milk
Instant coffee without milk

[a]*Note*: All fruits and vegetables contain some oxalate, but the above list details those with the highest content of oxalate

The main aim of this line of approach to the prevention of stone recurrence is to bring dietary oxalate below 1.5 mmol/day (135 mg/day).

Low Calcium Intake

For many years, a low-calcium diet was the only advice given to patients with calcium-containing stones, and some patients took this very seriously to the extent that they completely eliminated calcium-containing foods from their diet [19]. Unfortunately, this practice still continues in many clinics and family doctor practices today. The theory behind this form of treatment is as follows: (a) hypercalciuria was considered to be the main or only urinary risk factor for stones in most patients (this was in the days before the importance of mild hyperoxaluria was recognized and before it could be measured routinely in the laboratory), and (b) calcium was present in most stones. Therefore, it was concluded that stone recurrence should be preventable by reducing urinary calcium and the simplest way to achieve this was to put the patients on a low-calcium diet which usually meant them cutting down severely on their consumption of dairy produce. However, several studies have now shown that there is no beneficial effect of a low-calcium diet per se on the recurrence rate of stones [20, 21]. Indeed, in a cross-sectional study of many thousands of individuals in the USA, Curhan et al. showed that a low calcium intake was actually conducive to forming stones, whereas a normal or high calcium intake reduced the risk [22]. The probable reason for this is that a low intake of calcium leads to less calcium being available in the intestine to precipitate or complex with oxalate, and so more oxalate becomes "free" for passive absorption in the large bowel, in turn leading to an increase in urinary oxalate, whereas a normal or high intake of calcium reduces the intestinal absorption and urinary excretion of oxalate [9].

Similarly, any factor, such as vitamin D, that increases the ability of the intestine to absorb calcium may also lead to a secondary increase in the absorption of oxalate [23]. This additionally absorbed oxalate then spills out in the urine. Incidentally, this phenomenon may explain why there is an apparent increase in stone formation in the UK during the summer months when both urinary calcium and urinary oxalate have been shown to increase as a result of increased exposure to UV light, which stimulates the production of vitamin D in the skin [24]. On average, normal subjects absorb around 20 % of their intake of calcium but hyperabsorbers may absorb up to 50 or 60 % of their daily intake of the mineral. A diet high in refined sugars may also stimulate the intestine to absorb more calcium than normal and lead to an increased urinary excretion of calcium [25]. If a high-sugar diet is combined with a high intake of salt, which may cause a renal leak of calcium, this often leads to gross hypercalciuria. Usually, this may be corrected by reducing the intakes of both refined sugars and salt.

There is another group of patients who may benefit from a moderately reduced intake of calcium—those who congenitally have a higher than normal intestinal absorption of calcium and who also have a high intake of calcium, particularly calcium derived from dairy products, which is the most absorbable source of calcium in the diet [26]. This group often has marked hypercalciuria, which can be controlled to some extent by partially reducing the intake of calcium. Care must be taken, however, not to take this too far so as to cause stimulation of the parathyroids and possible bone resorption.

More recently, it has been shown that hypercalciuria is not the main risk factor for stones in the majority of calcium stone formers and that it is less important than a low urine volume, mild hyperoxaluria, and a high urinary pH for causing the formation of calcium-containing stones [2]. In fact, it is roughly equivalent to hypocitraturia in order of importance. It has also been shown that hypercalciuria is rarely the sole cause of stones and that there has to be an additional factor such as a low urine volume, mild hyperoxaluria, hypocitraturia, an alkaline urine, hyperuricosuria, or a low urinary magnesium excretion for stones to form [2].

The general aim in Western countries is to get the dietary intake of calcium in the range 20–25 mmol/day (800–1,000 mg/day) for normal absorbers of calcium and 15–20 mmol/day (600–800 mg/day) for hyperabsorbers of calcium. In the oil-rich countries of the Arabian Gulf, however, the picture is very different [27]. In that part of the world, the intake of calcium is only about one half of what it is in the West and the intake of oxalate is about three times of what it is in the West. As a result, the oxalate/calcium ratio in the diet is 5–6 times higher, leading to a very high incidence of mild hyperoxaluria and a low incidence of hypercalciuria. The latter is in part due to the (perhaps surprisingly) low levels of 25-OH vitamin D_3 in the Arabian Gulf [28]. The object then is to increase the dietary intake of calcium in order to precipitate oxalate in the intestine and reduce its availability for passive absorption in the large bowel. It has been shown that by adding 1 g (equivalent to 25 mmol) of additional calcium per day to the diet in the form of calcium citrate brings the abnormally high urinary oxalate values down into the normal range with little or no concomitant increase in urinary calcium excretion [13].

Low Meat + Fish + Poultry Intake

It has been clearly shown that populations that consume a diet that is high in meat + fish + poultry protein and in purine have a higher incidence of stones than more vegetarian populations [6]. This is due to the fact that a high-animal-protein diet adversely affects five of the seven main urinary risk factors for calcium oxalate (CaOx) stone formation and, concomitantly, also affects adversely two of the three main risk factors for uric acid (UA) stone formation. The risk factors concerned are increases in urinary calcium, oxalate, and uric acid and decreases in urinary pH and citrate. The mechanisms by which these urinary changes come about are summarized in Table 86.2. Basically, a high-animal-protein diet is highly acidogenic as a result of the high sulfur content of animal protein compared with that of protein from fruit, vegetables, and cereals. The high acid content of animal protein causes urine to become more acidic and the acidic urine, in turn, leads to an increase in urinary calcium (by interfering with the tubular reabsorption of calcium) and a decrease in urinary citrate (by causing an increase in the tubular reabsorption of citrate). Urinary oxalate increases via the mechanism detailed previously and urinary uric acid increases as a result of the high purine content of meat, fish, and poultry. These changes in urinary composition lead to an increase in the risk of forming both CaOx- and UA-containing stones, a phenomenon clearly seen in the oil-rich Gulf states, where the consumption of animal protein is even higher than in the USA and the incidence of stones is the highest so far identified in the world [13].

It has been shown that decreasing the intake of animal protein does decrease the recurrence rate of stone formation [20], although, as with all dietary restrictive means of controlling disease, it suffers from patient noncompliance [29].

Table 86.2 Biochemical effects of a high meat + fish + poultry diet

Causal factor	Metabolic effect	Effect on urine
↑ Dietary acid (sulfur amino acids)	↑ Urinary acid excretion	↓ pH
↑ Urinary acid excretion	↑ Tubular reabsorption of citrate	↓ Citrate
↑ Urinary acid excretion	↓ Tubular reabsorption of calcium	↑ Calcium
↑ Dietary hydroxyproline	↑ Partial metabolism to oxalate	↑ Oxalate tyrosine, tryptophan, and phenylalanine
↑ Dietary purine	↑ Metabolism to uric acid	↑ Uric acid

People like to eat what they like to eat and, since patients with urolithiasis tend to feel well most of the time, it is often difficult to motivate them to adhere to a restrictive diet over a long period. Indeed, this was shown in a study on stone patients followed up after removal of their stones [30]. Within 3 months, their urine volumes had dropped and their urinary calcium and oxalate excretions had increased until they had another attack of renal colic, which rekindled their motivation to adhere to their diet. Moreover, this study was conducted in the days of open surgery when one might think that the patients would be highly motivated to adhere to any preventative measures so as not to risk another episode of renal colic.

The general aim of an animal protein restriction diet is to reduce the consumption of meat, fish, and poultry to only once per day and then a helping of no more than 5–6 oz (140–160 g). For stone disease, I draw no distinction between red meat and white meat or between meat and fish and poultry. A high consumption of any of these products will increase the risk of forming stones. For heart disease, there may be a difference between these different forms of animal protein, but for stone disease none. However, there are some animal protein foods that should be completely avoided by stone patients, namely, foods that contain higher than the average quantity of purine such as oily fish, anchovies, caviar, and offal.

High Magnesium Intake

Magnesium is known to be a weak inhibitor of the crystallization of calcium salts in urine and is also known to bind to oxalate to form a complex that is many times more soluble in urine than the corresponding complex of oxalate with calcium. For this reason, some workers have proposed that magnesium supplements in the form of magnesium hydroxide or, more recently, potassium magnesium citrate might be useful in the prevention of the recurrence of calcium-containing stones [31, 32]. The main problem with magnesium supplements is that there is a limit to how much magnesium can safely be prescribed in supplement form because of possible gastrointestinal discomfort and diarrhea.

In my own experience in the UK, urinary magnesium has dropped by about 20–25 % over the past 40 years or so. This appears to be due to a decrease in the consumption of brown and wholemeal bread, bran-containing cereals, and certain fruits and vegetables, particularly those containing chlorophyll of which magnesium is a key constituent. Unfortunately, some high-magnesium-containing foods, such as nuts and spinach, also have a high content of oxalate.

Magnesium deficiency is rare and usually results from excessive losses through diarrhea or chronic alcoholism rather than from a low intake of the mineral. However, humans absorb about 25–30 % of our daily intake of the mineral, so any reduction in intake will have a noticeable effect on its excretion in urine. I normally advise patients to consume at least 16 mmol/day (approximately 400 mg/day) of magnesium.

High Potassium Intake

Potassium is known to inhibit the tubular reabsorption of citrate and thereby stimulate the urinary excretion of citrate. Since citrate is an inhibitor of the crystallization of calcium salts in urine and since it also forms a soluble complex with calcium, it is generally considered that a high urinary citrate is a protective factor against calcium stone formation. Conversely, hypocitraturia is a risk factor for the disorder. This is the basis of the wide use of potassium citrate supplements as preventative treatment for calcium stone formation [33, 34]. However, the dosage has to be rather high of the order of 60 mmol/day additional potassium equivalent to 20 mmol/day of potassium citrate (potassium citrate has three potassium ions for every citrate ion). This is claimed to correct the low excretion of citrate in patients with hypocitraturia, not through the 20 mmol of extra citrate ingested (which is largely metabolized) but through the effect of the markedly increased throughput of potassium on the renal excretion of citrate, as mentioned above. However, not all researchers agree with these findings [35]. Some patients have not responded to potassium citrate supplements and have shown little or no increase in their urinary excretion of citrate. Furthermore, as a result of the alkalinizing effect of potassium citrate on urinary pH, some have progressed from being "pure" calcium oxalate stone formers to form "mixed stones" containing a large proportion of calcium phosphate.

In my own experience in the UK, potassium excretion has not changed much over the past 40 years or so, the average excretion being about 50–60 mmol/day. For although there has been a reduction in the consumption of potassium derived from fruit and vegetables in the population, this has largely been compensated for by the concomitant increase in the consumption of meat, fish, and poultry, which also contain reasonable quantities of potassium. Although the net effect of these changes has little or no effect on potassium excretion (as noted above), the acidifying effect on urine of the transition towards a more acid-ash diet has caused a reduction in the urinary excretion of citrate through an increased tubular reabsorption of citrate.

My advice to both calcium and uric acid stone formers is to correct the imbalance between the acidifying and alkalinizing factors in a diet high in animal protein and low in fruit and vegetables in order to induce the patient to pass a 24-h urine with an average pH of around 6.0 and a normal urinary excretion of citrate of at least 2 mmol/day.

Low Salt Intake

A diet that is high in salt often leads to hypercalciuria by causing a renal leak of calcium [36]. This is because sodium and calcium share a common transport mechanism in the distal tubule and, therefore, a high throughput of sodium ions through that part of the nephron interferes with the tubular reabsorption of calcium. The degree of hypercalciuria increases proportionately with the amount of sodium excreted in the urine. The body usually compensates for this loss of calcium by absorbing more calcium from the intestine or by stimulating the parathyroid glands. Diets high in salt are a scourge of modern society, the problem being that children may develop a taste for salt at an early age and find it difficult to reduce their intake in adulthood.

I try to persuade patients living in a temperate climate to reduce their total intake of salt to no more than about 9–10 g/day. This includes all sources of salt in the diet such as salt inherent in the food concerned, salt added to preprepared foods or convenience foods, salty snacks, salt added during cooking, and salt added at the table. Since about 90 % of dietary sodium is absorbed through the intestine, this will produce a urinary sodium of around 140–150 mmol/day. However, patients who live or work in a hot environment or who participate in strenuous physical work or exercise may require a higher intake in order to compensate for salt losses through sweating.

Low Refined Sugar Intake

A diet high in refined sugars will stimulate the intestinal absorption of calcium and lead to hypercalciuria [25]. As with a high-salt diet, high-refined-sugar diets are another scourge of modern society since sugar is an ingredient of many products such as confectionery, cakes, biscuits, fruit juices and fruit squashes, ice cream, and desserts. Again, the problem is that children develop a "sweet tooth" at an early age and find it difficult to reduce their intake of sugary foods in adulthood. The combination of a diet high in salt and high in refined sugars (part of the so-called Bad Western Diet – see later) often leads to gross hypercalciuria since the renal leak of calcium induced by the former is fed by the increased intestinal absorption of that mineral induced by the latter.

I try to persuade patients to limit their total intake of refined sugars to no more than 120 g/day.

Fiber Intake

Dietary fiber appears to have a "Jekyll and Hyde" role as a risk factor for stone formation.

Firstly, most dietary fiber, particularly that containing phytate, has the ability to bind calcium and thereby making it less available for absorption in the intestine. Thus, a normal fiber diet (around 20 g/day) plays some role in limiting the absorption and urinary excretion of calcium. A low-fiber diet, on the other hand, binds less calcium than a normal fiber diet, thereby making more calcium available for absorption. This may aggravate hypercalciuria in some patients, particularly those who are hyperabsorbers of calcium.

On the other hand, a diet that is very high in fiber (>25 g/day) may increase the risk of stones by binding water in the intestine and making it less available for absorption, this being the principle by which high-fiber laxatives work. However, such a diet leads, in turn, to the patient passing a lower urine volume than expected from their fluid intake, thereby increasing the risk of forming stones.

I usually try to persuade the patient to consume a diet that contains around 20 g/day of fiber.

Role of Diet in Metabolic Syndrome

Over the past 33 years in the UK, there has been a continuing rise in the percentage of uric acid-containing stones in the stone-forming population. In 1975, the percentage of UA-containing stones was around 4.5 %, but this has increased to around 10.8 % in 2008 in National Health Service (NHS) patients. In Private Health Care patients, however, the figure has reached more than 15 %. This increase is at least partly attributable to a steady increase in the consumption of animal protein during that period which leads to the acidification of urine and to a higher incidence of hyperuricosuria. However, this is not the whole explanation as there is a group of patients whose urine is more acidic than would be expected from the composition of their diets [37]. This group has been found to be more obese, have a higher incidence of hypertension, and, most of all, a very high incidence of type 2 diabetes—a group of disorders collectively known as "metabolic syndrome" [38, 39]. Further studies have shown that the high acidity of urine from these patients is due to a defect in renal ammoniagenesis, which leads to a lower urinary excretion of ammonium ions than would be expected for the high renal acid load in these patients [37]. This defect in ammoniagenesis reduces the buffering of H^+ ion excretion and so urine becomes more acidic than normal, thereby increasing the risk of forming uric acid-containing stones. The defect in ammoniagenesis, in turn, appears to be more related to the type 2 diabetes in these patients rather than the tendency to obesity and hypertension, but the exact mechanism by which this occurs is not yet clear. It is also not yet clear whether or not this sequence of events can be reversed either through changes in diet and lifestyle or through medication.

The So-Called Bad Western Diet for Stone Formation

In recent years, the media in the UK have continually run stories about the effect of the so-called Bad Western Diet, which usually means a diet high in fat, salt, and refined sugars, on the general health of the population. In terms of urolithiasis, I would add to this combination of dietary abuses a high intake of meat + fish + poultry. The effect of this diet on the risk of forming both calcium oxalate and uric acid stones is shown in Fig. 86.3.

- If we start with an underlay of a high-animal-protein diet in the population, which leads to hyperuricosuria, an acidic urine, mild hyperoxaluria, hypocitraturia, and hypercalciuria, these combine to increase the risk of forming both calcium oxalate and uric acid stones.
- If we then add a high-fat diet to this (which might follow naturally from the aforementioned high-animal-protein diet), this will tend to increase body mass index (BMI). In turn, this will tend to accentuate the acidity of urine and further increase the risk of forming uric acid-containing stones in the population.
- If we then add a high intake of refined sugars, this will tend to increase BMI and increase the risk of type 2 diabetes. In turn, this will lead to reduced ammoniagenesis and a low urinary ammonium ion excretion and consequently a more acidic urine. The high intake of refined sugars will also increase the intestinal absorption and urinary excretion of calcium. These changes further increase the risk of forming both calcium oxalate and uric acid stones in the population.
- Finally, if we add a high intake of salt, this will increase the risk of hypertension. The high-salt diet will also cause the kidneys to leak calcium and accentuate the risk of gross hypercalciuria, thereby increasing the risk of forming calcium oxalate-containing stones in the population.

The effect of this diet, which increases BMI and the incidence of hypertension and type 2 diabetes in the population, will be to increase the incidence of metabolic syndrome, as discussed in the previous section.

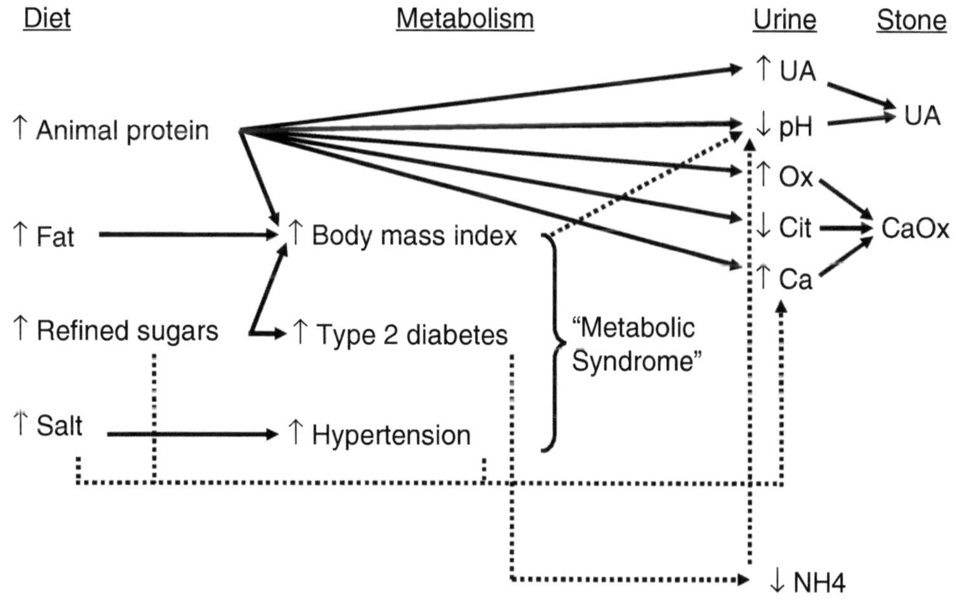

Fig. 86.3 Effect of "Bad Western Diet" on the risk of forming calcium oxalate and uric acid stones

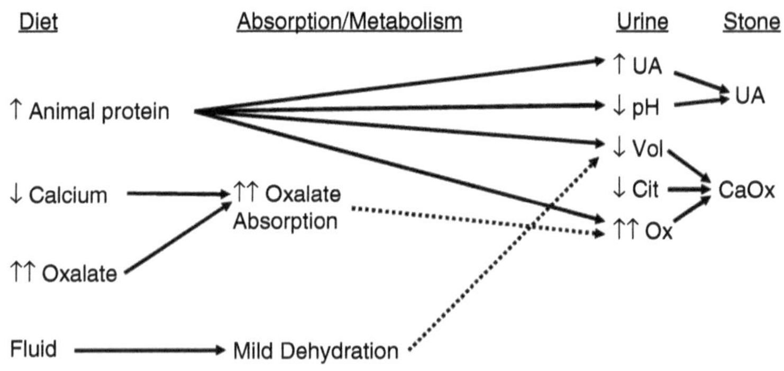

Fig. 86.4 Effect of "Bad Middle Eastern Diet" on risk of forming calcium oxalate and uric acid stones

The So-Called Bad Middle Eastern Diet for Stone Formation

A summary of the so-called Bad Middle Eastern Diet for stone formation is shown in Fig. 86.4. This shares some common factors with the "Bad Western Diet" for stone formation and also leads to the formation of both calcium oxalate- and uric acid-containing tones.

- If we start with a base of a very high-animal-protein diet in the Middle Eastern population, which leads to marked hyperuricosuria, a highly acidic urine, mild hyperoxaluria, and marked hypocitraturia, these combine to increase the risk of forming both calcium oxalate and uric acid stones. As previously mentioned, the incidence of hypercalciuria in the oil-rich states of the Arabian Gulf is very low because of the low intake of calcium and the low prevailing levels of vitamin D in the population. Even the high acid content of the Middle Eastern diet, which tends to cause a renal leak of calcium, is not enough to counter the low intestinal absorption of calcium in that population. So, hypercalciuria is not a major risk factor for stones in these countries.
- If we then add the combination of a low-calcium and very-high-oxalate diet to this, this leads to a very high incidence of marked hyperoxaluria and a further substantial increase in the risk of forming calcium oxalate-containing stones.
- If, finally, we add a tendency to mild dehydration because of the very hot, dry climate of the region, this will tend to reduce urine volume and further increase the risk of forming both calcium oxalate and uric acid stones.

My overall advice to both groups of patients in the West and Middle East is to consume a more balanced diet and to drink more water.

General Advice on the Dietary Management of Patients with Urolithiasis

In summary, there are some general pieces of advice that will work for most patients with idiopathic calcium and/or uric acid stones:

- Drink sufficient fluid to produce a urine volume of 2.2–2.5 l/day.
- Eliminate as far as possible foods that have a high content of oxalate.
- Reduce your intake of meat + fish + poultry protein to only once per day and then a helping of no more than 5–6 oz (140–160 g/day).
- Increase your intake of fresh fruit and vegetables, with the exception of those in Table 86.1, which have a high content of oxalate.
- Do not eliminate calcium from your diet, but keep your calcium intake at a reasonable level.
- Consider changing your consumption of white bread to brown bread and your consumption of cereals to bran-containing products in order to correct a low-fiber diet —but do not consume excessive quantities of high-fiber foods unless you compensate for this by simultaneously increasing your fluid intake.
- Decrease your intake of salt and salty foods.
- Decrease your intake of sugar and sugary foods.

Conclusion

It is important that the patients are given more specific advice that is tailored to their particular metabolism as defined by the risk factors identified by means of a detailed metabolic, nutritional, and lifestyle screening procedure. Although this may appear to be costly initially, in the long run it will save the health authority money by reducing the necessity for urologists to remove stones that will inevitably form in the future if the patient is not put on a specific prophylactic course of treatment. Calculations have shown that for every stone episode prevented, the health service will save about £2,000 [40]. In addition to the financial savings, it would clearly be of considerable benefit to the patient not to have to suffer the discomfort and inconvenience of further stone episodes. It would also save the Exchequer considerable sums in unclaimed sick pay and industry a significant number of days otherwise lost from work.

References

1. Robertson WG. Urinary tract stones. In: Shergill IS, Arya M, Grange PR, Mundy AR, editors. Medical therapy in urology. London/Dordrecht/Heidelberg/New York: Springer; 2010. p. 147–62.

2. Robertson WG. A risk factor model of stone-formation. Front Biosci. 2003;8:1330–8.
3. Robertson WG. A comprehensive screening procedure for the assessment of patients with recurrent stones. In: Borghi L, Meschi T, Briganti A, Schianchi T, Novarini A, editors. Kidney stones. Cosenza: Editoriale Bios; 1999. p. 407–10.
4. Pak CYC, Sakhaee K, Crowther C, Brinkley L. Evidence justifying a high fluid intake in treatment of nephrolithiasis. Ann Intern Med. 1980;93:36–9.
5. Robertson WG, Peacock M. The cause of idiopathic calcium stone disease: hypercalciuria or hyperoxaluria? Nephron. 1980;26:105–10.
6. Robertson WG, Heyburn PJ, Peacock M, Hanes F, Swaminathan R. The effect of a high animal protein intake on the risk of calcium stone-formation in the urinary tract. Clin Sci. 1979;57:285–8.
7. Caldwell EF, Mayor LR, Thomas MG, Danpure CJ. Diet and the frequency of the alanine:glyoxylate aminotransferase Pro11Leu polymorphism in different human populations. Hum Genet. 2004;115:504–9.
8. Jaeger P, Robertson WG. Role of dietary intake and intestinal absorption in calcium stone-formation. Nephron Physiol. 2004;98: 64–71.
9. Curhan GC, Willett WC, Rimm EB, Stampfer MJ. A prospective study of the intake of vitamins C and B_6, and the risk of kidney stones in men. J Urol. 1996;155:1847–51.
10. Savage GP, Charrier MJ, Vanhanen L. Bioavailability of soluble oxalate from tea and the effect of consuming milk with the tea. Eur J Clin Nutr. 2003;57:415–9.
11. Brogren M, Savage GP. Bioavailability of soluble oxalate from spinach eaten with and without milk products. Asia Pac J Nutr. 2003;12:219–24.
12. Gleeson MJ, Thompson AS, Mehta S, Griffith DP. Effect of unprocessed wheat bran on calciuria and oxaluria in patients with urolithiasis. Urology. 1990;35:231–4.
13. Robertson WG, Hughes H, Husain I, Al-Faqih S, Arafat A, Chakrabarti A, et al. Simultaneous treatment of calcium oxalate and uric acid stone disease in Saudi Arabia. In: Ryall R, Bais R, Marshall VR, Rofe AM, Smith LH, et al., editors. Urolithiasis 2. New York/London: Plenum Press; 1994. p. 581–6.
14. Hess B, Jost C, Zipperle L, Takkinen R, Jaeger P. High-calcium intake abolishes hyperoxaluria and reduces urinary crystallization during a 20-fold normal oxalate load in humans. Nephrol Dial Transplant. 1998;13:2241–7.
15. Siener R, Jahnen A, Hesse A. Influence of a mineral water rich in calcium, magnesium and bicarbonate on urine composition and the risk of calcium oxalate crystallization. Eur J Clin Nutr. 2004; 58:270–6.
16. Robertson WG, Hughes H, Walker V, Nisa M, Husain I, Al-Faqih S, et al. Risk factors for urolithiasis in the Arabian peninsula. In: Vahlensieck W, Gasser G, Hesse A, Schoeneich G, editors. Urolithiasis. Amsterdam: Excerpta Medica; 1990. p. 10–1.
17. Robertson WG, Hughes H. Importance of mild hyperoxaluria in the pathogenesis of urolithiasis – new evidence from studies in the Arabian Peninsula. Scanning Microsc. 1993;7:391–402.
18. Terris MK, Issa MM, Tacker JR. Dietary supplementation with cranberry concentrate tablets may increase the risk of nephrolithiasis. Urology. 2001;57:26–9.
19. Nordin BEC, Barry H, Bulusu L, Speed R. Dietary treatment of recurrent calcium stone disease. In: Cifuentes Delatte L, Rapado A, Hodgkinson A, editors. Urinary calculi. Basel: Karger; 1973. p.170–6
20. Borghi L, Schianci T, Meschi T, Guerra A, Allegri F, Maggiore U, et al. Comparison of two diets for the prevention of recurrent stones in idiopathic hypercalciuria. N Engl J Med. 2002;346:77–84.
21. Fuss M, Simon J, Fontinoy N, Coussaert E. High fluid – low calcium intake: not all stone-formers adhere to this simple treatment. Eur Urol. 1979;5:97–9.
22. Curhan GC, Willett WC, Rimm EB, Stampfer MJ. A prospective study of dietary calcium and other nutrients and the risk of symptomatic kidney stones. N Engl J Med. 1993;328:833–8.
23. Erickson SB, Cooper K, Broadus AE, Smith LH, Werness PG, Binder HJ, et al. Oxalate absorption and postprandial urine supersaturation in an experimental human model of absorptive hypercalciuria. Clin Sci. 1984;67:131–8.
24. Robertson WG, Peacock M, Marshall RW, Speed R, Nordin BEC. Seasonal variations in the composition of urine in relation to calcium stone-formation. Clin Sci Mol Med. 1975;49:597–602.
25. Barilla DE, Townsend J, Pak CYC. An exaggerated augmentation of renal calcium excretion after oral glucose in patients with renal hypercalciuria. Invest Urol. 1978;15:486–8.
26. Peacock M, Hodgkinson A, Nordin BEC. Importance of dietary calcium in the definition of hypercalciuria. Br Med J. 1967;3:469–71.
27. Walker VR, Bissada N, Qunibi W, Hughes H, Barkworth SA, Holbrow G, et al. Urinary calcium excretion in Saudi Arabia. In: Walker VR, Sutton RAL, Cameron ECB, Pak CYC, Robertson WG, editors. Urolithiasis. New York: Plenum Press; 1989. p. 717–8.
28. Sedrani SH. Low 25-hydroxyvitamin D and normal serum calcium concentrations in Saudi Arabia: Riyadh region. Ann Nutr Metab. 1984;28:181–5.
29. Robertson WG. Is it possible to motivate patients with recurrent stones to adhere to their treatment regimen? In: Rodgers AL, Hibbert BE, Hess B, Khan S, Preminger GM, editors. Urolithiasis 2000. Cape Town: University of Cape Town Press; 2000. p. 624–7.
30. Peacock M, Robertson WG, Norman R, Selby PL. Institution and management of a stone clinic. In: Schwille PO, Smith LH, Robertson WG, Vahlensieck W, editors. Urolithiasis and related clinical research. New York: Plenum Press; 1985. p. 259–66.
31. Johansson G, Backman U, Danielson BG, Fellström B, Ljunghall S, Wikström B. Biochemical and clinical effects of the prophylactic treatment of renal calcium stones with magnesium oxide. J Urol. 1980;124:770–4.
32. Lindberg J, Harvey J, Pak CYC. Effect of magnesium citrate and magnesium oxide on the crystallization of calcium salts in urine: changes produced by food-magnesium interaction. J Urol. 1990; 143:248–51.
33. Barcelo P, Wuhl O, Servitge E, Rousaud A, Pak CY. Randomized double-blind study of potassium citrate in idiopathic hypocitraturic calcium nephrolithiasis. J Urol. 1993;150:1761–4.
34. Pak CY, Sakhaee K, Fuller CJ. Physiological and physiochemical correction and prevention of calcium stone formation by potassium citrate therapy. Trans Assoc Am Physicians. 1983;96:294–305.
35. Jendle-Bengten C, Tiselius HG. Long-term follow-up of stone-formers treated with a low dose of sodium potassium citrate. Scand J Urol Nephrol. 2000;34:36–41.
36. Massey LK, Whiting SJ. Dietary salt, urinary calcium and kidney stone risk. Nutr Rev. 1995;53:131–9.
37. Robertson WG, Nair D, Laing C, Choong S, Jaeger P, Unwin RJ. The role of "metabolic syndrome" in the formation of uric acid-containing stones. Urol Res. 2008;36:177–8.
38. Maalouf NM, Sakhaee K, Parks JH, Coe FL, Adams-Huet B, Pak CY. Association of urinary pH with body weight in nephrolithiasis. Kidney Int. 2004;65:1422–5.
39. Maalouf NM. Metabolic syndrome and the genesis of uric acid stones. J Renal Nutr. 2011;21:128–31.
40. Robertson WG. The medical management of urinary stone disease. Eur Urol Update Ser. 1998;7:139–44.

87 Overview of Stone Prevention Strategies in China

Zhiqiang Chen

Abstract

Depending upon the type of stone formed, preventative strategies can be designed to assist the patient in preventing recurrences. However, the universally applicable principle is the production of large volumes of urine, through liberal water intake, and a judicious balanced diet.

Keywords

Water • Balanced diet • Calcium • Oxalate • Purines • Uric acid • pH • Sodium • Obesity • Proteins • Orthophosphate • Cellulose phosphate • Citrate • Aluminum • Magnesium • Meglumine GAG • Vitamin B6 • Chinese herbal medicine • Methionine • Acetylhydroxamic acid

The Prevention of Calcium Urolithiasis

Having a clear idea of the advantages and disadvantages of various prevention measures for calcium urolithiasis is very important, as there is some dispute as to what is the best treatment [1]. As patients might have to spend a lifetime taking these treatments, the preventive measure must be clinically effective, easy to implement, and have no side effects.

Modifying Lifestyles

Firstly, patients should modify their living habits and diet. It is important for them to maintain an ideal/appropriate body mass index, exercise regularly, balance their nutrition, and increase their intake of fruits, which are rich in citric acid [2, 3]. Medication should be considered only if the modification of living habits and diet is ineffective.

Z. Chen, M.D., Ph.D.
Department of Urology, Tongji Hospital,
Huazhong University of Science and Technology,
Wuhan, Hubei 430030, People's Republic of China
e-mail: zhqchen8366@163.com

Increasing the Intake of Water

Increasing the intake of water will increase urinary volume. Thus, the supersaturation of the composition of urinary stone will be reduced, and the probability of relapse of urolithiasis will be decreased. To keep the quantity of the urine above 2.0 ~ 2.5 l every day, the intake of fluid should exceed 2.5–3.0 l. Urolithiasis patients should be advised to measure the urinary specific gravity at home by themselves, and keep its value below 1.010, in order to maintain adequate water intake and dilution of urine [4, 5].

Generally, nondairy liquids that are lower in oxalic acid—such as orange juice, cranberry juice, and lemonade—are good for patients [6–8]. Whether hard water (water with a high calcium content) will increase the probability of the formation of calcium stones is still controversial. Patients should not drink an excess of coffee, tea, grape juice, apple juice, and cola.

The Need for a Balanced Diet

Calcium

When the calcium intake is below 800 mg (20 mmol), a negative calcium balance will be caused. The low calcium will

J.J. Talati et al. (eds.), *Urolithiasis*,
DOI 10.1007/978-1-4471-4387-1_87, © Springer-Verlag London 2012

decrease the urinary calcium excretion, but may lead to osteoporosis and increase in the urinary oxalic acid excretion. Having a normal calcium diet and limiting the intake of animal proteins and sodium are better ways to prevent the relapse of urolithiasis than the traditional low-calcium diet [9]. In some patients, a normal or an appropriate high-calcium diet has the clinical value for the therapy of the urolithiasis relapse [10]. Calcium supplements added to the daily diet, however, may cause a relapse of urolithiasis, because the over-intake of calcium without control will increase urinary supersaturation. Only for the patients with intestinal hyperoxaluria can supplementing calcium by medication be taken as a treatment to prevent urolithiasis relapse [11]. Orally taking 200–400 mg of calcium citrate will inhibit the urinary oxalate excretion and increase the urinary citrate excretion at the same time [12].

Patients should eat more tofu, fish, and dairy such as milk, cheese, and yogurt. The targeted calcium intake for adults is 800–1,000 mg, 20–25 mmol per day. The exception is patients with absorptive hypercalciuria who should be advised to have a low-calcium diet.

Limitation of Oxalic Acid Intake

Although only 10–15 % urinary oxalic acid derives from food, urinary oxalate excretion will increase significantly after the excessive intake of oxalic acid in food. Patients with calcium oxalate stone, especially those with hyperoxaluria, should avoid oxalic acid-rich food such as cabbage, almonds, peanuts, sugar beets, parsley, spinach, rhubarb, black tea, and cocoa. Among them, spinaches are richest in oxalic acid and should strictly not be taken by these patients [13].

A low-calcium diet can promote the intestinal absorption of oxalate and increase the urinary oxalate excretion. Calcium supplements, therefore, will be helpful for decreasing the intestinal absorption of oxalate. However, this therapy should only be taken by patients with intestinal hyperoxaluria (see also Chap. 19).

Limitation of Sodium Intake

A high-sodium diet will raise urinary calcium excretion. The daily sodium intake, therefore, should be less than 2 g.

Limitation of Protein Over-Intake

A low-carbohydrate and high-animal-protein content in diet promotes the formation of calcium stones. The high-protein diet will increase the urinary calcium and oxalate excretion and decrease the urinary citrate excretion and urinary pH [14]. Therefore, it is the major factor that causes the urinary calcium stones.

Keeping a balanced nutritional intake and eating three meals per day are very important. Patients should maintain their intake of protein to less than 150 g per day, and those with recurrent stones should consume less than 80 g.

Keeping Slim

According to the research, being overweight is a vital factor that causes urolithiasis. Patients with urolithiasis should keep their body mass index (BMI) between 11 and 18 [15].

Increasing the Intake of Fruits and Vegetables

Eating fruits and vegetables every day can reduce the risk of urinary stones and will improve the concentration of urinary potassium and citrate [16]. Therefore, for patients with hypocitraturia, the suitable ingestion of fruits and vegetables can prevent urolithiasis relapse.

Increasing the Intake of Coarse Grains and Cellulose

Rice bran can reduce the urinary calcium excretion and decrease the probability of urolithiasis relapse [17]. However, patients should avoid the intake of fiber foods that are rich in oxalic acid such as wheat bran.

Decreasing the Intake of Vitamin C

Vitamin C can be naturally transformed into oxalic acid by the body. Orally taking vitamin C will remarkably increase the urinary oxalate excretion and raise the risk of the calcium oxalate crystals formation [18]. Although there is no research showing that the over-intake of vitamin C has something to do with the recurrence of the calcium oxalate stones, patients with recurrent calcium oxalate stones are still advised not to exceed the recommended daily dosage of 1.0 g of vitamin C [19].

Limitation of the High-Purine Diet

Calcium oxalate stone patients with high uric acid urine disease should avoid a high-purine diet. The recommended daily intake of purine is less than 500 mg. The foods rich in purine are internal organs of animals, such as liver and kidney, poultry skin, herring skin, sardines, anchovies, and so on.

Drug-Based Prevention

There are a variety of drugs used in the preventive treatment of calcium stones. However, only a few of them—citrate salts, thiazide diuretics, and allopurinol—have definite effects.

Thiazide Diuretics

For patients with increased urinary calcium, thiazide diuretics (such as fluorobenzene thiophene, trichlorothiazole, hydrochlorothiazide, indapamide) can decrease the urinary calcium and oxalate excretion and inhibit the intestinal absorption of calcium. What is more, it can inhibit bone resorption and promote regeneration of bone cells. Therefore, it can prevent the osteoporosis of stone patients with hypercalciuria. It can help patients with both calcium stones and hypercalciuria by reducing their hypercalciuria [20]. The commonly used dosage is hydrochlorothiazide 25 mg twice a day, or trichlorothiazole 4 mg per day.

The major side effects of thiazide diuretics are hypokalemia and hypocitraturia. Adding potassium citrate to thiazide therapy can reduce the side effects and enhance the function that prevents stone recurrence. Low blood pressure, fatigue, and erectile dysfunction may occur in some patients after a long-term combined use of thiazide diuretics and potassium citrate. It should be noted that there is the possibility of causing hypomagnesemia and lowering magnesium excretion in the urine.

Orthophosphate

Orthophosphate can reduce the circulating concentrations of 1,25-dihydroxyvitamin D. Its main functions are decreasing the calcium excretion and increasing the urinary phosphate and citrate excretion. Therefore, it can inhibit the formation of stones. The neutral orthophosphate has a better effect than the acidic orthophosphate.

Orthophosphate is mostly used in patients with both urinary calcium stones and hypercalciuria. However, there is insufficient evidence to prove its effectiveness. Therefore, it is used selectively in some of the patients in a urinary stone clinic and is not the first choice of preventive treatments.

Cellulose Phosphate

Phosphate fiber and sodium phosphate fiber can restrain the intestinal absorption of calcium and reduce the urinary calcium excretion by bonding with calcium and forming complexes. It is mostly used in the urinary stone patients with absorptive hypercalciuria. Its clinical effects are still not fully known. Because of the possibility of causing hyperoxaluria, low magnesium excretion in the using, cellulose phosphate is not recommended in the prevention treatment of stone recurrence.

Citrate

Alkaline citrate will raise the urinary excretion of citrate and decrease the urinary supersaturation of calcium oxalate, calcium phosphate, and uric acid salt. Therefore, it can inhibit the crystallization and reduce the recurrence of calcium stones effectively [21, 22].

In the clinic, the citrate salts used to prevent the recurrence of calcium stones include hydrogen potassium sodium citrate, potassium citrate, sodium citrate, sodium potassium citrate, and potassium magnesium citrate [23]. Potassium citrate and sodium citrate both produce good therapeutic effects. However, sodium can promote the urinary excretion of calcium, which weakens its effect, while potassium does not. Clinical research indicates that the urinary alkalization of potassium citrate is better than sodium [24]. Therefore, potassium citrate is more effective than sodium in preventing stone recurrence. A hydrogen potassium sodium citrate, Uralyt-U® (Madaus GMBH, Cologne, Germany), is easy to take and has a good taste; therefore, it has high patient compliance.

Although the most suitable cases for alkaline citrate are patients with low citrate urine disease, these days the possibility of using it in all kinds of calcium stone patients is being considered. The commonly used dose is hydrogen potassium sodium citrate, Uralyt-U, 1–2 g three times per day, or potassium citrate 1–2 g or potassium sodium citrate 3 g twice to three times per day.

The main side effect of the alkaline citrate is diarrhea, which leads to poor compliance.

Allopurinol

Allopurinol can reduce the generation of urate and decrease the concentration of serum urate and the urinary excretion of urate and oxalate [25].

Allopurinol is recommended to be used in calcium oxalate stone patients with high uric acid urine disease to prevent uric acid stones. The commonly used dosage is 100 mg three times per day, or 300 mg once a day.

Magnesium

Magnesium can reduce the supersaturation of calcium oxalate by binding with it and then inhibit the formation of the calcium urolithiasis. Supplementing magnesium will promote the urinary magnesium and increase the content of citrate in urine and the urinary pH. Therefore, magnesium can prevent calcium oxalate stone recurrence effectively. It is suitable for oxalate stone patients with or without low magnesium urine disease.

Since only 4 % of calcium stone patients have a low urinary magnesium, it is now not recommended to use it alone to prevent recurrent calcium urolithiasis, except when prescribed as a citrate.

Glycosaminoglycan

Glycosaminoglycan can inhibit the growth of calcium oxalate stones. It is suitable for the treatment of recurrent calcium oxalate stones. However, at this point in time, there is insufficient evidence to recommend use of synthetic or semi-synthetic glycosaminoglycan in the prevention of recurrent calcium urolithiasis.

Vitamin B_6

The lack of vitamin B_6 will cause an increase in oxalate excretion. Large doses of vitamin B_6 (300–500 mg per day) have a therapeutic effect in patients with primary hyperoxaluria [26].

Chinese Herbal Medicine

Chinese herbal medicines that have some effect in preventing calcium stones are alisma, panda hai (the dry mature seeds of *Sterculiaceae Sterculia lychnophora*), money grass, maydis stigma (corn silk), and banana cores [27–29]. However, there are no clinical reports about their therapeutic effects.

The recommended drug treatments for calcium urolithiasis for patients with abnormal urine constituents are summarized in Table 87.1.

The Prevention of Uric Acid Stones

The key to the prevention of uric acid stones lies in increasing the quantity of urine, raising urinary pH, and decreasing the formation and excretion of uric acid [30].

Water intake needs to be increased to the level that produces >2,000 ml of urine/24 h.

Urinary alkalinization can be promoted by prescribing hydrogen potassium sodium citrate, Uralyt-U, 1–2 g three times per day or sodium bicarbonate 1.0 g three times per day to keep the urinary pH between 6.5 and 6.8.

The formation of uric acid can be reduced in patients with a raised blood or urinary uric acid by prescribing allopurinol 300 mg per day or folic acid 5 mg per day. Folic acid is recommended since it is more effective than allopurinol in inhibiting the activity of xanthine oxidase [31].

The Prevention of Stones

A low-calcium and low-phosphorous diet is recommended for infection stones. Aluminum chloride or aluminum carbonate gel can bind with phosphate ions and form into insoluble aluminum phosphate. Therefore, they can decrease the intestinal absorption of phosphorus and the urinary excretion of phosphorus. It is generally not recommended.

For magnesium ammonium phosphate and carbonate apatite stones, which are caused by urease bacterial infection, patients should have their stones cleared as completely as possible by surgery.

Based on the antimicrobial susceptibility testing, antibiotics are used to eliminate infection. Anti-infection treatment needs to be sustained over a long period. At the beginning of this treatment, the dose (the healing dose) of the antibiotics should be relatively large. After 1–2 weeks of treatment, when the urine is sterile, the dose, maintenance dose, can be reduced to half and be maintained for 3 months. Urine culture and sensitivity testing should be performed every month, reverting to the healing dose to control infection if a patient is infected again.

Acidification of the urine can raise the solubility of phosphate. To acidify urine, ammonium chloride 1 g, 2–3 times per day, or methionine 500 mg, 2–3 times per day, can be used.

For patients with severe infection, a urease inhibitor should be used. Acetylhydroxamic acid or hydroxyurea is recommended. The first dose can be 250 mg twice a day for 3–4 weeks. The dose can then be raised to 250 g three times per day if the patient can tolerate it.

Table 87.1 The recommended drug treatments for calcium urolithiasis for patients with abnormal urine constituents in China

Drugs	Treatment group
Thiazide diuretics[a]	Hypercalciuria
	Stones containing dicalcium phosphate dihydrate
	Other kinds of abnormal diseases
Alkaline citrate	Low citrate urine disease
	Renal tubular acidosis
	Intestinal hyperoxaluria
	Low inhibitory activity of crystal growth[b]
Allopurinol	High uric acid urine disease
Vitamin B_6 (pyridoxine)	Primary hyperoxaluria
	Mild hyperoxaluria
Calcium supplement	Intestinal hyperoxaluria
orthophosphate[c]	Calcium disorders

[a]Potassium supplement is needed to prevent hypokalemia and the secondary low citrate urine disease after the intracellular acidosis and hypokalemia

[b]Operates when the inhibitory activity of crystal growth is low

[c]Although orthophosphate drugs are not the first choice, they can be used in patients who cannot tolerate thiazide diuretics

The Prevention of Cystine Stones

Patients should drink lots of water, at least 150 ml/h, to increase the proportion of cystine in solution and keep the daily urine quantity above 3,000 ml.

Oral hydrogen potassium sodium citrate, Uralyt-U, 1–2 g three times per day may be used to alkalinize the urine and keep its pH above 7.5.

In order to reduce the excretion of cystine, patients should have a low-protein diet, which is mainly composed of vegetables and cereals, and avoid eating foods that are rich in methionine such as soybeans, wheat, fish, meat, beans, and mushrooms.

Patients should also limit the intake of sodium. The recommended quantity is less than 2 g per day.

When the urinary excretion of cystine is above 3 mmol per day, patients should take tiopronin, α(alpha)-mercaptopropionyl glycine, 250–2,000 mg per day, or captopril, 75–150 mg per day [32].

The Prevention of Other Rare Stones

Prevention of Drug Stones

Prevention of Calcium Drug Stones

Calcium and vitamin D supplements can cause stones because of increase in urinary calcium excretion.

A supplement of large doses of vitamin D may promote the urinary oxalate excretion. The keys of the prevention of calcium drug stones are decreasing the urinary calcium and oxalate excretion and reducing the calcium and oxalate urine saturation [12].

Prevention of Non-calcium Drug Stones

The best way to prevent indinavir stones is drinking enough water, above 3,000 ml per day. This can prevent the precipitation of drug crystals. What is more, when the urinary pH is acidified below 5.5, the dissolution of drug crystals will be raised.

The way to prevent triamterene, acetazolamide, and sulfonamide drug stones is by drinking a lot of water to dilute urine. In order to increase the solubility of drug crystals, patients should use basic drugs appropriately to raise the urinary pH.

Prevention of Purine Stones

Patients should eat a low-purine diet to prevent purine stones, mainly including 2,8-dihydroxy adenine stones and xanthine stones. Allopurinol can inhibit the activity of xanthine oxidase and reduce the excretion of 2,8-dihydroxy adenine. Therefore, it can be used to prevent these stones. Theoretically, alkalizing the urine can promote the solution of the 2,8-dihydroxy adenine stones. However, it is impossible to raise the urinary pH above 9 in clinic by using drugs; thus alkalization of urine has no value in practical application.

Conclusion

Stone prevention strategies are common across the world. While there is potential for investigating a number of indigenous drugs, there is yet insufficient scientific evidence for their effectiveness. In addition to a judicious diet and high water intake, specific targeted remedies have established their niche in prevention programs.

References

1. Hess B, Mauron H, Ackermann D, Jaeger P. Effects of a 'common sense diet' on urinary composition and supersaturation in patients with idiopathic calcium urolithiasis. Eur Urol. 1999;36(2):136–43.
2. Borghi L, Meschi T, Schianchi T, Briganti A, Guerra A, Allegri F, et al. Urine volume: stone risk factor and preventive measure. Nephron. 1999;81 Suppl 1:31–7.
3. Finkielstein VA, Goldfarb DS. Strategies for preventing calcium oxalate stones. CMAJ. 2006;174(10):1407–9.
4. McCormack M, Dessureault J, Guitard M. The urine specific gravity dipstick: a useful tool to increase fluid intake in stone forming patients. J Urol. 1991;146(6):1475–7.
5. Rodgers A. Effect of cola consumption on urinary biochemical and physicochemical risk factors associated with calcium oxalate urolithiasis. Urol Res. 1999;27(1):77–81.
6. Seltzer MA, Low RK, McDonald M, Shami GS, Stoller ML. Dietary manipulation with lemonade to treat hypocitraturic calcium nephrolithiasis. J Urol. 1996;156(3):907–9.
7. Wabner CL, Pak CY. Effect of orange juice consumption on urinary stone risk factors. J Urol. 1993;149(6):1405–8.
8. McHarg T, Rodgers A, Charlton K. Influence of cranberry juice on the urinary risk factors for calcium oxalate kidney stone formation. BJU Int. 2003;92(7):765–8.
9. Straub M, Hautmann RE. Developments in stone prevention. Curr Opin Urol. 2005;15(2):119–26.
10. Tiselius HG. Epidemiology and medical management of stone disease. BJU Int. 2003;91(8):758–67.
11. Delvecchio FC, Preminger GM. Medical management of stone disease. Curr Opin Urol. 2003;13(3):229–33.
12. Tiselius HG. Possibilities for preventing recurrent calcium stone formation: principles for the metabolic evaluation of patients with calcium stone disease. BJU Int. 2001;88(2):158–68.
13. Borghi L, Schianchi T, Meschi T, Guerra A, Allegri F, Maggiore U, et al. Comparison of two diets for the prevention of recurrent stones in idiopathic hypercalciuria. N Engl J Med. 2002;346(2):77–84.
14. Reddy ST, Wang CY, Sakhaee K, Brinkley L, Pak CY. Effect of low-carbohydrate high-protein diets on acid–base balance, stone-forming propensity, and calcium metabolism. Am J Kidney Dis. 2002;40(2):265–74.
15. Tiselius HG, Ackermann D, Alken P, Buck C, Conort P, Gallucci M. Guidelines on urolithiasis. Eur Urol. 2001;40(4):362–71.
16. Meschi T, Maggiore U, Fiaccadori E, Schianchi T, Bosi S, Adorni G, et al. The effect of fruits and vegetables on urinary stone risk factors. Kidney Int. 2004;66(6):2402–10.
17. Hiatt RA, Ettinger B, Caan B, Quesenberry Jr CP, Duncan D, Citron JT. Randomized controlled trial of a low animal protein, high fiber diet in the prevention of recurrent calcium oxalate kidney stones. Am J Epidemiol. 1996;144(1):25–33.
18. Baxmann AC, De O G Mendonça C, Heilberg IP. Effect of vitamin C supplements on urinary oxalate and pH in calcium stone-forming patients. Kidney Int. 2003;63(3):1066–71.
19. Auer BL, Auer D, Rodgers AL. The effect of ascorbic acid ingestion on the biochemical and physicochemical risk factors associated with calcium oxalate kidney stone formation. Clin Chem Lab Med. 1998;36(3):143–7.
20. Ohkawa M, Tokunaga S, Nakashima T, Orito M, Hisazumi H. Thiazide treatment for calcium urolithiasis in patients with idiopathic hypercalciuria. Br J Urol. 1992;69(6):571–6.
21. Ettinger B, Pak CY, Citron JT, Thomas C, Adams-Huet B, Vangessel A. Potassium-magnesium citrate is an effective prophylaxis against recurrent calcium oxalate nephrolithiasis. J Urol. 1997;158(6):2069–73.
22. Abdulhadi MH, Hall PM, Streem SB. Can citrate therapy prevent nephrolithiasis? Urology. 1993;41(3):221–4.
23. Jendle-Bengten C, Tiselius HG. Long-term follow-up of stone formers treated with a low dose of sodium potassium citrate. Scand J Urol Nephrol. 2000;34(1):36–41.
24. Whalley NA, Meyers AM, Martins M, Margolius LP. Long-term effects of potassium citrate therapy on the formation of new stones in groups of recurrent stone formers with hypocitraturia. Br J Urol. 1996;78(1):10–4.
25. Ettinger B, Tang A, Citron JT, Livermore B, Williams T. Randomized trial of allopurinol in the prevention of calcium oxalate calculi. N Engl J Med. 1986;315(22):1386–9.
26. Holmes RP. Pharmacological approaches in the treatment of primary hyperoxaluria. J Nephrol. 1998;11 Suppl 1:32–5.
27. Cao ZG, Liu JH, Zhou SW, Wu W, Yin CP, Wu JZ. The effects of the active constituents of Alisma orientatis on renal stone formation and bikunin expression in rat urolithiasis model. Natl Med J China. 2004;84(15):1276–9.
28. Li HY, Liu JH, Cao ZG, Wang SG, Cai D, Ye ZQ, et al. An in vitro and in vivo study of water and lipid soluble extracts from Alisma orientatis on urinary oxalate calcium stone formation. Chin J Urol. 2003;24(10):658–62.

29. Wang YQ, Zhu BJ, An RH, Qi YC, Li CC. Inhibitory effect of desmodium styracifolium injection on calcium oxalate renal stone formation. Chin J Urol. 1999;20(11):689–91.
30. Coe FL. Uric acid and calcium oxalate nephrolithiasis. Kidney Int. 1983;24(3):392–403.
31. Lewis AS, Murphy L, McCalla C, Fleary M, Purcell S. Inhibition of mammalian xanthine oxidase by folate compounds and amethopterin. J Biol Chem. 1984;259(1):12–5.
32. Barbey F, Joly D, Rieu P, Méjean A, Daudon M, Jungers P. Medical treatment of cystinuria: critical reappraisal of long-term results. J Urol. 2000;163(5):1419–23.

Management of Hypercalciuria and Oxalates in the Prevention of Stone Recurrence

88

John R. Asplin

Abstract

Urinary excretion of calcium and oxalate are two of the critical determinants of urine supersaturation of calcium oxalate salts and the risk of calcium oxalate stone formation. Therefore, treatment to reduce stone recurrence is focused on lowering the excretion of these lithogenic factors. Both diet and medication can lower urine calcium. Thiazide diuretics have been shown to reduce stone recurrence in randomized controlled trials and have the added benefit of improving bone mineral density. Citrate and bisphosphonates can lower urine calcium modestly but have not been well studied in hypercalciuric stone disease. Treatments to lower oxalate are not as well documented as are those for hypercalciuria. For idiopathic hyperoxaluria, pyridoxine and magnesium have been proposed as therapies, but there is conflicting data regarding their effectiveness. In enteric hyperoxaluria, low-oxalate diets and calcium supplements to bind dietary oxalate are the standard therapy. There is great interest in the use of oxalate-degrading bacteria as probiotics to treat hyperoxaluria, but human data is limited at this time.

Keywords

Hypercalciuria • Hyperoxaluria • Urolithiasis • Thiazide • Citrate • Bisphosphonate • Probiotic • Enteric hyperoxaluria • Supersaturation • Calcium • Oxalate

Introduction

Calcium is the most common component of human kidney stones. Approximately 85 % of calcium stones are predominantly calcium oxalate, either the monohydrate or dihydrate salt. Saturation is the physical chemical driving force for crystallization and can be expressed as the ratio of the ion activity products of the components of the salt of interest to its solubility [1]. A supersaturated solution is a requirement for crystals to form and grow. Urine concentrations of calcium and oxalate are the key determinants of saturation of calcium oxalate in the urine. Other urine components such as citrate, phosphate, and magnesium will affect saturation, but not to the level of either calcium or oxalate [2]. Prevailing urine saturation has been shown to correlate with the types of stones patients actually form [3]. Thus, our treatments to prevent stone formation are mainly focused on lowering saturation. Certainly, the standard recommendation to increase fluid intake to dilute urine will lower the concentration of all lithogenic components of the urine, lowering saturation and reducing stone risk. Reducing renal excretion of calcium and oxalate are the other primary goals in the treatment of calcium oxalate stones, both of which will reduce saturation. This chapter will address medical therapy to treat hypercalciuria and hyperoxaluria. Dietary therapy, which is of great importance in stone disease, has been covered in Chap. 86.

J.R. Asplin, M.D., FASN
Department of Medicine, University of Chicago, Litholink Corporation, 2250 W Campbell Park Dr., Chicago, IL 60612, USA

Department of Medicine, University of Chicago, Chicago, IL, USA
e-mail: asplinj@labcorp.com

J.J. Talati et al. (eds.), *Urolithiasis*,
DOI 10.1007/978-1-4471-4387-1_88, © Springer-Verlag London 2012

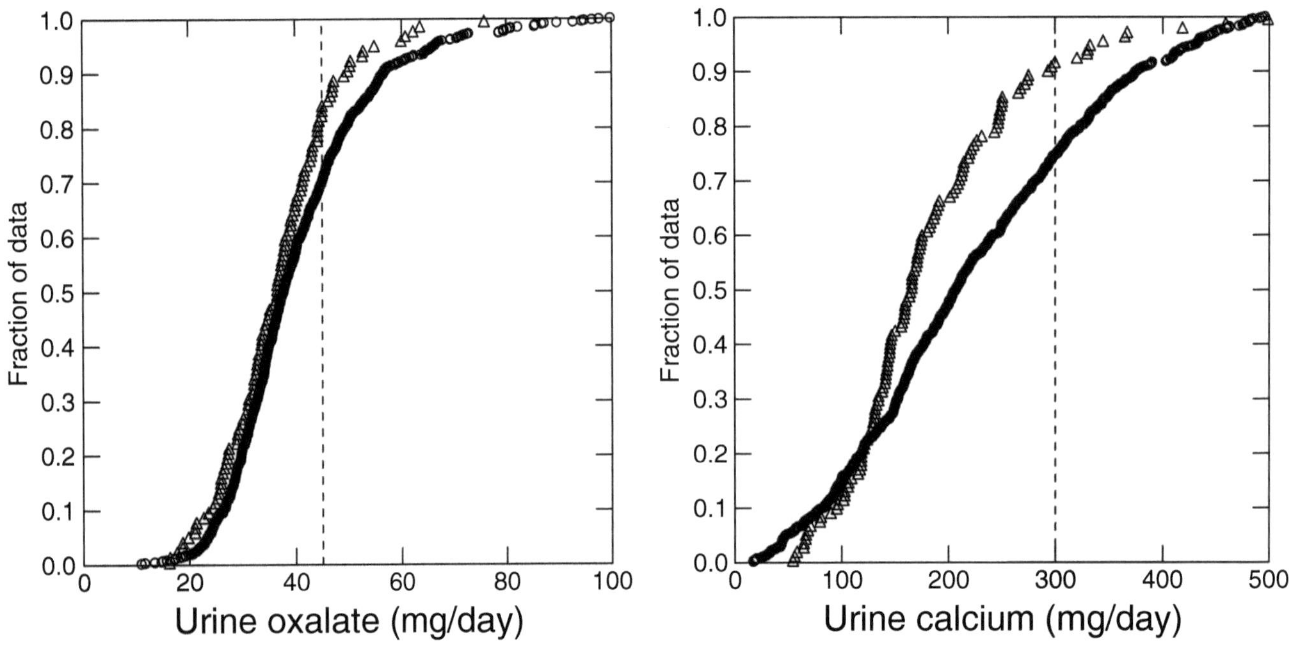

Fig. 88.1 Quantile plots of urine oxalate and urine calcium in men. Stone-forming patients (*circles*) have excretion rates shifted to the right of normal subjects (*triangles*). The right shift of patients is much greater for calcium excretion than that of oxalate excretion, where the distributions greatly overlap. The *vertical dashed line* identifies 45 mg/day for oxalate and 300 mg/day for calcium

Definition of Hypercalciuria and Hyperoxaluria

Most commonly, hypercalciuria is defined as an excretion of 300 mg/day in men or 250 mg/day in women, or as a ratio of the daily excretion to the patient's weight using 4 mg/kg as the upper limit. Other researchers use a definition of 200 mg/day when the patient is studied while consuming a low calcium, low sodium diet [4]. However, strict control of diet is required for this definition and is hard to achieve in routine clinical practice. For oxalate, a common definition of hyperoxaluria is greater than 45 mg/day (0.5 mmol/day), though some authors use a slightly lower value of 40 mg/day [5]. Overall, these definitions are useful in research in defining populations to be studied to understand pathophysiology and therapeutic interventions. In clinical practice, we need to recognize that reference ranges likely differ from one culture/country to another. Laboratory methods vary, particularly for oxalate, such that each lab should have ranges specific for the population and analytic method employed [6].

An important factor to recognize in the treatment of patients is that urine calcium and oxalate are not dichotomous variables and there is not a distinct level beyond which stone risk rises dramatically. Though hypercalciuria is the most common metabolic abnormality found in calcium stone formers, there is considerable overlap in urine calcium excretion in normal and stone-forming populations. For urine oxalate, there is only a mild difference between stone formers and normal subjects. As can be seen in Fig. 88.1, using data obtained from a commercial laboratory, the distribution of urine calcium is clearly shifted higher than non-stone-forming controls, though overlap is considerable. For oxalate, the shift is much less dramatic and overlap of the distributions is almost complete. Such data can lead to the conclusion that oxalate is not an important component of stone risk, but it needs to be recognized that stone risk is a continuous variable and increases as urine calcium and urine oxalate increase. Curhan et al. have reported that stone risk starts to increase well within the classically defined normal ranges for both oxalate and calcium [7]. It may be necessary to treat urine chemistries that are within the normal range, as lowering excretion to below the population mean may be required to lower saturation sufficiently to prevent stone formation. Historically, there has been more focus in treating urine calcium as both diet and medications were shown to lower urine calcium consistently. For hyperoxaluria, treatment effects have not been so clear but that does not mean lowering urine oxalate excretion would not be effective therapy for stone disease.

Throughout this chapter, the terms hypercalciuria and hyperoxaluria will be used but with recognition that stone risk increases as excretion of calcium and oxalate increases. Physicians may treat to lower urine calcium and/or oxalate even when they are within the "normal range."

Management of Hypercalciuria

Once hypercalciuria has been identified, the physician must determine the etiology. Idiopathic hypercalciuria is the most common cause of hypercalciuria in kidney stone patients. It is defined as excess urine calcium with normal serum

Table 88.1 Randomized prospective trials of thiazide and thiazide-like diuretics in calcium urolithiasis

Study	Drug[a]	*N*	Duration (years)	Control (%)	Drug (%)	*P* value
Scholz et al. [10]	HCTZ 25 mg bid	51	1	23	24	NS
Brocks et al. [9]	BFMT 2.5 mg tid	62	1.5	17	15	NS
Ohkawa et al. [12]	TCM 4 mg qd	175	2	14	8	$0.05<p<0.1$
Mortensen et al. [11]	BFMT 2.5 mg tid	22	2	40	0	$0.05<p<0.1$
Ettinger et al. [13]	CTD 25 or 50 mg qd	73	3	50	20	$p<0.05$
Laerum and Larsen [14]	HCTZ 25 mg bid	50	3	55	25	$p<0.05$
Borghi et al. [15]	IND 2.5 mg qd	50	3	43	16	$p<0.02$

Results of each study are expressed as the percent of subjects who had at least one stone during follow-up for the nonthiazide group (control) compared to the active treatment group (drug)

[a]*HCTZ* hydrochlorothiazide, *BFMT* bendroflumethiazide, *TCM* trichlormethiazide, *CTD* chlorthalidone, *IND* indapamide.

calcium, in the absence of systemic disorders known to affect calcium metabolism. If systemic disorders that lead to excess urine calcium excretion are present, such as primary hyperparathyroidism or sarcoid, then the treatment should be directed at the primary disorder, if possible.

The standard pharmaceutical treatment of hypercalciuria is the use of thiazide diuretics. Thiazide diuretics lower urine calcium excretion, mainly by inducing a state of volume depletion, which results in increased proximal tubule reabsorption of calcium [8]. There may also be a direct effect on tubule reabsorption in the distal convoluted tubule. Based on the hypocalciuric effect of thiazides, a number of prospective randomized trials of thiazide with reduction of stone formation as the primary endpoint have been performed. It has been said that the results of the thiazide trials are conflicting and that it is not clear if thiazides reduce stone recurrence. However, as can be seen in Table 88.1, though there are multiple studies of thiazide, there are only three trials that have lasted 3 years. This is a critical point, as studies with a stone formation outcome require sufficient time from entry to accumulate adequate stone events to detect a treatment effect. The two trials that were less than 2 years were negative [9, 10]; the trials of 2 years duration had a borderline statistical significance for the positive effect found for thiazides [11, 12]. The three 3-year prospective randomized trials all showed a significant reduction in stone events in the thiazide group [13–15]. Of note, the trials by Ettinger et al. and Laerum and Larsen used calcium stone formation, not hypercalciuria, as entry criteria. That they were able to show a reduction in stone events suggests that patients do not have to meet the standard criteria of hypercalciuria to receive benefits of treatment that lower urine calcium.

In the thiazide trials, note that two of the thiazides used were chlorthalidone and indapamide, both of which have very long half-lives, providing continuous action throughout the day. The positive study, which used a short-acting thiazide, was that of Laerum, who used hydrochlorothiazide but dosed the drug twice a day. In general, a long-acting drug like chlorthalidone or indapamide should be preferred, but if a short-acting thiazide is to be used, it should be used on a twice-a-day schedule. When using a thiazide, patients should be instructed to limit their sodium intake to 2,300–3,000 mg/day. Not only will salt restriction itself lower urine calcium excretion but it will enhance the action of the diuretic. If patients eat large amounts of salt while taking thiazide, they will prevent the volume depletion the drug needs to induce in order to work. Plus, the large salt load in combination with the diuretic will greatly enhance renal potassium wasting. Patients on thiazide should have blood potassium levels measured to monitor for hypokalemia. Hypokalemia can reduce urine citrate levels, blunting any benefit obtained from lowering urine calcium [16]. Not all the thiazide trials made an attempt to maintain serum potassium in the normal range. Attention to such detail in clinical practice may allow the physician to obtain even better results than the randomized trials. Repletion of potassium losses can be accomplished with oral potassium salts, with a goal of keeping serum potassium above 4.0 mmol/l. An alternative is to use a potassium sparing diuretic. Amiloride is the preferred potassium sparing diuretic since triamterene has been shown to crystallize in the urinary tract and can be a component of stones itself [17].

In addition to reducing stone formation, thiazides provide the added benefit of improving bone mineral density. Thiazides not only reduce urine calcium but also increase net calcium balance [18]. Patients with low bone mineral density from hypercalciuria have been shown to increase bone mineral density during treatment with thiazides [19]. Though there are no direct fracture outcomes for hypercalciuric patients treated with thiazide, large cohort studies of patients with hypertension who were treated with thiazide diuretics have been shown to have lower fracture rates than matched controls who did not receive thiazide [20, 21]. The well-documented reduction in stones and the overall benefit to bone health make thiazide diuretics the primary treatment for hypercalciuric patients with nephrolithiasis.

Though low sodium, low-protein diets, and thiazide diuretics are clearly the primary therapies for hypercalciuria,

Table 88.2 Effect of alendronate on urine calcium and bone mineral density in patients with hypercalciuria

Study	Subjects[a]	Duration	UCa baseline[b]	UCa on therapy	Spine BMD baseline (g/cm²)	Spine BMD on therapy (g/cm²)
Weisinger et al. [29]	18 HCSF	1 year	277 ± 28 mg/g	202 ± 26 mg/g*	1.16 ± 0.23	1.20 ± 0.25*
Heller et al. [28]	9 HCSF	17 days	140 ± 70 mg/g	60 ± 40 mg/g*	NA	NA
Giusti et al. [30]	25 HCPM	1 year	379 ± 79 mg/day	279 ± 68 mg/day*	0.76 ± 0.09	0.80 ± 0.08*

Urine calcium fell significantly with alendronate treatment in all studies. The bone mineral density increased significantly in both 1 year studies
[a]*HCSF* hypercalciuric stone formers, *HCPM* hypercalciuric postmenopausal women
[b]mg/g, mg of urine calcium per gram of creatinine
*$p < 0.05$

there are other drugs that may have beneficial effects in hypercalciuria. Alkali, usually provided in the form of potassium citrate salts, has a modest effect on urine calcium excretion. Since diets rich in animal protein result in a dietary acid load that increases renal calcium excretion, providing alkali to neutralize metabolic acid production can lower urine calcium excretion. In well-controlled studies where diet was fixed, potassium citrate in doses of 60–80 meq/day reduced calcium excretion by 20–25 % [22, 23]. In the prospective trials of citrate therapy, no significant fall in urine calcium was noted during the 3 years of follow-up, suggesting the magnitude of the alkali effect is modest and difficult to detect when diet is not fixed [24, 25]. Potassium citrate is not indicated as the primary treatment for hypercalciuria but may provide additional benefit in lowering urine calcium when used to maintain potassium stores in patients treated with thiazide [26]. The one caveat concerning use of alkali in hypercalciuric patients is that increasing urine pH above 6.3 can promote calcium phosphate stone formation. If alkali is used, the clinician needs to ensure that urine calcium excretion is being lowered sufficiently by therapy in order to offset the negative effects of a high urine pH.

Bisphosphonates reduce bone resorption and are the most common drugs used to treat osteoporosis. Since reduced bone mineral density and increased lability of bone mineral are frequent findings in hypercalciuric stone formers, it is reasonable to consider therapy directed at the bone component to hypercalciuria [27, 28]. There are a small number of papers that have reported the effects of bisphosphonates in hypercalciuric stone patients. The papers summarized in Table 88.2 do not include studies done with earlier forms of bisphosphonates such as etidronate, which is seldom used today. The studies have shown a modest improvement in urine calcium on bisphosphonates, and two of them have shown an improvement in bone mineral density after a year of treatment [28–30]. There are no studies where a reduction in kidney stone formation was used as an end point, and none of these studies included a control group. More research is necessary before the role of bisphosphonates in hypercalciuric stone disease is clearly established. At the present time, the use of these drugs should be restricted to hypercalciuric stone patients who have low bone mineral density that has not responded adequately to normal calcium diet and a thiazide diuretic.

Management of Hyperoxaluria

In most patients, urine oxalate is only modestly elevated and is likely dietary in origin. However, more severe forms of hyperoxaluria do exist and need to be identified as they can cause kidney damage and require more aggressive management. Enteric hyperoxaluria is seen with intestinal disease in which fat malabsorption leads to increased oxalate absorption in the colon. Enteric hyperoxaluria may be seen in Crohn's disease or with extensive small bowel resection. In recent years, it has been recognized that a significant number of patients who have had bariatric surgery, either Roux-en-y gastric bypass or biliopancreatic diversion, will develop enteric hyperoxaluria [31, 32]. Primary hyperoxaluria is an autosomal recessive disorder characterized by severe hyperoxaluria, kidney stones, and potentially loss of kidney function. To date, three types of primary hyperoxaluria have been identified [33]. When urine oxalate is greater than 80 mg/day in an adult without bowel disease, primary hyperoxaluria needs to be considered in the differential diagnosis. In children, significant hyperoxaluria (adjusted for body size or creatinine excretion) demands evaluation for primary hyperoxaluria. In reviewing treatment options for hyperoxaluria, idiopathic hyperoxaluria will be considered first, and then specific comments will be made concerning enteric and primary hyperoxaluria.

Pyridoxine has been recommended as a treatment of hyperoxaluria, because pyridoxine is a cofactor for the enzyme alanine-glyoxylate aminotransferase (AGT), which converts glyoxylate to glycine, reducing formation of oxalate. There are a number of trials of pyridoxine in stone disease, but none have prospectively shown a reduction in stone formation using an adequate control group. A few studies showed reduction in urine oxalate with pyridoxine, but this was not a universal finding [34–37]. In some studies pyridoxine therapy was combined with magnesium supplements, making it impossible to isolate the pyridoxine effect. Two large prospective studies found a relationship of low pyridoxine intake with incident stone formation in women, but not in men [38, 39]. More definitive studies are needed to define the role of pyridoxine in routine calcium oxalate stone disease. At modest doses of 5–25 mg/day, pyridoxine is well tolerated and can be used in patients who have hyperoxaluria unresponsive to dietary therapy, with recognition that there is not clear evidence favoring benefit.

Magnesium has been used as a treatment for urolithiasis because it may lower urine oxalate by complexing oxalate in the intestine [40], as well as acting as a calcium crystal inhibitor in the urine [41]. There are uncontrolled trials that report a benefit of magnesium therapy in reducing stone rates [42, 43], but there has been only one controlled trial of magnesium supplements in calcium stone disease, and it did not show a reduction in stone formation [13]. Unanswered is whether patients with hypomagnesuria [44] represent a subset of patients who may respond to magnesium supplements, since no trials have considered magnesium excretion as an entry criteria. Use of magnesium supplements is limited by diarrhea when magnesium dose exceeds 350–400 mg/day.

Oxalobacter formigenes is an anaerobic bacteria that is part of the normal intestinal flora and uses oxalate as its sole carbon source [45]. The potential of oxalate-degrading bacteria as a therapy for hyperoxaluria and calcium oxalate stones has been an area of active investigation. In a rat model of hyperoxaluria, Sidhu et al. showed *O. formigenes* delivered by gavage lowered urine oxalate excretion [46]. In a study using a rat model, Hatch et al. showed that the bacteria not only increase intestinal oxalate secretion by lowering luminal oxalate concentration but that bacterial homogenates can stimulate intestinal secretion of oxalate by upregulating transporters [47]. The secretory action of *O. formigenes* was confirmed in a mouse model of primary hyperoxaluria. No studies have been performed in humans to show if *O. formigenes* can stimulate intestinal oxalate secretion.

Lactic acid bacteria also have the capacity to degrade oxalate, though not as efficiently as *O. formigenes*. An uncontrolled trial of a probiotic preparation of lactic acid bacteria in six patients showed a significant reduction of urine oxalate [48]. In addition, a trial of escalating dose of the lactic acid preparation showed a modest reduction in urine oxalate excretion in patients with enteric hyperoxaluria [49]. However, a randomized control trial of the same probiotic did not show a lowering of urine oxalate in patients with hyperoxaluria and calcium oxalate stones [50]. Whether *O. formigenes* or lactic acid bacteria are truly effective therapies in hyperoxaluric stone, patients remain to be seen.

In patients with enteric hyperoxaluria, the control of oxalate is of utmost importance as loss of renal function is a risk. The pathophysiology of enteric hyperoxaluria depends on two alterations of intestinal function: (1) fat malabsorption leading to excess free fatty acids in the intestinal lumen which bind diet calcium, leading to more free oxalate available to be absorbed and (2) increased delivery of bile acids to the colon, leading to increased oxalate permeability of the colonic mucosa. Since excess urine oxalate is derived from the diet, intestinal oxalate absorption needs to be minimized. A low-oxalate diet limits oxalate available for absorption and low dietary fat will reduce free fatty acids to bind calcium. Increasing calcium intake increases intestinal calcium concentration, reducing oxalate bioavailability. Calcium supplements are usually required and need to be taken with meals to maximize binding to diet oxalate. Calcium citrate is preferred over calcium carbonate because patients who have altered stomach anatomy from bariatric surgery may not acidify stomach contents adequately to dissolve calcium carbonate pills. Though there is the concern that calcium excretion will increase, calcium absorption is often compromised in patients with small bowel disease, and the extra calcium provided will be essential to maintain skeletal integrity. Cholestyramine, which binds fatty acids and oxalate, has been shown to be useful in patients with hyperoxaluria from Crohn's disease but has not been studied in those with enteric hyperoxaluria from bariatric surgery.

Primary hyperoxaluria requires aggressive lifelong treatment in order to control recurrent stone formation and prevent progressive loss of kidney function. At one time, primary hyperoxaluria was felt to universally end in kidney failure, but data collected over the last two decades show that a large number of patients maintain adequate kidney function when treated early. Approximately, 25–30 % of patients with type 1 primary hyperoxaluria will respond to pyridoxine therapy with a significant reduction in urine oxalate excretion. In most patients with primary hyperoxaluria, we do not have a therapy to lower urine oxalate, so all effort is directed at minimizing the risk of calcium oxalate crystallization. Fluid intake is maximized and potassium citrate and neutral phosphate salts are prescribed [51, 52]. If kidney damage does develop, the patient should be considered for a liver transplant to correct the underlying metabolic defect. If kidney damage is severe, a kidney transplant may be done simultaneously.

Conclusion

Treatment of calcium oxalate stones is focused on lowering urine concentrations of calcium and oxalate, which can be accomplished by increasing fluid intake to create diluted urine or by lowering excretion rates of calcium and oxalate. Clinicians need to recognize that urine calcium and oxalate are continuous variables in regards to stone risk and patients often require treatment to lower excretion rates even though they do not meet a research definition of hypercalciuria or hyperoxaluria. Pharmacologic treatment is often needed in addition to diet to prevent stone recurrence. Thiazide diuretics lower urine calcium excretion and improve calcium balance.

There are three 3-year prospective randomized trials showing thiazide diuretics reduce calcium stone formation. Patients with urolithiasis and hypercalciuria are at increased risk of fracture; thiazides can improve bone mineral density in these patients. Citrate can lower urine calcium excretion by buffering metabolic acid production. The effect is modest so citrate is usually used as an adjunct to thiazide in the setting of hypercalciuria. Bisphosphonates reduce bone resorption and can lower urine calcium modestly. They have not been extensively studied in patients with urolithiasis so the role of bisphosphonates in treatment of urolithiasis is not well established. Medical therapy to lower urine oxalate is not well defined. Idiopathic hyperoxaluria has been treated with magnesium and/or pyridoxine supplementation. However, there are no prospective randomized trials to show that these therapies lower stone recurrence. Oxalate-degrading bacteria, used as probiotics, are an area of great interest. Though shown to be effective in animal models of hyperoxaluria, human trials are inconclusive at this time.

References

1. Werness PG, Brown CM, Smith LH, Finlayson B. EQUIL 2: a basic computer program for the calculation of urinary saturation. J Urol. 1985;134:1242–4.
2. Tiselius HG. An improved method for the routine biochemical evaluation of patients with recurrent calcium oxalate stone disease. Clin Chim Acta. 1982;122(3):409–18.
3. Asplin J, Parks J, Lingeman J, Kahnoski R, Mardis H, Lacey S, et al. Supersaturation and stone composition in a network of dispersed treatment sites. J Urol. 1998;159(6):1821–5.
4. Pak CY, Sakhaee K, Moe OW, Poindexter J, Adams-Huet B. Defining hypercalciuria in nephrolithiasis. Kidney Int. 2011;80(7):777–82.
5. Asplin JR. Hyperoxaluric calcium nephrolithiasis. Endocrinol Metab Clin North Am. 2002;31(4):927–49.
6. Maalouf NM, Adams HB, Pasch A, Lieske JC, Asplin JR, Siener R, et al. Variability in urinary oxalate measurements between six international laboratories. Nephrol Dial Transplant. 2011;26(12):3954–9.
7. Curhan GC, Willett WC, Speizer FE, Stampfer MJ. Twenty-four-hour urine chemistries and the risk of kidney stones among women and men. Kidney Int. 2001;59(6):2290–8.
8. Nijenhuis T, Vallon V, van der Kemp AW, Loffing J, Hoenderop JG, Bindels RJ. Enhanced passive Ca^{2+} reabsorption and reduced Mg^{2+} channel abundance explains thiazide-induced hypocalciuria and hypomagnesemia. J Clin Invest. 2005;115(6):1651–8.
9. Brocks P, Dahl C, Wolf H, Transbol I. Do thiazides prevent recurrent idiopathic renal calcium stones? Lancet. 1981;2(8238):124–5.
10. Scholz D, Schwille PO, Sigel A. Double-blind study with thiazide in recurrent calcium lithiasis. J Urol. 1982;128(5):903–7.
11. Mortensen JT, Schultz A, Ostergaard AH. Thiazides in the prophylactic treatment of recurrent idiopathic kidney stones. Int Urol Nephrol. 1986;18(3):265–9.
12. Ohkawa M, Tokunaga S, Nakashima T, Orito M, Hisazumi H. Thiazide treatment for calcium urolithiasis in patients with idiopathic hypercalciuria. Br J Urol. 1992;69(6):571–6.
13. Ettinger B, Citron JT, Livermore B, Dolman LI. Chlorthalidone reduces calcium oxalate calculous recurrence but magnesium hydroxide does not. J Urol. 1988;139:679–84.
14. Laerum E, Larsen S. Thiazide prophylaxis of urolithiasis: a double-blind study in general practice. Acta Med Scand. 1984;215:383–9.
15. Borghi L, Meschi T, Guerra A, Novarini A. Randomized prospective study of a nonthiazide diuretic, indapamide, in preventing calcium stone recurrences. J Cardiovasc Pharmacol. 1993;22 Suppl 6:S78–86.
16. Hamm LL. Renal handling of citrate. Kidney Int. 1990;38(4):728–35.
17. Ettinger B, Oldroyd NO, Sorgel F. Triamterene nephrolithiasis. JAMA. 1980;244(21):2443–5.
18. Coe FL, Parks JH, Bushinsky DA, Langman CB, Favus MJ. Chlorthalidone promotes mineral retention in patients with idiopathic hypercalciuria. Kidney Int. 1988;33(6):1140–6.
19. Adams J, Song C, Kantorovich V. Rapid recovery of bone mass in hypercalcuric, osteoporotic men treated with hydrochlorothiazide. Ann Intern Med. 1999;130:658–60.
20. Schoofs MW, van der Klift M, Hofman A, De Laet CE, Herings RM, Stijnen T, et al. Thiazide diuretics and the risk for hip fracture. Ann Intern Med. 2003;139(6):476–82.
21. LaCroix AZ, Wienpahl J, White LR, Wallace RB, Scherr PA, George LK, et al. Thiazide diuretic agents and the incidence of hip fracture. N Engl J Med. 1990;322(5):286–90.
22. Sakhaee K, Nicar M, Hill K, Pak CY. Contrasting effects of potassium citrate and sodium citrate therapies on urinary chemistries and crystallization of stone-forming salts. Kidney Int. 1983;24:348–52.
23. Sakhaee K, Alpern R, Jacobson HR, Pak CY. Contrasting effects of various potassium salts on renal citrate excretion. J Clin Endocrinol Metab. 1991;72(2):396–400.
24. Ettinger B, Pak CYC, Citron JT, Thomas C, Adams-Huet B, Vangessel A. Potassium-magnesium citrate is an effective prophylaxis against recurrent calcium oxalate nephrolithiasis. J Urol. 1997;158:2069–73.
25. Barcelo P, Wuhl O, Servitge E, Roussaud A, Pak C. Randomized double-blind study of potassium citrate in idiopathic hypocitraturic calcium nephrolithiasis. J Urol. 1993;150:1761–4.
26. Frassetto LA, Nash E, Morris Jr RC, Sebastian A. Comparative effects of potassium chloride and bicarbonate on thiazide-induced reduction in urinary calcium excretion. Kidney Int. 2000;58(2):748–52.
27. Pietschmann F, Breslau NA, Pak CY. Reduced vertebral bone density in hypercalciuric nephrolithiasis. J Bone Miner Res. 1992;7(12):1383–8.
28. Heller HJ, Zerwekh JE, Gottschalk FA, Pak CY. Reduced bone formation and relatively increased bone resorption in absorptive hypercalciuria. Kidney Int. 2007;71(8):808–15.
29. Weisinger JR, Alonzo E, Machado C, Carlini R, Martinis R, Paz-Martinez V, et al. Role of bones in the physiopathology of idiopathic hypercalciuria: effect of amino-bisphosphonate alendronate. Medicina (B Aires). 1997;57 Suppl 1:45–8.
30. Giusti A, Barone A, Pioli G, Girasole G, Siccardi V, Palummeri E, et al. Alendronate and indapamide alone or in combination in the management of hypercalciuria associated with osteoporosis: a randomized controlled trial of two drugs and three treatments. Nephrol Dial Transplant. 2009;24(5):1472–7.
31. Asplin JR, Coe FL. Hyperoxaluria in kidney stone formers treated with modern bariatric surgery. J Urol. 2007;177(2):565–9.
32. Patel BN, Passman CM, Fernandez A, Asplin JR, Coe FL, Kim SC, et al. Prevalence of hyperoxaluria after bariatric surgery. J Urol. 2009;181(1):161–6.
33. Belostotsky R, Seboun E, Idelson GH, Milliner DS, Becker-Cohen R, Rinat C, et al. Mutations in DHDPSL are responsible for primary hyperoxaluria type III. Am J Hum Genet. 2010;87(3):392–9.

34. Rattan V, Sidhu H, Vaidyanathan S, Thind SK, Nath R. Effect of combined supplementation of magnesium oxide and pyridoxine in calcium-oxalate stone formers. Urol Res. 1994;22(3):161–5.
35. Prien Sr EL, Gershoff SF. Magnesium oxide-pyridoxine therapy for recurrent calcium oxalate calculi. J Urol. 1974;112(4):509–12.
36. Edwards P, Nemat S, Rose GA. Effects of oral pyridoxine upon plasma and 24-hour urinary oxalate levels in normal subjects and stone formers with idiopathic hypercalciuria. Urol Res. 1990; 18(6):393–6.
37. Mitwalli A, Ayiomamitis A, Grass L, Oreopoulos DG. Control of hyperoxaluria with large doses of pyridoxine in patients with kidney stones. Int Urol Nephrol. 1988;20(4):353–9.
38. Curhan GC, Willett WC, Speizer FE, Stampfer MJ. Intake of vitamins B_6 and C and the risk of kidney stones in women. J Am Soc Nephrol. 1999;10(4):840–5.
39. Curhan GC, Willett WC, Rimm EB, Stampfer MJ. A prospective study of the intake of vitamins C and B_6, and the risk of kidney stones in men. J Urol. 1996;155(6):1847–51.
40. Berg W, Bothor C, Pirlich W, Janitzky V. Influence of magnesium on the absorption and excretion of calcium and oxalate ions. Eur Urol. 1986;12(4):274–82.
41. Bisaz S, Felix R, Neuman WF, Fleisch H. Quantitative determination of inhibitors of calcium phosphate precipitation in whole urine. Miner Electrolyte Metab. 1978;1:74–83.
42. Johansson G, Backman U, Danielson BG, Fellstrom B, Ljunghall S, Wikstrom B. Biochemical and clinical effects of the prophylactic treatment of renal calcium stones with magnesium hydroxide. J Urol. 1980;124(6):770–4.
43. Melnick I, Landes RR, Hoffman AA, Burch JF. Magnesium therapy for recurring calcium oxalate urinary calculi. J Urol. 1971;105: 119–22.
44. Preminger GM, Baker S, Peterson R, Poindexter J, Pak CYC. Hypomagnesiuric hypocitraturia: an apparent new entity for calcium nephrolithiasis. J Lithotr Stone Dis. 1989;1: 22–5.
45. Allison MJ, Dawson KA, Mayberry WR, Foss JG. *Oxalobacter formigenes* gen. nov., sp. nov.: oxalate-degrading anaerobes that inhabit the gastrointestinal tract. Arch Microbiol. 1985;141(1): 1–7.
46. Sidhu H, Allison MJ, Chow JM, Clark A, Peck AB. Rapid reversal of hyperoxaluria in a rat model after probiotic administration of *Oxalobacter formigenes*. J Urol. 2001;166(4):1487–91.
47. Hatch M, Cornelius J, Allison M, Sidhu H, Peck A, Freel RW. *Oxalobacter* sp. reduces urinary oxalate excretion by promoting enteric oxalate secretion. Kidney Int. 2006;69(4):691–8.
48. Campieri C, Campieri M, Bertuzzi V, Swennen E, Matteuzzi D, Stefoni S, et al. Reduction of oxaluria after an oral course of lactic acid bacteria at high concentration. Kidney Int. 2001;60(3): 1097–105.
49. Lieske JC, Goldfarb DS, De Simone C, Regnier C. Use of a probiotic to decrease enteric hyperoxaluria. Kidney Int. 2005;68(3): 1244–9.
50. Goldfarb DS, Modersizki F, Asplin JR. A randomized, controlled trial of lactic acid bacteria for idiopathic hypercalciuria. Clin J Am Soc Nephrol. 2007;2:745–9.
51. Leumann E, Hoppe B, Neuhaus T. Management of primary hyperoxaluria: efficacy of oral citrate administration. Pediatr Nephrol. 1993;7(2):207–11.
52. Milliner DS, Eickholt JT, Bergstralh EJ, Wilson DM, Smith LH. Results of long-term treatment with orthophosphate and pyridoxine in patients with primary hyperoxaluria. N Engl J Med. 1994;331(23): 1553–8.

Citrate Therapy for Calcium and Uric Acid Stones

89

Ephrem O. Olweny and Margaret S. Pearle

Abstract

Despite revolutionary advances in the surgical management of stone disease over the past three decades, recurrence rates without adjuvant medical therapy are high, underscoring the important role of metabolic evaluation and targeted medical therapy. Calcium and uric acid calculi comprise nearly 85–90 % of all kidney stones encountered in common clinical practice. Evidence from clinical trials suggests that alkali citrate pharmacotherapy, alone or in combination with other medical and dietary therapies, is effective for the metaphylaxis of calcium nephrolithiasis occurring in a wide range of clinical settings and of calcium nephrolithiasis-associated conditions. Clinical evidence also supports the use of alkali citrate therapy as first-line treatment of uric acid stones or mixed uric acid and calcium stones. Data from studies on dietary citrate therapy suggest that several beverages including vegetable juices, citrus juices, sports drinks, and various sodas with a high citrate content can induce a citraturic response to varying degrees, but concomitant alkalinizing effects appear to best be achieved with beverages containing potassium citrate rather than citric acid. Further studies on pharmacologic and dietary citrate therapies are needed to more comprehensively define their role in the management of calcium and uric acid nephrolithiasis.

Keywords

Kidney calculi • Urolithiasis • Citrate • Potassium citrate • Calcium oxalate • Lithotripsy • Bone density • Weightlessness • Uric acid • Diet therapy

Introduction and Historical Perspective

Experiments in thyroparathyroidectomized dogs in the 1920s led to the discovery of an organic compound within the serum that was critical for maintaining the ionic equilibrium of calcium [1]—a compound that was subsequently identified as citrate [2]. Later experiments demonstrated that citrate was an important inhibitor of calcium salt precipitation in urine [3]. This work eventually led to clinical studies in the early 1970s that demonstrated a link between hypocitraturia and nephrolithiasis [4]. A decade later, investigators demonstrated the role of oral alkali citrate supplementation in the prevention of stone formation in a group of recurrent calcium oxalate stone formers whose only identifiable metabolic abnormality was hypocitraturia [5].

Since these initial studies, the role of citrate, alone or in combination with other agents, in the pharmacotherapy of stone prevention has expanded considerably and currently includes urinary alkalinization in hyperuricosuria, prevention of stone formation in patients with thiazide-unresponsive hypercalciuria, treatment of idiopathic hypocitraturic calcium oxalate nephrolithiasis, prevention of stone recurrence and regrowth after shock wave lithotripsy, improvement in bone mineral density in patients with calcium nephrolithiasis and/or medullary sponge kidney, treatment of distal renal tubular acidosis, and decrease in stone formation

E.O. Olweny, M.D. • M.S. Pearle, M.D., Ph.D. (✉)
Professor of Urology and Internal Medicine, Department of Urology, University of Texas Southwestern Medical Center,
5323 Harry Hines Blvd., J8.106, Dallas, TX 75390-9110, USA
e-mail: margaret.pearle@utsouthwestern.edu

J.J. Talati et al. (eds.), *Urolithiasis*,
DOI 10.1007/978-1-4471-4387-1_89,

Table 89.1 Randomized controlled trials of evaluating alkali citrate for the prevention of recurrent calcium stone formation

Series	Treatment	Dose	Selection	Duration of study (years)	*N*	Pretreatment stones/pt/year	Posttreatment stones/pt/year	Remission rate (%)	*p*-value
Barcelo et al. [17]	KCit	60 mEq/day	Hypocitraturia	3	18	1.2	0.1	72.2	<0.05
	Placebo	–			20	1.1	1.1	20	
Ettinger et al. [18]	KMgCit	42 mEq/day potassium, 21 mEq/day magnesium, 63 mEq/day citrate	None	3	16	–	–	87.1	n/a (RR KMgCit / placebo = 0.16)
	Placebo	–			25	–	–	36.4	
Hoffbauer et al. [19]	NaKCit	30 g/day	None	3	16	2.1	0.9	31	0.65
	No Rx	–			22	1.8	0.7	27	

KCit potassium citrate, *KMgCit* potassium magnesium citrate, *NaKCit* sodium potassium citrate

risk after space flight [5–11]. In the ensuing chapter, we review the clinical role of alkali citrate therapy for the prevention of calcium and uric acid stones occurring in a variety of clinical settings, highlighting the available evidence supporting its use in each clinical scenario.

Alkali Citrate Therapy for Calcium Stones

Role in Idiopathic Hypocitraturic Calcium Nephrolithiasis

A number of mechanisms have been proposed to explain the inhibitory action of citrate on the growth of calcium stones, including formation of soluble calcium salts and inhibition of crystal growth and aggregation [3, 12–15]. Early uncontrolled clinical trials in patients with recurrent hypocitraturic calcium nephrolithiasis demonstrated the effectiveness of potassium citrate therapy in reducing rates of stone growth or recurrent stone formation, as well as the need for surgical treatment for newly formed stones [5, 16]. These findings prompted further investigation with randomized controlled trials (RCTs), of which three have been completed to date [17–19] (Table 89.1). Among these three RCTs, two were placebo-controlled, and participants were additionally provided with general dietary recommendations including increased fluid intake and salt restriction in the study by Barcelo and colleagues and protein, oxalate, and refined sugar restriction in the study by Ettinger and coworkers. Subjects in each of these trials were active stone formers, with a history of two or more stone events in the preceding 2–5 years, composed of 50 % or more calcium oxalate, calcium phosphate, or mixed calcium oxalate and calcium phosphate. At baseline metabolic evaluation, mean urinary citrate excretion ranged from 549 to 626 mg/day. In the Barcelo study, hypocitraturia was the sole metabolic selection criteria, while in the Ettinger study, metabolic background was unselective (i.e., subjects with a variety of metabolic derangements were included), but the prevalence of multiple abnormalities was similar in the treatment and placebo arms. Respective treatment interventions were 60 mEq potassium citrate in three divided doses daily in the study by Barcelo and colleagues, and two tablets of potassium magnesium citrate three times daily (for a total daily dose of 42 mEq potassium, 21 mEq magnesium, and 63 mEq citrate) in the study by Ettinger and coworkers. Treatment duration in each trial was 3 years. Combined, these two studies demonstrated remission rates of 72–87 % for the treatment arms, compared to 20–36 % for the placebo arms ($p<0.05$), with an unadjusted relative risk reduction of 84 % in the Ettinger study. Additionally, a significant increase in urinary citrate excretion (from 587 to 617 mg/day at baseline to 769–1,070 mg/day posttreatment), as well as a modest to significant increase in urinary pH (from a baseline level of 5.4–6.0 to a posttreatment level of 6.3–6.4), was observed in each of these trials (*p*-values for citrate and pH were <0.05 and 0.08, respectively, in the Ettinger study but were not reported in the Barcelo study). Despite the proven efficacy of potassium magnesium citrate in an unselected calcium stone-forming population, however, the drug has not yet been approved by the US Food and Drug Administration (FDA).

In contrast, the RCT by Hoffbauer and associates failed to demonstrate a benefit of sodium potassium citrate therapy with regard to reduction in stone formation, despite a significant increase in urinary citrate excretion (from 1.3 ± 0.8 mmol/l to 2.28 ± 1.09 mmol/l, *p*-value not reported) and a reduction in calcium excretion (48 % had hypercalciuria pretreatment compared to 25 % posttreatment, *p*-value not reported) [19]. In this study, subjects at baseline had experienced recurrent stone formation for a mean duration of 9.7 years in the control arm and 8.2 years in the citrate arm. Urinary metabolic abnormalities other than hypocitraturia were present in both treatment arms. Subjects in the treatment arm received three daily doses of 10 g sodium potassium citrate. A placebo control was not used. Rather, standard dietary measures were initiated in both arms, and patients in the treatment arm additionally received citrate therapy. After 3 years of intervention, remission rates in the control versus citrate arms were 27 versus 31 %, a statistically insignificant difference. Interestingly, elimination of pain during stone passage was observed for a significantly greater number of patients in the citrate arm ($p=0.001$). The authors suggested that the findings could be explained by spontaneous remission in stone formation in individual patients and that an unknown mechanism could be responsible for calcium oxalate stone formation [19]. It is also likely that sodium coadministration during alkali citrate therapy counterbalanced the beneficial effects of citrate, given the known role of increased sodium intake on calcium salt crystallization in the urine [20].

Role in Thiazide-Unresponsive Hypercalciuric Nephrolithiasis

Thiazides or thiazide-like diuretics (indapamide) are widely used in the treatment of nephrolithiasis associated with hypercalciuria, based on evidence from both randomized and non-randomized studies demonstrating their efficacy in reducing stone formation and recurrence rates in patients with hypercalciuric nephrolithiasis [20]. However, some patients with hypercalciuria are refractory to thiazide treatment, possibly because of thiazide-induced hypocitraturia. Pak and colleagues examined the role of potassium citrate therapy in a group of 13 patients with absorptive or renal hypercalciuria who continued to form stones after the initiation of thiazide treatment [7]. Among these patients, eight received potassium chloride supplementation, while five patients remained normokalemic without potassium supplementation. Mean duration of thiazide ± potassium chloride treatment was 2.1 ± 0.97 years/patient, and relapses occurred at 1.0–4.5 years into treatment. With addition of potassium citrate (30–60 mEq/day), 77 % of patients (10 of 13) demonstrated complete stone remission, and all patients had a significant decrease in the rate of new stone formation during a mean of 1.8 ± 0.5 SD years of potassium citrate treatment compared with stone formation rates in the preceding 3 years while on thiazide therapy [7].

Role in Distal Renal Tubular Acidosis (RTA)

Distal renal tubular acidosis results from a failure of distal renal tubular cells to acidify the urine in the face of an acid load, resulting in impairment of acid-base balance and ultimately metabolic acidosis. Secondary hypokalemia, hypercalciuria, and hypocitraturia ensue, leading to intractable calcium nephrolithiasis and nephrocalcinosis [10, 21]. Stone composition is typically calcium phosphate and less commonly calcium oxalate or mixed calcium oxalate and calcium phosphate.

Preminger and coworkers investigated the role of potassium citrate therapy in prevention of recurrent stone formation in nine patients with incomplete distal RTA [10]. Over a mean treatment duration of 34 months, all patients demonstrated complete cessation of new stone formation. Changes in urine biochemistry with treatment included significant increases in pH, potassium, and citrate levels and a significant decrease in calcium excretion. Correspondingly, a significant decrease in the relative saturation ratio (RSR) of calcium oxalate was observed, while that of brushite and sodium urate remained unchanged. The unchanged RSR for brushite despite an increase in urinary pH was thought to be due to the hypocalciuric effect of potassium citrate, which likely negated the effect of increased phosphate dissociation [10]. Other studies have similarly demonstrated high complete remission rates and reduced individual stone formation rates associated with potassium citrate therapy in the setting of distal RTA, but these involved heterogeneous patient populations [16, 22].

Role in Bone Mineral Density Preservation Among Calcium Stone Formers

Calcium nephrolithiasis has been associated with loss of bone mineral density (BMD) and an increased risk of osteoporotic fractures [23, 24]. Loss of bone mineral density has been identified in both hypercalciuric and normocalciuric stone formers, although the risk is higher among hypercalciuric stone formers [25]. The decrease in bone density among stone formers has been reported in those with idiopathic hypercalciuria and with medullary sponge kidney but has not been studied in those with distal RTA [25]. The underlying pathophysiologic mechanism has not been clarified.

RCTs in postmenopausal women with osteopenia have yielded conflicting results regarding the effects of potassium citrate treatment on bone mineral density. Jehle and associates compared the effect of 12 months of treatment with potassium citrate (30 mEq/day) versus potassium chloride (30 mEq/day) on BMD and found that the fractional increases in BMD measured in the lumbar spine, femoral neck, and total hip were significantly higher for the potassium citrate group compared to the potassium chloride group [26]. In contrast, McDonald and colleagues found no significant difference in spinal BMD loss in postmenopausal women among those who received placebo, low-dose potassium citrate (18.5 mEq/day), high-dose potassium citrate (55.5 mEq/day), or additional fruit and vegetable intake (estimated 18.5 mEq alkali equivalent) [27]. In a retrospective, uncontrolled study of 21 hypocitraturic stone formers treated solely with potassium citrate who underwent BMD testing before and after treatment, Pak and associates observed an overall 3.1 %

increase in lumbar spine BMD and a 3.8 % increase in Z-score (deviation of BMD compared to mean BMD of age- and gender-matched controls) over a mean treatment duration of 44 months (range 11–120 months) [28]. In a prospective, uncontrolled study, Vescini and colleagues studied BMD changes in 109 patients with idiopathic recurrent calcium oxalate nephrolithiasis who were treated with potassium citrate over a 2-year period of time [29]. Compared to baseline, mean BMD at the end of treatment increased by 0.04 g/cm^2 ($p=0.0001$) and mean T-score (deviation of BMD from mean BMD of healthy, young, adult controls) increased by 0.53 ($p=0.0001$). These trends held true both for the overall cohort and for individual subgroups of men, premenopausal women, and postmenopausal women [29].

Bone demineralization is also a feature of medullary sponge kidney (MSK), a disease entity estimated to be present in 3–5 % of recurrent stone formers, and characterized by recurrent calcium stone formation, osteopathy, kidney malformation, tubular functional abnormalities such as incomplete distal RTA, hypocitraturia, impaired renal concentrating ability, hypercalciuria, and cystic abnormalities of the ducts of Bellini [9]. Fabris and coworkers retrospectively compared 65 patients with MSK treated with potassium citrate therapy with 10 patients with the disorder who declined therapy. Bone densitometry data were available for 75 % of patients in the treatment group (49/65) and 100 % of patients in the control group. During a mean treatment duration of 78 months (range 12–96 months), lumbar spine T- and Z-scores, as well as total hip Z-scores, significantly improved from baseline in the treated group, while an insignificant trend toward further demineralization was observed in the control group [9]. Notably, the baseline BMD profile among all these MSK patients was consistent with osteopenia/osteoporosis [9].

Given these and other data linking bone disease and nephrolithiasis, along with proven beneficial effects of medical therapy for the treatment of both conditions, some authors have suggested that potassium citrate with or without hydrochlorothiazide constitutes a superior therapeutic regimen to conservative dietary therapy alone among patients with kidney stones [25]. Further studies including placebo-controlled RCTs will be invaluable in further defining the role of these therapies for prevention of both bone loss and stone recurrence.

Role in Preventing Growth or Recurrence of Calcium Stones After Shock Wave Lithotripsy

Soygur and colleagues treated 110 patients with lower pole renal calculi with shock wave lithotripsy (SWL) and, at 4 weeks posttreatment, randomized those rendered stone-free ($n=56$) and those left with <5-mm residual fragments ($n=34$) into two subgroups, one given potassium citrate (60 mEq/day) and the other no additional treatment. All patients had a history of calcium oxalate nephrolithiasis. At 12 months follow-up, none of the stone-free patients treated with potassium citrate (0 of 28) versus 28.5 % (8 of 28) of those in the control group demonstrated new stone growth ($p<0.05$) [30]. In the patients left with residual fragments, complete remission occurred in 45.5 % (8 of 18) of the potassium-citrate-treated group as compared to 12.5 % (2 of 16) of the control group ($p<0.05$). Growth arrest occurred in 54.5 % (10 of 18) in the potassium citrate group, while stone regrowth occurred in 62.5 % (10 of 16) in the control group. A similar randomized trial in calcium stone-forming children revealed that among those who were stone-free after SWL, the stone recurrence rate in the group treated with 1 mEq/kg/day potassium citrate for 12 months was significantly less than that in untreated controls (7.6 versus 34.6 %, respectively, $p<0.05$) [8]. Among children who had <5-mm residual fragments 4 weeks after SWL, the stone regrowth and recurrence rate in those treated with 1 mEq/kg/day potassium citrate for 12 months was significantly lower than in untreated controls (18.1 versus 72.7 %, $p<0.05$). Mean overall follow-up in this study was 24.4 months (range, 12–36.6 months) [8]. Combined, these studies suggest that potassium citrate administered as adjuvant therapy after SWL in patients with calcium stones may improve outcomes with regard to disease recurrence or progression.

Role in Counteracting Microgravity-Induced Kidney Stone Risk

Weightless environments during space travel cause a potential threat to the health of astronauts as a result of broad-ranging physiologic derangements including cardiovascular deconditioning, bone loss, muscle atrophy, and kidney stone formation [31]. A total of 14 stone episodes have been documented in 12 United States astronauts during space missions, 5 of which presumably occurred in-flight. Indeed, an in-flight stone episode is known to have nearly caused a mission abortion due to intractable symptoms in one astronaut, but spontaneous passage occurred just before an urgent deorbit was initiated [31]. Studies of urine composition during and just after short- and long-term missions, as well as during Earth bed-rest studies, have revealed that the most common alteration in urine composition that predisposes to an increased stone risk is an increase in calcium and phosphate excretion due to enhanced bone resorption [32].

Recently, placebo-controlled RCTs investigating the role of potassium citrate therapy in counteracting the increased stone risk associated with immobilization or space flight have been completed [11, 32]. Zerwekh and associates evaluated the effect of potassium magnesium citrate (KMgCit) therapy, containing 42 mEq potassium, 21 mEq magnesium, and 63 mEq citrate/day, versus placebo on the relative saturation ratio (RSR) of urine with respect to calcium oxalate, brushite, and undissociated uric acid. Study subjects were normal volunteers restricted to 5 weeks of bed rest, a valid Earth-based model to assess the effects of microgravity on the musculoskeletal system [32]. Relative to placebo, KMgCit therapy was found to decrease the urine RSR of calcium oxalate and undissociated uric acid but not brushite, despite a significant increase urinary pH. Part of the effect of KMgCit on the RSR of calcium oxalate was thought to be due to an increase in magnesium excretion, which binds oxalate in the urine, thereby preventing calcium oxalate crystallization [32]. The authors concluded that KMgCit, in combination with exercise or bisphosphonate therapy, could be an effective countermeasure to microgravity-induced renal stone risk [32].

Whitson and associates investigated the effects of potassium citrate (KCit) on 24-h urinary stone risk profiles of crew members who undertook missions to the Mir space station and International Space Station (ISS) [11] by randomizing 18 ISS cosmonauts to potassium citrate (KCit) 20 mEq/day ($n=12$) or to placebo ($n=6$). An additional 12 NASA-Mir crew members who did not ingest medication but also collected 24-h urine specimens served as additional no-treatment controls. No significant change from preflight baseline to after space flight was measured with regard to the urine RSR of calcium oxalate in the potassium citrate group. In contrast, the control group demonstrated higher-than-baseline calcium oxalate RSR values throughout each flight and postflight phase, although this difference was significant only on day 0 after landing ($p=0.006$). RSR for uric acid was also significantly lower for the KCit group compared to controls ($p=0.005$). RSR for brushite and sodium urate was not significantly altered by KCit treatment. The authors concluded that KCit supplementation decreased the risk of calcium oxalate renal stone formation during and after space flight [11].

Alkali Citrate Therapy for Uric Acid Stones

Pure uric acids stones comprise 5–10 % of renal calculi in Western countries, while uric-acid-related stone disease may be present in up to 40 % of cases [33, 34]. Acidic urine, rather than hyperuricosuria, is the primary pathophysiologic process that leads to precipitation of uric acid crystals in the urine [34]. Uric acid is a weak acid with two dissociation constants (pK_{a1} and pK_{a2}) of 5.3 and >10, respectively. At pH levels below $pKa1$, uric acid is present in its sparingly soluble, undissociated form, which can promote crystallization of uric acid or calcium stones through heterogeneous nucleation. The source of uric acid in the urine is excretion of the end products of purine metabolism; humans and Dalmatian dogs lack uricase, an enzyme that further metabolizes uric acid to allantoin, and are thus the only known mammals prone to uric acid stone formation [35]. Low urine pH has been epidemiologically linked to obesity, type II diabetes, and the metabolic syndrome and is also present in those with gouty diathesis, chronic diarrheal syndromes, and excessive consumers of meat-containing, high acid ash diets, suggesting that these patient subgroups may be most prone to uric acid stone formation [6, 34].

In a retrospective study, Pak and colleagues evaluated the effect of potassium citrate therapy (30–80 mEq/day) in 18 patients with pure uric acid ($n=6$) or mixed uric acid + calcium ($n=12$) stones [6]. Among this group, 11 of 18 patients took potassium citrate alone, while 7 patients took potassium citrate along with allopurinol or thiazide. The mean (± SD) duration of treatment was 2.8 ± 1.3 years. Compared to the 3 years prior to initiation of potassium citrate (when all patients experienced recurrent stones), complete stone remission occurred in 94.4 % of patients (17 of 18) after initiating potassium citrate therapy. Overall stone formation rate decreased from 1.2 ± 1.7 stones/patient/year to 0.1 ± 0.04 stones/patient/year ($p<0.001$). Individual stone formation decreased in 100 % of patients. Additionally, urinary volume, pH, potassium, and citrate levels significantly increased, while urinary calcium and oxalate did not significantly change, and the urine RSR of calcium oxalate significantly decreased during potassium citrate therapy [6]. Furthermore, a subset of five patients previously documented to have pure uric acid calculi and initially treated with other alkali agents (sodium citrate; sodium bicarbonate; a mixture of sodium bicarbonate, sodium citrate, and citric acid; and a mixture of sodium bicarbonate and potassium bicarbonate) developed recurrent calcium stones on these therapies. Initiation of potassium citrate in this group (duration 1–3.5 years) resulted in complete remission in all of them [6]. The authors concluded that potassium citrate was the ideal alkali therapy for uric acid nephrolithiasis occurring alone or in combination with calcium nephrolithiasis [6].

A related study by Trinchieri and coworkers in eight patients with uric acid calculi ≤15 mm in size demonstrated that an alkali mixture of potassium citrate (40 mEq) and potassium bicarbonate (20 mEq) daily was effective in completely dissolving stones in 62.5 % of patients (6 of 8), with up to 6 months of treatment. Partial stone dissolution occurred in the remainder [36]. In situations in which stone dissolution is nonurgent, some authors have proposed intermittent alkali therapy (once daily or thrice weekly), to avoid secondary deleterious effects of continuous base administration, such as calcium phosphate shell formation, transient systemic alkalosis, and gastrointestinal side effects [37].

The role of potassium citrate for the management of uric acid calculi refractory to primary treatment was investigated by Moran and associates [38]. Primary therapy included medical therapy or urgent endourologic intervention. Among

11 patients referred for secondary management, 7 of 11 patients (64 %) reported a history of antecedent medical therapy, but all were either noncompliant or only sporadically complaint due to intolerance. Additional therapies then included ureteroscopy, shock wave lithotripsy, or nephrostomy tube insertion. Potassium citrate, titrated to maintain urine pH between 6.0 and 6.5, was administered as salvage therapy in all patients. Complete dissolution of their stones occurred in 8 of 11 patients (73 %) on potassium citrate, and none of these patients required further endourologic intervention. Among the three patients who failed, two had impacted stones and the third was suspected to be noncompliant with therapy, as evidenced by persistently acidic urine on follow-up clinical evaluations [38].

Role of Dietary Citrate as an Alternative to Alkali Citrate Pharmacotherapy

Despite the evidence for efficacy of alkali citrate pharmacotherapy in the prevention of recurrence and progression of calcium and uric acid stones, a number of patients do not comply with long-term treatment for reasons that include high cost, cumbersome dosing regimens, and gastrointestinal intolerance [17–19, 39]. For these reasons, investigators have explored the use of dietary citrate therapy as a substitute for oral alkali citrate therapy. Citrus juices are a known, rich source of dietary citrate. The first clinical study on the role of dietary citrate in reducing the risk of stone formation was performed by Wabner and associates in 1993 [40]. In this study, 11 subjects, including 8 healthy volunteers with no history of nephrolithiasis and 3 patients with documented hypocitraturic nephrolithiasis, completed a three-phase metabolic study in which they received placebo, 1.2 l of orange juice (containing 60 mEq potassium and 190 mEq citrate) per day with meals, or potassium citrate (60 mEq/day) with meals. Orange juice ingestion resulted in an increase in 24-h urine pH (from a baseline of 5.71–6.75) and an increase in citrate excretion (from 571 to 944 mg/day)—treatment effects that were equivalent to those observed during the potassium citrate phase. Orange juice ingestion additionally increased urinary oxalate excretion but did not alter urinary calcium excretion, while potassium citrate decreased calcium excretion without altering urinary oxalate excretion [40].

In a related study, Seltzer and coworkers explored the use of lemonade as a citrate substitute in 12 patients with documented hypocitraturic calcium nephrolithiasis who were noncompliant with or intolerant of pharmacologic citrate therapy [41]. All patients were counseled on standard dietary recommendations including adequate fluid intake to ensure a urine volume of 2 l/day and salt and protein restriction. No other dietary intervention besides the addition of 2 l of reconstituted lemonade (containing 84 mEq citric acid) was instituted. After 1 week of lemonade therapy, significant increases in urinary citrate excretion (from 142 to 346 mg/day, $p<0.001$) and insignificant decreases in urinary calcium (from 131 to 92 mg/day) and urinary oxalate (from 53 to 42 mg/day) were observed. Lemonade therapy was well tolerated, with only two patients complaining of mild indigestion, which did not result in cessation of treatment [41].

Following these early, uncontrolled studies that suggested a probable benefit of dietary citrate in the reduction of stone-forming risk factors, several subsequent studies have investigated the effects of a variety of sources of dietary citrate on urine lithogenicity in stone formers [42–45] and non-stone formers [46–48]. One prospective, randomized metabolic study compared the effects of orange juice versus lemonade on the urinary profile of a mixed population of stone formers and non-stone formers [49]. Additionally, several studies have quantified the citrate and alkali levels in a variety of juices, sports drinks, and commercially available beverages [50–52].

Among the studies in stone formers, two were prospective, randomized metabolic studies [43, 45]. Koff and associates conducted a prospective, randomized, crossover study in 21 recurrent stone formers, 54 % of whom (11 of 21) had baseline hypocitraturia, comparing the effects of potassium citrate (60 mEq daily) and lemonade therapy (ReaLemon, 63 mEq citrate equivalent daily). Treatment duration per phase was 5 days, and the minimum washout period between phases was 2 weeks. During the lemonade phase, 24-h urine pH and urinary citrate excretion did not significantly change from baseline (pH increased from 5.51 to 5.63 and citrate decreased from 476 to 446 mg/day, *p*-value nonsignificant for each). In contrast, potassium citrate therapy resulted in significant increases in urine pH (5.51–5.89, $p=0.001$) and in citrate excretion (476–583 mg/day, $p=0.0015$) [43].

Aras and coworkers conducted a prospective, randomized, three-way trial in 30 patients with hypocitraturic calcium nephrolithiasis comparing the effects of 3 months of potassium citrate (60 mEq/day), fresh lemon juice (60 mEq/day citrate equivalent), or dietary restriction (3 l/day water, 1.2 g/day calcium, 5 g/day sodium chloride, and 1 g/kg/day protein) on urinary lithogenic risk factors [45]. Patients in the potassium citrate and lemon juice arms followed identical dietary recommendations as in the control arm. Compared to baseline levels, urinary citrate excretion in the lemon juice arm increased from 123 to 303 mg/day ($p=0.003$), in the potassium citrate arm from 86 to 324 mg/day ($p=0.001$), and in the dietary restriction arm from 103 to 187 mg/day ($p=0.001$). A significant increase in urine pH occurred in the potassium citrate group (5.9–6.5, $p=0.04$), but not the lemon juice (5.8–6.0, $p=0.65$) or diet-only arm (5.7–5.8, $p=0.72$). Urinary calcium and oxalate levels did not significantly change from baseline in any group ($p > 0.05$ for each), while urine volume increased from baseline in all three groups ($p < 0.05$ for each). The increase in urinary citrate excretion but not pH during lemon juice therapy was thought to be secondary to excretion of unmetabolized citrate without the co-delivery of alkali, given the acidic pH of lemon juice [45]. However, given excellent tolerance and low cost of fresh lemon juice, the authors felt that along with standard dietary measures, lemon juice could be recommended as an acceptable treatment alternative in patients with severe hypocitraturia [45].

In a prospective, randomized, crossover short-term metabolic study by Odvina and colleagues, 1 week of orange juice consumption (100 mEq citrate and 42 mEq potassium/day) in comparison to 1 week of lemonade therapy (100 mEq citrate/day) or control (400 ml distilled water/day) resulted in a significant increase in urine pH (+0.6 units in the orange juice phase compared with lemonade and control, $p < 0.05$ for each), an increase in urinary citrate (+367 mg/day compared with lemonade and +433 mg/day compared with control, $p < 0.05$ for each), and an increase in urinary oxalate (+5 mg/day compared with lemonade and +4 mg/day compared with control, ANOVA $p < 0.005$). However, RSR of calcium oxalate during the orange juice phase did not significantly change compared to lemonade or control (ANOVA $p = 0.06$). In addition, calculated undissociated uric acid was lowest during the orange juice phase (77 mg/day during orange juice, compared with 181 mg/day during lemonade and 184 mg/day during control; ANOVA $p < 0.0001$). The authors concluded that orange juice consumption resulted in greater alkalinizing and citraturic effects than lemonade and could result in biochemical modification of stone risk factors [49].

Only one long-term retrospective study has evaluated the role of dietary citrate therapy on actual stone formation [42]. Kang and coworkers compared outcomes of 11 patients with hypocitraturia treated with lemonade therapy for a mean of 44 months with 11 age- and sex-matched controls treated with potassium citrate therapy for a mean of 42.5 months. In the lemonade group, 10 of 11 patients demonstrated an increase in urinary citrate excretion averaging +383 mg/day ($p < 0.05$), while all patients in the potassium citrate group showed increase in urinary citrate, with a mean of +482 mg/day ($p < 0.0001$). In the lemonade group, stone burden decreased from 37.2 mm^2 pretreatment to 30.4 mm^2 posttreatment ($p > 0.05$), and pre- and posttreatment new stone formation decreased from 1.0 to 0.13 stones/patient/year ($p > 0.05$). The authors concluded that lemonade therapy was acceptable second-line therapy after potassium citrate, based on its pronounced citraturic effect [42].

Short-term metabolic studies in non-stone formers using alternative sources of dietary citrate demonstrated citraturic effects associated with grapefruit juice consumption [46, 47] and Performance (Shaklee Corp., Pleasanton, CA, USA) sports drink [48] although increased urinary citrate did not always translate into reduced urinary saturation of calcium stone-forming salts based on other non-favorable effects on urinary stone risk factors.

Investigators have determined the citrate content of a variety of juices, including fresh tomato juice (82.4 mmol/l citrate) and grapefruit juice (64.7 mmol/l citrate), which have higher citrate levels than lemon juice (38–48 mmol/l), orange juice (36–47 mmol/l), or reconstituted lemonade (39 mmol/l) [50, 51]. In addition, several commonly consumed diet sodas are known to contain an amount of citrate equal to or greater than that of a lemonade beverage commonly used to treat hypocitraturic calcium nephrolithiasis [52]. However, citrate content alone does not determine the citraturic response to fruit juices, and the form of citrate, whether potassium citrate or citric acid, and consequently the amount of alkali delivered, may be the determining factor in promoting a citraturic response. Additionally, other constituents of the juice may contribute positively or negatively to the stone-forming risk of a fruit juice.

Based on the conflicting data from the aforementioned studies, it is clear that additional prospective, randomized studies in well-selected patient populations, evaluating the effects of different sources of dietary citrate on both the urinary lithogenic risk as well as stone formation and recurrence rates, are needed so as to better define the clinical role of these therapies as alternatives to potassium citrate.

Conclusion

Calcium and uric acid stones comprise 85–90 % of all kidney stones encountered in common clinical practice. In addition to causing significant patient morbidity due to stone-related symptoms, current evidence suggests that stone disease may be associated with other conditions such as metabolic syndrome and bone disease via presently unknown mechanisms. A review of the literature to date on alkali citrate therapy for the treatment and/or prophylaxis of calcium nephrolithiasis, nephrolithiasis-associated bone disease, and uric acid nephrolithiasis suggests that it is perhaps the single most important therapy for the treatment of nephrolithiasis in a wide range of clinical settings and of nephrolithiasis-associated conditions. Further randomized studies, including investigation of its potential role in the primary prevention of stone disease, will be needed to help more completely define its role in the management of calcium and uric acid stones. Additionally, further studies on dietary citrate therapies will be needed to better define their role as potential alternatives to potassium citrate in the management of calcium and uric acid nephrolithiasis.

References

1. Greenwald I. The effect of the administration of calcium salts and sodium phosphate upon the calcium and phosphorus metabolism of thyroparathroidectomized dogs, with a consideration of the nature of the calcium compounds of blood and their relation to the pathogenesis of tetany. J Biol Chem. 1926;67:1–28.
2. Hastings AB, McLean FC, Eichelberger L, Hall JL, Da Costa E. The ionization of calcium, magnesium, and strontium citrates. J Biol Chem. 1934;107:351–70.
3. Fleisch H. Inhibitors and promoters of stone formation. Kidney Int. 1978;13:361–71.
4. Elliot JS, Ribeiro ME. The urinary excretion of citric, hippuric, and lactic acid in normal adults and in patients with calcium oxalate urinary calculus disease. Invest Urol. 1972;10:102–6.
5. Pak CY, Fuller C. Idiopathic hypocitraturic calcium-oxalate nephrolithiasis successfully treated with potassium citrate. Ann Intern Med. 1986;104:33–7.
6. Pak CY, Sakhaee K, Fuller C. Successful management of uric acid nephrolithiasis with potassium citrate. Kidney Int. 1986;30:422–8.
7. Pak CY, Peterson R, Sakhaee K, Fuller C, Preminger G, Reisch J. Correction of hypocitraturia and prevention of stone formation by combined thiazide and potassium citrate therapy in thiazide-unresponsive hypercalciuric nephrolithiasis. Am J Med. 1985;79: 284–8.
8. Sarica K, Erturhan S, Yurtseven C, Yagci F. Effect of potassium citrate therapy on stone recurrence and regrowth after extracorporeal shockwave lithotripsy in children. J Endourol. 2006;20:875–9.
9. Fabris A, Bernich P, Abaterusso C, et al. Bone disease in medullary sponge kidney and effect of potassium citrate treatment. Clin J Am Soc Nephrol. 2009;4:1974–9.
10. Preminger GM, Sakhaee K, Skurla C, Pak CY. Prevention of recurrent calcium stone formation with potassium citrate therapy in patients with distal renal tubular acidosis. J Urol. 1985;134:20–3.
11. Whitson PA, Pietrzyk RA, Jones JA, Nelman-Gonzalez M, Hudson EK, Sams CF. Effect of potassium citrate therapy on the risk of renal stone formation during spaceflight. J Urol. 2009;182:2490–6.
12. Nicar MJ, Hill K, Pak CY. Inhibition by citrate of spontaneous precipitation of calcium oxalate in vitro. J Bone Miner Res. 1987;2: 215–20.
13. Meyer JL, Smith LH. Growth of calcium oxalate crystals. II. Inhibition by natural urinary crystal growth inhibitors. Invest Urol. 1975;13:36–9.
14. Meyer JL, Thomas Jr WC. Trace metal-citric acid complexes as inhibitors of calcification and crystal growth. I. Effects of Fe(III), Cr(III) and Al(III) complexes on calcium phosphate crystal growth. J Urol. 1982;128:1372–5.
15. Meyer JL, Thomas Jr WC. Trace metal-citric acid complexes as inhibitors of calcification and crystal growth. II. Effects of Fe(III), Cr(III) and Al(III) complexes on calcium oxalate crystal growth. J Urol. 1982;128:1376–8.
16. Pak CY, Fuller C, Sakhaee K, Preminger GM, Britton F. Long-term treatment of calcium nephrolithiasis with potassium citrate. J Urol. 1985;134:11–9.
17. Barcelo P, Wuhl O, Servitge E, Rousaud A, Pak CY. Randomized double-blind study of potassium citrate in idiopathic hypocitraturic calcium nephrolithiasis. J Urol. 1993;150:1761–4.
18. Ettinger B, Pak CY, Citron JT, Thomas C, Adams-Huet B, Vangessel A. Potassium-magnesium citrate is an effective prophylaxis against recurrent calcium oxalate nephrolithiasis. J Urol. 1997;158: 2069–73.
19. Hofbauer J, Hobarth K, Szabo N, Marberger M. Alkali citrate prophylaxis in idiopathic recurrent calcium oxalate urolithiasis – a prospective randomized study. Br J Urol. 1994;73:362–5.
20. Pearle MS, Roehrborn CG, Pak CY. Meta-analysis of randomized trials for medical prevention of calcium oxalate nephrolithiasis. J Endourol. 1999;13:679–85.
21. Konnak JW, Kogan BA, Lau K. Renal calculi associated with incomplete distal renal tubular acidosis. J Urol. 1982;128:900–2.
22. Pak CY, Sakhaee K, Fuller CJ. Physiological and physiochemical correction and prevention of calcium stone formation by potassium citrate therapy. Trans Assoc Am Physicians. 1983;96: 294–305.
23. Lauderdale DS, Thisted RA, Wen M, Favus MJ. Bone mineral density and fracture among prevalent kidney stone cases in the Third National Health and Nutrition Examination Survey. J Bone Miner Res. 2001;16:1893–8.
24. Melton 3rd LJ, Crowson CS, Khosla S, Wilson DM, O'Fallon WM. Fracture risk among patients with urolithiasis: a population-based cohort study. Kidney Int. 1998;53:459–64.
25. Sakhaee K, Maalouf NM, Kumar R, Pasch A, Moe OW. Nephrolithiasis-associated bone disease: pathogenesis and treatment options. Kidney Int. 2011;79:393–403.
26. Jehle S, Zanetti A, Muser J, Hulter HN, Krapf R. Partial neutralization of the acidogenic Western diet with potassium citrate increases bone mass in postmenopausal women with osteopenia. J Am Soc Nephrol. 2006;17:3213–22.
27. Macdonald HM, Black AJ, Aucott L, et al. Effect of potassium citrate supplementation or increased fruit and vegetable intake on bone metabolism in healthy postmenopausal women: a randomized controlled trial. Am J Clin Nutr. 2008;88:465–74.
28. Pak CY, Peterson RD, Poindexter J. Prevention of spinal bone loss by potassium citrate in cases of calcium urolithiasis. J Urol. 2002;168:31–4.
29. Vescini F, Buffa A, La Manna G, et al. Long-term potassium citrate therapy and bone mineral density in idiopathic calcium stone formers. J Endocrinol Invest. 2005;28:218–22.
30. Soygur T, Akbay A, Kupeli S. Effect of potassium citrate therapy on stone recurrence and residual fragments after shockwave lithotripsy in lower caliceal calcium oxalate urolithiasis: a randomized controlled trial. J Endourol. 2002;16:149–52.
31. Pietrzyk RA, Jones JA, Sams CF, Whitson PA. Renal stone formation among astronauts. Aviat Space Environ Med. 2007;78:A9–13.
32. Zerwekh JE, Odvina CV, Wuermser LA, Pak CY. Reduction of renal stone risk by potassium-magnesium citrate during 5 weeks of bed rest. J Urol. 2007;177:2179–84.
33. Low RK, Stoller ML. Uric acid-related nephrolithiasis. Urol Clin North Am. 1997;24:135–48.
34. Kenny JE, Goldfarb DS. Update on the pathophysiology and management of uric acid renal stones. Curr Rheumatol Rep. 2010;12:125–9.
35. Shekarriz B, Stoller ML. Uric acid nephrolithiasis: current concepts and controversies. J Urol. 2002;168:1307–14.
36. Trinchieri A, Esposito N, Castelnuovo C. Dissolution of radiolucent renal stones by oral alkalinization with potassium citrate/ potassium bicarbonate. Arch Ital Urol Androl. 2009;81:188–91.
37. Rodman JS. Intermittent versus continuous alkaline therapy for uric acid stones and ureteral stones of uncertain composition. Urology. 2002;60:378–82.
38. Moran ME, Abrahams HM, Burday DE, Greene TD. Utility of oral dissolution therapy in the management of referred patients with secondarily treated uric acid stones. Urology. 2002;59:206–10.
39. Tracy CR, Pearle MS. Update on the medical management of stone disease. Curr Opin Urol. 2009;19:200–4.
40. Wabner CL, Pak CY. Effect of orange juice consumption on urinary stone risk factors. J Urol. 1993;149:1405–8.
41. Seltzer MA, Low RK, McDonald M, Shami GS, Stoller ML. Dietary manipulation with lemonade to treat hypocitraturic calcium nephrolithiasis. J Urol. 1996;156:907–9.

42. Kang DE, Sur RL, Haleblian GE, Fitzsimons NJ, Borawski KM, Preminger GM. Long-term lemonade based dietary manipulation in patients with hypocitraturic nephrolithiasis. J Urol. 2007;177:1358–62; discussion 1362; quiz 1591.
43. Koff SG, Paquette EL, Cullen J, Gancarczyk KK, Tucciarone PR, Schenkman NS. Comparison between lemonade and potassium citrate and impact on urine pH and 24-hour urine parameters in patients with kidney stone formation. Urology. 2007;69:1013–6.
44. Penniston KL, Steele TH, Nakada SY. Lemonade therapy increases urinary citrate and urine volumes in patients with recurrent calcium oxalate stone formation. Urology. 2007;70:856–60.
45. Aras B, Kalfazade N, Tugcu V, et al. Can lemon juice be an alternative to potassium citrate in the treatment of urinary calcium stones in patients with hypocitraturia? A prospective randomized study. Urol Res. 2008;36:313–7.
46. Goldfarb DS, Asplin JR. Effect of grapefruit juice on urinary lithogenicity. J Urol. 2001;166:263–7.
47. Trinchieri A, Lizzano R, Bernardini P, et al. Effect of acute load of grapefruit juice on urinary excretion of citrate and urinary risk factors for renal stone formation. Dig Liver Dis. 2002;34 Suppl 2: S160–3.
48. Goodman JW, Asplin JR, Goldfarb DS. Effect of two sports drinks on urinary lithogenicity. Urol Res. 2009;37:41–6.
49. Odvina CV. Comparative value of orange juice versus lemonade in reducing stone-forming risk. Clin J Am Soc Nephrol. 2006;1:1269–74.
50. Haleblian GE, Leitao VA, Pierre SA, et al. Assessment of citrate concentrations in citrus fruit-based juices and beverages: implications for management of hypocitraturic nephrolithiasis. J Endourol. 2008;22:1359–66.
51. Yilmaz E, Batislam E, Basar M, Tuglu D, Erguder I. Citrate levels in fresh tomato juice: a possible dietary alternative to traditional citrate supplementation in stone-forming patients. Urology. 2008;71:379–83; discussion 383–4.
52. Eisner BH, Asplin JR, Goldfarb DS, Ahmad A, Stoller ML. Citrate, malate and alkali content in commonly consumed diet sodas: implications for nephrolithiasis treatment. J Urol. 2010;183: 2419–23.

The Importance of Water and Other Fluids in the Prevention of Stone Recurrence

90

Tiziana Meschi, Antonio Nouvenne, and Loris Borghi

Abstract

The natural history of nephrolithiasis is characterized by a high recurrence rate making pharmacological and non-pharmacological secondary prevention measures necessary. Among these, dietary manipulations are of primary importance. Water therapy is one of the oldest therapeutic tools available: the increase in urinary flow reduces the concentration of urinary factors that promote stone formation without altering the effect of the inhibitors; it renders the urinary microenvironment less suitable for the formation and aggregation of crystals—and hence kidney stones—and prevents recurrences. Notwithstanding the widespread application and efficacy of this therapy, only one randomized controlled trial actually exists in literature. Except during acute episodes of renal colic, all patients suffering from stone disease should be prescribed a sufficient intake of water and other fluids to produce a urine volume of at least 2 L/24 h. Oligomineral water with a low NaCl content is preferable, associated to a diet with a high fruit and vegetable content, a low salt and protein intake, and a controlled calcium, fat, and carbohydrate intake.

Keywords

Nephrolithiasis • Kidney stones • Water therapy • Oligomineral water • Fluid intake • Stone recurrence • Prevention • Dietary manipulations • Urine volume

Everything comes from water! And everything is kept alive by water!

Goethe, Faust II, 1833

T. Meschi, M.D. • A. Nouvenne, M.D., Ph.D. (✉) • L. Borghi, M.D.
Department of Clinical and Experimental Medicine,
University of Parma,
Via A. Gramsci 14, Parma 43126, Italy
e-mail: tiziana.meschi@unipr.it; antonio.nouvenne@alice.it;
loris.borghi@unipr.it

J.J. Talati et al. (eds.), *Urolithiasis*,
DOI 10.1007/978-1-4471-4387-1_90, © Springer-Verlag London 2012

Introduction

The natural history of stone disease is characterized by a high recurrence rate. This is true both for the rare abnormalities such as primary hyperoxaluria and cystinuria, as well as for idiopathic calcium nephrolithiasis, which, as is well known, accounts for roughly 80 % of all cases of renal stone disease. It has, in fact, been documented that in idiopathic calcium nephrolithiasis, patients have a 50 % probability of having a second episode 5 years after an initial episode of renal colic [1, 2]. Obviously the high clinical and economic impact of such recurrences requires the implementation of pharmacological and non-pharmacological secondary prevention measures [3].

Among these, dietary manipulations are of fundamental importance as they have the power to modify the urinary stone risk factors involved in the crystallization process, both as promoters and inhibitors.

For calcium oxalate the risk factors are as follows: low urine volume (<2 L/day), hypercalciuria (>250 mg/day, 6.25 mmol), hyperoxaluria (>40 mg/day, 0.44 mmol), hyperuricosuria (>600 mg/day, 3.6 mmol), hypocitraturia (<320 mg/day, 1.7 mmol), and hypomagnesiuria (<50 mg/day, 2.1 mmol). For calcium phosphate, in addition to the aforementioned factors, hyperphosphaturia (>1,000 mg/day, 10.5 mmol) and urinary pH also acquires considerable importance because a pH>7 promotes the formation of stones predominantly composed of phosphates, while a pH between 6 and 7 associated with a urine volume <1 L/day can raise calcium phosphate supersaturation and leads to the formation of mixed calcium oxalate and calcium phosphate stones. Finally, for uric acid stone disease—with an incidence of 10–15 %—the decisive risk factors are hyperuricosuria and pH<5.5 [4].

Among the recommended dietary measures, as described later, hydration has a fundamental role. The role of water in kidney stone disease was already acknowledged in the writings of Hippocrates and Galen, and both during the classical era and the Renaissance, certain thermal water sources in the countries of the Mediterranean Sea basin were considered "magical" with healing properties for "disease of stone," otherwise known today as nephrolithiasis.

This chapter will deal with the role of water and other fluids in the prevention of stone recurrences, with particular reference to calcium and uric acid nephrolithiasis. We shall discuss the evidence existing in scientific literature as derived from (1) experimental pathophysiological studies, (2) epidemiological studies, and (3) clinical intervention studies. Finally, some handy hints and practical advice for stone-forming patients will be provided to heighten awareness and help increase compliance with the treatment.

Experimental and Pathological Studies

Using the Equil© computer program [5], it is possible to simulate the changes of the relative saturation for calcium oxalate, calcium phosphate, and uric acid when the urine volume increases from 0.5–3.0 L/day while keeping all the other urinary parameters constant. Such urine composition reflects that seen in a healthy subject on a Western-style diet. It may be seen that with diuresis below 1 L/day, even the urine of a normal subject reaches extremely high supersaturation levels, certainly high enough to promote spontaneous (heterogeneous or homogeneous) crystallization of the lithogenic salts. If, on the other hand, the volume is maintained over 2.5 L/day, the urine becomes undersaturated with calcium phosphate and uric acid (below 1) and only slightly supersaturated with calcium oxalate, making spontaneous crystallization impossible. Since, in the context of these physiological variations in diuresis, ion concentrations are largely dependent on urine volume, this example simulates very closely what actually happens when water intake is high. The increase in volume, moreover, does not change the activity of the inhibitory molecules naturally present in urine. We have demonstrated that in diluted urine the supersaturation value of calcium oxalate required to trigger crystallization is much greater compared with that in concentrated urine, while the aggregation capacity and quantity of crystals after an oxalate load are greatly reduced in diluted urine [6–8]. In addition to this, as highlighted in review from 2005 [9], all the "risk indices" proposed by various authors over the years assign an important role to urine volume. Last but not least, it has been demonstrated—in vitro as well as in experimental animals—that the load of water and the ensuing urine dilution have beneficial effects on the epithelium of the urinary tract. Increased activity and coordination of complex motor muscles was recorded. Moreover, there was a reduction in inflammatory substances, a reduction of bacterial adhesiveness, and an increased clearance of crystals [10].

Epidemiological Studies

It is well known that nephrolithiasis is more widespread in geographical areas with a hot/damp climate and that there is a seasonal variation of the onset of the disease correlated with environmental temperature. An increase in the incidence of stone disease has been observed in certain categories of people exposed to chronic dehydration such as soldiers posted to hot regions, steelwork welders, or marathon runners [11].

Extensive epidemiological studies have demonstrated, also in the general population, the protective effect of high urine volume on the lithogenic risk. In 280,000 patients

(32 % men) followed up for an average period of 10 years, it was demonstrated that a volume of >2,500 mL/24 h reduced the risk by 29–39 % compared with that seen in subjects who had a 24-h volume of <1,400 mL [12–15].

Finally, both the Mediterranean and the DASH diets were associated with a reduction in lithogenic risk, also in relation to a higher urinary output compared with patients not following these diets [16, 17].

Clinical Studies

Although, since many years, patients with stone disease have been advised to increase their water intake, only one randomized controlled trial has studied water therapy as the sole form of treatment in first-episode stone formers. In that study it was demonstrated that in patients who had a stable urine volume above 2 L/day, there was a significant reduction in the rate of recurrences (12.1 % versus 27 %, $p = 0.008$) and increase in the interval to recurrences (3.23 years versus 2.09 years, $p = 0.016$) [18, 19]. In 1966, Frank and De Vries [20] conducted an intervention study in two Israeli villages. An educational program was launched for the population of one of the two villages in order to stimulate water intake, whereas the second village was not subjected to any kind of program. After 3 years, the incidence of stone disease in the village subjected to the educational program was one-third compared with that in the control village, given an average difference in 24-h urine volume of only 267 mL.

Other intervention studies suggest the appropriateness of water therapy, although the results are not perfectly comparable, either because the effect of a high water intake on stone recurrences was not the main objective of the particular study [21] or because the water therapy was combined with other measures (e.g., low salt, low protein, normal calcium diet) [22, 23] making it difficult to distinguish the net effect of water intake [24].

What Kind of Water?

Over the years, numerous studies have investigated the effects of different types of water on urinary stone risk factors and on various kinds of stone disease [24]. The results cannot really be generalized, and additionally it is difficult to compare such studies for a variety of reasons: (1) difficulty in classifying the various types of water, (2) geo-specific characteristics of the water and difficulty in calculating the effect of the various dissolved and/or trace ions, (3) different legislation and regulatory standards, and (4) lack of comparative studies.

Very often, in fact, the studies simply record the difference between tap water, mineral water, and spring water, or between hard and soft water without specifying in detail the composition of the waters and the hardness of the same. Mineral waters can be classified either on the basis of their dry residue at 180 °C (minimum, low, medium, and high mineral content) or on the basis of their ion composition (bicarbonate waters, sulfate waters, saltwater, sulfurous waters) or on the basis of their biological effects (diuretic waters, cathartic waters, waters with anti-inflammatory properties). In Italy, the legislation on mineral waters is extremely strict and all the characteristics are strictly certified and controlled by the Ministry of Health [25].

It is clear, therefore, that while there may be a general consensus advocating the administration of a bicarbonate water to a patient with uric acid kidney stones in order to alkalinize urine, it may be difficult to recommend which type of water should be consumed by a patient affected by calcium stone disease. For example, two waters with the same quantity of calcium may have different effects on the absorption of calcium and on calciuria due to a different concentration of other accompanying ions such as Na, Cl, or Mg. Although no strong evidence actually exists, the choice of an oligomineral, low NaCl content water seems to offer a good compromise. Lastly, there are no differences between still and sparkling water, although some authors suggest that patients used to drinking sparkling water are likely to consume a smaller volume because the carbon dioxide might "anesthetize" the nerve endings of the tongue and palate that mediate the sensation of thirst [25].

The Role of Other Drinks

While the role of water is now accepted, there are contrasting opinions in the literature regarding the role of hydration by other drinks. The majority of the studies conducted have, in fact, evaluated a surrogate endpoint (i.e., urinary stone risk factors), and data from studies with a long follow-up designed to verify the impact of other drinks on the onset or recurrence of stone disease are few [11, 14, 15, 19].

Generally speaking, there are drinks that exert a positive effect since they increase pH and/or citrate and/or urine volume, such as freshly squeezed oranges or lemons, juices made from the same fruits, green tea, and wine. Cranberry juice is particularly useful in cases of infected stone disease, also due to its acidifying properties. Beer has been found to have a protective effect in calcium stone disease, while it seems to increase the risk of uric acid stone disease due to the uricosuric effect caused by its high purine-guanosine content [26, 27].

Table 90.1 Useful advice for water therapy, obtaining a urine volume of at least 2 L/day

1. Drink two glasses of water in the morning when you get up and in the evening before you go to bed
2. Keep a bottle of water in all places where you spend your time (at work, in the car, in the living room, on your bedside cabinet, etc.) and drink some once an hour
3. Drink a glass of water before leaving the house and on returning home
4. Drink at least three glasses with every meal
5. Choose low mineral content water and avoid mineralized waters or tap water rich in chlorine
6. Choose still as opposed to sparkling water and drink it cool but not cold
7. Eat foods with high water content (melon, water melon, citrus fruits) and centrifuged/freshly squeezed juice
8. Involve your family in these habits
9. Collect 24-h urine at home once a month in order to check the results in order to measure the volume
10. Change your brand of water once a year

Tea and coffee, on the other hand, increase oxalate; although it has been documented that this effect is canceled out if milk is added, the calcium of which binds with the oxalate thereby reduces its absorption. Other drinks are prolithogenic and have a mechanism that has not been fully understood (grapefruit and apple juices, cola). In this context, it is important to mention soft drinks, given the quantities and frequency with which they are consumed. Recent studies have identified an increased risk of both calcium and uric acid stone disease correlated with the consumption of soft drinks—probably due to their content of fructose, sucrose, and phosphoric acid—and have documented a reduction in the risk of recurrences of approximately 10 % in patients who were instructed to avoid soft drinks [24].

Sport and energy drinks, the consumption of which is growing in Western countries, are another matter. Very few studies exist in the literature, and those that do are often contradictory and conducted with the aim of evaluating urinary stone risk factors: energy/sport drinks—particularly rich in sodium, carbohydrates, and caffeine—could increase the risk of stone disease, although further studies are required for definite conclusions [28–33].

Conclusion

Apart from patients whose water balance must be strictly controlled (cardiac, hepatic, and renal failure), therapy with water and other drinks should be prescribed and recommended to all patients affected by nephrolithiasis. Table 90.1 summarizes the ten golden rules for increasing the effectiveness of and compliance with the treatment.

Increased fluid consumption is, therefore, effective because (1) it lowers urinary concentrations of calcium, oxalate, and urate, thereby reducing supersaturation with calcium oxalate, calcium phosphate, and uric acid; (2) it increases urinary tolerance to an oxalate load; (3) it reduces urinary concentration of macromolecules without altering their inhibitory power; and (4) it increases the clearance of crystals and reduces their retention.

Summary

- Water therapy is a valid tool for prevention of stone recurrences; it is simple and well tolerated.
- It is useful to drink oligomineral water with a low NaCl content in order to obtain a urine volume of more than 2 L/day.
- The effect is reinforced by diet with a low salt and protein content, rich in fruit and vegetables, and with a controlled calcium, fat, and carbohydrate content.

Acknowledgement This work was supported by Fondazione per la Ricerca Scientifica Termale (FoRST) grants.

References

1. Goldfarb DS. Increasing prevalence of kidney stones in the United States. Kidney Int. 2003;63:1951–2.
2. Soucie JM, Thun MJ, Coates RJ, et al. Demographic and geographic variability of kidney stones in the United States. Kidney Int. 1994;46:893–9.
3. Clark JY, Thompson IM, Optenberg SA. Economic impact of urolithiasis in the United States. J Urol. 1995;154:2020–4.
4. Worcester EM, Coe FL. Clinical practice. Calcium kidney stones. N Engl J Med. 2010;363:954–63.
5. Werness PG, Brown CM, Smith LH, Finlayson B. Equil 2: a basic computer program for the calculation of urinary saturation. J Urol. 1985;134:1242–4.
6. Borghi L, Guerra A, Meschi T, et al. Relationship between supersaturation and calcium oxalate crystallization in normals and idiopathic calcium oxalate stone formers. Kidney Int. 1999;55:1041–50.
7. Guerra A, Meschi T, Allegri F, et al. Concentrated urine and diluted urine: the effects of citrate and magnesium on the crystallization of calcium oxalate induced in vitro by an oxalate load. Urol Res. 2006;34:359–64.
8. Guerra A, Allegri F, Meschi T, et al. Effects of urine dilution on quantity, size and aggregation of calcium oxalate crystals induced in vitro by an oxalate load. Clin Chem Lab Med. 2005;43:585–9.
9. Sutton RAL. The use of risk indices: do they predict recurrence? Urol Res. 2005;34:122–5.
10. Pak CY, Sakhaee K, Crowther C, et al. Evidence justifying a high fluid intake in treatment of nephrolithiasis. Ann Intern Med. 1980;93:36–9.
11. Borghi L, Meschi T, Schianchi T, et al. Urine volume: stone risk factor and preventive measure. Nephron. 1999;81:31–7.
12. Curhan GC, Willet WC, Rimm EB, et al. A prospective study of dietary calcium and other nutrients and the risk of symptomatic kidney stones. N Engl J Med. 1993;328:833–8.
13. Curhan GC, Willett WC, Knight EL, et al. Dietary factors and the risk of incident kidney stones in younger women: Nurses' Health Study II. Arch Intern Med. 2004;164:885–91.
14. Taylor EN, Stampfer MJ, Curhan GC. Dietary factors and the risk of incident kidney stones in men: new insights after 14 years of follow-up. J Am Soc Nephrol. 2004;15:3225–32.

15. Curhan GC, Willett WC, Speizer FE, et al. Beverage use and risk for kidney stones in women. Ann Intern Med. 1998;128:534–40.
16. Taylor EN, Fung TT, Curhan GC. DASH-style diet associates with reduced risk for kidney stones. J Am Soc Nephrol. 2009;20:2253–9.
17. Taylor EN, Stampfer MJ, Mount DB, et al. DASH-style diet and 24-hour urine composition. Clin J Am Soc Nephrol. 2010;5:2315–22.
18. Borghi L, Meschi T, Amato F, et al. Urinary volume, water and recurrences in idiopathic calcium nephrolithiasis: a 5-year randomized prospective study. J Urol. 1996;155:839–43.
19. Qiang W, Ke Z. Water for preventing urinary calculi. Cochrane Database Syst Rev. 2004;(3):CD004292.
20. Frank M, De Vries A. Prevention of urolithiasis. Education to adequate fluid intake in a new town situated in the Judean Desert Mountains. Arch Environ Health. 1966;13:625–30.
21. Sarica K, Inal Y, Erturhan S, et al. The effect of calcium channel blockers on stone regrowth and recurrence after shock wave lithotripsy. Urol Res. 2006;34:184–9.
22. Hiatt RA, Ettinger B, Caan B, et al. Randomized controlled trial of a low animal protein, high fiber diet in the prevention of recurrent calcium oxalate kidney stones. Am J Epidemiol. 1996;144:25–33.
23. Borghi L, Schianchi T, Meschi T, et al. Comparison of two diets for the prevention of recurrent stones in idiopathic hypercalciuria. N Engl J Med. 2002;346:77–84.
24. Fink HA, Akornor JW, Garimella PS, et al. Diet, fluid, or supplements for secondary prevention of nephrolithiasis: a systematic review and meta-analysis of randomized trials. Eur Urol. 2009;56:72–80.
25. Petraccia L, Liberati G, Masciullo SG, et al. Water, mineral waters and health. Clin Nutr. 2006;25:377–85.
26. Jeong BC, Kim BS, Kim JI, et al. Effects of green tea on urinary stone formation: an in vivo and in vitro study. J Endourol. 2006;20:356–61.
27. Johri N, Cooper B, Robertson W, et al. An update and practical guide to renal stone management. Nephron Clin Pract. 2010;116:159–71.
28. Taylor EN, Curhan GC. Fructose consumption and the risk of kidney stones. Kidney Int. 2008;73:207–12.
29. Asselman M, Verkoelen CF. Fructose intake as a risk factor for kidney stone disease. Kidney Int. 2008;73:139–40.
30. Choi HK, Curhan G. Soft drinks, fructose consumption, and the risk of gout in men: prospective cohort study. BMJ. 2008;336:309–12.
31. Choi HK, Willett W, Curhan G. Fructose-rich beverages and risk of gout in women. JAMA. 2010;304:2270–8.
32. Passman CM, Holmes RP, Knight J, et al. Effect of soda consumption on urinary stone risk parameters. J Endourol. 2009;23:347–50.
33. Goodman JW, Asplin JR, Goldfarb DS. Effect of two sports drinks on urinary lithogenicity. Urol Res. 2009;37:41–6.

Orthophosphates

91

Renata Caudarella

Abstract

Hypercalciuria is the commonest metabolic alteration found in patients with idiopathic calcium disease, and the absorptive type is the most prevalent. Therapies for hypercalciuria include thiazides, thiazide-like drugs, alone or together with potassium citrate, and bisphosphonates. In the past, orthophosphates appeared to be highly indicated for absorptive hypercalciuria treatment since they reduce serum 1,25-dihydroxyvitamin D levels, urinary calcium excretion, and, perhaps, bone resorption. Inorganic phosphate salts include acid potassium phosphate, neutral mixtures of acid and alkaline potassium phosphate, and neutral mixtures of sodium and potassium phosphate. Moreover, neutral potassium orthophosphates include compounds characterized by fast or slow release. The effect is most pronounced for neutral orthophosphates, which not only reduce calcium and increase pyrophosphate excretion but also induce greater urinary citrate excretion; inhibitory power in urine against the crystallization process thus results as increased. The hypocalciuric response to the drug is probably the result of the combined effects of reduced intestinal calcium absorption, increased renal tubular calcium reabsorption, and diminished bone resorption. Positive effects of orthophosphate therapy have been described in several papers, although most of them consisted of open non-randomized studies. There are only two double-blind studies with orthophosphate treatment; in the first, no differences were observed between treated and untreated patients, whereas in the second, a reduced rate of stone formation was observed.

Common side effects of orthophosphate therapy include diarrhea, abdominal cramps, nausea, and vomiting. According to the type of orthophosphate, other side effects have been reported. Furthermore, alkaline phosphates promote dissociation of urinary phosphate and increase brushite saturation. In conclusion, orthophosphates have been proposed as an alternative for treating patients with hypercalciuria, especially of the absorptive type, but there are insufficient studies, above all clinical randomized trials, to confirm their efficacy beyond any shadow of a doubt. Their usefulness may thus be limited to being a second choice for the treatment of selected patients. In accordance with these indications, no mention of orthophosphates is reported for hypercalciuria treatment in the most recent guidelines on urolithiasis.

R. Caudarella, M.D.
Department of Mineral Metabolism,
Fondazione Ettore Sansavini per la Ricerca Scientifica
(Health Science Foundation) ONLUS,
Corso Garibaldi, 11, Lugo, Ravenna 48022, Italy
e-mail: rcauderella@gvm-val.it; renata.caudarella@alice.it

J.J. Talati et al. (eds.), *Urolithiasis*,
DOI 10.1007/978-1-4471-4387-1_91, © Springer-Verlag London 2012

Keywords
Hypercalciuria therapy • Absorptive hypercalciuria • Orthophosphate • Acid orthophosphate • Neutral orthophosphate • Calcium urolithiasis • Intestinal calcium and phosphate absorption • Bone resorption • Renal tubular calcium reabsorption • 1,25-dihydroxyvitamin D_3

Introduction

Idiopathic calcium stone disease is a common event in clinical practice, and kidney stones have shown a progressive increase worldwide, with a prevalence ranging between 2 and 20% [1]. Kidney stone disease shows a high recurrence as its main trait, but the number of patients undergoing metabolic evaluation is very scarce, although metabolic evaluation allows the identifications of about 97% of metabolic risk factors for stone formation [2]. Selective medical treatment appears to be an important tool in clinical prophylaxis and treatment of renal stone disease; in fact, surgical treatment such as extracorporeal shock-wave lithotripsy does not treat the underlying cause of stones and thus does not induce a decrease of recurrence. About 40% of patients presenting a first episode of kidney stones show a recurrence within 3 years if adequate prophylactic and medical treatment are not established. The positive effects of medical treatment pointed out by several authors [2–6] have been further confirmed by Parks and Coe [7], who observed that patients who were actively treated showed a significant decrease in stone recurrence and urological procedure rates. Several risk factors may induce the formation of kidney stones, which are mainly composed of calcium oxalate or calcium phosphate; hypercalciuria is the commonest metabolic alteration found in patients with idiopathic calcium disease [8–11], and its percentage is different according to the type of hypercalciuria as well as to whether hypercalciuria occurs singly or combined with other metabolic alterations. Hypercalciuria may favor stone formation by increasing the urinary saturation of calcium oxalate and calcium phosphate as well as by reducing inhibitor activity in urine by binding negatively charged inhibitors and inactivating them [8, 10]. At the moment the diagnostic tests for evaluating hypercalciuria types (absorptive, renal, resorptive, hypercalciuria linked to phosphate renal tubular leak) are not considered cost-effective; but, very recently, Pak et al. have suggested a very simple method for absorptive hypercalciuria diagnosis based on the documentation of high 24-h urinary calcium excretion on both free and restricted diets [12]. Several studies have indicated that in most patients hypercalciuria is due to an inappropriately increased intestinal absorption and that absorptive hypercalciuria is the commonest type [8, 13, 14]. Absorptive hypercalciuria is characterized by normocalcemia alongside hypercalciuria, normal to low levels of parathyroid hormone (PTH), and normal to high serum concentrations of 1,25-dihydroxyvitamin D [15, 16]. An excessive bone loss due to increased cytokine levels may contribute to hypercalciuria pathogenesis [17]. In these patients bone loss seems to influence mainly trabecular bone [18]. The pathogenetic aspects of absorptive hypercalciuria are not yet completely understood, although some authors have found an increased plasma level of 1,25-dihydroxyvitamin D in a large number of these patients [14–16]. An increased number of vitamin D receptors and/or sensitivity to them have also been proposed [14]. Other authors have suggested that the main alteration in patients with absorptive hypercalciuria may be a primary phosphate renal tubular leak inducing an increase of 1,25-dihydroxyvitamin D production and thus hypercalciuria [19]. Lau et al. [20] have shown that phosphate infusion in rats increases calcium reabsorption in the distal convoluted tubule, and possibly in the terminal part of the nephron independently of PTH, plasma calcium concentration, and renal handling of sodium. The authors' data suggest that these effects may be mediated by an increase in tubular fluid and/or plasma phosphate concentration. The commonest therapies for the treatment of hypercalciuria include thiazides or thiazide-like (indapamide) drugs, alone or in association with potassium citrate. In the past, of the drugs used in hypercalciuria treatment, orthophosphates have appeared to be the most indicated for idiopathic absorptive hypercalciuria treatment, above all when hypophosphatemia is present. Orthophosphates have also been proposed for resorptive hypercalciuria treatment and other conditions associated with renal stone formation (primary hyperoxaluria, type I renal tubular acidosis, sarcoidosis, immobilization, carbonic anhydrase inhibitor-induced stones). Orthophosphates have been widely used for the treatment of idiopathic calcium stone formers [21–27] as they induce both a decrease in urinary calcium excretion [20–24] and an increase in inorganic pyrophosphates [22, 25], which are among the most powerful urinary inhibitors of calcium crystal formation and aggregation [21, 22, 25].

Mechanism of Action

Urinary calcium decrease may be induced by several mechanisms.

First, orthophosphate may reduce intestinal calcium absorption by means of physiochemical binding of calcium by phosphate in the intestinal tract and by a decrease in

1,25-dihydroxyvitamin D_3 synthesis. Some authors have proved that orthophosphate therapy lowers plasma 1,25-dihydroxyvitamin D_3 concentration in patients with hypercalciuria [19].

Second, orthophosphate induces an increase in plasma phosphate and a contemporary decrease in plasma calcium concentration, which induces PTH secretion [28]. In turn, the PTH increase induces both a decrease in glomerular filtration rate and an increase in tubular calcium reabsorption with a consequent decrease in urinary calcium excretion. Otherwise, orthophosphates could, through a plasma phosphate concentration increase, induce an inhibition of 1,25-dihydroxyvitamin D_3 synthesis, thus reducing intestinal calcium absorption. Lau and Eby [29] have shown that phosphate infusion in rats increases calcium reabsorption in the distal convoluted tubule, and possibly in the terminal part of the nephron independently of PTH, plasma calcium concentration, and renal handling of sodium. The authors' data suggest that these effects may be mediated by an increase in tubular fluid and/or plasma phosphate concentration.

Third, orthophosphates may contribute to reducing urinary calcium excretion by decreasing bone resorption [26, 30]. Inorganic phosphate salts include the following: acid potassium phosphate (KH_2PO_4), a neutral mixture of acid and alkaline potassium phosphate ($KH_2PO_4 + K_2HPO_4$), and a neutral (pH 7) mixture of sodium and potassium phosphate ($Na_2HPO_4 + KH_2PO_4$) [31].

Differential Absorption from Available Preparations

Moreover, neutral potassium orthophosphates include compounds characterized by a fast or slow release [32]. Slow-release neutral-K-phosphate composition includes a mixture of mono-dibasic phosphate salts of potassium and does not contain sodium; this phosphate composition, maintaining a urinary pH of 7.0, avoids the problems linked to acidic or alkaline phosphates. The positive changes observed in urine chemistry include a decrease in calcium urinary excretion together with an increase in phosphate, potassium, citrate, and pyrophosphate; moreover, a decrease was observed in calcium-oxalate urinary saturation, brushite spontaneous nucleation, and calcium-oxalate crystal agglomeration [32]. In the plasma, a decrease of 1,25-dihydroxyvitamin D_3, alkaline phosphatase, and procollagen concentration was observed. The restricted phosphate release limits the high phosphate concentration in bowel lumen observed with rapid-release orthophosphates. Table 91.1 summarizes the therapeutic effects of slow- and rapid-release orthophosphates. From a theoretical point of view, neutral phosphates seem to be safer than acid phosphates, which induce a greater production of fixed acid that in turn increase rather than decrease urinary calcium excretion [33, 34]. Nevertheless, there is no general agreement about the therapeutical response to this treatment [21–27, 33]. Several authors (Table 91.2) have shown positive effects for orthophosphate therapy, although most of these papers consisted of open non-randomized studies with patients having different types of stone disease with nonhomogeneous criteria used for their enrolment. Furthermore, the authors describe several aspects of orthophosphate therapy such as plasma and urinary laboratory modifications, side effects, remission rates, and modifications in stone formation rate (Table 91.3). These contrasting results seem to be explained by the paper of Lau et al. [31] from 1979 detailing randomized studies of patients with hypercalciuria to compare the acute and chronic effects of acid phosphate and neutral phosphate on the excretion of stone-forming salts.

Table 91.1 Therapeutic effects of orthophosphates

	Rapid-release orthophosphate	Slow-release neutral-K phosphate
Plasma $1,25(OH)_2D_3$	↓	↓
Total alkaline phosphatase	n/a	↓
Procollagen	n/a	↓
Urinary calcium excretion	↓	↓
Urinary phosphate excretion	↑	↑
Urinary pyrophosphate excretion	↑	↑
Urinary citrate excretion	↑	↑
CaOx urinary saturation	↓	↑
CaP urinary saturation	=/↑	n/a
Brushite spontaneous nucleation	n/a	↓
Crystalluria	↓	n/a
CaOx crystal agglomeration	n/a	↓

Dosage

One gram of acid phosphate contains 9 mEq of potassium and 23 mEq of sodium as the monobasic salt; 1 g of neutral phosphate contains 28 mEq of sodium and 28 mEq of potassium, present as monobasic and dibasic forms of phosphate (dibasic to monobasic ratio 3:1; pH 7.3). The difference in the amount of fixed base (56–32 = 24 mEq) represents the hydrogen ion load per gram of elemental phosphorus that must be buffered and excreted when using the acid phosphate preparation. Lau et al. [31] proved that both acute and chronic acid and neutral phosphate treatment induce different effects on the excretion of some risk factors for stone formation. In fact, urinary calcium excretion was significantly higher during acid phosphate treatment, associated with an increased net acid excretion (titratable acid, ammonium, and net acid excretion). These results give a clear physiological

Table 91.2 Positive effects of orthophosphate therapy

Authors	Journal/book	Year	Volume	Pages
Fleisch and Bisaz [25]	*Lancet*	1964	ii	1065–1067
Edwards et al. [21]	*Br J Urol*	1965	37	390–398
Bernstein and Newton [22]	*Lancet*	1966	ii	1105–1107
Ettinger and Kolb [51]	*Am J Med*	1975	55	32–37
Smith et al. [24]	*Urinary Calculi*	1973	–	188–197
Thomas [52]	*Kidney Int*	1978	13	390–396
Van Den Berg et al. [39]	*J Clin Endocrinol Metab*	1980	51	998–1001
Pak et al. [40]	*Am J Med*	1981	71	615–662
Klein and Griffith [41]	*Urolithiasis: Clinical and Basic Research*	1981	–	253–258
Peacock et al. [42]	*Urolithiasis: Clinical and Basic Research*	1981	–	259–265
Broadus et al. [30]	*J Clin Endocrinol Metab*	1983	56	953–961
Smith [43]	*Urolithiasis: Clinical and Basic Research*	1984	–	483–489
Wilson et al. [44]	*Urolithiasis: Clinical and Basic Research*	1984	–	491–493
Wilkstrom et al. [45]	*Urolithiasis: Clinical and Basic Research*	1984	–	495–498
Insogna et al. [46]	*J Urol*	1989	141	269–273
Breslau et al. [47]	*J Urol*	1995	160	664–668
Heller et al. [32]	*J Urol*	1998	159	1451–1456

Table 91.3 Reported stone episode rates before and during treatment with orthophosphate

	Stone episode rate/patient/year	
Reference	Before	During
Pak et al. [40]	2.21±2.03	0.29±0.70
Peacock et al. [42]	0.74	0.24
Klein and Griffith [41]	8.35	1.5
Wilson et al. [44]	0.74	0.24
Wikstrom et al. [45]	0.56	0.07
Smith [43]	2.6	0.5

explanation of the reduced action of acid phosphate treatment in decreasing calcium urinary excretion, whether in normocalciuric subjects [26, 35] or in hypercalciuric stone formers [36–37]. Moreover, Lau et al. [31] have shown that both acid and neutral phosphates induce a decrease in urinary calcium excretion, but the amount of calcium decrease obtained with acid phosphate was sim ilar to that induced by dietary calcium restriction. These data are in agreement with the clinical observation that acid phosphate showed the same efficacy as dietary calcium restriction in producing stone disease remission [33]. A possible explanation for the different results after phosphate treatment described in the literature [22, 24, 26, 27, 30] may be found in the quantity of hydrogen ions present in the acid phosphate rather than in the slight difference in dosages [31]. Furthermore, the 64 mmol of acid phosphate ingested daily by the patients may produce 48 mEq of hydrogen ions, a sufficient amount to induce a decrease in urinary citrate excretion [31]. Both acid and neutral phosphates induce a similar phyrophosphate urinary excretion [31]. Finally, the relative urinary supersaturation was only decreased by neutral phosphate [31, 38]. Taken together, these results indicate that neutral salts may be preferred for stone formers with idiopathic hypercalciuria. Positive effects of orthophosphate therapy have been described in several papers (see Table 91.2), although most of them consisted of open non-randomized studies including patients with different enrollment and treatment criteria (types of stones, presence/absence of hypercalciuria, male/female ratio, acidic or neutral orthophosphate, drug dosage). In all the literature, there are only two double-blind studies with orthophosphate; in the first, no significant differences were observed between treated and untreated stone formers undergoing therapy with rapid-release orthophosphate [33]. The second study, testing a slow-release orthophosphate, showed a reduced rate of stone formation [32]. Orthophosphate preparations have a potential use in absorptive hypercalciuria since they reduce serum 1,25-dihydroxyvitamin D levels, urinary calcium excretion, and perhaps bone resorption. Absorptive hypercalciuric patients with hypophosphatemia should be particularly responsive. Unfortunately, the use of available preparations of rapid-release phosphate is often limited by the need for frequent dosing, as well as by gastrointestinal symptoms such as abdominal cramping and diarrhea. The only controlled trial using phosphate showed no benefit, but the acidic and sodium-containing forms of phosphate used in the trial may be expected to be less effective due to the potential hypercalciuric and hypocitraturic effects of the accompanying acid and sodium load [33]. The hypocalciuric response to the drug is probably the result of the combined effects of reduced intestinal calcium absorption, increased renal tubular calcium reabsorption, and diminished bone resorption. The decline in calcium intestinal absorption is in agreement with the reduction in serum 1,25-dihydroxyvitamin D_3. Renal calcium reabsorption is probably due either to PTH increase or the direct action of phosphate on the renal tubule. Decreased alkaline phosphatase and fasting urine calcium suggest that bone turnover was reduced by the treatment. Decreased skeletal resorption is to be expected since phosphate has been demonstrated in vitro to reduce bone resorption [48]. The absence of age-related bone loss over 4 years in hypercalciuric patients provides supportive evidence that calcium loss from bone may have diminished with treatment [24].

Side Effects of Orthophosphates

Finally, common side effects of orthophosphate therapy include diarrhea, abdominal cramps, nausea, and vomiting. According to the type of orthophosphate, other side effects have been reported: for example, the acidic and sodium-containing forms of phosphate used in some studies may be responsible for hypertension and may be expected to be less effective due to the potential hypercalciuric and hypocitraturic effects of the accompanying acid and sodium load. Furthermore, alkaline phosphates promote dissociation of urinary phosphate and increase brushite saturation. Possible effects on parathyroid hormone and metastatic calcifications are also reported.

Conclusion

In conclusion, orthophosphates have been proposed as an alternative for treating patients with hypercalciuria, especially of the absorptive type, but as debated by the members of the Advisory Board of European Urolithiasis Research (ABEUR) during the consensus conference organized in Mannheim on 23 January 1999, there are insufficient studies, above all clinical randomized trials, to confirm their efficacy beyond any shadow of a doubt. Their usefulness may thus be limited to being a second choice for the treatment of selected patients [49]. In accordance with these indications, over recent years the use of orthophosphates in hypercalciuria treatment has declined progressively, and no mention of them is reported in the most recent guidelines on urolithiasis [50].

Acknowledgment The author wishes to thank Dr. Luke Seaber for his linguistic advice in the preparation of this chapter.

References

1. Johri N, Cooper B, Robertson W, Choong S, Rickards D, Unwin R. An update and practical guide to renal stone management. Nephron Clin Pract. 2010;116:c159–71.
2. Preminger GM. Guidelines for the Medical Management of Urolithiasis. In: Business briefing: US kidney & Urological Disease 2005. Published by Touch Briefings. May 2005, pp.33–36.
3. Chandhoke PS. When is medical prophylaxis cost-effective for recurrent calcium stones? J Urol. 2002;168:937–40.
4. Vahlensiec W, Hesse A, Nolde A. Urolithiasis: the calculus is gone: what now? Principles of urinary calculus metaphylaxis. Urologe A. 1993;32:W347–57.
5. Strohmaier WL. Economic aspects of nephrolithiasis: a critical review and future outlook. In: Borghi L, Meschi T, Briganti A, Schianchi T, Novarini A, eds. Proc. 8th Eur Symp on Urolith, Parma, Italy, June 1999. Cosenza: Editoriale Bios, 1999: 111–118.
6. Caudarella R, Vescini F. Urinary citrate and renal stone disease: the preventive role of alkali citrate treatment. Arch Ital Urol Androl. 2009;81:182–7.
7. Parks JH, Coe FL. Evidence for durable kidney stone prevention over several decades. BJU Int. 2009;103:1238–46.
8. Pak CYC, Ohata M, Lawrence EC, Snyder W. The hypercalciurias: causes, parathyroid functions, and diagnostic criteria. J Clin Invest. 1974;54:387–400.
9. Nordin BEC, Peacock M, Wilkinson R. Hypercalciuria and calcium stone disease. In: McIntyre I, editor. Clinics in endocrinology and metabolism. Philadelphia: Saunders; 1972. p. 169–83.
10. Pak CYC, Britton F, Peterson R, Ward D, Northcutt C, Breslau NA, et al. Ambulatory evaluation of nephrolithiasis: classification, clinical presentation and diagnostic criteria. Am J Med. 1980;69:19–30.
11. Levy FL, Adams-Huet B, Pak CYC. Ambulatory evaluation of nephrolithiasis: an update of a 1980 protocol. Am J Med. 1995; 98:50–9.
12. Pak CYC, Sakhaee K, Pearle MS. Detection of absorptive hypercalciuria type I without the oral calcium load test. J Urol. 2011;185:915–9.
13. Bordier P, Ryckewaert A, Gueris J, Rasmussen H. On the pathogenesis of so-called idiopathic hypercalciuria. Am J Med. 1977;63:398–409.
14. Worcester EM, Coe FL. New insights into the pathogenesis of idiopathic hypercalciuria. Semin Nephrol. 2008;28:120–32.
15. Insogna KL, Broadus AE, Dreyer BE, Ellison AF, Gertner JM. Elevated production rate of 1,25- dihydroxyvitamin D in patients with absorptive hypercalciuria. J Clin Endocrinol Metab. 1985;61:490–5.
16. Breslau NA, Preminger GM, Adams BV, Otey J, Pak CYC. Use of ketoconazole to probe the pathogenetic importance of 1,25-dihydroxyvitamin D in patients with absorptive hypercalciuria. J Clin Endocrinol Metab. 1992;75:1446–52.
17. Weisinger JR, Alonzo E, Belloforin-Font E, Blasini AM, Rodriguez MA, Paz-Martinis R. Possible role of cytokines on the bone mineral loss in idiopathic hypercalciuria. Kidney Int. 1996;49:244–50.
18. Pietschmann F, Breslau NA, Pak CYC. Reduced vertebral bone density in hypercalciuric nephrolithiasis. J Bone Miner Res. 1992;7:1383–8.
19. Shen FH, Baylink DJ, Nielsen RL, Sherrard DJ, Ivey JL, Haussler MR. Increased serum 1,25-dihydroxyvitamin D in idiopathic hypercalciuria. J Lab Clin Med. 1977;90:955–62.
20. Lau K, Goldfarb S, Goldberg M, Agus ZS. Effects of phosphate administration on tubular calcium transport. J Lab Clin Med. 1982; 99:317–24.
21. Edwards NA, Russel RGGG, Hodgkinson A. The effects of oral phosphate in patients with recurrent renal calculus. Br J Urol. 1965;37:390–8.
22. Bernstein DS, Newton R. The effect of oral sodium phosphate on the formation of renal calculi and on idiopathic hypercalciuria. Lancet. 1966;2:1105–7.

23. Thomas Jr WC. Effectiveness and mode of action of orthophosphate in patients with calcareous renal calculi. Trans Am Clin Climatol Assoc. 1971;83:113–34.
24. Smith LH, Thomas Jr WC, Arnaud CD. Orthophosphate therapy in calcium renal litiasi. In: Cifuentes D, Rapado A, Hodgkinson A, editors. Trinary calculi: recent advances in aetiology, stone structure and treatment. Basel: Karger; 1973. p. 188–97.
25. Fleisch H, Bisaz S. Effects of orthophosphate on urinary pyrophosphate excretion and the prevention of urolithiasis. Lancet. 1964;ii: 1065–7.
26. Ettinger B, Kolb FO. Inorganic phosphate treatment of nephrolithiasis. Am J Med. 1973;55:32–7.
27. Oliver J, Weinberger A, Bar-Meir S, Sperling O, Jahav J, De Vries A. Orthophosphate treatment of calcium lithiasis associated with idiopathic hypercalciuria. Urol Int. 1974;29:414–20.
28. Reiss E, Canterbury JM, Bercovitz MA, Kaplan EL. The role of phosphate in the secretion of parathyroid hormone in man. J Clin Invest. 1970;49:2146–9.
29. Lau K, Eby BK. Tubular mechanism for the spontaneous hypercalciuria in laboratory rat. J Clin Invest. 1982;70(4):835–44.
30. Broadus AE, Magee JS, Mallette LE, Horst RL, Lang R, Jensen PS, et al. A detailed evaluation of oral phosphate therapy in selected patients with primary hyperparathyroidism. J Clin Endocrinol Metab. 1983;56:953–61.
31. Lau K, Wolf C, Nussbaum P, Weiner B, DeOreo P, Slatopolsky E, et al. Differing effects of acid versus neutral phosphate therapy of hypercalciuria. Kidney Int. 1979;16:736–42.
32. Heller HJ, Reza-Albarran AA, Breslau NA, Pak CYC. Sustained reduction in urinary calcium during long-term treatment with slow release neutral potassium phosphate in absorptive hypercalciuria. J Urol. 1998;159:1451–6.
33. Ettinger B. Recurrent nephrolithiasis: natural history and effect of phosphate therapy: a double-blind controlled study. Am J Med. 1976;61:200–6.
34. Lemann Jr J, Litzow JR, Lennon EJ. The effects of chronic acid loads in normal man: further evidence for the participation of bone mineral in the defense against chronic metabolic acidosis. J Clin Invest. 1966;45:1608–16149.
35. Adams ND, Gray RW, Lemann Jr J. The calciuria of increased fixed acid production in humans: evidence against a role for parathyroid hormone and 1,25$(OH)_2$-vitamin D. Calcif Tissue Int. 1979;28(3): 233–388.
36. Farquharson RF, Salter WT, Tibbetts DM, Aub JC. Studies of calcium and phosphorus metabolism: XII. The effect of the ingestion of acid-producing substances. J Clin Invest. 1931; 10:221–49.
37. Farquharson RF, Salter WT, Tibbetts DM, Aub JC. Studies of calcium and phosphorus metabolism: XIII. The effect of phosphate on the excretion of calcium. J Clin Invest. 1931;10:251–69.
38. Burdette DC, Thomas Jr WC, Fynlaison B. Urinary supersaturation with calcium oxalate before and during orthophosphate therapy. J Urol. 1976;115:418–22.
39. Van den Berg CJ, Kumar R, Wilson DM, Helath III H, Smith LH. Orthophosphate therapy decreases urinary calcium excretion and serum 1,25-dihydroxyvitamin D concentrations in idiopathic hypercalciuria. J Clin Endocrinol Metab. 1980;51:998–1001.
40. Pak CYC, Peters P, Hurt G, Kadesky M, Fine M, Reisman D, et al. Is selective therapy of recurrent nephrolithiasis possible ? Am J Med. 1981;71:615–62.
41. Klein AS, Griffith P. Neutral potassium phosphate and thiazide: combined treatment in recurrent stone formers. I. In: Smith LH, Robertson WG, Finlayson B, editors. Urolithiasis: clinical and basic research. New York: Plenum Press; 1981. p. 253–8.
42. Peacock M, Robertson WG, Heyburn PJ, Davies AEJ, Rutherford A. Phosphate treatment of idiopathic calcium stone disease. In: Smith LH, Robertson WG, Finlayson B, editors. Urolithiasis: clinical and basic research. New York: Plenum Press; 1981. p. 259–65.
43. Smith LH. The effects of orthophosphate and ion binders. In: Smith LH, Robertson WG, Schwille PO, editors. Urolithiasis: clinical and basic research. New York: Plenum Press; 1984. p. 483–9.
44. Wilson JWL, Werness PG, Smith LH. Effect of orthophosphate treatment on urine composition in idiopathic calcium urolithiasis. In: Schwille PO, Smith LH, Robertson WG, editors. Urolithiasis: clinical and basic research. New York: Plenum Press; 1984. p. 491–3.
45. Wikstrom B, Backman U, Danielson BG, Fellstrom B, Johansson G, Ljunghall S, et al. Phosphate treatment of calcium urolithiasis. In: Schwille PO, Smith LH, Robertson WG, editors. Urolithiasis: clinical and basic research. New York: Plenum Press; 1984. p. 495–8.
46. Insogna KL, Ellison AS, Burtis WJ, Sartori L, Lang RL, Broadus AE. Trichlormetazide and oral phosphate therapy in patients with absorptive hypercalciuria. J Urol. 1989;141:269–73.
47. Breslau NA, Heller HJ, Reza-Albarran AA, Pak CYC. Physiological effects of slow release potassium phosphate for absorptive hypercalciuria: a randomized double-blind trial. J Urol. 1995;160:664–8.
48. Yates AJ, Oreffo ROC, Mayor K, Mundy GR. Inhibition of bone resorption by inorganic phosphate is mediated by both reduced osteoclast formation and decreased activity of mature osteoclasts. J Bone Miner Res. 1991;6:473–8.
49. Tiselius HG. Possibilities for preventing recurrent calcium stone formation: principles for the metabolic evaluation of patients with calcium stone disease. BJU Int. 2001;88:158–68.
50. Turk CH, Knoll T, Petrick A, Sarica K, Seitz C, Straub M. Guidelines on Urolithiasis J Urol. 2007;178:2418–834 (Text update Apr 2010)
51. Ettinger B, Kolb FO. Inorganic phosphate treatment of nephrolithiasis. Am J Med. 1973 Jul;55(1):32–7.
52. Thomas WC Jr. Use of phosphates in patients with calcareous renal calculi. Kidney Int. 1978 May;13(5):390–6. Review.

Management of Cystinuria

92

Jan Peter Jessen and Thomas Knoll

Abstract

Cystinuria is an autosomal inherited disorder of dibasic amino acid transport in the proximal tubule and small intestine, being responsible for 1–2 % of urinary stones in adults and up to 10 % in children. Recurrent stone formation and repeated need of surgical intervention are typical for patients suffering from cystinuria and are possibly leading to an impairment of renal function and quality of life. Thus, an appropriate strategy for stone removal as well as medical recurrence prevention is of great importance but is also demanding. Another most important factor is the patient's compliance with conservative therapy. However, many of these patients, who require a lifelong therapy and regular follow-up, have problems achieving and maintaining a good adjustment. Traditionally, the disease was classified by the urine phenotype, measured by excretion of amino acids. Increased understanding of the underlying genetic characteristics has led to a revised classification based on the genotype. So far, two involved genes have been identified: SLC3A1 on chromosome 2 and SLC7A9 on chromosome 19. Their products form the $b^{o,+}$-transporter, which transports dibasic amino acids in exchange for neutral amino acids. Conservative therapy aims at reducing the frequency of urological intervention and is based on two principles: to reduce the saturation of urine with cystine and to increase the solubility of cystine in the urine. Interventional therapy focuses on minimally invasive techniques. Despite the increased pathophysiological and genetic knowledge regarding cystinuria, no new treatment modalities could be derived from that during the last years.

Keywords

Cystinuria • Urolithiasis • Prevention • Treatment • SLC3A1 • SLC7A9 • $b^{o,+}$-transporter • Autosomal recessive disorder • Dibasic amino acid transport

Introduction

Cystinuria is an autosomal recessive inherited disorder of dibasic amino acid transport in the proximal tubule and small intestine, being responsible for 1–2 % of urinary stones in adults and up to 10 % in children [1]. Recurrent stone formation and repeated need of surgical intervention are typical for patients suffering from cystinuria and are possibly leading to an impairment of renal function and quality of life [2]. Thus, an appropriate strategy for stone removal as well as medical recurrence prevention is of great importance but is also demanding [3]. Despite the increased pathophysiological

J.P. Jessen, M.D. (✉) • T. Knoll, M.D., Ph.D., M.Sc.
Department of Urology, Sindelfingen-Boeblingen Medical Center, Arthur-Gruber Str. 70, Sindelfingen, Baden-Wuerttemberg, 72076, Germany
e-mail: j.jessen@klinikverbund-suedwest.de; t.knoll@klinikverbund-suedwest.de

J.J. Talati et al. (eds.), *Urolithiasis*,
DOI 10.1007/978-1-4471-4387-1_92, © Springer-Verlag London 2012

and genetic knowledge regarding cystinuria, no new treatment modalities could be derived from that during the last few years [4].

Epidemiology

The estimated global prevalence of cystinuria is 1:7,000 [5]. Considering the genetic transmission of the disease, it is not surprising that the reported prevalence differs remarkably from country to country. Since regular screening programs are quite rare, the prevalence shown in Table 92.1 is approximate. Some of these prevalence rates were derived from urine screening in newborns. Since maturation of SLC3A1 gene expression between midgestation and 4.5 years postnatal age may account for transient neonatal cystinuria [5], these newborn screenings may have resulted in false high findings.

Pathophysiology

Cystinuria is characterized by a hyperexcretion of cystine and dibasic amino acids (lysine, ornithine, and arginine) into the urine [6, 7]. This is caused by an impaired transport of these amino acids across the apical membrane of epithelial cells of the renal proximal tubule and small intestine [4, 8, 9], thus hindering the reabsorption of the filtered amino acids (normally 98–99 %) [10]. Although all of these amino acids reach high concentrations in urine, only cystine is insoluble enough to form stones [1]. Due to this poor solubility, hyperexcretion and supersaturation lead to the development of cystine stones [11, 12]. The impairment of the intestinal transport does not result in malnutrition because the amino acids can be formed by metabolism or taken up by another transporter [13, 14].

The precipitation of characteristic hexagonal cystine crystals is influenced by urine pH with an acidic pH promoting it [15]. An alkaline pH > 8 leads to a threefold increase of cystine solubility [16]. Varying effect of pH on cystine solubility among patients suggests further influencing factors [17–19]. Besides known factors such as dietary intake of fluid, salt, and protein, other, yet unknown, genetic influences can be assumed to be contributory. This is supported by the observation that the proportion of cystine stone-producing mice increases from 40 % in the second filial generation of SLC7A9-knockout mice [20] to 85 % in the sixth filial generation [4]. Intake of dietary salt increases the cystine excretion. However, no prospective study has shown a decrease in stone activity resulting from sodium-restricted diets [17]. Another known factor is dietary intake of animal protein. Lowered intake of the cystine precursor methionine reduces urinary cystine excretion [21].

Table 92.1 Prevalence of cystinuria

Region/population	Prevalence	References
Average	1: 7,000	[10]
Turkey	1: 772–1,000	[74, 75]
Spain (east coast)	1: 1,887	[76]
Libyan Jews	1: 2,500	[77]
USA and Europe	1: 1,000–20,000	[1, 77]
Australia	1: 4,000	[78]
Czech Republic	1: 5,600	[79]
Quebec	1: 7,200	[80]
Japan	1: 16,000–50,000	[81, 82]
Sweden	1: 100,000	[1]

In patients with cystinuria, eventually, the cystine crystals will form stones with the corresponding typical clinical problems like obstruction, pain, or infection. Cystinuric patients are overrepresented among stone formers who have lost a kidney [22]. Histological examination of papillary biopsies of patients with cystine stones has shown cystine crystal-plugged ducts of Bellini, with the surrounding interstitium showing changes from inflammation to fibrosis. Also, many inner medullary collecting ducts will be seen to be dilated, some with and others without crystal plugs [22].

The main effector of cystine reabsorption in the kidney is the amino acid transport system $b^{o,+}$, belonging to the family of heterodimeric amino acid transporters (HAT). These transporters, which consist of a heavy chain linked by a disulphide bridge to a range of light chains, prefer antiport mechanisms which lead to exchange of amino acids [14]. In the case of $b^{o,+}$, the association of the light subunit called $b^{o,+}$AT (neutral and dibasic amino acid transporter) with the heavy chain called rBAT (related to basic amino transporter) forms the active transporter, which transports dibasic amino acids in exchange for neutral amino acids [14, 23]. Incorrect assembly of the subunits, caused by genetic mutations, can lead to clinical manifestation of cystinuria of varying severity, depending on the underlying mutation [24].

Genetics, Inheritance, and Classification

Positional genetics, genetic linkage studies, and mutational analysis helped to identify two genes whose mutations cause cystinuria [4]:

- SLC3A1 on chromosome 2 (gene locus 2p16), coding for the heavy rBat subunit of the $b^{o,+}$-transporter [25]
- SLC7A9 on chromosome 19 (gene locus 19q12–13), coding for the light $b^{o,+}$AT subunit of the $b^{o,+}$-transporter [26]

So far, 133 mutations have been identified in SLC3A1 and 95 in SLC7A9. Reported mutations include nonsense, missense, splicing, frameshifts, and large sequence rearrangements [4]. Five hundred seventy-nine mutated alleles in SLC3A1 have been reported in patients from 23 countries, frequencies varying regionally, and 436 mutated SLC7A9 alleles in patients from 18 countries [4].

Cystinuria is usually considered an autosomal recessive disorder. Classification of the phenotype was traditionally achieved by identifying the urinary excretion pattern of cystine and dibasic amino acid acids of the obligate heterozygous parents [4]. Three phenotypes have been described, heterozygous relatives of patients with type I showing normal aminoaciduria, those of type II cystinuric patients having a high hyperexcretion (not matching that of a homozygous patient), and type III relatives having a moderate hyperexcretion (Table 92.2) [27].

Observation of the varying extent of amino acid excretion in patients who carry the same mutation has led to a revised classification to type I, non-type I (includes former type II and III), and mixed type (type I/non-type I). Due to rare formation of cystine calculi with concomitant variable hyperexcretion of cystine in non-type I heterozygotes, an autosomal dominant inheritance with incomplete penetration for the cystine lithiasis trait is assumed for non-type I cystinuria [4]. A lack of genotype-phenotype correlation in some cystinuria cases has led to the recommendation of a new classification based on the genotype [24, 28], defining patients with mutations in SLC3A1 as type A, patients with mutations in SLC7A9 as type B, and patients with mutations in both SLC3A1 and SLC7A9 as type AB.

Diagnostics

The average onset of the disease is during the second decade of life, with male patients having a more severe evolution and an earlier onset of symptoms [28]. Every younger stone-forming patient should be suspected to have cystine stones, especially if he or she is a member of a known cystinuric family. Diagnosis of cystinuria is possible even before the first stone has been passed spontaneously or extracted (Table 92.3). For patients with stones, a diagnosis of cystine stone can be confirmed by noting an increased urinary excretion of dibasic amino acids or by identifying mutations on both alleles of one of the involved genes. An excretion of >1,300 μmol/g creatinine of cystine or >5,900 μmol total dibasic amino acids also confirms the diagnosis in those without stones. Genotyping analyses can also be made in relatives of cystinuric patients.

Stone Analysis

Stone analysis should always be carried out after stone expulsion or extraction. Cystine stones have a pale amber color and a waxy appearance. They often present as staghorn stones at first diagnosis, due to their often rapid growth. Pure cystine stones are identified in 60–80 % of cases. Potential diagnostic error may occur due to partial analysis of the stone [13]. A distinction between rough and smooth subtypes of cystine stones has been made by electron microscopic evaluation. Smooth calculi have an irregular, interlacing crystal structure and are thereby more resistant to fragmentation than those of the rough subtype [29].

Table 92.2 Cystine excretion in relatives (in μmol/g creatinine)

Type I	Type II	Type III
<100	>900	100–900

Radiological Appearance

Cystine stones are easily detectable by ultrasound. They appear poorly radio-opaque on plain film (Fig. 92.1). In case of large stone masses or a mixed stone composition, they may appear radio-opaque. In computed tomography (CT) cystine stones appear poorly attenuated, with CT-collimation and stone size influencing the attenuation [30]. The CT-based prediction of stone composition remains an interesting issue for research. Latest reports using a dual-energy multidetector CT with postprocessing techniques showed good results [31]. However, these findings are not yet generally transferred to routine clinical practice.

Urine Analysis

Microscopic morning urine examination may reveal typical hexagonal cystine crystals (Fig. 92.2) that confirm the diagnosis. However, their absence does not exclude the diagnosis because they are only detectable in 20–39 % of urine specimens from cystinuric patients [1, 32]. Since cystine contains sulfur, the urine may have the characteristic smell of rotten eggs. Quantitative daily cystine excretion is determined by ion-exchange chromatography from collected urine. Twenty-four-hour urine collection is not only important for determination of cystine excretion but also for other metabolic abnormalities like hyperuricosuria, hypocitraturia, and hypercalciuria, which can be found in up to 45 % of cystinuric patients [33]. It should be performed regularly to plan and monitor the therapy. For a proper determination of cystine excretion, sodium bicarbonate should be added to the urine to achieve a pH above 7.5. In this way, cystine dissolution is promoted and false reporting of low cystine values can be avoided. Patients excreting 1,300 μmol of cystine per g creatinine are presumed to be homozygous and need further evaluation and treatment [34].

Conservative Management of Cystinuria

Recurrent stone formation causes repeated need of urological intervention with typical associated risks. Due to ongoing improvement of minimally invasive techniques, these are today's preferential treatment modalities in case of existing

Table 92.3 Definition of cystinuria

Stone present			No stone present	
Increased urinary excretion of dibasic amino acids	*or*	Identification of mutations on both alleles of one of the involved genes	*Excretion in 24-h urine µmol/g creatinine*	
			Cystine only	>1,300
			Dibasic amino acids total	>5,900

Following Dello Strologo et al. [77]

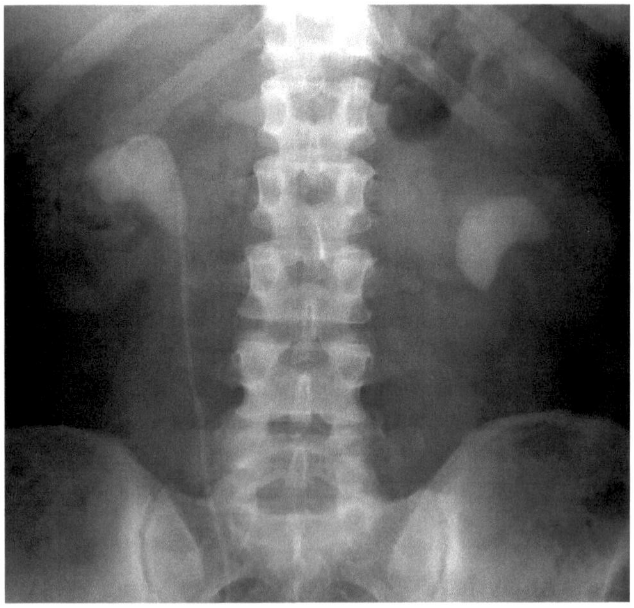

Fig. 92.1 Cystine stones on plain film

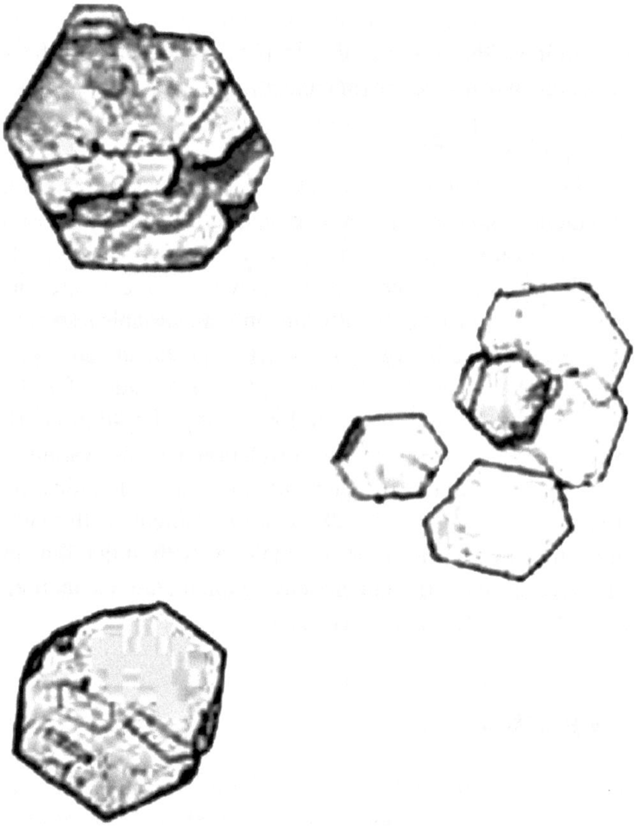

Fig. 92.2 Cystine crystals

stones. To reduce the frequency of intervention, conservative treatment plays a great role in the management of cystinuria. It is based on two main principles: to reduce the saturation of urine with cystine and to increase the solubility of cystine in urine. The former goal can be achieved by either lowering the excreted amount of cystine or by reducing the excreted cystine to better soluble cysteine or by increasing the total urine volume. Raising the urinary pH level entails an improved solubility of cystine.

Patient compliance is an important issue as patients often have problems to maintain the necessary high urinary flow, urine alkalinization, or the rigorous low-sodium, low-protein diets used to reduce cystine excretion [35]. Also, available pharmacological therapy often has adverse side effects that lower patient compliance with the therapy. Despite the increased pathophysiological and genetic knowledge regarding cystinuria, no methods to fix the transport-defect have been found as yet. Recently, an approach to retard cystine crystal growth was reported, by using new compounds in an in vitro environment [36]. However, it remains to be seen whether this can lead to an applicable in vivo therapy.

For all patients first-line therapy includes increased fluid intake, urine alkalinization, and low-salt diet. Other medical approaches are reserved for those patients who do not sufficiently respond to these measures.

Urine Dilution

The single most important factor for cystine-stone prevention is a constant hyperdiuresis to decrease the urine saturation with cystine. Up to pH 7 cystine solubility is approximately 250 mg/L (1 mmol/L); at a pH above 7.5, this is doubled to 500 mg/L (2 mmol/L); and at a pH above 8, it is tripled to 750 mg/L (3 mmol/L) [16]. Since a homozygous cystinuric patient excretes 600–1,400 mg of cystine per day, the needed urine volume ranges from at least 2.4–5.6 L. Usually, the total daily urine volume should be at least 3 L, thus making a daily intake of at least 4–4.5 L of fluid desirable. In children, fluid intake should be 1.5 L/m^2 body surface. Ideally, this should be evenly distributed in equivalent doses across 24 h. Therefore, it is important to advise the patient to drink before going to bed to provoke nocturia, as well as to drink during the night after micturition [37, 38]. The European Association of Urology recommends an hourly intake of at least 150 mL in its 2011 guidelines update

[39]. Urine neutral and alkalizing beverages like mineral water (preferably high in bicarbonate and low in sodium), herbal teas, and citrus juices are recommended. Dilution success can be evaluated by patient's use of dipstick tests, keeping the urine specific gravity below 1.010 [40].

Dietary Prevention

Although it was shown that reduced intake of animal protein lowers the urinary excretion of cystine [21], such restrictions to the menu are not accepted by most patients and are therefore not generally recommended. Adults should follow a mixed common sense diet with relatively low protein. Protein restriction is not recommended in children [1].

Reduction of dietary intake of sodium chloride has been shown to reduce urinary cystine concentration significantly [41, 42]. Therefore, a reduction to less than 2 g/day has been recommended for adolescents and grown-ups [43]. A low-salt diet is also effective in children [44]. However, compliance with dietary restriction is often poor.

Urine Alkalinization

As described previously, the solubility of cystine increases with higher urine pH values. Therefore, continuous urine alkalinization is another important measure to improve cystine solubility. This can be achieved by either administering potassium citrate or sodium bicarbonate [45]. The latter is only recommended in cases with severe renal insufficiency because sodium increases the urinary cystine excretion. Therefore, potassium citrate is the first-line treatment for alkalinization in cystinuric patients. It should be given in 2–4 single doses of 3–10 mmol. Monitoring of the urine pH should be performed at least three times a day to keep a constant pH of at least 7.5. After starting with low doses, careful adjustment should be carried out until therapeutic pH values are reached. Monitoring of serum potassium levels is advisable [45].

There are reports that azetazolamide, a sulfonamide, can be used to reinforce the alkalizing effect of other pH-increasing therapy [46]. But then, azetazolamide is known to increase the risk of calcium phosphate stone formation and long-term data is not yet available. No general recommendation can be made at the moment.

Pharmacological Therapy

In case of a urinary cystine excretion above 3 mmol/day or if the aforementioned measures fail to prevent cystine stone recurrence, further pharmacological intervention is needed. Thiol-containing compounds can cleave the disulfide bond of cystine, forming mixed disulfides with the cysteine monomers that are as much as 50 times more soluble than cystine [47] (Fig. 92.3). Most widely studied and used thiol agents are D-penicillamine (DP) and α(alpha)-mercaptopropionylglycine (MPG, thiopronin) [48, 49]. In one study, MPG was shown to be 50 % more effective than DP [35]. Although

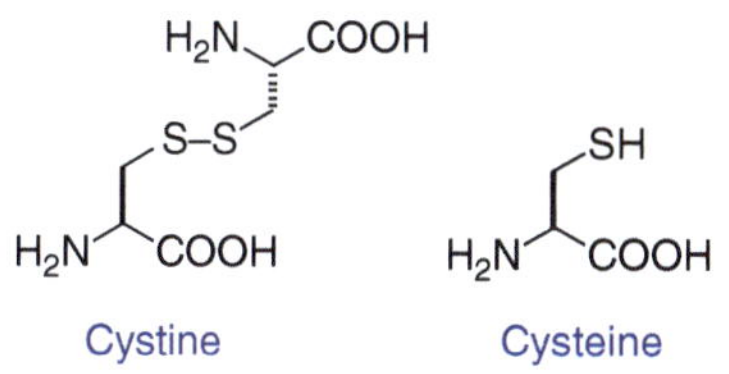

Fig. 92.3 Cystine – cysteine

both have the same side effect profile, MPG appears to have significantly lower frequency and severity of side effects [19], which is why it is the favored treatment option today. However, in a recent study, a good tolerance to DP was shown in a cohort of American children [50]. Typical side effects include rash, arthralgia, leukopenia, gastrointestinal intolerance, proteinuria, and nephrotic syndrome [43], thus occasionally limiting treatment success. It has been shown in a mouse model that the efficacy of MPG therapy is highly dependent on urinary pH [51] and should therefore always be based on a combination with urine alkalinization. The suggested initial MPG dose is 250 mg/day, which may be consecutively increased to a maximum dose of 2 g/day [39]. An early tachyphylaxia is possible. Treatment in children must be individualized as the required amount of drug is strictly dependent on body size [52]. The recommended dosage is 20–40 mg/kg body weight administered in two doses, which is important as cystine excretion is higher during the night [45].

Captopril, an angiotensin-converting-enzyme inhibitor, contains free sulfhydryl groups. Reported results regarding its therapeutic use in cystinuria are controversial [37, 48, 53–55]. Therefore, it remains a second-line therapeutic option, applicable when MPG therapy is unfeasible or unsuccessful [39].

Likewise, the use of ascorbic acid as a therapeutic agent for cystinuria is controversial [56, 57]. It has limited reductive power and is estimated to lower urinary cystine levels by about 20 % [56]. It was assumed that the positive effect on stone formation could be traced back to the fraction of sodium bicarbonate in the fizzy tablets used. High ascorbic acid supplementation may also increase urinary oxalate concentration and should therefore be avoided in patients with simultaneous calcium oxalate stone formation [58].

Many cystinuric patients form stones of mixed composition [29]. Hypercalciuria, hyperuricosuria, hyperoxaluria, hypocitraturia, or infections might accompany cystinuria and should be determined and treated if necessary.

Urological Intervention

Despite the prophylactic conservative treatment, recurrent stone formation is common in cystinuric patients, thus leading to a repeated need of urological intervention. Today, minimally invasive procedures are preferred in almost all cases. Indication criteria are generally the same as for any patient with urinary stones. The chosen technique does not influence stone recurrence, but being totally stone free after the procedure results in a longer time interval until stone recurrence [59].

Extracorporeal Shock Wave Lithotripsy

Cystine stones are usually considered to be relatively resistant to extracorporeal shock wave lithotripsy (SWL), which often leads to multiple treatments, especially in cases of larger stones. The classification in rough and smooth subtype in combination with a possible increasing clinical use of CT-based prediction of these subtypes could lead to a better selection of SWL-suited cystine stones. However, in regard to the low invasiveness and recurrent stone events in cystinuric patients, SWL remains the primary therapy option for all stone sites of the upper urinary tract and stone sizes below 1.5 cm, particularly in children [60–62]. Treatment success in case of lower pole stones might be limited due to remaining fragments, depending on anatomic characteristics (steep infundibular-pelvic angle, long lower pole, narrow infundibulum) [39, 63–66].

Ureterorenoscopy

Due to the development of new small semirigid and flexible scopes and the availability of the holmium:YAG laser, ureterorenoscopy (URS) offers a safe and efficient alternative for the treatment of cystine stones [67, 68], even in prepubertal children [69]. This applies especially to all ureteric sites and also to all localizations in the collecting system, although larger stone masses lead to long operative times, thus making a percutaneous approach or SWL more favorable. URS offers a good treatment opportunity for fragments refractory to prior SWL treatment.

Percutaneous Nephrolithotomy

For stones exceeding 1.5–2 cm or calyceal diverticular stones, percutaneous nephrolithotomy (PNL) is recommended and is also well suited for the treatment of cystine stones. Monotherapy (Fig. 92.4) with PNL is safe and efficient in the management of staghorn and complex renal calculi in one single hospital stay. It may be combined with

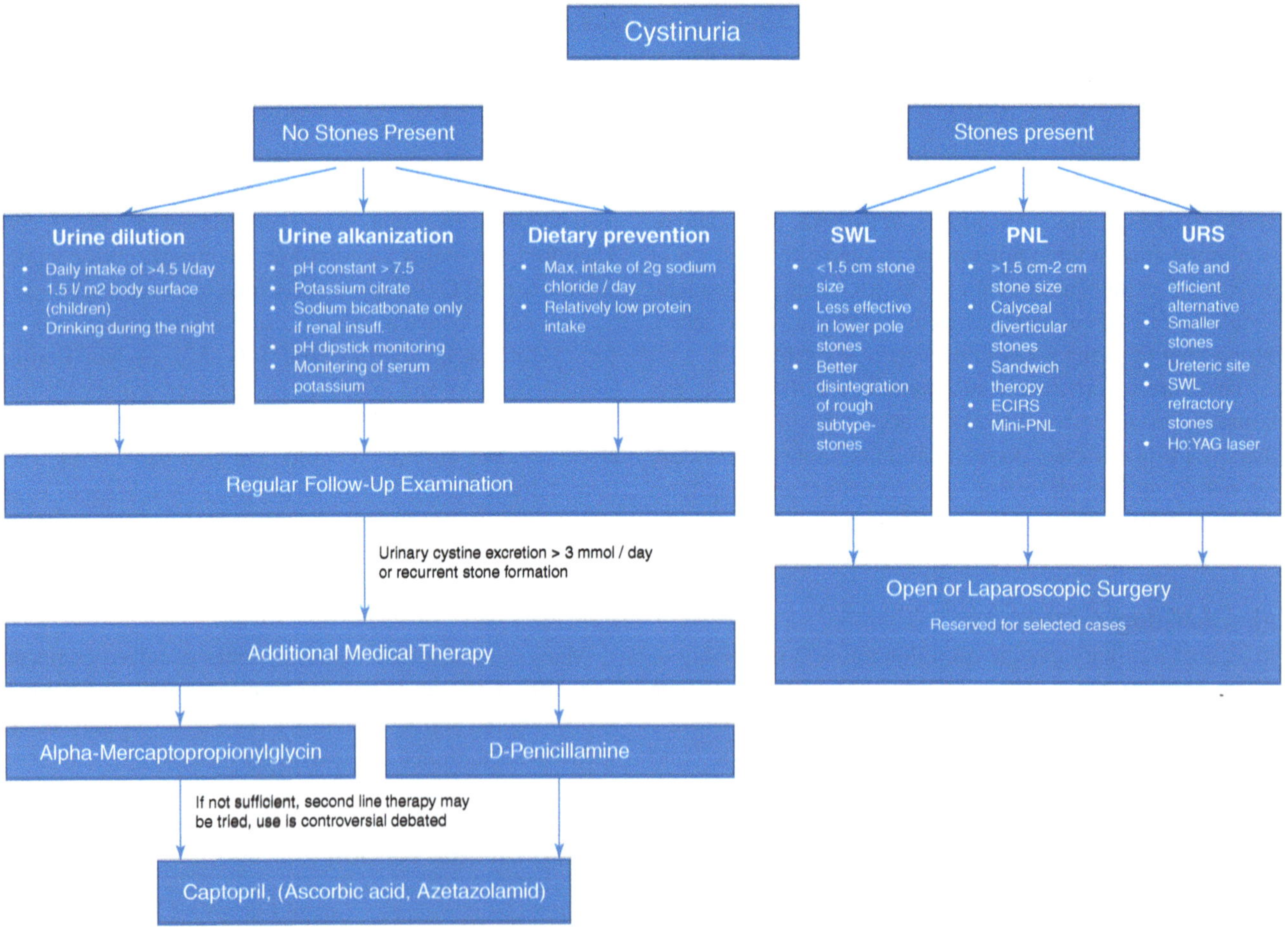

Fig. 92.4 Therapy overview

SWL, so-called sandwich therapy, or with URS, even in one procedure [70], if necessary. Simultaneous PNL and URS (endoscopic combined intrarenal surgery, ECIRS) allows circumvention of multiple tract access in case of large and complex stone situations. The use of miniaturized instruments (Mini-Perc) as an alternative to conventional PNL [71, 72] has facilitated the successful application of PNL in the pediatric population [73].

Conclusion

Cystinuria is responsible for 1–2 % of urinary stones in adults and up to 10 % of stones in children. The higher incidence reported in children might result from screening of newborn urines which detects transient cystinuria, which disappears as the SLC3A1 gene expression matures. Cystine stones are recurrent and impair renal function and the quality of life. The recurrent nature of the stone requires that definitive treatment be minimally invasive and active attempts be made to reduce recurrences by approaches that lower the saturation of urine with cystine and increasing the solubility of cystine in urine.

References

1. Knoll T, Zollner A, Wendt-Nordahl G, Michel MS, Alken P. Cystinuria in childhood and adolescence: recommendations for diagnosis, treatment and follow-up. Pediatr Nephrol. 2005;20:19–24.
2. Assimos DG, Leslie SW, Ng C, Streem SB, Hart LJ. The impact of cystinuria on renal function. J Urol. 2002;168:27–30.
3. Tiselius HG. New horizons in the management of patients with cystinuria. Curr Opin Urol. 2010;20:169–73.
4. Chillarón J, Font-Llitjos M, Fort J, Zorzano A, Goldfarb DS, Nunes V, Palacin M. Pathophysiology and treatment of cystinuria. Nat Rev Nephrol. 2010;6:424–34.
5. Boutros M, Vicanek C, Rozen R, Goodyer P. Transient neonatal cystinuria. Kidney Int. 2005;67(2):443–8.
6. Scriver CR, Beaudet AL, Sly WS, Valle D, Palacin M, Goodyer P, Nunes V, Gasparini P, editors. The metabolic and molecular bases of inherited disease. New York: McGraw-Hill; 2001. p. 4909–32.
7. Palacin M, Borsani G, Sebastio G. The molecular bases of cystinuria and lysinuric protein intolerance. Curr Opin Genet Dev. 2001;11:328–35.
8. Rosenberg LE, Durant JL, Holland JM. Intestinal absorption and renal extraction of cystine and cysteine in cystinuria. N Engl J Med. 1965;273:1239–45.
9. Their S, Fox M, Segal S, Rosenberg LE. Cystinuria: in vitro demonstration of an intestinal transport defect. Science. 1964;143:482–4.
10. Goodyer P. The molecular basis of cystinuria. Nephron Exp Nephrol. 2004;98(2):e45–9.
11. Coe FL, Favus MJ, Pak CYC, Parks JH, Preminger GM, Tiselius HG, editors. Kidney stones: medical and surgical management. Philadelphia: Lippincott-Raven Publishers; 1996. p. 33–64.
12. Evan AP. Physiology and etiology of stone formation in the kidney and the urinary tract. Pediatr Nephrol. 2010;25:831–41.
13. Biyani SB, Cartledge JJ. Cystinuria – diagnosis and management. EAU-EBU Update Series. 2006;4:175–83.
14. Wagner CA, Lang F, Broeer S. Function and structure of heterodimeric amino acid transporters. Am J Physiol Cell Physiol. 2001;281:C1077–93.
15. Wagner CH, Mohebbi N. Urinary pH and stone formation. J Nephrol. 2010;23 Suppl 16:165–9.
16. Dent CE, Senior B. Studies on the treatment of cystinuria. Br J Urol. 1955;27(4):317–32.
17. Goldfarb DS, Coe FL, Asplin JR. Urinary cystine excretion and capacity in patients with cystinuria. Kidney Int. 2006;69(6):1041–7.
18. Nakagawa Y, Asplin JR, Goldfarb DS, Parks JH, Coe FL. Clinical use of cystine supersaturation measurements. J Urol. 2000;164(5):1481–5.
19. Pak CY, Fuller C, Sakhaee K, Zerwekh JE, Adams BV. Management of cystine nephrolithiasis with alpha-mercaptopropionylglycin. J Urol. 1986;136:1003–8.
20. Feliubadaló L, Arbonés ML, Mañas S, Chillarón J, Visa J, Rodés M, et al. SLC7A9-deficient mice develop cystinuria non-I and cystine urolithiasis. Hum Mol Genet. 2003;12:2097–108.
21. Rodman JS, Blackburn P, Williams JJ, Brown A, Pospischil MA, Peterson CM. The effect of dietary protein on cystine excretion in patients with cystinuria. Clin Nephrol. 1984;22(6):273–8.
22. Evan AP, Coe FL, Lingeman JE, Shao Y, Matlaga BR, Kim SC, et al. Renal crystal deposits and histopathology in patients with cystine stones. Kidney Int. 2006;69:2227–35.
23. Feliubadalo L, Font M, Purroy J, Rosaud F, Estivill X, Nunes V, et al. Non-type I cystinuria caused by mutations in SLC7A9, encoding a subunit ($b^{o,+}$AT) of rBAT. International Cystinuria Consortium. Nat Genet. 1999;23:52–7.
24. Font-Llitjos M, Jimenez-Vidal M, Bisceglia L, Di Perna M, De Sanctis L, Rousaud F, et al. New insights into cystinuria: 40 new mutations, genotype-phenotype correlation, and digenic inheritance causing partial phenotype. J Med Genet. 2005;42:58–68.
25. Calogne MJ, Gasparini P, Chillaron J, Chillon M, Gallucci M, Rosaud F, et al. Cystinuria caused by mutations in rBAT, a gene involved in the transport of cysteine. Nat Genet. 1994;6:420–5.
26. Pras E, Kreiss Y, Frishberg Y, Prosen L, Aksentijevich I, Kastner DL. Refined mapping of the CSBU3 gene to a 1,8-Mb region on chromosome 19q13.1 using historical recombinants in Lybian Jewish cystinuria patients. Genomics. 1999;60:248–50.
27. Rosenberg LE, Downing S, Durant JL, Segal S. Cystinuria: biochemical evidence for three genetically distinct diseases. J Clin Invest. 1966;45:365–71.
28. Dello Strologo L, Pras E, Pontesilli C, Beccia E, Ricci-Barbini V, De Sanctis L, et al. Comparison between SLC3A1 and SLC7A9 cystinuria patients and carriers: a need for a new classification. J Am Soc Nephrol. 2002;13:2547–53.
29. Bhatta KM, Prien Jr EL, Dretler SP. Cystine calculi – rough and smooth: a new clinical distinction. J Urol. 1989;142:937–40.
30. Saw KC, McAteer JA, Monga AG, Chua GT, Lingeman JE, Williams Jr JC. Helical CT of urinary calculi: effect of stone composition, stone size, and scan collimation. AJR Am J Roentgenol. 2000;175:329–32.
31. Boll DT, Patil NA, Paulson EK, Merkle EM, Simmons WN, Pierre SA, et al. Renal stone assessment with dual-energy multidetector CT and advanced postprocessing techniques: improved characterization of renal stone composition – pilot study. Radiology. 2009;250(3):813–20.
32. Daudon M, Cohen-Solal F, Barbey F, Gagnadoux MF, Knebelmann B, Jungers P. Cystine crystal volume determination: a useful tool in the management of cystinuric patients. Urol Res. 2003;31(3):207–11.
33. Sakhae K, Poindexter JR, Pak CY. The spectrum of metabolic abnormalities in patients with cystine nephrolithiasis. J Urol. 1989;141(4):819–21.
34. Guillen M, Corella D, Cabello ML, Garcia AM, Hernandez-Yago J. Reference values of urinary excretion of cystine and dibasic amino

acids: classification of patients with cystinuria in the Valencian Community, Spain. Clin Biochem. 1999;32:25–30.
35. Pietrow PK, Auge BK, Weizer AZ, Delvecchio FC, Silverstein AD, Mathias B, et al. Durability of the medical management of cystinuria. J Urol. 2003;169(1):68–70.
36. Rimer JD, Zhihua A, Zhu Z, Lee MH, Goldfarb DS, Wesson JA, et al. Crystal growth inhibitors for the prevention of L-cystine kidney stones through molecular design. Science. 2010;330:337–41.
37. Monnens LA, Noordam K, Trijbels F. Necessary practical treatment of cystinuria at night. Pediatr Nephrol. 2000;14:1148–9.
38. Fjellstedt E, Denneberg T, Jeppson JO, Christensson A, Tiselius HG. Cystine analyses of separate day and night urine as a basis for the management of patients with homozygous cystinuria. Urol Res. 2001;29:303–10.
39. Türk C, Knoll T, Petrik A, Sarica K, Straub M, Seitz C. Guidelines on urolithiasis (update 2011) [online]. 2011. Link: http://www.uroweb.org/gls/pdf/18_Urolithiasis.pdf. Accessed on Aug 30.
40. Rutchik SD, Resnick MI. Cystine calculi: diagnosis and management. Urol Clin North Am. 1997;24:163.
41. Jaeger P, Portmann L, Saunders A, Rosenberg LE, Their SO. Anticystinuric effects of glutamine and of dietary sodium restriction. N Engl J Med. 1986;315:1120–3.
42. Jaeger P. Cystinuria: pathophysiology and treatment. Adv Nephrol Necker Hosp. 1989;18:107.
43. Ng CS, Streem SB. Contemporary management of cystinuria. J Endourol. 1999;13:647–51.
44. Rodriguez LM, Santos F, Malaga S, Martinez V. Effect of a low sodium diet on urinary elimination of cystine in cystinuric children. Nephron. 1995;71:416–8.
45. Fjellstedt E, Denneberg T, Jeppsson JO, Tiselius HG. A comparison of the effects of potassium citrate and sodium bicarbonate in the alkalinization of urine in homozygous cystinuria. Urol Res. 2001; 29(5):295–302.
46. Sterret SP, Penniston KL, Wolf Jr JS, Nakada SY. Azetazolamide is an effect adjunct for urinary alkalinization in patients with uric acid and cystine stone formation recalcitrant to potassium citrate. Urology. 2008;72:278–81.
47. Lotz M, Potts Jr JT, Holland JM, Kiser WS, Bartter FC. D-penicillamine therapy in cystinuria. J Urol. 1966;95:257.
48. Chow GK, Streem SB. Medical treatment of cystinuria: results of contemporary clinical practice. J Urol. 1996;156:1576–8.
49. Harbar JA, Cusworth DC, Lawes LC, Wrong OM. Comparison of 2-mercaptopropionylglycine and D-Penicillamine in the treatment of cystinuria. J Urol. 1986;136:146–9.
50. DeBerardinis RJ, Coughlin 2nd CR, Kaplan P. Penicillamine therapy for pediatric cystinuria: experience from a cohort of American children. J Urol. 2009;180:2620–3.
51. Wendt-Nordahl G, Meister L, Michel S, Knoll T. Evaluation of alkalinization and chelating agent therapy for cystinuria in animal model [abstract #340]. Eur Urol. 2009;S8:205.
52. DelloStrologo L, Laurenzi C, Legato A, Pastore A. Cystinuria in children and young adults: success of monitoring free-cystine urine levels. Pediatr Nephrol. 2007;22(11):1869–73.
53. Cohen TD, Streem SB, Hall P. Clinical effect of captopril on the formation and growth of cystine calculi. J Urol. 1995;154:164–6.
54. Perazella MA, Buller GK. Successful treatment of cystinuria with captopril. Am J Kidney Dis. 1993;21:504–7.
55. Michelakakis H, Delis D, Anastasiadou V, Bartsocas C. Ineffectiveness of captopril in reducing cystine excretion in cystinuric children. J Inherit Metab Dis. 1993;16:1042–3.
56. Birwe H, Schneeberger W, Hesse A. Investigations of the efficacy of ascorbic acid therapy in cystinuria. Urol Res. 1991;19(3):199–201.
57. Ragone R. Medical treatment of cystinuria with vitamin C. Am J Kidney Dis. 2000;35(5):1020.
58. Traxer O, Huet B, Poindexter JR, Pak CY, Pearle MS. Effect of ascorbic acid consumption on urinary stone risk factors. J Urol. 2003;170:397–401.
59. Chow GK, Streem SB. Contemporary urological intervention for cystinuric patients: immediate and long-term impact and implications. J Urol. 1998;160:341–4.
60. Kachel TA, Vijan SR, Dretler SP. Endourological experience with cystine calculi and a treatment algorithm. J Urol. 1991;145:25–8.
61. Brinkmann OA, Griehl A, Kuwertz-Broking E, Bulla M, Hertle L. Extracorporeal shock wave lithotripsy in children. Efficacy, complications and long-term follow-up. Eur Urol. 2001;39:591–7.
62. Muslumanoglu AY, Tefekli A, Sarilar O, Binbay M, Altunrende F, Ozkuvanci U. Extracorporeal shock wave lithotripsy as first line treatment alternative for urinary tract stones in children: a large retrospective analysis. J Urol. 2003;170:2405–8.
63. Argyropoulos AN, Tolley DA. Evaluation of outcome following lithotripsy. Curr Opin Urol. 2010;20(2):154–8.
64. Knoll T, Musial A, Trojan L, Ptashnyk T, Michel MS, Alken P, et al. Measurement of renal anatomy for prediction of lower-pole caliceal stone clearance: reproducibility of different parameters. J Endourol. 2003;17(7):447–51.
65. Preminger GM. Management of lower pole renal calculi: shock wave lithotripsy versus percutaneous nephrolithotomy versus flexible ureteroscopy. Urol Res. 2006;34(2):108–11.
66. Pearle MS, Lingeman JE, Leveillee R, Kuo R, Preminger GM, Nadler RB, et al. Prospective, randomized trial comparing shock wave lithotripsy and ureteroscopy for lower pole caliceal calculi 1 cm or less. J Urol. 2005;173(6):2005–9.
67. Ruggera L, Zanin M, Beltrami P, Zattoni F. Retrograde transureteral approach: a safe and efficient treatment for recurrent cystine renal stones. Urol Res. 2011;39(5):411–5.
68. Kourambas J, Munver R, Preminger GM. Ureterorenoscopic management of recurrent renal cystine calculi. J Endourol. 2000; 14(6):489–92.
69. Schuster TG, Russell KY, Bloom DA, Koo HP, Faerber GJ. Ureteroscopy for the treatment of urolithiasis in children. J Urol. 2002;167(4):1813.
70. Scoffone CM, Cracco CM, Cossu M, Grande S, Poggio M, Scarpa RM. Endoscopic combined intrarenal surgery in Galdakao-modified supine Valdivia position: a new standard for percutaneous nephrolithotomy? Eur Urol. 2008;54(6):1393–403.
71. Lahme S, Zimmermanns V, Hochmuth A, Janitzki V. Minimally invasive PCNL (Mini-perc). Alternative treatment modality or replacement of conventional PCNL? Urologe A. 2008;47(5):563–8. [Article in German].
72. Lahme S, Bichler KH, Strohmaier WL, Götz T. Minimally invasive PCNL in patients with renal pelvic and calyceal stones. Eur Urol. 2001;40(6):619–24.
73. Schuster TK, Smaldone MC, Averch TD, Ost MC. Percutaneous nephrolithotomy in children. J Endourol. 2009;23(10):1699–705.
74. Oezalp I, Coskun T, Tokol S, Demircin G, Moench E. Inherited metabolic disorders in Turkey. J Inherit Metab Dis. 1990; 13(5):732–8.
75. Tanzer F, Ozgur A, Bardakci F. Type I cystinuria and its genetic basis in a population of Turkish school children. Int J Urol. 2007;14(10):914–7.
76. Cabello ML, Guillen M. Pilot screening programme for cystinuria in the Valencian community. Eur J Epidemiol. 1999;15:681–4.
77. Dello Strologo L, Rizzoni G. Cystinuria. Acta Paediatr Suppl. 2006;95(452):31–3.

78. Turner B, Brown DA. Amino acid excretion in infancy and early childhood. A survey of 200,000 infants. Med J Aust. 1972; 1(2):62–5.
79. Hyanek J. Cystinurie. Dědičné metabolické poruchy. Praha: Avicenum. 1991; 53–58.
80. Scriver CR, Clow CL, Reade TM, Goodyer P, Auray-Blais C, Giguere R, et al. Ontogeny modifies manifestations of cystinuria genes: implications for counseling. J Pediatr. 1985;106(3):411–6.
81. Ito H, Murakami M, Miyauchi T, Mori I, Yamaguchi K, Usui T, et al. The incidence of cystinuria in Japan. J Urol. 1983;129(5):1012–4.
82. Scriver CR, Beaudet AL, Sly WS, Valle D, Segal S, Thier SO, editors. The metabolic and molecular bases of inherited disease. New York: McGraw-Hill; 1995. p. 3581–601.

The Detection and Management of Primary Hyperparathyroidism in Patients with Urolithiasis

93

Mumtaz Jamshed Khan, Syed Raziuddin Biyabani, Nuzhat Faruqui, and Jamsheer Jehangir Talati

Abstract

This chapter discusses the variable presentation of primary hyperparathyroidism and the association of this disease with urinary tract stone formation, methods for detection and screening of hyperparathyroidism and treatment of hypercalcemia, anatomical variations in position and number of parathyroids, parathyroid hyperfunction in pregnancy, and indications for parathyroidectomy.

Keywords

Primary hyperparathyroidism • Renal stones • Hypercalcemia • Bone disease • Diverse disease spectrum • Pregnancy • Vitamin D • Methylene blue • Parathyroidectomy • Pregnancy

Introduction

In the advanced industrialized world, primary hyperparathyroidism (PHPT) is detected through screening programs. It is treated early in the course of the disease, in about 1 % of the general population [1], often before stones develop.

Because of early diagnosis, PHPT is detected infrequently in stone formers—in 1972–1978, in only 0.178 % of stone formers in the USA [2] and in 1980, in 1.6 % of stone formers in Belgium. This is in contrast to the 8 % in whom stones were noted in 1934 [2].

The detection of PHPT is ordinarily difficult, because hypercalcemia (the initial test used to raise suspicion about its presence) can be intermittent and requires repeated tests over time to detect it. Additionally, in countries where vitamin D deficiency is widespread, patients do not always develop diagnostic levels of hypercalcemia. In such circumstances, diagnosis can be delayed for as many as 1–16 years [3, 4].

At other times, bizarre presentations with giant cell tumors of the maxilla and tibia and a raised parathyroid hormone level may yet again be associated with a normal calcium level [5].

Because of the role of parathyroid glands in stone formation and recurrence, knowledge of all aspects of parathyroid gland disease is essential for all urologists. This chapter therefore describes the disease spectrum, diagnostic tests, and options for management of hypercalcemia and hyperparathyroidism, including the specifics of managing the disease in pregnancy.

Definition

Primary hyperparathyroidism (PHPT) is a syndrome characterized by elevated serum calcium, low or low-normal serum phosphorus, and elevated parathyroid hormone (PTH).

M.J. Khan, M.D., FACS (✉)
Department of Otolaryngology, Head and Neck Institute, Cleveland Clinic Foundation, 9500 Euclid Ave., Cleveland, OH 44195, USA
e-mail: khanm6@ccf.org

S.R. Biyabani, M.B.B.S., FCPS (Urol), FEBU • N. Faruqui, M.B.B.S., FCPS(Urology), FEBU • J.J. Talati, M.B.B.S., FRCS
Section of Urology, Department of Surgery, The Aga Khan University, Stadium Road, 3500, Karachi, Sindh 74800, Pakistan
e-mail: raziuddin.biyabani@aku.edu; nuzhat.faruqui@aku.edu; jamsheer.talati@aku.edu

Electronic supplementary material The online version of this chapter (doi:10.1007/978-1-4471-4387-1_93) contains supplementary material, which is available to authorized users.

J.J. Talati et al. (eds.), *Urolithiasis*,
DOI 10.1007/978-1-4471-4387-1_93, © Springer-Verlag London 2012

Hypercalciuria is not an essential feature, as urinary calcium excretion is normal in 30 % of patients. This is because PTH increases reabsorption of calcium, and hypercalciuria occurs only when the amount of filtered calcium exceeds the reabsorptive capacity. The prefix primary denotes that the changes result from autonomous hypersecretion of PTH and are not secondary to vitamin D deficiency, renal failure, or other causes.

The Association Between Stone Formation and Primary Hyperparathyroidism

Frequency of Stones in Patients with PHPT

Stones were present in 60 % of PHPT patients in the 1940s [6]. At the end of the last century, there was a ~50 % chance that a patient with PHPT had an upper urinary tract stone [7, 8], although Bilezikian [6] suggests this had already dropped to 15–20 %. Purnell et al. [9] also agrees that stones are found in 50 % of PHPT patients but are metabolically active only in 10 %. In 2008, an ultrasound examination of all (271) PHPT patients disclosed stones in only 7 %, although this was four times more common than in controls [10].

Today, PHPT has widely different patterns of presentation across the world, with stones present in 40–60 % of PHPT patients in recently industrialized countries such as China (Bilezikian), Pakistan [11], and India (Table 93.1) [12].

But it is not just stones that the urologist/lithotomist will need to worry about. In addition to stones, HPT causes a number of symptoms: proximal muscle weakness, a general feeling of "not feeling well," abdominal pain, and a spectrum of mild to severe bone pain, accompanied by structural changes in bones. Some of these symptoms are dramatically reversed once the offending parathyroid tissue has been removed.

Most asymptomatic patients in the West also have numerous symptoms. These include fatigue, exhaustion, weakness, polydipsia, polyuria, nocturia, joint pain, bone pain, constipation, depression, anorexia, nausea, heartburn, and associated conditions. Moreover, hematuria was shown by Chan to occur more frequently in PHPT than in controls, and this abnormality disappeared after surgery [13].

In the countries, only recently emerging from poverty, associated bone disease is common. This pathology causes considerable problems in reestablishing calcium homeostasis following surgery. In Pakistan [11], two-thirds of patients have bone disease, and in Indian adolescents [14], this can be severe, with the full-blown picture of osteitis fibrosa cystica. The brown tumors of osteitis fibrosa cystica are still seen, albeit infrequently (8 cases in 15 years in 1 unit) in Adis Abbaba et al. [15] and Pakistan [11]. Less severe forms of bone changes, such as osteopenia/osteoporosis, are seen even in industrialized countries [16].

Whether or not the hyperparathyroid state is responsible for the stone has now become a subject of some debate. Diaz et al. [16] has shown that stone recurrence is rare after parathyroidectomy, except when there are residual stones. In Chan's series [13], only 5.3 % patients failed to have any improvement in symptoms or associated conditions following parathyroidectomy. This suggests that PHPT does play an important role in stone formation. However, Mollerup and Lindwald, studying 297 patients, showed that 30 % formed 1–4 stones in 5 years [7].

Why Are Stones Common in PHPT and Why Do Only Some PHPT Patients Form Stones?

Hypercalciuria is the most commonly provided explanation for stone formation in PHPT.

However, Berger et al. [17] has noted that there is no difference in the 24-h urinary excretion of metabolites between those with and without stone and that the vast majority of patients with hypercalcemia and hypercalciuria do not form stones. Rejnmark et al. [18] noted that while the risk for hospitalization for renal stone formation is increased in patients with PHPT (compared to those without PHPT) prior to surgery, surprisingly the risk for stone remains elevated for 10 years post parathyroidectomy but at a lower rate that is equivalent to that of calculi in other patients. Similarly, surgery reduces postoperative urinary calcium, but it still remains elevated beyond the normal [18].

Bilezikian, too, was unable to show any distinctive biochemical difference between those with and without stones, which were seen in only 18 % of his series. Broadus et al. [19] studying 50 PHPT patients noted that 63 % of those with hyperabsorption of calcium, hypercalciuria on the calcium tolerance test, and marked elevations in vitamin D had stones, as against only 15 % of those with normal levels of vitamin D and normocalciuria. Diaz et al. [16] found higher values of parathyroid hormone, alkaline phosphatase, osteocalcin, and Cl/P ratio in patients with stones versus stone-free PHPT patients.

Others have found differences in the single nucleotide polymorphisms (SNPs) of the calcium-sensing receptor (CASR) gene at the regulatory region known to be associated with idiopathic calcium nephrolithiasis. A study of 332 patients and 453 controls [20] showed that PHPT patients with the AA/AA or AA/GG genotype had an increased stone incidence and higher serum ionized calcium and parathyroid hormone than patients with the GG/GG diplotype ($P=0.049$). Patients with AA/AA or AA/GG diplotype were

Table 93.1 Presentation of primary hyperparathyroidism in cities in the USA, China, Pakistan, and India

	New York [6]	Beijing [6]	Karachi [11]	India [4]	India [12]	India [14]
Age	Within 10 years of menopause		38 ± 13 years	36.38 ± 12.73 years	33.5 + 8.82 (21–55 years)	Children and adolescents 17.73 (13–20) years
Serum calcium (mg/dL)	10.5 + 1	12 mg/dL	12.23 ± 1.92	(Elevated in 86.5 %)	12.55 ± 1.77 mg/dL	
Serum phosphorus (mg/dL)			2.3 ± 0.84		1.81 ± 0.682	
PTH × upper limit of normal value (pg/mL)	1.5–2 × *N* (118 + 9 pg/mL)	20 × *N*	Up to 2,900 × *N*		866 ± 799.15 (up to 3,820)	
Bone involvement	Detected by bone dexa scan	60 %	34 % bone disease alone, 28.5 % bone and stone disease together	46	In 75 %	86.7 % osteitis fibrosa cystica in 33.3 %
Kidney stones in vitamin D av	60 % in the 1940s now 15–20 %	42 % (21 % bilateral)	31 % stone disease alone, 28.5 % stone and bone disease together	21	40.50 %	40 %
	21 ng/mL	8.8 ng/mL	7.17 ng/mL			
Hungry bones	NA	NA	NA	59 %	30 % alkaline phosphatase 762 (50–4,930) IU/L	
Delay in diagnosis	NA	NA	NA	1 month to 16 years	1 month to 10 years	
Nodule in neck	NA	NA	0 % increase vascularity from enlarged inferior thyroid artery causes prominence of ipsilateral thyroid lobe	19 %	NA	13.30 %

Note: The figures in brackets refer to the references in the text

younger—their age groups were in the lowest tertile and their calcium in the highest tertile [20].

Tests to Detect Hyperparathyroidism

There is consensus that in countries with adequate supplementation of foods with vitamin D, estimating the ionized serum calcium level is an appropriate first step to detecting PHPT. As ionized calcium is not routinely measured in clinical laboratories, albumin is simultaneously estimated, and serum calcium is corrected upward by 0.8 mg/dL (0.2 mmol/L) for every 1 g depletion of serum albumin, as suggested by Bilezikian or by other formulae. As the parathyroid gland consists of discontinuously replicating cells [21], the serum calcium also fluctuates and can be in the normal range at the time the blood sample is drawn. Hence, repeated measurements of the calcium level are important. Once hypercalcemia (defined by a rise of 1 mg/dL—0.25 mmol/L—above the upper normal limit) is identified, the diagnosis is clinched by demonstrating concurrent elevated serum calcium and inappropriately raised PTH concentrations. Physiologically, the parathyroid is geared to reduce secretion when the calcium levels rise. Raised PTH levels in the presence of hypercalcemia indicate a degree of autonomy, and hence, a diagnosis of PHPT can be made with confidence. Serum phosphorous is low, but this is not diagnostic.

In a stone patient, when hypercalcemia is detected, it is probably due to PHPT, as the other causes such as vitamin D intoxication, malignancy, and sarcoidosis are infrequent. Nevertheless, they need to be excluded by the patient's medical history or by other tests.

Benign idiopathic familial hypocalciuric hypercalcemia (IFHH) should be considered in differential diagnosis of hypercalcemia, especially in children, as PHPT is rare at this age. In Chap. 95, Lynn provides a useful formula to identify these patients. From a urologist's standpoint, however, IFHH is not associated with urinary tract stones, and a raised serum calcium together with normal urinary calcium will be found in other family members as well. Rarely mutation of both alleles of the CaSR may result in infantile hyperparathyroidism, in which case urinary calcium is likely to be increased.

Of the different assays available, intact PTH molecule (IPTH) assay is the best, particularly in the presence of renal impairment. Renal failure delays the excretion of endocrinologically inactive fragments of PTH, which may be detected by other methods. The PTH estimation should be combined with a repeat serum calcium analysis as this will detect the occasional patient with hypercalcemia and normal—but inappropriately high— PTH levels, which clinch the diagnosis of PHPT.

Screening for PHPT

As shown earlier, operation on screened populations found to have PHPT has reduced the frequency of stone disease in PHPT. Screening of entire elderly female populations yields a high pickup rate and has definite advantages, by reducing the numbers of patients with severe forms of PHPT and stones. Such screening approaches in the elderly would not be cost-effective in developing countries from the point of view of preventing stone disease before it occurs, as stone disease occurs in younger patients, and is complicated by vitamin D deficiency. Nevertheless *every stone patient* should have ionized serum calcium measured.

Screening by serum calcium estimation costs well under USD 10 in the developing world and is more cost-effective than screening by PTH analysis. Abnormal values of calcium lead to estimation of serum PTH and simultaneously serum calcium and phosphorous to confirm PHPT. PTH estimation is an expensive test and cannot be used as the first-line test for screening, as it would detect a large number of vitamin D-deficient patients with secondary hyperparathyroidism, in addition to patients with HPT secondary to renal failure.

Mass screening for PHPT through serum calcium estimation will also not be effective unless care is taken to define the target population. For example, mass screening of hospitalized patients is ineffective. In this setting, the majority of hypercalcemics has a malignancy or is on calcium carbonate as an antacid because of chronic renal failure.

Mass screening in hospital practice when not clinically indicated has not only a poor yield, it is likely to be associated with a failure to seek out and note the result or take action if high calcium levels are found. Shek et al. [22] found hypercalcemia in 1.6 % of 29,107 hospitalized-patient samples, confirmed in a second sample from 183 (60 %) of 302 accessible patients. Only 5.5 % of these 302 patients had PHPT, yielding 15 patients from screening 29,107 samples.

We fail to detect more than five hyperfunctioning parathyroids a year. The frequency of PHPT detection is low in India too—one unit saw 79 patients in 22 years (1986–2008), an average of 4/year; another unit reported 52 cases in 13 years [4]. Western units commonly see 40–70/year. This raises the question: Are PHPT patients being missed in the developing world?

Tests for Screening Urolithiasis Patients in Vitamin D-Deficient Countries

Because of the low yield from serum calcium investigation, it has been suggested that patients in vitamin D-deficient countries should have their phosphate excretion index, fractional calcium excretion, and chloride/phosphate ratios estimated to enhance detection rates. Parks et al. [23] suggests that stone formers with even slight hypercalcemia and brisk hypercalciuria probably have this curable disease.

Clinical Spectrum of the Disease

Primary hyperparathyroidism is caused by a single parathyroid gland in up to 96 % of cases [24]. Most cases are due to single adenomas; some due to more than one adenoma or hyperplasia. Carcinoma is rare. In our initial series at Aga Khan University, PHPT was detected in 1.25 % of patients with stones, 88.6 % were from adenomas, 5.7 % from hyperplasia, and 5.7 % due to carcinomas.

Bilezikian draws attention to the divergent spectrum of this disease across the world [6] and states that in countries that have been industrialized for a long period of time, the typical PHPT patient has a serum calcium of 11.7 mg/dL (2.93 mmol/L) (normal up to 10.7 mg/dL or 2.68 mmol/L), a serum phosphorus of 2.8 mg/dL (0.90 mmol/L) (normal range 2.5–4.5 mg/dL; 0.81–1.45 mmol/L), and a PTH immunoradiometric assay of 119 ± 7 pg/mL (normal 10–65). Only 18 % have stones, 1 % have radiologically evident bone disease, and most are asymptomatic. Bone mineral density, however, shows the evidence for PHPT. In India and Pakistan, the picture is different (see Table 93.1).

In Pakistan [11], patients are younger (57 % <40 years—mean age 38 ± 13 years) as also in India (mean age 36.38 ± 12.73) [4]. Both India and Pakistan see few patients per unit—in India one unit recorded 52 cases in 13 years. In India, renal calculi were found in 40.5 % and proximal muscle weakness in 45.5 %. Biochemical features included hypercalcemia (total corrected calcium 12.55 ± 1.77 mg/dL; 3.14 ± 0.44 mmol/L), a very low inorganic phosphorus (1.81 ± 0.682 mg/dL; 0.58 ± 0.22 mmol/L), elevated total alkaline phosphatase (mean: 762.2; median: 559; range: 50–4,930 IU/L), and high parathyroid hormone (PTH) (mean ± SD: 866.61 ± 799.15; median: 639.5; range: 52–3,820 pg/mL). Postoperative hungry bone disease was seen in 30.3 %, and transient hypoparathyroidism developed in 62 % patients postoperatively [12].

Parathyroid surgery for all causes is infrequently done in Pakistan. In one series, 0.055 % of the total surgical output (67,566 operations) was for PHPT [11].

In China, the clinical picture is very similar to that in India and Pakistan [6] (see Table 93.1).

Another notable regional difference has been reported by George et al. from India who noted primary hyperparathyroidism (PHPT) in children and adolescents—normally a rather rare condition [14].

They found 15 children and adolescents (age <20 year) with PHPT in a period of 13 years. The mean age of the patients was 17.73 years (range: 13–20), with a M:F ratio of 1:4. Average duration of symptoms was 18.87 (range: 0–48) months. Clinical features at presentation included calculi in 40 %, bone pain in 86.67 %, palpable neck swelling in 13.3 %, proximal myopathy in 46.67 %, bony deformities in 53.33 %, fractures in 60 %, palpable osteitis fibrosa cystica in 33.3 %, and acute pancreatitis in 6.67 %. None had positive family history or features suggestive of multiple endocrine neoplasia (MEN). Histopathology confirmed adenoma in all cases. Postoperative hungry bone syndrome occurred in 33.3 %.

It is unusual to be able to palpate the enlarged parathyroid clinically. The mean weight of a normal parathyroid gland is 33.1 mg, and its mean measurements 6.7×3.9×2.0 mm [25] (it is easier to remember an approximation: 1–2×3–4×5–6 mm), and even large adenomas are seldom palpable because of their deep placement in the neck. However, the blood flow to the gland is increased many fold, and this causes the inferior thyroid artery to enlarge, and often the thyroid lobe on the side of the adenoma is felt on clinical examination to be enlarged. In George's series of below 20-year-old PHPT patients, 13 % had a palpable neck mass. And there is at least one other published report [26] where the gland was felt, and yet another reported in the appended case scenario (see later).

Management of Hypercalcemia in a Patient with Stone Disease and PHPT

Detection of hypercalcemia during metabolic investigation of a stone patient brings to attention the possibility that the patient may have primary hyperparathyroidism (PHPT).

The cause of hypercalcemia under such circumstances is most likely PHPT, and this is confirmed by estimation of PTH. In PHPT, it is raised. In hypercalcemia of malignancy, PTH is not elevated. Hypercalcemia with suppressed PTH might also be caused by vitamin D intoxication, milk alkali syndrome, and adrenal insufficiency. Secondary hyperparathyroidism is associated with a low serum calcium and not hypercalcemia.

While investigating the patients and preparing them for surgical or other options for treatment of calculi, the urgency of treating the hypercalcemia needs to be determined. Not all levels of serum calcium require urgent management. When the calcium has to be lowered, the approach depends upon the level of calcium and the symptoms. Calcium levels can be lowered by hydration, loop diuretics, and reduction of osteoclastic activity. All causes of severe hypercalcemia involve osteoclastic bone absorption, and calcium absorption from the gastrointestinal (GI) tract is usually not a major factor, except in cases associated with vitamin D [27].

At times, a rapid lowering of calcium level is required for a patient with hypercalcemia who needs urgent surgery for decompression of an obstructed kidney. The level at which intervention is required to lower calcium depends upon its rate of rise, the degree of symptoms, and the patient's age. Hypercalcemia has greater adverse effects on the elderly and in those in whom the calcium has risen rapidly. Patients vary in their response to elevated serum calcium. Symptoms usually start at 11.5–12 mg/dL (2.9–3 mmol/L). A serum calcium of <11.2 mg/dL (<2.8 mmol/L) requires assessment of symptoms, but most often does not require urgent treatment. Elevations above 15 mg/dL (3.75 mmol/L) need to be promptly brought down, as these levels are associated with coma and cardiac arrest. Readers are referred to Bilezikian's excellent review [27].

In Pakistani patients, PHPT often has existed for many months as patients delay visits to doctors. The patients therefore are active, alert, and unaffected by much higher calcium levels.

For nonurgent mild hypercalcemia, an increase in fluid intake (with no change in diet) is recommended. For moderately elevated levels >1 mg/dL (0.025 mmol/dL) above normal, furosemide or any other loop diuretic (which reduces the reabsorption of calcium, which is occurring under the influence of PTH) may be added to vigorous hydration, if necessary by intravenous drip. If the serum calcium is 13.5 mg/dL (3.38 mmol/L) or above, then in addition to adequate hydration and 10–20 mg of furosemide every 6–12 h, Bilezikian recommends the use of (1) pamidronate, 40–60 mg, intravenously over 2 h; (2) calcitonin, 4MRC U/kg; (3) plicamycin (mithramycin), 15–25 μg/kg over 4–6 h; or (4) glucocorticosteroids, 200–300 mg hydrocortisone intravenously for 3–5 days to further reduce the serum calcium by inhibiting osteoclastic resorption. Pamidronate could cause problems in postoperative management by causing a low serum calcium. Phitayakorn and McHenry [28] used bisphosphonates in 2.8 % of 292 patients needing parathyroidectomy and noted that it lowered mortality to 0 % as compared to the historical 7 % mortality in 1978–2008.

Which Patients with Renal Stones and PHPT Should Be Subjected to Parathyroidectomy?

As in every case of hypercalcemia, one has to additionally treat the underlying disorder. When due to PHPT, surgery (parathyroidectomy) is indicated. Endocrinology literature categorically supports surgical treatment for "virtually all" patients with PHPT who have specific end-organ signs or symptoms [1, 2].

The benefits of surgery in these patients have been well established, including improvements in bone density and fracture rates, cognitive function and quality of life, and reduction in kidney stone incidence [1, 2]. Lynn's chapter (Chap. 95) lists the indications for operation in asymptomatic patients.

Every patient with proven PHPT, even if they have no residual stones after stone surgery or only a small asymptomatic stone, must have a parathyroidectomy. While some authors have questioned the relationship between PHPT and stone disease and recurrence, liberal indications for parathyroidectomy are justified by the finding in longitudinal cohort studies that asymptomatic PHPT patients will exhibit significant decrease in bone density at 12 years follow-up. Silverberg et al. [29] found that 60 % of untreated patients will lose 10 % of their bone density.

Parathyroid surgery is a definitive treatment of PHPT and is cost-effective for patients with a life expectancy of 5 years. Pharmacological therapy is not a cost-effective option unless the annual cost of medication is <$221 (in 2005 dollars). Surgery is less costly than medical treatment when the time interval for medical treatment exceeds 5.5 years [2]. Granted, 10 % of patients may die within a year of parathyroidectomy [30]. But, patients with more severe forms of PHPT (55 % of the patients who had a hypercalcemic crises and 24 % of the patients with cystic bone changes) had died, while only 4 % of patients in the renal stone group died. Yet when not operated on, even the asymptomatic cases progress. Chan et al. [13], as mentioned, has shown that on questioning and after an ultrasound examination of the kidneys, few are "asymptomatic."

Parathyroidectomy Definitively Corrects Biochemical Abnormalities and Improves Bone Density. But Does It Prevent Further Stone Formation?

The consensus view is that parathyroidectomy in PHPT patients with stones is rewarding, as patients will remain stone-free or show a decrease in the number of stones formed. Nephrocalcinosis and preexisting stones may also disappear, and new stone formation has been shown to decrease from 0.36 to 0.02 per patient year in Deaconson's series and from 0.24 to 0.05 per patient year in McGeown's series [31, 32].

However, the results of surgery are not always excellent. Some may have double adenomas. Others feel that surgery does not guarantee freedom from recurrence—45 % of patients with hyperplasia may reform their stones, though patients with adenoma have a greater tendency to remain stone-free. Starr et al. report [33] that 2 of their 52 patients had appropriate intraoperative IPTH levels but yet had persisting hypercalcemia postoperatively, with 4.8 % failure rate in correction of serum calcium and 29 % failure rate in the normalization of postoperative IPTH. The evidence for incriminating PHPT as the cause of stone disease is now being reexamined. After parathyroidectomy, Mollerup found that the rate of stone formation may remain the same as in idiopathic stone formers. He therefore questioned the validity of considering stone disease as an outcome of PHPT [34]. He suggests that screening all stone patients by serum calcium could pick up PHPT—even though it is not a cause of stone disease—just coincidentally, because PHPT too is a common ailment in the elderly. The disease is, however, a different entity in Pakistan, where PHPT is seen in younger individuals [11, 34].

The younger the patient, the greater is the risk of stone formation after surgery. The risk for stone formation extended 10 years before surgery and continues 10 years thereafter. Being male increased the risks of stones before and after surgery. They found that the preoperative calcium and size of gland, skeletal pathology (fractures), and level of IPTH had no influence on stone recurrence. The stone-free rate was 90.4 % in operated cases and 98.7 % in controls. Patients with preoperative stones had 27 times higher risk of forming stones in comparison with others without stones [34].

Anatomy

Knowledge of embryology and the possible anatomical positions (Fig. 93.1) of the parathyroids are essential for successful and complete parathyroidectomy.

The parathyroids develop from the third and the fourth pharyngeal pouches. The superior parathyroid glands develop from the fourth pouch, while the inferior glands come from the third pouch [35]. Because the ultimobranchial body, from which the parafollicular or C-cells of the thyroid gland are evolved, also arises from the fourth pouch, the superior parathyroid glands may in some cases be intrathyroidal.

Similarly, because the thymus develops from the third pharyngeal pouch and descends in the neck to reach the anterior superior mediastinum, the inferior parathyroid glands may (instead of lying at the inferior border of the thyroid gland) descend into the superior mediastinum. Conversely, if the parathyroid gland fails to descend in the neck, then the inferior parathyroid glands may even settle at a level above the superior parathyroid glands.

The inferior parathyroid glands tend to have a greater variation in location, due to a longer migratory course. The superior parathyroid glands are comparatively more constant and predictable.

Taubman et al. [24] have aptly described the common position of the glands, summarize:

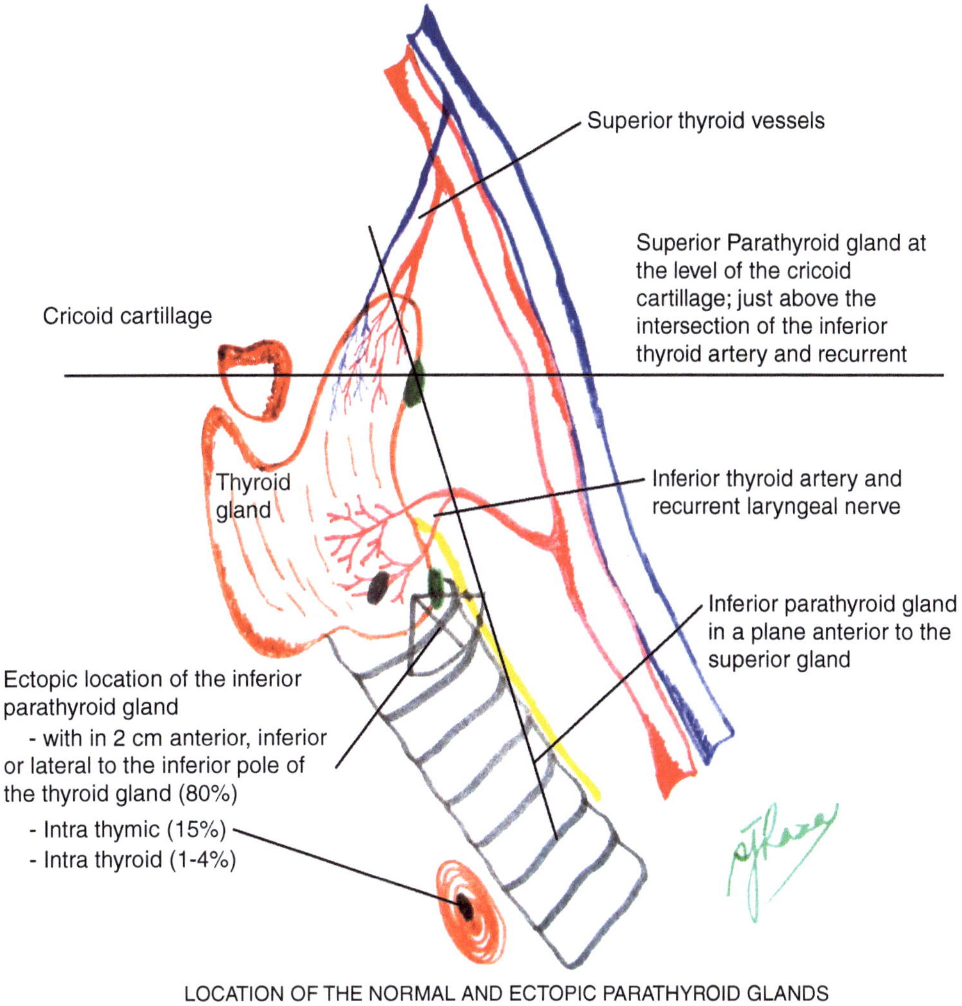

Fig. 93.1 Common sites for the parathyroid gland (Diagrammatic representation drawn by Johar Raza, Chief Resident Urology, Aga Khan University)

(The superior glands are found on the posteromedial aspect of the thyroid's superior poles approximately one centimeter above the intersection of the recurrent laryngeal nerve and inferior thyroid artery at the level of the cricoid cartilage. They are rarely ectopic; however, when they do occupy ectopic domains, the positions include the tracheoesophageal groove, posterior mediastinum, retroesophageal space, retropharyngeal space, and intrathyroid locations. The inferior parathyroid glands are typically located on the posterolateral surface of the inferior poles of the thyroid gland below the intersection of the recurrent laryngeal nerve and inferior thyroid artery. In about 80 % of the population, the inferior parathyroid glands reside anteriorly, inferiorly, or laterally within 2 cm of the inferior pole of the thyroid gland. They tend to lie at an anterior plane compared to the superior glands because of the anterior plane of descent of the third pouch. In the 20 % that have an ectopic inferior gland, the most common location is within the true sheath of the thymus (15 %); less frequently they are found in the intrathyroidal location (1–4 %), anterior mediastinum, submandibular location, tracheoesophageal groove, retroesophageal space, and carotid sheath).

The number of parathyroid glands is also of significance, especially when hyperfunction results from activity of multiple glands. Although, most commonly there are four glands (87 %), there may actually be only three glands (6 %) [36]. Basing his summary on an autopsy study of 503, Akerstrom et al. [37], however, noted that only 3 % had three glands, but their combined weight in any one patient was lower than expected, suggesting that a fourth might have been missed. Normally, the mean weight of a parathyroid gland is 33.1 mg, and its mean measurements 6.7×3.9×2.0 mm. It is however easier to remember their size as 1–2×3–4×5–6 mm, making them difficult to palpate even when enlarged, especially as they lie deep in the neck.

Having an extra parathyroid gland is rare, but this possibility must be considered when multiglandular disease is expected. When extra, they are usually found in the superior mediastinum within thymic tissue. Knowledge of ectopic sites is also important. Hojaij et al. [25] found that additional to 4 or more parathyroid glands in 89.3 % of 56 cadavers in a Brazilian autopsy study, 12.8 % of cases had at least 1 ectopic gland. These ectopic glands were sited in the mediastinum and thymus in 19.6 %, in the thyroid subcapsular space in 12.5 %, and in the thyroid parenchyma in 5.4 %.

Therefore, in case of parathyroid hyperplasia, bilateral neck exploration is performed, and all parathyroid glands are identified. Typically, the thymus is also removed since there is a 13–25 % chance of a fifth parathyroid gland within the thymus [37].

Thompson et al. [38] noted that 80 % had single adenomas, 2.6 % two adenomas, 15 % hyperplasia, and 2.6 % negative exploration.

Who Should Operate?

In the setting of renal stone disease, the urologist is primarily responsible for diagnosing concurrent PHPT if present. The exploration for PHPT, however, should be done by a person competent in surgery of the neck. While an endocrinological surgeon or head and neck surgeon is preferred, surgeons trained as a general surgeon in head and neck surgery, and who can be relied upon to respect the recurrent laryngeal nerve with all its variable courses and the variations in gland anatomy, could be certified for parathyroid surgery. The specialty of endocrine surgery is not well developed in developing countries. It is the urologist's responsibility to have the operation done by a competent person capable of international standards and outcomes and careful monitoring of postoperative problems.

The disease is infrequently picked up or uncommon in Pakistan, and most surgeons in Pakistan will be occasional operators performing fewer than five operations per year. In contrast, one unit has an experience of thousands. Infrequent operative experience of less than five procedures per year can place the patient at a disadvantage, and it is certainly preferable to send all patients with PHPT to one tertiary hospital. However, this is not logistically possible in Pakistan, as it involves disruption of family life and earning capacity and adds to expenses, as at least two other members travel into town. The vitamin D-deficient state of most hyperparathyroid patients in developing countries often results in prolonged postoperative hospital stay.

Few laboratories in the developing world can provide the rapid IPTH test for completeness of operation, but it would be very helpful under such circumstances to have a frozen section to confirm that the removed tissue is a parathyroid gland and not a lymph node. Fortunately, there is little difficulty in distinguishing a parathyroid adenoma, at operation, from its color, consistency, and rich blood supply. Surgery for parathyroid glands in situations where sestamibi scans show a single large 3-cm gland can be safe in the hands of an occasional operator with the competence outlined previously.

Intraoperative Management

Immediately preoperatively, on the operating room table, the gland site can be confirmed by ultrasound with Doppler and marked on the skin. In radio-guided parathyroidectomy, the patient can be given an injection of sestamibi 2 h before surgery and a handheld probe used to assist in defining the parathyroid intraoperatively.

Before the availability of sestamibi scans, we used methylene blue (MB) to localize the glands. Given intravenously in a dose of 6–8 mg/kg, diluted in 200 mL of normal saline, half to 1 h prior to operation, the glands stain gray-blue. The larger dose per kilogram is used for lean individuals with a higher muscle-to-fat ratio: muscle takes up more of the methylene blue than does fat. Infusion causes dark blue pigmentation of the skin and interferes with the pulse oximeter readings during infusion. The dye is eliminated by renal excretion but is retained in the parathyroid glands. We have had one episode of bradycardia and hypotension, in a patient who was prone to vasovagal attacks and had similar attacks when taken for her previous eye surgeries (at which time, methylene blue had not been used). We have abandoned the use of her dye since sestamibi was made available.

Pollack has reviewed the use of sestamibi over 30 years. Thirty-six cases of toxic encephalopathy have been reported and attributed to central serotonin toxicity, which occurs if given in patients with combined with drugs that increase central serotonin neurotransmission, as MB is a monoamine oxidase inhibitor [39].

Intraoperative Monitoring with Rapid IPTH to Test Completeness of Surgery

Serial intraoperative monitoring with rapid IPTH has been used in the West to detect the completeness of operation as results are available in 15 min. Blood should be drawn 10 min after the removal of all abnormal tissue. However, it has been shown that in patients with abnormal levels of IPTH prior to surgery, which levels fall after removal of the first adenoma, it is not therefore a substitute for bilateral exploration in such patients. In poor countries, one has to remember that the rapid IPTH is more expensive than the regular test pack and that the infrequency of PTH estimates in developing countries drives laboratories to have a scheduled day in the week on which the test is done. Rapid IPTH is economically not cost-effective.

Using the quick (rapid) parathyroid hormone assay, Carneiro et al. [40] noted that the Miami criterion gives the best guide to indicate completeness of operation. The Miami criterion is defined as a drop of IPTH *of more than* 50 % from the highest pre-incision or pre-excision level, 10 min after gland excision. Yet, Carneiro found that it correctly predicted only 329 of the 341 cases when followed up for 6 months—there were 3 false-positive and 9 false-negative results. Starr reports that 2 of 52 patients who had appropriate decreases on intraoperative monitoring of PTH had persistent hypercalcemia after 1 month [33]. There was a 4.8 % failure rate in the correction of postoperative serum calcium levels and a 29 % failure rate in the normalization of postoperative serum iPTH levels in his series.

Impact of 25-Hydroxyvitamin D Deficiency on Perioperative Parathyroid Hormone Kinetics and Results in Patients with Primary Hyperparathyroidism

Though vitamin D can affect many parameters in the care of PHPT patient, it does not alter the intraoperative kinetics of IPTH, so that successful parathyroidectomy can be predicted even in D-deficient patients by a 50 % drop in PTH intraoperatively. Untch found that the average drop in PTH level 5 min post resection was 79 ± 14 % in the deficient group and 72 ± 22 % in the non-deficient group ($P = 0.03$) [41].

Histological Proof of Identification

Seventy percent of surgeons questioned by Tiblin et al. [42] consider intraoperative histological confirmation necessary, but biopsy of the remaining glands is practiced regularly only in some countries. In difficult cases, histological confirmation by biopsy is necessary to ensure that fat lobules or thyroid nodules are not mistakenly identified as parathyroids. Figure 93.2 shows the distinctive architecture of a parathyroid gland on frozen section. In most cases, this examination cannot differentiate between an adenoma and hyperplasia, for which definitive sections are needed.

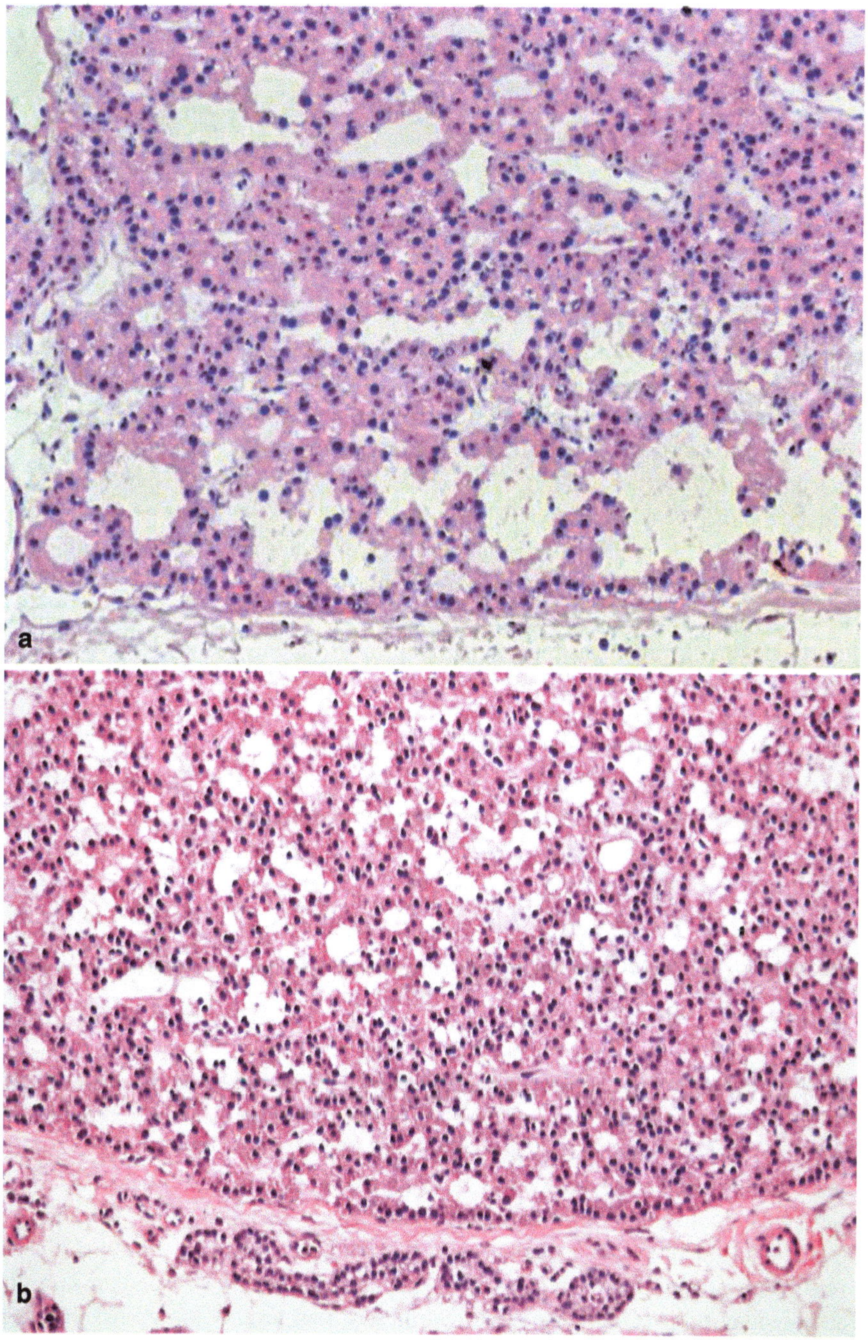

Fig. 93.2 Histological appearances of (**a**) intraoperative frozen section demonstrating the removed tissue is a parathyroid gland and not a lymph node or fat; and (**b**) the same tissue stained after definitive section

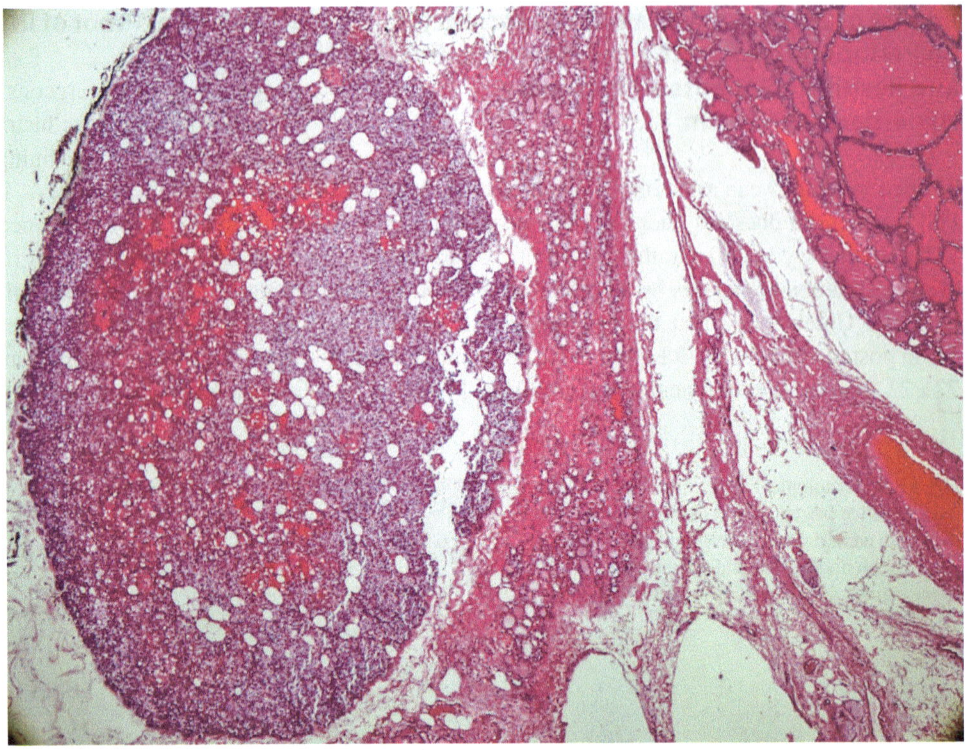

Fig. 93.3 Incidentally removed normal encapsulated parathyroid of 36-year-old female who underwent thyroidectomy. Note delicate septa and glandular elements with adipose tissue (H&E)

If the surgeon chooses to biopsy the remaining glands, a careful technique is warranted. Tenting up one pole of the gland by a 5/0 Prolene suture and snipping it off with an iris scissors can remove adequate tissue for biopsy confirmation (that the gland identified is a parathyroid gland) without lifting the entire parathyroid from its vascular bed. This will reduce the risk of hypoparathyroidism.

Figure 93.3 demonstrates the appearances of a normal gland on definitive histology examination (not frozen section). This is a gland that was removed inadvertently during thyroidectomy and demonstrates the proportion of fat/endocrine cell content. In a gland suppressed because of hyperfunction of an adenoma, the fat content will be even greater. In four-gland hyperplasia (Fig. 93.4a, b), the fat content will be significantly lower.

The histological appearance of an adenoma on definitive section and staining is shown in Fig. 93.5a, b and that of a carcinoma in Fig. 93.6a, b.

Simultaneous Operation for PHPT Along with Other Diseases

Though parathyroid surgery may occasionally take a long time, it does not involve sudden shifts in intravascular volume. It is therefore safe to combine surgery for PHPT simultaneously or sequentially, with operations for other diseases. Serum calcium should be monitored intraoperatively during the second operation, as a patient with hungry bones and renal stones, requiring surgery for PHPT and say, renal stones, may drop serum calcium to alarmingly low levels during the second surgical procedure (we noted a drop of 4 mg/dL [1 mmol/L] in one of our patients). In such cases where alkaline phosphatases and bone X-rays are suggestive of severe bone involvement, the surgeon may wish to do the additional procedure first, before the parathyroidectomy if the hypercalcemia has been controlled. Farley et al. [43] have combined parathyroid exploration in 117 patients with other operations: on the breast (in 25 patients) biliary tract (in 21), female genitourinary tract (in 19), as well as in intra-abdominal (in 18) and cardiothoracic (in 6) surgical procedures. The mean operating time was 155 min and hospital stay 7.6 days in their series.

Postoperative Management

Predicting Severe Postoperative Hypocalcemia

Facial tingling will alert the physician to the possibility of hypocalcemia, as will a Chvostek's sign (wherein there is twitching of the facial muscles on tapping the facial nerve as it exits from the stylomastoid foramen or in the pretragus area). Vitamin D deficiency and extensive bone disease, presence of osteitis fibrosa cystica, preoperative hypomagnesemia, and the postoperative hypomagnesemia of hungry bones can predict profound or prolonged hypocalcemia requiring continuous drip infusion replacement of calcium.

Postoperative hypocalcemia, which reaches its nadir around the morning of the first postoperative day in the West or around the second to third day in our experience, results

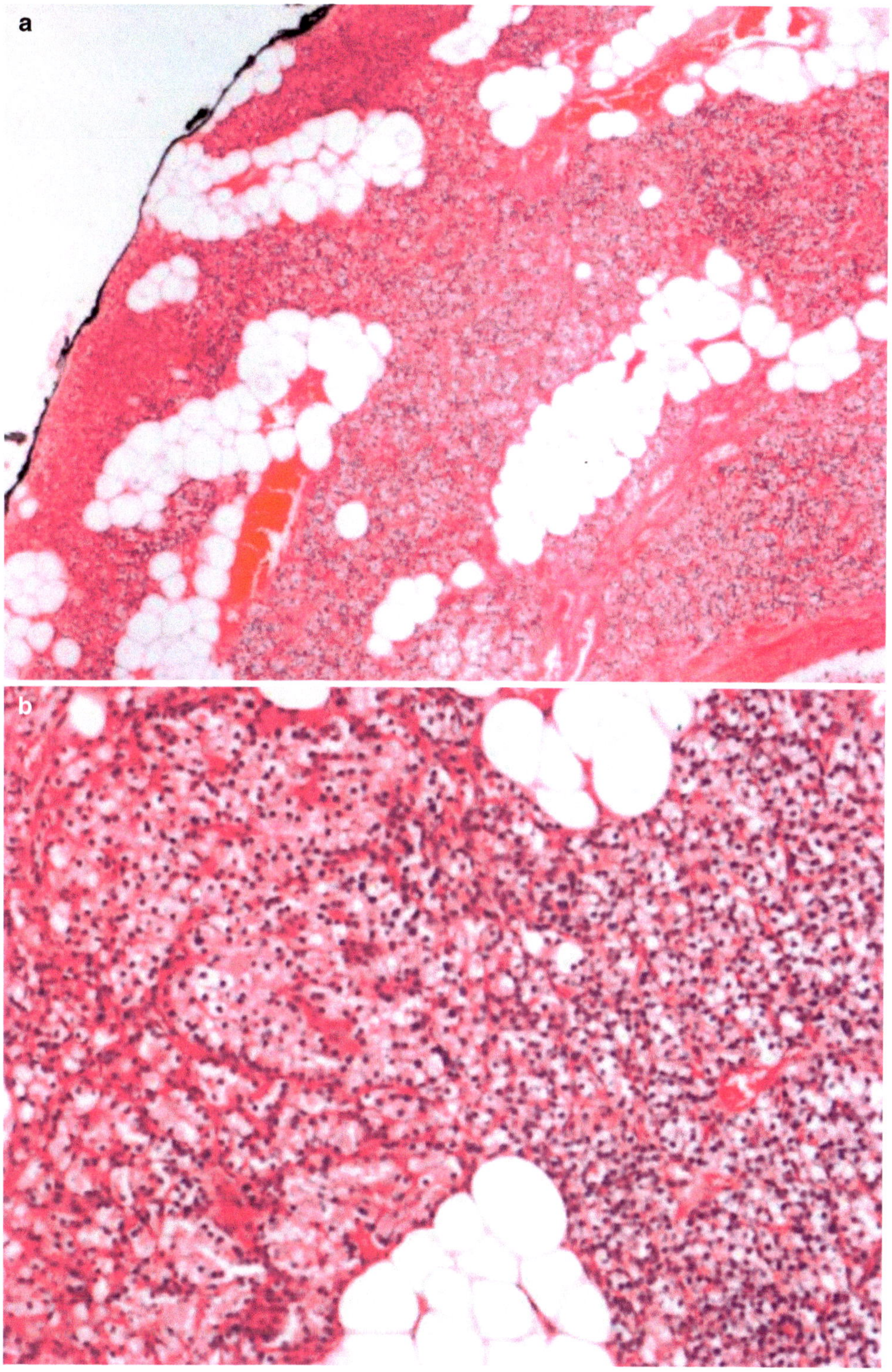

Fig. 93.4 Parathyroid gland hyperplasia (**a**) Shows a thinly encapsulated lesion and there is no rim of compressed or atrophic normal parathyroid surrounding it. (**b**) An admixture of chief and oxyphil cells and stromal fat (H&E, x 10 magnification)

from a drop in the PTH levels as the remaining suppressed glands struggle to produce more hormone.

The fat content of the remaining glands is indicative of the degree of suppression of the gland. On a histological section, up to 30 % of the section of normal parathyroid tissue will consist of fat cells. An increase in fat content of the remaining glands might produce a postoperative hypocalcemia more profound than when the remaining glands show little replacement of the gland by fat.

Hypocalcemia will be exaggerated by inadvertent interference with the blood supply of the remaining glands or removal of an excess amount of glandular tissue in patients with hyperplasia. Profound postoperative hypocalcemia is also seen in patients with hyperplasia, extensive coexisting

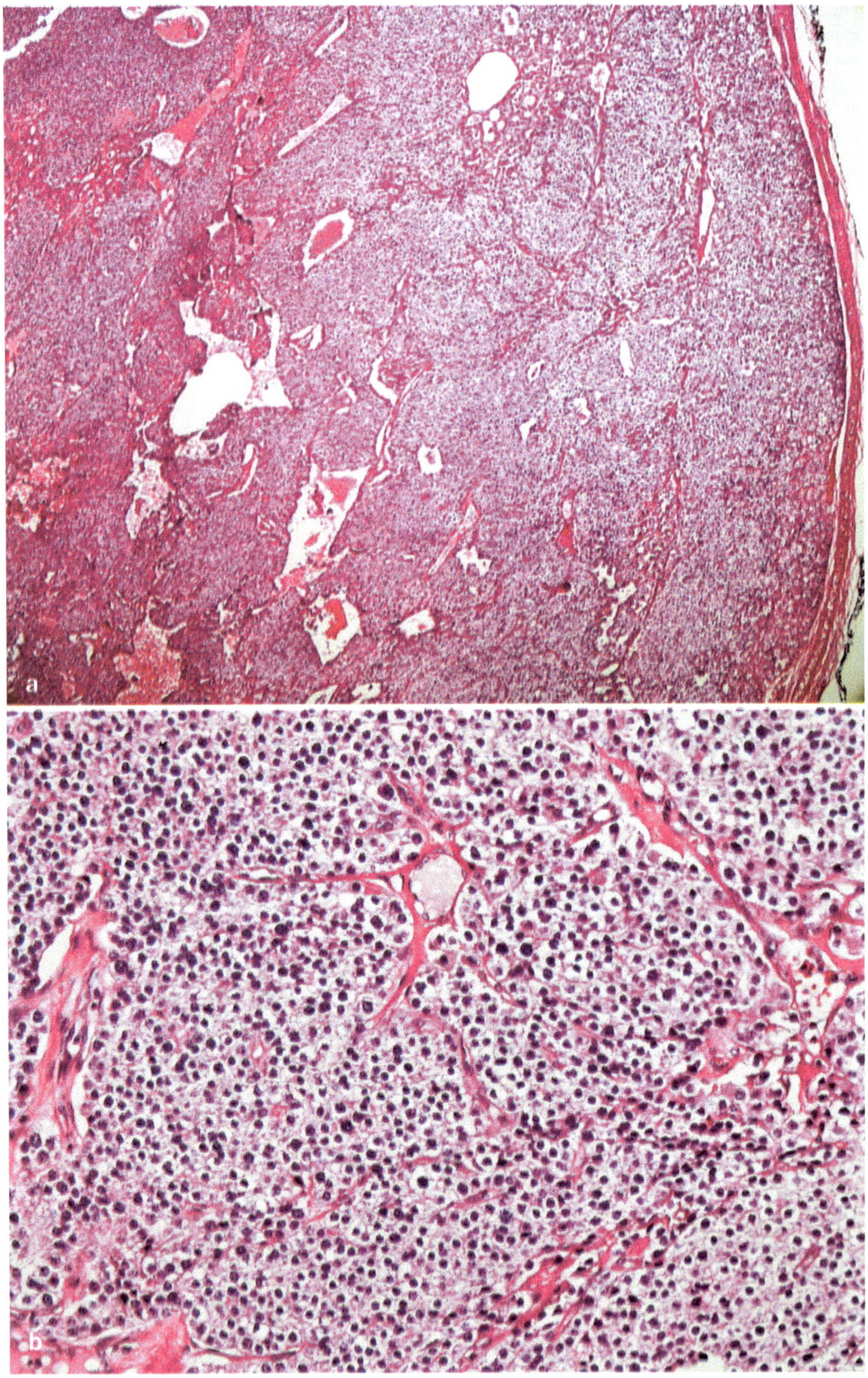

Fig. 93.5 Histopathological features of a parathyroid adenoma in a 46-year-old female. (**a**) This was an encapsulated lesion (The compressed rim of uninvolved/normal parathyroid tissue is not seen on this view. See also Figure 94.7). (**b**) Diffuse pseudofollicles with a predominance of chief cells

bone disease, and elevated serum alkaline phosphatase, which latter is a good predictor of the amount of calcium required to maintain normocalcemia.

Magnesium is essential for the manufacture, release, and peripheral action of PTH. Serum magnesium drops significantly in patients with hungry bone disease, and this also predicts more profound and prolonged hypocalcemia. Magnesium sulfate orally or intramuscularly is effective in combating hypomagnesemia. Bone remineralization takes a long time, and some noted no change in the dual photon absorptiometry in the bone density of lumbar spine at 1 year, though it increased in the femoral neck by 7.4 %.

Mittendorf noted that 42 % (of 132 patients with primary) and 29 (97 %) of 30 patients with renal HPT had postoperative hypocalcemia [44].

Generally in the West, PHPT manifesting as renal stones is associated with minor changes in serum calcium and small glands, normal bone status, and less marked changes in bone

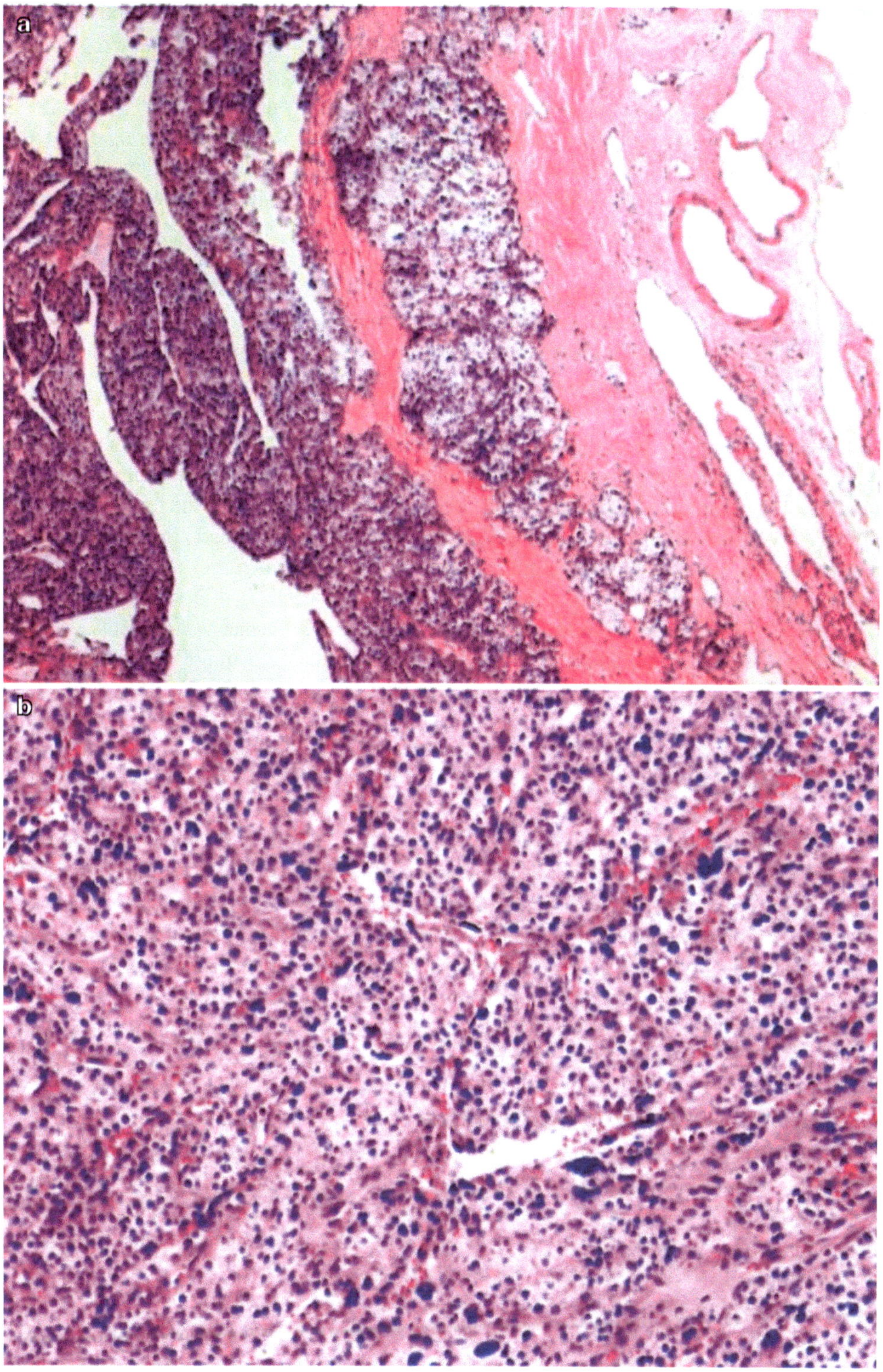

Fig. 93.6 Histopathological features of a parathyroid carcinoma in a 55-year-old female. (**a**) Low-power examination shows capsular invasion. (**b**) Cytological atypia is seen (H&E, ×10)

density. Patients are reported to return home by normal airline flight schedules the same day as surgery. Norman's group [45] found that the following findings were predictive of postoperative hypocalcemia, each item increasing the postoperative calcium requirement by 315 mg/day (7.9 mmol): preoperative serum calcium of >12 mg/dL (3.0 mmol/L), >13 mg/dL (3.25 mmol/L), and >13.5 mg/dL (3.38 mmol/L); bone mineral density z score of −3; removal of more than one gland; biopsy of other glands; and morbid obesity [45].

Does Biopsy of the Suppressed Glands Increase Chances of Making the Patient Hypoparathyroid?

Kaplan et al. [46] has shown that an aggressive biopsy policy leads to higher incidence of postoperative hypocalcemia. Search for the gland itself might increase the chance of devascularizing it. However, if caution is taken not to lift the gland out of its bed, then there is little reason to suspect that that will promote postoperative hypoparathyroidism.

Avoiding Long-Continuing Hypocalcemia

Persistent postoperative hypocalcemia is likely to occur on a long-term basis without an end point in patients with hyperplasia in whom too much tissue has been removed. It is therefore prudent to follow a procedure of removing all four parathyroid glands and then implanting a portion of one-half of a gland in the forearm or sternomastoid muscle.

This will prevent hypocalcemia, and if the remaining graft hyperfunctions, this can easily be detected by radioisotope scanning, and a part of the surviving transplant removed. It is preferable to transplant a portion of the parathyroid in the arm than to leave it behind a half gland in the neck.

Cryopreservation of parathyroid grafts is another useful adjunct in treatment of hyperplasia patients. It allows reimplantation in those cases where serum calcium does not return to normal. Cryopreserved tissue can also be used in those 10 % of cases of hyperplasia where the initial autograft into the forearm fails or malfunctions. Freezers used for storing bone marrow can be used. Tanaka et al. have shown that the ratio of PTH levels in veins draining the implanted tissue and veins in the contralateral arm will be 1.5 after 1 week if the graft has taken.

Mediastinal Parathyroids

Most mediastinal parathyroids are within the thymus, and most can be removed through the neck, as blood supply to the thymus is from the neck. However, if a radioisotope scan detects a parathyroid in the chest and a CT scan shows that this is a large, deeply seated mass or the planes of the capsule are not clearly defined, the primary exploration must be carried out through a median sternotomy.

Management of Hyperparathyroidism in Pregnancy

As 25 % of PHPT occurs in women during the childbearing age, pregnancy and hyperparathyroidism are not an unlikely combination. Yet, PHPT in pregnancy is rare. Even so, two of the authors of this chapter each with a small parathyroid experience have each had a case; one reported in the literature.

In one patient, PHPT had been diagnosed after the first child had tetany in the neonatal period but had not been treated before she became pregnant again. McMullen et al. [47] reported a series of seven patients, aged 20–39 years; Norman et al. [48] reported a series of 32 women (aged 19–40 years) seen over 6 years with 77 pregnancies. They constitute 0.7 % of his total pool of women with PHPT. As up to 80 % of pregnant patients with primary hyperparathyroidism are asymptomatic, many cases might remain undiagnosed.

PHPT is rarely detected in pregnancy, because physiological changes mask the symptoms or mislead physicians. These physiological changes include maternal blood volume expansion, hypoalbuminemia, increased fetal calcium requirements, and increased calcium clearance.

Physiological Changes in Pregnancy

During pregnancy, maternal serum calcium falls by about 10 %. As serum albumin falls by 20 %, the ionized calcium remains unchanged. Fetal 1, 25-dihydroxyvitamin D, synthesized in the fetal kidneys and placenta, acts as the major stimulus and regulator of calcium transfer across the placenta. It increases maternal gastrointestinal absorption of calcium by 150–400 mg (3.75–10 mmol) daily; additionally, maternal urinary excretion is also increased from 90 to 300 mg (2.25–7.5 mmol) daily. Major fetal calcium demands of approximately 25–30 g (0.63–0.75 mol) are required in the third trimester for skeletal tissue mineralization [49]. This requires an active transport of calcium across the placenta, and the fetal serum calcium remains higher than maternal blood.

It Is Now Recognized That Hyperparathyroidism Is Not a Normal Physiological Adaptation in Pregnancy

Initial parathyroid hormone assays measured biologically inactive fragments of PTH, hence the misconception that this condition exists. When measured with current assays, PTH falls during pregnancy to the low-normal range during the first trimester and may increase back to the mid-normal range by term. Most of these recent studies of PTH during pregnancy have examined women from North America and Europe who also consumed calcium-replete (often calcium-supplemented) diets. In contrast, in women from Asia and Gambia who have very low dietary calcium intakes, the PTH level did not suppress during pregnancy, and in some cases it increased significantly [49].

If a Patient with Stone Disease Is Discovered to Be Hyperparathyroid and Is Pregnant, the Patient Should Be Operated Upon to Remove the Offending Gland(s). Why?

Schnatz's [50] review of literature showed that medical treatment can only provide a suboptimal control of serum calcium, with a resulting higher fetal loss rate. If surgery is delayed up to the postpartum period, there are significant risks to the fetus and mother.

In the mother, complications associated with PHPT may occur in 67 %; up to 80 % of these pregnancies might end up in abortion, intrauterine death, or neonatal tetany. The mother may suffer a hypercalcemic crisis and die. The symptoms of hypercalcemic crisis, namely, nausea, vomiting, dehydration, weakness, and altered mental state are not readily diagnosed as being due to hypercalcemia. Fetal loss can occur at any level of serum calcium, but most losses occurred at maternal calcium of >11.4 mg/dL (2.85 mmol/L). The rate of fetal loss increases in direct proportion to the serum calcium level [48]—the risk of fetal death is 50 % when the calcium is above 11.5 mg/dL (2.88 mmol/L), but almost certainly 85 % when Ca nears 13 mg/dL (3.25 mmol/L) [48].

Fetal problems include intrauterine growth retardation, low birth weight, preterm delivery, intrauterine fetal demise, postpartum neonatal tetany, and permanent hypoparathyroidism. If lucky, the child may be born underweight and might suffer from hypocalcemic tetany on birth.

What Is the Best Time to Operate?

Earlier recognition and surgical cure before becoming pregnant is ideal. However, once pregnant, surgery should be offered in the latter part of the second or early part of the third trimester. Surgery should not be left to the postpartum period because of the significant risk to the fetus. Norman operates between 13 and 17 weeks of pregnancy, completing the operation in an average of <20 min. The choice of timing of the operation is determined by the fact that pregnancy loss occurred typically in the late first or early second trimester, with the 30 % second trimester losses being sixfold higher than expected.

Not all patients comply with a request to undergo surgery. In Norman's series, only 15 patients underwent parathyroidectomy with uneventful delivery of a healthy infant at 36 and 40 weeks gestation. There were no maternal or infant complications at surgery or during the subsequent delivery. Thirty (48 %) of the remaining unoperated upon 62 pregnancies were lost, a rate that is 3.5-fold higher than expected. Sadly, in those who did not have the HPT addressed after the first miscarriage, one third lost one or more additional pregnancies. Since 1993 2005, no complications were reported from surgery on women >27 weeks pregnant, barring hypocalcemia, which was easily correctable.

As Preoperative Imaging Reduces Operation Time, What Options for Imaging Can Be Used Safely in Pregnancy?

McMullen states that a Tc-99m sesta MIBI imaging may be used safely for localization of the parathyroids after negative cervical explorations.

The hypocalcemia in the neonate results from suppression of fetal parathyroid from the high maternal calcium and calcitonin. At birth, the neonate is suddenly deprived of this source of calcium and cannot mobilize calcium from bone due to low levels of PTH and high concentrations of calcitonin. Acute neonatal hypocalcemia results, with tetany and convulsions, usually at 5–14 days of age. Tetany may not manifest itself when the child is on breast feeds but would occur if formula feed high in phosphorous are used [48].

Conclusion

PHPT does cause stone and its cure relieves the patient of recurrence in most instances. Every stone patient should be screened through ionized calcium estimation followed by appropriate tests if found hypercalcemic. The clinical picture in patients from emerging industrial giants is one of vitamin D deficiency-dominated bone and stone disease, with greater hypocalcemia and a slower return to normal after surgery. Surgery is the best option and needs to be done even when no endocrinological surgeon is available.

Acknowledgments Photographs of all histopathological slides provided by Dr. Nasir Ud Din, Department of Pathology, Aga Khan University. Anatomical representation is drawn by Dr. Johar Raza, Chief Resident Urology, Aga Khan University.

References

1. Macfarlane DP, Yu N, Donnan PT, Leese GP. Should "mild primary hyperparathyroidism" be reclassified as "insidious": is it time to reconsider? Clin Endocrinol (Oxf). 2011. doi:10.1111/j.1365-2265.2011.04201.x.
2. Derrick Jr FC. Renal calculi in association with hyperparathyroidism: a changing entity. J Urol. 1982;127(2):226.
3. Jan MA, Falah SQ. Clinical aspects of primary hyperparathyroidism. J Postgrad Med. 2006;20(4):410–2. http://www.jpmi.org.pk/cms/PDF/21%20Mian%20Asadullah%20Jan.pdf. Last accessed 20 Nov 2011.
4. Bhansali A, Masoodi SR, Reddy KS, Behera A, Radotra B, Mittal BR, et al. Primary hyperparathyroidism in north India: a description of 52 cases. Ann Saudi Med. 2005;25(1):29–35. Full text http://www.ncbi.nlm.nih.gov/pubmed/15822491. Last accessed 20 Nov 2011.
5. Wasty SWH, Iqbal K, Beg MR, Mahida KH, Ali G, Tariq M. Giant cell tumor of the maxilla and tibia presenting concurrently as an

initial manifestation of primary parathyroid adenoma. J Pak Med Assoc. 2005;55(4):170–1. http://www.pakmedinet.com/printit.php?id=7164&choice=a. Last accessed 21 Nov 2011.
6. Bilezikian JP, Meng X, Shi Y, Silverberg SJ. Primary hyperparathyroidism in women: a tale of two cities – New York and Beijing. Int J Fertil Womens Med. 2000;45(2):158–65.
7. Mollerup CL, Lindewald H. Renal stones and primary hyperparathyroidism: natural history of renal stone disease after successful parathyroidectomy. World J Surg. 1999;23:173–6.
8. Diamond TH, Botha JR, Kalk WJ, Shires R. Primary hyperparathyroidism. A study of 100 patients in Johannesburg. S Afr Med J. 1986;69(2):94–7.
9. Purnell DC, Smith LH, Scholz DA, Elveback LR, Arnaud CD. Primary hyperparathyroidism: a prospective clinical study. Am J Med. 1971;50(5):670–8.
10. Suh JM, Cronan JJ, Monchik JM. Primary hyperparathyroidism: is there an increased prevalence of renal stone disease? Am J Roentgenol. 2008;191(3):908–11.
11. Biyabani SR, Talati J. Bone and renal stone disease in patients operated for primary hyperparathyroidism in Pakistan: is the pattern of disease different from the west? J Pak Med Assoc. 1999;49(8):194–8.
12. Gopal RA, Acharya SV, Bandgar T, Menon PS, Dalvi AN, Shah NS. Clinical profile of primary hyperparathyroidism from western India: a single center experience. J Postgrad Med. 2010;56(2):79–84.
13. Chan AK, Duh QY, Katz MH, Siperstein AE, Clark OH. Clinical manifestations of primary hyperparathyroidism before and after parathyroidectomy: a Case-control study. Ann Surg. 1995;222(3): 402–14.
14. George J, Acharya SV, Bandgar TR, Menon PS, Shah NS. Primary hyperparathyroidism in children and adolescents. Indian J Pediatr. 2010;77(2):175–8. Epub 2010 Jan 20.
15. Admassie D, Kebede T, Feleke Y. Brown tumor an uncommon and late manifestation of hyperparathyroidism: a case series done at Tikur Anbessa Specialized Hospital, Addis Ababa. Ethiop Med J. 2011;49(2):149–53.
16. Valle Díaz de la Guardia F, Arrabal Martín M, Arrabal Polo MA, Quirosa Flores S, Miján Ortiz JL, Zuluaga Gómez A. Renal lithiasis in patients with primary hyperparathyroidism. Evolution and treatment. Arch Esp Urol. 2010;63(1):32–40.
17. Berger AD, Wu W, Eisner BH, Cooperberg MR, Duh QY, Stoller ML. Patients with primary hyperparathyroidism – why do some form stones? J Urol. 2009;181(5):2141–5.
18. Rejnmark L, Vestergaard P, Mosekilde L. Nephrolithiasis and renal calcifications in primary hyperparathyroidism. J Clin Endocrinol Metab. 2011;96(8):2377–85.
19. Broadus AE, Horst RL, Lang R, Littledike ET. The importance of circulating 1, 25-dihydroxyvitamin D in the pathogenesis of hypercalciuria and renal-stone formation in primary hyperparathyroidism. N Engl J Med. 1980;302(8):421–6.
20. Vezzoli G, Scillitani A, Corbetta S, Terranegra A, Dogliotti E, Guarnieri V, et al. Polymorphisms at the regulatory regions of the CASR gene influence stone risk in primary hyperparathyroidism. Eur J Endocrinol. 2011;164(3):421–7. Epub 2010 Dec 23.
21. Dusso AS. Nodular parathyroid growth: role of vitamin D resistance. Kidney Int. 2002;62:1472–3. http://www.nature.com/ki/journal/v62/n4/full/4493247a.html. Last accessed on 21 Nov 2011.
22. Shek CC, Natkunam A, Tsang V, et al. Incidence, cause and mechanism of hypercalcemia in a hospital population in Hong Kong. Q J Med. 1990;77:1277–85.
23. Parks JH, Coe FL, Evan AP, Worcester EM. Clinical and laboratory characteristics of calcium stone-formers with and without primary hyperparathyroidism. BJU Int. 2009;103(5):670–8.
24. Taubman ML, Goldfarb M, Lew JI. Role of SPECT and SPECT/CT in the surgical treatment of primary hyperparathyroidism. Int J Mol Imaging. 2011;2011:141593. doi:10.1155/2011/141593. Published online 2011 June 21.
25. Hojaij F, Vanderlei F, Plopper C, Rodrigues CJ, Jácomo A, Cernea C, et al. Parathyroid gland anatomical distribution and relation to anthropometric and demographic parameters: a cadaveric study. Anat Sci Int. 2011;86(4):204–12.
26. Khan MK, Taous A, Sultana SZ, Sharif A, Hossain MM, Mostafa G, et al. Neck swelling with renal stone. Mymensingh Med J. 2010;19(4):622–6.
27. Bilezikian JP. Clinical review 51. Management of hypercalcemia. J Clin Endocrinol Metab. 1993;77(6):1445–9.
28. Phitayakorn R, McHenry CR. Hyperparathyroid crisis: use of bisphosphonates as a bridge to parathyroidectomy. J Am Coll Surg. 2008;206(3):1106–15. Epub 2008 Feb 21.
29. Silverberg SJ, Shane E, Jacobs TP, Siris E, Bilezikian JP. A 10-year prospective study of primary hyperparathyroidism with or without parathyroid surgery. N Engl J Med. 1999;341:1249–55.
30. Ronni-Sivula H. Causes of death in patients previously operated on for primary hyperparathyroidism. Ann Chir Gynaecol. 1985; 74(1):13–8.
31. McGeown MG. Effect of parathyroidectomy on the incidence of renal calculi. Lancet. 1961:1(7177):586–7.
32. Deaconson TF, Wilson SD, Lemann Jr J. The effect of parathyroidectomy on the recurrence of nephrolithiasis. Surgery. 1987; 102(6):910–13.
33. Starr FL, DeCresce R, Prinz RA. Normalization of intraoperative parathyroid hormone does not predict normal postoperative parathyroid hormone levels. Surgery. 2000;128(6):930–6.
34. Mollerup CL, Vestergaard P, Frøkjær VG, Mosekilde L, Christiansen P, Blichert-Toft M. Risk of renal stone events in primary hyperparathyroidism before and after parathyroid surgery: controlled retrospective follow up study. BMJ. 2002;325:807. doi:10.1136/bmj.325.7368.807.
35. Boyd JD. Development of the thyroid and parathyroid glands and the thymus. Ann R Coll Surg Engl. 1950;7:45.
36. Gilmour JR. The gross anatomy of the parathyroid glands. J Pathol. 1938;46:133.
37. Akerström G, Malmaeus J, Bergström R. Surgical anatomy of human parathyroid glands. Surgery. 1984;95(1):14–21.
38. Thompson NW, Eckhauser FE, Harness JK. The anatomy of primary hyperparathyroidism. Surgery. 1982;92(5):814–21.
39. Pollack G, Pollack A, Delfiner J, Fernandez J. Parathyroid surgery and methylene blue: a review with guidelines for safe intraoperative use. Laryngoscope. 2009;119(10):1941–6.
40. Carneiro DM, Solorzano CC, Nader MC, Ramirez M, Irvin III GL. Comparison of intraoperative iPTH assay (QPTH) criteria in guiding parathyroidectomy: which criterion is the most accurate? Surgery. 2003;134(6):973–9. doi:10.1067/msy.2000.110850. http://www.sciencedirect.com/science/article/pii/S003960600300480X.
41. Untch BR, Barfield ME, Dar M, Dixit D, Leight Jr GS, Olson Jr JA. Intraoperative kinetics of iPTH in vit d deficient states. Surgery. 2007;142(6):1022–6.
42. Tiblin S, Bondesson AG, Uden P, et al. Current trends in the surgical treatment of parathyroid adenoma, a questionnaire study from 53 surgical departments in 14 countries. Eur J Surg. 1991;157: 103–7.
43. Farley DR, van Heerden JA, Grant CS. Are concomitant surgical procedures acceptable in patients undergoing cervical explorations for PHPT. Mayo Clin Proc. 1991;66:681–5.

44. Mittendorf EA, Merlino JI, McHenry CR. Post-parathyroidectomy hypocalcemia: incidence, risk factors, and management. Am Surg. 2004;70(2):114–9.
45. Vasher M, Goodman A, Politz D, Norman J. Postoperative calcium requirements in 6000 patients undergoing outpatient parathyroidectomy: easily avoiding asymptomatic hypocalcemia. J Am Coll Surg. 2010;211(1):49–54.
46. Kaplan EL, Bartlett S, Sugimoto J, Fredland A. Relation of postoperative hypocalcemia to operative techniques: deleterious effect of excessive use of parathyroid biopsy. Surgery. 1982;92:827–34.
47. McMullen TP, Learoyd DL, Williams DC, Sywak MS, Sidhu SB, Delbridge LW. Hyperparathyroidism in pregnancy: options for localization and surgical therapy. World J Surg. 2010;34(8):1811–6.
48. Norman J, Politz D, Politz L. Hyperparathyroidism during pregnancy and the effect of rising calcium on pregnancy loss: a call for earlier intervention. Clin Endocrinol. 2009;71(1):104–9. doi:10.1111/j.1365-2265.2008.03495.x.
49. Kovacs CS. Calcium metabolism during pregnancy and lactation. http://www.endotext.org/pregnancy/pregnancy3/pregnancy3.html. Last accessed 11 Nov 2011.
50. Schnatz PF, Thaxton S. Parathyroidectomy in the third trimester of pregnancy. Obstet Gynecol Surv. 2005;60(10):672–82.

Normocalcemic Hyperparathyroidism: An Illustrative Case Scenario

94

Johar Raza, Jamsheer J. Talati, and Nasir Ud Din Yashkun

Abstract

In vitamin D-deficient countries, many cases of hyperparathyroidism are missed as the serum calcium may remain in normal range. The course of a patient with normocalcemic hyperparathyroidism is described.

Keywords

Normocalcemic hyperparathyroidism • Tetany • Bone changes • Hypercalcemia • Vitamin D deficiency

Introduction

The key laboratory investigation parameter that triggers the physician to estimate parathyroid hormone is hypercalcemia. We report a patient who was presented to us with a number of investigations that made it easy for us to diagnose her ailment and demonstrated that she did have primary and not secondary hyperparathyroidism.

The populations of India and Pakistan are vitamin D deficient. This case is presented to stimulate thought on cost-effective ways of detecting primary hyperparathyroidism among stone patients in countries that are vitamin D deficient.

J. Raza, M.B.B.S., FCPS (Urol)
Section of Urology, Aga Khan University, Stadium Road, Karachi, Sindh 74800, Pakistan

J.J. Talati, M.B.B.S., FRCS (✉)
Section of Urology, Department of Surgery, Aga Khan University, Stadium Road, P.O. Box 3500, Karachi, Sindh 74800, Pakistan
e-mail: jamsheer.talati@aku.edu

N. Ud Din Yashkun, M.B.B.S., FCPS (Histopathology)
Department of Pathology, Aga Khan University, Stadium Road, Karachi, Sindh 74800, Pakistan

Case Report

A 57-year-old female was referred for management of hyperparathyroidism from the orthopedic clinics where she had presented with persistent severe right hip pain. Her previous medical and surgical history was unremarkable. Physical examination was within normal limits except for marked clubbing of the fingernails (Fig. 94.1a, b) and a small swelling palpable in the left side of the neck, without any regional lymphadenopathy. Proximal muscle weakness was demonstrable when she got out of a chair, and she had a lurching gait.

Her laboratory workup was as follows:

- Hb—9.8 mg/dl
- Creatinine—0.5 mg/dl (44 μmol/l)
- Electrolytes—normal
- Serum Ca—9.9 mg/dl (2.48 mmol/l)
- Serum P—4.0 mg/dl (1.29 mmol/l)
- IPTH—2,330 pg/ml
- Vitamin D—9.25 ng/ml
- Serum Mg—1.6 mg/dl (0.67 mmol/l)
- Urinary Mg—108 mg (4.5 mmol)/24 h
- Urinary Ca—54 mg (1.35 mmol)/24 h

X-ray examinations of the hand and skull are shown in Figs. 94.2a, b and 94.3. In view of her raised serum IPTH levels, she had undergone a sestamibi scan (Fig. 94.4) and ultrasound examination of her neck (Figs. 94.5 and 94.6). On sestamibi scan, a single area of intense accumulation of

J.J. Talati et al. (eds.), *Urolithiasis*,
DOI 10.1007/978-1-4471-4387-1_94, © Springer-Verlag London 2012

radioactivity was seen, suggesting an adenoma. Following the localization, the patient underwent left inferior parathyroidectomy through a small central incision (Fig. 94.7).

Perioperative frozen section confirmed that the removed tissue was a parathyroid gland, and postoperative IPTH levels in the recovery room (rapid IPTH is not available at our center, as it would be cost ineffective to use it) declined to 166 pg/ml (from 2,330 pg/ml). In order to combat anticipated postoperative hypocalcemia, she was started on calcium gluconate infusion along with oral calcium, vitamin D, and magnesium replacement. The patient did not develop any signs of hypocalcemia (see chart in Fig. 94.6) while admitted and was sent home on the seventh postoperative day. On follow up, she stated that she had experienced two episodes of symptomatic hypocalcemia and Chvostek's sign could be elicited. She, however, recovered well following aggressive calcium replacement and oral 1-alpha vitamin D.

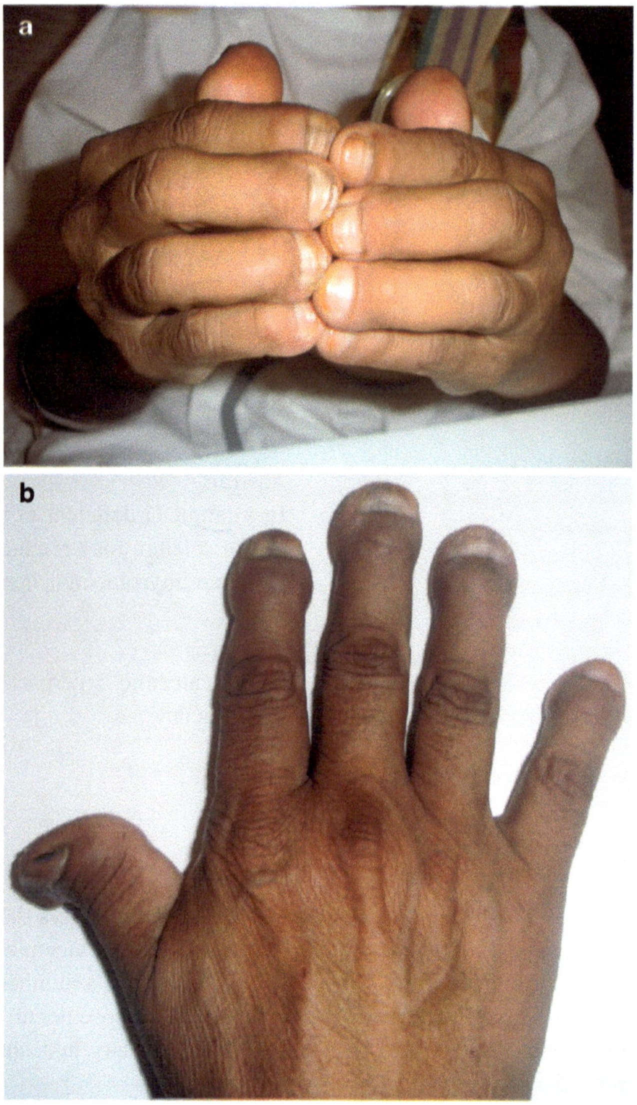

Fig. 94.1 Clubbing of the fingernails

Discussion

This patient's low serum calcium is probably the outcome of long-standing aggressive hyperparathyroidism in the presence of insufficient vitamin D. How then does one categorically determine that the patient has primary and not secondary hyperparathyroidism? Using Harvey's formula, it becomes clear that the patient's PTH was very much higher than expected. In Harvey's formula (1), the expected PTH-level (pg/ml) is calculated as 120 – (6×calcium [mg/dl]) – (0.52×25-hydroxy vitamin D (ng/ml))+(0.26×patient age [years]). In her case, the calculation is 120 – (6×9.9) – (0.52×9.25)+(0.26×45)=120–(59.4)–(4.81)+11.7=77.11. Thus, her PTH was much higher than this figure and hence indicates primary hyperparathyroidism. This was confirmed by ultrasound and sestamibi scans. There was no doubt that this patient had an adenoma.

Acknowledgements Radiological images from the Department of Radiology, Aga Khan University, courtesy of Dr. Zafar Sajjad, Chair of the Department of Radiology.

Histological specimens for this patient and comparative hyperplastic gland from the Department of Pathology, Aga Khan University, courtesy of Dr. Nasir Ud Din and Dr. Rashida Ahmed.

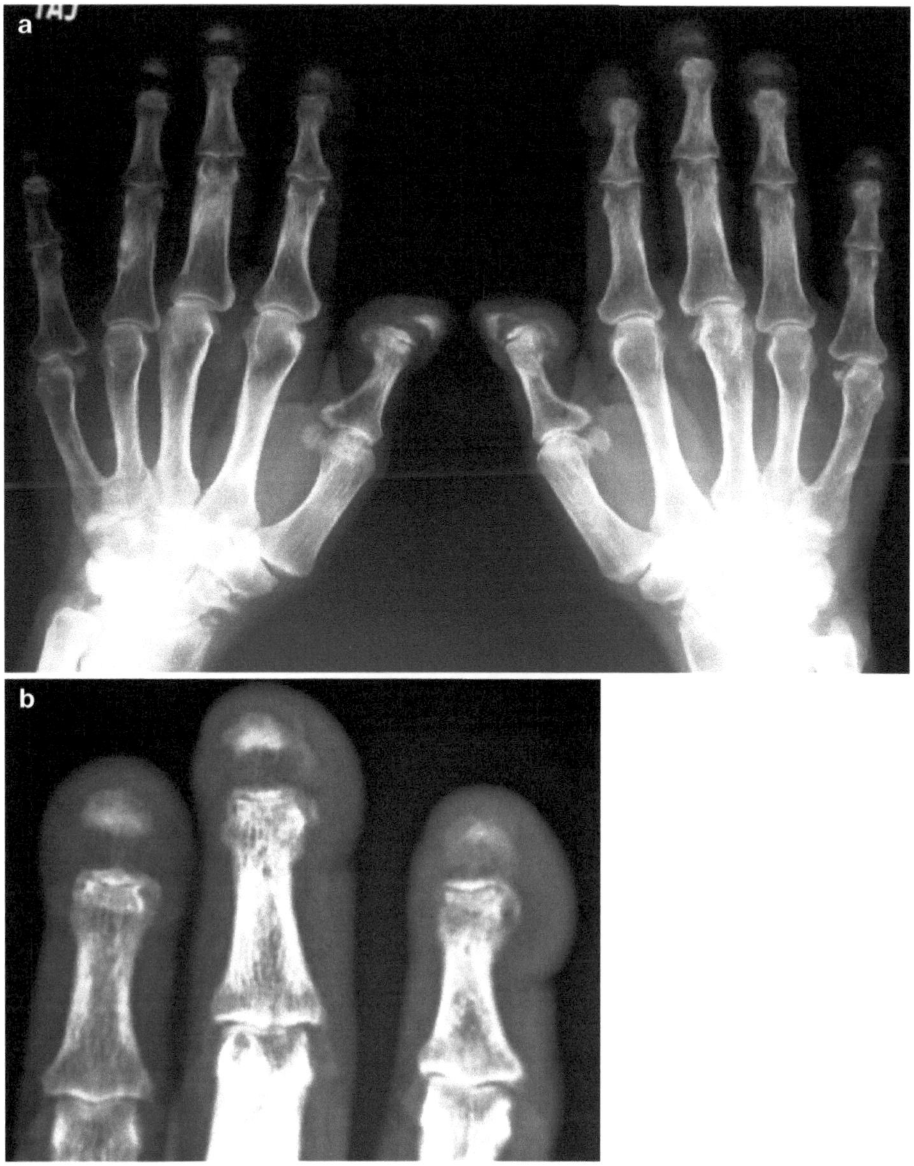

Fig. 94.2 X-rays of the hands showing resorption of bone in the terminal phalanges

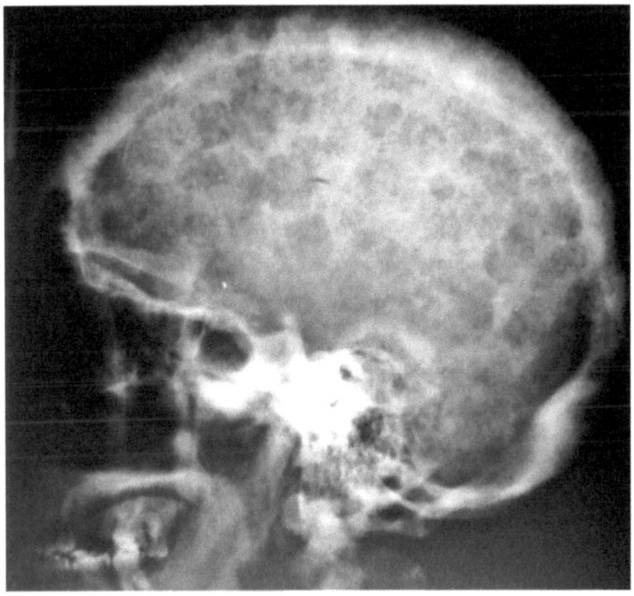

Fig. 94.3 X-ray of the skull (lateral view)

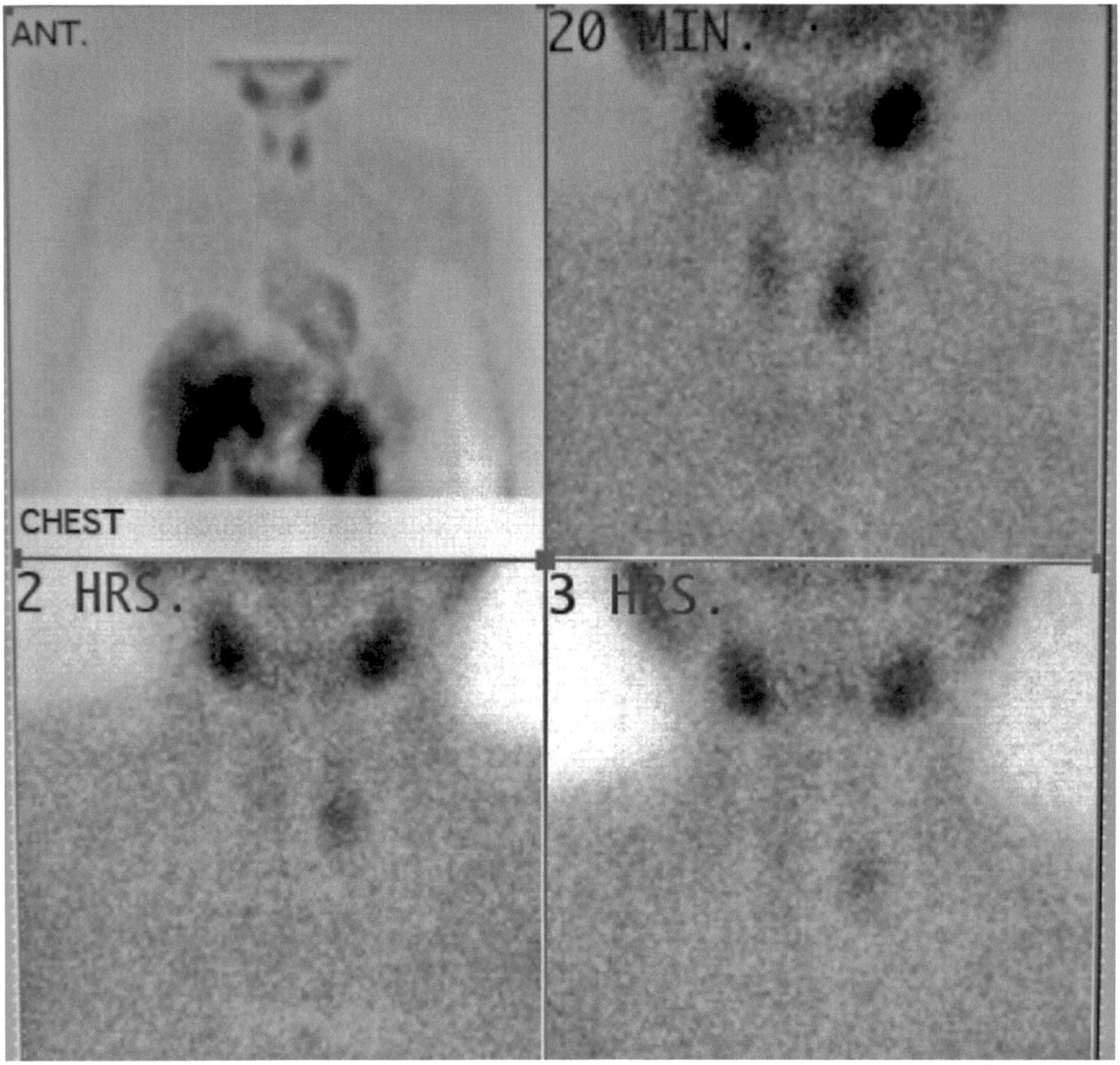

Fig. 94.4 Sestamibi scan of the patient showing increased and retained uptake in the *left* lower parathyroid gland. The submandibular glands, seen here in the upper part of each figure, retain the radioactivity longer than thyroid tissue

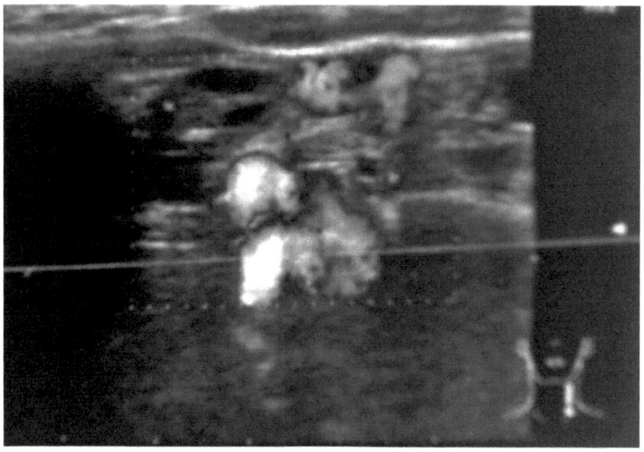

Fig. 94.5 Doppler ultrasound scan of the neck showing the enlarged parathyroid gland with increased vascularity

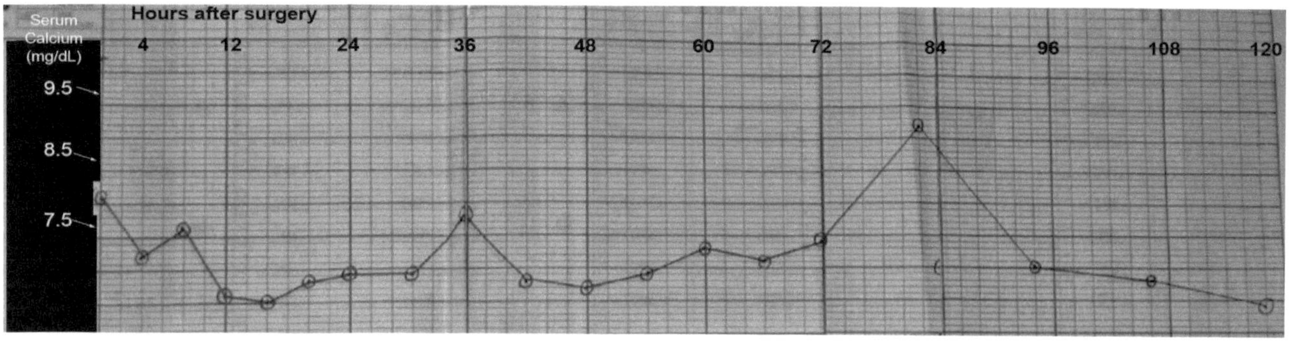

Fig. 94.6 Graph of serum calcium levels plotted postoperatively to demonstrate the trend of variance. In this graph, serum Ca is represented on the y-axis, and hours elapsed from operation are represented on the x-axis. This patient required a calcium infusion

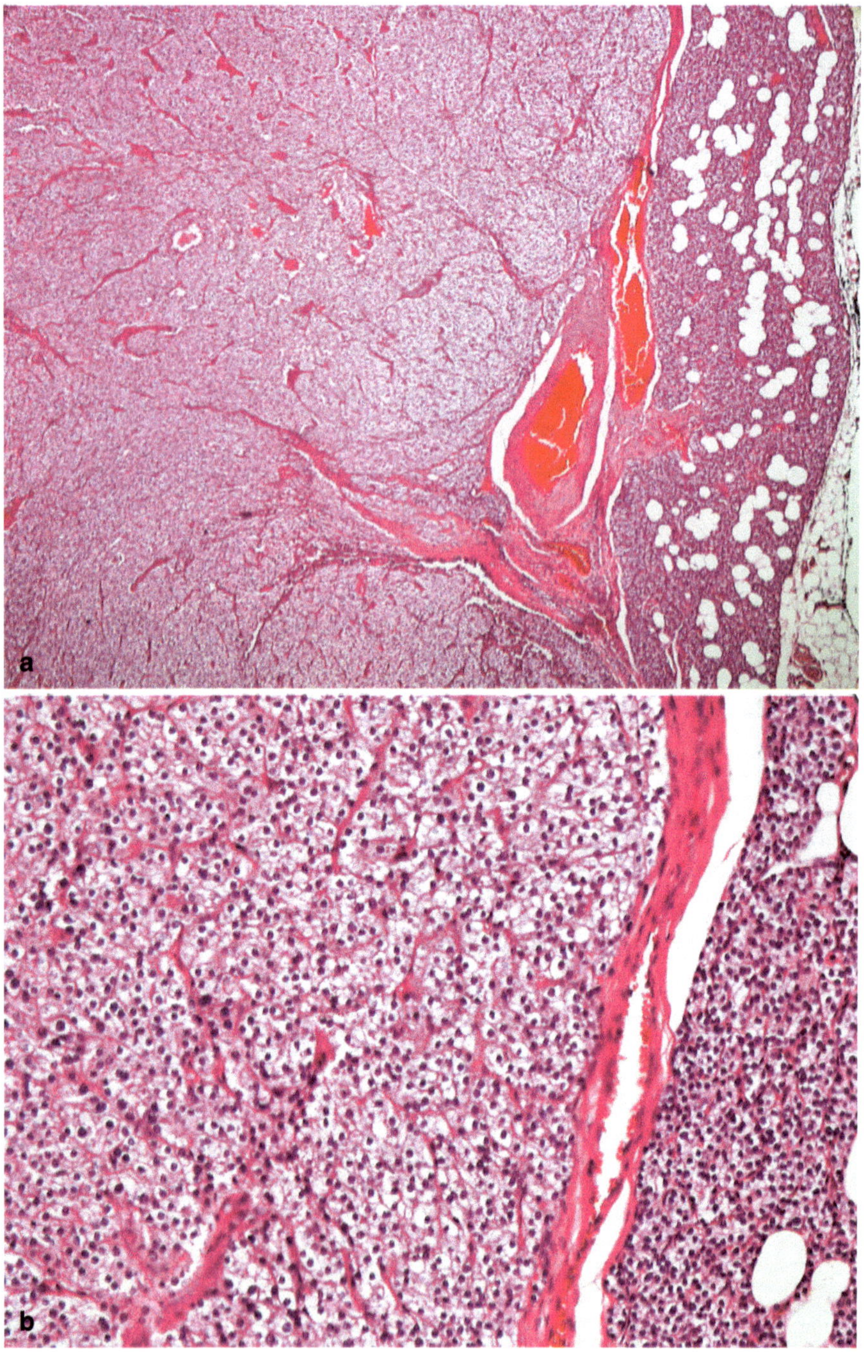

Fig. 94.7 Histopathology of the excised gland. This was an adenoma. In this patient, compressed normal parathyroid tissue can be seen in the periphery. Note predominance of chief cells with clear cytoplasm and fine vasculature. Note absence of fat

Reference

1. Harvey A, Hu M, Gupta M, Butler R, Mitchell J, Berber E. A new, vitamin D-based, multidimensional nomogram for the diagnosis of primary hyperparathyroidism. Endocr Pract. 2012;18(2):124–31. Accessed on 23 Nov 2011.

How to Perform a Successful Exploration of the Neck for Primary Hyperparathyroidism

95

William R. Lynn and John A. Lynn

Abstract

This chapter explains in detail how to perform a successful parathyroidectomy. If the technique suggested is followed closely, one would expect in excess of 95 % success rate for the management of primary hyperparathyroidism.

Keywords

Bilateral neck exploration (BNE) • Familial hypocalciuric hypercalcemia (FHH) • Hyperparathyroidism • Hypoparathyroidism • Minimally invasive parathyroidectomy • Parathyroid adenoma • Parathyroid cancer • Parathyroid hyperplasia • Parathyroid surgery • Sestamibi scan • Vitamin D deficiency

Introduction

For a successful parathyroid exploration for primary hyperparathyroidism (PHPT), surgeons must ask themselves five important questions:

1. Is the diagnosis of primary hyperparathyroidism correct?
2. Have the abnormal parathyroid adenoma or hyperplastic parathyroid glands been successfully localized?
3. Does the patient need surgery?
4. Has the patient been safely prepared for the surgical procedure?
5. Should a localized, scan-directed or traditional open technique be used?

W.R. Lynn, M.B.B.S., B.Sc. (Hons), MRCS
Department of General Surgery, Barnet and Chase Farm Hospital NHS Trust, London Deanery, London, UK

J.A. Lynn, M.S. FRCS (✉)
Department of General Surgery, Barnet and Chase Farm Hospital NHS Trust, Bupa Cromwell Hospital, Cromwell Road, London SW5 0TU, UK
email: john.lynn@endocrinesurgeon.co.uk

Department of Endocrinology, Hammersmith and Ealing Hospitals, London, UK

Is the Diagnosis of Primary Hyparathyroidism Correct?

Primary hyperparathyroidism is a common disease. The diagnosis is made by a persistently raised calcium level outside the local reference range combined with an inappropriate secretion of parathyroid hormone (PTH) with normal renal function. Patients with primary hyperparathyroidism will excrete normal or increased amounts of calcium in their urine. Vitamin D deficiency is widespread throughout the world and complicates the diagnosis [1]. Patients with vitamin D deficiency and primary hyperparathyroidism may have a normal calcium level, which, when they are made vitamin D replete, rises above the reference range. They will then continue to have a persistently raised PTH and excrete large amounts of calcium in the urine. One diagnostic problem occurs when the patient is suffering from the rare entity of familial hypercalcemic hypocalciuria (FHH) (Fig. 95.1). These patients, like patients with primary hyperparathyroidism, have a raised serum calcium with an inappropriate PTH but excrete little or no calcium in their urine. If FHH is not excluded in a patient, repeated unnecessary parathyroid explorations may result. FHH is not a surgical condition.

J.J. Talati et al. (eds.), *Urolithiasis*,
DOI 10.1007/978-1-4471-4387-1_95, © Springer-Verlag London 2012

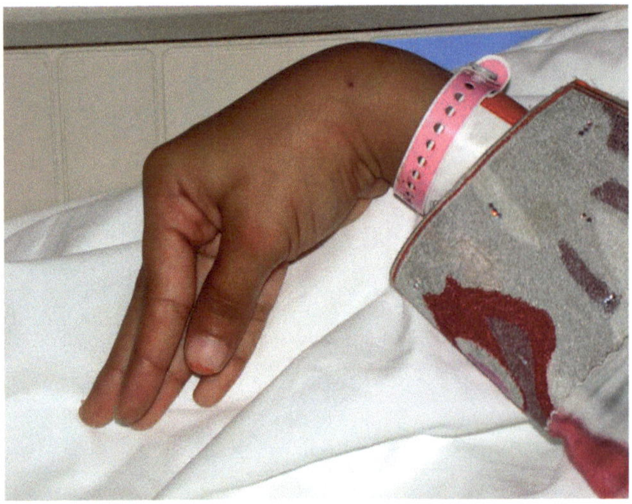

Fig. 95.1 Carpopedal spasm due to severe hypocalcemia

A ratio to diagnose FHH has been developed and is calculated as follows:

$$\frac{\text{Urine calcium }(\text{mmol}/\text{l})\times[\text{plasma creatinine }(\mu\text{mol}/\text{l})/1{,}000]}{\text{Plasma calcium }(\text{mmol}/\text{l})\times\text{ urinary creatinine }(\text{mmol}/\text{l})}$$

A ratio <0.01 is diagnostic of FHH, and ratios of >0.01 confirm pHPT.

Where necessary, genetic studies will confirm the genetic defect.

Has the Abnormal Parathyroid Adenoma or Hyperplastic Parathyroid Glands Been Successfully Localized?

In 1978 at the start of the senior consultant author's career, preoperative localized techniques were inadequate. Endocrine surgeons made no preoperative attempt to localize parathyroid tumors and went straight to four gland open parathyroidectomy. The enormous improvement in technology has now completely changed the situation. Whenever possible, attempts should be made preoperatively to localize exactly the parathyroid abnormality. It must be remembered that in primary hyperparathyroidism (1HPT), 80 % of cases will be due to a single adenoma and the remaining 20 % will be mainly parathyroid hyperplasia with an incidence of parathyroid carcinoma at less than 1 % [2].

High-resolution ultrasound with a probe of 7.5 or 10 mHz will demonstrate 90 % of adenomas weighing 1 g or more. This is an inexpensive technique but highly operator dependant. Ultrasound can only assess the tumor in the neck and is therefore of no value in assessing tumors of the mediastinum. Parathyroid tumors can also be visualized by sestamibi (Metroxyl – isobutyronitrile) radio-labeled with 99 mtc-pertechnetate. Unlike ultrasound, sestamibi scans can detect tumors in the mediastinum. It is recommended that wherever possible, both scans are performed in patients with primary hyperparathyroidism (Fig. 95.2). It is wise to add to the sestamibi scan photon emission tomography (PET) since this will give a three-dimensional view. This is helpful in evaluating tumors in the mediastinum and will demonstrate whether the tumor is in the anterior or the posterior mediastinum.

For the first exploration, computerized tomography (CT) is not routinely used unless the sestamibi and ultrasound are unhelpful. Invasive tests such as venous sampling or angiography are used only in reoperative cases. Magnetic resonance imaging (MRI) of the neck and anterior mediastinum is used only in reoperative cases. Ultrasound-guided biopsy of the parathyroids is not recommended as this may cause disruption of the parathyroid tumor with seeding. This can subsequently cause small pockets of parathyroid tissue to grow around the tumor bed. This leads to the condition known as disrupted parathyroid syndrome (parathyromatosis), characterized by local regrowth of parathyroid tissue.

Does the Patient Need Surgery?

Modern parathyroid surgery is so effective and safe that the diagnosis in any patient who is symptomatic may be considered for surgery.

It has been well established that patients with asymptomatic primary hyperparathyroidism have a better quality of life if they undergo surgery than if they remain untreated. In the past, this has been a controversial area, but the indications for surgery in the asymptomatic patient are now considered to be:

1. A serum calcium 0.25 mol/L above the local reference range
2. A urinary calcium greater than 200 mg over 24 h
3. A 30 % reduction in creatinine clearance for age, sex, and racial matching of normal individual.
4. Patients less than 50 years old
5. Patients with a bone mineral density score 2.5 standard deviations below the gender age and race-matched controls
6. Patients where medical surveillance is likely to be difficult

Has the Patient Been Safely Prepared for the Surgical Procedure?

Prior to the consideration of surgery, all patients should be vitamin D replete (patients operated on who are deficient in vitamin D have a higher risk of symptomatic postoperative hypocalcaemia). Most patients will have mild hypercalcemia with a serum calcium less than 3.0 mmol/L. It should be ensured that patients are well hydrated prior to surgery but other measures are unnecessary. If the calcium exceeds

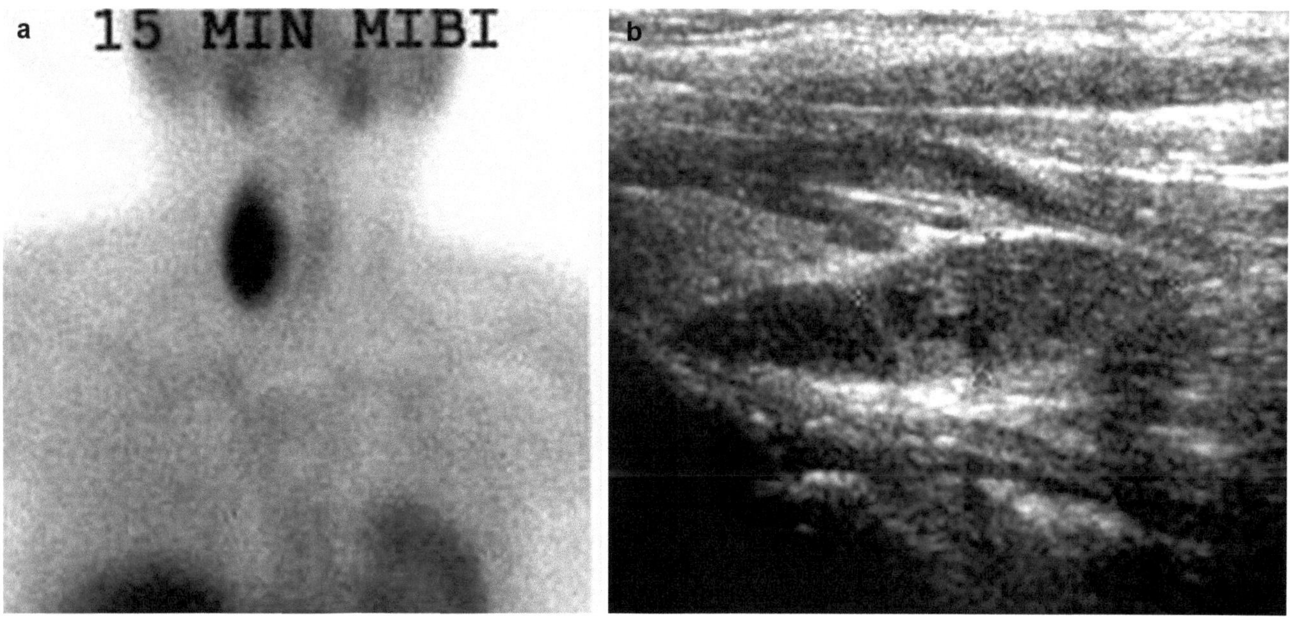

Fig. 95.2 Concordant scans: (**a**) sestamibi and (**b**) ultrasound

3.0 mmol/L, the patient should be admitted preoperatively for at least 24 h or more prior to surgery and be hydrated with 3 L of 0.9 % saline over 24 h using, in addition, a loop diuretic such as a furosemide to obtain a forced diuresis. If the calcium is above 3.5 mmol/L, several days of forced diuresis may be necessary to obtain a preoperative calcium of 3.0 mm/L or less. If this is not successful, then 90 mg intravenously of disodium pamidronate in 500 mL of 0.5 % saline over 4 h should be administered. This is usually successful, but on occasions, this dose may need to be repeated prior to surgery. Whenever possible, the use of pamidronate should be avoided as it leads to persistent postoperative hypocalcemia, which can prove very difficult to manage. Some clinicians have used the type two calcimimetic drug (cinacalcet) to prepare patients for surgery. This is an expensive way of preparing patients and is almost certainly unnecessary and is not recommended in patients with parathyroid adenoma or hyperplasia. However, it may be of value in preparing patients for surgery who have parathyroid carcinoma. Intravenous phosphate should be used rarely as it is likely to cause widespread soft tissue and kidney calcium deposition. In the rare event that one is considering using this drug, renal dialysis is a much better option. There is absolutely no role for the use of steroids, calcitonin, or mithramycin in the preparation of patients for parathyroidectomy.

Should a Localized, Scan-Directed or Traditional Open Technique Be Used?

It must never be forgotten that bilateral neck exploration (BNE) for primary hyperparathyroidism (pHPT) is a safe, easy-to-teach operation, the results of which are the gold standard for every other procedure. Worldwide rates of successful BNE have been reported in the region of 95 % [3]. The original BNE approach used was to identify all four parathyroid glands, remove the enlarged glands, and biopsy the remaining normal or suppressed glands. The philosophy was to confirm whether or not there was multiple gland disease or single gland disease. Over the years, the methodology of BNE has changed and there is now a tendency not to biopsy normal or suppressed glands. If biopsy is undertaken, there is a significant risk of damage to the parathyroids and a subsequent high incidence of postoperative hypocalcemia. Modern BNE consists, therefore, of removal of the adenoma or hyperplastic glands and the visualization of normal or the suppressed glands but not biopsying them. Intraoperative frozen section and intraoperative iPTH (IOPTH) estimation is desirable. If facilities are limited, these are not essential in BNE.

The Technique of Bilateral Neck Exploration (BNE)

Most patients are operated on under general anesthesia, although the author has done BNE using local anesthetic and the short-acting analgesic remifentanil. In patients undergoing general anesthesia, endotracheal anesthesia is used with the nerve monitoring equipment. The skin incision is based 2–4 cm above the sternal notch, and care is taken to gently extend the neck (pain in the neck following BNE is a common complication). Infiltration of the wound with 40–50 cc of Marcaine 0.25 % with 1:200,000 adrenaline can be performed before making the incision; however, the authors leave this until the end of the procedure as the local anesthesia may make the identification of a subcutaneous tissue plane difficult. Bipolar or monopolar diathermy is also less effective when local anesthetic has been used. There is no need when making the incision and raising the flaps to stray outside the confines of the sternocleidomastoid muscles. Staying within the confines of the muscles reduces the risk of damaging the cutaneous branches of the cervical plexus and minimizes the loss of sensation in the front of the neck. When raising the flaps, one should raise the flap laterally, as laterally the platysma is thicker and easy to separate from the underlying strap muscles (Fig. 95.3). If the dissection is started centrally, there is little in the way of platysma, and it can be difficult to raise the flap leading to a risk of buttonholing the skin (Fig. 95.4). Strap muscles are separated in the midline and are rarely divided. Before any structure is divided, apart from the middle thyroid vein, it is mandatory that the recurrent laryngeal nerve is identified (Figs. 95.5 and 95.6). It must be remembered that in approximately 1 % of patients, the recurrent laryngeal nerve on the right side can be nonrecurrent. The authors believe that the recurrent laryngeal nerve must always be identified; the old technique of intracapsular dissection of the thyroid in our view is outdated. We would always recommend the use of a nerve stimulator, which aids in the identification of the recurrent laryngeal nerve and is also of prognostic value as it will indicate that the nerve is anatomically intact at the end of the procedure (Figs. 95.7 and 95.8).

The surgeon should start looking for the parathyroid tumor on the side indicated by the imaging. Normal parathyroids are the size of a grain of rice: 5 mm in length, 3 mm wide, and, when normal, weigh no more than 40 mg. Any parathyroid that looks more than 40 mg in weight must be considered abnormal. Most normal parathyroids are bean shaped or spherical but may be bilobed or multilobed, although sometimes they are just flat structures lying in a fascial layer separate from the thyroid capsule. Normal parathyroids vary in color from pale yellow to brown. A typical normal parathyroid has a fatty surround and is soft, unlike a lymph node (Fig. 95.9). Small thyroid nodules look very different to parathyroid tissue, and thyroid nodules can be felt. It must be remembered that more than four glands may exist, and glands may also be found within the thymus. The recurrent laryngeal nerve may in part indicate the position of the parathyroid. The upper parathyroid in 80 % of cases is located behind the recurrent laryngeal nerve, in an area 2 cm in diameter, centered on the intersection of the recurrent laryngeal nerve and the inferior thyroid artery. The superior gland is remarkable as regards its symmetry. Once a superior gland has been found, it should be clipped so it can be identified at a later date—this acts as a marker for the contralateral upper parathyroid. Never remove a normal-sized parathyroid gland and be careful when clipping a normal parathyroid not to damage the blood supply. If the blood supply is damaged and the parathyroid goes a dark brown color, it should be transplanted into muscle pocket.

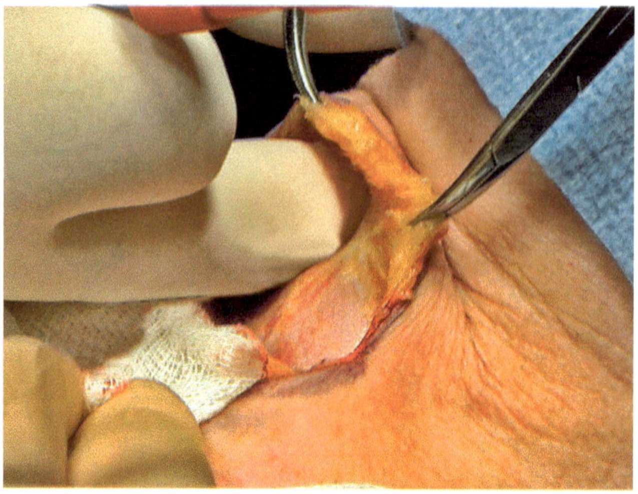

Fig. 95.3 Lateral dissection: platysma

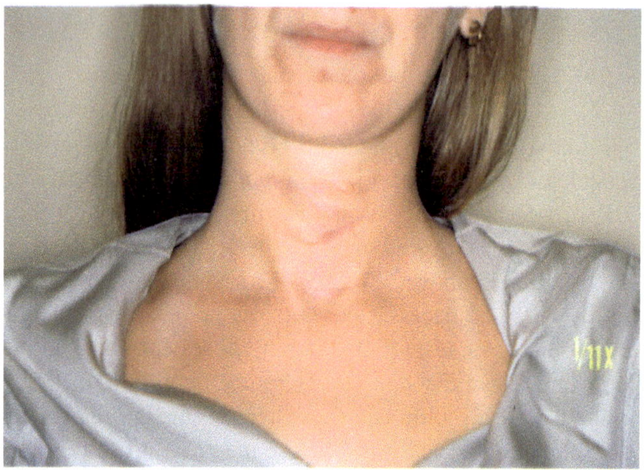

Fig. 95.4 Buttonholing of skin

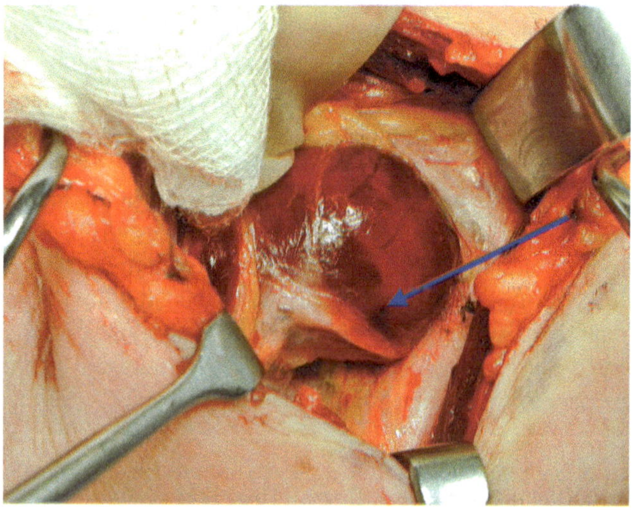

Fig. 95.5 Demonstrates the attachment of recurrent laryngeal nerve to large parathyroid tumour

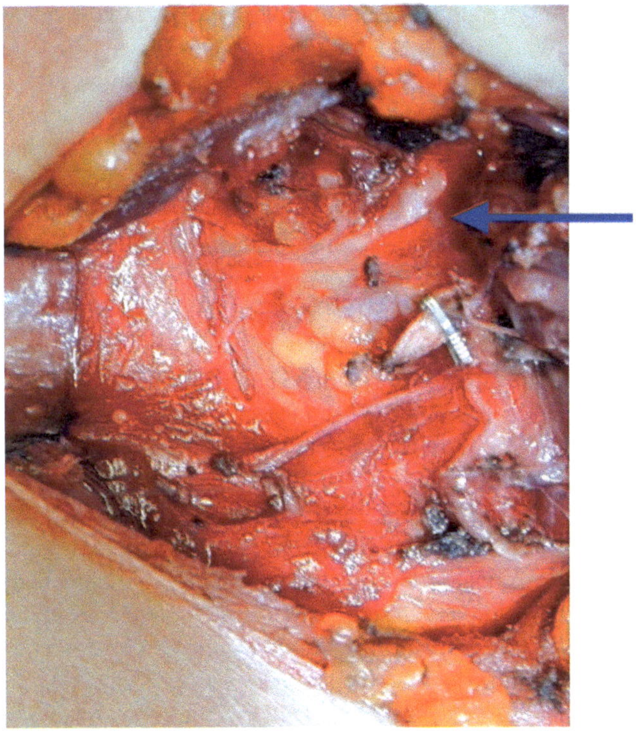

Fig. 95.6 Nonrecurrent laryngeal nerve. The arrow points to the nerve

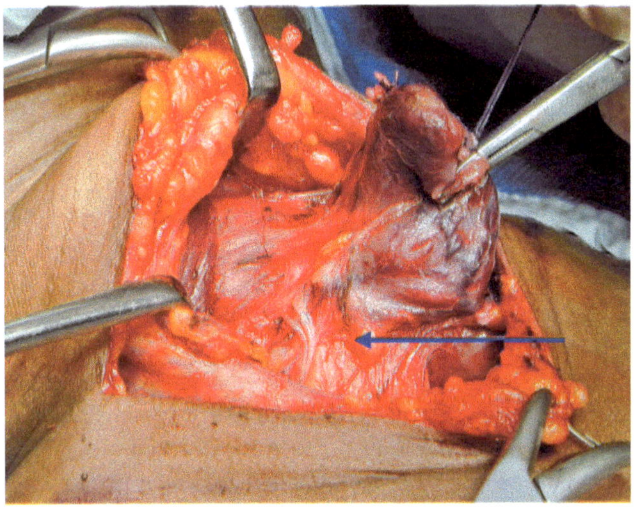

Fig. 95.7 Typical anatomical position of the recurrent laryngeal nerve

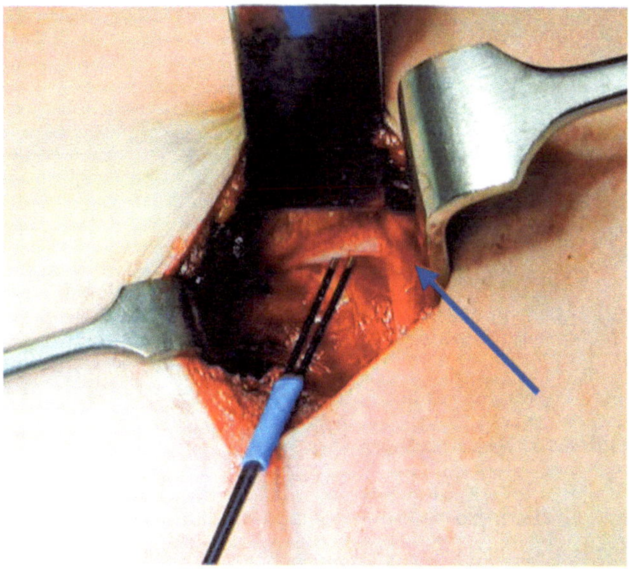

Fig. 95.8 Use of the nerve stimulator to assess the recurrent laryngeal nerve

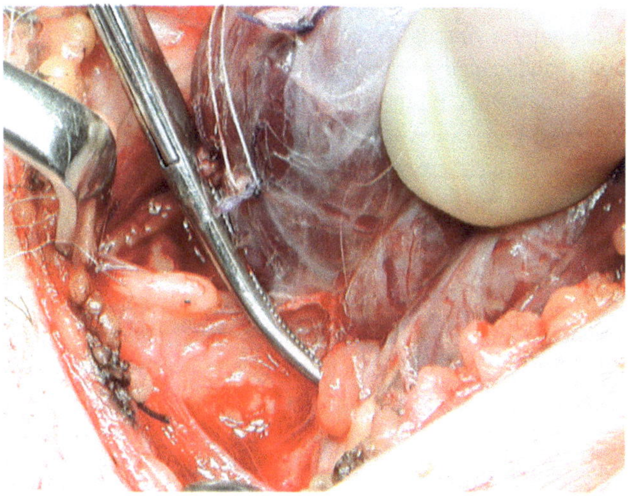

Fig. 95.9 Small lymph node

On occasions, a superior parathyroid gland that is enlarged is pushed down behind the esophagus by deglutition and can lie lower than the true lower parathyroid in the neck. Very rarely a true upper parathyroid derived from the 4th branchial pouch lies very high in the neck within the substance of the pharynx. Mediastinal parathyroids from the upper parathyroid position are always in the posterior mediastinum and can be paraesophageal or very low behind the pericardium.

The lower parathyroids are unkind to the surgeon. They are derived from the 3rd branchial pouch, and as they have a long developmental course, they can be anywhere from the angle of the mandible or bifurcation of carotid to the lower anterior mediastinum. They migrate with the thymus (parathymic complex), and in 1–5 % of cases, a parathyroid is truly intrathyroidal—when this occurs it is derived from the inferior glands. Fortunately, most lower parathyroids are within the thyrothymic ligament or thymus and are easily retrievable from the neck.

Careful hemostasis is essential, and one may come across an abnormal gland during one's dissection (Fig. 95.10). It is wise not to remove any enlarged parathyroid glands until all the other glands have been identified and clipped. If on one side there is a missing inferior gland despite a meticulous search, an intrathyroidal adenoma must be considered, and a thyroid lobectomy or lobotomy should also be considered. Often, parathyroids are wrapped around by thyroid tissue and are not truly intrathyroidal. If the surgeon is meticulous

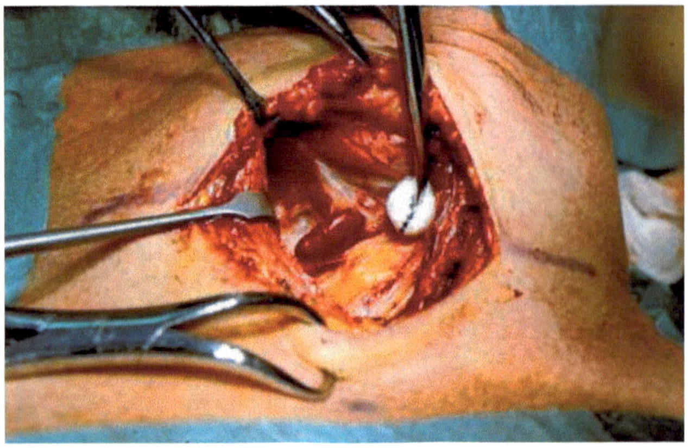

Fig. 95.10 Typical adenoma

and an abnormal parathyroid gland has not been found, it is likely the diagnosis is wrong or the adenoma is in the rare position under the aortic arch. It is best in these circumstances not to split the sternum but to reevaluate the patient and once more to review the diagnosis.

Missing lower parathyroids are usually within the thymus. The thymus is a tough structure in the lower neck, yellow in color, and usually drained by a single vein into the left innominate vein. It obtains its blood supply from the inferior thyroid artery. Lower parathyroid tumors low in the anterior mediastinum can usually be easily harvested by a transcervical thymectomy. This is carried out by simply just pulling up the thymus out of the mediastinum using traction with Spencer Well forceps having previously divided the vascular attachments. Apart from the blood vessels mentioned, there are no other vessels involved and the procedure is totally bloodless. One must always remember that in 80 % of cases reexplored for recurrent or persistent primary hyperparathyroidism that the missing abnormal gland is in a common anatomic position. In 20 % of cases of BNE for primary [4] hyperparathyroidism, there will be parathyroid hyperplasia; this may be asymmetric, also when it occurs five or more glands are common and accessory glands in the thymus are particularly common. This means that in these circumstances, apart from always identifying all the glands in the neck, the thymus should also be routinely removed (Fig. 95.11).

When single gland disease is found, only the adenoma should be removed, and the normal gland should be clipped but should not be biopsied. Great care must be taken, as already stated, not to break a parathyroid adenoma as spilled parathyroid tissue grows like weeds and can cause parathyromatosis (the disrupted parathyroid syndrome). This can subsequently be extremely difficult to treat and almost behaves like a parathyroid carcinoma.

While the management of single gland disease is relatively easy by BNE, the management of hyperplasia is difficult. A surgeon must always consider the possibility of the MEN1 syndrome if parathyroid hyperplasia is found at BNE. When managing multiple gland disease, there are really two main plans. The most radical is to remove all the parathyroid tissue and the thymus maintaining a normal serum calcium by the use of calcium and vitamin D supplements for life. This has the advantage of a definite cure of the hypercalcemia; it does mean lifelong replacement with tablets and does not really fill the tenants of endocrine surgery of returning the patient to a normal situation. A more elegant approach is to combine total parathyroidectomy with parathyroid transplantation of tissue into a nondominant forearm. Autotransplantation is performed into a muscular pocket (Fig. 95.12). It is quite difficult to judge the amount of parathyroid tissue to leave in place. Facilities in some units are available to cryopreserve parathyroid tissue, which can be used at a later date if not enough parathyroid tissue has been transplanted at the first operation. If the parathyroid transplant overproduces PTH and as long as the area has been carefully marked with titanium clips, it is quite easy under local anesthetic to remove small bits of parathyroid so as to obtain normocalcemia. The second approach to parathyroid hyperplasia is to do a subtotal parathyroidectomy, removing three glands and the major part of a fourth, taking the thymus while leaving behind 50 mg of parathyroid tissue in the neck, ensuring that it is well vascularized. This technique has an incidence of hypoparathyroidism and a significant incidence of recurrent hypercalcemia. It is best to leave behind a lower parathyroid that lies well away from the recurrent laryngeal nerve and mark it clearly with titanium clips so it can be easily identified if reoperation is necessary.

Parathyroid carcinoma is rare, and the approach is radical. At surgery, there is a hard mass involving the ipsilateral thyroid lobe, and local lymph nodes at level 4 and 3 may be involved. The management is an en bloc resection of the malignant mass, the ipsilateral thyroid lobe, and regional lymph node dissection. Titanium ligaclips should be placed to localize the area for subsequent postoperative radiotherapy, which has been shown to reduce the risk of local recurrence.

Double adenoma occurs in 2 % of cases, and [2] only the adenomas should be removed. The normal parathyroid should not be biopsied but left intact.

While the results of BNE are considered the gold standard for the treatment of primary hyperparathyroidism, modern technology with imaging has allowed less extensive procedures to be used with excellent results. Collectively, these techniques are known as minimally invasive parathyroidectomy. There are five main types:

1. Open scan-directed parathyroidectomy
2. Video-assisted parathyroidectomy with external retraction, gasless (Fig. 95.13)
3. Endoscopic parathyroidectomy using gas and a lateral approach

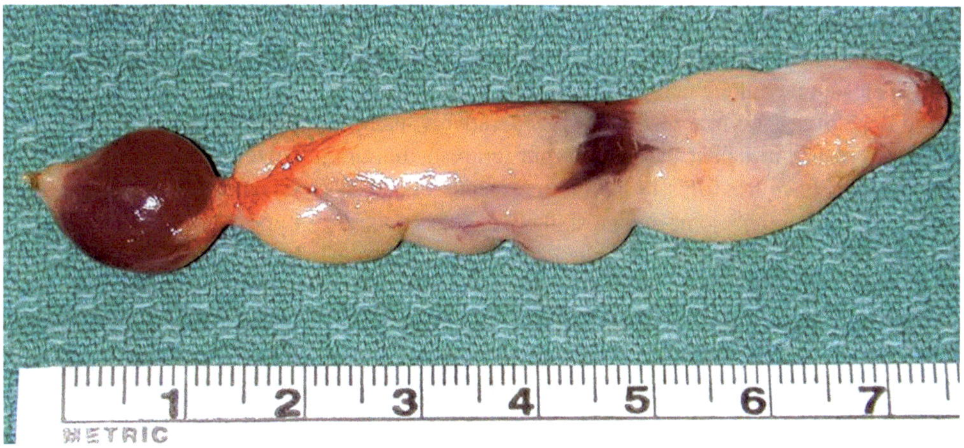

Fig. 95.11 Adenoma in thymus

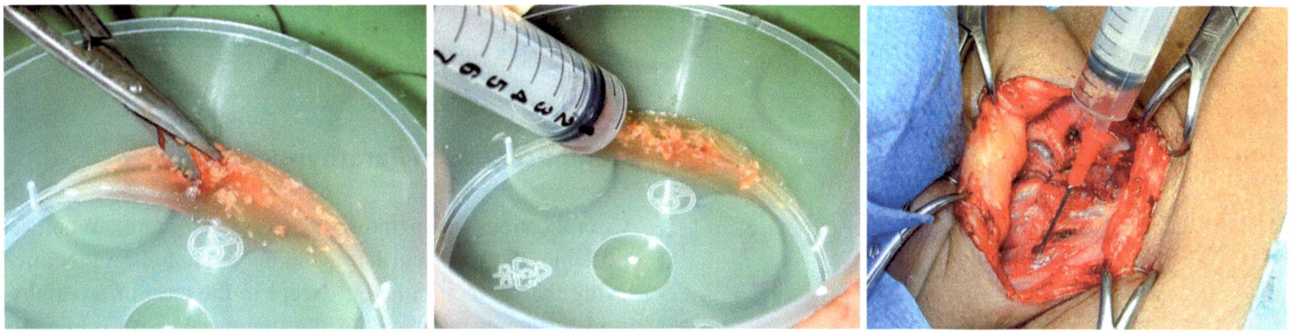

Fig. 95.12 Parathyroid transplantation

4. A trans-axillary endoscopic parathyroidectomy (this may be robotic assisted)
5. Sestamibi-directed parathyroidectomy

The most important principle of all these methods is that with a concordant sestamibi and ultrasound that the chance of missing a second parathyroid tumor or parathyroid hyperplasia is low (less than 5 %).[1] If in addition intraoperative PTH measurement is added, the results are almost as good as BNE. This has a great advantage to the patient as the incision is small. It is claimed that the complications are less, and minimally invasive parathyroidectomy can easily be done as a day case. This, of course, reduces costs.

An open concordant scan-directed parathyroidectomy is very simple. A small incision is made over where the skin has been marked, the recurrent laryngeal nerve is identified and the small parathyroid tumor is removed. If possible, the other ipsilateral parathyroid is visualized, intraoperative frozen section is performed and, if available, IOPTH is used. This procedure can be done under local anesthetic. Where possible, the recurrent laryngeal nerve should be identified, but if the parathyroid lies just within the thymus, it would be permissible not to identify the recurrent laryngeal nerve. The video-assisted technique is open and is gasless. It uses a central incision in the neck and allows all four parathyroids to be visualized. It is an excellent technique if one is concerned about parathyroid hyperplasia. It has, however, a very steep learning curve but has been developed extensively in Pisa, Italy [5], and results are equal to those of BNE.

Jean-Francois Henry [6] developed the endoscopic parathyroidectomy technique in Marseilles and uses gaseous inflation of the tissues and a lateral approach. This technique has a very steep learning curve and has the disadvantage that one can only look at one side of the neck at once. One would need, if one is unsuccessful on one side, to insert extra ports on the opposite side. Although popular in France, it has obtained little popularity in the United Kingdom or the United States of America.

The concern for having no neck scar has led surgeons to develop the trans-axillary approach. This can either be done with gas or gasless and uses a large incision in the axilla and has a steep learning curve. It has the advantage that there is no scar in the neck, which is very important in certain cultures. However, one cannot really call this a minimally invasive approach. It is really a highly invasive approach, although

[1] Personal unpublished observation by John Lynn, 2011.

not giving a scar in the neck. We do not believe this approach should be recommended or indeed is inappropriate.

An elegant technique that is quite complicated is to use a large dose of sestamibi a few hours preoperatively, using a gamma counter to detect the parathyroid tumor or tumors. The authors have used this on several occasions but, to be frank, found it cumbersome and most likely no longer necessary. It is widely used in certain units in the United States of America but has not gained great favor in the United Kingdom or Europe. In essence, we use ultrasound sestamibi scanning, intraoperative PTH, and intraoperative frozen section. In this method, the surgeon confirms that all the abnormal parathyroid tissues are removed by a combination of a fall in intraoperative PTH and a fall in radiation in the neck.

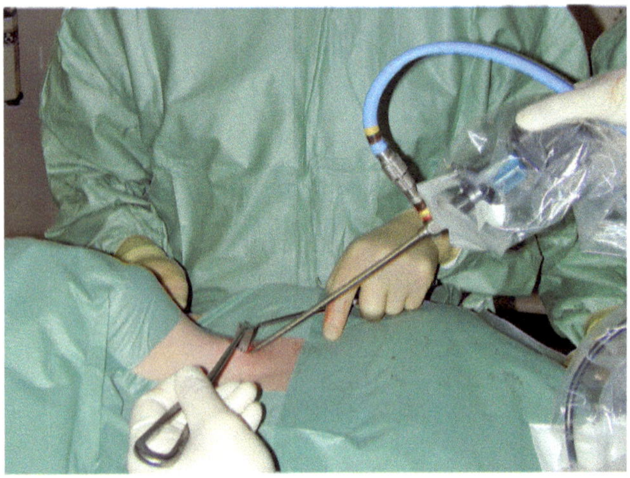

Fig. 95.13 Video-assisted

Where possible, frozen section pathology of the removed parathyroid tissue should be performed. The role of the frozen section is to do no more than confirm that the tissue is parathyroid tissue. Distinction between an adenoma, hyperplastic, or carcinoma is based not on frozen section but on the naked eye operative findings. IOPTH measurement is in many ways more useful than frozen section. Intact PTH has a half-life of some 3 min, and successful removal of diseased parathyroid tissue is confirmed by an intraoperative fall of a 50 % reduction in baseline PTH level as long as the post-excision level is low in the normal range. False positives are rare. On occasions a contralateral adenoma that is small may be missed by this technique, but this can easily be retrieved at a later date. The risk of this is less than 0.5 %.[2]

Complications of Parathyroidectomy

Complications of parathyroidectomy are rare. Wherever possible, the recurrent laryngeal nerve should be identified using the nerve stimulator, except in the case of a parathyroid adenoma lying within the thymus when a minimally invasive approach is being used. Hypocalcemia can be a major problem. Often the hypocalcemia is aggravated by low magnesium, and all patients with hypocalcaemia should be made magnesium replete. Surgery in patients with vitamin D deficiency should be avoided if

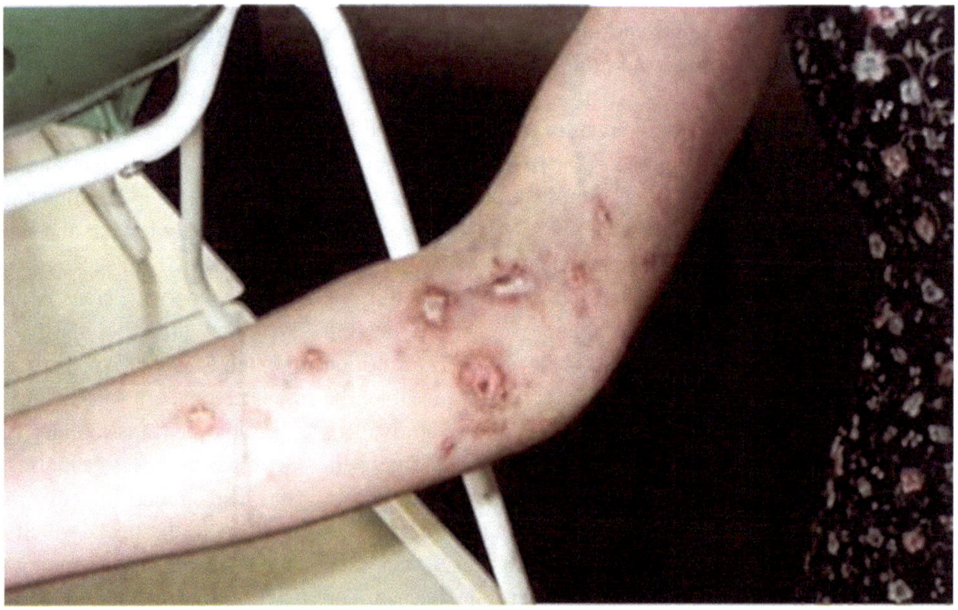

Fig. 95.14 Effects of extravasated calcium infusion

[2] Personal observations by John Lynn, 2011.

possible, as this increases the risk of postoperative hypocalcaemia. In some cases, vast amounts of calcium and vitamin D may be needed to be given to patients to maintain their serum calcium due to hungry bone disease and the massive flow of calcium into the bones. When this occurs, it may be necessary to give a continuous infusion of calcium gluconate 10 %. Under no circumstances should such an infusion be given in a peripheral vein as if the fluid extravasates; there is the chance of damage to the tissues (Fig. 95.14). In all patients with hungry bone disease, intravenous calcium must be administered through a central line.

Therefore, there is now a trend, because of excellent imaging, combined with the widespread use of IOPTH for minimally invasive parathyroid surgery. Most surgeons in the United Kingdom perform open incision parathyroidectomy under local or general anesthetic with intraoperative frozen section. Where possible, people are also using, in addition, IOPTH.

Conclusion

The surgeon should never forget that the gold standard for results is BNE, and, if in any doubt, a minimally invasive procedure should be converted to a BNE to obtain satisfactory results. It must also be remembered that if a procedure failed in inexpert hands, the most likely reason is that the tumor is in the neck and has been overlooked. In expert hands, it means that either a diagnosis was incorrect, possibly FHH, or that there is a tumor deep in the mediastinum.

References

1. Jean-François H, David T, van Slycke S. Parathyroid localization and imaging. In: Hubbard JGH, editor. Endocrine surgery, Springer specialist surgery series. London: Springer; 2009. p. 235.
2. Lewis PD. Surgical pathology of the parathyroids in primary and secondary hyperparathyroidism. In: Lynn J, Bloom SR, editors. Surgical endocrinology. Oxford: Butterworth Heinemann; 1993. p. 370.
3. Delbridge LW, Younes NA, Guinea AI. Surgery for primary hyperparathyroidism 1962–1996: indications and outcomes. Med J Aust. 1998;168(4):153–6.
4. Olubowale OO, Harrison BJ. Reoperative parathyroid surgery. In: Hubbard JGH, editor. Endocrine surgery, Springer specialist surgery series. London: Springer; 2009.
5. Miccoli P, Berti P, Materazzi G. Results of video-assisted parathyroidectomy: single institution's six-year experience. World J Surg. 2004;28:1216–8. Endocrine Surgery Principles and Practice. Series: Springer Specialist Surgery Series, Hubbard J, Inabnet WB, Lo, C-Yu (eds.). 2009, London: Springer-Verlag London Limited.
6. Henry JF, Raffaelli M, Iacobone M, et al. Video-assisted parathyroidectomy via the lateral approach v conventional surgery in the treatment of sporadic primary hyperparathyroidism: results of case–control study. Surg Endocsc. 2001;15:1116–9.

Part IX

Education, Training, Assessment, and Development

Professional Development and Competence of Physicians

96

Camer W. Vellani

Abstract

Technically enabled clinical specialization has enhanced the scope of clinical care. Moreover, with longevity grows the complexity of patients' illnesses and the need for expertise from various clinical disciplines. All the more important, therefore, is the need for holistic consideration of health care from the perspective of the patient's needs and circumstances.

Optimal care requires interpretation of the patient's complaints and careful observation, at times assisted by additional knowledge and special investigation. Crucially important is the fact that technical operative skills are of greater value when combined with a reasoned, rational approach to diagnosis and management.

Knowledge is the basis of all action but has limited practical value without thoughtful analysis of clinical observations and consideration of the world of the patient. Communication with the patient should relate to the person as a whole and must be attuned to the capacity of the recipient to understand.

The trainee learning from today's role models becomes tomorrow's model with critical potential to influence many in the practice of medicine.

Keywords

Professional development • The age of specialists • Knowledge • Technical skills • Role models • Assessment • Coordinated care

Introduction: The Age of Specialists

Currently physicians are raised in a world awash with information that grows exponentially by the day. Their readiness for practice is assessed by tests probing acquisition of specific facts and performance of focused procedures in the manner prescribed by a curriculum. Certification of satisfactory performance qualifies for basic professional practice.

Professional maturation follows, strongly conditioned by the nature of the health service where the young physician is employed, the filtration of clinical problems referred for a specialist's or subspecialist's opinion, the performance of role models and peers [1], the guidelines and algorithms for management of specific clinical conditions, and the susceptibility to litigation for alleged negligence, alongside intensive learning and search for the latest information. Such information is greater in volume than one's ability to assimilate, assess, and use rationally, even for the seemingly limited scope of a clinical subspecialty.

Knowledge that is useful for diagnosis and management of diverse clinical conditions, however, requires understanding of the basis of knowledge, beyond facts, and synthesis of elements of knowledge that has greater meaning than the elements considered individually. The process of deriving widely applicable synthesis of knowledge rather than just acquiring facts requires thought, reflection on the validity of an application, in the context of clinical problems that one is entrusted with for solutions, and time.

C.W. Vellani, MD (Wales), FRCP (London)
Department of Medicine, Aga Khan University, Stadium Road, Karachi 74800, Sindh, Pakistan
e-mail: camer.vellani@aku.edu

J.J. Talati et al. (eds.), *Urolithiasis*,
DOI 10.1007/978-1-4471-4387-1_96, © Springer-Verlag London 2012

By contrast, knowledge is commonly used differently for diagnosis in the process of pattern recognition and reliance on special investigation. Advantages of this method include reduction of the physician's time for clinical decisions and optimal use of resources for professional practice. Norman et al. [2] summarized evidence to support experience-based pattern recognition as the basis of a nonanalytical process leading to hypotheses for diagnostic consideration, practiced by both experts and novices. Useful knowledge for this purpose would comprise many clinical examples supplemented by "analytical de-biasing strategies."

This mode of practice assumes that diagnosis can be recognized by proximity to classical presentations of clinical conditions, conditioned by known associates of coexistent chronic illnesses; indeed, the latter must be considered always for management although they may not necessarily be the cause of the clinical problem at hand. Programmed management of the diagnosis follows. Too often this happens without clear understanding of the problem beyond the diagnostic label, or the difficulty experienced by the patient, or the familial, social, cultural, and economic consequences of his or her illness.

Recipients of Clinical Care

Coexistence of multiple diseases often requires referral to other clinical specialists. Frequently in such circumstances, a recipient of clinical care is confronted with fragmented opinions, investigations, communications, and interventions, and suffers from the absence of a coordinator who has a holistic understanding of the patient as a reactive person.

In such conditions, the patient seldom communicates his or her concern to the clinician, partly because the time for consultation is so limited and partly because the patient does not fully understand the expert physician's message. However, the patient does sense the experts' concerns with components of the organism rather than the whole person and questions the physician's competence to be a valid advocate for his or her good overall, even when the technical performance of the physician is at the highest level.

Patients function confidently in their own world, molded by their upbringing and society. Disbelief in interventions of almost any kind is compounded by information gleaned from the Internet, the usually unrelated experiences of relatives, friends, and acquaintances, and lack of any knowledge of health sciences. This leads to confused notions of science-supported interventions and apparent effectiveness of alternative remedies. Concerns generated by such information are often masked by the urge for multiple professional opinions.

Difficulty is multiplied when a physician presents different interventional options and asks the patient to choose, without the realization that often, in most parts of the world, a patient has little notion of how the body works, what the choices of interventions might mean for the outcome of the illness, and whether or not his or her systems can tolerate an internal assault on the body. Moreover, most patients across the world do not understand statistics; consequently the physician's oft-cited statistical "evidence" serves to confound the patient further.

The sufferer's anxiety then escalates to focus on the prognosis for life and functional ability and the impact of the illness on commitments to his or her family and unfinished work.

Surely, recruitment of the patient's compliance with the physician's advice requires confidence in the physician. Clear communication in carefully selected, understandable terms about the basis of the diagnosis and rationale for the plan of management, the prognosis for life and functionality, and the measures to prevent or ameliorate progression and disability is a crucial determinant of confidence [3]. More so when the plan of management takes into consideration the social and economic dimensions of the health care required, as well as provisions for long-term care, especially to prevent complications of the illness.

Application of Knowledge

Knowledge is the basis for understanding the structure, functions, and mechanisms of organ systems; the homeostasis that sustains functioning of the organism as a whole; and the nature of reproduction and differentiation of cells and their response to injury, as well as the rationale and complications of investigations and therapeutic interventions. Information about these elements is growing exponentially. Also growing is information concerning social and economic determinants of health and the burden of disease in the local, regional, and interconnected global population.

Preoccupation with knowledge, however, is unhelpful for solving clinical problems unless it can explain observations of the clinical state. Therefore, a major task for educators and assessors of physicians is to facilitate learning the skills of understanding the patient's thoughts and the significance of accurate clinical observations, in terms not only of the structures and functions of various organ systems but also the social and economic contexts of the clinical problem at hand.

Clinical observation and deductive reasoning provide a clearer understanding of the interrelated conditions of pathology and its functional consequences than pattern recognition and diagnostic label as the objective for management of illness. The basic knowledge required for deduction requires integration of crucial elements distributed across multiple disciplines, with recent additions that may or, as is often the case, may not be applicable in a given situation.

Equally important for the learner is the discipline of unbiased review of all the clinical observations of a patient, not just the faulty organ system or a fragment of it that is the subject of focus at a particular moment, and unbiased evaluation of the outcome of one's conclusions and actions. The process of review extends naturally to continuity of care that is supported by succinct and accurate written communication of the nature of the clinical state, the considerations leading to the management, the residual matters for further review, and the plan of management until progress or the lack of it is determined either by the primary team or another professional. Not often realized by the learner is the importance of this phase of care not only for the patient's future but also for enrichment of the physician's learning from experience of the natural history of an illness and the outcomes of interventions.

The discipline of critical review brings to notice matters of etiology and aspects of management of a clinical problem, especially in communities with limited resources, and triggers search for knowledge of that which is known and that which is not, individually and in collaboration with others as determined by complexity and need for diverse expertise.

The search leads to clearer understanding of a specific problem, stimulates discovery of new knowledge, and synthesis of knowledge that provides greater insights than its elements considered separately. Such outcomes form the basis of inductive reasoning that is broadly applicable and beneficial for patients, profession, and society at large, as well as intellectually satisfying for the physician, even though clarity of one's thought might have evolved over many years of critical clinical experience.

Technical Skills

Technical competence is generally considered for interventional procedures, but it applies equally to accuracy of observation, measurement, and consideration of error. Technical skill is required also for successful management of a patient's condition and reflection on the validity of decisions, with concern for constructive functional outcomes related to the individual's needs and socioeconomic circumstances.

Competent execution of instrumental procedures without harm requires learning by observation and one-on-one interaction with a skilled operator who is also an assessor of a learner's decisions and technical performance, through a process of graded responsibility and opportunity to practice under supervision. Advances in virtual technology have enhanced the ability to manage clinical problems, on the one hand, and challenge both the established physician and the learner to acquire expertise in new procedural skills, on the other [4].

A crucial element of competence and maturity is the ability to take decisions about the need for an interventional procedure in a given clinical situation. Assessment of technical competence is the function of the supervisors of a physician's period of learning, in relation to management of the problems that have been observed.

Role Model

Considerations of a physician's competence generally overlook the fact that today's learner will be tomorrow's educator. In clinical practice, a physician's professional behavior, resulting in efficient decisions under pressure, achieved with tireless empathy, technical skill, and accurate, comprehensible communication, will be the model for a learner's professional development [5]. Learning professional behavior is not restricted to an academic setting or program; a model of behavior also profoundly entrains other members of a health-care team. The educator and the learner of today should be wary at all times of the crucial but silent and unconscious influence of a physician's behavior and clinical performance on the intellectual development of a wide range of professionals in a health-care setting.

Conclusion

The nature of health services and performance of all its actors are essential determinants of the professional development and competence of a physician. Maturation of thoughtful decisions and skillful performance of technical skills requires time, opportunities to practice under supervision, close interaction with competent physicians, and constructive assessment of performance, taking into consideration observations of the health-care team and recipients of service. Much of professional competence is observable but not measurable.

If followed reliably with conviction by all assessors, the process should provide a more comprehensive assessment of professional competence than reliance on probes for awareness of factual information and performance of tasks according to specified method.

References

1. Irvine D. The performance of doctors: the new professionalism. Lancet. 1999;353:1174–7.
2. Norman G, Young M, Brooks L. Non-analytical models of clinical reasoning: the role of experience. Med Educ. 2007;41(12):1140–5.
3. Taylor I. Maintaining surgical professionalism. Ann R Coll Surg Engl. 2011;93:423.
4. McCulloch P. Surgical professionalism in the 21st century. Lancet. 2006;367:177–81.
5. Watkins PJ. Learning professionalism: a personal view. Clin Med. 2011;11(4):327–8.

Assessment in Postgraduate Training

97

Zareen Zaidi and John Norcini

Abstract

This chapter provides an overview of the assessment strategies used in postgraduate education. Assessment methodologies commonly used like the mini-clinical evaluation exercise (mini-CEX), direct observation of procedural skills (DOPS), objective structured clinical examination (OSCE), and portfolios are discussed.

No single assessment methodology serves as a panacea, and triangulation of multiple assessment methodologies based on the curriculum design are required. The reliability, the validity, and the educational impact of an assessment are of paramount importance. Quality assurance, staff training, and trainee insight into assessment tools used are imperative, and feedback should be a part of the assessment process rather than a separate entity. Assessment that focuses on the higher levels of the Miller's pyramid (shows how and does)—i.e., assessment of trainees as they work—is known as workplace-based assessment. As a formative tool, workplace-based assessment has the ability to influence the behavior of trainees by informing and advising them about their learning needs and motivating them to progress, thus steering learning down the right road.

Keywords

Postgraduate training • Workplace-based assessment • Examination • Certification • Miller's pyramid • Mini-clinical evaluation exercise (mini-CEX) • Clinical encounter card (CEC) • Direct observation of procedural skills (DOPS) • Objective structured clinical examination (OSCE) • Objective structured assessment of technical skills (OSATS) • nonoperative technical skills for surgeons (NOTSS) • Case-based discussion (CbD) • Multi-source feedback (MSF) • Mini-peer assessment tool (mini-PAT) • Portfolios

Introduction

Worldwide there has been a call for improving the assessment methodologies used to evaluate postgraduate trainees in medicine [1–3]. The age-old methodologies used including open-ended written questions and viva voce examinations have been criticized for not being standardized and for invoking examiner bias [4, 5, 6]. There has been an increased awareness that assessment should not be used only for summative purposes (i.e., examinations/certification) but should also be used to provide feedback, which is "the heart of medical education" as it informs and advises trainees about their learning needs and motivates them to progress [7, 8].

In 1990, Miller proposed a hierarchy of learning (Fig. 97.1) [9]. The lowest level of the pyramid is knowledge (knows), followed by competence (knows how), performance (shows how), and demonstration of action (does). In 2002, Van der Vleuten added assessment methodologies commonly used for each level of the Miller's pyramid; for

Z. Zaidi, M.B.B.S., M.D. (✉) • J. Norcini, Ph.D.
FAIMER Fellow (Philadelphia Institute), Foundation for Advancement of International Medical Education and Research (FAIMER), Philadelphia, PA, USA
e-mail: zzfaimer@gmail.com; jnorcini@faimer.org

J.J. Talati et al. (eds.), *Urolithiasis*,
DOI 10.1007/978-1-4471-4387-1_97, © Springer-Verlag London 2012

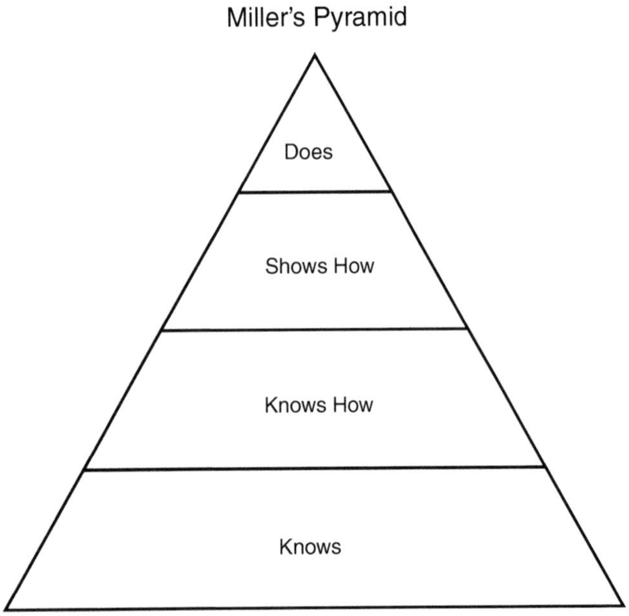

Fig. 97.1 The Miller's pyramid hierarchy of learning [9]

example, multiple-choice questions assess "knows" and "knows how" levels; observed clinical skills assessment exams like the mini-clinical evaluation exercise (mini-CEX), the direct observation of procedural skills (DOPS), and the objective structured clinical examination (OSCE) assess the "shows how" level; and peer assessments and patient outcomes assess the "does" level.

Over time, there has been growing emphasis on assessment that focuses on the higher levels of the Miller's pyramid (shows how and does), i.e., assessment of trainees as they work, also known as *workplace-based assessment* [10, 11]. Further, no single assessment methodology can "do it all." The concept of workplace-based assessment is to combine several assessment methodologies longitudinally, interspersed over a training period, such that snapshot pictures of the performance of the trainee from different perspectives are obtained. These snapshot pictures also provide opportunities to give feedback to the trainee throughout their training period instead of just at the end.

Judging the Assessment

To judge if the assessment tool used is robust, several different frameworks have been proposed. One of the commonly used ones looks at the psychometric properties of the test (validity, reliability) as well as the acceptability, educational impact, and cost of the test [3].

The *reliability* of an assessment method describes the reproducibility, generalizability, or consistency of its results, or the likelihood of the method producing similar scores, if repeated over time or if assessment is conducted by different examiners [12]. There are many different measures of reliability, often reported as coefficients, and some of which focus on particular sources of error. For instance, *inter-rater reliability* is the level of agreement between two or more independent assessors for the same trainee, measured as the Cohen's kappa (categorical data) or Pearson's correlation coefficient (interval data). *Internal consistency* evaluates if the results on two or more parts of the assessment agree with each other, often measured as Cronbach's alpha. The overall reliability coefficient is often obtained through a calculation based on generalizability theory, which takes into account several sources of error simultaneously. Reliability coefficients range from 1 (no error) to 0 (all error).

Validity is an aggregation of evidence indicating whether the scores from an assessment reflect the intended purpose [13]. Although this is now thought of as unitary judgment, it has several aspects. *Content validity* provides evidence that items on the test represent the content domain that is being tested, *predictive validity* provides evidence about the ability to predict future performance, and *concurrent validity* consists of evidence that the scores are related to those based on measures of the same domain.

The reliability and validity of an assessment are necessary but not sufficient; the educational impact of the assessment is of paramount importance [14]. The assessment methodology can "steer learning down the right road" [15]. Summative assessment alone misses the powerful opportunity to promote learning, while relying too heavily on self-assessment and self-directed learning fails to respond to the need for accountability. A fine balance is needed in assessment, with care to provide ample opportunity for feedback on performance. Additionally, the assessment method has to be acceptable to the trainers and trainees, and the costs incurred have to be kept in mind.

Workplace Assessment Methods

Workplace-based assessment is a combination of several tools, each measuring different competencies laid out by the General Medical Council, Association of American Medical Colleges (AAMC), Accreditation Council for Graduate Medical Education (ACGME), and CanMEDS [16–18]. Today's doctor is not just required to be knowledgeable and skillful but also must possess good communication skills, demonstrate an ability to work in a team, be compassionate, aware of the latest advances in their field, produce scholarly work, and demonstrate thorough professionalism. Knowledge may be assessed during summative written examinations, but several of the other competencies previously described require assessment during training. Here we discuss some of the commonly used instruments, all of which stress formative assessment.

Mini-CEX

This was first described in the USA, and it is an observed encounter of a trainee by an assessor, while the trainee undertakes a focused history and physical examination in a clinical setting [19]. The assessor uses a form to document the performance of the trainee along six dimensions: history taking, physical examination, humanistic qualities/professionalism, clinical judgment, counseling/communication skills, and organization and efficiency [20]. Once the trainees have completed the focused task, they are asked to summarize their findings. Depending on the level of the trainees, the assessor can ask them to discuss the provisional diagnosis and management plan. The assessor then marks the overall clinical competence/care (Fig. 97.2). The total duration of the encounter is 15 min followed by at least 5 min of feedback time. Trainees are expected to be assessed several times in a year by multiple assessors on different patients. The mini-CEX has strong construct, predictive, and concurrent validity; with 12–14 encounters, a reliability coefficient of 0.8 can be achieved [21, 22]. Good inter-rater reliability has been reported [23]. There is a concern about leniency in scoring and a requirement for faculty training to help standardize the results [24].

Clinical Encounter Card System (CEC)

The clinical encounter card (CEC) system is a variation of the mini-CEX that was developed in Canada [25]. Like the mini-CEX, the trainee is scored and given feedback during an observed encounter on history taking, physical examination, professional behavior, technical skill, case presentation, problem formulation, and problem solving skills.

Direct Observation of Procedural Skills (DOPS)

Structured like the mini-CEX and CEC, direct observation of procedural skills (DOPS) is an assessment tool, developed in the UK, which is used to evaluate trainee's procedural skills while observing them perform a procedure (Fig. 97.3) [26]. DOPS differs from logbooks in that assessors observe and provide trainees with immediate feedback on the procedure performed. Most commonly DOPS is used to evaluate competence in placing nasogastric tubes, intravenous lines, performing arterial blood gases, and endotracheal intubations. In the future, the focus of initial procedural skills training and assessment may move from bench simulators toward virtual reality simulators [27, 28].

Objective Structured Assessment of Technical Skills (OSATS)

Objective structured assessment of technical skills (OSATS) offers an assessment of technical skills [29]. The first component of OSATS is a checklist of specific competencies required to perform a particular procedure. The second component assesses generic skills, such as instrument handling and communication with the team (Fig. 97.4a, b). OSATS has been shown to have strong concurrent, construct, and face validity and inter-rater reliability of up to 0.8 [30–32]. For procedure-based training programs, it is recognized that some "higher-order" skills—such as situation awareness, decision-making, team working, and leadership—should be assessed other than procedural skills. For this purpose, the nonoperative technical skills for surgeons (NOTSS) tool have been developed in Edinburgh [33].

Case-Based Discussion (CbD)

Initially described in the USA and called chart-stimulated recall, case-based discussion (CbD) requires the trainee to select two case records of patients in which they made notes and present them to an assessor [34]. The assessor selects one and then discusses the management of the patient including investigations, treatment, and discharge plans (Fig. 97.5). Medical record keeping and overall professionalism of the trainee can also be assessed during the encounter. CbD has been found to have strong construct and concurrent validity, with good inter-rater reliability [35].

Multi-source Feedback (MSF)

Multi-source feedback (MSF), also known as 360 ° assessment, is a systematic collection of performance data and feedback for an individual trainee by a number of stakeholders who are asked to fill the form anonymously [26]. Several structured questionnaires have been developed for this purpose. A commonly used tool developed in the UK is the mini-peer assessment tool (mini-PAT), which gathers data on clinical care and practice, teaching and training ability, relationships with patients and colleagues, ability to work in a team, and an overall assessment (Fig. 97.6a, b) [36]. Collated data is presented to the trainee by an assessor, discussed, and an action plan drawn up, at least twice in the year. Satisfactory reliability requires several different assessors, and specialty-specific use of MSF has documented good concurrent validity [37].

Mini-Clinical Evaluation Exercise (CEX)

F2

Assessor: have you been trained in assessment methodology and feedback?
☐ Yes ☐ No

Please complete the questions using a cross ☒ Please use black ink and CAPITAL LETTERS

Doctor's Surname: ☐☐☐☐☐☐☐☐☐☐☐☐☐☐☐☐☐☐☐☐☐☐☐☐

Forename: ☐☐☐☐☐☐☐☐☐☐☐☐☐☐☐☐☐☐☐☐☐☐☐☐

GMC number: ☐☐☐☐☐☐☐ **YOUR GMC NUMBER MUST BE COMPLETED**

Clinical setting: A&E ☐ OPD ☐ In-patient ☐ Acute Admissions ☐ GP Surgery ☐ Other (please specify)

Clinical problem category: Airway/ Breathing ☐ CVS/ Circulation ☐ Gastro ☐ Neuro & visual ☐ Pain ☐ Psychiatric/ Psychological ☐ Other (please specify)

New or FU: New ☐ FU ☐ **Focus of Clinical encounter** History ☐ Diagnosis ☐ Management ☐ Explanation ☐

Assessor's rating of complexity of case: (F2) Low ☐ Average ☐ High ☐

Assessor's position: Consultant ☐ GP ☐ ST/CT 1-2 ☐ ST 3 or above/SPR ☐ Specialty Doctor/SASG ☐ Other (please specify)

Please rate the following areas	Well below expectations for F2 completion	Below expectations for F2 completion	Borderline for F2 completion	Meets expectations for F2 completion	Above expectations for F2 completion	Well above expectations for F2 completion	U/C*
	1	**2**	**3**	**4**	**5**	**6**	
1 History Taking	☐	☐	☐	☐	☐	☐	☐
2 Physical Examination Skills	☐	☐	☐	☐	☐	☐	☐
3 Communication skills	☐	☐	☐	☐	☐	☐	☐
4 Critical Judgement	☐	☐	☐	☐	☐	☐	☐
5 Professionalism	☐	☐	☐	☐	☐	☐	☐
6 Organisation/Efficiency	☐	☐	☐	☐	☐	☐	☐
7 Overall clinical care	☐	☐	☐	☐	☐	☐	☐

* U/C Please mark this if you have not observed the behaviour and therefore feel unable to comment.

Anything especially good?

Suggestions for development:

Agreed action:

Would you like to link this assessment as evidence to the foundation doctors PDP? *(If yes; drop down menu will appear; you can select up to 10 outcomes)* ☐ Yes ☐ No

Time taken for observation: (in minutes) ☐☐

Date (mm/yy) ☐☐ / ☐☐

Time taken for feedback (in minutes) ☐☐

Assessor's signature:

Assessor's surname: ☐☐☐☐☐☐☐☐☐☐☐☐☐☐☐☐☐☐☐☐☐☐☐☐

Assessor's registration number*: ☐☐☐☐☐☐☐☐

Appendix 1: Mini-Clinical Evaluation Exercise (CEX)
Source: http://www.foundationprogramme.nhs.uk/pages/trainers/assessment-guidance

Fig. 97.2 Mini-clinical evaluation exercise form (Adapted with permission of the Foundation Programme, National Health Service, UK. http://www.foundationprogramme.nhs.uk/pages/trainers/assessment-guidance)

Direct Observation of Procedural Skills (DOPS)

F1

Assessor: have you been trained in assessment methodology and feedback?
☐ Yes ☐ No

Please complete the questions using a cross ☒ Please use black ink and CAPITAL LETTERS

Doctor's Surname:

Forename:

GMC number: **YOUR GMC NUMBER MUST BE COMPLETED**

Clinical setting:	A&E ☐	OPD ☐	In-patient ☐	Acute Admissions ☐	GP Surgery ☐	Other (please specify)

Procedure (Please specify)

Assessor's position: Consultant ☐ GP ☐ ST3 or above/SpR ☐ Speciality Doctor/SASG ☐ Other (please specify)

Please grade the following areas	Well below expectation for F1 completion	Below expectation for F1 completion	Borderline for F1 completion	Meets expectation for F1 completion	Above expectation for F1 completion	Well above expectation for F1 completion	U/C*
	1	2	3	4	5	6	
1 Demonstrate understanding of indications, relevant anatomy, technique of procedure	☐	☐	☐	☐	☐	☐	☐
2 Obtains informed consent	☐	☐	☐	☐	☐	☐	☐
3 Demonstrates appropriate preparation pre-procedure	☐	☐	☐	☐	☐	☐	☐
4 Appropriate analgesia or preparation pre-procedure	☐	☐	☐	☐	☐	☐	☐
5 Technical ability safe sedation	☐	☐	☐	☐	☐	☐	☐
6 Aseptic technique	☐	☐	☐	☐	☐	☐	☐
7 Seeks help where appropriate	☐	☐	☐	☐	☐	☐	☐
8 Post procedure management	☐	☐	☐	☐	☐	☐	☐
9 Communication skills	☐	☐	☐	☐	☐	☐	☐
10 Consideration of patient/professionalism	☐	☐	☐	☐	☐	☐	☐
11 Overall ability to perform procedure	☐	☐	☐	☐	☐	☐	☐

* U/C Please mark this if you have not observed the behaviour and therefore feel unable to comment.

Please use this space to record areas of strength or any suggested development:

Would you like to link this assessment as evidence to the foundation doctors PDP? *(If yes; drop down menu will appear; you can select up to 10 outcomes)* ☐ Yes ☐ No

Date (mm/yy) /

Time taken for observation: (in minutes)

Time taken for feedback (in minutes)

Assessor's signature:

Assessor's surname:

Assessor's registration number*:

*if appropriate Please note failure of return of all completed forms to your administrator is a probity issue

Appendix II: Directly observed procedural skills form
Source: http://www.foundationprogramme.nhs.uk/pages/trainers/assessment-guidance

Fig. 97.3 Directly observed procedural skills form (Adapted with permission of the Foundation Programme, National Health Service, UK. http://www.foundationprogramme.nhs.uk/pages/trainers/assessment-guidance)

a

DIAGNOSTIC LAPAROSCOPY

Trainee Name:		StR Year:		Date:	
Assessor Name:		Post:			
Clinical details of complexity/ difficulty of case					

	Performed independently	Needs help	Not Applicable
	PLEASE TICK RELEVANT BOX		
Preparation of the patient:			
Ensures correct positioning of the patient			
Checked or observed catheterisation, pelvic examination and insertion of uterine manipulator where appropriate			
Establishing pneumoperitoneum			
Demonstrates knowledge of instruments and can trouble shoot problems			
Check patency and function of Veress (if used)			
Correct incision			
Controlled insertion of Veress (if used)			
Insufflation to at least 20 mmHg			
Controlled insertion of primary port			
Controlled insertion of secondary port under direct vision			
Operative procedure			
Maintains correct position of optics			
Clear inspection of pelvic and abdominal structures			
Movements: fluid and atraumatic			
Appropriate use of assistants (if applicable)			
Correct interpretation of operative findings			
Removal of ports under direct vision			
Deflation of pneumoperitoneum			
Appropriate skin closure			

Both sides of this form to be completed and signed

Appendix III: Objective structured assessment of technical skills form

Source: http://www.rcog.org.uk/education-and-exams/curriculum/core

Fig. 97.4 (**a, b**) Objective structured assessment of technical skills form (Reproduced from http:www.rcog.org.uk/education-and-exams/curriculum/core with the permission of the Royal College of Obstetricians and Gynaecologists. All rights reserved)

b

GENERIC TECHNICAL SKILLS ASSESSMENT

Assessor, please ring the candidate's performance for each of the following factors:

Respect for tissue	Frequently used unnecessary force on tissue or caused damage by inappropriate use of instruments.	Careful handling of tissue but occasionally causes inadvertent damage.	Consistently handled tissues appropriately with minimal damage.
Time, motion and flow of operation and forward planning	Many unnecessary moves. Frequently stopped operating or needed to discuss next move.	Makes reasonable progress but some unnecessary moves. Sound knowledge of operation but slightly disjointed at times.	Economy of movement and maximum efficiency. Obviously planned course of operation with effortless flow from one move to the next.
Knowledge and handling of instruments	Lack of knowledge of instruments.	Competent use of instruments but occasionally awkward or tentative.	Obvious familiarity with instruments.
Suturing and knotting skills as appropriate for the procedure	Placed sutures inaccurately or tied knots insecurely and lacked attention to safety.	Knotting and suturing usually reliable but sometimes awkward.	Consistently placed sutures accurately with appropriate and secure knots and with proper attention to safety.
Technical use of assistants **Relations with patient and the surgical team**	Consistently placed assistants poorly or failed to use assistants. Communicated poorly or frequently showed lack of awareness of the needs of the patient and/or the professional team.	Appropriate use of assistant most of the time. Reasonable communication and awareness of the needs of the patient and/or of the professional team.	Strategically used assistants to the best advantage at all times. Consistently communicated and acted with awareness of the needs of the patient and/or of the professional team.
Insight/attitude	Poor understanding of areas of weakness.	Some understanding of areas of weakness.	Fully understands areas of weakness.
Documentation of procedures	Limited documentation, poorly written.	Adequate documentation but with some omissions or areas that need elaborating.	Comprehensive legible documentation, indicating findings, procedure and postoperative management.

Based on the checklist and the Generic Technical Skills Assessment, Dr ....

☐ is competent in all areas included in this OSATS.

☐ is working towards competence.

Needs further help with: * *	Competent to perform the entire procedure without the need for supervision
Date	Date
Signed (trainer)	Signed
Signed (trainee)	Signed

Appendix III: Objective structured assessment of technical skills form
Source: http://www.rcog.org.uk/education-and-exams/curriculum/core

Fig. 97.4 (continued)

Case-based Discussion (CbD)

F1

Assessor: have you been trained in assessment methodology and feedback?
☐ Yes ☐ No

Please complete the questions using a cross ☒ Please use black ink and CAPITAL LETTERS

Doctor's Surname:

Forename:

GMC number: **YOUR GMC NUMBER MUST BE COMPLETED**

Clinical setting: A&E ☐ OPD ☐ In-patient ☐ Acute Admissions ☐ GP Surgery ☐ Other (please specify)

Clinical problem category: Airway/ Breathing ☐ CVS/ Circulation ☐ Gastro ☐ Neuro & visual ☐ Pain ☐ Psychiatric/ Psychological ☐ Other (please specify)

Focus of clinical encounter: Medical record keeping ☐ Clinical Assessment ☐ Management ☐ Professionalism ☐

Assessor's rating of complexity of case: (F1) Low ☐ Average ☐ High ☐ **Assessor's position:** Consultant/GP ☐ ST3 or above/ SpR ☐ Specialty Doctor/SASG ☐

Please grade the following	Well below expectations for F1 completion	Below expectations for F1 completion	Borderline for F1 completion	Meets expectations for F1 completion	Above expectations for F1 completion	Well above expectations for F1 completion	U/C*
	1	2	3	4	5	6	
1 Medical record keeping	☐	☐	☐	☐	☐	☐	☐
2 Clinical assessment	☐	☐	☐	☐	☐	☐	☐
3 Investigation and referrals	☐	☐	☐	☐	☐	☐	☐
4 Treatment	☐	☐	☐	☐	☐	☐	☐
5 Follow-up and future planning	☐	☐	☐	☐	☐	☐	☐
6 Professionalism	☐	☐	☐	☐	☐	☐	☐
7 Overall clinical judgement	☐	☐	☐	☐	☐	☐	☐

* U/C Please mark this if you have not observed the behaviour and therefore feel unable to comment.

Anything especially good?

Suggestions for development:

Agreed action:

Would you like to link this assessment as evidence to the foundation doctors PDP? *(If yes; drop down menu will appear; you can select up to 10 outcomes)* ☐ Yes ☐ No

Date (mm/yy) ☐☐/☐☐

Time taken for observation: (in minutes)

Time taken for feedback (in minutes)

Assessor's signature:

Assessor's surname:

Assessor's registration number*:

*if appropriate

Appendix IV: Case-based assessment form
Source: http://www.foundationprogramme.nhs.uk/pages/trainers/assessment-guidance

Fig. 97.5 Case-based assessment form (Adapted with permission of the Foundation Programme, National Health Service, UK. http://www.foundationprogramme.nhs.uk/pages/trainers/assessment-guidance)

a

The Yorkshire Deanery

Department for NHS Postgraduate Medical and Dental Education

mini-PAT (peer assessment tool)

Please complete the questions using a ☒ Please use black ink and CAPITAL LETTERS
A doctor who is performing at the expected level for the grade scores a 4

Doctor's surname

Doctor's forename

Doctor's GMC No. Grade Year in Grade Form No.

How do you rate this Doctor in their:	1 Below expectations for grade	2	3 Borderline for grade	4 Meets expectations for grade	5	6 Above expectations for grade	U/C*
Good clinical care							
1. Ability to diagnose patient problems	☐	☐	☐	☐	☐	☐	☐
2. Ability to formulate appropriate management plans	☐	☐	☐	☐	☐	☐	☐
3. Awareness of their own limitations	☐	☐	☐	☐	☐	☐	☐
4. Ability to respond to psychosocial aspects of illness	☐	☐	☐	☐	☐	☐	☐
5. Appropriate utilisation of resources e.g. ordering investigations	☐	☐	☐	☐	☐	☐	☐
Maintaining good medical practice							
6. Ability to manage time effectively/prioritise	☐	☐	☐	☐	☐	☐	☐
7. Technical skills (appropriate to current practice)	☐	☐	☐	☐	☐	☐	☐
Teaching and training, appraising and assessing							
8. Willingness and effectiveness when teaching/training colleagues	☐	☐	☐	☐	☐	☐	☐
Relationship with patients							
9. Communication with patients	☐	☐	☐	☐	☐	☐	☐
10. Communication with carers and/or family	☐	☐	☐	☐	☐	☐	☐
11. Respect for patients and their right to confidentiality	☐	☐	☐	☐	☐	☐	☐
Working with colleagues							
12. Verbal communication with colleagues	☐	☐	☐	☐	☐	☐	☐
13. Written communication with colleagues	☐	☐	☐	☐	☐	☐	☐
14. Ability to recognise and value the contribution of others	☐	☐	☐	☐	☐	☐	☐
15. Accessibility/reliability	☐	☐	☐	☐	☐	☐	☐
16. Overall, how do you rate this doctor compared to another doctor of the same grade?	☐	☐	☐	☐	☐	☐	☐

Do you have any concerns about this doctor's probity or health? ☐ Yes ☐ No

If yes please state your concerns:

*U/C Please mark this if you have not observed the behaviour and therefore feel unable to comment

Please turn over ......

Appendix V: Mini-peer assessment questionnaire
Source: http://www.mmc.nhs.uk

Fig. 97.6 (**a**, **b**) Mini-peer assessment questionnaire (Adapted with permission of the Foundation Programme, National Health Service, UK. http://www.mmc.nhs.uk)

b

Anything especially good?

Please describe any behaviour that raised concerns or should be a particular focus for development:

Your Gender: ☐ Male ☐ Female

Your ethnic group?:

☐ British
☐ Irish
☐ Other White Background
☐ Caribbean
☐ African
☐ Any other Black Background
☐ Indian
☐ Pakistani
☐ Bangladeshi
☐ Other Asian Background
☐ White and Black Caribbean
☐ White and Black African
☐ White and Asian
☐ Any other mixed background
☐ Chinese
☐ Any other ethnic group

Which environment have you primarily observed the doctor in?
(Please choose one answer only)

☐ Inpatients
☐ Outpatients
☐ Both In and Out-patients
☐ A&E/Admissions
☐ Community Speciality
☐ Laboratory/Research
☐ Intensive Care
☐ Theatre
☐ General Practice
☐ Other (Please Specify)

Your position:

☐ Consultant ☐ SASG ☐ Allied Health Professional
☐ Nurse ☐ SHO ☐ Foundation/PRHO
☐ GP ☐ SpR
☐ Other (Please specify)

If you are a Nurse or AHP how long have you been qualified?: years

Length of working relationship: months

Have you had training in the use of this assessment tool?:

How long has it taken you to complete this form (in minutes)?:

☐ No
☐ Yes: Have Read Guildelines
☐ Yes: Face-to-Face
☐ Yes: Web/CD rom

Your Signature: Date: / /

Your Surname:

Your GMC No: **(doctors only)**

Appendix V: Mini-peer assessment questionnaire
Source: http://www.mmc.nhs.uk

Acknowledgements: mini-PAT is derived from SPRAT (Sheffield Peer Review Assessment Tool)

Fig. 97.6 (continued)

Portfolios

Unlike logbooks, which provide evidence of completion of technical tasks, portfolios show the professional growth and learning of the trainee through a collection of material over time [38]. The collection can be in paper form or Web-based, with assessors providing feedback to the trainee and encouraging reflective practice. Due to the qualitative nature of the assessment, portfolios are subject to assessor bias, which renders their use difficult in summative assessment. Various authors have studied the validity and reliability of portfolios, the results of which are disparate [39]. However, there is evidence that if portfolios are well implemented and triangulated with other assessment methodologies, they can support the professional development of trainees.

Conclusion

In conclusion, assessment design has to match the curriculum design, and triangulation of multiple assessment methodologies achieves the best results. Quality assurance of assessment is necessary to ensure quality; therefore, staff training as well as trainee insight into assessment tools used is imperative. Providing feedback should be a part of the assessment process rather than a separate entity; unfortunately trainees often go through long periods without directly observed assessment and structured feedback [40]. In order to give constructive feedback and help develop action plans with trainees, faculty requires training for which an ongoing faculty development plan is helpful [41].

Workplace-based assessment tools are best used for formative assessment rather than summative high-stake assessments. This is because it is difficult to ensure that all trainees encounter patients of equivalent difficulty, standards vary across institutions, and there is the potential for examiner bias [8]. However, because of the power of being able to influence behavior through feedback, workplace-based assessment remains instrumental in shaping the performance of young doctors.

References

1. ABIM Foundation, ACP–ASIM Foundation, ACP–ASIM Foundation, European Federation of Internal Medicine. Medical professionalism in the new millennium: a physician charter. Ann Intern Med. 2002;136(3):243–6.
2. Panel on the General Professional Education of the Physician and College Preparation for Medicine (GPEP). Physicians for the twenty-first century: The GPEP Report. Washington, D.C.: Association of American Medical Colleges; 1984.
3. Van der Vleuten CPM. The assessment of professional competence: development, research and practical implications. Adv Health Sci Educ. 1996;1(1):41–67.
4. Chikwe J, de Souza AC, Pepper JR. No time to train surgeons. Br Med J. 2004;328:418–9.
5. Wragg A, Wade W, Fuller G, et al. Assessing the performance of specialist registrars. Clin Med. 2003;3(2):131–4.
6. Newble D, Jolly B, Wakeford R. The certification and recertification of doctors. Issues in the assessment of clinical competence. Cambridge: Cambridge University Press; 1994:231–43.
7. Branch WT, Paranjape A. Feedback and reflection: teaching methods for clinical settings. Acad Med. 2002;77:1185–8.
8. Norcini J, Burch V. Workplace-based assessment as an educational tool: AMEE guide No 31. Med Teach. 2007;29:855–71.
9. Miller GE. The assessment of clinical skills/competence/performance. Acad Med. 1990;65(9):S63–7.
10. Norcini JJ. ABC of learning and teaching in medicine: work based assessment. Br Med J. 2003;326(7392):753–5.
11. Postgraduate Medical Education and Training Board Assessment Sub-group (2003). Principles and Standards for Assessment. Postgraduate Medical Education and Training Board, London 2005.
12. Schuwirth LWT, van der Vleuten CPM. How to design a useful test: the principles of assessment. In: Swanwick T, editor. Understanding medical education: evidence, theory and practice. Oxford: Wiley-Blackwell; 2010.
13. Sheskin DJ. Handbook of parametric and nonparametric statistical procedures. 4th ed. Washington, D.C.: Chapman and Hall/CRC; 2004. ISBN 1584888148.
14. Shumway JM, Harden RM. The assessment of learning outcomes for the competent and reflective physician: AMEE guide N0.25. Med Teach. 2003;25(6):569–84.
15. Norman G, Neville A, Blake JM, Mueller B. Assessment steers learning down the right road: impact of progress testing on licensing examination performance. Med Teach. 2010;32(6):496–9.
16. AAMC. Report I: learning objectives for medical student education. Medical Schools Objectives Project. Washington, D.C.: AAMC; Jan 1998.
17. ACGME. Accreditation Council for Graduate Medical Education[Online]. [cited Nov 1 2010]. 2003. Available from: http://www.acgme.org.
18. CanMEDS. Extract from the CanMEDS 2000 project societal needs working group report. Med Teach. 2000;22(6):549–54.
19. Norcini JJ, Blank LL, Arnold GK, Kimball HR. The mini-CEX (clinical evaluation exercise): a preliminary investigation. Ann Intern Med. 1995;123:795–9.
20. Norcini JJ, Blank LL, Duffy FD, Fortna G. The mini-CEX: a method for assessing clinical skills. Ann Intern Med. 2003;138: 476–81.
21. Torre DM, Simpson DE, Elnicki DM, et al. Feasibility, reliability and user satisfaction with a PDA-based mini-CEX to evaluate the clinical skills of third-year medical students. Teach Learn Med. 2007;19(3):271–7.
22. Kogan JR, Bellini LM, Shea JA, et al. Feasibility, reliability, and validity of the mini-clinical evaluation exercise (mCEX) in a medicine core clerkship. Acad Med. 2003;78(10 Suppl):S33–5.
23. Norcini JJ, Blank LL, Arnold GK, et al. Examiner differences in the mini-CEX. Adv Health Sci Educ. 1997;2(1):27–33.
24. Hawkins RE, Margolis MJ, Durning SJ, Norcini JJ. Constructing a validity argument for the mini-clinical evaluation exercise: a review of the research. Acad Med. 2010;85(9):1453–61.
25. Hatala R, Norman GR. In-training evaluation during an internal medicine clerkship. Acad Med. 1999;74:S118–20.
26. Wragg A, Wade W, Fuller G, Cowan G, Mills P. Assessing the performance of specialist registrars. Clin Med. 2003;3:131–4.
27. Taffinder N, McManus I, Jansen J, Russell R, Darzi A. An objective assessment of surgeon's psychomotor skills: validation of the MIST-VR laparoscopic simulator. Br J Surg. 1998;75:281.
28. Kneebone R. Simulation in surgical training: educational issues and practical implications. Med Educ. 2003;37:267–77.

29. Martin JA, Regehr G, Reznick R, Macrae H, Murnaghan J, Hutchison C, et al. Objective structured assessment of technical skill (OSATS) for surgical residents. Br J Surg. 1997;84:273–8.
30. Hance J, Aggarwal R, Stanbridge R, et al. Objective assessment of technical skills in cardiac surgery. Eur J Cardiothorac Surg. 2005;28(1):157–62.
31. Ault G, Reznick R, MacRae H, et al. Exporting a technical skills evaluation technology to other sites. Am J Surg. 2001;182(3): 254–6.
32. Setna Z, Jha V, Boursicot KA, Roberts TE. Evaluating the utility of workplace-based assessment tools for speciality training. Best Pract Res Clin Obstet Gynaecol. 2010;24:767–82.
33. Yule S, Flin R, Paterson-Brown S, Maran N, Rowley D. Development of a rating system for surgeons' non-technical skills. Med Educ. 2006;40:1098–104.
34. Maatsch JL, Huang R, Downing S, Barker B. Predictive validity of medical specialist examinations. Final report for Grant HS 02038-04. East Lansing: National Center of Health Services Research. Office of Medical Education Research and Development, Michigan State University; 1983.
35. Norman GR, Davis D, Painvin A, Lindsay E, Rath D, Ragbeer M. Comprehensive assessment of clinical competence of family/general physicians using multiple measures. Proceedings of the research in medical education conference, 1989;7:75–9.
36. Archer JC, Norcini JJ, Davies HA. Peer review of pediatricians in training using SPRAT. Br Med J. 2005;330:1251–3.
37. Archer J, Norcini J, Southgate L, Heard S, Davies H. Mini-PAT (peer assessment tool): a valid component of a national assessment programme in the UK? Adv Health Sci Educ Theory Pract. 2008;13:181–92.
38. Tochel C, Haig A, Hesketh A, Cadzow A, Beggs K, Colthart I, et al. The effectiveness of portfolios for post-graduate assessment and education: BEME guide No 12. Med Teach. 2009;31:299–318.
39. Dannefer EF, Henson LC. The portfolio approach to competency-based assessment at the Cleveland clinic Lerner college of medicine. Acad Med. 2007;82(5):493–502.
40. Day SC, Grosso LG, Norcini JJ, Blank LL, Swanson DB, Horne MH. Residents' perceptions of evaluation procedures used by their training program. J Gen Intern Med. 1990;5:421–6.
41. Holmboe ES, Yepes M, Williams F, Huot SJ. Feedback and the miniclinical evaluation exercise. J Gen Intern Med. 2004;19: 558–61.

Assessment of Competence

98

Edward Matsumoto and Jen Hoogenes

Abstract

Accrediting bodies worldwide are now requiring residents to be deemed clinically competent in their specialty before certification is granted. Over time, residency training has shifted from the unstructured apprenticeship model to a more practice-based systems approach that includes ensuring that residents are competent to practice safe, effective medicine and surgery in practice. Surgical residency programs are adopting competency-based curricula with specialty-specific objectives that must be met by all residents. Although "medical competence" has yet to be defined in the literature, several governing bodies throughout the world have developed and implemented core competency frameworks designed for uptake by residency programs. Multiple valid and reliable assessment measures are now widely used to evaluate a resident's ability to meet core competency requirements. These measures can be tailored to a specific specialty. In surgery, the assessment of technical skills is vital to ensuring competency, and various tools are available for this purpose. Although surgical educators are faced with numerous barriers, the development and implementation of a competency-based curriculum is fundamental to ensuring that surgical residents are capable of working as safe, certified surgeons.

Keywords

Competency assessment • Surgical education • Urology • Technical skills assessment Competency-based curriculum • Residency • Educational measurement • CanMEDS ACGME core competencies • UK Foundation Programme

A skilled surgical practitioner requires a depth of cognitive knowledge, an appropriate surgical judgment, and an ability to act quickly but thoughtfully and when necessary in a decisive manner. The surgeon must have compassion and be a good communicator and must be perceptive and dedicated. Surgeons must also be skilled in the surgical craft to perform particular technical tasks which are often the centerpiece of the care of the surgical patient.

Wanzel, Ward, and Reznick [1]

E. Matsumoto, M.D., MEd, FRCSC (✉)
Division of Urology, St. Joseph's Healthcare, McMaster University, 50 Charlton Ave. E. G343, Hamilton, ON L8N 4A6, Canada
e-mail: matsumo@mcmaster.ca

J. Hoogenes, M.S., Ph.D.(c)
Department of Clinical Epidemiology and Biostatistics and Department of Surgery, McMaster University, St. Joseph's Healthcare, 50 Charlton Ave. E. G826, Hamilton, ON L8N 4A6, Canada
e-mail: reamja@mcmaster.ca

J.J. Talati et al. (eds.), *Urolithiasis*,
DOI 10.1007/978-1-4471-4387-1_98, © Springer-Verlag London 2012

Introduction

Clinical competence and demonstration of professional excellence are requisites for the majority of accreditation processes for the recognition or certification of skills worldwide. Embedded in many surgical residency programs is a competency-based curriculum that is designed to challenge, observe, and measure residents' performance as they progress through their respective programs. Before accreditation is granted, surgical residents are expected to successfully demonstrate their proficiency to perform tasks set forth by their local program and its governing agencies. The development of educational objectives, curricula, and means of assessment is an ongoing process and a primary focus for surgical educators in ensuring the competence of surgical residents.

Defining Competence

Currently, there is no agreed-upon definition of medical competence in the literature; however, Epstein and Hundert (2002) have proposed that professional medical competence is "the habitual and judicious use of communication, knowledge, technical skills, clinical reasoning, emotions, values, and reflection in daily practice for the benefit of the individual and community being served" [2]. Leach (2002) adds that skill acquisition is a developmental process, and that although insights may occur suddenly while training, competence develops over time and is "nurtured by reflection on experiences" [3], and as Epstein and Hundert suggest, competence is a habit [2]. "To be competent, residents must be involved enough to be accountable" [3].

Historical Significance

Medical systems worldwide have been charged with consistent reexamination of their educational programs and processes for licensing and accreditation purposes and to ensure that residents are equipped with the competencies required of them to practice safe, effective medicine and surgery in practice. There has been a recent paradigm shift in medicine that has gone from a generally unstructured apprenticeship model to a more practice-based systems approach [4].

In the late 1800s, Sir William Halstead established the modern American surgical residency program at Johns Hopkins School of Medicine, based on the German system of regimen and discipline and graded responsibility [1, 5]. Still, a single system that actually worked for each medical institution did not exist. In an effort to regulate medical training, the American Medical Association (AMA) commissioned Abraham Flexner, who in turn published the *Flexner Report* in 1910, a summary of his investigation of medical schools in the United States and Canada, which contained quality ratings of each institution. Flexner was critical of the process of medical education, citing that only 10 % of approximately 300 medical schools would be worth maintaining, but recommended that medical schools become affiliated with universities [4]. Throughout the years, due to slow advancement in the practice of medicine, growing skepticism among the public about the competence of doctors, and the increasing responsibilities of residents [6], in 1999 the Accreditation Council for Graduate Medical Education (ACGME) established their Outcomes Project to improve the quality of graduate medical education and focus on educational outcomes [4].

Based on their Outcomes Project, the ACGME mandated that, prior to accreditation, each resident's performance be assessed across six competency domains: patient care, medical knowledge, practice-based learning and improvement, professionalism, interpersonal and communication skills, and systems-based practice [7]. The American Board of Medical Specialties (ABMS), including the American Board of Surgery (ABS) and the American Board of Urology (ABU), now must prove that certification and competence are interrelated, when the assumption in the past has been that, intuitively, this relationship already exists, without ever having a concrete process for demonstrating it [8].

Alongside the work in the United States, the Canadian competency initiative, known as the CanMEDS framework (Canadian Medical Education Directives for Specialists), was created in 1996 by the Royal College of Physicians and Surgeons in Canada (RCPSC) [9] out of a perceived need to improve the medical training process across Canada. This reform was initiated due to a shift in societal expectation, which generated questions about patient consumerism, patient safety, quality of care, technological advances, fiscal constraint, government regulation, physician competence, and maintenance of training [10, 11]. The most recent CanMEDS (2005) framework measures seven core competencies: medical expert, communicator, collaborator, manager, health advocate, scholar, and professional. The CanMEDS program has been adopted in at least 17 jurisdictions worldwide (including European and Asian countries) and been used in the frameworks of at least eight professions [12].

In the United Kingdom, the Foundation Programme curriculum [13], updated in 2007, focuses on measuring seven competencies: good clinical care, maintaining good medical practice, teaching and training, relationships with patients and communication, working with colleagues, professional behavior and probity, and acute care.

Table 98.1 CanMEDS, ACGME, and UK Foundation Programme core competencies

CanMEDS	ACGME	UK Foundation Programme
1. Medical expert	1. Medical knowledge	1. Maintaining good medical practice
2. Communicator	2. Communication and interpersonal skills	2. Relationships with patients and communication
3. Collaborator	3. Patient care	3. Working with colleagues
4. Manager	4. System-based practice	4. Good clinical care
5. Health advocate	5. Practice-based learning and improvement	5. Teaching and training
6. Scholar	6. Professionalism	6. Acute care
7. Professionalism		7. Professional behavior and probity

The CanMEDS Framework

When comparing the CanMEDS, ACGME, and UK-based competency frameworks (Table 98.1), it is clear that similarities exist across many of the core competencies. The means of assessing these competencies are also somewhat comparable. However, because of the widespread use of the CanMEDS framework [12], it will be used here as the primary example in describing the assessment and measurement of competency. The structure of each core competency (also called a "role") contains a brief definition, a more detailed description of the role, a list of key competencies, and then a section entitled "enabling competencies," which takes each of the key competencies and provides a very detailed list of what the physician should be able to do to satisfy each key competency. Following are the seven core competencies and their definitions [9]:

1. *Medical Expert*

As *medical experts*, physicians integrate all of the CanMEDS roles, applying medical knowledge, clinical skills, and professional attitudes in their provision of patient-centered care. *Medical expert* is the central physician role in the CanMEDS framework.

2. *Communicator*

As *communicators,* physicians effectively facilitate the doctor-patient relationship and the dynamic exchanges that occur before, during, and after the medical encounter.

3. *Collaborator*

As *collaborators*, physicians effectively work within a health-care team to achieve optimal patient care.

4. *Manager*

As *managers*, physicians are integral participants in health-care organizations, organizing sustainable practices, making decisions about allocating resources, and contributing to the effectiveness of the health-care system.

5. *Health Advocate*

As *health advocates*, physicians responsibly use their expertise and influence to advance the health and well-being of individual patients, communities, and populations.

6. *Scholar*

As *scholars*, physicians demonstrate a lifelong commitment to reflective learning, as well as the creation, dissemination, application, and translation of knowledge.

7. *Professional*

As *professionals*, physicians are committed to the health and well-being of individuals and society through ethical practice, profession-led regulation, and high personal standards of behavior.

The CanMEDS framework is designed to be applied to multiple specialties; however, it does not specifically address surgical competencies, as these are thought to be part of the hidden curriculum within the competencies in the "medical expert" role [14]. Although the CanMEDS framework has been distributed and used widely, the uptake into practice has been somewhat slow. Mickelson and MacNeily [10] suggest that this could be due to barriers such as a lack of understanding of what the core competencies actually represent, a lack of tools available to teach them, and an inability to quantify residents' performance. Further, they believe that urology programs have struggled to incorporate the competencies into existing curricula, and that urology faculty may be unsure how to assess performance [10]. This is especially true when it comes to the assessment of technical skills. In an attempt to assist program directors and educators in the assessment process, the ACGME Outcomes Project included a "toolbox" for instruction and assessment methods for their competencies [15], and CanMEDS has produced the assessment tools handbook [16]. Both provide methods for assessing and measuring competencies in each domain, and some overlap does exist between publications with respect to assessment methods.

Assessment and Measurement of Competencies

Background

Assessment strategies vary based on the purpose of the test or action being evaluated. Some tests may be used to provide feedback to trainees, some assess a trainee's ability to progress to the next level of training, while others will be used to issue licenses to practice medicine or to certify specialty competence [1]. Tests can be cognitive-based (knowledge) or technical-based (skills). In 2002, Wanzel and colleagues asserted that there are two main categories of assessment: formative and summative [1].

Formative assessment is conducted primarily to provide constructive feedback to residents and focuses on individual progress. It measures progress toward meeting objectives and helps identify those who require additional assistance and instruction. Summative assessment findings are designed to accumulate all relevant information in order to make the decision to pass or fail a resident. These are used to determine whether a resident qualifies to continue on to the next level of training, whether he or she should be dropped from the residency program, or if the resident should be recommended for board certification.

Cutoff scores for determining pass or fail are determined either by comparison to peers in norm-referenced standard settings or comparison to objectives or test content in criterion-referenced standard settings.

When assessing residents, the tools used to assess performance must be valid and reliable measures. Reliability ensures that the test is reproducible, and results would be expected to be the same upon repeated administration to the same person. The notion of validity is more complex than that of reliability, as multiple factors play into determining whether the interpretations made (based on test scores) are valid. These include measures of construct, criterion, and content validity, all of which are important to consider when determining if the test is measuring what it sets out to measure. Each of the assessment measures described in this chapter have been found to be reliable and valid; although as with any test, it is important to consider that certain biases introduced during the assessment process may jeopardize reliability and validity. In the next section, we briefly describe types of assessments and how these are incorporated into examination programs.

Assessment Measures

Written Examinations: Short-Answer (SAQ), Multiple-Choice (MCQ), and Open-Ended Questions

Written exams with short-answer, multiple-choice, and open-ended questions evaluate factual knowledge and abstract problem solving [17]. These exams are one of the most effective means for evaluating medical knowledge and are widely used [15]. These types of questions are often used along with other measures as part of an examination program.

Objective Structured Clinical Examinations (OSCE)

The OSCE is a performance-based multi-station clinical examination developed in 1975 by Harden and colleagues and is widely used in residency competency assessment. The OSCE uses direct observation (by a physician-examiner) with a criteria assessment technique [1]. Each station is between 5 and 10 min in length and has a different examiner. OSCEs generally use standardized patients to simulate clinical scenarios. A global score is used to determine if the candidate either passes or fails the station.

360-Degree Evaluations

The 360-degree evaluations use measurement tools completed by multiple people in a resident's sphere of influence [10]. These evaluators can include physicians from other specialties who have worked with the resident, nurses, allied health-care workers, patients, the senior resident evaluating a junior resident and vice versa, and a senior resident evaluating a medical student and vice versa.

The United States Medical Licensing Examination (USMLE)

The USMLE assesses the ability to apply knowledge, concepts, and principles and to demonstrate fundamental patient-centered skills that are important in health and disease and that constitute the basis of safe and effective patient care. This is a three-step examination to determine whether medical students possess the medical knowledge sufficient to become a physician [18]. It is unclear whether USMLE results can predict who will become a proficient surgeon, but studies are looking at this potential correlation.

The Medical Council of Canada Qualifying Examination (MCCQE)

The MCCQE (part I) is a one-day, computer-based test that assesses the competence (knowledge, clinical skills, and attitudes) of candidates who have obtained their medical degree, for entry into supervised clinical practice in postgraduate training programs. The MCCQE (part II) is a three-hour OSCE that assesses the competence of candidates—specifically the knowledge, skills, and attitudes essential for medical licensure in Canada—prior to entry into independent clinical practice [19]. Competencies assessed by the MCCQE are comparable to those measured by the USMLE.

Urology-Specific Assessments: American Urology Association In-Service Examination (AUA ISE), the Queen's Urology Examination Skills Training (QUEST), and the European Board of Urology (EBU) In-Service Assessment

The American Urology Association provides North American urology programs the opportunity for their residents to take the AUA ISE (MCQ test), which provides a yearly review of a residents' performance when compared with other North American cohorts. In Canada, in addition to the AUA ISE, toward the end of resident training, the QUEST program serves to assess knowledge and practice via the use of SAQs and OSCEs. Both the AUA ISE and the QUEST performance correlate well with results on RCPSC certifying examinations

[10]. The ACGME Residency Competency Evaluation System-Urology [15] also provides a Web-based system of competency evaluations for urology residents that include the Global Resident Competency Rating Form, 360° Rating Form, Operative Performance Rating Form, and the Observed Patient Encounter Rating Form.

Mickelson and MacNeily have proposed a summary of potential instruction methods and assessment strategies for urology residents, based on the CanMEDS competencies [10]. For each core competency, or role, the authors suggest certain instruction methods that may help residents achieve competence, followed by different assessment strategies (some of which are not noted above) for each role. Table 98.2 is an adaptation of the authors' summary and may be very helpful for curriculum design and program implementation.

The European Board of Urology (EBU) administers annual in-service examinations to residents as part of the European Urology Residency Curriculum. As a section of the European Union of Medical Specialists (UEMS), the EBU collaborates with the European Association of Urology (EAU) to promote high-quality urological training and assessment. The in-service assessment is designed to provide feedback to program directors and residents about training progress and to identify deficiencies in areas that require further study. Residents' results are compared with those of other trainees with the same level of experience (duration of training). The assessment allows residents to test their theoretical knowledge and clinical competence across 23 main urology subjects. It consists of 100 MCQs covering all fields of urology and can be completed either online or via a written/paper assessment. It must be completed within 2 h time. The EBU recommends that practicing urologists also take these annual assessments as part of their continuing medical education (they are assigned a separate peer group) [20].

Technical Skills Competency Assessment

With the changes and advances in surgical techniques, tools, and technologies over time, surgical educators are faced with multiple challenges when ensuring residents' technical skills competency. In urology, as with other specialties, the achievement of the objectives of training is hampered by various factors, such as limited hours in the workweek, regulations on the necessity for attending surgeon participation in all procedures, pressure on faculty surgeons to increase their productivity, operating room costs, and an increased awareness in the general public of medical errors [21]. For the most part, technical skills assessment is subjective and therefore may not always be highly reliable in terms of assessing competency. The development of the Objective Structured Assessment of Technical Skills (OSATS) aimed to reduce the variability among assessments and has proven to increase reliability and validity of the assessment process [22].

Table 98.2 Instruction methods and potential assessment strategies for urology residents using the CanMEDS framework

Competency (role)	Instruction method	Potential assessment strategy
Medical expert	Academic half-day teaching	Written exams (MCQ, SAQ, open-ended)
	Grand rounds	AUA ISE
	Case presentations	QUEST
	Seminars	Standardized oral exams
	Review courses	Standardized patient exams
	Surgical simulators	Chart-simulated recall oral exams
		OSATS
Communicator	Transdisciplinary workshops	Faculty evaluation
	Small-group role-play activities	OSCE
		Standardized patient exams
		360° evaluations
		Patient surveys
Collaborator	Interdisciplinary collaboration and empathy workshops	Faculty evaluation
		360° evaluations
		Patient surveys
Manager	Interactive seminars with health-care administrators	Faculty evaluation
	Money management seminars (invite accountants/financial planners)	360° evaluation
Health advocate	Faculty modeling	Faculty evaluation
	Faculty and resident seminars on health advocacy	Portfolios
Scholar	Faculty mentorship	Faculty evaluation
	Journal clubs	Evaluation of grand rounds, journal club, and meeting presentations
	Local and national urology meetings	
	Seminars on scholarship	
Professionalism	Faculty mentorship	Global Resident Competency Rating Form
	Professionalism seminars (residents and faculty)	

Objective Structured Assessment of Technical Skills (OSATS)

Martin and colleagues (1995) [23] developed the OSATS as a tool to ensure technical competence of graduates of surgical programs [24]. The OSATS consists of multiple (usually 6–8) individual tasks that the resident performs over a 90-min period. A qualified surgeon assesses each task, using two separate marking methods: a task-specific checklist and a global rating scale. Each task is measured (Was it done effectively?), and when using the global rating scale, seven general operative competencies are rated on a five-point Likert scale.

Fundamentals of Laparoscopy Program (FLS)

The Fundamentals of Laparoscopy Program (FLS) was developed to address the need for educating surgeons on the underlying principles and basic skills of laparoscopic surgery and also to attend to the growing demand to document competency in surgical practice [25]. The Society of American Gastrointestinal and Endoscopic Surgeons (SAGES) and the FLS committee members have developed a technical skills curriculum specifically designed for use in residency training programs. This is a proficiency-based curriculum, and trainees are oriented to the materials and self-practice until expert-derived performance levels are reached. The FLS has partnered with ongoing national (US) initiatives, making this curriculum a part of the Basic and Advanced Laparoscopic Skills Modules included in the American College of Surgery (ACS) and Association of Program Directors in Surgery (APDS) National Skills Curriculum Project [26]. The overall goal of the FLS program is to teach a standard set of cognitive and psychomotor skills to practitioners of laparoscopic surgery to ensure a minimum standard of care for all patients undergoing laparoscopies [25]. The McGill Inanimate System for Training and Evaluation of Laparoscopic Skills (MISTELS) was developed as an educational instrument to train and evaluate basic laparoscopic skills outside of the operating room and is used in the FLS [27]. Dauster and colleagues (2005) studied the MISTELS with urology residents and determined that it has construct validity and therefore supports the use of MISTELS in evaluating urology residents in fundamental laparoscopic skills [27]. Studies are currently being conducted that assess the value of MISTELS in training urology residents to perform laparoscopy. The FLS assessment component is a two-part, proctored exam that covers cognitive knowledge and manual skills and is designed to test the understanding and application of the basic fundamentals of laparoscopy with emphasis on clinical judgment and intraoperative decision making [26]. The FLS can be taken and evaluated at the levels of resident and fellow, and is also available for surgeons who wish to complete it for continuing education purposes. As of 2010, the American Board of Surgery (ABS) requires all surgeons undertaking the certification process to pass the FLS Program [28].

To our knowledge, a competency assessment measure has yet to be developed and tested with regard to technical skills at the high-stakes level. Although the need for this has been clearly demonstrated in the literature, an appropriate test has not been devised. There is an ever-increasing necessity for further development in this area.

Conclusion

Ensuring the competency of surgical residents as they progress through training is essential to the development of the resident as a surgeon, favorable patient outcomes, and the success of residency programs. A competency-based curriculum is designed to measure the proficiency of its trainees and provides a framework for ensuring that residents are able to meet the standards required for accreditation. The core competencies that comprise the CanMEDS, ACGME, and the UK Foundations Programme frameworks can be integrated into a surgical residency curriculum to provide guidelines for measuring residents' competency in multiple domains associated with a given specialty. Multiple tools exist to assess certain competencies and can provide for formative or summative evaluations. Established tools have been found to be both reliable and valid, although additional research regarding the relationship between these measures and competence is warranted. Additional research and development of technical skills assessment measures for use at the high-stakes level is necessary. As surgery continues to advance, society and other key stakeholders will need assurance that surgeons are competent to practice in a safe and sound manner.

References

1. Wanzel KR, Ward M, Reznick RK. Teaching the surgical craft: from selection to certification. Curr Probl Surg. 2002;39:573.
2. Epstein RM, Hundert EM. Defining and assessing professional competence. JAMA. 2002;287:226.
3. Leach DC. Competence is a habit. JAMA. 2002;287:243.
4. Joyner BD. An historical review of graduate medical education and a protocol of Accreditation Council for Graduate Medical Education compliance. J Urol. 2004;172:34.
5. Niederee MJ, Knudtson JL, Byrnes MC, et al. A survey of residents and faculty regarding work hour limitations in surgical training programs. Arch Surg. 2003;138:663.
6. Zinner MJ. Surgical residencies: are we still attracting the best and the brightest? Bull Am Coll Surg. 2002;87:20.
7. Miller DC, Montie JE, Faerber GJ. Evaluating the Accreditation Council on Graduate Medical Education core clinical competencies: techniques and feasibility in a urology training program. J Urol. 2003;170:1312.
8. Ritchie Jr WP. The measurement of competence. Current plans and future initiatives of the American Board of Surgery. Bull Am Coll Surg. 2001;86:10.
9. The Royal College of Physicians and Surgeons of Canada: CanMEDS framework. Available: http://rcpsc.medical.org/canmeds/about_e.php. Accessed 20 May 2011.
10. Mickelson JJ, Macneily AE. Translational education: tools for implementing the CanMEDS competencies in Canadian urology residency training. Can Urol Assoc J. 2008;2:395.

11. Frank JR, Langer B. Collaboration, communication, management, and advocacy: teaching surgeons new skills through the CanMEDS project. World J Surg. 2003;27:972.
12. Frank JR. Canadian urology programs can be leaders in competency-based education. Can Urol Assoc J. 2008;2:405.
13. Academy of Medical Royal Colleges: The Foundation Programme: Curriculum. 2007. Available: http://www.foundationprogramme.nhs.uk/pages/home/training-and-assessment. Accessed 2 May 2011.
14. Mickelson J, Macneily A. Author's reply. Can Urol Assoc J. 2008;2:497.
15. Accreditation Council for Graduate Medical Education (ACGME) and American Board of Medical Specialties (ABMS): Toolbox of assessment methods version 1.1. Chicago: The Council and the Board; 2000. Available: www.acgme.org/Outcome/assess/Tollbox.pdf. Accessed 2 May 2011.
16. Bandiera G, Sherbino J, Frank J. The CanMEDS assessment tools handbook. Ottawa: The Royal College of Physicians and Surgeons of Canada; 2006.
17. Newble D, Dawson B, Dauphinee D. Guidelines for assessing clinical competence. Teach Learn Med. 1994;6:213.
18. United States Medical Licensing Examination: About USMLE: General information. Available: http://www.usmle.org/General_Information/general_information_about.html. Accessed 2 May 2011.
19. Medical Council of Canada: About the examinations. Available: http://www.mcc.ca/en/exams/. Accessed 2 May 2011.
20. European Board of Urology. EBU in-service assessment. 2011. Available: http://ebu.com/examinations/in-service-assessment/. Accessed 31 Aug 2011.
21. McDougall EM, Clayman RV. Rapid communication: minimally invasive urologic surgery curricula. J Endourol. 2007;21:197.
22. Ault G, Reznick R, MacRae H, et al. Exporting a technical skills evaluation technology to other sites. Am J Surg. 2001;182:254.
23. Martin J, Regehr G, Reznick R. An objective, structured assessment of technical skill for surgical residents. Gastroenterology. 1995;108: A1231.
24. Faulkner H, Regehr G, Martin J, et al. Validation of an objective structured assessment of technical skill for surgical residents. Acad Med. 1996;71:1363.
25. Peters JH, Fried GM, Swanstrom LL, et al. Development and validation of a comprehensive program of education and assessment of the basic fundamentals of laparoscopic surgery. Surgery. 2004;135:21.
26. Society of American Gastrointestinal and Endoscopic Surgeons (SAGES): Fundamentals of laparoscopic surgery (FLS). Available: http://www.flsprogram.org/. Accessed 3 June 2011.
27. Dauster B, Steinberg AP, Vassiliou MC, et al. Validity of the MISTELS simulator for laparoscopy training in urology. J Endourol. 2005;19:541.
28. Autorino R, Haber GP, Stein RJ, et al. Laparoscopic training in urology: critical analysis of current evidence. J Endourol. 2010;24: 1377.

Modern Concepts on Cognito-Psychomotor Skill Development

99

Rebecca L. Tregunna, Matthew F. Bultitude, and Muhammad Shamim Khan

Abstract

Urological training has advanced in line with the introduction of new techniques and technologies in modern urological practice. Out-of-date apprenticeship models have been replaced with a focus on attainment of appropriate cognitive and psychomotor skills relevant to practice.

To facilitate acquisition of these skills, a number of simulation training models have been developed for out of operating room education and practice. Animal and cadaver models as well as bench and virtual reality computer simulation range in both fidelity and price, and all have a role in both the learning and assessment of techniques and procedures in a safe environment. As well as simulation, mentor training still has an important role to play, and intensive training has been shown to both shorten the learning curve and lead to a higher rate of retention of technical skills. Appropriate assessment of these skills is also crucial in ensuring proficiency, and several different methods have been introduced to ensure fair, unbiased evaluation.

This chapter discusses both the principles of cognitive and psychomotor skill development as well as methods to develop these skills prior to exposure to the pressures of the operating room.

Keywords

Educational assessment • Training • Cognitive science • Computer simulation

Introduction

The Halstedian principle of "see one, do one, teach one" is a concept far outdated in the current climate of litigation and media coverage. With rapidly advancing technologies requiring that consultants continually learn new skills, urological trainees undoubtedly need a place in which to train outside of the operating room [1]. With limitations such as the European Working Time Directive (EWTD) and similar regulations in other countries, the hours in which junior doctors can work have been significantly reduced. Thus newer formats for intensive training as well as opportunities to refine operating skills are critical for the production of the next generation of urological surgeons.

The operating room is a high-stress, high-price environment and there are heavy costs incurred in spending time training juniors: Bridges and Diamond found that if they extrapolated their figures to a national level in the United States, training juniors in the operating room was at a cost of $53 million, predominantly due to lengthier operation times [2].

Expanding areas such as laparoscopy and endourological surgery requires interpretation of a three-dimensional space on a two-dimensional screen [3]. Having a reduction in both

R.L. Tregunna, M.B.B.S., B.Sc. (Hons.) (✉) • M. F. Bultitude, M.B.B.S., MRCS, M.Sc., FRCS (Urol) • M. S. Khan, M.B.B.S., MCPS, FRCS (Urol), FEBU
Department of Urology, Guy's and St. Thomas' NHS FoundationTrust, Great Maze Pond, London SE1 9RT, UK
e-mail: rebecca.tregunna@doctors.org.uk; matthew.bultitude@gstt.nhs.uk; shamim.khan@gstt.nhs.uk

J.J. Talati et al. (eds.), *Urolithiasis*,
DOI 10.1007/978-1-4471-4387-1_99, © Springer-Verlag London 2012

visual field and haptic feedback compared with open surgery means that the learning curve is steep and that the operating room should no longer be the sole environment in which to learn. Steep learning curves could mean higher risks to the patient [4, 5], but the risks could be reduced by initiating intensive training to acquire and refine appropriate psychomotor skills outside of the operating room [3, 5].

This chapter discusses emerging developments in urological training, with a focus on psychomotor skill acquisition and operative practice.

Principles of Cognitive and Psychomotor Skill Development

Although technical skill may not be the most important ability of a surgeon, certainly complications do occur as a direct result of procedural failure [6]. It is believed that in successful execution of any surgical procedure, the proportionate contribution of technical skills is only 25 %, whereas cognitive decision making has the major share of 75 % [7]. Hence it is important that both cognitive and psychomotor aspects of surgical skills are addressed during training.

There are several theories pertaining to the acquisition of surgical skills, the most widely studied of which is Kopta's theory [6]. This proposes that skill acquisition involves three stages [6]:

Stage One: Cognitive Phase

This period involves observation and "meaningful receptive learning," which includes both trainer and trainee in active demonstrations of the task, as well as autonomous reading, attendance at conferences, and assisting or being assisted in the operating room [8, 9]. This "intellectualizes" the task and ensures the planning of steps in order to complete it [6].

Stage Two: Integrative Phase

During this phase, the cognitive element of the task is coupled with appropriate psychomotor skills and must take in feedback while practicing. This phase is led by the "meaningful guided inquiry" where the trainee explains the procedure along with the reasoning behind, for example, the choice of instruments and options for techniques [8, 9].

A study using positron emission tomography (PET) has revealed that approximately five-and-a-half hours after a skill is learned, there is reorganization of memory from the temporary storage area of the prefrontal cortex to the contralateral dorsal premotor cortex, ipsilateral anterior cerebellar cortex, and contralateral posterior parietal areas, indicating stability of memory [10].

Consequently, feedback at this stage is vital as much of the learning occurs in the psychomotor domain and bad habits are difficult to unlearn once established [6].

Stage Three: Autonomous Phase

This is where automatic, smooth performance of the skill is achieved. At this stage little cognitive input is required to complete the task [6, 11]. Leff et al., having reviewed the literature, showed that as novices become experts, areas of high attention such as the prefrontal cortex and anterior cingulate cortex are recruited less often [12].

Supporting Kopta's theory is a study by Keehner et al. who reported on spatial ability, a cognitive function of great importance in surgical skill performance [13]. In this study a group of experienced and another of less experienced laparoscopic surgeons were assessed on their spatial ability. The authors found a wide range of spatial abilities in both of the groups. Although there was a significant correlation between spatial ability and operative skills among inexperienced laparoscopic surgeons, no such association was found in the experienced group. This is in keeping with Kopta's theory of skill acquisition, which proposes that higher levels of cognitive function are less likely to be involved in the latter stages of attainment as the process becomes automatic [6, 13]. However, to prevent the "plateau" that occurs after the autonomous phase of learning, there must be more challenging exercises to ensure that there is continuous improvement [16].

This background leads us on to the teaching of psychomotor skills, which involves four stages listed in Table 99.1 [14, 15].[1]

Variability in the rate of acquisition of skill may result from the complexity of the task to be performed, the learner's ability, and quality of the training that they have received [16].

Juniors tend to have "declarative knowledge," that is, they know what to do but do not have the "procedural knowledge," that is, how to do it [17]. They need to be taught this explicitly, step by step. Experts are often unaware of the cognitive processes involved in procedures as they have become autonomous and consequently struggle to deconstruct [6, 18] and explain this to the resident. This is where courses such as the "training the trainers" and equivalent are vital in developing consultant mentors to aid training.

A study by Cauraugh et al. reviewed the difference in performance of a McVay inguinal hernia repair between two groups; the control group had only read about the procedure, while the experimental group underwent cognitive modeling, videotape

[1] Personal communication with J. W. R. Peyton

Table 99.1 Psychomotor skills teaching as described by Peyton

Stage 1	*Demonstration*	The instructor demonstrates the skill at normal speed
Stage 2	*Deconstruction*	The instructor demonstrates the skill by breaking it down into simple steps and adding commentary
Stage 3	*Formulation*	The instructor demonstrates the skill while being "talked through" the steps by the student. This stage also includes passive and active visualization of the technique before carrying it out
Stage 4	*Performance*	The student performs the skill and describes the steps

Adapted from [14, 15]

analysis, and auditory deconstruction of the procedure [17]. They found that the experimental group were significantly faster at performing the procedure and had better instrument control, more purposeful movements, and superior knot tying.

Didactic teaching, educational conferences, operating room exposure, clinical courses, and clinical skills laboratories are therefore crucial in the development of both cognitive and psychomotor domains of procedural development.

Assessment of these skills is also of paramount importance to ensure surgical competence. However, according to the American Board of Medical Specialties, competency encompasses not just technical ability but knowledge, professionalism, practice-based learning and development, interpersonal and communication skills, patient care, and systems-based practice [19].

Surgical proficiency is a measurement of performance in each category, and overall competence is the sum of all levels. Consequently, one may be proficient in technical skill but not be deemed overall competent due to lacking in feats of communication and professionalism [19, 20]. Many qualitative assessment tools such as multisource feedback, surgical audit, patient complaint records, and board certification exams are used to assess these nontechnical skills and to ensure certification of clinically competent surgeons [20]. A proficiency-based curriculum thus ensures that certain criteria are achieved as opposed to a curriculum that is based on time frame and number of cases completed [21]. This ensures that a reduction in working hours does not impact on patient safety [22].

Simulation

Simulation has been used for decades in the aerospace and military for both training and assessment to demonstrate proficiency [1]. The medical profession has recognized this as an invaluable tool and has begun to incorporate simulation into courses such as life support and medical emergency. Transfer of training is the transfer of basic surgical skills to new, more complex skills, with the aim of shortening the learning curve. However, a study by Figert et al. found that transfer of training from open surgical skills to laparoscopic skills did not occur and consequently there should be specific laparoscopic skills training [23].

Laparoscopy and endourological surgery can be ideally taught by simulation. Psychomotor skills and procedures can be taught in a safe, nonthreatening environment with higher-fidelity models being able to replicate the stresses of the operating room with regard to time constraints and complications such as bleeding.

The British Association of Urological Surgeons (BAUS) published guidelines for training in laparoscopy because, in urology, as the technology was being introduced, laparoscopic procedures were rare, with few centers performing large numbers [24]. This led to concerns over patient safety as surgeons rushed to take up the procedures. They advised both "dry" (bench models and virtual reality simulators) and "wet" (animal and cadaver) laboratory simulation courses, as well as observation and mentorship, to ensure competent techniques are acquired.

There are three stages to laparoscopic and endourological simulation: The first is to enable the user to work in a two-dimensional zone working on basic tasks. The second comprises simple surgical tasks such as suturing and knot tying. The third is simulating the entire procedures [25].

There are many new and exciting developments in urological simulation, some of which are outlined below. Vehicles such as high-fidelity bench models and virtual reality (VR) simulators are being incorporated into clinical skills centers worldwide allowing trainees to be able to practice their skills outside of the operating room.

Animal Models

Large animal models for urological training have been used for some time for both laparoscopic and endourological simulation. Anesthetized porcine models allow the trainee to operate on a live replica of the human body and consequently are ideal for training as the tissues correlate more than synthesized material with that of human tissue [26]. An additional advantage of using such models is that complications such as time constraints, bleeding, and surrounding anatomical structures must be dealt with.

However, most animal training is a one-time experience, which is very costly to the individual as veterinary services, housing, and disposal must be organized [4]. As well as this, many countries have ethical concerns with using a large number of animals for training [27].

Van Velthoven and Piechaud performed a survey-based study on urology trainees attending courses from 1997 to 2007 at the European Institute of Telesurgery in Strasbourg, France, a 3–5-day course involving theory, surgical demonstrations, and anesthetized large animal practice sessions [28]. They found that 85 % of trainees were satisfied with the course, with the main concerns being that trainees wanted further technical and written support, wanted further supervision, or wanted to practice basic skills on box trainers, indicating a need for continuous teaching. This indicates that although an invaluable experience, further work is required to improve the course, especially given the cost to the individual ranges from approximately €1,686 to €2,887 (US $2,340–$3,990).

In an attempt to abate ethical concerns and reduce cost, Hammond et al. explored the option of using tissue removed from animals killed for food such as a porcine urological tract [29]. This was used in a study looking at percutaneous renal access surgery where pebbles were implanted into the pelvicaliceal system and the kidney was then placed inside an empty chicken carcass. Residents were then taught percutaneous renal access using fluoroscopy. All residents found this session worthwhile and rated it as a "valuable experience," indicating that haptic feedback is useful during simulation of procedures.

Cadaver Models

There are few papers looking at the use of cadaveric models for urological training. Certainly there is a shortage of cadavers; they are expensive and must be stored in an appropriate facility [30]. In addition, cadaveric tissue has poor compliance [31] and cannot be used to replicate operative scenarios such as hemorrhage control, thus reducing the authenticity.

A rare paper looking at cadaveric versus porcine models in urological laparoscopic training [32] used a survey of groups attending either a porcine or a cadaveric laparoscopy session. Both groups were satisfied with either training, but the cadaveric group expressed a significantly higher appreciation of anatomy, laparoscopic technique, and instruments, suggesting that cadaveric training may be superior to animal models [32].

Bench Models

Bench models are dry models that allow the trainee to practice some or all skills required for a specific procedure. They are used in resuscitation exercises as well as for practicing an exhaustive list of skills such as suturing, chest drain insertion, central catheter access placement, and intubation. The fidelity of bench models increases with more realistic tissue texture, correct anatomy, and replication of important steps of the procedure [33]. Models for simulation must be validated to ensure that carrying out the procedure on the bench model will have impact on improving skills relevant to performing the procedure in the medical field.

There are many different facets of validity that must be reviewed before a simulator can be deemed a valuable training tool (Table 99.2) [34].

Several authors have shown improvement in urological skills when practicing on bench models: Matsumoto et al. found that practice on genitourinary bench models when combined with didactic teaching led to an improvement in endourological skills on a global rating scale and checklist [35]. Brehmer and Tolley tested 14 trainees and consultants in rigid ureteroscopy on both a ureteroscopic bench model and a patient [36]. Both groups performed as well on the patient as they did with the model, demonstrating predictive validity.

Low-Fidelity Bench Models

Low-fidelity bench models have poor realism. They do not replicate the procedure visually and often have unrealistic tissue quality and anatomical relation. These trainers are both cheap and portable but can only teach skills rather than procedures [31]. However, these devices may help to develop the trainee in a multilevel process such as in the URobotics Laboratory at John Hopkins University, which has stages to its low-fidelity trainers, with stage one using three-dimensional vision of the task and the second stage having the equipment in a closed box trainer to develop two-dimensional training [37].

High-Fidelity Bench Models

High-fidelity trainers are much more realistic and have the added ability to teach basic skills using the correct instruments as well as higher level skills such as dissection and suturing [37]. However, high fidelity comes with high cost, meaning that the models have to be versatile at teaching several skills or procedures to justify a clinical skills center purchasing them.

More advanced trainers can also aid training in more difficult areas such as partial nephrectomy, and some high-fidelity mechanical trainers, such as the pulsatile organ perfusion (P.O.P.) trainer (OPTIMIST, Bregenz, Austria) at a cost of €5,434 ($7,540), even have the advantage of simulating the blood supply of organs to aid training of hemorrhage control [37].

Table 99.2 Assessing validity of training tools [34]

Face validity	The model replicates the real task
Content validity	The individual steps that make up the task replicate the steps of the real procedure
Construct validity	A significant difference in performance on the model is demonstrated between groups of differing levels of experience
Concurrent validity	There is a correlation between assessment on the simulator and assessment using an already established training tool
Predictive validity	There is equivalence of performance on the simulator with performance of the real task

The Uro-Scopic Trainer (Limbs and Things, Bristol, UK) is a high-fidelity trainer at a cost of $4,350 replicating the male genitourinary tract, which allows endoscopic procedures such as cystoscopy and both diagnostic and therapeutic ureteroscopy. Watterson and Denstedt also describe another high-fidelity ureteroscopy trainer called the Scope Trainer (Mediskills Ltd, Edinburgh, UK), a realistic trainer that can be connected with a percutaneous-access trainer to aid training in several aspects of upper urinary tract surgery [30].

Matsumoto et al. compared two models differing in fidelity for ureteroscopy training. The first was a cheap, low-fidelity model costing approximately $20 consisting of a Penrose drain, inverted polystyrene cup, and two straws embedded into a molded latex case [38]. This was compared with the more expensive, high-fidelity Uro-Scopic Trainer (Limbs and Things, Bristol, UK). The authors trained 40 novice medical students, following a 15-min video looking at surgical instruments and demonstrating removal of a mid-ureteric stone on the high-fidelity model. The students were split into three groups, with either a 1-h didactic teaching session, a 1-h training session on the low-fidelity trainer, or a 1-h teaching session on the high-fidelity trainer. Both training sessions were combined with feedback from an experienced endourologist. The students were then asked to remove a mid-ureteric stone from the high-fidelity bench model and were assessed by two blinded examiners using a checklist and global rating scale. The results demonstrated that the group in the low-fidelity bench model performed significantly better than those in the didactic teaching group. However, there was no difference in performance between those in the low-fidelity group and those in the high-fidelity group. The authors postulate that it is therefore practice combined with feedback that aids development of the appropriate psychomotor skills required for the procedure and that the low-fidelity bench model demonstrated the key skills necessary.

Virtual Reality Models

Virtual reality (VR) simulators such as the URO Mentor (Simbionix, Cleveland, OH, USA) are the latest in simulation medicine. They comprise computer-generated simulations of procedures and have the added benefit of having an instructional system, being able to give educational, instant feedback to the trainee, have the ability to record procedures, and also have virtual patient data with anatomical variants and differing complexity of cases to aid training at all levels [4]. Some simulators are even further advanced and can reproduce haptic feedback to the user [30].

Face and content validity of these trainers have been validated in previous studies [30]. A recent review of the literature by Thijssen and Schijven looked at validation of VR trainers with regard to construct, concurrent, and predictive validities [39]. Authors reviewed 42 publications and found that if the parameter of time to complete a task was used, the VRs did achieve construct validity but did not reach full construct validity when different parameters such as number of errors made were used.

Concurrent validity was tested in five publications, and although the VR showed good validity when tested with the fundamentals of laparoscopic surgery score in one paper, others showed less convincing results [39].

Predictive validity was tested in five publications looking at VR training compared with real-life laparoscopic surgery on either human or animal models. None used a validated system for assessment and only one used human models, and this study had the least correlation [39].

In a study comparing medical students who had no previous laparoscopic experience who were trained on the VR and subsequently performed on human cadavers, predictive validity was shown [40]. However, predictive validity in procedures on human cadavers was not shown in urology residents who had some laparoscopic experience and were then trained on the VR, indicating that the VR may be most useful in early training.

In comparing the usefulness of bench models with VR simulators, a number of factors must be addressed. High-fidelity bench models are cheaper ($3,000–$5,000) than VR simulators ($60,000–$85,000) and are more portable but with the addition of expensive equipment such as cameras, flexible cystoscopes, flexible ureteroscopes, and guidewires, which will require frequent replacement; the costs can in fact be equivocal [4]. VR simulators can also provide a large number of different scenarios with instant feedback, critical to establishing the integrative phase of skill acquisition, whereas the bench model requires a trainer to be present to provide coaching and evaluation.

A number of papers have compared and contrasted bench models with VR simulators in the field of urology. No significant difference was found in basic ureteroscopy skills when assessed using the Objective Structured Assessment of Technical Skill (OSATS) (discussed later) on an animal model in a group of 16 novice medical students randomized into training on a high-fidelity bench model (Uro-Scopic trainer) versus a VR simulator (URO Mentor) [4] ($p=0.38$).

McDougall et al. recruited 20 novice medical students into a study to compare the low-fidelity silicone box trainers versus the high-fidelity VR LAP Mentor (Simbionix) involving suturing and knot-tying skills on a porcine 2-cm cystostomy [31]. No significant difference was found in the OSATS scores in either group ($p=0.24$), and the only significant difference found was that the group in the VR group felt that their training had been too short. The authors concluded from this that basic surgical skills training in the early stages may be better taught on the more "user-friendly" box trainer.

Hybrid Models

A randomized controlled trial by Knudsen et al. looked at a hybrid model comprising a VR simulator as well as a percutaneous-access bench model [41]. The PERC Mentor (Simbionix) can be either a stand-alone model or purchased as an addition to the VR URO Mentor. Sixty-three subjects received didactic teaching on percutaneous access and then performed a case scenario on the PERC Mentor. The subjects were then randomized into either a control group that received no further training or a training group that received 230-min sessions on the hybrid model. Two days later the subjects all then performed a different case scenario of percutaneous renal access on the PERC Mentor. The subjects were tested using a 5-point scale previously validated, evaluating both cognitive and psychomotor domains of renal anatomical knowledge, planning, instructor assistance, use of instruments, and overall performance. Face validity was achieved, as all subjects were able to orientate themselves to the system. The authors found that the trained group improved on their pretest scores in most of the parameters compared with the untrained group ($p<0.001$). The untrained group only improved on their pretest scores in one parameter. This demonstrates content validity for the PERC Mentor, as scores relating to percutaneous access improved in the trained group suggesting that the steps involved relate to the genuine task of percutaneous access.

Mishra et al. also found in a small study that the PERC Mentor gained both face and content validities [42]. The authors reviewed construct validity and found that experts were faster at completing the task of percutaneous renal access, took a shorter amount of time introducing the needle into the collecting system, and had a fewer number of attempts at puncturing the collecting system ($p<0.005$) when compared with novices, demonstrating construct validity in these domains.

Predictive validity was also achieved in five novices who initially performed percutaneous renal access on a porcine model before any training. Here, only one novice was successful in obtaining access and there were three complications (extravasation, infundibular tear, and vessel injury) [42]. Following on from 230-min supervised training sessions on the PERC Mentor, the novices reattempted percutaneous renal access on the porcine model. All five subjects were successful in achieving access with no complications.

Mentor Training

"Proficiency" in surgery is an ill-established marker of expertise and relates to the autonomous phase of cognito-psychomotor learning. The absolute number of procedures to be performed to become proficient in laparoscopic procedures, for example, is widely variable and has not been clearly defined [43].

An illustration of this is in percutaneous nephrolithotomy (PCNL). PCNL involves a steep learning curve. Recent surveys in the United States found that only 11 % of urologists gain renal access by themselves, indicating that more training is required [44].

The number of PCNLs undertaken to gain "proficiency" by a novice urologist performing solo PCNL was reviewed by Allen et al. who used criteria such as stone clearance, complications, screening time, and radiation dose as markers of proficiency [45]. The suggested number to become proficient is more than 60, with excellence comparable with a senior surgeon with a subspecialist interest in PCNL achieved after 115 procedures.

Those who had PCNL training during residency were more likely to be comfortable with this procedure at consultant level, even if they had only been in training for a short while, and they were more likely to offer PCNL as a treatment modality over other stone treatments such as shock wave lithotripsy [44]. Consequently, in addition to simulation, a number of urologists have formulated their own training programs to allow intensive training in complicated aspects of urology such as laparoscopy and endourology. Programs consisting of a 1–2-year fellowship involving research, laparoscopy, and robotics are included in most programs offered by the Endourological Society and the Society of Urologic Oncology in the United States [27, 46].

Corica et al. constructed a 5-day mini-residency program for urologists in laparoscopic ablative or reconstructive training [47]. Here, the trainees received mentor-to-trainee direct supervision with simulation, animal models, operating room observation, and skills assessment. The authors found that this program led to a significant increase in the uptake of laparoscopic surgery in the trainees' future practice compared with previous shorter courses. As well as this, fewer trainees were using hand-assisted approaches and were performing more complex procedures ($p=0.008$). The cost of this course was $10,000 and, although subsidized, meant that $3,850 was still payable by the trainee [5].

More intensive training over longer periods, such as the fellowship instituted by Rané [48], involve a nine-phase curriculum over a period of approximately 6 months from basic training to independent practice (Table 99.3).

Following 36 months with nine participants, six had completed the course and had independent practice, two were at phase eight, and one at phase seven [48]. However, issues with this program include a large amount of time away from clinical practice at a significant cost to the provider. In addition a low caseload at smaller hospitals may mean that the trainee has a lengthy process to achieve the desired number of cases.

Table 99.3 A fellowship training model in laparoscopic surgery instituted by Rané [5, 48]

Phase 1	Fellows attend both a basic and advanced training course
Phase 2	Fellows practice on pelvic trainers
Phase 3	Fellows practice on animal models
Phase 4	Fellows observe laparoscopic cases at tertiary centers
Phase 5	Fellows observe mentors performing laparoscopic cases
Phase 6	Fellows are observed performing hand-assisted cases at mentor's hospital
Phase 7	Fellows are observed performing laparoscopic cases at mentor's hospital
Phase 8	Fellows perform laparoscopic procedures at own hospital with mentor as assistant
Phase 9	Independent practice at fellow's own hospital

Assessment of Technical Skills

Assessment of operative skills is crucial for patient safety, especially given that training time has been dramatically reduced [49]. Crude measurements such as time to complete procedure are unable to judge technical ability, and for subjective ratings to be accurate, a number of assessors must be used to ensure reliability [50]. Bias is often an underlying issue in assessment of junior colleagues, and so an objective assessment tool is necessary for accurate appraisal. It is consequently important that consultants must be developed into mentors and assessors mutually; programs such as the "training the trainer" course can aid development of both teaching skills and assessment [51].

Several clinical assessment means such as OSATS have roles in today's training and evaluation [49]. The OSATS examination [52] is a technical skills examination consisting of several 15-min stations assessing surgical skills such as abdominal wall closure, insertion of tracheostomy, and control of IVC hemorrhage, which are evaluated by two reviewers who have a task checklist of stages that should be completed as well as a global rating scale zero to four.

In a Canadian study involving 48 general surgical residents, the inter-rater reliability scores were found to be 0.78 for the checklist and 0.80 for the global rating scale using Cronbach's coefficient alpha, indicating good reliability [52]. Construct validity of the score showed significant differences in all levels of training except those in their fourth year of training in comparison with those in their fifth and sixth year.

Matsumoto et al. found that a checklist alone did not have construct validity when looking at a group of junior and senior residents performing removal of a mid-ureteric stone on a bench model with regard to pretest scores, as junior residents usually have "declarative knowledge" [35]. However, the global rating scale did have construct validity, indicating that "procedural knowledge" is gained with experience, and therefore, both list and scale must be used in conjunction for valid overall assessment.

The McGill Inanimate System for Training and Evaluation of Laparoscopic Skills (MISTELS) is a series of standardized tasks performed in a box trainer (peg transfer, pattern cutting, placement of ligating loop, extracorporeal knot, and intracorporeal knot). These skills are used to help in the acquisition of laparoscopic skills relevant to clinical practice. Vassiliou et al. found that the MISTELS system had excellent reliability when looking at inter-rater (0.998 [95 % CI 0.985–1.00]) and retest (0.892 [95 % CI 0.665–0.968]) reliabilities [53].

Fraser et al. found that giving a "pass/fail" score on the MISTELS system did discriminate between noncompetent and competent surgeons ($p<0.0001$) [54]. However, a pass/fail system did lead to a situation where 18 % of clinically noncompetent surgeons would be able to pass and 20 % of clinically competent surgeons would not pass this examination.

Dauster et al. looked at MISTELS with regard to construct validity comparing 13 urology residents, one fellow, and three laparoscopic urologists [55]. They found that the experienced surgeons performed better in all tasks, although the difference was only statistically better in two of the five tasks (peg transfer and intracorporeal suture). The authors comment on their small study size and that the residents assessed had a broad range of experience. However, overall there was a significant difference between the junior trainees and the senior surgeons, indicating that the MISTELS assessment tool does have construct validity.

For assessing minimally invasive surgery, the Global Operative Assessment of Laparoscopic Skills (GOALS) developed by Vassiliou et al., consisting of a ten-item task-specific checklist, has been shown to have construct validity in laparoscopic cholecystectomy and appendicectomy [56]. As well as this, the inter-rater validity was excellent with Cronbach's alpha ranging 0.91–0.93. In this assessment tool, trainees are scored by their mentors in five areas: depth perception, bimanual dexterity, efficiency, tissue handling, and autonomy, with scores from one to five. Each score has a description related to the area being assessed to ensure accurate scoring. Gumbs et al. use the GOALS assessment at the end of every case with a computerized form at the end of the operation note, allowing low-cost, regular assessment of trainees [57].

Videotape assessment is a low-cost way of reviewing trainees' skills as it does not require referees to be present in the hospital operating room and allows unbiased assessment as referees can be blinded to the name of the trainee. Scott et al. looked at assessing skills from *edited* videotapes of laparoscopic cholecystectomy [58]. They found poor inter-rater reliability and did not find that the assessment correlated with direct observation, suggesting that edited videotape analysis is not a good predictor of operative technique.

An interesting, unbiased assessment tool has been studied by a group of Japanese urologists who have looked at reviewing *unedited* videotapes of laparoscopic nephrectomies and adrenalectomies to assess the operative skill of trainees [59]. A set of six expert referees was established following videotaped assessment of each other performing laparoscopic surgery. These surgeons originally pioneered laparoscopic urological surgery in the early 1990s. Following on from this, a subset of 23 referees was created following video assessment by the original expert referees. These referees then went on to assess urological trainees for accreditation with the Endoscopic Surgical Skill Qualification (ESSQ) using unedited tapes of a laparoscopic procedure with a pass rate of 66 %. Two referees per trainee were blinded to the applicant's name and provided individual scores. Those disqualified by one or more referee were discussed at a committee level. A perfect score of a laparoscopic procedure was 75, with marks deducted following dangerous maneuvers based on a checklist. No global score was used as this would be difficult to comment on in a videotaped situation, but the ESSQ was focused on reducing complication rates, and therefore dangerous maneuvers were considered the more important parameter to assess. However, some may argue that good communication and attitude during a procedure may itself reduce the complication rate. The authors recognized that they had a marked significant difference in inter-rater results, but they believe that this was due to lack of training of the referees and poor guidelines, and so hope this can be improved.

Retention of Skills

Of course, learning a particular skill is of no use unless it is retained. Likelihood of retention of a skill has been found to be related to how well the skill was initially perfected [15]. Following on from training, the maintenance of competency can only be achieved by performing a certain number of procedures per year [60].

A small study looking at the impact on urological residents of a 2-day intensive endourological course with a high-fidelity model showed significant improvement in global ratings scores and time to complete task 1–2 years later [61]. Although those who had performed a larger number of ureteroscopic cases in practice had a greater improvement, this did not reach statistical significance, perhaps due to small sample size.

Lee et al. looked at graduated urology residents and found that if the resident had been trained in percutaneous renal access surgery they were more likely to continue to perform percutaneous surgical procedures than those who were untrained, performing a mean of 14.0 per year compared with 3.3 in those who were untrained ($p = 0.02$) [62].

Cadeddu et al. reviewed 13 surgeons from different centers who had all received at least 12 months of laparoscopic training either through a dedicated fellowship or as part of training [63]. They looked at all cases performed as a consultant up until March 2000. The authors found that the surgeons had been part of 71 (±24) laparoscopic cases and had been the principal surgeon in 37 (±19). They found no difference in complication rate in the first 20–30 cases performed compared with subsequent cases (approximately 12 %). This indicates that intensive laparoscopic training may have helped to flatten the learning curve. They did, however, find a difference in elective conversion of laparoscopic procedures due to a failure to progress between the first 40 cases compared with subsequent cases (6.6 % versus 1.5 %, $p < 0.05$). The authors suggest that perhaps better patient selection or better skills and/or confidence may have led to this discrepancy. Overall, the study showed a good uptake of laparoscopic surgery in consultant practice following intensive training, indicating that this training helped these surgeons to achieve competence.

Conclusion

The training of urological trainees has dramatically changed over the past 10 years due to barriers such as reduction in working hours and the length of training time. There is also a heightened expectation of competence from the public. With an increase in the technical aspects of surgery, such as complex laparoscopic procedures, there is appreciation of the learning curves needed to achieve "competence." The old adage that "practice makes perfect" holds true for surgery, and the "practice" element should not initially occur on patients. It is therefore recognized by training bodies that there is a need for training and assessment on models and simulators to occur prior to performing real procedures. As a result, there has been an increase in the availability of simulation centers and the quantity and quality of simulators available. There is, however, a need for continued improvement in the realism of simulators in order to allow appropriate training. It is important that these are correctly validated to ensure that the model reproduces the real task in the different domains of validity.

Assessment of skills should be regular and unbiased, with clinical courses and examinations providing feedback and learning opportunities. Increasingly, curricula are competency-based whereby trainees have to demonstrate ability in a wide range of tasks. The role of the trainer and assessor is also vital with formal courses on how to train, education degrees, and set time for training becoming mandatory.

In summary, the future of training and development of cognitive and psychomotor skills depends on out of operating room experience with simulators, combined with the expertise and guidance of consultant mentors to ensure that clinical competence and surgical proficiency are attained prior to independent practice.

References

1. Wignall GR, Denstedt JD, Preminger GM, Cadeddu JA, Pearle MS, Sweet RM, et al. Surgical simulation: a urological perspective. J Urol. 2008;179(5):1690–9.
2. Bridges M, Diamond DL. The financial impact of teaching surgical residents in the operating room. Am J Surg. 1999;177(1):28–32.
3. Hedican SP, Nakada SY. Videotape mentoring and surgical simulation in laparoscopic courses. J Endourol. 2007;21(3):288–93.
4. Chou DS, Abdelshehid C, Clayman RV, McDougall EM. Comparison of results of virtual-reality simulator training model for basic ureteroscopy training. J Endourol. 2006;20(4):266–71.
5. Gamboa AJR, Box GN, Preminger GM, McDougall EM. NOTES: education and training. J Endourol. 2009;23(5):813–9.
6. Kopta JA. The development of motor skills in orthopaedic education. Clin Orthop Relat Res. 1971;75:80–5.
7. Spencer F. Teaching and measuring surgical techniques: the technical evaluation of competence. Bull Am Coll Surg. 1978;63:9–12.
8. Barnes RW. Surgical handicraft: teaching and learning surgical skills. Am J Surg. 1987;153(5):422–7.
9. Lippert III FG, Farmer JA. Psychomotor skills in orthopedic surgery. Baltimore: Williams & Wilkins; 1984.
10. Shadmehr R, Holcomb HH. Neural correlates of motor memory consolidation. Science. 1997;277(5327):821–5.
11. Wanzel KR, Ward M, Reznick RK. Teaching the surgical craft: from selection to certification. Curr Probl Surg. 2002;39(6): 573–659.
12. Leff DR, Leong JJ, Aggarwal R, Yang GZ, Darzi A. Could variations in technical skills acquisition in surgery be explained by differences in cortical plasticity? Ann Surg. 2008;247(3):540–3.
13. Keehner MM, Tendick F, Meng MV, Anwar HP, Hegarty M, Stoller ML, et al. Spatial ability, experience, and skill in laparoscopic surgery. Am J Surg. 2004;188(1):71–5.
14. Peyton JWR. Teaching and learning in medical practice. Rickmansworth: Manticore Europe; 1998.
15. Hamdorf JM, Hall JC. Acquiring surgical skills. Br J Surg. 2000;87(1):28–37.
16. Sachdeva AK. Acquiring skills in new procedures and technology: the challenge and the opportunity. Arch Surg. 2005;140(4): 387–9.
17. Cauraugh JH, Martin M, Martin KK. Modeling surgical expertise for motor skill acquisition. Am J Surg. 1999;177(4):331–6.
18. Perry RE. Laying the foundation of surgical skills for trainees (residents). ANZ J Surg. 2009;79(3):122–6.
19. Satava RM, Gallagher AG, Pellegrini CA. Surgical competence and surgical proficiency: definitions, taxonomy, and metrics. J Am Coll Surg. 2003;196(6):933–7.
20. Ahmed K, Jawad M, Dasgupta P, Darzi A, Athanasiou T, Khan MS. Assessment and maintenance of competence in urology. Nature reviews. Urology. 2010;7(7):403–13.
21. Stefanidis D, Korndorffer Jr JR, Black FW, Dunne JB, Sierra R, Touchard CL, et al. Psychomotor testing predicts rate of skill acquisition for proficiency-based laparoscopic skills training. Surgery. 2006;140(2):252–62.
22. Kishore TA, Pedro RN, Monga M, Sweet RM. Assessment of validity of an OSATS for cystoscopic and ureteroscopic cognitive and psychomotor skills. J Endourol. 2008;22(12):2707–11.
23. Figert PL, Park AE, Witzke DB, Schwartz RW. Transfer of training in acquiring laparoscopic skills. J Am Coll Surg. 2001;193(5): 533–7.
24. Keeley Jr FX, Eden CG, Tolley DA, Joyce AD. The British association of urological surgeons: guidelines for training in laparoscopy. BJU Int. 2007;100(2):379–81.
25. Hasson HM. Core competency in laparoendoscopic surgery. J Soc Laparoendosc Surg. 2006;10(1):16–20.
26. Strohmaier WL, Giese A. Porcine urinary tract as a training model for ureteroscopy (abstract only). Urol Int. 2001;66(1):30–2.
27. Kommu SS, Dickinson AJ, Rané A. Optimizing outcomes in laparoscopic urologic training: toward a standardized global consensus. J Endourol. 2007;21(4):378–85.
28. van Velthoven RF, Piechaud PT. Training centers: an essential step to developing skills in urolaparoscopy. Curr Urol Rep. 2009;10(2):93–6.
29. Hammond L, Ketchum J, Schwartz BF. A New approach to urology training: a laboratory model for percutaneous nephrolithotomy. J Urol. 2004;172(5 pt 1):1950–2.
30. Watterson JD, Denstedt JD. Ureteroscopy and cystoscopy simulation in urology. J Endourol. 2007;21(3):263–9.
31. McDougall EM, Kolla SB, Santos RT, Gan JM, Box GN, Louie MK, et al. Preliminary study of virtual reality and model simulation for learning laparoscopic suturing skills. J Urol. 2009;182(3): 1018–25.
32. Katz R, Hoznek A, Antiphon P, van Velthoven R, Delmas V, Abbou CC. Cadaveric versus porcine models in urological laparoscopic training (abstract only). Urol Int. 2003;71(3):310–5.
33. Matsumoto ED. Low-fidelity ureteroscopy models. J Endourol. 2007;21(3):248–51.
34. Gallagher AG, Ritter EM, Satava RM. Fundamental principles of validation and reliability: rigorous science for the assessment of surgical education and training. Surg Endosc. 2003;17(10):1525–9.
35. Matsumoto ED, Hamstra SJ, Radomski SB, Cusimano MD. A novel approach to endourological training: training at the surgical skills center. J Urol. 2001;166(4):1261–6.
36. Brehmer M, Tolley DA. Validation of a bench model for endoscopic surgery in the upper urinary tract. Eur Urol. 2002;42(2):175–80.
37. Rassweiler J, Klein J, Teber D, Schulze M, Frede T. Mechanical simulators for training for laparoscopic surgery in urology. J Endourol. 2007;21(3):252–62.
38. Matsumoto ED, Hamstra SJ, Radomski SB, Cusimano MD. The effect of bench model fidelity on endourological skills: a randomized controlled study. J Urol. 2002;167(3):1243–7.
39. Thijssen AS, Schijven MP. Contemporary virtual reality laparoscopy simulators: quicksand or solid grounds for assessing surgical trainees? Am J Surg. 2010;199(4):529–41.
40. Ogan K, Jacomides L, Shulman MJ, Roehrborn CG, Cadeddu JA, Pearle M. Virtual ureteroscopy predicts ureteroscopic proficiency of medical students on a cadaver. J Urol. 2004;172(2): 667–71.
41. Knudsen BE, Matsumoto ED, Chew BH, Johnson B, Margulis V, Cadeddu JA, et al. A randomized, controlled prospective study validating the acquisition of percutaneous renal collecting system access skills using a computer based hybrid virtual reality surgical simulator: phase I. J Urol. 2006;176(5):2173–8.
42. Mishra S, Kurien A, Patel R, Patil P, Ganpule A, Muthu V, et al. Validation of virtual reality simulation for percutaneous renal access training. J Endourol. 2010;24(4):635–40.
43. Dagash H, Chowdhury M, Pierro A. When can I be proficient in laparoscopic surgery? A systematic review of the evidence. J Paediatr Surg. 2003;38(5):720–4.
44. Bird VG, Fallon B, Winfield HN. Practice patterns in the treatment of large renal stones. J Endourol. 2003;17(6):355–63.
45. Allen D, O'Brien T, Tiptaft R, Glass J. Defining the learning curve for percutaneous nephrolithotomy. J Endourol. 2005;19(3): 279–82.
46. Yap SA, Ellison LM, Low RK. Current laparoscopy training in urology: a comparison of fellowships governed by the Society of Urologic Oncology and the Endourological Society. J Endourol. 2008;22(8):1755–60.
47. Corica FA, Boker JR, Chou DS, et al. Short-term impact of a laparoscopic "mini-residency" experience on postgraduate urologists' practice patterns. J Am Coll Surg. 2006;203(5):692–8.

48. Rané A. A training module for laparoscopic urology. J Soc Laparoendosc Surg. 2005;9(4):460–2.
49. Thomas WEG. Teaching and assessing surgical competence. Ann R Coll Surg Engl. 2006;88(5):429–32.
50. Darzi A, Smith S, Taffinder N. Assessing operative skill. Needs to become more objective. Br Med J. 1999;318(7188):887–8.
51. Godfrey J, Dennick R, Welsh C. Training the trainers: do teaching courses develop teaching skills? (abstract only). Med Educ. 2004;38(8):844–7.
52. Reznick R, Regehr G, MacRae H, Martin J, McCulloch W. Testing technical skill via an innovative "bench station" examination. Am J Surg. 1997;173(3):226–30.
53. Vassiliou MC, Ghitulescu GA, Feldman LS, Stanbridge D, Leffondré K, Sigman HH, et al. The MISTELS program to measure technical skill in laparoscopic surgery. Surg Endosc. 2006;20(5):744–7.
54. Fraser SA, Klassen DR, Feldman LS, Ghitulescu GA, Stanbridge D, Fried GM. Evaluating laparoscopic skills: setting the pass/fail score for the MISTELS system. Surg Endosc. 2003;17(6):964–7.
55. Dauster B, Steinberg A, Vassiliou MC, Bergman S, Stanbridge DD, Feldman LS, et al. Validity of the MISTELS simulator for laparoscopy training in urology. J Endourol. 2005;19(5):541–5.
56. Vassiliou MC, Feldman LS, Andrew CG, Bergman S, Leffondré K, Stanbridge D, et al. A global assessment tool for evaluation of intraoperative laparoscopic skills. Am J Surg. 2005;190(1):107–13.
57. Gumbs AA, Hogle NJ, Fowler DL. Evaluation of resident laparoscopic performance using global operative assessment of laparoscopic skills. J Am Coll Surg. 2007;204(2):308–13.
58. Scott DJ, Rege RV, Bergen PC, Guo WA, Laycock R, Tesfay ST, et al. Measuring operative performance after laparoscopic skills training: edited videotape versus direct observation (abstract only). J Laparoendosc Adv Surg Tech. 2000;10(4):183–90.
59. Matsuda T, Ono Y, Terachi T, Naito S, Baba S, Miki T, et al. The endoscopic surgical skill qualification system in urological laparoscopy: a novel system in Japan. J Urol. 2006;176(5): 2168–72.
60. de la Rosette JJ, Laguna MP, Rassweiler JJ, Conort P. Training in percutaneous nephrolithotomy – a critical review. Eur Urol. 2008;54(5):1003.
61. Chatterjee S, Radomski SB, Matsumoto ED. Durability of endourological skills: two-year follow-up study. J Endourol. 2007;21(8): 843–6.
62. Lee CL, Anderson JK, Monga M. Residency training in percutaneous renal access: does it affect urological practice? (abstract only). J Urol. 2004;171(2 pt 1):592–5.
63. Cadeddu JA, Wolfe Jr JS, Nakada S, Chen R, Shalhav A, Bishoff JT, et al. Complications of laparoscopic procedures after concentrated training in urological laparoscopy. J Urol. 2001;166(6): 2109–11.

Integration of Competences

100

Munir Ahmed

Abstract

The first segment of this chapter explores the importance and relevance of imparting and assessing an ability to integrate competences within and beyond the "competencies-based" curriculum for the training. The second part expands the concept (based on complex organization functioning principles/systems approach) to argue for the integration of complementary and "continuous" competencies between the healthcare professionals, in the context of health economics, equity of care, and patient-focused outcomes to develop an "integrated" healthcare model in urolithiasis management.

Keywords

Integration of competences • Competence • Integrated care • Care pathways • Reflective practice

Introduction

The General Medical Council of the UK, responsible for undergraduate and postgraduate medical education, expects "tomorrow's doctors" to be "fit for practice" and be prepared "for the changing needs and requirements for medical practice in today's world," i.e., "competent and reflective practitioners" [1]. This desire for competence (maintained by lifelong learning through reflective practice) and, particularly, demand from stakeholders (constituted by patient groups, health providers, regulatory bodies, and governments), over the past two decades or so, to prove and document "competence," has led to the development of "competency-based" curricula for the training of doctors [2].

M. Ahmed, M.Sc. (Med Ed. Cardiff), MAcaMed, FRCS, FRCS(Urol) (✉)
Department of Urology, Kings College of Medicine, University of London, Doll House, 48A Murray Avenue, Bromley, Kent BR1 3DQ, UK
e-mail: munirahmed@urologyandhealthcare.com

Competence

Different perspectives on "competence," when translated into an educational and vocational vocabulary, have resulted in a confusing taxonomy, which includes terms such as competent, competency, capability, expertise, novice, performance, and competence-based [3]. This confusion, however, should not get in the way of how we train our workforce to achieve the best outcomes for an individual patient and the population at large. Therefore, the intended outcome of professional training for doctors is to be able to deal with the uniqueness of each individual patient's problems in their own context, integrating all the competences in ways that provide the best possible outcomes, thus preparing the physician to deal with "uniqueness" and "uncertainty" of clinical practice [4]. Such models of training, at times called "vocational models," based on the outcomes, and requiring the ability to demonstrate integration of competences, are well established in nursing, police training, and construction management [5].

Competences, in competences-based medical curriculum, are an anchor for training and assessment and not an outcome in itself [6]. However, the assessment structures always seem to drive the training system. As assessment methods

J.J. Talati et al. (eds.), *Urolithiasis*,
DOI 10.1007/978-1-4471-4387-1_100, © Springer-Verlag London 2012

are expected to be valid, reliable, and feasible, the assessment structures, in order to meet those objectives, require disintegration of competencies in to smaller measurable tasks. *These competencies or assessed tasks, in a competences-based curriculum assessment structure, become proxy competences.* Assessment methods are modeled on technical skills, which are easy to fragment for the learning and assessment of individual elements. Traditional perspectives on "competency-based curriculum," therefore, use a framework of domains in knowledge, skill, and attitudes, in various combinations, to define "competencies" for a particular curriculum [7]. Interesting examples of this approach are the curricula for urological training of the American Urological Association (AUA), European Association of Urology (EAU), and the British Association of Urological Surgeons (BAUS) (available on the Internet for members). In these "competency-based curricula," competencies provide a useful checklist for curriculum delivery and assessment. For urologists, "competencies" in these domains will continue to expand. It is quite conceivable that for urologists in the twenty-first century, not only technical skills (e.g., microrobotics, imaging), but knowledge (e.g., genetics, nanotechnobiology) and skilled use of information technology, human skills, and communication systems will be incorporated into urological training. The "competency base" provides a structure to allow incorporation of "new" and "emerging" competences into the curriculum.

The challenge, however, is to ensure that assessment of these competencies translates into a performance in the career framework that leads to better patient outcomes. Performing meaningful clinical activity requires integration (vertical, horizontal, internal, external, real, and virtual) of competences and appropriate application in the context of a clinical situation, to achieve the ultimate outcome from a patient perspective [8]. With new advances in medicine (and competencies in the skill and knowledge domains), the professional skills for the practice will get even more complex. That "the whole is a lot bigger than the parts" is an apt expression to articulate the problem. The issue of integrating competencies, throughout the continuum of curricula, from undergraduate to subspecialist, and even within the narrow confines of within each training grade (e.g., post graduate, undergraduate, and specialist), needs to be addressed. Could these integrated competencies be "taught" and assessed?

Take the example of urolithiasis. In a curriculum, diagnostic work-up, choosing appropriate treatment modality, technical skills for treatment application, assessing treatment results, follow-up, prevention of further stone formation, etc., could be taught and assessed as individual aspects using a variety of teaching methods and formats. However, a real-life situation of a patient presenting with features of ureteric colic raises issues of diagnostic uncertainty, choice of total patient and pain management, decision on whether to admit or not, and advice on work and recreation among others. These come into play alongside specifics of the stone size, location, presence or otherwise of infection, obstruction, availability of treatment modalities, available expertise, and best and critical times for intervention, all of which require formulation of thought and actions that goes much beyond curricular-assessed competencies. "Knowing in action" (tacit knowledge)—i.e., the context for applying these competencies—defines the outcome from a patient's perspective. *Knowing what to do in an unfamiliar, changing clinical situation, using elements of previous learning, requires a higher level of learning and functioning, using a flexible integration of competences.* Institutional guidelines and protocols are an articulation and formalized way of expressing some of these elements for making clinical decisions. Is it possible to map "untidiness" and variability in day-to-day practice to the curriculum? Is it possible to learn the wisdom of practice though the curriculum?

Confucius stated, "by three methods we may learn wisdom: first, by reflection, which is the noblest; second by imitation, which is the easiest; and third by experience, which is the bitterest"—an ancient wisdom which remains as importantly relevant today.

In experiential adult learning during service, reflective practice integrates all of the above three into a formalized educational process in a constructivist approach to learning. Donald Schön [4] has been instrumental in introducing reflective practice into professional learning in a practice (experiential) setting as a formalized learning technique. Schön suggests that reflection links the reality of practice (what Schön described as the "swampy lowlands," reflecting the untidy, unpredictable, and unique nature of professional practice) with the theory. Experience triggers reflection, leading to a better integration of "competences," which over a period of time expands into "capability" and improved "performance." Reflective practice has constructivist underpinning in professional learning [9]. *As a trainee gains more and more experience, reflecting and learning from each individual experience (patient), he/she builds higher and higher level of integration over a period of time.*

The reflection could be individual (e.g., it could be recorded in personal learning journals), collective (e.g., interprofessional action learning sets, ALS), or mentored (e.g., clinical supervision). *Interprofessional ALS*, originally developed in industry and commerce, are forums for team *involving all the professionals working in a team, analyzing and reflecting on each other's perspective, role, competences, contributions, attitudes,* etc., *in a given clinical situation or problem, to develop integrated team learning plans.* Can the curriculum design incorporate integration of competences as a learning objective, both as an individual practitioner and as a team? Although the answer may be in the delivery aspect of the curriculum design, an interesting way of "evidencing" this level of integration of competences has been proposed as Entrustable Professional Activities (EPAs) [10]. Alongside assessing competences in the curriculum, an assessment of developing clinical responsibility can potentially demonstrate an ability to integrate these competences. EPAs mapped on the curriculum alongside the competences for each level of training can provide a useful framework. In the pure apprenticeship model of training, the training was only regarded as complete when the trainee has reached a certain level of clinical responsibility, irrespective of time, mostly based on the observations of the trainer. The competences-based curriculum is time-lined and evidence-based. A competences-based curriculum that incorporates EPAs as assessment can be delivered using an apprenticeship model of training in a specified time. For the assessment and learning, when a real-life situation is not available (i.e., limited time for delivering the curriculum) or not desirable as a learning situation (e.g., life-threatening sepsis following lasertripsy of a renal pelvis stone), a simulation model can be used to teach multilevel and interprofessional skills of Crisis Resource Management (CRM). *CRM, originally developed in the aviation industry to learn, integrate, and practice human factors in an emergency, has been adopted and adapted for training healthcare professional working in a team in a simulated situation.* Although these educational concepts have developed separately (and often viewed as such), they are linked by the same thread of a need to integrate competences for a safe, effective, and efficient practice. It could be argued that a competency-based curriculum that uses the reflective practice strategies, in actual or simulated clinical situations, measuring the integration ability by using assessable EPAs in a "time-lined" apprenticeship model, may be the best way of integrating "competences" relevant to the complexity of the medical practice. In this sense, the construct of competence is behaviorist- or performance-based, i.e., the competencies are a description of an action, behavior, or outcome in a form that is capable of demonstration, observation, and assessment (i.e., something that a person is able to do in a real clinical situation). The competence is therefore judged against a set of defined "competencies." In this holistic approach, the competence is dynamic in application (applying in different clinical contexts), evolutionary (developing with increasing experience), and relational (applying knowledge, skills, attitudes, and values in the complexity and untidy setting of a real-life situation) [11].

So far, this chapter has focused on the ability to integrate competences within the medical practitioner for each patient presentation. In real-life practice, a number of professionals and systems work in conjunction for the patient care. The eventual outcome for the patient, like any complex system, depends on the collective of organizational performance [12]. Work on patient safety [13] has produced ample evidence that the best outcomes for patients are achieved not by the individual competence and expertise but by how the teams and organizational structures and functions integrate in delivering an effective, efficient, safe, quality-controlled, cost-effective, equitable, acceptable, patient-centric, and self-improving service—a "learning organization" (where research, development, and audit integrate with day-to-day service). This concept, translated into an operational model, provides the framework for integrated care, which combines an integration of competences between different health and social care professionals, with health economics and healthcare systems, from a patient perspective. In the context of this chapter, it is an exercise in competences matching as appropriate to the patient journey. Good evidence exists for integrated care in state-run healthcare systems [14]. Integrated healthcare systems are mostly a policy decision. However, healthcare professionals are the prime movers in any such decisions, as many aspects require competency matching, understanding patient journeys, education of health professional in all core issues, removing duplication and obstacles, shared responsibility, understanding shared values and outcomes, communication systems, and, above all, putting the patient at the center [15]. How this could be achieved is well demonstrated by the Cancer Networks in the UK, which aim to provide a complete integration model (i.e., clinical, professional, functional, and organizational) for better patient outcomes [16]. The patient care is also integrated with research, training, service development, sharing good practice, and patient involvement in the delivery of care. Urological training in integrated healthcare, therefore, will require teaching and assessing integration and matching of competences at various levels, beyond the immediate care of patients. Admittedly, the state-run healthcare allows for easy integration due to its central policy-making ability, but eventually a better understanding and "preparedness" of professionals is the key to the success and continuing development.

Could a model like this be applied to urolithiasis in all its presentations and management? In the management of urolithiasis, variability of care within one healthcare system, even in the same organization, has been well reported [17]. In the United States, over one million emergency room visits are made every year with urolithiasis-related problems. Such variability of care will clearly have national consequences (e.g., in productivity). Most of the published literature on integrated care in urolithiasis has focused on streamlining care within one stone center or a group of hospitals. These integration attempts are purely focused around the technical expertise housed in a single facility and/or decision making relating to technical expertise required to solve a clinical problem. The focus, therefore, has been on technological developments to achieve "integrated" care on a single aspect of patient care [18]. This limits the wider perspective on "integrated care." Much less has been written on the training of both the urological and non-urological trainees (such as community practitioners, who are the primary point of contact in most acute urolithiasis presentations) and other professional involved in delivering care in urolithiasis. Attempts at integrating from bottom-up approach, in form of developing clinical care pathway across the primary and the secondary care, have been described [19].

Conclusion

Do we have to wait for a healthcare system to make policy decisions on integrated care? It could be argued that integration does not have to be provided at a high level of policy from the outset. Training of the urologists of the future in integrated care concepts and application is achievable even today. The advances in the care of urolithiasis are not going to be only technological; service and care delivery systems will be a major factor in giving a patient-focused, equitable, and optimal care. This chapter started with an exploration of integration of competences as the main element of urological training and has now expanded the concept to include integrated healthcare as the ultimate example of "integrating" competences for improving healthcare. In the context of urolithiasis, research, innovation, learning, training, and quality improvement will follow with integrated care. This may not just be sky gazing. Complexity of patient features, new and evolving treatments, costs, equitable healthcare, desire to reduce variability of care, etc., [20] are all working toward an integrated care model that will lead to curricula that are geared toward trainees being able to function effectively in such systems.

References

1. The General Medical Council of UK. Tomorrow's doctors. London: GMC; 2003.
2. PMETB. Appendix 1: key principles and standards for postgraduate medical education training programmes. London: DOH; 2005.
3. Manley KG. Paying Peter and Paul: reconciling concepts of expertise with competency for a clinical career structure. J Clin Nurs. 2000;9:347–59.
4. Schön DA. Educating the reflective practitioner: towards a new design for teaching and learning in the professions. San Francisco: Jossey-Bass; 1996.
5. Hill C. The integration of professional competences into construction management degrees. http://ctiweb.cf.ac.uk/learning/casestudies/case_pdf/hillc.pdf. Accessed 12 Apr 2011.
6. Miller G. The assessment of clinical skills, competence and performance. Acad Med. 1990;65 suppl 9:S63–7.
7. Shumway JHR. AMEE Medical Education Guide No. 25: the assessment of learning outcomes for the competent and reflective physician. Med Teach. 2003;25(6):569–84.
8. Carraccio C, Burke AE. Beyond competencies and milestones: adding meaning through context. J Grad Med Educ. 2010;2(3): 419–22.
9. Kinsella EA. Constructivist underpinning in Donald Schon's theory of reflective practice: echoes of nelson Goodman. Reflect Pract. 2006;7(3):277–86.
10. Ten Cate O, Scheele F. Competency-based postgraduate training: can we bridge the gap between theory and clinical practice? Acad Med. 2007;82(6):542–7.
11. Evans K, Hodkinson P, Unwin L, editors. Working to learn: transforming learning in workplace. London: Kogan Page; 2002.
12. Swanson RA, editor. The purpose of human resource development is to improve organizational performance. In: Debating the future of educating adults in the work place. San Francisco: Jossey-Bass; 1996.
13. Department of Health Expert Group. An organisation with memory. London: DOH; 2000.
14. Ramsay A, Fulop N. Evidence base for Integrated Care. London: DOH; 2008. http://www.dhcarenetworks.org.uk/_library/Resources/ICN/ICN_advice/The_evidence_base_for_Integrated_care.pdf. Accessed on 12 Apr 2011.
15. Lloyd J, Wait S. Integrated care: a guide for policy makers. London: Alliance for Health and the Future, DOH; 2005. http://www.ilcuk.org.uk/files/pdf_pdf_7.pdf. Accessed 12 Apr 2011.
16. DOH. 2007. Cancer networks. http://www.ncat.nhs.uk/what-is-ncat/cancer-networks. Accessed 12 Apr 2011.
17. Sterrett S, Moore NW, Nakada SY. Emergency room follow-up trends in urolithiasis: single-center report. Urology. 2009;73(6): 1195–7.
18. Hayes WS, Tohme W, Komo D, Dai H, Persad SG, Benavides A, et al. A telemedicine consultative service for the evaluation of patient with urolithiasis. Urology. 1998;51(1):39–43.
19. Wright PE, English PJ, Hungin AP, Marsden SN. Managing acute renal colic across the primary-secondary care interface: a pathway of care based on evidence and consensus. BMJ. 2002;325: 1408–12.
20. Williams R. Urologic disease in America project. J Urol. 2005;173:679.

Education and Training of an Academic Urologic Surgeon

101

Farhat Abbas and Michael Coburn

Abstract

… this chapter describes the training systems in USA, UK and Pakistan; paradigm shifts in medical education, competency based education, assessment; and the impact of the proposed health reforms suggested by the Lancet Commission.

Keywords

Urology • Postgraduate medical education (PGME) • Self-directed learning • Evidence-based practice • Certification • Competency-based curricula • Endoscopy • Laparoscopy • Minimally invasive procedures • Continuing medical education (CME) • Continuing professional development (CPD) • Proposed reforms

Introduction

Today, we are living in a world that is going through rapid change. The demographics of populations are changing, people are living longer, and the spectrum of diseases is changing. This requires that the health system and the education system must adjust themselves and adapt to the changing environment. New and exciting developments in medical technology are revolutionizing the way education and health care is delivered; the global financial scenario and resource requirements and allocations for health and education are undergoing significant change; major disparities exist between the developing and the developed world. This creates major challenges, especially in the context of ever-changing needs. As physicians are now required to be leaders and managers in addition to being medical experts, it is essential that they are equipped to handle these challenges.

Keeping pace with changes in the way health care is delivered, paradigm shifts are also taking place in the way the medical education is imparted. The current focus is on assessing whether the structure and processes of existing systems are appropriately designed for outcomes that best meet the current and future societal health care needs. Today recommendations are being formulated (in terms of required adjustments in health care and education systems) to address these societal priorities [1].

Postgraduate Medical Education

Postgraduate medical education (PGME) is the period of learning undertaken by medical graduates after successful completion of basic studies in medicine and is targeted toward developing specialists who are leaders, researchers, and practitioners in a specialty/discipline of medicine.

PGME is by and large a time when the resident gets hands-on training. Traditionally it was meant to transfer a set of cognitive and psychomotor skills to the trainee by virtue of him/her being associated with an expert in the field. In the nineteenth century, the tradition expanded to include theoretical grounding in the discipline, whereby the trainee was required to demonstrate a grasp over the knowledge

F. Abbas, M.B.B.S., FCPS, FRCS, FRCSEd, FEBU, FACS (✉)
Department of Surgery, Medical college, Aga Khan University, Stadium Road, Karachi, Sindh 74800, Pakistan
e-mail: farhat.abbas@aku.edu

M. Coburn, M.D., FACS
Scott Department of Urology, Ben Taub General Hospital, Baylor College of Medicine,
6620 Main Street, Suite 1325, Houston, TX 77030, USA

J.J. Talati et al. (eds.), *Urolithiasis*,
DOI 10.1007/978-1-4471-4387-1_101, © Springer-Verlag London 2012

base. In the twentieth century, we witnessed a greater structuring of the PGME with increasing emphasis on written curriculum identifying the requisite knowledge and skills important for the specialty and a structured program which would gradually enable students to move from the level of advanced beginner to a proficient practitioner [2]. By the middle of the twentieth century, aspects of self-directed learning, evidence-based practice, and professionalism [3] were added to medical education with a major change in written PGME curricula. We are now in the era when PGME is no longer considered "training" but "education," which helps in developing critical and creative thinkers with clinical reasoning and problem-solving skills [4].

A major impetus for this change came from a better understanding of learning, especially the constructivist theory [5], and the process of clinical reasoning and decision making [6]. In addition to these, the emergence of regulatory and accrediting bodies for PGME laid down policies [7] that have resulted in better structuring of these programs.

Education and Training in Urology

Urology is a surgical specialty, which deals with diseases of the male and female urinary tract and the male reproductive organs [8]. Medical professionals specializing in the field of urology are called urologists and are trained to diagnose, treat, and manage patients with urological disorders. The organs covered by urology include the kidneys, adrenal glands, ureters, urinary bladder, urethra, and the male reproductive organs (testes, epididymis, vas deferens, seminal vesicles, prostate, and penis).

There is a long tradition of education, training, and skill acquisition in the field of urology. The early history of urology and more specifically the treatment for stones is considered to be the first surgical specialty dating back to ancient times. References to urine diagnosis exist in the Babylonian, Egyptian, and Indian medical writings [9]. It appears that imparting relevant education and training was established way back with recognition of so-called experts—the Hippocratic Oath referred to "cutting for stone," which should not be done by all medical practitioners but be left to those who are skilled in this—thus, recognizing the role of specialists for stone disease treatment [10]. Bladder stones were discovered in Egyptian mummies several millennia BCE, while the rite of circumcision in Egypt were established as early as 4000 BCE. The Hippocratic and Alexandrian schools promoted the early urology teachings, practices, and innovations with wonderful references about techniques, instruments, and practices [11]. The specialty continued to evolve with development of modern urology of today with a preserved culture of investment in teaching, education, research, and innovation, which defines the core values of academic urology, strongly influencing the quality of application of knowledge in the form of service delivery.

Modern urology as a specialty with a number of well-developed subspecialties (pediatric urology, urologic oncology, renal transplantation, male infertility and andrology, urinary tract stones, female urology, neurourology, and various advancements in technologies such as minimally invasive urology including robotics) is now well established. Education and structured training in urology is now generally well organized globally with support of governments, higher educational institutions, and professional bodies and the dedicated efforts of faculty and staff. The modern urologist of today owes a great deal to the visionary, innovative, and tremendously resourceful contributions of the academic leaders, educationists, program directors, faculty, and administrative leaders in elevating the specialty to its current level of preeminence.

Current Status of Postgraduate Medical Education in Urology

Following completion of undergraduate medical education, postgraduate medical education in urology generally follows the pattern of PGME for other disciplines. Entry into a medical school for undergraduate medical education is usually following 12–16 years of education depending on different parts of the world. The undergraduate medical education programs (MBBS, MD, etc.) usually last between 4 and 6 years. The medical students learn in various settings, and the undergraduate medical education program varies significantly across the world in terms of the structure, content, duration, pedagogies, assessment methodologies, and certification processes. In most part of the world, however, following graduation and receiving a basic medical degree such as MBBS or MD, the fresh graduates usually cannot practice independently, and they tend to enter into a postgraduate medical education program (structured or unstructured) in a variety of disciplines which lends them to eventually qualify as so-called specialist in a defined specialty. The postgraduate medical education programs vary significantly again in terms of the variables as cited above and could last from as little as 2 years for family physicians to as long as 8 or 9 years for certain subspecialty training programs.

Following successful completion of the training program, the residents and fellows are usually required to be certified as a specialist by independent bodies such as colleges of physicians and surgeons, boards, etc. In most of the developed world, postgraduate medical education is overseen by bodies outside the universities, such as the royal colleges in the UK, Canada, and Australia, the colleges in South Africa and Pakistan, and the Accreditation Council for Graduate Medical

Education (ACGME) and American Board of Medical Specialties (ABMS) in the USA, which award (and are responsible for the quality of) the postgraduate qualifications, generally diplomas. However, in India, East Africa, and many other countries, universities have been responsible for awarding clinical postgraduate medical degrees—MD or DM in India and MMed (in Nairobi, Dar es Salaam, or Kampala—Makerere) in East Africa. It should be noted that some universities in Pakistan do offer a clinical postgraduate degree equivalent to FCPS, e.g., the MD degrees of Karachi and Lahore universities, which are clinical, and not equivalent to a UK MD degree, which is a research (thesis-based) degree comparable with a PhD.

In most parts of the world, the certified postgraduates have to register themselves to a licensing body, a mandatory credential that along with discipline-specific certification enables them to practice as an independent specialist practitioner. In many developed countries, they must demonstrate evidence of continuing education, and at certain intervals (usually by 10 years) they must clear the recertification examination to demonstrate up-to-date knowledge base and skill set, requisite for a safe and competent specialist. Table 101.1 provides a summary of the structures of training and education in urology in many parts of the world.

Structure of Urology Education and Certification in the USA

To practice at the majority of hospitals in the United States, MD-trained urologists must achieve recognition of the American Board of Urology (ABU) that they are appropriately trained and competent to practice in their field. This designation is called board certification. The ABU consists of 12 experienced and practicing urologists who serve 6-year terms and whose mission is to assure the public that all urologists are practicing in a competent manner. While the board has some independence, it is a member board at present of the American Board of Medical Specialties, which provides overriding guidelines within which the ABU must function. A mandatory element for consideration for certification as urologist by the ABU is that a candidate must complete an accredited training program. Urology training programs are accredited by the Residency Review Committee for Urology, which is a working committee of the Accreditation Council for Graduate Medical Education. One of the fundamental responsibilities of the ABU is to work with the urology RRC to construct standards for how urology training programs are organized and conducted [22].

Medical residency training programs in the United States are conducted under the auspices of the ACGME. This is the oversight organization that sets the guidelines for residency review committees and reviews the conduct of those committees.

The Urology Residency Review Committee (RRC) is 1 of 28 review committees of ACGME and is responsible for setting accreditation standards and providing peer evaluation of all urology and pediatric urology training programs. The evaluation assesses the degree to which the program complies with a published set of educational standards and confers an accreditation status on programs meeting or failing to meet those standards. The RRC reviews training programs on a regular basis to ensure that urology residents are being appropriately trained and become competent urologists at the end of successful completion of their residency programs. While the RRC has some autonomy in deciding policy and standards for urology training, it must adhere to the general guidelines and regulations of the ACGME. It is the ACGME that delegates the responsibility to the urology RRC to accredit training programs just as the ABMS delegates the responsibility to the ABU to certify urologists.

Programs must adhere to the common requirements and the specialty specific requirements. These requirements are structured with the objective of assuring the public that residents are competently trained and with the goal of protecting the educational needs of residents. Common requirements include duty hours, regulations about evaluations of programs and residents, and core competencies. These requirements are identical for training programs across all core specialties and cannot be modified by individual RRCs. The specialty specific training requirements are determined by the specialty specific RRC with approval of the ACGME. These requirements include core content education areas (e.g., fertility, stones, genitourinary cancer), surgical case loads, and faculty duties and qualifications. The urology RRC periodically undergoes review by the monitoring committee of the ACGME to ensure that it is conducting business in a manner consistent with ACGME policies and regulations.

UK System

In the UK, doctors have to enter a first (intern) year, also called foundation year one, in which there is a structured and protected job training, monitored by regular assessments. This is divided into three 4-month hospital-based rotations in various disciplines like medicine, surgery, pediatrics, obstetrics, and gynecology. In the foundation year 2, a further three posts of 4 months duration are followed in wider ranges of specialties.

Following these 2 years, doctors enter into specialty training. The time to complete such training is generally 4–6 years. After satisfactory completion of designated training, Certificate of Completion of Specialist Training (CCST) is awarded to those who have satisfactory appraisals at the end of each year and who pass their specialty examination from the appropriate college. They are then automatically added to the specialist registrar [23].

Table 101.1 Structure of urology training and education

S. no.	Country	Eligibility criteria	Duration of residency	Certification	Graduating authority	Specialized fellowships
1.	Pakistan	Basic medical qualification (MBBS) with 1-year house job Entry exam (FCPS part 1)	Five years – 2 years general surgery training (passing intermediate module) and 3 years training in urology	Fellow College of Physicians and Surgeons Pakistan (FCPS Urology) MS Urology	College of Physicians and Surgeons Pakistan Health sciences universities	Offered by individual institutions with certification No subspecialty certification by College of Physicians and Surgeons Pakistan
2.	India [12]	Basic medical qualification + house job	Six years (3 years general surgery and 3 years in urology)	MS Mch (Master of Chirurgical) DNB (Diplomate National Board of Urology)	Health sciences universities	SIU-accredited regional centers Offered by individual institutions with certification No subspecialty certification by Board of Urology
3.	United States [13, 14]	Basic medical qualification (4 + 4 years)	Minimum 5 years (1–2 years general surgery + 3–4 years urology)	Diplomate American Board of Urology	ABU (American Board of Urology)	Many AUA (American Urological Association) endourology society and SIU-accredited centers offering in the field of minimally invasive urological oncology, female and reconstructive urology, pediatric urology, etc.
4.	United Kingdom [15, 16]	Basic medical qualification + house job	6 years (5 years clinical training + 1 year flexible training)	FRCS (urol) can only be taken after completion of 4-year assessment RITA C CCST (Certificate of Completion of Specialist Training)	Royal colleges of Surgeons General Medical Council	Many fellowship programs (BAUS and endourology society accredited) in uro-oncology, reconstructive urology, minimally invasive urology, etc.
5.	Canada [17]	Graduation from medical school	5 years (2 years core surgery + 3 years in urology)	Fellow of Royal College of Physicians and Surgeons of Canada	Royal College of Physicians and Surgeons of Canada Canadian Urological Association (CUA) Societe Internationale d Urologie	SIU- and endourology society-accredited fellowship programs
6.	Australia and New Zealand [18]	Basic medical qualification	5–6 years	Fellow of Royal Australasian College of Surgeons	Royal Australasian College of Surgeons (RACS) Surgical Education and Training (SET) Program	Many accredited fellowship programs in various disciplines
7.	Other European countries [19]	Basic medical qualification	Variable (from 2 to 7 years)	FEBU	European Board of Urology	SIU- and other European societies-accredited fellowship programs
8.	Middle East countries [20]	Doctor of Medicine (M.D.)	5 years	CAB Urol (Certified Arab Board of Urology)	Arab Board of Medical Sciences	–
9.	Egypt [21]	Doctor of Medicine (M.D.)	4 years	Masters (MS) Doctorate (Ph.D.)	Health science universities	SIU-accredited fellowships
10.	Japan	Basic medical qualification	5–6 years	Ph.D.	Japanese Urological Association	

Table 101.2 Curricular reforms in undergraduate medical education [30]

The apprenticeship model	(1765–)
The discipline-based model	(1871–)
The organ-system-based model	(1951–)
The problem-based-learning model	(1971–)
The clinical presentation-based model	(1991–)

Pakistan System

Currently, there are two coexisting urology licensing bodies with separate training formats. Among the two, the one offered by the College of Physicians and Surgeons Pakistan (CPSP) is more widely popular and recognized [24]. The college runs a fellowship program at the end of completion of which a fellowship diploma (FCPS) is offered to successful candidates. The other program is university-based Master's degree (MS).

College of Physicians and Surgeons Pakistan has developed a competency-based curricula. The candidate has to complete a 1-year house job (internship). He/she then has to pass an entry exam (FCPS part 1) in order to get registered and start training from an accredited institute. Most of the institutions offer a 5–6-year program, which involves core training in general surgery for 2 years, after completion of which the candidate has to pass a mid-training exam (intermediate module). Following this, focused education and training in urology of 3–4 years duration is started. The candidates have to attend a number of short courses and workshops, complete an independent research project, continuously maintain a log of cases performed, and pass an exit exam conducted by CPSP.

Paradigm Shift in Medical Education

New developments in medical education reflect changing societal needs, health care needs, changes in provision of health care, and developments in the field of education [1, 25]. The objective of medical education is to prepare the individuals for effective acquisition, integration, and application of knowledge (independent professional functioning) in a defined area, primarily through development of knowledge, skills, and attitudes, whereas the scope of education focuses on acquisition of "personal and professional attributes, characteristics, and competencies" [26–29].

The way the undergraduate medical education delivery models have changed over time (Table 101.2) has also influenced the postgraduate medical education. In essence, the PGME had always been largely based on problem-based and clinical presentation-based model. Enhanced understandings of the knowledge-based structure and cognitive processes that characterize and distinguish medical experts and novices have influenced the curricular reforms. Also there is growing realization that medical educators must call upon and utilize the literature, research methods, and theoretical perspective of cognitive science for effective and efficient forward movements of curricular reforms.

The medical universities and colleges are unique institutions as they (1) impart training to the medical graduates, (2) provide services for the communities, and (3) advance science. They have a mandate from the society to provide quality service, impart high-quality training to the future health care providers of the society, and to excel in research [31]. With the changing times, the health sciences institutions are now becoming increasingly aware and are playing their due role toward "social responsibility" (duties regarding society) and "social responsiveness" (engagement in a course of actions responding to social needs) [32] as expected from them. Within this paradigm of "social responsibility, social responsiveness, and social accountability," the health sciences institutes can and should enhance their role to influence the nature, quality, and attributes of the health care force being groomed and developed. The leadership as well as each faculty member can contribute to making its institution more socially accountable by reorienting education, research, and service delivery programs toward priority health needs and aiming to address specific challenges of the given society in which their graduates are going to work. They must also ensure that their efforts have achieved intended outcomes and the required impact.

Tables 101.3 and 101.4 show some salient changes that have occurred in medical education in order to address the emerging needs.

The Curriculum

The postgraduate medical education curriculum has progressed from an initial complete apprenticeship-based model to an organized educational curriculum in most programs. The current curricula are primarily focused on the duration of total training and the time spent in different clinical rotations or attachments to obtain desired exposure and experience. It is generally assumed that by going through such a syllabus, the trainee will acquire the required educational needs and exposure [34].

In recent times, however, there is a greater emphasis to move to an outcome-based educational model which takes into account the attributes, competencies, and aptitude of the trainee with desired expected learning outcomes. By using such an approach, the learning outcomes are more clearly and specifically defined. The education and training schedules are then adjusted to the desired learning outcomes; pedagogies and the educational strategies are adjusted, the infrastructure is contextually adjusted, and the assessment methodologies are based on the desired outcome [35].

Table 101.3 Shifting paradigms of medical education

Drivers of change in medical education	Paradigm changes in medical education
Medical education should be designed to serve the needs of the population that is ultimately being served	Societal needs concept
The societal needs are ever changing	Educational programs must be flexible
Widely diversified and increasing societal needs	Broadening of education
Better understanding of principles of learning/acquisition of knowledge	Curricular reforms
Desirable characteristics/attributes/competences of graduating students better defined	Focused and refined educational strategies and assessment methodologies
Desirable characteristics of medical educators/teachers	Redefined "role profile" of teachers; evidence-based medical education versus opinion based
Integration and application of knowledge, problem solving, and skills development	Refined assessment methodologies, outcome-based education, curricular mapping, skills labs, and e-learning
Emergence of innovative learning technologies	Integration of learning technologies with education —simulators, information and communication technologies (ICT), e-learning, etc.

Table 101.4 Shifting paradigms of medical education [33]

Traditional	Revised paradigm
The individual	The community
Cure of disease	Preservation of health
Episodic care	Continuous care
Physician provider	Teams of providers
Paternalism	Partnership with patients
Provider centered	Patient-family centered
Anecdotal care	Evidence-based medicine
Inpatient focused	Ambulatory/home centered
Individual accountability	System accountability

Competency Framework in Postgraduate Medical Education

Medical competence is defined by Epstein [36] as "the habitual and judicious use of communication, knowledge, technical skills, clinical reasoning, emotions, values and reflection in daily practice for the benefit of individuals and communities being served." The institutions/organizations involved in postgraduate medical education, certification, and licensure have responded by defining a framework of desired competencies and adopting a competence-based approach to medical education. The ACGME Outcomes Project which is the Joint Initiative of the Accreditation Council for Graduate Medical Education (ACGME) and American Board of Medical Specialties (ABMS) has identified five outcomes to be assessed [37] (Tables 101.5 and 101.6). Royal College of Physicians and Surgeon Canada (RCPSC) has identified similar competencies in the seven CanMEDS roles [38] and the General Medical Council, UK [39]. In Pakistan, the general instructional objectives of the fellowship programs defined by the College of Physicians and Surgeons Pakistan provide a framework for the desired competencies. The Aga Khan University Medical College, Karachi, has also defined seven competencies for its postgraduate medical education (PGME) programs.

It is important that the medical education in the context of undergraduate, postgraduate, and continuing education should be seen as a true continuum extending through school through college, medical school, postgraduate medical education, and medical practice [40]. Medearis and Kinney [41] propagated this concept and argued against compartmentalization of medical education into different blocks. While a number of principles and strategies of medical education are now interchangeably used between undergraduate and postgraduate as well as continuing education, there is still a lot to be desired to see this as a true continuum of education.

While urology remains a male-dominated specialty, in recent times it is slowly becoming an increasingly popular career choice for women. It was not until 1962 that Dr. Elisabeth Pickett became the first board certified urologist in the USA, and by the mid-1980s there were only 22 female urologists in the United States [42]. At present, about 20 % of all residents in urology training programs are females in the United States [43]. In a recent study, the females opted for urology as a career choice because of diversity of procedures and the breadth of experience that this specialty provides. Most women in-training in urology seek subspecialty training in pediatrics or female/reconstructive urology. More than half of all trainees were confronted with negative behavior by male patients or by male colleagues in relation to their gender. It is important that the system and programs understand the women's perspective and concerns in order to maximize the contributions women can make to the specialty and to its patients [44].

Technology in Postgraduate Medical Education

Rapid expansion and availability of innovative technology and learning resources has revolutionized the teaching and learning in postgraduate medical education. While there are many technologies that are being used, there is no consensus on the nature and type of educational and technical tools that must be integrated in the medical, including postgraduate medical educational curricula (Table 101.7). The existing

Table 101.5 Outcomes and competencies for postgraduate medical education

Royal College of Physicians and Surgeons of Canada (RCPSC)	Accreditation Council for Graduate Medical Education (ACGME& ABMS)	General Medical Council, UK (GMC)	College of Physicians and Surgeons, Pakistan (CPSP)	Aga Khan University, Pakistan (AKU)
Medical expert	Medical knowledge	Good clinical care	Clinically competent	Medical expert
Communicator	Interpersonal and communication skills	Relationship with patient	Effective team member/leader	Communication and interpersonal skills
Collaborator	Systems-based practice	Working with colleagues	Evidence-based practice	Systems-based practice
Manager	Patient care	Maintaining good medical practice	Health promotion and prevention	Evidence- and Practice-based learning and improvement
Professional	Professionalism	Probity		Professionalism
Scholar	–	–	Educator	Scholar
Health advocate	Practice-based learning and improvement	Teaching, training, appraising, and assessing	Research and publications	

Table 101.6 Competency common to all

Biomedical ethics
Communication skills
Teaching skills
Quality assurance/improvement
Research and critical appraisal
Management skills
Advocacy
Collaboration

and emerging technology tools will, however, influence the future of PGME in a major way and call for a careful review by everyone involved in PGME.

Various advancements have been done in technology especially with regard to training of urology residents. There are not only improvements in optics and imaging for the training of endourological procedures but also advancements in communication via incorporation of internet and telemedicine for patient care to take place from a remote location [47]. These include synchronous and real-time motion video-conferencing as well as an asynchronous or store-and-forward system by which information is transmitted via Internet [48].

A major component of urology training comprises of mastering skills in endoscopic, laparoscopic, and other minimally invasive procedures, which requires a certain skill sets. Many factors such as cost, supply, infrastructure, and ethical dilemmas including the animal and cadaveric models may lead to reduced training opportunities for urology trainees [49].

This has led to the development of virtual reality simulation which overcomes the moral and ethical dilemmas associated with patients and animal models, and with advancements in computer software, this technology reproduces the real-time anatomy much more naturally [47].

Integrating technology for education not only assists the learning curve and rapid acquisition of skills required for routine and complex urological procedures, but the requisite skills can also be tested and validated. A virtual reality (VR) endoscopic simulator (URO Mentor system, Simbionix, Tel Aviv, Israel) provides realistic anatomic projections and simulations of most of the endoscopic urological procedures such as cystoscopy, retrograde pyelography, and ureteroscopy including simulations for guidewire placement and stone fragmentation and removal [50, 51].

Desai et al. [52] showed better outcomes with respect to management of staghorn stones by percutaneous nephrolithotomy (PCNL), a procedure that requires considerable expertise, with the advancement in technologies. They compared their own results in three different periods with regard to changes in treatment policy, global trends, and advances in equipment and imaging and showed that by incorporation of many technology-related strategies into the training led to improved outcomes. Some of these were three-dimensional (3D) assessments of renal anatomy via computed tomography (CT) scans, training of ultrasound-guided puncture to urologists, optimal use of flexible endoscopes including retrograde intrarenal surgery, etc.

Assessment in Postgraduate Medical Education

Developers of any assessment system are faced with the following questions:

- Why is assessment required?
- What is it that is to be assessed?
- How will the student be assessed?
- How to decide what to use?
- What is the utility of assessment?

Table 101.7 Use of technology in postgraduate medical education

No.	Technology	Example	Comments
1.	Learning management systems	Institutional centralized and integrated learning infrastructure and tools, e.g., courses, assessment/reporting tools, Moodle, WebCT, etc.	More used in UGME than PGME
2.	Computer-based learning resources	Information searching such as MEDLINE, web, online tutorials, and self-study package	Contains journal citations and abstracts for biomedical literature from around the world Independent exploration of complex phenomena with easy access and relatively low cost
3.	Video technologies	Web-conferencing, video-conferencing, video-based educational rounds, video-learning patients, etc.	Allows conferencing events to be shared from remote locations. WEBINAR [45] (web-based seminar is used for a lecture, presentation, workshop, or seminar that is transmitted over the web) Can be one way (webcast) from the speaker to the audience with limited audience interaction May be more collaborative (including polling and question and answer sessions to allow full participation)
4.	Clinical systems/clinical educational systems	Electronic medical records, picture archiving and communication systems (PACS), clinical encounter recording system, e-portfolios, etc.	Economical storage and convenient access Eliminates the need to manually file, retrieve, and transport data Images and patient health-related information could be sent electronically from one caregiver to another and from multiple modalities
5.	Virtual patients	American Board of Family Medicine (ABFM) virtual patients exercises	Specific type of computer-based program that simulates real-life clinical scenarios Encompasses multiple aspects of clinical encounter but has limited physical interactivity and limited fidelity
6.	Simulators [46]:	Procedural simulations, e.g., Vasovasostomy and laparoscopic nephrectomy in animals	Effective for objective assessment of junior and intermediate trainees
	Bench	Cystoscopy, semirigid ureteroscopy, and basket extraction of a distal ureteric stone in human cadavers	Transferability of skills from simulation to patients can be incorporated and assessed
	Animal models Human cadavers Virtual reality	Laparoscopic nephrectomy, flexible cystoscopy in virtual reality.	Forms part of a comprehensive curriculum (including knowledge attained alongside the technical skills required)

The Purpose of Assessment in PGME

One of the main purposes of assessment in PGME is to certify competence assuring the society that the newly certified consultant will perform safely as an independent practitioner and train juniors in his/her field. The certification process takes place upon the completion of the residency program. However, for the required learning to take place, it is imperative that the resident is frequently assessed during the years of residency education and provided constructive feedback, reinforcing what has been learned correctly and improving areas needing attention. Another purpose of assessment is to monitor the growth and promote residents to next levels of education or remediate [53].

The principles of assessment guiding all assessment processes place great emphasis on defining what is to be assessed so that the assessors select the most appropriate instruments and identify assessment situations. In addition the assessment should give reliable results, should be considered fair, be feasible, and provide validity evidence for decisions that are made on the basis of the scores [54].

Assessing the Competence

The fundamental principle of competency-based residency education is that residents must demonstrate achievement of the desired outcomes before they are considered fit for advancement to the next phase of education [55]. It is therefore required that purposes and details of every component of the assess-

Table 101.8 Assessment methodologies

Case logs
Patient surveys
Portfolios
Record review
Objective structured clinical examination (OSCE)
Simulations and models
Standardized oral examination
Standardized patient examination (SP)
Written examinations (essays, MCQ)
360° evaluation instrument
Chart-stimulated recall oral exam (CSR)
Checklist evaluation of live or recorded performance
Global rating of live or recorded performance

ment system is specified and available to all interested parties, including residents and their supervisor. Sequential multimodal assessments help gauge progress of required competencies in the desired direction, with appropriate documentation and a system of verbal constructive feedback.

A number of instruments are being used to assess the desired skills ranging from written tests for assessment of cognition to high-tech simulations for assessing complex skills. The selection of the most appropriate instrument is dependent on their suitability for assessing the targeted skill with good reliability, assessors' knowledge of instrument development and use, agreed upon standards of performance, and their relevance to actual practice. Adequate sampling of the outcome of interest by multiple assessors, in varying clinical situations and on a diverse set of patients, gives validity to the decisions made on the basis of these assessments [56]. Good quality assessments help in identification, diagnosis, and remediation of problem residents at an early stage.

The commonly used instruments [57] are direct observation of time-limited performance measures using mini-clinical examination, direct observation of procedural skills, objective structured assessment of technical skills, daily-encounter cards, or observation across a range of time using multisource feedback, in-training evaluation record, etc. Other methods that are employed use longitudinal, comprehensive judgment of performance using portfolios and logbooks (Table 101.8).

The utility of assessment during residency education is improved with clear goals and objectives, alignment of assessment to practice and patient safety, and when it is perceived to be of educational benefit rather than documentation of competence [58]. In a study done by Snell et al. [59], residents strongly appreciated the feedback that they received as a result of their assessment and found it to be useful for their further learning.

In conclusion, therefore, assessments during PGME will be useful only when residents see the value of the assessment in improving learning, the assessment instruments are content and construct valid, multiple observations are made, structured feedback is given, and opportunities for improvement are provided.

Continuing Education and Professional Development

As physicians continue on with their practice, they rely more and more on their prior experiences. But as new information and techniques become available, these physicians must update their "memories." Physicians who have been in practice for long could be at risk for providing lower quality care [60].

With the perspective of lifelong learning, continuing medical education (CME), continuing professional development (CPD), and evidence-based medicine (EBM) have become established ways of enhancing one's ability of remaining up to date in knowledge base and skill sets in order to enhance clinical reasoning and the quality of care [61–64]. The CME, CPD, and EBM aim to address the needs of the practicing physicians and offer opportunities for ongoing intellectual stimulation and professional renewal.

There is however differing evidence about the impact of formal CME programs in bringing about the anticipated changes in physician's performance [65, 66]. Using a meta-analysis of the formal CME interventions, Davis et al. [67] concluded that interactive CME sessions that enhance participant activity and provide the opportunity to practice skills could effect change in physicians' practice and at time, health care outcomes. The pure didactic sessions are least likely to bring about the desired changes.

Davis et al. [68] recommended four steps for effective CPD experience both for the teacher as well as for the learner:

1. Knowing the audience—composition, background, practice patterns, expertise, and experience
2. Knowing the topic—the subject area, the objective, and goals of the given session
3. Knowing the format—choosing the educational processes with interactive sessions, with post-intervention reinforcing material and methods
4. Knowing the outcome—and preferably measuring it

The mission of the CME and CPD activities, most importantly, is that the physician must alter their practice, if so required, and thus the content of such sessions must be relevant, as simple as possible, and enjoyable to the physicians. A number of urology-specific resources are now available to support evidence-based urology including journals, electronic tools, and live training opportunities, and they must be selectively integrated in the training, education, and continuing education for the urologists.

Table 101.9 Proposed reforms by the Lancet Commission on Education of Health Professionals for the Twenty-First Century [69]

Instructional reforms
1. Adoption of competency-based curricula that are repsonsive to rapidly changing needs rather than being dominated by static coursework.
2. Promotion of interprofessional and transprofessional education that breaks down professional silos while enhancing collaborative and nonhierarchial relationships in elective teams.
3. Exploitation of the power of information technology (IT) through development of evicdence, capacity for data collection and analysis, simulation and testing, distance learning, collaborative conectivity, and management of the increase in knowledge.
4. Adaptation locally but harnessing of resources globally in a way that confers capacity to flexibly address local challenges while using global knowledge, experience, and shared resources, including faculty, curriculum, didactic materials, and students linked internationally through exchange programs.
5. Strengthening of educational resources, since faculty, syllabuses, didactic materials, and infrastructure are necessary instruments to achieve compentencies.
6. Promote a new professionalism that uses compentencies as the objective criterion for the classification of health professionals, transforming present conventional silos.
Institutional reforms
7. Establishment of joint planing mechanisms in every country to engage key stakeholders, especially ministries of education and health, professional associations, and the academic community, to overcome fragmentation by assessment of national conditions, setting priorities, shaping policies, tracking change, and harmonizing the supply and demand for health professionals to meet the health needs of the population.
8. Expansion from academic centers to academic systems, extending the traditional discovery-care-education continuum to the community setting.
9. Linking together through networks, alliances, and consortia between educational institutions worldwide and across to allied sectors such as governments, civil society organizations, business, and media.
10. Nurturing of a culture of critical inquiry as a central function of universities and other institutions of higher learning.

Proposed Reforms for Health Professionals Education

The Lancet Commission on Education of Health Professionals for the Twenty-First Century

The Lancet Commission on Education of Health Professionals for the Twenty-First Century published their report in 2010. They used a global outlook with a multiprofessional perspective and a system approach considering the connection between education and health systems. The summary recommendations as given in Table 101.9 attempt to describe a global strategy for postsecondary education in medicine, nursing, and public health. The focus is to groom educated, ethical, and critical health professionals who are competent to participate in patient-centered and population-centered health systems as members of locally responsive and globally connected teams. These generic strategies are applicable to all educational programs, including urology.

Medical Education and Training Regulation Policy Review, Lord Patel Report, UK

In 2010, the General Medical Council and Postgraduate Medical Education and Training Board, UK, published a draft report of the Medical Education and Training Regulation Policy Review, led by Lord Naren Patel (the Patel Review) [70].

The draft report makes 27 proposed recommendations for the future regulation of education and training for the medical profession in the UK. Its recommendations address the different stages of education and training (undergraduate, postgraduate, and continuing practice) and the links between them, as well as the handling of medical graduates from other countries. The recommendations have implications not only for doctors and those involved in their training but also for patients and for health care organizations throughout the UK.

With the assimilation of Postgraduate Medical Education and Training Board, UK, in 2011, the General Medical Council has now become a single organization responsible for the regulation of the entire spectrum of medical education in the UK. This will allow GMC to take a long-term look at the future regulation of medical education and training as a whole and to consider how this fits in with its other responsibilities for registration, setting and maintaining standards, and ensuring fitness to practice.

Information and Educational Technology in Postgraduate Medical Education: Future of Medical Education in Canada Postgraduate (FMEC PG) Project

In 2011, the Association of Faculties of Medicine of Canada (AFMC) published their project report on "information and educational technology in postgraduate medical education" consisting of a literature review and interviews of seven key stakeholders from across the country [71]. They identified that though Canadian postgraduate medical education (PGME) has incorporated the digital technologies, it needs to be addressed more broadly to meet the requirements of trainees and health care system as a whole. They identified several problems in Canadian system including handling and managing the strategic direction of technology integration at institutional levels professionally and nationally. They also identified a significant problem of working with and within the digital environments and lack of integration of digital methods into the curricula. A series of challenges were presented as:

1. Need for a digital competency framework for physicians in training
2. Need for improved research, scholarship, and critical appraisal of the role of digital media and methods in PGME
3. Need for a more digitally informed leadership in PGME

The report identified several core steps to address the shortcomings around the use of digital media and methods in Canadian PGME. These include developing a national digital literacy and professionalism curriculum, creating common educational and technical standards, and creating better opportunities for digital educators to collaborate and align PGME with the development of Canada's digital health care system.

The Future of Urology and Urologic Education in America

In 2006, American Urological Association published the report "The Future of Urology and Urologic Education in America" based on the work of a group of experts assessing the existing strengths and weaknesses and current and future challenges related to urology education and training in America [72]. The group was charged with this task given a rising concern that the American urological training was evolving more toward a "two-tiered system," similar to the trend in many European countries, of separate paths for "office-based urologists" versus "specialty urologic surgeons." The major disadvantage of such a model is decreased broad-based capabilities of graduating urologists.

The planning group observed that comprehensive training of general urologists is vital to meet the needs of the patients and communities, while the enhancement and expansion of subspecialty fellowship training in various areas is crucial for the long-term health of both academic and private practice. They concluded that the two-tiered model was not in the best interest of the patients or the specialty. The changing environment calls for the programs to adapt to the emerging technologies, newer ways of treating patients, and to continue to offer comprehensive care for all urological disorders, both medically and surgically. They made the following specific recommendations:

1. Develop a national core curriculum for urologists to include both cognitive and manipulative skills.
2. Urologic subspecialty societies should define the knowledge and skills to be acquired during core versus fellowship training.
3. Put urology program directors in charge of postgraduate year 1.
4. Make the last 2 years of residency flexible (to allow for electives) after core competencies are developed.
5. Move away from all residents needing equal surgery logs; focus more on the minimal number of total cases than specific type of cases.
6. Partially integrate chief residency year into fellowship.
7. Fellowship program directors must develop common fellowship standards.
8. Reinforce the importance of the research experience to all trainees, irrespective of their career goals.
9. Develop electives for those interested in academic career to develop skills in teaching, research, writing, and craftsmanship.
10. Put ongoing assessment of urologic training more into a continuous quality improvement model and repeat national assessment periodically (e.g., 5 years).

Establishment of Postgraduate Medical Education at an Institution

Establishing PGME programs at an institutional level requires that there must be a firm commitment to offer high-quality educational opportunity to all program entrants and that in turn requires that careful attention must be paid to ensure provision of and compliance with both "institutional standards and requirements" as well as that of "program standards and requirements" (Table 101.10). These standards must take into account the national/regional and international standards as applicable as well as attempt to adopt best practices based on available evidence.

Some of the learning points that we gathered at our institution (Aga Khan University) in terms of successful establishment of PG programs include the following:

1. The Health Sciences Education including the PG education at the institution must be aligned with the mission/vision of the institution.
2. The education strategy must take into account the changing health care needs, societal needs, changes in provision of health care, and development in the field of education.
3. The primary focus of PG education of the development of knowledge, skills, and attitudes must be broadened to include secondary and tertiary considerations.
4. The individuals must be prepared for effective acquisition, integration, and application of knowledge.
5. For establishment of quality PG education, equal emphasis must be placed on defining and maintaining both the institutional as well as the programmatic standards.
6. A strong institutional commitment for excellence in both education and health care provision is the key for achieving an overall excellence in Health Sciences Education.

Opportunities and Challenges in PGME in Developing World Scenario

Establishing high-quality PGME programs in the developing world poses both opportunities as well as particular challenges when compared with the developed world scenario. Many of the particular challenges in the developing world scenario also act as potential opportunities (such as large populations and widened disease burden) as they provide a base for broad exposure and diverse experience for the trainees:

Table 101.10 Minimum considerations toward establishment of PG program at an institution

Institutional standards/requirements	Program standards/requirements
Institutional commitment	Scope of specialty
Excellence in education and medical care	Duration and scope of education
Scholarly environment	Administrative structure
Commitment exhibited by provision of leadership and resources to help programs achieve their objectives:	Goals and objectives (written curriculum)
Governance	Structure and organization of program
Educational administration—establishment and implementation of policies (selection, evaluation, promotion, dismissal, grievances, complaints, funding, work environment, monitoring, curriculum, etc.)	Resources
Liaison with appropriate personnel	Clinical, academic, and scholarly content of program
Reviews—internal, external	Assessments/evaluations
Educational organization	Accreditation/certification
Teaching faculty and staff	Other
Standards: (e.g., PG Med. Education)	
Accreditation of patient care	
Credentialing of faculty	
Quality assurance	
Standards of facilities and resources	
Hospital facilities (diagnostic/therapeutic)	
Space and equipment	
Patient population	
Medical library/learning resources	
Medical records/support Services	
Other	

1. Large populations
2. Wide disease burden
3. Socioeconomic challenges
4. Limitations of infrastructure, education, finance, and natural resources
5. Varying commitment and support of governments and key institutions toward PGME
6. Challenges related to status of women
7. Social, cultural, linguistic, and religious variations
8. Availability of resourceful human resource (faculty, technical staff, etc.)
9. Maintenance of balance among educational, research, and service throughputs
10. Quality of academic programs and research with quality assurance mechanisms
11. Technology, equipment, and innovation
12. Cost of education
13. Networking
14. Sustainability of the high-quality academic programs

Given these specific challenges, it is important that the PGME programs in developing world are contextually aligned to address the specific needs. This should be done while maintaining the objectives of providing the highest possible level of postgraduate training structure in the country/region with international standards. It obviously requires thoughtful deliberations of the academic leadership in consultation with leading academic institutions/organizations. It is particularly important that the PGME programs prepare the individuals for focused interventions in the following areas:

1. Promotion of social justice through addressing health disparities
2. Collaborations between the basic scientists and other scholars—interdisciplinary and multidisciplinary collaborations and research
3. Implementation or application of research—"translational and applied research"
4. Attracting the talented faculty and students with diversity
5. Task shifting
6. Advocacy and influencing national policy
7. Sustainability

Conclusion

With the ever-expanding new horizons and dimensions in medical education, the education and training of an academic urologist remains a challenge for both the trainees as well as the trainers. It is important that the education systems across the globe are ready to embrace the newer and refined ways of inculcating the right knowledge base, skill sets, attitudes, and attributes to the emerging group of urologists as well as to continue to build on existing strengths. Given the plethora of existing resources to support the educational mandate, the training environment had never been more conducive and is likely to grow even further. Thus, it is important that the system as a whole, including the trainees and trainers, must take maximum advantage of the existing supportive environment and leverage the situation in their favor. At the same time, they must grow much beyond being a urologist to play a much larger role of being a leader, a change agent, a role model for addressing social and economic challenges, and above all, an ethical, morally correct, and just human being.

Unless we start producing graduates who have some depth of understanding of our ecology, of what history teaches us about the consequences of large scale inequity, of what riches there are in this world that can't be found at a shopping center, of how much social change depends on personal choices, what chance do we have?

Keith Bezanson [73]

Acknowledgments For their contributions to the chapter, we thank Syed Muhammad Nazim, MBBS, MCPS, MRCS, FCPS, senior instructor, Section of Urology, Department of Surgery, and Syeda Kausar Ali, MBBS, MhPE, Ph.D., senior lecturer, Department for Educational Development, Aga Khan University, Karachi, Pakistan.

References

1. Shifting public perceptions of doctors and healthcare. Submitted to Association of Faculties of Medicine of Canada. Ontario: Ekos Research Associates; 2011.
2. Dreyfus HL, Dreyfus SE. Mind over machine: the power of human intuition and expertise in the age of the computers. Oxford: Blackwell Scientific; 1986.
3. Association of American Medical Colleges. A flag in the wind: educating for professionalism in medicine. Washington, D.C.: Association of American Medical Colleges; 2003.
4. Maudsley RF. Training, education and scholarship. Ann R Coll Physicians Surg Can. 1997;30(4):201–2.
5. Bruning RH, Schraw GJ, Norby MM. Cognitive psychology and instruction. 5th ed. Saddle River: Pearson Merrill Prentice Hall; 2010.
6. Elstein AS. Thinking about diagnostic thinking: a 30-year perspective. Adv Health Sci Educ Theory Pract. 2009;14(S1):7–18.
7. Southgate L, Grant J. Principles and standards for an assessment system for postgraduate medical training. PMETB subgroup on assessment. 2003. http://evavalpa.org/modulos/modulo_04/principles__assessment.pdf. Last accessed September 14, 2012.
8. Excerpts from What Is Urology: Information for Medical Students and Prospective Urology Residents, prepared by the AUA Graduate Medical Education Committee. http://www.auanet.org/content/about-us/what-is-urology.cfm. Accessed 16 Jan 2012.
9. Neuberger M, Phil DM, Riesman D. The early history of urology. Bull Med Libr Assoc. 1937;25(3):147–65.
10. Greenspan R. A brief history of urology: collectmedicalantiques.com. 2011.
11. Wishard WMN. History of urology. Baltimore: Williams and Wilkins; 1943.
12. Aron M. Urology training in India: balancing national needs with global perspectives. Indian J Urol. 2009;25(2):254–6.
13. American Urological Association. What is urology? Available from: www.auanet.org/content/residency/what-is-urology.cfm. Last accessed on 16 Jan 2012.
14. Amling CL. Changes in training and education. J Urol. 2011;186(4):1185–6. Epub 2011 Aug 17.
15. Higher surgical training in urology. Urology_grey_manual – UK and Ireland. A guide for trainers and trainees in the UK and Ireland. 2003. Available from: www.jcst.org/publications/Curriculum/.../urology_grey_manual.pdf. Last accessed September 14, 2012.
16. The Biritish Association of Urological surgeons. Training and workforce. Available from:www.baus.org.uk/Sections/female/workforce. Last accessed on 16 Jan 2012.
17. Royal College of Physicians and Surgeons of Canada. Urology. Available from: http://rcpsc.medical.org/residency/accreditation/arps/urology_e.php. Last accessed on 16 Jan 2012.
18. Urological Society of Australia & New Zealand. Surgical education and training (SET). Available from: http://www.usanz.org.au/surgical-education-and-training-set/. Last accessed on 16 Jan 2012.
19. Parkar SP, Fuglsig S, Nunes P, Keskin S, Kniestedt WJ, Sedelaar JP. European society of residents in urology. Urological training in Europe: similarities and differences. BJU Int. 2005;96(2):207–11.
20. The Arab Board of Health Specializations. Urology specialty. Available from: http://arab-board.org/node/43218. Last updated on 12 Jan 2012.
21. Kasr Al-Ainy. Urology, Cairo University. Training and education. Available from: http://www.kasralainyurology.net/pgedu.php. Last accessed on 16 Jan 2012.
22. Accreditation Council for Graduate Medical Education. Urology menu. Available from: http://www.acgme.org/acWebsite/navPages/nav_480.asp. Last Accessed on 16 Jan 2012.
23. Ahmed K, Jawad M, Dasgupta P, Darzi A, Athanasiou T, Khan MS. Assessment and maintenance of competence in urology. Nat Rev Urol. 2010;7:403–13. doi:10.1038/nrurol.2010.81.
24. College of Physicians and Surgeons of Pakistan. Training program. Available from: http://www.cpsp.edu.pk/index.php?code=NnxUb3B8dHJhaW5pbmcucGhwfDA=. Last accessed on 16 Jan 2012.
25. CanMEDS 2000 Project. Skills for the new millennium – societal needs working group. Ann RCPSC. 1996;29(4):206–16.
26. Learning objectives for medical students education – guidelines for medical schools: report 1 of the Medical School Objectives Project. Acad Med. 1999;74(1):13–8.
27. Maudsley RF. Content in context: medical education and society's needs. Acad Med. 1999;74(2):143–5.
28. Fundamental issues in specialty education-task force to review fundamental issues in specialty education. Annals RCPSC. 1996;29(5).
29. Bickel J. Proceedings of the AAMC conference on students' and residents' ethical and professional development. Acad Med. 1996;71(6):622–40.
30. Papa FJ, Harasym PH. Medical curriculum reform in North America, 1765 to the present: a cognitive science perspective. Acad Med. 1999;74(2):154–64.
31. The social accountability of medical schools. Changing Medical Education and Medical Practice. WHO News Lett. 1996:1–3.
32. Boelen C. Social accountability: the extra leap to excellence for educational institutions. Med Teach. 2011;33:614–9.
33. South-Paul JE. Proceedings of advancing diversity and excellence in science and engineering. Ann Arbor: University of Michigan; 2007.
34. Holm HA. Postgraduate education. In: Norman GR, van der Vleuten CPM, Newble DI, editors. International handbook of research in medical education. Dordrecht: Kluwer; 2002. p. 381–413.
35. Harden RM, Crosby JR, Davis MH. An introduction to outcome-based education. Med Teach. 1999;22(1):7–14.

36. Norcini J. Standards and reliability in evaluation: when rules of thumb don't apply. Acad Med. 1999;74:1088–90.
37. ACGME. Outcome project: enhancing residency education through Outcome Project. https://dconnect.acgme.org/outcome/comp/compMin.aspCanMEDS. Accessed 16 Jan 2012.
38. Frank JR, Jabbour M, Tugwel P, et al. Skills for the new millennium: report of the societal needs working group, CANMEDS 2000 project. Ann R Coll Physicians Surg Can. 1996;26:206–16.
39. General Medical Council. Good medical practice. London: General Medical Council; 2001.
40. Harden RM. Trends and the future of postgraduate medical education. Emerg Med J. 2006;23(10):798–802.
41. Medearis DN, Kinney TD. On creating a true continuum of medical education. In: Anlyan WG, Austen WG, Beck JC, et al., editors. The future of medical education. Durham: Duke University Press; 1973. p. 133.
42. Lerner BH. Urology field slowly altered by women. The New York Times, Sept 8 2008.
43. Lightner DJ, Terris MK, Tsao AK, Naughton CK, Lohse CM. Status of women in urology: based on a report to the society of university urologists. J Urol. 2005;173(2):560–3.
44. Jackson I, Bobbin M, Jordan M, Baker S. A survey of women urology residents regarding career choice and practice challenges. J Womens Health (Larchmt). 2009;18(11):1867–72.
45. Webinar definition. PC Magazine Encyclopedia. Available at: http://www.pcmag.com/encyclopedia_term/0,2542,t=Webinar&i=54380,00.asp. Last accessed on 16 Jan 2012.
46. Ahmed K, Jawad M, Abboudi M, Gavazzi A, Darzi A, Athanasiou T, et al. Effectiveness of procedural simulation in urology: a systematic review. J Urol. 2011;186(1):26–34. Epub 2011 May 14.
47. Marguet CG, Springhart WP, Preminger GM. New technology for imaging and documenting urologic procedures. Urol Clin North Am. 2006;33(3):397–408. Review.
48. Goldberg MA. Teleradiology and telemedicine. Radiol Clin North Am. 1996;34(3):647–65. Review.
49. Shah J, Mackay S, Vale J, Darzi A. Simulation in urology – a role for virtual reality? BJU Int. 2001;88(7):661–5. Review.
50. Kuo RL, Delvecchio FC, Preminger GM. Virtual reality: current urologic applications and future developments. J Endourol. 2001; 15(1):117–22.
51. Arora S, Lamb B, Undre S, Kneebone R, Darzi A, Sevdalis N. Framework for incorporating simulation into urology training. BJU Int. 2011;107(5):806–10. doi:10.1111/j.1464-410X.2010.09563.x. Epub 2010 Sep 24.
52. Desai M, Jain P, Ganpule A, Sabnis R, Patel S, Shrivastav P. Developments in technique and technology: the effect on the results of percutaneous nephrolithotomy for staghorn calculi. BJU Int. 2009;104(4):542–8; discussion 548. Epub 2009 Mar 6.
53. Ogrinc G, Headrick LA, Foster T. Teaching and assessing resident competence in practice-based learning and improvement. J Gen Intern Med. 2004;19(5pt 2):496–500.
54. Epstein RM, Dannefer EF, Nofziger AC, Hansen JT, Schultz SH, Jospe N, et al. Comprehensive assessment of professional competence: the Rochester experiment. Teach Learn Med. 2004;16(2): 186–96.
55. Caverzagie KJ, Aagaard EM, Chick DA, Smith CD. Measuring resident progress: competency milestones in internal medicine. Acad Intern Med Insight. 2010;8(1):4–5.
56. Landy FJ, Farr JL. The measurement of work performance methods, theory and application. Orlando: Academic; 1983.
57. ACGME. Tool box of assessment methods. https://dconnect.acgme.org/outcome/assess/toolbox.asp. Accessed 16 Jan 2012.
58. Ringsted C, Henriksen AH, Skaarup AM, Van der Vleuten CP. Educational impact of in-training assessment (ITA) in postgraduate medical education: a qualitative study of an ITA programme in actual practice. Med Educ. 2004;38:767–77.
59. Snell L, Tallett S, Haist S, Hays R, Norcini J, Prince K, et al. A review of the evaluation of clinical teaching: new perspectives and challenges. Med Educ. 2000;34:862–87.
60. Lloyd FJ, Reyna VF. Clinical gist and medical education: connecting the dots. JAMA. 2009;302(12):1332–3.
61. Leach DC, Fletcher SW. Perspective on continuing education in the health professions. Chest. 2008;134(6):1299–303.
62. Peck C, McCall M, McLaren B, Rotem T. Continuing medical education and continuing professional development: international comparisons. BMJ. 2000;320:432–5.
63. Brown CA, Belfield CR, Field SJ. Cost effectiveness of continuing professional development in health care: a critical review of the evidence. BMJ. 2002;324(7338):652–5.
64. Scales Jr CD. Education and training in evidence-based urology. World J Urol. 2011;29:325–9.
65. Grimshaw JM, Russel IT. Effect of clinical guidelines on medical practice: a systematic review of rigorous evaluations. Lancet. 1993;342:1317–22.
66. Lau J, Antman EM, Jimenez-Silva J, Kupelnick B, Mosteller F, Chalmers TC. Cumulative meta-analysis of therapeutic trials for myocardial infarction. N Engl J Med. 1992;327:248–54.
67. Davis D, O'Brien MA, Freemantle N, Wolf FM, Mazmanian P, et al. Impact of formal continuing medical education: do conferences, workshops, rounds, and other traditional continuing education activities change physician behavior or health care outcomes? JAMA. 1999;282:867–74.
68. Davis DA, Goldman J, Perrier L, Silver IL. Continuing professional development. In: Dent JA, Harden RM, editors. A practical guide for medical teachers. 3rd ed. New York: Churchill Livingstone; 2009. p. 46–54.
69. Frenk J, Chen L, Bhutta ZA, Cohen J, Crisp N, Evans T, et al. Health professionals for a new century: transforming education to strengthen health systems in an interdependent world. Lancet. 2010;376(9756):1923–58. Epub 2010 Nov 26.
70. General Medical Council. Lord Patel seeks views on recommendations for the future regulation of medical education and training. 2010. Available from: http://www.gmc-uk.org/news/5546.asp. Last accessed on 16 Jan 2012.
71. Ellaway RH, Topps M, Bahr T. Information and educational technology in Postgraduate medical education. 2011 AFMC. http://www.afmc.ca/pdf/fmec/14_Ellaway_Information%20Technology.pdf. Accessed 16 Jan 2012.
72. McConnell JD, et al. The future of urology and urologic education in America. Future of urologic residency strategic planning committee. AUA News. 2006;11(8):1–4.
73. Bezanson KA. Education in an automated society. (Cited at: education for a new century conference. May 15–17, 1994, Winnipeg, Manitoba). Available at: http://idl-bnc.idrc.ca/dspace/bitstream/10625/13261/1/99060.pdf. Last accessed on 16 Jan 2012.

Advanced Training of a Practicing Urologist in Stone Disease Management

102

Tamer El-Husseiny and Noor N.P. Buchholz

Abstract

Surgical training encourages the development of cognitive, clinical, and technical skills that are acquired traditionally through mentoring. Increasing pressures from the demands on clinicians to increase productivity, the resident work hour restrictions, the increased cost associated with trainee involvement in the operating room, the complexity of patients seen in tertiary care centers, and the overall goal of decreasing patients' morbidity and mortality all make the acquisition of the necessary technical skills in the operating room more difficult nowadays.

Therefore, in an effort to address this aspect of learning for minimally invasive surgery techniques such as endourology and laparoscopy, alternative methods of training including simulated teaching environments that allow for acquisition of technical skills outside the operating room and also new educational programs, courses, workshops, observerships, and fellowships have been developed to overcome these educational challenges.

Keywords

Advanced training • Urology • Endourology • Laparoscopy • Simulation • Low-fidelity simulator • High-fidelity simulator • Courses • Workshops • Observerships • Fellowships

Introduction

Since the initial description of the Halstedian model as a traditional method of acquiring surgical skills a century ago, surgical education has faced significant reforms, mainly as a direct result of the rapidly expanding technological developments in the field of surgery in general and urology in particular.

T. El-Husseiny, MBBCh (Hons), M.Sc. (Urol), MRCS (Ed.) (✉)
Department of Urology, Queen Elizabeth Hospital Birmingham, University Hospitals Birmingham NHS Foundation Trust, Birmingham, UK
e-mail: d_tamer@hotmail.com

N.N.P. Buchholz, M.B.B.S. (D), M.D. (CH), FSSU (CH), FKNMG (NL)
Department of Endourology and Stone services, Barts and The London School of Medicine and Dentistry, Barts and the London NHS Trust, West Smithfield, London, EC1A 7BE, UK
e-mail: nb@londonurologyconsultant.com

Concerns regarding the preparation of the next generation of surgeons and the reexamining of the classical surgical training methods have become a common denominator of all surgical specialties dealing with endoscopic and laparoscopic techniques.

Surgical training consists of developing cognitive, clinical, and technical skills that are acquired traditionally through mentoring [1]. However, there are certain inherent risks with this type of training for the patient during the initial stages of the trainees' learning curve, which may be more pronounced with the highly complex skills required for minimally invasive surgery such as in endourology. Therefore, the concept of trial and error learning in the clinical environment has been revised for the benefit of both the trainee and the patient.

Increasing pressures from the demands on clinicians to increase productivity, the resident work hour restrictions, the increased cost associated with trainee involvement in the operating room, the complexity of patients seen in tertiary

J.J. Talati et al. (eds.), *Urolithiasis*,
DOI 10.1007/978-1-4471-4387-1_102, © Springer-Verlag London 2012

care centers, and the overall goal of decreasing patients' morbidity and mortality all make the acquisition of the necessary technical skills in the operating room more difficult nowadays [2, 3].

The decreasing time available for training stresses the need to improve surgical skills in an efficient way within a minimum time. Urology, with an important case load on endoscopic or laparoscopic surgery, is one of the surgical specialties whose training programs suffer from the results of time, financial, and social constraints. As a result, some educational changes have resulted in an increase in the length of residency training programs or the necessity for subspecialty fellowship training programs such as in endourology [3–5].

For these reasons, the Halstedian model can hardly be applicable to the new surgical skills, and the earlier stages of technical skills acquisition should take place outside the operating room [6].

The general consensus today among surgical educators is that the traditional Halstedian paradigm of "see one, do one, teach one" is not applicable anymore to modern surgery as this concept of training has been challenged over the past few years, shifting to the paradigm of "see several, simulate many, do one perfectly" instead.

Therefore, in an effort to address this aspect of learning for minimally invasive surgery techniques such as endourology and laparoscopy, alternative methods of training including simulated teaching environments that allows for acquisition of technical skills outside the operating room and also new educational programs, courses, workshops, observerships, and fellowships have been developed to overcome these educational challenges.

Surgical Simulation

Simulation has been defined as "....an imitation of the conditions of (a situation), e.g., for training" [7].

Surgical simulation, whether model based or computer based, provides a unique opportunity for repetitive skills training, thus having the potential to reduce the learning curve required in a number of operations, which can maximize the educational experience, reduce the cost, and reduce the length of surgical training in complex surgical techniques.

Repetition of a task improves performance in terms of efficiency, error-free performance, and better outcomes. However, volume alone is not the only factor accounting for proficiency. Repetitive, deliberate (focused) practice instead may be more important to determine the level of expertise [8]. Simulation provides the ideal frame to develop deliberate practice at least in initial stages and for basic skills. Consequently, practice on a simulator may allow for reaching a given proficiency level in a safer and cost-effective way. Therefore, and as a consequence of reduced training

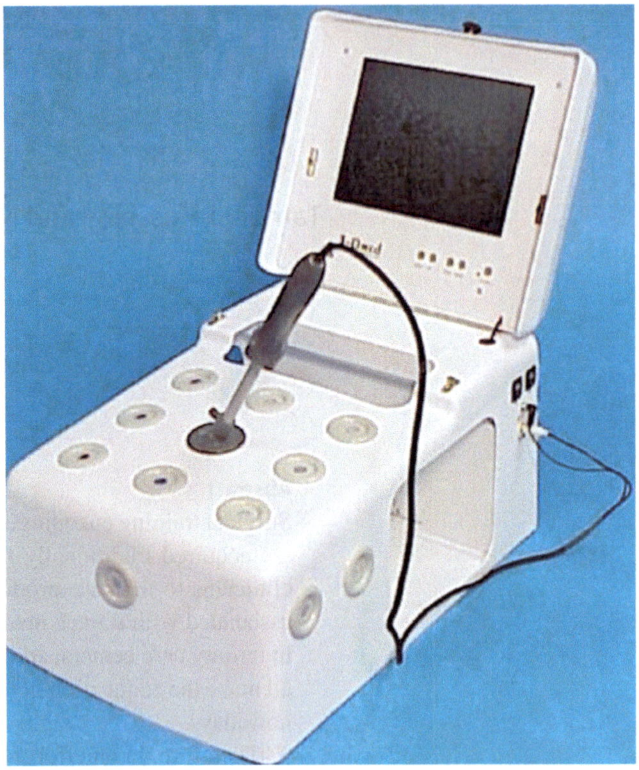

Fig. 102.1 Low-fidelity box trainer (Courtesy Limbs & Things Ltd, Bristol, UK)

time and an increasing number of complex endourological and laparoscopic procedures, surgical simulation has developed considerably over the past 10 years.

Simulators can be classified on the basis of fidelity to low- and high-fidelity simulators. *Low-fidelity* simulators are those that are not very lifelike, such as silicone or rubber representatives of tissues. Examples of low-fidelity simulators include mechanical simulators such as box trainers (Fig. 102.1) and some virtual reality (VR) simulators such as the MIST VR™ (Mentice AB, Gothenburg, Sweden) during which the trainee has to move, transfer, or do diathermy of objects. There is generally a better evidence for the use of low-fidelity simulators compared with high-fidelity simulators, as they have been available on the market for longer time. The advantages of low-fidelity simulators include lower cost and portability. The main disadvantages are the lack of realism and the inability to teach entire operations [9].

High-fidelity simulators more accurately represent real surgery; they require basic skills but also simulate complex tasks or complete operations. These simulators are, however, significantly more expensive than low-fidelity models and usually require more maintenance. Traditional high-fidelity simulators have included animal models, cadavers, and several computer-based virtual reality simulators, such as the LAP Mentor (Simbionix USA Corporation, USA) (Fig. 102.2).

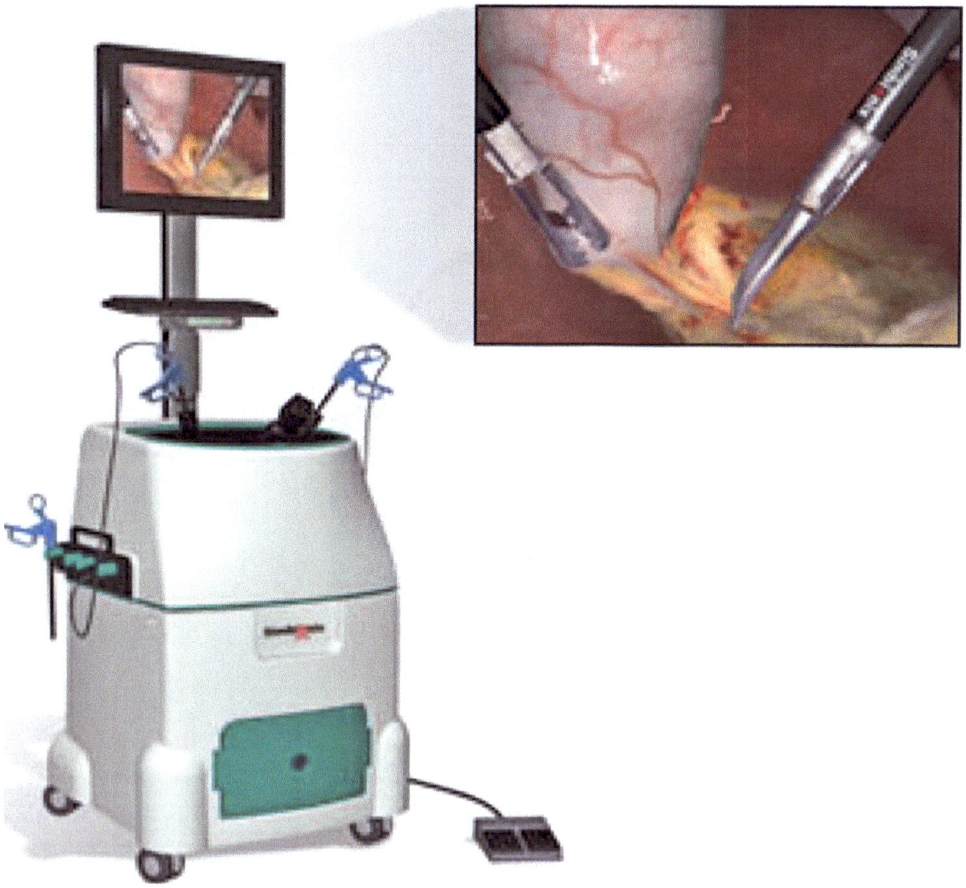

Fig. 102.2 LAP mentor (Courtesy of Simbionix USA, Cleveland, OH)

TURP Simulators

Learning opportunities for transurethral resection of the prostate (TURP), the current gold standard in the treatment of benign prostatic hyperplasia (BPH), are somewhat limited, and the skills required to perform the procedure are difficult to learn and teach as the surgeon has to coordinate the scope, the loop, the diathermy current, and the flow of the irrigation fluid. In addition, there are key surgical landmarks that must be avoided, and vision can vary throughout the procedure because of bleeding or debris. Historically, this training problem was addressed with sheer case volume, but the number of procedures performed during the average residency period has declined [10].

Limbs & Things™ (Bristol, UK) created a disposable mechanical simulator of the prostate that allows the user to practice basic cutting skills (the Bristol TURP Trainer™). As a mechanical simulator, it lacks the ability to measure metrics of performance, but the user is able to look at the synthetic prostate to evaluate their resection.

Several virtual reality TURP simulators have been developed to train and assess the skills necessary to perform this procedure using a logical, step-by-step approach for skills development while also providing the performance tracking needed to objectively assess proficiency, such as the University of Washington VR TURP Trainer (METI, Sarasota, FL) and the SurgicalSIM TURP simulator.

Cystoscopy and Ureteroscopy Simulators

There are several high-fidelity mechanical simulators available for upper and lower urinary tract endoscopy such as the Uro-Scopic Trainer™ (Limbs & Things, Bristol, UK) (Fig. 102.3), the Scope Trainer™ (Mediskills Ltd., Edinburgh, UK) (Fig. 102.4), and the kidney-ureter-bladder (KUB) model LapED™ (Irvine, CA, USA) (Fig. 102.5).

They accurately simulate the urinary tract, and the user can perform cystoscopy, ureteroscopy, stent insertion, and lithotripsy. The trainee uses the same instruments as in the operating room, and depending on the quality of the model, there is realistic haptic feedback. However, the models do not simulate bleeding and cannot measure performance [11].

Several cystoscopic and ureteroscopic virtual reality simulators are currently commercially available. The best-studied urological simulator is the URO Mentor™ (Simbionix USA, Cleveland, OH) (Fig. 102.6), which is able to simulate many cystoscopic and ureteroscopic procedures. It is also able to measure performance patterns, and this was found to correlate with the surgeon's skills [12].

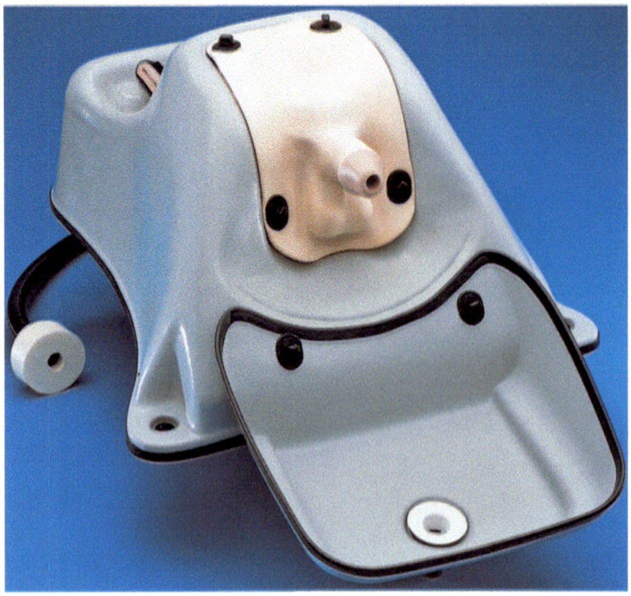

Fig. 102.3 Uro-Scopic Trainer™ (Courtesy Limbs & Things Ltd, Bristol, UK)

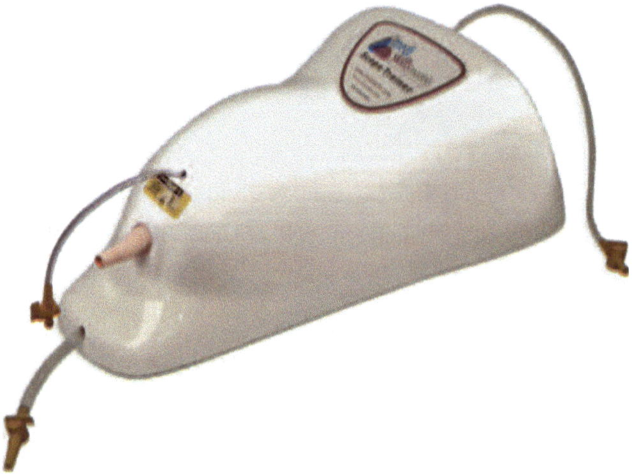

Fig. 102.4 The Scope Trainer™ (Courtesy of Mediskills Ltd., Edinburgh, UK)

The Uro-Trainer™ (Karl Storz, GmbH Tuttlingen, Germany) is another new virtual reality endourology trainer which incorporates haptic feedback; however, only initial validation studies have been performed [13].

PCNL Simulators

PCNL is currently the most complicated stone surgery technique to teach. The steep learning curve is mainly related to obtaining a percutaneous renal access where the surgeon (or radiologist) must integrate information gained from imaging (fluoroscopy, ultrasound, or a combination), knowledge of renal anatomy, and haptic feedback from the needle.

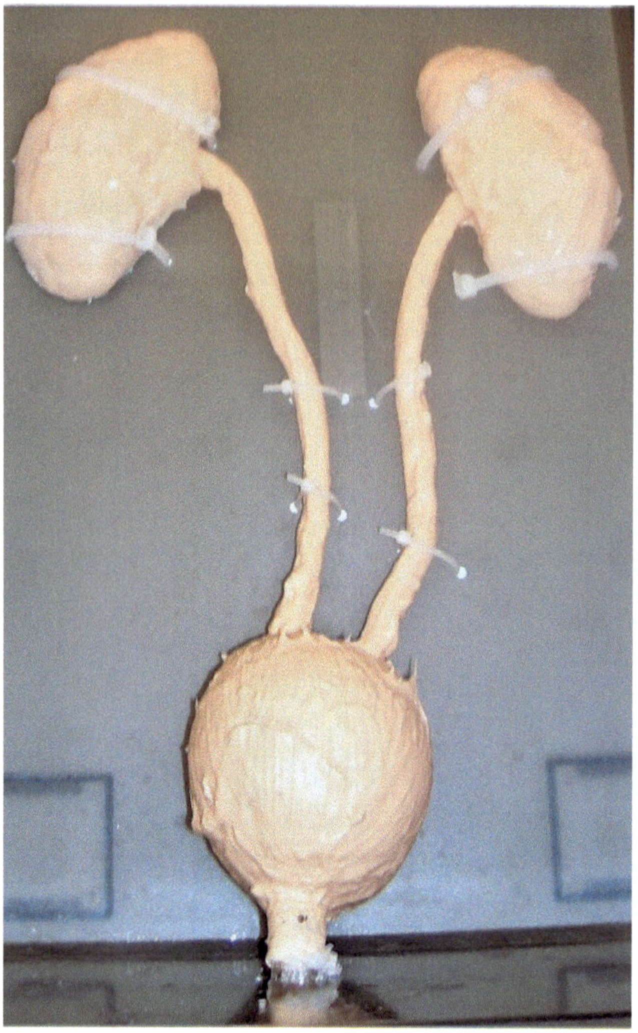

Fig. 102.5 The kidney-ureter-bladder (KUB) model LapED™ (Courtesy of LapED, Irvine, CA, USA)

Synthetic models available for percutaneous tract simulation includes the Percutaneous Nephrolithotomy Trainer™ (Limbs & Things Ltd. Bristol, UK) (Fig. 102.7) that allows for simulated needle puncture, guidewire insertion, tract dilatation, nephroscopy, and stone removal [14].

The Perc Trainer™ (Mediskills Ltd. Edinburgh, UK) (Fig. 102.8) is a similar synthetic model that simulates ultrasound- or fluoroscopic-controlled percutaneous renal access.

The main advantage of these synthetic models is that they allow the trainee to practice with the actual endoscopic instruments used clinically in the model platform, mimicking the in vivo scenario. However, they lack the realism of the reaction of normal tissue to the instrument manipulation, such as bleeding. Also the expenses of the maintenance of the fragile endoscopes and the added cost of replacement of the ancillary equipment and the time needed by an expert surgeon for providing feedback and guidance to the trainee are all considered disadvantages related to that type of training models [15, 16].

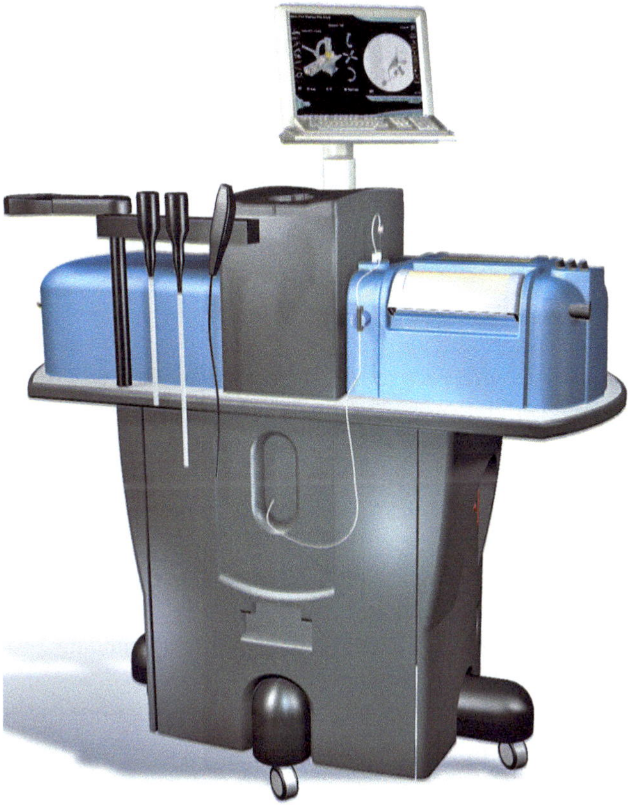

Fig. 102.6 URO Mentor™ (Courtesy of Simbionix USA, Cleveland, OH)

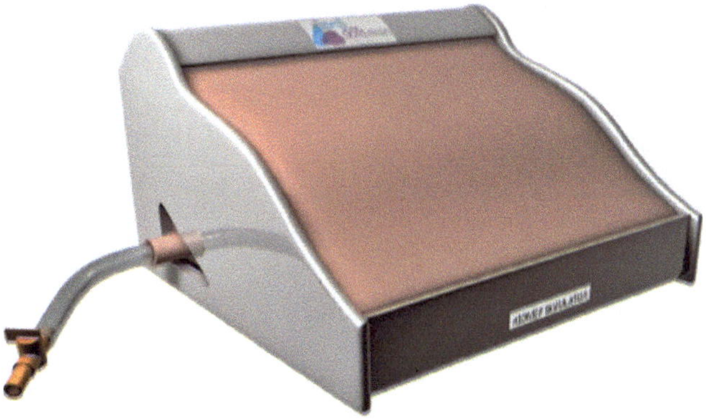

Fig. 102.8 Perc Trainer™ (Courtesy of Mediskills Ltd. Edinburgh, UK)

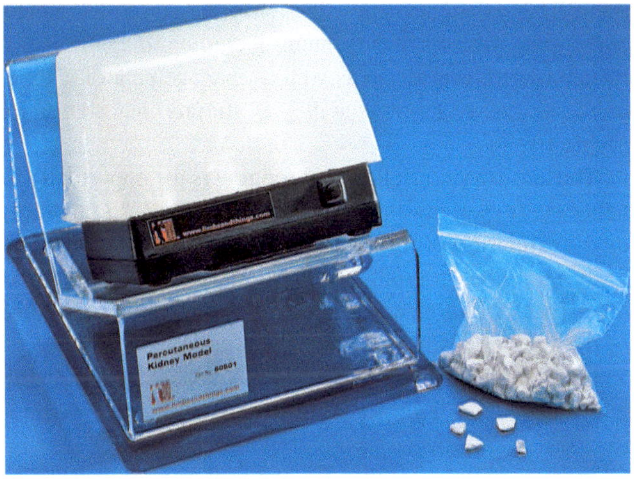

Fig. 102.7 Percutaneous Nephrolithotomy Trainer™ (Limbs & Things Ltd. Bristol, UK)

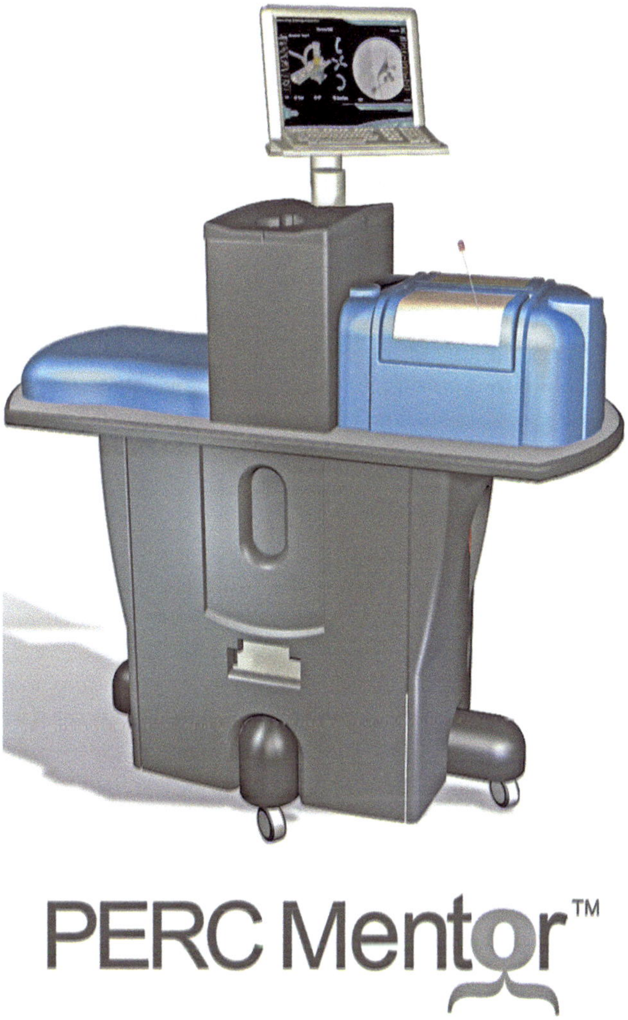

Fig. 102.9 PERC Mentor™ (Courtesy of Simbionix USA, Cleveland, OH)

Two models using porcine kidneys have also been described; in one model, the kidney is placed in a chicken carcass, and in the other it is embedded in silicone. These ex vivo porcine kidney models may provide a more realistic "feel" than the synthetic competitors [17].

The PERC Mentor™ (Simbionix, Cleveland, OH, USA) provides virtual reality simulation for percutaneous renal access (Fig. 102.9). This percutaneous renal access simulator consists of a mannequin representing the human flank including simulated skin and palpable ribs. It provides training under simulated fluoroscopic guidance for advancing the

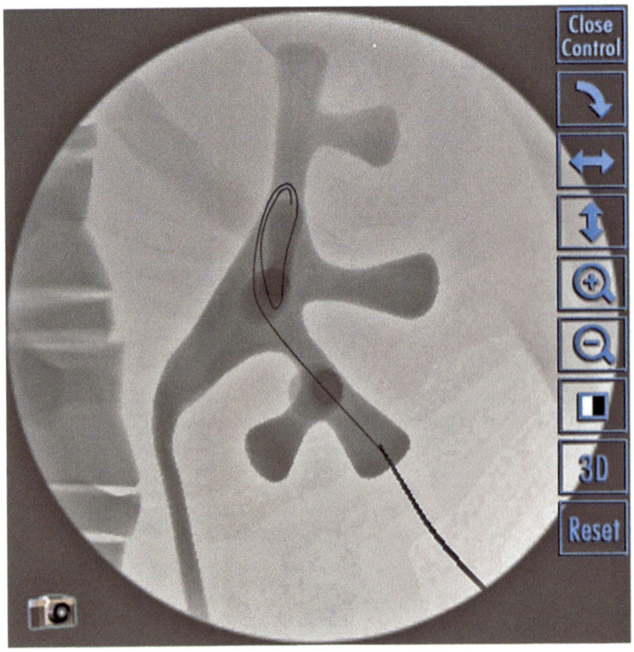

Fig. 102.10 PERC Mentor™ – Simulation of guidewire insertion under fluoroscopy (Courtesy of Simbionix USA, Cleveland, OH)

access needle through muscle, fascia, and kidney capsule to puncture the collecting system. It also simulates advancing a guidewire through the needle and into the collecting system, the ability to perform retrograde or antegrade pyelography, needle aspiration, and rotation of the C-arm (Fig. 102.10).

Animal Models

They have been used extensively to develop new surgical techniques and provide trainees with the necessary platform for expansion of skills. They provide the best tactile and anatomic feedback as it allows realistic tissue conditions that more accurately simulate the human patient. However, law enforcement regulations limit their use, and in some countries, it is now impossible to practice surgical skills in living animals. Breeding, maintenance, and anesthetic requirements make this model extremely expensive for its routine use.

Cadavers

Cadavers, whether fresh or embalmed, represent the most reliable anatomical model and have been used for centuries to teach human anatomy. Cadavers have also been used as teaching models for endourologic procedures such as ureterorenoscopy and transurethral resection of the prostate as they offer a very realistic surgical training environment. The procedure can be performed similar to the clinical situation but is limited by the lack of bleeding and the tissue distortion when preserved in formalin. Trainer's presence during the procedure is required to assess performance, which can be considered as another difficulty that can hamper its use in some training facilities. The potential risk of transmission of communicable diseases is a concern when working with human cadavers and therefore requires the same protective procedures as clinical endourology [18].

Fellowships

At its core, irrespective of personal motivation, fellowship training in endourology, laparoscopic surgery, and robotic surgery represents an important opportunity to concentrate intensively on a specific area of urology and to become proficient beyond what might ordinarily be attained during residency [19].

Societies, such as the International Endourological Society (IES) founded in 1984 (New York, USA) have created and developed endourology fellowship training programs with defined guidelines.

Current internationally recognized fellowships are either 1- or 2-year programs. As of 2010, all fellowships recognized by the IES are required to be 2 years except some selected European centers. The main benefit to a 2-year fellowship program is to allow the fellow long enough periods to develop both clinical skills and perform meaningful and productive research from both a clinical and research standpoint. This would also allow the fellow to gain skills in general stone disease management including diagnosis and metabolic risk evaluation as well as management of a stone unit as these fellows will be future team leaders (Table 102.1).

The key aspect of fellowship training is the opportunity to become an expert in a chosen subspecialty. Because endourology is primarily a surgical field, the most important aspects of an accredited training center should be the breadth and diversity of the surgical volume, in addition to the credibility of the training institution to meet the training requirements and aspirations of the fellow. On the other hand, and from the fellow's point of view, applying for a fellowship program involves an informed and possibly high-standard choice on where to spend his/ her next few years of training, especially if this means being far away from home with all the associated personal and financial implications such as obtaining the appropriate medical licensure and completing the necessary institutional paperwork. It should be the role of standardization programs by educational bodies, such as the "certification in subspecialty training" and "center of excellence certification" awarded by the European Board of Urology (EBU) and the "approved fellowship center" by the International Endourological Society (IES) to validate and approve training centers and thus provide guidance and to

Table 102.1 IES fellowship and certification requirements

IES endourology fellowship requirements
Fellowship program and director must be approved by the Fellowship Review Committee of the Endourological Society
Each program is reviewed annually and must demonstrate a minimum of three publications in peer-reviewed journals, with the fellow as first author on at least two of such publications
Program will be 2 years with equal distribution of research and clinical activity. A 4-year transition period (starting from 2006) will be given to allow current 1-year fellowship programs to develop a 2-year program
Program must be in association with an ACGME-accredited urology residency program (or equivalent for international program) providing sufficient clinical volume and variety of endourologic cases to develop clinical competence
Based on the median index cases from submitted case logs as of 2006, it has been determined that the following are minimum index cases in each category over 2 years:
Total percutaneous renal procedures 45 cases
Total ureteroscopy 60 cases
Total laparoscopy 60 cases
Listing of other technologies and techniques such as:
Shockwave lithotripsy
Needle ablative therapy
Robotic surgery
Percutaneous access to kidney
Others
Program should have adequate research facilities, with PhD support preferably, to develop and stimulate scholarly research that can qualify for extramural funding. The ongoing research should include basic science and bench projects
Program should have access to state-of-the-art radiologic, endoscopic, laparoscopic, and preferably robotic facilities
Requirements for certification
A paper to the Endourological Society Essay Contest
A list of all operative cases performed during the fellowship
A three-ring binder with all manuscripts, videos, abstracts, and any projects that have been worked on during the fellowship. Also include here a list of teaching conferences that the fellow has conducted during the past year to medical students, residents, grand round talks, etc.
A letter of recommendation from the program director

Available at: http://www.endourology.org/fellowship/credential.html

some extend a guarantee for the future fellow that these centers meet standardized training program requirements.

Creating and establishing a standardized curriculum for application to fellowship training programs is of major importance, and therefore both the American Urological Association (AUA) and the International Endourological Society (IES) have agreed to create a training curriculum that has a basic cognitive component, technical skills training guidelines, and an objective evaluation process. These curricula are aimed at facilitating the fellow's training while complying with regulations for accreditation.

Courses and Workshops

Short-term courses and workshops (usually ranging from 1 to 4 days) can provide an introduction to basic endourological skills and build on core techniques. The format is usually either laboratory or theater based. The benefit of such short courses as an educational tool can be maximized when "hands-on" experience using simulators or models is offered and when individual tuition and feedback in small groups or individual training sessions are included.

Industry-sponsored workshops on international and national meetings have a limited value since groups are often larger and the individual's time on a simulator is short. However, they may serve as an introduction in theory and practice for delegates who then wish to proceed to more in-depth learning.

Live surgery sessions can be educational but do lack the "hands on" experience. In small groups, attendance in theaters for live surgery can be a valuable option providing the delegates with unrestricted views of the operation and one-to-one question and answer sessions with the operating surgeon.

Individual so-called mini-fellowships such as that offered by the University of California Los Angeles (UCLA) in USA, in several subdisciplines of endourology, i.e., robotic urology, combine one-to-one teaching, individual dry-lab sessions and wet-lab sessions with the robot on anesthetized pigs. However, tuition fees of several thousand US dollars plus accommodation and travel costs may make such an option unaffordable to most trainees.

Observerships

Observerships of various duration in internationally recognized specialist centers can be another option to familiarize oneself with the workings of an endourology unit. However, it cannot replace in-depth training. In some countries, health regulations may prohibit a guest doctor from patient contact altogether. Nevertheless, such a short visit cannot only be very educational but also inspirational for aspiring endourologists. For that reasons, several national (i.e., British Association of Urological Surgeons BAUS) and international (i.e., European Association of Urology EAU) urological societies have established funds and bursaries to enable suitable urologist to travel abroad.

Conclusion

The field of endourology, which encompasses urinary tract endoscopy, percutaneous, laparoscopic, and robotic surgery including all stone surgery, has advanced rapidly over the past quarter century, thus allowing endourology to be considered a subspecialty of urology.

The development of fellowship programs, surgical simulation, postgraduate courses, workshops, and observerships is now providing the cornerstone for subspecialty training in stone disease as they provide an opportunity for urologists worldwide to improve existing skills and acquire new endourologic techniques.

References

1. Knudsen B, Matsumoto E, Chew B, et al. Randomized, controlled, prospective study validating the acquisition of percutaneous renal collecting system access skills using a computer based hybrid virtual reality surgical simulator: phase I. J Urol. 2006;176(5): 2173–8.
2. Bridges M, Diamond D. The financial impact of teaching surgical residents in the operating room. Am J Surg. 1999;177(1):28–32.
3. Schneider J, Coyle J, Ryan E, et al. Implementation and evaluation of a new surgical residency model. J Am Coll Surg. 2007;205(3): 393–404. Grillo H. To impart this art: the development of graduate surgical education in the United States. Surgery. 1999;125(1): 1–14.
4. Gawande A. Creating the educated surgeon in the 21st century. Am J Surg. 2001;181(6):551–6.
5. Hammond DL, Ketchum J, Schwatz B. Accreditation council on graduate medical education technical skills competency compliance: urologic surgical skills. J Am Coll Surg. 2005;201(3):454–7.
6. Reznick RK, MacRae H. Teaching surgical skills: changes in the wind. N Engl J Med. 2006;355:2664–9.
7. The concise Oxford dictionary of current English. 9th ed. By Della Thompson. New York: Oxford University Press; 1995.
8. Leape L. Error in medicine. JAMA. 1994;272(23):1851–7.
9. Gamboa AJR, McDougall EM. Training implications for stone management in urinary tract stone disease. London: Springer; 2011. p. 577–87.
10. Sweet RM. Review of trainers for transurethral resection of the prostate skills. J Endourol. 2007;21(3):280–4.
11. Brewin J, Nedas T. Simulation in urology. In: Dasgupta P et al., editors. New technologies in urology. London: Springer; 2010. p. 259–67.
12. Wignall GR, Denstedt JD, Preminger GM, et al. Surgical simulation: a urological perspective. J Urol. 2008;179(5):1690–9.
13. Reich O, Noll U, Gratzke C, et al. High-level virtual reality simulator for endourologic procedures of lower urinary tract. Urology. 2006;67:1144–8.
14. Strohmaier W, Giese A. Ex vivo training model for percutaneous renal surgery. Urol Res. 2005;33(3):191–3.
15. Opppenheimer P, Gupta A, Weghorst S, et al. The representation of blood flow in endourologic surgical simulations. Stud Health Technol Inform. 2001;81:365–71.
16. Strohmaier W, Giese A. Porcine urinary tract as a training model for ureterorenoscopy. Urol Int. 2001;66(1):30–2.
17. Stern J, Zeltser IS, Pearle MS. Percutaneous renal access simulators. J Endourol. 2007;21(3):270–3.
18. Trindale J, Lauenschlager M, de Araujo C. Endoscopic surgery: a new teaching method. J Urol. 1981;126(2):192.
19. Koh CJ, Freeman MR, Retik AB. Increasing the ranks of physician scientists in urology through the promotion of fellowship training: the example of pediatric urology. J Urol. 2005;173:2110–1.

Across Semantic Turfs: The Need for Broader Education

103

Syed Nomanul Haq

Abstract

This chapter constitutes a reasoned plea for broadening the educational base of medical researchers. Through a conceptual analysis of the nature of scientific knowledge, the author draws upon a large body of data from the history of science to argue the case. He points out that science is not unrelated to humanistic disciplines such as philosophy, history, or even arts and literature; nor can it grow in an intellectual vacuum. Emphasizing the distinction between science and technology, the chapter reiterates that medical sciences are an embodiment of a critical *attitude* to biological investigation, and this critical attitude is common between the natural sciences and humanistic modes of expression and inquiry, and can therefore nourish one another.

Keywords

Broader education • Philosophy • Background knowledge • Cognitive valence • Integration • Science • Technology • Scientism • Logic • Imagination • Eye to detail • Creative arts

Philosophical Considerations

A reflection on the nature of human knowledge renders the case for broader education compelling—compelling in all modes of discourses and practices, whether in the field of the humanities or of the sciences. Indeed, the reflection throws into sharp relief what with hindsight seems to have been obvious all along: that human knowledge is an integrated entity, not a bag of isolated bits of cognitive acquisitions, each bit with its own ontologically fixed boundaries, hermetically sealed away from all others. When we acquire empirical data, say, of the motion of stars, we integrate these data into the whole range of that epistemological corpus we call "background knowledge"—relating it, for example, to what at the time we know of geometry and astronomy, of motion and rest, of space and time, of light and optics, and even of beauty and ugliness. It is only through this integration that a specific item of knowledge is admitted into the cognitive pool of our minds.

All of this happens to be rather abstract. But before moving to the concrete, allow me to add one more remark in the same vein: It is true that in both empirical and theoretical research we often study a particular entity or a process analytically—that is, in *isolation* from other entities or processes—and this way of study can certainly be most fruitful. But then, this separation is a methodological device (as Aristotle would say, this separation is only a separation in thought [1][1]); it does not embody any ontological stance. A cardiologist studying the heart as a muscle may for research purposes set aside the physiology of the gastrocnemius, but this is an investigative posture with no claim as to the essential duality or incommensurability of the two muscular systems. On the contrary, analytical investigations may lead to the determination of the place of the isolated entity in the totality of the universe to which it belongs in its relation to other entities. In

S.N. Haq, Ph.D.
Social Sciences and Humanities, Lahore University of Management Sciences (LUMS), DHA, Lahore 54792, Pakistan
e-mail: noman@lums.edu.pk

[1] Aristotle discusses conceptual analysis particularly in his *Categories* and *Metaphysics*. For a lucid account, see Richard Sorabji. *Matter, Space, and Motion*. Ithaca: Cornell University Press, 1988.

J.J. Talati et al. (eds.), *Urolithiasis*,
DOI 10.1007/978-1-4471-4387-1_103,

the world of perception, for example, we receive a piece of music as a totality in terms of the overall effects it yields. But when a critic analytically separates its elements, the aim is none other than to explain this very totality.

Abstract though it is, the foregoing discourse is aimed at pointing out something very straightforward: that when we consider the process of education philosophically, we must arrive at the conclusion that our differentiated learning modes, our academic disciplines, are related to one another in some ultimate conceptual sense. Our scientific body of knowledge helps us make sense of the world—or, in other words, has cognitive valence—only insofar as it is a *coherent* body of knowledge. Thus, for instance, biological theories are not supposed to contradict laws of mathematics nor are these theories posited in violation of the accepted principles of physics or chemistry; similarly, what we consider statistical truths cannot be flouted in drug trials or in economics and finance or in anthropology. If, indeed, there is a piece of research that does not accord with and cannot be integrated into the established body of background scientific knowledge, we call it ad hoc, an anomaly. Faced with ad hoc, anomalous research data, it becomes incumbent upon the scientific community to make adjustments and changes, sometimes so drastic as to lead even to the overthrow of some hitherto reigning theoretical structure—a phenomenon famously dubbed "paradigm change" by Thomas Kuhn [2].

From the Abstract to the Concrete

Let us now consider some down-to-earth practical questions. In the actual context of education, if one takes the claim literally that the cosmos is given to us as a totality and so everything in the world is related to everything else, the task of higher education becomes utterly unwieldy. In fact, it is rendered virtually impossible since the all-embracing claim would mean that each and every academic subject is linked to each and every other—from anthropology and evolutionary biology to literature and physics and from physics and philosophy to statistics and zoology; these are all mutually connected to one another; therefore, all of these must be taught to every student. Given the rise in our times of highly specialized and minutely differentiated research disciplines, this sounds preposterous in practical terms—but only in practical terms.

The world academia seems to have accepted the principle, decisively admitting it at the conceptual plane. Thus, we see moves in top universities toward integrated studies and curricular interdisciplinarity, a broad-based educational approach whereby the semantic turfs of various disciplines are no longer locked in their own particularities. Indeed, these interdisciplinary thrusts must have limitations and, in actual fact, can only be narrowly conceived in order for them to be made practicable. Here there are two considerations that provide a concrete, narrowed -down, and realizable substance to our philosophical observations. These considerations are historical in nature, illuminated by the empirical evidence that we gather when looking at the growth of scientific knowledge over time.

So we move from philosophy to history. Let us recall the text *On the Sacred Disease* belonging to the Hippocratic corpus, composed in the latter part of the fifth or the early part of the fourth century BCE. This is a decisive text in the history of scientific medicine, a landmark, since it embodies a rapturous break from the past. The text dethrones the doctrine that epilepsy is a result of divine intervention—and this means that it thereby rejects occult, magical, or transcendental explanations of diseases. And, on the constructive side, it explicitly proposes a naturalistic explanation of epilepsy in terms of natural forces. This, in turn, is grounded upon a metaphysical presupposition—that there are immutable, uniform laws of nature and that these laws are intelligible. What is most significant here is that "[b]y and large, the medical doctors of the Hippocratic School appealed to naturalistic causes *without* possessing a real positivist methodology or an efficacious technology of curing, including pharmacopeia … Thus we may note that 'nature' as the ground of explanation was accepted theoretically *before* efficacious medicine and medical technology were developed" [3]. Here we have a momentous methodological and doctrinal watershed in the history of medicine, a watershed whose undercurrents lie *outside* the region of medicine. It ushers in a new *philosophical* attitude to the real world, an attitude in which an altogether new belief system is enshrined.

Similar is the case of the Copernican Revolution. The heliocentric system of Copernicus (d. 1543), mathematically based as it was on the works of Muslim astronomers Nasir al-Din al-Tusi (d. 1274) and Mu'ayyad al-Din al-'Urdi (d. 1266) and on the planetary models of a Damascus mosque *muwaqqit* ("timekeeper") Ibn al-Shatir (d. 1375), was largely accepted on aesthetic grounds. The revolutionary system was accepted on grounds of mathematical elegance, conceptual simplicity, and internal harmony—all of these characteristics making it much more beautiful than the messy Ptolemaic geocentric astronomy which had become, to quote Copernicus himself, "a monster!" [4, 5] We ought to recognize very carefully that the defense of the new system provided by our monumental Polish astronomer in his *De Revolutionibus* is indeed an aesthetic plea, almost "poetic" in nature. Note also that on pragmatic grounds, the earlier Ptolemaic system was just as serviceable and could make just as accurate predictions of planetary positions. And more, the Copernican astronomy was already running into empirical difficulties: it predicted certain stellar parallaxes which were never observed! But then the scientific world espoused Copernicus and irreversibly discarded Ptolemy, and we know with hindsight that it did the right thing [6]. Here again, the explanation of the success of the Copernican Revolution, a revolution in astronomy, lies *outside* astronomy.

Examples like these can be multiplied from the history of science. William Harvey, for example, who is credited with the discovery of the systemic circulation of blood, argued for his case on Aristotelian, teleological grounds—"nature does nothing in vain," he would keep crying [7]. Galileo had worked out his inverse square law by analytical mathematical reasoning *before* his famous dropping of balls from the Tower of Pisa [8]. Newton was obsessed with alchemy, and with this mysterious entity "ether," which was thrown out once and for all from the world of science by Einstein [9][2]—from Einstein we finally learned on purely *theoretical* (not experimental) grounds that no such entity exists in the physical cosmos; thus, "ether," as a *physical* entity and as an explanatory principle, was laid to rest by virtue of *mathematical* and *logical* reasoning [10].

The Case for Broader Education

We can go on. But the point here is that philosophical, conceptual, and methodological considerations are the motors of scientific progress. And this means that foundational issues in any scientific field are of prime importance. In concrete terms, then, the educational preparation of the scientists —including particularly those working in medical/surgical field—should include some philosophical training, sharpening in them the ability to ask fundamental questions and to develop critical analytical skills. Such abilities and skills are nurtured not only by studying some philosophy proper —particularly the philosophy of science, a field that claims such great names as Sir Karl Popper [11] and Quine [12][3] —but also by the study of history, history of science in particular. The principle is simple: science cannot grow in an intellectual vacuum. Note that by "science" here I do not mean unexplained, ad hoc, often commercially generated, technological innovations.

I have always felt that history of science should really be part of any scientific education. The staggering success of the Scientific Revolution of the sixteenth and seventeenth centuries, coupled with the social, political, economic, and commercial developments in imperial Europe, led to discourses on science becoming more and more ideological in nature. Enlightenment epistemologies, with their colonial confidence, spoke of science as a thoroughly "rational" enterprise, based exclusively on observations and experiments, out of which theories were derived through a formal inductive logical process—this is what we call the positivistic view of science. Of course, contemporary Western intelligentsia has rejected this positivism or rather this ideological reconstruction of the story of science, but this is a stance that still reigns supreme in developing countries, such as Pakistan and nearly all countries belonging to the Islamic world—in this world it appears in the guise of "scientism."

What is scientism as opposed to science? Scientism is a malady which has three types of interrelated essential symptoms: logical, epistemological, and political. Logically, scientism presupposes that all disciplines of human knowledge, when sufficiently purified and developed, will reduce to "hard" sciences, such as physics or biology. This reductionism thereby denies any logical independence to the humanities and the social sciences. The second type of symptom of scientism is related to the first—it creates an epistemological hierarchy wherein "hard" sciences are found at the peak and humanistic studies somewhere at the lowest rungs. And this means that while hard sciences have much to teach, for example, a literary critic, a literary critic has nothing to teach the hard sciences. An art critic or a historian or a sociologist must emulate and strive to approximate as closely as possible biologists and physicists and astronomers—but not vice versa.

Then, there is the politics of scientism. It is this politics that leads to an obfuscation of the crucial distinction between science and technology. For an average science teacher in countries which are in the throes of scientism, science *is* technology, and workshops that teach repair and maintenance of cell phones are institutions of *science*, and vocational centers that produce graduates for pharmaceutical industries or glass-making factories are centers of *science*. One far-reaching consequence of this politics is the high status given to those identified as "scientists"—who are in fact industry-oriented applied scientists or, to put it bluntly, high order technicians. This means more government funding for them, more corporate grants, and more participation of these "experts" in the decision-making process of an educational policy. On the other hand, the liberal arts disciplines wither on the periphery with scant money and little dignity [13].[4]

We have seen the result—almost no scientific achievement in scientistic societies like Pakistan! The treatment of this malady comes from history. There is overwhelming evidence that, for example, metaphysics in its purest forms has played a direct role in scientific development—the example of the famous physician-philosopher Avicenna's (d. 1037)

[2] A new chapter in the understanding of Newton was opened by the ground-breaking studies of Betty Jo Dobbs. See her *The Janus Faces of Genius: the Role of Alchemy in Newton's Thought*. Cambridge: Cambridge University Press, 1991.

[3] The Harvard philosopher Quine is the father of contemporary logic. Some of his seminal essays are to be found in his *From a Logical Point of View*. Cambridge, MA: Harvard University Press, 1953.

[4] I have discussed scientism somewhat fully in my article "Science vs. Scientism," Daw*n*, Karachi, July 31, 2005.

speculations on the question of "the one and the many" generating the mathematical system of what is called combinatorial analysis constitutes a case in point [14]. The career of the logical studies of George Boole (d. 1864), unencumbered by any physical (or technological) considerations, is another glowing instance [15]. Surely, the application of Boolean algebra to digital electronics is an amazing story of pure imaginative work in formal logical structures finding a pride of place in contemporary solid-state physics. And then, of course, we have already looked at many examples from classical Greek medicine to Copernicus and William Harvey, pressing upon us the historical truth that the roots of numerous paradigmatic scientific moments lie in extrascientific considerations. So, history teaches us that humanistic disciplines are not irrelevant to biological or physical sciences—indeed, these disciplines can teach science fundamental lessons, lessons of a decisive kind.

Then, one must carve this in one's historical consciousness: that science and technology are two different things. Historically, technology has existed without science and science has moved without any considerations of "applications." The steam engine was developed by traders, not university-educated scientists of the Newtonian world, and it was operative before Nicolas Carnot (d. 1832) could explain its operation in terms of his famous "Carnot's cycle." But it must be admitted that the relationship between science and technology has become way more complex in our times; indeed, the separation is not as neat as it was in earlier phases of history. And yet the two—science and technology—must be conceived apart from each other on the conceptual plane. We learn from history, as we learn through philosophical reflection, that science is a free, imaginative, and creative enterprise controlled and reigned in only by a single set of bridles—real nature itself. Science operates not in an intellectual vacuum nor in semantic isolation but in an intellectual fullness, drawing upon a cognitive pool whose waters come from all kinds of modes of thought—logic, metaphysics, language, religious discourse, and, yes, even art and poetry.

I just spoke of human imagination. It hardly needs arguing that the most powerful faculty possessed by human beings, qua human beings, is their power of imagination. So, any subject in their education that enhances, nurtures, and organizes this faculty must be of prime importance, not only in medical curricula but in any field of study whatsoever. And there is nothing more enriching to imagination than the poetic, musical, and visual arts. These arts provide more than an aesthetic experience, more than an experience in the beauty of proportions, colors, and rhythms; they also play a role in organizing and ordering human imagination. For example, they give us an *eye to detail*—and this is the crux of the matter both in the arts and the sciences.

When in their creative moments, Shakespeares or Ghalibs work with language in a piece of writing, they have in their minds all the nuances, imageries, usages, and rhythms of the language being used; its relationship with the other elements of the work is not obscured from their eyes either; then, they also keep in the sphere of their creative judgments the overall effects of this language in the totality of the poem or the play or the narrative. In other words, a great writer keeps in his view—consciously or unconsciously—every nook and corner of his particular treatment of language, every *detail* that is. Compare him with a surgeon who deals with a complex network of very tiny nerves: while touching one particular nerve, he has in view all the details of the nerve system—how will his touching a specific nerve affect this one and that one, and what consequences does it have for the totality of, say, the limb to which it belongs: these are the overwhelming issues of surgical consideration. And a careless handling of a single invisibly small nerve may have disastrous consequences—it can, for example, make the whole limb irreversibly incapacitated! The analogy here with poetry is most instructive—one inelegant or incorrect use of a single word is enough to destroy a whole piece of poetry! This *attitude* of an eye to detail is shared by a good surgeon and a good poet. In a way, then, poets and scientists have their abode in the same camp. And by this token, the poet Ghalib is phenomenologically a surgeon, and a surgeon is a Ghalib. So we see: apart from their deep enriching value in their own right, all creative arts are science's analogues; they cannot be overlooked in any system of education.

References

1. Sorabji R. Matter, space, and motion. Ithaca: Cornell University Press; 1988.
2. Kuhn T. The structure of scientific revolutions. Chicago: Chicago University Press; 1996.
3. Tambiah S. Magic, science, religion, and the scope of rationality. Cambridge: Cambridge University Press; 1990. p. 10.
4. Copernicus N. On the revolution of heavenly spheres, tr. Charles Wallis. Amherst: Prometheus Books; 1995.
5. Saliba G. Islamic science and the making of the European renaissance. Cambridge: MIT Press; 2007.
6. McClellan III JE, Dorn H. Science and technology in world history. Baltimore: The John Hopkins University Press; 1999.
7. Pagel W. New light on William Harvey. New York: S. Karger; 1976.
8. McClellan III JE, Dorn H. The crime and punishment of Galileo. In: McClellan III JE, Dorn H, editors. Science and technology in world history. Baltimore: Johns Hopkins University Press; 2006. p. 223–47.
9. Dobbs BJ. Janus face of genius: the role of alchemy in Newton's thought. Cambridge: Cambridge University Press; 1991.
10. McClellan III JE, Dorn H. Science and technology in world history. Baltimore: The John Hopkins University Press; 1999. p. 343–9.
11. Popper K. Conjectures and refutations. New York: Basic Books; 1965.

12. Quine WVO. From a logical point of view. Cambridge: Harvard University Press; 1953.
13. Haq SN. "Science vs. scientism". *Dawn*, Karachi, July 31, 2005.
14. Haq SN. "Science in Islam". In: Robert B, editor. Oxford dictionary of the middle ages. 4th ed. Oxford: Oxford University Press; 2010.
15. *Grattan-Guinness I*. The search for mathematical roots. Princeton: Princeton University Press; 1870–1940.

Stimulating Research and Innovation in Residents

104

Scott Leslie and Mihir Desai

Abstract

The integration of research into residency training benefits the resident, institution and community. Residents develop a better understanding of research methodology, evidence based medicine, practical approaches to generating research questions, and successful publication; all of which lead to better job prospects. Establishment of research requires apportioning of time, provision of training, support staff, funds and mentors. A dedicated research team can go a long way in establishing research in a departmental training program. Assessment of residents' progress can be made in departmental presentations which lead to international presentations.

Keywords

Evidence based medicine-research-assessment-support for research

The integration of scholarly activity during residency holds tangible benefits for both the resident and the institution. Exposure to research at an early stage of a physician's training promotes critical appraisal of the scientific literature and provides the opportunity to develop investigative skills that may benefit the resident, the department, and the wider community. Indeed, research remains a fundamental part of most surgical residency programs. Requirements of residency programs as outlined by the Accreditation Council for Graduate Medical Education (ACGME) stipulate that the "curriculum must advance residents' knowledge of the basic principles of research, including how research is conducted, evaluated, explained to patients, and applied to patient care" [1].

As a faculty member, it is important to provide the necessary encouragement, resources, and mentoring so that residents may achieve these research goals. The ACGME guidelines state that the "sponsoring institution and program should allocate adequate educational resources to facilitate resident involvement in scholarly activities." By stimulating research among residents, the skills to analyze scientific publications and lifelong curiosity in clinical enquiry can be fostered.

S. Leslie, M.D. • M. Desai, M.D. (✉)
Robotic Urological Surgery, USC Institute of Urology,
Keck School of Medicine, University of Southern California,
Los Angeles, CA, USA
e-mail: mihir.desai@usc.edu

Benefits of Undertaking Research

In this era of evidence-based medicine, an understanding of research methods and the ability to critically appraise the literature are of paramount importance [2]. Physicians who have received research training have a greater appreciation for evidence-based medicine and are better able to assimilate scientific evidence into their clinical practice and subsequently provide the highest standard of care to their patients [3].

Research involvement by residents at an early stage of their training promotes the acquisition of skills necessary to conduct research and answer relevant clinical questions. It provides the resident with an opportunity to challenge the limitations of what is known on a subject, potentially contributing knowledge to a field. This is particularly relevant for those pursuing an academic career as a physician-scientist. However, even for those whose goal is private practice, realization of a particular subspecialty interest may be facilitated

J.J. Talati et al. (eds.), *Urolithiasis*,
DOI 10.1007/978-1-4471-4387-1_104, © Springer-Verlag London 2012

by involvement in research projects during residency [4]. Furthermore, publications may improve a resident's chance of successfully applying for a job or fellowship position in the future [5]. Resident's ability to publish during their training correlates with their ability to continue to publish as attending physicians, a fact that may make a candidate more attractive to a potential employer.

Residency is an ideal period to undertake research with readily available resources and greater access to experts and mentors. By actively promoting research activity, benefits to the institution may also be realized, including recognition at national and international meetings, securing funds, and attracting academically oriented residents to the program.

Requirements for Achieving Research Goals During Residency

Time

Competing priorities during residency may hinder resident's ability to undertake research. These include the demands of clinical work, work hour reforms that limit hours worked per week, and balancing family and social needs [6, 7]. Given these obligations, dedicated periods of "protected" research time may facilitate successful involvement in research projects. Tasks requiring protected time include accessing medical records, preparing manuscripts, or collaborating with other members of a research team. Dedicated time may range from a block of a few hours per week up to a whole year of research.

Training

Some residents may lack the knowledge or confidence to undertake research, and structured training during residency may improve their research skills. Lectures on appropriate research topics such as clinical study design and biostatistics, critically evaluating the literature and ethical principles of research, may enhance residents ability to participate and contribute to research [8].

Support

Successful implementation of a research program requires the expertise of many individuals. Research coordinators, scientists (M.D. or Ph.D.), database managers, and statisticians all contribute to a department's research productivity. Their skills can compliment the work of the resident and assist with all aspects of research including study design, data analysis, manuscript writing, and presentations. Through this collaborative, team approach, an increase in research productivity can be achieved [9].

Mentors

A mentor can be an invaluable resource for a resident embarking on research. They can guide a resident toward achieving their research goals by providing constructive advice, being approachable, and inspiring all members of the research team [10]. Qualities recognized of a good mentor include being committed to the role, providing appropriate critique of a residents progress, demonstrating a desire for continuous learning, and remaining optimistic [11]. A mentor can best assess the merits and feasibility of a study and therefore helps the resident set achievable research goals. Assigning an appropriate mentor to a resident can be a difficult task. Program directors are in an ideal position to identify a suitable mentor for a resident by recognizing similar areas of interest. An available list of faculty, their interests, and possible projects can broaden a resident's knowledge about what research topics are available and which mentors would be best suited to guide them.

Funds

No matter what the source (grants, endowed funds, departmental money), funds are an important aspect of any research program. Funds are required for the day-to-day costs of performing research. Furthermore, residents often require financial support for travel and accommodation to present their research at meetings.

Facilitating Research Ideas in Residents

Finding an appropriate research topic can be elusive, and residents may have trouble identifying a relevant topic to study. Research ideas come from many sources, including clinical observation, knowledge of the relevant literature, and conversations with other colleagues. Faculty are therefore perhaps in the best position to guide the resident toward novel ideas that are worth exploring. Appropriate projects for residents tend to be focused and aim to answer a simple clinical question. If the study involves a well-defined study population and a well-defined outcome, then the resident is more likely to successfully complete the research.

Practical Measures of Promoting Compliance with Research

Fisher et al. demonstrated that simple measures such as making research a priority within the department, faculty submission of research topics, and making themselves available as mentors improved the participation and quality of research by residents [8].

More structured resident scholar programs that involve the implementation of a dedicated research curriculum have also been shown to increase research productivity [12, 13]. Structured resident research curriculum establishes expectations, gives examples, develops timelines, and supports the development of hypotheses and project development. Within the curricula are structured learning topics including trial design and biostatistics that further enhance the resident's scope for completing their research goals. Institutions that offer this type of structured support have seen increased participation by residents in research. Furthermore, the research is more likely to be of better quality, and faculty research productivity increases in parallel with the residents' own research endeavors [13].

Lohr et al. demonstrated that the introduction of a dedicated "research team" comprising residents, mentors, and other research staff significantly increased the output of scholarly work (presentations and publications) within established residency programs [14]. One of the benefits of a research team was to stimulate critical thinking about projects that subsequently lead to improvements in study design, analysis, and eventual publication.

Assessment of a Resident's Progress in Research

Regular review by mentors should be conducted to assess whether a resident is meeting their research objectives. A running list of projects within a department including the stage and outcomes (abstracts, presentations, publications) also provides a measure of a resident's progress with their research. Regular departmental research meetings allow discussion of a resident's work and troubleshooting of individual projects to facilitate successful completion. The final goal is to encourage quality research that can be refined as they present their work either at grandrounds dedicated departmental research forums, and national or international meetings or submit a manuscript for publication [15].

Conclusion

There are many barriers to conducting research, and programs that aim to address these issues are likely to see the benefits of greater resident participation and increased research productivity. Availability of infrastructural facilities, maybe even centralized, also helps translate concepts to end results in the relatively short time residents spend in research activities during the duration of their training. These issues should be taken up by residency governing bodies to streamline the research process.

References

1. ACGME Program Requirements for Graduate Medical Education in Surgery. cited 2012. Available from: http://www.acgme.org/. Accessed Sep 13, 2012
2. Timmermans S, Mauck A. The promises and pitfalls of evidence-based medicine. Health Aff. 2005;24(1):18–28.
3. Smith M. Research in residency: do research curricula impact post-residency practice? Fam Med. 2005;37(5):322–7.
4. Hayward RA, Taweel F. Data and the internal medicine houseofficer: alumni's views of the educational value of a residency program's research requirement. J Gen Intern Med. 1993;8(3):140–2.
5. Byrnes AB, et al. The resident scholar program: a research training opportunity for internal medicine house staff. J Cancer Educ. 2007;22(1):47–9.
6. Parsa CJ, Organ Jr CH, Barkan H. Changing patterns of resident operative experience from 1990 to 1997. Arch Surg. 2000;135(5):570–3; discussion 573–5.
7. Whang EE, et al. Work hours reform: perceptions and desires of contemporary surgical residents. J Am Coll Surg. 2003;197(4):624–30.
8. Fisher C, Baker MK. Improving participation and quality of clinical research in a university-based general surgery residency program. Am Surg. 2010;76(7):741–2.
9. Konstantakos EK, et al. Assuring the research competence of orthopedic graduates. J Surg Educ. 2010;67(3):129–34.
10. Steiner JF, et al. Assessing the role of influential mentors in the research development of primary care fellows. Acad Med. 2004;79(9):865–72.
11. Rowley JB. Becoming a high-performance mentor: a guide to reflection and action. Thousand Oaks: Corwin Press; 2006. p. xx. 180 p.
12. Gaspar MJ, Ely TL. Research in a busy family practice training program. Fam Med. 1987;19(6):463–5.
13. Hebert RS, et al. A systematic review of resident research curricula. Acad Med. 2003;78(1):61–8.
14. Lohr J, et al. Stimulating resident research in a general surgery residency community program. Curr Surg. 2006;63(6):426–34.
15. Dengel LT, et al. Resident research forums stimulate novel research within general surgical training programs. J Surg Educ. 2009;66(3):146–51.

Part X

Equitable Management of Stone Disease

Bringing Sophisticated High-Technology Surgical Care to the Rural Masses: What Is India Doing?

105

Tehemton E. Udwadia

Abstract

The demands for sophisticated high-technology surgical care are growing at a furious pace. The staggering cost of surgical advance is so far, somehow, met by the developed world. In India, 41 % of the population earns less than $1.25 per day and 75 % less than $2 per day. The government spending on health care for more than one billion people is less than 1 % of the gross domestic product (GDP), and an appreciable percentage never gets to see a surgeon in their lifetime. The country's economic boom ensures the opulent 20 % have attained a degree of sophisticated high-technology surgical care, which could outdo that in any part of the world. On the other hand, to talk about sophisticated high-technology surgical care in rural India would sound like a utopian fantasy.

Fortuitously, there is emerging in rural India a degree of sophisticated surgical care that goes beyond and belies the hard facts of resources and poverty. "Sophistication" and "high technology," like all else in life, are relative. If in their village hospital a patient receives care, compassion, and cure, while being looked after in the hospital by their relatives and untrained nurses, that to the patient is sophistication enough. If by the forces of humanism, ingenuity, and improvisation the rural surgeons in India can offer the same gold standard of surgical care to their patients by affordable, available, accessible, and acceptable locally generated materials and equipment, be it for routine surgery like repair of hernia or for advanced minimal access to surgery, that to the rural surgeon is applicable high-technology surgical care. With appreciation of their ability and dedication, rural surgeons in India are increasingly recognized as essential superspecialists and with the support of some national surgical associations are endeavoring to bring with their own brand of high technology the benefits of surgical advance to their communities.

Keywords

High-technology surgical care • Developing countries • Rural surgery • Attain gold standards • Appropriate affordable surgical care • Minimal access surgery (MAS)

T.E. Udwadia, M.S., FCPS, FRCS (Eng.), FRCS (Edin.), FAMS, FACS (Hon.), FICS (Hon.), FARSI (Hon.) (✉)
Department of Surgery, Grant Medical College & J.J. Hospital, Mumbai, Maharashtra, India

Department of M.A.S., P.D. Hinduja National Hospital, Mumbai, Maharashtra, India and
Parsee General Hospital, Breach Candy Hospital, Cook's Building, 4th Floor, D.N. Road, Mumbai, Maharashtra 400 001, India
e-mail: t_udwadia@hotmail.com

J.J. Talati et al. (eds.), *Urolithiasis*,
DOI 10.1007/978-1-4471-4387-1_105, © Springer-Verlag London 2012

Of all the forms of inequality, injustice in health care is the most shocking and inhumane.

Martin Luther King Jr.

Introduction

The practice of surgery in any country is a part and reflection of the total medical care and health delivery system in that country. Health and medical care are but a segment of the socioeconomic fabric of any country. Before one can even consider the possibility of sophisticated high-technology surgery in rural India, it is essential to have an overall bird's-eye view of surgery in India—not as hyped by the media, by the exclusive 5-star corporate or private hospitals, or by the few cutting-edge teaching hospitals, but as it functions in factual reality under the existing socioeconomic pressures that create opulent luxury for some and deplorable deprivation for many. India has a population well over one billion, greater than the combined populations of North America and Western Europe. Seventy percent of this population resides in rural India. Accepting the World Health Organization (WHO) criterion that an income of less than $1 per day would be considered below the poverty line, it is estimated that about 40 % (more than 400 million people) of the Indian population would be below the poverty line. It is a myth that all of the poor live only in rural India—30 % of the urban population is likewise below the poverty line. With inadequate provisions for health care or medical insurance in this group, the cost of health care lowers a further 2.2 % of the population (40 million) below the poverty line annually (World Bank estimates). India has 60 doctors and 90 hospital beds per 100,000 population (against WHO-recommended 150 doctors and 300 beds). Doubling the number of beds from 90 to 180 would require an infrastructure expenditure of more than $80 billion US dollars. As against this, for the last three decades, India's spending on health care has been below 1 % of its gross domestic product (GDP), among the lowest in the developing world, well below that of neighboring countries like Bangladesh, Sri Lanka, and Pakistan and one-tenth of China. Hence, in spite of being one of the world's highest and fastest growing economies, weighted down by its poor health-care indices, India's Human Development Index score ranks 119th out of 169 countries. If these figures sound grim, the reality is much worse. About 70 % of the country's doctors and 80 % of its hospital bed strength serve 30 % of its urban population, leaving the remaining inequitable 30 % of doctors and 20 % of beds for the succor of 70 % of rural India. This brief and bare data is fundamental in the appreciation and understanding of the growth of sophisticated high-technology surgical care in rural India.

There are some fundamental requirements for the entry, growth, and sustenance of sophisticated high-technology surgical care anywhere:

1. An awareness and desire in the community for such surgical care
2. The financial strength for the long-term sustained growth of this technology
3. An infrastructure of hospitals and clinics
4. An availability of trained and qualified doctors, nurses, and supportive paramedical staff to ensure safe and large volume use of this technology
5. A population that, through private funding, corporate funding, and insurance, can pay for this surgery

In today's urban India, all these requirements are met in totality. With the world becoming a global village, awareness and desire to be part of the global village led to the affluent community demanding such technological advance. Private enterprise, quick to scent the tremendous financial returns boosted by India's exploding economy, was more than willing and able to finance this sophisticated high-technology surgery. Over the last two decades, humongous state-of-the-art private, trust, and corporate hospitals—administered and functional with the utmost efficiency, on a par, if not better, than the best in the world—are mushrooming all over India not only in the large, metropolitan cities but also in smaller cities and towns all over so that the medical industry is one of the fastest growing industries in the country.

The disproportionately distributed 70–80 % of India's surgeons who work in urban India have always kept abreast with the cutting edge of surgical advance over the past several decades so that there is a capable, aggressive, indigenous workforce of safe and competent surgeons and support staff capable of sustaining and improving urological surgery. The excellence with which this surgery is done, at one-fifth or less of the cost in the developed world, is reflected in the large number of patients coming for this surgery to India, ensuring that medical tourism into India is growing at 15–20 % annually. There can be no arguing the fact that high-technology surgery is here to stay and grow in India. With a large proportion of the benefits of the growing economy captured by 20 % (200 million) of the population, the opulent urban sector in India can well afford to pay for this surgery.

Rural Surgery

I have worked for more than 30 years in a welfare teaching hospital looking after the poor in Mumbai and more than 40 years in tertiary care hospitals where sophisticated high-technology surgery is practiced. Fortunately, my urge to spread the benefits of diagnostic laparoscopy and, later over the last 20 years, minimal access surgery (MAS) into small towns and rural India gave me the eye-opening opportunity (not often granted to city surgeons) to see, experience, and be humbled by the ingenuity and quality of surgery in small town and rural India.

Surgery in rural India is astounding (and to me inspiring), occurring against a kaleidoscopic backdrop of almost insurmountable difficulties, infrastructure inadequacies, economic deprivation, poor communication and transport, and absence of essential qualified support system and staff such as anesthetists, nurses, radiologist, pathologists, and blood bank facilities. Further, the entire education and training of the surgeon in India has been directed solely to the care of the urban population, with complete oblivion to the reality of Indian surgery. The most astounding element in this kaleidoscope is India's rural surgeons. They have thrown themselves into the battle with total commitment, rising above all difficulties, training to be the most difficult superspecialists—the true general surgeons—training junior colleagues and encouraging them to do more advanced surgery, and training the local unqualified population to fulfill requirements of the support system while remaining aware of the financial constraints of the majority of patients who need surgery at their doorstep. Rural surgeons are the last bastion of hope for the deprived and destitute. Surely the surgeon in rural India is the spine and soul of Indian surgery.

None of the five criteria mentioned previously for the entry, growth, and sustenance of sophisticated high-technology surgery into rural India would be applicable. A population where nutrition, drinking water, sanitation, malaria, tuberculoses, diarrhea, and preventive medicine are of immediate concern could not dream of, let alone desire, sophisticated surgery. A major motivating factor for private finance to build hospitals and import expensive technology is profit. Profit can only come from patients who can pay. The poor cannot pay. The solely-for-profit vast multinational manufacturers have little time for the poor. The government, through the National Rural Health Mission in India and similar schemes, very rightly has its priorities to concentrate on health at all basic grassroot level interventions. In such a vast country, the impact of active motivated nongovernmental organizations (NGOs) can only be productive in a few areas. It would appear from all that is written so far that the battle to bring and sustain sophisticated high-technology surgery into rural India is forever lost.

Strange and surprising as it may seem, the battle has begun and is progressing well. The pundits, the government, the health and hospital industry, multinational manufacturers, and all who monitor and manipulate health care in India are involved, enthusiastic, and euphoric over the magnificent growth of high-technology surgery in the large hospitals. The entry of sophisticated surgery into rural India is so gradual, so smooth, so quiet, and so natural as to be almost imperceptible. There are a few identifiable factors responsible for the entry and growth of high-technology surgery into rural India:

1. The overall growth in economy
2. Involvement of national surgical associations and NGOs, and the awakening of the Medical Council of India
3. The Indian rural surgeon

The strong sustained growth of the Indian economy over the last two decades has a clear impact into rural India—an impact below Western norms, but nonetheless significant. Improvement in roads and transport, communication (the mobile phone miracle and Internet), schools, education and literacy, and preventive health—all of which attract more surgeons into rural India—have contributed to the foundation necessary for the entry of sophisticated surgery. In the Indian economy, the spotlight is so strong on the two extremes—the 20 % absurdly affluent and 40 % desperately deprived—that a large segment, the 40 % in-between, is in the shadows. While the effect of the economy is to make the rich even more disproportionally richer, it percolates into this intermediate section of the Indian population, and this gives a greater purchasing power to a large segment of Indian society, a boost to more sophisticated surgery in rural India.

Surgical associations like the Association of Rural Surgeons of India (ARSI), an association devoted to the propagation of need-based, ethical rural surgery, the Association of Surgeons of India (ASI), the Indian Association of Gastrointestinal Endoscopic Surgery (IAGES), and several similar associations have all pitched in strongly for the sophistication and growth of rural surgery. The revamped, new caretaker Medical Council of India has the vision to see the full spectrum of Indian surgery, the honesty to accept the glaring deficiencies in our surgical education as directed toward care of the vast majority of our population, and the will and courage to make comprehensive changes in the rigid archaic system of surgical education.

The ground for the entry of sophisticated surgery into rural India is being assiduously prepared so that rural surgeons will no longer remain unseen, unheard, remote individuals struggling in the backwaters. They have gained recognition and respect for their dedication and surgical prowess and are far from being an endangered species [1]. Rural surgery is now accepted as a superspecialty in India. In conjunction with ARSI, the Indira Gandhi National Outreach University (IGNOU) offers a long-distance course diploma [2–4] and the National Board of Examination has created a superspecialty status for rural surgery [5]. Even so, the rural surgeons have their feet firmly on the ground. Having no desire to keep up with the Joneses in the metropolis or engage in futile exercises of one-upmanship, their thrust is the practice of need-based, multi-specialty surgery under resource constraints to make quality surgical care affordable and accessible to the community [6]. Still, they also have their aspirations and their dreams and their indignant questions. They ask, "Why in one country or world must there forever and ever be perpetuated a class system with a second tier of humans fit only for second-rate care and facilities?" [7] If health is a fundamental human right as professed by all governments, they ask: Surely, the poorest of the poor have as much right as anyone to advanced sophisticated surgery? This strong sentiment is the springboard of rapidly spreading sophisticated surgery in rural areas.

High technology is making a deafening roar in the cities with surgeons there trying to outdo their colleagues (competitors) with smaller incisions, less punctures, a plethora of investigations, and newer, costlier equipment. In the quiet of the village, the rural surgeon has time to ponder and evaluate, keeping the patient the priority. The rural surgeon will assess and evaluate sophisticated high-technology surgery as an analysis of the outcome of his work in relation to society [8] and will endeavor to achieve the results of high technology with homegrown equipment created through ingenuity, improvisation, and financial necessity. They know their strength and limitations—no heart or liver transplants for them. However, if in their daily practice rural surgeons can offer the same gold standard of treatment for various ailments as can be given by the high-technology surgery of the developed world, what they use is adequate sophisticated surgery for them.

The commonest surgical procedure, repair of inguinal hernia, was until recently done all over the developing world only by tissue repair, as the commercially available mesh was totally unaffordable to the rural population. Tension-free open mesh repair is the gold standard of hernia repair worldwide [9]. Enterprising surgeons in India, and later in Africa, started using mosquito net—freely available—that is affordable with similar properties and identical results over follow-up of several years as commercial mesh [10, 11]. The of cost ratio of this mosquito net to commercial mesh is 1:2,000, helping introduce simple "gold standard" sophistication to routine rural surgery.

Laparoscopy came to surgery in India in 1972 as a diagnostic modality with the use of a simple sigmoidoscope pump to create pneumoperitoneum using atmospheric air [12].

From that small beginning, MAS has spread all over rural India [13]. More than 80 % of the members of ARSI practice MAS, many of them doing safe advanced MAS in adverse conditions [14, 15]. Sophisticated surgery is defined by the result, not the equipment. Single-incision laparoscopic surgery is a method under trial. The high-cost technology of this surgery has been reduced to the cost of one surgical glove and four reusable trocars, making it as efficient and completely affordable [16].

A surgeon in a small town of India created abdominal wall lift equipment out of bathroom piping [17] and went on to make a perfect surgeon-friendly robot for laparoscopic surgery at a fraction of the cost of comparable robots [18]. The "Jaipur foot"—easy to fabricate in a small garage, low in cost, and light in weight—is the ultimate sophisticated technology for the rural Indian amputee [19]. One surgeon in a very small town starting from a seven-bed missionary-run hospital (a mission hospital), in the course of more than 10,000 lip and palate repairs, created a world-renowned center for this abnormality, his unmatched sophisticated high-technology care being cost-free dedication to the poor and meticulous perfection of surgical technique [20].

There is no end to the list of such improvised, affordable sophisticated high-technology rural surgeries. These explode the myth that sophisticated high-technology surgical care comes only in multimillion dollar crates so avidly desired and purchased by health-care providers. To maintain a sense of proportion, to recount the first foray into initiating the surgical revolution of MAS, the first closed cholecystectomy was performed in a small village by an unheard-of German surgeon using equipment made from the aluminum tubing of his daughter's bicycle. To the Indian rural surgeon, surgery is defined not by the cost of equipment but by the end result of surgical care. A vital role is being played by Indian surgical instrument manufacturers who have realized their duty to maintaining quality at affordable cost [21]. One finds it difficult to comprehend the thought process of multinational manufacturers of high-technology equipment whose entire research and development (R & D) is solely directed to the one billion world's wealthy, be it in the developed or developing world, for the immense immediate financial benefits they reap. Would it perhaps make financial sense to devote part of their R & D toward the affordable care of the remaining five billion in the world? And doing so express some sentiment of humanism?

Conclusion

A final thought. Could the most expensive, very latest, burgeoning with high technology equipment ever bring, in the least measure, the surgical care of rural surgeons to their patients: empathy, caring, commitment, and undifferentiated devotion and skill for both rich and poor patients? Surgery is a humanitarian science. This attribute is not unique to the Indian rural surgeon—it is the hallmark of rural surgeons worldwide, for they are the answer to the 2,000-year-old question: "What would it avail a man if he gain the world but lose his soul?"

References

1. Semir J. The rural surgeon on endangered species. World J Surg. 2006;30:267–8.
2. Agarwal AK, Jena TK. Multiskilling the surgeons through a distance education programme (certificate in rural surgery) of 'IGNOU' 8th annual conference of rural surgeons of Indian. Manipal, 2000.

3. Panda S, Jena TK. Changing the pattern: towards flexible learning, learner support and mentoring. In: Lockwook F, Gooley A, editors. Innovations in open and distance learning. London: Kogan Page Limited; 2001.
4. Prabhu RD. Editorial. Indian J Surg. 2003;65:22–3.
5. Mukerjee S. Surgery in India. Arch Surg. 1997;132(6):571–8.
6. Udwadia TE. Surgical care for the poor. A personal Indian perspective. Indian J Surg. 2003;65:504–9.
7. Udwadia TE. One world, one people, one surgery. Surg Endosc. 2001;15:337–43.
8. Banerjee JK. Analysing outcome of surgical development – rural surgery as an example. Indian J Surg. 2003;65:68–72.
9. Lichstenstein IL, Shulman AG, Amid PK. The tension free hernioplasty. Am J Surg. 1989;157:188–93.
10. Tongaonkar RR, Reddy BV, Mehta VK. Preliminary multicentre trial of cheap indigenous mosquito net cloth for tension free hernia repair. Indian J Surg. 2003;65:89–95.
11. Freudenberg S, Sono D, Ouengre E, Weiss C, Wilhelm JS. Commercial mesh versus nylon mosquito net for hernia repair – a randomized double blend study in Burkina Faso. World J Surg. 2006;30:1784–9.
12. Udwadia TE. Pentoneoscopy for surgeons. Ann R Coll Surg Engl. 1986;68:125–9.
13. Engelking EJ. Development of laparoscopic surgery in rural India – how do we proceed? Rural Surg. 2010;6(1):11–2.
14. Udwadia TE. Laparoscopy in India – personal perspective. J Min Access Surg. 2005;1(2):51–2.
15. Gnenhraj J. Laparoscopic fundoplication in rural area. The lesson learnt. Rural Surg. 2010;6(2):10–14f.
16. Khrangte R, Newme I, Phicken P, Medhi S. Improvised trans-umbilical glove port – cost effective method for single port laparoscopic surgery. Indian J Surg. 2011;73:142–5.
17. Deshpande SV. Abdominal wall lift. In: Udwadia TE, editor. Laparoscopic surgery in developing countries. New Delhi: Joypee Medical Publishers; 1997. p. 326–8.
18. Deshpande S. Invited international faculty on "Low Budget Technology"-indigenous robot. In: 10th world congress of endoscopic surgery, Berlin, 2006.
19. Mohan D, Seth PK, Ravi R. Mathematical modeling and field trials of an inexpensive endoskeletal above-knee prosthesis. Prosthet Orthot Int. 1992;16:118–23.
20. Adenwalla HS. International update. Indian society of cleft lip, palate and cranio-fascial anomalies, Madras, 2003.
21. Muhe E. Roadblocks to surgical progress. Dr. Karl Storz Lecture on new technology. Society of american gastrointestinal endoscopic surgeons (SAGES) annual congress 1999. In Reynolds W. The first laparoscopic cholecystectomy journal of society of laparoendoscopic surgeons 2001;5(1):89–94.

106 Bringing Highly Technological Urolithiasis Care to a Billion People: What Is China Doing?

Guo-Min Wang and Jian-Ming Guo

Abstract

Currently, lithotripter development is in a very advanced stage in China, and there are a large number of lithotripter centers in China. However, compared to the number of people in China, the number of lithotripter centers is insufficient to meet the needs of the population. Even if all patients who require such treatment went to the urban hospitals, the capacity in those centers is inadequate. The fee for such surgery is not high, and in urban areas most of the fee is covered by medical insurance. However, for peasants in rural areas, medical insurance does not adequately cover their treatment costs. This becomes problematic for these peasants as their salaries in comparable occupations are lower compared to those in urban areas. China is now working on models that will provide medical insurance for patients from rural areas.

Keywords

China • Population • Income • Insurance • Lithotripter distribution • Rural • Urban • Urolithiasis • Shock wave lithotripsy (SWL) • Percutaneous nephrolithotomy (PCNL) • Ureteroscopy (URS) • Calculi • Technology • Health-care program

Introduction

As technology advances, the practice of medicine also advances. However, not all parts of the world will be able to enjoy the benefits of advanced technologies. These past few years, China is attempting to bring the best technological care to the whole nation, spreading the best care possible to the entire population.

Currently, the most popular treatments for urolithiasis are shock wave lithotripsy (SWL), ureteroscopy (URS), and percutaneous nephrolithotomy (PCNL). In China, since the late 1980s, SWL has become the most common intervention for patients suffering from upper urinary tract calculi. However, since the start of the twenty-first century, endourologic techniques such as URS and PCNL radically changed the treatment paradigm for renal and ureteral calculi. Even so, some of the patients still receive an open surgical procedure in some towns where the hospital does not have any lithotripters or sophisticated technology, such as URS or PCNL.

Each of the provinces of China has a variable number of lithotripter centers equipped with different combinations of sophisticated technology. The greater the prosperity of the city (as is seen in the cities of Beijing, Shanghai, and Guangzhou), the better the technology. On the other hand, the cities that are more rural (e.g., Hainan, Ningxia, and Qinghai) have much less technology available. Table 106.1 [1] explains the situation more clearly, where it can be seen that the lithotripter-to-population ratio varies from 1:~40,000 to 60,000 population (in Xinjiang and Jiangsu) to 1:~250,000 (in Beijing and Shanghai) and to 1:1.5 million people (in Tibet).

As shown in Table 106.1, in some parts of China, people with stones have very little access to technology [1].

G.-M. Wang (✉) • J.-M. Guo, M.D., Ph.D.
Department of Urology, Zhongshan Hospital, Fudan University, 180 Fenglin Road, Shanghai, 200032, China
e-mail: guo.jianming@zs-hospital.sh.cn; guojm@sina.com

J.J. Talati et al. (eds.), *Urolithiasis*,
DOI 10.1007/978-1-4471-4387-1_106,

Table 106.1 Comparison of available stone treatment technology in Chinese provinces [1]

Province	Population (million)	Population density (sq/km)	Number of lithotripter centers	Number of centers with sophisticated technology	Centers-to-population ratios
Beijing	19.612	1167.4	29	73	1:192,275
Shanghai	23.019	3712.76	34	80	1:201,921
Tianjin	12.938	1144.97	12	25	1:347,796
Chongqing	28.846	351.78	20	54	1:389,811
Guangdong	104.303	560.77	100	114	1:488,310
Shandong	95.793	627.27	84	82	1:578,460
Jiangsu	78.659	766.67	60	108	1:468,208
Zhejiang	54.426	537.28	60	83	1:381,134
Henan	94.023	563.02	107	50	1:598,111
Hebei	71.854	378.18	73	53	1:570,270
Liaoning	43.746	300.25	90	35	1:350,529
Sichuan	80.418	164.79	77	80	1:511,565
Fujian	36.894	307.45	49	49	1:374,939
Hubei	57.237	309.9	54	74	1:445,771
Hunan	65.683	312.78	77	88	1:399,532
Heilongjiang	38.312	81.69	97	26	1:309,968
Anhui	59.500	428.06	53	60	1:527,482
Guangxi	46.026	194.78	91	42	1:345,541
Inner Mongolia	24.706	20.88	35	24	1:420,170
Shanxi	35.712	230.4	23	14	1:960,000
Jiangxi	44.567	267.51	90	65	1:287,901
Shanxi	37.327	182.08	38	28	1:565,561
Jilin	27.462	146.86	43	34	1:357,578
Yunnan	45.956	116.64	42	58	1:461,406
Xinjiang	21.813	13.63	25	35	1:363,550
Guilin	34.746	204.39	56	31	1:396,644
Gansu	25.575	56.83	67	22	1:288,007
Hainan	8.671	255.04	10	11	1:425,049
Ningxia	6.301	94.9	10	8	1:350,056
Qinghai	5.626	12.5	12	7	1:293,021
Tibet	3.002	2.46	2	2	1:682,273
Total	1,332.764		1,619	1,516	

This is at least in part due to the cost of such technology. Not all Chinese people are able to afford such sophisticated surgeries, least of all the people from rural areas. The earnings from different professions and employment (e.g., government officials, factory workers, and farmers) differ even within the profession or job, depending upon their town of placement. Statistics show that the salary of government officials varies according to location: in eastern China it averages 42,810 RMB/year; in the middle parts of China, 31,594 RMB/year; in western China, 33,130 RMB/year; and in northeastern China, 31,882 RMB/year.

The cost of ureteroscopic (URS) treatment and SWL for stone disease also differs from the cost in the United States. In China, the cost of URS is around 10,000 RMB/surgery, and the cost of external shock wave lithotripsy is around 2,000 RMB. Some people in China who are in desperate need of such surgeries are, because of their low income, unable to pay for the treatment needed.

However, the government is trying to provide health treatment to all citizens of China. Through its health-care programs, the government is providing money for 80 % of the cost for such treatment in urban areas, with the citizen only having to pay 20 % of the cost themselves. On the other hand, in rural parts of China, the government healthcare program only pays for 50 % of the cost of treatment, and the citizens have to pay the remaining 50 % by themselves.

Conclusion

Provision of sophisticated care to more than a billion people is fraught with many complexities. In addition to the provision of equipment, and placement of services, government subsidies are required to offset the costs of technology-dependent treatment. Despite a large number of lithotripters, population needs have not been met because of the very large population size. The capacity of individuals to pay for treatment is unfortunately limited by not just the citizen's profession but by the location of residence, which also determines salary. The effects of living in rural areas are further compounded by reduced government subsidy for treatment.

Reference

1. http://www.stats.gov.cn/tjgb/rkpcgb/qgrkpcgb/t20110429_402722510.htm.

Lithotripter Sharing

107

André van der Merwe, Nicole Ebinger Mundorff, and Rian Nieuwoudt

Abstract

The sharing of expensive medical equipment, such as extracorporeal shock wave lithotripters, between hospitals is not often considered, though there are significant advantages to the patient and the hospital. Choosing an appropriate business model is essential for success. Reliability of a mobile service depends on a number of factors such as transport and operating theater (OR) interface with the vending company. Appropriate training of the technical team ensures minimal breakdown and safety. A plan of action must be in place for emergency after-hours work and breakdown periods.

Keywords

Lithotripter • Sharing • Extracorporeal shock wave lithotripsy • SWL • Laser • Mobile • Vendor

Introduction

Sharing lithotripters generally means to share extracorporeal shock wave lithotripsy (SWL) equipment between hospitals. However, other types of lithotripsy machines (e.g., laser) may also be shared and will be discussed briefly. To make this chapter as practical as possible, the authorship includes two urologists (one using stationary and one using a mobile lithotripsy service) and a successful vendor of lithotripsy services (SWL as well as laser lithotripsy).

A. van der Merwe, MB Ch B, MRCS (Eng), MRCS (Ed) MMed (Urology), UCT, FC (Urol)SA (✉)
Department of Urology, Faculty of Health Sciences, University of Stellenbosch and Tygerberg Hospital, 19063 Tygerberg, Cape Town, 7505 South Africa
e-mail: arvdm@sun.ac.za

N.E. Mundorff, M.D.
Department of Urology, University Hospital Basel, Spitalstrasse 21, Basel 4031 Switzerland
e-mail: nebinger@uhbs.ch

R. Nieuwoudt, Pr.Eng, M.Eng, B.Eng (Stell)
Managing Director at Spectra-Medic, AHG Group of Companies, 6 Arun Place, Sir Lowry's Pass Road, Somerset West, Western Cape, 7130, South Africa
e-mail: rian.nieuwoudt@spectra-medic.co.za

As economic conditions change, renal stones become more frequent in Third World countries [1]. To have a sustainable healthcare service, it is important to offer cost-effective healthcare treatment. Overservicing of lithotripter service is seen when lithotripsy units are installed and then not regularly utilized as seen in some hospitals. This contrasts with areas like sub-Saharan Africa (excluding South Africa) where there are only six lithotripter machines for countries with a combined population of 954 million people. Countries such as Ethiopia, Kenya, Tanzania, Nigeria, Mauritania, and Senegal had only one lithotripsy unit each in 2010.

The Rationale of Sharing a Lithotripsy Service

In the United States, the cost of healthcare related to urinary calculi is US $1.2 billion. About 3 % of the population suffers from renal stones accounting for 10 % of hospital admissions [2]. This indicates that funding for expensive capital equipment will be available as most patients in the United States have some form of medical insurance. However, in the Third World, the cost that can be recovered from patients is much less. This will mean that many more patients have to be treated

J.J. Talati et al. (eds.), *Urolithiasis*,
DOI 10.1007/978-1-4471-4387-1_107,

to justify and offset the cost of expensive equipment. The lithotripter would then have to be used every day, and as this is not always possible due to limited patient numbers, sharing a lithotripter between hospitals makes financial sense.

Economics

It may not be economical to treat a first stone episode medically [3]. The major contributor to viability of mobile lithotripsy services is the dominant health financing system within a specific country. In order to make the supply of the service viable, it is essential that there is a fee that can cover the costs of a specific visit. Another aspect is the type of ownership of a hospital, for example, is it private or state owned, and the approach of treating the patients—that is, in the case of SWL, to aim for treatments where the patient should be stone-free after the first treatment in contrast to treatment schedules where patients may need to return for up to eight treatments on a low-intensity approach. In South Africa, there is insufficient manpower and monetary resources to follow the last approach. Other factors playing a role in the viability are the weather (e.g., risk of severe snow storms) and road/geographical conditions, the distances between patients and nearest hospitals, the availability of specialists (medical and technical), and density of patient distribution.

Listed below is a summary of the trends in a few countries:

1. Canada: The insurance system is essentially a national health system sponsored by the state. Mostly, the hospitals aim to purchase their own machines (stationary), and patients travel to a specialized site to be treated for renal stones. There are mobile units in existence but not to the level found in South Africa.
2. Germany and United Kingdom: Essentially state-sponsored insurance systems, but private insurance systems are also significant contributors. Here mobile units are found in a higher percentage than, for example, in Canada.
3. South Africa: It is one of the countries with the highest number (among all the countries of the world) of renal stones that are treated by mobile units. This is due to the positive combination of the aforementioned factors.
4. Other African countries: Very low to almost no incidence of mobile lithotripsy units mostly due to lack of funds and specialists.

Business Models for Sharing Lithotripters

The cost of a new lithotripter is significant. In 2011, the cost of the Storz® Modulith lithotripter (Karl Storz GmbH, Tuttlingen, Germany), which is available worldwide, ranges between US $425,000 and $600,000. However, there are more economical mobile units from around US $100,000, such as the electrohydraulic units from Direx® (Direx Corp., Natick, MA, USA). Choosing the correct business model is therefore essential. The following are a few examples of different models:

1. Hospital owned: The advantage of this model is a greater guaranteed availability of the lithotripter as the agreement to share this expensive equipment is between no more than 6 hospitals and generally fewer. This is in contrast to a contract with a vendor who might service 20 or 30 hospitals, and the lithotripter may not be available on short notice. When hospital owned, the administrative effort to run this service may be cumbersome, as extra personnel may have to be appointed, and costly as the capital cost of the equipment is significant. Maintenance and insurance costs too would have to be borne by the hospitals. Breakage would mean interruption of service to the hospital until the equipment is repaired; and the cost of repair would have to be borne by the hospital.
2. Vendor owned: The advantage of this type of agreement is that the risk is borne by the vendors, who become specialists in setup, maintenance, and transport of the expensive equipment. Downtime (i.e., nonavailability of the equipment during breakdowns) means less financial turnover for the vendor; so every effort is made by the vendor to keep the unit functional. Consequently, this type of service is generally very reliable. In the vendor-owned system, the vendor, hospital, and urologist (where applicable) charge a "fee for service."
3. Selling extra SWL capacity: Hospitals with underutilized SWL machines may sell capacity to nearby hospitals making it cost-effective to have, maintain, and update a lithotripter. The broader patient population benefits by this. The lithotripter may not be mobile, making the transport of the patients to the lithotripter imperative.
4. Gaining extra SWL capacity: Hospitals without SWL service may seek a service agreement with hospitals that own lithotripters. A negative financial effect is that the total cost of hospitalization (charges for admission, laboratory services, etc.) is gained by the remote hospital, incurring a loss for the referring hospital.

Requirements for Sharing a Lithotripsy Service

The particular business model followed will dictate the details needed to set up a lithotripter-sharing service. Some general principles, however, apply to all models.

The lithotripter needs to satisfy the needs of the client, first. Therefore, the strength of the energy delivered must be maximal for a mobile unit, fragmenting as many calculi as possible. In South Africa, a spark gap generator is used with great success. This type of generator requires general anesthesia as a larger amount of energy is delivered. The latest-generation electrohydraulic and electromagnetic generators may not need general anesthesia for all the patients. Intensity can be reduced to allow more comfort, but more treatments may be needed to pulverize a stone. However, if as high as possibly energy is to be delivered to the calculus, then severe discomfort may be experienced, hence needing a general anesthetic. Breathing can also be more easily controlled while under general anesthetic, making it easier to continuously target the stone. Some electromagnetic lithotripters have an oval focal area to compensate for the effect of breathing.

A stone localization technique has to be agreed upon and established within the sharing hospitals: image intensifier or ultrasound guided. Ultrasound has the disadvantage that a fragment closest to the ultrasound probe may cast acoustic shadows that interfere with identifying and focusing on the possible desired calculus more distally. All hospitals sharing a single lithotripter would preferably need to use the same stone-locating modality to make the treatment standard for the technician and surgeon operating the lithotripter.

Current lithotripters have suffered from inferior fragmentation rates compared with the original Dornier HM3 lithotripter (Dornier MedTech GmbH, Wessling, Germany) [4]. This may be due to decreased energy released (as in piezoelectric generators) or decreased f2 focal area (e.g., electromagnetic generators) making the effect of breathing significant as the calculus moves cyclically, with each breath, out of the sharp, smaller, focus area. An experienced operator can compensate for this to a large degree. This level of experience is often only reached after many cases of treatment are performed and unlikely to be reached by a hospital's own stationary unit operator who will not be exposed to a high-volume caseload.

To have ultrasound in addition to fluoroscopy as localization technique may be convenient but expensive for developing countries. Fluoroscopy for radiolucent stones may be possible with a retrograde contrast study helping to locate and target the filling defect caused by the calculus to be treated.

Reliability

The reliability of a mobile service is absolutely essential to attain cost-effective treatment of renal stones [5]. The reliability is defined by the certainty that a mobile unit will be ready on time in the operating room (OR) and that all equipment as well as operators will be 100 % functional. Factors playing a role are:

1. Reliability of the transport: Here the type of vehicle used is very important. The way that the equipment is loaded and off-loaded is fundamental to protecting the equipment (Fig. 107.1). The drivers must be trained to drive carefully and cautiously and to observe the equipment and the way it is handled. They must have a proper understanding of the importance of punctuality and timely communication in times of trouble on the road or otherwise.
2. Reliability of the equipment: Holmium YAG lasers, for example, are very sensitive to vibrations and shocks. In the case that it is not handled well, the alignment of the light bundle shifts, with the effect that the machine arrives in a dysfunctional condition with huge financial implications and disruption to the hospital and patients' schedules. It is therefore essential to design systems to protect the laser during transport. Certain brands of equipment are designed to be more robust, and therefore, it is wise to investigate the robustness and after-sales service before investing in a specific brand. The technical team and systems that are covering the mobile team also play an essential role.
3. Reliability of the operator of the equipment: The heart of the mobile unit in the hospital is not the equipment but the level of experience, training, and commitment of the specialized operator handling the equipment. Imagine what will happen if an Airbus A380 with all its wonderful advanced systems develops severe technical problems in flight while its pilots are not properly trained and experienced enough to handle this crisis!
4. Reliability of the host hospital and its OR to interface with the mobile unit: It is essential that the host hospital's OR and equipment are 100 % reliable and compatible with the equipment of the mobile unit. The OR staff must be trained on all aspects that have a bearing on the compatibility of all equipment and must be able to properly communicate, understand, and support the mobile unit operator.

Technical Team/Training

Mobile lithotripsy services are not so well organized that the team traveling with the lithotripter remains the same group of people, as would be expected. To make this high-cost-capital equipment service cost-effective, equipment transporting teams deliver, set up, and prepare the lithotripters. Operators travel independently between booked patients and are therefore more mobile to move on to the next hospital where patients are waiting to receive lithotripsy treatment and the machines have been set up.
The advantage of this is that the team becomes very efficient in handling, setting up, caring for, and troubleshooting the complex equipment.

A doctor experienced in the treatment of renal stones should be available at all times to make sure the correct stones are treated. The operator using the shared lithotripter should be trained in recognizing the contraindications for lithotripsy. This is not to take any responsibility away from

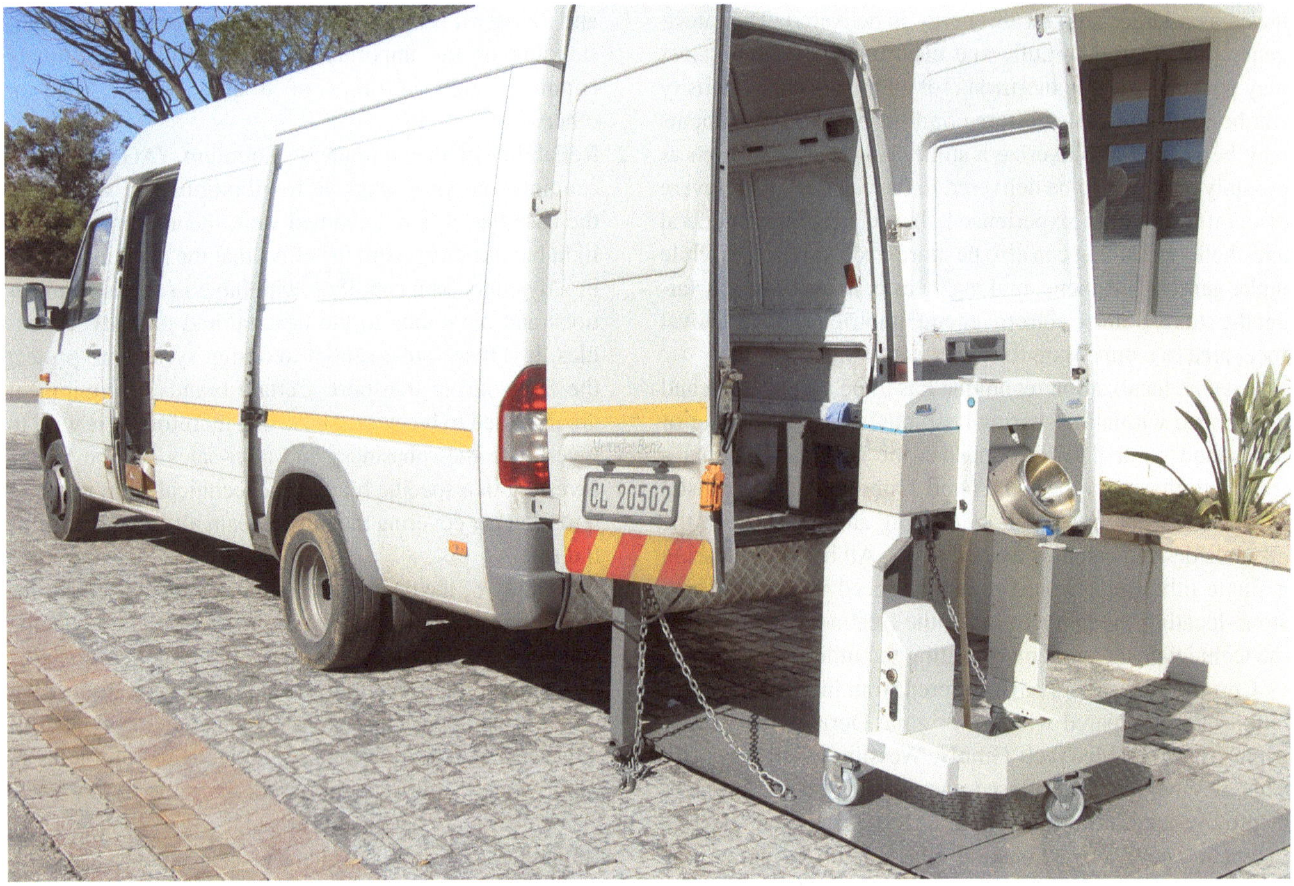

Fig. 107.1 Dedicated, safe, efficient transport with lifting equipment is needed to maintain a mobile SWL service

the medical team but rather to have an extra safety measure. Easily recognized problem patients such as pregnant females, children, and patients with spinal deformities could be identified and the medical team alerted.

Since the operator has to be specially trained in SWL, the quality of treatment will be high and time effectively used, especially important when the number of treatments done increases.

Disadvantages for lithotripter sharing may arise if distances between the hospitals are far and travel time is significant for the mobile lithotripter or if patients have to travel long distances. This time lost will impact negatively on the minimal invasive nature of the procedure.

Emergency Equipment

To maintain a lithotripsy service, spare parts and servicing expertise should be available in case of breakdown. It is not possible to repair high-technology equipment such as SWL machines in an operating theater. Therefore, patients who are receiving treatment during breakdown of equipment have to be re-treated at a later stage when a backup lithotripter is available and brought to the theater.

The vendor (the entity who is marketing a mobile lithotripsy service) would probably have more than one machine in working condition. The vendor might therefore be able to circumvent the effect of equipment failure by providing at least a scaled down service spreading existing machines wider while the broken machine is repaired.

Transport

Specialized equipment such as lithotripters should be transported by specialized transportation methods using minimal physical effort.

Sharing Other Forms of Lithotripsy

Any lithotripter that can be moved safely can be shared if carefully transported and if the setup is done by experienced personnel. This includes laser lithotripsy, electrokinetic lithotripsy, and pneumatic lithotripsy. The risks involved in moving these expensive machines are significant, so vendor-based lithotripsy possibly makes more sense. This provides a direct motivation for the technician to maintain the machines in working order.

Outcomes

The ultimate success and continued use of programs utilizing a shared lithotripter will be dependent on the success with which the stones are cleared. It is essential that the renal stones are successfully targeted and adequately fragmented by the visiting mobile unit. The right patient selection is fundamental when ordering a mobile unit. It does not help to order an SWL machine if the right method should have been a percutaneous stone removal for larger than 2-cm stones. Mobile units are seldom able to transport all types of equipment like SWL, laser, and percutaneous nephrolithotomy (PCNL) systems. Often the operators are super specialized only in their specific equipment. It is essential to know up front what method will be the correct one. Different urologists also have different approaches and preferences. It is essential that the machine operator is well acquainted with the urologist and that they have a good working relationship to ensure good and timely outcomes.

The following are the most important factors in outcomes:

1. Correct patient selection and equipment application as per previous example.
2. Skill of the urologist with, for example, a flexible ureterenoscope. For example, an unskilled urologist can easily damage a flexible scope if not properly trained.
3. Training and level of experience of the operators. For example, in the case of SWL, a kidney stone needs to be localized and properly focused upon; otherwise, it will be missed by the shock waves.
4. Type and capacity of equipment used. For example, in South Africa in certain regions, it is essential to have a 30-W Holmium YAG laser available for hard stones.
5. Using well-serviced and reliable equipment. For example, if the shock wave strength is not measured and calibrated, it can lead to a bad outcome with regard to low energy on the one side and kidney damaged with too high energy on the other side.
6. Regular feedback on statistical and practical outcomes to urologists and companies operating equipment is essential in order to correct problems as soon as they surface.

Conclusion

Careful planning and teamwork is essential to ensure excellent results with mobile or shared services. This can be done successfully in most economical situations, and mobile/shared lithotripsy services have been provided to government hospitals too. Shared lithotripsy has the potential for providing better results in situations where each hospital has only a limited number of patients, as in mobile lithotripsy services, a single operator across hospitals gains greater expertise. It may also ultimately be safer, as vendors will strictly adhere to maintenance and calibration schedules as it makes economical sense to do so. However, as far as we can determine, no prospective randomized trials are available looking at the success rate and safety of owner versus vendor lithotripsy.

References

1. Trinchieri A. Epidemiological trends in urolithiasis: impact on our healthcare systems. Urol Res. 2006;34(2):151–6.
2. Pearle MS, Calhoun EA, Curhan GC. Urologic diseases in America project: urolithiasis. J Urol. 2005;173(3):848–57.
3. Chandhoke PS. When is medical prophylaxis cost-effective for recurrent calcium stones? J Urol. 2002;168(3):937–40.
4. Lingeman J, Lifschitz D, Evan A. Surgical management of urinary lithiasis. In: Wein A, Walsh P, editors. Campbell's urology, vol. 4. 8th ed. Philadelphia: Saunders; 2002. p. 3361–451.
5. Lotan Y. Economics and cost of care of stone disease. Adv Chronic Kidney Dis. 2009;16(1):5–10.

Choosing and Purchasing Expensive Medical Equipment: A Hospital Perspective

108

Nadeem Kamal Mustafa Khan and Farhan Bhayani

Abstract

Rapid innovations in material, laboratory, and computer-based diagnostic and therapeutic technology have improved outcomes of interventional treatment of urinary tract stones. However, costs and risks have increased disproportionately, and machines face obsolescence as newer inventions replace them. The higher the costs and shorter the life span, the greater the risk, as the value of the machine can decrease by 30–35 % immediately upon purchase. To ensure effective and financially feasible plans for treatment of stones, a number of questions must be addressed before purchasing expensive equipment. This chapter provides a framework for an appropriate decision-making process involved in the acquisition of high-value medical equipment. While readership of this chapter primarily includes urologists and other related health-care professionals, the process defined here can be easily applied to the purchase of any high-value high-cost medical, therapeutic, or diagnostic equipment.

Keywords

Equipment purchase • Financing • Lithotriptors • Decision-making • High-cost equipment

Introduction

Expensive medical equipment purchases in a volatile, rapidly changing world are fraught with risks. Such decisions require a thorough process and careful analysis of all factors to ensure that the decision will be a sound one.

Current trends in technology for health care show rapid innovations with respect to material-based, laboratory-based, or computer-based technology. While such medical advancement in technology has helped improve medical care, costs have increased disproportionately and so have risks. The highest risk factor is obsolescence occurring at different times for different machines. The higher the costs, the greater the risk, as the value of the machine decreases by 30–35 % immediately upon purchase [1]. The life of the machine is also a strong determining factor. The more stretched out the life cycle, the less risky the option. Therefore, the following questions must be addressed: Does it make sense for the institution to invest, at this point in time, in such a high-cost item, and does it make sense within the overall strategy of the institution?

This chapter deals with all aspects of the decision-making process involved in the acquisition of high-value medical equipment. While readership of this chapter primarily includes urologists and other related health-care professionals, the process defined here can be easily applied to the purchase of any high-value medical, therapeutic, or diagnostic equipment.

N.K.M. Khan, B.A., B.Sc. (Econ), FCA (✉)
Regional CEO, Health Services, Asia,
The Aga Khan University Hospital,
Stadium Road, Karachi 74800, Sindh, Pakistan
e-mail: nadeem.khan@aku.edu

F. Bhayani, B.E. (Mech.), MBA, CPM
Division of Materials Management, Aga Khan University,
Stadium Road, Karachi 74800, Sindh, Pakistan
e-mail: farhan.bhayani@aku.edu

J.J. Talati et al. (eds.), *Urolithiasis*,
DOI 10.1007/978-1-4471-4387-1_108, © Springer-Verlag London 2012

Equipment Acquisition Process

The equipment acquisition process begins with the following steps:

- Definition of needs
- Technology analysis
- Market analysis
- Financial feasibility
- Evaluation of risk
- Funding

The following is a detailed explanation of the preceding steps.

Definition of Needs

While the need for equipment might originate from faculty, patients, or staff, a logical and critical first step in the process of equipment acquisition is to review the long-term operational plans of the organization. If the proposed investment is for equipment that fits into the stated goals and long-term service plans of the organization, it can be considered for acquisition provided it is financially feasible for the organization to acquire and operate it.

Technology Analysis

The next step is to assess how the technological aspects of that particular equipment have "fared" and are "going to fare" over a period of time. Review of recent developments in hardware and software functionalities will be important. Moreover, discussions with relevant clinicians and vendors who can predict trends in technology should also be undertaken. Literature is replete with benefits of early supplier involvement (ESI) [2] at this stage of acquisition. When in-house knowledge is not readily available for specialized equipment, a "request for information"(RFI) letter can be developed and sent to a few leading vendors asking for specific information related to technology, preparation of the site where the equipment will be housed, regulatory requirements, ballpark cost estimates, etc. Alternatively, vendors can also be asked to make detailed presentations covering these aspects so that any queries from staff and faculty can be addressed promptly. Moreover, third-party firms who specialize in compiling such information, such as Emergency Care Research Institute (ECRI), which prepares and periodically updates the Healthcare Product Comparison System (HPCS), can also be contacted for the same purpose. HPCS can also serve as a useful guide in developing equipment specifications as well as identifying potential suppliers who can offer the required equipment.

Certain large organizations generally have completely centralized purchasing functions preventing clinicians from directly approaching vendors. Such organizations should establish mechanisms and forums for direct interaction of clinicians with vendors to enable them to stay updated on recent technological advancements. If this is not taken care of, the buying organizations will find it extremely difficult to effectively undertake a technology analysis.

Market Analysis

It is equally important at this stage to gather information regarding one's competitors, i.e., providers of similar services to the same target population. Data regarding their target markets, product niche, volumes, and charges will help the organization plan, position, and market their offering appropriately. Moreover, the organization can also learn from others' experience of acquiring, operating, and maintaining similar equipment as well as designing appropriate facilities instead of "reinventing the wheel."

Financial Feasibility

Financial feasibility will primarily determine the payback period as well as whether the program will generate enough cash to plow back into the program for ongoing operational needs and capital replacement when the equipment becomes obsolete. This chapter should include total cost of ownership (TCO) [3] of the equipment instead of just focusing on the up-front capital investment. TCO considers the total cost of acquisition, operations (including additional staff and disposable costs), maintenance/service contracts, and disposal of a given equipment. TCO modeling does not actually require precise calculation of all costs but looks at major cost issues that may be relevant to the decision at hand. TCO analysis should include the following cost elements (see sample table later):

- Capital cost (including cost of packaging, transportation, duties and taxes, clearance, etc.)
- Warranty and expected life of equipment
- Cost of peripheral equipment and other utilities
- Site visits, if needed
- Site preparation cost (including installation and commissioning costs)
- Staff recruitment and training costs (clinicians, operators as well as biomedical engineers)
- Cost of associated consumables (especially in case of "closed systems" where one has to use consumables offered by the same manufacturer who is supplying the equipment)
- Post-warranty maintenance cost (including parts and labor)
- Costs associated with disposal of the equipment

Evaluation of Risks

With all investments involving major capital outflows, it is important that the organization evaluates all its risks. These risks relate to the market, technology, human factors, finances, and the fact whether the expectations will be fulfilled or not. In fact, the risks ought to be mitigated as much as possible, and some of them relate to the supplier and are dealt with in detail later in this chapter.

Funding

Once the organization develops an idea of capital costs involved in establishing a new service, potential funding options must be reviewed. These may include up-front investment by the buying organization, leasing or borrowing from external financial institutions, and other funding mechanisms, which may be offered by vendors including deferred payment, payment in installments, or pay-as-you-earn basis. Many "closed" diagnostic equipment are also available on placement (also called reagent/rental) basis whereby the buying organization agrees to purchase consumables from the vendor at an agreed price against free-of-cost placement of equipment as long as it continues to operate the equipment.

In case the organization decides to adopt any funding mechanism involving capital borrowing, interest payments must be included in the TCO calculations while conducting the financial feasibility of the equipment.

Acquisition Follow-Through

Once the decision to purchase is made and all the related approvals received from hospital management, the next steps in the purchase acquisition include:

- Formation of working group
- Site selection
- Request for proposals (RFP)
- Supplier prequalification
- Evaluation of received bids
- Negotiations
- Negotiating risks
- Approvals and sign-offs
- Closing the deal

Formation of Working Group

A preliminary report is made to the appropriate authority for approval and guidance on how to proceed further. Once approval is received, a working group with clearly defined terms of reference and timelines should be formed to formally start the acquisition process. The working group should have representation from users, biomedical engineering, construction, and purchasing departments.

Site Selection

It is important to keep in mind the dynamics of patient flow, adjacencies of other related services, and availability of required utilities while selecting the site for installing any equipment. Moreover, there may be regulatory requirements for certain equipment that the organization must adhere to while designing the facility.

Developing Request for Proposals (RFP)

Development of a complete, clear, and concise RFP is essential in order to get an accurate and comprehensive response from potential vendors. RFP may include the following sections:

- Technical and operational specifications comprehensively defining required performance of the equipment
- Site drawings with dimensions
- Schedule including milestones that must be achieved, including final delivery requirements
- Other terms and conditions
- Any other data requirements such as warranty period and post-warranty maintenance contract costs

Data gathered during technology analysis phase should be extensively used while developing the RFP.

Supplier Prequalification

It is advisable that an objective criterion is established to prequalify an adequate number of suppliers who could be invited to participate in the bidding process. Factors used in the prequalification process could include:

- Technology offered
- Suppliers' background (number of years in business, financial position, market share, etc.)
- Availability of after-sales support including trained engineers
- Previous satisfactory experience of the organization and other users in the region
- Standardization

In order to ensure that the process of acquisition can be carried out in a smooth and transparent manner, the number of prequalified suppliers should be kept at a manageable level. While everyone who could offer the required equipment should not be included, it should be ensured that at least three suppliers are prequalified so that the buying organization can negotiate price and other commercial and contractual terms from a position of strength at later stages of acquisition.

Evaluation of Received Bids

Evaluation of received bids involves the following reviews that can be carried out simultaneously:

Operational Review

Operational review will be carried out by users to ascertain that the offered unit includes necessary hardware and software to fulfill all operational requirements defined in the RFP. Subsequently, a comparative statement of features offered by different vendors should be drawn up. If needed, appropriate weightings can be assigned to each feature depending on their relative importance. This will allow users to prioritize various available options.

If needed, vendors can be asked to facilitate visits to sites where similar equipment are installed. While selecting such sites, it is important to ensure that the installed equipment is in operational condition for at least a few months and has volumes and setup similar to that of the buying organization. While many suppliers may offer to sponsor such visits, the buying organization should be willing to pay for such trips as accepting vendors' sponsorship is likely to compromise negotiation leverage at later stages of the acquisition. Accordingly, such costs should be factored in while finalizing the equipment acquisition budget.

During the review, users should also be able to furnish a list of consumables that will be required to ensure continuity of operations. In case these consumables will be required on an ongoing basis, the user department should initiate necessary protocols to ensure that the organization always keeps adequate stock of these items to ensure continuity of service provision.

Technical Review

While conducting a technical review, biomedical engineers should ensure that the supplier has adequate capability to provide after-sales support and services during the warranty as well as post-warranty periods. Availability of trained engineers and critical spares as well as requisite tools for maintenance and calibration must be checked. Moreover, some thought should also be given at this stage whether the organization would like to outsource the maintenance of the equipment once the warranty of the unit comes to an end. This will help the organization to get agreement from the vendor regarding post-warranty maintenance contract costs and/or comprehensive training of the organization's engineer(s).

Table 108.1 Total cost of ownership (TCO) analysis

Assumptions
Product life
Discount factor/inflation rate for service and consumables
Warranty
Annual post-warranty maintenance contract cost
Annual value of projected consumption of consumables
Capital cost
Cost of equipment
Cost of optional accessories
Freight, duties, and clearance charges
Installation and commissioning charges
Operating cost (net present value [NPV] of each component over the life of equipment)
Cost of consumables projected to be used
Cost of future planned upgrades
Post-warranty maintenance (labor and parts) cost
Cost of utilities and manpower
Total cost of ownership: capital cost + NPV of operating cost over life of the equipment

Here again, biomedical engineering should prepare a comprehensive matrix comparing technical features offered by different vendors and assign weightings to each feature based on their relative importance. Subsequently, order of priority can be assigned to each potential vendor.

This is one of the most important stages of the equipment acquisition process. An equipment with state-of-the-art technical and operational specifications available at a very attractive price but without adequate after-sales support is likely to give perpetual headaches to hospital administrators in the long run. Hence, the organization should be willing to compromise on equipment specifications or pay a little extra to acquire equipment with availability of adequate after-sales support.

To facilitate operational and technical reviews, vendors can be asked to make detailed presentations on their offerings. This will allow users and other technical members to seek clarifications on any query they might have.

Commercial Review

The purchasing department should undertake comprehensive TCO analysis of offers received from prequalified suppliers. Vendors who have been classified as "unacceptable" during operational and technical reviews by users and biomedical engineers can be excluded from this analysis. Moreover, costs that are not likely to change irrespective of which vendor is selected can also be excluded from this analysis as they are not going to influence the supplier selection. Moreover, payment, shipment, and other technical terms should also be taken into account during commercial reviews. A sample matrix for calculating TCO is produced in Table 108.1.

Table 108.2 Technology risks versus mitigation strategies

Risks	Mitigation strategies
Obsolescence due to rapid pace at which technology advances	Include clauses in contract that allows for automatic upgrades (especially software updates) as part of the post-warranty maintenance. In most cases, this will be limited to minor hardware and software updates that can be done in the field. Some companies, however, may allow for major hardware upgrades in factory as well
Risks associated with "new" technology	It is generally preferable to select tried and tested technology in order to avoid risks involved when dealing with new and untried equipment
Ability to retrofit developments in the future	Wherever possible, preference should be given to equipment that is built on a modular design and in which it is easier to retrofit new developments on the same machine. This is likely to be cheaper than replacing an obsolete machine with another costly machine in the future in order to avoid becoming out-of-date due to advancements in technology

Negotiations

Based on the previous reviews, the buyer should, in consultation with users and biomedical engineers, select two to three top vendors for negotiations. In order to obtain maximum value out of negotiation meetings, the buyer must spend an appropriate amount of time in preparation for the same. This involves reviewing strengths and weaknesses of the selected vendors as well as that of the buying organization. This will allow the buyer to systematically evaluate all issues that may have bearing on the outcome of the negotiations. Clear-cut objectives must be set for the negotiation meeting with each of the selected vendors, which may include reduced price, warranty, early delivery, contractual terms, and other items included in the aforementioned TCO analysis.

"Failing to plan" for negotiation is a sure recipe of "planning to fail." Without adequate planning, a negotiation meeting turns into a mere bargaining event where the buying organization negotiates from an extremely weak position due to absence of any negotiation leverage.

It should be noted that throw-ins such as training sponsorships are negotiated once all the commercial aspects are agreed upon by both the parties.

Negotiating Risks

An important part of the negotiations is also to work with the suppliers and ascertain how the risks related to technology could be minimized. Table 108.2 presents some risks in this regard and the related mitigation strategies as well.

Approvals and Sign-Offs

Once the buyer and other members of the negotiation team are satisfied with the outcome of negotiations, necessary documents should be prepared as per institutional policies to seek approval from relevant authorities. It is important that recommendations and their rationale are clearly spelt out in these documents and that each stakeholder physically signs off on these recommendations. In many organizations, decisions involving purchasing of equipment above a certain value are approved by a specially designated high-level purchase committee.

Closing the Deal

Subsequently, a purchase order should be placed and a letter of credit established. For all major equipment, especially ones that require substantial site modifications, it is advisable to prepare a formal contract clearly defining responsibility and timelines for each party during the phase of installation and commissioning.

Conclusions and Recommendations

Acquisition of equipment is a complex process involving multiple stakeholders with each bringing something unique to the table. The entire process is likely to run into several months and, in some cases, more than a year. While efforts can be made to expedite the process, it should be remembered that there are no shortcuts. Missing any of the steps outlined previously will not only compromise the outcome but also the integrity and transparency of the whole exercise, resulting in lack of accountability on the part of relevant stakeholders.

Our advice to all institutions considering investments in major pieces of equipment is to approach the decision scientifically: Marry the program with the strategic plan, do a thorough technology and market analysis and evaluation of risks, and complete a financial feasibility and funding plan. Then follow-through with the formation of a work group that should go through with the detailed steps outlined previously.

It is our view that by meticulously following such a thorough process, the decision, almost inevitably, will be a sound and effective one.

References

1. Khan NM, Dhanani M. Selecting a lithotripter: hospital perspectives. In: Talati J, Sutton RAL, Moazzam F, Ahmed M, editors. The management of lithiasis. Dodrecht: Kluwer Academic Publishers; 1997.
2. Handfield RB, editor. CPSM (certified professional in supply management) study guide 2. Task 2-A-3. Tempe: Institute for Supply Management; 2008. p. 33–6.
3. Ellram LM. Total cost of ownership. The purchasing handbook. 6th ed. New York: McGraw-Hill; 1999.

Comparative Costs of Various Treatment Strategies and Preventive Measures

109

Roswitha Siener and Albrecht Hesse

Abstract

The impact of urolithiasis as an economic factor in health care systems is steadily increasing. Replacement of open surgery with noninvasive and minimally invasive techniques (i.e., ESWL, PCNL, and URS) for the treatment of stones of different sizes and locations has greatly reduced morbidity and the period of hospitalization. Although ESWL, PCNL, and URS are effective treatment options, direct and indirect costs are substantial. Moreover, severe complications and recurrences may occur with varying frequency. Specific metaphylactic measures, including metabolic evaluation, dietary, and drug therapy, have been demonstrated to be cost-effective and efficacious.

Keywords

Urinary calculi • Recurrence rate • Metaphylaxis • Diet • Drug therapy • Metabolic evaluation • Cost analysis • Economics

Introduction

The prevalence and incidence of urinary stone disease worldwide have increased during the last decades. The prevalence of urolithiasis in the Unites States was estimated to be 5.2 % in 1988–1994 [1]. It has been estimated that approximately 12 % of men and 5 % of women in the United States will have at least 1 episode during their lifetimes [2]. The rates of hospital discharge for stone disease have been estimated to 140/100,000 of the population, but as many as 70 % of the patients will not require hospitalization [2]. In Japan, the prevalence was 5.4 % in 1985, compared to 4.0 % in 1975, with the annual incidence of urolithiasis increasing from 53.8/100,000 in 1965 to 92.5/100,000 people in 1985 [3]. In Germany, a marked increase in the prevalence from 4.0 to 4.7 % and a rise in the incidence of stone disease from 0.54 to 1.47 % were observed between 1979 and 2001 [4]. The peak prevalence of first stone episode occurred in both men and women in the 25–49-year age group, i.e., in patients at the most active stages of their careers. The high incidence of urolithiasis of 1.47 % corresponds to approximately 1.2 million stone episodes per year in Germany.

Although more than 40 % of the stones are passed spontaneously, often intervention is required [4]. For patients requiring treatment, various procedures are available. Medical treatment strategies for urolithiasis include dietary measures, drug therapy, and surgical intervention. Noninvasive and minimally invasive treatments, such as extracorporeal shock wave lithotripsy (ESWL) and endourologic procedures ureterorenoscopy (URS) or percutaneous nephrolithotomy (PCNL), are effective treatment options. When compared with PCNL and ureteroscopy, the data on ESWL support the finding that complications occur less frequently with ESWL than with the other two procedures [5]. However, Steinstrasse, an obstructing accumulation of stone fragments or gravel in the ureter, occurs in 4–7 % of cases after ESWL. The relationship between ESWL and hypertension or diabetes is

R. Siener, Ph.D. (✉)
Department of Urology, University Stone Centre, University of Bonn, Sigmund-Freud-Strasse 25, D-53105 Bonn, Germany
e-mail: roswitha.siener@ukb.uni-bonn.de

A. Hesse, Ph.D.
Urinary Stone Analysis Centre Bonn, Theaterplatz 14, D-53177 Bonn, Germany
e-mail: beratung@harnsteinanalysezentrum-bonn.de; albrecht-hesse@web.de

J.J. Talati et al. (eds.), *Urolithiasis*,
DOI 10.1007/978-1-4471-4387-1_109, © Springer-Verlag London 2012

unclear. Published data are contradictory and no conclusion can be attained [5]. The recurrence rate of stone formation was found to be higher after ESWL treatment due to residual fragments or microscopic sand particles that may act as foci for new stone formation [6, 7].

Without appropriate metaphylaxis, many patients have recurrent stones. The recurrence rate of urinary stones is estimated to be up to 40 % [4, 8, 9]. In Germany, about 600,000 stone recurrences occur per year [4]. About 20 % of the patients experience three or more stone episodes during their life [4].

Apart from medical reasons for recurrence prevention, an important consideration in the choice of treatment strategy is cost-effectiveness. Besides routine patient care costs of stone removal, it has to be considered that depending on the applied method, complications are to be expected, which may involve a considerable increase in costs. Moreover, indirect costs such as those associated with lost work time should be taken into consideration. It has been estimated that these expenses would add an additional 15–20 % to the computed costs [10]. Because structures and expenses in the different health care systems vary considerably, cost-effectiveness analyses should be performed for specific countries and practice patterns.

Stone Removal

ESWL

Since its introduction in the 1980s, ESWL has become the most frequently used treatment option for the renal and ureteric stones requiring removal. Although ESWL is the least invasive method of managing stones, other factors must be considered when applying this technique. Stone-free rates for calculi in renal pelvis and upper/middle calices were 56–94 % and 79–85 %, respectively, for ESWL [11]. Therefore, ESWL may require some time before the patient is stone-free, making frequent outpatient assessments and/or re-treatments necessary. For proximal ureteral stones, the stone-free rate of ESWL ranged from 62 to 100 % but was negatively correlated with stone size [11, 12]. Residual fragments after ESWL for ureteric calculi remain a problem as such patients are at risk for complications such as obstruction, hydronephrosis, and urosepsis [13]. These findings indicate that the stone size must be considered to improve cost-effectiveness.

For the United States, the estimated costs of ESWL, URS, and PNL were obtained from the mean cost of >100 cases performed at a large, metropolitan county hospital [14]. In this trial, cost centers included the operating room, operating room supplies, day surgery, recovery room, laboratory costs, and anesthesia along with professional fees. ESWL was assumed to be an outpatient procedure. The total average cost of ESWL was $6,620 (4,598 €). Strohmaier reported for the Klinikum Coburg, Germany, a reimbursement to the hospital for ESWL of 1,394 € [15].

URS

Although most patients require general anesthesia, URS has become an attractive option for ureteric stone removal. The overall rate of complications after URS has been reported to be between 9 and 25 % [5]. Most complications are minor and do not require intervention. Previous perforations of the ureter were found to be the most important risk factor for complications. For all distal stones, URS yields better stone-free rates overall as compared to other methods for active stone removal, independent of stone size.

For the United States, the mean cost of URS, carried out as an outpatient procedure, was $4,773 (3,315 €) [14]. Strohmaier reported for the Klinikum Coburg, Germany, that the reimbursement for URS of kidney stones was 1,532 €, for URS of ureteral stones 1,632 €, and for URS of complicated cases of ureteral stones 2,771 € [15].

The progress in endoscopic stone therapy that followed the introduction of flexible scopes has increased success rates and lowered morbidity. On the other hand, the expenses for flexible ureteroscopes and disposable instrumentation are considerable [15]. Collins et al. assessed the cost for 100 procedures of flexible ureteroscopy including ancillary equipment to 52,130 £ (59,530 €) [16].

PCNL

PCNL, a minimally invasive surgical procedure, is especially suitable for removal of large renal stone volumes. PCNL has replaced open procedures in removing complex urinary calculi almost completely. Rigid and flexible nephroscopes of different sizes have been developed. In the majority of cases, PCNL is performed in the prone position under general anesthesia with the additional cost associated with that type of anesthesia.

Common and significant complications associated with PCNL are systemic inflammatory response syndrome, bleeding, pelvic perforation, and adjacent organ injury. Further complications include fluid overload, hypothermia, inward migration of working sheath, strictures of the collecting system, nephrocutaneous fistula, and mortality [17]. The frequency of major complications was 0.9–4.7 % for septicemia, 0.6–1.4 % for renal hemorrhage requiring intervention, 2.3–3.1 % for pleural injury, and 0.2–0.8 % for colonic injury [18].

The efficacy of PCNL is hardly affected by stone size. A study conducted by Bagrodia et al. revealed that a large stone burden independently predicts higher costs in patients who undergo PCNL despite no associated increase in the complication or transfusion rate [19]. For the United States, the mean costs of PCNL were estimated to $11,530 (8,009 €) [14]. PCNL thereby was considered an inpatient procedure. Strohmaier reported a reimbursement for PCNL between 3,107 € and 4,487 €, with the latter amount for complicated cases [15].

Open and Laparoscopic Surgery for Removal of Renal Stones

Indications for open surgery for renal stones have decreased significantly over the past 20 years. Laparoscopic or open surgical stone removal may be considered in rare cases where ESWL, URS, and percutaneous URS fail or are unlikely to be successful [5]. No figures regarding costs are available for these procedures.

Residual Stones

Residual fragments are commonly seen after both ESWL and sometimes after intracorporeal lithotripsy, and the fragments most frequently are present in the lower calyx [5]. Irrespective of stone composition, 21–59 % of patients with residual stones require another treatment within 5 years. The indication for active stone removal and selection of the procedure is based on the same criteria as for primary stone treatment and also includes repeat ESWL [5]. Active removal of residual fragments will add to costs.

Metabolic Evaluation and Metaphylaxis

Although ESWL is a noninvasive and efficient method for stone therapy, the results of ESWL treatment of some stone locations are sobering. Moreover, the initial assumption that ESWL could lower the costs of stone therapy was soon disproved. Although cost savings of 40–140 million DM (approximately 20–72 million €) have been assumed in Germany, mainly due to a decrease in the length of hospital stay, the usage of ESWL caused additional expenses of 42 million DM (21 million €) already in 1986 largely owing to an increased number of treatment sessions, enlarged indications, and treatment of residual stone fragments [20, 21].

Due to the increasing prevalence and incidence of urolithiasis and predicted changes in climate, a high recurrence rate is expected during the next years [4, 14]. A representative study conducted in Germany revealed a recurrence rate of 600,000 stones per year [4]. More than half of recurrent stone formers experience three or more stone episodes during their life. Interventions that prevent recurrence among stone formers may be a cost-effective component of secondary preventive treatment strategies in a working-age population due to reduction of direct and indirect costs [10].

Table 109.1 Patients at high risk for recurrent stone formation

Highly recurrent stone formation (≥3 stones in 3 years)
Infection stones
Uric acid and urate stones (gout)
Brushite stones
Genetically determined stones
Cystinuria (types A, B, AB)
Primary hyperoxaluria (PH)
Renal tubular acidosis type I
2,8-dihydroxyadenine (APRT deficiency)
Xanthine
Cystic fibrosis
Children and teenagers
Hyperparathyroidism
Gastrointestinal diseases (e.g., Crohn's disease, malabsorption, colitis)
Solitary kidney
Residual stone fragments (3 months after stone therapy)
Nephrocalcinosis
Bilateral vast stone burden
Family history of stone disease

According to [22]

Stone patients at high risk for recurrent stone formation (e.g., patients with residual stones 3 months after stone therapy and patients with cystine, brushite, struvite, uric acid, and urate stones) always require a specific metabolic evaluation and metaphylaxis (Table 109.1) [22]. The evaluation of cost-effectiveness of various medical and surgical treatment options for urolithiasis revealed that medical prevention programs are indicated for individuals with a stone recurrence rate of at least 0.3 per year (corresponding to one stone episode every 3 years) [23]. Accurate analysis of urinary stone composition by infrared spectroscopy or X-ray diffraction is the most crucial laboratory diagnostic procedure for the treatment and recurrence prevention in stone formers and should be performed in each patient [24, 25].

Nolde et al. have demonstrated that specific metabolic evaluation and metaphylaxis can lower the recurrence rate by 46 % [26]. Other investigations confirmed that both dietary [27, 28] and drug therapy are effective in reducing recurrence rates [29–31]. International experience has indicated that the costs of an extensive metabolic evaluation were estimated to be between 250 € and 350 € [33, 34], while the costs of pharmacological therapy were 130 €, 350 €, and 13 € per patient per year [15, 32–34]. For Germany, the annual costs of a simple metabolic evaluation were estimated to about 90 € and the annual expenses for special metaphylaxis 280 € per patient [15]. For highly recurrent stone formers, a comprehensive program for metabolic evaluation is offered at the University Stone Centre, Department of Urology, Bonn University, Germany. The costs of this metabolic program for a patient with urolithiasis are 2,864 €, including analysis of a 7-day dietary record and 24-h urine on individual diet, urinary stone analysis, Bonn Risk Index, ammonium chloride loading test, calcium loading test, [$^{13}C_2$]oxalate absorption test, where appropriate, serum, and 24-h urines during a 12-day hospital stay on standardized dietary conditions [22]. If we assume that at least one to two stones per patient can be prevented, expenses for stone intervention procedures such as ESWL, URS, or PCNL are saved.

Conclusion

The cost-effectiveness of stone metaphylaxis depends on the stone recurrence rate and the efficacy of the recurrence prevention strategy. It has been demonstrated that specific metabolic evaluation and metaphylaxis can lower the recurrence rate significantly. Accurate analysis of urinary stone composition is the most important laboratory diagnostic procedure for the treatment and recurrence prevention in stone formers. In first-time stone formers, dietary measures are cost-effective and efficacious [35]. In recurrent stone formers, additional drug therapy, based on the results of specific metabolic evaluation, may lower cost due to a reduction of recurrence rate. The evaluation of cost-effectiveness of various medical and surgical treatment options for urolithiasis revealed that medical prevention programs are indicated for individuals with a stone recurrence rate of at least 0.3 per year or about once every 3 years, respectively [23]. Repeat surgical interventions are associated with risks and complications. Metabolic evaluation is therefore mandatory in recurrent stone formers.

References

1. Stamatelou KK, Francis ME, Jones CA, Nyberg LM, Curhan GC. Time trends in reported prevalence of kidney stones in the United States: 1976–1994. Kidney Int. 2003;63:1817–23.
2. Resnick MI, Persky L. Summary of the National Institutes of Arthritis, Diabetes, Digestive and Kidney Diseases Conference on Urolithiasis: state of the art and future research needs. J Urol. 1995;153:4–9.
3. Yoshida O, Okada Y. Epidemiology of urolithiasis in Japan: a chronological and geographical study. Urol Int. 1990;45:104–11.
4. Hesse A, Brändle E, Wilbert D, Köhrmann KU, Alken P. Study on the prevalence and incidence of urolithiasis in Germany comparing the years 1979 vs. 2000. Eur Urol. 2003;44:709–13.
5. Türk C, Knoll T, Petrik A, Sarica K, Straub M, Seitz C. Guidelines on urolithiasis. Arnhem: European Association of Urology; 2011.
6. Carr LK, Honey RJD, Jewett MAS, Ibanez D, Ryan M, Bombardier C. New stone formation: a comparison of extracorporeal shock wave lithotripsy and percutaneous nephrolithotomy. J Urol. 1996; 155:1565–7.
7. Streem SB, Yost A, Mascha E. Clinical implications of clinically insignificant stone fragments after extracorporeal shock wave lithotripsy. J Urol. 1996;155:1186–90.
8. Ahlstrand C, Tiselius HG. Recurrences during a 10-year follow-up after first renal stone episode. Urol Res. 1990;18:397–9.
9. Trinchieri A, Ostini F, Nespoli R, Rovera F, Montanari E, Zanetti G. A prospective study of recurrence rate and risk factors for recurrence after a first renal stone. J Urol. 1999;162:27–30.
10. Saigal CS, Joyce G, Timilsina AR. Direct and indirect costs of nephrolithiasis in an employed population: opportunity for disease management? Kidney Int. 2005;68:1808–14.
11. S2-Leitlinien zur Diagnostik, Therapie und Metaphylaxe der Urolithiasis. Teil 1: Diagnostik und Therapie [S2 guidelines on diagnostic, therapy and metaphylaxis of urolithiasis. Part 1: Diagnostic and therapy]. Urologe. 2009;48:917–24.
12. Lingeman JE, Coury TA, Newman DM, Kahnoski RJ, Mertz JHO, Mosbaugh PG, et al. Comparison of results and morbidity of percutaneous nephrostolithotomy and extracorporeal shock wave lithotripsy. J Urol. 1987;138:485–90.
13. Bierkens AF, Hendrikx AJM, de la Rosette JJMCH, Stultiens GNM, Beerlage HP, Arends AJ, et al. Treatment of mid- and lower ureteric calculi: extracorporeal shock-wave lithotripsy vs laser ureteroscopy. A comparison of costs, morbidity and effectiveness. Br J Urol. 1998;81:31–5.
14. Brikowski TH, Lotan Y, Pearle MS. Climate-related increase in the prevalence of urolithiasis in the United States. PNAS. 2008; 105:9841–6.
15. Strohmaier WL. Economic implications of medical and surgical management. In: Rao PN, Preminger GM, Kavanagh JP, editors. Urinary tract stone disease. London: Springer; 2011. p. 245–50.
16. Collins JW, Keeley FX, Timoney A. Cost analysis of flexible ureterorenoscopy. BJU Int. 2004;93:1023–6.
17. Desai M, Symons SJ. Percutaneous nephrolithotomy. In: Rao PN, Preminger GM, Kavanagh JP, editors. Urinary tract stone disease. London: Springer; 2011. p. 481–95.
18. Skolarikos A, de la Rosette J. Prevention and treatment of complications following percutaneous nephrolithotomy. Curr Opin Urol. 2008;18:229–34.
19. Bagrodia A, Gupta A, Raman JD, Bensalah K, Pearle MS. Predictors of cost and clinical outcomes of percutaneous nephrostolithotomy. J Urol. 2009;182:586–90.
20. Bruckenberger E. Beispiel Nierenlithotripter: Ursachen des Kostenbooms. Dtsch Ärztebl. 1988;85:383–4.
21. Strohmaier WL. Economic aspects of evidence-based metaphylaxis. Urologe. 2006;45:1406–9.
22. Hesse A, Tiselius HG, Siener R, Hoppe B. Urinary stones: diagnosis, treatment, and prevention of recurrence. 3rd ed. Basel: Karger; 2009.
23. Chandhoke PS. When is medical prophylaxis cost-effective for recurrent calcium stones? J Urol. 2002;168:937–40.
24. Hesse A, Sanders G. Atlas of infrared spectra for the analysis of urinary concrements. Stuttgart, New York: Thieme; 1988.
25. Hesse A, Kruse R, Geilenkeuser WJ, Schmidt M. Quality control in urinary stone analysis: results of 44 ring trials (1980–2001). Clin Chem Lab Med. 2005;43:298–303.
26. Nolde A, Hesse A, Scharrel O, Vahlensieck W. Modellprogramm zur Nachsorge bei rezidivierenden Harnsteinpatienten (Model program for follow-up of recurrent urinary stone formers). Urologe B. 1993;33:148–54.
27. Borghi L, Meschi T, Amato F, Briganti A, Novarini A, Giannini A. Urinary volume, water and recurrences in idiopathic calcium nephrolithiasis: a 5-year randomized prospective study. J Urol. 1996; 155:839–43.
28. Borghi L, Schianchi T, Meschi T, Guerra A, Allegri F, Maggiore U, et al. Comparison of two diets for the prevention of recurrent stones in idiopathic hypercalciuria. N Engl J Med. 2002;346:77–84.
29. Barcelo P, Wuhl O, Servitge E, Rousaud A, Pak CYC. Randomized double-blind study of potassium citrate in idiopathic hypocitraturic calcium nephrolithiasis. J Urol. 1993;150:1761–4.

30. Ettinger B, Tang A, Citron JT, Livermore B, Williams T. Randomized trial of allopurinol in the prevention of calcium oxalate calculi. N Engl J Med. 1986;315:1386–9.
31. Ohkawa M, Tokunaga S, Nakashima T, Orito M, Hisazumi H. Thiazide treatment for calcium urolithiasis in patients with idiopathic hypercalciuria. Br J Urol. 1992;69:571–6.
32. Hesse A, Nolde A, Scharrel O. Qualitätssicherung mit Diagnostik-Standards und wirtschaftliche Aspekte der Nachsorge bei Urolithiasis (Quality assurance through diagnostic standards and economic aspects of follow-up in urolithiasis). Urologe B. 1993;33:155–9.
33. Parks JH, Coe FL. The financial effects of kidney stone prevention. Kidney Int. 1996;50:1706–12.
34. Robertson WG. Medical management of urinary stone disease. Eur Urol Update Ser. 1998;7:139–44.
35. Lotan YL, Cadeddu JA, Roerhborn CG, Pak CYC, Pearle MS. Cost-effectiveness of medical management strategies for nephrolithiasis. J Urol. 2004;172:2275–81.

Financial Options for Purchase, Lease, and Hire of Lithotripters

110

Faridun K. Dadachanji

Abstract

Loaning and leasing are the two primary methods of financing a lithotripter device. Leasing can be advantageous for tax purposes; however, a deferred payment letter of credit is more commonly used. Paperwork that is required to obtain a business loan includes a business plan, cash flow statements and projections, balance sheets, past business tax returns, and a credit rating report. Loan practices in the United States, United Kingdom, India, and Pakistan are analogous. Pakistan and India however slightly differ from their Western counterparts in several ways. In India and Pakistan, the relationship between the borrowing institution and the credit-extending agency plays a much larger role in whether a loan will be extended or not. In the United States and United Kingdom, on the other hand, a company's previous 2-year cash flows and balance sheets reign supreme in deciding whether a borrowing institution will obtain a loan.

Of all the nations examined (United Kingdom, United States, China, Pakistan, India), China seems to be the most distinct in terms of its loan practices. China is unique as it is a communist country with capitalistic attributes. China's banks are subject to governmental intercession, and loans are determined by fund availability rather than borrower profitability. Although Chinese banks are beginning to be privatized, state-owned Chinese banks lack comprehensive credit risk analysis.

When deciding to lease or loan, an institution must look at the tax implications, loan rates, as well as duration of the payments. It is important to note that medical institutions must carefully look at all the implications of financing options in order to make an informed decision.

Keywords

Lease • Loan • Lithotripter • Borrow • Debt • Equity • Medical • Equipment • Pakistan • Credit

Introduction

Since the onset of the financial crisis, bank and lending practices have changed dramatically. Banks are now more stringent with loan allowances, and financial institutions are making it significantly more difficult to obtain financing on business loans. Debt to equity levels has dropped to what have been historically low levels while even the most creditworthy borrowers are having difficulty receiving loans from credit-extending institutions.

Different lending practices are common among different countries; however, there are a few general "rules of thumb" that all countries' financial institutions abide by. In turn, there are several general factors that determine whether a bank will extend out a loan or not. In this chapter, I will

F.K. Dadachanji, B.A., Economics
Advisory Services, Advanced Equities, First Allied Security,
655 W. Broadway, 12th floor, San Diego, CA 92101, USA
e-mail: fkdadacha@gmail.com; fdadachanji@firstallied.com

J.J. Talati et al. (eds.), *Urolithiasis*,
DOI 10.1007/978-1-4471-4387-1_110, © Springer-Verlag London 2012

define "sponsor" as the institution that is borrowing the money from a credit-extending institution.

Factors Determining Whether a Financial Institution Will Extend a Loan

Credit Risk/Default Risk

Default risk is an investor's risk of loss arising from a borrower who does not make payments as contracted [1]. Risk can be categorized as diversifiable or non-diversifiable. Non-diversifiable risk occurs when the sponsor has no control over whether the business loan will default or not. Factors contributing to non-diversifiable risk include the current (global and domestic) economic, political, and environmental situations.

Diversifiable risk is the risk that the sponsor is capable of mitigating. Factors of diversifiable default risk include the amount of the loan taken by the sponsor, the sponsor's knowledge on the business he or she is running, the resale value of the equipment (for which the business loan is taking out for), the liquidity of the collateral goods given to the leaser, and the reputation of the sponsor taking the lease (this can be measured by a credit score) [2].

Typically, commercial risk will be evaluated by a banker's feasibility study. The analysis will include the threats of new entrants, existing competitors, political influence, supply shock, etc. In the United States and United Kingdom, a banker will complete a cash flow profitability and projection analysis using the balance sheet and cash flows of the sponsor's operations during the previous 2 years. In Pakistan, a chartered accountant is required to audit loans that are greater than ten million rupees.

Timeline

The time frame for which a loan is due also plays a significant role whether a loan is extended or not. Typically, banks will extend out a short-term loan for equipment, for up to 1 or 2 years. The longer the time frame for which the sponsor has to repay the loan, the higher the interest rate [2]. In the United States and United Kingdom, large loans are given in smaller installments. In order to receive all payments of a loan, the sponsor has to display profitability on a monthly basis to confirm an ability to repay the loan. Bankers in the United States and United Kingdom typically use a debt service cover ratio analysis to determine whether an entity is able to repay its loans or not [2]. The debt to service coverage ratio (DSCR) (also known as "debt coverage ratio") is the proportion of cash undertaken for debt servicing on lease payments. It is popularly used as a metric for an entity's ability to produce enough liquidity to cover its debt (including all liabilities such as lease payments). The higher the DSCR ratio is, the easier it is to obtain a loan [2]. The DSCR also displays the minimum ratio that is acceptable to a lender. The DSCR is calculated using the following formula:

DSCR = (Annual Net Income + Amortization/Depreciation + Interest Expense + other non-cash and discretionary items (such as non-contractual management bonuses)) / (Principal Repayment + Interest payments + Lease payments)

A DSCR of less than one indicates that there is a negative cash flow. This means that the sponsor would have to draw onto personal savings every month to keep the undertaking operation afloat. In the United States/United Kingdom, lenders will only give loans to individuals with negative cash flow if the sponsor has strong outside income. In the United States, commercial bankers require a DSCR ratio of approximately 1.35 (previously 1.15 was considered acceptable; however, since the onset of the financial crises of 2008, the value has increased significantly) [3].

How Are Interest Rates Determined by Banks?

There are several factors that banks use when calculating the interest rate of a loan being extended. The first and primary factor is the risk involved. The banker will examine how credible the borrowing institution is (usually calculated using balance sheets, cash flow statements, and credit scores) and whether the sponsor firm has the collateral necessary to borrow the funds. A banker will also analyze any contingency plans that the borrowing institution has. The second factor that determines the interest rate of the loan is the current prime rate. The prime rate is the general interest rate assigned by the government to issue loans. The real interest rate is the rate of interest that takes into account the inflation rate of the nation in question. The nominal interest rate refers to the rate of interest before the adjustment of inflation. It is important to note that when looking at a loan, one should examine the real interest rate rather than the nominal interest rate [2].

Globally, the LIBOR (London Interbank Offered Rate) is used by credit-extending agencies as the gold standard for measuring real interest rates. The LIBOR is the reference rate that London-based banks use to borrow unsecure funds from other banks in the wholesale money market [2]. In other words, the LIBOR is the interest rate at which banks will lend to each other. It is also used as a metric for the "offer amount" for a loan for differing currencies as well as differing time periods.

What Paperwork Is Needed to Obtain a Business Loan?

To obtain a business loan, several documents will be needed to provide to a banker.

A Business Plan

The business plan will be needed to demonstrate why the sponsored institution needs the loan. The business plan should also state through what venues and what sources the sponsored firm will be able to pay back the loan.

Cash Flow Statements and Projections

The cash flow statement will help the banker calculate the revenues and short-term liquidity of the sponsored institution. Typically, bankers will look at the previous 2-year cash flow statements as well as projected future cash flows.

Balance Sheet

This is a statement of the sponsored institutions' personal assets and debts. The lender will view these statements to examine the sponsored institution's financial health.

Past Business Tax Returns

The banker will examine the past 3 years of the sponsored firms' tax returns. This is to verify the profitability of the sponsored institution's operations.

Credit Rating Reports

A credit rating report will display the sponsored institutions loan repayment history. The credit history will be a key determinant in calculating the interest rate of the loan and whether a loan will be extended or not. It is important to note that each country has its own proprietary credit rating system. In order to obtain a loan in the United States, one must have an American credit rating.

A high credit rating is obtained by purchasing items on credit and paying back liabilities in a timely manner. Repayment history plays a major role in establishing one's credit rating.

How Each Country's Loan Practices Differs

Each country has its own nuances regarding loan practices. This chapter examines the lending practices in the United States, United Kingdom, India, Pakistan, and China. Lending practices in the United States, United Kingdom, India, and Pakistan are analogous. Pakistan and India, however, slightly differ from their Western counterparts in some ways. In India and Pakistan, the relationship between the borrowing institution and the credit-extending agency plays a much larger role in determining whether a loan will be extended or not. In the United States and United Kingdom, on the other hand, a company's previous 2-year cash flows and balance sheets reign supreme in deciding whether a borrowing institution will obtain a loan.

Of all the nations examined, China seems to be the most distinct in terms of its lending practices. China has a unique paradigm as it is a communist country with capitalistic attributes. In China, politics play a much larger role in whether an institution will obtain a loan or not. The Chinese government intercedes on loan decisions that Chinese banks make based on political special interests. Although Chinese state banks are becoming more privatized (Chinese state banks have sold a large number of shares to international investors), state-owned Chinese banks continue to lack comprehensive credit risk analysis [4].

Methods of Financing a Lithotripter

There are two primary methods of financing lithotripter devices, namely, by lease or by a deferred payment letter of credit (standard loan). In Pakistan, a deferred payment letter of credit is almost exclusively used to finance lithotripter machines. Pakistani financial institutions will only lend to organizations that have a 40 % minimum stake in the project (meaning that the borrowing organization must have at least 40 % of the long-term debt). It is important to note that in an event of liquidation, senior debts will be paid before any subordinate debt. In Pakistan and other developed countries, loans can also be taken from export credit agencies. Export credit agencies include the World Bank or host governments. A primary advantage of taking from an export agency is that the loan terms will be significantly less costly to the borrowing firm. The primary disadvantage, however, is that the approval procedures are often cumbersome.

Possible Advantages of Leasing Systems in Pakistan

Due to the nature of the Islamic banking system, leasing is the most financially economical way to acquire medical equipment in Pakistan. In Pakistan, both the interest rate and the depreciation of the leased equipment are tax deductible. Depreciation can deduct up to 50 % of the cost of the equipment in the first year alone of the user firms' tax returns. These deductions, however, are only allowed with equipment that is leased out by a Pakistani company. If the company leasing out the equipment is not domestically situated in Pakistan, tax deductions are not permitted.

Conclusion

Lending and leasing are the two primary methods of financing lithotripter devices. When deciding to lease or loan, an institution must look at the tax implications, loan rates, as well as duration of the payments. It is also important to note that medical institutions must carefully look at all the implications of financing options before making an informed decision.

Acknowledgements The author thanks Don Nguyen, banker for Wells Fargo, and Jamshed Kakalia, investment banker.

References

1. Duffie D. Measuring corporate default risk. New York: Oxford University Press; 2011.
2. Tavakoli J. Structured finance and collateralized debt obligations: new developments in cash and synthetic securitization. New York: Wiley Finance Press; 2008.
3. Heffernan S. Modern banking. Chichester: Wiley; 2005.
4. Brown C, Serdar D. The politics of bank failures: evidence from emerging markets. Q J Econ. 2005;120:1413–44.

The Engagement of Philanthropy

111

Shamsh Kassim-Lakha

Abstract

This chapter notes the increasing role of philanthropy in health care and discusses how it can be engaged more effectively to aid the treatment of kidney diseases whose case has not been made strongly enough in the past. It explains that while greater use of technology continues to raise the cost of treatment, partnerships between the state and private resources have softened the impact both in the industrialized and developing countries. This chapter uses the example of Pakistan to illustrate how, even in a low-income country, philanthropy can successfully aid patients with this affliction. Finally, the chapter suggests ways in which philanthropists can be motivated to support this important cause.

Keywords

Aga Khan • Ask • Awareness • Cancer • Cardiac • Charities • Costs • Civil society organizations (CSOs) • Culture • Dialysis • Diseases • Foundations • Fundraising • Health care • Hemodialysis • India • Kidney • Pakistan • Peritoneal • Philanthropy • Religion • Sindh Institute of Urology and Transplantation (SIUT) • Stone • Trust • United States • Urinary • Urolithiasis

Introduction

While philanthropy as we understand it today may have become everyday parlance in the last century, because of the humane work supported by charities and foundations, humankind's diversion of resources to benefit the disadvantaged in society is an age-old practice. Philanthropic groups existed in the ancient civilizations of the Middle East, Greece, and Rome. An endowment supported Plato's Academy (circa 387 BCE) for some 900 years; the Islamic *waqf* (religious endowment) dates to the seventh century CE, and the medieval Christian church administered trusts for benevolent purposes [1]. European merchants in the seventeenth and eighteenth centuries founded organizations for worthy causes. Starting in the late nineteenth century, large personal fortunes led to the creation of private foundations that bequeathed gifts totaling millions and then billions of dollars in support of education, arts, medical research, public policy, social services, environmental causes, and other special interests.

"Philanthropy" is perhaps best defined as "activities of voluntary giving and serving, primarily for the benefit of others beyond one's family" [2]. Philanthropy in the contemporary setting is associated with giving for social causes by non-state individuals and entities.

This chapter notes the increasing role of philanthropy in health care and discusses how it can be engaged more effectively to aid the treatment of kidney diseases whose case has not been made strongly enough in the past. It explains that while greater use of technology continues to raise the cost of treatment, partnerships between the state and private resources have softened the impact both in the industrialized and developing countries. This chapter uses the example of

S. Kassim-Lakha, MBA
Founding President, Aga Khan University and Chairman, Board of Directors of Pakistan Centre for Philanthropy, Islamabad, Pakistan

Aga Khan University,
39B, South Sea View Ave., DHA2, Karachi, Sindh, 75500, Pakistan
e-mail: skassim.lakha@gmail.com

J.J. Talati et al. (eds.), *Urolithiasis*,
DOI 10.1007/978-1-4471-4387-1_111, © Springer-Verlag London 2012

Pakistan to illustrate how, even in a low-income country, philanthropy can successfully aid patients with this affliction. Finally, the chapter suggests ways in which philanthropists can be motivated to support this important cause.

Rising Health-Care Costs Enhance Importance of Philanthropy

Unfortunately, in this age of competing social needs and limited resources, health care has become increasingly expensive, because of its dependence on technology, which advances rapidly with every passing year. Many treatments are now beyond the capacity of average citizens. While the state is often considered primarily responsible for the health care of its citizens, financial constraints of most countries make it difficult, if not impossible, to fulfill this obligation. Even in those industrialized states with reasonable budgets for health care, policy makers have often found it difficult to make equitable allocations between primary, secondary, and tertiary care and between various expensive technology-driven cures such as heart by-pass surgeries and kidney transplants. Citizens and health-care providers in almost every setting have therefore been obliged to look beyond government funding. Consequently, nongovernment sources including charities have gradually become major players in this arena. Anecdotal experience from many countries shows that after giving to religious causes, contributions in support of the sick carry the strongest appeal for donors. In fact, over the last 100 years, philanthropy has provided an exceptionally important source of support for health care including the establishment of facilities for health care and health sciences education. This is as true of the industrialized countries as it is of developing economies.

In its March 2004 report "Update on Foundation Health Policy Grant making," the US-based Foundation Center, which is the world's leading source of information on philanthropy, fundraising, and grant programs, reported that "the number of foundations making health policy grants increased by more than half between 1995 and 2002 and grant dollars more than tripled" [3]. According to the 2009 Million Dollar List™ by the center on philanthropy at Indiana University, more than 80 separate gifts of \$1 million or more were donated to hospitals and health systems in the United States in 2009. A more recent, impressive pacesetting example is the Bill & Melinda Gates Foundation's contribution of US \$1.5 billion in support of the Global Alliance for Vaccines and Immunizations to reach an additional 115 million children in developing countries to help prevent 1.7 million deaths annually [4].

India's giving, which totaled ~\$5 billion in 2006 [5] and constituted 0.2 % of the gross domestic product (GDP), grew to make up between 0.3 and 0.4 % of GDP. Giving for a religious cause far surpassed all other causes [6], and Indian philanthropists made a subtle shift from a previous focus on funding education to a targeting of health as their priority. This shift in private sector spending is occurring at a time when the Indian government too is trying to increase health spending from 1.1 % of gross domestic product to at least 2 % [7].

Over all, it is reasonable to conclude that whereas economic realities of industrialized and developing countries differ significantly, philanthropy is playing an increasingly important role in extending health services to the citizens in both settings. This is notwithstanding the fact that a significant portion of philanthropic giving in industrialized countries tends to focus on research and development of new drugs and degenerative diseases, while in developing countries such benevolence is mostly applied toward subsidizing the treatment of the needy. In fact, philanthropy for health-care support—including the introduction of new, expensive medical technology—becomes even more important in developing countries where weak economic conditions force governments to make difficult choices in how to allocate public expenditures.

Thus, we find that in developing countries financial support for health care has become a partnership between public resources and private philanthropy. This is not novel in the history of many nations. We see evidence of this in the nascent days of American statehood where the nation's first hospital, Pennsylvania Hospital was established in 1751 by Dr. Thomas Bond and Benjamin Franklin, "to care for the sick-poor and insane who were wandering the streets of Philadelphia" [8]. It was funded by both the state assembly and private donors [8, 9]. Later, several other medical institutions were funded by private philanthropy. The most notable examples of this are Johns Hopkins' bequeath of a prestigious hospital and nursing school founded in 1889, followed by a medical school in 1893 and school of hygiene and public health in 1916 [9]. Meanwhile, in 1901, John D. Rockefeller Sr. established the Rockefeller Institute for Medical Research, which was the first medical research institute in the United States [9]. By the dawn of the twentieth century, medicine in the United States was rapidly evolving from a craft and a vocation to a scientific profession. That transition was cemented—and modern medicine was in large part created by interventions from the nation's large philanthropic foundations in the early twentieth century. The Rockefeller Foundation undertook a series of hugely ambitious campaigns to fight killer diseases around the globe, namely, hookworm, yellow fever, and malaria [9].

Interestingly, as noted by the *Forbes* survey of the super rich in 2010 [10], many rapidly growing developing countries are now experiencing similar support from their own philanthropists whose ranks are increasing at a much faster pace than their counterparts in industrialized nations. In Pakistan, for example, donations by public listed companies has increased tenfold in 9 years [11]. It is therefore opportune for these countries to encourage their rich to direct their philanthropy toward those sectors including health care, where the need is huge.

Kidney Diseases and the Engagement of Philanthropy

Having looked at philanthropy as a source of health care support, it is important to note that health care is not a first priority among many philanthropists. Interestingly, charity throughout the world has a strong religious foundation and probably for this reason, faith-related and faith-based themes attract the bulk of philanthropic resources. This is true both across religions and cultures. According to Giving USA, a report compiled annually by the American Association of Fundraising Counsel, health care received only 7 % of the total US $307.75 billion philanthropy generated in the United States in 2009, whereas religious organizations received 33 % of the total pie [12].

Similarly in India, where both public and private investment in the health sector has shown a rising trend in the past few years, the largest portion of philanthropic money in 2002–2003 was directed to religious causes, which accounted for 29 % of giving whereas health was able to attract just 7 % [13]. The position is not very different in Pakistan where, according to the 1999 Aga Khan Development Network commissioned study on "indigenous philanthropy," 94 % of giving is for faith-based or faith-related causes [14].

The challenge thus is twofold, convincing philanthropists to consider health care as an option for giving and more importantly making it a higher priority sector.

With this setting in perspective, we turn to the treatment of urinary diseases, including urolithiasis as a beneficiary of philanthropic giving. In the wide spectrum of noncommunicable but proliferating ailments, poor and rich alike experience medical problems associated with kidneys. The treatment of kidney diseases is both technical and expensive. If not treated properly and in time, most urinary tract ailments have the potential to lead to other medical complications. The treatment of kidney diseases is both technical and complex. Long-term hemodialysis is the most costly treatment option at approximately US $60,000 per year at a center and US $40,000 at home in industrialized countries [15]. It is most cost-effective if used as an interim measure before kidney transplant. Peritoneal dialysis is less expensive but still costs approximately US $20,000 per year [16]. Clearly, dialysis is not a viable long-term solution in places where health budgets are limited. Despite this, dialysis programs proliferate in many middle-income countries of Asia such as Thailand and Turkey and in middle-income countries of Latin America [17]. Surprisingly, such programs are also found in some low-income countries. For example, in 2003, Pakistan had 110 centers with 2,400 patients on hemodialysis; India had 100 centers with 6,000 patients mostly on hemodialysis; and China had 75,000 patients on dialysis [15].

According to WHO, "of the 57 million global deaths in 2008, 36 million, or 63 %, were due to noncommunicable diseases (NCD), principally cardiovascular diseases, diabetes, cancers, and chronic respiratory diseases". Renal failure is an outcome of many NCDs. Importantly, WHO underlines "The delivery of effective NCD interventions is largely determined by the capacity of health-care systems. Gaps in the provision of essential services for NCDs often result in high rates of complications such as heart attacks, strokes, renal disease, etc. This results in catastrophic spending on health care and impoverishment for low-income families" [18], as approximately 15–20 % of persons 40 years of age or older have a reduced estimated glomerular filtration rate (GFR) [19].

In Pakistan, every year more than 150,000 persons suffer from chronic kidney disease, of whom more than 15,000 patients have end-stage renal failure [20]. In such cases, patients have only two options: either a kidney transplant or regular dialysis. Both modes of treatment are very expensive. Patients undergoing dialysis have difficulty maintaining regular employment and have to pay Pakistan Rupees (PKR) 2,000–3,000 ($25–$38 at 2010 US $/PKR parity) for one-time dialysis treatment [20]. As most patients are not in a position to bear the recurring financial burden of long-term dialysis or of a kidney transplant, cultural norms oblige that the resources of the entire extended family be made available, requiring significant adjustment of spending priorities for the other members.

In India and Pakistan, less than 10 % of all patients receive any kind of renal replacement therapy [21]. In most developing countries, government allocations for chronic treatment of kidney disease are quite limited and almost unavailable in support of kidney transplant. However, these very attributes of the disease provide a rather strong case for financial appeals to donors when explaining the desperate helplessness of needy patients. To illustrate this point and to learn from its experience, let us examine the case study of Pakistan, a country of 180 million located in a challenging political and economic neighborhood of the world, with 40 % of its population subsisting below the poverty line.

Philanthropic Partnerships: A Case Study of Pakistan

Despite the poor availability of kidney treatment facilities in Pakistani government hospitals, and perhaps because of this, kidney disease seems to attract larger philanthropic support than many other serious medical conditions. It is encouraging to note that public-spirited citizens and dedicated medical practitioners have been particularly successful in mobilizing both private philanthropy and state funds, collected as Zakat (obligatory Islamic giving), for the treatment of kidney patients.

How was such support mustered? It was quite an uphill task and required two major vectors. The first was galvanizing the spirit of some outstanding, dedicated individuals who established and effectively managed health-care institutions. The second was the fostering of trust. The competence of the leadership of these institutions and trust in them resulted in the unprecedented mobilization of donors. Their generosity has not only helped to establish and expand treatment facilities but also to sustain their ongoing operations—despite significant portions of patients receiving free care. Interestingly, in several cases, the state has also been persuaded by philanthropists and medical leaders in this field to supplement their own resources for the treatment of needy patients. The following examples illustrate this observation and provide insight into how philanthropy has been mustered in support of medical treatment of the needy, kidney patients among them.

The Pakistan Kidney Patients Association (PKPA) a not-for-profit organization commenced operation in 1997 with just two physicians treating approximately 60–70 needy patients daily. In just 14 years, with recurring support from donors, the association now conducts more than 5,000 dialyses free of charge annually. With donor support, the association contributes 25 % toward the treatment of poor patients, while the government of Pakistan, through its *Baitulmaal* (Zakat repository), bears the remaining 75 % [22].

Rehman Foundation, established in 2004 and operating from six cities in Pakistan, provides services to the destitute suffering from chronic renal failure, diabetes, and diseases of the liver. In just 6 years, the center grew from three dialysis machines performing 1,000 procedures per year to nine machines performing more than 35,000 dialysis procedures annually. Nearly 60 % of the annual cost of free treatment is generated through donations from the foundation's directors and from individual philanthropists [20].

The Kidney Center was established in 1985 as an exclusive hospital for kidney patients in Karachi, the industrial and business capital of the country. Of more than 35,000 patients receiving care, 55 % are treated for kidney stones. Most patients are treated for free or are heavily subsidized. To meet its philanthropic objectives, the Kidney Center established a society in 1989 to raise funds in support of free treatment. A Patients' Welfare Association (PWA) was also created in the hospital to mobilize funds for patient welfare. The association's *Istehqaq* certificate is a unique mode for confirming the eligibility of needy patients who are required to fill out a form and get it certified by the chairman of the local Zakat committee—associated with the local municipality. This exercise in verification of the needy and deserving lends reasonable transparency to the system [23].

The Sindh Institute of Urology and Transplantation (SIUT) is an internationally acclaimed institution that provides free medical treatment for kidney and liver diseases as well as cancers. SIUT has developed a model of partnership with the government and the community to fund the needs of poor patients. It depends substantially on contributions from citizens and corporations to provide this free treatment. In 2009, SIUT treated 690,000 patients, performed more than 144,000 dialysis procedures, and carried out 544 renal transplants [24]. No patient is charged any fee, but those who wish to do so voluntarily contribute a donation within their means.

Perhaps the most interesting example is that of the Aga Khan University Hospital (AKUH), Karachi, Pakistan, a tertiary care teaching institution. In 2010, it spent US $5.3 million for the treatment of needy and deserving patients. Of this, AKUH provided US $1.9 million from its own resources while the hospital's fundraising volunteers raised an additional US $3.4 million from citizens and corporations. As a result, the hospital was able to provide treatment for kidney and heart diseases, maternal child care, as well as cancer, including bone marrow transplants. Within the total $3.4 million raised for patient welfare, approximately $2 million was Zakat contributed through voluntary giving by individuals to the Patients Behbud (*welfare*) Society for AKUH. In addition to this, the Aga Khan University and AKUH periodically mount multimillion dollar fundraising campaigns for the support of their academic and patient welfare endowments and for the construction and operation of new physical facilities. One might ask how it was possible to attract this exceptional level of support in a country under great economic hardship and where there is a major deficit of public trust in most institutions. Fundraising volunteers believe this is due to public recognition of AKUH's high quality of care that matches international standards and a genuine trust in the integrity of its founder and its professional management.[1]

One of the most striking features of AKUH's fundraising strategy is to appeal to individual philanthropists and corporations to support large fundraising targets, such as for the construction of the hospital's cancer treatment center. Of the capital cost of more than $6.9 million for this facility, AKUH contributed $2.7 million from its own resources. As it was difficult to identify a single donor who could give the remaining $4.2 million needed, it sought the support of dozens of individual and corporate donors to contribute units of $83,000 each. These donors found an appeal of this size quite manageable, especially as the funds were to be payable over 3 years—the time it took to build the cancer center. This hugely successful approach to fundraising has since been deployed for the hospital's cardiac care unit and the expansion of its emergency room services.[1]

[1] Anecdotal, Dr. Shamsh Kassim-Lakha (Founding President) Aga Khan University.

These case studies in mobilizing philanthropic funds in a developing country are not unique to Pakistan. While such strategies and methods have been tried and tested in industrialized countries, many developing countries are using these and other methods. However, it is important that these strategies are suitably adapted to local needs, cultural sensitivities, and economic circumstances.

What Are the Factors That Motivate Philanthropists?

Having reviewed different ways in which indigenous resources are mobilized in developing countries in support of treatment for kidney and other diseases, it is useful to analyze what motivates potential donors to give. Three factors stand out. The first is the culture of giving in a society. The second relates to what fundraising experts call defining "the case for support" and creating an awareness of the cause, that is to say why a donor should support the appeal, and the different options for supporting a given appeal. The third factor is the trust that donors have in the credibility, integrity, and quality of the institution.

Culture of Giving

It is said that while the quantum of giving may be affected by one's financial position, the act of giving goes beyond one's wallet. This comes as a positive note to the millions requiring medical care in poor countries. This phenomena is illustrated in the Charities Aid Foundation's *The World Giving Index* for 2010, "...the link between the giving of money and happiness is stronger (a coefficient of 0.69) than the link between the giving of money and the GDP of a nation (0.58). It would be reasonable to conclude that giving is more an emotional act than a rational one... The ranking of the countries in the World Giving Index underlines that the countries whose citizens 'give' the most are not necessarily the countries that might have been expected. Based on an average of their giving of money, volunteering, and helping strangers, around half of the 20 most charitable countries might be seen as traditional economic 'powerhouses,' but the other half (countries such as Guinea, Guyana and Turkmenistan) almost certainly would not"[25].

Case for Support

In developing the "case for support" for kidney diseases, it should be recognized that in comparison with such afflictions as cardiac diseases, cancer, and human immunodeficiency virus/acquired immune deficiency syndrome (HIV/AIDs), the impact of kidney diseases is neither as striking nor their cure as dramatic. Consequently, they are not an instinctively attractive proposition for potential donors. Creation of awareness about them and building up of a "kidney diseases constituency" is therefore a most important strategy to focus the attention of philanthropists. This includes the forging of partnerships whose importance is evident from the several Pakistani examples previously cited. Most kidney treatment centers there receive considerable support from philanthropists and the government, as well as private citizens, individually and through the contribution of Zakat. Partnerships where civil society can demonstrate that its endeavors are supplementing government efforts for health care will be better able to access state funds meant for general welfare. In addition, it is important to provide the option of various "gift opportunities" to which donors (of various capacities) can direct their generosity. Such gift opportunities may range from support for the care of a single patient to education of a critical mass of health professionals, to the building of a new facility or introduction of the latest technology.

Trust

It is increasingly recognized that a society's capacity for social investment is closely related to the credibility and effectiveness of philanthropy-receiving institutions. Even in emerging countries where incomes are low and national economies weak, credible institutions have achieved remarkable success in raising charitable funds. It would not be out of place to suggest that a due diligence mechanism for such institutions would greatly enhance their attractiveness to donors. One strikingly successful example of this is the certification of civil society organizations (CSOs) by the Pakistan Center for Philanthropy. In evaluating CSOs that voluntarily offer themselves for certification, the center assesses them on multiple parameters, including programmatic performance and impact on beneficiaries as well as financial and management probity [26]. This process assures in donors that the certified entities as transparent and effective spenders of philanthropic donations. A similar certification regime for CSOs is undertaken by the Philippines Council for NGO Certification for Philanthropy [27].

As a side note, it is interesting that sponsors of charitable causes in developing countries are often quick to appeal to overseas donors among whom the diaspora of a country are the first to be solicited. The propensity of overseas donors to give is often higher, possibly due to a greater ability to give. However, it is important to recognize that the effectiveness of a fund raising campaign is best established by an indigenous donor base, which provides greater credibility and eventually larger support from overseas.

Finally, those wishing to mobilize philanthropic support must recognize that *trust* remains the magic word in any philanthropic interaction—people give and will give more when there is trust between contributors and users of philanthropy. It is a well-known adage in fundraising that "people give to people." The cause is of course important, but the outcome is almost always depends on who does the asking.

While philanthropy can provide an important source of support for the treatment of diseases of the kidney, significant efforts are required to develop a strong "case for support." This would keep the issue alive in front of busy philanthropists who each year are inundated by multiple appeals. No matter who might lead fundraising efforts, there is no doubt that physicians themselves must remain important players in this endeavor. They know the disease and its impact on society and can best articulate the need for redirecting the focus and priority of donors. Equally important, they inspire a strong sense of trust on behalf of the organizations receiving donations. For the same reasons, physicians themselves are particularly well placed to lead the "ask" because society reposes considerable faith in them.

Conclusion

This chapter notes the historic role of philanthropy in health care and how it can be engaged more effectively in aid of kidney diseases, whose case has not been made strongly enough in the past. Whereas economic realities of the industrialized and developing countries differ significantly, philanthropy is playing an increasingly important role in extending health services to the citizens in both settings. Although kidney diseases are debilitating and their treatment expensive, government allocations for chronic treatment in most developing countries are quite limited and almost unavailable in support of kidney transplant. However, these very attributes of the disease provide a strong case for support for appeal to donors. In many emerging economies, philanthropic support has tended to increase in keeping with economic growth, and in several of these countries, support for health care needs has become a partnership between public resources and private philanthropy. The case of Pakistan, a country of 180 million demonstrates how private initiatives have successfully managed to secure the support of philanthropists and government in aid of needy kidney disease patients and new treatment facilities. Three major factors motivate potential donors to give. They are a culture of giving in a society, a well-defined "case for support," and trust in the recipient institution. As to who might lead the effort to access philanthropic support, the author suggests that physicians themselves are among the most important players in this endeavor. They can best articulate the need for redirecting the focus and priority of donors to the support of debilitating kidney afflictions, and they do inspire a strong sense of trust on behalf of organizations receiving philanthropy.

References

1. Philanthropic Foundation. Encyclopedia Britannica, Inc., http://www.britannica.com/EBchecked/topic/455867/philanthropic-foundation. Last accessed on 27 Sept 2011.
2. Payton RL. Philanthropy: voluntary action for the public good. New York: American Council on Education; 1988. p. 32.
3. Lawrence S. Update on Foundation Health Policy Grantmaking. The Foundation Centre. 2004. p. 1–12. http://foundationcenter.org/gainknowledge/research/pdf/update_health_policy.pdf. Last accessed on 27 Sept 2011.
4. Global Alliance for Vaccinations and Immunization, newsletter. 2007. http://www.gavialliance.org/library/news/press-releases/2-007/five-nations-and-the-bill-and-melinda-gates-foundation-launch-advance-market-commitment-for-vaccines/. Last accessed on 27 Sept 2011.
5. Sheth A. State of Indian Philanthropy. http://www.asianphilanthropyforum.org/2010/03/stateofindianphilanthropy.html. Last accessed on 22 Sept 2011.
6. Wharton College at University of Pennsylvania, Today Knowledge @ Wharton – treasure trail: private philanthropy in India proves no match for religious giving. 2011. http://knowledgetoday.wharton.upenn.edu/2011/07/treasure-trail-private-philanthropy-in-india-proves-no-match-for-religious-giving/. Last accessed on 27 Sept 2011.
7. Anecdotal – Surya Prakash Loonker, Catalyst – Social Development Consultants Pvt Ltd. Alaknanda, New Delhi – 110 019, India. www.catalystindia.net.
8. History of Pennsylvania Hospital. In the beginning the story of the creation of the Nation's First Hospital. http://www.uphs.upenn.edu/paharc/features/creation.html. Last accessed on 22 Sept 2011.
9. Keiper A. Medical research is dominated by government and corporate funding. How can philanthropic dollars find a distinctive niche? Philanthropy Roundtable. 2010. http://www.philanthropyroundtable.org/article.asp?article=1617&cat=147. Last accessed on 27 Sept 2011.
10. http://www.forbes.com/2010/03/09/worlds-richest-people-slim-gates-buffett-billionaires-2010-intro.html. Last accessed on 23 Sept 2011.
11. Pakistan Centre for Philanthropy. Corporate philanthropy in Pakistan: survey of public listed companies. 2009. p. ii. http://pcp.org.pk/documents/corporate%20survey%202008.pdf. Last accessed on 23 Sept 2011.
12. Giving Statistics, National Park Service. US Department of the Interior. http://www.nps.gov/partnerships/fundraising_individuals_statistics.htm. Last accessed on 27 Sept 2011.
13. India's Charity Sector. An overview and analytical approach COPOL partners research. 2006. http://www.oneworldtrust.org/csoproject/images/documents/INDA5.pdf. Last accessed on 26 Sept 2011.
14. Aga Khan Development Network. Enhancing indigenous philanthropy for social investment. 1999. http://www.akdn.org/akf_indigenous.asp. Last accessed on 12 Sept 2011.
15. Dirks J, Remuzzi G, Horton S, Schieppati A, Rizvi SAH. Diseases of the kidney and the urinary system. In: Jamison DT, Bremen JT, Measham AR, Alleyne G, Claeson M, Evans DB, et al., editors. Disease control priorities in developing countries. 2nd ed. Washington, D.C.: World Bank Publications; 2006. p. 695–706. Oxford University Press (free full text at http://www.ncbi.nlm.nih.gov/pubmed/21250363. Last accessed on 23 Sept2011).
16. Winkelmayer WC, Weinstein MC, Mittleman MA, Glynn RJ, Pliskin JS. Health economic evaluations: the special case of end-stage renal disease treatment. Medical Decision Making. 2002;22:417–30.
17. Zatz R, Romão Jr JE, Noronha IL. Nephrology in Latin America, with special emphasis on Brazil. Kidney Int. 2003;Suppl 83:S131–4.

18. WHO Non-communicable diseases report. Executive summary. http://www.who.int/nmh/publications/ncd_report_summary_en.pdf. Last accessed on 22 Sept 2011.
19. Jafar TH, Hatcher J, Chaturvedi N, Levey AS. Prevalence of reduced estimated GFR (eGFR) in Indo Asian population. J Am Soc Nephrol. 2005;16:323A. Abstract.
20. Rehman Foundation. http://www.rehmanfoundation.org/intro.php. Last accessed on 26 Sept 2011.
21. Sakhuda V, Sud K. End-stage renal disease in India and Pakistan: Burden of disease and management issues. Kidney Int. 2003;63 Suppl 83:115–8.
22. Report; Pakistan Kidney Patients Association. http://www.pkpa.org.pk/index.html. Last accessed on 26 Sept 2011.
23. The Kidney Center. http://www.kidneycentre.com/patient-welfare-department.html. Last accessed on 23 Sept 2011.
24. Sindh Institute of Urology and Transplantation. http://www.siut.org/services/statistics. Last accessed on 27 Sept 2011.
25. Charities Aid Foundation. The world giving index. 2010. https://www.cafonline.org/pdf/WorldGivingIndex28092010Print.pdf. Last accessed on 27 Sept 2011.
26. Pakistan Centre for Philanthropy. www.pcp.org.pk. Last accessed on 27 Sept 2011.
27. Phillipine Council for NGO Certification. http://www.pcnc.com.ph/. Last accessed on 27 Sept 2011.

The Impact on Health Care of the Recent Global Epidemiological Trends in Urolithiasis

112

Alberto Trinchieri

Abstract

Urolithiasis had previously been endemic, due to a condition of malnutrition, with prevalent localization in the bladder and composition of ammonium urate and calcium oxalate. Over the years, this type of stone disease has been gradually disappearing in western countries to be replaced by stones of the urinary upper tract, consisting of oxalate and/or calcium phosphate and typical of adulthood.

A trend toward globalization of urinary upper tract stone disease has been recently observed, probably as a result of the rapid economic development in many regions of the world. In some developing countries (Eastern Europe, India, China, Brazil, South Africa), the incidence of stone disease is still increasing, and it could reach higher peaks as a consequence of hot climate in some geographical areas. This increase of incidence of renal stones will have a relevant impact on health-care systems.

Assessing the economic cost of urinary stone disease is very complex because it must take into account the incidence of stone episodes, the direct cost of treatment of each episode and the indirect cost in terms of loss of work, the cost of treating complications, and finally the cost of preventing recurrence. Although the care of individuals with urolithiasis has shifted from the inpatient to the outpatient setting and the hospital length of stay has decreased, however, the social cost for managing stone disease will still increase due to the further increase of costs for diagnosing and treating each single stone episode.

Keywords

Urinary calculi • Incidence • Economics • Costs • Global epidemiology

Introduction

Assessing the economic cost of urinary stone disease is very complex because it must take into account the annual number of stone episodes (incidence), the direct cost of treatment of each episode and the indirect cost in terms of loss of work, the cost of treating complications, and finally the cost of preventing recurrence.

A. Trinchieri, M.D., FEBU
Department of Urology, A. Manzoni Hospital,
Via Dell'Eremo 9/11, Lecco, 23900, Italy
e-mail: a.trinchieri@ospedale.lecco.it

These parameters vary locally and over the years in each country in relation to the changes in the epidemiology of the disease and the evolution of the procedures used for its diagnosis and treatment.

Incidence

In epidemiological terms, the most important aspect observed in recent years is the trend toward globalization of the disease, probably as a result of the rapid economic development in many regions of the world [1–3].

Since the beginning of the past century, a trend of gradual increase of the disease had been described. The urolithiasis

J.J. Talati et al. (eds.), *Urolithiasis*,
DOI 10.1007/978-1-4471-4387-1_112, © Springer-Verlag London 2012

had previously been endemic with prevalent localization in the bladder and composition of ammonium urate and calcium oxalate. Over the years, this type of stone disease, due to a condition of malnutrition, was gradually disappearing to be replaced by stones of the urinary upper tract, consisting of oxalate and/or calcium phosphate and typical of adulthood.

This epidemiological trend was first described in Scandinavia, and then spread gradually in the United Kingdom and Central and Southern Europe, and lately in the countries of Eastern Europe. A similar trend was observed in North America, Japan, and Australia.

At the beginning of the new century, the spread of the disease had taken on global dimensions, affecting large areas of Asia, North Africa, and South America, where previously the disease had less frequently been described.

However, there are still some regions, particularly in Sub-Saharan Africa, where urolithiasis is still rarely observed, and regions in Asia where the endemic pediatric vesical stones still occur with some frequency.

These variations in the incidence of the disease are related to the change in lifestyle and, most likely, dietary habits but also to the improvement of health care that allows more frequent diagnosis of stones that would have been kept unrecognized or not subjected to active treatment.

Variations in the incidence of the disease are also associated to changes in its clinical presentation with the gradual disappearance of ammonium urate/calcium oxalate bladder stones associated to a progressive increase of calcium renoureteral stones. The incidence of infection stones is instead decreased as a result of health improvements in terms of improved diagnosis and treatment of urinary tract infections.

As a result of these changes, especially in western countries, the size of the stones treated was reduced, not only for the disappearance of large staghorn stones, but also as consequence of earlier diagnosis of the stones. In addition, there is a tendency to treat actively stones of smaller size that previously were followed conservatively until spontaneous expulsion. This tendency to treat smaller stones often originated by the choice of the patient who wants to avoid the suffering during the spontaneous passage of the stone along the ureter and the consequent loss of working activity with consequent missed days at work.

In short, in western countries, very frequent stones of smaller size mainly composed of calcium oxalate and uric acid are now seen, while in more recently developed countries, larger stones are still observed, as demonstrated by the report of large series of stones treated with percutaneous or laparoscopic surgery from these regions.

Emergency Treatment

Renal colic is a common emergency department (ED) presentation, and trend data indicate that the volume of visits for renal colic is still increasing during the last years.

ED visits with a primary diagnosis of renal calculus or colic represent an approximate rate of 1 % [4–6]. On this basis, an annual number of more than one million ambulatory care visits to hospital EDs for renal colic in the United States could be estimated.

Most patients in the United States are managed on an outpatient basis and ED visits end in hospital admission in fewer than 13 % of cases [5], but there is more variability worldwide with respect to the type of ancillary testing offered to patients with renal colic and especially to the percent admitted to the hospital. The severity of the pain symptom and the fear for potential renal damage is a possible explanation for the relatively high rate of hospitalization observed.

In a study by Lotan et al. [7] on ED costs of treatment modalities in ten countries in Europe and America, the costs ranged from US $80 to $750.

Protocols for emergency work-up of patients presenting with a renal colic attack are different in any institution. Emergency visit can consist in a simple physical examination with prescription or administration of analgesic treatment or imply a complete diagnostic evaluation including lab testing, renal ultrasound, or X-ray. As a consequence, the estimated cost of the emergency room visit for a stone episode could range from $30 to $400 in different countries [8].

The reason for this difference can be also related to possible regional variations of the nature of the disease.

Radiological investigations are the greatest contributors in the ED costs (40.5 %) followed by treatment costs (19.7 %). Size and location of the stone were independent variables affecting the costs. Renal stones caused lower costs compared to ureteral stones, and ureteral stones larger than 5 mm augmented costs due to the longer time to achieve pain control and a tendency to cause more severe obstruction or hydronephrosis [9].

More investigations and a more severe pain were associated with stones equal to and larger than 6 mm and stones situated in middle ureter [10].

A number of studies have shown unenhanced computed tomography (CT) to be superior to intravenous pyelography (IVP) in the diagnosis of renal colic. Unenhanced CT has a sensitivity of approximately 97 % and specificity of 98 % compared to IVP with 69 and 94 %, respectively [11].

It is a common opinion that unenhanced CT scan is the more expensive study and that the tendency to employ unenhanced CT as the first choice radiological investigation for renal colic would augment costs in the ED.

Chandoke et al. [8] reported an estimated cost for unenhanced CT ranging from $50 to $686 in different countries. Non-contrast CT was estimated more expensive than IVP ($256 vs. $92 respectively), although the cost of IVP rises to $240 when nonionic contrast was used [12, 13].

However, CT scan ordered as the initial diagnostic modality reduces the need for further imaging and consultation, total time spent in the hospital, and inappropriate admissions. This leads to an overall reduction in health-care cost, despite the difference between each imaging study. In a study in patients with renal colic, unenhanced CT saved the hospital $265,000 every 6 months compared to the use of IVU by savings outside the radiology department [14].

The combination of plain film and ultrasound remains an alternative to unenhanced CT with a lower sensitivity but a lower radiation dose that still has a good practical value and helps to yield significant cut-off in the expenditure.

Plain film radiography in combination with ultrasound has shown a sensitivity of 77–79 % and specificity of 90–92.7 % for stone detection and greater than 90 % sensitivity and specificity for the detection of urinary tract obstruction [15, 16].

Observation is the least costly treatment strategy for ureteral stones.

The use of pharmacological medical expulsive therapy (MET), including the use of alpha-adrenergic antagonists or calcium channel blockers in combination with corticosteroids, may increase the likelihood of spontaneous passage of ureteral stones. A meta-analysis of nine trials demonstrated that patients given alpha-adrenergic antagonists or calcium channel blockers had a 65 % greater likelihood of stone passage than those not given such treatment [17].

MET is a cost-effective strategy for the management of distal ureteral stones, even those with a low rate of spontaneous passage. A survey demonstrated that MET maintained its cost advantage even in countries where the cost of ureterorenoscopy (URS) is much lower than in the United States [18].

Treatment Costs

Due to the high incidence of stone disease, active treatment is required for a large percentage of patients with urinary stones. In the United States, about 4 out of 1,000 population required surgery for stone disease (54 % shock wave lithotripsy, 41–42 % ureterorenoscopy, 4–6 % percutaneous nephrolithotomy) [19].

The reported costs of surgical management of stones vary in consideration of the method applied for estimating costs: billing charges, evaluation of institutional costs, or reimbursement by national health care or maximal insurance reimbursement.

An international survey [8] reported highly variable costs in ten different countries. In Europe, costs for shock wave lithotripsy (SWL) and ureterorenoscopy (URS) ranged $360 to 2,740 (mean $1,311) and $160 to $1,900 (mean $1,154), respectively, whereas the costs estimated in the United States were much higher ($9,924 and $8,108 for SWL and URS respectively) and in Canada lower ($750 for both SWL and URS). Finally, costs in Japan and Turkey were $2,490 and $373 for SWL and $1,527 and $491 for URS, respectively.

Accordingly to these huge variations, comparisons of the costs of the different methods of stone treatment seem to be reliable only within the institution in which they were computed and their extrapolation to a broader context is difficult due to the lack of reproducibility of the evaluation. It was a general consensus that the SWL was more costly than endoscopic procedures [20].

Among surgical options for ureteral stones at all locations, URS was evaluated less costly than SWL.

Percutaneous nephrostolithotomy resulted in being more cost-effective than SWL only for renal stones greater than 2 cm in any dimension, while SWL may be cost-effective for smaller stones.

The high cost of purchasing and maintaining a lithotripter is responsible for the high treatment cost associated with SWL. In more recent years, the evolution of the technology of lithotripsy led manufacturers to produce more manageable equipments that do not require the use of anesthesia, are small, easily transportable, and less expensive. On the other hand, this technological change has reduced the effectiveness of lithotripsy, in comparison to first-generation lithotripters, with the need for multiple treatments. Conversely, the endoscopic instrumentation has improved with the production of instruments of smaller caliber, semirigid or flexible, better vision, operating channels of greater diameter, and improvement of accessories for lithotripsy and retrieval of the fragments. These characteristics make intracorporeal lithotripsy more competitive, even for stones of the upper ureter and of kidney stones. The growing use of flexible instrumentation, however, affects the costs for the acquisition and maintenance of instruments and the increased consumption of disposable accessories. Endoscopic techniques still maintain the disadvantage of the need for anesthesia but have the advantage of a more rapid resolution of the disease.

On this basis, the cost-benefit should be reassessed because the costs for the SWL may have become more favorable and SWL may be more expensive just in case of repeated treatments for the same stone.

On the other hand, the evaluations acquired in western countries may not be applicable in other health systems. In fact, in many countries, large stones are still very frequent, as demonstrated by several series of percutaneous nephrolithotomies for large kidney stones reported from Iran, Egypt, India, and other Asian countries. Endourologic treatments are rapidly spreading in those countries where these procedures were also optimized in order to minimize the cost in terms of equipment and disposable accessories.

Finally, in many countries, open surgery is still a very common option that has an alternative laparoscopic (rather than endourological) approach.

Follow-up and Prevention

The cost effectiveness of medical prophylaxis is controversial.

Parks and Coe [21] estimated that medical stone prevention could result in an average saving of 2,158 ±500 USD/patient/year. This figure was derived from the savings in medical costs (from not needing to treat a patient with stone) of USD 3,226/patient minus an expected expenditure of USD 1,068/patient on yearly drugs and testing in stone prevention regimes.

Some authors calculated the various stone recurrence rates at which medical prophylaxis becomes cost-effective. Chandoke et al. [8] calculated 0.32 stone episodes/years, the lowest stone recurrence rate at which medical prophylaxis become cost-effective, whereas we [22] previously reported that pharmacological prevention is cost-effective only for patients with a recurrence rate >0.5 stone episodes/year/patient. Tiselius calculated an annual saving of 1,875 euro/year/patient for patients with an annual stone rate of 0.2 [23].

Also Strohmaier and Robertson demonstrated that medical management of recurrent stone formers could be cost-effective [24, 25].

In first-time stone formers, conservative therapy (dietary measures alone) demonstrated to be cost-effective and efficacious, whereas in recurrent stone formers, it is unsatisfactory despite its low cost because of a high recurrence rate. In fact, drug treatment strategies are more costly than conservative treatment ($885 to $1,187 vs. $258 yearly) but decrease recurrence rates by 60–86 % [26].

Complications and Outcomes

In past years, conservatively treated infection stone disease was associated with a mortality rate of 28–30 % [27, 28]. Chronic renal insufficiency was a relatively frequent complication of infection stones and metabolic stones associated with cystinuria, oxalosis, and renal tubular acidosis. It was estimated that end term renal failure of 1.4–2.5 % of patients on dialytic treatment has been caused by infection stones [29, 30].

The improvement of medical and surgical treatment of renal stones and particularly the application of newer endoscopic and extracorporeal treatments reduced the risk of chronic renal insufficiency associated with stone disease, although in less developed countries or in people who cannot afford appropriate medical treatment, the risk of developing chronic renal insufficiency secondary to infection staghorn stones still persists [31].

The individual and social cost of dialitic treatment or of transplantation for such patients should be included when computing the costs of renal stone disease.

Conclusion

The increase of incidence of renal stones will have different impact on health-care systems of different countries. In Scandinavia and North America, the peak of incidence was reached in 1980s, while in other European or non-European (Australia, Japan, Korea, Taiwan, Saudi Arabia), about 10–20 years after.

Although the care of individuals with urolithiasis has shifted from the inpatient to the outpatient setting and the hospital length of stay has decreased, however, the social cost for managing stone disease will still increase due to the further increase of costs for diagnosing and treating each single stone episode. For this reason, the actual objective should be to optimize protocols avoiding redundant or expensive diagnostic procedures or inappropriate treatments.

In other developing countries (Eastern Europe, India, China, Brazil, South Africa), the incidence of stone disease is still increasing, and it could reach peaks even higher as a consequence of hot climate in some geographical areas. In those countries, the demand for treatment of symptomatic stones could dramatically increase involving a huge financial outlay.

Educational campaigns with the intent of modifying dietary habits in order to prevent stone formation could be a way for reducing the economic impact of the disease on our health-care systems.

References

1. Trinchieri A. Epidemiology of urolithiasis. Arch Ital Urol Androl. 1996;68:203–50.
2. Trinchieri A, Coppi F, Montanari E, Del Nero A, Zanetti G, Pisani E. Increase in the prevalence of symptomatic upper urinary tract stones during the last ten years. Eur Urol. 2000;37:23–5.
3. Trinchieri A, Curhan G, Karlsen S, Wu JK. Epidemiology. In: Segura J, Conort P, Khoury S, Pak C, Preminger GM, Tolley D, editors. Stone disease – 1st international consultation on stone disease. Editions 21. Paris; 2003.
4. Caballero Alcantara J, Padilla Leon M, Marchal Escalona C, Garcia Penit J. Changes in frequency of external office visits for diseases. Analysis of trends in 6 years. Actas Urol Esp. 2004;28:95–100.
5. Brown J. Diagnostic and treatment patterns for renal colic in US emergency departments. Int Urol Nephrol. 2006;38:87–92.
6. Trinchieri A, Cappoli S, Esposito N, Acquati P. Epidemiology of renal colic in a district general hospital. Arch Ital Urol Androl. 2008;80(1):1–4.
7. Lotan Y, Cadeddu JA, Pearle MS. International comparison of cost effectiveness of medical management strategies for nephrolithiasis. Urol Res. 2005;33:223–30.

8. Chandoke PS, Honey RJDA, Mardis H, Montanari E, Munch L. Economics. In: Segura J, Conort P, Khoury S, Pak C, Preminger GM, Tolley D, editors. Stone disease – 1st international consultation on stone disease. Editions 21. Paris; 2003.
9. Turkcuer I, Serinken M, Karcioglu O, Zencir M, Keysan MK. Hospital cost analysis of management of patients with renal colic in the emergency department. Urol Res. 2010;38:29–33.
10. Papa L, Stiell IG, Wells GA, Ball I, Battram E, Mahoney JE. Predicting intervention in renal colic patients after emergency department evaluation. CJEM. 2005;72:78–86.
11. Worster A, Preyra I, Weaver B, Haines T. The accuracy of noncontrast helical computed tomography versus intravenous pyelography in the diagnosis of suspected acute urolithiasis. Ann Emerg Med. 2002;40:280–6.
12. Mill OF, Rineer SK, Reichard SR, Buckley RG, Donovan MS, Graham IR, et al. Prospective comparison of unenhanced spiral computed tomography and intravenous urogram in the evaluation of acute flank pain. Urology. 1998;52:982–7.
13. Li J, Kennedy D, Levine M, Kumar A, Mullen J. Absent hematuria and expensive computerized tomography: case characteristics of emergency urolithiasis. J Urol. 2001;165:782–4.
14. Lauritsen J, Andersen JR, Nordling J, Thomsen HS. Unenhanced computed tomography in acute renal colic reduces cost outside radiology department. Acta Radiol. 2008;49(10):1182–6.
15. Shokier AA, Abdulmaaboud M. Prospective comparison on nonenhanced helical computerized tomography and Doppler ultrasonography for the diagnosis of renal colic. J Urol. 2001;165:1082–4.
16. Morales M. Suspected ureteral colic: plain film radiography and sonography vs unenhanced helical CT – a prospective study in 66 patients. Eur Radiol. 2004;14:129–36.
17. Hollingsworth JM, Rogers MA, Kaufman SR, Bradford TJ, Saint S, Wei JT, et al. Medical therapy to facilitate urinary stone passage: a meta-analysis. Lancet. 2006;368(9542):1171–9.
18. Bensalah K, Pearle M, Lotan Y. Cost-effectiveness of medical expulsive therapy using alpha-blockers for the treatment of distal ureteral stones. Eur Urol. 2008;53:411–8.
19. Pearle MS, Calhoun EA, Curhan GC. Urologic diseases of America Project. Urologic diseases in America project: urolithiasis. J Urol. 2005;173:848–57.
20. Chandoke PS, DeAntoni E. Cost-effectiveness analysis: application to endourology. J Endourol. 1998;12:485–91.
21. Parks JH, Coe FL. The financial effects of kidney stone prevention. Kidney Int. 1996;50:1706–12.
22. Pisani E, Trinchieri A, Mandressi A, Luongo P, Zaatar A, Longo G. New guidelines for the prevention of renal stone recurrence. In: Giuliani L, Puppo P, editors. Controversies on the management of urinary stones international course, Genoa 1987. Basel: Karger; 1988. p. 213–8.
23. Tiselius HG. Comprehensive metabolic evaluation of stone formers is cist effective. In: Rodgers AL, Hibbert BE, Hess B, Khan SR, Preminger GM, editors. Urolithiasis 2000: proceedings 9th international symposium on urolithiasis. Cape Town: University of Cape Town; 2000. p. 349–55.
24. Strohmaier WL. Economic aspects of urolithiasis and metaphylaxis in Germany. In: Rodgers AL, Hibbert BE, Hess B, Khan SR, Preminger GM, editors. Urolithiasis 2000: proceedings 9th international symposium on urolithiasis. Cape Town: University of Cape Town; 2000. p. 406–9.
25. Robertson WG. Medical management of urinary stone disease. EBU Update Ser. 1998;7:139–44.
26. Lotan Y, Cadeddu JA, Roerhborn CG, Pak CY, Pearle MS. Cost-effectiveness of medical management strategies for nephrolithiasis. J Urol. 2004;172:2275–81.
27. Blandy JP, Singh M. The case for a more aggressive approach to staghorn stones. J Urol. 1976;115:505.
28. Rous SN, Turner WR. Retrospective study of 95 patients with staghorn calculus disease. J Urol. 1977; 18:902.
29. Mebel M, Brien G, Bick C, Gremske D, Fahlenkamp D, Eger E. Results of surgical and conservative therapy on patients with nephrolithiasis and chronic renal insufficiency. Eur Urol. 1982; 8:150.
30. Holmgren K, Danielson BG, Fellstrom B. Infection-induced urinary calculi and renal failure. Scand J Urol Nephrol. 1987;21:219.
31. Sitprija V. Nephrology in South East Asia: fact and concept. Kidney Int. 2003;83:S128–30.

113 Societal Changes and the Etiology of Stone Disease

Dorit E. Zilberman, Tyler Luthringer, Daniel Young and David M. Albala

Abstract

Significant advances have taken place in medicine over the past century. In addition, increasing rates of obesity, diabetes mellitus, and metabolic syndrome have resulted in increasing rates of stones among men and women. Within 1 year of forming a calcium oxalate stone, 10 % of men will form another calcium oxalate stone, and 50 % will form another stone within 10 years.

Males are affected three times as frequently as females for stones. Testosterone clearly has an impact on this; however, the rates of nephrolithiasis among women are increasing. Urine studies have demonstrated a decrease in urinary pH (>5.5) and an increase in uric acid supersaturation. This has resulted in increased rates of uric acid stones. In addition, obesity surgery has increased the risk of calcium oxalate stone formation.

All of these factors combined have had a profound influence on the patterns of stone disease. Lifestyles have significantly affected the prevalence of kidney stone disease. In this chapter, we will review the impact of societal changes on stone patterns.

Keywords

Metabolic syndrome • Stone formation rates • Obesity surgery • Urolithiasis

Introduction

Momentous advances in the field of medicine have taken place over the past century. The discovery of penicillin, other pharmaceutical and technological advancements that have followed, and the ongoing growth of our medical knowledge have continuously extended life expectancy throughout society. These progressions have set the ground for a rapid expansion of the world's population, which has nearly tripled from 2.5 to approximately seven billion in the past 50 years. This swift growth has created an increasing demand and need for more food sources, consequently leading to both the development and consumption of greater amounts of canned and processed products. These products, which are both cheap and easy to produce in large quantities, are inherently less healthy than their non-processed alternatives. Although the caloric and salt content of most of today's food has increased tremendously, there has been no downsizing of meals to compensate. In addition, advances in computer and communications technology have piloted individuals of both genders toward a more sedentary lifestyle, diminishing the amount of daily physical activity for the average individual. The combination of this inactivity level and larger, less healthy diets has spurred an increasing prevalence of metabolic syndrome—namely, obesity, hypertension, and type II diabetes—across the world. This chapter will consider the

D.E. Zilberman, M.D.
Department of Urology, Chaim Sheba Medical Center, Tel-Hashomaer, Ramat Gan 52621, Israel
e-mail: dorit1e@yahoo.com

T. Luthringer, B.A. • D.M. Albala, M.D. (✉)
Division of Urology, Associated Medical Professionals, 1226, East Water Street, Syracuse, NY 13104, USA
e-mail: tluthringer@ampofny.com; dalbala@ampofny.com

D. Young, M.D.
Division of Urology, Duke University Medical Center, 200 Trent Drive, Durham, NC, USA
e-mail: daniel.young@duke.edu

J.J. Talati et al. (eds.), *Urolithiasis*,
DOI 10.1007/978-1-4471-4387-1_113,

growing incidence of nephrolithiasis in the global population and how worldwide changes in lifestyle are heavily correlated with origin of this disease.

Rising Numbers

Numerically speaking, more than 346 million people worldwide had diabetes in 2011, and this number is likely to more than double by 2030 [1]. In 2008, approximately 1.5 billion adults aged 20 years and older—who together comprise more than 20 % of the worldwide population—were overweight (i.e., Body Mass Index [BMI] ≥ 25), and at least 500 million of them were obese (i.e., BMI ≥ 30). Since 1980, international obesity has more than doubled; current trends suggest that 2.3 billion adults will be overweight before 2015, while more than 700 million will be obese [2]. In similar fashion, hypertension is currently estimated to affect one billion people across the globe, but that number is predicted to continue to rise to 1.5 billion in the next 15 years [3].

Each of these aforementioned trends, all of which are attributable to lifestyle changes in society, has been found to influence patterns of stone disease. In particular, these new standards of living have led to a rising prevalence of nephrolithiasis, as well as alterations in its societal distribution.

Scales et al. [4] reviewed the Nationwide Inpatient Samples (NIS) database to examine changes in the prevalence of stone disease in the United States over the 5-year period from 1997 to 2002. The investigators showed that the total number of hospital discharges for stone disease had increased by 5.7 % throughout that time. Similarly, the quantity of hospitalizations for renal calculi has also increased by almost 20 %. Stratifying their results by sex revealed that female discharges increased by 22 %, whereas male discharges did not change significantly over the 5-year period.

These alterations have decreased the male-to-female ratio of treated stone diseases from 1.7:1 to a ratio of 1.3:1. Scales and his colleagues attributed this shift to global changes in lifestyle that have been associated with rising rates of overweight and obese individuals since 1960, which have apparently been more prominent in women than in men.

Obesity

The association between nephrolithiasis and weight gain, BMI, and waist circumference was well established by a recent large prospective study [5] that reviewed three large cohorts:

1. Health Professional Follow-up Study (HPFS) that consisted of 51,529 male dentists, osteopathic physicians, pharmacists, podiatrists, and veterinarians between the ages of 40 and 75 years, who in 1986 completed and returned a questionnaire regarding diet, medical history, and medications.
2. Nurses' Health Study (NHS) I that included 121,700 female registered nurses aged 30–55 years who completed the questionnaire in 1976.
3. Nurses' Health Study (NHS) II that included 116,671 female registered nurses aged 25–42 years who completed the questionnaire in 1989.

The investigators excluded those participants who had a baseline history of kidney stone disease from the analysis. In these studies, participants reported the presence of kidney stones on a 2-year interval, and the database was updated regularly regarding any changes in the medical status of the subjects—a total of 4,827 incidents of kidney stones were reported overall in a combined 46 years of follow-up.

All three cohorts revealed that greater weight was associated with an increased risk of kidney stone formation. The relative risk (RR) for men weighing more than 100 kg compared with men weighing less than 68.2 kg was 1.44. In a similar comparison for older and younger women, the RR for these overweight categories were 1.89 and 1.92, respectively. Weight gain, occurring in early adulthood, was also associated with increased risk of kidney stone formation across both genders. The RR for men who gained more than 15.9 kg compared to those who did not was 1.39. In the same category of weight gain, the RR were 1.7 and 1.82 for old and young women, respectively.

Both waist circumference and BMI were also positively correlated with a greater risk of renal lithiasis. The RR for men with a waist circumference of more than 109.2 cm compared with that of less than 86.4 cm was 1.48. For waist circumferences of more than 101.6 cm versus less than 78.7 cm in older and younger women, the RR were 1.71 and 1.94, respectively. Regarding BMI, the RR in men with a BMI of at least 30 compared with that of 21–22.9 was 1.33. While in older and younger women, the corresponding RR were 1.9 and 2.09, which respectively increased to 2.27 and 2.28 when comparing BMI of at least 35 to BMI of 21–23. All of these indicators of obesity proved to be significant risk factors for the development of stone disease. Furthermore and of important consideration, the magnitude of this increased risk may be greater for the female population.

Urinary Composition and Nephrolithiasis

In a subsequent analysis, the investigators examined the same three cohorts for a possible relationship between body size and 24-h urine sample composition [6]. Twenty-four-hour urine samples from participants with a history of kidney stones and randomly selected controls were collected in two cycles. The examined group consisted of 2,176 white stone formers and 1,097 white non-stone formers overall. The analysis showed BMI to be positively associated with urinary oxalate, uric acid, sodium, and phosphate excretion in each of the three cohorts. Moreover, the relative urinary supersaturation of uric acid increased with greater BMI. Inversely, urinary pH decreased as BMI rose.

In female stone formers, a positive correlation was seen between BMI and both urinary potassium and citrate excretion. An association between increasing BMI and urinary calcium excretion was additionally observed in stone-forming men and young women. In the study, participants with lower BMIs were concluded to consume less animal protein and less sodium than participants with higher BMIs; across all three cohorts, beef and other foods high in animal protein represented a major contributor to total dietary and urinary phosphate. The inverse relationship between body size and urinary pH was attributed to insulin resistance, which decreases ammonia excretion and impairs hydrogen ion buffering. The study data also suggests that the increase in stone risk for the overweight and obese patient may actually represent a rising incidence of uric acid nephrolithiasis rather than calcium nephrolithiasis.

In 2008, the same group conducted an addition analysis on the same three cohorts [7]. In this study, the influence of various factors on 24-h urinary oxalate excretion was investigated further. Overall, higher BMIs were associated with increased 24-h urinary oxalate excretion, and every 5-kg increase in body weight was correlated with a 0.6 mg/day increase in urinary oxalate. The investigators found additional factors to be linked with increased oxalate excretion including younger age, presence of diabetes, and increased consumption of vitamin C (beyond the recommended daily allowance of 90 mg/day). Higher dietary calcium and consumption of calcium supplements were conversely associated with decreased oxalate excretion, while hypertension was found to have no influence on urinary oxalate excretion patterns. A strong relationship between non-dietary factors (i.e., age, diabetes) and patterns of oxalate excretion was found; the assumption reached was that the restriction of dietary oxalate may be relatively ineffective in reducing urinary oxalate levels for many stone formers.

Obesity's influence on lithiasis risk factors and stone reoccurrence was investigated in a study of 704 Korean subjects with stone formation—467 first-time formers (FSFs) and 247 recurrent stone formers (RSFs) underwent a complete metabolic assessment [8]. An analysis of stone composition was further available in 150 of the participants and revealed that uric acid stone formation was more common among obese individuals. Serum and urine chemistry was collected for all individuals in the sample. By and large, obese stone formers (i.e., BMI≥5) had higher serum levels of potassium, uric acid, urea nitrogen, and creatinine compared to non-obese subjects. Obese FSFs had decreased urinary pH, whereas obese RSFs did not; the precise reason for this observation, however, remains unclear. Among FSFs, stone recurrence rates were more frequent in obese stone formers compared with the non-obese ones; however, this rule did not hold true for RSFs. Moreover, FSFs were found to experience stone recurrence more quickly if they were obese, whereas time to recurrence was not affected by obesity for RSFs. Obesity was the strongest predictor for stone recurrence in the case of FSFs; however, among RSFs, the strongest predictor proved to be hypercalciuria. The results of this study reveal that obesity is interconnected with both metabolic alterations and recurrent lithiasis and further conclude that weight control may effectively prevent stone recurrence.

BMI and Stone Composition

To investigate the types of stones most commonly produced by obese individuals, 2,100 calculi were obtained from patients for whom information on both height and weight was available [9]. Stones from patients with diabetes mellitus were excluded, as were struvite and cystine stones, ultimately yielding 1,931 calcium and uric acid calculi to examine the influence of BMI on stone composition. Of the sample population, 672 patients had a BMI greater than 25 (34.8 %), 24.9 % were overweight (BMI 25–29.9), and 9.9 % were obese (BMI≥30). Out of the patients with a BMI of at least 25, a significantly higher proportion fell into the category of uric acid stone formers (UASFs) rather than calcium stone formers. In general, a higher frequency of calcium stones was observed across both genders. As BMI rose, however, uric acid stones became more dominant—a phenomenon more prominent in males compared with the female group.

In addition, age was found to be an independent factor in uric acid stone formation. Among those of less than 60 years of age, BMI had the strongest influence on uric acid stone prevalence, although beyond the age mark, there was a decrease in uric acid stone proportion attributable to differences in BMI. Similar findings were reported in a smaller study [10] investigating the biochemical profiles of 30 patients with "pure" uric acid nephrolithiasis and 29 patients with "pure" calcium oxalate stones. That is, overweight and obese patients of increasing age tended to have higher serum levels of uric acid and lower urinary pH, and had a predisposition toward "pure" uric acid stone formation.

Nephrolithiasis Following Modern Bariatric Surgery

Jejunoileal bypass, a surgery used to treat morbid obesity until 1980, resulted in severe complications of hyperoxaluria, oxalate-containing nephrolithiasis, and renal failure [11].

Modern techniques that have since replaced jejunoileal bypass most commonly include gastric banding and Roux-en-Y gastric bypass (RYGB).

To our knowledge, Asplin and Coe [11] were the first to review hyperoxaluria patterns in patients with nephrolithiasis postmodern bariatric surgery. Oxalate excretion was reportedly two or three times higher in their sample of 132 patients when contrasted with other stone formers and normal individuals of the same sex.

Compared to their counterparts, this modern patient group had higher urinary calcium oxalate supersaturation as well as lower urinary pH and calcium levels. Interestingly, calcium oxalate supersaturation was higher in the modern bariatric surgery group compared to patients who underwent jejunoileal bypass, thus serving to further augment their risk of calcium oxalate nephrolithiasis.

Duffey et al. [12] attempted to detect risk factors for stone formation in candidates for gastric bypass surgery by collecting 24-h urine samples from 12 men and 32 women with a mean BMI of 49.5 (range 30–70) and mean age of 47 prior to their operations. Their daily diet was recorded and further translated to daily calcium, sodium, protein, and caloric consumption. Of all the subjects, nearly 98 % were identified to have at least one lithogenic risk factor. The most frequent anomaly recorded was a low total urinary volume (<2 l/24-h). Over 50 % of participants had increased uric acid relative supersaturation, and a BMI of more than 45 was found to be the strongest predictor for hypercalciuria. Within the sample, diuretics were found to be likely indicators for increased uric acid excretion. In addition, obese stone formers tended to excrete more oxalate and had higher relative Na-Urate supersaturation, while they also had more urinary abnormalities compared to non-stone formers (6.2 vs. 4.4).

In attempt to determine any associated risk of RYGB and calcium oxalate stone formation, Duffey and colleagues reported on a prospective longitudinal study in which 24 patients underwent 24-h urinary analysis both 7 days prior and 90 days after RYGB surgery [13]. Following the procedure, 25 % of patients were found to have increased urinary oxalate excretion and relative supersaturation of calcium oxalate, leading to de novo oxalate lithiasis. Future investigation on risk factors for hyperoxaluria development post-RYGB and long-term effects of the surgery are still necessary.

Diabetes Mellitus and Metabolic Syndrome

An increased prevalence of uric acid stones in type II diabetics has been proven by past cross-sectional studies [14, 15]. Insulin resistance frequently increases the acidity of the urine through impaired renal ammoniagenesis; as seen elsewhere, the resulting low urinary pH acts as a significant contributing factor to uric acid nephrolithiasis. Cameron et al. [16] obtained and analyzed 24-h urine sample composition from three sample groups: normal volunteers, diabetic patients without nephrolithiasis, and diabetic patients who were known UASFs. General findings concluded that, when compared with normal volunteers, the diabetic patients tended to be more obese and hypertensive and had lower urinary pH levels, higher serum insulin levels, and higher urinary undissociated uric acid content. Further, diabetics were found to have a higher level of titratable acidity in the urine, and a greater net acid excretion that could be resultant of abnormally low ammonia excretion, or higher plasma lactate levels. The study identified the primary risk factor for uric acid nephrolithiasis among type II diabetics as low urinary pH.

Another comparative study [17] explored 2,464 stones obtained from 272 patients with diabetes and 2,192 non-diabetics. Generally, the diabetic stone formers tended to be older (≥50 years), more overweight, or obese and had a strikingly higher proportion of uric acid stones (three times higher compared with non-diabetic individuals) in comparison with the non-diabetic subjects. Obesity, old age, and male sex did appear to increase the percentage of uric acid stones in both groups; however, in combination with diabetes, this effect was even more pronounced.

Other epidemiological studies have examined the relationship between diabetes and nephrolithiasis via a different approach [18]. Lieske et al. [18] attempted to establish the probability of a certain individual having a concurrent diagnosis of diabetes mellitus by reviewing the medical records of kidney stone patients. After viewing the records of 3,561 individuals diagnosed with nephrolithiasis from 1980 and 1999, the associated odds ratio (OR) for diabetes was calculated to be 1.44; for BMI it was 1.05 and for hypertension, 1.71. As has been shown by other studies, diabetic patients had a greater proportion of uric acid stones and vice versa.

A sample of 14,670 men and women of 20 or more years of age who participated in the National Health and Nutrition Examination Survey (NHANES III) between 1988 and 1994 was recently evaluated for a study on metabolic syndrome and nephrolithiasis [19]. The study defined the diagnosis of metabolic syndrome by the presence of three of the following five traits: abdominal obesity (waist circumference >102 cm in men and >88 cm in women), increased serum triglycerides (>50 mg/dl), decreased serum high-density lipoprotein (HDL; < 40 mg/dl for men, < 50 mg/dl for women), hypertension (SBP medications), and impaired glucose tolerance or diabetes (fasting serum glucose >100 mg/dl or use of antidiabetic medications or self-reported diabetes). The incidence of metabolic syndrome was associated with a two-fold increase in the OR of self-reported kidney stone disease (2.13, 95 % confidence interval (CI) 1.74–2.62). After adjustment for age, sex, and race, this OR decreased to 1.52 (95 % CI 1.22–1.89) but remained considerable.

A more recent observational study tracked the effect of metabolic syndrome on nephrolithiasis specific to gender in a population of 40,687 Korean individuals from 1995 to 2009 [20]. Physical examination, anthropometric and biochemical measurements, and kidney ultrasonography were used to examine the subjects prior to retrospective data analysis. The cohort averaged 45 years of age and was comprised of 55.4 % men and 44.6 % women; 19.2 % of the participants had metabolic syndrome, defined by having three of the five below criteria, and 1.5 % had nephrolithiasis. In the study, both metabolic syndrome and each of its components—that is, elevated blood pressure (systole BP≥130 mmHg and/or diastole BP≥85 mmHg), abnormal glucose metabolism (≥110 mg/dl), high serum triglyceride levels (≥150 mg/dl), low HDL cholesterol level (≤40 mg/dl in men, ≤50 mg/dl in women), and BMI (>25 kg/m^2 for Asian populations)—were all found to be lithogenic risk factors. Overall, a significant correlation between the prevalence of metabolic syndrome and stone disease was observed. In this Korean study, it was men over women who exhibited an increased tendency toward traits of metabolic syndrome. Consistently, this gender distribution was also reflected in the heightened risk of nephrolithiasis among Korean males [20].

Melamine Nephrolithiasis

Over recent decades, a rapidly expanding population and societal changes in lifestyle have placed a mounting pressure on the food industry to provide an adequate supply of food products that meet daily nutritional criteria. Not before September of 2008 did the food industry's phenomenon of falsifying of nutritional content come to the public's attention. At a press conference on September 17 of that year, China's health minister announced that "three babies [which rose to four the following day] died of kidney failure, 158 more had acute kidney failure, and 1,372 babies remained in a hospital" as a result of melamine-contaminated infant formula ingestion [21].

An organic base commercially synthesized from urea, melamine is 66 % nitrogen by molecular weight and is widely used in commercial products such as dry erase boards, fabrics, glues, housewares, and flame retardants [22]. The addition of 1 g of the substance to 1 l of milk will deceptively increase the protein content by 0.4 %. Adding melamine to milk powder can further enhance this protein percentage, as a greater amount of the compound can be used without precipitation [22]. This dangerous technique has been abused to falsely boost the protein concentration of cow's milk when it was tested prior to sale to milk product manufacturers [21].

Melamine toxicity is already well recognized from previous experiments with animal subjects. Direct contact with melamine will cause irritation of the skin, eyes, and respiratory tract, while oral ingestion may cause nausea, vomiting, and diarrhea. Long-term exposure has been documented to reduce fertility and cause fetal toxicity, although the most commonly noted detriment to health is nephrotoxicity [22]. Despite the fact that the mechanism of toxic action remains unknown, melamine has been shown to precipitate and crystallize in the distal renal tubules [23]. The calculi most frequently formed consist of either a combination of melamine and uric acid, or a matrix of protein, melamine, uric acid, and phosphate [22].

In a large observational study, 589 infants 36 months and younger were screened for possible melamine exposure [24]. Another study of similar interest screened 1,091 children of ages 4 and under, who were suspected to have consumed melamine-contaminated milk formulas [25]. The first study [24] assessed patients by ultrasonography and had participants complete questionnaires regarding possible signs and symptoms of nephrolithiasis. The majority of stones observed were localized to the renal pelvis and situated in clusters, were sand-like, and did not cause sonographic shadowing. The vast proportion of babies eventually diagnosed with stones showed no typical signs or symptoms of urolithiasis [24, 25].

Abnormal glomerular function was only seen in four patients, and none of the subjects had tubular dysfunction [24]. Sporadic signs of hematuria, leukocyturia, dysuria, polyuria, and proteinuria were reported in both studies [24, 25]. Stone presence was strongly associated with the consumption of high melamine content formula, as well as preterm birth. The high melamine formula was found to increase the risk of stone presence by 5.4–7 times compared to non-exposure. Consumption of moderate melamine formula, however, did not increase the likelihood of stone formation in the young subjects. Additionally, preterm infants were concluded to have 3.7–4.5 times the chance of stone formation compared with term infants [24].

Both studies recommended prompt hydration and urinary alkalinization to facilitate stone passage. Ultrasound was the recommended screening test in effort to minimize radiation exposure, and none of the affected infants required surgical intervention for stone removal.

In a 2011 analysis, Liu et al. reported findings of a previously unidentified link between melamine exposure and kidney stone formation in adults [26], which—contrary to prior beliefs—suggests that not only high but also low levels of melamine exposure might be harmful to humans. The authors suggest that the melamine-related stones in adults may consist of calcium and melamine, lending to the possibility of melamine being a contributing factor in the etiology of calcium nephrolithiasis—the most common type of lithiasis worldwide [26, 27]. However, some potential shortcomings of Liu et al.'s findings have been noted. These include the timing at which urine melamine was measured, which was at the point of diagnosis rather than during stone formation [27].

Yuan et al. analyzed the content of 49 melamine-related urinary calculi from children of 4–82 months of age qualitatively and quantitatively, by Fourier transform infrared, and both high-performance liquid chromatography and flame atomic absorption spectrum, respectively [28]. This study identified unprecedented results in that 51 % of the melamine stone samples contained calcium compounds; uric acid remained the predominant calculus component. Of the calcium compounds, 92 % of the stones contained calcium oxalate, and a positive correlation between stone calcium level and child's age was found to be statistically significant [28]. Due to the calcium content of these melamine-related calculi, this study suggested that alkalization alone may not be enough to treat lithiasis in older children, as their stones will likely contain a higher percentage of calcium, which does not disintegrate in alkaline substance. Many valuable questions surrounding melamine toxicity and its contribution to nephrolithiasis remain unanswered and ought to be examined in the near future.

Indinavir Nephrolithiasis

Since protease inhibitors were introduced as a treatment for human immunodeficiency virus (HIV) infection, a previously unknown urinary calculus has appeared—indinavir stones. The pharmaceutical agency that manufactures these compounds reports an overall prevalence of nephrolithiasis among recipients as high as 8.7 % [29]. Studies of larger populations, however, have proven these rates to be as high as 13–28 % [30–32].

Kidney stone formation has been reported in HIV patients after consumption of a standard 800 mg dose of indinavir three times daily for 1–102 days [30–34] with a cumulative incidence of nephrolithiasis being 43.2 % at the 78-week interval [30]. While the exact mechanism of stone formation is unknown, it has been postulated to result from precipitation of indinavir crystals in the renal tubules caused by diminished solubility due to low urinary pH and volume [35].

All of the following factors—age, high baseline serum level of alanine aminotransferase (ALT), low baseline cholesterol level, high drug load calculated as daily indinavir dose/BMI, and baseline urine alterations including proteinuria, leukocyturia, hematuria, and crystalluria—were found to be significant predictive measures for the development of nephrolithiasis and colic events in subjects undergoing indinavir therapy [30, 31]. One study found hypocitraturia to be a universal metabolic abnormality in all patient-subjects with indinavir stones [33]. Chemical analysis of these calculi has revealed indinavir sulfate, a radiolucent compound [33, 34]; intravenous pyelography (IVP) imaging, rather than non-contrast-enhanced computed tomography (CT), was consequently the recommended diagnostic approach of these studies.

Non-contrast CT scanning does not routinely reveal the presence of indinavir stones [33]. Calculi of this composition are reportedly soft, yellow in color, gelatinous in consistency, and can be disintegrated with minimal manipulation [33]. The literature also suggests that conservative therapy with intravenous hydration, analgesics, and temporary cessation of indinavir therapy be the first-line of treatment for this form of nephrolithiasis [33, 34].

In more severe cases complicated by persistent high fever, intractable pain, oliguria, or anuria, endoscopic stenting for a 2-week duration is recommended. Due to the soft, gelatinous consistency of indinavir stones as well as their radiolucent nature, such calculi are not amenable to ureteroscopy and stone basketing or to shock wave lithotripsy [33].

Conclusion

Societal changes and the resultant health factors have had a tremendous effect over stone prevalence and composition. Continuously rising rates of stone formation have been recorded among the general population. Unfortunately, due to the increasing incidence of obesity and diabetes worldwide, these trends are only predicted to persist. As time continues, we may encounter increasing numbers of unknown stone types caused by offending agents intentionally or unintentionally incorporated in our food and drug supply. Prompt education of a healthier lifestyle, and better quality control in the food and drug industry, is the key to reducing nephrolithiasis rates as well as its consequences.

References

1. Diabetes. Fact sheet #312. www.who.int/mediacentre/factsheet/fs312/en/index.html. In: World Health Organization, editor; 2011.
2. Obesity and over-weight. Fact sheet #311. www.who.int/mediacentre/factsheet/fs311/en/index.html. In: World Health Organization, editor; 2011.
3. Kearney PM, Whelton M, Reynolds K, Muntner P, Whelton PK, He J. Global burden of hypertension: analysis of worldwide data. Lancet. 2005;365:217–23.
4. Scales Jr CD, Curtis LH, Norris RD, Springhart WP, Sur RL, Schulman KA, et al. Changing gender prevalence of stone disease. J Urol. 2007;177:979–82.
5. Taylor EN, Stampfer MJ, Curhan GC. Obesity, weight gain, and the risk of kidney stones. JAMA. 2005;293:455–62.
6. Taylor EN, Curhan GC. Body size and 24-h urine composition. Am J Kidney Dis. 2006;48:905–15.
7. Taylor EN, Curhan GC. Determinants of 24-h urinary oxalate excretion. Clin J Am Soc Nephrol. 2008;3:1453–60.
8. Lee SC, Kim YJ, Kim TH, Yun SJ, Lee NK, Kim WJ. Impact of obesity in patients with urolithiasis and its prognostic usefulness in stone recurrence. J Urol. 2008;179:570–4.

9. Daudon M, Lacour B, Jungers P. Influence of body size on urinary stone composition in men and women. Urol Res. 2006;34:193–9.
10. Negri AL, Spivacow R, Del Valle E, Pinduli I, Marino A, Fradinger E, et al. Clinical and biochemical profile of patients with 'pure' uric acid nephrolithiasis compared with 'pure' calcium oxalate stone formers. Urol Res. 2007;35:247–51.
11. Asplin JR, Coe FL. Hyperoxaluria in kidney stone formers treated with modern bariatric surgery. J Urol. 2007;177:565–9.
12. Duffey BG, Pedro RN, Kriedberg C, Weiland D, Melquist J, Ikramuddin S, et al. Lithogenic risk factors in the morbidly obese population. J Urol. 2008;179:1401–6.
13. Duffey BG, Pedro RN, Makhlouf A, Kriedberg C, Stessman M, Hinck B, et al. Roux-en-Y gastric bypass is associated with early increased risk factors for development of calcium oxalate nephrolithiasis. J Am Coll Surg. 2008;206:1145–53.
14. Daudon M, Lacour B, Jungers P. High prevalence of uric acid calculi in diabetic stone formers. Nephrol Dial Transplant. 2005;20:468–9.
15. Pak CY, Sakhaee K, Moe O, Preminger GM, Poindexter JR, Peterson RD, et al. Biochemical profile of stone-forming patients with diabetes mellitus. Urology. 2003;61:523–7.
16. Cameron MA, Maalouf NM, Adams-Huet B, Moe OW, Sakhaee K. Urine composition in type 2 diabetes: predisposition to uric acid nephrolithiasis. J Am Soc Nephrol. 2006;17:1422–8.
17. Daudon M, Traxer O, Conort P, Lacour B, Jungers P. Type 2 diabetes increases the risk for uric acid stones. J Am Soc Nephrol. 2006;17:2026–33.
18. Lieske JC, de la Vega LS, Gettman MT, Slezak JM, Bergstralh EJ, Melton 3rd LJ, et al. Diabetes mellitus and the risk of urinary tract stones: a population-based case-control study. Am J Kidney Dis. 2006;48:897–904.
19. West B, Luke A, Durazo-Arvizu RA, Cao G, Shoham D, Kramer H. Metabolic syndrome and self-reported history of kidney stones: the national health and nutrition examination survey (NHANES III) 1988–1994. Am J Kidney Dis. 2008;51:741–7.
20. Jung HS, Chang IH, Kim KD, Moon YT, Kim TH, Myung SC, et al. Possible relationship between metabolic syndrome traits and nephrolithiasis: incidence for 15 years according to gender. Korean J Urol. 2011;52:548–53.
21. Parry J. Contaminated infant formula sickens 6200 babies in China. BMJ. 2008;337:a1738.
22. Hau AK, Kwan TH, Li PK. Melamine toxicity and the kidney. J Am Soc Nephrol. 2009;20:245–50.
23. Bhalla V, Grimm PC, Chertow GM, Pao AC. Melamine nephrotoxicity: an emerging epidemic in an era of globalization. Kidney Int. 2009;75:774–9.
24. Guan N, Fan Q, Ding J, Zhao Y, Lu J, Ai Y, et al. Melamine-contaminated powdered formula and urolithiasis in young children. N Engl J Med. 2009;360:1067–74.
25. Zhu SL, Li JH, Chen L, Bao ZX, Zhang LJ, Li JP, et al. Conservative management of pediatric nephrolithiasis caused by melamine-contaminated milk powder. Pediatrics. 2009;123:e1099–102.
26. Liu CC, Wu CF, Chen BH, Huang SP, Goggins W, Lee HH, et al. Low exposure to melamine increases the risk of urolithiasis in adults. Kidney Int. 2011;80:746–52.
27. García López FJ, Quereda C. Melamine toxicity: one more culprit in calcium kidney lithiasis. Kidney Int. 2011;80:694–6.
28. Yuan L, YiRong C, Wei Z, Huang X, Li W, Ru X, et al. Study of stone composition changes in melamine-related urinary calculi and its clinical significance. J Urol. 2011;78:417–21.
29. Merck Frosst Canada Ltd. Product Monograph Crixivan. Indinavir sulfate capsules 200 and 400 mg (as indinavir). HIV protease inhibitor. Date of last revision: 27 Mar 2009.
30. Saltel E, Angel JB, Futter NG, Walsh WG, O'Rourke K, Mahoney JE. Increased prevalence and analysis of risk factors for indinavir nephrolithiasis. J Urol. 2000;164:1895–7.
31. Meraviglia P, Angeli E, Del Sorbo F, Rombolà G, Viganò P, Orlando G, et al. Risk factors for indinavir-related renal colic in HIV patients: predictive value of indinavir dose/body mass index. AIDS. 2002;16:2089–93.
32. Hirsch MS, Steigbigel RT, Staszewski S, McMahon D, Fischl MA, Hirschel B, et al. Long-term efficacy, safety, and tolerability of indinavir-based therapy in protease inhibitor-naive adults with advanced HIV infection. Clin Infect Dis. 2003;37:1119–24.
33. Kohan AD, Armenakas NA, Fracchia JA. Indinavir urolithiasis: an emerging cause of renal colic in patients with human immunodeficiency virus. J Urol. 1999;161:1765–8.
34. Rich JD, Ramratnam B, Chiang M, Tashima KT. Management of indinavir associated nephrolithiasis. J Urol. 1997;158:2228.
35. Tashima KT, Horowitz JD, Rosen S. Indinavir nephropathy. N Engl J Med. 1997;336:138–40.

Part XI

Case Scenarios

Case Scenarios and Interesting Images in Urolithiasis

114

M. Hammad Ather, Zafar Sajjad, Basit Salam and M. Nasir Sulaiman

Case 1: Parathyroid Adenoma and Urolithiasis

Figure 114.1 is a Doppler ultrasound (US) study of the neck, demonstrating a vascular well-circumscribed mass in a patient with recurrent, bilateral urolithiasis and a raised serum calcium level (>2.96 mmol/l). What does it represent?

A patient with recurrent or bilateral urolithiasis and elevated calcium (and PTH 3.9 or more times as normal) should be suspected as having primary hyperparathyroidism. A (99m) TC-MIBI image functions best in preoperative localization of the abnormal gland. Some surgeons perform an ultrasound examination in the operating room just preceding the surgery. Parathyroidectomy is the curative approach for the disease. See Chaps. 94 and 95.

Selected Bibliography

Fujii T, Yamaguchi S, Yajima R, Tsutsumi S, Uchida N, Asao T, Oriuch N, Kuwano H. Use of a handheld, semiconductor (cadmium zinc telluride)-based gamma camera in navigation surgery for primary hyperparathyroidism. Am Surg. 2011;77(6):690–3.

Katz SC, Wang GJ, Kramer EL, Roses DF. Limitations of technetium 99m sestamibi scintigraphic localization for primary hyperparathyroidism associated with multiglandular disease. Am Surg. 2003;69(2):170–5.

Uller W, Jung EM, Hornung M, Ross C, Jung W, Schlitt HJ, Stroszczynski C, Agha A. Evaluation of the microvascularization of pathologic parathyroid glands in patients with primary hyperparathyroidism using conventional ultrasound and contrast-enhanced ultrasound. Clin Hemorheol Microcirc. 2011;48(1):95–103.

Yabuta T, Tsushima Y, Masuoka H, Tomoda C, Fukushima M, Kihara M, Inoue H, Higashiyama T, Takamura Y, Ito Y, Kobayashi K, Miya A, Miyauchi A. Ultrasonographic features of intrathyroidal parathyroid adenoma causing primary hyperparathyroidism. Endocr J. 2011;58(11):989–94.

M.H. Ather, M.B.B.S., FCPS (Urol), FEBU (✉)
Department of Surgery, Aga Khan University,
Stadium Road, P.O. Box 3500, Karachi, Sindh 74800, Pakistan
e-mail: hammad.ather@aku.edu

Z. Sajjad, M.B.B.S., MRCP (UK), FRCR
Department of Radiology, Aga Khan University,
Stadium Road, Karachi, Sindh 74800, Pakistan
e-mail: zafar.sajjad@aku.edu

B. Salam, M.B.B.S., FCPS
Department of Radiology, Aga Khan University Hospital,
Stadium Road, Karachi, Sindh 74800, Pakistan
e-mail: basit.salam@aku.edu

M.N. Sulaiman, M.B.B.S., FRCS, FRCS (Urol)
Section of Urology, Department of Surgery,
Aga Khan University Hospital,
Stadium Road, P.O. Box 3500, Karachi 74800, Pakistan

J.J. Talati et al. (eds.), *Urolithiasis*,
DOI 10.1007/978-1-4471-4387-1_114, © Springer-Verlag London 2012

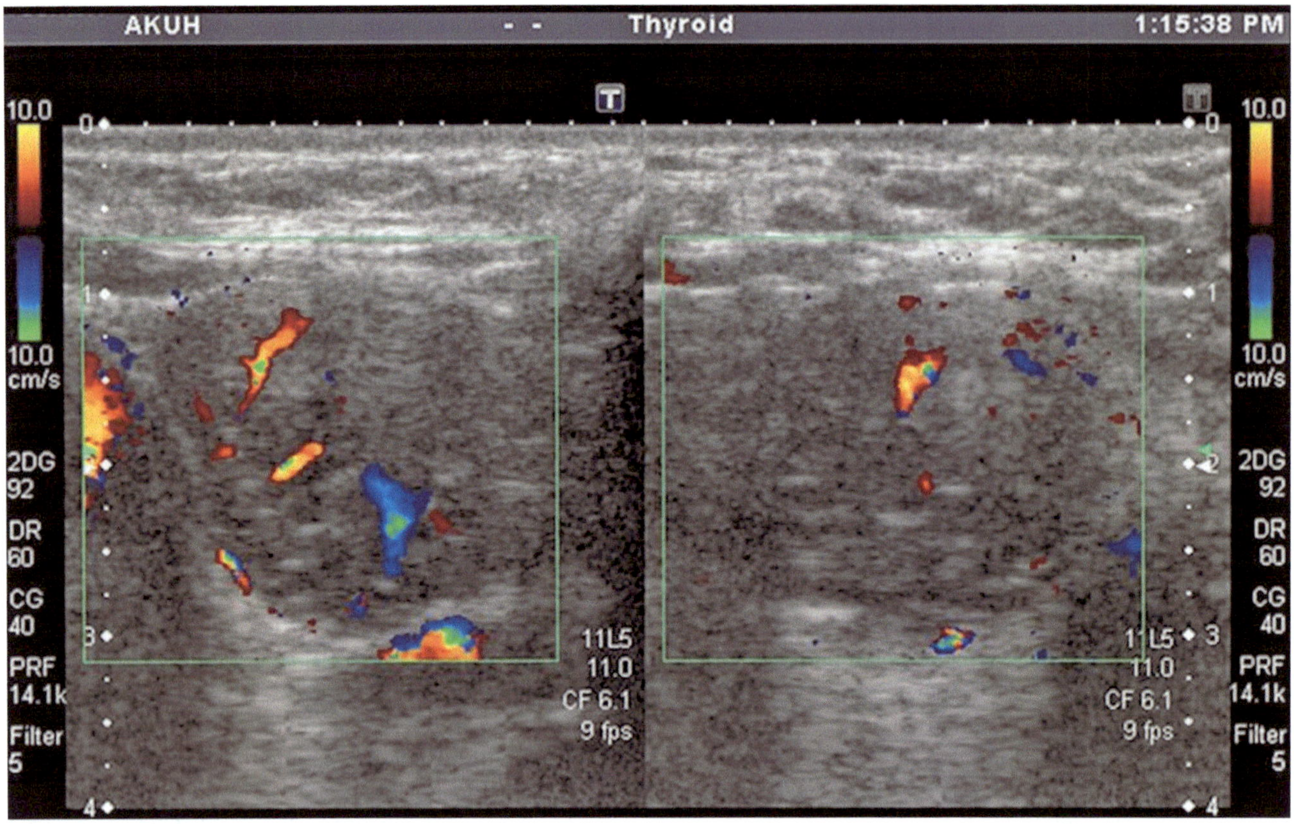

Fig. 114.1 Parathyroid adenoma and urolithiasis

Case 2: Heminephrectomy and Calculus Disease

A primary physician referred to the urologist a 66-year-old male with a history of symptomatic urinary tract infection (UTI). He is a known case of urolithiasis and had open surgery some 20 years back for left renal stone. He has lower urinary symptoms suggestive of benign prostatic obstruction. His ultrasound showed a 1.2-cm stone in the left kidney with associated scarring (Fig. 114.2a). Doppler showed well-perfused parenchyma caudal to the stone. His computed tomography (CT) kidneys-ureters-bladder (KUB) scan (Fig. 114.2b) showed that he had a stone and had had an upper polar nephrectomy.

How would you treat this patient?

How We Treated This Patient

The patient was successfully treated by shockwave lithotripsy (SWL). He required two sessions and was stone free. Neglected urolithiasis presenting with parenchymal scarring and loss of polar region of the kidney is less frequently seen now. This is primarily due to the widespread use of imaging, in particular ultrasound imaging, which leads to early definitive treatment of stone. This patient has had a partial nephrectomy. Parenchymal scarring associated with an infundibulocalyceal stone, which was usually branched, is often the indication for such resection. Often, these patients have stones and hydrocalix, and the associated cortex is scarred. Surgery is performed under cold or warm ischemia. More recently, partial nephrectomy is being performed through laparoscopic surgery rather than open surgery.

Selected Bibliography

Bates RJ, Heaney JA, Kerr WS Jr. Segmental calculus disease: potential of partial nephrectomy. Urology. 1981;17(5):409–14.

Nambirajan T, Jeschke S, Albqami N, Abukora F, Leeb K, Janetschek G. Role of laparoscopy in management of renal stones: single-center experience and review of literature. J Endourol. 2005;19(3):353–9.

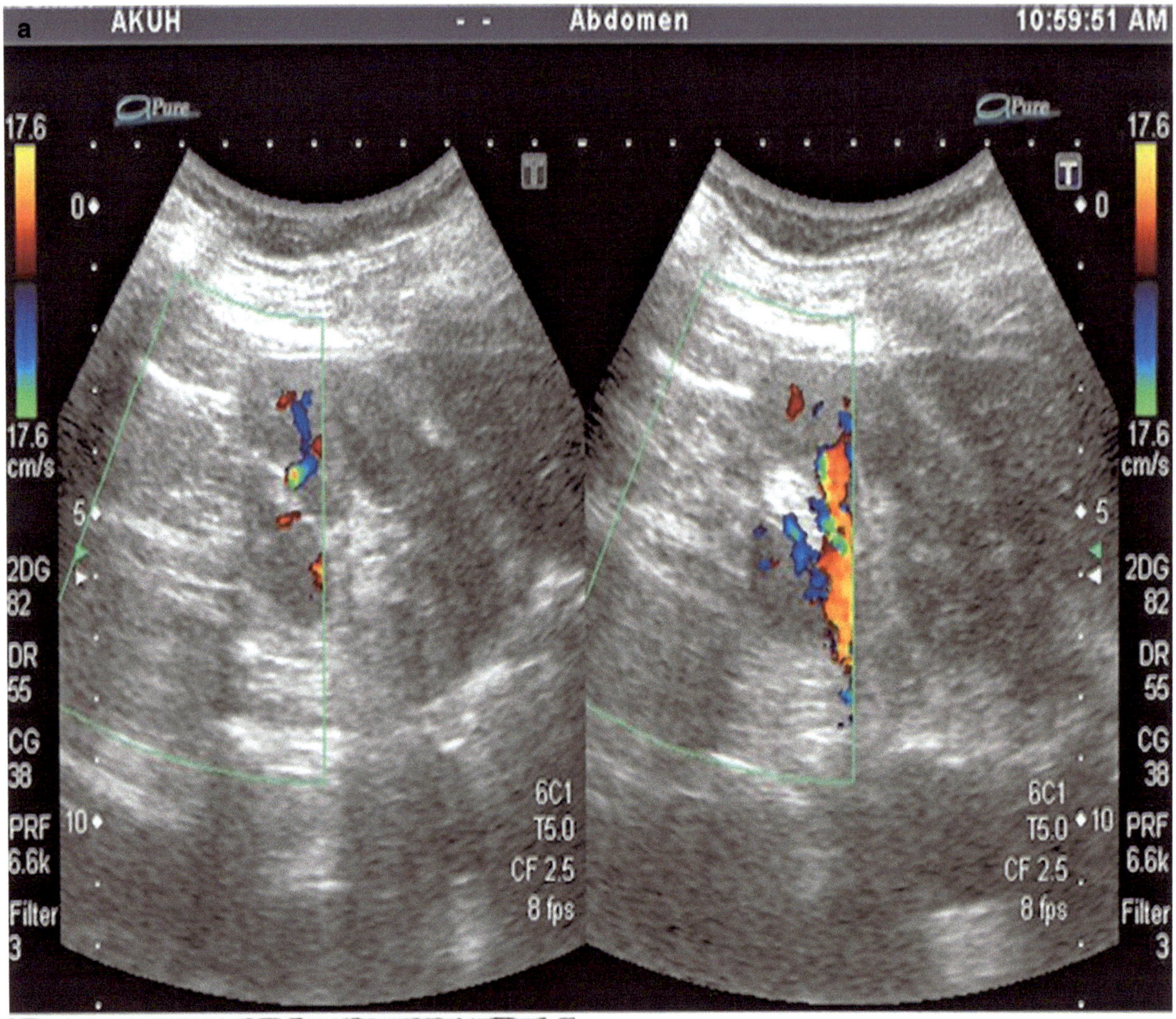

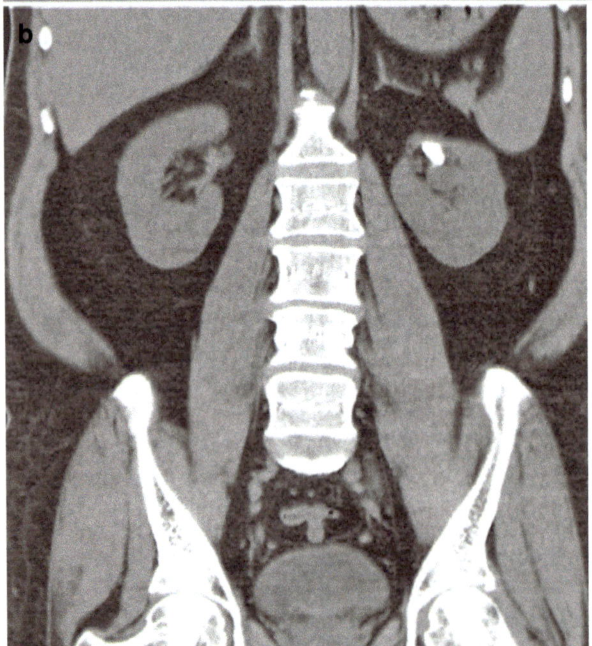

Fig. 114.2 (**a**) Ultrasound and (**b**) CT KUB scan showing stones

Case 3: Nephrocalcinosis

A 46-year-old male has a history of spontaneous passage of stones for the past 14 years. Seven years back, he was also treated with SWL for a 1.4-cm right renal stone. His ultrasound showed medullary nephrocalcinosis (Fig. 114.3). In view of colic at the time of presentation, a CT KUB was also performed, which showed no ureteral stone and similar stone burdens in both the kidneys.

How would you treat this patient, and what is the current definition of nephrocalcinosis?

This patient was treated by SWL and had subjective improvement. The radiological diagnosis using ultrasound, plain X-ray KUB, and CT shows that there is low level of concordance between various modalities. This renders the radiological diagnosis of NC difficult. Nephrocalcinosis should be confirmed by CT combined with either US or KUB. It is at times difficult to differentiate between a stone and nephrocalcinosis until a flexible endoscopy demonstrates there is no stone in the collecting system. Symptomatic patients with nephrocalcinosis resulting from medullary sponge kidneys are often treated by SWL.

Selected Bibliography

Cheidde L, Ajzen SA, Tamer Langen CH, Christophalo D, Heilberg IP. A critical appraisal of the radiological evaluation of nephrocalcinosis. Nephron Clin Pract. 2007;106(3):c119–24.

Miller NL, Humphreys MR, Coe FL, Evan AP, Bledsoe SB, Handa SE, Lingeman JE. Nephrocalcinosis: re-defined in the era of endourology. Urol Res. 2010;38(6):421–7. Epub 2010 Nov 6.

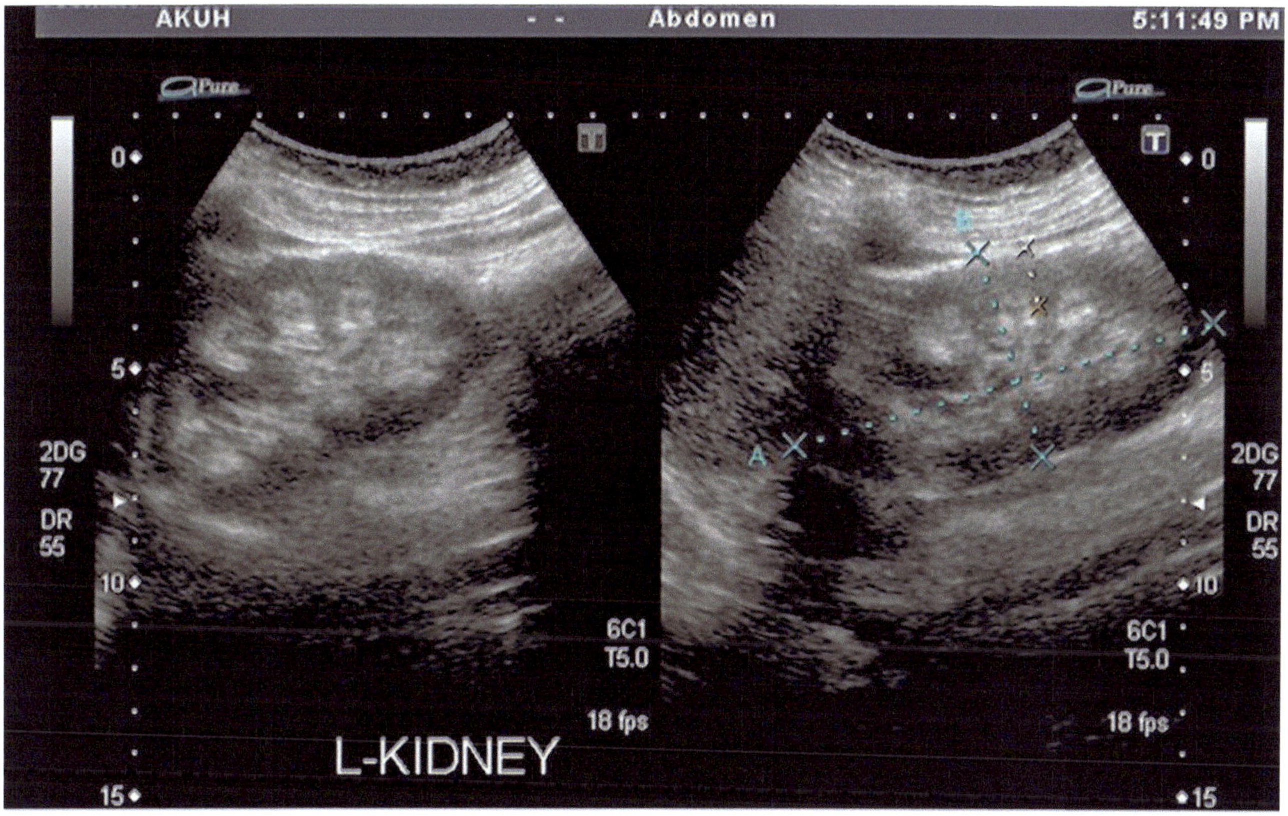

Fig. 114.3 Ultrasound showing medullary nephrocalcinosis

Case 4: Xanthogranulomatous Pyelonephritis (XGPN)

A 46-year-old diabetic woman presented with left flank pain, fever, and hematuria. She was a poorly controlled diabetic and had a past history of open pyelolithotomy some 20 years back in the same (left) renal unit. She was initially managed by percutaneous drainage and antibiotics. What would you do next?

This patient had xanthogranulomatous pyelonephritis (XGPN). In view of poor renal function of the right renal unit, she underwent open nephrectomy. She made an unremarkable recovery.

Renal stone with obstruction and diabetes mellitus are often associated with development of XGPN. Although presence of xanthoma cells in urine is suggestive of XGPN, imaging is often diagnostic. CT scan is particularly useful (Fig. 114.4). Demographic data, comorbidities, predisposing factors, and biochemical as well as roentgenological features are significant but nonspecific indicators of preoperative diagnosis of XGPN.

Selected Bibliography

Afgan F, Mumtaz S, Ather MH. Afgan F, Mumtaz S, Ather MH. Preoperative diagnosis of xanthogranulomatous pyelonephritis. Urol J. 2007;4(3):169–73.

Saavedra Jo S, Pow-Sang Godoy M, Benavente Corrales V, Morante Deza C, Meza Montoya L, Taxa Rojas L, Cisneros Guerrero F. Xanthogranulomatous pyelonephritis: clinical, radiological and pathologic characteristics. Arch Esp Urol. 2004;57(6):595–600.

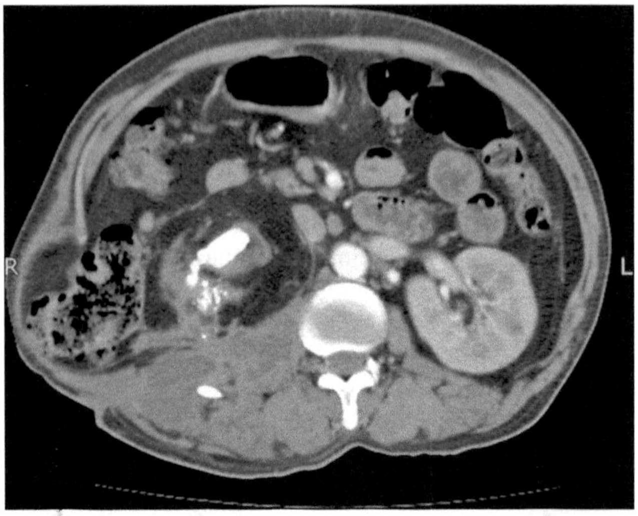

Fig. 114.4 CT scan

Case 5: Bilateral Staghorn Stones

A 48-year-old male with a known case of urolithiasis for the past 15 years presented with recurrent UTI and right flank pain. He was previously treated by open surgery about 15 years back. Since then, he was once treated by SWL. His serum creatinine was 1.4 (0.6–1.1 mg/dl).

How would you manage this patient?

How would you approach removal of his right and left renal calculi?

The right side was initially treated by PCNL (and subsequently the left kidney also by PCNL) followed by SWL for residual stones. What would be the other alternative approach?

Bilateral staghorn stones (Fig. 114.5) are often managed by staged percutaneous nephrolithotomy (PCNL). Small volumes stones can however be managed by simultaneous procedure. In a randomized study, Wang and colleagues noted that simultaneous bilateral tubeless PCNL is a safe, efficacious, and cost-effective option in bilateral renal staghorn calculi, which is associated with low morbidity, short hospital stay, high stone-free rate, and early return-to-normal activity.

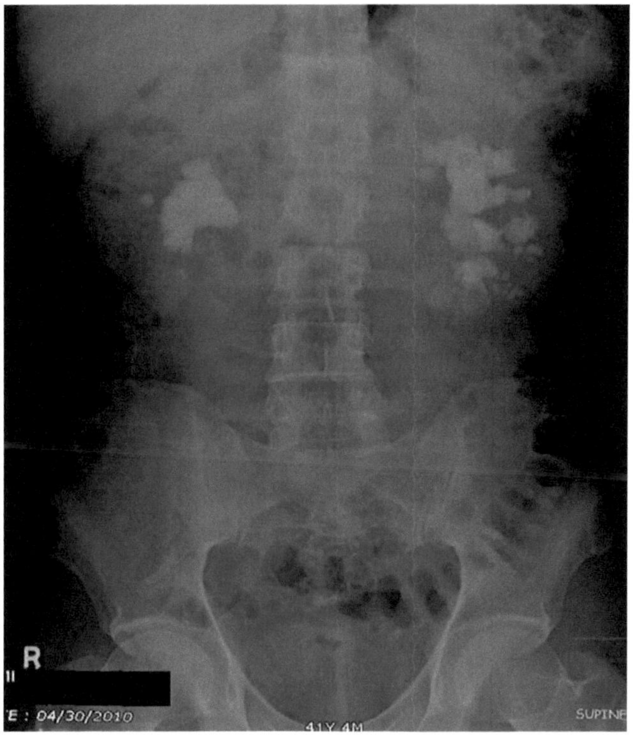

Fig. 114.5 Bilateral staghorn stones

Selected Bibliography

Falahatkar S, Khosropanah I, Roshani A, Neiroomand H, Nikpour S, Nadjafi-Semnani M, Akbarpour M. Tubeless percutaneous nephrolithotomy for staghorn stones. J Endourol. 2008;22(7):1447–51.

Wang CJ, Chang CH, Huang SW. Simultaneous bilateral tubeless percutaneous nephrolithotomy of staghorn stones: a prospective randomized controlled study. Urol Res. 2011;39(4):289–94.

Case 6: Sestamibi Scan

The classic treatment approach for primary hyperparathyroidism has been bilateral neck exploration with identification of all parathyroid glands. Recent work has shown benefits of more selective approaches, including better cosmesis and decreased risk of nerve injury. Both ultrasound and CT-guided FNA are well-described, successful techniques for the definitive diagnosis of lesions in the neck. Both techniques can provide a diagnosis in >90 % of patients. Sestamibi scan (Fig. 114.6) and surgeon-performed ultrasound are currently considered the best imaging modalities.

Selected Bibliography

Marcheix B, Brouchet L, Berjaud J, Dahan M. Recurrent hyperparathyroidism: a sixth mediastinal parathyroid gland. Eur J Cardiothorac Surg. 2006;30(5):808–10.

Pesenti M, Frasoldati A, Azzarito C, Valcavi R. Parathyroid incidentaloma discovered during thyroid ultrasound imaging. J Endocrinol Invest. 1999;22(10):796–9.

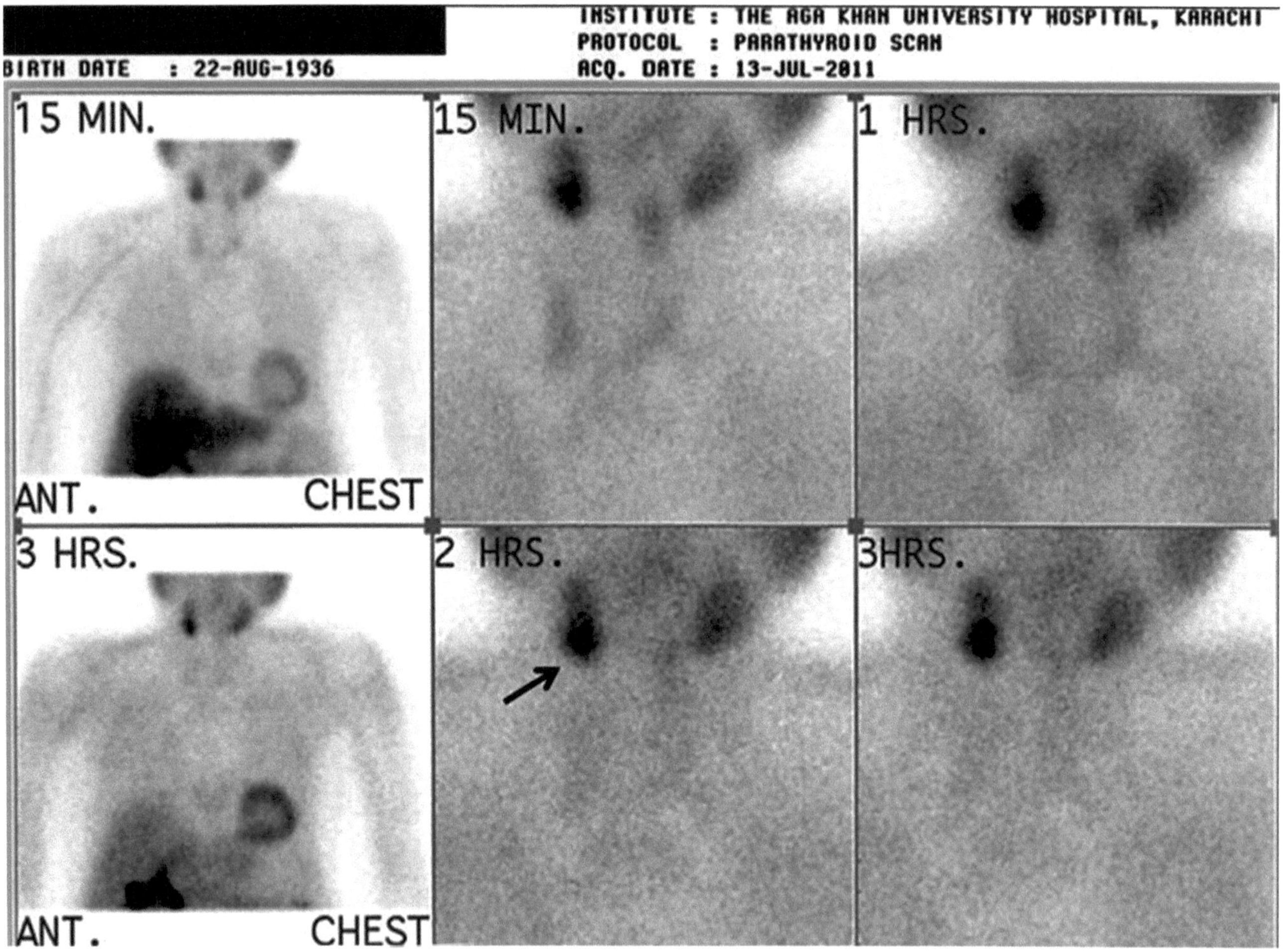

Fig. 114.6 Sestamibi scan

Case 7: Broken Stent

A 48-year-old male presented to the clinic with right flank pain and was found to have partial staghorn stone. He underwent PCNL, following which a JJ stent was placed in an antegrade fashion. Later he required one session of SWL for a small residual stone. JJ stent removal was attempted under local anesthesia with flexible scope, which failed. A subsequent attempt under general anesthesia also failed and the stent broke (Fig. 114.7). He was positioned for percutaneous access in the same sitting. On percutaneous access, the stent was found to be burying in the parenchyma. It was freed by laser resection of the surrounding parenchyma. The remaining portion of the stent was retrieved. Nephroscopy and ureteroscopy (flexi cystoscope) were performed in an antegrade fashion to see if any portion of the stent or residual stone was left. The patient was discharged home the same day.

Literature Search

Forgotten implants pose a significant management dilemma for physicians. The tracking system significantly lowers the incidence of overdue JJ stents from 12.5 to 1.2 % and 1.5 % in the first and second years of the program, respectively ($p = .00039$). In a report by Ather et al., it was proposed that this technically simple program should be used for all implants placed in patients. Successful management of retained ureteral stents requires careful planning and may entail a combination of endourologic approaches. It is imperative to avoid using significant force, which can result in severe ureteral injury or breakage of the stent. If encrustations are present along the stent, we believe in treating the distal component prior to managing any proximal or ureteral components.

Selected Bibliography

Ather MH, Talati J, Biyabani R. Physician responsibility for removal of implants: the case for a computerized program for tracking overdue double-J stents. Tech Urol. 2000;6(3): 189–92.

Lam JS, Gupta M. Tips and tricks for the management of retained ureteral stents. J Endourol. 2002;16(10):733–41.

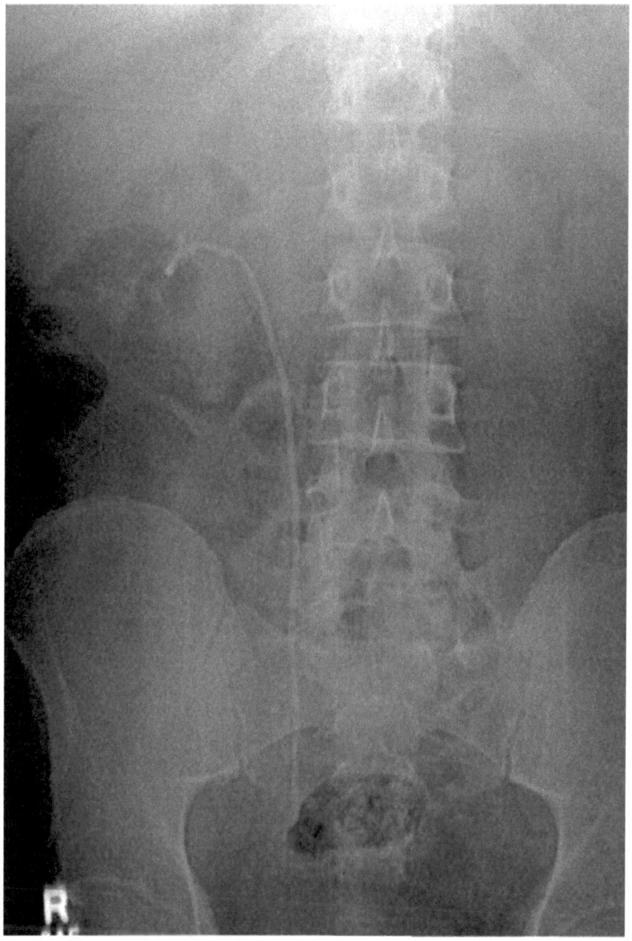

Fig. 114.7 Broken stent

Case 8: Bladder Stones

A 65-year-old man presented to the clinic with hematuria and intermittent urinary retention for the past 4 years. He had been on Ayurvedic medicine for the past few years with some relief of symptoms. His ultrasound indicates, besides two moderately large vesical stone and significant post-void residue, a large median lobe. What are the various management options available provided he is medically fit?

The incidence of bladder stones (Fig. 114.8) has decreased worldwide, particularly in the western world. Classically vesical stones in the adults are seen in the elderly with neglected benign prostatic obstruction and neurogenic bladder. Presence of vesical stones along with benign prostatic obstruction is an absolute indication of intervention. Both stones and prostate can be dealt with endoscopically. However, there are reports of dealing with smaller vesical stone by SWL and prostatic obstruction medically in selected cases. There is a significant incidence of vesical urolithiasis in reconstructed urinary tract. Three-dimensional CT is helpful for better displaying the morphology of a new renovesical anatomy, and some features seem to be indicative of a predisposition to develop possible complications. It may be useful for surgeons to plan a reintervention to obviate or prevent complications.

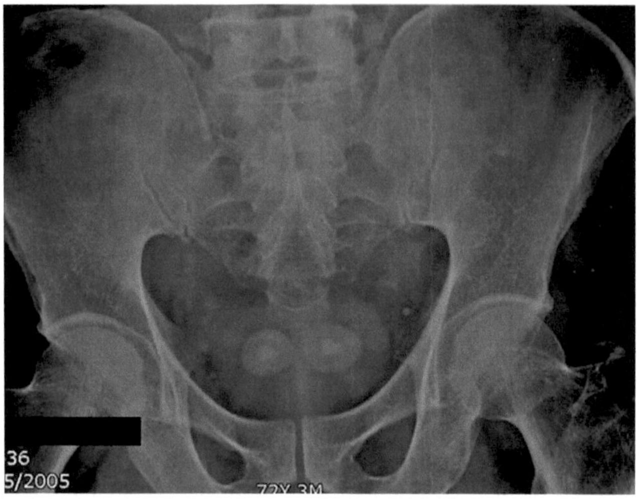

Fig. 114.8 Bladder stones

Selected Bibliography

Ather MH, Faruqui N, Abid F, Sulaiman MN. Is there a difference in early perioperative morbidity in transurethral resection of prostate (TURP) versus TURP with cystolitholapaxy and TURP with inguinal herniorrhaphy? Int Urol Nephrol. 2002;33(1):69–72.

De la Torre CG, Barusso GH, Chernobilsky VG, Borghi MO, Montes de Oca LF, Becher EF. Outpatient simultaneous treatment of benign prostatic hyperplasia and bladder lithiasis with GreenLight® and Holmium laser. J Endourol. 2012;26(2):164–7. Epub 2012 Jan 16.

Philippou P, Moraitis K, Masood J, Junaid I, Buchholz N. The management of bladder lithiasis in the modern era of endourology. Urology. 2012;79(5):980–6. Epub 2011 Nov 25.

Sassi C, Santilli L, Concetti S, Schiavina R, Amadori E, Severini E, Martorana G, Battista G. Three-dimensional computed tomography of the orthotopic ileal neobladder reconstruction: normal and abnormal findings. Urol Int. 2009;82(3):301–5.

Case 9: Ureteral Jet

A 35-year-old male was seen in the consulting clinic with a 10-day history of flank pain. Urinalysis showed microscopic hematuria. Examination showed tenderness in the flank. He had a CT KUB performed that indicated a 5-mm ureterovesical junction stone with mild hydroureter. Planning plain film of the CT did not show a stone. He was advised medical expulsive therapy (α[alpha] adrenergic blocker) and follow-up imaging with ultrasound. Ultrasound performed 2 weeks later indicated no evidence of stone and ureteral jet (see Fig. 114.9).

Discussion

With the widespread use of CT KUB in the routine evaluation of ureterolithiasis and level 1 evidence in favor of use of medical expulsive therapy in the management of ureteral stone, the use of follow-up imaging has become a major issue. It is recommended to use a plain X-ray KUB with a CT to define the radio-opacity of the stone. This facilitates the ordering of correct imaging during follow-up. The majority of ureteral stones at the time of presentation are in the distal ureter. Ultrasound is a safe and efficacious follow-up for such patients. Moesbergen and colleagues recently observed that ureteral calculi within 35 mm of the UVJ can be accurately followed-up by using transabdominal US, which substantially reduces patient radiation burden.

Selected Bibliography

Mitterberger M, Pinggera GM, Pallwein L, Gradl J, Feuchtner G, Plattner R, Neururer R, Bartsch G, Strasser H, Frauscher F. Plain abdominal radiography with transabdominal native tissue harmonic imaging ultrasonography vs unenhanced computed tomography in renal colic. BJU Int. 2007;100(4):887–90.

Moesbergen TC, de Ryke RJ, Dunbar S, Wells JE, Anderson NG. Distal ureteral calculi: US follow-up. Radiology. 2011;260(2):575–80.

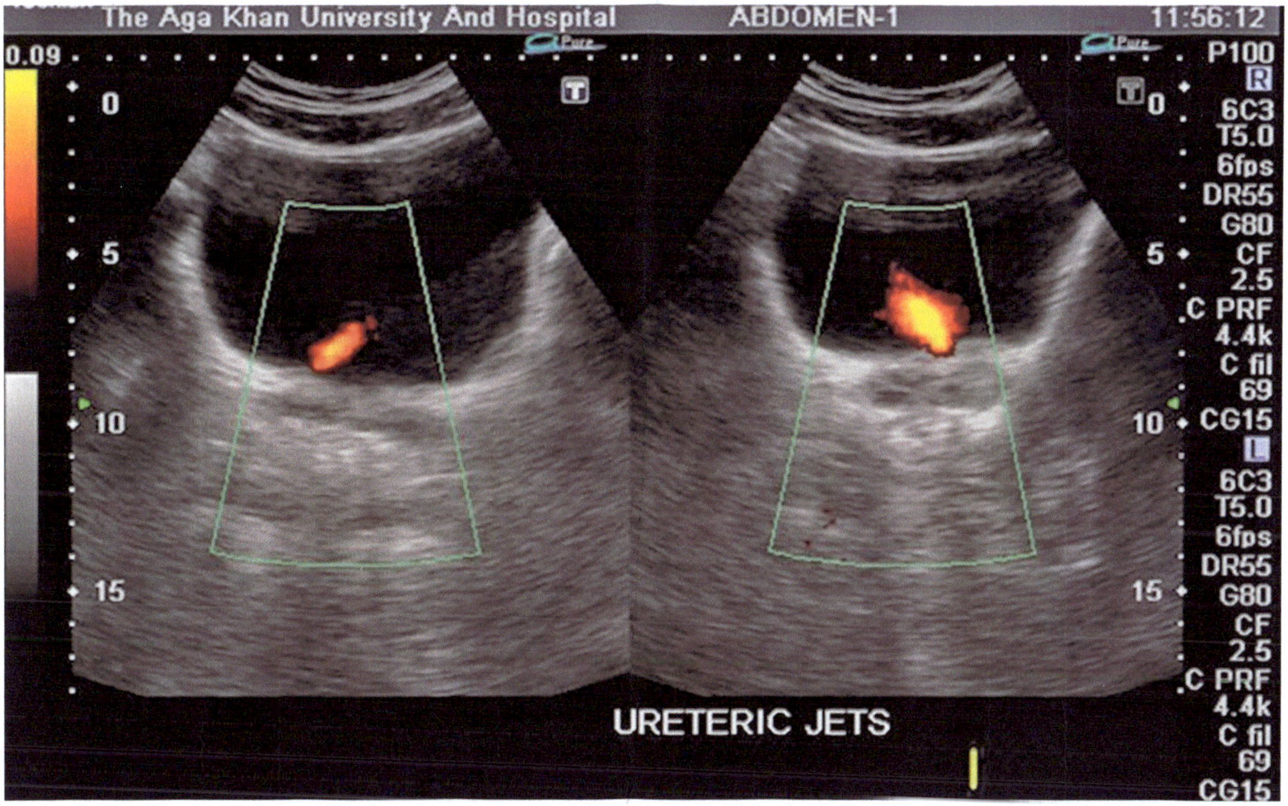

Fig. 114.9 Ultrasound showing ureteral jets

Case 10: Staghorn Stones

A 42-year-old male recurrent stone former presented to the clinic with bilateral flank pain more on the right side. Ultrasound (Fig. 114.10) showed a large staghorn stone in the right kidney. There was a small distal ureteral stone in the left side. The left-sided stone passed with medical expulsion therapy (MET). For the right side, a PCNL was planned followed by SWL for residual stones if needed.

An unremarkable PCNL followed by stented SWL was performed for residual stone. He needed three sessions to clear three 8–10-mm calculi in various calyces. Subsequently, his stent was removed and the patient is stone free.

Selected Bibliography

Chen S, Zhu L, Yang S, Wu W, Liao L, Tan J. High- vs low-power Holmium laser lithotripsy: a prospective, randomized study in patients undergoing multitract minipercutaneous nephrolithotomy. Urology. 2012;79(2):293–7. Epub 2011 Oct 15.

Desai M, De Lisa A, Turna B, Rioja J, Walfridsson H, D'Addessi A, Wong C, Rosette on Behalf of the Croes Pcnl Study Group J. The clinical research office of the endourological society percutaneous nephrolithotomy global study: staghorn versus nonstaghorn stones. J Endourol. 2011; 25(8):1263–8.

Viprakasit DP, Sawyer MD, Herrell SD, Miller NL. Changing composition of staghorn calculi. J Urol. 2011; 186(6):2285–90. Epub 2011 Oct 20.

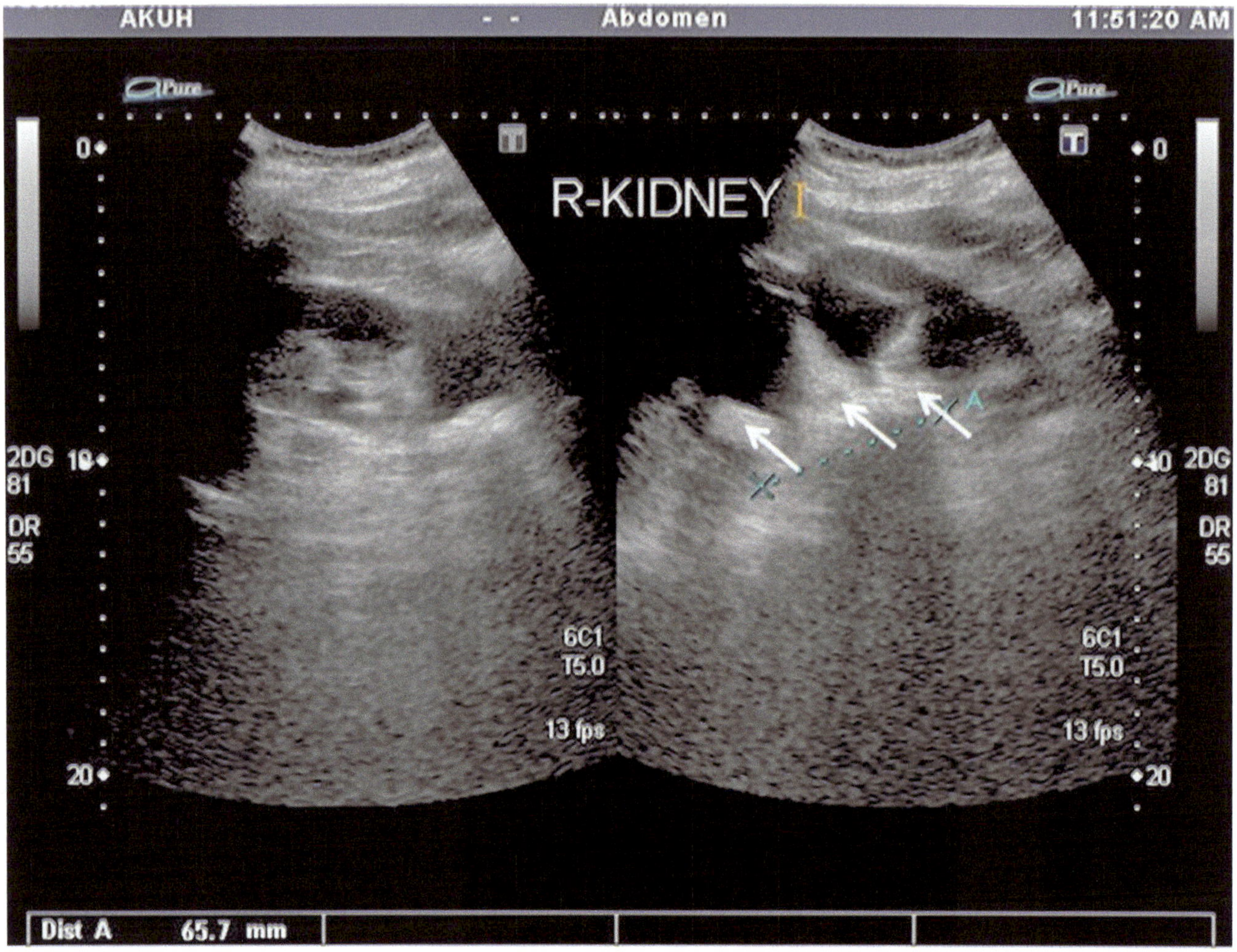

Fig. 114.10 Staghorn stone indicated by hyperechoic head and acoustic shadowing (*arrow*)

Case 11: Renal Stones and Pyelonephritis

A 65-year-old woman, with a known case of diabetes mellitus, ischemic heart disease, and rheumatoid arthritis, presented to the emergency room with acute onset flank pain, fever, and vomiting. Her initial evaluation indicated a raised total leukocyte count of 12.3 (4–11), raised serum creatinine 2.5 (0.7–1.1 mg/dl), and urinalysis showing leukocyturia, nitrite, and red cells. Her initial ultrasound (Fig. 114.11) showed parenchymal swelling, multiple renal stone, and hydronephrosis with signs of pyelonephritis. She was initially managed by antibiotics and percutaneous drainage and later had SWL for the stone.

Selected Bibliography

Miwa S, Yamamoto H, Sugata T. Antibiotics therapy was effective in preventing bilateral staghorn renal matrix stones. Urol Res. 2011;39(1):69–72.

Ramsey S, Robertson A, Ablett MJ, Meddings RN, Hollins GW, Little B. Evidence-based drainage of infected hydronephrosis secondary to ureteric calculi. J Endourol. 2010;24(2):185–9

Rule AD, Krambeck AE, Lieske JC. Chronic kidney disease in kidney stone formers. Clin J Am Soc Nephrol. 2011;6(8):2069–75.

Zanetti G, Paparella S, Trinchieri A, Prezioso D, Rocco F, Naber KG. Infections and urolithiasis: current clinical evidence in prophylaxis and antibiotic therapy. Arch Ital Urol Androl. 2008;80(1):5–12.

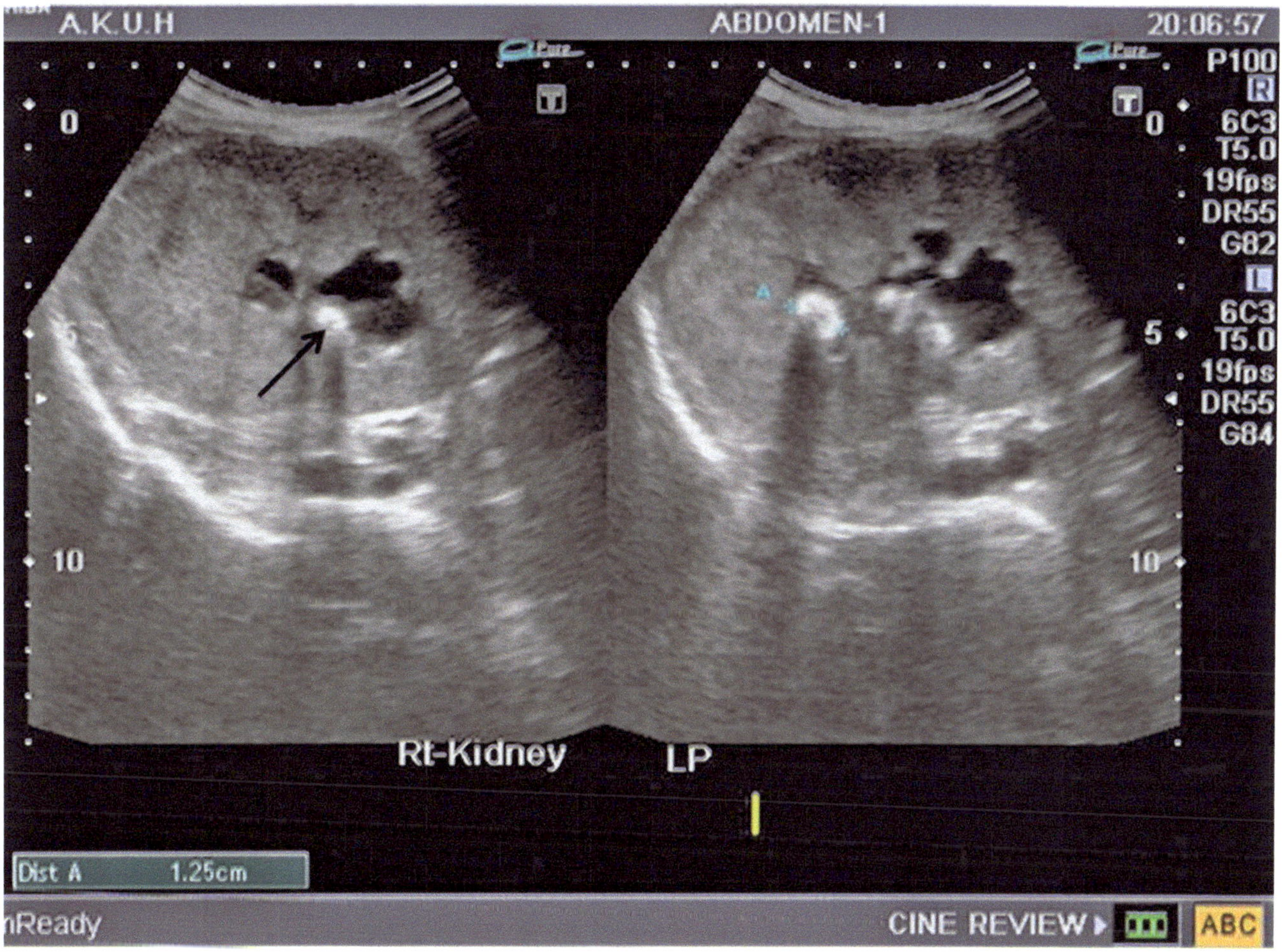

Fig. 114.11 Ultrasound showing renal stones and pyelonephritis (*arrow*)

Case 12: Obstruction

Ultrasound examinations often provide the first imaging for clinically suspected stone and obstruction. Fullness of the collecting system without an obvious cause (most commonly a renal stone) is often half the story. Presence of hydroureter with clinical picture of acute pain often indicates ureteral stone (see Fig. 114.12). Non-contrast-enhanced CT, plain X-ray, and sometimes contrast studies (intravenous urogram, CT urogram, and MRU) are often required to delineate the cause of obstruction. Renal scintigraphy using radioisotope scan differentiates between obstruction and nonobstructive dilatation.

Selected Bibliography

Benson AD, Taylor ER, Schwartz BF. Metal ureteral stent for benign and malignant ureteral obstruction. J Urol. 2011;185(6):2217–22. Epub 2011 Apr 17.

Sinescu I, Surcel C, Mirvald C, Chibelean C, Gîngu C, Avram D, Hîrza M, Manu M, Lazar R, Savu C, Udrea A. Prognostic factors in retroperitoneal fibrosis. J Med Life. 2010;3(1):19–25.

Vittori M, D'Addessi A, Pinto F, Tartaglione G, Bassi P. 99mTc-MAG3 diuretic renography in assessment of obstructive uropathy. The new test F + 10sp: a step ahead in the differential diagnosis. Urologia. 2011;78(3):221–6. doi: 10.5301/RU.2011.8633.

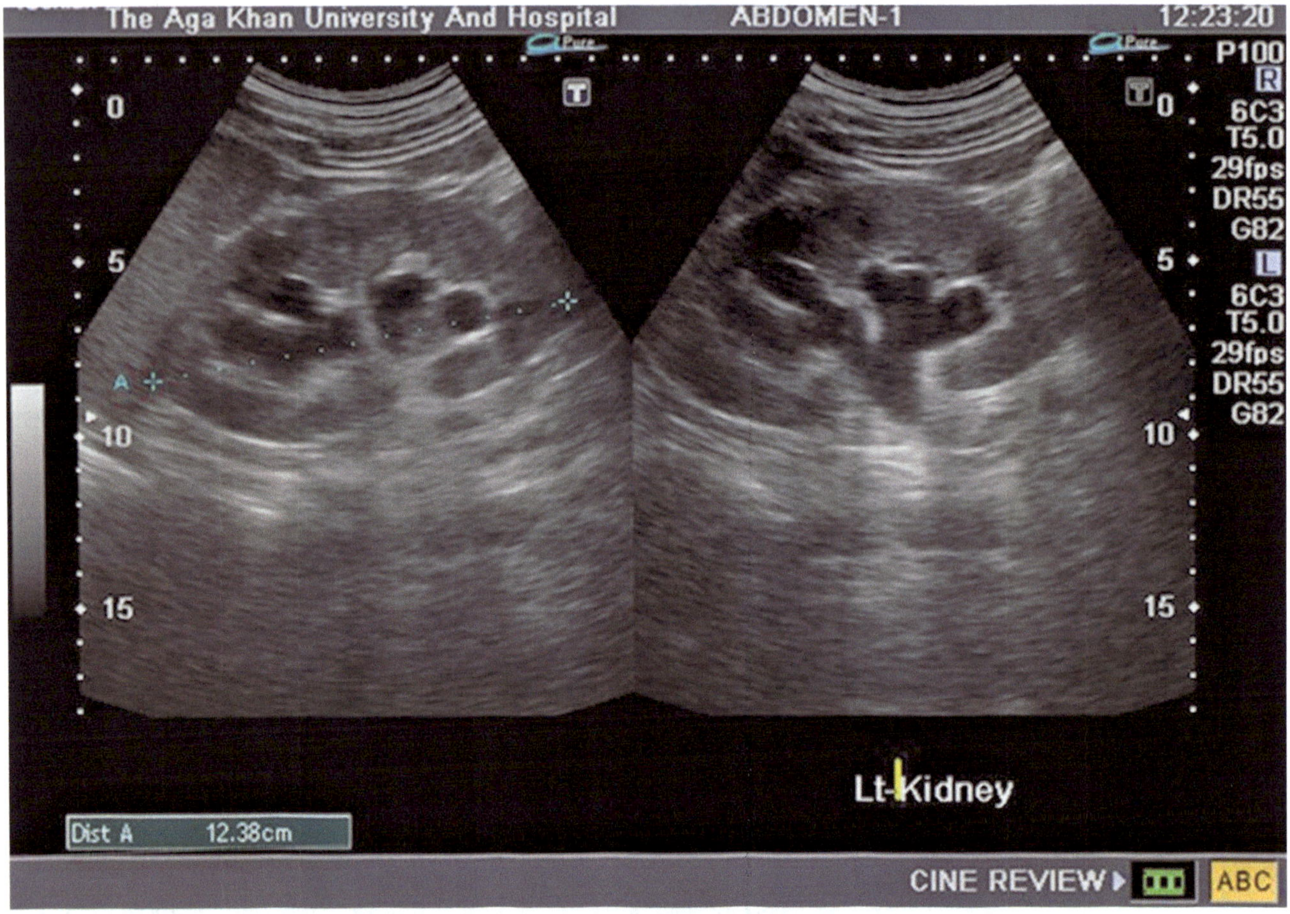

Fig. 114.12 Ultrasound indicating ureteral stone

Case 13: Distal Ureteral Stone

A 24-year-old male presented with acute left ureteral colic. Initial ultrasound (Fig. 114.13a, b) and plain X-ray KUB (not shown) showed a distal ureteral stone with hydroureter and hydronephrosis. He was initially managed conservatively; he passed stone in 12 days. Follow-up ultrasound showed resolution of hydronephrosis and no evidence of stone and ureteral jet.

Selected Bibliography

Moesbergen TC, de Ryke RJ, Dunbar S, Wells JE, Anderson NG. Distal ureteral calculi: US follow-up. Radiology. 2011;260(2):575–80.

Pichler R, Skradski V, Aigner F, Leonhartsberger N, Steiner H. In young adults with a low body mass index ultrasonography is sufficient as a diagnostic tool for ureteric stones. BJU Int. 2012 Mar;109(5):770–4.

Turkcuer I, Serinken M, Karcioglu O, Zencir M, Keysan MK. Hospital cost analysis of management of patients with renal colic in the emergency department. Urol Res. 2010;38(1):29–33.

Zehri AA, Ather MH, Abbas F, Biyabani SR. Preliminary study of efficacy of doxazosin as a medical expulsive therapy of distal ureteric stones in a randomized clinical trial. Urology. 2010;75(6):1285–8.

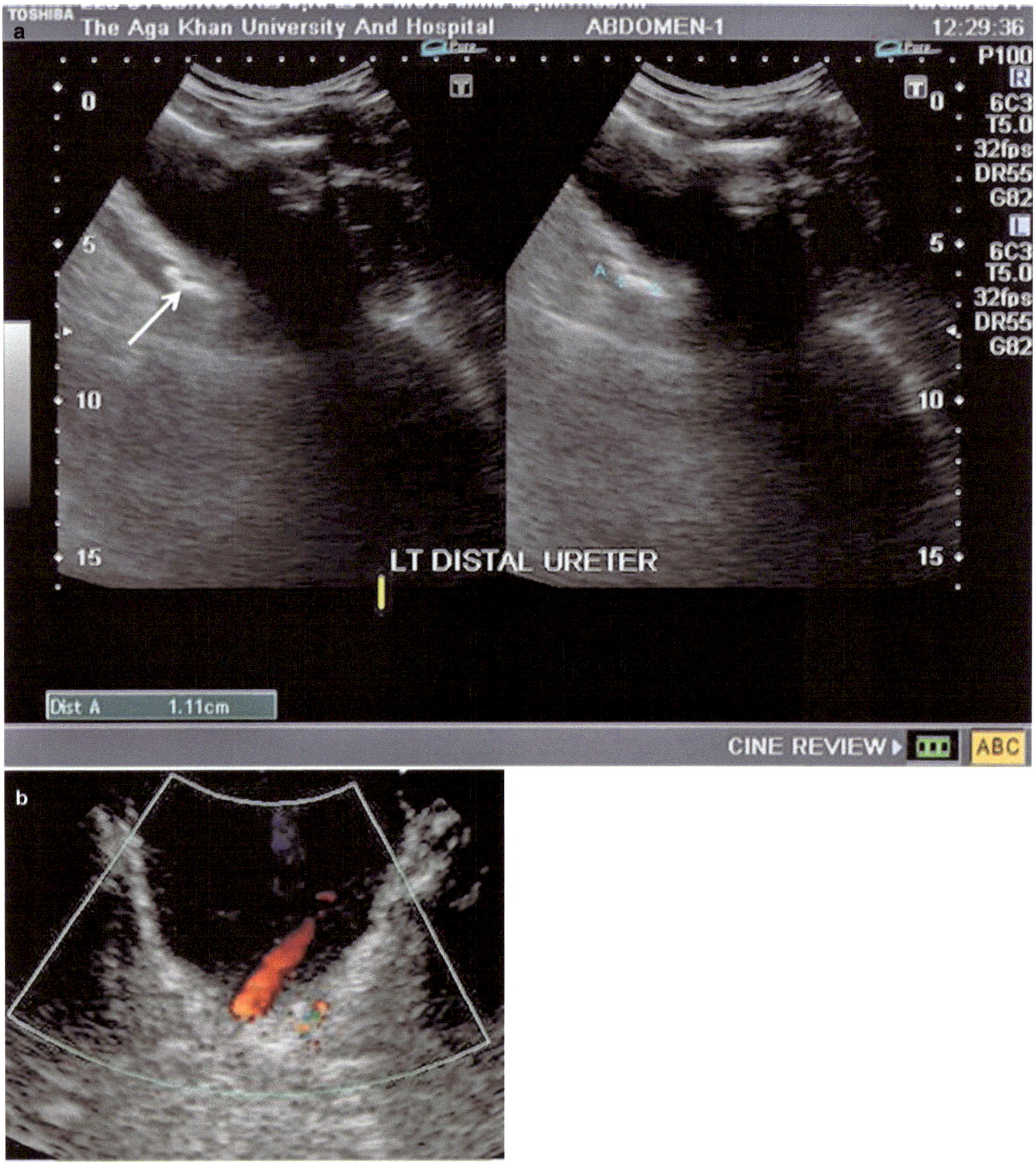

Fig. 114.13 (**a**, **b**) Ultrasound showing distal ureteral stone indicated by a hyperechoic head and acoustic shadowing (*arrow*)

Case 14: Vesical Stone

A 65-year-old woman with a history of fall resulting in spinal cord injury with paraplegia and LUTS some 3 years back. The neurosurgeon and vascular surgeon due to the suspicion of DVT initially evaluated her. In the course of work-up for LUTS, she was found to have large bladder stones (Fig. 114.14). She underwent cystolitholapexy, following which urodynamic investigation were performed in order to devise long-term care of the lower urinary tract. More recently, it has also been identified in patients with reconstructed bladder.

Selected Bibliography

Pavlica P, Gaudiano C, Barozzi L. Sonography of the bladder. World J Urol. 2004;22(5):328–34.

Vaidyanathan S, Hughes PL, Soni BM. A comparative study of ultrasound examination of urinary tract performed on spinal cord injury patients with no urinary symptoms and spinal cord injury patients with symptoms related to urinary tract: do findings of ultrasound examination lead to changes in clinical management? ScientificWorldJournal. 2006;6: 2450–9.

Volkmer BG, Nesslauer T, Kuefer R, Engel O, Kraemer SC, Gottfried HW. Visualization of urinary stones by 3-D ultrasound with surface rendering. Ultrasound Med Biol. 2002;28(2):143–7.

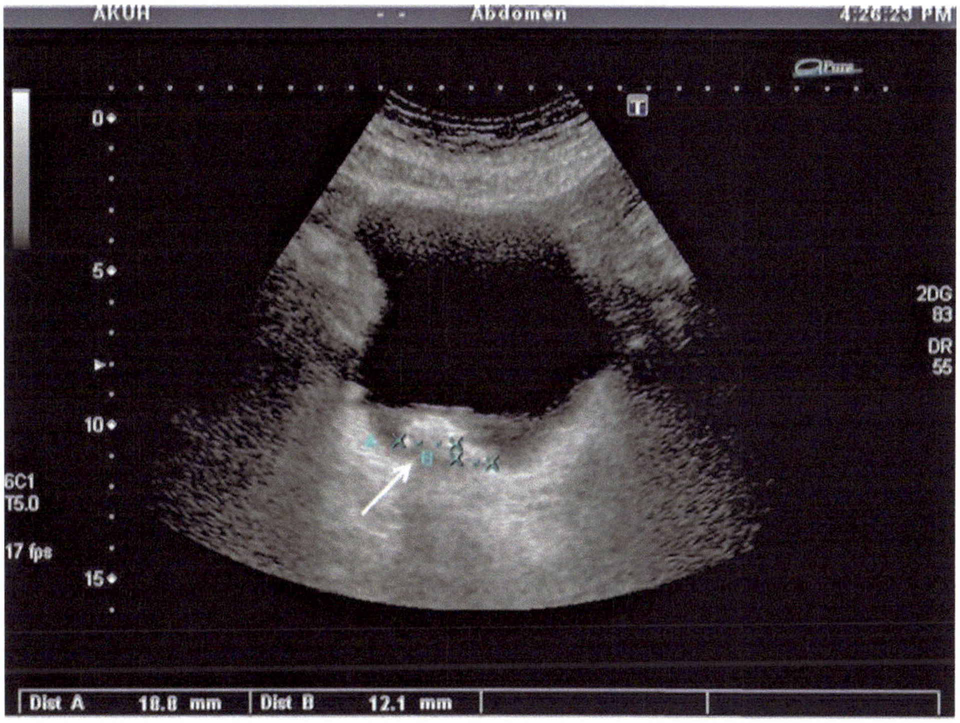

Fig. 114.14 Vesical stone indicated by hyperechoic head and acoustic shadowing (*arrow*)

Case 15: Steinstrasse with Stent

A 42-year-old male presented to the clinic with a history of left flank pain. He is a known case of urolithiasis and had an open surgery some 15 years back. At the time of presentation, he had a 2.0-cm proximal ureteral stone with hydronephrosis. His work-up did not show any ongoing infection. Options of management including percutaneous surgery were discussed; he wished to avoid interventional procedure. He agreed to undergo JJ stent placement followed by SWL. Following two sessions of SWL, he again presented to the clinic with mild flank pain. His repeat hemi-KUB X-ray showed a steinstrasse (Fig. 114.15). He was managed initially by medical expulsive therapy followed by ureteroscopy due to nonprogression of the fragments on conservative treatment.

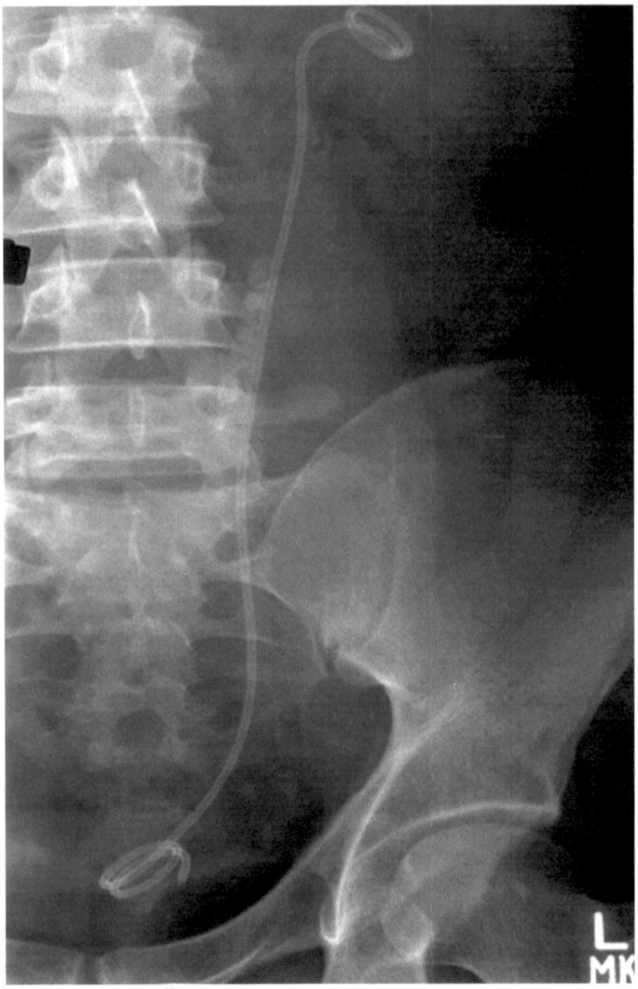

Fig. 114.15 Static steinstrasse with JJ stent in place

Case 16: Dynamic Steinstrasse (SS)

An 18-year-old male, first-time stone former, presented to the emergency room with acute right ureteral colic in the middle of the night. Ultrasound showed a right proximal ureteral stone 9 mm and proximal hydroureter and hydronephrosis. Plain X-ray KUB confirmed the radio-opaque nature of the stone. He was treated with in situ SWL follow-up scan 4 days later when he presented to emergency again with fever and vomiting, and flank pain showed a Steinstrasse. Medical expulsive treatment was instituted, and he passed all the fragments with conservative treatment (Fig. 114.16a, b).

Steinstrasse seen in routine follow-up scan following SWL in asymptomatic patients is categorized as dynamic SS. It is the state of stones in transition through the ureter and often does not require any active intervention. Static SS on the contrary is a state in which stone fragments fail to progress through the ureter, and they are often associated with lead fragment, ureteral wall edema, and infection.

Selected Bibliography

Ather MH, Shrestha B, Mehmood A. Does ureteral stenting prior to shock wave lithotripsy influence the need for intervention in steinstrasse and related complications? Urol Int. 2009;83(2):222–5.

Moursy E, Gamal WM, Abuzeid A. Tamsulosin as an expulsive therapy for steinstrasse after extracorporeal shock wave lithotripsy: a randomized controlled study. Scand J Urol Nephrol. 2010;44(5):315–9.

Puppo P. Steinstrasse 20 years later: Still a problem after ESWL? Eur Urol. 2006;50(4):643–7.

Sulaiman MN, Buchholz NP, Clark PB. The role of ureteral stent placement in the prevention of Steinstrasse. J Endourol. 1999;13(3):151–5.

Talati J, Khan S, Biyabani R, Khan RA, Naz I, Abbas F, Buchholz NP. Reduction of radiation exposure to patients in the follow-up of shockwave lithotripsy. BJU Int. 2000;85(4): 404–7.

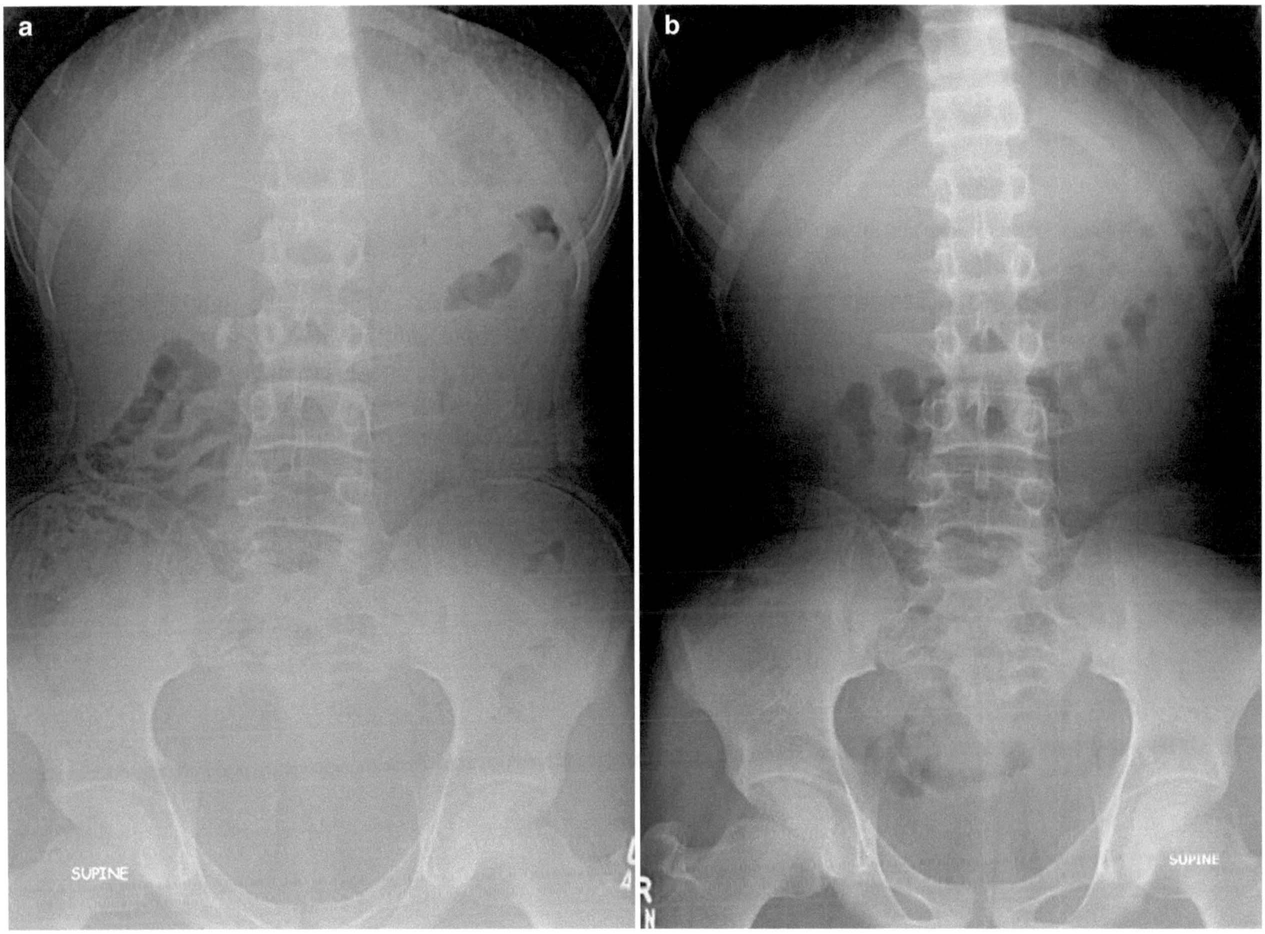

Fig. 114.16 (**a**, **b**) Dynamic steinstrasse

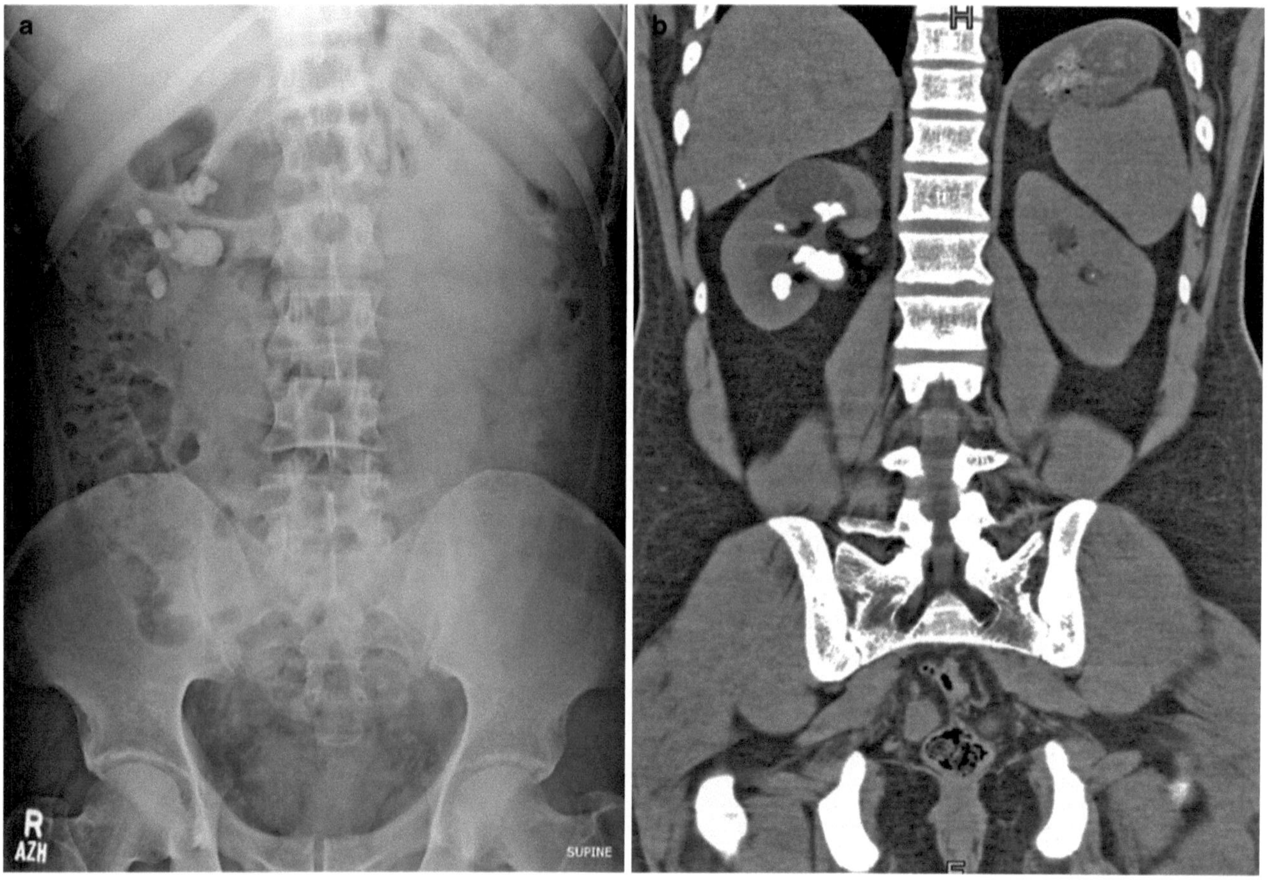

Fig. 114.17 (**a**) Partial staghorn stone and (**b**) small calculi

Case 17: Partial Staghorn Stones

A 31-year-old male presented to the outpatient clinic with a 2-month history of bilateral flank pain. Physical examination showed right flank tenderness. Urinalysis showed leukocyturia and with negative urine culture. His initial plain X-ray KUB (Fig. 114.17a) showed a partial staghorn stone with multiple secondary calculi in the right kidney. CT KUB (Fig. 114.17b) in addition showed few small stones in the left kidney as well. He underwent right PCNL with post-procedure scan showing couple of 3–4-mm residual stone at 1 month. He was placed on potassium citrate, and a 3-month scan showed complete clearance of stone bilaterally.

Case 18: Staghorn Stones and Immobilization

Recurrent urinary tract infections, indwelling catheters, vesicoureteral reflux, and immobilization hypercalciuria are a few of the major risk factors for the development of urolithiasis among patients who are immobilized, particularly following spinal cord injury (Fig. 114.18a, b).

Endourological open surgical interventions are all associated with significant complication. Retrograde intrarenal surgery is inadequate to clear the stone burden and is also technically difficult due to lower extremity contractures, spinal curvature, and pelvic tilt. SWL success rates are effective in stone fragmentation provided patients could be adequately positioned, but clearance rates are often delayed. Percutaneous surgery is often used, and the success rate is similar to the general population but at the expense of a higher complication rate. Meticulous planning with regard to appropriate prophylactic antibiotics and body position will maximize efficacious outcomes.

Early identification and treatment of urolithiasis in spinal cord injury patients will aid in preserving renal function and minimizing associated complications. Despite variation in common urological practices between spinal cord injury units and the lack of clear-cut guidelines for follow-up, the increased incidence of risks associated with urolithiasis lends support for routine genitourinary imaging in order to identify and treat those individuals at highest risk.

Selected Bibliography

Ganpule AP, Mishra S, Desai MR. Multiperc versus single perc with flexible instrumentation for staghorn calculi. J Endourol. 2009;23(10):1675–8.

Honeck P, Wendt-Nordahl G, Krombach P, Bach T, Häcker A, Alken P, Michel MS. Does open stone surgery still play a role in the treatment of urolithiasis? Data of a primary urolithiasis center. J Endourol. 2009;23(7):1209–12.

Malcolm JB, Derweesh IH, Brightbill EK, Mehrazin R, DiBlasio CJ, Wake RW. Tubeless percutaneous nephrolithotomy for complex renal stone disease: single center experience. Can J Urol. 2008;15(3):4072–6; discussion 4076–7.

Ost MC, Lee BR. Urolithiasis in patients with spinal cord injuries: risk factors, management, and outcomes. Curr Opin Urol. 2006;16(2):93–9.

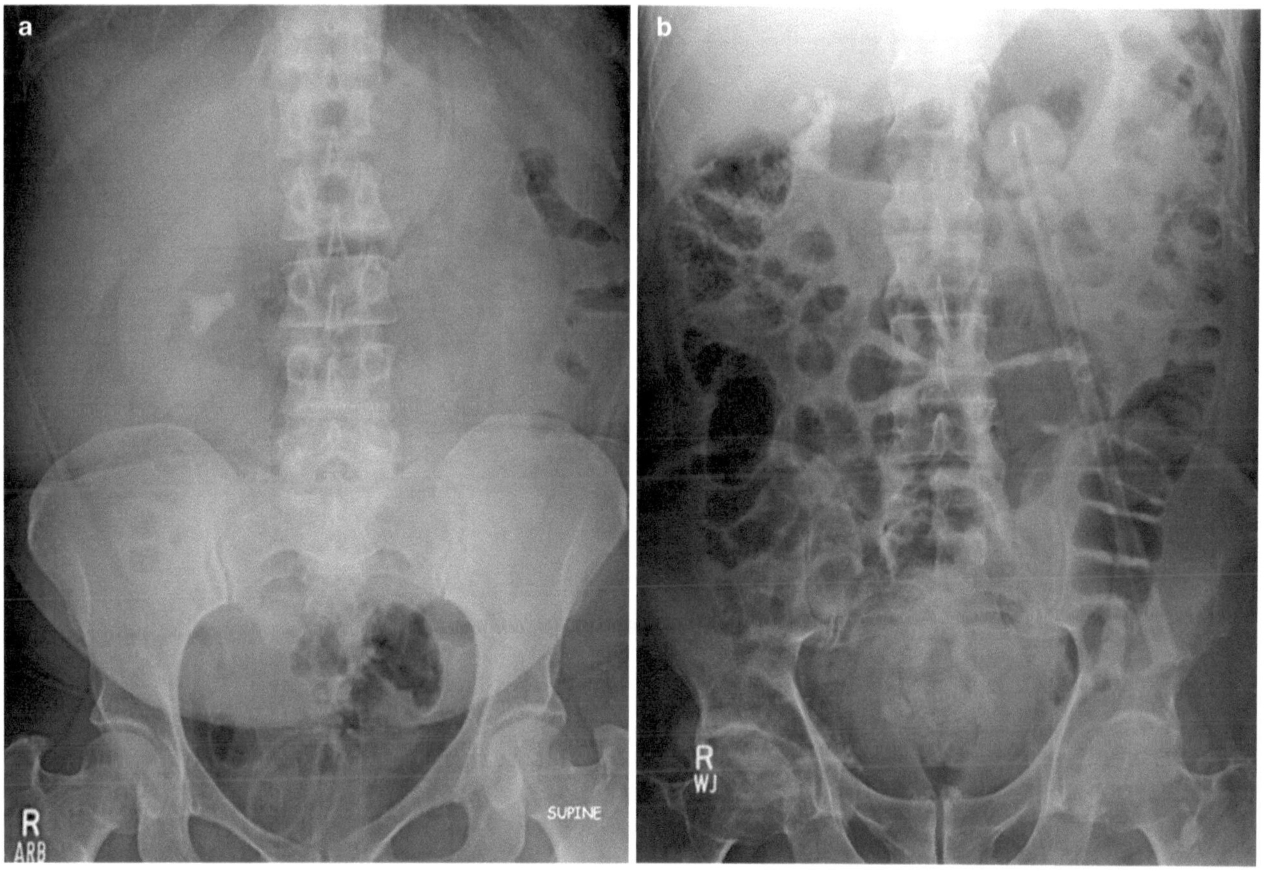

Fig. 114.18 (a, b) Staghorn stones in immobilized patients

Soucy F, Ko R, Duvdevani M, Nott L, Denstedt JD, Razvi H. Percutaneous nephrolithotomy for staghorn calculi: a single center's experience over 15 years. J Endourol. 2009;23(10):1669–73.

Thomas K, Smith NC, Hegarty N, Glass JM. The Guy's stone score – grading the complexity of percutaneous nephrolithotomy procedures. Urology. 2011;78(2):277–81.

Case 19: Renal Stone and Ureterocele

A 25-year-old woman with no comorbidities, resident of Hyderabad, working in a bank, presented with hematuria, strangury, and left renal colic. There was no prior history of tuberculosis or lower urinary tract symptoms and no accompanying fever. Examination was unremarkable. She brought her previous investigations, which showed that she has *a left renal stone and a left ureterocele.* We advised a non-contrast CT KUB (Fig. 114.19a–c), urine analysis and culture, a serum calcium, albumin, and uric acid.

We explained that in view of the ureterocele, post-ESWL fragments might form a Steinstrasse. We advised endoscopic deroofing of the ureterocele, a JJ stent insertion, and then ESWL. We also explained that the deroofing may not be a permanent solution and that if serious reflux occurred, she might require a reimplantation. We explained that reimplantation is a more major procedure, and incision of the ureterocele is an acceptable first option.

The patient and relatives were overwhelmed with the amount of information received, perplexed by the additional finding of the ureterocele, and uncertain of why the incision was necessary. Further explanations were provided and the patient wished to think it over with her relatives. She did not return for surgery. When talking to patients, the amount of information given needs to be tailored to the patients' understanding and needs to be couched in terms the individual can understand (see Chap. 96) and tailored to the society in which the individual has grown up. At times the options need to be framed in terms of definitive outcomes. Nevertheless, in an ebullient society such as ours in Karachi, Pakistan, a full detailed explanation of what is going on is one way of also developing society. Would you have offered a ureteroneocystostomy to this patient, and in a country which has so much stone disease, which technique would you use? (Case submitted by Dr. Mazher Ali.)

Selected Bibliography

Vijay MK, Vijay P, Dutta A, Gupta A, Tiwari P, Kumar S, Bera MK, Das RK, Kundu AK. The safety and efficacy of endoscopic incision of orthotopic ureterocele in adult. Saudi J Kidney Dis Transpl. 2011;22(6):1169–74.

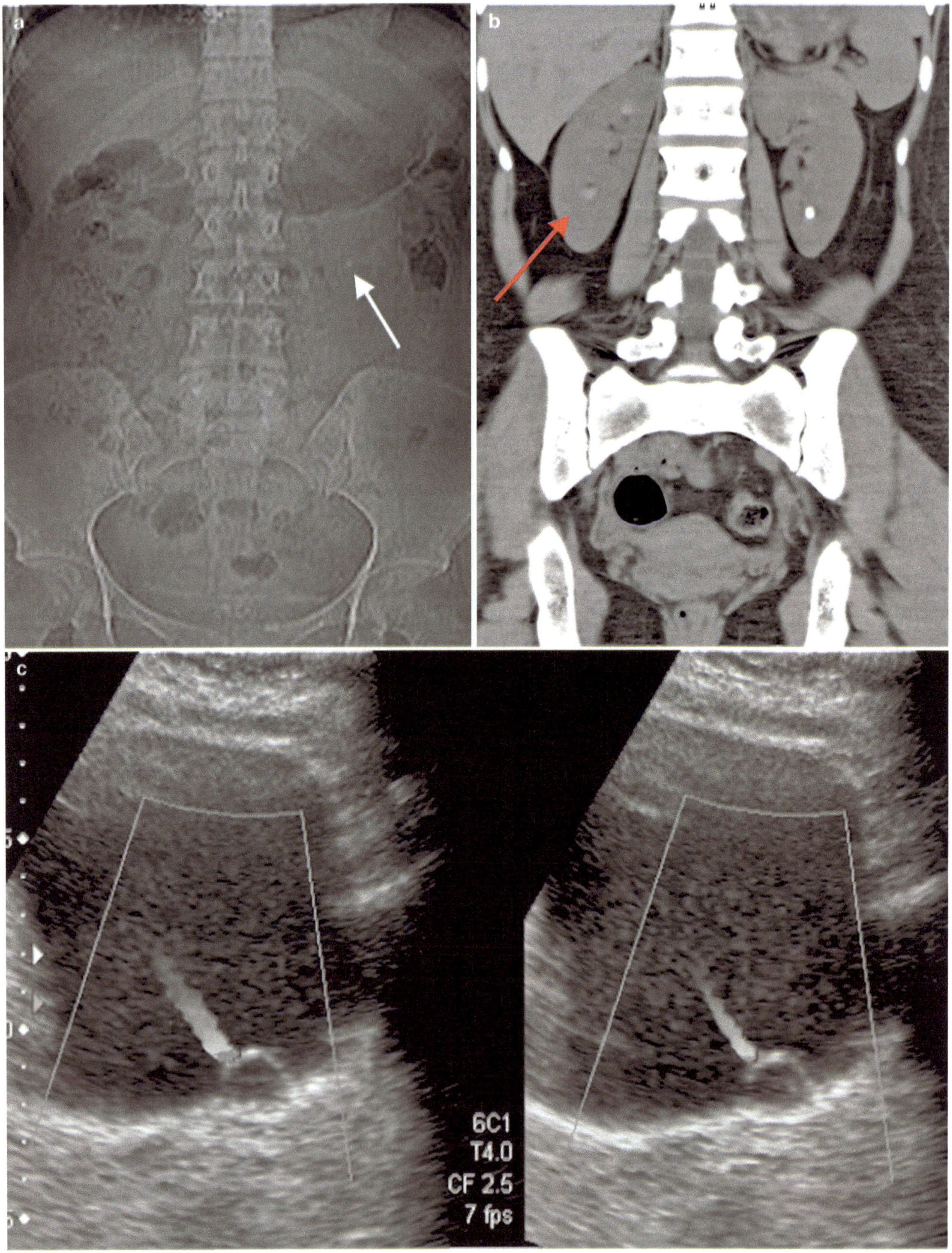

Fig. 114.19 CT KUB. (**a**) The *arrow* points to nephrocalcinosis. (**b**) There is a faintly radio-opaque left renal stone (*arrow*). An interesting point is that the ureterocele was not detectable on this NCCT and would have been missed but for a previous ultrasound (**c**)

Case 20: Medical Expulsive Therapy

A 54-year-old male on treatment for hypertension and hypercholesterolemia, presented with bilateral flank pain and hematuria for 1 week. The pain was felt more on the right side and radiated to the right testes. It was severe in intensity (pain score about 9/10). On examination, the renal punch was positive on the right but otherwise unremarkable.

An ultrasound KUB showed a right proximal 0.6-cm ureteric stone. The plain film KUB and the NCCT are shown in Fig. 114.20a, b.

The serum creatinine was 0.9 mg/dl, and urine culture did not grow any organisms. Options of treatment including ureteroscopic fragmentation and medical expulsive therapy (MET) were explained. He opted for MET. A day later, he returned with severe right colic. In view of repeated colics, he was advised to have a ureterorenoscopy (URS) for stone fragmentation. The patient again declined.

Subsequently he returned yet again, asking how we would know that he had not passed the stone before subjecting him to URS. He was advised to continue MET and urinate in a jug each time (easily said, difficult to do) to check whether a stone had been passed. He was also informed that we would repeat an X-ray KUB and U/S bladder looking for ureteric jets on the morning of surgery.

The X-ray on the morning of the operation day showed radio-opacities in the pelvis, one of which was in the line of right ureter. On ultrasound the same morning, bilateral small renal stones were noted. During this ultrasound examination, he asked the sonologist about the stone, and he was told "you have no stone in the ureter now, so there is no need for the procedure." The patient was convinced he did not need a ureteroscopy and refused to get admitted. The X-rays were discussed with him and the stone location, now in the pelvis near the anatomical ischial spine was pointed out and explained to him (Fig. 114.20c). In view of the stone and continuing pain, the patient was advised day-care ureteroscopy.

The patient refused surgery, saying he has no stone.

What would you have done?

The patient's stone had moved down a considerable distance within a week. He appeared to be compliant in taking MET. We therefore allowed him to continue MET; in actual fact, he refused URS. The same evening he passed a stone into the jug which served as a urinal, and he let us know of the event, on our mobile phone.

The stone was 0.6 cm and causing significant pain requiring frequent intramuscular/intravenous analgesia. Should the decision have been first to try medical treatment and not discuss ureteroscopy? That too would be wrong. If we had done the URS, then would it have been an unnecessary procedure?

Stones in our part of the world are often neglected by patients when they become silent. This probably drives an aggressive approach to stone removal, in an effort to lower the incidence of calculus renal failure.

The case also indicates that verbal communication with the patient who is already averse to procedures needs to be couched in careful terms. Patients value highly the ability to contact residents, and the mobile phone has transformed the service and improved patient satisfaction. (Case submitted by Dr. Mazher Ali)

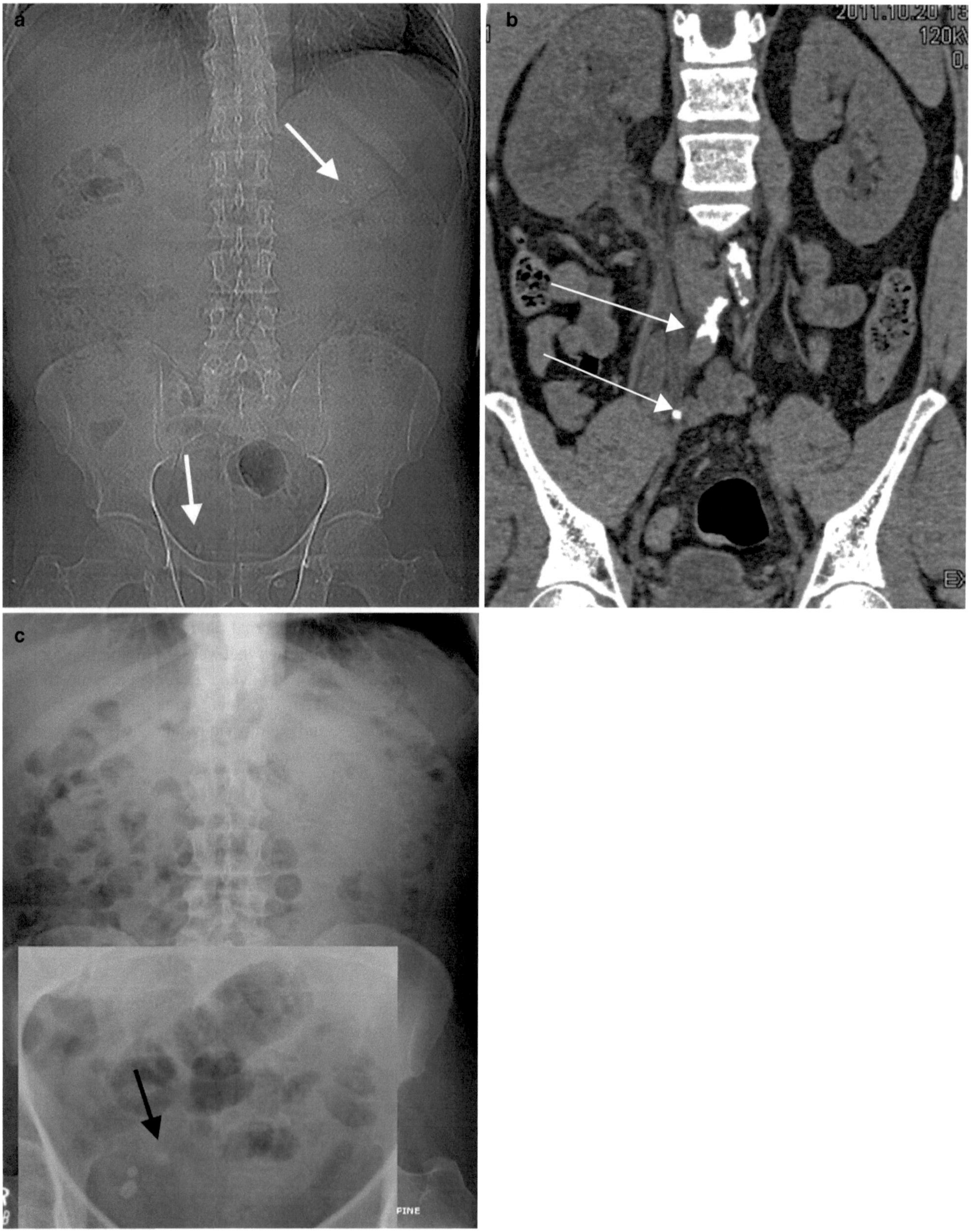

Fig. 114.20 NCCT (**a**)) Pain film: notice the arrow in pelvis pointing to a radio-opaque shadow, which could be a phlebolith, and a small radio-opaque stone in the left kidney. (**b**) Coronal view of scan: right middle ureteric stone, (see lower *arrow*) which cannot be seen on the plain KUB film), with mild hydronephrosis and proximal hydroureter (Upper *arrow*). (**c**) The morning of the proposed URS, the stone had migrated down the ureter (see *arrow*)

Case 21: Angulated and Tortuous Ureter

An elderly woman with no known comorbidities presented with left flank pain. A CT KUB was done which showed mid-ureteric stone measuring 9 mm.

A ureteroscopic stone fragmentation was planned. Preoperatively the ureter was noted to be angulated and tortuous. There was difficulty negotiating the URS and reaching the stone. A JJ stent was introduced over the guidewire and left in place for 6 weeks (Fig. 114.21).

A repeat URS was done 6 weeks later, and we removed both the stone and JJ stent successfully (See Chap. 58). (Case submitted by Mahwish Nadeem)

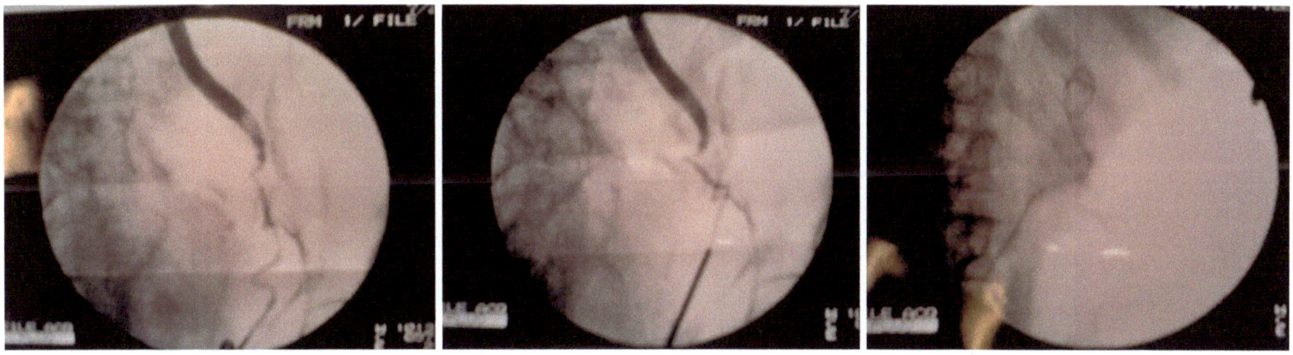

Fig. 114.21 An angulated and tortuous ureter made it difficult to perform URS and reach a mid-ureteric stone, so a JJ stent was inserted for 6 weeks prior to URS

Epilogue

Do we really need another book on the management of Urolithiasis, a condition that has plagued men and women for centuries? With the numerous texts on medical and surgical stone management, one's first impulse would be, certainly not. Yet, Talati, Tiselius, Albala and Ye, should be congratulated on this innovative volume. Not only does it update the basic pathophysiology of nephrolithiasis, metabolic stone management, as well as describe the indications and use of new and innovative minimally invasive techniques for stone diagnosis and removal, but it addresses many of the social concerns and potential economic solutions for managing this endemic disease.

Urolithiasis continues to affect a large percentage of the world population and incurs increasing costs in both the Western world and in underdeveloped societies. In fact, the incidence of renal stone disease continues to increase, mainly due to changes in diet and lifestyle. Metabolic syndrome, diabetes, and obesity have increased in all parts of the world, bringing with them an increased incidence of nephrolithiasis. Can the innovations described within this text in metabolic stone management, shock wave lithotripsy, and endourology provide us with the tools we need to reduce or eliminate this significant health problem? Perhaps changes in health care financing, resource sharing, and evidence-based therapy, all described in this volume, will address many of these issues.

Nowhere in medicine have we seen such dramatic enhancements over one generation in diagnosis, therapy, and prevention as we have in urolithiasis. What will the next generation bring? The purpose of this compilation is to stimulate the reader to further develop a better understanding of the epidemiology and pathogenesis of nephrolithiasis. Advances in genetic and gene-based therapy may ultimately reduce the incidence of renal stone disease and play a major role in stone prevention. Enhancements in shock wave technology continue to provide new algorithms to improve renal and ureteral stone fragmentation, while reducing tissue injury. Superlative developments in endoscopic imaging and intracorporeal stone fragmentation continue to improve the efficiency and decrease the morbidity of renal and ureteral stone removal. Ultimately continued focus on health care disparities and improvements in funding the health enterprise will bring many of these solutions to fruition, thereby changing the management of urolithiasis even more over the next generation.

Glenn M. Preminger

G.M. Preminger, M.D. (✉)
Division of Urologic Surgery, Duke University Medical Center, RM 1573 White Zone, Duke South, DUMC 3167, Durham, NC, 27710, USA and
Duke Comprehensive Kidney Stone Center, Durham, NC, USA
e-mail: glenn.preminger@duke.edu; premi001@mc.duke.edu

J.J. Talati et al. (eds.), *Urolithiasis*,
DOI 10.1007/978-1-4471-4387-1, © Springer-Verlag London 2012

Index

A

Accreditation Council for Graduate Medical Education (ACGME), 820, 821, 869
Acetohydroxamic acid (AHA), 534
ACGME. *See* Accreditation Council for Graduate Medical Education (ACGME)
Acute renal failure (ARF), 220
Advanced training, urology. *See* Stone disease management
Aga Khan University Hospital (AKUH), 910
AKUH. *See* Aga Khan University Hospital (AKUH)
Alanine-glyoxylate aminotransferase (AGT) enzyme, 625
ALARA. *See* As low as reasonably achievable (ALARA)
Alkali citrate therapy
- calcium stones
  - bone mineral density (BMD), 737–738
  - counteracting microgravity, 738–739
  - distal renal tubular acidosis (RTA), 737
  - idiopathic hypocitraturic calcium nephrolithiasis, 736–737
  - shock wave lithotripsy (SWL), 738
  - thiazide-unresponsive hypercalciuric nephrolithiasis, 737
- dietary, 740–741
- uric acid stones, 739–780

Alkaline therapy
- calcium, renal parenchymal tissue and renal injury, 198
- RTA patients, 197
- urinary potassium excretion, 197

American Urological Association (AUA), 258
American Urology Association In-Service Examination (AUA ISE), 822–823
Ammonium urate stones, 238
Anesthesia
- agents
  - LA, 552–553
  - non-opioid, 552
  - NSAIDs, 552
  - opioid, 552
  - paracetamol, 552
- children
  - PCNL, 660
  - URS, 664
- description, 548
- ESWL (*see* Extracorporeal shock wave lithotripsy (ESWL))
- PCNL (*see* Percutaneous nephrolithotomy (PCNL))
- postoperative pain
  - assessment, 550–551
  - management, 551–552
- preoperative evaluation, 548
- SWL, children, 657

Animal models, urological training, 829–830
Animal protein intake, stone formation, 714–715
Antegrade stent placement, 441–442
Antegrade ureteroscopy. *See* Nephrolithotripsy
Antibiotic therapy, 233, 234
Anticoagulation therapy, 388
Anti-inflammatory proteins, kidney stone matrix
- constituents, 177–178
- defined, 177
- and noninfection kidney stones
  - calgranulin (calprotectin), 179–180
  - defensin, 179
  - injury and inflammation, 178, 179
  - MCP-1, 180
  - MPO, 178–179

Antiplatelet medication, ESWL, 558–559
Antiplatelet therapy, 558–559
AP(CaOx) index
- excretion, 677
- urine collection, 679–680
- values, 678

AP(CaP) index
- ion-activity products, 677
- urine collection, 679–680
- values, 678

ARF. *See* Acute renal failure (ARF)
ARSI. *See* Association of Rural Surgeons of India (ARSI)
ASI. *See* Association of Surgeons of India (ASI)
As low as reasonably achievable (ALARA), 274
Assessment, postgraduate training
- age-old methodologies, 807
- Miller's pyramid hierarchy, 807, 808
- portfolios, 817
- quality assurance, 817
- validity and reliability, 808
- workplace assessment methods (*see* Workplace assessment methods)

Association of Rural Surgeons of India (ARSI), 877
Association of Surgeons of India (ASI), 877
Atkins diet, 188
AUA. *See* American Urological Association (AUA)
AUA ISE. *See* American Urology Association In-Service Examination (AUA ISE)
Australia
- aboriginal and non aboriginal population, 76
- renal colic, 73
- treatment modalities, 74, 75
- upper urinary tract stones, 73, 74

B

Balanced diet
- calcium, 721–722
- coarse grains and cellulose, 722
- fruits and vegetables, 722
- high-purine, 722

J.J. Talati et al. (eds.), *Urolithiasis*,
DOI 10.1007/978-1-4471-4387-1, © Springer-Verlag London 2012

Balanced diet (*cont.*)
  overweight and BMI, 722
  oxalic acid, 722
  protein, 722
  sodium, 722
  Vitamin C, 722
Balloon dilatation system, 660
Bariatric surgery, 188
Bartter's syndrome, 142–143
Bench models, 830
Bilateral neck exploration (BNE)
  adenoma
    thymus, 796, 797
    typical, 795–796
  anatomical position, 794, 795
  biopsy, 793
  extravasated calcium infusion effects, 798, 799
  general anesthesia, 793
  lower parathyroids, 795
  methodology, 793
  nerve stimulator access, 794, 795
  nonrecurrent laryngeal nerve, 794, 795
  parathyroidectomy (*see* Parathyroidectomy)
  platysma lateral dissection, 794
  procedure, 793–794
  recurrent laryngeal nerve, 794
  skin buttonholing, 794
  small lymph node, 794, 795
  transplantation, 796, 797
Bilateral percutaneous nephrolithotomy, 662
Bilateral staghorn stones, 937
Biochemical risk evaluation
  calcium stone disease, 676–680
  cystine, 675–676
  diagnosis, DRAT, 681
  infection stone disease, 676
  medical history
    blood analyses, 374–375
    identification, abnormalities, 374
    stone formation(*see* Stone formation)
    uric acid, 375
  nonsurgical treatment, 671
  procedure, stone removal, 671
  stone age index (SAI), 680
  stone composition
    analysis, 672
    calcium stone, 672
    cystine, 673
    KUB and NCCT, 672
    microscopic identification, 673
    pH measurements, 673
    procedure, 672–673
    uric acid formation, 673
  stone formation, unrinary tract, 671
Bisphosphonates, 730
Bladder stones, 940
Blood analysis, 374–375
BMI. *See* Body mass index (BMI)
Body mass index (BMI)
  defined, 86
  and stone composition, 923
Bone density
  biochemical abnormalities, 772
  prevention, calcium stone formers, 737–738
Broader education
  Boolean algebra, 866
  cosmos, 864
  creative arts, 866
  eye to detail, 866
  heliocentric system, Copernicus, 864
  historical consciousness, 866
  human imagination, 866
  medical/surgical field, 865
  metaphysical presupposition, 864
  nerve system, 866
  philosophical considerations, 863–864
  Ptolemaic system, 864
  sacred disease, 864
  scientific revolution, 865
  scientism, 865
  square law, 865
Brushite, 190–193, 214

C

Cadaver models, 830
Cadavers, 860
Calcium
  human kidney stones, 727
  hypercalciuria (*see* Hypercalciuria)
  hyperoxaluria (*see* Hyperoxaluria)
  saturation, 727
  urine concentration, 727
Calcium channel antagonists, 529
Calcium homeostasis
  absorption and transport, renal tubule, 202
  CaSR, 201–202
  nephrolithiasis, 203
  parathyroid hormone, 202
  vitamin D, 202–203
Calcium intake, stone formation, 713–714
Calcium oxalate
  and brushite, 192, 193
  citrate (*see* Alkali citrate therapy)
  SI and RSR, 191–192
  urinary saturation, 188
Calcium oxalate dihydrate (COD)
  gender, 5
  idiopathic calcium nephrolithiasis, 9
Calcium oxalate dihydrate (COD) stones, 132
Calcium oxalate monohydrate (COM), 180
Calcium oxalate (CaOx) stones
  COM and COD, 5, 9
  defined, 129
  idiopathic, 129–133
  Randall's plaque, 9, 10
Calcium phosphate stones
  carbonation rate, 135
  dRTA, 134
  primary hyperparathyroidism, 134
  weddellite and carbapatite, 134
Calcium-sensing receptor (CASR)
  CATTCA haplotype and stone-forming condition, 143
  defined, 142
Calcium stones
  AP(CaOx) and AP(CaP) index, 677, 679–680
  biochemical risk evaluation, 677
  Bonn Risk Index, 677
  bottom line analysis, 677
  creatinine excretion, 678, 679
  disadvantages, 677
  formation, urinary tract, 676
  inhibition activities, 678
  ion-activity products, 677–678

oxalate, 676, 678
pH measurements, 678
phosphate, 676, 677
risk factors, 679
urine collections, 677
variables analysis, 678–679
Calculus renal failure in Pakistan
Alma-Ata Declaration, 595
bilateral renal stones, 598
CKD, 596
consequences, 596
dialysis centers, 596, 597
differences, 595
education, 595
end-stage renal disease (ESRD), 596, 597
health care, 595–596
hypertension, 597–598
kidney foundation, 596
left kidney operation, 598
renal replacement therapy (RRT), 596
and stones, 596–597
Calgranulin (calprotectin), 179–180
CanMEDS, 820, 821
CaOx stones. *See* Calcium oxalate (CaOx) stones
Cardiac resynchronization devices (CRT), 565
Cardiac rhythm management devices
CRT, 565
description, 563
ICD, 565
pacemakers (*see* Pacemakers)
Case-based discussion (CbD), 809, 814
CaSR. *See* Calcium-sensing receptor (CaSR)
CbD. *See* Case-based discussion (CbD)
CEC. *See* Clinical encounter card (CEC)
China
nationalities, 56
prevalence, 57
urolithiasis, 53–56
Chinese MPCNL. *See* Minimally invasive percutaneous nephrolithotomy (MPCNL)
Chloride channel 5 (CLCN5), 143
Chronic kidney disease (CKD)
description, 587–588
economic implications, 587
ESRD Medicare-funded program, 587
management and prevention, 592
pathophysiology
obstructive nephropathy, 590, 591
tubular thyroidization, 590–591
prevalence, 588
risk factors
anatomic and urodynamic abnormalities, 588
drugs, 589, 590
environment, 588
genetics, 590
metabolic, 588
temperature and sunlight levels, 589
ultrasound, 588, 589
CIRF. *See* Clinically insignificant residual fragments (CIRF)
Citrate
alkali therapy (*see* Alkali citrate therapy)
calcium oxalate stone formation, 735
early 1970s, 735
hyperoxaluria, 730
identification, 735
shock wave lithotripsy, 735
Civil society organizations (CSOs), 911
CKD. *See* Chronic kidney disease (CKD)
Claudin, 143
CLCN5. *See* Chloride channel 5 (CLCN5)
Clearance rates, SWL, 657
Clinical encounter card (CEC), 809
Clinically insignificant residual fragments (CIRF), 390
CME. *See* Continuing medical education (CME)
Coagulation disorders, 558, 560
COD. *See* Calcium oxalate dihydrate (COD)
Cognito-psychomotor skill
animal models, 829–830
autonomous phase, 828–829
bench models, 830
cadaver models, 830
cognitive phase, 828
Halstedian principle, 827
high-fidelity bench models, 830–831
hybrid models, 832
integrative phase, 828
laparoscopy and endourological surgery, 827–828
low-fidelity bench models, 830
mentor training
fellowship training model, 832, 833
PCNL, 832
retention, skills, 834
technical skills, 833–834
VR models, 831
COM. *See* Calcium oxalate monohydrate (COM)
Competency assessment
CanMEDS, 821
cutoff scores, 822
definition, 820
360-degree evaluations, 822
FLS, 824
formative assessment, 822
historical significance, 820
MCCQE, 822
OSATS, 823–824
OSCE, 822
technical skills, 823
tests, 821
urology, 822–823
USMLE, 822
written examinations, 822
Complications of ureteric stone treatment, 470–471
Comprehensive stone analysis
identification, stone disease, 121
types, calculi, 121–124
Computed tomography (CT)
cystinuria, 759
low-dose (*see* Low-dose CT)
pediatric vesicle calculus, 650
Continuing medical education (CME), 849
Continuing professional development (CPD), 849
Contrast enhancing methods, 287
CPD. *See* Continuing professional development (CPD)
CSOs. *See* Civil society organizations (CSOs)
CT. *See* Computed tomography (CT)
Cystine stones, 675–676, 724
Cystinuria
alkalinization, urine, 761
autosomal recessive inherited disorder, 757
classification, 759
crystals, 759, 760
CT, 759
diagnosis, 759
dietary, 761

Cystinuria (*cont.*)
epidemiology, 758
extracorporeal SWL, 762
genetics and inheritance, 758–759
management, 759–760
pathophysiology, 758
pharmacological therapy, 761
PNL, 762–763
prevalence, 758
radiopaque stones, 625
SLC3A1 and SLC7A9 gene, mutations, 625
stone analysis, 759
stone formation and surgical intervention, 757
treatment, 628
urine analysis, 759
urine dilution, 760–761
urological intervention, 761–762
URS, 762
Cystolitholapaxy, 521–522
Cystolithotomy, 522–523, 651–652
Cystolithotripsy, 522
Cystoscopic lithotripsy, 637
Cystoscopic stenting method
cannulation, ureteric orifice (UO), 493, 494
pusher, 494, 495
sliding, 493, 495
upper pole and renal pelvis, guidewire, 493, 494

D
da Vinci Surgical System, 516
Debt to service coverage ratio (DSCR), 904
Defensin, 179
Diabetes and obesity, 43
Diathermal techniques, tubeless PCNL, 430–431
Dietary
cystinuria, 761
factors, 43–44
Dietary management, kidney stones
bad middle eastern diet, 718
bad western diet, 717
calcium stone formation, 709–710
LITHOSCREEN procedure, 710
metabolic syndrome, 716–717
prevention, stone recurrence
fiber, 716
high magnesium and potassium intake, 715–716
low calcium intake, 713–714
low salt and sugar, 716
meat, fish and poultry intake, 714–715
modalities, 711
oxalate intake, 712–713
reduce biochemical risk, 711
supersaturation, urine, 709
treatment, 710
uric acid stone formation, 710, 711
urolithiasis, 709, 718
variation, hormonal and vitamin status, 711
Dietary manipulations, stone recurrences, 746
Diet therapy, citrate, 740–741
Dilatation
balloon system, PCNL, 660
URS
passive ureteral, 665
ureteric orifice, 665
Dilution, cystinuria, 760–761
Direct observation of procedural skills (DOPS), 809, 811
Distal renal tubular acidosis (dRTA), 134, 144–145
Donor and kidneys transplantation
acceptance, stone-bearing kidneys, 601–602
stone-bearing kidneys
acceptance, 601–602
contraindications, 602
stone disease management, 602
Doppler ultrasonography (DUS), 246
Doppler ultrasound (US)
neck, hyperparathyroidism, 785, 789
pregnancy, 568–569, 573
DOPS. *See* Direct observation of procedural skills (DOPS)
dRTA. *See* Distal renal tubular acidosis (dRTA)
Drug-based stone prevention, China
allopurinol, 723
calcium, 724–725
cellulose phosphate, 723
citrate, 723
glycosaminoglycan, 723
herbal medicine, 723–724
magnesium, 723
non-calcium, 725
orthophosphate, 723
recommendations, 724
thiazide diuretics, 722–723
vitamin B_6, 723
Drug therapy, 899, 900
DSCR. *See* Debt to service coverage ratio (DSCR)
DUS. *See* Doppler ultrasonography (DUS)

E
EBM. *See* Evidence-based medicine (EBM)
EBU. *See* European Board of Urology (EBU)
Ectopic and fused kidneys, PCNL
laparoscopy guidance, 424
ultrasound guidance, 424
ED. *See* Effective dose (ED)
Effective dose (ED), 272
EHL. *See* Electrohydraulic lithotriptor (EHL)
Electrohydraulic lithotriptor (EHL), 335, 337
Electrohydraulic shock wave generation, 302–303
Electromagnetic shock wave generation, 304–305
Encrustation
bacterial biofilm
bacterial activity, 498
description, 497–498
formation, steps, 498
catheter blockage symptoms, 499
dental plaque, 497
health economics, 498–499
knotted stents, 500, 501
lost/neglected stent, 499–500
strategies, combat biofilm, 498
ureteric stents, 499
Endoirrigation systems, 297
Endoscopic stone treatment, pregnancy
indications, 570
lithotripsy, 570
URS, 570, 571
Endoscopic Surgical Skill Qualification (ESSQ), 834
Endoscopic techniques, 917
Endoscopy, 847

End-stage renal disease (ESRD)
calculus renal failure in Pakistan, 596, 597
CKD, 588, 591
Energy flux density (ED), 306–307
Energy sources for ureteric stone fragmentation, 468–469
Enteric hyperoxaluria, 730
Epidemiological and etiological considerations
ammonium urate stones, 239
calcium oxalate stones, 237–238
patient data, 239
p^H-measurements, 239
prevalence and male/female quotients, 237, 238
prophylactic treatment, 239
stone disease, 237
uric acid, 239
urine abnormalities, 238, 239
Epidemiology of stone diseases
in Australia (*see* Australia)
in China (*see* China)
in European Union (*see* European Union)
in Iran (*see* Iran)
in Japan (*see* Japan)
in Kerala, South India (*see* Kerala, South India)
in North America (*see* North America)
in Northern India (*see* Northern India)
in Russian Federation and post-Soviet area (*see* Russian Federation and post-Soviet area)
in Saudi Arabia (*see* Saudi Arabia)
in South Africa and sub-Saharan Africa (*see* South Africa and sub-Saharan Africa)
in South America (*see* South America)
Epidural anesthesia, 549, 550
Equil2 program, 190
Erbium:yttrium aluminum garnet (Er:YAG) laser, 484
ESRD. *See* End-stage renal disease (ESRD)
ESSQ. *See* Endoscopic Surgical Skill Qualification (ESSQ)
ESWL. *See* Extracorporeal shock wave lithotripsy (ESWL)
ETFE. *See* Ethylene tetrafluoroethylene (ETFE)
Ethylene tetrafluoroethylene (ETFE), 322
European Board of Urology (EBU), 822–823
European Union
age and gender, 4–5
description, 3–4
eliminating procedures, 10–11
idiopathic calcium nephrolithiasis, 9–10
MIAF-urolithiasis, 7–9
prevalence and incidence, 4
prevention, 11
recurrence, 6
risk factors, 6–7
stone composition, 5–6
Evidence-based medicine (EBM), 849
Extracorporeal shock wave lithotripsy (ESWL)
acute and long-term side effects, 391
adequate analgesia, 388–389
anesthesia, 548–549
anomalous kidneys treatment
ADPKD, 576, 577
complications, 578
duplex and malrotated kidneys, 576–578
ectopic, 576, 577
horseshoe, 576, 577
indications, 576
stone-free rate, 576–578
technique, 576
anticoagulation therapy, 388
application., 383
asymptomatic small caliceal stones, 386
bladder calculi, 523
bypassing disturbing structures, 389
defined, 898
disintegration efficacy, 388
endoscopic stone removal, 385
fragment passage, 390–391
laparoscopic/open surgery, 899
large and solid stone, right kidney, 397, 398
left distal ureter, 399
lithotripsy device, 384
lower caliceal stones, 385–386
mid-ureteral stone, 398, 399
multilayered morphology, 396
obesity, 387
optimized coupling, 389
parameter selection, 389
patient fixation, 389
patient monitoring, 390
pediatric urolithiasis, 388
pediatric URS, 666
percutaneous stone removal, 398
PNL, 396
power, transmission, 398
pregnancy, 387
preoperative stenting, 385
pretreatment, low energy, 390
prevention, tissue injury, 390
removal, stones, 395
renal anomalies, 387
renal calculi, 385
right distal ureter, 399
RIRS, 398
stone composition, 387
target stability, 388
technical developments, 384–385
therapy, kidney stones, 383
tissue trauma, 390
transverse process, 398
treatment, pregnancy, 570
ureteral calculi, 386–387
urinary tract calculi
antiplatelet therapy(*see* Antiplatelet therapy)
chronic urinary retention, 560
description, 557
hemostasis(*see* Hemostasis)
LMWH, 558
management, 558
minimal invasive procedures, 557
retention, 560
right staghorn renal calculus, 560
Vitamin K antagonists, 557–558
warfarin therapy, fatal hemorrhage, 558
X-ray film, 397

F

Family history
calcium, 151
clustering, genetic/dietary factors, 153
frequency, stones, 152
monogenetic/polygenic inheritance, 153–154
parents and siblings percent, propositi and controls, 152
Fiber intake, stone formation, 716

Fibrin sealants
Evicel™, 428–430
preparation, Tisseel, 428, 430
safety and efficacy, 431
splenic trauma, cardiac and liver surgery, 428, 429
Flexible ureterorenoscopy (F-URS)
indications, 578
outcomes, 578, 580
techniques, 578, 579
FLS. *See* Fundamentals of Laparoscopy Program (FLS)
Fluid intake, 711–712, 747–748
Fluoroscopy, 273, 274
FMEC PG. *See* Future of Medical Education in Canada Postgraduate (FMEC PG)
Forgotten and retained stents, 506–507
Fourier transform infrared spectroscopy (FTIR)
absorption spectra, 686
calcium oxalate, 685
chemical structures and features, 685
drawback, 699
energy scale, 685
function, 685
infrared spectra components, urinary calculi, 686–692
vibrational motions, chemical bonds, 685
FREDDY lasers, 483
Freehand stent placement method, 494–496
FTIR. *See* Fourier transform infrared spectroscopy (FTIR)
Fundamentals of Laparoscopy Program (FLS), 824
F-URS. *See* Flexible ureterorenoscopy (F-URS)
Future of Medical Education in Canada Postgraduate (FMEC PG), 850–851

G

GAGs. *See* Glycosaminoglycans (GAGs)
Gastric bypass, 214–215
Gated SWL, 657
General anesthesia
ESWL, 548, 549
PCNL, 550
Genetics, kidney stones
citrate, 146
cystinuria, 146
genes and environment, nephrolithiasis, 146–147
hypercalciuric nephrolithiasis, 142–145
hyperoxaluria, 145
hyperuricosuria, 146
monogenic disorders, idiopathic nephrolithiasis, 147
nephrolithiasis, 141
Global Operative Assessment of Laparoscopic Skills (GOALS), 833
Glucocorticoids, 530
Glycosaminoglycans (GAGs), 45
GOALS. *See* Global Operative Assessment of Laparoscopic Skills (GOALS)
Gonadal hormones, 530
Graft and transplanted ureter calculi treatment
conservative, 604
PNL and antegrade ureteroscopy
advantages, 605
difficulties, 605–606
open surgery, 606
postoperative complications, 606
SWL
complications, 605
indications and outcome, 604–605
limitations, 605
retrograde endoscopy, 605
Grayscale ultrasound (US), 568, 573

H

Health Professional Follow-up Study (HPFS), 922
Hematuria
hypercalciuria, 623, 624
hyperuricosuria, 623, 626
urinalysis, 626
Heminephrectomy and calculus disease, 933, 934
Hemodialysis, 909
Hemorrhagic complication, PCNL, 442–443
Hemostasis
assessment, 559
description, 559
perioperative hemorrhage management, 559
Hemostatic agents
defined, 428
description, 431
diathermal techniques, 431
FloSeal, 431
liquid and flowable products, 428, 429
High-fidelity bench models, 830–831
High-fidelity simulator, 856
High-technology surgical care
fundamental requirements, 876
GDP, 876
medical care and health delivery system, 876
rural (*see* Rural surgery)
HIV. *See* Human immunodeficiency virus (HIV)
Holmium YAG laser, 887, 889
Holmium:yttrium aluminum garnet (Ho:YAG) laser, 484
HOX. *See* Hyperoxaluria (HOX)
HPFS. *See* Health Professional Follow-up Study (HPFS)
HPT. *See* Hyperparathyroidism (HPT)
Human immunodeficiency virus (HIV), 926
Hybrid models, 832
Hypercalcemia, 32–33, 204–205
Hypercalcemic hyperparathyroidism, 204
Hypercalciuria
causes, 625
defined, 62, 624
definition, 728
Dent's disease, 624–625
idiopathic, 62
management, 627, 728–730
types, 624
Hyperoxaluria (HOX)
AGT enzyme, 625
definition, 728
diagnosis, 625
enteric, 169–170
idiopathic calcium oxalate stone former
dietary management, 170–171
identification, 170
pathogenesis, 170
management
bisphosphonates, 730
citrate therapy, 730
diets, 729–730
etiology, 728–729, 730
PHT, 729
standard treatment, 729
thiazide trials, 729

oxalate, 625
pyridoxine, 625
treatment, 627
Hyperparathyroidism (HPT), 215, 216
Hypertension, 597–598
Hyperuricosuria, 44, 146
Hypocitraturia
bariatric surgery, 188
calcium stones, 185
causes, 187
dietary-environmental factors, 187–188
high-animal protein low-carbohydrate diet, 188, 189
potassium depletion, 186
topiramate therapy, 188
Hypothermia risk, 660

I
IAGES. *See* Indian Association of Gastrointestinal Endoscopic Surgery (IAGES)
ICSF. *See* Idiopathic calcium oxalate stone formers (ICSF)
Idiopathic calcium nephrolithiasis, 8–10
Idiopathic calcium oxalate stone formers (ICSF)
Randall's plaque, 210–212
stone formation, non-ICSF patients (*see* Stone formation, non-ICSF patients)
unattached stones, 212–213
Idiopathic Caox stones
COD, 132
enteric hyperoxaluria, 131–132
hypercalciuria and oxalate concentration, 131
PH and "Type Ic" calculi, 131
umbilicated calculi and Randall's plaque, 132–133
Idiopathic hypercalciuria (IH), 203–204
IFIS. *See* Intraoperative floppy iris syndrome (IFIS)
IH. *See* Idiopathic hypercalciuria (IH)
Indian Association of Gastrointestinal Endoscopic Surgery (IAGES), 877
Infection stones
description, 231
formation, 92
infrared spectroscopy, 115
metabolic abnormalities, 80
PCNL, 233
Proteus mirabilis and *Pseudomonas aeruginosa*, 87
renal function, 234
signs and symptoms
antibiotic therapy, 233
clinical presentation, 232–233
CT, 233
diagnosis, 231–232
staghorn calculi, 231, 232
SWL, 233
treatment, 233, 234
urinary tract infection, 234
Integration, competences
adult learning, 838
assessment methods, 837–838
competency-based curriculum, 838
educational and vocational vocabulary, 837
EPAs, 838–839
healthcare system, 840
medical education, 837
operational model, 839
urological training, 839
Internal cardiac defibrillator (ICD), 565
Intracorporeal lithotripsy, 337
Intracorporeal lithotriptors, 412
Intraoperative floppy iris syndrome (IFIS), 457
Intravenous pyelography (IVP), 634, 916
Intravenous urogram (IVU), 246–247, 266–268
Invasive techniques
anatrophic pyelo-nephrolithotomy, 367–368
bench surgery and autotransplantation, 371
CT, 365
ileal replacement, ureter, 369
ileocecal junction, 370
isotope renogram, 365
management, residual stones, 372
PCNL, 363
preoperative preparation, 369
pyelolithotomy, Gil-Vernet, 365–366
radial nephrotomy, Doppler ultrasound, 368–369
renal ischemia, 366–367
RIRS, 363
surgical approach, 365
urine culture, 365
X-Ray, abdomen and IVU, 365
Iran
geographical specifications, 85–86
kidney stone, 85, 86
urolithiasis, research, 86–87
Irrigative therapy
chemolytic agent, 535
cystine stones, 535
flexible nephroscopy, 535
hemiacidrin, 535
struvite stones, 536
uric acid dissolution, 535
IVP. *See* Intravenous pyelography (IVP)
IVU. *See* Intravenous urogram (IVU)

J
Japan
abnormalities, urinary tract, 94–95
composition, 91–93
description, 89
factors, 93–94
geographical distribution, urolithiasis, 92
lower and upper urinary tract stones, 90
pharmacological treatment, 94
removal, stone, 90–91
uric acid stones, 93
JESS program, 190

K
Kerala, South India
chemical constituents, calculi, 57, 58
composition, 49
epidemeology, 47–48
factors, stone formation, 49, 50
metabolic assessment, 49, 50
retrieval, 48–49
Kidney stones etiopathogenesis
calcifications, 683–684
chemical constituents, 684
ectopic calcification, 684
genetics (*see* Genetics, kidney stones)
infrared spectroscopy, 685–686

Kidney stones etiopathogenesis (*cont.*)
nucleation, 684
prevalence, disease, 684
Randall's plaque, 684
Randall's plaque characterization, 700
stone characterization
calcium oxalate, 699
calcium phosphate, 699–700
trace elements classification, 700
techniques, routine analysis (*see* Routine analysis techniques)
water therapy (*see* Stone recurrences, prevention)
Kidneys-ureters-bladder (KUB)
CT, 934, 950, 953, 954
and NCCT, 955, 956
radiographs, 244–245
Kidney-ureter-bladder (KUB) model LapED™, 857, 858
KUB. *See* Kidneys-ureters-bladder (KUB)

L
Laparoscopic and retroperitoneoscopic stone surgery
advantages, 512
diverticulum, calyx, 511
double-J stenting, 512
endourologic stone treatment, 513
financial resources and medical infrastructure, 513
indications, 510
kidney and ureter, 511
laparoscopic ureterolithotomy, 512
pelvic and horseshoe kidneys, 511–512
preparation, 510
size and shape, stone, 511
stone-free rates, 512–513
stones, renal pelvis, 511
stricture rate, 512
Laparoscopic-assisted PCNL
indications, 584
outcomes, 584–585
technique, 584
Laparoscopic pyelolithotomy
indications, 583
outcomes, 584
technique, 583–584
Laparoscopic stone surgery, 645
Laparoscopy, 847, 878
Laryngospasm, 665
Laser fibers, 482
Laser lithotripsy
amplification, 313
clinical application, 324
compilation, bubble expansion and collapse, 318, 319
CT, 318, 320
debris ejection, short-pulse, 320, 322
dye, 314
erbium and holmium, 321
fiber, stone particles, 320, 321
fluoride fibers, 321
gas, 314
in-phase photons, 314
kidney stone applications, 314
optical fibers, 322–324
photothermal interaction, 315
pressure transients, 318
pulsed dye, 317
retropulsion, 320
skin components, optical absorption coefficients, 315
solid-state, 315
stone retropulsion distance *vs.* recoil momentum, 320, 321
-tissue interaction
distribution, tissues, 316
fragmentation, 316
photochemical interactions, 315
tissue pigmentation, 317
transient stress waves, 316
types, 315
ureteronephroscopy, 317
YAG, 315
Lasers
Er:YAG, 484
fibers, 482
FREDDY, 483
history, 481
Ho:YAG, 484
instruments and devices, 482
photoacoustic, 483
photothermal, 483
physics, 481–482
pulsed-dye, 483
systems, 482
Lasertripsy and URS, 664
Leasing systems, Pakistan, 905
Lesch-Nyhan syndrome (LNS), 146
Linear no-threshold model (LNT), 272
Lithotripsy, 738
Lithotripters
adeferred payment letter, 905
leasing systems, Pakistan, 905
loan, 904–905
Lithotripter sharing
business models, 886
economics, 886
emergency equipment, 888
movements, 888
outcomes, 889
reliability, 887
requirements, 886–887
SWL, 885
technical team/training, 887–888
transport, 888
United States, 885–886
LNS. *See* Lesch-Nyhan syndrome (LNS)
LNT. *See* Linear no-threshold model (LNT)
Loan, finance lithotripter devices
business, 904–905
country, 905
credit/default risk, 904
interest rates, 904
timeline, 904
Low-dose CT
ALARA, 280
beam collimation width/pitch, 278
disadvantages, 278–280
ionizing radiation-based testing, 277
medical imaging studies, 278
radiation exposure, 277–278
renal calculus, 278, 279
Lower caliceal stones, 385–386
Lowe's oculocerebrorenal syndrome, 144
Low-fidelity bench models, 830
Low-fidelity simulator, 856

Lysimachia christina
calcium oxalate stones, 540
clinical efficacy and practical experience, 540–541
herb preparation, 540
Niao Shitong soluble granules, 541
Pai Shi granules, 541
Lysimachia christinae, 530

M
Magnesium and potassium intake, 715–716
Magnetic resonance urography (MRU), 248, 569–570, 573
MAS. *See* Minimal access surgery (MAS)
MCCQE. *See* Medical Council of Canada Qualifying Examination (MCCQE)
McGill Inanimate System for Training and Evaluation of Laparoscopic Skills (MISTELS), 833
MCP-1. *See* Monocyte chemoattractant protein-1 (MCP-1)
MCUG. *See* Micturating cystourethrogram (MCUG)
Mean annual temperature (MAT), 17
Medical Council of Canada Qualifying Examination (MCCQE), 822
Medical equipment
acquisition, 895
approvals and sign-offs, 895
financial feasibility, 892
funding, 893
market analysis, 892
mitigation strategies *vs.* technology risks, 895
needs, definition, 892
negotiations, 895
purchases, 891
received bids
commercial review, 894
operational review, 894
technical review, 894
RFP, 893
site selection, 893
supplier prequalification, 893–894
technology analysis, 892
working group, 893
Medical errors and informed consent, 544
Medical expulsive therapy (MET)
alpha blocker therapy, 456
calcium channel antagonists, 529
Chinese medicine, 530
drug side effects, 457
factors, 528
glucocorticoids, 530
gonadal hormones, 530
IFIS, 457
MIS, 522
multivariate analysis, 456
nonsteroidal anti-inflammatory drugs, 529–530
pain management and antiemetic therapy, 456
pharmacologic agents, 456
prostaglandin synthesis inhibitors, 529–530
$\alpha 1$ receptor blocker agents, 528–529
tamsulosin *vs.* nifedipine trials, 456–457
Medullary sponge kidney (MSK), 8, 145
Melamine
animals and toxicity, 219–220
broken stones, 220, 224
CT scan, 221, 225
description, 219
diagnosis, 221
IVU, 221
milk powder tainted, 220, 224
treatment, 222–224
ultrasound screening, 221, 225
uric acid, 225–226
urinary stone formation
animals, 220–223
children, 220
urothelial tumor, 225
Melamine-associated urinary stone (MAUS). *See* Melamine
MET. *See* Medical expulsive therapy (MET)
Metabolic acidosis, 43
Metabolic-related diagnostic methods, 248–249
Metabolic screening, 716–717
Metabolic stone disease, children
clinical presentation, 623
cystinuria, 625
diagnostic evaluation, 626–627
factors, 621–622
hypercalciuria, 624–625, 627
hyperoxaluria, 625, 627
hyperuricosuria, 625–626
medical treatment, 627
stone formation, 622–623
uric acid lithiasis, 627–628
Metabolic syndrome (MS)
and diabetes mellitus, 924–925
and UA nephrolithiasis, 155–156
Metaphylaxis
cost-effectiveness, stone, 900
and metabolic evaluation, 899–900
Methylene blue, 774
MIAF-urolithiasis
Danish survey, 7, 8
metabolic causes, 7, 9
MSK, 8
screening program, 7–8
Micturating cystourethrogram (MCUG), 272
Miller's pyramid, 807–808
mini-CEX. *See* Mini-clinical evaluation exercise (mini-CEX)
Mini-clinical evaluation exercise (mini-CEX), 809, 810
Minimal access surgery (MAS), 876, 878
Minimally invasive percutaneous nephrolithotomy (MPCNL)
calyceal puncture, 434–435
description, 436–437
endoscopic pump, 434, 435
fascial dilators, 434, 435
modern instrumentation and technical improvement, 436
"neutral position", midcalyceal puncture, 434
procedures, general anesthesia, 434
RPP, 435–436
sheath sizes and instruments, 434
sonography guidance and X-ray fluoroscopy, 434, 436
stone fragments removal, 435
Minimally invasive surgery (MIS), 527
mini-PAT. *See* Mini-peer assessment tool (mini-PAT)
Mini-peer assessment tool (mini-PAT), 809
Miniperc PCNL, 424–425
MIS. *See* Minimally invasive surgery (MIS)
MISTELS. *See* McGill Inanimate System for Training and Evaluation of Laparoscopic Skills (MISTELS)
Monitored anesthesia care (MAC), 549
Monocyte chemoattractant protein-1 (MCP-1), 180
Monogenetic inheritance, 153–154
Morpho-constitutional stone analysis method, 124, 137
MPCNL. *See* Minimally invasive percutaneous nephrolithotomy (MPCNL)

MPO. *See* Myeloperoxidase (MPO)
MRU. *See* Magnetic Resonance Urography (MRU)
MS. *See* Metabolic syndrome (MS)
MSF. *See* Multi-source feedback (MSF)
MSK. *See* Medullary sponge kidney (MSK)
Multimodal pain management, 551
Multi-source feedback (MSF), 809, 815–816
Myeloperoxidase (MPO), 178–179

N
Nanobacteria, 43
NCCT. *See* Non-contrast-enhanced computed tomography (NCCT)
Nephrocalcinosis, 935
Nephrolithiasis
  bariatric surgery, 923–924
  hypercalciuric
    CASR, 142–143
    claudin, 143
    CLCN5, 143
    genes, dRTA, 144–145
    locus on 9q33.2-q34.2, 144
    MSK, 145
    phosphatidylinositol 4,5-bisphosphate 5-phosphatase, 144
    SAC, 143
    serine/threonine kinase, 144
    sodium/phosphate transporter, 144
    VDR, 143
  idiopathic calcium, 745
  indinavir, 926
  melamine, 925–926
  uric acid, 745
  and urinary composition, 922–923
Nephrolithotomy, 661–662
Nephrolithotripsy
  AUA, 258
  echogenic-tipped needles, 259, 262
  interventional radiology, 258
  mandril/stylet, 261
  needle placement, 258–259, 261
  PCNL, 258
  renal pelvis, 262
  stone and kidney, 259
Nephroscopy, 661–662
NHS. *See* Nurses' Health Study (NHS)
Non-contrast-enhanced computed tomography (NCCT)
  bilateral renal staghorn stones, 247
  CT, 247
  disadvantage, 247
  Hounsfield units, 457–458, 460
  pediatric vesicle calculus, 650
  SSD, 458, 460
  stone burden, 455
  stone disease, 248
  stone size, 456
Nonoperative technical skills for surgeons (NOTSS), 809
Nonsteroidal anti-inflammatory drugs (NSAIDs), 246, 355–356, 529–530, 552
Normocalcemic hyperparathyroidism
  Doppler ultrasound scan, neck, 785, 789
  fingernails clubbing, 785, 786
  graph, serum calcium levels, 786, 789
  Harvey's formula, 786
  histopathology, adenoma, 786, 790
  hormone, 785
  lab test, 785
  physical examination, 785
  sestamibi scan, left lower parathyroid gland, 785, 788
  severe right hip pain, 785
  vitamin D deficient countries, 785
  X-ray
    lateral view, skull, 785, 787
    terminal phalanges, hands, 785, 787
North America
  description, 13
  dietary/environmental factors, 17–18
  incidence, 13–14
  medical, surgical and genetic factors, 17
  prevalence, 14–16
  stone composition, 16
  treatment, 15–16
  urinary parameters, 16
Northern India
  description, 39
  dietary factors, 43–44
  drinking water, 44
  environmental factors, 43
  fluoride and magnesium, 44
  frequency, urinary risk factors, 42, 43
  GAGs, 45
  genetic factors, 42–43
  geographic distribution, 40, 41
  hyperuricosuria, 44
  hypocitraturia, 45
  incidence and prevalence, 40
  metabolic acidosis, 43
  nanobacteria, 43
  Oxalobacter formigenes, 43
  protein, calcium and phosphate, 44
  site of occurrence, 40, 42
  socioeconomic status, 40
  stone composition, 40, 42
  systemic disorders, 43
  urinary tract infection (UTI), 43
  zinc, copper and manganese, 44
NOTSS. *See* Nonoperative technical skills for surgeons (NOTSS)
NSAIDs. *See* Nonsteroidal anti-inflammatory drugs (NSAIDs)
Nurses' Health Study (NHS), 922

O
Objective structured assessment of technical skills (OSATS), 809, 812–813, 823–824
Objective Structured Clinical Examinations (OSCE), 822
Oligomineral water, kidney stones, 747
Open stone surgery, SWL, 655
Operating room
  PCNL, 344
  postprocedure instrument care
    endoscope channel, 344, 345
    equipment, lubricated, 344, 346
    PPE, 344, 345
    proper storage, lens, 344, 346
  preparation for cystolitholapaxy, 344
  preparation for ureterorenoscopy, 344
  procedure day
    role, circulator, 343–344
    scrub nurse, 344
Operating theater (OR), 887
Optical fibers
  collimated laser emission, 323
  ETFE, 322

evanescent waves, 324
silica, 322
Optimal coupling, 389
OR. *See* Operating theater (OR)
Oral chemolytic therapy
calcium oxalate, 535
cystine stones, 534–535
struvite stones, 534
uric acid stones, 533–534
Orthophosphates
contribution, 753
dosage
bone resorption, 755
calcium intestinal absorption, 755
fixed base, acid phosphate preparation, 753
hypercalciuric stone formation, 754
positive effects, 754
rapid-release phosphate, 754
reabsorption, renal calcium, 755
slow-release test, 754
stone episode rate, 754
urinary calcium excretion, 753
excessive bone loss, 752
hypercalciuria treatment, 752
idiopathic calcium disease, 752
intestinal calcium reduction, 752–753
medical treatment, 752
plasma phosphate and PTH increase, 752, 753
side effects, 755
therapeutic effects, 753
OSATS. *See* Objective structured assessment of technical skills (OSATS)
OSCE. *See* Objective Structured Clinical Examinations (OSCE)
Osteopenia, 196
Osteoporosis, 18, 200, 248, 674, 722, 730
Oxalate and urolithiasis
absorption, 166
bacterial degradation, intestine, 167–169
defined, 165–166
dietary calcium and supplements, 167
enteric hyperoxaluria, 169–170
excretion, 166
hyperoxaluria, idiopathic calcium oxalate stone former, 170–171
PH (*see* Primary hyperoxaluria (PH))
transport, 166
Oxalate intake, stone formation, 712–713
Oxalobacter formigenes
ability, 168–169
colonization, 168, 169
fecal culture, 168

P

Pacemakers
causes, 564
extrinsic electrical activity, 564
postoperative management, 565
preoperative assessment, 564
pulse generator, 563
rate responsive (R) mode, 563
sensing function, 563
SWL shocks, 564
Pain management, 357
Pakistan
advantages, leasing systems, 905
chartered accountant, 904
deferred payment letter, credit, 905
distribution, 25
gender differences, stone site and transitions, 25
hospital operating room statistics, 22, 23
hypercalcemia, 32–33
hypocitraturia, 33–34
pediatric patients, 24
pediatric stone, 23
population and health-care systems, 24
population-based data, 34
practice patterns, 26–30
prevalence, 22–23
provinces and major cities, 22, 23
silent stones, 24
socioeconomic, dietary and nutritional status, 34–35
soil, salinity, irrigation and water, 34
stone burden and surgical workloads, 24
stone composition (*see* Stone composition)
transitions, 25–26
urinary and blood chemistry, 32, 33
urinary tract infection (UTI), 24
urinary tract obstruction, 24
vitamin D deficiency, 33
Paracellin-1 (PCLN1), 143
Parathyroid adenoma and urolithiasis, 931, 932
Parathyroidectomy
complications, 798–799
description, 796–797
endoscopic, 797–798
gasless external retraction, 797
open scan-directed parathyroidectomy, 797
sestamibi, 798
Parathyroid hormone (PTH)
IH, 203–204
primary hyperparathyroidism, 204
renal calcium absorption and transport, 202
tertiary hyperparathyroidism, 204
Patient safety
clinical care, 543, 545
description, 544
health-care providers, 545
medical errors and informed consent, 544
"respect for person", 543, 545
teach-back, 544–545
well-understood informed consent, 545
PCCL. *See* Percutaneous cystolithotomy (PCCL)
PCLN1. *See* Paracellin-1 (PCLN1)
PCNL. *See* Percutaneous nephrolithotomy (PCNL)
PCNL procedure
fluoroscopy-guided access, 419
insertion, safety wire, 421
management, complications, 423
optical puncture system, 420–421
positioning, 418, 420
postoperative drainage, 423
prevention, complications, 423
retrograde percutaneous access, 420
retrograde ureteric catheter, 418, 420
selection, calyx, 418–419
stone fragmentation, 422–423
tract dilatation
Amplatz dilator, 422, 423
balloon dilators, 422
telescopic metal dilators, 422–423
ultrasound guidance, 419, 421
ureteroscopic guidance, 419

Pediatric stone disease
  anatomic abnormalities, 639
  bladder stones, 639
  components frequency, urinary calculi, 119, 120
  imaging, 640
  influence, age, 120–121
  laparoscopic surgery, 645
  open surgery, 645
  PCNL, 642–644
  stone analysis, 641
  stone composition, 120, 121
  SWL, 641–642
  symptoms, 639–640
  urine and blood analyses, 640
  URS, 644
Pediatric urolithiasis in China
  anatomical abnormalities, 633
  B-ultrasound (B-US), 634
  clinical manifestations, 633
  computed tomography (CT), 634
  conservative and medical treatment, 635
  cystoscopic lithotripsy, 637
  description, 631
  emergency management, 635
  Escherichia coli, 633
  feeding modality, 633
  imaging, 634
  investigations, 633
  KUB and IVP, 634
  laboratory tests, 633–634
  laparoscopic and retroperitoneoscopic surgery, 636
  magnetic resonance (MR), 634–635
  metabolic disorders, 632
  nuclear imaging, 635
  open surgery, 636
  PCNL, 637
  prevalence, 631–632
  stone composition, 632
  SWL, 635–636
  ureteroscopy, 636
Pediatric vesicle calculus
  association, urinary stasis, 647
  bladder, 647
  clinical trials, 649
  diagnosis
    complete blood cell count, 649
    comprehensive metabolic panel, 649
    CT, 650
    MRI, 650
    NCCT, 650
    radiopaque, 649, 650
    urinalysis, 649
    urine culture and sensitivity, 649
  epidemiology, 647–648
  etiopathogenesis, 648–649
  treatment
    cystolithotomy, 651–652
    ESWL, 651
    PCCL, 651
    surgical, 651
    therapy, 650–651
    transurethral cystolitholapaxy, 651
Pelviureteric junction obstruction (PUJO), 517
PERC Mentor™, 859–860
Perc Trainer™, 858, 859
Percutaneous cystolithotomy (PCCL), 651
Percutaneous nephrolithotomy (PCNL)
  anatomy, 440
  anesthesia
    complications, 550
    general and regional, 550
    intraoperative, 550
    periodical bilateral auscultation, 550
    prone position achieving, 549–550
    spinal-epidural, 550
    surgical treatment, larger stones, 549
  anomalous kidneys
    ADPKD, 580, 582
    complications, 582
    duplex, 580–582
    ectopic, 580, 582
    horseshoe, 580, 582
    indications, 580
    laparoscopic-assisted(*see* Laparoscopic-assisted PCNL)
    malrotated, 582
  antegrade stent placement, 441–442
  antibiotic prophylaxis and anesthesia, 660
  balloon dilatation system, 660
  bilateral, 662
  Chinese MPCNL (*see* Minimally invasive percutaneous nephrolithotomy (MPCNL))
  complications
    fluid absorption, 663
    long-term effects, 663
    postoperative fever, 662
    renal hemorrhage, 662
    urinary leakage, 663
  congenital renal anomalies, 662
  cystinuria, 762–763
  defined, 898–899
  description, 417
  double-J stent (DJS), 439
  ectopic and fused kidneys, 424
  effectiveness
    steep learning curve, 664
    stone clearance rates, 663–664
  hemorrhagic complication, 442–443
  horseshoe kidneys, 424
  hypothermia risk, 660
  indications, 417–418, 660
  infection stones, 233, 234
  late 1970s, 660
  "mini-PCNL", 433–434
  miniperc, 424–425
  nephroscopy, 661–662
  patient position, 660–661
  patient preparation
    complications, 440
    CT scan guidance, 440, 441
    guide wires, 440, 441
    post-placement care, 440, 442
    prophylactic antibiotics, 440
    serial dilatation, 440
  pediatric stone disease, 642–644
  pediatric urolithiasis, China, 637
  pregnancy
    clinical outcomes, 571–572
    Doppler US, 573
    general anesthesia, 571
    grayscale ultrasound, 572, 573

vs. internal stent, obstructed kidney, 571
MRI-MRU, 573
open surgery, 572
pelviureteric junction obstruction, 573–574
preoperative evaluation, 418
preoperative imaging, 418, 419
procedure (*see* PCNL procedure)
renal drainage, 662
staghorn stones
bilateral, 451
children, 451
drainage, 449
fluoroscopy, 449
percutaneous access, 449, 450
residual stones, 450–451
retrograde ureteroscopy, 449
supine/prone position, 449
supracostal puncture, 449
ureteric catheter, 449
stone extraction, catheter and vascular access sheath, 660
stone removal, 433
supine, 424, 425
tract site size and dilatation, 661
training, 425
tubeless (*see* Tubeless PCNL)
Percutaneous Nephrolithotomy Trainer™, 858, 859
Percutaneous nephrostolithotomy (PNL), 396
Percutaneous nephrostomy (PCN), 506
Periodic paralysis, 196
Personal protective equipment (PPE), 344, 345
PH. *See* Primary hyperoxaluria (PH)
Philanthropy, health care
costs, 908–909
defined, 907
factors, philanthropists
culture of giving, 911
support, 911
trust, 911–912
kidney diseases and engagement, 909
Pakistan, 909–911
Philosophy
broader education compelling, 863
cognitive valence, 864
integration, 863
process analytically, 863
Photoacoustic lasers, 483
Photothermal lasers, 483
PHPT. *See* Primary hyperparathyroidism (PHPT)
Physicians knowledge, 804–805
Piezoelectric shock wave generation, 303–304
Plain films radiography, 265
PND. *See* Powder neutron diffraction (PND)
Polygenetic inheritance, 153–154
Post-data acquisition protocols, 280
Postgraduate medical education (PGME)
assessment, 847–849
challenges, developing world, 852
curriculum, 845
description, 841–842
education and certification, USA, 843
FMEC PG project, 850–851
MBBS/MD, 842
medical competence, 846, 847
Pakistan system, 845
programs, 851, 852
technology, 846–848
UK system, 843
urology training and education, 843, 844
Potassium citrate
brushite and calcium oxalate, 192, 193
citrate therapy (*see* Alkali citrate therapy)
Equil2 program, 190
and Equil2 *vs.* JESS Program, 190–191
JESS program, 190
p^H, SI and RSR, 191–192
physiological action, 190
Powder neutron diffraction (PND)
beamline G4.1, Orphée reactor, 696, 697
description, 696
intensity, different synthetic and biological apatites, 696, 697
peaks, 696
PPE. *See* Personal protective equipment (PPE)
Pregnancy
PHPT
asymptomatic, 780
calcium-supplemented diets, 780
hypocalcemia, neonate, 781
physiological changes, 780
stone disease, 780–781
surgery, 781
Tc-99m sesta MIBI imaging, 781
stone disease
anatomy and physiological changes, urinary tract, 567–568
clinical presentation, 568, 569
Doppler US, 568–569
glomerular filtration rate (GFR), 567
grayscale ultrasound, 568
MRU, 569–570
nephrolithiasis, 568
premature rupture, 568
treatment, 570
urolithiasis, 567
X-ray, 568
Primary hyperoxaluria (PH)
PH1 and PH2, 171–172
renal replacement therapy, 172
Primary hyperoxaluria (PHO)
calcium oxalate, 612
clinical manifestations, 612
deficiency, 612
diagnosis, 612
glomerular filtration rate (GFR), 612
in India
costs, transplant surgery, 615
kidney transplantation, 615
liver transplant center, 616
noncontrast computed tomogram, 615, 616
organ transplant program, 615
private sector, 615–616
type I and II, 615
kidney stones, 612
liver-kidney transplantation, 614–615
management, 613
obstructive uropathy urinary tract infection, 613
renal transplantation, 613–614
type II, 613
urolithiasis, 611–612

Primary hyperparathyroidism (PHPT)
anatomy, 772–774
definition, 767–768
detection
CaSR, 769
IFHH, 769
PTH estimation, 770
renal failure delays, 770
screening programs, 767, 770
serum albumin, calcium and phosphorous, 769
urolithiasis screening, 770
diverse disease spectrum
bone disease, 770
hyperplasia, 770
India, 771
Pakistan and China, 770
parathyroid glands, 767
stone formation(*see* Stone formation)
early diagnosis, 767
intraoperative management
adenoma, 776, 778
carcinoma, 776, 779
four-gland hyperplasia, 776, 777
frozen section, parathyroid gland removal, 775
25-hydroxyvitamin D deficiency, 775
monitoring, IPTH, 774
normal encapsulated parathyroid removal, thyroidectomy, 776
operations, 776
radio-guided parathyroidectomy, 774
sestamibi scans, 774
skin mark, 774
mediastinal parathyroids, 780
neck exploration
BNE(*see* Bilateral neck exploration (BNE))
diagnosis, 791–792
preoperative localized techniques, 792
surgeons, 791
surgery and procedure, 792–793
postoperative management
cryopreservation, 780
hypocalcemia, 776–779
hypoparathyroid, 779
pregnancy (*see* Pregnancy)
rewsponsibility, endocrinological surgeon, 774
sestamibi scan, 938
stone disease
biochemical abnormalities and bone density, 772
endocrinology literature, 771–772
fluid intake, 771
hypercalcemia, 771
Pakistani patients, 771
pamidronate, 771
surgery, 771, 772
treatment, 771
Primary oxaluria, renal transplant
antegrade pyeloureterography, 608, 609
biplanar fluoroscopy, upper calyceal graft PNL, 607, 608
gray scale ultrasonography, hyperechoic stone, 607
non-contrast computerized tomography scan, 607, 608
static graft function, 607
Professional development, physicians
assessment, 805
clinical care, 804
knowledge, 804–805
role models, 805
specialists age, 803–804
technical competence, 805
Prostaglandin synthesis inhibitors, 529–530
Protein intake, 678
PTH. *See* Parathyroid hormone (PTH)
PUJO. *See* Pelviureteric junction obstruction (PUJO)
Pulsed-dye lasers, 483
Pulse wave Doppler, 257
Purine stones
ammonium urate, 135
prevention, China, 725
uric acid, 135
Pyelonephritis and renal stones, 943
Pyeloplasty-pyelolithotomy, 516

Q
Queen's Urology Examination Skills Training (QUEST), 822–823
QUEST. *See* Queen's Urology Examination Skills Training (QUEST)

R
Racial differences, renal stone disease
black and Caucasian populations, 108
defined, 107–108
gender, 109
metabolic abnormalities and stone types, 108–109
stone composition, 109
Radial nephrotomy
contact X-ray, 368, 369
Doppler ultrasound, 369, 370
extraction, stone, 369, 370
Radiation exposure, uroradiology
ALARA, 274
biological damage, 272
biological effects, 271
diagnosis and treatment, 275
ED, 272
fluoroscopy, 273, 274
LNT, 272
MCUG, 272
pregnant or potentially pregnant patient, 274
radionuclide imaging procedures, 273–274
stochastic effects, 271–272
X-ray-based imaging modalities, 271
Radiological imaging
CT, 267–270
IVU, 266–268
plain abdominal films, 265–266
renal stones, 269
SWL/medical expulsion therapy, 266
RALP. *See* Robotic-assisted laparoscopic pyeloplasty (RALP)
Randall's plaque (RP)
calcium oxalate stone growth, 210–212
characterization
advantage, 701
calcium oxalate dihydrate crystallites, 701–702
calcium oxalate monohydrate, 701
endoscopic procedures, 701
epidemiological data, 701
mesoscopic scale, SEM, 701
observation, calcium deposits, 700
oligoelements map, 702, 703
phosphate phases, 702–703
renal papilla observation, 704, 705
XANES spectra, 704
crystalline composition, 210
description, 209–210
ductal deposit, 217

ICSF, 210, 211
papillary mapping and biopsy protocol, 210
stone formation (*see* Stone formation, non-ICSF patients)
tubular deposits, 217
unattached stones, ICSF patients, 212–213
RC. *See* Renal colic (RC)
Recurrent stone formers (RSFs), 923
Relative saturation (RSR), 191–192
Reliability, mobile service
equipment, 887
host hospital and OR, 887
operator, equipment, 887
transport, 887
Renal calculi
children (*see* Percutaneous nephrolithotomy (PCNL))
minimally invasive treatment
congenital renal anomalies, 575
ESWL(*see* Extracorporeal shock wave lithotripsy (ESWL))
F-URS(*see* Flexible ureterorenoscopy)
guidelines, 575
laparoscopic-assisted PCNL(*see* Laparoscopic-assisted PCNL)
laparoscopic pyelolithotomy(*see* Laparoscopic pyelolithotomy)
open surgery, 575
Renal colic (RC)
acute stone problems, special patients
pregnancy, 358
stones, children, 358
drainage, obstructed infected kidneys, 357
epidemiology and economic burden, 354
MET, 357–358
nonpharmacological treatment, renal pain
acupuncture, 357
heat therapy, 357
sterile water and forced hydration, 357
pathophysiology, 354–355
pharmacological treatment, pain relief
combination therapy, 356
desmopressin, 356–357
nonopiate analgesics, 356
NSAIDs, 355–356
opiate analgesics, 356
parasympatholytics, 356
standardization, pain management protocol, 357
stone impaction and renal function, 358–359
Renal drainage, 662
Renal handling, citrate
calcium nephrolithiasis, 183
filtration and reabsorption, 184
metabolism, 183–184
metabolism, tubular cells, 184, 185
regulators, 184–186
tubular transport, 184
urinary organic anion, 186
Renal hemorrhage, 662
Renal hypercalciuria, 170
Renal ischemia
nephrolithotomy, 367
open pyelo-nephrolithotomy, 366
staghorn stone, 367
Renal pelvic pressure (RPP), 435–436
Renal replacement therapy (RRT), 596
Renal stone disease, 199–200
Renal transplant
bladder calculi
cystolitholapaxy, 606
development, 606
impact, graft stones and survival, 607
primary oxaluria, 607–609
ureteroneocystostomy, 606
clinical presentation, 604
description, 601
donor (*see* Donor and kidneys transplantation)
recipient (*see* Renal transplant recipients)
treatment (*see* Graft and transplanted ureter calculi treatment)
X-ray and CT, 604
Renal transplant recipients
de novo development stones, 603
donor-gifted nephrolithiasis, 602–603
pathogenesis, stone development
calcium oxalate, 603
calcium phosphate, 603
uric acid, 603
urological risk factors, 603
Renal tubular acidosis (RTA)
alkaline therapy, 198
categories, 195
clinical manifestation, 196
diagnosis, 196–197
hydrogen ion secretion, 215
papillae and dilated ducts, 216
pathogenesis, 196
sodium thiosulfate, 198
treatment, 197
Renal/ureteric colic, 252–253
Request for proposals (RFP), 893
Residents, research and innovation
ACGME, 869
assessment, 871
benefits, 869–870
facilitation, 870
investigative skills, 869
practical measures, 870–871
requirements
funds, 870
mentors, 870
support, 870
time, 870
training, 870
Retrograde intrarenal surgery (RIRS)
description, 411
flexible ureteroscope, 412
guidewire, 412
intracorporeal lithotriptors, 412
irrigation, 412
postoperative care, 413–414
procedure (*see* RIRS procedure)
stone retrieval devices, 412–413
treatment, 414
ureteral access sheath, 412
ureteral avulsion, 414
ureteral balloon dilator, 412
ureteral stricture, 414
ureteroscopy, children, 41
urosepsis, 414
RFP. *See* Request for proposals (RFP)
RIRS. *See* Retrograde intrarenal surgery (RIRS)
RIRS procedure
antibiotic prophylaxis, 413
cystoscopy, 413
patient preparation, 413
positioning, 413
safety guidewire, 413
ureteral stenting, 413
ureteroscope insertion, 413

Robotic-assisted laparoscopic pyeloplasty (RALP), 516
Robotic-assisted surgery
  calculus removal, 517
  clinical assessment, 517
  development, 516
  endoscopic equipment, 515
  laparoscopic reconstruction, 515–516
  PUJO, 517
  pyeloplasty-pyelolithotomy, 516
  RALP, 516
  robotic-assisted extended pyelolithotomy, 517
  robotic systems, 516
Routine analysis techniques
  chemical analysis, 684, 685
  elemental analysis, X-ray fluorescence (XRF), 693–694
  field-effect scanning electron microscope, 693
  FTIR microspectroscopy, 699
  generalities, 684–685
  infrared spectroscopy, 685–692
  scattering techniques, 686, 692–693, 695–696
  SEM, 694–695
  synchrotron radiation, 696–698
  X-ray absorption spectroscopy, 698–699
RP. *See* Randall's plaque (RP)
RPP. *See* Renal pelvic pressure (RPP)
RSFs. *See* Recurrent stone formers (RSFs)
RSR. *See* Relative saturation (RSR)
RTA. *See* Renal tubular acidosis (RTA)
Rural surgery
  ARSI, 877
  ASI, 877
  high-technology surgery, 878
  IAGES, 877
  Indian economy, 877
  kaleidoscope, 877
  laparoscopy, 878
  MAS, 878
  NGOs, 877
  strange and surprising, 877
  tertiary care hospitals, 876
  tissue repair, 878
Russian Federation and post-Soviet area
  chemical composition, urinary stones, 100, 104
  composition, 105
  data and methods, 99
  objectives, research, 99, 103
  official statistics, urolithiasis, 97, 98, 100
  oxalate stones, 100, 103
  prevalence, urolithiasis, 97–99
  prostate diseases, 99, 101–102
  recurrence preventive treatment, 105
  sex distribution, 100, 104
  sex ratio, 105
  stones identification, mineral composition, 100

S

SAC. *See* Soluble adenylyl cyclase (SAC)
SAI. *See* Stone age index (SAI)
Salt intake, stone formation, 716
Saudi Arabia
  childhood urolithiasis, 80–81
  climate conditions and fluid intake, 79
  diabetes and obesity, 79
  diet and urine composition, 78
  drinking water, 78–79
  healthcare systems, 81
  lithogenic factors, 77
  prevalence, 78
  stone composition, 78
  urinary stone management, 81
  urolithiasis, region, 79
Scanning electron microscopy (SEM)
  biological apatite crystals display, 695, 696
  FEI/Philips XL40 ESEM, 694
  spherical morphology, apatite crystallites, 695, 696
  Zeiss SUPRA55-VP, 694–695
Scientism, 865
Scope Trainer™, 857, 858
SEM. *See* Scanning electron microscopy (SEM)
Sharing, lithotripter. *See* Lithotripter sharing
Shock wave lithotripsy (SWL)
  acoustic coupling, 330–331
  acoustic impedance, 375
  adverse effects
    chronic injury, 328
    diabetes mellitus and hypertension, 329
    diastolic pressure, 329
    new-onset hypertension, 328
    parenchymal bleeding, 327
    PCNL, 329
    physical mechanism, 328
    shear forces, 328
    SPECT, 328
  alkali citrate therapy, 738, 739
  calyceal diverticular calculi, 378
  changes, lithotripter, 379
  children *vs.* adults, 642
  Chinese lithotripters
    clinical comparison, lithotripters, 406, 407
    electrohydraulic and electromagnetic, 402, 403
    generation, 402
    imaging systems, 402
    low-moderate pressure and focal zone, 402
    low-pressure and wide-focus lithotripter, 404
    low voltage and high capacitance, circuit, 402–404
    operative technique, 404–406
    patient selection, 404
    real-time tracking lithotripter, 404
    Sans analgesia/sedation, 404
    tandem-pulse, 404
    UTI, 407
  collapse, cavitation bubble, 307, 309
  configuration, 309
  contraindications, 457
  cost-benefit, 917
  defined, 301
  diabetes mellitus and hypertension, 642
  distal ureteral stone, 408
  ED (*see* Energy flux density (ED))
  electrohydraulic shock wave generation, 302–303
  electromagnetic shock wave generation, 304–305
  energy, 306
  extracorporeal, 81, 885
  extracorporeal, pediatric URS, 666
  fragmentation forces, 307, 308
  fundamental physics, 375–376
  gaining extra capacity, 886
  hydronephrosis, bladder dysfunction and vesicoureteral reflux, 642
  in-line localization, 309, 310
  instrumentation, 376–377
  internal ureteral stenting, 81
  large calculi/staghorn calculi, 378

lithotripter, 917
management, pediatric urolithiasis, 408
medical training, diagnosis, 309
middle and distal ureters, 642
mobile service, 888
multifunctional urological workstation, 310
NCCT, 457–458
noninvasive modalities, 81
pacemakers, 564
and PCNL therapy, 81, 402
pediatric stone management
anesthesia, 657
clearance rate, 657
efficacy and safety, 656
gated *vs.* ungated, 657
incidence and characteristics, nephrolithiasis, 656
minimal invasive management, 655
open stone surgery, 1980s, 655
percutaneous and endourological access, 655
preoperative stent placement, 656–657
types, 657
pediatric urolithiasis, China, 635–636
piezoelectric shock wave generation, 303–304
postgraduate fellowship programs, 81
rate, 329–330
renal and ureteral stones, 327, 402
renal calculi, 377–378
selling extra capacity, 886
staghorn stones, 451
steepening, pressure rise, 302
stent placement, 642
stone-free rates, 458
stone-free status, 641–642
structural and functional consequences, 327
tensile trail, 307, 308
time profile, pressure, 302
training and level, operators, 889
treatment strategy, 379–380
upper tract calculi, 327
ureteral calculi, 378
vs. URS, 459, 917
SI. *See* Supersaturation index (SI)
Sindh Institute of Urology and Transplantation (SIUT), 909, 910
Single-photon emission computed tomography (SPECT), 328
SIUT. *See* Sindh Institute of Urology and Transplantation (SIUT)
Skin-to-stone distances (SSD), 458, 460
Soluble adenylyl cyclase (SAC), 143
Solution chemistry
cystine, 675–676
uric acid, 675
South Africa and sub-Saharan Africa
distribution, urinary, 67, 68
stone analysis, 69
stone prone and free, 68
urine analysis, 69–70
South America
causes and metabolic abnormalities, 62
characteristics and composition, 62
costs, 65
description, 61
distribution, Brazilian population, 63
distribution, hospital admissions, 64
ethnicity, 62
treatment, 64–65
Specialists age, 803–804
SPECT. *See* Single-photon emission computed tomography (SPECT)
Spora lygodii, 540, 541
SSD. *See* Skin-to-stone distances (SSD)
Staghorn stones
bilateral, 937
definition, 445
etiology, 446, 447
and immobilization, 951
open surgery, 448
PCNL, 448–451
pre-therapeutic evaluation, 447–448
prevalence, 445–446
removal, stone segments, 446, 448
retrograde ureteroscopic intrarenal surgery, 451
SWL, 451
symptoms, 446
treatment and follow-up, 452
treatment strategy, 447
ultrasound, 942
X-ray KUB, 950
Steinstrasse, 469
Stenting
postoperative, URS, 666
SWL, children, 656–657
Stent placement
extrinsic compression, 504–505
open surgical procedures, 505
protocol, 503, 504
urinary diversion, 505–506
Stent removal
difficulty, 506
open surgery, bladder, 506
PCN, 506
Stone age index (SAI), 680
Stone analysis
cystinuria, 759
in South Africa and Sub-Saharan Africa, 69
Stone characterization
calcium oxalate, 699
calcium phosphate, 699–700
classification, 700
Stone clearance efficacy
children
PCNL, 663–664
URS, 666
SWL, 657
Stone composition
complex stones, 30
core and shell, 30, 31
European Union (EU)
age, 5–6
gender, 5
regional variations, 6
Japan
areas, 93
calcium, 91, 92
infection, 92
lower and upper urinary tract calculi, 91
Kerala, 49
magnesium and trace elements, 32
pediatric patients, 32
phosphate, 31
practice patterns, 28–30
racial differences, 109
Saudi Arabia, 78
single component, 30
struvite, 31–32
uric acid, 32

Stone composition and morphology
age, 118
calcium oxalate stones, 114
calcium phosphate stones, 133–135
CaOx (*see* Calcium oxalate (CaOx) stones)
carbapatite, 114–115
components identification, urinary calculi, 114–116
comprehensive stone analysis, 121–124
diagnostic orientations, 135, 136
differences, countries, 118, 119
distribution, 117
factors, 129, 131
gender, 117–118
morpho-constitutional stone analysis method, 124
morphological classification
calcium/magnesium phosphates, 124, 128
COD/weddellite, 124, 126
COM/whewellite, 124, 125
cystine, 124, 129
pure/abundant proteins, 124, 130
uric acids/urate salts, 124, 127
urinary calculi, mixed types, 129, 130
pediatric stone formers
age, 120–121
components frequency, urinary calculi, 119, 120
physical and chemical methods, 114
purine stones, 115–116, 135
relationships, types and stones, 136, 138
stone formation, 116–117
Stone disease management
classical surgical training methods, 855
donor and renal transplantation
advantages and disadvantages, 602
shock wave lithotripsy, 602
techniques, 602
endourology, 862
Halstedian model, 855
health regulations, 862
IES fellowship and certification, 860–861
short-term courses and workshops, 861–862
surgical simulation (*see* Surgical simulation)
training stresses, 856
Stone diseases
Aha moment, 349–350
BMI and composition, 923
diabetes mellitus and metabolic syndrome, 924–925
failure, rejection, and persistence, 349
hypertension, 922
indinavir nephrolithiasis, 926
innovation, 348
inspiration and building, 348–349
male-to-female ratio, 922
melamine nephrolithiasis, 925–926
methods, treatment, 349–350
nephrolithiasis, bariatric surgery, 923–924
obesity, 922
PCNL, 347
SWL, 347
urinary composition and nephrolithiasis, 922–923
Web-based survey, 348
Stone dissolution
chemolytic agent, 533
irrigative therapy, 535–536
minimally invasive procedures, 533
oral chemolytic therapy, 533–535
Stone extraction, 660
Stone formation
cystinuria, 757
diseases association
cystinuria, 674
dRTA and pRTA, 674
enteric hyperoxaluria, 673
hypercalcemia, 673
hyperparathyroidism, 673
ileostomy, 673
intestinal malfunction, 673
Lesch-Nyhan syndrome, 673–674
primary hyperoxaluria, 673
ulcerative colitis, 673
non-ICSF patients
brushite stone formers, 214
cystinuria, 213–214
gastric bypass, 214–215
HOX, 216–217
HPT, 215, 216
ileostomy patients, 215
phenotypes, 213, 214
Randall's plaque, 213
RTA, 215–216
tubular deposits/ductal plugging, 213
pharmacological agents
calcium and vitamin D, 674
calcium phosphate, 674
corticosteroids, 674
sulfonamides and triamterene, 674
vitamin C, 674
PHPT
hypercalcemia and hypercalciuria, 768
industrialized countries, 768, 769
osteitis fibrosa cystica, 768
SNPs, CASR, 768–769
symptoms, 768
upper urinary tract stone, 768
Stone fragmentation, 422–423, 665–666
Stone prevention strategies, China
calcium urolithiasis
advantages and disadvantages, 721
balanced diet(*see* Balanced diet)
drug(*see* Drug-based stone prevention, China)
lifestyles, 721
water intake, 721
cystine, 724
infection stones, 724
purine, 725
uric acid, 724
Stone recurrences, prevention
calcium oxalate, 746
clinical trails, 747
dietary, 746
epidemiology, 746–747
Equil© computer program, 746
fluid intake, 747–748
hyperoxaluria and cystinuria, 746
nephrolithiasis, 746
physiology, 746
water therapy, 747
Stone removal methods
ESWL, 898
open and laparoscopic surgery, renal stones, 899
PCNL, 898–899
residual stones, 899
URS, 898
Stone retrieval devices, 296, 412–413

Stone retrieval methods, 48–49
Stone surgeon/lithotomists armamentarium
  C-arm monitors, 293, 294
  endoirrigation systems, 297
  guidewires, 294–295
  intracorporeal ithotrites, 295–296
  stone retrieval devices, 296
  ureteral access sheaths, 295
  ureteral balloon dilators, 295
  ureteral occlusion devices, 296
  ureteroscopes, 296–297
Stone treatment technology, 881, 882
Sugar intake, stone formation, 716
Supersaturation index (SI), 191–192
Supine PCNL, 424, 425
Suprapubic cystolitholapaxy, 522
Surgical simulation
  animal models, 860
  cadavers, 860
  cystoscopy and ureteroscopy, 857–859
  description, 856
  high-fidelity, 856
  LAP mentor, 856, 857
  PCNL, 858–860
  TURP, 857
SWL. *See* Shock wave lithotripsy (SWL)
Synchrotron radiation
  cartography, 697
  description, 696–697
  emitted continuous spectrum, 697
  ESRF and SOLEIL, France, 697, 698
  properties, 697

T
Tamm-Horsfall protein (THP), 146
TCO. *See* Total cost of ownership (TCO)
Teach-back, 544–545
THI. *See* Tissue harmonic imaging (THI)
Thiazide, 729
THP. *See* Tamm-Horsfall protein (THP)
Tips and tricks, ureteroscopy
  ancillary equipment, 474–475
  clinical experience
    KUB and IVP, 478, 479
    laparoscopic ureterolithotomy, 479
    PCNL, 478
    URSL, 479
    YAG laser lithotripsy, 479–450
  description, 473
  flexible ureteroscopes
    characteristics, 474, 475
    step-by-step maneuver, 477–478
  intracorporeal lithotriptors, 475
  preoperative preparation, 475
  semirigid ureteroscopes
    antegrade passage, 477
    characteristics, 474
    retrograde passage, 475–476
    retropulsion, 476–477
Tissue harmonic imaging (THI), 287
Tissue injury, 390
Topiramate therapy, 188
Total cost of ownership (TCO), 892, 894
Trace elements, urolithiasis
  fluorine, 229
  inorganic nutritional components, 227
  iron, 228
  stone types, 228
  strontium, 229
  urinary stone phases, 229
  zinc, 228
Traditional Chinese medicine
  diagnosis and treatment, 539
  etiology and pathogenesis, 539–540
  Herba lysimachiae, 540
  Lysimachia christina (*see Lysimachia christina*)
Transurethral cystolitholapaxy, 651
Transurethral resection of the prostate (TURP), 857
Tubeless PCNL
  diathermal techniques, 430–431
  fibrin sealants, 428–430
  flowable products, 430
  hemostatic agents, 428
  sizes and types, nephrostomy tubes
  vs. standard PCNL, 428
  "totally", 428
Tubular deposits/ductal plugging, 213
Tubular reabsorption, citrate, 184
TURP. *See* Transurethral resection of the prostate (TURP)

U
UA nephrolithiasis. *See* Uric acid (UA) nephrolithiasis
UASFs. *See* Uric acid stone formers (UASFs)
UK foundation programme, 821
Ultrasonography (US), 245–246, 287
Ultrasound
  change, frequency, 284
  contrast enhancing methods, 287
  crystals, 287–288
  CT scan, 256, 259
  exponential attenuation, 285
  imaging modalities, 256
  imaging systems, 288
  kidneys and bladder, 256, 258
  light waves, 283
  nephrolithotripsy/antegrade ureteroscopy, 258–259, 261–262
  piezoelectric crystals, 256
  radiography, 285–286
  renal calculi
    hydronephrosis, 256
    indicators, urinary stone, 256, 259
    pulse wave Doppler, 257, 260–261
    transvaginal, 258
  sound waves, 283
  specular and diffuse reflection, 284–285
  terminology, 283–284
  tomography, 286
  transabdominal and transvaginal sonographic imaging, 256, 257
  ultrasonography, 287
United States Medical Licensing Examination (USMLE), 822
Ureaplasma urealyticum, 43
Ureteral balloon dilation, 412
Ureteral balloon dilators, 295
Ureteral occlusion devices, 296
Ureteral stone management
  medical expulsive therapy, 456–457
  preoperative/postoperative evaluation, 455–456
  procedures, 459
  SWL, 457–458
  URS, 458–459

Ureteric orifice dilatation, 665
Ureteric stents
catheters and devices, 488–489
double-J stent, 489–490
"double pigtail" design, 487, 488
encrustation (*see* Encrustation)
endoscopic equipment, upper urinary tract, 493
exchanging, 505
forgotten and retained stents, 506–507
grooves, 490
hollow tube, 490
materials, 490–491
Memokath® stent, 487, 489
PCN, 506
placement (*see* Ureteric stents placement)
relief, renal obstruction, 491–492
removal, stents (*see* Stent removal)
safe healing, 493
side holes, 490
solid metal coil stent, 487, 488
stent length, 503–504
stent placement (*see* Stent placement)
tips and tricks, 504, 505
upper curl, JJ stent, 487, 488
Ureteric stents placement
antegrade stent placement, 495
cystoscopic stenting method, 493–494
difficult stent insertion easier, 496–497
freehand stent placement method, 494–496
Ureterorenoscopy (URS)
in 1929, 664
complications, 666
contraindication, UTI, 664
cystinuria, 762
cystoscopes, 413
defined, 898
deflecting mechanism, 336, 339
deflection, flexible ureteroscopes, 335, 338
description, 664
EHL, 335, 337
ESWL, 666
fiber-optic imaging bundle, 337, 340
flexible, 412
flexible ureteroscopes, 339, 341
indications, 664
instrument designs, 333
intracorporeal lithotripsy, 337
intrarenal collecting system, 335, 338
laparoscopic/open surgery, 899
laser lithotripsy development, 338
and lasertripsy, 1988, 664
late 1980s, 664
pediatric stone disease, 644
procedure
anesthesia and caudal block, 664
fragmentation, 665–666
laryngospasm, 665
passive ureteral dilatation, 665
patient position, 664
postoperative stenting, 666
prophylactic antibiotics, 664
ureteric orifice dilatation, 665
renal pelvis, 334, 335
sizing, urologic instruments, 339, 340
stone clearance efficacy, 666
stone-free rates, SWL, 458–459
stone treatment, 337
tips and tricks (*see* Tips and tricks, ureteroscopy)
ultrasonic lithotripsy, 335, 337
ultrasound probe, 335
ureteral access sheaths, 412
ureteral injury, 666
ureteral stricture, 414
visualized calculus, 335, 336
wire-guided bougie dilation, 334
Ureteroscopic surgery (URS)
anesthesia, 466
angiocatheter, 466–467
contraindications, 465
description, 463
essential procedural steps, 466, 467
indications, 464–465
instrumentation, 465–466
management, complications, 471
"optical dilation", 467–468
postoperative care, 470
preoperative preparation, 466
prevention, 470
skeletal abnormalities, 469
Steinstrasse, 469
treatment, 468–469
upper tract reconstruction, 469–470
ureteral healing, 470
visualization, ureter, 468
Uric acid (UA) lithiasis, 627–628
Uric acid (UA) nephrolithiasis
acidic urinary pH, 158
alkali citrate therapy (*see* Alkali citrate therapy)
conservative treatment, 160–161
defined, 155
differential diagnosis, 160
homeostasis, 156
hyperuricosuria, 157–158
impaired NH_4+ excretion, 158
increased endogenous acid production, 159–160
low urine volume, 157
metabolic evaluation, 160
MS (*see* Metabolic syndrome (MS))
pathogenesis and etiologies, 157
pharmacological treatment, 161
physicochemical scheme, stone formation, 156
renal handling, 156–157
renal lipotoxicity, 158–159
Uric acid stone formers (UASFs), 923, 924
Uric acid stones
prevention, 724
prevention, China, 724
Urinary bladder calculi
clinical presentation, 520
cystolitholapaxy, 521–522
cystoscopy, 521
diagnosis, 520
ESWL, 523
etiology, 520
history, 519–520
imaging modalities, 521
incidence, 519
KUB X-rays, 524
medical therapy, 521
open cystolithotomy, 522–523
pathophysiology, 520
suprapubic cystolitholapaxy, 522

surgical treatment, 521
transurethral cystolithotripsy, 522
urinalysis, 521
urine culture and sensitivity, 521
Urinary citrate
calcium-citrate complexes, 188–190
crystal growth and crystal agglomeration, 189
hypocitraturia (*see* Hypocitraturia)
inhibitor activity, 188
kidney stones, 187
and magnesium excretion, 33–34
potassium citrate (*see* Potassium citrate)
Urinary leakage, 663
Urinary stone formation
animals, 220–223
children, 220
Urinary tract infection (UTI), 43, 407
Urinary tract stones
blood analysis and urine, patient, 248
clinical presentation, 243–244, 251
costovertebral angle tenderness, 251
crystallization, 249
CT, 247–248
differential diagnosis, 252–253
flank pain, 251
investigatory procedures, 252
IVU, 246–247
KUB radiographs, 244–245
MRU, 248
NCCT, 248
physical examination, 244
pyuria, 244
renal colic, 252, 254
spot urine samples, 249
ultrasonograph, 252
ureteric colic and renal pain, 254
uric acid crystals, 244
US, 245–246
Urine analysis, South Africa and Sub-Saharan Africa
compositions, 70
risk factors, black and white males, 69, 70
stone formation, 69
Urine pH
acidic, 158
differential diagnosis, 160
lower, 158–159
monitoring, 161
treatment, alkali salts, 161
Urine preservation, 675, 678
Urine volume, 746–747
Urolithiasis
angulated and tortuous ureter, 957
bladder stones, 940
broken stent, 939
calcium (*see* Calcium)
citrate (*see* Citrate)
diagnosis (*see* Urinary tract stones)
distal ureteral stone, 945, 946
distribution
age, 55, 56
gender, 55
geographic, 53–55
occupational, 55–56
dynamic steinstrasse (SS), 949
heminephrectomy and calculus disease, 933, 934
highly technological care, China
health-care programs, 882–883
sophisticated surgeries, 882
stone treatment technology, 881, 882
urolithiasis, 881
immobilization and staghorn stones, 951
MET, 955, 956
nephrocalcinosis, 935
obstruction, 944
outcomes, 918
and parathyroid adenoma, 931, 932
prevalence, 57
prevenention, 918
renal stone and ureterocele, 953, 954
renal stones and pyelonephritis, 943
sestamibi scan, PHPT, 938
staghorn stones, 937, 942, 950
steinstrasse, stent, 948
treatment
costs, 917
CT, 916–917
MET, 917
renal colic, 916
ultrasound (*see* Ultrasound)
ureteral jets, 941
vesical stone, 947
XGPN, 936
Urology
assessments, 822–823
challenges, developing world, 852
CME, CPD, and EBM, 849
curriculum, 845
education and training, 842
health professionals education
American Urological Association, 851
information and educational technology, 850–851
Lancet Commission, 850
medical education and training regulation policy, 850
PGME programs, 851, 852
medical education, 845, 846
PGME (*see* Postgraduate medical education (PGME))
trainees and trainers, 853
URO Mentor™, 857–859
Uroradiology. *See* Radiation exposure, uroradiology
Uro-Scopic Trainer™, 857, 858
URS. *See* Ureterorenoscopy (URS); Ureteroscopic surgery (URS)
US. *See* Ultrasonography (US)
USMLE. *See* United States Medical Licensing Examination (USMLE)
UTI. *See* Urinary tract infection (UTI)

V
VDR. *See* Vitamin D receptor (VDR)
Virtual reality (VR) models, 831
Vitamin D
deficient (*see* Normocalcemic hyperparathyroidism)
hypercalcemia, 204–205
mechanism, 201
metabolism, 200–201
PHPT (*see* Primary hyperparathyroidism (PHPT))
production, 200
renal calcium absorption and transport, 202–203
replacement therapy and stone, 203
transport, 201
Vitamin D receptor (VDR), 143
VR models. *See* Virtual reality (VR) models

W

Weddellite calculi, 228, 229
Whewellite zinc, 228
Workplace assessment methods
  CbD, 809, 814
  CEC, 809
  DOPS, 809, 811
  mini-CEX, 809, 810
  MSF, 809, 815–816
  OSATS, 809, 812–813

X

Xanthogranulomatous pyelonephritis (XGPN), 936
XGPN. *See* Xanthogranulomatous pyelonephritis (XGPN)
X-ray absorption spectroscopy, 698–699
X-ray fluorescence (XRF)
  advantages, 693
  biological apatite, kidney stones, 694, 695
  elemental composition, 693
  implementation, LPS, 694
  physical process, 693–694
  quantitative analysis, geometric parameters, 694
X-ray scattering
  Bragg diffraction, 692
  calcium tartrate tetrahydrate, rat kidney calculus, 692
  chemical parameters, 692
  Debye function analysis, 692
  determination, crystal structure, 686
  LPS, 2D detector, 692–693
  Randall's plaque, 693
  spatial arrangement, atoms, 686
  yielding, 692
XRF. *See* X-ray fluorescence (XRF)

Y

YAG. *See* Yttrium aluminum garnet (YAG)
Yttrium aluminum garnet (YAG)
  laser crystal, 315
  photothermal mechanism, 316
  retropulsion, 320

MIX
Papier aus verantwortungsvollen Quellen
Paper from responsible sources
FSC® C105338

If you have any concerns about our products,
you can contact us on
ProductSafety@springernature.com

In case Publisher is established outside the EU,
the EU authorized representative is:
Springer Nature Customer Service Center GmbH
Europaplatz 3, 69115 Heidelberg, Germany

Printed by Libri Plureos GmbH
in Hamburg, Germany